NEURAL BLOCKADE

IN CLINICAL ANESTHESIA AND MANAGEMENT OF PAIN

THIRD EDITION

NEURAL BLOCKADE

IN CLINICAL ANESTHESIA AND MANAGEMENT OF PAIN

THIRD EDITION

EDITORS

Michael J. Cousins, A.M., M.B., B.S., M.D. (SYD), F.A.N.Z.C.A., F.R.C.A.
Professor and Head
Department of Anaesthesia and Pain Management
Royal North Shore Hospital
University of Sydney
St. Leonards, New South Wales
Australia

Phillip O. Bridenbaugh, M.D.
Professor and Chairman
Department of Anesthesia
University of Cincinnati College of Medicine
Cincinnati, Ohio

Lippincott - Raven
PUBLISHERS
Philadelphia • New York

Acquisitions Editor: R. Craig Percy
Developmental Editor: Anne Snyder
Manufacturing Manager: Dennis Teston
Production Manager: Jodi Borgenicht
Production Editor: Raeann Touhey
Cover Designer: Alan Bentley
Indexer: Nancy Newman
Compositor: Maryland Composition
Printer: Quebecor Kingsport

Printed in the United States of America

9 8 7 6 5 4 3 2 1

Library of Congress Cataloging-in-Publication Data

Neural blockade in clinical anesthesia and management of pain /
editors, Michael J. Cousins, Phillip O. Bridenbaugh.—3rd ed.
p. cm.
Includes bibliographical references and index.
ISBN 0-397-51159-0
1. Nerve block. 2. Anesthesia. 3. Analgesia. I. Cousins, Michael J. II. Bridenbaugh, Phillip O., 1932– .
[DNLM: 1. Nerve Block. 2. Pain—therapy. WO 300 N494 1998]
RD84.N48 1998
617.9′6—dc21
DNLM/DLC
for Library of Congress

To patients with acute, chronic non-cancer and cancer pain

The theoretical and practical information in this text is dedicated to more enlightened and effective use of neural blockade for the management of all types of pain and for the prevention of the harmful sequelae of severe unrelieved pain

Contents

B. Extremities

C. Thorax and Abdomen

D. Head and Neck

PART 3. NEURAL BLOCKADE IN THE MANAGEMENT OF PAIN

Contributing Authors

Stephen E. Abram, M.D.
Professor
Department of Anesthesiology and Critical Care
University of New Mexico School of Medicine
2701 Frontier Northeast
Albuquerque, New Mexico 87131-5216

C. Richard Bennett, D.D.S., Ph.D.
Professor
Department of Anesthesiology
University of Pittsburgh
School of Dental Medicine
3501 Terrace Street
Pittsburgh, Pennsylvania 15261

John J. Bonica, M.D., D.Sc. *(Deceased)*
Professor Emeritus
Department of Anesthesiology
University of Washington
Seattle, Washington 98195

Harald Breivik, M.D., Ph.D.
Professor and Chairman
Department of Anaesthesiology
The National Hospital (Rikshospitalet)
N-0027 Oslo
Norway

Phillip O. Bridenbaugh, M.D.
Professor and Chairman
Department of Anesthesia
University of Cincinnati College of Medicine
231 Bethesda Avenue
Cincinnati, Ohio 45267-0531

L. Donald Bridenbaugh, M.D.
Clinical Professor
Department of Anesthesiology
Virginia Mason Medical Center
1100 Ninth Avenue
Seattle, Washington 98111

Lynn M. Broadman, M.D.
Professor
Departments of Anesthesiology and Pediatrics
West Virginia University School of Medicine
3618 Health Sciences Center
Morgantown, West Virginia 26506

David L. Brown, M.D.
Professor and Head
Department of Anesthesia
University of Iowa
6618 John Colloton Pavillion
200 Hawkins Drive
Iowa City, Iowa 52242-1079

Peter Brownridge, M.B., Ch.B., D.R.C.O.G, F.R.C.A., F.A.N.Z.C.A
Senior Lecturer and Director of Obstetric Anaesthesia
Department of Anaesthesia and Intensive Care
Flinders Medical Center
The Flinders University of South Australia
Adelaide, South Australia 5042
Australia

Sorin J. Brull, M.D.
Associate Professor
Department of Anesthesiology
Yale University School of Medicine
Chief, Section of General Anesthesia
Yale-New Haven Hospital
333 Cedar Street
New Haven, Connecticut 06510

Daniel B. Carr, M.D.
Saltonstall Professor of Pain Research
Departments of Anesthesia and Medicine
Tufts University School of Medicine
New England Medical Center
750 Washington Street
Boston, Massachusetts 02111

J. Edmond Charlton, M.B., B.S., F.R.C.A., D.Obst.R.C.O.G.
Department of Pain Management and Anaesthesia
Royal Victoria Infirmary
Queen Victoria Road
Newcastle upon Tyne NEI 4LP
United Kingdom

Sheila E. Cohen, M.B., Ch.B., F.R.C.A.
Professor and Director of Obstetric Anesthesia
Department of Anesthesia
Stanford University School of Medicine
300 Pasteur Drive
Stanford, California 94305

Michael J. Cousins, A.M., M.B., B.S., M.D.(SYD), F.A.N.Z.C.A., F.R.C.A.
Professor and Head
Department of Anaesthesia and Pain Management
Royal North Shore Hospital
University of Sydney
St. Leonards, New South Wales 2065
Australia

Benjamin G. Covino, M.D., Ph.D. *(Deceased)*
Professor Emeritus
Department of Anesthesia
Harvard Medical School
Brigham and Women's Hospital
75 Francis Street
Boston, Massachusetts 02115

James C. Crews, M.D.
Associate Professor
Department of Anesthesia
University of Cincinnati College of Medicine
231 Bethesda Avenue
Cincinnati, Ohio 45267-0531

Marianne E. Feitl, M.D.
Assistant Professor
Department of Ophthalmology
University of Chicago
939 East 57th Street
Chicago, Illinois 60614

B. Raymond Fink, M.D.
Professor Emeritus
Department of Anesthesiology
University of Washington School of Medicine
1959 Northeast Pacific Street
Seattle, Washington 98195-6540

Joseph A. Giovannitti, Jr., D.M.D.
Adjunct Associate Professor
Departments of Oral and Maxillofacial Surgery and Pharmacological Sciences
Baylor College of Dentistry
3302 Gaston Avenue
Dallas, Texas 75246

Nicholas M. Greene, M.D., M.A., F.R.C.A.
Professor Emeritus
Department of Anesthesiology
Yale University School of Medicine
333 Cedar Street
New Haven, Connecticut 06520-8051

J. David Haddox, M.D.
Associate Professor
Center for Pain Medicine
Emory University Medical Center
1327 Clifton Road Northeast
Atlanta, Georgia 30322

Quinn H. Hogan, M.D.
Associate Professor
Department of Anesthesiology
Director, Pain Management Center
Medical College of Wisconsin
Froedtert Memorial Hospital
9200 West Wisconsin Avenue
Milwaukee, Wisconsin 53226-3569

Charles McK. Holmes, M.D., B.Ch., F.A.N.Z.C.A.
Anaesthetist
Department of Anaesthesia
Mercy Hospital
Dunedin
New Zealand

Henrik Kehlet, M.D., Ph.D.
Professor of Surgery
Department of Surgical Gastroenterology
Hvidovre University Hospital
Kettegård Allé 30
DK-2650 Hvidovre
Denmark

Dan J. Kopacz, M.D.
Staff Anesthesiologist
Department of Anesthesiology
Virginia Mason Medical Center
1100 Ninth Avenue
Seattle, Washington 98111

Theodore Krupin, M.D.
Professor
Department of Ophthalmology
Northwestern University School of Medicine
300 East Superior, Tarry 5-715
Chicago, Illinois 60611

J. Bertil Löfström, M.D., Ph.D.
Professor Emeritus
Department of Anesthesiology
Linkoping University
S-581 85 Linkoping
Sweden

William A. Macrae, F.R.C.A.
Consultant Anaesthetist
The Pain Clinic
Ninewells Hospital
Dundee DD1 9SY
United Kingdom

Donald C. Manning, M.D., Ph.D.
Assistant Professor
Department of Anesthesiology
Pain Management Center
University of Virginia Health Sciences Center
Charlottesville, Virginia 22908

Laurence E. Mather, Ph.D., F.A.N.Z.C.A.
Professor of Anaesthesia and Analgesia (Research)
Department of Anaesthesia and Pain Management
Royal North Shore Hospital
University of Sydney
St. Leonards, New South Wales 2065
Australia

Kathryn E. McGoldrick, M.D.
Professor
Department of Anesthesiology
Yale University School of Medicine
333 Cedar Street
New Haven, Connecticut 06510;
and Section of Ambulatory Surgery
Yale-New Haven Hospital
New Haven, Connecticut 06520

Ronald Melzack, Ph.D.
Professor
Department of Psychology
McGill University
1205 Dr. Penfield Avenue
Montreal, Quebec, H3A 1B1
Canada

Michael F. Mulroy, M.D.
Staff Anesthesiologist
Department of Anesthesiology
Virginia Mason Medical Center
1100 Ninth Avenue
Seattle, Washington 98111

Terence M. Murphy, M.D. *(Deceased)*
Professor Emeritus
Department of Anesthesiology
University of Washington School of Medicine
1959 Northeast Pacific Street
Seattle, Washington 98195-6540

Robert R. Myers, Ph.D.
Professor of Anesthesiology and Pathology (Neuropathology)
Department of Anesthesiology Research-0629
University of California at San Diego
9500 Gilman Drive
La Jolla, California 92093-0629

Richard B. Patt, M.D.
Director, Anesthesia Pain Programs
Deputy Chief, Pain and Symptom Management Section
Associate Professor of Anesthesiology and Neuro-Oncology
University of Texas
M. D. Anderson Cancer Center
1515 Holcombe Boulevard
Houston, Texas 77030

Linda Jo Rice, M.D.
Director of Pain Management
Department of Anesthesiology
All Children's Hospital
565 21st Avenue Northeast
St. Petersburg, Florida 33704-4641

John C. Rowlingson, M.D.
Professor
Department of Anesthesiology
Director, Pain Management Center
University of Virginia Health Sciences Center
Charlottesville, Virginia 22908

Philip J. Siddall, M.B., B.S., Ph.D.
Clinical Lecturer
Department of Anaesthesia and Pain Management
Royal North Shore Hospital
University of Sydney
St. Leonards, New South Wales 2065
Australia

Raymond S. Sinatra, M.D., Ph.D.
Professor
Department of Anesthesiology
Yale University School of Medicine;
Director of Acute Pain Management Service
Yale-New Haven Hospital
333 Cedar Street
New Haven, Connecticut 06510

Gary R. Strichartz, A.M. (Hons), Ph.D.
Professor of Anesthesia (Pharmacology)
Department of Anesthesia
Harvard Medical School
Brigham and Women's Hospital
75 Francis Street
Boston, Massachusetts 02115

Ronald R. Tasker, M.D., F.R.C.S.(C)
Professor
Department of Surgery
Division of Neurosurgery
University of Toronto
The Toronto Hospital, Western Division
399 Bathurst Street, Suite 2-431 Mc1
Toronto, Ontario M5T 2S8
Canada

Gale E. Thompson, M.D.
Staff Anesthesiologist
Department of Anesthesiology
Virginia Mason Medical Center
1100 Ninth Avenue
Seattle, Washington 98111

Geoffrey T. Tucker, B.Pharm., Ph.D.
Professor of Clinical Pharmacology
Departments of Medicine and Pharmacology
Section of Molecular Pharmacology and Pharmacogenetics
University of Sheffield
The Royal Hallamshire Hospital
Glossop Road
Sheffield S10 2JF
United Kingdom

Bernadette T. Veering, M.D., Ph.D.
Staff Anesthesiologist
Department of Anesthesiology
University Hospital Leiden
2300 RC Leiden
The Netherlands

Suellen M. Walker, M.B., B.S., F.A.N.Z.C.A.
Clinical Lecturer and Staff Specialist
Department of Anaesthesia and Pain Management
Royal North Shore Hospital
University of Sydney
St. Leonards, New South Wales 2065
Australia

Patrick D. Wall, F.R.S., D.M., F.R.C.P.
Professor
Department of Physiology
United Medical and Dental Schools
St. Thomas Campus
Lambeth Palace Road
London SE1 7EH
United Kingdom

M. Elizabeth Ward, M.D., F.R.C.P.C.
Senior Lecturer and Specialist Anaesthetist
Department of Anaesthesia and Pain Management
Royal North Shore Hospital
University of Sydney
St. Leonards, New South Wales 2065
Australia

Denise J. Wedel, M.D.
Professor
Department of Anesthesiology
Mayo Clinic
200 First Street Southwest
Rochester, Minnesota 55905

John A. W. Wildsmith, M.D., F.R.C.A., F.R.C.P.Ed.
Professor
University Department of Anaesthesia
Ninewells Hospital and Medical School
Dundee DD1 9SY
United Kingdom

Richard J. Willis, M.B., B.S., F.A.N.C.Z.A.
Director of Clinical Anaesthesia
Department of Anaesthesia and Intensive Care
Royal Adelaide Hospital
Adelaide, South Australia 5000
Australia

Tony L. Yaksh, Ph.D.
Professor of Anesthesiology and
Adjunct Professor of Pharmacology
Department of Anesthesiology
University of California at San Diego
9500 Gilman Drive
La Jolla, California 92093-0818

Foreword to the Second Edition

Neural Blockade in Clinical Anesthesia and Management of Pain must be the most ambitious project of its kind ever undertaken. This book ranges from a consideration of the physiology, pharmacology, and toxicology of the local analgesic agents in common use to a number of the less orthodox methods of relieving suffering of various origins. The book is indeed encyclopedic in its coverage, and, like encyclopedias in other sciences, each section has been entrusted to a recognized world authority in his own special field. No book on local analgesia could have a sounder pedigree.

There are situations in which, manifestly, local anesthesia is preferable to general. Apart from these, improved sedation and longer-acting analgesic drugs have improved patient acceptance, but the practitioner still has to acquire the necessary "know-how" to deposit the solution with reasonable accuracy for it to be effective. Both editors are renowned for their practical teaching, which should be a sound guarantee that both the expert and the tyro can turn to this book for guidance and profit.

Neural blockade offers far more to the patient than merely analgesia during surgery. Rapid growth in application of neural blockade to postoperative, post-traumatic, and obstetric pain management is extensively covered in this textbook. Even more extensive is the breadth and depth of scientific information and clinical application of neural blockade in chronic pain; this is presented as completely and concisely as possible.

Sir Robert Macintosh, D.M., F.R.C.S. (EDIN), HON F.E.A.R.C.S.
Emeritus Nuffield Professor of Anaesthetics, University of Oxford

Preface

In just under a decade, since the publication of the Second Edition of *Neural Blockade,* there have been substantial developments in the knowledge of anatomy, physiology, and pharmacology of regionally applied drugs, including local anaesthetics and substantial advances in the techniques of neural blockade, with respect to their use in clinical anesthesia. In contrast to these steady advances, there has been a major increase in knowledge about acute, chronic and cancer pain, in some areas with the evolution of new concepts which have opened up completely new treatment options.

The overall structure of the Third Edition of *Neural Blockade* remains the same as in the Second Edition, however, each chapter of the text has been extensively revised. There are 52 authors from 10 different countries, with 28 new authors.

In the Introduction, Chapter 1 has been retitled *History of Neural Blockade and Pain Management* and is now authored by Dr. David Brown of the University of Iowa. The Chapter contains much new material about the more recent history of local anesthesia and there is a significantly expanded section on the history of pain management.

In **Part 1** on Pharmacology and Physiology of Neural Blockade, Chapter 2, the *Physiology of Neural Blockade,* is again entrusted to Dr. Gary R. Strichartz, from Harvard University, Boston, who has been preeminent in investigating the site and mechanisms of action of local anesthetics.

Chapter 3, the *Properties, Absorption, and Disposition of Local Anesthetic Agents,* remains in the hands of Dr. Geoff Tucker, University of Sheffield, and Dr. Laurie Mather, University of Sydney, who have pioneered this field. They have provided a very concise and understandable summary of this complex and large area of important information for the safe and effective use of neural blockade.

Chapter 4, the *Clinical Pharmacology of Local Anesthetics,* has been updated by Dr. Tony Wildsmith, Ninewells Medical School, Dundee, United Kingdom, building on the excellent prior version by the late Dr. Ben Covino.

The final chapter in this Part, Chapter 5, the *Modification of Responses to Surgery by Neural Blockade: Clinical Implications,* has again been authored by the leader of this field, Dr. Henrik Kehlet, Hvidovre, Denmark. Dr. Kehlet has drawn from a vast amount of his own and other recent work in this area. He has provided a new chapter with major implications for the perioperative management of surgical patients.

In **Part 2**, on Techniques of Neural Blockade, Chapter 6, *Perioperative Management of Patients for Neural Blockade,* is again written by Dr. Phillip O. Bridenbaugh, with the addition of Dr. Jim Crews, from the University of Cincinnati, Cincinnati, Ohio.

Chapter 7, *Spinal, (Subarachnoid) Neural Blockade,* has again been written by Dr. Phillip O. Bridenbaugh, in the company of the author of the classic monograph on this subject, Dr. Nicholas M. Greene, and his colleague Dr. Sorin Brull from Yale University, New Haven, Connecticut. The chapter has been extensively rewritten to accommodate a large amount of new material, which is surprising given the long history of this technique.

Chapter 8, *Epidural Neural Blockade,* is authored by Dr. Michael J. Cousins, in the company of a new author, Dr. Bernadette T. Veering from the University of Leiden, the Netherlands. This chapter has been a major challenge for the authors, since much new anatomical, physiological, and pharmacological information has emerged since the Second Edition. Thus, the authors have devised new illustrations and tables and have taken a strict "evidence-based" approach to editing previous material, in order to present a concise summary of this area, which has been the subject of substantial textbooks in its own right.

Chapter 9, *Caudal Epidural Blockade,* is again written by Dr. Richard J. Willis, from the University of Adelaide, Australia, who remains one of the leading exponents of this technique in the adult population. He has again provided the reader with the appropriate background knowledge and technical details to carry out this valuable technique.

Chapter 10, the *Upper Extremity: Somatic Blockade,* is written by Dr. David Brown, formerly of the Mason Clinic and now at the University of Iowa. He is joined by Dr. Don Bridenbaugh, also formerly of the renowned Mason Clinic "regional school." New illustrations have been developed by artist Alan Bentley to give further insights into existing techniques. Some new approaches to upper extremity blocks have also been included and new illustrations are provided to give the reader a clear insight into the anatomical basis and technique required to perform these blocks.

Chapter 11, the *Lower Extremity: Somatic Blockade,* is written by Dr. Phillip O. Bridenbaugh, in the company of Dr. Denise Wedel of the Mayo Clinic. Although techniques have remained reasonably constant, this chapter has been substantially rewritten, with the benefit of new publications on the subject.

Chapter 12, *Intravenous Regional Neural Blockade,* is again written by this century's pioneer of this technique, Dr. Charles McK. Holmes of New Zealand. Dr. Holmes' authoritative account of this subject is updated, including the addition of drugs other than local anesthetics.

Chapter 13, *Sympathetic Neural Blockade of Upper and Lower Extremity,* is written by a new author, Dr. Harald Breivik from the University of Oslo, Norway, and Dr. Michael J. Cousins, in the company of the pre-eminent investigator of the scientific basis of these techniques, Dr. J. Bertil Löfström, from the Linkoping University, Sweden.

Chapter 14, *Celiac and Hypogastric Plexus, Intercostal, Interpleural, and Peripheral Neural Blockade,* is written by one of the Mason Clinic advocates for these techniques, Dr. Dan Kopacz, with his colleague, Dr. Gale Thompson. The new techniques of interpleural and hypogastric blockade are presented with some innovative and clear illustrations in the classic style of Alan Bentley. New illustrations are also provided to clarify some of the existing techniques. This chapter is a clear and concise source for those who wish to perform these techniques, which have wide application in acute, chronic, and cancer pain.

Chapter 15, *Somatic Blockade of Head and Neck,* is authored by the pre-eminent exponent of these techniques, the late Dr. Terence Murphy from the University of Washington, Seattle, Washington. Sadly, this was the last major contribution by Dr. Murphy prior to his untimely death. In his inimitable style, it presents a wonderful exposition of the entire range of neural blockade techniques for head and neck regional anesthesia and for pain management. We are indebted to Dr. Murphy for his unique contributions to this field.

Chapter 16, *Neural Blockade for Oral and Circumoral Structures: Intraoral Approach,* is again written by Dr. C. Richard Bennett from the University of Pittsburgh, Pittsburgh, Pennsylvania, drawing upon his own classic monograph and including much updated material. His colleague Dr. Joseph A. Giovannitti, Jr. is his co-author.

Chapter 17, *Neural Blockade for Ophthalmologic Surgery,* is an entirely new chapter with a complete new set of color illustrations drawn by Alan Bentley. Dr. Kathy McGoldrick of Yale University, New Haven, Connecticut, has taken over primary responsibility for this chapter, in collaboration with prior authors Dr. Theodore Krupin of Northwestern University, Chicago, Illinois, and Dr. Marianne Feitl of the University of Chicago, Illinois. Much new information about the anatomical basis, refinements in technique, and potential complications has been drawn together from a wide range of sources in the world literature. Its presentation is based on illustrations that are clear, even to those unfamiliar with this now frequently used application of neural blockade.

Chapter 18, *Neural Blockade for Obstetrics and Gynecologic Surgery,* is again co-authored by Dr. Peter Brownridge, of Flinders University, Australia, and Dr. Sheila Cohen of Stanford University, Stanford, California. This vast area of practice of neural blockade, the subject of many textbooks, is superbly summarized by the authors. The enormous job of achieving this condensation of material necessitated adding a new author, Dr. M. Elizabeth Ward of Sydney University, Australia.

Chapter 19, *Neural Blockade for Outpatients,* was entrusted to Drs. Michael Mulroy and L. Donald Bridenbaugh from the Mason Clinic. The increasing emphasis on ambulatory surgery and rapid return to normal function of surgical patients, has placed new demands for the use of neural blockade, as described in this chapter.

Chapter 20, *Neural Blockade for Pediatric Surgery,* is a completely new chapter co-authored by Dr. Lynn Broadman of West Virginia University, Morgantown, West Virginia, and Dr. Linda Jo Rice of the All Children's Hospital, St. Petersburg, Florida. The previous superb illustrations by Alan Bentley have been retained. However, in the 10 years since the Second Edition there has been a major upsurge in the use of neural blockade for pediatric surgery and postoperative pain relief which is reflected in the chapter.

Chapter 21, *Complications of Non-Neurolytic Neural Blockade,* continues to be authored by Dr. Phillip O. Bridenbaugh, in the company of Dr. Denise J. Wedel. This chapter presents a very well-balanced and precise account of this important area, which is often the subject of anecdote and confusion.

Chapter 22, *Complications of Neurolytic Neural Blockade,* is a completely new chapter co-authored by Dr. Ed Charlton of the Royal Victoria Infirmary, Newcastle upon Tyne, United Kingdom, and Dr. William A. Macrae of Ninewells Hospital, Dundee, United Kingdom. A rigorous approach is taken to the evaluation of complications and their possible mechanisms.

In **Part 3**, Neural Blockade in the Management of Pain, the text continues to deal in a concise manner with the use of neural blockade in acute, chronic, and cancer pain.

Chapter 23.1, *Introduction to Pain Mechanisms: Implications for Neural Blockade,* is authored by a new contributor, Dr. Philip Siddall of the University of Sydney, Australia, in the company of Dr. Michael J. Cousins. The chapter has been completely rewritten to include the new knowledge of pain mechanisms. This is presented in a very concise manner with the assistance of a large number of specially designed illustrations, aimed at clarifying this complex material, not only for the pain specialists, but also for the anesthesiologist who is unfamiliar with this subject matter. The chapter continues to present an overview of the International Association for the Study of Pain, Taxonomy of Chronic Pain Syndromes, Definitions of Pain Terms, Classification, and Coding.

Chapter 23.2 is a completely new chapter entitled *Introduction to Pain in Pediatric and Neonatal Patients.* It is authored by a pediatric anesthesiologist and pediatric pain specialist, Dr. Suellen M. Walker of the University of Sydney, Australia, who presents an excellent summary of this new field of knowledge.

Chapter 24, *Physiologic and Pharmacologic Substrates of Nociception and Nerve Injury,* is authored by the preeminent research worker in this field, Dr. Tony L. Yaksh of the University of California, San Diego, California. As in the previous edition, Dr. Yaksh produces an extraordinary condensation of the vast literature on this subject. This chapter represents a "treasure trove" of references for both clinicians and research workers.

Chapter 25, *Psychological Aspects of Pain: Implications for Neural Blockade,* is again written by the renowned psychologist and pain researcher Dr. Ronald Melzack from McGill University, Canada, a prolific contributor to our understanding of pain, commencing with his proposal of the "gate control theory of pain."

Chapter 26, *Acute Pain Management and Acute Pain Services,* is written by Dr. Raymond S. Sinatra from Yale University, New Haven, Connecticut, author of the highly acclaimed monograph on this subject. This chapter has been completely rewritten to include a concise summary of the enormous amount of new information that has become available since the Second Edition.

Chapter 27 is a new chapter entitled *Diagnostic and Prognostic Neural Blockade.* It is written by two new authors, Dr. Quinn Hogan of the Medical College of Wisconsin, Milwaukee, Wisconsin and Dr. Stephen E. Abram of the University of New Mexico, Albuquerque, New Mexico. This chapter builds on the critical approach taken in the Second Edition. Readers will be interested to see how we have advanced in our attitude to "evidence based medicine" and how Drs. Hogan and Abram have successfully applied this approach to diagnostic and prognostic neural blockade.

Chapter 28, *Back Pain and the Role of Neural Blockade,* is also a new chapter written by Drs. Donald C. Manning and John C. Rowlingson of the University of Virginia, Charlottesville, Virginia. Since the Second Edition there has been a major shift in our understanding and approach to the diagnosis and treatment of back pain. This chapter provides an excellent summary of anatomical, clinical, psychological, and environmental aspects of back pain and the implications that this presents for the use of neural blockade. Any anesthesiologist contemplating contributing to the treatment of back pain would be well advised to read this chapter prior to embarking on any neural blockade technique for such patients.

Chapter 29, *Spinal Route of Analgesia: Opioids and Future Options,* is authored by a new author, Dr. Daniel B. Carr of Tufts University, Boston, Massachusetts, in the company of Dr. Michael J. Cousins. The major advances in understanding spinal mechanisms of pain and pharmacologic options for the use of the spinal route has necessitated a major revision of this chapter. It takes the reader back to the cellular level and then builds an understanding that carries through into the safe and effective clinical use of spinal opioid and nonopioid drugs. The substantial advances in knowledge and techniques have also required the provision of a substantial number of new tables and figures, particularly relating to spinal infusion system implantation.

Chapter 30, *Neuropathology of Neurolytic Agents,* has again been entrusted to Dr. Robert R. Myers of the University of California, San Diego, California. Dr. Myers has essentially pioneered the rigorous investigation of the scientific basis and clinical implications of neuropathology associated with neurolytic agents. He also provides the reader with some "new horizons," which give some fascinating insights in this rapidly evolving field.

Chapter 31, *Techniques for Neurolytic Neural Blockade,* is written by Dr. Michael J. Cousins, along with a new author, Dr. Richard B. Patt of the M. D. Anderson Cancer Center; Dr. Patt draws upon the extensive material from his own monograph on cancer pain. The scientific and technical information available for this chapter has evolved substantially since the Second Edition and is reflected in an expanded chapter and a significant number of new illustrations.

Chapter 32, *Neurostimulation and Percutaneous Neural Destructive Techniques,* is again written by preeminent neurosurgeon, Dr. Ronald Tasker from the University of Toronto, Canada. Dr. Tasker has the benefit of drawing upon his recently completed, extensive text on neurosurgical techniques. In view of controversy surrounding the efficacy of neurostimulation procedures, Dr. Tasker takes a very objective view of the evidence for the application of this rapidly growing technology for the treatment of severe pain. A superb new set of illustrations for neurostimulator implantation technique is provided by Alan Bentley. This chapter also explores in substantial detail the various percutaneous neural destructive techniques, apart from the use of neurolytic agents.

Chapter 33, the *Evolution of the Specialty of Pain Medicine and Multidisciplinary Approach to Pain,* is a new chapter written by Dr. J. David Haddox of Emory University, Atlanta, Georgia. It draws on material from the Second Edition, written by the late Dr. John J. Bonica, the father of the specialty of pain management. This chapter provides a timely summary of the magnitude of the problem of pain, some particular challenges arising from the evolution of the specialty of pain management, and the importance of the multidisciplinary approach to diagnosis and treatment of pain for the safe and effective use of neural blockade.

Chapter 34 is entitled *New Horizons: An Essay* and is written by the pre-eminent pain researcher and coauthor of the "gate control theory of pain," Dr. Patrick D. Wall, of United Medical and Dental Schools, London, United Kingdom. With the benefit of his own extraordinarily diverse research contributions and his editorship of the journal, *Pain,* Dr. Wall is well placed to take a view of the future horizons for pain therapy.

Since the Second Edition of *Neural Blockade,* some major changes in *surgical milieu* in most countries have had an impact on the use of neural blockade: (i) increased use of day stay and short stay surgery; (ii) emphasis of rapid rehabilitation, even after major surgery; (iii) development of "acute postoperative pain services" and other acute pain services, including obstetric analgesia in most parts of the world; and (iv) a gradual move towards recognizing acute pain relief as "a basic human right." There has been a steady growth of Regional Anesthesia societies, including the American Society (ASRA), European Society (ESRA), Latin American Society (LASRA), and the Asian and Oceanic Society (AOSEA). All of these societies joined forces to organize an International Symposium on Regional Anesthesia (ISRA) in Auckland, New Zealand, at the time of the World Congress of Anesthesiologists in April 1996. It was a privilege for one of the editors, Michael J. Cousins, to act as President of ISRA, which attracted over 1,000 registrants from 43 countries around the world.

Pain management has "come of age" in the past 10 years: publication by the IASP of the "Core Curriculum on Pain for Health Professionals;" publication by the USA Agency for Health Care Policy and Research (AHCPR) of Clinical Practice Guidelines on *Acute Pain Management in Adults: Operative and Medical Procedures; Acute Pain Management in Children: Operative and Medical Procedures; Cancer Pain Management;* and *Acute Low Back Pain;* publications by the American Society of Anesthesiologists, the American Pain Society, and Surgical, Neurologic, Oncologic, Nursing, and other organizations of recommendations for improved pain management; and publication of major reports on pain by governments of many countries. The development of an added qualification in "Pain Management" independently by the American Board of Anesthesiologists and by the Australian and New Zealand College of Anaesthetists; the development of an examination and certification by the American Academy of Pain Medicine; the publication by the IASP of *Desirable Characteristics of Pain Management Facilities,* of *The Taxonomy of Chronic Pain Syndromes, Second Edition,* and of *A Manual of Acute Pain Management;* and other significant national and international publications and initiatives have acknowledged that severe pain is a major health problem.

The massive financial costs, lost work days, erosion of lifestyles, disruption of families, and devastating human suffering associated with severe pain, have finally been recognized as an unacceptable medical, economic, and social problem. Persisting pain has now become a "hidden epidemic" with costs rising exponentially in all industrialized countries; the costs of pain exceed the combined costs of AIDS, cancer and heart disease. Because of the diverse physical and psychological effects of severe pain, it is appropriate to view it as a "disease entity." It is now one of the most costly diseases in most countries.

The diagnosis and treatment of severe persisting pain of subacute, chronic-noncancer, or cancer origin, is best carried out in a Multidisciplinary Pain Center as described by IASP. In this, and other settings, neural blockade techniques play an important part. This text aims to give a balanced view, with a critical analysis of the literature, of the safe and effective use of neural blockade in the treatment of acute, chronic, and cancer pain.

Acknowledgments

The Third Edition of *Neural Blockade in Clinical Anesthesia and Management of Pain* has been an even larger undertaking than the Second Edition. As indicated in the Preface, extraordinary growth in this exciting field over the past years has made it necessary to add 28 new authors, out of a total of 52 contributors from 10 different countries. The administrative and logistical exercise of developing this book and bringing it to the final stage has placed great demands on the Editors, their staff, and their families. The Editors wish to thank their professional colleagues in the Department of Anaesthesia and Pain Management, Royal North Shore Hospital and University of Sydney, and the Department of Anesthesia, University of Cincinnati, for their support, interest, and understanding. In Sydney, particular thanks are due to Pat Gray, Susan Ulstrup, and Dr. Margaret Wilkins; and in Cincinnati to Louella Canning.

The love and support of the Editors' families made it possible for the Editors to cope with the demands of the Third Edition; it helped greatly to know that the families believed their work was worthwhile.

To their teachers and peers, the Editors owe their early interest in the scientific basis and clinical aspects of neural blockade and pain management. Professor Cousins developed his interest in neural blockade while working with Professor Philip Bromage at McGill University, Montreal, Canada. While at McGill, his interest in pain was kindled by the lectures of Professor Ronald Melzack on the new Melzack-Wall "gate control theory of pain." He subsequently developed a commitment to the multidisciplinary approach to pain management as a result of working closely with Professor John J. Bonica on the Council of the International Association for the Study of Pain. Editorial skills can, to a degree, be learned "on the job;" however, a term on the editorial board of *Anesthesia and Analgesia* provided superb experience under the masterly leadership of Nicholas M. Greene. Experience as an Associate Editor of the journal, *Pain,* under the leadership of Patrick D. Wall was invaluable. At Stanford University a keen appreciation was gained of scientific method and critical appraisal of the scientific literature from Professors Richard Mazze, John P. Bunker, Ellis Cohen, and C. Philip Larson, Jr.

Professor Bridenbaugh began his clinical and academic involvement in neural blockade at the very start of his specialist career while at the Virginia Mason Clinic in Seattle, Washington, with Drs. L. Donald Bridenbaugh and Daniel C. Moore. He subsequently began a commitment to scientific work in this field while at Stanford University, then at Oxford University, with Sir Robert Macintosh, and also in association with Professor Benjamin G. Covino at Harvard University. His knowledge and his perspective of neural blockade have been greatly influenced by his colleagues in the American Society of Regional Anesthesia and by his experience as an editor and then as Editor-in-Chief of *Regional Anesthesia.*

The Editors have been fortunate to have the services of a medical illustrator of extraordinary talent. Alan Bentley of the Department of Medical Illustrations and Media, Flinders Medical Centre, prepared the artwork for the cover and drew all of the color illustrations, and many of the black and white anatomic illustrations. Each one of these figures resulted from observation of actual block procedures and anatomic dissections, careful study of many original source materials, and long hours of discussion. The Editors thank Alan Bentley for his artistic skill, while preserving anatomic integrity, and his willingness to persevere with the Editors' and authors' attempts to explain the practical points they wished to illustrate.

Many authors and publishers gave permission for their works to be quoted or reproduced, and due acknowledgment has been given in the text.

The First Edition of *Neural Blockade in Clinical Anesthesia and Management of Pain* was started by Professor Michael J. Cousins and the then Editor-in-Chief of medical books at the J.B. Lippincott Company, Mr. Lewis Reines. Soon afterward Professor Phillip Bridenbaugh began working on the book, and both Editors rapidly appreciated the benefits of a running partner. The Second and Third Editions have been the result of a very close and rewarding collaboration between the two Editors. The staff of Lippincott–Raven Publishers have been of great assistance. Particular thanks are due to Craig Percy, Anne Snyder, and Raeann Touhey.

Michele Cousins, B.A. provided editorial assistance to Professor Cousins and proofread a substantial portion of the manuscript.

It is now a quarter of a century since the concepts and early planning for the First Edition of this text began in 1973, while Professor Cousins was at Stanford University, with publication of this edition in 1980. The gestation periods for the Second Edition (1988) and Third Edition (1998) were somewhat longer, reflecting the growth of knowledge in this field. Over the 18 years spanning the first three editions, a large number of readers have expressed their appreciation of the text. For this, the editors wish to say thank you, especially to those who have made suggestions for subsequent editions.

Introduction

Neural Blockade in Clinical Anesthesia and Management of Pain, Third Edition,
edited by M.J. Cousins and P.O. Bridenbaugh.
Lippincott–Raven Publishers, Philadelphia © 1998.

CHAPTER 1

The History of Neural Blockade and Pain Management

David L. Brown and B. Raymond Fink

The father of the field of pain management as we know it today was John J. Bonica, who tirelessly pioneered the development of the multidisciplinary concept of pain research and treatment from the end of World War II until his death in 1994. Among his many contributions, John Bonica founded the International Association for the Study of Pain (IASP) in 1974, which quickly led to the publication of the first issue of the journal Pain in 1975. From its first exciting meeting in Issaquah, Washington, the IASP has grown to a large international body bringing together pain scientists and clinicians from over 50 countries. The IASP and its World Congress on Pain have stimulated relevant basic and clinical research, which has resulted in major advances in our knowledge of pain and its treatment (see also Part 3).

PHYSIOLOGY OF PAIN

Fundamental to modern neural blockade is the concept that pain is a sensory warning conveyed by specific nerve fibers, amenable, in principle, to modulation or interruption anywhere in the nerve's pathway. This outlook may be traced back to developments in the study of physiology that finally supplanted the view first expressed by Plato and Aristotle that pain, like pleasure, is a passion of the soul, that is, an emotion and not one of the senses (see Appendix A at the end of this chapter). Philosophical changes from the great revolutions of the 18th century and the birth of biology gradually, although not entirely, effaced the religious connotations of pain in Western civilization.[29] These revolutions of the 18th century were in part based on the mechanistic concepts of biologic function that Descartes developed during the 17th century. Descartes matured the concept of a neural connection from the periphery to the brain (Fig. 1-1). James Moore (1762–1860), a London surgeon (Fig. 1-2), used these mechanistic concepts to promote neural compression as a useful technique for the provision of surgical anesthesia (see Appendix B at the end of this chapter). As illustrated in Figure 1-3, Moore developed techniques for both upper and lower extremity nerve compression and wrote his monograph, "A Method of Preventing or Diminishing Pain in Several Operations of Surgery," only after experimenting upon himself.[14,100]

The doctrine of specific energies of the senses was first promulgated by Johannes P. Müller (1801–1858) in 1826.[114] This doctrine, although it did not posit specificity for the conduction of pain, initiated the movement of scientific thought toward analysis and classification of the specific characters of different nerves. Earlier, in 1803, Charles Bell defined important functions of the dorsal roots of the spinal nerves as distinct from those of the ventral roots, and initiated a rigorous search for a more complete understanding of the sensory phenomena. Bell highlighted that dorsal root function is sensory and ventral root function is motor.[12] It was in 1851 when von Helmholtz succeeded in measuring the velocity with which the nerve impulse travels and opened the way for the development of modern electrophysiology.[136]

The theory that pain was a separate and distinct sense was first definitely formulated by Moritz S. Schiff (1823–1896) in 1858, following experiments on animals.[37] A rival theory, the intensity theory, was stated explicitly by Erb in 1874 but had been anticipated by Erasmus Darwin (1731–1802), who said that pain results "whenever the sensorial motions are stronger than usual."[37] Attempts to influence neuralgic pain by applying a drug to the transmitting nerve appear to have been published first by Francis Rynd (1801–1861).[116] Rynd's idea may be said to have foreshadowed both nerve block and, more remotely, opioid regional analgesia.

According to some accounts of the 1850s, Pravaz in Lyon

D. L. Brown: Department of Anesthesia, University of Iowa, Iowa City, Iowa 52242.
B. R. Fink: Department of Anesthesiology, University of Washington School of Medicine, Seattle, Washington 98195-6450.

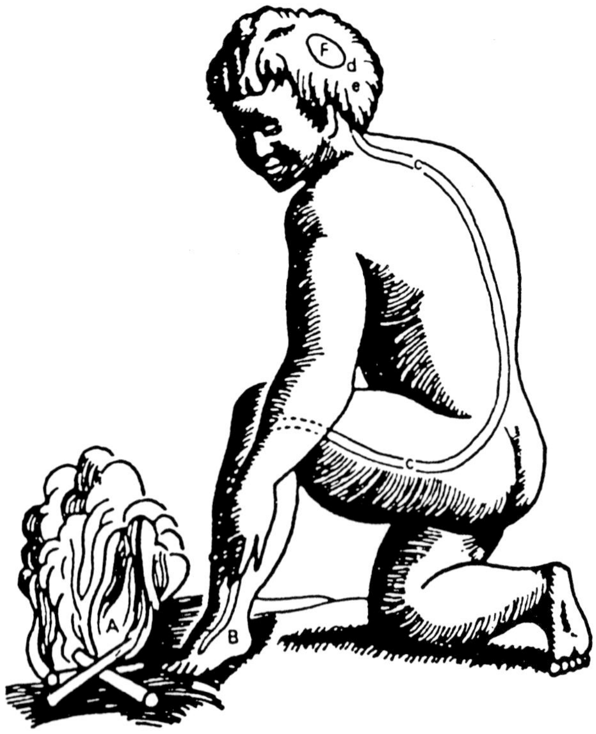

FIG. 1-1. The path of sensation according to Descartes. He wrote: "If for example fire (A) comes near the foot (B), the minute particles of this fire, which as you know move with great velocity, have the power to set in motion the spot on the skin of the foot which they touch, and by this means pulling upon the delicate thread CC, which is attached to the spot of the skin, they open up at the same instant the pore, d, e, against which the delicate thread ends, just as by pulling at one end of a rope one makes to strike at the same instant a bell which hangs at the other end." (With permission from Procacci, P., and Maresca, M.: Evolution of the concept of pain. *In:* Sicuteri, F., Terenius, L., Veccheit, L., and Maggi, C. A. (eds.): Pain Versus Man. Raven Press, New York, 1992.)

and Wood in Edinburgh invented the syringe and hypodermic hollow needle, respectively (see Appendix B at the end of this chapter). A thorough sifting of the historical evidence[72] and independent reexamination of the sources support the following outline of the facts. Rynd in 1845 described the idea of introducing a solution of morphine hypodermically in the neighborhood of a peripheral nerve,[116] with the intention of allaying neuralgic pain in that nerve. However, he introduced the solution not by syringe but by means of gravity, allowing it to enter passively through a cannula after removal of the trocar. The invention of the syringe is lost in the mists of several centuries preceding Alexander Wood (1817–1884). Wood's contribution was his procedure of subcutaneous injection, which he performed in 1855 with a graduated glass syringe and hollow needle supplied by Ferguson.[141] This equipment had been manufactured by Ferguson for a different purpose, namely the injection of ferric perchloride into an aneurysm to produce a coagulum as proposed by Charles-Gabriel Pravaz (1791–1853) in 1853 following experiments in animals.[109] Pravaz himself had used a syringe and trocar (*trois-carre*). Wood thus originated the practice of percutaneous subcutaneous injection to medicate locally a peripheral nerve. His technique was adopted by C. Hunter and renamed hypodermic injection, ostensibly because Hunter had in view a different purpose, namely, systemic absorption of the drug.

Carl Koller (1857–1944) (Fig. 1-4) searched for a surgical local surface anesthetic and hit upon cocaine in 1884, and immediately demonstrated its startling effectiveness on the cornea.[77] This opened the vast new world of local and regional analgesic therapy. James Leonard Corning (1855–1923)[32] conceived and attempted the direct application of an analgesic to the spinal cord, but a defective rationale and unserviceable technique stultified his approach to the management of chronic pain (Fig. 1-5). A deeper knowledge of the underlying mechanisms was requisite. Understanding of these mechanisms remained relatively superficial until the era of electrophysiologic and neuropharmacologic microexploration following World War II.

Melzack and Wall's hypothesis that a spinal gate controls the cephalad transmission of nociception[98] was based on evidence suggesting that the intensity and quality of pain perceived do not bear a push-button, straight-through, one-to-one relationship to the intensity of the stimulus, but are instead determined by a multiplicity of physiologic and psychologic variables (Fig. 1-6). This led directly to the reintroduction of electrical stimulation as a method of treating

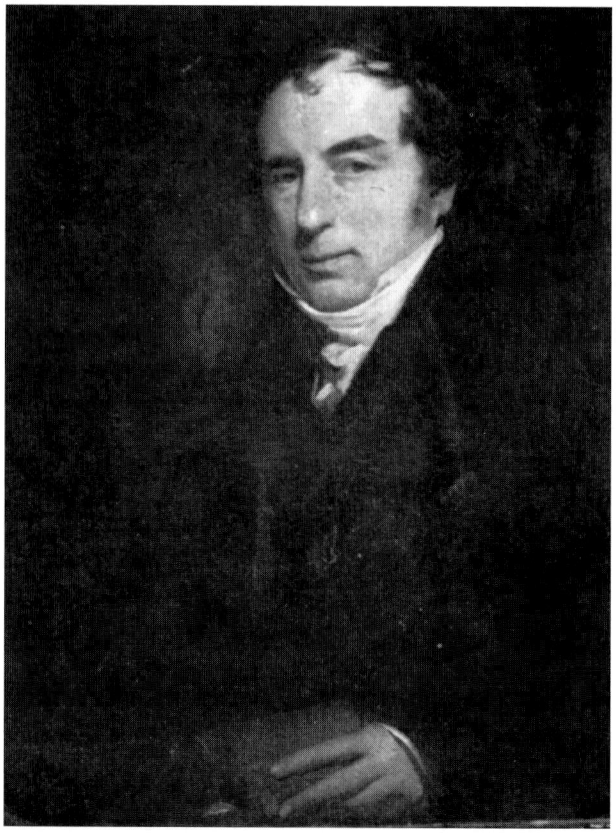

FIG. 1-2. James Moore (1762–1860)

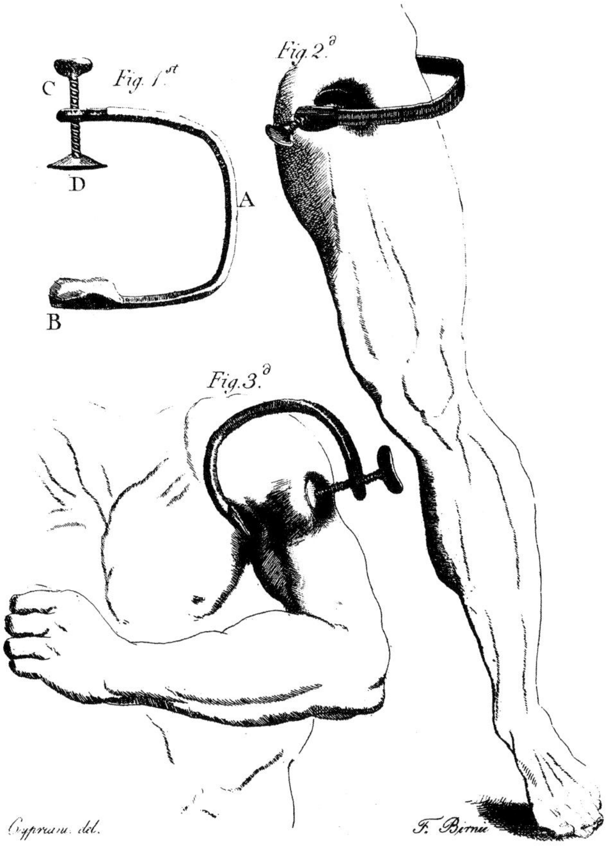

FIG. 1-3. James Moore's compression instruments for upper and lower extremities. (With permission from Moore, J.: A Method of Preventing or Diminishing Pain in Several Operations of Surgery. London, T. Cadell, 1784.)

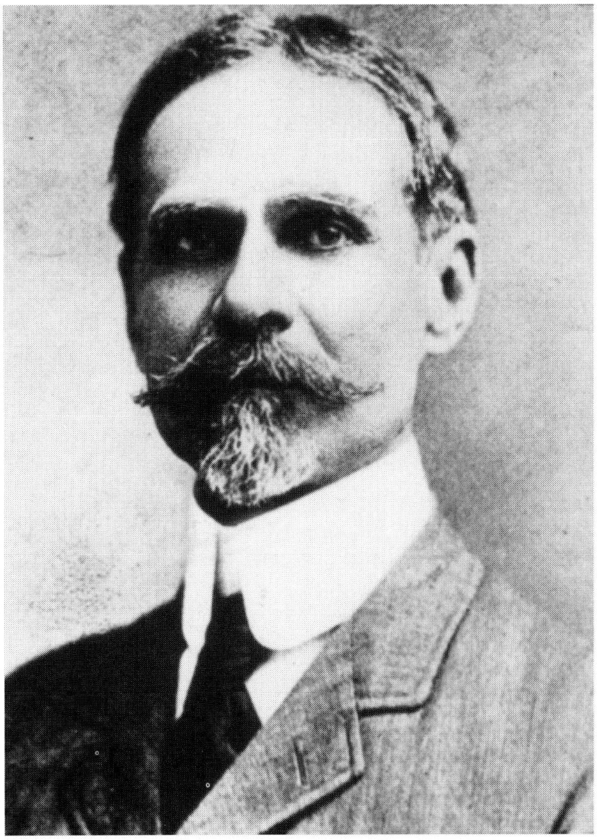

FIG. 1-5. James Leonard Corning (1855–1923)

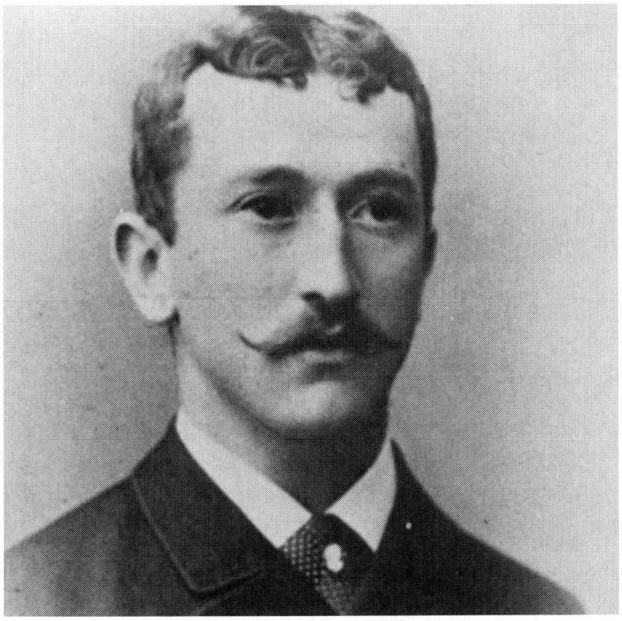

FIG. 1-4. Carl Koller (1857–1944)

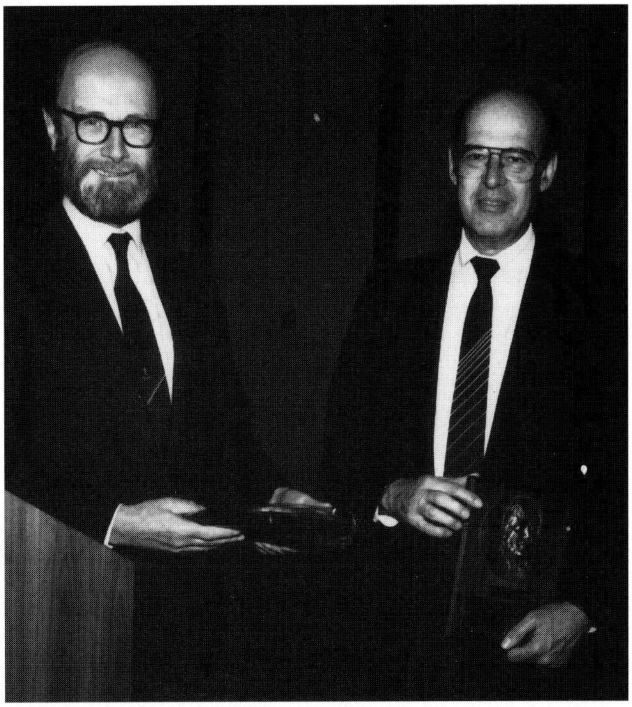

FIG. 1-6. Patrick Wall *(left)* and Ronald Melzack *(right)* receiving awards at 1989 annual meeting of the American Society of Regional Anesthesia.

chronic pain. Although their gate control theory has been shown to be conceptually incomplete with today's understanding, it did provide the framework for most of the advances in understanding spinal cord nociceptive processing.

The search for the mechanism of opiate analgesia and opiate addiction resulted in Reynolds' spectacular demonstration in 1969 of the analgesic effect of electrical stimulation of the periaqueductal gray matter.[113] This seminal discovery gave enormous impetus to pain research and led to the uncovering of a system of descending neurons that inhibit pain and are activated by opiate drugs acting at endorphinergic synapses. Brilliant experimental work by many researchers conceptualized analgesia via a direct spinal action of narcotics, a landmark advance from which important clinical developments have sprung.[76,83,143] Further experimental studies have now been extended to define, with isolated nerve techniques, the concept of "neuroplasticity" and how multiple spinal cord receptors may be modulated by preemptive analgesia techniques.[42] The progression of clinical applications sharply illustrates the process and value of basic medical research. (see Appendix A at the end of this chapter).

COCAINE

The mid-19th century was a period of growth in Western science and technology. In 1865, six years after the publication of Charles Darwin's epochal book, Lister opened a new era in surgery by applying Pasteur's proof of nonspontaneous generation to the elimination of sepsis. Pflüger showed that the seat of respiration was in the tissues and not in the blood, and in 1882, the same year that produced the world's first electrical power station (in New York), Ringer demonstrated the need for calcium and potassium salts to maintain the excitability of the heart. The establishment of the coal tar industry in Germany led to large-scale production of pharmaceuticals, of which the marketing of cocaine by Merck was one result. The year 1886 saw the introduction of steam sterilization of dressings by von Bergmann, and the year 1890, the use of surgical rubber gloves, initially for the purpose of protecting the hands of Halsted's instrument nurse from disinfectant.

Koller's demonstration of ocular surface anesthesia with cocaine[77] had antecedents almost as numerous as those of general anesthesia 40 years earlier. Dr. Scherzer, an Austrian explorer and a member of an expedition to South America, returned with coca leaves to Vienna. Some were sent to Friedrich Wohler for analysis, and subsequently to his pupil, Albert Niemann. Niemann (1834–1861) was successful in isolating and naming the alkaloid from the leaves of *Erythroxylon coca,* as first recorded in 1860 in a report signed W. (for H. Wofler 1800–1882), which also related the passionate chewing of the leaves by the *coqueros* of Peru and the deleterious mental effects this had on them.[103,132] Nobody paid a great deal of attention to the benumbing effects of cocaine on the tongue and the lips until the Peruvian army surgeon Moreno y Mayz remarked in 1868 that the sensory paralyzing effects of cocaine might be put to use in medicine.[121] A thorough pharmacologic investigation of the properties of the alkaloid in frogs was presented by von Anrep, a Baltic surgeon. In 1880, von Anrep published an extensive article on the physiologic and pharmacologic effects of cocaine. It is clear that he understood that cocaine had a locally numbing effect on the tongue and that it dilated the pupil upon local application, and he did suggest that this drug might some day become of medical importance.[134] He ended the report as follows: "The animal experiments have no practical application; nevertheless I would recommend trying cocaine as a local anesthetic in persons of melancholy disposition."[134] Plainly, von Anrep was most impressed by the stimulating properties of cocaine, and these seem also to have been uppermost in the mind of Sigmund Freud (1856–1939) when he suggested a study of the drug to Koller.[9]

Freud wanted to know more about the analeptic action of cocaine, which, he hoped, because of reports from the United States, might be useful in curing one of his great friends of addiction to morphine. This friend was a pathologist who had developed an unbearably painful thenar neuroma after accidentally cutting himself while performing an autopsy. Freud obtained a supply of cocaine from the manufacturing firm of Merck and shared it with Koller, who was to help him investigate its effects on the nervous system. Koller was a junior intern in the Ophthalmological Clinic at the University of Vienna and longed to obtain the coveted appointment of assistant in the clinic, on the strength of a worthy piece of research. In 1884, Koller met Dr. Joseph Gartner at Stricker's Institute for Pathological Anatomy. They dissolved a trace of the white coca powder in distilled water and instilled it in the conjunctival sac of a frog, which allowed its cornea to be touched with no evidence of reflex action or defense. Identical tests were performed on a rabbit and a dog, and the results were equally favorable. Koller wrote: "One more step had now to be taken. We trickled the solution under each other's lifted eyelids, then placed a mirror before us, took pins, and with the head tried to touch the cornea. Almost simultaneously we were able to state jubilantly 'I can't feel anything.'"[9,132] After these experiments he then performed an operation for glaucoma with topical cocaine anesthesia on September 11, 1884, just 4 days before the Congress of Ophthalmology was due to meet in Heidelberg. Koller immediately wrote a paper for the Congress, but, being an impecunious intern, he could not afford the train fare to Heidelberg so he gave the paper to a visiting ophthalmologist from Trieste, Dr. Brettauer, who had stopped in Vienna on his way to the Congress. Brettauer's news from Heidelberg reached New York in a letter from H. D. Noyes, an American ophthalmologist who had attended the Heidelberg Congress.[105]

Noyes's letter to the New York Medical Record excited numerous readers to test the new wonder drug and many of them rushed into print with astounding experiences. One of the most striking, published within 5 weeks of Noyes's communication, was that of N. J. Hepburn, a New York ophthalmologist.[66] There were no standards for drug trials in those days, and the tradition of self-experimentation was inviolate. If a researcher or physician wanted to know whether a drug was safe, he tried it on himself. Hepburn describes how on October 16, 1884, he experimented with a 2% solution of cocaine, giving himself a series of subcutaneous injections of 0.4 ml (8 mg) at intervals of 5 minutes. He noted that by the time of the eighth injection, the agreeable stimulating effects of the drug—rapid respiration and pulse, a feeling of warmth, pleasant hallucinations—had reached such a point that he felt it best to stop. For reasons that Hepburn does not state, he repeated the performance 2 days later, and then found it possible to carry the number of 0.4 ml injections to 16 before the general disturbance persuaded him to cease. He records that four days later he was at it again, and this time he tried a larger unit volume and amount (10 mg), and was able to tolerate 16 of these doses. It seems likely that Hepburn was already in the grip of addiction.

By November 29, 1884, the ophthalmologist Bull was able to report that he had used the drug to produce anesthesia of the cornea and conjunctiva in more than 150 cases.[25] He gave sound reasons for his enthusiasm: He saved the time required for complete etherization and avoided the enormous engorgement of the ocular blood vessels produced by the ether, the danger of vomiting, and the disadvantage that almost any apparatus for producing anesthesia by inhalation was a physical interference for the operator.

One evening in January 1885, while he was on duty in the emergency room, a workman with an injured finger was brought in. Koller noticed there was a tourniquet applied to the base of the finger. Zinner, Billroth's intern, asked Koller to admit the man to Billroth's service and Koller did so but he himself urgently removed the tourniquet in order to save the finger. This act aroused Zinner's ire. Zinner called Koller an impudent Jew. Koller in return slapped Zinner's face. Zinner thereupon challenged Koller to a duel. Billroth specified that all duels were strictly prohibited, but both parties were officers in the reserve and members of the Patriotic German Student Society, whose unwritten code dictated that honor must be avenged. The duel was fought with swords the next day, and Koller wounded his opponent. The law impartially charged both parties with the crime. Koller received an official pardon a few months later, but his prospects for advancement in German-speaking Europe were wrecked, destroyed by the first and last duel known to have been fought over a tourniquet. Soon he immigrated to the Netherlands, and, with Freud's and others' advice, in 1885, to the United States.[51] This series of events seems to be in character for Koller, whose own daughter said he was "a difficult tempestuous young man, one who could never be compelled to speak diplomatically even for his own good."[139]

CONDUCTION ANESTHESIA

After the publication of Noyes's 1884 letter, the idea of injecting cocaine directly into tissues in order to render them insensible occurred simultaneously to several American surgeons. William C. Burke injected 5 minims (drops) of 2% solution close to a metacarpal branch of the ulnar nerve and painlessly extracted a 22-caliber bullet from the base of his patient's little finger.[26] But it was William Stewart Halsted (1852–1922) and Richard John Hall (1856–1897) and their associates who most clearly saw the great possibilities of conduction block (Fig. 1-7).[63–65] The term was introduced by François-Franck in 1892,[53] though he may well have borrowed part of it from Corning, for in 1886 Corning was writing that "the thought of producing anaesthesia by abolishing conduction in sensory nerves, by suitable means, should have been rife in the minds of progressive physicians."[32] Corning himself quite possibly got the idea from Halsted, for Halsted later attested that Corning was a frequent observer at the Roosevelt Hospital in New York, where Halsted, assisted by Hall, performed his teaching. In 1884 Hall described how he blocked a cutaneous branch of the ulnar nerve in his own forearm.[62] He and Halsted made injections into the musculocutaneous nerve of the leg and the ulnar nerve. Hall noted the appearance of marked constitutional symptoms, giddiness, severe nausea, cold perspiration, and dilated pupils, but this did not daunt these bold pioneers, and the same evening

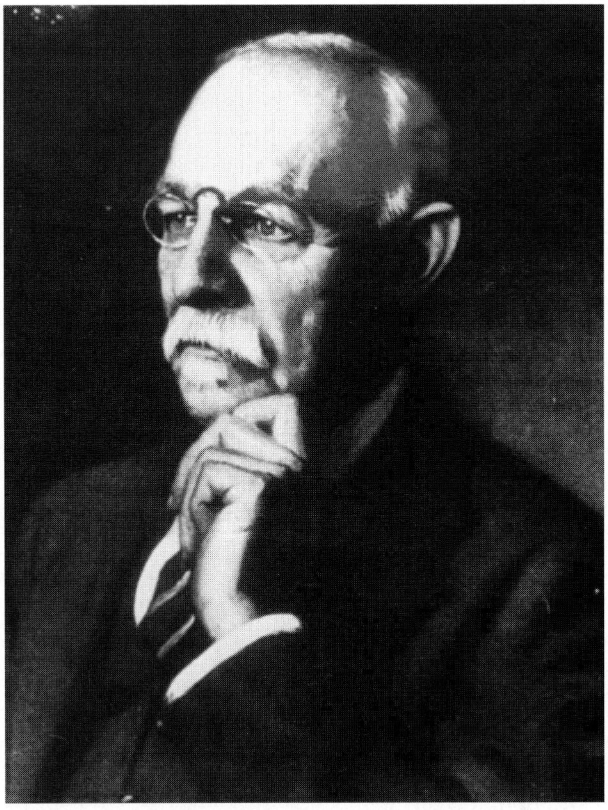

FIG. 1-7. William Stewart Halsted (1852–1922)

Halsted blocked Hall's supratrochlear nerve and removed an adjoining congenital cystic tumor. He also induced Nash, a dental surgeon, to tend to Hall's own upper incisor tooth after injection of cocaine into the infraorbital nerve at the infraorbital foramen, and Halsted thereafter performed an inferior dental nerve block on a medical student volunteer and later did the same to Hall. Hall's report was quite explicit in predicting that, once the limits of safety had been determined, this mode of administration would find very wide application in the outpatient department.

The daring experimenters at the Roosevelt Hospital unfortunately became addicted to the new drug, and no more was heard from them about its use in surgery. It appears that Dr. Halsted with the help of his friend, Dr. William H. Welch, was the only one of the group able to overcome the addiction. It was in 1886, that Halsted, upon an invitation from Dr. Welch, moved to Baltimore. In 1889, after his final recovery from cocaine addiction, he was appointed acting surgeon and head of the outpatient department of the newly established Johns Hopkins Hospital, and in 1890 he became professor of surgery at the new Johns Hopkins Medical School.[50] But that Hall and Halsted were the true progenitors of conduction anesthesia can hardly be doubted.[62,95]

The great advantage of local anesthesia with cocaine was, of course, that it anesthetized only the part of the body on which the operation was to be performed. However, a price was paid in toxicity and time. Rapid absorption limited the safe quantity of cocaine to 30 mg and the useful duration of anesthesia to 10 to 15 minutes. In 1885 Corning sought a means of prolonging the local anesthetic effects for surgical and other purposes, although he was primarily interested in the application of the drug to the therapeutics of neurologic disease.[31] His notion of pharmacokinetics was that after the introduction of cocaine beneath the skin, a certain period of time elapsed during which the anesthetic agent was diffused throughout the surrounding tissue, the capillary circulation having a dual effect, first as a distributor and afterward as a dilutor and rapid remover of the anesthetic substance. In his first article of 1885 Corning described how he experimentally injected 0.3 ml of a 4% solution of cocaine into the lateral antebrachial nerve and obtained immediate anesthesia of the skin supplied by this nerve as far as the wrist. He found that simple arrest of the circulation in the involved part by compression or constriction proximal to the point of injection intensified the anesthesia and prolonged it indefinitely. He used an Esmarch bandage for this purpose and pointed out that the method was readily applicable to surgery of all the extremities. The Riva-Rocci cuff tourniquet had not yet been invented. Esmarch had introduced his elastic bandage in 1874 for the purpose of producing a bloodless field in major amputations.[48]

As has briefly been mentioned, François-Franck was the first to apply the term nerve blocking to the infiltration of a nerve trunk in any part.[53,95] He found that the effect of the blocking drug was not limited to the purely sensory fibers because it paralyzed all nerves, whether motor or sensory, and that the sensory anesthesia was manifested much more promptly than was the motor paralysis, a confirmation of von Anrep's observations of 1879 to 1880. François-Franck spoke of the action of cocaine as a "physiological section," transitory and noninjurious.

Corning's principle of prolonging the local anesthetic action of cocaine by arresting the circulation in the anesthetized area inspired Heinrich F. W. Braun (1862–1934) to dispense with the elastic tourniquet and substitute epinephrine, a "chemical tourniquet" as he called it.[21] Epinephrine had become available in pure form after Abel isolated it from the suprarenal medulla in 1897.[1]

The suggestion for this use of epinephrine came from ophthalmologic practice, in which it had been introduced to limit hemorrhage and to render the conjunctiva bloodless, as well as to treat certain diseases, notably glaucoma, in which it was found to prolong the local effect of other drugs in general and of cocaine in particular. This observation had been confirmed by rhinologists and had enabled them to reduce the concentration and dose of cocaine and correspondingly to limit the hazard of toxicity.[96] Initially, in Braun's solution, the epinephrine was present in concentrations from 1:10,000 to 1:100,000. The first experiments to determine the dosage to be injected subcutaneously were made by Braun on himself. He found his limit of tolerance was 0.5 mg (0.5 ml of 1:1000 solution), after which general symptoms occurred and he had to lie down.

Braun introduced the term *conduction anesthesia*, and he felt that the use of epinephrine rendered conduction anesthesia in other parts of the body as effective as that in an extremity. In 1905 Braun published a textbook on local anesthesia, giving detailed descriptions of the technique for every region (see Appendix B at the end of this chapter).

INFILTRATION ANESTHESIA

Some 10 years earlier, a different approach, termed *infiltration anesthesia*, had been advocated by Karl Ludwig Schleich (1859–1922).[119] Schleich's interest in infiltration anesthesia appeared to stem from poor effects that often followed general anesthesia in that era. Schleich stated: "For however great the improvement that our methods in the treatment of narcosis may undergo in the course of time, it will always remain a dangerous and uncertain interference with the brain mechanism the working of which we are unable to fathom . . . What a blessing, then, if narcosis can be avoided in so great a proportion of cases!"[50,119] Schleich applied the principle that pure water has a weak anesthetic effect but is painful on injection, whereas physiologic saline is not. Although Schleich's initial report on infiltration anesthesia before the Congress of Surgeons in Mainz, Germany, was unfavorably received, by the early 20th century, this technique of anesthesia was widely used. It is reported that Schleich was a meticulous technician who gave great attention to detail, and this likely explains his success over time.[50]

The observation that subcutaneous injection of water produced local anesthesia was apparently first made by Potain in 1869. Halsted, in a short letter to the editor of the New York Medical Journal, dated September 19, 1885,[64] baldly asserted that "the skin can be completely anesthetized to any extent by cutaneous injections of water;" he had of late used water instead of cocaine in skin incisions, and the anesthesia did not always vanish just as soon as hyperemia supervened.

Schleich believed that there must be a solution of such a concentration between "normal" (0.6% salt solution) and pure water that would not provoke pain on injection and yet be usefully anesthetic, and he thought a 0.2% solution of sodium chloride was ideal. To this, he added cocaine to a concentration of 0.02% and employed the mixture to produce a field of cutaneous anesthesia in the surgery of hydrocele, sebaceous cyst, hemorrhoids, and small abscesses.

The reason why Schleich's hypotonic solutions containing a minuscule amount of cocaine produced impairment of sensation does not appear to have been explained. In the light of later work, it seems possible that loss of electrolyte from nerve fibers may have been involved. Braun dismissed Schleich's solutions as nonphysiologic and insisted that injections into the tissues for whatever purpose must be composed of fluids of the same osmotic tension as the body fluids. Inasmuch as most local anesthetic solutions are hypotonic, a corresponding amount of an indifferent salt, such as sodium chloride, must be added to prevent any injurious action upon the tissue.

Nevertheless, Schleich's infiltration technique was an important advance in that it extended the field of usefulness of a small quantity of anesthetic. Schleich was probably indebted to Paul Reclus for the idea of using a weak solution of cocaine to avoid toxic reactions and fatalities. Enthusiasm for local anesthesia had diminished owing to casualties, but Reclus clearly understood that the basic cause of accidental deaths was overdose from the use of unnecessarily high concentrations.[112] He realized that undue absorption could be avoided by using lower concentrations, and he eventually reduced the strength of his cocaine solutions to 0.5%.

LOCAL ANESTHETICS

The toxicity of cocaine, coupled with its vast potential for usefulness in surgery, led to an intensive search for less toxic substitutes. However, decreased toxicity without increased irritancy—or impractically brief effectiveness—proved elusive until the synthesis of procaine (Novocaine) by Einhorn in 1904. No specific report to that effect appears in the literature, so it fell to the lot of the surgeon Heinrich Braun to make the report in 1905, along with descriptions of two other agents, stovaine and alypin.[33] Procaine's short duration of activity limited clinical utility; thus, research focused on dibucaine (1925). Meischer synthesized dibucaine, a quinoline derivative, which Uhlmann introduced clinically. In 1928, Eisleb synthesized tetracaine, which was then introduced into clinical practice in 1932. Although dibucaine and tetracaine proved to be potent, long-acting local anesthetics, their increased systemic toxicity limited the usefulness of these agents for many of the regional anesthetic techniques in which large volumes of drugs were required. Thus, these agents found their primary use in the field of spinal anesthesia and even today continue to be used. Most of the chemical compounds synthesized during this first pharmaceutical period were amino ester derivatives similar in most respects to cocaine. Most of these amino ester agents were relatively unstable and could not be subjected to repeated autoclaving for sterilization. In addition, the hydrolysis of amino esters by the enzyme plasma pseudocholinesterase resulted in the formation of para-aminobenzoic acid which was responsible for reported allergic reactions.[22] Additional crucial properties for wider use of local anesthetics, chemical stability and absence of sensitization, were achieved with lidocaine, which was introduced in 1947 (see Appendix C at the end of this chapter).[89]

Lidocaine, synthesized in 1943 by Löfgren and Lundqvist, was a stable compound that was not influenced by repeated exposures to high temperatures and thus, could be resterilized often. In addition, the metabolites of lidocaine did not include *P*-aminobenzoic acid; thus, allergic reactions were avoided.

Lundqvist, like many early investigators, started using lidocaine on his own toes and fingers and even for spinal anesthesia. In August 1943, Lundqvist called another friend Lagergreen and said that a friend of his had synthesized a new local anesthetic. They arranged a meeting with representatives of the drug company Pharmacia and asked if Lagergreen would come as their medical expert and demonstrate finger blocks on volunteers. This he did, performing five to ten of the blocks, and the results were demonstrated for the executives of Pharmacia. They were to be given a decision within 2 weeks, but Löfgren and Lundqvist never heard from them. Since there had been no response after the respite time, Lundqvist called Lagergreen and said that a Mr. Jordan, science attaché at the U.S. embassy, wanted to meet them. Lagergreen went with them more as an interpreter. Mr. Jordan made an immediate offer of $15,000 for the rights to the discovery, but nothing was decided. The gossip spread like wild fire, and soon Ciba, Roche, and Bayer were out to get this new wonder drug. Also, ICI was interested and it is said that Löfgren went to London in the tail of a Mustang, a plane which flew ball bearings from Sweden to England, by night during the war. However, again no decision was made. This happened between August 23 and September 10, 1943, when Astra laboratories bought the method and patent.[58] At this point, the clinical testing of lidocaine was conducted by Gordh (Fig. 1-8) with the assistance of his wife, Ulla, also a physician. Volunteer patients were given 5 crowns (60 cents) for their help. Students were given a copy of Gordh's thesis (1945) or a package of American cigarettes, which were very difficult to obtain during the war. Most of them chose the cigarettes. Gordh made his first presentation of clinical results in 1947 at a meeting of the Swedish Anesthesia Club, the predecessor of the Swedish Society of Anesthesiologists.

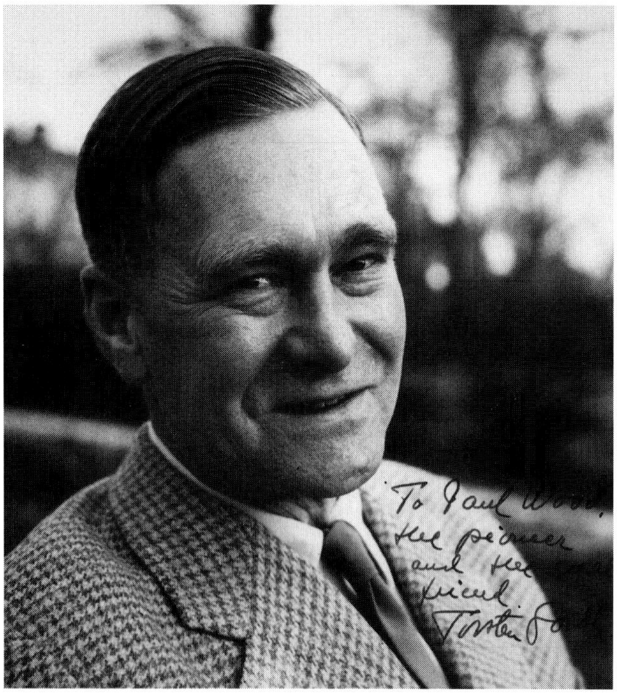

FIG. 1-8. Torsten Gordh (1907–)

In the same year, it was also presented at the Scandinavian Surgical Society's first meeting after the war. The results were published in Svenskja Lakartidningen in 1948.[58]

Subsequent to lidocaine's release, a number of amino amide compounds were synthesized and four eventually found their way into clinical practice. In 1956, Ekenstam in Sweden synthesized mepivacaine, whose anesthetic properties were similar to lidocaine. In 1959, Löfgren and co-workers synthesized prilocaine in an attempt to produce a local anesthetic whose clinical potency was similar to that of lidocaine, but which was less toxic. Lidocaine and mepivacaine were tertiary amide compounds while prilocaine was a secondary amide. Bupivacaine had been synthesized by Ekenstam at approximately the same time as mepivacaine. However, bupivacaine was not introduced into clinical practice until 1963 by Telivuo. Following the initial reports by Widman concerning the prolonged duration of action of bupivacaine, it gained wide acceptance because of its potency and ability to provide significantly longer anesthesia than was possible with either lidocaine or mepivacaine. In 1971, Takman synthesized etidocaine, which was another amino amide compound similar in structure to lidocaine but with a duration of action comparable to bupivacaine. Unlike bupivacaine, which provided only partial blockade of motor fibers, etidocaine provided profound motor blockade. The most recent amide local anesthetic to be introduced is ropivacaine. The drug was synthesized by Ekenstam in 1957 and is structurally related to bupivacaine and mepivacaine. It is a chiral drug and exists as two stereoisomers (*S* or *R* form) and is manufactured as a single enantiomer, rather than a racemic mixture. Interest in the drug stems from experimental work suggesting it has less potential for cardiotoxicity than bupivacaine.

INTRAVENOUS REGIONAL ANESTHESIA

In 1908, August K. G. Bier (1851–1949), a surgeon and physiatrist, and first assistant to Johann Friedrich August von Esmarch, devised a very effective method of bringing about complete anesthesia and motor paralysis of a limb (Fig. 1-9).[16] He injected a solution of procaine into one of the subcutaneous veins that were exposed between two constricting bands in a space that had previously been rendered bloodless by an elastic rubber (Esmarch) bandage extending from the fingers or toes. The injected solution permeated the entire section of the limb very quickly, producing what Bier called *direct vein anesthesia* in 5 to 15 minutes. The anesthesia lasted as long as the upper constricting band was kept in place. After it was removed, sensation returned in a few minutes. Heinrich Braun reports that Bier suggested limiting this "vein anesthesia" to those cases in which local anesthesia was not possible.[23] Direct vein anesthesia (intravenous regional anesthesia) was not widely used until Holmes reintroduced the technique with lidocaine in 1963 (see Appendix D at the end of this chapter).[70,85]

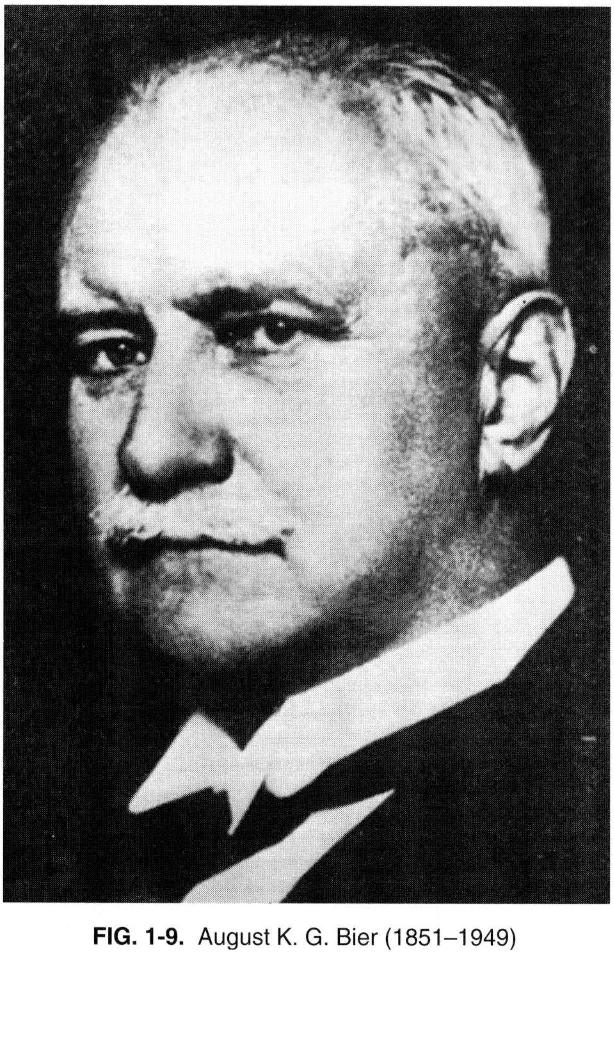

FIG. 1-9. August K. G. Bier (1851–1949)

SPINAL ANESTHESIA

Somewhat paradoxically, the first spinal anesthesia occurred 5 years before the first lumbar puncture. The term *spinal anesthesia* was introduced by Corning in his famous second paper of 1885.[32] It was the fruit of a brilliant yet erroneous idea, because what he had in mind was neither spinal nor epidural anesthesia as currently understood. Corning was under the mistaken impression that the interspinal blood vessels communicated with those of the spinal cord, and his intention was to inject cocaine into the minute interspinal vessels and have it carried by communicating vessels into the spinal cord. He made no mention of the cerebrospinal fluid, nor of how far he introduced the needle into the spinal space.

Corning's objective was clearly expressed by the title of his article, "Spinal Anaesthesia and Local Medication of the Cord with Cocaine."[32] There is no doubt that Corning was quite literally aiming directly at the spinal cord, as he introduced a hypodermic needle—he does not say of what size—between the spinous processes of the T11 and T12 vertebrae. He wrote:

> I reasoned that it was highly probable that, if the anesthetic was placed between the spinous processes of the vertebrae, it would be rapidly transported by the blood to the substance of the cord and would give rise to anaesthesia of the sensory and perhaps also of the motor tracts of the same. To be more explicit, I hoped to produce artificially a temporary condition of things analogous in its physiological consequences to the effects observed in transverse myelitis or after total section of the cord.

Corning's report was based on a series of two: one dog and one man. In the case of the man, he injected a total of 120 mg of cocaine, about four times the potentially lethal dose, in a period of 8 minutes. Corning implies that he was using the procedure partly as a treatment for masturbation. What he achieved in the man was probably what is now called *epidural* or *extradural anesthesia*, and, in the dog, which received 13 mg, *spinal anesthesia*, as judged by the rates of onset. Corning certainly did have an original idea, as he was at no small pains to indicate, but the results were a lucky accident because the experiment could easily have been fatal and was conceived on the basis of an entirely erroneous notion of the local circulation.

There is, of course, no direct communication between the extradural capillaries and those of the spinal cord so it is rather difficult to understand on what Corning based his expectations. At least as early as 1870, Gray's Anatomy[59] had a section on the meninges, including the subarachnoid space and cerebrospinal fluid,[4] but Corning apparently was unaware of its existence. He kept the syringe connected to the needle with rubber tubing and thus would not have seen cerebrospinal fluid drip from the needle. Although English language anatomy books clearly delineated the spinal meninges and cerebrospinal fluid, the contemporary German and French language textbooks did not. Corning had a long line of New England ancestors, but he received his medical education in Europe at the University of Wurtzburg,[17] and so possibly never learned the basic facts of meningeal anatomy. In any case, how he got the idea that there were vascular channels between the spinous processes of the vertebrae which were a direct avenue into the spinal cord remains unclear.

Lumbar Puncture

Corning was a neurologist, not a surgeon, and he thought of his spinal use of cocaine as a new means of managing neurologic disorders. He did foresee that it would probably find application as a substitute for etherization in genitourinary or other branches of surgery. However, nothing came of his suggestion until 14 years later, perhaps because conceptual errors flawed his technique at a time when the procedure of lumbar puncture had not yet been invented, let alone standardized. It fell to Heinrich Irenaeus Quincke (1842–1922) to do this, by basing his approach on the anatomical ground that the subarachnoid spaces of the brain and spinal cord were continuous and ended in the adult at the level of S2, whereas the spinal cord extended only to L2.[30] Thus, a puncture effected in the third or fourth lumbar intervertebral space would not damage the spinal cord. Quincke's principal claim to fame was his introduction and popularization of lumbar puncture, first as a method of treatment for tubercular meningitis in children, then as a simple, safe, and necessary clinical development in the investigation of diseases of the nervous system.[85]

Lumbar puncture, as the title of Quincke's article indicated,[111] was invented as a treatment for hydrocephalus. Quincke acknowledged in his communication that he followed in the steps of Essex Wynter, who 6 months earlier had described the use of a Southey's tube and trocar for a similar purpose.[142] This device was originally designed to drain edema fluid in cases of dropsy. Wynter introduced the tube between the lumbar vertebrae, after making a small incision in the skin, for the purpose of instituting drainage of the fluid in two cases of tuberculous meningitis. Quincke's method was a vast improvement and became the standard technique, thanks to a detailed description that is still up to date. Quincke prescribed bed rest for the 24 hours following the puncture. Quincke's needles had an internal diameter of 0.5 to 1.2 mm, and only the larger ones were equipped with a stylet. It is interesting to note that he entered the skin 5 to 10 mm from the midline. Thus, the paramedian approach is and has always been the classic one, and not the median approach as is sometimes taught.

It took 8 years for Quincke's technique to be applied to the production of what is now called *spinal anesthesia*. No doubt, great courage was required to introduce a drug as toxic as cocaine directly into the nervous system, as Corning had attempted in 1885. Unfortunately, Corning's audacity had no direct sequel unless the title of Bier's paper is taken as an implied tribute to Corning. (Bier does not mention him by name.) August Bier published his celebrated paper on spinal anesthesia in 1899, under the title "Versuche über Cocainisirung des Rückenmarkes" (Research on Cocainization of the Spinal Cord).[15] Apparently Bier also assumed that intrathecal injection of cocaine produced anesthesia by a direct action on the spinal cord. Bier had a certain amount of luck on his side; he worked at the same institution as Quincke and would have been familiar with his technique and might even have borrowed his needles.

Bier, of course, was a surgeon, and it is noticeable that for many years virtually all the extensions of technique in the use of local anesthetics were developed by surgeons. They first performed the block and then performed the operation. This makes Corning's interest in cocaine all the more remarkable because he was genuinely an outsider in the field and may well have been viewed as such. He seems to have eluded the hazard to which several of the American surgical pioneers of regional anesthesia fell victim when their conscientious zeal led them to experiment on themselves before trying their ideas on patients. Apparently the first surgeons in the United States to use spinal anesthesia were Tait and Caglieri of San Francisco. On October 26, 1899, they performed an osteotomy of the tibia after the patient received spinal anesthesia (see Appendices B and D at the end of this chapter).[128]

Bier wanted to apply cocaine anesthesia for major operations and saw spinal anesthesia as a way to safely produce a maximum area of anesthesia with a minimum amount of drug. It was his opinion that the spectacular insensitivity to pain evoked by small amounts of cocaine injected into the dural sac resulted from its spread in the cerebrospinal fluid and that it acted not only on the surface of the spinal cord but especially on the unsheathed nerves that traverse the intramembranous space. However, this understanding was not conclusive. The extent of the anesthesia produced was somewhat unpredictable, so Bier decided to obtain an improved insight by experimenting on himself. His assistant, Hildebrandt, performed the lumbar puncture on Bier, but when the time came to attach the syringe to the needle, a crisis developed; the needle did not fit. A considerable amount of cerebrospinal fluid and most of the cocaine dripped onto the floor. To salvage the experiment, Hildebrandt volunteered his own body. This time there was a good fit and complete success. However, the success was not without sequel. The experimenters celebrated with wine and cigars, and the next day Bier suffered an oppressive headache that lasted for 9 days. Hildebrandt's "hangover" developed even before the night ended. Moreover, while he was anesthetized, Hildebrandt had been scientifically kicked in the shins to demonstrate the depth of the analgesia, and in the aftermath he duly developed painful bruises in places where no pain had been. As Bier emphasized in his paper, his experiences proved that by the injection of extraordinarily small amounts of cocaine (5 mg) into the dural sac, about two-thirds of the entire body could be made insensible enough for the painless performance of major operations. Complete loss of sensation lasted about 45 minutes. Bier decided that the escape of a considerable amount of cerebrospinal fluid was probably responsible for the after effects. He believed that in his own case some type of circulatory disturbance was present, because he felt absolutely well in a supine position but had a sensation of very strong pressure in the head and felt dizzy only if he sat up. Bier concluded that the escape of cerebrospinal fluid should be avoided if possible, and strict bed rest should be observed. Bier said that the size of the needle should be very fine and that, after the dural sac had been entered, the stylet should be withdrawn and the opening immediately closed with a finger so that as little cerebrospinal fluid as possible escaped.

Halsted had introduced the use of rubber gloves at operations in the winter of 1889 to 1890, as noted earlier in this chapter, but not with the intention of avoiding wound infection. That consequence was actually serendipitous. His motive was to spare the hands of his operating room nurse (whom he later married), who had developed a dermatitis from mercurous chloride. Soon the operators took to wearing them as well, but only out of convenience. It was not until 1894 that the wearing of gloves was recommended as part of aseptic technique.[65] It surely is a fortunate coincidence that Bier did not start his work on spinal anesthesia until after this important prophylactic measure had become generally available.

The news of Bier's work, published in April 1899, spread quickly, and, although he abandoned it himself, his method of subarachnoid spinal anesthesia was soon brought into prominence by Théodore Tuffier (1857–1929) (Fig. 1-10).[129] In the spring of 1900, in a report on 63 operations, Tuffier enunciated the rule: "Never inject the cocaine solution until the cerebrospinal fluid is distinctly recognized."[84,130] The sensation caused by Tuffier's demonstrations is well conveyed by Hopkins, who wrote: "To be able to converse with a patient during the performance of a hysterectomy, the patient all the while evincing not the slightest indication of pain (and even being unable to tell where the knife was being applied) was certainly a marvel, and was well worth crossing the Atlantic to see."[71]

In the United States, spinal anesthesia was adopted for obstetrics by Marx and for general surgery by a number of surgeons, most prominently Rudolph Matas (1860–1957) (Fig. 1-11).[94] Matas's article begins with a critical historical review of older methods of local and regional anesthesia. In his description of spinal anesthesia, cocaine hydrochloride, in the amount of 10 to 20 mg, was dissolved in distilled water. The solution instilled was therefore clearly hypotonic. Fowler preferred to have his patients in the sitting position for the injection and not surprisingly was often astonished by the rapidity and completeness of the anesthesia.[52] Gravity methods were not yet understood.

Aseptic precautions were strictly observed, and E. W. Lee mentions that the injection he used consisted of 12 to 20 minims of a 2% sterilized solution prepared in hermetically sealed tubes by Truax, Green and Company of Chicago.[84] This appears to be the earliest published reference to this

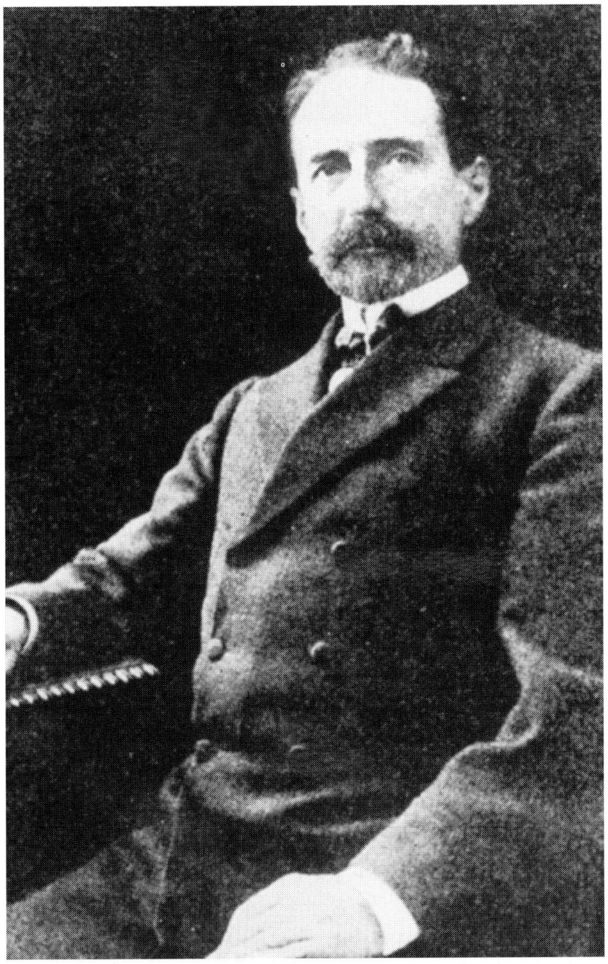

FIG. 1-10. Theodore Tuffier (1857–1929)

method of packaging, an important advance because previously it was necessary for the surgeon to prepare his own solution from tablets and sterilize it.

In 1912, Gray and Parsons of Birmingham, England, undertook an extensive study of variations in blood pressure associated with the induction of spinal anesthesia.[60] They concluded that the bulk of the fall in arterial blood pressure during high spinal anesthesia is attributable to the diminished negative intrathoracic pressure during inspiration, which is dependent on abdominal and lower thoracic paralysis. They noted that when the negative pressure in the thorax is increased, the arterial blood pressure rises (see Appendices B and E at the end of this chapter).

It was by then quite clear that one of the principal dangers of spinal anesthesia is the lowering of the blood pressure. Believing this to be the primary hindrance to its more universal adoption among urologists, Smith, working with Porter, reported in 1915 the results of 50 experiments on cats.[124] They found that the quantity of anesthetic solution was more important for diffusion than its concentration, dilute solutions usually spreading farther than concentrated ones. The introduction of procaine beneath the dura in the region in which the splanchnic nerves arise caused as profound a fall in blood pressure as was caused by complete resection of the cord in the upper thoracic region. This, they thought, proved that the fall in blood pressure was not due to toxicity of the drug or to paralysis of the bulbar vasomotor center but to paralysis of the vasomotor fibers that regulate the tonus of the blood vessels in the splanchnic area. Since these nerve roots originate between T2 and T7, Smith and Porter believed that the main clinical objective was to prevent cephalad diffusion of the drug from reaching this height and paralyzing these nerve roots.

Gaston Labat (1877–1934)[80] emphasized that the danger of spinal anesthesia was not the fall in blood pressure *per se* but rather the associated cerebral anemia, both being attributable to the increased volume of blood in the viscera caused by splanchnic vascular paralysis and vasomotor collapse (Fig. 1-12). He expressed the belief that this cerebral anemia could be avoided by placing the patient in the Trendelenburg position immediately following the intraspinal injection and that, by this procedure, the brain would be kept amply supplied with blood, and irremediable respiratory failure would be avoided. To ensure that the blood pressure would not drop during spinal anesthesia, the practice of administering ephedrine subcutaneously was introduced. The idea of making the injected solution hyperbaric with glucose,

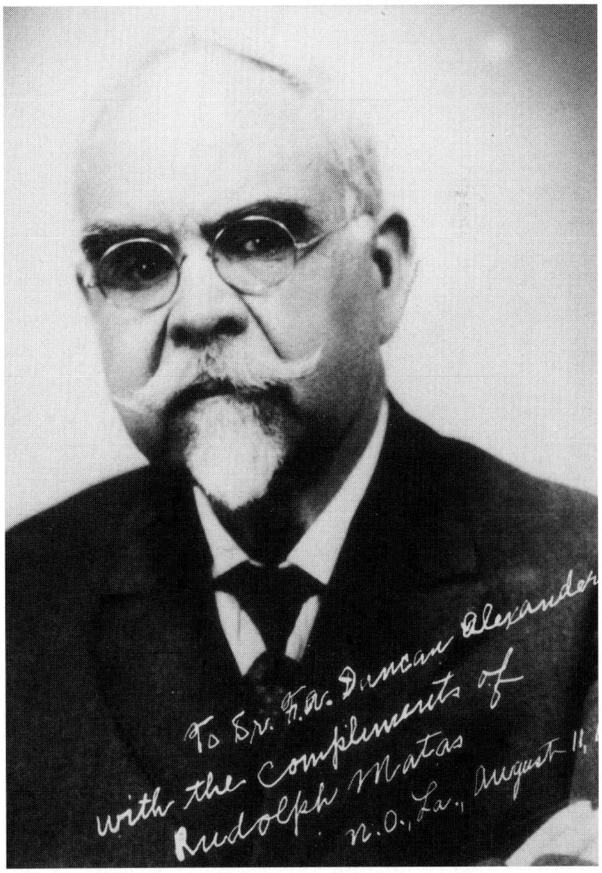

FIG. 1-11. Rudolph Matas (1860–1957)

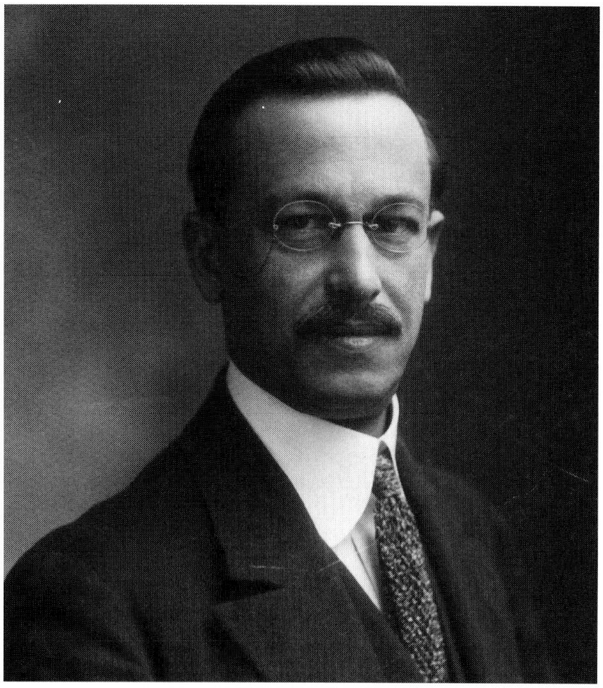

FIG. 1-12. Gaston Labat (1876–1934)

in order to obtain control over the intrathecal spread of the solution, originated with Arthur E. Barker.[7] Barker employed stovaine, euphoniously so called from the English translation of its inventor's name, Fourneau.[41] Stovaine was less toxic than cocaine but was very slightly irritating and was eventually superseded by procaine. Barker's stovaine came directly from the laboratory of Billon in Paris, where it was made up in 5% glucose especially for Barker and packaged in sterile ampules. Barker was a professor of surgery at the University of London, and his article is exceedingly thoughtful, based on some 80 cases. He describes experiments with a glass model of the spinal canal, conforming to the shape seen in a mesial section of a cadaver and bearing a T-junction in the lumbar region to simulate the injection site.

Years later, Pitkin, in 1928, and Etherington-Wilson, in 1934, experimented with a similar apparatus but without acknowledging any debt to Barker.[108] Their goal was the opposite of Barker's, to obtain control over the rate of ascent of the drug by making the injected solution hypobaric. Control was achieved by varying the time the patient was kept sitting upright after the injection. Pitkin did this by mixing alcohol with the procaine solutions, a mixture he called *spinocaine*, but he categorically warned against having the patient in the sitting position during injection. He controlled level of blockade by tilting the table and illustrated this with a figure showing an "altimeter" attachment.

Barker stressed such points of technique as raising the head on pillows: Whenever he injected a heavy fluid intradurally, he kept the level of analgesia below the transverse nipple line. At times, he seated the patient on the edge of the table with the feet on a low chair to make the fluid run into the sacral end of the dural sac, where it quickly affected the roots of the nerves supplying the anus and the perineum.

Barker advocated puncture in the midline as being easier and allowing more even spread of the injected fluid than the paramedian approach. He, too, emphasized that in no case should the analgesic solution be injected unless the cerebrospinal fluid ran satisfactorily. Above all else, perfect asepsis throughout the entire procedure was absolutely necessary. Moreover, no trace of germicides should be left on the skin, because they could be conveyed by the needle into the spinal canal, where their irritating qualities were particularly undesirable. Barker enjoined that all needles, syringes, and other instruments for the procedure were to be kept apart for this sole use, including the little sterilizer in which they were boiled. Billon's sterilized, sealed ampules were to be opened only a moment before use.

Barker's rational approach to the use of a hyperbaric solution for spinal anesthesia was apparently forgotten when stovaine was replaced by improved drugs and had to be rediscovered after trials of quasi-isobaric solutions of several new drugs led to unsatisfactory control of spinal level. The lessons of the past were ignored or forgotten by surgeons and not yet learned by anesthesiologists. Indeed, at that time there were few anesthesiologists to learn. In 1920, W. G. Hepburn[67] revived Barker's technique with stovaine, and Sise, an anesthesiologist at the Lahey Clinic, applied it to procaine in 1928 and to tetracaine in 1935 (Fig. 1-13).[122,123]

Tetracaine's great advantage as a spinal anesthetic was its relatively prolonged duration of action without undue toxic effects, but this advantage was partially negated by the vagaries of its segmental spread, which resulted from its being used in an approximately isobaric solution. Therefore, Sise mixed the solution with an equal or greater volume of 10% glucose and injected it while the patient lay on his side on a table tilted head down 10°. The patient was then turned on his back and a good-sized pillow inserted under his head and shoulders to flex the cervical spine forward as much as possible; the slope of the table was adjusted during the next few minutes as dictated by the level of analgesia needed.

A refinement of this technique was the "saddle-block" described in detail by Adriani and Roman-Vega.[4] Anesthesia deliberately confined to the perineal area was obtained by performing the lumbar puncture and injection of hyperbaric solution with the patient sitting on the operating table and remaining so for 35 to 40 seconds after the injection.

An article that announced a hypobaric solution and the associated modifications in the technique of spinal anesthesia was published by W. W. Babcock in 1912.[5] He dissolved 80 mg of stovaine in 2 ml of 10% alcohol, thus obtaining a solution whose specific gravity was less than 1.000, well below that of the cerebro-spinal fluid, which he took to be 1.0065. He believed that the anesthesia that resulted was chiefly a nerve root anesthesia and not the "true spinal cord anesthesia" obtained with the standard solutions. Babcock said that the lightness of this particular anesthetic solution caused it to rise rapidly within the cavity of the arachnoid. He stressed that the patient should promptly have the head and shoulders lowered after the injection, but he rather perversely insisted that during the injection the patient should be sitting on the operating table, the legs hanging over the side of the table. He further remarked: "In most cases spinal anesthesia enables me to operate entirely free from the worry and watchfulness associated with etherization by an untrained assistant . . . I have thus been able to operate successfully upon the neck, face, and even the cranium. . ." But let us not fail to note that Babcock also promulgated the following dictum: *"Death from spinal anesthesia usually indicates inefficient or insufficiently prolonged methods of resuscitation."* The emphasis is his. Further, Babcock's dictum must be considered in light of the report that he was so depressed over the death rate (1 per 500) associated with general anesthetics administered by interns at his Philadelphia institution (Temple University) that spinal anesthesia was preferred over general anesthesia for almost all patients.[46]

One of the first lumbar puncture needles was that devised by James Corning and it was fashioned of either gold or platinum alloy to prevent rusting and fracture. It was by necessity very expensive, and came with an introducer, rather like the introducer described by Sise of Boston in 1928. Other early spinal needles were manufactured from carbon steel "nickeled over," but this stained and rusted on repeated boiling, and occasionally fractures occurred in these needles. Stainless steel, which was really rust-resistant steel, made its appearance in about 1928 following the work of Brearley of Sheffield in England and was known as the hard type or martensitic steel. In the 1930s, the German firm of Krupp and Essen produced a truly stainless alloy steel that was given the name austenitic steel of V2A, but it was not until the 1940s that this material was used in the production of spinal needles. By 1945, nearly all needles used for spinal analgesia were made from rust-proof or true stainless steel. Fine bore needles were employed by Hoit in 1922 and by Green of the University of Oregon in 1923 in attempts to prevent post–lumbar puncture headache. Green's needle also included a pencil-point smooth needle tip which he hoped would reduce dural trauma and thus development of postdural puncture headaches.

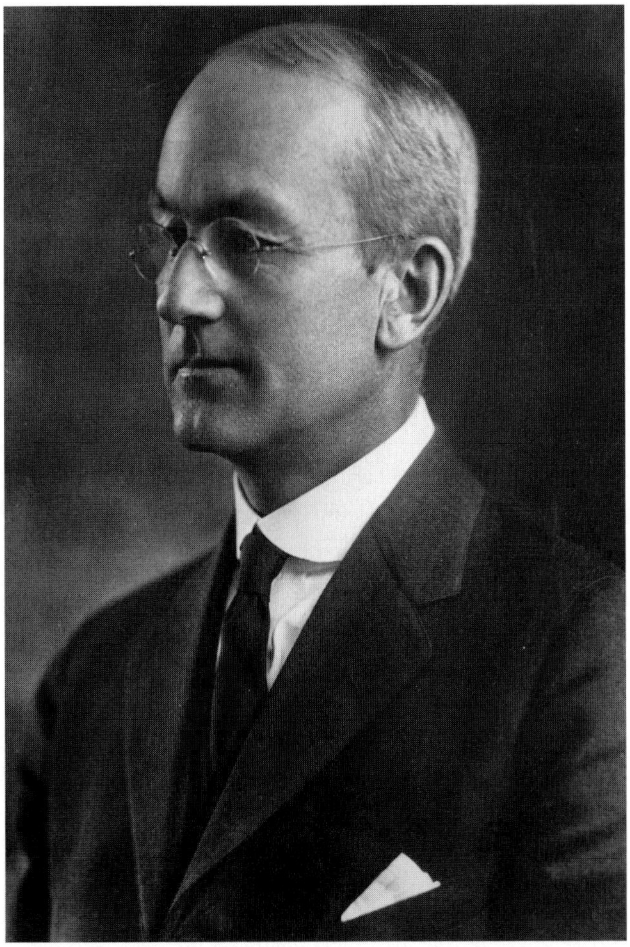

FIG. 1-13. Lincoln F. Sise (1874–1942)

A method for continuous spinal anesthesia was described by W. T. Lemmon in 1940.[87] It was performed with the aid of a special mattress, a malleable needle, and special tubing, and was proposed for long operations that required abdominal relaxation. The equipment was original but not the main idea. In 1907, H. P. Dean wrote of having so arranged the exploring needle that it could be left *in situ* during the operation and another dose injected without moving the patient beyond a slight degree.[39] He proposed that additional injections be made postoperatively to treat pain or abdominal distention. Whether anything ever came of his proposal, he did not say. Lemmon's ponderous technique was quickly simplified by E. B. Tuohy.[131] He performed continuous spinal anesthesia by means of a ureteral catheter introduced in the subarachnoid space through a needle with a Huber point.

There were also surgeons who purposely attempted to achieve widespread regional block via the spinal route to perform a wide variety of surgical procedures. Koster in 1928 detailed the types of procedures he was carrying out during spinal anesthesia.[78] Koster reported:

> The purpose of this paper is to describe a technique for safely producing surgical anesthesia of the entire body by the injection of an anesthetic solution into the spinal subarachnoid space. In my clinic, in a general surgical service, spinal anesthesia has been used almost exclusively for the past 3½ years in all cases needing operation on structures below the diaphragm. The only exceptions have been where the anesthesia was needed for such a short period as to make not worth while, e.g., ambulatory cases needing incision, drainage of fingers, abscesses, etc.

Koster went on to include a section on mortality in this report.

> Is the anesthesia safe? We have not as yet had a fatality directly attributable to the anesthesia. Nevertheless: another death occurred in a highly toxic diabetic patient of 62 with a rapid spreading gangrene of the foot and leg. During the course of the guillotine operation at the middle third of the thigh, his pulse suddenly became imperceptible, and stimulation failed to restore his circulation.

TABLE 1-1. *Listing of surgical procedures promoted by Koster as suitable for spinal anesthesia, circa 1928*

Amputation of lower extremity up to hip
Embolectomy of external iliac artery
Herniotomy
Reduction of fractures and dislocations
Operation for osteomyelitis, lower and upper extremity
Appendectomy
Excision of rectum for carcinoma
Colectomy
Enterectomy
Hemorrhoidectomy
Anterior and posterior colporrhaphy
Tracheoplasty
Interposition operation
Repair of vesicovaginal and rectovaginal fistulae
Salpingo-oophorectomy
Hysterectomy
Hysteropexy
Nephropexy
Nephrectomy
Nephrolithotomy and pyelotomy
Uretotomy
Prostatectomy
Cholecystectomy, choledochotomy, and cholecystenterostomy
Splenectomy
Gastrectomy, pylorectomy, pyloroplasty, and gastroenterostomy
Costectomy and thoracotomy
Radical mastectomy
Embolectomy of the axillary artery
Thyroidectomy
Resection of cervical glands
Excision of tumors of the tongue, face, and scalp
Craniectomy
Mastoidectomy
Nasal plastic
Cesarean section

One must wonder if this may have been one of the predictable bradycardias that have accompanied spinal anesthesia since its introduction. The variety of procedures carried out under spinal anesthesia in Koster's clinic is indicated in Table 1-1. Koster's work followed an earlier work by Jonnesco who was an early proponent of the wide use of spinal anesthesia for surgical procedures.

As with many new ideas, proponents are often characterized as zealots, and such is the case with Thomas Jonnesco of Bucharest.[73]

> At a meeting of the German Society of Surgery in Berlin in April, 1909, Professor Beir of Berlin is reported to have said that the method of general spinal analgesia described by me at the Congress of the International Society of Surgery in Brussels, in September, 1908, must be rejected, and Professor Rehn of Frankfurt is reported to have said that experiments on animals showed that considerable danger attended such injections if made higher than the lumbar region as recommended by me. These pronouncements, which seem to be without appeal, prove once more that the method described by myself and my assistant, Dr. Amza Jiano was too novel and too hearty to be accepted without opposition . . . During the eight months subsequent to October, 1908, I used spinal analgesia in all my operations, whether performed in the University Clinic, in the Cultza Hospital, or in my private practice; I have never once had recourse to anesthesia by inhalation. There are two essential points of novelty in the method: (1) The puncture is made at the level of the spinal column appropriate to the region to be operated upon; (2) An anesthetic solution is used which, thanks to the addition of strychnine, is tolerated by the higher nervous centers.

OBSTETRIC AND EPIDURAL ANESTHESIA

Tuffier's favorable experience with spinal anesthesia for operative interventions on the lower limbs and urogenital organs led O. Kreis of Basel to give the method a trial in childbirth.[79] He injected 10 mg of cocaine at the L4–5 level, in five parturients, and claimed that this alleviated pain with little impairment of muscular power or uterine motility; however, he recommended the method particularly for forceps delivery. S. Marx[93] in the United States quickly followed with several reports praising the ability of lumbar cocainization to still "the agonizing and maniacal shrieks of these poor women" for 1 to 5 hours, without cessation of uterine contractions; spontaneous bearing down was eliminated, although when told to do so the patient was capable of bringing her abdominal muscles into play as powerfully as under normal conditions. All of this occurred in the year 1900, but the enthusiasm soon waned.

Interest in obstetrical regional anesthesia was revived when W. Stoeckel[125] developed what he termed *sacral anesthesia* with procaine. The feasibility of injecting a local anesthetic by the caudal route was demonstrated by Fernand Cathelin (1873–1945) in 1901. Cathelin based his approach on a thorough anatomical study of the sacral canal and its contents.[28] He found that fluids injected into the extradural space through the sacral hiatus rose to a height proportional to the amount and speed of injection. His objective was to develop a method that would be less dangerous but just as effective as subarachnoid lumbar anesthesia. He was successful in reducing the danger, but his efforts to demonstrate the efficiency of the caudal injection for surgical operations were disappointing, and indeed Cathelin himself thought its principal sphere of usefulness lay in the treatment of bladder incontinence and of enuresis in children. Of further interest is that Cathelin's promotion of epidural anesthesia via the sacral route came only a week after Sicard had presented a paper on extradural injections at the Society of Biology meeting in Paris (Fig. 1-14). It seems clear from Cathelin's remarks that competition for priority of publication was well established even at the turn of the century. Quoting Dr. Cathelin, "We believe we should present our results now, remarking only that setting aside all questions or priority, Dr. Sicard and I carried out our experiments simultaneously and independently, one from another." Despite Dr. Cathelin's position that priority was not an issue, in his brief report dates that preempted Dr. Sicard's paper were presented five times.[28]

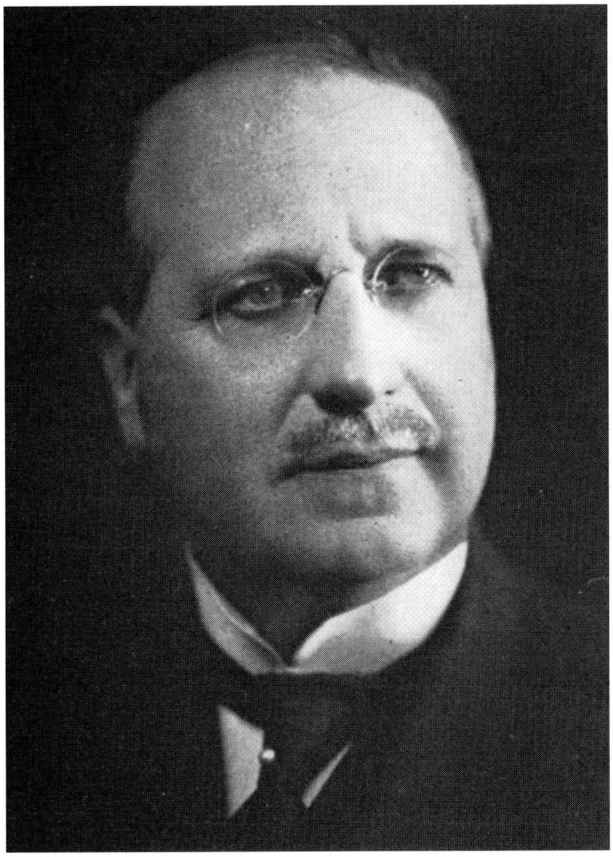

FIG. 1-14. John Sicard (1872–1929)

Reflecting on the similarities in the innervation of the bladder and uterus, the gynecologist W. Stoeckel thought that if the pain of childbirth was largely uterine in origin, as seemed probable, the caudal epidural method of the urologist Cathelin offered an ideal approach to painless obstetrics. Cathelin himself had considered pregnancy a contraindication to epidural injection because of the hazard of toxic absorption of cocaine. Stoeckel, however, had begun to use procaine and considered the reduced toxicity of the new drug acceptable. Stoeckel gave the method careful study. He injected colored fluid into the sacral canal of cadavers and noted its extensive spread upward and, contrary to Cathelin's observations, also through the sacral foramina. In 1909 Stoeckel described his experience with caudal anesthesia in the management of labor. He wrote that various concentrations of procaine and epinephrine produced predictably varying degrees of success after a single injection. Pain relief averaged 1 to 1½ hours in duration, but, warned Stoeckel, the greater the analgesic effect, the greater the hazard of impairing the forces of labor. These reservations, of course, would not apply to the use of caudal anesthesia for surgical operations, and Läwen, in 1910, described how he used Stoeckel's experience and Cathelin's ideas to perform a variety of interventions in the vicinity of the perineum.[81]

Läwen had tested the effectiveness of various concentrations and volumes of procaine–sodium chloride solutions with indifferent success, until he took to preparing and using the bicarbonate salt, as recommended by O. Gros.[61] Gros, in the pharmacology laboratory, had established that bicarbonate salts penetrated the nerve sheaths more rapidly than the hydrochloride salts. Läwen exploited this discovery by using increased volumes and stronger concentrations (20 to 25 ml of a 1.5% to 2% solution) to produce anesthesia in the gluteal region, rectum, anus, skin of the scrotum, penis, upper and inner parts of the thigh, and the vulva and vagina. The anesthesia developed after a delay of 20 minutes and lasted for 1½ to 2 hours. He performed all the common operations on these parts and, hence, was the first to employ sacral anesthesia for operative work, reporting 47 cases with an incidence of failure of 15%.

Pauchet, in 1914, prior to becoming Labat's mentor, was credited with overcoming this incidence of failure by injecting the sacral nerves individually through the posterior sacral foramina, a method that has become known as transsacral anesthesia (Fig. 1-15).

The duration of satisfactory anesthesia from a single peridural injection was limited to a few hours. After Lemmon's demonstration of continuous spinal anesthesia in 1940,[87] it was not long before the "continuous" technique (actually replenishments at half-hour intervals) was transferred by Edwards and Hingson to obstetrical delivery, in which it had an important sphere of usefulness (Fig. 1-16).[47] This was a rational development, following on the seminal work of Cleland, which identified the pathways of uterine pain and clarified the sources of failure and success of regional obstetric block.[30] Cleland had determined that all the sensory fibers that supply the fallopian tubes and uterus enter the spinal cord through T11 and T12, and he blocked

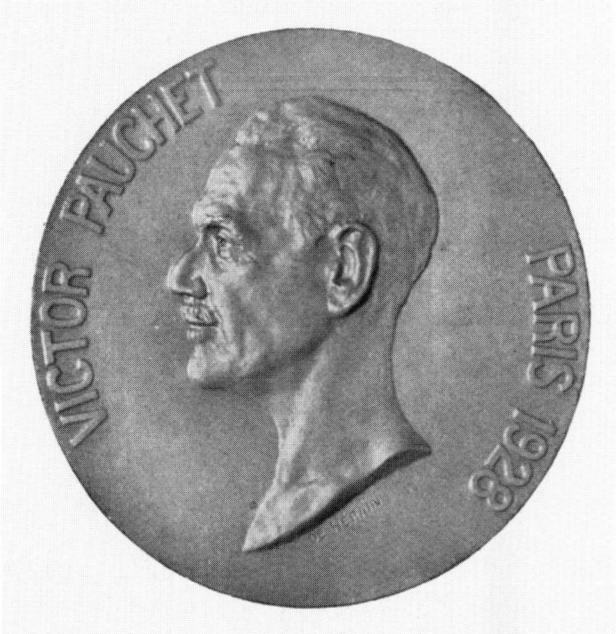

FIG. 1-15. Likeness of Victor Pauchet, imprinted in Paris in 1928 upon his death.

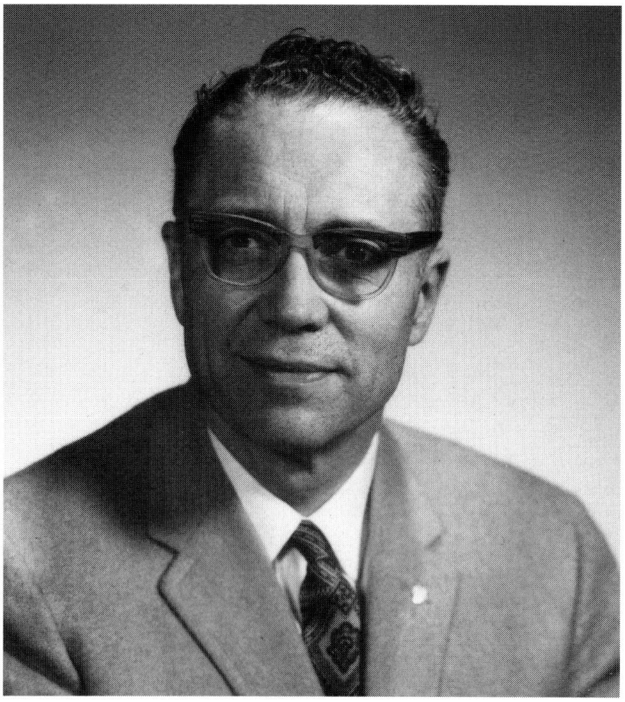

FIG. 1-16. Robert A. Hingson (1913–)

them paravertebrally, while those from the cervix and perineum were interrupted by caudal block.[30] Edwards and Hingson realized that the continuous method enabled them to start the anesthesia early and to continue it for as long as necessary, 5 or 6 hours on the average, to the completion of labor and repair of an episiotomy or laceration. An initial dose of 30 ml of 1.5% metycaine in physiologic saline produced freedom from pain within 5 minutes.

Caudal block by catheter in obstetrics was announced by Manalan in 1942,[91] independently of Hingson's group, but his described technique of injection was not "continuous." He introduced a No. 4 ureteral silk catheter through the lumen of a 14-gauge needle, advanced the catheter until stopped by the dura, and then withdrew the needle, leaving the catheter in place. The injection, 30 ml of 1% procaine with epinephrine, was withheld until required. Later he substituted a nylon catheter for the silk catheter because the nylon one could be sterilized more easily. Block and Rochberg devised a continuous gravity drip of procaine and instituted it from the outset, so as to detect any untoward symptoms before a large amount of the drug had been introduced.[18] However, the earliest intimation of continuous regional anesthesia in the practice of obstetrics came from Eugene Aburel of Romania.[3] For the first stage of labor he used a specially made combination of catheter and needle: He introduced the needle paravertebrally into the lumbosacral plexus, injected 30 ml of 0.05% dibucaine solution, and then introduced an elastic silk catheter similar to a ureteral catheter through the needle, before withdrawing the needle and fixing the catheter with adhesive tape. Repeated paravertebral injections were given through the catheter, which was "tolerated well, during a rather long period of time." For the second stage he administered a single (caudal) injection of 30 to 35 ml or infiltrated the perineum. He declared that continuous local anesthesia for obstetrics was henceforth a proven practical procedure but this claim apparently failed to persuade contemporary obstetricians (see Appendix D).

PARAVERTEBRAL CONDUCTION ANESTHESIA

Matas, the eminent American pioneer and historian of regional anesthesia, recorded that Sellheim, injecting close to the posterior roots of T8 to T12, in addition to the ilioinguinal and iliohypogastric nerves, was able to perform abdominal operations successfully.[95] Sellheim was, therefore, credited by Matas as being the originator of the paravertebral method of anesthesia. It was 6 years later, Kappis having in the meantime greatly improved on Sellheim's technique, that the method was first used in urologic surgery. According to Kappis, success with conduction anesthesia of the trigeminal nerve led him to seek an anatomically reliable approach to conduction anesthesia of the spinal nerves at their exit from between the vertebrae.[74] In his paper, he described posterior approaches to the lower seven cervical nerves for the purposes of cervical and brachial plexus block. He cautioned against blocking C4 bilaterally at the same time. He made up his own solution of procaine-epinephrine and let it stand for an hour because he believed this improved its effectiveness. The method for paravertebral block of the thoracic nerves and the first four lumbar nerves was given in this same paper, and was used in a great many upper abdominal operations. Finally, Kappis pointed out that these techniques could also be used to treat acute and chronic pain with procaine, or even with alcohol if motor function could be disregarded. Two years later, Kappis described his posterior approach to the splanchnic plexus.[75] In 1922, Läwen found unilateral paravertebral block of selected spinal nerves useful in the differential diagnosis of intra-abdominal disease.[82] For example, he observed that a 10-ml injection of 2% procaine at T10 could completely relieve the pain of a severe biliary colic for 3 hours. The use of segmental paravertebral block for the differential diagnosis of painful conditions was an original idea of Läwen's. At the suggestion of Pal, it was then tried by Brunn and Mandl in 1924[24] as a therapeutic measure in the hopes of obtaining pain relief in acute cholecystitis, but without significant success. Kappis had treated a case of angina pectoris in this manner in 1923, and von Gaza used 0.5% procaine diagnostically prior to resection of the affected paravertebral nerves.[135] In 1925 Mandl reported 16 cases of angina pectoris in which he injected procaine, 0.5%, paravertebrally with excellent results.[92] The next year Swetlow attempted to destroy the afferent sensory fibers altogether by substituting 85% alcohol for the procaine and for the most part obtained satisfactory relief of pain for several months.[81]

The pioneer of alcohol injection for the purpose of producing a long-lasting interruption of neural conduction was

Schloesser.[120] Schloesser presented the method as a means of managing convulsive facial tic; he obtained paralysis that lasted from days to months, according to the quantity of alcohol injected. He suggested that the method would also be useful for supraorbital neuralgia and tic douloureux. Like many a pioneer, he was too far ahead of his time to gain an immediate following.

Segmental peridural anesthesia, under the name of metameric anesthesia, was used for the first time in 1921 by Fidel Pagés, a Spanish military surgeon (Fig. 1-17).[106] It is of note that Pagés, reported in his original metameric anesthesia manuscript that the epidural space diameter varies at different levels of the spinal column: "These dimensions are not fixed, and in part, depend on movement of the body." Thus, another early report contains an issue which continues to be highlighted by researchers even today.[69] To Dogliotti, however, belongs the credit for systematizing and popularizing the peridural principle to produce what he termed *segmental peridural spinal anesthesia* (Fig. 1-18).[43–45] In the light of later theory, which requires that three consecutive internodes be blocked to prevent saltatory conduction, it is interesting to note Dogliotti's iteration of the need to bathe a sufficient length of the spinal nerves. He emphasized that if the anesthetic solution is injected in sufficient quantity (50 to 60 ml) and under adequate pressure, it will be quite easy to subject the spinal nerves to the action of the injected fluid throughout their length in the spinal canal and the intervertebral foramina, and even beyond. Dogliotti's method was easier and, without question, simpler than paravertebral regional block, since only one puncture was needed. He stressed the sudden loss of resistance when the point of the needle, having pierced the ligamentum flavum, entered the epidural space. The usefulness of this technique was extended further when Curbelo decided to apply the Tuohy armamentarium for continuous spinal anesthesia to continuous segmental peridural anesthesia.[35] In one case, he left the catheter in place for as long as 4 days and administered a total of 10 injections of 15 ml each of 2% procaine solution for the production of a continuous sympathetic lumbar block.

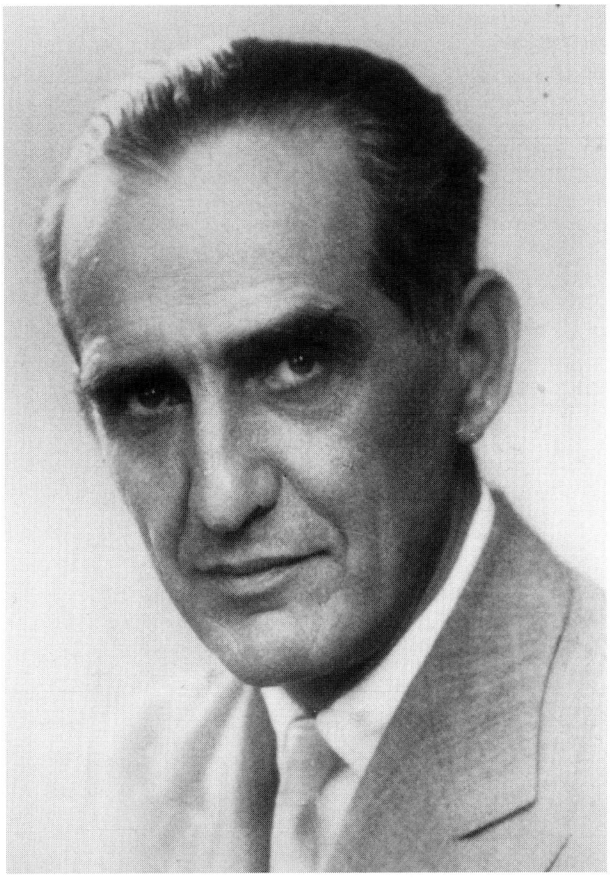

FIG. 1-18. Achile Mario Dogliotti (1897–1966)

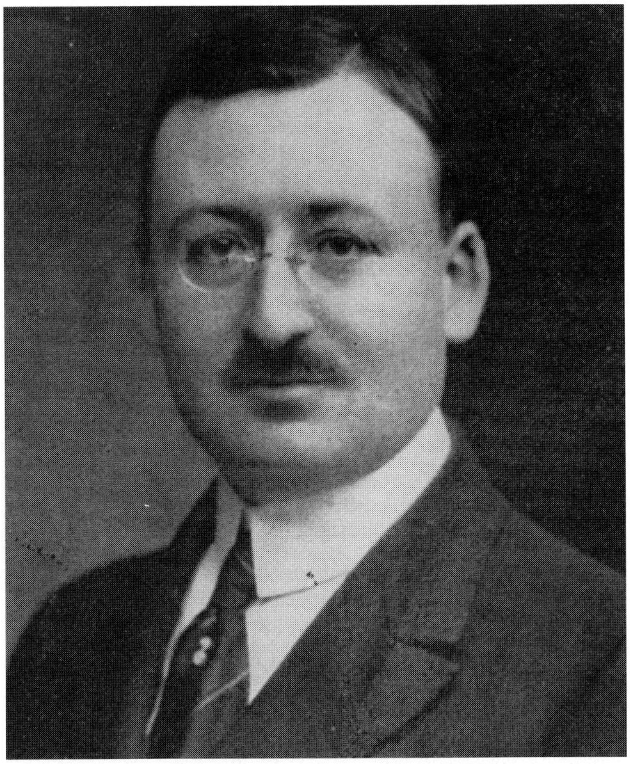

FIG. 1-17. Fidel Pagés (1886–1923)

DEVELOPMENT OF PAIN MEDICINE

The treatment of pain is one of the oldest of human needs. An understanding of neural pathways of pain necessarily waited for development of local anesthetics, which allowed anatomic pathways to be clarified. As outlined earlier in this chapter, until the 19th century, many concepts of pain were tied to Greek and Roman philosophy, which sought to provide a conceptual framework for the site of the soul, the means of pain transmission, mechanisms of external sensation, and balancing of pain, pleasure, and sensory input.[110]

The scientific study of sensation and more specifically pain began when Bell and Magendie demonstrated in animals that the function of ventral roots is motor and that of dorsal roots sensory.[90] Müller's concept of specific nerve energies, that is the idea that the brain receives information on external objects and body structures only by way of sensory nerves, fit with Bell and Magendie's observations and thus was widely accepted.[101] Müller's concept of a "straight-through" system from sensory organ to the brain appears to have been embraced in part because of its simplicity.[110] Schiff performed animal experiments and noted that pain and touch were independent, further supporting the specificity theory of pain.[118] Finally, Gasser and Erlanger demonstrated in 1929 that peripheral nerve conduction velocity was a function of fiber type, adding support to the specificity theorists (see also Chapter 33, Table 33-4).[54]

A competing theory on pain was the intensive theory of pain, originally proposed by Erasmus Darwin (1751–1802), who suggested that pain resulted "whenever the sensorial motions are stronger than usual."[38] This theory received support from Naunyn[102] and Goldscheider[57] who developed the theory that stimulus intensity and central summation of pain impulses were critical determinants of pain.

Overlaid on these two competing theories was one from the anatomical school of Oxford promoted by Weddell, who proposed the pattern theory.[86] The pattern theory suggested that there are no specific cutaneous receptors for the different sensory modalities, rather, the different stimuli provoke excitation of nonspecific receptors according to different spatiotemporal patterns of activation; the different spatiotemporal patterns induce the onset of various kinds of sensations in the central nervous system. Weddell's theory was accepted especially by clinicians, who found it suitable to interpret some complex clinical conditions, such as postherpetic neuralgia, sympathetically maintained pain, and central pain. It also gained support from Beecher[11] who described and popularized the concept of transient loss of perception of pain even when fully adequate painful stimulation was occurring. He described this in soldiers wounded in battle at Anzio, and it was readily apparent that the same phenomenon occurred in athletes hurt during sport.

In 1959, Noordenbos promoted the "sensory interaction" theory of pain, derived from Goldscheider's original concept.[104] It was only years later that Melzack and Wall outlined their gate control theory of pain (Fig. 1-19), which again supported clinical observations (that is external stimuli on the skin can often inhibit pain), and this introduced a dynamic and adaptable concept of pain.[98] This theory outlined the following concepts:

1. All primary afferents, large and small, were activated by noxious stimulation of the skin.
2. Both large and small fibers activated the nociceptive neurons deeper in the dorsal horn, which they named transmission neurons.
3. Large fibers activated, but small fibers inhibited, the neurons of the substantial gelatinosa.
4. Substantia gelatinosa neurons, when active, inhibited the input onto transmission neurons from both large and small primary afferents by a presynaptic mechanism ("close the gate").
5. Higher brain centers could also activate this inhibitory system to close the gate.
6. Pain perception, thus, was influenced by the net effect of large primary afferents, small primary afferents, and higher brain function, via their pattern of activity on substantia gelatinosa neurons.[70]

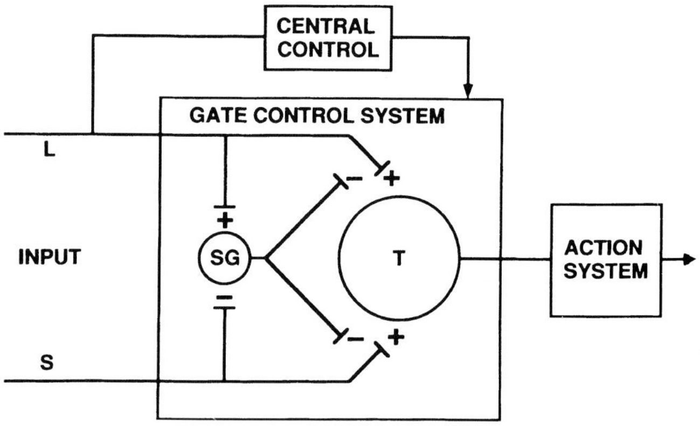

FIG. 1-19. Schematic representation of the gate control theory of pain mechanisms: *L*, large diameter fibers; *S*, small diameter fibers. The fibers project to the substantia gelatinosa *(SG)* and first central transmission *(T)* cells. The inhibitory effect exerted by SG on the afferent fiber terminals is increased activity in L fibers and decreased activity in S fibers. The central control trigger is represented by a line running from the large-fiber system to the central control mechanisms. These mechanisms, in turn, project back to the gate control system. The T cells project to the entry cells of the action system. +, excitation; −, inhibition. (Reprinted with permission from Melzack, R., and Wall, P.D.: Pain mechanisms. Science, *150*:971, 1965. Copyright by the AAAS).

These six points of the gate control theory emphasized that sensory input is subject to modulation by afferent, intrinsic (interneuronal), and descending (bulbospinal) activity. Further, it proposed that modulation could be either excitatory or inhibitory.[2] Although this theory has been shown to be an incomplete and sometimes erroneous hypothesis, it remains likely that it was the most important work of the 20th century on the neurophysiology of pain.[68]

Much of the early work with pain perception focused on nociceptive impulse transmission from periphery to the brain. Nonetheless, shortly following the introduction of the gate control theory, another important observation was made, but this time focusing on descending modulation of pain perception. Reynolds reported in 1969 that rats tolerated laparotomy without an anesthetic if their periaqueductal gray matter was electrically stimulated, but not if adjacent brain areas were stimulated.[113] Over the intervening 25 years considerable research into descending modulation has been performed, and it is clear that activation of certain brain sites results in inhibition of nociceptive neurons in the spinal cord.[8] These descending pathways involve chemicals ranging from opiates to cathecholamines, and dorsal horn neurons including nociceptive-specific to wide dynamic range neurons.

Parallel to the interest in nociceptive neurophysiology was a developing interest in clinical relief of often obscure painful conditions. As outlined, wartime often "concentrated" chronic pain patients, allowing physicians to see patterns otherwise too infrequent for tabulation. For example, Weir Mitchell and associates G. R. Moorehouse and W. W. Keen observed during the American Civil War that many men experienced "causalgia" from war-related nerve injury. At that time they published their monumental work, *Gunshot Wounds and Other Injuries of Nerves*, which contained their observations of injuries in the Unionist soldiers at Turners Lane Hospital for Nervous Diseases in Philadelphia.[99] During and following World War I, a number of physicians, including Meige and Athanassio[97] and Leriche,[88] continued to investigate sympathetically mediated pain, as did others involved in caring for patients in nerve injury centers during World War II.[20] Similarly, Beecher's observation of pain modulation occurring during the invasion of Anzio probably would not have been possible without the "concentration" of large numbers of injured men. Nevertheless, anesthesiologists did not always wait for wars to concentrate patients; rather, many began early diagnostic work with nerve blocks and local anesthetics, once maturity of block techniques and drug manufacturing existed.

Von Gaza pioneered the use of procaine for determining the pathways of obscure pain.[135] But it was left to White to discover and demonstrate the wide diagnostic utility of procaine block of sensory or sympathetic nerves, as the case may be, in determining the pathways of peripheral pain.[138] White emphasized the advantage to the surgeon and the patient of knowing exactly how much relief of suffering or improvement of circulation might be expected from an operation. Conceptually, it was but a short step from diagnostic block to therapeutic block, and indeed the step was taken by von Gaza and by Brunn and Mandl in 1924[24] in the management of visceral pain. In the same year, Royle in Australia demonstrated that relief of deforming contractions and spastic paralyses (Little's disease) could be obtained by interrupting the sympathetic nerve supply to the musculature of the affected parts.[115] Long-term pain relief by neurolytic injection of alcohol was developed by Swetlow for the interruption of cardiac afferent inflow and subsequently applied to paravertebral sympathetic block in the treatment of severe intractable pain, particularly the pain of malignant disease (see Appendix D).[127]

Dogliotti, in 1930, took the bold step of injecting absolute alcohol into the subarachnoid space, hoping to produce by simple chemical means a posterior rhizotomy equivalent to that previously attainable only by surgery.[122] At the opposite end of the local anesthetic concentration spectrum, Sarnoff and Arrowood exploited the continuous subarachnoid injection of dilute procaine (0.2%) to obtain a differential block limited to efferent sympathetic fibers and afferent fibers subserving pain.[117]

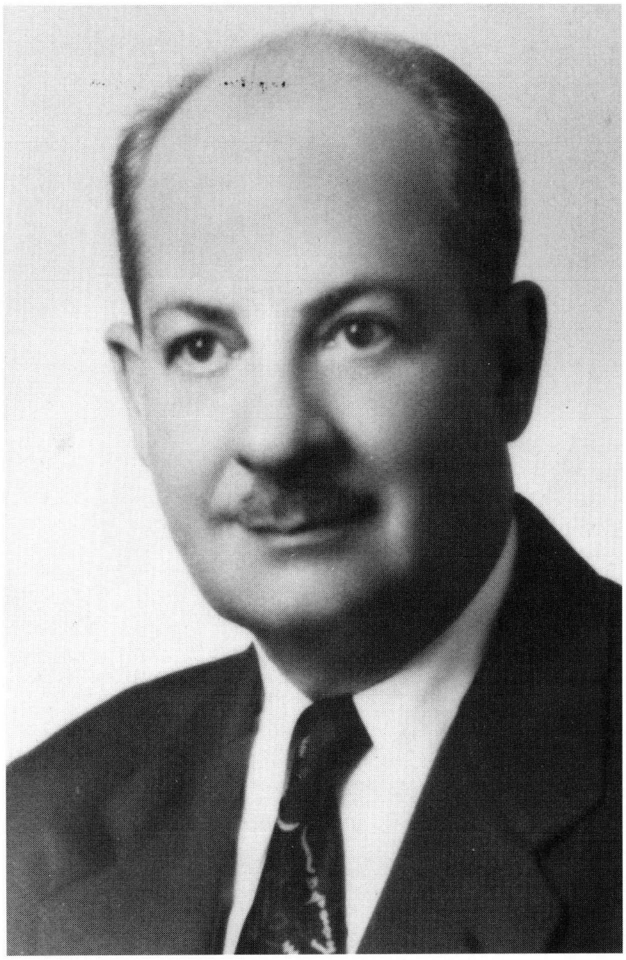

FIG. 1-20. Emery Andrew Rovenstine (1895–1960)

Wertheim and Rovenstine, anesthesiologists at the New York University College of Medicine, devised and described a technique of suprascapular nerve block in the treatment of intractable shoulder pain, such as subacromial bursitis.[137] They reported that the analgesic effect of a 2% procaine injection may continue for 4 to 6 weeks. In 1948, Papper and Rovenstine (Fig. 1-20) collaborated in publishing the description of the obligation of the anesthesiologist to participate in the therapeutics of pain. They said: "Events in the changing medical world have made it imperative that our functions be broadened and we accept the challenge of pain occurring outside the surgical amphitheater. Such a concept fully justifies an anesthesia clinic on the therapy of pain." [107]

Seemingly taking this recommendation to heart, John Bonica (Fig. 1-21) nurtured an interest in pain medicine and published a seminal work, *The Management of Pain,* in 1953, at a time when he was an anesthesiologist at Tacoma General Hospital in Tacoma, Washington, and before he became chair of the newly formed Department of Anesthesiology at the University of Washington School of Medicine in Seattle, Washington. At this time, much of pain medicine care still focused on nerve block clinics, and Vandam (Fig. 1-22) and Eckenhoff in 1954 suggested the focus should not

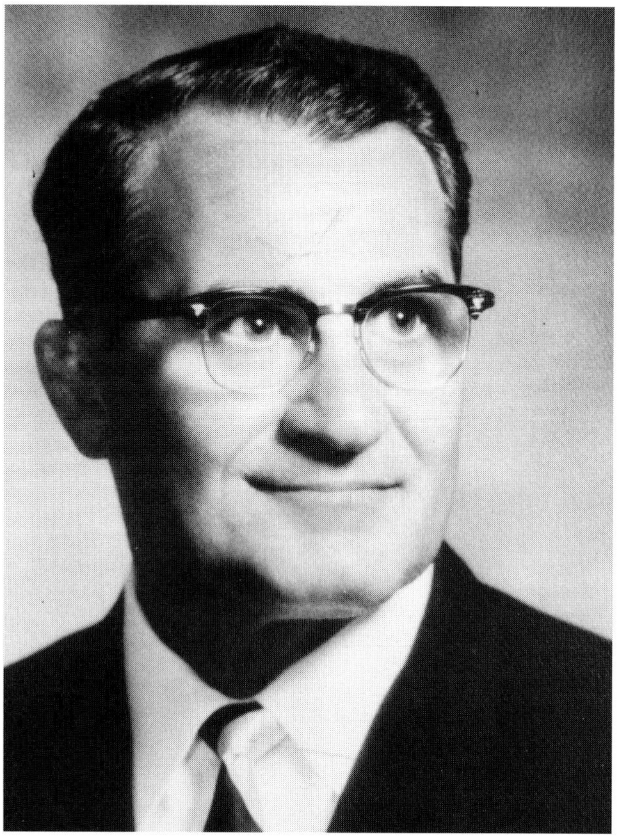

FIG. 1-21. John J. Bonica (1917–1994)

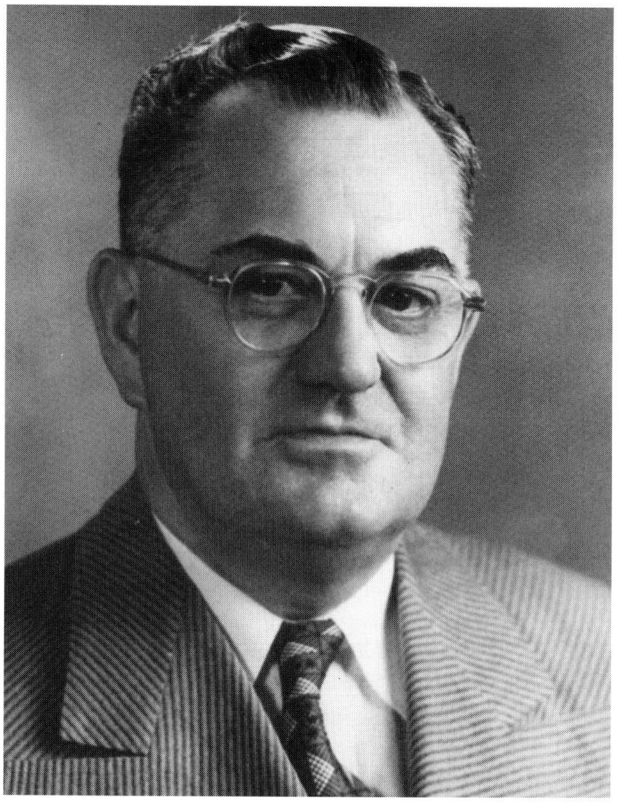

FIG. 1-23. John S. Lundy (1894–1973)

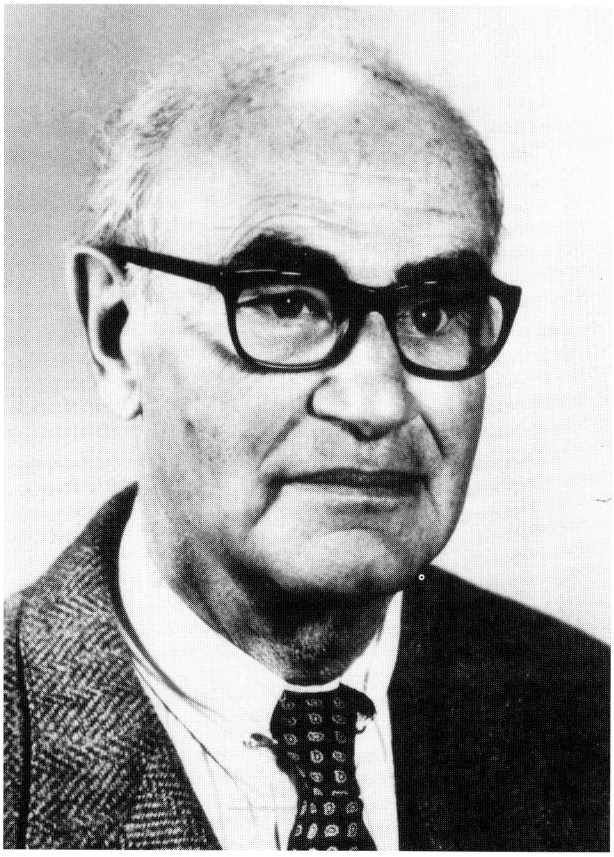

FIG. 1-22. Leroy D. Vandam (1914–)

only be on pain relief from nerve blocks, but also on the basic nature of pain, and an integrated approach to treatment.[133] Once Bonica accepted his position at the University of Washington, he and Lowell White, a neurosurgeon, and other colleagues in 1960 collaborated to create the first multidisciplinary pain clinic in the United States. This small group began to see patients with chronic pain and hold weekly conferences. As a result, the group gradually attracted orthopedists, psychologists, surgeons, and other specialists.[19]

Pain care in other countries also seemed to follow the suggestions of Papper and Rovenstine and following World War II, B. G. B. Lucas, of the University College Hospital in London, spent a month at the Mayo Clinic with John Lundy (Fig. 1-23). There he learned pain therapy nerve blocks and returned to London to develop the first nerve block pain clinic in the United Kingdom.[126]

ANESTHESIOLOGY AS A SPECIALTY PRACTICE

One of the more noticeable and surprising features in the history of the first 50 years of neural blockade is the almost total lack of involvement by anesthesiologists. Virtually all the developments were devised by surgeons and basic scientists. Also surprising is the miniscule nature of the contribution from Britain, the country of Snow and Lister and pioneering investigation in general. This was not a case of noncommunication, since the very first notice of Koller's discovery in the foreign press had appeared in the London

Lancet. There is no easy explanation. In most of the medical world, the practice of anesthesia was considered a poor relation, comparatively unhonored and unskilled, seemingly offering little opportunity or incentive for innovative work. In the British quarter of the globe, general anesthesia was administered by physicians and perhaps generated a certain sense of security and a tendency to leave well enough alone. Everywhere, if local anesthesia was the choice, the surgeon did both the choosing and the injecting. It was not until nerve block began to be perceived as an independent diagnostic and therapeutic tool that a demand arose for regional anesthetic skill independent of surgical operation. One must wonder whether the "choosing and injecting" by the surgeon allowed a more complete view of the perioperative period. The concepts of preemptive analgesia, currently receiving considerable research attention, have many of their foundations in work by George W. Crile (Fig. 1-24).[34] Crile advanced the thesis that general anesthesia alone was insufficient for shielding patients from the harmful stress of major operations, and he proposed the term *anociassociation* to describe an ideal combination of sedation, local and regional anesthesia, and general anesthetic techniques that protected patients from surgical stress (Fig. 1-25). He subsequently showed that anesthetic prescription affected physiologic variables not only intraoperatively and immediately postoperatively, but also for several days thereafter. In the United States, this period saw the beginnings of anesthesiology as an individual specialty, welcomed by forward-looking surgeons such as William Mayo, who established Labat, one of the first regional anesthesiologists, as a lecturer at the renowned Mayo Clinic in Minnesota.

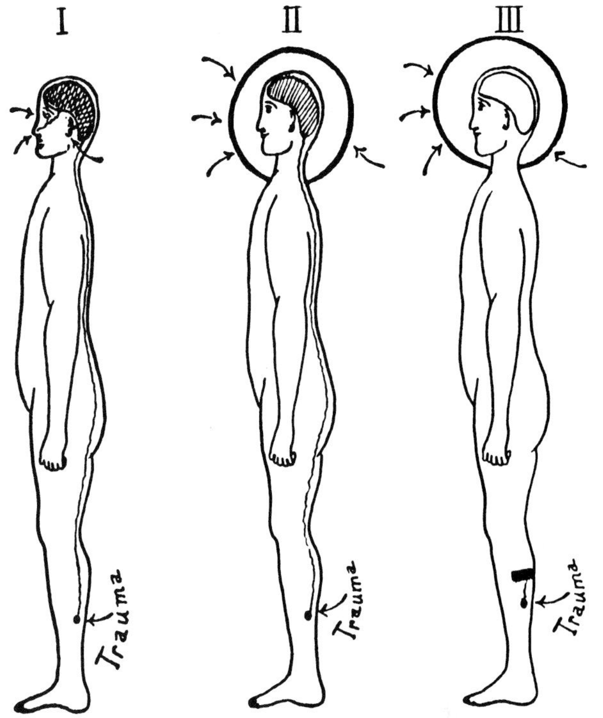

FIG. 1-25. (**I**) Crile's concept of anociassociation. Schematic drawing illustrating protective effect of anociassociation. (**II**) Patient under inhalational anesthesia in whom traumatic noci-impulses only reach the brain. (**III**) Patient under complete anoci-association. Auditory, visual, and olfactory impulses are excluded from the brain by inhalational anesthesia. Traumatic impulses from the seat of injury are blocked by Novocain.

Not least of the services rendered by the development of regional anesthesia was the stimulation of a higher level of vigilance and physiologic awareness in anesthetic practice as a whole. No better proof of this trend could be desired than that provided by anesthesia records. Charted records of the vital signs during an operation were apparently being kept by Dr. Codman at the Massachusetts General Hospital at the close of the 19th century, stimulated by the recommendations of Cushing. It must be remembered that a convenient method of measuring the blood pressure of a patient was not available until Riva-Rocci invented the arm cuff in 1896, and that 10 years were to elapse before Korotkoff, a Russian army surgeon, discovered the auscultatory method. Thus, the analgesia charts of Codman at first showed only the pulse rate, and when blood pressure was added, only the systolic pressure. Cushing's insistence on charted records demonstrated his greatness as a medical scientist and surgeon.[10] Following the lead of Crile, he sought to combat shock in major amputations by cocainizing the large nerve trunks before dividing them and he kept graphic track of the patient's condition by having the vital signs measured every 5 minutes.[36] The first publication, however, of a chart for recording the progress of a patient during anesthesia should be credited to Sydney Ormond Goldan (1869–1944), who presented a facsimile of one in the *Philadelphia Medical Journal,* November 3, 1900.[56] It was designed specifically for registering the course of "intraspinal cocainization" and provided for the recording of three vital signs, pupil, pulse, and respiration, every 10 minutes (Fig. 1-26). Goldan's paper has

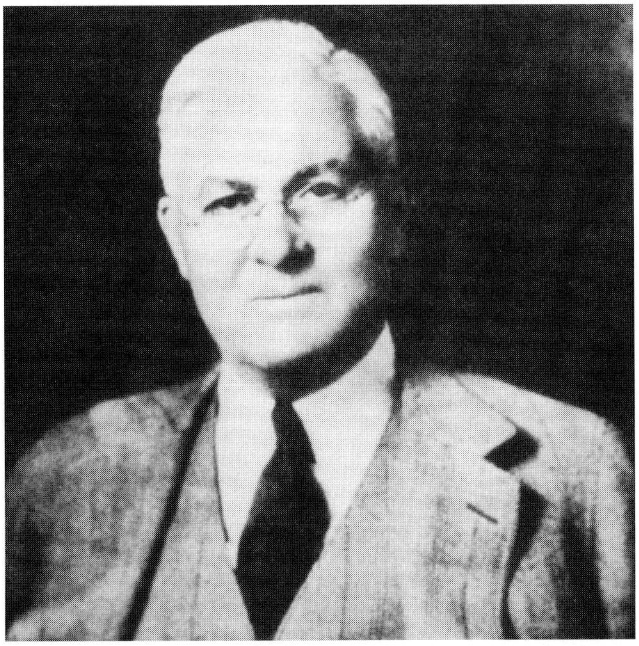

FIG. 1-24. George W. Crile (1864–1943)

a further title to scholarly distinction; it seems to have been the earliest article in the literature of local anesthesia to include a list of bibliographic citations. Historically, Goldan's contribution is also of interest for his concluding remark: ". . . a remedy for the headache may be found not in simple analgesics, but drugs exerting their influences upon the circulation. . . Increasing the blood pressure favors an increased tension in the veins retarding absorption."

Goldan gave full details of 16 cases of spinal anesthesia, a large series for that time, and explicitly described himself as an anesthetist. Thus, the practice of careful record-keeping in the operating room, an indispensable foundation to the progress of anesthesiology, was initiated publicly by the first physician to describe himself as an anesthetist in the United States. It is worth noting that Goldan, a much forgotten trailblazer, was also incontrovertibly the first anesthetist to practice regional block anywhere in the world. Goldan disagreed with the approach to anesthetic care that was prevalent in the early 20th century. He objected to the philosophy of one individual performing both the anesthetic and operative procedures. Goldan's beliefs may have contributed to the brevity of his tenure (1896–1903) as a full-time anesthetist. He was an outspoken man, as evidenced by his comments on the question of who should be responsible for the consequences of anesthesia: "There can be but one correct way of viewing this subject, and that is the administrator, whether experienced or not, is responsible for narcosis. . . The surgeon should divest himself of the idea that he is doing the anesthetist a favor by having him administer the anesthetic, as he (the anesthetist) is far more important to the patient and the success of the operation." [55]

The interest in regional anesthesia stimulated the formation of the first American Society of Regional Anesthesia (ASRA) on August 2, 1923. The ASRA was founded (i) to develop the methods of local and regional and spinal anesthesia; (ii) to promote and further research work along these lines; and (iii) to encourage clinical investigations and spread the use of these methods.[140] The Society had been a direct outgrowth of a postgraduate course of surgery given at the New York University in Bellevue Hospital Medical College, and, according to notes kept by Dr. Paul Wood, the founders had intended to name this society The Labat Regional Anesthesia Society, but Dr. Labat refused. During the first 10 years of the society's existence, regional anesthesia for surgery took great strides, and toward the end of the decade regional anesthesia had even extended beyond the scope of surgical anesthesia. It was utilized effectively for diagnostic and prognostic blocks, and with the advent of neurolytic agents, for therapeutic blocks as well. However, as the ASRA (original version) entered its second decade, the role of the physician-anesthetist as a specialist was evolving more rapidly, so surgeons became less interested and less involved in anesthesia. In the late 1930s as the specialty of anesthesiology gained momentum, the New York Society became the American Society of Anesthesiologists (ASA), the American Board of Anesthesiology was founded, and the section on anesthesia of the American Medical Association became a separate entity. Indicative of the stature of the ASRA at the time when the American Board of Anesthesiology was founded is the fact that the Board consisted of two representatives from the ASA, two representatives from the section on surgery of the American Medical Association, and two representatives from the ASRA. To this day, the first paragraph of the *Booklet of Information* of the American Board of Anesthesiology and the logo of the Board contain the letters ASRA along with ASA and American Medical Association Board of Specialties. Unfortunately, with the increasing scope of the role of the ASA and the decreasing size of the membership of the ASRA (due to the withdrawal of most of the surgeons), ASRA decided to merge with the ASA and ceased to exist, that is, until its reintroduction in 1976.[6] As Winnie detailed in his 1981 Labat address[140]:

> But when we anesthesiologists accepted the regional block needle from the surgeon-anesthetist, we did not take with it the body of knowledge that the surgeon-anesthetist had developed to render the use of the needle simple, safe, and effective. We ignored it, or forgot it, or perhaps, even refused to accept it, and, as a result, again and again we have rediscovered and reintroduced techniques which were described accurately and succinctly 50, 60, or 70 years ago.

As of this writing, societies of regional anesthesia, and likely other national societies, have been formed in Europe, Latin America, and Asian and Pacific countries.

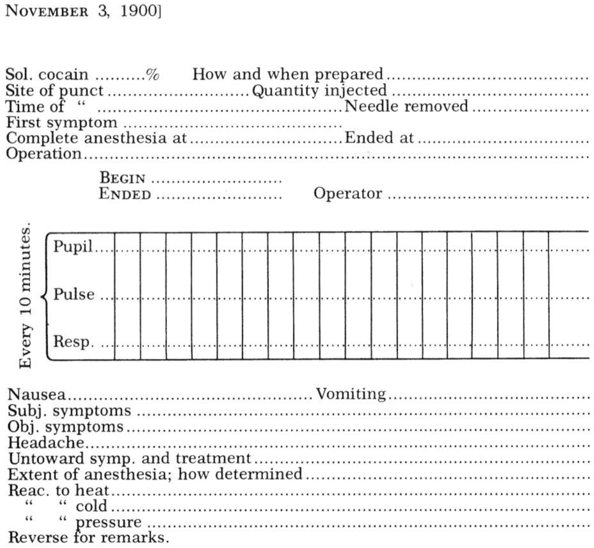
NOVEMBER 3, 1900]
Sol. cocain ....% How and when prepared
Site of punct Quantity injected
Time of " Needle removed
First symptom
Complete anesthesia at Ended at
Operation
BEGIN
ENDED Operator
Every 10 minutes. Pupil / Pulse / Resp.
Nausea Vomiting
Subj. symptoms
Obj. symptoms
Headache
Untoward symp. and treatment
Extent of anesthesia; how determined
Reac. to heat
" " cold
" " pressure
Reverse for remarks.

FIG. 1-26. Facsimile of Goldan's chart, the earliest published anesthesia chart. (From Goldan, S.O.: Intraspinal cocainization for surgical anesthesia. Philadelphia Med. J. *6:*850, 1900.)

REFERENCES

1. Abel, J.J.: On the blood-pressure-raising constituent of the suprarenal capsule. Johns Hopkins Hosp. Bull., *8:*151, 1897.

2. Abram, S.E.: Advances in chronic pain management since gate control. Reg. Anesth., *18:*66–81, 1993.
3. Aburel, E.: L'anesthésie locale continue (prolongée) en obstétrique. Bull. Soc. Obstét. Gynecol., *20:*35, 1931.
4. Adriani, J., and Roman-Vega, D.: Saddle block anesthesia. Am. J. Surg., *71:*12, 1946.
5. Babcock, W.W.: Spinal anesthesia; with report of surgical clinics. Surg. Gynecol. Obstet., *15:*606, 1912.
6. Bacon, D.R., deLeon-Casasola, O.A., Myers, D.P., Peppriell, J. and Lema, M.J.: Minutes of the American Society of Regional Anesthesia: 1924–1939. Anesthesiology *79:*A1028, 1993.
7. Barker, A.E.: Clinical experiences with spinal analgesia in 100 cases and some reflections on the procedure. Br. Med. J., *1:*665, 1907.
8. Basbaum, A.I., and Fields, H.L.: Endogenous pain control mechanisms: Review and hypothesis. Ann. Neurol., *4:*451, 1978.
9. Becker, H.K.: Carl Koller and cocaine. Psychoanal. Quart., *32:*309, 1963.
10. Beecher, H.K.: The first anesthesia records (Codman, Cushing). Surg. Gynecol. Obstet., *71:*789, 1940.
11. Beecher, H.K.: Relationship of significance of wound to the pain experienced. J.A.M.A., *161:*1609, 1956.
12. Bell, C.: Anatomy of the Human Body, 3rd Edition, T.N. Longman & O. Rees, London, *3:*224, 1803.
13. Bell, C.: Idea of a New Anatomy of the Brain Submitted for the Observations of his Friends. London, Strahan and Preton, 1811.
14. Bergman, N.A.: James Moore (1762–1860) An 18th century advocate of mitigation of pain during surgery. Anesthesiology, *80:*657–662, 1994.
15. Bier, A.: Versuche über Cocainisirung des Rückenmarkes. Dtsch. Z. Chir., *5151:*361, 1899.
16. Bier, A.: Ueber einen neuen Weg Localanästhesie an den Gliedmassen zu erzeugen. Arch. Klin. Chir., *86:*1007, 1908.
17. Biographical sketch of Doctor James Leonard Corning of New York City, and his recent remarkable discoveries in local anesthesia. Va. Med. Mon., *12:*713, 1886.
18. Block, N., and Rochberg, S.: Continuous caudal anesthesia in obstetrics. Am. J. Obstet. Gynecol., *45:*645, 1943.
19. Bonica, J.J.: Basic principles in managing chronic pain. Arch. Surg., *112:*783, 1977.
20. Bonica, J.J.: Causalgia and other reflex sympathetic dystrophies. *In* Bonica, J.J. (ed.): The Management of Pain, 2nd ed. pp. 220–221. Philadelphia, Lea and Febiger, 1990.
21. Braun, H.: Ueber den Einfluss der Vitalität der Gewebe auf die örtlichen und allgemeinen Giftwirkungen localanästhesirender Mittel und über die Bedeutung des Adrenalins für die Localanästhesie. Arch. Klin. Chir., *69:*541, 1903.
22. Braun, H.: Ueber einige neuer örtliche Anaesthetica (Stovain, Alypin, Novocain). Dtsch. Klin. Wochenschr., *31:*1667, 1905.
23. Braun, H.: Local Anesthesia: Its Scientific Basis and Practical Use, 3rd ed. Philadelphia, Lea & Febiger, 1914.
24. Brunn, F., and Mandl, F.: Die paravertebral Injektion zur Bekäampfung visceraler Schmerzen. Wien. Klin. Wochenschr., *37:*511, 1924.
25. Bull, C.S.: The hydrochlorate of cocaine as a local anaesthetic in ophthalmic surgery. N.Y. Med. J., *40:*609, 1884.
26. Burke, W.C. Jr.: Hydrochlorate of cocaine in minor surgery. N.Y. Med. J., *40:*616, 1884.
27. Calvillo, O., Henry, J.L., and Neuman, R.S.: Effects of morphine and naloxone on dorsal horn neurons in the cat. Can. J. Physiol. Pharmacol., *52:*1207–1211, 1974.
28. Cathelin, F.: Une nouvelle voie d'injection rachidienne. Méthodes des injections épidurales par le procédé du canal sacré. Applications à l'homme. C.R. Soc. Biol. (Paris), *53:*452, 1901.
29. Caton, D.: The secularization of pain. Anesthesiology, *62:*493, 1985.
30. Cleland, J.G.: Paravertebral anesthesia in obstetrics. Surg. Gynecol. Obstet., *57:*57, 1938.
31. Corning, J.L.: On the prolongation of the anesthetic effect of the hydrochlorate of cocaine, when subcutaneously injected. An experimental study. N.Y. Med. J., *42:*317, 1885.
32. Corning, J.L.: Spinal anaesthesia and local medication of the cord with cocaine. N.Y. Med. J., *42:*483, 1885.
33. Covino, B.: One hundred years plus two of regional anesthesia. Reg. Anesth., *11:*105, 1986.
34. Crile, G.W.: Nitrous oxide anesthesia and a note on anoci association, a new principle in operative surgery. Surg. Gynecol. Obstet., *13:*170, 1911.
35. Curbelo, M.M.: Continuous peridural segmental anesthesia by means of a ureteral catheter. Anesth. Analg. (Cleve.), *28:*13, 1949.
36. Cushing, H.: On the avoidance of shock in major amputations by cocainization of large nerve-trunks preliminary to their division. Ann. Surg., *36:*321, 1902.
37. Dallenbach, K.M.: Pain: History and present status. Am. J. Psychol., *52:*331, 1939.
38. Darwin, E.: Zoönomia, or the Laws of Organic Life. London, Johnson, 1794.
39. Dean, H.P.: Relative value of inhalation and injection methods of inducing anaesthesia. Br. Med. J., *2:*869, 1907.
40. DeLange, J.J., Cuesta, M.A., and Cuesta de Pedro, A.: Fidel Pagés Miravé (1886–1923). The pioneer of lumbar epidural anaesthesia. Anaesthesia, *49:*429, 1994.
41. De Lapersonne, F.: Un nouvel anesthésique local, la stovaïne. Presse Med., *12:*233, 1904.
42. Dickinson, A.H., and Sullivan, A.F.: Subcutaneous formaline-induced activity of dorsal horn neurons in the rate: differential response to an intrathecal opiate administered pre- or postformaline. Pain, *30:* 349–360, 1987.
43. Dogliotti, A.M.: Eine neue Methode der regionaren Anästhesie. Zentralbl. Chir., *58:*3141, 1931.
44. Dogliotti, A.M.: Proposta di un nuovo metodo di cura delle algie periferiche. L'alcoolizzazione sottomeningea delle radici posteriori. Considerazioni sulle prime 30 osservazione cliniche. Minerva Med., *1:*536, 1931.
45. Dogliotti, A.M.: A new method of block anesthesia. Segmental peridural spinal anesthesia. Am. J. Surg., *20:*107, 1933.
46. Eckenhoff, J.E.: A wide angle view of anesthesiology: Emory A. Rovenstein Memorial Lecture. Anesthesiology, *48:*272, 1978.
47. Edwards, W.B., and Hingson, R.A.: Continuous caudal anesthesia in obstetrics. Am. J. Surg., *57:*459, 1942.
48. Esmarch, F.: Ueber künstliche Blutleere. Arch. Klin. Chir., *17:*292, 1874.
49. Etherington-Wilson, E.: Intrathecal nerve root block. Some contributions and a new technique. Proc. R. Soc. Med., *27:*325, 1934.
50. Faulconer, A. Jr., and Keys, T.E.: Foundations of Anesthesiology, Vol. II. Springfield, Ill, Charles C. Thomas, 1963.
51. Fink, B.R.: Leaves and needles: the introduction of surgical local anesthesia. Anesthesiology, *63:*77, 1985.
52. Fowler, R.G.: Cocaine analgesia from subarachnoid injection, with a report of forty-four cases together with a report of a case in which antipyrine was used. Philadelphia Med. J., *6:*843, 1900.
53. Francois-Franck, C.A.: Action paralysant locale de la cocaïne sur les nerfs et les centres nerveux. Applications à la technique expérimentale. Arch. Physiol. Norm. Pathol., *24:*562, 1892.
54. Gasser, H.S., and Erlanger, J.: The role of fiber size in the establishment of a nerve block by pressure or cocaine. Am. J. Physiol., *88:*581, 1929.
55. Goldan, S.O.: Anesthetization as a specialty: Its present and future. Am. Med., *2:*101, 1901.
56. Goldan, S.O.: Intraspinal cocainization for surgical anesthesia. Philadelphia Med. J., *6:*850, 1900.
57. Goldscheider, A.: Ueber den Schmerz in physiologischer und klinischer Hinsicht. Berlin, Hirschwald, 1894.
58. Gordh, T.: Anesthesiology Topics/January-February. pp. 7. Karolinska Hospital, Stockholm, Sweden, 1986.
59. Gray, H.: Anatomy: Descriptive and Surgical, 5th ed. pp. 572–574. Philadelphia, Henry C. Lea, 1870.
60. Gray, H.T., and Parsons, L.: Blood pressure variations associated with lumbar puncture and the induction of spinal anesthesia. Quart. J. Med., *5:*339, 1912.
61. Gros, O.: Ueber die Narkotika und Localanästhetika. Arch. Exp. Pathol. Pharmakol., *63:*80, 1910.
62. Hall, R.J.: Hydrochlorate of cocaine. N.Y. Med. J., *40:*643, 1884.
63. Halsted, W.S.: Practical comments on the use and abuse of cocaine; suggested by its invariably successful employment in more than a thousand minor surgical operations. N.Y. Med. J., *42:*294, 1885.
64. Halsted, W.S.: Water as a local anesthetic. N.Y. Med. J., *42:*327, 1885.
65. Halsted, W.S.: Surgical Papers by William Steward Halsted, Vol. 1. pp. 37–39. Baltimore, Johns Hopkins Press, 1924.
66. Hepburn, W.G.: Some notes on hydrochlorate of cocaine. Med. Record, *26:*534, 1884.

67. Hepburn, W.G.: Stovain spinal analgesia. Am. J. Surg., *34:*87, 1920.
68. Hoffert, M.J.: The neurophysiology of pain. *In* Potenoy, R.K. (ed.): Pain: Mechanisms and Syndromes. Neurol. Clin., *7:*183–203, 1989.
69. Hogan, Q.H.: Lumbar epidural anatomy. Anesthesiology, *75:* 767–775, 1991.
70. Holmes, G.M.: Intravenous regional anesthesia: A useful method of producing analgesia of the limbs. Lancet, *1:*245, 1963.
71. Hopkins, G.S.: Anesthesia by cocainization of the spinal cord. Philadelphia Med. J., *6:*864, 1900.
72. Howard-Jones, N.: A critical study of the origins and early development of hypodermic medication. J. Hist. Med., *2:*201, 1947.
73. Jonnesco, T.: Remarks on general spinal anesthesia. Br. Med. J., 2:1396, 1909.
74. Kappis, M.: Ueber Leitungsanästhesie an Bauch, Burst, Arm und Hals durch Injektion ans Foramen intervertebrale. Münch. Med. Wochenschr., *1:*794, 1912.
75. Kappis, M.: Erfahrungen mit Lokalanästhesie bei Bauchoperationen. Verh. Dtsch. Ges. Chir., *43:*87, 1914.
76. Kitahata, L.M., Kosaka, Y., Taub, A., Bonikos, K., and Hoffert, M.: Lamina-specific suppression of dorsal-horn unit activity by morphine sulfate. Anesthesiology, *41:*39, 1974.
77. Koller, C.: On the use of cocaine for producing anaesthesia on the eye. Lancet, *2:*990, 1884.
78. Koster, H.: Spinal anaesthesia, with special reference to its use in surgery of the head, neck, and thorax. Am. J. Surg., *5:*554, 1928.
79. Kreis, O.: Ueber Medullarnarkose bei Gebärenden. Zentralbl. Gynakol., *24:*724, 1900.
80. Labat, G.: Circulatory disturbances associated with subarachnoid nerve block. Long Island Med. J., *21:*573, 1927.
81. Läwen, A.: Ueber die Verwertung der Sakralanästhesie fur chirurgische Operationen. Zentralbl. Chir., *37:*708, 1910.
82. Läwen, A.: Ueber segmentäre Schmerzaufhebung durch papavertebrale Novokaininjektionen zur Differentialdiagnose intra-abdominaler Erkrankungen. Med. Wochenschr., *69:*1423, 1922.
83. Le Bars, D., Guilbaud, G., Jurna, I., and Besson, J.M.: Differential effects of morphine on response of dorsal horn lamina V type cells elicited by A and C fibre stimulation in the spinal cat. Brain Res., *115:*518, 1976.
84. Lee, E.W.: Subarachnoidean injections of cocaine as a substitute for general anesthesia in operations below the diaphragm, with report of seven cases. Philadelphia Med. J., *6:*865, 1900.
85. Lee, J.A.: Labat Lecture: Some foundations on which we have built. Reg. Anesth., *10:*99, 1985.
86. Lele, P.P., Weddell, G., and Williams, C.: The relationship between heat transfer, skin temperature and cutaneous sensibility. J. Physiol. (London), *126:*206–234, 1954.
87. Lemmon, W.T.: A method for continuous spinal anesthesia. Ann. Surg., *111:*141, 1940.
88. Leriche, R.: De la causalgie envisagée comme une nevrité du sympathique et son traitement par la dénudation et l'excision de plexus nerveux périartériels. Presse Med., *24:*178, 1916.
89. Löfgren, N.: Studies on Local Anesthetics. Xylocaine: A New Synthetic Drug. Inaugural dissertation, Stockholm, Hoeggstroms, 1948.
90. Magendi, F.: Expériences sur les fonctions des racines des nerfs rachidiens. J. Physiol. Exp., *2:*276–279, 1822.
91. Manalan, S.A.: Caudal block anesthesia in obstetrics. J. Indiana State Med. Assoc., *35:*564, 1942.
92. Mandl, F.: Die Wirkung der paravertebralen Injektion bei "Angina pectoris." Arch. Klin. Chir., *136:*495, 1925.
93. Marx, S.: Analgesia in obstetrics produced by medullary injections of cocain. Philadelphia Med. J., *6:*857, 1900.
94. Matas, R.: Local and regional anesthesia with cocaine and other analgesic drugs, including the subarachnoid method, as applied in general surgical practice. Philadelphia Med. J., *6:*820, 1900.
95. Matas, R.: Local and regional anesthesia: A retrospect and prospect. Am. J. Surg., *25:*189, 1934.
96. Mayer, E.: Clinical experience with adrenaline. Philadelphia Med. J., *7:*819, 1901.
97. Meige, H., and Athanassio-Benisty, P.: Les signes cliniques des lesions de l'appareil sympatheque et de l'appareil vasculaire dans les blessures de membres. Presse Med., *24:*153, 1916.
98. Melzack, R., and Wall, P.D.: Pain mechanisms: A new theory. Science, *150:*971, 1965.
99. Mitchell, S.W., Moorehouse, G.R., and Keen, W.W.: Gunshot wounds and other injuries of nerves. Philadelphia, J.B. Lippincott, 1864.
100. Moore, J.: A method of preventing or diminishing pain in several operations of surgery. London, T. Cadell, 1784.
101. Müller, J.: Handbuch der Physiologie des Menschen für Vorlesungen. Koblenz, Hollscher, 1840.
102. Naunyn, B.: Ueber die Auslosung von Schmerzempfindung durch Summation sich zeitlich folgender sensibler Erregungen. Arch. Exp. Pathol. *25:*275, 1889.
103. Niemann, A.: Ueber eine organische Base in der Coca. Ann. Chem., *114:*213, 1860.
104. Noordenbos, W.: Pain. Amsterdam, Elsevier, 1959.
105. Noyes, H.D.: The ophthalmological congress in Heidelberg. Med. Record, *26:*417, 1884.
106. Pagés, F.: Anestesia metamerica. Rev. Sanid. Milit. Argen., *11:*351–356, 1921.
107. Papper, E.M.: Regional anesthesia: A critical assessment of its place in therapeutics. Anesthesiology, *28:*1074, 1967.
108. Pitkin, G.: Controllable spinal anesthesia. Am. J. Surg., *5:*537, 1928.
109. Pravaz, C.G.: Sur un nouveau moyen d'opérer la coagulation du sang dans les artères, applicable à la guérison des anéurismes. C.R. Acad. Sci. (Paris), *36:*88, 1853.
110. Procacci, P., and Maresca, M.: Evolution of the concept of pain. *In* Sicuteri, F., Terenius, L., Veccheit, L., and Maggi, C.A. (eds.): Pain Versus Man. pp 1–18. New York, Raven Press, 1992.
111. Quincke, H.: Die Lumbalpunction des Hydrocephalus. Ber. Klin. Wochenschr., *28:*929, 1891.
112. Reclus, P.: Analgésie locale par la cocaïne. Rev. Chir., *9:*913, 1889.
113. Reynolds, D.V.: Surgery in the rat during electrical analgesia induced by focal brain stimulation. Science, *164:*444, 1969.
114. Riese, W., and Arrington, G.E., Jr.: The history of Johannes Müller's doctrine of the specific energies of the senses: Original and later versions. Bull. Hist. Med. *37:*179, 1963.
115. Royle, N.D.: A new operative procedure in the treatment of spastic paralysis and its experimental basis. Med. J. Aust., *1:*77, 1924.
116. Rynd, F.: Neuralgia—Introduction of fluid to the nerve. Dublin Med. Press, *13:*167, 1845.
117. Sarnoff, S.J., and Arrowood, J.G.: Differential spinal block. Surgery, *20:*150, 1946.
118. Schiff, M.: Lehrbuch der Physiologie. Schauenburg, Lahr, 1848.
119. Schleich, C.L.: Zur Infiltrationsanästhesie. Therapeutisch Monathefte, *8:*429, 1894.
120. Schloesser, Heilung peripherer Reizzustände sensibler und motorischer Nerven. Klin. Monatsbl. Augenheilkd., *41:*255, 1903.
121. Seelig, M.G.: History of cocaine as a local anesthetic. J.A.M.A., *117:*128, 1941.
122. Sise, L.F.: Spinal anesthesia for upper and lower abdominal operations. N. Engl. J. Med., *199:*61, 1928.
123. Sise, L.F.: Pontocainglucose for spinal anesthesia. Surg. Clin. North. Am., *15:*1501, 1935.
124. Smith, G.S., and Porter, W.T.: Spinal anesthesia in the cat. Am. J. Physiol., *38:*108, 1915.
125. Stoeckel, W.: Ueber sakrale Anästhesie. Zentralbl. Gynaekol., *33:*1, 1909.
126. Swerdlow, M.: The early development of pain relief clinics in the UK. Anesthesia, *47:*977–980, 1992.
127. Swetlow, G.I.: Paravertebral alcohol block in cardiac pain. Am. Heart J., *1:*393, 1926.
128. Tait, D., and Caglieri, G.: Experimental and clinical notes on the subarachnoid space. Transactions Medical Society of California, Abstracted. J.A.M.A., *35:*6, 1900.
129. Tuffier, T.: Analgésie chirurgicale par l'injection sous-arachnoidienne lombaire de cocaïne. C.R. Soc. Biol., 11th Series, *1:*882, 1899.
130. Tuffier, T.: Anesthésie medullaire chirurgicale par injection sous-arachnoidienne lombaire de cocaïne; technique et resultats. Semaine Medicale, *20:*167, 1900.
131. Tuohy, E.B.: Continuous spinal anesthesia: Its usefulness and technic involved. Anesthesiology, *5:*142, 1944.
132. Vandam, L.D.: Some aspects of the history of local anesthesia. *In* Strichartz, G.R. (ed.): Local Anesthetics. pp. 1–19. Berlin, Springer-Verlag, 1987.
133. Vandam, L.D., and Eckenhoff, J.E.: The anesthesiologist and therapeutic nerve block: technician or physician? Anesthesiology, *15:*89, 1954.

134. von Anrep, B.: Ueber die physiologische Wirkung des Cocain. Pflugers Arch., *21:*38, 1880.
135. von Gaza, W.: Die Resektion der paravertebralen Nerven und die isolierte Durchschneidung des Ramus communicans. Arch. Klin. Chir., *133:*479, 1924.
136. von Hemholtz, H.: Ueber di Dauer, und, den Verlauf der durchstonesschwankungen inducierten elektrischen Strome. Poggendorf's Annalen Physik Chemie, *83:*505, 1851.
137. Wertheim, H.M., and Rovenstine, E.A.: Suprascapular nerve block. Anesthesiology, *2:*541, 1941.
138. White, J.C.: Diagnostic novocaine block of the sensory and sympathetic nerves. A method of estimating the results which can be obtained by their permanent interruption. Am. J. Surg., *9:*264, 1930.
139. Wildsmith, J.A.W.: Carl Koller (1857–1944) and the introduction of cocaine into anesthetic practice. Reg. Anesth., *9:*161, 1984.
140. Winne, A.P.: Nothing new under the sun—Labat address. Reg. Anesth., *7:*95, 1982.
141. Wood, A.: New method of treating neuralgia by the direct application of opiates to the painful points. Edinburgh Med. Surg. J., *82:*265, 1855.
142. Wynter, W.E.: Four cases of tuberculosis meningitis in which paracentesis of the theca vertebralis was performed for the relief of fluid pressure. Lancet, *1:*981, 1891.
143. Yaksh, T.L., and Rudy, T.A.: Analgesia mediated by a direct spinal action of narcotics. Science, *192:*1357, 1976.

APPENDIX A: CHRONOLOGY OF IDEAS CONCERNING PAIN AND NEURAL BLOCKADE[a]

ca. 500 B.C. **Alcmaeon (Croton)**
The brain is associated with the organs of sense

ca. 375 B.C. **Plato (Athens)**
Pain is an emotion that dwells in the brain

ca. 200 **Galen (Pergamon)**
Recognized the functional unity of the brain, spinal cord, and peripheral nerves

1752 **Haller (Germany)**
Only certain specific parts of the body react to pain, disclosing sensibility

1826 **Müeller (Germany)**
Asserted the doctrine of specific sensory energies, that there is no direct correlation between the external stimulation and the impression received.

1855 **Wood (UK)**
Neuralgic pain can be treated by circumneural injection of pain-relieving drug

1885 **Corning (USA)**
Pain can be treated by "medication of the spinal cord"

1900 **Cushing (USA)**
Nerve block to prevent pain and "shock" of amputation

1908 **Crile (USA)**
"Anociassociation"—neural blockade to prevent noxious stimulation

1929 **Gasser and Erlanger**
Nerve fiber size and function

1933 **Brouwer (Netherlands)**
Proposed centrifugal influence on centripetal systems in the brain

1934 **O'Shaughnessy and Slome (UK)**
Spinal anesthesia decreased mortality in dogs with limb trauma

1953 **Bonica (USA)**
Publication of an encyclopedic treatise on the management of acute pain and chronic pain

1957 **Hagbarth and Kerr (Australia)**
Evidence of descending control of sensory input

1958 **Bromage (Canada)**
Epidural block restored respiratory function after abdominal surgery

1963 **Hume and Egdahl**
Spinal lesions or spinal anesthesia modified the stress response to surgery in man

1965 **Melzack and Wall (Canada and UK)**
A spinal gate in the dorsal horn controls the transmission of nociceptive messages

1969 **Reynolds (USA)**
Pain-inhibitory impulses descend from the midbrain to the spinal cord. The pathway is activatable by electrical stimulation and morphine

1971 **Bromage (Canada)**
Epidural block in humans modifies stress response during and after surgery

1976 **Yaksh and Rudy (USA)**
Spinal application of morphine inhibits nociceptive transmission

1979 **Cousins and colleagues (Australia)**
Epidural administration of opioids in humans results in "selective spinal analgesia" on the basis of studies of pharmacokinetics and neural effects

1981 **Duggan (Australia)**
More than one population of opioid receptors in spinal cord

1983 **Yaksh (USA)**
Several different spinal receptor systems mediating antinociception

---

[a]See also Chapter 33, Table 33-4.

APPENDIX B: CHRONOLOGY OF LOCAL ANESTHESIA

1564 **Paré (France)**
Local anesthesia by nerve compression

1600 **Valverdi (Italy)**
Regional anesthesia by compression of nerves and blood vessels supplying operative area

1646 **Severino (Italy)**
Refrigeration anesthesia by use of freezing mixtures of snow and ice

1656 **Wren (England)**
First experiments with intravenous injection

1784 **Moore (England)**
Local anesthesia of extremity by compression of nerve trunks

1839 **Taylor and Washington (USA)**
Hypodermic injection

1843 **Wood (Scotland)**
Morphine injection (published 1855)

1845 **Rynd (Dublin)**
Hypodermic Needle

1853 **Pravaz (France)**
Hypodermic Syringe

1855 **Gaedcke (Germany)**
Isolation of alkaloid from leaves of cocoa plant

1860 **Niemann (Germany)**
Purification and naming of cocaine

1873 **Bennett (Scotland)**
Anesthetic properties of cocaine

1878 **von Anrep (Germany)**
Pharmacologic effects of cocaine (published 1879–1880)

1884 **Koller (Austria)**
First topical use of cocaine (eye surgery)
Halsted and Hall (USA)
Neural blockade with cocaine (in each other)
Burke (USA)
Removal of bullet from finger under nerve block with cocaine

1885 **Corning (USA)**
"Spinal anesthesia" (actually injected epidurally)

1890 **Reclus (France)**
Early use of infiltration anesthesia

1891 **Quincke (Germany)**
Lumbar puncture technique

1892 **Schleich (Germany)**
Introduced infiltration anesthesia
François-Franck
Coined term nerve blocking

1897 **Braun (Germany)**
Cocaine toxicity related to absorption; advocated use of epinephrine

1898 **Bier (Germany)**
First planned spinal anesthetic

1899 **Tuffier (France)**
Report of 125 spinal anesthetics
Tait and Caglieri (USA)
First use of spinal anesthesia in USA (". . . never . . . inject . . . until CSF . . . recognized")

1900 **Tait and Caglieri (USA)**
Detailed studies of subarachnoid space and spinal anesthesia in animals and humans

1901 **Cathelin and Sicard (France)**
Independently discovered caudal epidural block using cocaine

1902 **Braun (Germany)**
Use of epinephrine in nerve blocking—term conduction anesthesia

1904 **Einhorn (Germany)**
Synthesis of procaine (Novocaine)

1905 **Braun (Germany)**
Text Local Anesthesia

1907 **Barker (UK)**
Introduction of hyperbaric spinal anesthetic solutions

1908 **Crile (USA)**
Anociassociation: regional block plus light general anesthesia

1912 **Gray and Parsons (UK)**

1915 **Smith and Porter (USA)**
Blood pressure changes during spinal anesthesia

1922 **Labat (USA)**
Text Regional Anesthesia: Its Technique and Clinical Application
Founded American Society of Regional Anesthesia (1923)

1942 **Allen (USA)**
Refrigeration anesthesia for amputation
Edwards and Hingson (USA)
Continuous caudal anesthesia in obstetrics

APPENDIX C: CHRONOLOGY OF LOCAL ANESTHETIC AGENTS

Cocaine

1860 Purification and naming by Niemann (Germany)

1884 First clinical use, topical, by Koller (Germany)

First clinical use, nerve block, by Halsted (USA)

Procaine

1904 Synthesis by Einhorn (Germany)

1905 Clinical introduction by Braun (Germany)

Stovaine[a]

1904 Synthesis by Fourneau (France)

Cinchocaine (Nupercaine, dibucaine)

1925 Synthesis by Meischer

1930 Clinical introduction by Uhlmann

Amethocaine (Pontocaine, Tetracaine)

1928 Synthesis by Eisleb

1932 Clinical introduction

[a]Discarded, too toxic.

Lignocaine (Lidocaine)

1943 Synthesis by Löfgren and Lundqvist

1947 Clinical introduction (Gordh)

Mepivacaine

1956 Synthesis by Ekenstam and Egner

1957 Clinical introduction (Dhunér)

Prilocaine

1959 Synthesis by Lofgren and Tegner

1960 Clinical introduction by Wielding

Bupivacaine

1957 Synthesis by Ekenstam

1963 Clinical introduction by Widman and Telivuo

Etidocaine

1971 Synthesis by Takman

1972 Clinical introduction by Lund

Ropivacaine

1957 Synthesis by Ekenstam

1997 Clinical introduction

APPENDIX D: CHRONOLOGY OF INDIVIDUAL NEURAL BLOCKADE TECHNIQUES

Spinal analgesia

1898 Bier (Germany)
First use for surgery in humans

1940 Lemmon (USA)
Continuous spinal anesthesia

1946 Adriani and Roman-Vega (USA)
Saddle block spinal

Lumbar epidural analgesia

1921 Pagés (Spain)
First use for surgery

1931 Dogliotti (Italy)
Popularized surgical use

1949 Curbelo
Used Tuohy equipment for continuous blockade

Caudal epidural analgesia

1901 Sicard, Cathelin (France)
First use for surgery

1909 Stoeckel
Use in obstetrical pain

1910 Läwen (Germany)
Popularized surgical use

1913 Danis (Belgium)
Transsacral approach

1942 Edwards and Hingson (USA), Manalan
Continuous caudal

"Continuous" regional techniques

1931 Aburel (Romania)
Continuous paravertebral lumbosacral plexus block

Paravertebral somatic block

1906 Sellheim
Thoracic paravertebral block

1912 Kappis
Paravertebral block for surgery and also for pain relief

1922 Läwen
Use in diagnosis of abdominal disease

Celiac block

1906 Braun
Anterior surgical approach

1914 Kappis
Posterior approach

Paravertebral lumbar sympathetic block

1926 Mandl

Stellate ganglion (cervicothoracic sympathetic) **block**

1930 Labat
Posterior approach

1934 Leriche and Fontaine
Anterior approach (used for cerebrovascular accidents)

1948 Apgar
Anterior approach

1954 Moore
Paratracheal approach

Brachial plexus block

1884 Halsted
Injection under direct vision

1897 Crile

1911 Hirschel
"Blind" axillary injection
Kulenkampff
Supraclavicular technique

1940 Patrick
Basis of current supraclavicular technique

1958 Burnham
Axillary perivascular technique

1964 Winnie and Collins
Subclavian

1970 Winnie
Interscalene

Cervical plexus block

1939 Rovenstine and Wertheim

Intravenous regional analgesia

1908 Bier
Injection between two cuffs

1963 Holmes
Injection below a single cuff after exsanguination

Intra-arterial regional anesthesia

1912 Goyanes (Spain)
Arterial injection below a cuff

Diagnostic blockade in pain management

1924 von Gaza
Procaine blockade in investigation of pain pathways

1930 Mandl
Paravertebral procaine block in diagnosis of angina pectoris

1930 White
Blockade of sensory and sympathetic nerves in pain diagnosis

Therapeutic nerve block in pain management

1899 Tuffier
Spinal cocaine for pain of sarcoma of leg

1901 Cushing
Regional anesthesia used to describe pain relief by nerve block

1903 Schloesser
Trigeminal alcohol block

1924 von Gaza, Braun, Mandl
Local anesthetic neural blockade for management of visceral pain

1924 Royle
Surgical sympathectomy for pain of spastic paralysis

1926 Swetlow
Neurolytic sympathetic block with alcohol for angina pectoris and abdominal pain

1930 Dogliotti
Neurolytic subarachnoid alcohol block

1941 Wertheim and Rovenstine
Suprascapular local anesthetic nerve block for shoulder pain

APPENDIX E: CHRONOLOGY OF THE STUDY OF COMPLICATIONS OF NEURAL BLOCKADE

1884 Halsted and associates (USA)
Cocaine addiction

1889 **Reclus (France)**
Toxicity due to systemic absorption defined
Bier and colleagues (Germany)
Severe postlumbar puncture headache

1900 **Goldan (USA)**
Development of anesthetic record of "intraspinal" cocainization

1901 **Dandois (Belgium)**
Paraplegia after subarachnoid cocaine

1906 **Koenig (USA)**
Permanent neurologic sequelae in several patients following spinal cocaine

1907 **Barker (UK)**
Recognition of need to control level of block

1912 **Gray and Parsons (UK)**
Recognition of vascular pooling due to sympathetic blockade

1927–1928 **Labat (USA)**
Emphasis on maintenance of cerebral perfusion

1952 **Sancetta and colleagues**
Cardiovascular effects of "low and high" spinal anesthesia

1953 **Gillies (UK)**
Studies of cardiovascular effects

1953– **Green (USA)**
Studies of physiologic effects of spinal anesthesia

1954 **Dripps and Vandam (USA)**
Long-term follow-up of 10,098 spinal anesthetics; failure to discover major neurologic sequelae
Importance of meticulous technique and safe handling of drugs stressed

1960– **Bromage and colleagues (Canada)**
Studies of physiology and pharmacology of epidural blockade

1965– **Braid and Scott (UK); Tucker and Mather (USA); Boyes and Covino (USA); Harrison and colleagues (USA); De Jong and colleagues (USA)**
Studies of pharmacokinetics and toxicity of local anesthetics

1970– **Bonica and colleagues (USA)**
Studies of cardiovascular effects of central neural blockade

PART I

Pharmacology and Physiology of Neural Blockade

Neural Blockade in Clinical Anesthesia and Management of Pain, Third Edition,
edited by M.J. Cousins and P.O. Bridenbaugh.
Lippincott–Raven Publishers, Philadelphia © 1998.

CHAPTER 2

Neural Physiology and Local Anesthetic Action

Gary R. Strichartz

BASIC PHYSIOLOGY AND PHARMACOLOGY

Overview of the Neuron

Local anesthetic drugs reversibly block conduction of nerve impulses at the level of the axonal membrane. In this overview we review briefly the structure and function of neurons, the impulse generating and conducting units of the nervous system.[53] A typical neuron is composed of a cell body, dendrites, with multiple small branches close to cell bodies, and a single axon for each neuron (Fig. 2-1).

Sensory neurons have their cell bodies in dorsal root ganglia. Only one axon is attached, with its longer branch extending to the periphery and a shorter branch to the spinal cord. Impulses are generated in the small peripheral axon branches at the "receptor" component of the neuron. The nerve endings reside in skin, joints, muscles, viscera, or connective tissue. Impulses may be selectively initiated by mechanical, thermal (hot or cold changes in skin temperature), or tissue-damaging (*noxious*) stimuli at the nerve endings which anatomically define the "receptive field" for that particular neuron. Intense mechanical and thermal stimuli result in the release of excitatory chemicals (e.g., bradykinin) from tissues closely surrounding the endings of specifically *nociceptive* afferent axons. The resulting local excitation of the nociceptor nerve endings leads to trains of impulses with average discharge frequencies that are proportional to the stimulus intensity above the threshold level for impulse generation. Axons then conduct these impulses to the spinal cord, although impulses also invade the soma.

Several axons usually *innervate* a particular receptive field. As these axons have branches with receptive fields overlapping those of neighboring axons, and each branch alone generates trains of impulses, there is a convergence in the spinal cord resulting in both spatial and temporal summation of afferent impulses. However, the dorsal horn, where primary afferent fibers synapse, is not merely a station for transmitting sensory signals. Complex interactions between incoming tactile and nociceptive fibers as well as modulation by axons descending from the brain impress sophisticated processing on pain-related activity. As a result, many specifically acting drugs are targeted to synapses in the spinal cord to exert a selective analgesia (see Chapter 23.1).

Motor neurons have their cell bodies in the ventral horn of the spinal cord gray matter (Fig. 2-1). They are *multipolar* in that they have many dendrites in addition to one axon which follows a long course to the periphery. The dendrites and cell body of the motor neuron are specially developed for integrating postsynaptic currents in order to determine the output activity, which occurs as impulse generation. The axon conducts these impulses to its branched, distal terminal enlargements, which contain neurotransmitters to activate effector organs.

Axons and Peripheral Nerves

Axons are cylinders of axoplasm encased in the axonal membrane, which is similar to other plasma membranes (Fig. 2-2). Axons are always enveloped by a Schwann cell. Many unmyelinated axons lie within invaginations of a single Schwann cell (Fig. 2-2C), in contrast to the thick myelin sheath of a myelinated axon which is formed by a single Schwann cell wrapped many times around the axon (Fig. 2-2B). This myelin sheath is interrupted periodically at the *nodes of Ranvier*, where the extracellular medium has access to the axolemma (Fig. 2-2A).

Nerve impulses travel along nonmyelinated axons as a uniform wave, similar to the way a flame progressively ignites the fuse of a firecracker. The nerve impulse, or *action potential*, is a change in the electrical voltage across the membrane which is due to changes in the permeability of ionic channels in the axon membrane (see following).[51] In nonmyelinated axons these permeability changes occur uniformly along the axon, supporting a wave of inward ion current that underlies the depolarization of the nerve impulse. In

G. R. Strichartz: Department of Anesthesia, Harvard Medical School, Brigham and Women's Hospital, Boston, Massachusetts 02115.

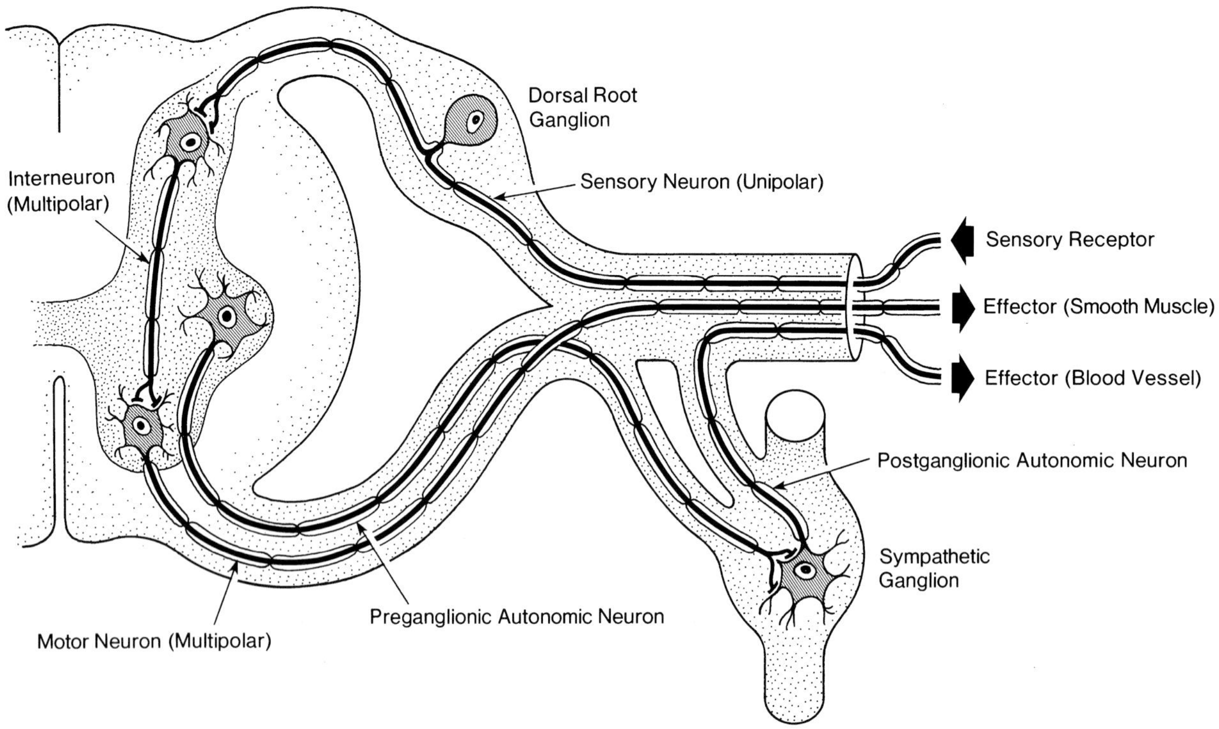

FIG. 2-1. The neuron. *Sensory neuron*, with a cell body (perikaryon) and an axon with long peripheral and short central branches ("unipolar" neuron). *Interneuron* with numerous dendrites, a cell body, and one short axon ("multipolar" neuron). *Motor* neuron with a great many dendrites, a cell body, and a long peripheral axon ("multipolar" neuron). Two *sympathetic neurons*, one with a cell body in the spinal cord and the other with its cell body in the sympathetic chain, are also shown. Each has several dendrites and a medium-length axon.

myelinated axons, however, changes in the membrane permeability and the associated inward currents occur only at the nodes of Ranvier; the myelinated *internode* of the axon is depolarized by the *passive* spread of current from the nodes. Thus, impulse conduction in these axons is continuous but not homogeneous.

Nerve Membranes

The *modern fluid mosaic model* depicts the plasma membrane as a bilayer of phospholipid molecules with their fatty acyl chains facing each other, thus making the inner portion of the membrane hydrophobic (Fig. 2-3). The surfaces of the membrane facing the cytoplasm and extracellular fluid are formed by the charged and polar hydrophilic groups of the phospholipid molecules. Globular proteins are also present and some of these penetrate through the entire thickness of the membrane. Ionic channels are composed of such transmembrane proteins.[1]

Organization of a Peripheral Nerve

In clinical practice local anesthetics must diffuse across a number of structures before reaching their site of action in the axonal membrane.[82] Peripheral nerves contain both afferent and efferent axons (Figs. 2-1 and 2-4). These axons and their Schwann cells are surrounded by a delicate layer of fine connective tissue (endoneurium) which permits easy diffusion of most local anesthetics.

Bundles of axons are enclosed in a squamous cellular sheath, the *perineurium*, which comprises several layers of cells and acts as a semipermeable barrier to local anesthetics.[3,38,90] One or more perineurial bundles are covered by an outermost, easily permeable, connective tissue layer, the *epineurium*. This layer also carries the nutritional blood vessels of larger nerves. Factors that have an important influence on local anesthetic diffusion to the axons include the perineurium, the presence or absence of myelin, the size of the axons, and the anatomical position of the axons, either in the outer or inner sections of the nerve.

Nerve Membranes and Impulses

The generation and propagation of impulses in excitable nerve and muscle cells depend on the flow of specific ionic currents through channels that span the plasma membrane.[50] These channels open and close in response to the electrical potential of the cell membrane and are the targets for local anesthetics as they block impulse propagation. This chapter describes the role of ion channels in impulse behavior that account for many of the physiological effects of local anesthetics.

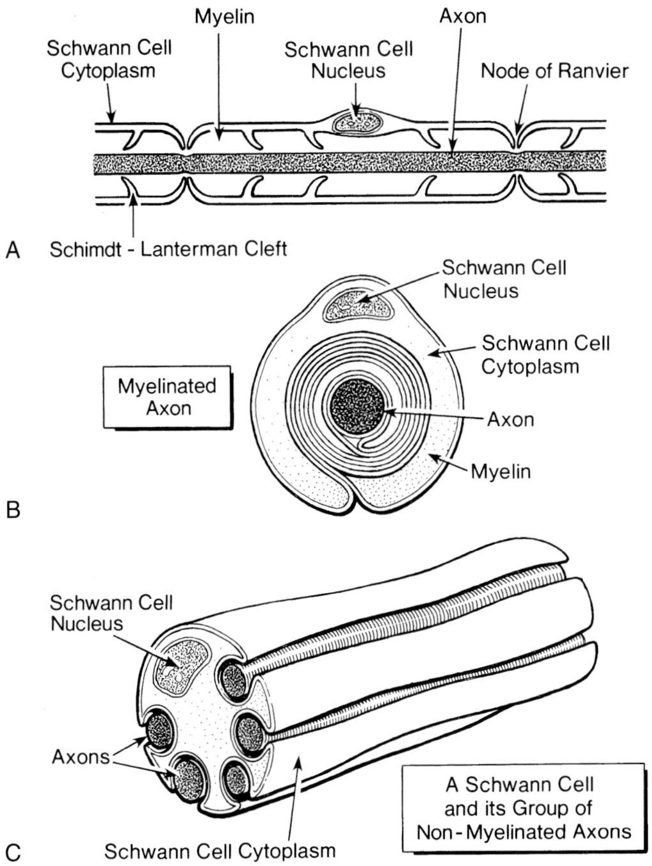

FIG. 2-2. Diagram of axon. *Myelinated axon.* **A:** Longitudinal section shows the relation of the myelin sheath to the nodes of Ranvier where myelin is absent, but one overlying Schwann cell and a thin layer of "gap substance" are present. The extranodal area is highly specialized and, because of anionic charges bound within it, tends to attract cationic substances such as local anesthetics. **B:** Transverse section of a myelinated fiber shows how the Schwann cell wraps around one axon many times to form the multiple layers of the myelin sheath. **C:** In transverse section many nonmyelinated axons can be seen embedded in the folds of a single Schwann cell. The Schwann cell surrounds the axon loosely, thus allowing uniform spread of depolarization directly along the axon.

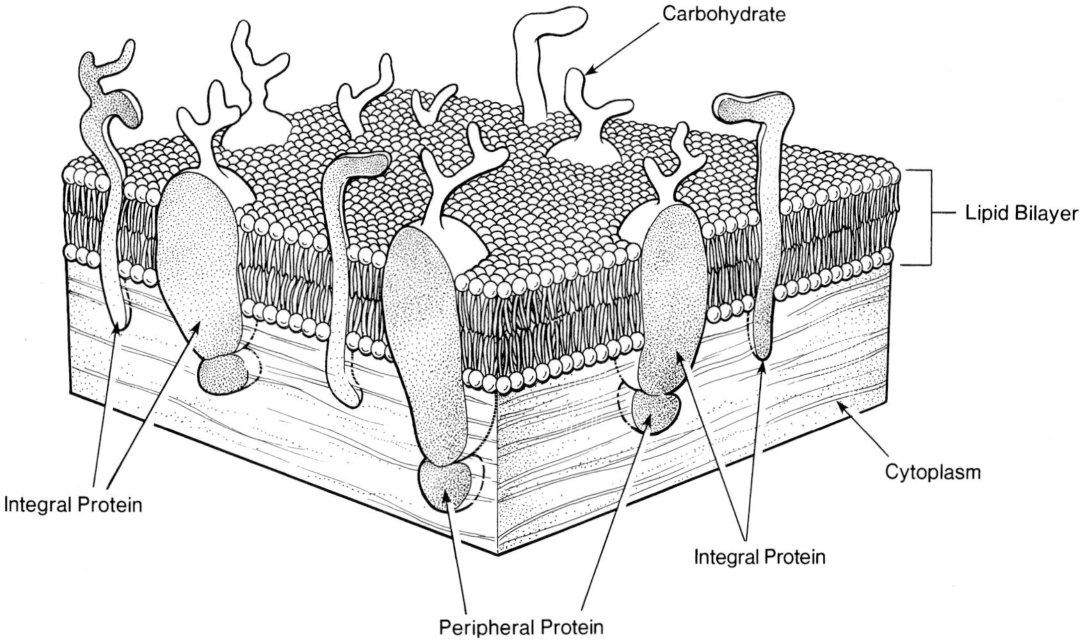

FIG. 2-3. Axonal membrane. The axonal membrane is similar to the plasma membrane of other cells. This diagram is modified from the classic Singer-Nicholson fluid-mosaic model (Singer, S.J. and Nicholson, G.L.: The fluid mosaic model of the structure of cell membranes. Science, *175*:720, 1972). Carbohydrate molecules attached to proteins and lipids on the extracellular surface of the membrane form a "cell coat." The lipid bilayer comprises densely packed phospholipids which, nevertheless, freely diffuse laterally in the plane of the membrane. Integral proteins of varying shapes and peripheral protein only on the cytoplasmic surface are associated with enzymatic and receptor functions.

Most ion channels appear to be very similar in the peripheral and central nervous systems, and in cell bodies as well as axons. Thus a single description will serve to characterize the actions of local anesthetics associated with blockade of axonal conduction.

Ionic Currents of the Nerve Impulse

Two factors contribute to electric potentials in cells: concentration gradients of ions across membranes and selective permeation of ions through membranes. The gradients are diffusional forces that tend to move the ions; the selective changes in permeability permit that tendency to be manifested as ionic current. Energy from the cell's metabolism is used to create and maintain the gradients.

The concentration of potassium ions (K^+) inside a cell is about 10 times greater than the extracellular K^+ concentration, and *vice versa* for sodium ions (Na^+). A special protein in the membrane (the Na/K pump) actively transports K^+ into the cell and Na^+ out of the cell, using ATP as the source of energy.[74] In the resting cell membrane there is a selective permeability to K^+ ions, permitting the net efflux of a small number of K^+ ions and leaving the axoplasm electrically

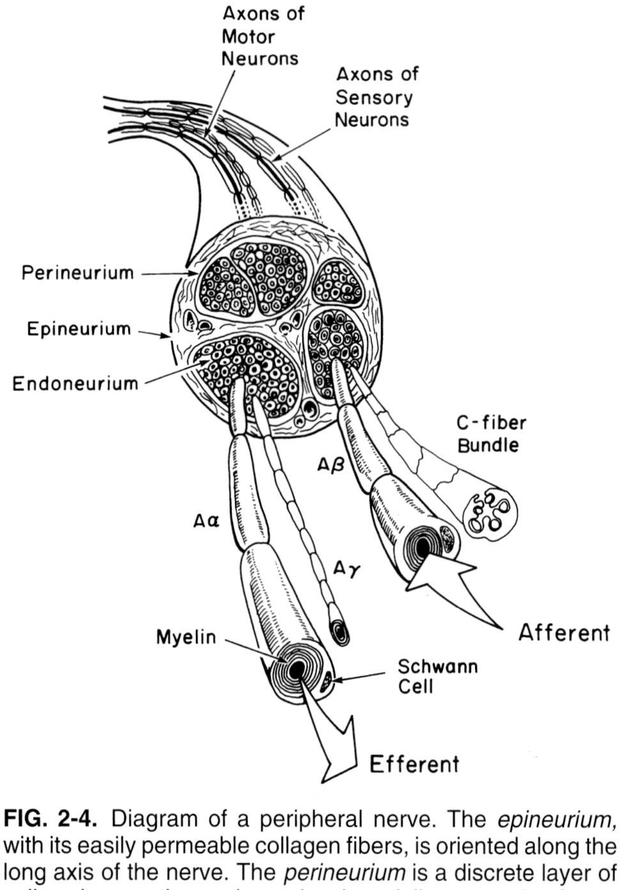

FIG. 2-4. Diagram of a peripheral nerve. The *epineurium,* with its easily permeable collagen fibers, is oriented along the long axis of the nerve. The *perineurium* is a discrete layer of cells, whereas the *endoneurium* is a delicate matrix of connective tissue embedding bundles of axons. Both afferent (sensory) and efferent (motor) axons are shown. Sympathetic efferent axons (not shown) are also present in mixed peripheral nerves.

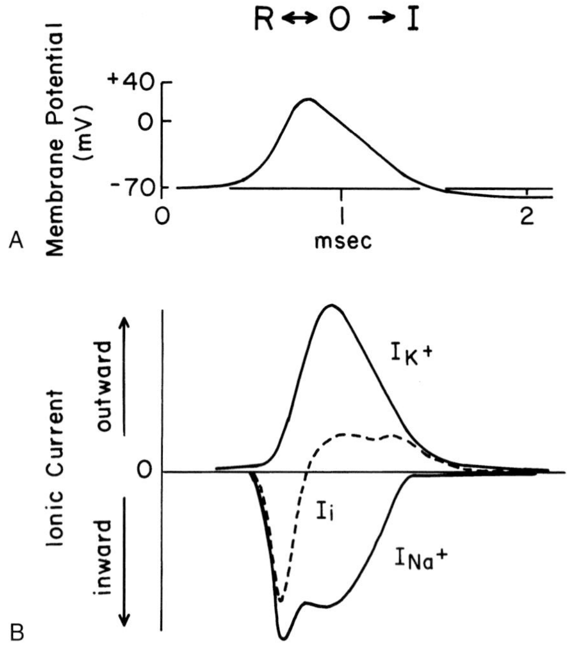

FIG. 2-5. A propagating action potential and the membrane currents that produce it. **A:** The membrane potential rises from its resting value, about −70mV in this squid axon, to reverse its sign, becoming positive inside, and then repolarizes. A hyperpolarization actually follows the impulse in this, but not in all, axons. **B:** Inward sodium current (I_{Na^+}) and outward potassium current (I_{K^+}) together yield the net ionic current across the membrane (I_i). The maximum rate of depolarization corresponds to the peak of net inward current, that of repolarization to the largest net outward current. The letters at the top of the figure describe the dominant state of the Na^+ channel during the underwritten phase of the impulse.

negative (polarized) while making the outside electrically positive. This accounts, for the most part, for the cell's "resting potential," which typically equals −70 to −80 mV (Fig. 2-5).

At rest Na^+ ions tend to flow into the axon, both because the axon is now electrically negative inside and because the Na^+ ions are more concentrated outside. A selective permeability to Na^+ arises when specific "sodium channels" in the axon membrane are opened.[50,51] Figure 2-5 shows the contributions of ionic currents during a conducted nerve impulse. The large inward Na current (I_{Na^+}) accounts for the *depolarizing phase* of the impulse. Opening of Na^+ channels occurs as the membrane is initially "depolarized" from the resting potential, that is, as the potential becomes less negative. This opening or "activation" is an intrinsic behavior of Na^+ channels, due to charged moieties that are part of their molecular structure.[99] As the membrane potential becomes less negative, more Na^+ channels open and they open more rapidly; and as more channels open, more Na^+ ions enter the cell and depolarization is accelerated (Fig. 2-6). This cycle accounts for the regenerative behavior of nerve impulses.[51]

Action potentials are brief, transient events. Repolarization of the membrane to the negative resting value occurs be-

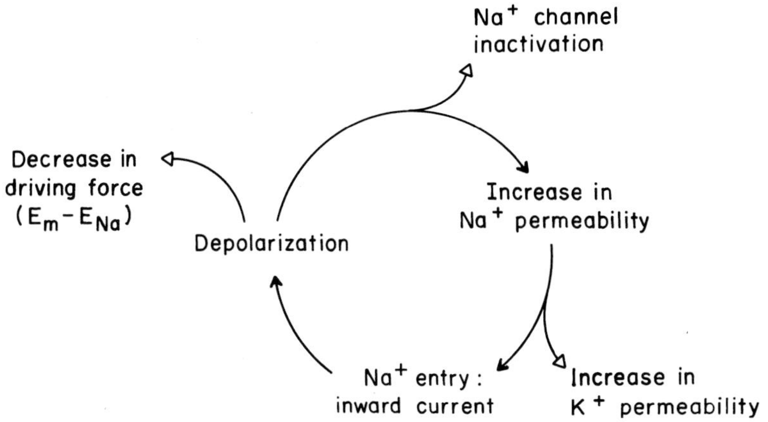

FIG. 2-6. The positive feedback cycle that underlies the depolarization phase of regenerative action potentials. Each of the three components in the cycle (*filled arrowhead*) is increased by the preceding one and, in turn, increases the subsequent one. Each outlying element (*open arrowhead*) reduces membrane excitability and terminates the action potential. The cycle is initiated by a source of current "external" to the membrane area being studied, for example, an adjacent excited region, a sensory ending depolarized by a physiologic stimulus, or a dendritic arbor that collects postsynaptic currents.

cause of three factors: (i) The driving force moving Na^+ into the cell diminishes as the axoplasmic potential becomes less negative and approaches the Nernst potential for Na^+; (ii) the sodium channels eventually close (inactivate) during a depolarization; and (iii) voltage-dependent potassium channels open and permit a large, outward K^+ current which returns the axoplasmic potential to its resting value, or beyond (Fig. 2-5). In simple terms, impulses have a depolarization phase and a repolarization phase. Inward currents, carried by Na^+ ions, depolarize the cell whereas outward currents, carried by K^+ ions, repolarize the cell. The integrated result of all these factors is diagrammed in Figure 2-6, which summarizes the ionic contribution to the nerve impulse.

With each nerve impulse, a pulse of Na^+ ions enters a cell and a pulse of K^+ leaves it. Small changes in the concentrations of these ions can build up during repeated discharge and lessen the driving force of the ion gradients. However, the Na^+/K^+-ATPase (Na^+/K^+ pump), which is activated by elevation of intracellular Na^+, will remove the Na^+ and restore the extracellular K^+, using the energy of ATP. This pump generates an outward current during this process and thereby hyperpolarizes the cell, contributing to an "after-potential"[74] and shaping the patterns of impulses that occur in constant or intermittent trains of discharge.

Impulse Propagation

Inward current entering the axon during the depolarizing phase of an impulse flows within the conducting medium of the axoplasm and thereby spreads to adjacent, inactive regions. These adjacent regions are depolarized by this "local circuit" current, usually to levels far in excess of those for threshold conditions, and the regenerative impulse "invades" this region, generating its own inward current. Figure 2-7 shows how the propagating potential wave is spread over myelinated and nonmyelinated axons during one instant. The spatial spread of the potential change is large compared to the nerve diameter. For example, if the impulse lasts for 1

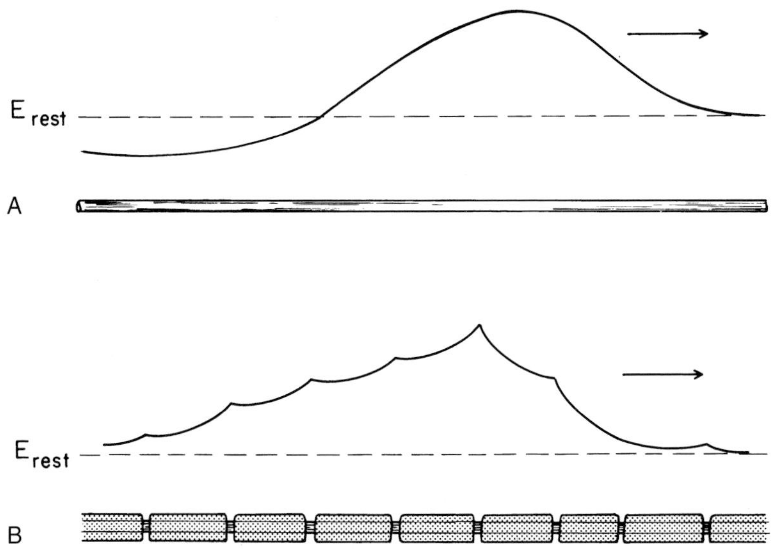

FIG. 2-7. Instantaneous spatial distribution of the membrane potential change during the propagation of an action potential conducted to the right, as shown by the arrows. **A:** In the smaller, nonmyelinated axon (e.g., a mammalian C fiber) the potential changes in the same smooth, continuous shape that it has when measured in time at one *narrow* region of the axon. This occurs because the axon is a cable with uniform properties along its length and the impulse propagates at a constant velocity. **B:** Conduction in a myelinated axon is also characterized by continuous potential changes along the axon. Regions in which large inward currents flow into the axon, the nodes of Ranvier, depolarize the adjacent internodes, which have no sodium channels and generate no active inward ionic current. (The lengths of nodes and internodes are not drawn to scale.) Note that during an impulse many nodes of Ranvier are simultaneously at some level of depolarization; thus the impulse travels much further in the same time in a myelinated axon (see text).

msec, and is conducted at a velocity of 1 m/sec in the small, nonmyelinated C fibers (of less than 1 μm diameter) then the potential change extends over 1 mm along the axon, 1000 times the axon's diameter. For large myelinated axons 20 μm in diameter, impulses travel at 60 to 100 m/sec and thus extend over distances of 60 to 100 mm. Inward currents from all the active nodes integrate as they spread toward inactive regions, ensuring that impulse propagation will continue. Therefore, complete block of impulses in about three to five nodes in sequences is necessary for the total prevention of impulse propagation.[76,80] Furthermore, the "action current" flowing into the nerve under the impulse is five to ten times that required to depolarize the next segment to threshold; this ratio is referred to as the *margin of safety* for impulse conduction. Due to this large margin of safety, about 80% of the sodium channels must be inhibited in order to block a propagated impulse fully.

In the face of reduced membrane excitability due to disease, altered metabolism, or drug action, impulses may still occur but will be conducted more slowly. When the net inward current is decreased, the action potential amplitude will be smaller, the rate of impulse depolarization slower, and the velocity of conduction lower. This condition often worsens as an impulse attempts to propagate through a diseased or drugged axon, a situation termed *decremental impulse conduction*. If the decrement is sufficiently great, conduction failure occurs; if not, then only conduction slowing in the affected axon region occurs and normal impulse conduction resumes if the decremented action potential is able to excite the contiguous normal region of the axon. This condition almost certainly applies to nerve conduction during the onset and regression of a local anesthetic block.

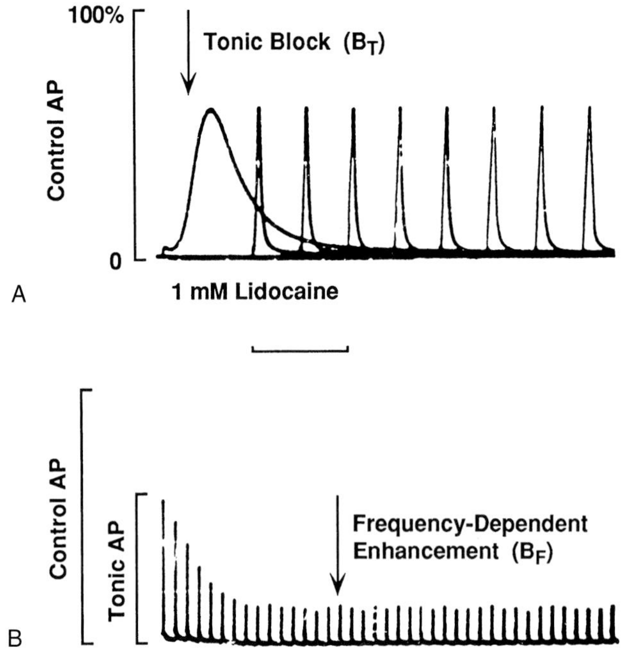

FIG. 2-8. Tonic (B_T) and use-dependent (B_F) inhibition of action potentials by local anesthetic. **A:** Tonic inhibition is the relative decrease in amplitude of the compound action potential (CAP) in the presence of drug with the nerve stimulated at low frequency (0.016Hz = 1/min). **B:** Frequency-dependent block (B_F) is the further decrease in amplitude of the action potential during a high-frequency pulse train (40 Hz here) which is completely reversible to the level of B_T when stimulation is slowed. The horizontal bar calibrates the time scale: 2 and 20 msec for the broad and narrow action potentials, respectively, in **A** and 200 msec in **B.** (Reprinted with permission from Bokesch, P. M., Post, C., and Strichartz, G. R.: Structure activity relationship of lidocaine homologues on tonic and frequency-dependent impulse blockade in nerve. J. Pharmacol. Exp. Ther., *237*:773, 1986.)

Mechanisms of Anesthetic Action

Local anesthetics block impulses by interfering with the function of sodium channels.[17,46,100] In the presence of local anesthetics sodium channels are less likely to open in response to a stimulating depolarization,[19] the resulting Na^+ current is decreased, and at sufficiently high anesthetic concentrations enough channels are impaired to prevent impulse generation. When a local anesthetic containing solution is applied to a *desheathed* peripheral nerve *in vitro*, inhibition is detected in a minute and a steady-state level of block is usually achieved in 10 minutes or less. At low frequencies of impulse firing, 1 Hz (1/sec) or less, this "tonic block" has a constant value (Fig. 2-8). Higher frequencies result in an increase in the degree of block, the so-called phasic or use-dependent block, which quickly reaches a new steady state (Fig. 2-8) and quickly reverses to the tonic block level when stimulation is slowed.

These changes in impulse behavior are caused by drug-induced changes in the inward Na^+ current. Figure 2-9 shows the tonic and phasic inhibitions of Na current caused by local anesthetics acting on a myelinated nerve membrane. Both lidocaine and bupivacaine yield about 50% tonic block, with bupivacaine being about eight times more potent. Despite its lower concentration, however, bupivacaine produces a phasic block equal to or greater than lidocaine's. A kinetic analysis of these actions suggests that bupivacaine is more potent for tonic block because it has a *faster* rate of binding to the Na^+ channel site (perhaps because it is more concentrated in the membrane than lidocaine). Bupivacaine also is more potent for phasic block because it dissociates *more slowly* from the closed channel than does lidocaine.[23]

Since they lessen the probability that channels will open, local anesthetics have an effect like that of a preceding depolarization. They shift channels toward an "inactivated" state which cannot be directly opened by stimulation.[18,47,49]

As a brief comment aside, compare the effective concentrations of lidocaine required for inhibition of Na^+ current and action potential. Lidocaine's IC_{50} for tonic channel inhibition is about 0.2 mM, but for inhibition of the action potential amplitude it is about 0.8 to 1.0 mM. (These numbers are in the ratio predicted by the 80% channel blockade needed for impulse failure.) By comparison, the molar concentration of 1% lidocaine often used for clinical peripheral

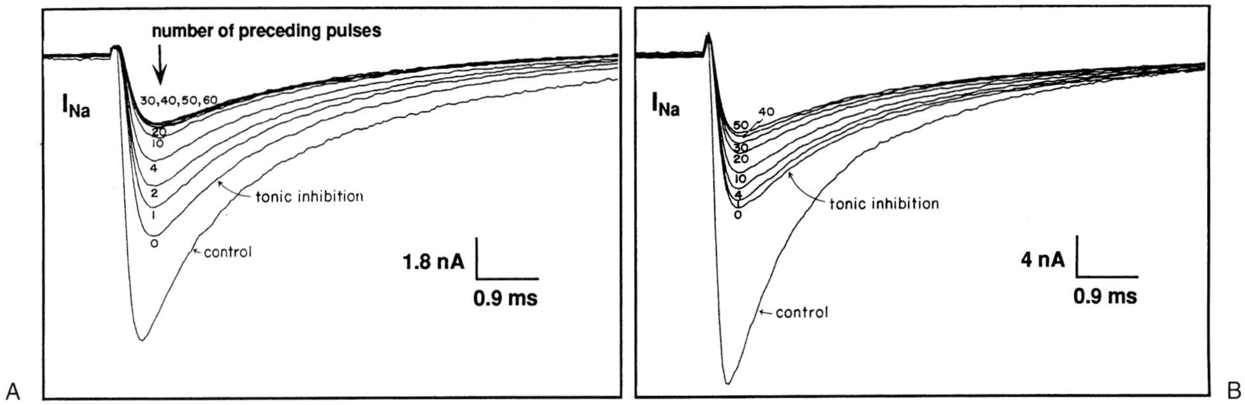

FIG. 2-9. Phasic inhibition of Na^+ currents in a myelinated nerve. In the presence of 200 μM lidocaine **(A)** or 25 μM R-bupivacaine **(B)** Na^+ currents are elicited by repetitive depolarization of the nodal membrane to −20 mV. About half the current is blocked tonically, that is, when measured with infrequent depolarizations. Further inhibition occurs when pulses are applied at a frequency of 10 Hz. Selected traces are shown, with numbers indicating the sequence in the pulse train.

nerve blocks is about 40 mM, about 50 times the desheathed nerve impulse blocking concentration! From laboratory experiments on rats we know that 0.1 ml of 1% lidocaine injected around the sciatic nerve gives complete motor block and analgesia but that 0.75% (30 mM) of the same volume (0.1 ml) yields an incomplete functional block of much briefer duration.[101] Why is so much more drug needed for impulse blockade *in vivo* than in isolated nerve? It is because the perineurial sheath is such an effective barrier against the diffusion of local anesthetics that under clinical conditions, only about 5% of the anesthetic dose that is injected actually penetrates into the nerve.[71]

Basic Pharmacology

Exploration of the mechanism of local anesthetic action raises three fundamental questions: Which species of the drug, neutral or protonated, is the active form? Where does the anesthetic molecule act? What is the molecular mechanism of channel interference?

Active Species: The Role of Ionization

Under physiological conditions, most local anesthetics exist in rapid equilibrium between the neutral and protonated, charged species (Fig. 2-10). The ratio of ionized (LH^+) to nonionized (L) molecules is given by the Henderson-Hasselbach equation

$$\frac{[LH^+]}{[L]} = 10^{pK_a - pH}$$

where the pK_a is the value of pH at which the concentrations of the two species are equal. The pK_a values of clinically used local anesthetics range from about 7.7 to 9.5,[96] so in solution all these drugs are charged more of the time than they are uncharged.

Both ionized and un-ionized drug species can inhibit Na^+ channels. Quaternary derivatives of local anesthetics, which are permanently charged, when directed into the axoplasmic space are potent blockers of impulses and of Na^+ currents.[39,93] Interestingly, these drugs have very slowly developing effects when placed outside of the axon; their charge and low hydrophobicity (see below) greatly restrict their passage into and through the membrane.

Perpetually uncharged local anesthetics also effectively block impulses and sodium channels,[22,81] demonstrating that ionization is not essential for pharmacological activity. The ability of tertiary amine local anesthetics to block sodium channels in single cells is faster and greater when the drug is applied externally at alkaline external pH,[48] or when it is applied by direct internal perfusion at neutral or slightly acidic internal pH.[66] Both of these observations are consistent with a model where the neutral form of the anesthetic dissolves in and passes through the axon membrane and, having reached a cytoplasmic region, becomes protonated (see Fig. 2-10). The experimental observations to date do not provide infor-

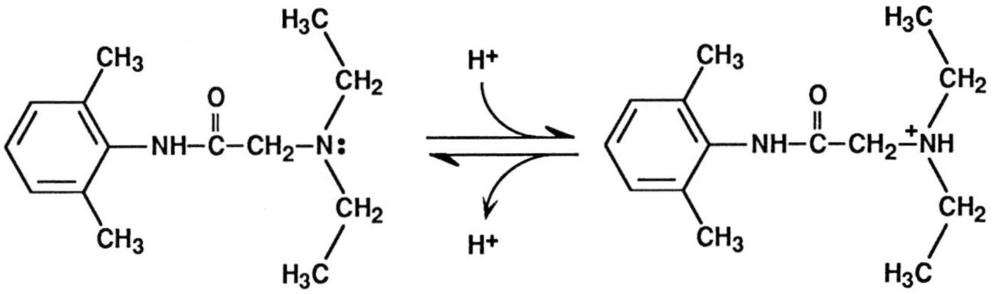

FIG. 2-10. The ionization (protonation and deprotonation) of lidocaine.

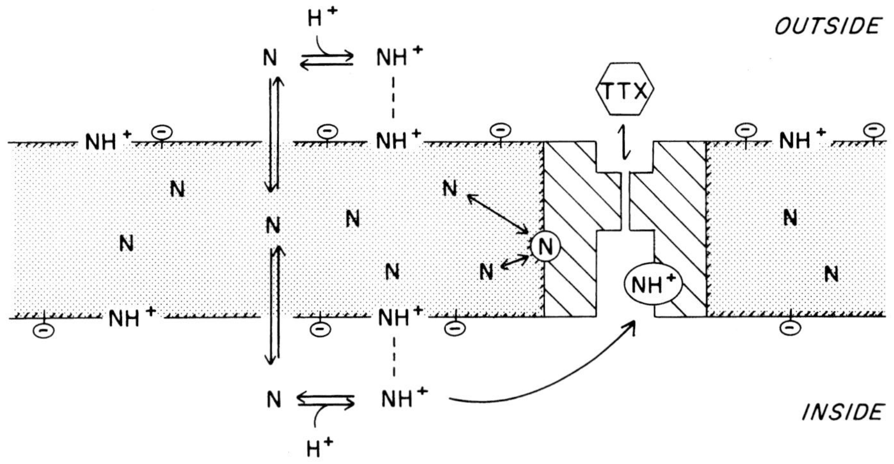

FIG. 2-11. Tertiary amine local anesthetics exist as neutral base *(N)* and protonated (*NH*$^+$) species in physiologic solution. These forms interact in various modes with phospholipids and proteins in nerve membranes: *N* preferentially partitions into the hydrophobic membrane interior, whereas NH$^+$ adsorbs at the negatively charged membrane surface, through hydrophobic and electrostatic interactions. Two primary reactions with Na$^+$ channel proteins are shown: rapid binding of the neutral form at the lipid:protein interface and slower binding of the charged form by means of the inner mouth of the channel; the latter depends on the conversion of the channel to open or activated conformations (see text). The natural "local anesthetics" tetrodotoxin *(TTX)* and saxitoxin bind at the external surface of the channel and have no obvious interactions with local anesthetics.

mation to choose between a membrane-associated binding site or one within the "pore" of the Na channel (Fig. 2-11). One intriguing finding is that dissociation of anesthetic molecules from the closed channel is clearly sensitive to the pH outside the nerve, but relatively insensitive to the intracellular pH.[88] Thus, wherever it is bound in the Na$^+$ channel, a blocking local anesthetic molecule can equilibrate with extracellular protons.

Hydrophobicity and Potency

Drug hydrophobicity is also a determinant of potency at the level of isolated nerves. The more hydrophobic drugs are more potent blockers of action potentials[12,91] and of sodium currents.[23,28,30] This increased potency results from a faster apparent association rate, not from a slower dissociation rate, for the binding of the local anesthetics to their channel sites.[23] In other words, the more hydrophobic local anesthetics can reach the site more easily, but do not appear to leave the site more slowly than the less hydrophobic drugs. Molecular mass of the anesthetics, however, does influence the leaving rate for the charged local anesthetics, but not the neutral ones. These results support the concept of two pathways to and from the anesthetic site.[47] One pathway may be through the channel's pore (*hydrophilic* route) and the other may be through the membrane (*hydrophobic* route), selectively favored by charged and neutral drug species, respectively (see following). Whether these separate routes lead to one or several sites of action is unclear at this time.

Thus, pH affects anesthetic potency on single fibers by two, conflicting means. An extracellular alkaline pH favors the neutral, membrane-permeant form of the drug, but an acidic extracellular pH favors the more potent blocking species at the site of action. Both neutral and charged forms of anesthetics participate in impulse blockade. Of course, during most clinical procedures, the functional potency of local anesthetics is determined largely by the fraction of injected drug that actually passes into the nerve bundle, and conditions that favor the penetrating, neutral species are desirable.[82] This situation is discussed in detail later in this chapter.

Locus of Action

In principle, local anesthetics can act at any of three phases in nerve membranes: (i) at the membrane:solution interface, (ii) in the membrane's hydrocarbon interior, or (iii) at the sodium channel itself. The last possibility is probably the case for traditional local anesthetic agents (Fig. 2-11). Increasing evidence shows that local anesthetics specifically associate with the sodium channel itself. First, the quaternary derivatives act on nerves only from the axoplasmic surface. Thus a general perturbation of the membrane cannot be a mechanism for nerve block. Second, as noted above, the inhibition of channels is enhanced by the application of patterns of membrane potential which favor the opening or inactivation of sodium channels by so-called use-dependent or phasic block.[26,88,93] This potentiation of anesthetic block by repetitive depolarizations is called use-dependent or phasic block. Local anesthetics also are more potent, tonically, on channels in depolarized membranes than on those in normally polarized membranes.[47,49]

Third, there is a weak yet significant stereoselective block by anesthetic enantiomers.[113] The presence of asymmetric carbons in the aromatic moiety, or in the cyclic amine of molecules like bupivacaine, results in a potency difference of two to five between stereoisomers.[2,61] Interactions of the anesthetic molecules with membrane lipids do not show stereoselectivity.

In addition, the effects of local anesthetics are modified by other drugs and treatments that specifically affect Na^+ channels. Activator compounds, which permit channels to open at the resting potential, and thus produce spontaneous depolarizations of the cell, are competitively antagonized by local anesthetics.[56,73] Enzymatic digestion of a proteinaceous portion of the channel facing the axoplasm greatly reduces the phasic blocking action of anesthetics, although tonic block is little affected.[18]

An emphatic observation favoring the Na^+ channel as anesthetic receptor is the modification of local anesthetic blocking actions by the intentional mutation of single amino acids of the channel protein. In particular, alterations of amino acid residues that probably line the channel's pore have potent and specific consequences for the tonic and phasic components of channel blockade.[72] These observations all point to the sodium channel itself as a *specific receptor* for local anesthetic molecules.

Molecular Actions of Local Anesthetics

Exactly how do local anesthetics interfere with the operation of Na^+ channels? All the information about mechanisms of local anesthetics comes from physiological studies. Much of it is anchored on the observation that anesthetics inhibit stimulated channels (phasic block) more than resting channels (tonic block).[23,28] A single explanation for tonic and phasic block has been formalized as the Modulated Receptor Hypothesis (MRH)[47,49] (see Fig. 2-12). The hypothesis rests on the accepted notion that sodium channels normally respond to membrane depolarizations by passing through defined conformational "states," beginning at rest (R), activating through closed intermediate forms (C) to reach an open (O) form, and then closing to an inactivated (I) state. According to the MRH, local anesthetics have a higher affinity for open and, especially, inactivated Na^+ channels than for resting channels.[23,26] During stimulation, channels that are opened and inactivated bind local anesthetics more tightly. This binding thus stabilizes the channels in a nonconducting state, and increasingly so with each stimulating pulse. Eventually some anesthetic-bound channels will return to the resting equilibrium, and a steady-state level of phasic block will be reached wherein increased inhibition during a depolarization is exactly reversed by drug dissociation in the time between pulses.

The normal inactivated state is not essential for block.[97,106] It appears that open and activated channels react most rapidly with anesthetic molecules and that inactivated channels react more slowly but still have a greater equilibrium drug affinity than resting channels.[21] Clinically, during one relatively brief nerve impulse (0.5 msec) the formation of inactivated channels is limited and drug binding to this state probably contributes little to the observed inhibition. The concept of selective, state-dependent binding of anesthetics lies at the core of the MRH.

Does an anesthetic molecule inhibit the channel by "plugging" the pore and preventing ions from passing, or by interfering with the conformational changes that underlie channel opening? Both possibilities may occur during the blockade of impulses by tertiary amine drugs. It is possible that tertiary amine drugs have two binding sites on the channel (Fig. 2-11). One site is near enough to the pore to permit the anesthetic molecule to become protonated directly from the solution and this site favors the charged anesthetic species. Binding and unbinding of drug molecules from this site are slow reactions, with rates that approximate those of the channel gating processes. The other site is in a hydrophobic milieu where the probability of encountering a proton donor is low. This second site is bound during tonic block and local anesthetics can bind to and dissociate from it, into the membrane, relatively rapidly and easily. During phasic block, anesthetic molecules bind to the first site, from which dissociation is much slower. Interestingly, the stereoisomers that show the greater potency for phasic block are all relatively long, planar molecules compared to their less potent enantiomers which show an acutely angled conformation.[30,61] The planar isomer probably slides easily into the phasic blocking site while the angled one is sterically restricted from that locus. Our knowledge about molecular mechanisms of anesthetic

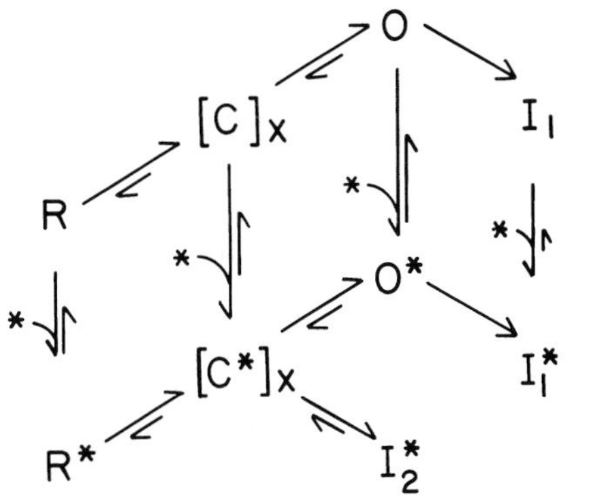

FIG. 2-12. The revised modulated receptor model. Each letter represents a state of the sodium channel: *R,* resting; C_x, any one of several intermediate, closed states between *R* and *O,* which is the open, ion-conducting state; I_1, an inactivated (nonopenable) state that is formed from *O;* and I_2, a different inactivated state that is formed from the anesthetic-bound *C** states, without going through *O.* The *vertical arrows* indicate binding reactions of a local anesthetic molecule (*asterisk*). States *C* and *O* and *I* have higher affinities for anesthetics than does *R.* The $[C^*]_X \rightarrow I_2^*$ reaction may account for much of the resting, tonic blocking activity of local anesthetics, and thus favor the neutral, more hydrophobic drugs. Anesthetic binding reactions of *O* and *I* conformations are activated by rapid depolarizations (e.g., action potentials), with the former being faster than the latter. Charged drugs bound to *O** and I_1 and I_2* dissociate slowly, accounting for much of the phasic blocking behavior.

action will expand greatly with the detailed structural analysis of purified sodium channels.[72]

CLINICAL APPLICATIONS FOR PERIPHERAL AND REGIONAL NERVE BLOCKS

Peripheral Nerve Anatomy and Function

Anatomical and chemical factors determine the susceptibility of fibers to block by local anesthetics. The particular nerve being blocked and the nature of the agent used and its formulation are important for the rate of onset, the maximum degree and duration of nerve block, and the differential actions of local anesthetics.

Fiber Size and Function

The diameter and myelination of a nerve fiber are correlated with its impulse physiology as well as its message-carrying function. Nerve fibers are categorized into three major anatomical classes (Table 1): myelinated somatic nerves (A fibers); myelinated preganglionic autonomic nerves (B fibers); and nonmyelinated axons (C fibers). The B and C fibers are small, ranging in diameter from about 2 μm to less than 1 μm, respectively, whereas the A fibers vary in diameter from 4 to 20 μm approximately.

The A fibers are divided further into four groups according to decreasing impulse conduction velocity and diameter: alpha, beta, gamma, and delta. Largest are the alpha fibers, related to motor function, and reflex activity. A-beta fibers also innervate muscle and transmit touch and pressure sensations, while gamma fibers control muscle spindle tone. The thinnest A fibers—the A-delta group—subserve pain and temperature sensations.

The thinly myelinated B fibers are preganglionic autonomic axons that ultimately control vascular smooth muscle, among others; B fibers thus assume cardinal importance during spinal or peridural anesthesia. The nonmyelinated C fibers, like the myelinated A-delta fibers, subserve pain and temperature transmission, as well as postganglionic autonomic functions. C fibers are thinner than myelinated fibers (less than 1 μm diameter) and have a much lower conduction velocity than even A-delta fibers, less than 1 m/sec.

It is evident from this summary that humans are equipped with two separate conducting systems that convey pain-related messages. One system (fast pain) conducts signals rapidly and is composed of myelinated A-delta fibers: the other system (slow pain) is composed of slowly conducting, nonmyelinated C fibers.

Both sensory perception and normal motor activity depend on the integrated actions of afferent and efferent impulses. Sensation is the result of patterns of impulses coding for several different modalities in different primary afferent fiber types, and sensation is tonically modulated by activity in efferent sympathetic nerve fibers.[106] Similarly, coordinated gross and deft motor activity depends on efferent impulses in axons of alpha motoneurons that are being *tuned* constantly by proprioceptive and muscle spindle afferent input to the spinal cord. Recognizing this inherent requirement for integrated afferent and efferent activity in the conduct of normal behavior leads to a realization of the complex pharmacology of peripheral nerve block that underlies clinical anesthesia. Equating small fiber inhibition with "sensory" (nociceptive) block and large fiber inhibition with "motor" block is nonsensical.[41]

Impulse Inhibition and Functional Impairment

Minimum Blocking Concentration (C_m)

The minimum blocking concentration (C_m) is the lowest concentration of local anesthetic *in vitro* that blocks all impulse activity in a given nerve within a reasonable period of time (commonly 10–15 min). For blockade of mixed somatic nerve function an *administered concentration* of 1% (40 mM) lidocaine *in vivo* appears to be necessary to achieve the measured C_m of approximately 0.5 to 1.0 mM lidocaine at all the axons.[41,84,98] The concept is important clinically, for only drug concentrations greater than C_m will reliably anesthetize a nerve. Because the pharmacologic potency of different local anesthetics varies greatly (see preceding section), each agent has its own C_m. Drug behavior also depends on the environment, so C_m must be further defined by the prevailing solution conditions, such as pH and temperature.[84,112]

The C_m of an axon is the same whether it runs in a peripheral nerve or in a spinal rootlet. The local anesthetic pool *in vivo*, however, is subject to numerous influences that act to reduce the final anesthetic concentration reaching the nerve

TABLE 2-1. *Classification and physiologic characteristics of nerve fibers*

	A-alpha	A-beta	A-gamma	A-delta	B	C
Function	Motor	Touch/pressure	Prociception/ motor tone	Pain/temperature	Preganglionic autonomic (sympathetic)	Pain/temperature
Myelin	+ + +	+ + +	+ +	+ +	+	—
Diameter (μm)	12–20	5–12	5–12	1–4	1–3	0.5–1
Conduction speed (m/sec)	70–120	30–70	30–70	12–30	14.8	1.2

+ + +, heavily myelinated; + +, moderately myelinated; +, lightly myelinated; —, nonmyelinated.

membrane. Dilution by tissue fluid, fibrous tissue barriers, absorption by fat and uptake into the vasculature, and local metabolism are all factors that determine the clinical potency. The final concentration of drug eventually arriving at the axon depends on the relative magnitude of these factors and on the length of nerve exposed to drug solution. For example, much less local anesthetic need be applied for subarachnoid than for peridural block, not because the C_m changes when an axon traverses the vertebral canal, but because spinal roots are weakly protected in the subarachnoid space. In addition, the drug is absorbed faster into the bloodstream from the vascular extradural space than from the marginally perfused intradural space.[11] As noted above, pharmacokinetic factors are major determinants of the clinical potency of local anesthetics because only a small fraction of the applied dose actually reaches the nerve tissue.

Differential Nerve Block

When clinically anesthetizing a peripheral nerve, it is sometimes observed that pain can be obtunded completely while motor function and touch are less affected.[45] This situation is one example of "differential block." Depending on the circumstance, it may be desirable or not to have this type of differential block. The presence of motor activity might be disconcerting to a surgeon accustomed to equating anesthesia with limp muscles, but is not always necessarily undesirable. Further, as touch and light pressure sensations are conveyed by large fibers, an anxious patient might misinterpret the mechanical perception of incision and tissue manipulation as pain.

Differential blockade, observed clinically, has its basis in several possible sources.[75] First, it may be a temporal rather than equilibrium phenomenon, impulses in small fibers being blocked *faster* than those in large ones because of the time course of drug diffusion into *as well as along the length of* nerve sufficient to block propagation through the anesthetized region.[71,76] Second, some fibers may be slightly more subject to impulse blockade by anesthetics than others because of anatomical features, such as the presence of myelin which can effectively pool anesthetic molecules near the axon membrane during the dynamics of nerve block. Third, axons *per se* may be differentially sensitive to block because, for example, some have potassium channels and some do not,[13,33] or the sodium channel types differ,[35] or the membrane lipids differ[94] and thus also the membrane concentration of anesthetics.

However, these categories to explain differential block are speculations about a complex behavior observed clinically. The situation is not much clarified by experimental studies. The relationship between C_m and fiber diameter is far more complex than usually appreciated. Despite widespread belief, C_m does not increase simply as a function of fiber diameter.[75] This is especially true when comparing myelinated and nonmyelinated fibers. In separate experiments, it has been shown that nerve signals associated with both B fibers and A-delta fibers are reduced at slightly lower concentrations of local anesthetics than those required to block the smaller C fibers.[44,98]

In almost all such studies, however, the amplitude of compound action potentials (CAP) was measured; this signal represents the summed response of thousands of similar but nonidentical individual axons. Reduction of the maximum CAP amplitude occurs because impulses in some fibers are *slowed* more than those in others, in addition to the total blockade present in yet other fibers. The consequences of this dispersion of conduction for synaptic integration of afferent information in the spinal cord are unknown,[55] whereas the effect of total impulse inhibition is clear.

When the ability of individual axons to propagate single action potentials is titrated by local anesthetics directly, *in vivo*, the results are contrary to long-held beliefs. A good example is seen in Figure 2-13 where the conducting probability of the larger A-beta fibers in rat sciatic nerve is slightly more susceptible to lidocaine than that of the smaller A-delta fibers. The susceptibility of impulses in C fibers is significantly less.

The responses during trains of impulses, which are the actual *units of information transfer*, may differ between these fiber types during partial block by local anesthetic.[77,101] Temporal summation in the spinal cord or at effector organs may be altered in significant or in subliminal ways by use-dependent block. In order to appreciate the relationship of impulses to behavior, it is important to avoid thinking that functional deficits are proportional to neurophysiological deficits; these two measures are not necessarily linearly related.

Partial impulse dropout, as a result of phasic block, has more intriguing effects on perception and paralysis, the im-

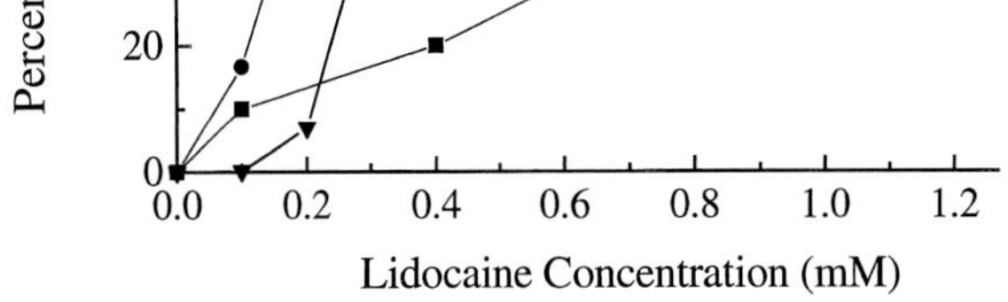

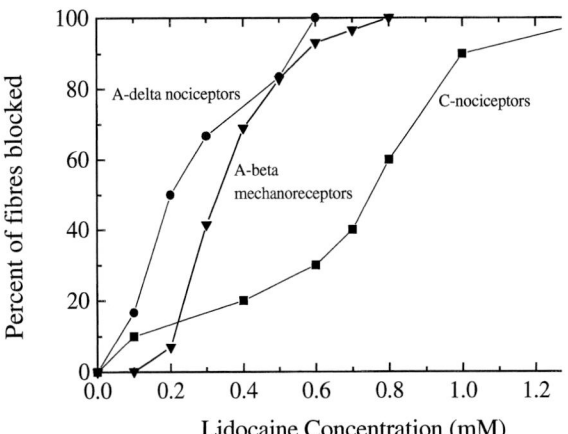

FIG. 2-13. Impulse blockade by lidocaine of individual axons of rat sciatic nerve *in vivo*. The percentage of fibers conducting at different concentrations of lidocaine for C fibers (CV <2.0 m/sec, n = 8), A-delta fibers (CV 2.1–30 m/sec, n = 15), and A-beta fibers (CV >30 m/sec, n = 18) shows that fibers in all categories are blocked over a range of concentrations from 0.2 to 0.8 mM but that nociceptive C fibers are significantly less susceptible (J. Huang *et al.*: J. Pharmacol. Exp. Ther. 1997, In press.)

portant behavioral end points. The effective reduction in impulses frequency that accompanies partial neural blockade may *distort the afferent impulse pattern* to a degree where it is unrecognizable to the central nervous system (CNS).[77] Thus, functional numbness or analgesia may occur without the need for total ablation of all afferent impulses.[9,104] This is vividly demonstrated in Figure 2-14 where the somatosensory evoked potentials recorded from the scalps of three different subjects, all given epidural injections of lidocaine yielding total regional numbness, show a range of reductions. Apparently neural activity can reach the brain without causing sensory perception. How such responses of the CNS persist in the face of regional nerve "block" is a provocative question.

Pharmacokinetics of Nerve Block

Delivery Phase

Because the local anesthetic is generally injected into the fluid medium surrounding a nerve, the drug molecules must diffuse through layers of fibrous and other tissue barriers before they ultimately reach individual axons. The density of non-neural tissue components in a peripheral nerve varies. The sciatic nerve contains much fibrous tissue, and even some fat; other peripheral nerves contain considerably less. An exception to this is the spinal rootlets, which are enclosed in the cerebral spinal fluid of the subarachnoid space by only a thin perineurium[90]; drug diffusion and penetration of these nerves accordingly is rapid, so that just a small amount of local anesthetic produces blockade quickly and fully. However, the length of unsheathed nerve in the roots also renders them vulnerable to mechanical and chemical insult.

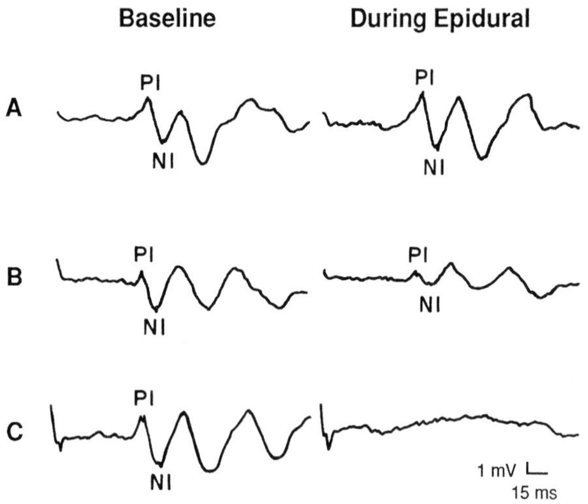

FIG. 2-14. Human somatosensory evoked potential (SSEP) during epidural lidocaine block in the presence of complete numbness on sensory examination of three different subjects. Depression of the S1 dermatomal SSEP ranged from 0% **(A)**, to greater than 50% **(B)**, to 100% **(C)**. Data are representative of examples. (Reprinted with permission from Benzon, H. T., Toleikis, J. R., Dixit, I., Goodman, I., and Hill, J. A.: Onset, intensity of blockade and somatosensory evoked potential changes of the lumbosacral dermatomes after epidural anesthesia with alkalinized lidocaine. Anest. Analg., *76*:328, 1993.)

The first step in moving the anesthetic to its neural target site is mass movement (spread) of the injected solution. A large injected volume spreads farther and exposes more nerves to the anesthetic (but, of course, also increases the vascular absorption surface). Mass movement is particularly important in subarachnoid (spinal) anesthesia, with the drug spreading upward and downward in the spinal fluid according to the specific gravity of the fluid that contains the local anesthetic and the patient's posture.

Diffusion, the movement of drug molecules away from the site of injection, is governed by concentration gradients and the viscosity of the surrounding liquid. Molecules move from an area of high concentration to one of low concentration, the rate of diffusion increasing with slope of the concentration gradient. Diffusion through solution also depends on the drug's molecular mass, varying with the square root of molecular weight. All local anesthetics are of similar mass, however (e.g., procaine = 236; bupivacaine = 288), and thus diffuse at about the same rate. Since diffusion is a relatively slow process, the local anesthetic solution is continually being diluted with tissue fluid. At the same time, drug is continuously absorbed by vascular and lymphatic channels. In addition, a substantial portion of the supply of available anesthetic is bound to tissue elements encountered along the diffusion path. Since this uptake is due largely to hydrophobic absorption,[91] generally, the more lipophilic the agent, the more it is bound and the slower is its effective diffusion. More potent drugs are used at lower concentrations, and also are more hydrophobic; both factors result in more slowly developing blocks. The most important factor in onset, however, is probably penetration through the perineurial sheath.

Permeation of the Nerve Sheath

The encasing perineurial sheath presents the major diffusion barrier to local anesthetics reaching the nerve axons (Fig. 2-4).[82] In the spinal cord this structure correlates with the arachnoid membrane. The major route of passage through this network of squamous cells connected by tight junctions[38] is via the cell membranes themselves. Because the lipid bilayer character of plasma membranes is common to almost all mammalian cells, drug penetration through the sheath is similar to penetration into nerve membranes.

Protonated anesthetic molecules have about 1:1000 the membrane permeability of the neutral anesthetic species, not because the charged molecules do not bind to the outer surface of the membrane, but because they cannot penetrate across to the other surface. The electrostatic forces that prevent this transport are largely absent in the unprotonated drug forms and neutral anesthetic molecules pass across the membrane much more easily.[82,47]

Formulations of local anesthetics for clinical use are always at acid pH. Not only are the anesthetic molecules more stable for storage in acid solutions, the antioxidants often added to protect the included vasoconstrictors are themselves weak acids. It is good practice and common sense to raise the pH of local anesthetic solutions before injection. This is easily accomplished by the addition of sterile sodium bicarbonate. The provisos in this procedure are twofold: (i) The bicarbonate volume added to an anesthetic should not be so much as to reduce its concentration to an impotent level (e.g., diluting 1% lidocaine to 0.5%); (ii) The pH should not be increased so much that the base form of the local anesthetic, which is considerably less soluble than the protonated form, precipitates from solution.[70] Even if it does not form a visible precipitate in the solution before injection, it may still come out of solution once in the body. Within these confines, there are valid clinical reasons to raise the pH; onset is briefer and drug requirements are less.

Hydrophobic adsorption provides much of the membrane binding energy for local anesthetics. Some hydrophobic quality is necessary for the drug to adsorb to the membrane at all, but too much hydrophobicity actually sticks the molecules at one surface and slows their transport to the other side. For example, lidocaine has only one-tenth the hydrophobicity of bupivacaine (by octanol:buffer partition coefficients),[96] but is 2.5 times as permeant through the peridural sheath.[85]

Comparison of the relationship between the published values of membrane permeability of hydrophobic bases, including local anesthetics, and their measured octanol:buffer distribution coefficients shows a bell-shaped curve (Fig. 2-15).[10] It is noteworthy that the most permeant drug is lidocaine, despite the fact that with its relatively low pK_a (7.7 at 37°C) it tends to be more ionized at physiological pH than most of the other compounds (pK_a range S = 8.2–9.5).

When the amount of lidocaine in a peripheral nerve *in vivo* is measured at times that correspond to observed behavioral end points, three noteworthy facts emerge (Fig. 2-16).[71] First, the total amount of lidocaine in the nerve is less than 5% of the total anesthetic injected (0.1 ml, 1% lidocaine, pH 6.5). Second, the peak neural concentration (ca. 8 nmol/mg wet nerve) equals only one fifth of the value that would be reached if the nerve had been *equilibrated* with 1% lidocaine. Third, the longitudinal distribution of drug along the nerve changes little during the course of the block. These results show how effective a barrier the sheath is and yet, that most visible movement of drug is across the sheath and not along the length of the nerve. Interestingly, the amount of lidocaine in the most concentrated segment of the nerve at a time when "deep pain" sensation returns (45–50 min) corresponds to the amount that would be present at equilibrium in a desheathed nerve bathed by lidocaine just at the marginal blocking concentration (ca. 0.4 mM; Fig. 2-13). Injection of less lidocaine (0.1 ml, 0.75%) gives an incomplete functional block; injection of more lidocaine prolongs the block.

Although proximity to the nerve is important, blockade can be further enhanced by limiting local vascular drug absorption, usually by incorporating a vasoconstrictor into the local anesthetic solution. The vasoconstrictor (with epinephrine still considered most efficacious) restricts the local cir-

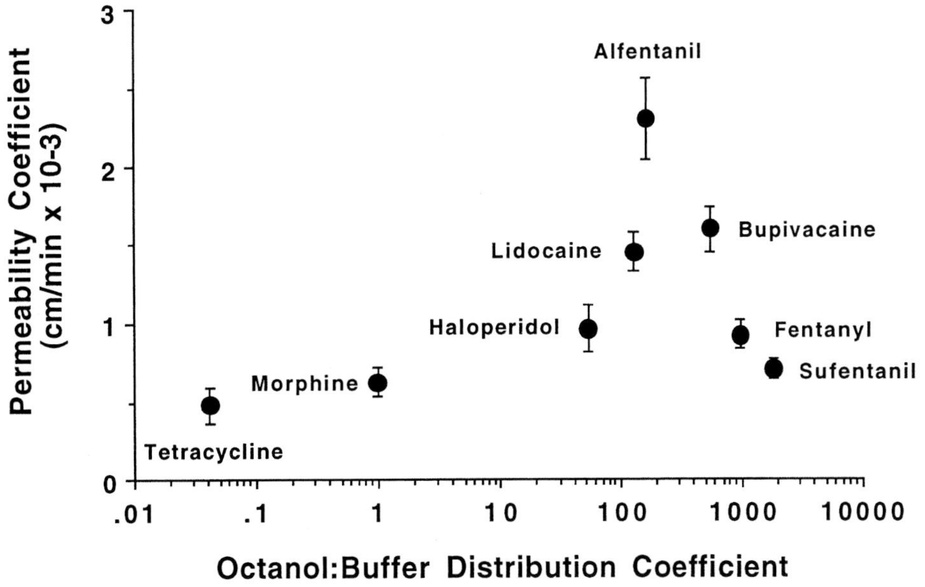

FIG. 2-15. Plot of octanol: buffer (pH = 7.4) distribution coefficient versus the experimentally determined permeability coefficient of a variety of neuroactive compounds. The individual data points are as follows: a, alfentanil; b, bupivacaine; c, lidocaine; d, haloperidol; e, fentanyl; f, sufentanil; g, morphine; h, tetracycline. (Reprinted with permission from Bernards, C. M., and Hill, H. F.: Physical and chemical properties of drug molecules governing their diffusion through the spinal meninges. Anesthesiology, *77*:750, 1992.)

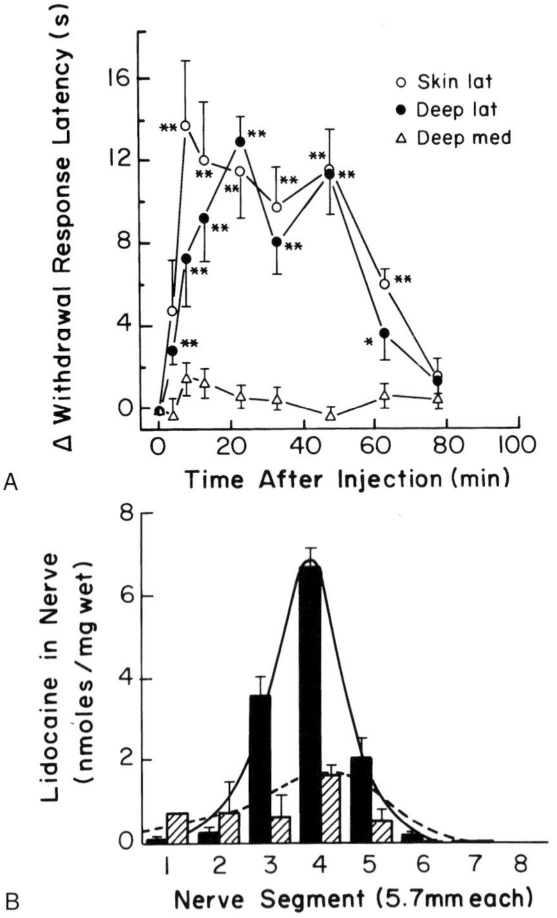

FIG. 2-16. Time course of analgesia **(A)** and intraneural lidocaine distribution **(B)** corresponding to blockade of rat sciatic nerve by 0.1 ml of 1% radiolabeled lidocaine injected near the pelvic notch. **A:** Time course of changes in withdrawal response latency (WRL) to pinch of a skin fold on the lateral foot ("skin lat") and deep pinch at the first ("deep med") and fifth toe ("deep lat") during nerve block. Plotted values represent mean values ± standard errors; $^{*}p < 0.05$, $^{**}p < 0.01$, relative to baseline (pre-drug) values (n = 12) (Thalhammer, J. G., Vladimora, M., Bershadsky, B., and Strichartz, G. R.: Neurological evaluation of the rat during sciatic nerve block with lidocaine. Anesthesiology, *82*:1013, 1995.) **B:** Distribution of lidocaine along the sciatic nerve removed from rats at two different behavioral end points: during profound block (15–20 min after injections; *solid bars*) and when movement response to deep pain (toe pinch) had returned (45–55 min; *striped bars*). At full block the total of all lidocaine in the nerve, exclusive of the sheath, is less than 5% of the injected dose.

culation so that the rate of local anesthetic vascular absorption is reduced.[108] Similarly, drug injected into highly perfused tissue (e.g., peridural space) is absorbed much faster than is drug injected into a marginally perfused region, such as the lumbar subarachnoid space.[31]

Highly fat-soluble local anesthetics, such as etidocaine and bupivacaine, are extensively bound to local tissue depots as well as to plasma proteins. Vascular uptake appears to be relatively less affected by the addition of epinephrine to solutions of these local anesthetics than to lidocaine, for example, and thus is less of an influence on the amount of drug available for action on the nerve.

Induction Phase

After the local anesthetic has been deposited near a nerve trunk, it diffuses from the nerve's outer surface toward the nerve's center.[58] Accordingly, axons that reside in the outer layers of the nerve (mantle fibers) are anesthetized well before axons that course through the nerve's inner layers (core fibers). Topographically, the fibers in a nerve trunk are arrayed in concentric layers. Fibers that innervate a limb's distal parts assume a central position in the nerve's core, whereas those that innervate the limb's proximal parts lie in the nerve's mantle.

As the local anesthetic diffuses through a nerve trunk from mantle to core, functional anesthesia tends to spread along the limb in a proximal to distal direction (Fig. 2-17). This can easily be observed during axillary block; the subject first notes that the upper arm becomes numb, anesthesia and analgesia spreading from there down the arm to reach the fingers last. Furthermore, motor block, corresponding to blockade of motor axons residing in the mantle, precedes sensory blockade arising from core fibers that innervate the distal receptive field.[109,110]

The rapidity of onset of nerve block is (roughly) proportional to the logarithm of the concentration of the drug. This means that doubling the drug concentration will only modestly hasten the onset of block, although, of course, the more concentrated solution also will block the nerve fibers more effectively. Thus, concentrated anesthetic solutions increase the maximum extent of nerve penetration, have a lesser ef-

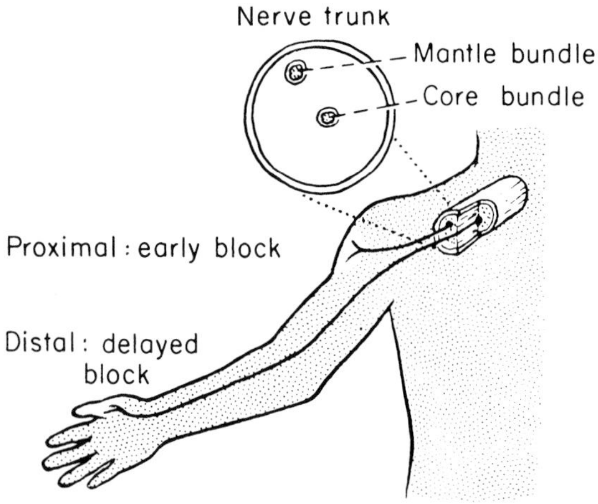

FIG. 2-17. Somatotopic distribution in peripheral nerve. Axons in large nerve trunks (*e.g.,* axillary terminus of brachial plexus) are arranged so that the outer (*mantle*) fibers innervate the more proximal structures, and the inner (*core*) fibers, the more distal parts of a limb. With the local anesthetic diffusing inward down the mantle-to-core gradient, the analgesia salient sweeps down the limb in proximal-to-distal fashion. (de Jong, R.H.: Physiology and Pharmacology of Local Anesthesia. Springfield, Ill., Charles C Thomas, 1970.)

fect on the speed of onset of block, and certainly increase the duration of block. It must be remembered, however, that increasing the concentration also increases the total dose of the drug being given and, therefore, the risk of systemic toxicity.

Recovery from Nerve Block

Diffusion from the nerve and absorption into the vascular bed mainly account for termination of blockade. It has been found empirically that the duration of the block is related linearly to the logarithm of the anesthetic concentration. Thus, repeated doubling of the anesthetic concentration will have progressively less effect on duration. This is probably because with repeated injections steady-state distributions of drug are achieved from which the duration of block is completely dependent on the saturation of local tissue depots. More important is the lipophilic solubility of the individual local anesthetic agents; for example, agents with high lipid solubility, such as bupivacaine and etidocaine, are highly concentrated in local tissue, such as cells around the nerve trunk as well as myelin sheaths around individual axons, and dislodge slowly from neural tissue. Blockade therefore persists for a long time. Dissociation times of local anesthetics from Na^+ channels are on the order of seconds and do not contribute to the kinetics of recovery from block.

Lipophilic uptake by local tissues is also slow, accounting for the fact that maintenance of block by repeated drug injections does increase the time for recovery, albeit to a limited extent. In addition, more lipophilic drugs have a lower sheath permeability and are thus retained longer within the nerve.

Vascular removal of local anesthetics is an important determinant of block duration. Not only is block duration enhanced by the addition of vasoconstrictors (see above) but the dynamics of peripheral nerve block recovery can be explained by uptake by the intraneural vasculature.[109,110] Thus, in a subclavian block in man the sensory fibers at the core of the nerve recover function before the motor fibers located in the mantle, apparently because of the rapid vascular removal of drug from the nerve core.[110]

Tachyphylaxis with Local Anesthetic

Tachyphylaxis, a drug's declining effectiveness when it is given repeatedly, is often observed when a nerve block is attempted over a long period of time. It is less liable to occur if a blocking agent is reinjected soon after the first signs of returning sensation; in fact, the aforementioned augmentation of blockade is more likely to occur than not under these conditions.[15] When the block is allowed to lapse, however (as when attempting to provide postoperative pain relief), tachyphylaxis frequently occurs. Hallmarks of tachyphylaxis are ever shorter duration of action, fading anesthetic potency, and shrinking analgesic field. Timing, evidently, is a prime consideration that determines whether augmentation or tachyphylaxis follows reinjection.

In the laboratory, *in vivo* nerve block does not seem to lessen with time or become less effective with repeated reapplication. Clinical tachyphylaxis may well prove to be the result of several independent factors. Important in this regard are anatomical causes such as perineural edema, microhemorrhage, or miniclots that may result from irritation by the catheter or from the anesthetic solution. Each, singly or combined, tends physically to shield the nerve from total contact with the anesthetic. In addition, the nerve's epineurium itself may become swollen. Other plausible causes are hypernatremia (from the anesthetic solution's saline carrier) and accumulating acidosis from anesthetic solutions at pHs well below 7. In addition, sensitization of the CNS from persistent or repeated nociceptive input, possibly involving the NMDA receptor, may explain why tachyphylaxis occurs with less frequent injections, at intervals that allow pain to recur.[60] Indeed, if tachyphylaxis resulted from desensitization due to continual presence of the drug, then less frequent injections should disfavor, not promote, its appearance.

Regional Anesthesia: Epidural and Intrathecal Mechanisms

Blockade of large regions of the body by epidural and intrathecal administration of local anesthetics shares many of the characteristics of peripheral nerve blocks. Drugs applied epidurally reach their target tissues by crossing the arachnoid barrier that is anatomically homologous with the perineurial sheath. These anesthetic molecules not only surround the nerve roots but penetrate deeply into the spinal cord tissue,[14] as do intrathecally administered drugs.[24] The same features of drug molecules and formulations that govern the potency and kinetics of peripheral nerve block are also determinants of epidural block with the additional aspect that larger injected volumes spread further along the rostrocaudal axis and thus effect a more extensive block of adjacent dermatomes.

Delivery of anesthetics by the epidural or spinal route also distributes them well into the sympathetic paravertebral ganglia and thus can have profound effects on autonomic tone and reflexia.[64] (Sympathetic nerve block also occurs during peripheral nerve procedures, of course, but there the consequences are more anatomically restricted.)

The locus and mechanism(s) of spinal/epidural anesthesia are not known with certainty. Clearly, local anesthetics delivered thus can block impulses in spinal roots.[40] There is also evidence that other loci are involved and, indeed, that the site of functionally effective block may shift during the course of a procedure.[103] More diverse targets are available to local anesthetics in the spinal cord than in peripheral nerve, because local anesthetics, at the concentrations that occur in cerebrospinal fluid (CSF) during spinal[24] and epidural[14] procedures, are able to inhibit not only Na^+ channels but also various K^+ channels,[5,29,42] Ca^{2+} channels,[68,69] and transmitter-gated ion channels such as β-adrenergic coupled[105] and substance P receptors.[63] Neurotransmission in the spinal cord is such a complex, integrated result of afferent and supraspinal inputs,[7,55] often involving spinal interneurons (Fig. 2-1), that the possible influences of the relatively nonselective and ubiquitously distributed local anesthetics are intriguing. Future pharmacological and physiological analysis should begin to reveal which of the many possible actions are important for regional anesthesia.

Toxicity of Local Anesthetics

Local anesthetic toxicity may occur systemically or locally. Allergic or inflammatory reactions have been reported but these are probably due to a component of the vehicle solution or to a local metabolite of ester-linked local anesthetics, for example, para-aminobenzoate.[4] Myonecrosis is a well-documented sequel of intramuscular injection of local anesthetic,[8] but muscle is an actively restored tissue and, aside from minor pain, no problems arise from this procedure (see also Chapters 4 and 30).

Toxicity from systemic local anesthetics has major manifestations in the CNS and in the cardiovascular system.[89] The CNS effects, including tinnitus, dizziness, fainting and, sometimes, convulsions, can be reversed by postural adjustment, waiting until a bolus dose is diluted, or the intravenous delivery of benzodiazepines. CNS actions for most local anesthetics occur at lower intravenous (IV) concentrations than the cardiovascular complications,[78,86] so the nervous system effects are useful alarms of toxic IV local anesthesia. Injection of small volumes of epinephrine-containing solutions provides a useful indicator of intravenous needle locations before massive doses of local anesthetic are injected.

Cardiovascular collapse has been reported when certain local anesthetics, most notoriously bupivacaine are accidentally injected intravenously. The collapse appears to result from direct actions of the drug on the myocardial impulse-conducting tissue[32,57] and on structures in the CNS,[43] as well as actions on vascular tissue. Prompt resuscitation can often prevent death,[54] but the normal stimulatory actions of adrenergic agents may be blocked by the local anesthetics themselves,[16,52] and direct cardiac massage may be required.[37]

Nerves of the spinal roots may be irreversibly distressed by high concentrations of local anesthetics. The delivery of 5% lidocaine in hyperbaric dextrose solutions through continuous spinal catheters has spawned several reports of "cauda equina syndrome," as the drug appears to pool around the sacral roots due to inadequate mixing.[79] Similar neurological sequelae have also been reported after multiple[83] and even single[87] intrathecal bolus injections of concentrated local anesthetics. Direct exposure to 5% lidocaine of a desheathed peripheral nerve, a "model" of spinal nerve roots, leads to rapid, complete, and irreversible ablation of the nerve impulse.[6,59,92] Irreversible block has been observed in both A and C fibers in mammalian nerve *in vitro*,[95] and some clinical deficits of cauda equina syndrome have been simulated by intrathecal infusion of lidocaine in the rat *in vivo*.[34,62]

The mechanism of this neurotoxic effect is unknown. However, since an equally effective block can be achieved clinically with larger volumes of less concentrated drug it is prudent to avoid use of 5% lidocaine at this time.

Cardiac Versus Neuronal Actions of Local Anesthetics

The same drug is often used regionally as a local anesthetic and systemically as an antiarrhythmic. In what ways are the actions of these agents on nerve and heart similar? To what extent do they differ?

Action potentials differ among the myocardial tissues. In atrial and ventricular musculature and in the fast conducting system of His bundle and Purkinje fibers, there is a rapid phase of depolarization, primarily due to, as in nerve, inward current through sodium channels; a plateau phase due to the near balance of inward calcium currents and outward potassium currents; and a repolarization phase due to the eventual dominance of outward potassium currents (Fig. 2-18).[67] By comparison, action potentials in the sino-atrial (S-A) and atrioventricular (A-V) nodes have slower rising depolarizations primarily due to inward currents through calcium channels alone.[20]

At the doses of local anesthetic drugs administered systemically as antiarrhythmics (e.g., 10–20 μmol lidocaine in blood), the primary target is the sodium channel. The other channels are affected by local anesthetics but at considerably higher (toxic) concentrations.[5,42,68,69] Inhibition of the sodium channel in heart under these conditions acts primarily to limit the rate of firing in ventricular tissue by raising the action potential threshold in a phasic manner. As in nerve, threshold is controlled by several factors, the availability of Na^+ channels being one important contributor. But two salient differences can occur in heart: (i) At the ventricular resting potential, or the mean diastolic potential, few of the channels are inactivated, whereas in nerve nearly 30% may be in that state; and (ii) the cardiac action potential produces a depolarization that endures for several hundred milliseconds, whereas the neuronal impulse is over in about 1 msec.[27] Therefore, in the absence of impulses, myocardial channels are neither activated nor inactivated and thus have a lower anesthetic affinity than do the partially inactivated channels in nerve. In the presence of impulses, myocardial channels stay opened or inactivated for relatively long times, and thereby greatly enhance the effective channel affinity of local anesthetics. After a cardiac action potential, the anesthetics dissociate from the channels, eventually returning the membrane threshold to near the normal value. A drug that dissociates in only tens of milliseconds does not elevate threshold long enough to be an effective antiarrhythmic. One that dissociates in several seconds will be bradycardiogenic, reducing ventricular contraction rates to unhealthy values. Lidocaine, fortuitously, has just the right kinetics to be an effective antiarrhythmic.[28]

Cardiotoxicity from systemic local anesthetics has two forms. One is the bradycardia just mentioned; the other is an arrhythmogenic action, particularly evident with bupiva-

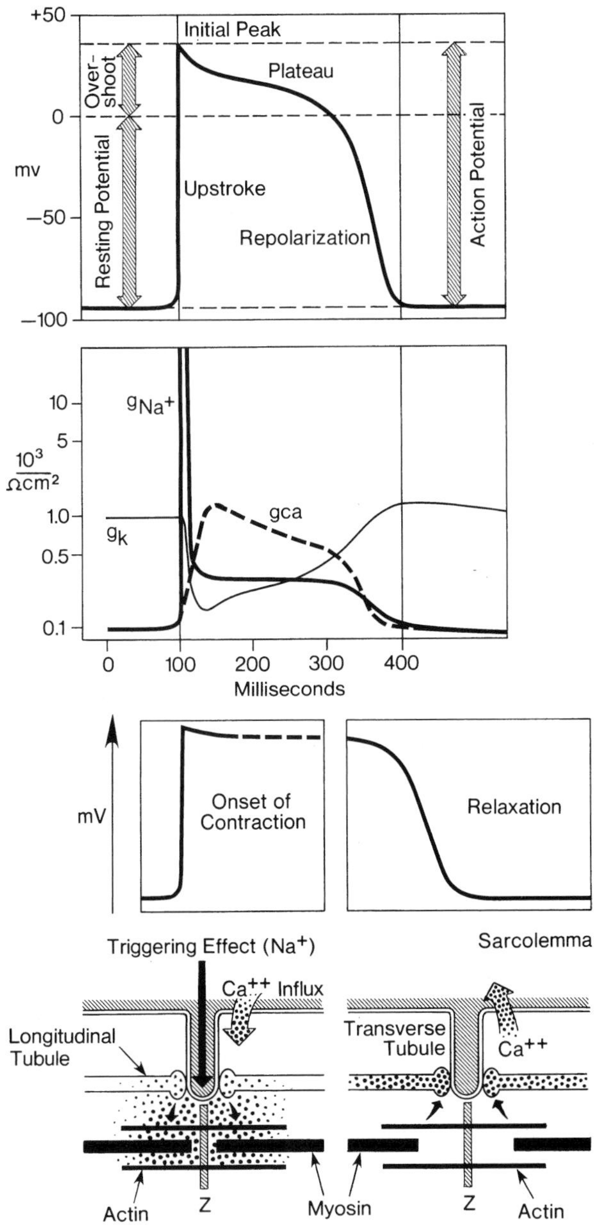

FIG. 2-18. Electrical and ionic events in myocardial muscle action potential (AP) leading to contraction. **Upper panel**. The AP of cardiac ventricular muscle cells begins with a very rapid depolarization of membrane potential to the "initial peak." This is followed by a characteristic feature of cardiac muscle (and also bundle of His and Purkinje tissue), a prolonged "plateau" responsible for the AP lasting more than 100 times longer than that of a peripheral nerve fiber. **Middle panel**. Changes in Na^+, Ca^{2+}, and K^+ conductance *(g)* that are responsible for the various phases of the AP: resting potential (G_K); initial peak ($G_{Na} + G_{Ca}$); plateau ($G_{Ca} + G_{K^+}$; and repolarization (gradual decrease in G_{Ca} and increase in G_K). Local anesthetics block the "fast Na^+ channel" except at very high concentrations where they may also block the "slow Ca^{2+} channel" (see text). **Lower two panels**. Diagram of relationship of excitation, rapid triggering (Na^+), Ca^{2+} movement, and action of contractile apparatus of cardiac muscle. During the AP there is an influx of Ca^{2+}, which not only prolongs the AP, but also triggers the release of internal Ca^{2+} for sarcoplasmic reticulum. Release of Ca^{2+} leads to activation of the actin/myosin contractile apparatus.

caine and leading to the rare but potentially lethal episode of cardiac collapse[111] (see Chapter 4). The origins of this arrhythmogenic action are unknown, but several recent reports suggest that bupivacaine may have more of an effect on calcium metabolism in heart than other local anesthetics.[65,107]

The increase in sarcoplasmic Ca^{2+} that is essential for tension development occurs through a Ca^{2+}-dependent Ca^{2+} release process; a relatively small amount of Ca^{2+} that enters the muscle through the plasma membrane triggers the release of a far greater amount of Ca^{2+} from sarcoplasmic reticular stores (Fig. 2-18).[36] An inward Ca^{2+} current through the plasma membrane, which can be selectively expressed by a combination of elevated external K^+ and isoproterenol, was not altered by bupivacaine, although contractile tension was significantly reduced.[65] Apparently bupivacaine effects the storage or release of cytoplasmic Ca^{2+}. It is known that divalent cations, particularly in the cytoplasm, can strongly modulate membrane excitability.[50] Perhaps bupivacaine's arrhythmogenic toxicity derives from its ability to interfere with Ca^{2+} storage inside the heart, and thereby to influence, indirectly, membrane excitability (see also Chapter 4).

SUMMARY

The impulse-blocking action of local anesthetics rests on their ability to interfere with the opening of voltage-gated sodium channels of excitable membranes. When enough channels cannot open, insufficient inward Na^+ current flows into the cell to elicit or sustain a regenerative action potential. If this situation occurs along a sufficient length of axon, then impulse propagation will terminate within the anesthetized region of that axon.

Although the final details remain to be specified, the molecular mechanisms of anesthetic block have many known features. Both neutral and protonated versions of the tertiary amine anesthetics can block Na^+ channels, although not necessarily by identical mechanisms. Anesthetic molecules appear to bind to and act directly on the Na^+ channels themselves. Changes of channel conformation, such as appear during an impulse, often potentiate anesthetic block in a use-dependent manner.

The potency of anesthetics in clinical situations depends as much on their ability to reach the nerve fibers as it does on their intrinsic blocking activities. Factors such as sheath penetration, vascular absorption, and local tissue binding are all important determinants of functional potency. Volume and pH and buffering capacity of the injected anesthetic solution are also important.

Although local anesthetics are usually reliable drugs, they can be improved in several respects. Predictable reversibility, to produce block of controlled duration, is desirable. Drugs of very long, but reversible action would be useful for nerve blocks such as intercostal block for postoperative pain. Selective block of functionally defined fiber types also would be a desirable clinical feature, permitting a differential titration of sensory and motor activities. In addition, reduced toxicity, both from accidental intravascular injection as well as from systemic accumulation following repeated injections, is a highly sought objective. As our knowledge about the relationship between molecular properties of local anesthetics and their pharmacological actions increases, we come closer to the reality of designing drugs and procedures to fulfill these clinical criteria.

REFERENCES

1. Agnew, W.S., Levinson, S.R., and Raftery, M.A.: Purification of the tetrodotoxin-binding component associated with the voltage-sensitive sodium channel from *electrophorus electroplax* membranes. Proc. Natl. Acad. Sci. U.S.A., *75*:2606, 1978.
2. Akerman, S.B., Camougis, G., and Sandberg, R.V.: Stereoisomerism and differential activity in excitation block by local anesthetics. Eur. J. Pharm., *8:*337, 1969.
3. Akert, K., Sandri, C., Weibel, R., Peper, K., and Moor, N.: The fine structure of the perineural endothelium. Cell Tissue Res., *165:*281, 1976.
4. Aldrete, J.A., and Johnson, D.A.: Evaluation of intracutaneous testing for investigation of allergy to local anesthetic agents. Anesth. Analg., *49:*173, 1970.
5. Arhem, P., and Frankenhaeuser, B.: Local anesthetics: effects on permeability properties of nodal membrane in myelinated nerve fibres from *Xenopus*. Potential clamp experiments. Acta Physiol. Scand., *91:*11, 1974.
6. Bainton, C.R., and Strichartz, G.R.: Concentration dependence of lidocaine-induced irreversible conduction loss in frog nerve. Anesthesiology, *81:*657, 1994.
7. Basbaum, A.I.: Functional analysis of the cytochemistry of the spinal dorsal horn. *In* Fields, H.L., *et al.* (eds.): Advances in Pain Research and Therapy. Vol. 9. New York, Raven Press, 1985.
8. Benoit, P.W., and Belt, W.D.: Some effects of local anesthetic agents on skeletal muscle. Exp. Neurol., *34:*264, 1972.
9. Benzon, H.T., Toleikis, J.R., Dixit, P., Goodman, I., and Hill, J.A.: Onset, intensity of blockade and somatosensory evoked potential changes of the lumbosacral dermatomes after epidural anesthesia with alkanized lidocaine. Anesth. Analg., *76:*328, 1993.
10. Bernards, C.M., and Hill, H.F.: Physical and chemical properties of drug molecules governing their diffusion through the spinal meninges. Anesthesiology, *77:*750, 1992.
11. Bernards, C.M., and Sorkin, L.S.: Radicular artery blood flow does not redistribute fentanyl from the epidural space to the spinal cord. Anesthesiology, *80:*872, 1994.
12. Bokesch, P.M., Post, C., and Strichartz, G.R.: Structure activity relationship of lidocaine homologues on tonic and frequency-dependent impulse blockade in nerve. J. Pharmacol. Exp. Ther., *237:*773, 1986.
13. Bostock, H., Sears, T.A., and Sherratt, R.M.: The effects of 4-amino pyridine and tetraethylammonium ions on normal and demyelinated mammalian nerve fibres. J. Physiol. (London), *313:*301, 1981.
14. Bromage, P.R., Joyal, A.C., and Binney, J.C.: Local anesthetics drugs: Penetration from the spinal extradural space into the neuraxis. Science, *140:*292, 1963.
15. Bromage, P.R., Pettigrew, R.T., and Crowell, D.E.: Tachyphylaxis in epidural analgesia. I. Augmentation and decay of local anesthesia. J. Clin. Pharmacol., *9:*30, 1969.
16. Butterworth, J.F. IV, Brownlow, R.C., Lieth, J.P., Prielipp, R.C., and Cole, L.R.: Bupivacaine inhibits cyclic 3′,5′-adenosine monophosphate production. A possible contributing factor to cardiovascular toxicity. Anesthesiology, *79:*88, 1993.
17. Butterworth, J.F., and Strichartz, G.R.: Molecular mechanism of local anesthesia: A review. Anesthesiology, *72:*711, 1990.
18. Cahalan, M.: Local anesthetic block of sodium channels in normal and pronase-treated squid giant axons. Biophys. J., *23:*285, 1978.
19. Cahalan, M., Shapiro, B.I., and Almers, W.: Relationship between inactivation of sodium channels and block by quaternary derivatives of local anesthetics and other compounds. *In* Fink, B.R. (ed.): Molecular Mechanisms of Anesthesia (Progress in Anesthesiology. Vol. 2). New York, Raven Press, 1980.
20. Carmeliet, E., and Vereecke, J.: Electrogenesis of the action potential and automaticity. In Berne, R.M., Sperelakis, N., and Geiger, S. (eds.): Handbook of Physiology, Section 2: The Cardiovascular System. Vol. 1, The Heart. pp. 269–334. Bethesda, MD, American Physiological Society, 1979.
21. Chernoff, D.M.: Kinetic analysis of phasic inhibition of neuronal sodium currents by lidocaine and bupivacaine. Biophys. J., *58:*53, 1990.
22. Chernoff, D.M., and Strichartz, G.R.: Tonic and phasic block of neuronal sodium currents by 5-hydroxyhexano-2′,6′,-xylidide, a neutral lidocaine homologue. J. Gen. Physiol., *93:*1075, 1989.
23. Chernoff, D.M., and Strichartz, G.R.: Kinetics of local anesthetic inhibition of neuronal sodium channels: pH- and hydrophobicity-dependence. Biophys. J., *58:*69–81, 1990.
24. Cohen, E.N.: Distribution of local anesthetic agents in the neuraxis of the dog. Anesthesiology, *29:*1002, 1968.
25. Condouris, G.A., Goebel, R.H., and Brady, T.: Computer simulation of local anesthetic effects using a mathematical model of myelinated nerve. J. Pharmacol. Exp. Ther., *196:*737, 1976.
26. Courtney, K.R.: Mechanism of frequency-dependent inhibition of sodium currents in frog myelinated nerve by the lidocaine derivative GEA-968. J. Pharmacol. Exp. Ther., *195:*225, 1975.
27. Courtney, K.R.: Antiarrhythmic drug design: Frequency-dependent block in myocardium. *In* Fink, B.R. (ed.): Molecular Mechanisms of Anesthesia. pp. 111–118. New York, Raven Press, 1980.
28. Courtney, K.R.: Structure-activity relations for frequency-dependent sodium channel block in nerve by local anesthetics. J. Pharmacol. Exp. Ther., *213:*114, 1980.
29. Courtney, K.R., and Kendig, J.J.: Bupivacaine is an effective potassium channel blocker in heart. Biochim. Biophys. Acta, *939:*163, 1988.
30. Courtney, K.R., and Strichartz, G.R.: Structural elements which determine local anesthetic activity. *In* Strichartz, G.R. (ed.): Handbook of Experimental Pharmacology: Local Anesthetics. Heidelberg, New York, Springer-Verlag, 1985.
31. Covino, B.G.: Pharmacokinetics of local anesthetic drugs. *In* Prys-Roberts, C., and Hug, C. Jr. (eds.): Pharmacokinetics of Anesthesia. pp. 202. Oxford, Blackwell Scientific Publications, 1984.
32. Coyle, D.E., and Speralakis, N.: Bupivacaine and lidocaine blockade of calcium mediated slow action potentials in guinea pig ventricular muscle. J. Pharmacol. Exp. Ther., *242:*1001, 1987.
33. Drachman, D., and Strichartz, G.R.: Potassium channel blockers potentiate impulse inhibition by local anesthetics. Anesthesiology, *75:*1051, 1991.
34. Drasner, K., Sakura, S. Chan, V.W.S., Bollen, A.W., and Ciriales, R.: Persistent sacral sensory deficit induced by intrathecal local anesthetic infusion in rat. Anesthesiology, *80:*842, 1994.
35. Elliott, A.A., and Elliott, J.R.: Characterization of TTX-sensitive and TTX-resistant sodium currents in small cells from adult rat dorsal root ganglia. J. Physiol. (London), *463:*30, 1993.
36. Fabiato, A., and Fabiato, F.: Contractions induced by a calcium-triggered release of calcium from the sarcoplasmic reticulum of single skinned cardiac cells. J. Physiol. (London), *249:*469, 1975.
37. Feldman, H.S., Arthur, G.R., Pitkanen, M., *et al.*: Treatment of acute systemic toxicity after the rapid intravenous injection of ropivacaine and bupivacaine in the conscious dog. Anesth. Analg., *73:*373, 1991.
38. Feng, T.P., and Liu, Y.M.: The connective tissue sheath of the nerve as effective diffusion barrier. J. Cell Comp. Physiol., *34:*1, 1949.
39. Frazier, D.T., Narahashi, T., and Yamada, M.: The site of action and active form of local anesthetics. II. Experiments with quaternary compounds. J. Pharmacol. Exp. Ther., *171:*45, 1970.
40. Frumin, M.J., Schwartz, H., Burns, J.J., Brodie, B.B., and Papper, E.M.: Sites of sensory blockade during segmental spinal and segmental peridural anesthesia in man. Anesthesiology, *14:*576, 1953.
41. Gissen, A.J., Covino, B.G., and Gregus, J.: Differential sensitivity of mammalian nerves to local anesthetic drugs. Anesthesiology, *53:*467, 1980.
42. Guo, X., Castle, N.A., Chernoff, D.M., and Strichartz, G.R.: Comparative inhibition of voltage-gated cation channels by local anesthetics. In Miller, K., Roth, Se., and Rubin, E. (eds.): Molecular and Cellular

Mechanisms of Alcohol and Anesthetics, Annals of the New York Academy of Sciences. Vol. 625. pp. 181–199. New York, New York Academy of Sciences, 1991.
43. Heavner, J.E.: Cardiac dysrhythmias induced by infusion of local anesthetics into the lateral cerebral ventricle in cats. Anesth. Analg., *65:*444, 1986.
44. Heavner, J.E., and deJong, R.: Lidocaine blocking concentration for B- and C-nerve fibers. Anesthesiology, *40:*228, 1974.
45. Heinbecker, P., Bishop, G.H., and O'Leary, J.: Pain and touch fibers in peripheral nerves. Arch. Neurol. Psychiatr., *20:*771, 1933.
46. Hille, B.: The common mode of action of three agents that decrease the transient change in sodium permeability in nerves. Nature, *210:*1220, 1966.
47. Hille, B.: Local anesthetics: Hydrophilic and hydrophobic pathways for the drug-receptor reaction. J. Gen. Physiol., *69:*497, 1977.
48. Hille, B.: The pH-dependent rate of action of local anesthetics on the node of Ranvier. J. Gen. Physiol., *69:*475, 1977.
49. Hille, B.: Local anesthetic action on inactivation of the Na channel in nerve and skeletal muscle: possible mechanisms for antiarrhythmic agents. *In* Morad, M. (ed.): Biophysical Aspects of Cardiac Muscle. pp. 55–74. New York, Academic Press, 1978.
50. Hille, B.: Ionic Channels of Excitable Membranes, 2nd ed. Sunderland, MA, Sinauer Associates, 1991.
51. Hodgkin, A.L., and Huxley, A.F.: A quantitative description of membrane current and its application to conduction and excitation in nerve. J. Physiol., *117:*500, 1952.
52. Hurley, R.J., Feldman, H.S., Latch, C., and Arthur, G.R.: The effects of epinephrine on the anesthetic and hemodynamic properties of ropivacaine and bupivacaine after epidural administration in the dog. Reg. Anaesth., *16:*303, 1991.
53. Kandel, E.R., Schwartz, J.H., and Jessell, T. (eds.). Principles of Neural Science. 2d ed. New York, Elsevier/North-Holland, 1992.
54. Kasten, G.W., and Martin, S.T.: Bupivacaine cardiovascular toxicity: comparison of treatment with bretylium and lidocaine. Anesth. Analg., *64:*491, 1985.
55. Kelley, D.D.: Somatic sensory system IV: Central representations of pain and analgesia. *In* Kandel, E.R., and Schwartz, J.H. (eds.): Principles of Neural Science. New York, Elsevier/North-Holland, 1981.
56. Khodorov, B.I., Peganov, E., Revenko, S., and Shishkova, L.: Sodium currents in voltage clamped nerve fiber of frog under the combined action of batrachotoxin and procaine. Brain Res., *84:*541, 1975.
57. Komai, H., and Rusy, B.F.: Effects of bupivacaine and lidocaine on AV conduction in the isolated rat heart: modification by hyperkalemia. Anesthesiology, *55:*281, 1981.
58. Kristerson, L., Nordenram, Å., and Nordqvist, P.: Penetration of radioactive local anaesthetic into peripheral nerve. Arch. Int. Pharmacodyn., *157:*148, 1965.
59. Lambert, L.A., Lambert, D.H., and Strichartz, G.R.: Irreversible conduction block in isolated nerve by high concentrations of local anesthetics. Anesthesiology, *80:*1082, 1994.
60. Lee, K.C., Wilder, R.T., Smith, R.L., and Berde, C.B.: Thermal hyperalgesia accelerates and MK-801 prevents the development of tachyphylaxis to rat sciatic nerve blockade. Anesthesiology, *81:*1284, 1993.
61. LeeSon, S., Wang, G.K., Concus, A., Crill, E., and Strichartz, G.R.: Stereoselective inhibition of neuronal sodium channels by local anesthetics: Evidence for two sites of action? Anesthesiology, *77:*324, 1992.
62. Li, D.F., Bahar, M., Cole, G., and Rosen, M.: Neurological toxicity of the subarachnoid infusion of bupivacaine, lignocaine or 2-chloroprocaine in the rat. Br. J. Anaesth., *57:*424, 1985.
63. Li, Y.-M., Wingrove, D., Too, H.P., *et al.*: Local anesthetics inhibit substance P binding and evoked increases in cell Ca^{2+}. Anesthesiology, *82:*166, 1995.
64. Löfström, J.B., and Cousins, M.J.: Sympathetic neural blockade of upper and lower extremity. *In* Cousins, M.J., and Bridenbough, P.O. (eds.): Neural Blockade. 2nd ed. pp. 461–500. Philadelphia, J.B. Lippincott, 1987.
65. Lynch, C.: Local anesthetic effects upon myocardial excitation-contraction (E-C) coupling. Reg. Anaesth., *10:*38, 1985.
66. Narahashi, T., Frazier, D., and Yamada, M.: The site of action and active form of local anesthetics, I. Theory and pH experiments with tertiary compounds. J. Pharm. Exp. Ther., *171:*32, 1970.
67. Noble, D.: The Initiation of the Heartbeat. Oxford, Oxford University Press, 1975.
68. Oyama, Y., Sadoshima, J.-I., Tokutomi, N., and Akaike, N. Some properties of inhibitory action of lidocaine on the Ca^{2+} current of single isolated frog sensory neurons. Brain Res., *442:*223, 1988.
69. Palade, P.T., and Almers, W.: Slow calcium and potassium currents in frog skeletal muscle: their relationship and pharmacological properties. Pflugers Arch., *405:*91, 1985.
70. Peterfreund, R.A., Datta, S., and Ostheimer, G.W.: pH adjustment of local anesthetic solutions with sodium bicarbonate: laboratory evaluation of alkalinization and precipitation. Reg. Anesth., *14:*265, 1989.
71. Popitz-Bergez, F.A., Lee-Son, S., Thalhammer, J.G., and Strichartz, G.R.: Intraneural lidocaine uptake and distribution during sciatic nerve block neurologically assessed in the rat. Reg. Anesth., *19:*20, 1994.
72. Ragsdale, D.S., McPhee, J.C., Scheuer, T., and Catterall, W.A.: Molecular determinants of state-dependent block of Na^+ channels by local anesthetics. Science, *265:*1724, 1994.
73. Rando, T., Wang, G.K., and Strichartz, G.R.: The interaction of alkaloid neurotoxins, batrachotoxin and veratridine, with the gating processes of neuronal sodium channels. Mol. Pharmacol., *29:*467, 1986.
74. Rang, H.P., and Ritchie, J.M.: On the electrogenic sodium pump in mammalian non-myelinated nerve fibers and its activation by various cations. J. Physiol. *196:*183, 1968.
75. Raymond, S.A., and Gissen, A.J.: Mechanisms of differential block. *In* Strichartz, G.R. (ed.): Handbook of Experimental Pharmacology. Vol. 81. Berlin, Heidelberg, Springer-Verlag, 1987.
76. Raymond, S.A., Steffensen, S., Gugino, L.D., and Strichartz, G.R.: The role of length of nerve exposed to local anesthetics in impulse blocking action. Anesth. Analg., *68:*563, 1989.
77. Raymond, S.A., Thalhammer, J.G., and Strichartz, G.R.: Axonal excitability: endogenous and exogenous modulation. *In* Dimitrievic, M.R. (ed.): Recent Achievements in Restorative Neurology 3. Altered Sensation and Pain. pp. 112–127. Basel, Karger, 1990.
78. Reiz, S., Häggmark, S., Johansson, G., and Nath, S.: Cardiotoxicity of ropivacaine—a new amide local anaesthetic agent. Acta Anaesthesiol. Scand., *33:*93, 1989.
79. Rigler, M.L., Drasner, K., Krejcie, T.C., *et al.*: Cauda equina syndrome after continuous spinal anesthesia. Anesth. Analg., *72:*275, 1991.
80. Ritchie, J.M.: Physiological basis for conduction in myelinated nerve fibers. In Morell, P. (ed.): Myelin. 2d ed. pp. 117–145. New York, Plenum Press, 1984.
81. Ritchie, J.M., and Ritchie, B.R.: Local anaesthetics: effect of pH on activity. Science, *162:*1394, 1968.
82. Ritchie, J.M., Ritchie, B., and Greengard, P.: The effect of the nerve sheath on the action of local anesthetics. J. Pharmacol. Exp. Ther., *150:*160, 1965.
83. Rosen, M.A., Baysinger, C.L., Shnider, S.M., *et al.*: Evaluation of neurotoxicity after subarachnoid injection of large volumes of local anesthetic solutions. Anesth. Analg., *62:*802, 1983.
84. Rosenberg, P.H., and Heavner, J.E.: Temperature-dependent nerve-blocking action of lidocaine and halothane. Acta Anaesth. Scand., *24:*314, 1980.
85. Rosenberg, P.H., Heavner, J.E., Kovach, K., Pacinda, M., and Racz, G.: Dural permeability to epinephrine, bupivacaine, lidocaine and phenol. *In* Wüst, H.J., and Stanton-Hicks, M.D. (eds.): New Aspects in Regional Anaesthesia 5. Heidelberg, Springer-Verlag, 1986.
86. Sage, D., Feldman, H., Arthur, G., *et al.*: The cardiovascular effects of convulsant doses of lidocaine and bupivacaine in the conscious dog. Reg. Anaesth., *10:*175, 1985.
87. Schneider, M., Ettlin, T., Kaufmann, M., *et al.*: Transient neurologic toxicity after hyperbaric subarachnoid anesthesia with 5% lidocaine. Anesth. Analg., *76:*1154, 1993.
88. Schwarz, W., Palade, P.T., and Hille, B.: Local anesthetics: Effect of pH on use-dependent block of sodium channels in frog muscle. Biophys. J., *20:*343, 1977.
89. Scott, D.B.: Evaluation of the toxicity of local anaesthesia agents in man. Br. J. Anaesth., *47:*56, 1975.
90. Shanthaveerappa, T.R., and Bourne, G.H.: The 'perineural epithelium,' a metabolically active, continuous, protoplasmic cell barrier surrounding peripheral nerve fasiculi. J. Anat. London, *96*(4):527, 1962.
91. Skou, J.C.: Local anesthetics: VI. Relation between blocking potency and penetration of a monomolecular layer of lipoids from nerves. Acta Pharmacol. Toxicol., *10:*325, 1954.

92. Skou, J.C.: The toxic potencies of some local anaesthetics and of butyl alcohol, determined on peripheral nerves. Acta Pharmacol. Toxicol., *10:*292, 1954.
93. Strichartz, G.R.: The inhibition of sodium currents in myelinated nerve by quaternary derivatives of lidocaine. J. Gen. Physiol., *62:*37, 1973.
94. Strichartz, G.R.: The composition and structure of excitable nerve membrane. *In* Jamieson, G.A., and Robinson, D.M. (eds.): Mammalian Cell Membranes. Vol. 3. pp. 173–205. London, Butterworths, 1977.
95. Strichartz, G.R., Manning, T., and Datta, S.: Irreversible conduction block in mammalian nerves by direct application of 2% and 5% lidocaine. Reg. Anesth., *19:*20, 1994.
96. Strichartz, G.R., Sanchez, V., Arthur, G.R., Chafetz, R., and Martin D.: Fundamental properties of local anesthetics. II. Measured octanol:buffer partition coefficients and pK_a values of clinically-used drugs. Anesth. Analg., *71:*158, 1990.
97. Strichartz, G., and Wang, G.K.: The kinetic basis for phasic local anesthetic blockade of neuronal sodium channels. *In* Miller, K.W., and Roth, S. (eds.): Molecular and Cellular Mechanisms of Anesthetics. pp. 217–226. New York, Plenum Publishing, 1986.
98. Strichartz, G., and Zimmermann, M.: Selective conduction blockade among different fiber types in mammalian nerves by lidocaine combined with low temperature. Society for Neuroscience, Annual Meeting Abstracts, p. 675, 1983.
99. Stühmer, W., Conti, F., Harukazu, S., *et al.*: Structural parts involved in activation and inactivation of the sodium channel. Nature, *339:*597, 1989.
100. Taylor, R.E.: Effect of procaine on electrical properties of squid axon membrane. Am. J. Physiol., *196:*1071, 1959.
101. Thalhammer, J.G., Raymond, S.A., and Strichartz, G.R.: Changes of response pattern of sensory afferent in rats exposed to sub-blocking concentrations of lidocaine. Soc. Neurosci. Abstr., *17:*440, 1991.
102. Thalhammer, J.G., Vladimirova, M., Bershadsky, B., and Strichartz, G.R.: Neurological evaluation of the rat during sciatic nerve block with lidocaine. Anesthesiology, *82:*1013, 1995.
103. Urban, B.J.: Clinical observations suggesting a changing site of action during induction and recession of spinal and epidural anesthesia. Anesthesiology, *39:*496, 1973.
104. Valbo, A.B., Hagbarth, K.E., Torebjörk, H.E., and Hallin, B.G.: Somatosensory, proprioceptive and sympathetic activity in human peripheral nerves. Physiol. Rev., *59:*919, 1975.
105. Voeikov, V.V., and Lefkowitz, R.J.: Effects of local anesthetics on guanyl nucleotide modulation of the catecholamine-sensitive adenylate cyclase system and β-adrenergic receptors. Biochim. Biophys. Acta, *629:*266, 1980.
106. Wahren, L.K., Torebjörk, E., and Nyström, B.: Quantitative sensory testing before and after regional guanethidine block in patients with neuralgia in the hand. Pain, *46:*23, 1991.
107. Wang, G.K., Brodwick, M.S., Eaton, D.C., and Strichartz, G.R.: Inhibition of sodium currents by local anesthetics in cloramine-T treated squid axons: The role of Na channel activation. J. Gen. Physiol., *89:*645, 1987.
108. Wildsmith, J.A.W., Tucker, G.T., Cooper, S., *et al.*: Plasma concentrations of local anaesthetics after interscalene brachial plexus block. Br. J. Anaesth., *49:*461, 1977.
109. Winnie, A.P., LaVallee, D.A., Sosa, B.P., *et al.*: Clinical pharmacokinetics of local anaesthetics. Can. Anaesth. Soc. J., *24:*252, 1977.
110. Winnie, A.P., Tay, C.-H., Patel, K.P., Ramamurthy, S., and Durrani, Z.: Pharmacokinetics of local anesthetics during plexus blocks. Anesth. Analg., *56:*852, 1977.
111. Wojtczak, J.A., LaVallee, D.A., Pesosa, B., and Masud, Z.K.: Bupivacaine cardiotoxicity: "Power failure" and its mechanisms. Reg. Anaesth., *10:*43, 1985.
112. Wong, K., Strichartz, G.R., and Raymond, S.A.: On the mechanism of potentiation of local anesthetics by bicarbonate buffer: Drug structure-activity studied on isolated peripheral nerve. Anesth. Analg., *76:*131, 1993.
113. Yeh, J.Z.: Blockage of sodium channels by stereoisomers of local anesthetics. Prog. Anesthesiol., *2:*35, 1980.

Neural Blockade in Clinical Anesthesia and Management of Pain, Third Edition,
edited by M.J. Cousins and P.O. Bridenbaugh.
Lippincott–Raven Publishers, Philadelphia © 1998.

CHAPTER 3

Properties, Absorption, and Disposition of Local Anesthetic Agents

Geoffrey T. Tucker and Laurence E. Mather

The ideal use of regional anesthesia requires administration of sufficient local anesthetic agent to be effective but not so much that toxicity develops. The anesthesiologist must have a thorough knowledge of the anatomical and physical landmarks to perform neural blockade in addition to a thorough knowledge of the pharmacology of the individual agents to be used. This includes familiarization with the disposition in the body of local anesthetic agents and, in particular, knowledge of their systemic absorption after the various methods of neural blockade.

In reviewing this aspect of the pharmacology of local anesthetic agents, it is important to examine relationships between the physicochemical properties of the agents (Table 3-1) and their fate in the body and to delineate the role of pharmacokinetics in the overall response to regional anesthesia. This response is a complex function of pharmacokinetics, pharmacodynamics, the physiological consequences of neural blockade, and the pathophysiological status of the patient. Each of these factors can influence the others.

STRUCTURE OF LOCAL ANESTHETICS

Local anesthetic agents can be classified with respect to their chemical structures in two principal ways—by functional groups and by physicochemical properties.

The functional groups contained in "classical" local anesthetic agents were established nearly 100 years ago. These are an aromatic (i.e., benzene-ring derived) head which conveys lipophilicity, an amino group which conveys hydrophilicity by way of its ability to form a charged species (or conjugate acid, see below), and a chain which joins the two. The original local anesthetic agent, cocaine, had an ester group in the chain and this group was used in other agents until subsequent experience showed that it could be replaced with an amide group (which has similar spatial and other characteristics). Thus, the principal classification used until relatively recently was into agents containing ester groups and agents containing amide groups. As ester-type local anesthetic agents are now used much less frequently, this division has more historical than pharmacological importance for contemporary anesthesiologists.

Ester Caines

As noted above, the grandfather of all local anesthetics was cocaine (Fig. 3-1). This naturally occurring compound was discovered in South America by German scientists during the 1850s and was first introduced into clinical medicine in the latter part of the 19th century. Note the aromatic "hydrophobic head," the ester linkages at the "neck" and "hand," and the amino group dangling down in front. The essential features of this "noble savage" were subsequently handed down to his more sophisticated son, procaine (Fig. 3-2), who was born just in time to take part in the First World War. After the war, procaine, in turn, became the father of a large family of ester caines; of these, chloroprocaine and tetracaine (Fig. 3-3) still remain popular with some anesthesiologists.

Amide Caines

The early 1930s saw the introduction of dibucaine (Fig. 3-4), a "two-headed" compound with the ester linkage replaced by a carbamoyl group. This agent is rather toxic, and its use was confined mainly to spinal anesthesia.

The next major development occurred in Sweden, where

G. T. Tucker: Departments of Medicine and Pharmacology, Section of Molecular Pharmacology and Pharmacogenetics, University of Sheffield, The Royal Hallamshire Hospital, Sheffield S10 2JF United Kingdom.

L. E. Mather: Department of Anaesthesia and Pain Management, Royal North Shore Hospital, University of Sydney, St. Leonards, New South Wales 2065 Australia.

TABLE 3-1. *Physicochemical properties of local anesthetics*

Agent	Chemical configuration (Aromatic lipophilic / Intermediate chain / Amine hydrophilic)	Physicochemical properties: Molecular weight (Base)	pK^a (25° C)	Partition coefficient[b]	Aqueous solubility[c]	Percent protein binding	Biologic properties: Equieffective[d] anesthetic concentration	Approximate anesthetic duration (min)[d]	Site of metabolism
Esters									
Benzocaine	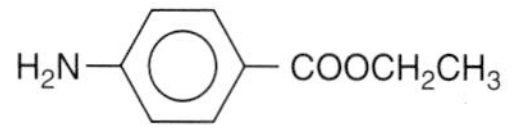	165	2.5	81	very low	?	?	?	widely
Butamben	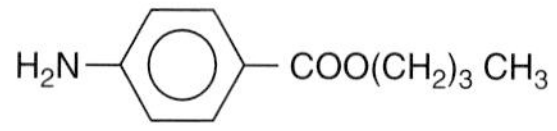	193	2.3	1028	0.1	?	?	?	?
Procaine	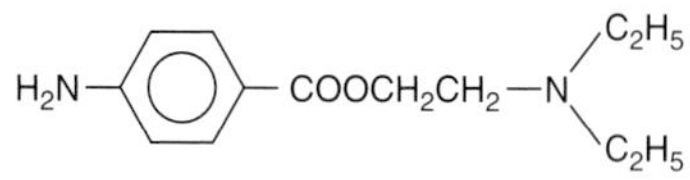	236	9.05	1.7	?	6	2	50	Plasma, liver
Chloroprocaine	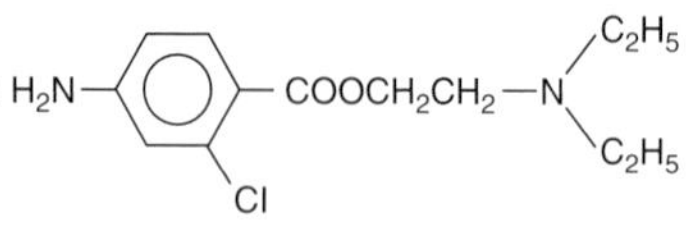	271	8.97	9.0	?	?	2	45	Plasma, liver
Tetracaine	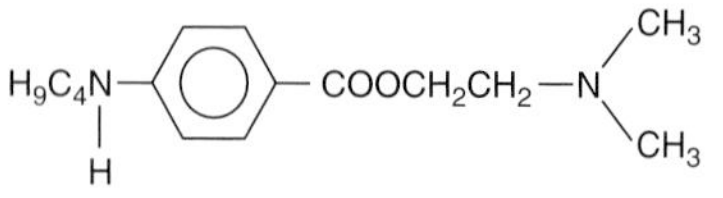	264	8.46	221	1.4	75.6[e]	0.25	175	Plasma, liver
Amides									
Prilocaine	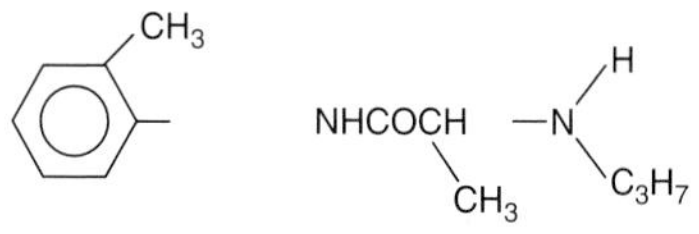	220	7.9	25	?	55 approx.	1	100	Liver, extra-hepatic tissues
Lidocaine	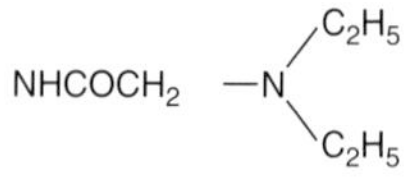	234	7.91	2.4	24	64[f]	1	100	Liver
Etidocaine	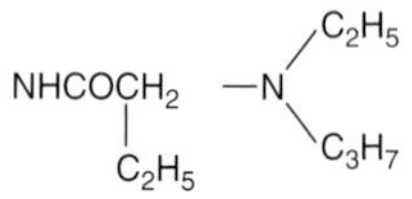	276	7.7	800	?	94[f]	0.25	200	Liver
Mepivacaine	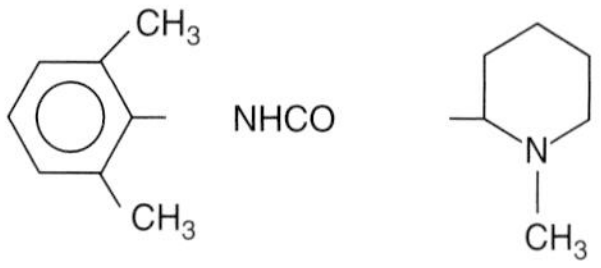	246	7.76	21	15	77[f]	1	100	Liver
Ropivacaine	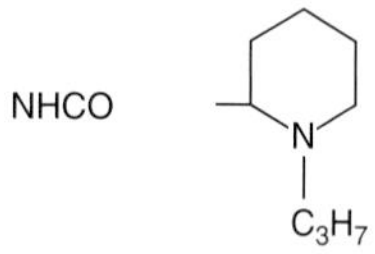	262	8.2	115	?	95	0.5	150	Liver
Bupivacaine	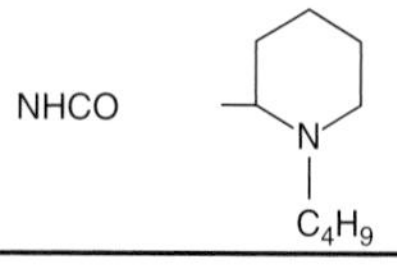	288	8.16	346	0.83	96[f]	0.25	175	Liver

[a] pH corresponds to 50% ionization.
[b] n-octanol/pH 7.4 buffer
[c] Aqueous solubility (mg HCl salt/ml at pH 7.37 and 37°C).
[d] Data derived from rat sciatic nerve blocking procedure.
[e] Nerve homogenate binding.
[f] Plasma protein binding—2μg/ml.

[Data from Ekenstam, B.: The effect of the structural variation on the local analgetic properties of the most commonly used groups of substances. Acta Anaesthesiol. Scand., 25 (Suppl.): 10, 1966; Truant, A. P., and Takman, B.: Differential physical-chemical and neuropharmacologic properties of local anesthetic agents. Anesth. Analg. (Cleve.), *38*:478, 1959; Tucker, G. T.: Biotransformation and toxicity of local anaesthetics. Int. Anesthesiol. Clin., *13*:33, 1975; L. E. Mather, Unpublished data; Kamaya, H., Hayes, J. J., and Ueda, I.: Dissociation constants of local anesthetics and their temperature dependence. Anesth. Analg. (Cleve.), *62*:1025, 1983; Dudziak, R., and Uihlein, M.: Loslichkeit von Lokalanaesthetika im Liquor cerebrospinalis und ihre Abhangigkeit von der Wasserstoffion-enkonzentration. Anaesthesist, *27*:32, 1978; Strichartz, G. R., Sanchez, V., Arthur, G. R., Chafetz, R., and Martin, D.: Fundamental properties of local anesthetics. II. Measured octanol: buffer partition coefficients and pK_a values of clinically used drugs. Anesth. Analg. (Cleve.) *71:*158, 1990; and Grouls, R. J. E., Ackerman, E. W., Machielsen, E. J. A., and Korsten, H. H. M.: Butyl-p-aminobenzoate. Preparation, characterization and quality control of a suspension injection for epidural analgesia. Pharm. Wkbl., *13*:13, 1991.]

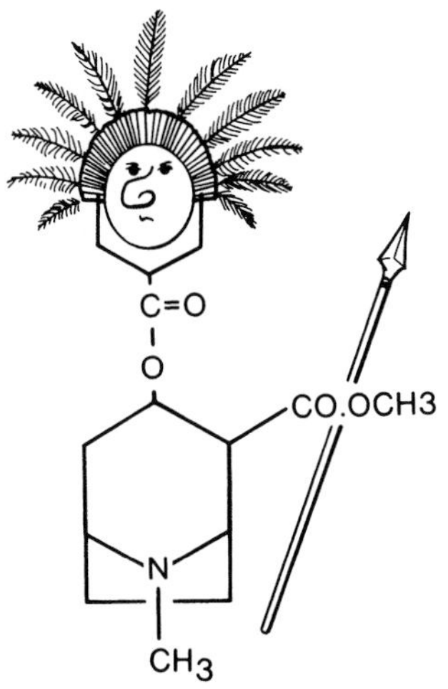

'Co' Sth. America (1850)

FIG. 3-1. Cocaine. (Tucker, G.T.: Biotransformation and toxicity of local anaesthetics. Acta Anaesthesiol. Belg., 26 [Suppl.]: 123, 1975.)

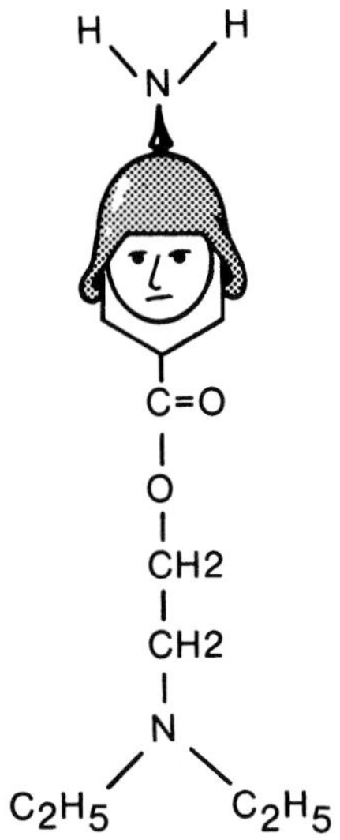

'Pro' Germany (1905)

FIG. 3-2. Procaine. (Tucker, G.T.: Biotransformation and toxicity of local anaesthetics. Acta Anaesthesiol. Belg., 26 [Suppl.]: 123, 1975.)

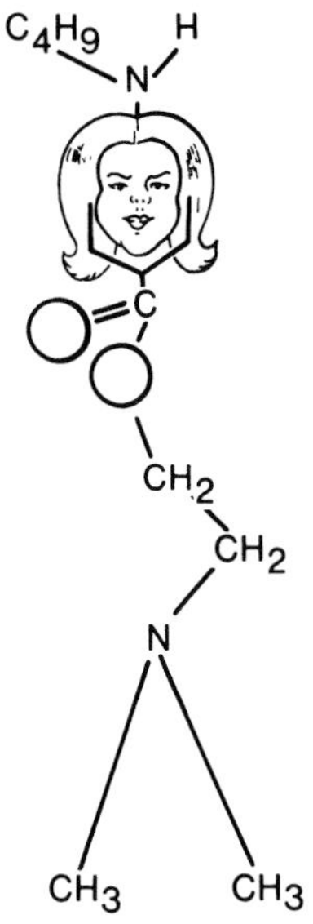

'Tetra' Germany (1933)

FIG. 3-3. Tetracaine. (Tucker, G.T.: Biotransformation and toxicity of local anaesthetics. Acta Anaesthesiol. Belg., 26 [Suppl.]: 123, 1975.)

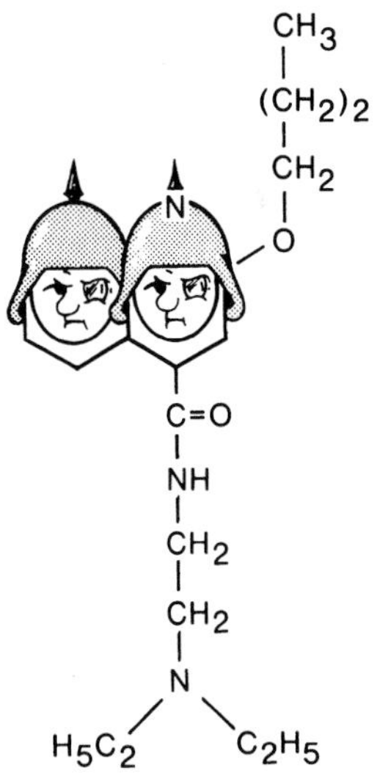

'Dibu' Germany (1932)

FIG. 3-4. Dibucaine.

some significant mutations resulted in a new, hardier breed of amide caines (Fig. 3-5). Thus, the labile ester linkage was replaced, this time by the chemically sturdier amide group, the reverse of the carbamoyl link. Lidocaine was the first of these "Viking maidens," followed by mepivacaine, bupivacaine, prilocaine, etidocaine, and, more recently, ropivacaine. Notice that prilocaine looks a little sad. This is because she has only one pigtail. The *o*-toluidine moiety, unlike the 2,6-xylidine ring found in the other amides, is associated with methemoglobinemia at high doses. Prilocaine differs also in having one leg—the amino group is secondary rather than tertiary as in her near-relatives.

Chiral Caines

The third major development came with the introduction of ropivacaine (Fig. 3-6)—the first synthetic "chirally clean caine." Many drugs used clinically, including the important general anesthetic agents halothane, enflurane, isoflurane, and thiopental and the local anesthetic amides mepivacaine, bupivacaine, prilocaine, etidocaine, and ropivacaine (but not lidocaine), have a *chiral center* (from the Greek, *cheir*, meaning hand). This is also referred to as an *asymmetric carbon atom* because it has bonded to it four different functional groups and imparts a particular type of stereoisomerism known as enantiomerism. *Enantiomers* (also referred to as *enantiomorphs*) are *stereoisomers* having nonsuperimposable mirror image relationships, and are sometimes referred to as *optical isomers* because of their ability to rotate plane polarized light. *Racemates* are drugs synthesized, prepared, and used as equal mixtures of two enantiomers. Chiral drugs found in nature, for example, atropine and morphine, are usually single enantiomers because they are synthesized enzymically and such reactions are usually stereospecific, but most synthetic chiral drugs are racemates. Cocaine, a natural product, is a single enantiomer; mepivacaine, bupivacaine, prilocaine, and etidocaine are made and used as racemates;

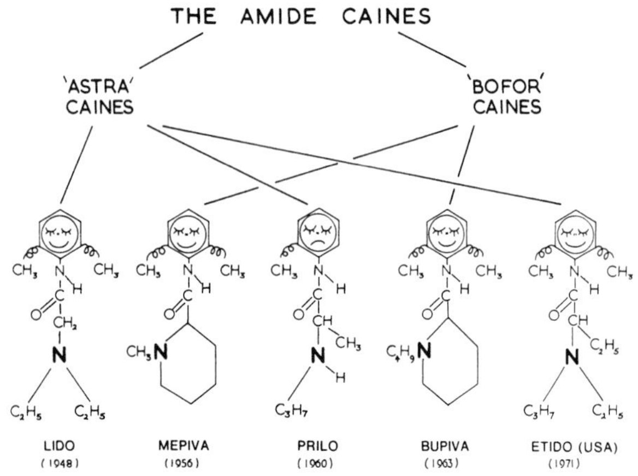

FIG. 3-5. The "amide caines." Left to right. Lidocaine, mepivacaine, prilocaine, bupivacaine, and etidocaine. (Tucker, G.T.: Biotransformation and toxicity of local anaesthetics. Acta Anaesthesiol. Belg., 26 [Suppl.]: 123, 1975.)

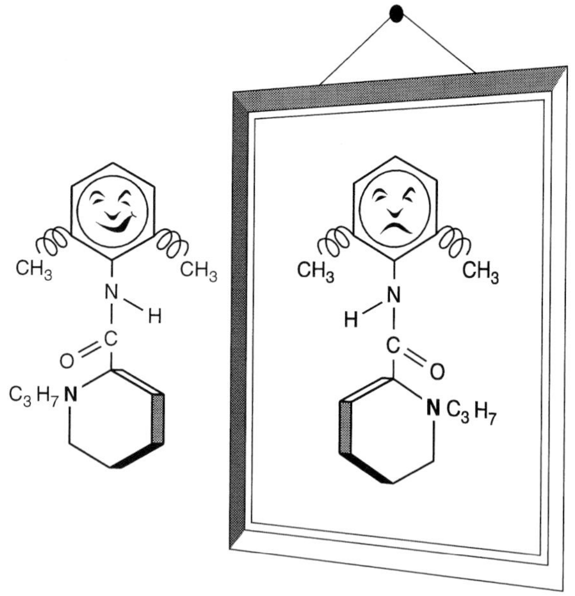

FIG. 3-6. Ropivacaine and her "mirror image." Chiral drugs bear mirror image relationships such that optical isomers have different pharmacological and pharmacokinetic properties.

ropivacaine is alone among the synthetic local anesthetic agents in being made and used as a single enantiomer from its inception. Lidocaine is achiral. Although many racemates may be used clinically, their component enantiomers can, and frequently do, have different pharmacological and pharmacokinetic properties.[432] It is only relatively recently that enantiomerism in anesthesiology has been "rediscovered"[272]; the extent of its clinical significance is, as yet, largely unknown.

Three notations are used to describe chirality and associated optical activity. First, (+) and (−), or *dextro* (or *d*) and *levo* (or *l*) are associated with the pairs of enantiomers that rotate plane polarized light, respectively, to the right and left. However, the direction of rotation is a phenomenological feature only: a molecule may rotate plane polarized light in one direction when dissolved in one solvent but in the other direction in another solvent. Second, a systematic method of associating the stereochemistry with the direction of optical rotation was developed in 1919 by Emile Fischer. The Fischer convention is based upon a molecule's configuration relative to (+)-glyceraldehyde, which was arbitrarily assigned a D configuration (note upper case D, compared with lower case *d* for *dextro*). The configuration of a molecule would be assigned this configuration if it (or a chemical degradation product that retained the chiral center) had the same direction of rotation as the model substance (+)-glyceraldehyde, and the L configuration if the direction of rotation was the reverse. The direction of rotation, (as in D[−]-bupivacaine) also may be added. Third, in 1955, the sequence rules of Cahn, Ingold, and Prelog[90] introduced a method for the unequivocal designation of molecular configuration by giving a sequence of priority to the four atoms or groups at-

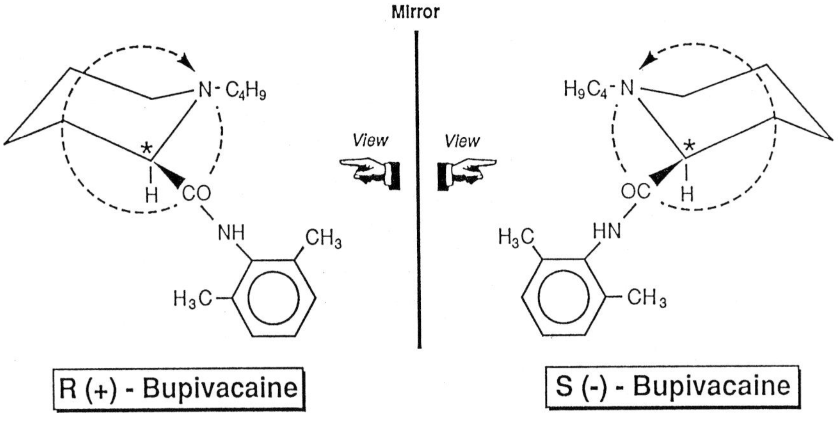

FIG. 3-7. Application of the Sequence Rules of Cahn, Ingold, and Prelog to the enantiomers of bupivacaine. The chiral carbon is marked*. The smallest attached group, hydrogen, is projected away from the viewer; the other groups, nitrogen of N-butyl, carbon of carbonyl, and carbon of piperidine ring methylene, are arranged in clockwise order of decreasing size to give *R*-bupivacaine which is *dextro*rotatory; its antipode, *S*-bupivacaine, has the opposite order and is *levo*rotatory.

tached to a tetrahedral chiral center. With the smallest atom or group extending away from the viewer, the arrangement of the largest to smallest groups proceeding clockwise is designated as *R* (for *rectus*); the antipode is designated *S* (for *sinister*) (Fig. 3-7, Table 3-2). Contemporary literature contains all three notations, depending upon the amount of information available, but only the Cahn-Ingold-Prelog notation denotes the absolute configuration. Racemates or racemic mixtures are designated (±)-, *dl*-, DL-, *rac*-, or *RS*-.

PHYSICOCHEMICAL PROPERTIES OF LOCAL ANESTHETICS

Basically, three mechanisms are involved in the movement of local anesthetic molecules within the body: bulk flow of the injected solution at the site of administration; diffusion into and through aqueous and lipoprotein barriers; and vascular transport. Of these, diffusion is most directly dependent on the physicochemical properties of the agent.

According to Fick's Law, the rate of passive diffusion (dQ/dt) of a drug through a biologic membrane at steady state may be approximated by equation 1, in which D is the diffusion coefficient of the drug in the membrane; A and δ are, respectively, the area and the thickness of the membrane; K is the partition coefficient of drug between the aqueous and membrane phases; and ΔC is the concentration gradient.

$$\frac{dQ}{dt} = \frac{D \cdot A \cdot K \cdot \Delta C}{\delta} \qquad [1]$$

Inasmuch as they determine D, K, and C, physicochemical properties will influence the rate of transport of local anesthetic agent at the membrane level, and potentially, therefore, the time course of anesthetic and pharmacologic effects. By influencing the equilibrium distribution of the drugs between fluids and tissues, physicochemical properties also modulate activity and overall drug movement in the bloodstream.

Equation 1 can be simplified to equation 2 in which the term comprising the constants, D, A, K, and δ is combined into a permeability constant P; this equation indicates that the concentration difference across a membrane, ΔC, is the driving force for drug movement.

$$\frac{dQ}{dt} = P \cdot \Delta C \qquad [2]$$

Some physicochemical properties of the clinically used local anesthetics are shown in Tables 3-1 and 3-3. As Table 3-1 shows, structural changes in the aromatic portion of the esters and in the amine group of the amides markedly alter physical properties such as lipid/aqueous partition coefficients and protein binding. These, in turn, have significant effects on potency, onset time, and duration of anesthesia.

TABLE 3-2. *Applications of stereochemical nomenclature to mepivacaine and bupivacaine*

Fischer	Cahn-Ingold-Prelog	$[\alpha]_{25}^{D}$
D(−)-mepivacaine	*R*(−)-mepivacaine	−18.6
L(+)-mepivacaine	*S*(+)-mepivacaine	+18.9
DL(±)-mepivacaine[a]	*RS* or *rac*-mepivacaine	0
D(+)-bupivacaine	*R*(+)-bupivacaine	+12.7
L(−)-bupivacaine	*S*(−)-bupivacaine	−12.0
DL(±)-bupivacaine[a]	*RS* or *rac*-bupivacaine	0

$[\alpha]_{25}^{D}$ = rotation of sodium spectrum D-line at 25°.

[a] denotes a racemate, that is, an equal mixture of enantiomers and is rotatory neutral because of canceling rotations of the enantiomers. Both of these racemates are the clinically used forms of these agents.

Data from Friberger, P., and Aberg, G.: Some physicochemical properties of the racemates and the optically active isomers of two local anaesthetic compounds. Acta Pharmaceut. Suec., *8*:361, 1971.

TABLE 3-3. *Features common to most local anesthetics*

- Weak bases with $pK_a > 7.4$. (Free base poorly water-soluble)
- Thus dispensed as acidic solution of hydrochloride salts (pH 4–7), which are more highly ionized and thus water-soluble
- Exist in solution as equilibrium mixture of nonionized, lipid-soluble (free base) and ionized, water-soluble (cationic) forms
- Body buffers raise pH and therefore increase amount of free base present
- Lipid-soluble (free base) form crosses axonal membrane
- Water-soluble (cationic) form is active blocker for most agents

For example, addition of a four-carbon *n*-butyl group to the lipophilic aromatic amino end with subtraction of two carbons from the hydrophilic amino end of the ester procaine gives tetracaine and results in a 200-fold increase in partition coefficient, a 10-fold increase in protein binding, and a marked increase in potency. With the amide mepivacaine, substitution of a four-carbon *n*-butyl group for the one-carbon methyl group on the amine function gives bupivacaine with a 35-fold increase in partition coefficient, increased protein binding, and increased potency. Similarly, substitution in the lidocaine molecule of an *n*-propyl for an ethyl group at the amine end and addition of an ethyl group at the *alpha*-carbon in the intermediate chain yields etidocaine. This results in a 50-fold increase in partition coefficient, increased protein binding and potency, and a duration of local anesthetic action at least twice that of lidocaine. Differences in molecular weight among drugs from homologous series are usually also associated with parallel differences in lipophilicity. Under these circumstances, differences in diffusibility and permeability occur as second-order effects.[82]

Molecular Weight

Molecular weights of the clinically useful local anesthetic agent bases vary from 220 to 288 (Table 3-1). Because the diffusion coefficient is inversely proportional to the square root of the molecular weight, and differences in molecular weight among related local anesthetic agents are relatively small, the diffusion coefficient does not contribute significantly to differences in their rates of diffusion.

Dural permeability has been claimed to be more dependent on molecular weight than lipid solubility (see below), but the relationship within a series of opioids having similar physicochemical properties to the amide local anesthetics[294] is unconvincing. Moreover, when tested with an *in vitro* preparation of the spinal meninges of the monkey, the permeability coefficients of a series of drugs including lidocaine and bupivacaine were found to be independent of molecular weight (and molecular axis and molecular volume). However, a "bell-shaped" relationship was found with lipophilicity (as measured by octanol:pH 7.4 buffer distribution coefficient).[43] The permeability of human dura mater *in vitro* to a variety of opioids and local anesthetic agents was found to be a simple diffusion process, independent of molecular weight, and driven by the concentration gradient.[258] There is, however, evidence to suggest that molecular weight might be relevant to the diffusion of local anesthetics in the sodium channel of the nerve membrane.[105]

Ionization

The inclusion of an amino group in the structure of most local anesthetics confers upon them the "split personality" of a weak base, meaning that they exist in solution partly as the unionized free base and partly as the ionized cation (conjugate acid) (equation 3):

$$\underset{\text{unionized base}}{\overset{|}{\underset{/\ \backslash}{N\!:}}} \quad + \quad \underset{\text{hydrogen ion}}{H^+} \quad \underset{K_a}{\rightleftharpoons} \quad \underset{\text{ionized cation (conjugate acid)}}{\overset{|}{\underset{/\ \backslash}{N\!:^+H}}} \qquad (3)$$

The position of equilibrium depends on the dissociation constant (K_a) of the conjugate acid and on the local hydrogen ion concentration (equation 4). Thus,

$$K_a = \frac{[H^+][\text{base}]}{[\text{conjugate acid}]} \qquad (4)$$

where the square brackets indicate concentration or, more properly, activity. By rearranging equation 4 and taking logarithms, the Henderson-Hasselbach equation (equation 5) is obtained:

$$pK_a = pH - \log \frac{[\text{base}]}{[\text{conjugate acid}]} \qquad (5)$$

where pK_a is defined, by analogy to pH, as the negative logarithm of the dissociation constant of the conjugate acid under particular conditions of solvent and temperature.[376,404,442]

Equation 5 shows that the pK_a is equal to the pH at which the local anesthetic is 50% ionized, that is, when

$$\frac{[\text{base}]}{[\text{conjugate acid}]} = 1, \text{ and } \log 1 = 0.$$

The greater the pK_a of a base, the stronger is the base and the smaller is the proportion of un-ionized form at any pH. Ester-type agents have higher pK_a values (8.5–9.1) than the amide types (7.6–8.2) (Table 3-1), which accounts, in part, for relatively poor penetrance and the need to inject these agents close to neural tissue. The effect on pK_a values of differences in structure within the two main types of agents is complex, involving steric factors as well as the inductive effects of alkyl substituents on the amine nitrogen. For example, the greater pK_a of bupivacaine compared with mepivacaine is explained by the effect of greater alkyl substitution making the nitrogen atom relatively more negative. In contrast, the lower pK_a of etidocaine and of prilocaine seems to reflect the effect of alkyl substituents on the bridging carbon atom in sterically hindering the approach of hydrogen ions to form the conjugate acid and in decreasing stabilization of the resultant cation by hydration.

Ionization is relevant to the solubility and activity of local anesthetics (Table 3-1) and their equilibrium distribution in various body compartments. Because the ionized forms are more water-soluble than the free bases, the drugs are dispensed as their hydrochloride salts in acidic solutions. This also helps to stabilize the esters since they are more readily hydrolyzed in alkaline conditions. The pH of plain solutions of the ester-type agents may be as low as 2.8 compared to 4.4 to 6.4 for those of the amides.[288] The drugs are much more lipid-soluble in their free-base forms than in their conjugate acid forms. Thus, the un-ionized fraction becomes essential for passage through lipoprotein diffusion barriers to the site of action on the nerve membrane. Decreasing ionization by alkalinization of the solution for injection will effectively raise the initial concentration gradient of diffusible drug,[441] thereby increasing the rate of drug transfer. This maneuver has been successful in decreasing the latent period of a peripheral nerve block[108,343,416] but has not been universally successful for epidural or caudal nerve block.[17,104,392,415] Once at the nerve membrane, ionization is again necessary for complete anesthetic activity.[409] Increasing the pH of aqueous local anesthetic solution also increases the surface tension[251] and this has been shown to decrease the drop rate when lidocaine solution was being delivered under gravity feed.

The aqueous phases on either side of many body membranes differ in their pH values. Consequently, although un-ionized drug concentrations in these phases will be the same at equilibrium, different concentrations of ionized and, therefore, of total drug will exist on either side of the membrane if there is a pH gradient. For a weak base, the equilibrium ratio (R) of total drug concentration across a membrane is given by equation 6. Thus,

$$R = \frac{1 + 10pK_a - pH_1}{1 + 10pK_a - pH_2} \qquad (6)$$

where the subscripts 1 and 2 refer to the two aqueous compartments. Total drug concentration will be greater in the compartment having the lower pH because a greater proportion will be in the ionized form. Thus, for example, lowered pH owing to infection in tissues surrounding a nerve results in less un-ionized drug, which is the form that can cross the axonal membrane. Similarly, local anesthetics will diffuse from blood to acidic gastric contents thereby maintaining a concentration gradient due to "ion trapping."[213]

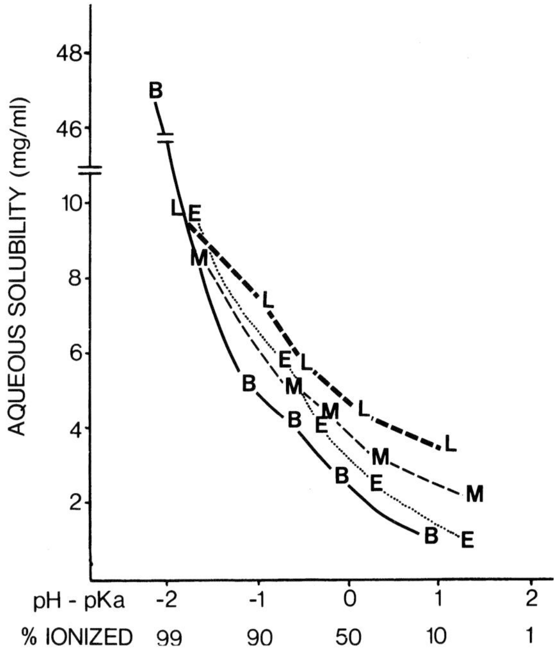

FIG. 3-8. Solubilities of lidocaine *(L)*, mepivacaine *(M)*, etidocaine *(E)*, and bupivacaine *(B)* in aqueous buffer in relation to their pKa and degree of ionization. (Mather, L. E.: unpublished data.)

Aqueous Solubility

The aqueous solubility of a local anesthetic is related directly to its extent of ionization and inversely to its lipid solubility (Table 3-1). Despite quite large differences in the lipid solubility of the amide local anesthetic bases, the differences in aqueous solubility of the conjugate acids are smaller (Fig. 3-8). Benzocaine, which lacks an amino group, is almost insoluble in water. For this reason its use is essentially confined to topical anesthesia, although it has been injected for prolonged intercostal nerve block after solubilization with dextran.

The aqueous solubilities of the clinically used racemic forms of mepivacaine and bupivacaine have been compared to those of their respective enantiomers. As expected, it was found for both agents that the *R* and *S* enantiomers each had the same aqueous solubility. However, over the range from pH 3 to 7.4, the solubility of *rac*-mepivacaine was nearly twice that of its component enantiomers, whereas over the range from pH 6 to 7.4 the solubility of *rac*-bupivacaine was nearly one half that of its component enantiomers.[166] While such findings are not known to have any special significance for clinical practice, they indicate that there can be complex physicochemical interactions between drugs and, it is presumed in this instance, buffer ions used in their solvents.

A low aqueous solubility was thought to be a limiting factor when selecting an agent for subarachnoid block. Thus, there has been concern over the possible neurotoxicity of 1% solutions of bupivacaine HCl since they become opalescent on mixing with cerebrospinal fluid (CSF) in vitro.[137] Clinical experience has not borne this out. Although precipitation of the compound may occur *in vivo*,[125,283,399] animal studies indicate that morphologic effects of the less water-soluble agents on the spinal cord are apparent only after intrathecal injection of concentrations greater than 2%.[9,10] Mixtures of local anesthetic agents with bicarbonate will lead to precipitation of the local anesthetic base after the acid of the solubilizing acid (normally hydrochloric acid) has been neutralized by the inorganic base.

Recent discussion about transient neurological disturbances after subarachnoid administration of hyperbaric 5% lidocaine solution has generated much speculation as to the possible cause(s).[124,418] De Jong[124] suggested that lumbosacral nerve root damage might be caused by caudad direction of a catheter tip (if used) depositing a pool of relatively concentrated lidocaine sacrally. He further suggested that, among other possible causes, this deposition might be more prominent for "highly water-soluble" drugs such as lidocaine and tetracaine whereas use of a low solubility agent such as bupivacaine might preclude a "potentially harmful buildup" of drug in the CSF. It is known that the aqueous solubility differs among agents[137] and is a function of pH (Fig. 3-8). However, it is not clear logic that neurotoxicity from hyperbaric 5% lidocaine solution might be avoided by substituting an agent with lower aqueous solubility (than lidocaine) which presumably will precipitate from solution when injected into CSF (at a higher pH), thereby leaving a lower concentration in the aqueous medium. Indeed, the problem might vanish if hyperbaric 2% lidocaine solution were substituted.[413]

The stability of local anesthetic agents in aqueous solution is related to their structure and to the pH of the solution. Ester-type local anesthetic agents have a maximum resistance to chemical hydrolysis in aqueous solutions of pH 3 to 4. Procaine, for example, stored at pH 3.7 to 3.8 undergoes hydrolysis at a rate of 0.5 to 1% per year; at pH 4.5 to 5.5 this increases to 1% to 1.5% per year and at pH 7.5 to 1% per day.[134] Amides are chemically stable in both conjugate acid and base forms even during sterilization and storage.[18,214,311,340,422,466] Although there is the potential for all drugs to undergo adsorptive losses into medical plastics, such as polyvinyl chloride catheters and polypropylene syringes, this has not been found to be a significant problem with the amide-type agents.[214,444,445] Similarly, there is no evidence of instability or of precipitation when solutions of the amide local anesthetic agents are premixed with other organic bases such as opioids, as long as the pH of the solution is no higher than neutral.[422] There is no evidence of significant inversion of ropivacaine to its antipode during storage.[168]

Lipid Solubility

The partition coefficients of drugs measured in aqueous/organic solvent systems *in vitro* are commonly used to reflect their relative *in vivo* partition characteristics or degree of lipid solubility.[404,421] The values obtained may differ quantitatively between systems[211,442] such that their best use is in making comparisons between drugs within the same system. For example, Rosenberg and colleagues[356] have shown good rank order correlation between the *n*-heptane/buffer partition coefficients of bupivacaine, etidocaine, ropivacaine, and lidocaine and their *in vitro* partition into rat sciatic nerve and human epidural and subcutaneous fat. The uptake into rat brain of a series of ester-type local anesthetics was found to be linearly related to the logarithmic value of the partition coefficients obtained in *n*-heptane/water or *n*-octanol/water.[301]

Net lipid solubility, as reflected by organic solvent (such as *n*-heptane or *n*-octanol)/buffer partition coefficients is independent of ester or amide grouping. Tetracaine (ester) is regarded as being highly lipid-soluble, as are ropivacaine, bupivacaine, and etidocaine (amides) (see Table 3-1).[404] The intrinsic potencies of amino ester, amino amide, and piperidine amide local anesthetics have been found to be inversely proportional to their calculated solubility in nerve fibers as determined from their lipid solubility.[243] The relationships for the three classes of agent are essentially parallel but, for the same degree of calculated solubility of the local anesthetic base, the intrinsic potencies were found to be in the order amino ester > amino amide > piperidine amide.[459] However, the relationship between potency and properties is complex. The partition coefficients were calculated on the basis of summing the effects of the composite chemical groups: A different relationship might apply *in vivo*, especially for the chiral agents. The relative proportions of base and conjugate acid of the individual agents depends on their pK_a: The relationship is developed in terms of base concentrations only when it is known that both forms are required for effect. Overall, a high lipid solubility would be expected to promote drug entry into membranes by increasing diffusion rate but this has to be balanced with a high fraction of drug in the un-ionized state.[459–461] The net effect on onset of maximum anesthetic action is difficult to predict, however, because a faster rate of diffusion is offset by a greater capacity for uptake into a membrane.

It has been found that a high lipid solubility alone also does not predict the relative rate of transfer of local anesthetics and chemically similar drugs through meninges in *in vitro* models.[42,258] Moreover, even when lipid solubility and unionized fraction are taken into account, the intrinsic potency of the agents is subject to differences in preferred molecular geometry for fit to the local anesthetic receptor site.[461] However, it is generally found that by promoting interaction with hydrophobic components of receptors, a high lipid solubility will increase potency and duration of effect.

Protein Binding

Besides being more lipid-soluble, the longer-acting local anesthetics also exhibit higher degrees of binding to plasma and tissue proteins (Table 3-1). This suggests that the binding forces are predominantly hydrophobic, which is also consistent with greater plasma binding at higher pH values.[89]

Adsorption of local anesthetics to binding sites or solubility within membranes or tissues, while producing relatively high apparent partition coefficients, may result in slower net penetration rates. This may be considered either as a lowering of diffusion coefficient or as a decrease in ΔC, the effective concentration gradient of diffusible drug (equation 2). Binding of the drugs to proteins associated with the aqueous phases on either side of a membrane will affect the transfer and equilibrium distribution of total drug, analogously to ionization. Only the unbound drug will diffuse readily and, again, this will modify net drug transfer rate by an influence on ΔC.

At equilibrium, the concentration of unbound, un-ionized drug will be the same on either side of the membrane, but total drug concentrations will differ depending on the relative capacities of the binding sites associated with the two aqueous phases and the pH values of these phases.[423] This mechanism has been used to explain, in large measure, the distri-

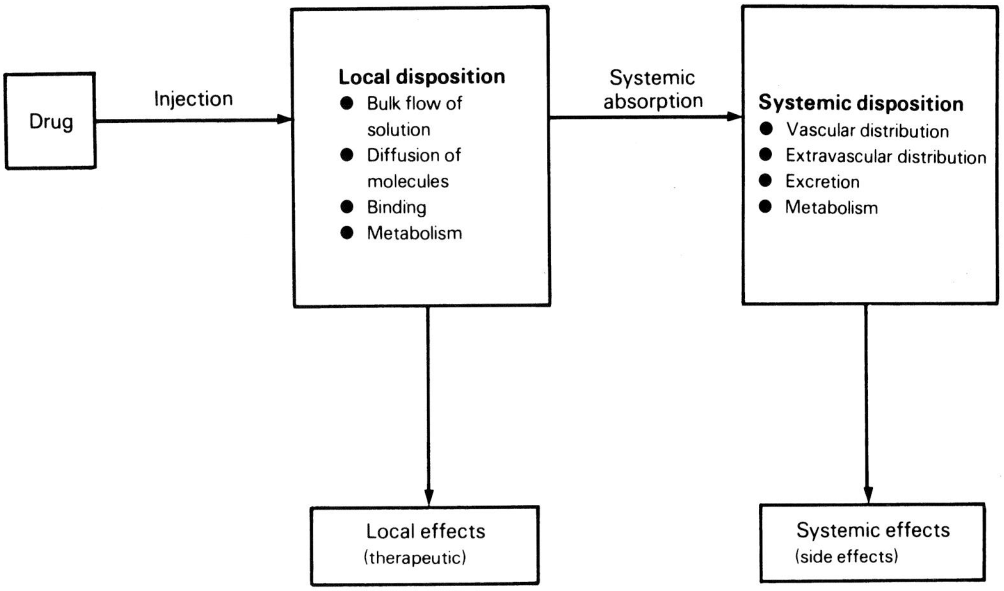

FIG. 3-9. Fate of local anesthetic agents. (Mather, L.E., and Cousins, M.J.: Local anaesthetics and their current clinical use. Drugs, *18*:185, 1979.)

bution of local anesthetic agents across the placenta.[221,223,269,430]

On the basis of an appreciation of the different structures and physicochemical properties of local anesthetics and the expected consequences of these differences,[74] it is possible to inquire more specifically into their absorption and disposition in various parts of the body. In doing so, the fate of the agents is best divided into consideration of their local disposition, systemic absorption, and systemic disposition and regional disposition (Fig. 3-9).[268] The term *disposition* has a special meaning; it refers collectively to the processes of *drug distribution* into and out of tissues and *drug elimination* by excretion and/or metabolism, while specifically excluding the process of absorption into the bloodstream.

LOCAL DISPOSITION

In contrast to many drugs, the primary effects of local anesthetics at both the pharmacological level (neural blockade) and clinical level (analgesia and anesthesia) can be measured fairly objectively. The anesthesiologist is concerned particularly with the onset, spread, quality, and duration of nerve block. Ultimately, however, these variables depend on the distribution and dissipation of the drugs at the site of injection. Therefore, it would be valuable to have chemical measurements of the agents at these sites as a function of time in order to establish pharmacodynamic relationships. Regrettably, such data are sparse, even from animals. Therefore, knowledge of the local disposition, or neurokinetics, of local anesthetics remains largely theoretical and is deduced from observation of the spatiotemporal changes in anesthetic effect, rather than from direct measurements of intraneural and perineural drug concentrations.

Factors that affect local disposition of local anesthetics include dispersion by bulk flow of the injected solution, diffusion, and binding of the agent. Metabolic breakdown seems less important. Local blood supply is critical, as this is responsible for local clearance of drug. It has been suggested that the local blood supply is responsible for delivery of drug to deeper structures of the spinal cord via the radicular arteries[41,107] but recent evidence suggests that this is unlikely.[46] Uptake into blood vessels leading to the systemic circulation also is important and this is discussed primarily in the context of systemic absorption. In addition to these factors, the pharmaceutical presentation of the agent (see above) can be manipulated so that the rate of release of agent controls the balance between local and systemic uptake of the agent.

Although lipophilicity is an intrinsic physicochemical property of a drug resulting from its molecular structure, the effective lipophilicity can be altered by pharmaceutical presentation. For example, opioid drugs have been combined with cyclodextrins to make them more hydrophilic[208] and with liposomes to make them more lipophilic.[45] Both combinations have been found to be longer-acting after subarachnoid administration in rats than the simple aqueous solutions of the same drugs. The mechanisms of prolongation of action are presumed to differ but have in common the alteration of the rate of drug diffusion. Drugs combined with cyclodextrins are believed to have a slower rate of vascular absorption than aqueous solutions. Liposome encapsulation provides a depot from which drug is released slowly. Liposomal preparations of local anesthetic agents have been found to have both a longer duration of action and a lower propensity for systemic toxicity than equivalent doses in aqueous media injected perivascularly, epidurally, or intrathecally in experimental animals[55,57,179,197,244,265,379] and in epidural anesthesia in humans.[56] Moreover, liposomal preparations of local anesthetic agents have a higher rate of penetration of the dermis than equivalent aqueous solutions.[163,336]

Bulk Flow

The extent of spread of the injected solution might be expected to depend on its volume, the force (rate) with which it is injected, and the turbulence generated, the size of the injected space, the physical resistance offered by tissues and fluids, gravity, and the position of the patient during and after injection. Bulk flow of local anesthetic solutions has been assessed by the use of marker dyes, radiographic contrast media, external counting techniques, and spinal canal models.[71,87,290,295,309,350,359,402] Although the spread of analgesia may also indicate the extent of bulk flow, these are not necessarily equivalent because spread of effect is also determined by solute diffusion and local perfusion. The observation that the epidural injection of bupivacaine in glycerol produced longer duration of analgesia than when injected in normal saline was interpreted as being due to a bupivacaine depot.[225] While this may be so, it also may be that the higher viscosity of the glycerol solution reduced the rate of bulk flow thereby increasing the concentration of bupivacaine diffusing into the nerve structures.

Subarachnoid Block

Hydrodynamic considerations are more important after subarachnoid injection than after any other regional anesthetic procedure. Using ^{131}I as a marker, Kitahara and colleagues[227] documented the spread of isobaric and hyperbaric local anesthetic solutions in relation to the level of analgesia and with patients in various positions. Hyperbaric solutions spread more cephalad than did isobaric ones; however, there was no difference in the spread of analgesia between isobaric and hypobaric solutions.[78] A head-down position does not cause extra-cephalad spread in most patients.[234,394] Unilateral block can be obtained by maintaining the lateral position, but the block rapidly becomes bilateral when the patient is turned supine.[462] In contrast, in a spinal canal model *in vitro,* solutions of bupivacaine mixed with methylene blue dye and equilibrated at 37°C became relatively hypobaric and were found to diffuse more cephalad than did solutions equilibrated at 22°C which became relatively hyperbaric.[402] Similarly, solutions of 0.5% bupivacaine, equilibrated at 37°C and injected rapidly (0.5 ml/sec), produced higher levels of subarachnoid blockade in patients initially sitting than the same solutions injected slowly (0.05 ml/sec). The difference may be explained by the fact that the solutions are slightly hypobaric at the higher temperature but that the slow injection allowed cooling so that the density effect was lost.[306,403] In these studies, the effect of decreased density overcame the anticipated greater effect of higher turbulence obtained from the faster injection rate in both the *in vitro* model and the patients undergoing subarachnoid block.[402,403] In another study in patients undergoing subarachnoid block, there were no differences in the spread of block with patients in the sitting position and injected with 0.5% bupivacaine equilibrated at 19° or 37°C.[234]

It has been found that the turbulence created upon rapid injection of local anesthetic solutions does not seem to convey any clinical advantage in increasing the spread of subarachnoid block.[359] Moreover, a slower speed of injection (3 ml/180 sec) was found to produce a median 2.5-segment higher level of block compared to subarachnoid injection of the same volume over 10 seconds to patients in the lateral horizontal position.[440] The results of this study suggest that turbulence as generated by rapid injection through a small-gauge spinal needle cannot be a prime factor determining the spread of subarachnoid block. Furthermore, comparison of the same dose of local anesthetic in different volumes indicated no difference in the spread of analgesia in the supine position produced by 15 mg of bupivacaine given as 0.5% and 0.75% hyperbaric solutions, but less cephalad spread when 10 mg was given as the 0.75% compared to the 0.5% solution.[96] Increased spread of analgesia resulting from increased abdominal pressure is thought to result from a decreased CSF volume.

Removal of 5 ml CSF was found to increase the cephalad spread resulting from subarachnoid injection of 2 ml 0.5% bupivacaine solution without evidence of increased abdominal pressure, suggesting that bulk flow is a major determinant of spread of analgesia.[210] Overall, spread of analgesia may or may not be influenced when concentration is constant and volume is varied, depending on the concentration of hyperbaric bupivacaine and the posture of the patient.[26,96,406]

Epidural Block

Studies using radiopaque markers indicate that increasing the volume of injectate causes a disproportionately smaller increase in cephalad spread.[87,289] This may reflect greater spillage into the paravertebral spaces with larger volumes and is consistent with volume spread of analgesia relationships.[71,182] Thus, below a limiting volume (constant dose), the spread and intensity of block become independent of volume, indicating that factors other than bulk flow are more important for the ultimate dispersion of the local anesthetic agent.

Neither Burn et al. nor Nishimura et al. could demonstrate any effect of the rate of injection on spread of solutions in the epidural space.[87,309] The results of studies on the spread of analgesia vary but, in general, indicate a minor influence of injection speed.[101,146,204,358] It has been suggested that, for comparisons, the dose/segment is a more useful outcome variable than spread alone.[111] Confounding cofactors include the drug used, the age and size of the patient, the range of injection pressures, and the direction of the needle bevel. It has been claimed that the presence or absence of epinephrine is not a significant factor.[111]

The cephalad spread of radiolabeled injectate vastly exceeds the caudad spread in supine patients. Spread has been found to parallel both the force of injection and the degree of negative pressure in the epidural space.[310] Posture has a minimal influence on the spread of analgesia. No significant differences in cephalad spread occur in the sitting and lateral positions.[281,309,324] An exception is the obese patient who achieves a lower block when seated.[195] Caudad spread may be marginally less when the patient is sitting.[281] The lateral position favors spread of analgesia to the dependent side in both nonpregnant and pregnant patients, but this does not appear to be of great clinical significance.[20,183,204,281,386]

Increases in the duration and longitudinal spread of epidural anesthesia with increasing age have been attributed to reduced lateral leakage of solution, owing to progressive sclerotic closure of the paravertebral foramina.[71] This is supported by the finding of increased residual epidural pressure after injection in older people, evidence from epidurograms, and more extensive cephalad spread shown by an external counting method.[75,309] In contrast, although Burn and co-workers[87] found evidence of reduced lateral spread of solution with age using 20-ml lumbar injections, this was not seen with 40-ml solutions and, when there was less lateral spread, it was not accompanied by greater longitudinal flow. Further, while verifying a decline in dose requirements with age, recent studies have shown that the relationship is more complex than originally proposed.[183,325,326,388,450,451]

Intercostal and Interpleural Block

The distribution of marker substances after injection into the costal grooves of cadavers has been investigated. It has been pointed out that variations in anatomy of this region are far more common than has been commonly believed[299] and that information about the spread of solutions derived from studies in cadaver studies may be misleading because of changes occurring postmortem.[295] Whereas Nunn and Slavin[314] concluded that spread occurs to the nerves above and below the target one, Moore[287,290,291] found that spread was exclusive to the injected intercostal groove. Interpleural injection of bupivacaine mixed with radiopaque dye into patients in either the supine or lateral positions indicated that there was no difference in rostrocaudal spread of dye (T3–L1 supine, T5–L1 lateral) although, in the supine group, there was a greater medial spread along the mediastinum than laterally.[396] From studies of bupivacaine mixed with methylene blue dye in patients undergoing thoracotomy, Moorthy[295] concluded that the spread of anesthesia depends on the volume injected: A 5-ml injection spread through one intercostal space but a 10-ml injection was more likely to spread to two or more intercostal spaces.

Brachial Plexus Block

The brachial plexus sheath contains a complex of fascial septa which, hypothetically, would impede the spread of solutions injected into it, leading to poor predictability in neural blockade.[385,419] Nevertheless, the spread of solutions within the sheath is not readily impeded[327] although it is known that it is not a continuous, single fascial compartment surrounding the brachial plexus from its origins and extending peripherally as far as the axilla, as described by Winnie and co-workers.[469] In this volume, Brown and Bridenbaugh[76] have made specific recommendations on technical and mechanical factors designed to improve the flow in the desired direction.

Diffusion

Once the local anesthetic has been deposited and spread physically in the extraneural fluids, it finds its way to sites of action in and on the nerve membrane largely by the process of diffusion.

Subarachnoid Block

After subarachnoid injection, the relatively high lipid solubility of local anesthetic bases will promote local cord uptake rather than extensive cephalad spread via CSF flow. Thus, drug concentrations in the CSF decline rapidly in both directions from the point of injection and exponentially at the site of injection as uptake proceeds.[232,283,339] Direct diffusion along the concentration gradient from CSF through the pia mater directly into the cord delivers drug only to the superficial parts of the structure. Access to deeper areas is effected by diffusion in the CSF contained in the spaces of Virchow-Robin which connect with perineural clefts surrounding the bodies of nerve cells within the cord.[180]

The pattern of drug distribution within the cord is a complex function of accessibility by diffusion from the CSF, the relative myelin (lipid) content of various tracts, and the rate of drug removal by local perfusion. Studies in animals using radiolabeled local anesthetics have shown their accumulation along the posterior and lateral aspects of the spinal cord as well as in the spinal nerve roots, but not to such a degree in the dorsal root ganglion or in the more central parts of the cord. Uptake of drug was higher in the gray matter than in the white matter of the cord, and posterior nerve roots had higher concentrations than anterior roots.[75,99,198] Overall, the model (Fig. 3-10) proposed for subarachnoid injection of opioids[107] may be viewed as a reasonable representation of the fate of local anesthetics because, in general, these agents have similar physicochemical properties.

Epidural Block

Local anesthetics appear rapidly in the CSF after epidural injection.[464] Thus, peak drug concentrations in the CSF occur within 10 to 20 minutes and are sufficient to produce blockade of spinal nerve roots. By 30 minutes high drug concentrations are also achieved in the peripheral cord and in the spinal nerves in the paravertebral space.[75]

Apart from direct diffusion of drug across the dura, access to the cord, particularly the dorsal horn region, may be mediated by diffusion; by uptake into the posterior radicular branch of spinal segmental arteries[41], although subsequent work has suggested that this might be more a source of clearance from the cord rather than uptake[46]; by centripetal subneural and subpial spread from the remote paravertebral nerve trunks[69,71] and by bulk flow through the arachnoid via the dural root sleeves, although the latter has not been supported in recent studies[42] using dura *ex vivo*. These suggestions are consistent with clinical observations of the distribution of analgesia during induction and regression of epidural block. A segmental pattern of analgesia during onset may be related to the initial drug diffusion into spinal nerves and roots, with subsequent nonsegmental regression resulting from ultimate diffusion to structures within the cord.[446] Again, the model (Fig. 3-10) proposed for epidural administration of opioids[107] may also represent the fate of local anesthetic agents. It is also clear that even a very small hole made during the introduction of an epidural needle can give rise to spuriously high "rates of diffusion" into the subarachnoid space of drugs injected epidurally.[44]

Electrophysiologic studies in monkeys indicate that the depth of penetration of the cord varies considerably with the agent used, chloroprocaine being limited to dorsal horn gray matter, bupivacaine reaching both the dorsal horn and white matter, and etidocaine concentrating predominantly in the white matter.[114] These differences are, however, concentration-dependent. Thus, increased concentration of bupivacaine was shown to influence penetration at the dorsal root entry zone and, to a lesser degree, at the white tracts of the spinal cord.[115] A marked effect of etidocaine on lower limb reflexes after thoracic epidurals in humans is consistent with blockade of relatively deep motor tracts within the cord using this agent.[70]

Much of an epidural dose of local anesthetic may be sequestered temporarily in extraneural tissues at the site of injection. This nonspecific "binding" may have two effects. By lowering the amount of agent free to diffuse onto the nerves, it effectively lowers clinical potency. On the other hand, by providing a depot from which drug is slowly dissociated to maintain anesthetic concentrations in the nerve, it could prolong duration of block. Prolonged sequestration of local anesthetic drugs in epidural fat, particularly those that are more lipid-soluble, has been demonstrated in sheep (Fig. 3-11).

Brachial Plexus Block

Progression of blockade from upper arm to hand and then to fingers is explained by more rapid diffusion of local anesthetic into mantle fibers that innervate more proximal regions than do the core fibers.[123] To explain why the onset of motor block often precedes that of sensory loss, Winnie and colleagues[468] have suggested that the effect of the larger diameter of the motor fibers is offset by their more peripheral location in the median nerve compared to sensory fibers. According to the classical view, the sequence of recovery should be the same as that of onset: arm first, then hand and fingers.[123] This follows if the concentration gradient within

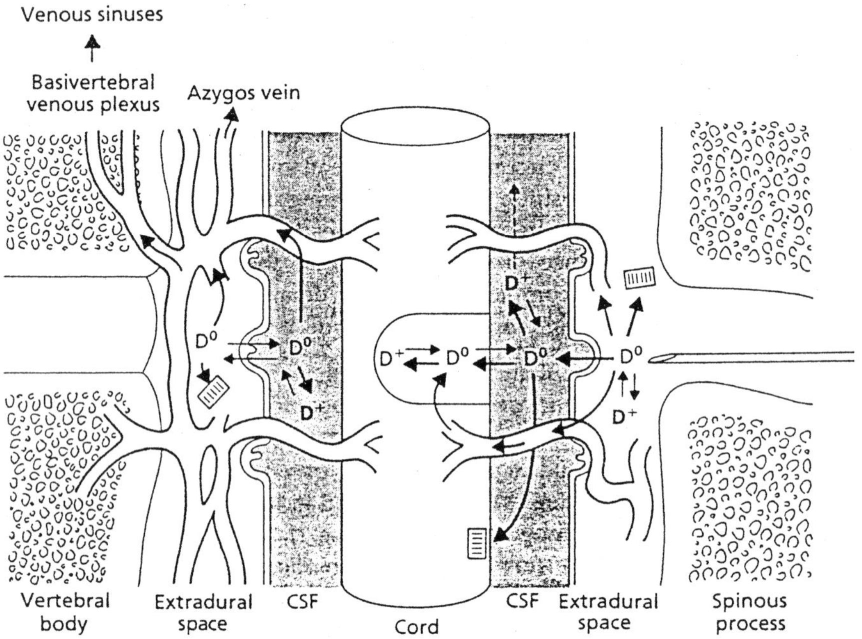

FIG. 3-10. A model of spinal drug disposition following epidural injection. Drug will exist in an equilibrium mixture of diffusible uncharged unbound form (D°) and charged water-soluble form (D^+). Equilibrium also exists with nondiffusible drug bound to macromolecules (⊟). The Law of Mass Action pertains, whereby alteration in the concentrations of any form reestablishes a new equilibrium. (From Cousins, M.J. and Mather, L.E.: Intracathel and epidural administration of opiods. Anesthesiology, *61*:276, 1984.)

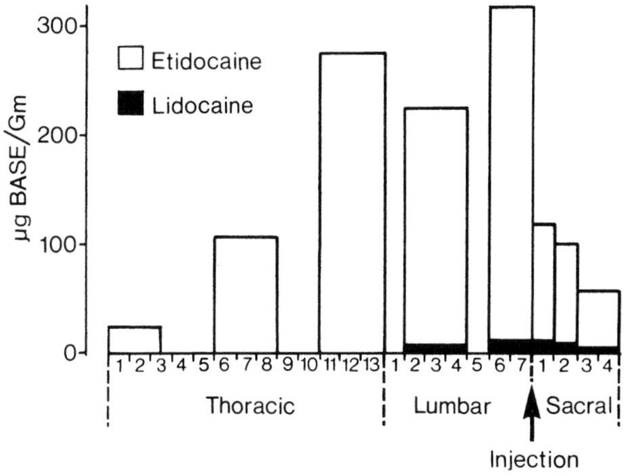

FIG. 3-11. Mean local anesthetic concentrations in peridural fat of sheep 12 hours after peridural injection. Dose was 80 mg of etidocaine hydrochloride, 50 mg of lidocaine hydrochloride, and 50 µg of epinephrine; n was 6. (M. Lebeaux and G.T. Tucker, unpublished data.)

the nerve now becomes reversed, decreasing from core to mantle. However, this has been challenged by Winnie and colleagues,[470] who observed the reverse order of recovery with significant motor block that outlasted analgesia. To account for these findings it was proposed that a more rapid vascular uptake of agent occurs near the more distally innervating sensory fibers located in the core of the nerve. As intraneural blood vessels pass from mantle to core they become increasingly branched and thus offer a larger surface area for drug absorption.

Differential Block

The propensity to produce a marked differential blockade is a characteristic of some local anesthetic agents, particularly tetracaine and etidocaine, which produce profound motor blockade, as well as bupivacaine, which provides a balance of analgesia and motor loss, and ropivacaine which can be used to provide analgesia with a minimum of motor loss.[298] In the case of epidural block, Bromage[70] has suggested that this phenomenon may be due to deeper penetration of the spinal cord by more lipid-soluble agents causing interference with long descending motor pathways. Bupivacaine, however, is more lipid-soluble than tetracaine and lidocaine, which produce less differential sensory loss, and the differences in sensory-motor dissociation seen with the various agents are also apparent after peripheral nerve block procedures, in which penetration of the cord is not a factor.[253,344] To accommodate the latter, differences in the ability of the agents to diffuse into individual sensory and motor fibers have been postulated.[459] Thus, from electrophysiologic studies with isolated rabbit vagus nerve, Gissen and coworkers[176] concluded that, compared to etidocaine, less lipid-soluble bupivacaine diffuses relatively slowly into fast-conducting A (motor) fibers at low concentrations. This is supported by other electrophysiologic studies,[164,323,355] although Fink and Cairns[157] discount diffusion within a nerve as a contributory factor to differential block. Nevertheless, when comparisons were made between a wide variety of agents, it was found that *in vitro* blockade of A fibers occurred before that of C fibers with procaine, ropivacaine, and bupivacaine and *vice versa* with tetracaine, etidocaine, and mepivacaine; blockade occurred at the same time with lidocaine. In summarizing the results of their studies, Wildsmith *et al.*[459] noted that equipotent concentrations of the various drugs blocked C fibers at the same rate but that blockade of A fibers was more dependent, as expected, on the physicochemical properties (see above). The contribution of frequency-dependent block to differential nerve block is discussed in Chapter 2.

pH Effects

Any factor that creates local extracellular acidosis should retard net diffusion of local anesthetic to the nerve by increasing and sustaining drug ionization (see equation 5). A low pH may be preexisting, for example, as a result of infection, or may be induced by injection of the anesthetic solution. A number of studies have indicated that raising the pH of local anesthetic solutions to near neutral hastens the onset of effects, sometimes prolongs the duration of effects, and usually decreases the local irritation or pain on injection. Likely effects of the injection on local pH have been reviewed by Rowland,[367] and the mechanisms suggested are summarized in Table 3-4. Of these, movement of carbon dioxide is probably fleeting; dilution of local bicarbonate stores is readily avoided; acidic solutions are rapidly counteracted by the buffer capacity of most tissues; and stabilizers may be circumvented by adding concentrated epinephrine before the injection rather than using a premixed acidic solution. The importance of vasoconstrictor and metabolic effects of epinephrine is indicated by the observation that whereas injection of a plain lidocaine solution lowers tissue pH for 30 minutes, solutions containing epinephrine (5 µg/

TABLE 3-4. *Mechanisms for lowering local extracellular pH by local anesthetic solutions*

Movement of intracellular carbon dioxide into solutions deficient in carbon dioxide
Dilution of local bicarbonate stores by large volumes of solution
Use of acidic solutions
To dissolve agents as their salts (pH 5–7)
To stabilize ester-type agents
To stabilize added epinephrine with addition of sodium bisulfite (pH 3–4)
Effect of added epinephrine, causing local ischemia and increased cellular metabolism

(Data from Rowland, M. Local anesthetic absorption, distribution and elimination. *In* Eger, E. (ed.): Anesthetic Uptake and Action. pp. 332–366. Baltimore, Williams & Wilkins, 1974.)

ml) maintain tissue acidosis for 90 minutes or more. This effect of epinephrine was the same, however, whether the pH was 3.5 or 6.5.[457]

Despite these considerations, it has been shown that the addition of epinephrine to local anesthetic solutions at the time of injection does not prolong the onset of clinical epidural or subarachnoid nerve block with lidocaine or bupivacaine.[83] In fact, with etidocaine, the opposite has been found.[67]

Cohen and colleagues suggested that increasing local acidosis could explain the development of tachyphylaxis to local anesthetics during multidose subarachnoid and epidural block.[100] They showed that repeated spinal injections of local anesthetic solutions in dogs resulted in a progressive decrease in pH of the poorly buffered CSF from pH 7.4 to 6.8. This has been confirmed by others after single doses and would be accompanied by a reduction in the fraction of unionized agent, and hence should decrease access of drug to the site of action (Table 3-5). Tachyphylaxis is not, however, explained adequately by pH effects alone.[266] In sheep, for example, duration of motor block after subarachnoid injections of local anesthetics was either longer or similar and showed a greater frequency when the pH of the solution was decreased from 6.5–7 to 4–4.5, although sensory blockade showed the expected opposite trend.[7,8,15] It has been suggested that tachyphylaxis is not explained by detectable differences in the spread of local anesthetic agent–containing solutions injected epidurally. Mogensen and colleagues[285] reported that neither the distribution of radio-technetium added to epidurally administered lidocaine solutions nor the systemic absorption of lidocaine was altered with four successive injections, despite the development of tachyphylaxis in most of the patients. Unfortunately, this conclusion cannot be substantiated from the experimental design used because the distribution of label and lidocaine may differ and systemic plasma drug concentrations alone do not indicate the absorption rate of local anesthetics administered epidurally.

Replacement of the hydrochloride salt solution of local anesthetic by carbonated solutions should obviate the movement of carbon dioxide out of the nerve. In contrast, rapid penetration of carbon dioxide into the nerve to cause a lowering of intraneural pH could promote a more rapid production of active ionized drug at the point where it is needed.[94] Open clinical studies have shown that carbonation of lidocaine significantly decreases onset time after epidural,[72] caudal,[106] and brachial plexus blocks. However, double-blind investigations, while showing that carbonation improves the quality of epidural analgesia, have not confirmed an effect on the onset of action of lidocaine.[264,286] Similarly, this process does not appear to hasten the effects of bupivacaine after epidural injection,[77] although it does so when this agent is used for brachial plexus block using the interscalene approach.[257]

Metabolism

The evidence suggests that local metabolism has a negligible influence on the neurokinetics of local anesthetics and the time course of conduction blockade. Thus when procaine is incubated with nerve tissue, it is hydrolyzed only to the extent of 2% to 4% per hour, which can be accounted for largely by nonenzymatic breakdown.[313,395] Hydrolysis of ester-type agents in CSF and in the vicinity of the nerve seems to be unimportant clinically, since the pseudocholinesterase activity of CSF was found to be only 1/20 to 1/100 that of plasma[217] and addition of a cholinesterase inhibitor to chloroprocaine solution did not prolong blockade.[255] On the other hand, the pseudocholinesterase activity of CSF of patients known to have recent hemorrhage into the CSF was one-fourth to one-half that of plasma. The dibucaine number of normal CSF is nearly 75% that of plasma while the dibucaine number of CSF subjected to recent hemorrhage is essentially the same as that of plasma.[217] Subarachnoid injection of exogenous cholinesterase has been shown to reverse a tetracaine block in rabbits.[456] Significant local metabolic alteration of the amide-type agents is most unlikely.

SYSTEMIC ABSORPTION

A knowledge of the rates of systemic absorption of local anesthetics helps to set confidence limits on the likelihood of systemic toxic reaction after the various block procedures. Indirectly, these rates suggest also the relationship between block and the amount of drug remaining at the site of injection.

In humans, measurement of drug concentration–time profiles in the peripheral circulation has been widely used to as-

TABLE 3-5. *pH of cerebrospinal fluid in dogs after subarachnoid injection of local anesthetic solutions*

Time after injection (min)	10% Dextrose in saline control (pH 5.5)	5% Lidocaine hydrochloride + 7.5% dextrose (pH 4.5)	0.75% Etidocaine hydrochloride + 5% dextrose (pH 4.2)	2% Procaine hydrochloride (pH 4.2)	4% Tetracaine hydrochloride (pH 4.2)
0	7.41	7.34	7.40	7.36	7.37
2	7.26	6.10	6.20	6.40	6.80
5	7.36	6.40	6.89	6.74	6.93
15		6.90	7.24	7.23	7.10
30		7.10	7.27	7.32	7.21

(Based on unpublished data from L.E. Mather, E. Pavlin, and M. Middaugh, 1975.)

TABLE 3-6. *Relationship between plasma concentrations of local anesthetics after intravenous administration and CNS toxicity*

Agent	Author	Number of subjects	Infusion rate (mg/min)	Infusion time (min)	Number of subjects with symptoms: Subjective[a]	Objective[b]	Convulsions	Plasma drug concentration (mean—range or SD μg/ml)[c]	Sampling site[d]	Assay[e]
Procaine	Usubiaga *et al.* (1966)	5	3–9/kg	To convulsions	5	5	5	38 (21–81) M	V	C
Lidocaine	Foldes *et al.* (1965)	10	0.50/kg	12.8	10	10	1	5.29 ± 0.55 M	V	C
	Jorfeldt *et al.* (1968)	4	0.25/kg	20	Most	Most	1	4.9 M	A	C
	Scott (1975)	5	20	12.5	5	2	0	~2.2 M	V	GC
Mepivacaine	Jorfeldt *et al.* (1968)	11	0.25/kg	20	Most	Most	0	6.0 M	A	C
Bupivacaine	Jorfeldt *et al.* (1968)	5	0.06/kg	20	Some	0	0	2.1 M	A	C
	Mather *et al.* (1971b)	3	Avg. 5.6	14–18	3	0	0	2.6–4.5 M	V	GC
	Scott (1975)	5	10	8–12.5	5	4	0	2.24 ± 0.48 M	V	GC
	Wiklund and Berlin-Wahlen (1977)	7	2	150	6	2	0	~2.3 T	A	GC
	Mather *et al.* (1979)	8	7.5	10	7	0	0	2.2–4.2[f] T	A	GC
	Scott *et al.* (1989)	12	15	to 15	Most	0	0	1.5 ± 0.6 M	V	GC
Ropivacaine	Scott *et al.* (1989)	12	15	to 15	Some	0	0	1.9 ± 0.5 M	V	GC
Etidocaine	Scott (1975)	5	10	12.5	4	0	0	2.27 ± 0.24 M	V	GC
		5	20	6.8–11	5	5	0	~2.2 M	V	GC
	Wiklund and Berlin-Wahlen (1977)	8	2	150	2[g]	0	0	1.96 ± 0.25 M	A	GC
	Mather *et al.* (1979)	8	7.5	10	6	0	0	2.1–5.3[f] T	A	GC

[a] For example, light-headedness, circumoral numbness, disorientation.
[b] For example, muscular twitching, nystagmus, slurred speech.
[c] M, maximum; T, threshold.
[d] V, peripheral venous; A, arterial.
[e] C, colorimetric; GC, gas chromatography.
[f] Venous levels about 50% lower.
[g] Fatigue only.

(Tucker, G.T., and Mather, L.E.: Clinical pharmacokinetics of local anaesthetic agents. Clin. Pharmacokinet, *4*:241, 1979, Foldes, F.F., Davidson, G.E., Duncalf, D., and Kuwabarra, S.: The intravenous toxicity of local anesthetic agents in man. Clin Pharmacol. Ther., *6*:328, 1965.)

sess systemic uptake of the different agents. Because these profiles are the net result of both systemic absorption and disposition, they are of value mainly to determine relative changes in drug uptake. Variables affecting absorption are assumed not to influence disposition. Thus, it is emphasized that measurements of the maximum plasma drug concentration (C_{max}) and the time at which C_{max} occurs (T_{max}) are not absolute indicators of the absorption kinetics of local anesthetic agents administered perineurally. Nevertheless, measures of C_{max} and T_{max} are useful in making clinically relevant comparisons between drugs, between procedures, and between patients.

To assess safety margins, vascular drug concentrations after perineural injection are compared with estimates of threshold values associated with the onset of significant CNS toxicity. These range from 5 to 10 μg/ml plasma for lidocaine and from 2 to 4 μg/ml plasma for bupivacaine (Table 3-6). Although these values are useful guidelines, they refer to the mythical "average subject" and should be interpreted in the light of a number of considerations. These include whether measurements are made of plasma or blood, total or unbound drug, ionized or nonionized species, enantiomers, active drug metabolites, and, most importantly, the rate of drug administration. The values in Table 3-6 are most relevant when concentrations are not changing rapidly and there is time for equilibration between drug concentrations in plasma and in brain. After an accidental intravenous dose the concentrations change rapidly so that those in the blood do not accurately reflect those in the brain.[372] The site of blood sampling (artery or vein) is critical when drug concentrations are changing rapidly.[425,436]

If blood drug concentration–time profiles are available also after intravenous administration, it becomes possible to calculate drug absorption rates by numerical deconvolution.[425]

TABLE 3-7. *Mean fractions and half-lives, characterizing the absorption of lidocaine and bupivacaine after subarachnoid and epidural administration*

	Lidocaine		Bupivacaine	
	Subarachnoid	Epidural	Subarachnoid	Epidural
F_1[a]	—	0.38	0.35	0.29
$T_{1/2}$ fast (min)	—	9.3	50	8
F_2[a]	—	0.58	0.61	0.64
$T_{1/2}$ slow (min)	71	82	408	371
F	1.03	0.96	0.96	0.91

[a] F_1 and F_2 are fractions of the doses absorbed in initial faster and subsequent slower phases proceeding with respective half-lives $T_{1/2}$ fast and $T_{1/2}$ slow. F is total systemic availability compared with intravenous injection.

(Burm, A.G.: Pharmacokinetics and clinical effects of lidocaine and bupivacaine following epidural and subarachnoid administration in man. Ph.D. thesis, University of Leiden, 1985.)

Because local anesthetics are relatively lipid-soluble compounds, their diffusion across the capillary endothelium is not likely to be rate-limiting. Hence their vascular absorption rates will primarily be related directly to blood flow and inversely to local tissue binding.

Important determinants of systemic absorption include the physicochemical and vasoactive properties of the agent, the site of injection, dosage factors, the presence of additives such as vasoconstrictors, other formulation factors intended to modify local drug residence and release, the influence of nerve block, and pathological features of the patient.

Agent

The extensive data on C_{max} and T_{max} of the amide local anesthetics after various routes of injection have been tabulated elsewhere.[436] This shows, for example, that after epidural injection of plain solutions, the increment in peak whole blood drug concentration per 100 mg of dose is about 0.9 to 1.0 μg/ml for lidocaine and mepivacaine, slightly less for prilocaine, and approximately 50% as much for bupivacaine and etidocaine. The increment for ropivacaine appears to be similar to that for bupivacaine.[220] Although differences in disposition kinetics contribute to this order (see below), it appears that, despite similar peak times, net absorption of the long-acting, more lipid-soluble agents is slower. This is consistent with data on residual concentrations of the agents in epidural fat after injection into sheep (Fig. 3-11)[436] and is confirmed by pharmacokinetic calculations of the time course of drug absorption in humans.[86,435] These calculations show that systemic uptake after epidural injection is a biphasic process, the contribution of the initial rapid phase being greater for lidocaine than for the long-acting analogs (Table 3-7; Fig. 3-12). This slower net absorption of the latter compounds adds to their systemic safety margins after accurate injection.

Differences in the absorption rates of the various agents have implications for their accumulation during repeated and continuous administration. Whereas systemic accumulation is most marked with the short-acting amides, extensive local

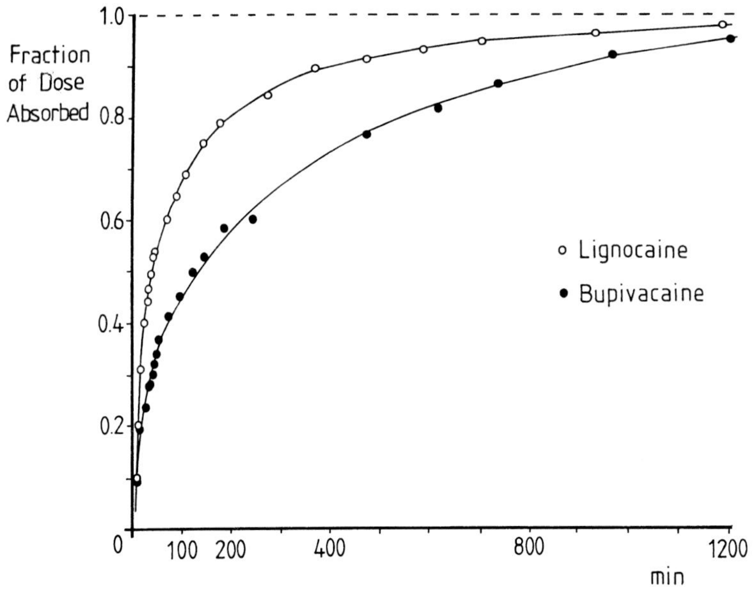

FIG. 3-12. Fraction of dose absorbed into the systemic circulation plotted as a function of time for epidural injection of lidocaine or bupivacaine. The data points represent values obtained by deconvolution of the measured plasma drug concentrations in representative subjects against the intravenous unit impulse curve in each subject. The curves represent biexponential functions fitted to the data points by nonlinear least squares regression. Data from Burm, A.G.L.: Clinical pharmacokinetics of epidural and spinal anaesthesia. Clin. Pharmacokinet., *16*:283, 1989.

accumulation is predicted for the longer-acting compounds, despite their longer dosage intervals.[205,431,433]

Observations of relatively low blood concentrations of prilocaine with respect to the toxic threshold, particularly after brachial plexus block (Fig. 3-13) and intravenous regional anesthesia, support the claim that this compound should be the agent of choice for such single-dose procedures.[463] In this case, however, a high systemic clearance, rather than slow absorption, is responsible mainly for the relatively low blood drug concentrations.

Although the rate of systemic absorption of local anesthetics is controlled largely by the extent of local binding, their intrinsic vasoactive properties could also modulate local perfusion and hence uptake.[21,22,48,151,212] However, the effects are a complex function of drug, dose, enantiomer, and type and tone of blood vessel, and their relevance to the relative absorption of drugs after peripheral and central nerve blocks is difficult to evaluate.[84] Nevertheless, it has been suggested, for example, that an increase in epidural blood flow (whether mediated locally or by change in cardiac output or both), with assumed increase in the systemic absorption rate of bupivacaine, is an important factor leading to regression of analgesia during continuous epidural infusion of

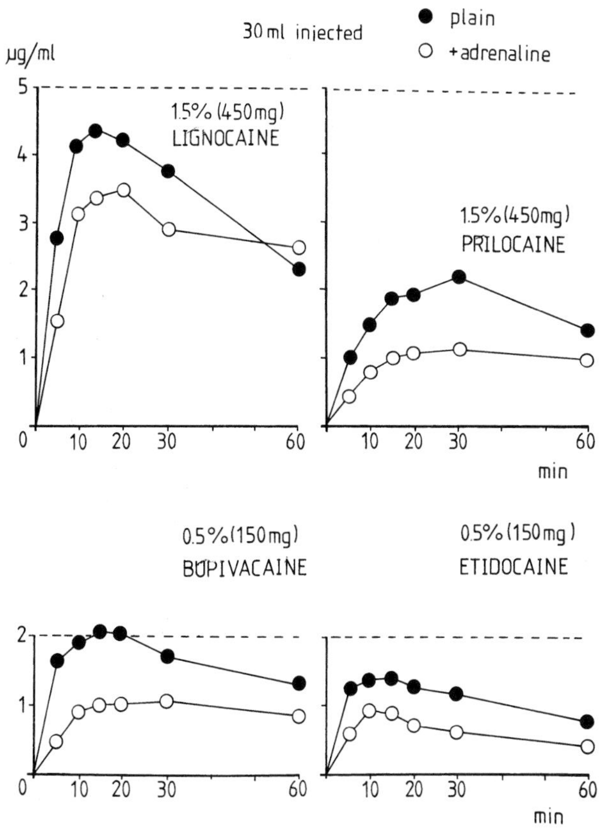

FIG. 3-13. Plasma concentrations of local anesthetic agents after interscalene brachial plexus block (30 ml volume) with or without added epinephrine. Data from Wildsmith, J.A.W., Tucker, G.T., Cooper, S., *et al.*: Plasma concentrations of local anaesthetics after interscalene brachial plexus block. Br. J. Anaesth., *49*:461, 1977.

bupivacaine.[284] Furthermore, the vasodilatory effect of *rac*-bupivacaine on both cutaneous and epidural blood vessels contrasts strikingly with the vasoconstrictor effect of ropivacaine, a difference which may contribute to their relative anesthetic profiles.[116,231] Although *R*(+)-bupivacaine was found to be two to three times more potent than *S*(−)-bupivacaine in blocking nerve fibers *in vitro*,[248] this intrinsic difference in action may be modulated by stereoselective effects of bupivacaine on blood vessels. Thus, the *S* enantiomers of amide local anesthetics are longer acting than their antipodes after subcutaneous injection, reflecting a greater vasoconstrictor activity and, therefore, a presumed slower systemic absorption.[3,12,13,22,151]

Site of Injection

Vascularity and the presence of tissue and fat that can bind local anesthetics are primary influences on their rate of removal from specific sites of injection. In general, and independent of the agent used, absorption rate decreases in the order: intercostal block > caudal block > epidural block > brachial plexus block > sciatic and femoral nerve block (Fig. 3-14).[436]

Intercostal Block

Maximum circulating concentrations of the agents after intercostal blocks using plain solutions may exceed toxic thresholds, but adverse systemic effects in patients, presumably, may be obtunded by light general anesthesia and/or premedication. Since sustained high plasma drug concentrations are achieved during continuous intercostal infusions, supplementary bolus injections are likely to be dangerous.[374]

Epidural Block

The effect of fat deposits within the epidural space in delaying the absorption of local anesthetics has been discussed above. Vascular uptake will take place into the extradural veins and from there to the azygos vein. In the presence of raised intrathoracic pressure, absorbed drug could be redirected also up the internal vertebral venous system to cerebral sinuses (Fig. 3-14). Vascular absorption of local anesthetic from different regions of the epidural space (cervical, lumbar, thoracic) appears to be similar.[276]

As noted above, Mogensen et al.[285] concluded that changes in drug absorption from the epidural space during continuous dosage do not account for tachyphylaxis since they found no time-dependent changes in the epidural distribution of radiocontrast medium nor in the rate of rise of plasma lidocaine after each injection. Unfortunately, neither of these measurements is a valid index of systemic drug absorption rate. However, others have shown that the accumulation of plasma concentrations of lidocaine and etidocaine measured after five successive doses (1- and 2-hour dosage interval, respectively) is predictable from first-dose data.[431]

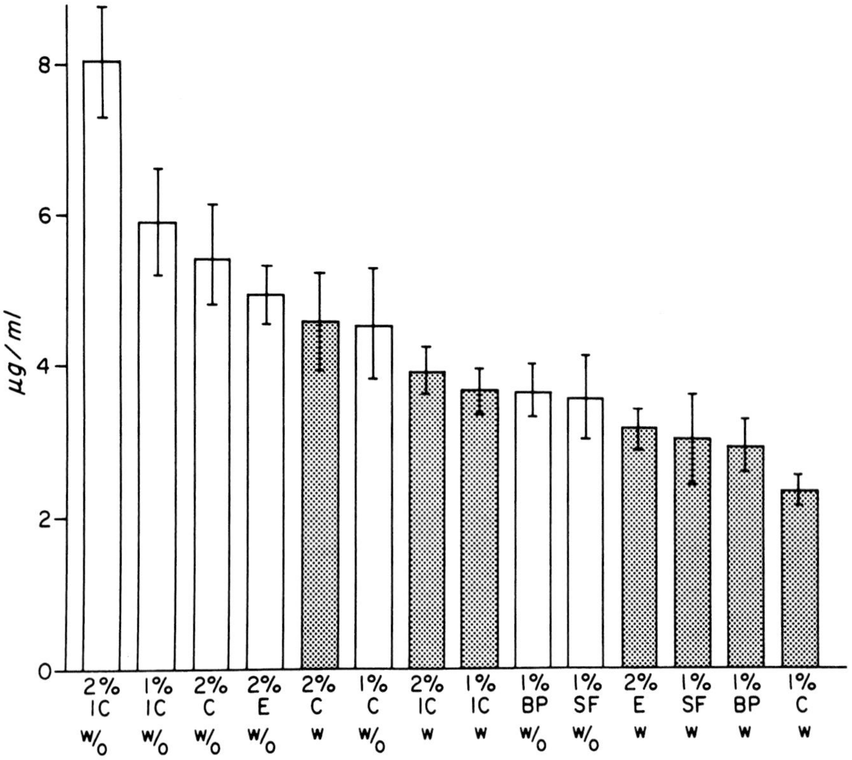

FIG. 3-14. Systemic absorption of mepivacaine in humans after various regional block procedures as indicated by mean maximum plasma drug concentrations. (± SEM) *IC*, intercostal block; *C*, caudal block; *E*, epidural block; *BP*, brachial plexus block; *SF*, sciatic/femoral block; *w/o*, solution without epinephrine; *w*, plus epinephrine 1:200,000 *(stippled blocks)*. (Tucker, G.T., Moore, D.C. Bridenbaugh, P.O., et al.: Systemic absorption of mepivacaine in commonly used regional block procedures. Anesthesiology, 37:277, 1972.)

Subarachnoid Block

Systemic uptake after subarachnoid injection is believed to occur predominantly after passage of drug across the dura into the more vascular epidural space,[99] as well as from blood vessels within the spinal space, in the pia mater, and in the cord itself (Fig. 3-10). Extensive diffusion into the epidural space would be expected to result in sequestration in fat, thereby retarding the absorption of the longer-acting agents to a greater extent than the shorter-acting ones. Deconvolution analysis shows that there are differences in the pattern of systemic absorption after subarachnoid and epidural injection, and confirms that there is a slower net absorption of bupivacaine compared to lidocaine (Table 3-7). The slower initial uptake from the subarachnoid space may reflect delay imposed by dural diffusion. The similarity of the slower uptake phase for subarachnoid bupivacaine and the overall monoexponential uptake of subarachnoid lidocaine with the corresponding slow phases of uptake after epidural injection suggests a common rate-limiting removal from epidural fat.

Brachial Plexus Block

The various techniques for blocking the brachial plexus are not associated with significant differences in local anesthetic absorption rate.[259,453]

Plasma concentrations of prilocaine after multiple injections for brachial plexus block were found to be predictable from first-dose data.[246]

Intravenous Regional Anesthesia

A pharmacokinetic analysis of plasma lidocaine concentrations measured after intravenous regional anesthesia[428] indicated that, if the cuff is inflated correctly for at least 10 minutes after injection, only about 20 to 30% of the dose enters the systemic circulation during the first minute after cuff release. This is consistent with the observation that only about 12% of the dose can be aspirated from veins shortly after injection.[109] The bulk of the dose remains in arm tissue, 50% remaining in the limb 30 minutes after cuff release.[428] Direct experimental support for this comes from observations of sustained high concentrations of local anesthetic in the venous drainage from the blocked arm after cuff release.[148] Longer application of the cuff delays wash-out of drug from the arm.[428] Intermittent deflation of the cuff for 10 to 30 seconds followed by reinflation appears to have little effect on the ultimate maximum plasma drug concentration but does prolong the time to maximum concentration.[405]

Endotracheal and Endobronchial Administration

Endotracheal doses of lidocaine up to 400 mg are associated with plasma drug concentrations which are well below the toxic threshold.[436] The concentrations are significantly lower in spontaneously breathing patients than in paralyzed patients since the former are more likely to swallow some of the dose, which then undergoes first-pass hepatic metabolism following absorption from the gut.[383] Application only to areas below the vocal cords may result in excessive plasma drug concentrations because of reduced transfer to the gut.[112] Plasma concentrations of lidocaine were found to be significantly lower when using an ultrasonic nebulizer compared to a conventional spray.[241]

Systemic absorption of local anesthetic from the respiratory tree is biphasic; an initial very rapid peak is followed by a second one at 5 to 30 minutes. The first phase appears to be less prominent after deep endobronchial administration of lidocaine compared to endotracheal instillation.[341]

Interpleural Block

Exposure of drug to a relatively large surface area of tissue, resulting in rapid systemic drug absorption, emphasizes the potentially small safety margin of this technique. Maximum plasma concentrations of bupivacaine are higher but occur later than when the same dose is injected for intercostal block.[448] Dosage and plasma drug concentrations measured after interpleural injection of bupivacaine vary widely among studies. However, in patients undergoing cholecystectomy or laparotomy, van Kleef et al.[449] advocate the use of an initial bolus dose of 100 mg followed by continuous infusion of 5 ml/h of 0.25% bupivacaine with epinephrine. This has been shown to be safe, with no further gain in analgesic effect on increasing the dose. Although Laurito et al.[245] observed that plasma bupivacaine concentrations often increased above the putative toxic threshold of 2 μg/ml using the same infusion rate as van Kleef et al.,[449] no adverse effects were observed since this probably reflects the postoperative rise in plasma drug binding. In contrast to van Kleef et al.[449] and Laurito et al.[245] who measured continually rising plasma drug concentrations throughout prolonged infusion, Kastrissios et al.[218] observed a steady state.

Subcutaneous Infiltration

The subcutaneous infiltration of large doses of lidocaine is an essential component of the technique of liposuction. When properly applied, the procedure is associated with remarkably slow systemic drug absorption. Thus, Klein[228] indicates 35 mg/kg as a conservative estimate of the safe maximum dose, based on the observation of maximum plasma drug concentrations well below the toxic threshold at 10 to 15 hours after injection. He emphasizes the use of a dilute solution with added epinephrine, injected slowly over 45 minutes. Injection of large doses over less than 5 minutes results in dangerously rapid drug absorption. About 30% of the dose of lidocaine is recovered with the removal of the subcutaneous fat tissue.

Dosage Factors

Concentration and Volume

There is some evidence that the absorption rates of local anesthetics after central and peripheral nerve blocks and after intravenous regional anesthesia are faster from concentrated solutions than from more dilute solutions containing the same dose (Fig. 3-14).[428,438] These differences presumably reflect saturation of local binding sites and/or greater vasodilator effects produced by more concentrated solutions. Both of these mechanisms should result in disproportionate increases in plasma drug concentrations when concentration and mass of drug are increased but volume is held constant. Up to a 300-mg epidural dose (constant volume) of etidocaine, plasma concentrations increase linearly with dose, but beyond this they become disproportionately higher.[66,256]

Speed of Injection

Compared to epidural injections given over 1 minute, those injected in 15 seconds resulted in 16% higher maximum plasma concentrations of lidocaine.[382] Plasma bupivacaine concentrations were not influenced by varying epidural injection speed from 20 to 100 seconds.[358]

Perivascular axillary injection of mepivacaine as a divided dose with an interval of 20 minutes resulted in slightly lower plasma drug concentrations up to 90 minutes than those after a single bolus dose, with no difference in sensory or motor blockade.[454] In contrast, the staged administration of an epidural injection of bupivacaine in two aliquots given 15 seconds apart resulted in a prolongation of block, although again there was only a trend for a decrease in the maximum plasma drug concentration.[390]

Additives

Vasoconstrictors

Vasoconstrictor agents are often added to local anesthetic solutions to slow the systemic absorption rate, thereby prolonging duration of action and increasing the intensity of neural blockade.

The degree to which epinephrine decreases the systemic absorption rate of local anesthetic is a complex function of the type, dose, and concentration of local anesthetic and of the characteristics of the injection site. Although peak plasma concentrations of local anesthetics after most of the common regional blocks are lowered by epinephrine, it does not always prolong the time to peak.[436] In general, the greatest effects are seen after intercostal blocks (Fig. 3-14) and with short-acting rather than long-acting agents. This suggests that the greater local binding of the latter tends to offset the vasoconstriction caused by epinephrine. These differences also seem to extend to subarachnoid block. Thus, the addition of epinephrine to hyperbaric lidocaine solutions lowers peak plasma drug concentration by 30 to 50%, without altering the time to peak,[27,86] whereas addition to hyperbaric bupivacaine has no significant effect on plasma concentrations of the local anesthetic.[86]

In addition to local binding the inherent vasoactivity of local anesthetics may modulate the vasoconstrictor effect of epinephrine on systemic drug absorption. Thus, vasoconstrictor effects would be expected to augment or override the action of epinephrine at low concentrations of local anesthetic and antagonize it at high concentrations associated with vasodilation. This might explain why epinephrine has a greater influence on peak plasma concentrations of prilocaine as the epidural dose is raised from 400 to 900 mg.[61,62] A lack of influence of epinephrine on plasma concentrations of ropivacaine after brachial plexus injection[193] might reflect the potent vasoconstrictor effect of this agent overriding that of added epinephrine. Paradoxically, the combined intradermal injection of ropivacaine and epinephrine resulted in less vasoconstriction than injection of epinephrine alone.[95] This antiepinephrine effect of ropivacaine would be consistent with a tendency toward longer duration of nerve blockade observed with plain compared to epinephrine solutions after brachial plexus injection.[192]

Studies of lidocaine and prilocaine[62,382] suggest that the use of epinephrine concentrations greater than 5 μg/ml produces only marginally greater decreases in maximum plasma local anesthetic concentration and should, therefore, be avoided in view of side effects associated with excessive systemic levels of epinephrine.[132] However, although a concentration of 5 μg/ml epinephrine is commonly employed, the decrease in peak plasma lidocaine concentrations after epidural injection has been shown to be independent of epinephrine concentration between 1.7 and 5 μg/ml.[321] The effect of epinephrine on plasma lidocaine concentrations was shown to be attenuated considerably during continuous epidural infusion compared to that observed after the initial loading injection.[408]

Alternative vasopressor agents to epinephrine include octapressin[229] and the pure alpha-adrenoceptor agonist phenylephrine. Addition of the latter, at a concentration of 50 μg/ml, to lidocaine for epidural block was found to be less effective than epinephrine (5 μg/ml) in lowering blood concentrations of the local anesthetic.[398] Phenylephrine had no effect on lidocaine absorption after subarachnoid injection in monkeys, yet it prolonged neural blockade.[130] Like epinephrine, phenylephrine prolongs useful clinical blockade after spinal tetracaine[23,103] possibly because of alpha-agonist activity at spinal regions involved in antinociception.

Alkalinization and Carbonation

Alkalinization of lidocaine solutions for epidural anesthesia was found to have no effect on plasma concentrations of the local anesthetic.[133] However, studies of intravenous (IV) regional anesthesia in dogs have shown that the release of bupivacaine into the circulation after deflation of the tourniquet is slowed significantly by prior IV injection of sodium bicarbonate into the occluded limb.[135] The effect of the latter is presumably to correct the acidosis caused by ischemia, thereby facilitating tissue uptake of the lidocaine.

Depot Formulations

As discussed previously, several delivery systems have been shown to prolong epidural and subarachnoid block in animals by providing a depot from which local anesthetic is slowly released. This slow local release should also be accompanied by a decrease in the rate of systemic drug absorption. Thus, lower and more prolonged plasma concentrations of lidocaine and bupivacaine have been measured in animals after injection of liposomal and other formulations compared to aqueous solutions.[57,147,247,249,265,379] Furthermore, Boogaerts et al.[55] demonstrated that this is accompanied by less risk of systemic toxicity.

In humans, dextran (6%–10%) has been shown to attenuate markedly the systemic absorption rate of lidocaine and epinephrine after injection into the scalp.[6,443]

Factors Related to Nerve Block

The hypotension that may accompany epidural anesthesia might prolong the duration of blockade owing to decreased perfusion of the epidural space and a slower systemic uptake of local anesthetic. This is supported by the observation that prophylactic subcutaneous or intravenous injection of ephedrine results in shorter durations of anesthesia and elevated blood concentrations of some local anesthetic agents.[143,275]

Physical and Pathophysiological Factors

An overview of the influence of some patient-related variables on the disposition of the principal local anesthetic agents is given in Table 3-9.

Weight and Height

In adults, plasma concentrations of local anesthetics after epidural and other nerve blocks are correlated poorly with body weight and height.[292,293,334,382,438]

Age

The effects of old age on the duration of nerve block and their mechanisms are unclear. For example, Veering and colleagues[451,452] observed decreased duration of subarachnoid and epidural block with increase in age, whereas Nydahl et al.[315] reported the opposite finding after epidural injection. On the basis that the rate of the late phase of bupivacaine absorption after subarachnoid block increased with age (22–81 years) although no change in absorption occurred after epidural block, Veering et al.[451,452] suggested that the increased duration of analgesia in elderly patients that they observed reflected changes in pharmacodynamics or local disposition rather than changes in systemic drug absorption. In contrast, a faster systemic absorption rate in elderly patients would be compatible with the data of Nydahl et al.[315]

Limited data are available in infants and children which indicate somewhat faster systemic absorption of local anesthetics than in adults.[64,140,149,150,361,407,436]

Pregnancy

Although engorgement of vertebral veins and a hyperkinetic circulation might be expected to enhance absorption of local anesthetics after epidural block, plasma drug concentration–time profiles appear to be similar in pregnant and nonpregnant women.[296,335]

Disease and Surgery

Changes in local perfusion associated with altered hemodynamics as a result of disease or surgery may modify absorption of local anesthetics and hence duration of anesthesia. For example, acute hypovolemia slows lidocaine absorption after epidural injection in dogs[297] and prolongs anesthesia in patients undergoing thoracotomy with regional block.[342] Conversely, a decreased duration of brachial plexus block in patients with chronic renal failure was suggested to reflect a hyperkinetic circulation and enhanced systemic uptake of local anesthetic.[73] However, this hypothesis is not supported by the results of subsequent studies.[348]

SYSTEMIC DISPOSITION

After absorption from the site of administration, local anesthetic drugs are distributed by the bloodstream to the organs and tissues of the body and cleared, mostly by metabolism and to a small extent by renal excretion. In pregnant women a small proportion of the dose also crosses the placenta into the fetus.

DISTRIBUTION

The Role of the Lung

The first capillary bed to be exposed to local anesthetic once it has entered the systemic circulation is that in the lung. This structure acts as a capacitor, sequestering temporarily a large quantity of drug because of a high lung:blood partition coefficient. Hence, after rapid intravenous input, the arterial blood drug concentration which hits the target organs for toxicity, the brain and the heart (via the coronary circulation), is attenuated considerably compared with the drug concentration in the pulmonary artery (Fig. 3-15).[215,254,428]

Arthur[24] has shown that lung uptake of prilocaine in humans exceeds that of lidocaine and this contributes to its greater systemic safety margin. Others have also found a greater uptake of prilocaine than of mepivacaine and bupivacaine in the isolated perfused rat lung, with little evidence of pulmonary metabolism.[171] The rank order of uptake in rat lung slices was found to be bupivacaine > etidocaine > lidocaine.[337]

The extravascular pH of the lung is low relative to plasma pH and this encourages ion trapping of local anesthetic.[338] Conversely, a relative decrease in plasma pH impairs uptake.[322] Other basic drugs, such as propranolol, may compete with local anesthetics for pulmonary binding sites,

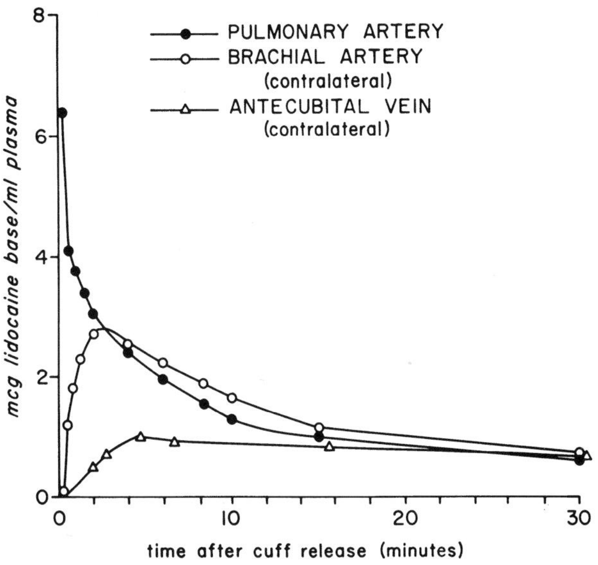

FIG. 3-15. Plasma lidocaine levels in a subject following cuff release after intravenous regional anesthesia with 3 mg/kg lidocaine hydrochloride (0.5% solution; 45 minutes cuff time). (Tucker, G.T., and Boas, R.A.: Pharmacokinetic aspects of intravenous regional anesthesia. Anesthesiology, 34:538, 1971.)

thereby decreasing their first-pass extraction.[363] Similarly, a bolus injection of bupivacaine has been shown to displace lidocaine from rabbit lung.[320] General anesthesia and severe respiratory deficiency do not appear to have a marked effect on the pulmonary extraction of local anaesthetics.[216]

Local anesthetic drugs injected into patients with intracardiac right-left shunts,[53] or injected inadvertently into the carotid or vertebral artery during attempted stellate ganglion block, bypass the lung, resulting in a high probability of CNS toxicity. Furthermore, Aldrete et al.[14,15] have shown that the introduction of local anesthetics, under pressure, into the lingual, brachial, or femoral artery of baboons and the facial artery of dogs can produce a retrograde flow facilitating direct access of high concentrations of drug to the cerebral circulation.

Blood Binding

The long-acting amides are bound in plasma to a greater extent than the short-acting ones (Table 3-8), and binding decreases at total plasma concentrations above about 2 μg/ml (Fig. 3-16). There are two main classes of binding sites: a high-affinity, low-capacity site on alpha$_1$-acid glycoprotein and a quantitatively less important low-affinity, high-capacity site on albumin.[126,233,269,274,332,364,429]

The extent of binding varies with the plasma concentration of alpha$_1$-acid glycoprotein, and both are elevated considerably in patients with cancer,[207] chronic pain,[167] trauma,[142] inflammatory disease[80] and uremia,[177] and in postoperative[189] and post–myocardial infarction patients[30] (Fig. 3-17). Low plasma concentrations of alpha$_1$-acid gly-

TABLE 3-8. *Pharmacokinetic variables describing the disposition kinetics of amide-type local anesthetics in adult males*

	Prilocaine	Lidocaine	Mepivacaine	Ropivacaine	Bupivacaine	Etidocaine
λ	1.1	0.8	0.9	0.7	0.6	0.6
F_u	0.45	0.30	0.20	0.05	0.05	0.06
$V_{ss}{}^a$ (liters)	191	91	84	61	73	134
Vu_{ss} (liters)	?	253	382	742	1028	1478
CL^a (liters/min)	2.37	0.95	0.78	0.73	0.58	1.11
E_H	?	0.65	0.52	0.49	0.38	0.74
$t_{1/2,z}$(h)	1.6	1.6	1.9	1.9	2.7	2.7
MBRT(h)	1.3	1.6	1.8	1.4	2.1	2.0

[a] Specified with respect to arterial total blood drug concentrations, with the exception of prilocaine data, which are specified with respect to peripheral venous blood drug concentration.

Key: λ, blood/plasma concentration ratio; V_{ss}, volume of distribution at steady state; Vu_{ss}, volume of distribution at steady state based on unbound drug concentrations in plasma water; CL, mean total body clearance; E_H, estimated hepatic extraction ratio; $t_{1/2,z}$, terminal "elimination" half-life; MBRT, mean body retention time.

[Tucker, G.T.: Pharmacokinetics of local anaesthetics: Role in toxicity. In Scott, D.B., McClure, J., and Wildsmith, J.A.W. (eds.): Regional Anaesthesia 1884–1984. pp. 61–71. Sodertalje, ICM AB, 1984; Lee, A., Fagan, D., Lamont, M., Tucker G.T., Halldin M., and Scott, D.B.: Disposition kinetics of ropivacaine in humans. Anesth. Analg (Cleve.), *69*:736, 1989.]

coprotein in neonates are associated with much lower binding of local anesthetics compared with that in adult plasma.[331,333,430,471] The plasma concentration of alpha$_1$-acid glycoprotein increases while the free fraction of lidocaine decreases from early infancy to adolescence.[252] In healthy adults, increasing age is not associated with a change in alpha$_1$-acid glycoprotein levels or in the extent of plasma binding of local anesthetic.[452] One study suggested an increase in plasma lidocaine binding in smokers,[262] but this has not been confirmed by others.[120] Most studies indicate lower plasma binding of local anesthetics during pregnancy and at term.[165,471,472] Decreases in binding may also occur acutely during and shortly after surgery.[373] This may be due to competition for binding sites by temporarily increased plasma concentrations of free fatty acids or disturbances to acid-base or electrolyte status. Binding decreases significantly as pH decreases.[28,89,110,261] The plasma protein binding of *R*(+)-bupivacaine was found to be greater than that of

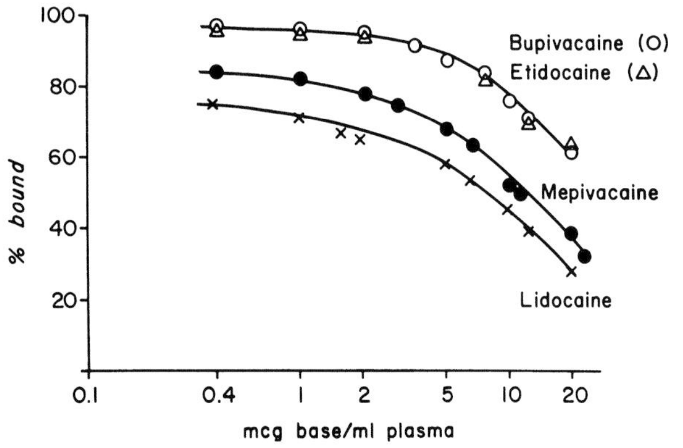

FIG. 3-16. Plasma binding of amide-type local anesthetics. (Tucker, G.T., and Mather, L.E.: Pharmacokinetics of local anaesthetic agents. Br. J. Anaesth., *47*::213, 1975.)

S(−)-bupivacaine in sheep plasma and less than that of *S*(−)-bupivacaine in plasma from healthy human subjects.[85,373]

The order of binding of local anesthetics to sites in or on erythrocytes is similar to that for plasma binding.[429] However, in the presence of plasma proteins, plasma binding competes with binding to the red cells. Hence, blood:plasma drug concentration ratios are related inversely to plasma binding (Table 3-8).

The role of plasma binding in local anesthetic toxicity has been discussed by Tucker.[426] It is important to allow for this phenomenon when interpreting measurements of plasma drug concentrations. For example, marked accumulation of total plasma drug concentrations postoperatively[349,360] may not signify a risk of toxicity. This change reflects the postoperative increase in alpha$_1$-acid glycoprotein and therefore plasma drug binding. Unbound (active) drug concentrations, which are likely to be a better index of effect, are similar before and after surgery (Fig. 3-18). When systemic drug input is gradual, as after perineural injection, distribution of the dose is spread over time and a large extravascular distribution space and extensive tissue binding (see below) ensures that only a small percentage remains in the blood. Under these conditions, any changes in plasma binding are buffered effectively by a high volume of distribution. Also, for drugs like bupivacaine, that have a relatively low hepatic extraction ratios, any increase in free drug concentration will be compensated by a faster elimination.

Theoretically, plasma binding could limit the first-pass uptake of local anesthetic into the brain and myocardium following rapid, inadvertent, intravenous injection, thereby modulating toxicity. However, it is likely that a toxic dose, delivered rapidly, would produce sufficiently high local blood drug concentrations to overwhelm the blood binding capacity on first pass through the brain and heart. Further-

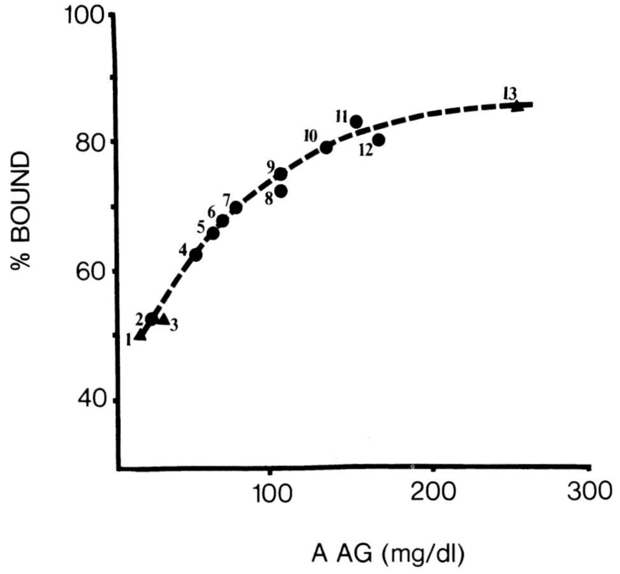

FIG. 3-17. Relation between the mean percentage of lidocaine bound and the concentration of alpha$_1$-acid glycoprotein in plasma in various clinical conditions. ●, patient group data; ▲, individual patient data; 1, patient with nephrotic syndrome; 2, neonates; 3, patient with carcinoma of prostate receiving high-dose estrogens; 4, females on oral contraceptives; 5, women under 40 years; 6, men under 40 years; 7, adults over 70 years; 8, epileptic subjects; 9, renal transplantation patients; 10, chronic renal failure patients; 11, cancer patients; 12, myocardial infarction patients; 13, patient with myocardial infarction. (Data from Jackson, P.R., Tucker, G.T., and Woods, H.F.: Altered plasma binding in cancer. Role of alpha$_1$-acid glycoprotein and albumin. Clin. Pharmacol. Ther., *32*:295, 1982; and Routledge, P.A., Stargel, W.W., Barchowsky, A., *et al.*: Control of lidocaine therapy: new perspectives. Ther. Drug. Monit., *4*:265, 1982.)

more, studies of the initial brain uptake of local anesthetics in rats indicate that there is an enhanced dissociation from plasma binding sites in the microcirculation.[414] The latter observation contrasts with findings in the dog, showing that at a few minutes after rapid intravenous injection of lidocaine, the extent of drug distribution into brain tissue and CSF was entirely governed by the equilibrium free concentration of drug in plasma.[263] Therefore, it appears important to distinguish events after even a few recirculations from those during first pass through an organ. In either case it should not be assumed that plasma binding modulates the extent of tissue drug uptake, thereby "protecting" against toxicity. A careful distinction should be made between the consequences of a change in free *fraction* and changes in free drug *concentration*.[426]

Tissue Distribution

In the amide series of local anesthetics, a greater extent of plasma binding is accompanied by a parallel increase in affinity for tissue components. Thus, steady-state volumes of distribution based on unbound drug in plasma (Vu_{ss}), which reflect net tissue binding, vary over a fivefold range, being greatest for the more lipid-soluble agents (Table 3-8). Distribution volumes based on total drug concentration in blood vary only twofold reflecting the balance between blood and tissue binding. Differences in tissue:blood partition coefficients of the enantiomers of local anesthetics, and hence volumes of distribution based on total drug concentration, may be explained by stereoselectivity in plasma binding rather than in tissue binding.[85,371]

The rate of tissue uptake of local anesthetic is not reflected accurately in either arterial or venous drug concentrations. Thus, in sheep the calculated time course of mean myocardial lidocaine concentration was found to be intermediate between those in arterial and coronary sinus blood.[199,200] Similarly, the time course of myocardial depressant effects are better correlated with those of the calculated myocardial drug concentrations than with those of arterial or coronary sinus blood drug concentrations.[199,200] The greater cardiotoxicity of bupivacaine and ropivacaine compared to lidocaine is not explained by a greater fraction of the dose partitioning into the myocardium[304]; similarly the greater toxicity of *R*(+)-bupivacaine compared to *S*(−)-bupivacaine is not adequately explained by stereoselectivity in myocardial drug uptake in the isolated perfused rabbit heart.[277]

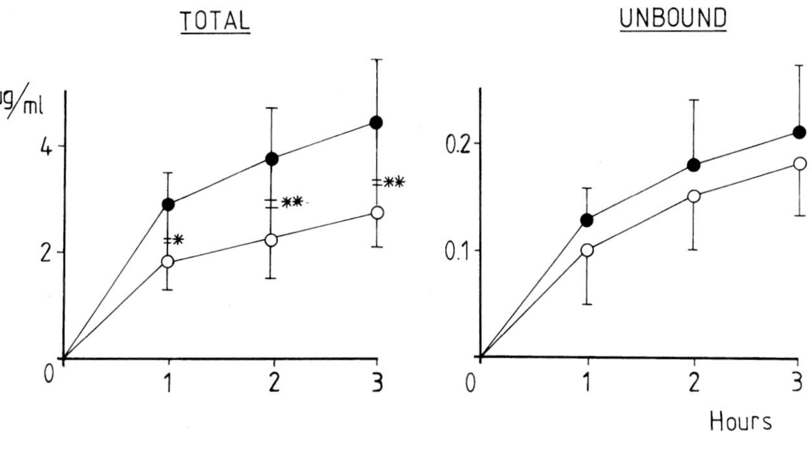

FIG. 3-18. Mean total and unbound plasma concentrations of bupivacaine during intravenous infusions of 2 mg/min of bupivacaine HCl in seven cholecystectomy patients studied 3 hours before surgery (○) and 72 hours postoperatively (●). Total concentrations differ but unbound concentrations do not.

EXCRETION

Renal excretion of unchanged local anesthetics is a minor route of elimination, accounting for less than 1 to 6% of the dose under normal conditions.[435] Depending on the agent, acidification of the urine increases this proportion to 5–20%, which is consistent with less tubular reabsorption as a result of greater ionization. However, this increase is insufficient to warrant the use of a forced acid diuresis in treating toxicity.

Secretion of unchanged local anesthetics down the pH gradient between blood and gastric juice is also a potential route of excretion. However, most of the drug that appears in the stomach contents is subsequently reabsorbed from the intestine and undergoes first-pass metabolism in the liver. Although evacuation of stomach contents has been advocated for treatment of local anesthetic toxicity, especially in neonates,[119] it is unlikely that this is of value. Gastric juice:blood drug concentration ratios may be high, but the proportion of the dose recycled by way of the stomach is unlikely to be significant.

METABOLISM

Esters

Clearance

These compounds are cleared in both the blood and the liver. *In vitro* half-lives in plasma reflect the action of pseudocholinesterase (Fig. 3-19) and in normal adults they vary from 10 to 20 seconds for chloroprocaine[237,316] to 40 seconds for procaine[138,347] to several minutes for tetracaine[162]

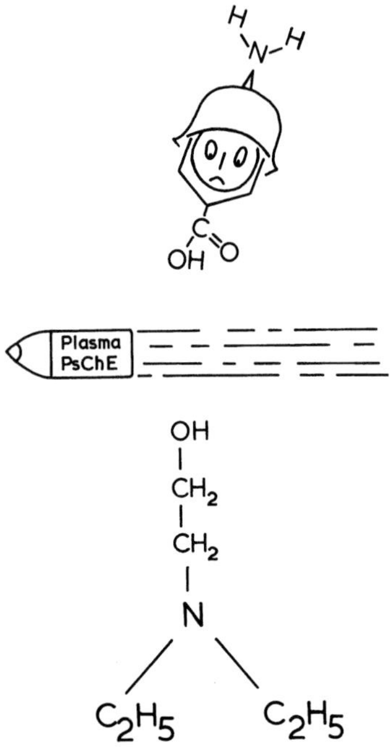

FIG. 3-19. Hydrolysis of procaine. (Tucker, G.T.: Biotransformation and toxicity of local anaesthetics. Acta Anaesthesiol. Belg., 26*[Suppl.]*:123, 1975)

(Table 3-9). Red cell esterases contribute also to blood clearance.[91]

In vivo half-lives are longer than those measured *in vitro* (*e.g.*, that of chloroprocaine after epidural injection is about 3 min).[237] However, this value probably reflects rate-limiting re-distribution from tissue rather than metabolic clearance. After high intravenous doses of procaine, clearances of 0.04 to 0.08 L/min/kg and elimination half-lives of 7 to 8 minutes have been observed, probably reflecting some saturation of the enzyme systems.[384] The clinical implication of the rapid clearance of the esters is that if a toxic concentration is attained after inadvertent intravenous injection, the ensuing reaction should be relatively short-lived. Values of the mean plasma elimination half-life of cocaine in humans vary from 40 to 150 minutes.[32,209]

Metabolites

The hydrolysis products of procaine, chloroprocaine, and tetracaine have been measured in human plasma but appear to be inactive pharmacologically,[68,235,238,280,316] although the aminobenzoic acids may contribute to the rare allergic reaction. The main routes of metabolism of cocaine in humans are ester hydrolysis and N-demethylation.[38] The former involves loss of the methyl group to give benzoylecgonine, enzymatic loss of the benzoyl group in plasma and liver yielding ecgonine methyl ester, and further hydrolysis of both of these compounds to ecgonine. Norcocaine, the product of N-demethylation, undergoes an analogous series of hydrolysis steps.[400,401] Of these metabolites, only norcocaine is believed to have significant pharmacological activity, but it is not a major product.[190,305] N-oxidized products of norcocaine are proposed as hepatotoxic metabolites.[230,351]

Amides

Clearance

The amide linkage is stable in blood, and most of the clearance of these agents occurs in the liver. Mean blood clearance values vary in the order: bupivacaine < ropivacaine < mepivacaine (reflecting the size of the N-methyl substituent in this homologous series) < lidocaine < etidocaine < prilocaine (Table 3-8). Over the whole series, there is no relationship to anesthetic potency, lipid solubility, or protein binding. Etidocaine clearance is dependent mostly on liver perfusion, whereas that of bupivacaine should be more sensitive to changes in intrinsic hepatic enzyme function. The clearance of lidocaine, which has an intermediate extraction ratio, should be dependent on both hepatic perfusion and enzyme activity.[425] Although clearance of etidocaine is twice that of bupivacaine and they are intrinsically equitoxic, any advantage this might offer for etidocaine is offset by the fact that twice the dose is needed to establish the same quality of sensory block as that produced by bupivacaine. The blood clearance of prilocaine exceeds liver blood flow indicating that some extrahepatic metabolism of this drug oc-

TABLE 3-9. *In vitro plasma $t_{1/2}$s of chloroprocaine and procaine (sec ± SD)*

	Author	Reference	Normals[a]	Pregnant	Liver disease	Renal disease	Pulmonary disease	Heart failure	Neonates
Chloroprocaine	Finster *et al.* (1973)	159	21 ± 2 (M) 25 ± 1 (F)						43 ± 2
Procaine	Reidenberg *et al.* (1972)	347	39 ± 8		138 ± 54	84 ± 50			84 ± 30
	DuSouich and Erill (1977)	138	43 ± 6				83 ± 16	92 ± 11	

[a] M, male; F, female.

Tucker, G.T., and Mather, L.E.: Clinical pharmacokinetics of local anaesthetic agents. Clin. Pharmacokinet., *4*:241, 1979.

curs. There is also evidence, from studies in anhepatic patients, that some of the N-deethylation of lidocaine may occur at extrahepatic sites.[375] There is also evidence that N-deethylation of lidocaine can take place in microsomes from rat lung and, to a lesser extent, from rat kidney.[412] Other studies have found that, *in vivo*, bupivacaine and ropivacaine clearance is essentially confined to the liver in sheep.[370,372]

The mean terminal elimination half-lives and mean body residence times are between 1.5 and 3 hours for all of the agents in humans, reflecting a balance between their distribution and clearance characteristics (Table 3-8). In humans, the total plasma clearance of *R*(+)-bupivacaine, the enantiomer intrinsically more toxic to the heart[447] and brain,[267] is about 20% to 30% greater than that of *S*(−)-bupivacaine.[85,270] Estimates of the relative unbound clearances of the enantiomers differ markedly. Whereas Burm et al.[85] reported less extensive plasma binding of *R*(+)-bupivacaine compared to *S*(−)-bupivacaine and a lower clearance of unbound drug, Blake et al.[49] found that both the total and unbound clearances of *R*(+)-bupivacaine exceeded those of *S*(−)-bupivacaine. However, because of enantiomeric differences in plasma binding, the order of unbound clearances of the isomers is reversed.[85] *R*(−)-mepivacaine is more toxic than *S*(+)-mepivacaine in animals,[3] yet appears to be cleared twice as fast in humans.[455] Since the systemic clearances of *S*(+)- and *R*(−)-prilocaine are similar, and the isomers have comparable anesthetic activity and acute toxicity in animals, a higher margin for systemic CNS toxicity is not likely to be achieved by substituting racemic prilocaine with one of its enantiomers.[437]

With the increasing use of techniques involving the prolonged administration of local anesthetics, it is important to assess any dose or time dependence in their systemic clearance. Under these conditions, the site of injection and drug absorption rate have no effect on the eventual steady-state plasma drug concentration. Following short-term intermittent epidural injections of lidocaine and etidocaine given over 5 to 10 hours, increases in plasma drug concentration were consistent with single-dose data.[431] As discussed previously, following more prolonged administration in postoperative patients, a time-dependent decrease in systemic clearance (based upon measurement of total bound plus free plasma drug concentration) is expected as levels of alpha$_1$-acid glycoprotein and plasma binding increase. In addition, there is evidence, mostly from animal studies, for a progressive decrease in the intrinsic ability of hepatic enzymes to clear lidocaine,[250,411] mepivacaine, and bupivacaine,[267,279] presumed to be due to product inhibition by metabolite(s). However, evidence that bupivacaine showed no time-dependent decrease in clearance when infused intravenously for 24 hours in sheep[370] is consistent with recent observations that the plasma concentrations of bupivacaine measured during prolonged interpleural infusion indicated no decrease in clearance with time: Such evidence is not consistent with either time-dependent increase in plasma binding or decrease in intrinsic hepatic clearance.[218,381] On the contrary, mobilization of patients at the end of the treatment period appears to be associated with an increase in the clearance of bupivacaine[381] perhaps mediated by a redistribution of cardiac output between central and peripheral pools.

Metabolites

Identification of the biotransformation products of the amides in human urine indicates three major sites of metabolic attack, namely aromatic hydroxylation, N-dealkylation, and amide hydrolysis[329,357,410,411,436] (Table 3-10). Monoethylgylcinexylidide (MEGX), glycinexylidide (GX), and the 4-hydroxy products formed from lidocaine and bupivacaine; pipecolylxylidide (PPX) from mepivacaine, ropivacaine, and bupivacaine; and the monodealkylated derivatives of etidocaine have all been measured in human plasma. Of these products, it is likely that MEGX contributes to the systemic effects of the parent drug. On continuous infusion, unbound plasma concentrations of MEGX are 70% of those of lidocaine,[136] and studies in rodents indicate that it is about 70% as toxic.[52] Plasma concentrations of PPX of about one third those of parent bupivacaine have been observed on continuous infusion of the latter.[357] This metabolite has about half the cardiotoxic potency of bupivacaine in the rat.[354] Additional biotransformation products of the piperidine amides include isomeric piperidine ring hydroxylation products and their possible conjugates.[436]

Studies using human liver microsomes and recombinant cytochromes P450 indicate that the N-dealkylation of lidocaine to MEGX and of ropivacaine to PPX is mediated by the CYP3A4 isoform.[31,319] The 3′-hydroxylation of ropivacaine by human liver microsomes appears to be mediated principally by CYP1A2.[319]

TABLE 3-10. *Renal excretion of amide-type local anesthetics and their metabolites (% dose)*

			Aromatic Hydroxylation		N-Dealkylation		Amide Hydrolysis		
Agent	Subject	Unchanged	3-Hydroxy*	4-Hydroxy*	Mono-	Di-	2,6-Xylidine*	40H-Xylidine*	Total
Lidocaine	Adult	1.9^{a}	$<1^{b,c}$	$<1^{b,c}$	2.6^{a}	2.3	2.2^{a}	65.1^{a}	
		(0.6–4.7)			(0.9–4.8)		(1.6–2.4)	(53.1–74.4)	~74
	Neonate	19.7^{a}	ND	ND	19.7^{a}	ND	2.7^{a}	8.9^{a}	~51
					(4.2–48.9)		(1.2–4.3)	(0–22.2)	~34
Mepivacaine	Adult	4.0^{a}	15.9^{d}	11.5^{d}	2.5^{d}	Not possible	ND	ND	~34
		(2.8–5.2)	(11.9–20.3)	(8.5–14.3)	(1.8–3.1)				
	Neonate	43.3^{e}	$<2^{e}$	$<2^{e}$	11.4^{e}	Not possible	ND	ND	~55
		(21.8–64.9)			(6.5–17.2)				
Bupivacaine	Adult	$2.6^{f} \pm 0.3$	$\sim 2^{g}$	$\sim 2^{g}$	$0.2^{f} \pm 0.3$	Not possible	$\sim 0^{g}$	$\sim 0^{g}$	~10
					$(5–20^{g})$				
Etidocaine	Adult	$0.3^{h} \pm 0.3$	$\sim 5^{h}$	$\sim 5^{h}$	$2.6^{h} \pm 4.3$	$13.1^{h} \pm 4.0$*	$0.9^{h} \pm 0.7$	$3.2^{h} \pm 2.3$	~30
Ropivacaine	Adult	1.0 ± 0.6	37 ± 3†	<1	2	Not possible	ND		

* Free and conjugated.
† 2 = Hydroxy also tentatively identified as 4–15% of dose.
[a] Mihaly, G.W., Moore, R.G., Thomas, J., *et al.*: The pharmacokinetics of the anilide local anaesthetic in neonates. I: Lignocaine. Eur. J. Clin. Pharmacol., *13*:143, 1978; 4 adults, 8 neonates.
[b] Keenaghan, J.B., and Boyes, R.N.: The tissue distribution, metabolism and excretion of lidocaine in rats, guinea pigs, dogs and man. J. Pharmacol. Exp. Ther., *180*:454, 1972; 2 adults, orally.
[c] Nelson, S.D., Garland, W.A., Breck, G.D., and Trager, W.F.: Quantification of lidocaine and several metabolites utilizing chemical-ionization mass spectrometry and stable isotope labelling. J. Pharm. Sci., *66*:1180, 1977; 3 adults, orally.
[d] Meffin, P., Long, G.J., and Thomas, J.: Clearance and metabolism of mepivacaine in the human neonate. Clin. Pharmacol. Ther., *14*:219, 1973; 3 adults, IV.
[e] Moore, R.G., Thomas, J., Triggs, E.J., *et al.*: The pharmacokinetics and metabolism of the anilide local anaesthetics in neonates. III: Mepivacaine. Eur. J. Clin. Pharmacol., *14*:203, 1978. 5 neonates, subcutaneous.
[f] Reynolds, F.: Metabolism and excretion of bupivacaine in man: A comparison with mepivacaine. Br. J. Anaesth., *43*:33, 1971; 4 adults, IV acid urine.
[g] Mather, L.E., Long, G.J., and Thomas, J.: The intravenous toxicity and clearance of bupivacaine in man. Clin. Pharmacol. Ther., *12*:935, 1971 and unpublished data; 3 adults, IV acid urine.
[h] Morgan, D.J., Smyth, M.P., Thomas, J., and Vine, J.: Cyclic metabolites of etidocaine in humans. Xenobiotica, *7*: 365, 1977; 9 adults, epidural, and IV.

(Tucker, G.T., and Mather, L.E.: Clinical pharmacokinetics of local anaesthetic agents. Clin. Pharmacokinet., *4*:241, 1979.)

Metabolism of prilocaine to *o*-toluidine and subsequent N-hydroxylation of this product is responsible for methemoglobinemia at doses above 600 mg.[194] There is also concern about this side effect in children less than 3 months of age receiving continuous applications of a cream containing a eutectic mixture of prilocaine and lidocaine bases.[169] Although cases of methemoglobinemia have also been reported with lidocaine,[122] its 2,6-xylidine product is less potent in this respect than *o*-toluidine.[260] Both of these aromatic amines are known to be genotoxic in rats, and 2,6-xylidine–hemoglobin adducts have recently been detected in human blood after low doses of lidocaine.[81]

EFFECTS OF PATIENT VARIABLES AND OTHER DRUGS

Much of the information on likely effects of patient variables and other drug therapy on the disposition kinetics of local anesthetics has been obtained from studies with intravenous lidocaine, and it may not be possible always to extrapolate these findings to patients receiving regional anesthesia. This is a problem especially when hemodynamic factors are involved, since the cardiovascular effects of sympathetic nerve block may complicate the issue, and changes in drug elimination may be offset by opposing changes in drug absorption.[424] For example, although hypovolemia decreases lidocaine clearance,[37] plasma drug concentrations are lower following epidural block in the presence of blood loss as a result of an impaired systemic absorption rate.[297]

Of the variables considered below, the evidence suggests that cardiovascular disease and liver cirrhosis are associated with clinically more significant alterations in kinetics.

Weight

Limited data on the amide-type agents indicate poor correlations between body weight, surface area, or lean body mass and parameters of drug disposition kinetics in young male subjects with normal height:weight ratios.[366,433] In obese subjects of either sex with no evidence of cardiac dysfunction, a 50% increase in the terminal elimination half-life of lidocaine was noted. This was explained by an expanded volume of distribution rather than a decreased clearance.[5]

Age

There is some evidence that the clearance of local anesthetics decreases with age in healthy subjects. A weak to moderate correlation was seen with bupivacaine.[450–452] Decreased clearance and a prolonged elimination half-life of lidocaine was observed in elderly men but not women.[4] Earlier studies had found no change in clearance in geriatric patients but longer half-lives associated with increased volumes of distribution.[113,304]

Elimination half-lives of the amide-type agents are prolonged two- to threefold in neonates, reflecting increased volumes of distribution, decreased clearance, or both (Table 3-11). The renal clearance of lidocaine and mepivacaine was found to be increased in neonates compared to adults, whereas the hepatic clearance of mepivacaine, but not of lidocaine, was considerably decreased. The first observation may be due to decreased protein binding in neonatal blood and decreased tubular reabsorption owing to higher urine flow rates and lower urine pH in newborns. Less impairment of hepatic lidocaine clearance might be explained by a greater dependence on hepatic perfusion compared to mepivacaine, the elimination of which should be affected more by the function of immature liver enzymes. The plasma half-life of 2-chloroprocaine is doubled in neonates compared to adults[159] (Table 3-9).

Along with suggestions that absorption is faster in children than in adults, the unbound clearance (corrected for body weight) appears to be similar (lidocaine) or greater (bupivacaine). Corresponding volumes of distribution seem to be similar or higher, such that half-lives are comparable with those in adults.[140,141,156,278,362]

Sex

There are suggestions that lidocaine may have up to a 50% longer half-life in women than in men. One study assigns this to a significant (64%) difference in volume of distribution,[467] whereas another found small (15%) differences in clearance.[5]

Race

No differences in the disposition kinetics and plasma binding of lidocaine have been found among white, Oriental, and black subjects.[177]

Posture

Prolonged bed rest is associated with increases in plasma and extracellular fluid volumes, and hepatic blood flow is less when standing. Thus, posture might be expected to alter drug disposition. However, although the clearance of lidocaine was observed to decrease on standing,[36] no influence of prolonged recumbency on its disposition and plasma binding was found.[219]

TABLE 3-11. *Comparison of the disposition kinetics of amide-type local anesthetics in adults and neonates*

	Lidocaine		Mepivacaine		Bupivacaine		Etidocaine	
Parameter	Adult	Neonate	Adult	Neonate	Adult	Neonate	Adult	Neonate
$t_{1/2,z}$(h)	1.8[a] (1.2–2.2)	3.2[b] (3.0–3.3) 3[c]	3.2[d] (1.7–7.9)	8.7[d] (6.2–12.2) 9[c]	2.7 ± 1.3[e]	8.1 ± 2.5[f] 18 ± 6[g]	2.6 ± 1.1[e]	6.42 ± 2.73[h]
V_{ss}[i] (liters/kg)	1.11[a] (0.58–1.91)		1.02[d] (0.68–1.52)					
V[i] (liters/kg)		2.75[b] (1.44–4.99)		1.71[d] (1.14–2.77)				
CL[i] (ml/min/kg)	9.2[a]	10.2[b] (5.3–12.1)	5.5[d] (5.1–19.0)	2.3[d] (2.9–8.9)	(1.7–3.1)			
f_e[j]	0.019[b] (0.006–0.047)	0.160[b] (0.015–0.313)	0.038[d] (0.021–0.057)	0.357[d] (0.197–0.527)				

[a] Rowland, M., Thomson, P., Guichard, A., and Melmon, K.L.: Disposition kinetics of lidocaine in normal subjects. Ann. N.Y. Acad. Sci., *179*:383, 1971.
[b] Mihaly, G.W., Moore, R.G., Thomas, J., *et al.*: The pharmacokinetics of the anilide local anaesthetic in neonates. I: Lignocaine. Eur. J. Clin. Pharmacol., *13*:143, 1978.
[c] Brown, W.U., Bell, G.C., Lurie, A.O., *et al.*: Newborn blood levels of lidocaine and mepivacaine in the first postnatal day following maternal epidural anesthesia. Anesthesiology, *42*:698, 1975.
[d] Moore, R.G., Thomas, J., Triggs, E.J., *et al.*: The pharmacokinetics and metabolism of the anilide local anaesthetics in neonates. III: Mepivacaine. Eur. J. Clin. Pharmacol., *14*:203, 1978.
[e] Tucker, G.T., Wiklund, L., Berlin, A., and Mather, L.E.: Hepatic clearance of local anesthetics in man. J. Pharmacokinet. Biopharm., *5*:111, 1977.
[f] Magno, R., Berlin, A., Karlsson, K., and Kjellmer, I.: Anesthesia for Cesarean section IV: Placental transfer and neonatal elimination of bupivacaine following epidural analgesia for elective Cesarian section. Acta Anaesthesiol. Scand., *20*:141, 1976.
[g] Caldwell, J., Moffatt, J.R., Smith, R.L., *et al.*: Determination of bupivacaine in human fetal and neonatal blood samples by gas liquid chromatography mass spectrometry. Biomed. Mass Spectrom., *4*:322, 1977.
[h] Morgan, D.J., Cousins, M.J., McQuillan, D., and Thomas, J.: The pharmacokinetics and metabolism of the anilide local anaesthetics in neonates. II: Etidocaine. Eur. J. Clin. Pharmacol., *13*:365, 1978; (urine data).
[i] Specified with respect to venous plasma concentrations.
[j] Fraction dose excreted unchanged in urine.

(Tucker, G.T., and Mather, L.E.: Clinical pharmacokinetics of local anaesthetic agents. Clin. Pharmacokinet., *4*:241, 1979.)

Pregnancy

Pregnancy is associated with decreases in the plasma half-lives of 2-chloroprocaine and procaine[159,238,316,347] (Table 3-9).

A trend toward lower clearance of bupivacaine in healthy parturients at term compared to controls was noted by Pihlajamaki et al.[335] They also observed higher plasma concentrations of the N-desbutyl metabolite of bupivacaine (PPX) in the pregnant patients. The clearance of lidocaine was decreased, with no change in plasma binding, in preeclamptic relative to normal parturients.[58,346] Pregnant ewes were found to clear lidocaine more rapidly and ropivacaine less rapidly than nonpregnant ewes.[51,377,378] This apparent inconsistency may be explained by differences in the determinants of the kinetics of lidocaine and ropivacaine. Thus, clearance of the former is more dependent on hepatic blood flow, which may be raised during pregnancy, while that of the latter is more dependent on the activity of hepatic enzymes, which may be inhibited during pregnancy.

Cardiovascular Disease

Plasma concentrations of lidocaine after intravenous injection in patients with congestive heart failure were found to be about twice as high as those in control subjects receiving the same dose.[39,420] Concentrations of MEGX formed from lidocaine may also be elevated.[185] These findings reflect significant decreases in the volume of distribution and clearance of the compounds (Table 3-12). Changes in the rate of drug distribution are a consequence of autoregulatory redistribution of blood from the periphery to vital organs. However, an increase in the extent of distribution (as measured by volume of distribution of steady state [V_{SS}]) presumably reflects altered tissue:blood partition or vascular shunting. The impaired clearance appears to be associated with diminished hepatic blood flow secondary to a low cardiac output or impaired hepatic extraction secondary to hepatocellular dysfunction or intrahepatic shunting.[37,420] Hypovolemia,[37] hypotension,[154] and cardiopulmonary resuscitation[97,98] are associated with changes in the disposition of lidocaine similar to those seen in heart failure.

Only minor decreases in the clearance and volume of distribution of lidocaine were observed in patients studied immediately after cardiopulmonary bypass surgery.[196] More marked changes seen in the postoperative period were explained, in part, by an increase in plasma binding accompanying the rise in alpha$_1$-acid glycoprotein levels.

TABLE 3-12. *Lidocaine disposition in various groups of patients*

	$t_{1/2,z}$ (h)	V_{ss} (liters/kg)	CL (ml/min/kg)
Normal	1.8	1.32	10.0
Heart failure	1.9	0.88^a	6.3^a
Liver cirrhosis	4.9^a	2.31^a	6.0^a
Renal disease	1.3	1.2	13.7

^{a} Values differ significantly in comparison to normal subjects.
(Data from Thompson, P., Melmon, K.L., Richardson, J.A. and Rowland, M. Lidocaine pharmacokinetics in advanced heart failure, liver disease, and renal failure in humans. Ann. Intern. Med., 78:499, 1973.)

Liver Disease

Although the plasma half-life of procaine is longer in patients with liver disease (Table 3-9), presumably owing to decreased synthesis of pseudocholinesterase, normal esterase activity is preserved in their erythrocytes.[91] This, and the fact that the absolute rate of plasma hydrolysis remains high, suggests that these patients may not be much more susceptible to toxicity.

The clinical significance of altered disposition of the amides in liver disease is greater than that of the esters and depends on the type of liver disease. In severe cirrhosis there are considerable increases in the half-life and volume of distribution and a decrease in the clearance of lidocaine (Table 3-12). The mechanism of the change in distribution may be related to altered plasma or tissue binding, or both.[33] The lowered clearance reflects decreased enzyme activity and hepatic blood flow.[203] Clearly, systemic accumulation of the amides will be more extensive and prolonged in patients with cirrhosis and the regression of systemic effects will be slower.[11] In contrast, chronic hepatitis appears to be associated with a higher lidocaine clearance than normal,[202] although V_{SS} is also increased secondary to a decreased plasma drug binding.[201] The acute phase of viral hepatitis is accompanied by increases in lidocaine half-life and volume of distribution and a trend toward lower clearance. No differences in the plasma binding of the drug were seen in the acute and recovery phases of the disease.[465]

Renal Disease

Procaine hydrolysis in sera from patients with impaired renal function is slowed[347] (Table 3-9). A decreased synthesis of pseudocholinesterase, rather than inhibition or inactivation of the enzyme by other components of uremic serum, appears to be responsible for this effect.[92] As in patients with liver disease, red cell esterase is preserved in renal disease,[91] and the change in plasma hydrolysis rate may be of little clinical significance.

As might be expected of drugs that are eliminated mostly by the liver, the disposition kinetics of the amides are unaffected by renal disease[420] (Table 3-12). However, in contrast to the parent drugs, more polar metabolites will tend to accumulate in patients with renal insufficiency. This is true of GX, formed from lidocaine, although the evidence suggests that the plasma concentrations reached are not likely to cause major toxicity.[102]

Diabetes

Patients with non-insulin-dependent diabetes were found to have a significantly lower clearance (60%) of lidocaine after epidural injection compared to controls.[328] Although the plasma binding of lidocaine was observed to be less in insulin-dependent diabetics, it was unchanged from normal in type II patients.[317]

Acidosis and Hypoxia

The toxicity of local anesthetics is increased significantly by acidosis and hypoxia.[144,145,191,353] In theory, an increased brain and myocardial concentration of free ionized drug could contribute to this through hemodynamic changes and ion-trapping.

Despite the known effect of arterial CO_2 tension on hepatic blood flow, studies in animals have shown that hypercarbia or hypocarbia does not alter the clearance of lidocaine or bupivacaine based on total plasma concentrations.[16,302] However, a decrease in plasma binding accompanying acidosis indicates an elevation of free drug concentration under this condition, with the implication of increased toxicity. During metabolic acidosis of the type associated with convulsions, this increase in free drug concentration does not appear to be augmented by an increase in ion trapping within the tissue. Thus, the partition coefficients of local anesthetics between whole brain or myocardial tissue and blood are similar[393] or reduced[302] compared to normal. This is because the lowering of blood pH is similar to, or greater than, the lowering of tissue pH. On the other hand, Simon et al.[393] have suggested that treatment of convulsions by paralysis and artificial ventilation will tend to exacerbate entry of local anesthetic into the brain, because prevention of the systemic acidosis, but not the cerebral acidosis, promotes ion trapping of drug in the organ (Fig. 3-20). This does not imply that ventilation with oxygen is deleterious, but it may require the use of anticonvulsants for continuation of ventilation until the drug is cleared from the brain.

Although the hepatic clearance of lidocaine has been shown to be sensitive to hypoxia in the isolated perfused organ,[282] studies in dogs with both acute and chronic moderate hypoxia and without hypocapnia indicated no effect on lidocaine clearance or liver blood flow. However, acute moderate hypoxia was shown to increase the plasma concentrations of the lidocaine metabilites MEGX and GX.[139]

Drug–Drug Interactions

Ideally, interpretation of pharmacokinetic data on drug–drug interactions should be based on measurement of unbound plasma drug concentrations because these are believed to relate more closely to drug effects than total concentrations. It becomes especially important in this context to stress the following point: Although the unbound *fraction* of local anesthetic in plasma may be increased by a second drug, this does not necessarily mean that its unbound plasma *concentration* will be significantly greater *in vivo*, and, therefore, that the risk of toxicity will be increased.[426] Failure to appreciate this point has led to confusion in the literature.

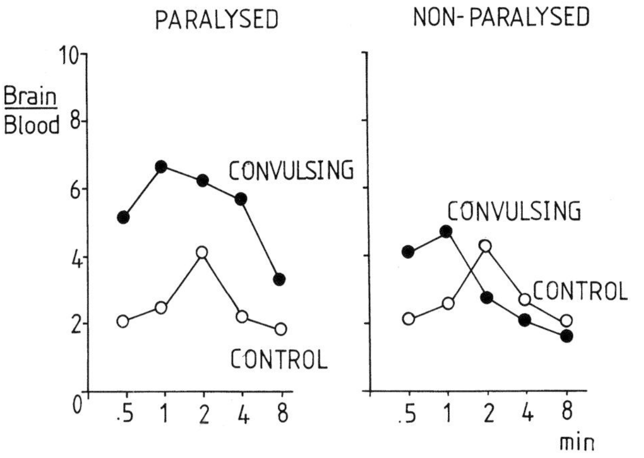

FIG. 3-20. Brain tissue: femoral artery blood partition ratios of lidocaine after intravenous injection into convulsing and nonconvulsing rats. The left panel shows data for animals that were paralyzed with gallamine and ventilated with nitrous oxide/oxygen; the right panel shows data for nonparalyzed animals. Data from Simon, R.P., Benowitz, N.L., and Culala, S.: Motor paralysis increases brain uptake of lidocaine during status epilepticus. Neurology, *34*:384, 1984.

An increasing number of drugs have been shown to alter the disposition kinetics of local anesthetics, but the clinical significance of the changes is largely unknown.

Local Anesthetics

There is *in vitro* evidence that plasma concentrations of etidocaine and bupivacaine in the clinical range can inhibit the hydrolysis of chloroprocaine by 10% to 40%.[242,345] Clinically relevant concentrations of bupivacaine may also increase the free *fractions* of lidocaine[178,262] and mepivacaine[187] in plasma. However, the suggestion that a toxic reaction to a combined block with bupivacaine and mepivacaine was due to such a displacement reaction increasing the free concentration of mepivacaine is unlikely.[188]

No differences in plasma concentration–time profiles of etidocaine were observed when intercostal block was performed with etidocaine alone and when it was given with bupivacaine for bilateral block.[65,66] Similarly, the plasma concentration–time profiles of lidocaine and bupivacaine were independent of whether they were used alone or in combinations for epidural block.[387] However, whether there are clinically significant enantiomer–enantiomer interactions of the chiral caines remains to be determined. Preliminary evidence obtained from sheep suggests that there may be, since the mean total body clearance of *R*(+)-bupivacaine was 65% greater than that of *S*(−)-bupivacaine when both enantiomers were administered separately, but only 20% greater when they were administered together as *rac*-bupivacaine.[267,273,370]

A bolus injection of bupivacaine has been shown to displace lidocaine from binding sites in rabbit lung[320] with possible implications for transient toxicity.

General Anesthetics

The rate of elimination of lidocaine in dogs was slower under halothane anesthesia than while breathing nitrous oxide[88] or air.[60] Similarly, a 34% lower clearance of lidocaine and a trend toward a smaller V_{SS} were found in patients receiving maintenance anesthesia with halothane and nitrous oxide–oxygen compared with a control group given fentanyl, thiopental, and nitrous oxide–oxygen. Pharmacokinetic parameters for the latter were similar to those for unanesthetized subjects.[40] All of these results are consistent with the effects of halothane in decreasing hepatic blood flow[271,368] and mixed-function oxidase activity.[129,369] In view of the profound effects of most general anesthetics on drug clearance,[369] it is surprising that plasma lidocaine concentrations in dogs were unaltered by methoxyflurane–nitrous oxide[131] or by thiopental-halothane anesthesia.[271] No difference in plasma lidocaine concentrations was noted in patients receiving isoflurane compared to halothane as general anesthetic.[308] Addition of sodium thiopental to human serum did not alter the protein binding of bupivacaine.[25]

Premedicants

Arteriovenous concentration differences of amide local anesthetics across the arm were found to be less in premedicated patients than in volunteers receiving similar epidural injections. It was suggested that the administration of premedicants, such as meperidine, to the patients caused a generalized vasodilation and opening of cutaneous shunts, which antagonized the compensatory vasoconstriction in the upper limbs produced by lumbar sympathetic block (T. M. Murphy, L. E. Mather, P. Zachariah, et al., unpublished observations).[433] At clinically relevant plasma concentrations, meperidine does not significantly influence the free fractions of lidocaine or bupivacaine in plasma.[127,178,434]

Although it has been suggested that diazepam may influence plasma concentrations of etidocaine and bupivacaine through alterations in plasma binding,[173] others have found no binding interaction.[128] As diazepam binds to albumin and the local anesthetics bind preferentially to alpha$_1$-acid glycoprotein, a binding interaction is not expected. Giaufre *et al.*[174,175] claim that diazepam but not midazolam inhibits the clearance of bupivacaine, whereas midazolam increases the clearance of lidocaine but has no effect on the clearance of bupivacaine.

Sympathomimetics

Benowitz et al.[37] have documented the effects of norepinephrine (alpha-adrenoceptor stimulation) and of isoproterenol (beta-adrenoceptor stimulation) on the disposition kinetics of lidocaine in monkeys. The former decreased initial volume of distribution, decreased clearance by lowering hepatic blood flow, and increased half-life; the latter had the opposite effects.

Inclusion of epinephrine in solutions for epidural block often results in a significant increase in cardiac output and decrease in peripheral resistance and arterial blood pressure over a period of about an hour.[54] These effects, together with an increase in liver blood flow (mediated partly through the increase in cardiac output and also by direct action on intrahepatic beta$_2$-receptors), could influence the systemic disposition of local anesthetics. Studies in monkeys[19] and in healthy humans[224] showed that epinephrine absorbed from the epidural space offsets temporarily the lowering of hepatic blood flow caused by sympathetic blockade. In patients receiving epidural injections of bupivacaine, Sharrock et al.[390] observed significantly lower plasma drug concentrations during concomitant intravenous infusion of epinephrine (maintained cardiac output) compared to phenylephrine (decreased cardiac output). Thus, epinephrine may protect against high systemic exposure to local anesthetic both by decreasing absorption rate and by maintaining or increasing clearance. Intravenous injection of ephedrine (20 mg) was also found to increase the clearance of lidocaine by stimulating hepatic blood flow.[458]

Beta-adrenoceptor Antagonists

In therapeutic doses, propranolol lowers the clearance of lidocaine in humans by about 40%, mainly by direct inhibition of mixed-function oxidase activity and partly by decreasing liver blood flow, through its effect on cardiac output and by intrahepatic beta$_2$ blockade. Other beta-adrenoceptor antagonists have less marked effects, depending on their lipid solubility, cardioselectivity, and intrinsic sympathomimetic activity.[35,427] Propranolol also impairs the clearance of bupivacaine.[59] The first-pass pulmonary extraction of bupivacaine in rabbits is decreased (10%) by injection of propranolol.[363]

H_2 Antagonists and Proton-Pump Inhibitors

Many studies of the potential effect of H_2 antagonists on the pharmacokinetics of local anesthetics have been reported, with various permutations of agents, dosage, routes of administration, and duration of treatment.[34,63,153,155,160,161,206,226,240,312,318,352,467] In isolation all of these studies suffer from low statistical power owing to the use of small numbers of subjects. However, in general, it seems that in single doses for premedication, ranitidine has no effect and cimetidine has little or no effect on the kinetics of either epidural lidocaine or bupivacaine. On continuous dosage, cimetidine lowers the clearance of lidocaine significantly but ranitidine has little effect. The effects of multiple doses of cimetidine and ranitidine on bupivacaine clearance have not been determined.

Omeprazole appears not to change the clearance of lidocaine.[29]

Enzyme-Inducing Agents

The systemic clearance of unbound lidocaine was found to be about 25% greater in epileptic patients than in controls.[330,365] This is presumed to be a consequence of the enzyme-inducing properties of the anticonvulsant. Long-term therapy with phenytoin also induces the synthesis of alpha$_1$-glycoprotein leading to increased plasma binding of lidocaine.[365] In contrast, the enzyme inducer rifampicin appears not to influence alpha$_1$-acid glycoprotein levels and plasma lidocaine binding in humans.[152]

Other Drugs

Administration of inhibitors of plasma pseudocholinesterase, for example, neostigmine and echothiophate, should be avoided in patients receiving ester-type local anesthetics, as should acetazolamide, which blocks hydrolysis by the red cell esterase.[91] Nitroprusside in hypotensive doses was shown to have no effect on lidocaine clearance in dogs.[391]

Many basic drugs have been shown to displace lidocaine from plasma binding sites, but only when added at supratherapeutic concentrations.[172,178,261,434] The pre-anesthetic use of oral clonidine does not impair the clearance of lidocaine.[307]

Placental Transfer

Esters

After maternal injection, 2-chloroprocaine appears in both maternal and cord plasma in very low concentrations.[1,2,238] Thus, even though elimination half-lives of chloroprocaine and procaine are twice as long in cord plasma as in maternal plasma, and pregnancy is associated with a decrease in pseudocholinesterase activity[159,238,316,347] (Table 3-10), the absolute rate of hydrolysis in the mother remains fast and helps to reduce placental transfer and the risk of fetal intoxication. Cocaine is transferred rapidly and passively across the isolated perfused human placenta.[380]

Amides

At delivery, mean values of cord:maternal plasma concentration ratios of the amides decrease in the order: prilocaine (1.0–1.1), lidocaine (0.5–0.7), mepivacaine (0.7), bupivacaine (0.2–0.4), and etidocaine (0.2–0.3).[435] These differences reflect differential maternal and fetal plasma binding of the drugs owing to relatively low fetal concentrations of alpha$_1$-acid glycoprotein (Fig. 3-21). Equilibrium cord:maternal total plasma ratios of the agents are predicted in humans and sheep from plasma binding data, with allowance for ion trapping due to fetal acidosis.[221,223,417,438] As such, therefore, these ratios are not direct predictors of relative fetal toxicity, as corresponding ratios of unbound (active) drug across the placenta are close to unity irrespective of the drug. (Negative followed by positive deviations from unity are expected with time as the transplacental concentration gradient reverses during the rise and fall of maternal drug concentrations). Nevertheless, a high maternal:fetal binding ratio should delay equilibration of drug in fetal tissues, despite rapid equilibration across the placenta.[121,186] On the other hand, similar umbilical artery:umbilical vein concentration ratios observed for the various agents argue against large differences in their equilibration rates in the fetus.[430] As a result of ion trapping, fetal acidosis increases both the cord:maternal ratio of unbound drug and the rate of placental transfer of local anesthetic.[47,79,118,170,222,430]

It has been suggested[158,239] that relatively low cord:maternal ratios of bupivacaine, based on total plasma drug concentrations, are due to more extensive uptake of this drug by the fetal tissues. Such an explanation is kinetically unsound, and certainly cannot explain low umbilical venous:maternal ratios.[93]

In the event of inadvertent maternal intravascular injection of local anesthetic, it is advisable to effect the delivery immediately before maximum fetal uptake occurs. Alterna-

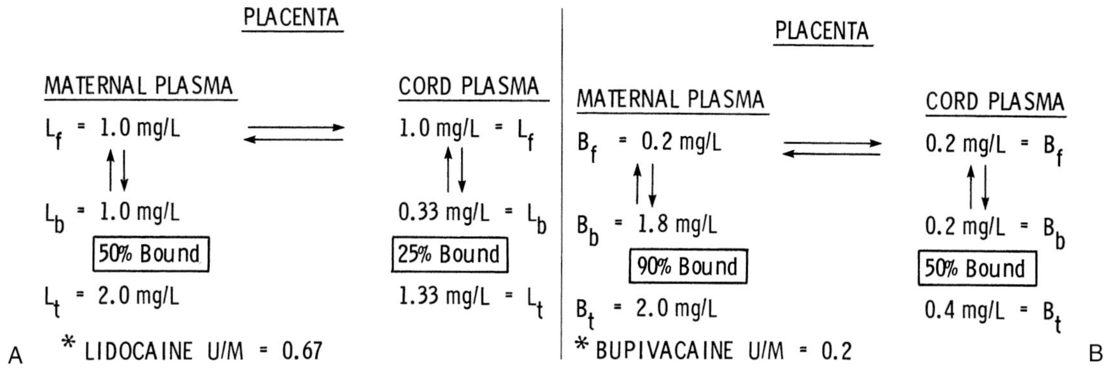

FIG. 3-21. Schematic showing how transplacentral distribution of local anesthetics may be predicted from differences in binding of the drugs in maternal and cord plasma. **A:** Lidocaine. **B:** Bupivacaine; *f, b,* and *t* represent free, bound, and total drug concentrations, respectively.

tively, providing that clinical conditions allow, there is a theoretical advantage in delaying delivery until significant back-transfer of drug to and clearance by the mother has taken place.[184] An intermediate window will exist in which the body burden to the newborn, whose capacity to eliminate the drug may be impaired, is relatively high. Net back-transfer of bupivacaine but not of lidocaine from fetus to mother was observed after a short intravenous infusion of the agents into ewes.[221,223] The interpretation of this difference with respect to relative rates of equilibration of the drugs in fetal tissues is complicated by the possibility of differential extraction on first pass through the fetal liver. Thus, a higher extraction ratio of lidocaine would amplify its transplacental gradient during infusion, thereby accelerating drug transfer to the fetal circulation. If these findings can be extrapolated to humans, they suggest that back-transfer, which was observed with bupivacaine, might be exploited after an inadvertent injection in the mother by delaying delivery to reduce the burden of drug in the neonate. In contrast, a significant fetal clearance of lidocaine might help to protect against toxicity, and the lack of net back-transfer of this agent would suggest no benefit in delaying delivery.

Metabolites of local anesthetics have been measured in fetal blood after maternal injection of the parent drugs.[50,236,239] The significance of this in relation to fetal toxicity is not known.

REFERENCES

1. Abboud, T.K., Afrasiabi, A., Sarkis, F., *et al*: Continuous infusion epidural analgesia in parturients receiving bupivacaine, chloroprocaine, or lidocaine—Maternal, fetal, and neonatal effects. Anesth. Analg. (Cleve.) *63:*421, 1984.
2. Abboud, T.K., Kim, K.C., Noueihed, R. *et al.*: Epidural bupivacaine, chloroprocaine, or lidocaine for Cesarian section—Maternal and neonatal effects. Anesth-Analg. (Cleve.), *62:*914, 1983.
3. Aberg, G.: Toxicological and local anaesthetic effects of optically active isomers of two local anaesthetic compounds. Acta Pharmacol. Toxicol., *31:*273, 1972.
4. Abernethy, D.R., and Greenblatt, D.J.: Impairment of lidocaine clearance in elderly male subjects. J Cardiovasc. Pharmacol., *5:*1093, 1984.
5. Abernethy, D.R., and Greenblatt, D.J.: Lidocaine disposition in obesity. Am. J. Cardiol., *53:*1183, 1984.
6. Adams, H.A., Biscoping, J. Kafurke, H., *et al.*: Influence of dextran on the absorption of adrenaline-containing lignocaine solutions: A protective mechanism in local anaesthesia. Br. J. Anaesth. *60:*645, 1988.
7. Adams, H.J.: Effect of pH on spinal anaesthesia with lidocaine in sheep. Pharmacol. Res. Commun., *7:*551, 1975.
8. Adams, H.J., Charron, D.M., and Takman, B.H.: Spinal anesthesia in sheep with local anesthetic solutions at pH 4 and pH 7. Acta. Anaesthesiol. Scand. *28:*270, 1984.
9. Adams, H.J., Mastri, A.R., and Doherty, J.: Bupivacaine: Morphological effects on spinal cords of cats and durations of spinal anesthesia in sheep. Pharmacol. Res. Commun., *9:*847, 1977.
10. Adams, H.J., Mastri, A.R., Eicholzer, A.W., and Kilpatrick, G.: Morphological effects of intrathecal etidocaine and tetracaine on the rabbit spinal cord. Anesthesiology, *53:*904, 1974.
11. Adjepon-Yamoah, K.K., Nimmo, J., and Prescott, L.F.: Gross impairment of hepatic drug metabolism in a patient with chronic liver disease. Br. Med. J., *4:*387, 1974.
12. Akerman, B., Hellberg, I.-B., and Trossvik C.: Primary evaluation of the local anaesthetic properties of the amino amide agent ropivacaine (LEA 103). Acta. Anaesth. Scand., *32:*571, 1988.
13. Akerman, B., Persson, H. and Tegner, C.: Local anaesthetic properties of the optically active isomers of prilocaine (Citanest). Acta. Pharmacol. Toxicol. *25:*233, 1967.
14. Aldrete, J.A., Nicholson, J., Sada, T., *et al.*: Cephalic kinetics of intraarterially injected lidocaine. Oral Surg. *44:*167, 1977.
15. Aldrete, J.A., Romo-Salas, F., Arora, S., *et al.*: Reverse arterial blood flow as a pathway for central nervous systemic toxic responses following injection of local anesthetics. Anesth. Analg. (Cleve.), *57:*428, 1978.
16. Alexander, G.M., Berko, R.S., Gross, J.B., Kagle, D.M., and Shaw, I.M.: The effect of changes in arterial CO_2 tension on plasma lidocaine concentration. Can. Anaesth. J. *34:*343, 1987.
17. Ali, Z. Chandola, H.C. Misra, M.N., and Chatterjee, S.: Effect of pH adjustment on onset and duration of epidural anaesthesia. J. Indian Med. Assoc. *91:*204–5, 1993.
18. Allen, L.V., Jr., Stiles, M.L., Wang, D.P., and Tu, Y.H.: Stability of bupivacaine hydrochloride, epinephrine hydrochloride, and fentanyl citrate in portable infusion-pump reservoirs. Am. J. Hosp. Pharm. *50:*714, 1993.
19. Amory, D.W., Sivarajan, M., and Lindbloom, L.E.: Systemic and regional blood flow during epidural anesthesia with epinephrine in the rhesus monkey. Acta. Anaesthesiol. Scand. *21:*423, 1977.
20. Apostolou, G.A., Zarmakoupis, P.K., and Mastrokostopoulos, G.T.: Spread of epidural anesthesia and the lateral position. Anesth. Analg. (Cleve.) *60:*584, 1981.
21. Aps, C., and Reynolds, F.: The effect of concentration on vasoactivity of bupivacaine and lignocaine. Br. J. Anaesth. *48:*1171, 1976.
22. Aps, C. and Reynolds, F.: An intradermal study of the local anaesthetic and vascular effects of the isomers of bupivacaine. Br. J. Clin. Pharmacol. *6:*63, 1978.
23. Armstrong, I.R., Littlewood, D.G., and Chambers, W.A.: Spinal anesthesia with tetracaine—Effect of added vasoconstrictors. Anesth. Analg. (Cleve.), *62:*793, 1983.
24. Arthur, G.R.: Distribution and elimination of local anaesthetic agents: The role of lung, liver and kidney. Ph.D. thesis, University of Edinburgh, 1981.
25. Arthur, G.R., Denson, D.D., and Coyle, D.E.: Effect of sodium thiopental on the serum protein binding of bupivacaine. Reg. Anesth. *9:*171, 1984.
26. Axelsson, K.H., Edstrom, H.H., Sundberg, A.E.A., and Widman, G.B.: Spinal anaesthesia with hyperbaric 0.5% bupivacaine: Effects of volume. Acta. Anaesthesiol. Scand. *26:*439, 1982.
27. Axelsson, K., and Widman, B. Blood concentration of lidocaine after spinal anaesthesia using lidocaine and lidocaine with adrenaline. Acta. Anaesthesiol. Scand. *25:*240, 1981.
28. Bachmann, B., Biscoping, J., Sinning, E., and Hempelmann, G.: Protein binding of prilocaine in human plasma: influence of concentration, pH and temperature. Acta Anaesthesiol. Scand. *34:*311, 1990.
29. Bannister, J., Noble, D.W., Lamont, M., and Scott, D.B.: Lack of effect of omeprazole on the disposition of lignocaine and its active metabolite in healthy subjects. Abstracts—World Congress of Gastroenterology, Sydney 1990, Abstract PP1363.
30. Barchowsky, A., Shand, D.G., Stargel, W.W., *et al.*: On the role of alpha-l-acid glycoprotein in lignocaine accumulation following myocardial infarction. Br. J. Clin. Pharmacol. *13:*411, 1981.
31. Bargetzi, M.J., Aoyama, T., Gonzalez, F.J., and Meyer, U.A.: Lidocaine metabolism in human liver microsomes by cytochrome P450IIIA4. Clin. Pharmacol. Ther. *46:*521, 1989.
32. Barnett, G., Hawks, R., and Resnick, R.: Cocaine pharmacokinetics in humans. J. Ethnopharamacol., *3:*353, 1981.
33. Barry, M., Keeling, P.W.N., Weir, D. and Feely, J.: Severity of cirrhosis and the relationship of α_1-acid glycoprotein concentration to plasma protein binding of lidocaine. Clin. Pharmacol. Ther., *47:*366, 1990.
34. Bauer, L.A., Edwards, W.A.D., Randolph, F.P., and Blouin, R.A.: Cimetidine-induced decrease in lidocaine metabolism. Am. Heart J., *108:*413, 1984.
35. Bax, N.D.S., Tucker, G.T., Lennard, M.S., and Woods, H.F.: The impairment of lignocaine clearance by propranolol–Major contribution from enzyme inhibition. Br. J. Clin. Pharmacol., *19:*597, 1985.
36. Bennett, P.N., Aarons, L.J., Bending, M.R., *et al.*: Pharmacokinetics of lidocaine and its deethylated metabolite: Dose and time dependency studies in man. J. Pharmacokinet. Biopharm., *10:*265, 1982.
37. Benowitz, N., Forsyth, R.P., Melmon, K.L., and Rowland, M.: Lidocaine disposition kinetics in monkey and man: II. Effects of hemor-

rhage and sympathomimetic drug administration. Clin. Pharmacol. Ther. *16:*99, 1974.
38. Benowitz, N.L.: Clinical pharmacology and toxicology of cocaine. Pharmacol. Ther. *72:*3, 1993.
39. Benowitz, N.L., and Meister, W.: Clinical pharmacokinetics of lignocaine. Clin. Pharmacokinet., *3:*177, 1978.
40. Bentley, J.B., Glass, S. and Gandolfi, A.J.: The influence of halothane on lidocaine pharmacokinetics in man. Anesthesiology, *59:*A246, 1983.
41. Bernards, C.M.: Flux of morphine, fentanyl and alfentanil through rabbit arteries in vivo: Evidence supporting a vascular route for redistribution of opioids between the epidural space and the spinal cord. Anesthesiology, *78:*1126, 1993.
42. Bernards, C.M., and Hill, H.F.: The spinal nerve root sleeve is not a preferred route for redistribution of drugs from the epidural space to the spinal cord. Anesthesiology, *75:*827, 1991.
43. Bernards, C.M., and Hill, H.F.: Physical and chemical properties of drug molecules governing their diffusion through the spinal meninges. Anesthesiology, *77:*750, 1992.
44. Bernards, C.M., Kopacz, D.J., and Michel, M.Z.: Effect of needle puncture on morphine and lidocaine flux through the spinal meninges of the monkey *in vitro.* Implications for combined spinal-epidural anesthesia. Anesthesiology, *80:*853, 1994.
45. Bernards, C.M., Luger, T.L., Malmberg, A.B., Hill, H.F., and Yaksh, T.L.: Liposome encapsulation prolongs alfentanil spinal analgesia and alters systemic redistribution in the rat. Anesthesiology, *77:*529, 1992.
46. Bernards, C.M., and Sorkin, L.S.: Radicular artery blood flow does not redistribute fentanyl from the epidural space to the spinal cord. Anesthesiology, *80:*872, 1994.
47. Biehl, D., Shnider, S.M., Levinson, G., and Callender, K.: Placental transfer of lidocaine: Effects of acidosis. Anesthesiology, *48:*409, 1978.
48. Blair, M.R.: Cardiovascular pharmacology of local anaesthetics. Br. J. Anaesth. *47:*247, 1975.
49. Blake, D.W., Bjorksen, A. Dawson, P. and Hiscock, R.: Pharmacokinetics of bupivacaine enantiomers during interpleural infusions. Anaesth. Intensive Care, *22:*521, 1994.
50. Blankenbaker, W.L., DiFazio, C.A., and Berry, F.A.: Lidocaine and its metabolites in the newborn. Anesthesiology, *42:*325, 1975.
51. Bloedow, D.C., Ralston, D.H., and Hargrove, J.C.: Lidocaine pharmacokinetics in pregnant and non-pregnant sheep. J. Pharm. Sci. *69:*32, 1980.
52. Blumer, J. Strong, J.M., and Atkinson, A.J.: The convulsant potency of lidocaine and its N-dealkylated metabolites. J. Pharmacol. Exp. Ther. *186:*31, 1973.
53. Bokesch, P.M. Castaneda, A.R., Ziemer, G., and Wilson, J.M.: The influence of right-to-left cardiac shunt on lidocaine pharmacokinetics. Anesthesiology, *67:*739, 1987.
54. Bonica, J.J., Akamatsu, T.J., Berges, P.U., *et al.*: Circulatory effects of peridural block: II. Effects of epinephrine. Anesthesiology, *34:*514, 1971.
55. Boogaerts, J. Declercq, A., Lafont, N., *et al.*: Toxicity of bupivacaine encapsulated into liposomes and injected intravenously: Comparison with plain solutions. Anesth. Analg. (Cleve.), *76:*553, 1993.
56. Boogaerts, J.G., Lafont, N.D., Declercq, A.G., *et al.*: J Epidural administration of liposome-associated bupivacaine for the management of postsurgical pain—a first study. J. Clin. Anesth. *6:*315, 1994.
57. Boogaerts, J.G., Lafont, N.D., Luo, H.W., and Legros, F.J.: Plasma concentrations of bupivacaine after brachial plexus administration of liposome-associated and plain solutions to rabbits. Can. J. Anaesth. *40:*1201, 1993.
58. Bottorf, M.B. Pieper, J.A., Boucher, B.A., Hoon, T.J. Ramanathan, J., and Sibai, B.M.: Lidocaine protein binding in preeclampsia. Eur. J. Clin. Pharmacol. *31:*719, 1987.
59. Bowdle, T.A., Freund, P.R., and Slattery, J.T.: Propranolol reduces bupivacaine clearance. Anesthesiology, *66:*36, 1987.
60. Boyce, J.R., Cervenko, F.W., and Wright, F.J.: Effects of halothane on the pharmacokinetics of lidocaine in digitalis-toxic dogs. Can. Anaesth. Soc. J., *25:*323, 1978.
61. Braid, D.P., and Scott, D.B.: The systemic absorption of local analgesic drugs. Br. J. Anaesth., *37:*394, 1965.
62. Braid, D.P., and Scott, D.B.: The effect of adrenaline on the systemic absorption of local anaesthetic drugs. Acta Anaesthesiol. Scand., *23:*334, 1966.
63. Brashear, W.T., Zuspan, K.J., Lazebnik, N., Kuhnert, B.R., and Mann, L.I.: Effect of ranitidine on bupivacaine disposition. Anesth. Analg. (Cleve.) *72:*369, 1991.
64. Bricker, S.R.W., Telford, R.J., and Booker, P.D.: Pharmacokinetics of bupivacaine following intraoperative intercostal nerve block in neonates and in infants aged less than 6 months. Anesthesiology, *70:*942, 1989.
65. Bridenbaugh, P.O.: Intercostal nerve blockade for evaluation of local anaesthetic agents. Br. J. Anaesth. *47:*306, 1975.
66. Bridenbaugh, P.O., Tucker, G.T., Moore, D.C., *et al.*: Preliminary clinical evaluation of etidocaine (Duranest): A new long-acting local anesthetic agent. Acta Anaesthesiol. Scand. *18:*165, 1974.
67. Bridenbaugh, P.O., Tucker, G.T., Moore, D.C., *et al.*: Role of epinephrine in regional block anesthesia with etidocaine: A double-blind study. Anesth. Analg. (Cleve.) *53:*430, 1974.
68. Brodie, B.B., Lief, P.A., and Poet, R.: The fate of procaine in man following its intravenous administration and methods for the estimation of procaine and diethylaminoethanol. J. Pharmacol. Exp. Ther. *94:*359, 1948.
69. Bromage, P.R.: Physiology and pharmacology of epidural analgesia. Anesthesiology, *28:*592, 1967.
70. Bromage, P.R.: Lower limb reflex changes in segmental epidural analgesia. Br. J. Anaesth., *46:*504, 1974.
71. Bromage, P.R.: Mechanisms of action of extradural analgesia. Br. J. Anaesth., *47:*199, 1975.
72. Bromage, P.R., Burfoot, M.E., Crowell, D.E., and Truant, A.P.: Quality of epidural blockade: III. Carbonated local anaesthetic solutions. Br. J. Anaesth., *39:*197, 1967.
73. Bromage, P.R., and Gertel, M.: Brachial plexus anesthesia in chronic renal failure. Anesthesiology, *36:*488, 1972.
74. Bromage, P.R., and Gertel, M.: Improved brachial plexus blockade with bupivacaine hydrochloride and carbonated lidocaine. Anesthesiology, *36:*479, 1972.
75. Bromage, P.R., Joyal, A.C., and Binney, J.C.: Local anesthetic drugs: Penetration from the spinal extradural space into the neuraxis. Science, *140:*392, 1963.
76. Brown, D.L., and Bridenbaugh, L.D.: The upper extremity: somatic block. *In* Cousins, M.J., and Bridenbaugh, P.O. (eds.): Neural Blockade, 3rd ed. Philadelphia, Lippincott, 1998.
77. Brown, D.T., Morison, D.H., Covino, B.G., and Scott, D.B.: Comparison of carbonated bupivacaine and bupivacaine hydrochloride for extradural anaesthesia. Br. J. Anaesth., *52:*419, 1980.
78. Brown, D.T., Wildsmith, J.A.W., Covino, B.G., and Scott, D.B.: Effect of baricity on spinal anaesthesia with amethocaine. Br. J. Anaesth., *52:*589, 1980.
79. Brown, W.U., Bell, G.C., and Alper, M.H.: Acidosis, local anesthetics and the newborn. Obstet. Gynecol., *48:*27, 1976.
80. Bruguerolle, B., Philip-Joet, F., Arnaud, C., and Arnaud, A.: Consequences of inflammatory processes on lignocaine protein binding during anaesthesia in fibreoptic bronchoscopy. Br. J. Clin. Pharmacol., *20:*180, 1985.
81. Bryant, M.S., Simmons, H.F. Harrell, R.E., and Hinson, J.A.: 2,6-dimethylaniline-hemoglobin adducts from lidocaine in humans. Carcinogenicity, *15:*2287, 1994.
82. Buchi, J. and Perlia, X: Structure-activity relations and physicochemical properties of local anesthetics. *In* Lechat, P. (ed.): Local Anesthetics (International Encyclopedia of Pharmacology and Therapeutics, Vol. 1). pp. 39. Oxford, Pergamon Press, 1971.
83. Burm, A.G.: Pharmacokinetics and clinical effects of lidocaine and bupivacaine following epidural and subarachnoid administration in man. Ph.D. thesis, University of Leiden, 1985.
84. Burm, A.G.: Clinical pharmacokinetics of epidural and spinal anaesthesia. Clin. Pharmacokinet., *16:*283, 1989.
85. Burm, A.G.L., Van der Meer, A.D. Van Kleef, J. W., Zeilmans, P.W.M., and Groen, K.: Pharmacokinetics of the enantiomers of bupivacaine following intravenous administration of the racemate. Br. J. Clin. Pharmacol. *38:*125, 1994.
86. Burm, A.G.L., Vermeulen, N.P.E. Van Kleef, J.W., *et al.*: Pharmacokinetics of lidocaine and bupivacaine in surgical patients following epidural administration. Simultaneous investigation fo absorption and disposition kinetics using stable isotopes. Clin. Pharmacokinet. *13:*191, 1987.
87. Burn, J.M., Guyer, P.B., and Langdond, L.: The spread of solutions injected into the epidural space. A study using epidurograms in patients with the lumbosciatic syndrome. Br. J. Anaesth.: *45:*338, 1973.

88. Burney, R.G., and DiFazio, C.A.: Hepatic clearance of lidocaine during N_2O anesthesia in dogs. Anesth. Analg. (Cleve.), *55:*322, 1976.
89. Burney, R.G., DiFazio, C.A., and Foster, J.H.: Effects of pH on protein binding of lidocaine. Anesth. Analg. (Cleve.), *57:*478, 1978.
90. Cahn, R.S., Ingold, C.K., and Prelog, V.: The specification of asymmetric configuration in organic chemistry. Experientia, *12:*81, 1956.
91. Calvo, R., Carlos, R., and Erill,S.: Effects of disease and acetazolamine on procaine hydrolysis by red cell enzymes. Clin. Pharmacol. Ther., *27:*175, 1980.
92. Calvo, R., Carlos, R., and Erill, S.: Procaine hydrolysis defect in uraemia does not appear to be due to carbamylation of plasma esterases. Eur. J. Clin. Pharmacol., *24:*533, 1983.
93. Carson, R.J., and Reynolds, F.: Maternal-fetal distribution of bupivacaine in the rabbit. Br. J. Anaesth. *61:*332, 1988.
94. Catchlove, R.F.H.: The influence of CO_2 and pH on local anesthetic action. J. Pharmacol. Exp. Ther., *181:*298, 1972.
95. Cederholm, I. Evers, H., and Lofstrom, J.B.: Skin blood flow after interdermal injection of ropivacaine in various concentrations with and without epinephrine evaluated by laser doppler flowmetry. Reg. Anesth., *17:*322, 1992.
96. Chambers, W.A., Littlewood, D.G., Edstrom, H.H., and Scott, D.B.: Spinal anaesthesia with hyperbaric bupivacaine: Effects of concentration and volume administered. Br. J. Anaesth., *54:*75, 1982.
97. Chow, M.S.S, Ronfeld, R.A., Hamilton, R.A., *et al.*: Effect of external cardiopulmonary resuscitation on lidocaine pharmacokinetics in dogs. J. Pharmacol. Exp. Ther., *224:*531, 1983.
98. Chow, M.S.S., Ronfeld, R.A., Ruffet, D., and Fieldman, A.: Lidocaine pharmacokinetics during cardiac arrest and external cardiopulmonary resuscitation. Am. Heart J. *102:*799, 1981.
99. Cohen, E.N.: Distribution of local anesthetic agents in the neuraxis of the dog. Anesthesiology, *29:*1002, 1968.
100. Cohen, E.N., Levine, D.A., Colliss, J.E., and Gunther, R.E.: The role of pH in the development of tachyphylaxis to local anesthetic agents. Anesthesiology, *29:*994, 1968.
101. Cohen, S., Luykx, W.M., and Marx, G.F.: High versus low flow rates during lumbar epidural block. Reg. Anaesth., *9:*8, 1984.
102. Collinsworth, K.A., Strong, J.M., Atkinson, A.J., *et al.*: Pharmacokinetics and metabolism of lidocaine in patients with renal failure. Clin. Pharmacol. Ther., *18:*59, 1975.
103. Concepcion, M., Maddi, R., Francis, D., *et al.*: Vasoconstrictors in spinal anesthesia with tetracaine—A comparison of epinephrine and phenylephrine. Anesth. Analg. (Cleve.), *63:*134, 1984.
104. Copoga, G., Celleno, D., Constantino, P., *et al.*: Alkalinization improves the quality of lidocaine-fentanyl ananesthesia for caesarean section. Can. J. Anaesth., *49:*425, 1993.
105. Courtney, K.R.: Structure-activity relations for frequency-dependent sodium channel block in nerve by local anesthetics. J. Pharmacol. Exp. Ther., *213:*114, 1980.
106. Cousins, M.J., and Bromage, P.R.: A comparison of the hydrochloride and carbonated salts of lignocaine for caudal analgesia in outpatients. Br. J. Anaesth., *43:*1149, 1971.
107. Cousins, M.J., and Mather, L.E.: Intrathecal and epidural administration of opioids. Anesthesiology, *61:*276, 1984.
108. Coventry, D.M., and Todd, J.G.: Alkalinization of bupivacaine for sciatic nerve blockade. Anaesthesia, *44:*467, 1989.
109. Cox, P.: Intravenous regional analgesia—a new modification. Acta Anaesthesiol. Scand., *33:*336, 1989.
110. Coyle, D.E., Denson, D.D., Thompson, G.A., *et al.*: The influence of lactic acid on the serum protein binding of bupivacaine: Species differences. Anesthesiology, *61:*127, 1984.
111. Curatolo, M. Orlando, A. Zbinden, A.M. Scaramozzino, and P. Venuti, F.S.: A mutifactorial analysis of the spread of epidural analgesia. Acta Anaesth. Scand., *38:*625, 1994.
112. Curran, J., Hamilton, C., and Taylor, T.: Topical analgesia before tracheal intubation. Anaesthesia, *30:*765, 1975.
113. Cusack, B., Kelly, J.G., Lavan, J, *et al.*: Pharmacokinetics of lignocaine in the elderly. Br. J. Clin. Pharmacol., *9:*293P, 1980.
114. Cusick, J.F., Myklebust, J.B., and Abram, S.E.: Differential neural effects of epidural anesthetics. Anesthesiology, *53:*299, 1980.
115. Cusick, J.F., Myklebust, J.B., Abram, S.E., and Davidson, A.: Altered neural conduction with epidural bupivacaine. Anesthesiology, *57:*31, 1982.
116. Dahl, J.B., Simonsen, L., Mogensen, T. Henkinsen, J.H., and Kehlet, H.: The effect of 0.5% ropivacaine on epidural blood flow. Acta Anaesthesiol. Scand., *34:*308, 1990.
117. Datta, S., Alper, M.H., Ostheimer, G.W., *et al.*: Effects of maternal position on epidural anesthesia for Cesarian section, acid-base status, and bupivacaine concentrations at delivery. Anesthesiology, *50:*205, 1979.
118. Datta, S., Brown, W.U., Ostheimer, G.W., *et al.*: Epidural anesthesia for Cesarian section in diabetic parturients: Maternal and neonatal acid-base status and bupivacaine concentration. Anesthesiology, *60:*574, 1981.
119. Datta, S., Houle, G.L., and Fox, G.S.: Concentration of lidocaine hydrochloride in newborn gastric fluid after elective Caesarian section and vaginal section and vaginal delivery with epidural analgesia. Can. Anaesth. Soc. J. *22:*79, 1975.
120. Davis, D., Grossman, S.H., Kitchell, B.B., *et al.*: The effects of age and smoking on the plasma protein binding of lignocaine and diazepam. Br. J. Clin. Pharmacol., *19:*261, 1985.
121. Dawes, G.S.: A theoretical analysis of fetal drug equilibrium. In Boreus, L. (ed.): Fetal Pharmacology. p. 381. New York, Raven Press, 1973.
122. Deas, T.C.: Severe methemolgobinemia following dental extractions under lidocaine anesthesia. Anesthesiology, *17:*204, 1956.
123. deJong, R.H.: Local Anesthetics. pp. 63–83. Springfield IL, Charles C Thomas, 1977.
124. deJong, R.H.: Last round for a "heavyweight"? Anesth. Analg. (Cleve.), *78:*3, 1994.
125. Dennhardt, R. and Ammon, K.: Untersuchungen zur Loslichkeit von Bupivacain im Liquor cerebrospinalis. Anaesthesist, *29:*10, 1980.
126. Denson, D.D., Coyle, D.E., Thompson, G., and Myers, J.A.: $Alpha_1$-acid glycoprotein and albumin in human serum bupivacaine binding. Clin. Pharmacol. Ther., *35:*409, 1984.
127. Denson, D.D., Myers, J.A., and Coyle, D.E.: The clinical relevance of the drug displacement interaction between meperidine and bupivacaine. Res. Commun. Chem. Pathol. Pharmacol., *45:*323, 1984.
128. Denson, D.D., Myers, J.A., Thompson, G.A., and Coyle, D.E.: The influence of diazepam on the serum protein binding of bupivacaine at normal and acidic pH. Anesth. Analg. (Cleve.), *63:*980, 1984.
129. Denson, D.D., Myers, J.A., Watters, C., and Raj, P.P.: Selective inhibition of the aromatic hydroxylation of bupivacaine by halothane. Anesthesiology, *57:*A242, 1982.
130. Denson, D.D., Tumer, P.A., Bridenbaugh, P.O., and Thompson, G.A.: Pharmacokinetics and neural blockade after subarachnoid lidocaine in the rhesus monkey: III. Effects of phenylephrine. Anesth. Analg. (Cleve.), *63:*129, 1984.
131. DeRick, A., Rossel, M.T., Belpaire, F., and Bogaert, M.: Lidocaine plasma concentrations obtained with a standardized infusion in the awake and anaesthetized dog. J. Vet. Pharmacol. Ther., *4:*129, 1981.
132. Dhuner, K.G.: Frequency of general side reactions after regional anaesthesia with mepivacaine with and without vasoconstrictors. Acta Anaesthesiol. Scand. *48:*23, 1972.
133. DiFazio, C.A., Carron, H., Grosslight, K.R., *et al.*: Comparison of pH-adjusted lidocaine solutions for epidural anesthesia. Anesth. Analg. (Cleve.), *65:*760, 1986.
134. Doerge, R.F.: Local anesthetic agents. *In* Wilson, C.O., and Gisvold, O. (eds.): Textbook of Organic Medicinal and Pharmaceutical Chemistry. p. 507. Philadelphia, J.B. Lippincott, 1962.
135. Donchin, Y., Ramu, A., Olshwang, D., *et al.*: Effect of sodium bicarbonate on the kinetics of bupivacaine in i.v. regional anaesthesia in dogs. Br. J. Anaesth., *52:*969, 1980.
136. Drayer, D.E., Lorenzo, B., Werns, S., and Reidenberg, M.M.: Plasma levels, protein binding, and elimination data of lidocaine and active metabolites in cardiac patients of various ages. Clin. Pharmacol. Ther., *34:*14, 1983.
137. Dudziak, R., and Uihlein, M.: Loslichkeit von Lokalanaesthetika in Liquor cerebrospinalis und ihre Abhangigkeit von der Wasserstoffionenkonzentration. Anaesthesist, *27:*32, 1978.
138. DuSouich, P., and Erill, S.: Altered metabolism of procainamide and procaine in patients with pulmonary and cardiac diseases. Clin. Pharmacol. Ther., *21:*101, 1977.
139. DuSouich, P., Saunier, C., Hartemann, D., and Allam, M.: Effect of acute and chronic moderate hypoxia on the kinetics of lidocaine and its metabolites and on regional blood flow. Pulmon. Pharmacol., *5:*9–16, 1992.
140. Ecoffey, C., Desparmet, J., Berdeaux, A., *et al.*: Pharmacokinetics of lignocaine in children following caudal anaesthesia. Br. J. Anaesth., *56:*1399, 1984.
141. Ecoffey, C., Desparmet, J., Maury, M., *et al.*: Bupivacaine in children:

pharmacokinetics following caudal anesthesia. Anesthesiology, *63:*447, 1985.
142. Edwards, D.J., Lalka, D., Cerra, F., and Slaughter, R.L.: Alpha$_1$-acid glycoprotein concentration and protein binding in trauma. Clin. Pharmacol. Ther., *31:*62, 1982.
143. Engberg, G., Holmdahl, M.H., and Edstrom, H.H.: A comparison of the local anesthetic properties of bupivacaine and two new long-acting agents, HS-37 and etidocaine, in epidural analgesia. Acta Anaesthesiol. Scand., *18:*277, 1974.
144. Englesson, S.: The influence of acid-base changes on central nervous system toxicity of local anaesthetic agents: I. An experimental study in cats. Acta Anaesthesiol. Scand., *18:*79, 1974.
145. Englesson, S., and Grevsten, S.: The influence of acid-base changes on central nervous system toxicity of local anaesthetic agents: II. Acta Anaesthesiol. Scand., *18:*88, 1974.
146. Erdemir, H.A., Soper, L.E., and Sweet, R.E.: Studies of the factors affecting peridural anesthesia. Anesth. Analg. (Cleve.), *44:*400, 1966.
147. Estbe, J.P., Lecorre, P., Chevanne, F., and Leverge, R.: Prolongation of spinal anesthesia with bupivacaine-loaded (DL-lactide) microspheres. Anesth. Analg. (Cleve.), *81:*99, 1995.
148. Evans, C.J., Dewar, J.A., Boyes, R.N., and Scott, D.B.: Residual nerve block following intravenous regional anaesthesia. Br. J. Anaesth., *46:*668, 1974.
149. Eyres, R.L., Bishop, W., Oppenheim, R.C., and Brown, T.C.K.: Plasma bupivacaine concentrations in children during caudal epidural analgesia. Anaesth. Intensive Care, *11:*20, 1983.
150. Eyres, R.L., Kidd, J., Oppenheim, R., and Brown, T.C.K.: Local anaesthetic plasma levels in children. Anaesth. Intensive Care, *6:*243, 1978.
151. Fairley, J.W., and Reynolds, F.: An intradermal study of the local anaesthetic and vascular effects of the isomers of mepivacaine. Br. J. Anaesth., *53:*1211, 1981.
152. Feely, J., Clee, M., Pereira, L., and Guy, E.: Enzyme inhibition with rifampicin: lipoproteins and drug binding to alpha1-acid glycoprotein. Br. J. Clin. Pharmacol., *16:*195, 1983.
153. Feely, J., and Guy, E.: Lack of effect of ranitidine on the disposition of lignocaine. Br. J. Clin. Pharmacol., *15:*378, 1983.
154. Feely, J., Wade, D., McAllister, C.B., *et al.*: Effect of hypotension on liver blood flow and lidocaine disposition. N. Engl. J. Med., *307:*866, 1982.
155. Feely, J., Wilkinson, G.R., McAllister, C.B., and Wood, A.J.J.: Increased toxicity and reduced clearance of lidocaine by cimetidine. Ann. Intern. Med., *96:*592, 1982.
156. Finholt, D.A., Stirt, J.A., DiFazio, C.A., and Moscicki, J.C.: Lidocaine pharmacokinetics in children. Anesth. Analg. (Cleve.), *65:*279, 1986.
157. Fink, B.R., and Cairns, A.M.: Diffusional delay in local anesthetic block in vitro. Anesthesiology, *61:*555, 1984.
158. Finster, M., and Pedersen, H.: Placental transfer and fetal uptake of drugs. Br. J. Anaesth., *51:*25S, 1979.
159. Finster, M., Perel, J.M., Hinsvark, O.N., and O'Brien, J.E.: Reassessment of the metabolism of 2-chloroprocaine hydrochloride (Nesacaine). *In* Abstracts of Scientific Papers, Annual Meeting, San Francisco. Chicago, American Society of Anesthesiologists, 1973.
160. Flynn, R.J., Moore, J., Collier, P.S., and Howard, P.J.: Single dose oral H2-antagonists do not affect plasma lidocaine levels. Acta Anaesthesiol. Scand., *33:*93S, 1989.
161. Flynn, R.J., Moore, J., Collier, P.S., and McClean, E.: Does pretreatment with cimetidine and ranitidine affect the disposition of bupivacaine? Br. J. Anaesth., *62:*87, 1989.
162. Foldes, F.F., Davidson, G.N., Duncalf, D., and Kuwabarra, S.: The intravenous toxicity of local anesthetic agents in man. Clin. Pharmacol. Ther., *6:*328, 1965.
163. Foldvari, M., Gesztes, A., and Mezei, M., *et al.*: Topical liposomal local anesthetics—design, optimization and evaluation of formulations. Drug Dev. Indl. Pharm., *19:*2499, 1993.
164. Ford, D.J., Raj, P.P., Regan, K.M., and Ohlweiler, D.: Differential peripheral nerve block by local anesthetics in the cat. Anesthesiology, *60:*28, 1984.
165. Fragneto, R.Y., Bader, A.M., Rosinia, F., Arthur, G.R., and Datta, S.: Measurements of protein binding of lidocaine throughout pregnancy. Anesth. Analg. (Cleve.), *79:*295, 1994.
166. Friberger, P., and Aberg, G.: Some physicochemical properties of the racemates and the optically active isomers of two local anaesthetic compounds. Acta Pharm. Suec., *8:*361, 1971.
167. Fukui, T., Hameroff, S.R., and Gandolfi, A.J.: Alpha$_1$-acid glycoprotein and beta-endorphin alterations in chronic pain patients. Anesthesiology, *60:*494, 1984.
168. Fyhr, P., and Hogstrom, C.: A preformulation study of the kinetics of the racemization of ropivacaine hydrochloride. Acta Pharm. Suec. *25:*121, 1988.
169. Gajraj, N.M., Pennant, J.H., and Watcha, M.F.: Eutectic mixture of local anesthetics (EMLA) cream. Anesth. Analg. (Cleve.), *78:*574, 1994.
170. Gaylard, D.G., Carson, R.J., and Reynolds, F.: Effect of umbilical perfusate pH and controlled maternal hypotension on placental drug transfer in the rabbit. Anesth. Analg. (Cleve.), *71:*42, 1990.
171. Geng, W.P., Ebke, M., and Foth, H.: Prilocaine elimination by isolated perfused rat lung and liver. Naunyn Schmeid. Arch. Pharmakol. *351:*93, 1995.
172. Ghoneim, M.M., and Pandya, H.: Plasma protein binding of bupivacaine and its interaction with other drugs in man. Br. J. Anaesth., *46:*435, 1974.
173. Giasi, R.M., D'Agostino, E., and Covino, B.G.: Interaction of diazepam and epidurally administered local anesthetic agents. Reg. Anaesth., *3:*8, 1980.
174. Giaufre, E., Bruguerolle, B., Morrison-Lacombe, G., and Rousset-Rouviere, B.: The influence of diazepam on the plasma concentrations of bupivacaine and lignocaine after caudal injection of a mixture of the local anaesthetics in children. Br. J. Clin. Pharmacol., *26:*116, 1988.
175. Giaufre, E., Bruguerolle, B., Morrison-Lacombe, G., and Rousset-Rouviere, B.: The influence of midazolam on the plasma concentrations of bupivacaine and lidocaine after caudal injection of a mixture of the local anesthetics in children. Acta Anaesthesiol. Scand., *34:*44, 1990.
176. Gissen, A.J., Covino, B.G., and Gregus, J.: Differential sensitivity of fast and slow fibers in mammalian nerve: III. Effect of etidocaine and bupivacaine on fast/slow fibers. Anesth. Analg. (Cleve.), *61:*570, 1982.
177. Goldberg, M.J., Spector, R., and Johnson, G.F.: Racial background and lidocaine pharmacokinetics. J. Clin. Pharmacol., *22:*391, 1982.
178. Goolkasian, D.L., Slaughter, R.L., Edwards, D.J., and Lalka, D.: Displacement of lidocaine from serum alpha$_1$-acid glycoprotein binding sites by basic drugs. Eur. J. Clin. Pharmacol., *25:*413, 1983.
179. Grant, G.J., Vermeulen, K., Langerman, L., Zakowski, M., and Turndorf, H.: Prolonged analgesia with liposomal bupivacaine in a mouse model. Reg. Anesth., *19:*264, 1994.
180. Greene, N.M.: Uptake and elimination of local anesthetics during spinal anesthesia. Anesth. Analg. (Cleve.), *62:*1013, 1983.
181. Grossman, S.H., Davis, D., Kitchell, B.B., *et al.*: Diazepam and lidocaine plasma protein binding in renal disease. Clin. Pharmacol. Ther., *31:*350, 1982.
182. Grundy, E.M., Ramamurthy, S., Patel, K.P., *et al.*: Extradural analgesia revisited. Br. J. Anaesth., *50:*805, 1978.
183. Grundy, E.M., Rao, L.N., and Winnie, A.P.: Epidural anesthesia and the lateral position. Anesth. Analg. (Cleve.), *57:*95, 1978.
184. Gupta, N., Kennedy, R.L., Vicinie, A., *et al.*: Fetal uptake of bupivacaine following bolus intravenous injection. Anesthesiology, *65:*382A, 1986.
185. Halkin, H., Meffin, P., Melmon, K.L., and Rowland, M.: Influence of congestive heart failure on blood levels of lidocaine and its active monodeethylated metabolite. Clin. Pharmacol. Ther., *17:*669, 1975.
185a Halldin, M.M., Bredberg, E., Angelin, B., *et al.*: Metabolism and excretion of nopivacaine in humans. Drug Metab. Disp., *24:*962, 1996.
186. Hamshaw-Thomas, A., Rogerson, N., and Reynolds, F.: Transfer of bupivacaine, lignocaine and pethidine across the rabbit placenta: Influence of maternal protein binding and fetal flow. Placenta, *5:*61, 1984.
187. Hartrick, C.T., Dirkes, W.E., Coyle, D.E., *et al.*: Influence of bupivacaine on mepivacaine protein binding. Clin. Pharmacol. Ther., *36:*546, 1984.
188. Hartrick, C.T., Raj, P.P., Dirkes, W.E., and Denson, D.D.: Compounding of bupivacaine and mepivacaine for regional anesthesia. A safe practice? Reg. Anaesth., *9:*94, 1984.
189. Hasselstrom, L., Nortved-Sorensen, J., Kehlet, H., *et al.*: The influence of systemically administered bupivacaine on cardiovascular function in cholecystectomised patients. Acta Anaesthesiol. Scand., *29:*76A, 1985.
190. Hawks, R.L., Kopin, I.J., Colburn, R.W., and Thoa, N.B.: Norcocaine: A pharmacologically active metabolite of cocaine found in brain. Life Sci., *15:*2189, 1974.

191. Heavner, J.E., Dryden, C.F., Sanghani, V., *et al.*: Severe hypoxia enhances central nervous system and cardiovascular toxicity of bupivacaine in lightly anesthetized pigs. Anesthesiology, *77:*142, 1992.
192. Hickey, R., Blanchard, J., Hoffman, J., Sjovall, J., and Ramamurthy, S.: Plasma concentrations of ropivacaine given with or without epinephrine for brachial plexus block. Can. J. Anaesth., *37:*878, 1990.
193. Hickey, R., Candido, K.D., Ramamurthy, S., *et al.*: Brachial plexus block with a new local anesthetic: 0.5% ropivacaine. Can. J. Anaesth., *37:*732, 1990.
194. Hjelm, M., and Holmdahl, M.H.: Biochemical effects of aromatic amines: II. Cyanosis, methaemoglobinaemia and Heinz-body formation induced by a local anaesthetic agent (prilocaine). Acta Anaesthesiol. Scand., *9:*99, 1965.
195. Hodgkinson, R., and Husain, F.J.: Obesity, gravity and spread of epidural anesthesia. Anesth. Analg. (Cleve.), *60:*421, 1981.
196. Holley, F.O., Ponganis, K.V., and Stanski, D.R.: Effects of cardiac surgery with cardiopulmonary bypass on lidocaine disposition. Clin. Pharmacol. Ther., *35:*617, 1984.
197. Hou, S.M., and Yu, H.Y.: Comparison of absorption of aqueous lidocaine and liposome lidocaine following topical application on rabbit vessels. J. Orthopaed. Res., *12:*294, 1994.
198. Howarth, F.: Studies with a radioactive spinal anaesthetic. Br. J. Pharmacol., *4:*333, 1949.
199. Huang, Y.F., Upton, R.N., and Runciman, W.B.: I.V. bolus administration of subconvulsive doses of lignocaine to conscious sheep: Myocardial pharmacokinetics. Br. J. Anaesth., *70:*326, 1993.
200. Huang, Y.F., Upton, R.N., and Runciman, W.B.: Relationships between myocardial pharmacokinetics and pharmacodynamics. Br. J. Anaesth., *70:*556, 1993.
201. Huet, P.-M., Arsene, D., and Richer, D.: The volume of distribution of lidocaine in chronic hepatitis: Relationship with serum alpha$_1$-acid glycoprotein and serum protein binding. Clin. Pharmacol. Ther., *29:*252, 1981.
202. Huet, P.-M., and LeLorier, J.: Effects of smoking and chronic hepatitis B on lidocaine and indocyanine green kinetics. Clin. Pharmacol. Ther., *28:*208, 1980.
203. Huet, P.M., and Villeneuve, J.-P.: Determinants of drug disposition in patients with cirrhosis. Hepatology, *3:*913, 1983.
204. Husemeyer, R.P., and White, D.C.: Lumbar extradural injection pressures in pregnant women. An investigation of relationships between rate of injection, injection pressures and extent of analgesia. Br. J. Anaesth., *52:*55, 1980.
205. Inoue, R., Suganuma, T., Echizen, H., Ishizaki, T., Kushida, K., and Tomono, Y.: Plasma concentrations of lidocaine and its principal metabolites during intermittent epidural anesthesia. Anesthesiology, *63:*304, 1985.
206. Jackson, J.E., Bentley, J.B., Glass, S.J., *et al.*: Effects of histamine-2-receptor blockade on lidocaine kinetics. Clin. Pharmacol. Ther. *37:*544, 1985.
207. Jackson, P.R., Tucker, G.T., and Woods, H.F.: Altered plasma binding in cancer: Role of alpha$_1$-acid glycoprotein and albumin. Clin. Pharmacol. Ther., *32:*295, 1982.
208. Jang, J., Yaksh, T., and Hill, H.F.: Use of 2-hydroxypropyl-beta-cyclodextrin as an intrathecal drug vehicle with opioids. J. Pharm. Exp. Ther. *261:*592, 1992.
209. Javaid, J.I., Musa, M.N., Fischman, M., *et al.*: Kinetics of cocaine in humans after intravenous and intranasal administration. Biopharm. Drug. Dispos., *4:*9, 1983.
210. Jawan, B., and Lee, J.H.: The effect of removal of cerebrospinal fluid on cephalad spread of spinal analgesia with 0.5% plain bupivacaine. Acta Anaesthesiol. Scand., *34:*452, 1990.
211. Johansson, P.A.: Liquid-liquid distribution of lidocaine and some structurally related antiarrhythmic drugs and some local anaesthetics. Acta Pharm. Suec., *19:*137, 1982.
212. Johns, R.A., DiFazio, C.A., and Longnecker, D.E.: Lidocaine constricts or dilates rat arterioles in a dose-dependent manner. Anesthesiology, *62:*141, 1985.
213. Jonderko, K.: Partitioning of intravenous lidocaine into gastric juice. Chung Kuo Yao Li Hsueh Pao., *11:*463, 1990.
214. Jones, J.W., and Davis, A.T.: Stability of bupivacaine hydrochloride in polypropylene syringes. Am. J. Hosp. Pharm., *50:*2364, 1993.
215. Jorfeldt, L., Lewis, D.H., Lofstrom, B., and Post, C.: Lung uptake of lidocaine in healthy volunteers. Acta. Anaesthesiol. Scand. *23:*567, 1979.
216. Jorfeldt, L., Lewis, D.H., Lofstrom, B., and Post, C.: Lung uptake of lidocaine in man as influenced by anaesthesia, mepivacaine infusion or lung insufficiency. Acta Anaesthesiol. Scand., *27:*5, 1983.
217. Kambam, J.R., Horton, B., Parris, W.C., *et al.*: Pseudocholinesterase activity in human cerebrospinal fluid. Anesth. Analg., *68:*486, 1989.
218. Kastrissios, H., Triggs, E.J., Mogg, G.A.G., and Higbie, J.W.: The disposition of bupivacaine following a 72h interpleural infusion in cholecystectomy patients. Br. J. Clin. Pharmacol. *32:*251, 1991.
219. Kates, R.E., Harapat, S.R., Keefe, D.L.D., *et al.*: Influence of prolonged recumbency on drug disposition. Clin. Pharmacol. Ther., *27:*624, 1980.
220. Katz, J.A., Bridenbaugh, P.O., Knarr, D.C., Helton, S.H., and Denson, D.D.: Pharmacodynamics and pharmacokinetics of epidural ropivacaine in humans. Anesth. Analg. (Cleve.), *70:*16, 1990.
221. Kennedy, R.L., Bell, J.U., Miller, R.P., *et al.*: Uptake and distribution of lidocaine in fetal lambs. Anesthesiology, *72:*483, 1990.
222. Kennedy, R.L., Erenberg, A., Robilliard, J.E., *et al.*: Effects of the changes in maternal-fetal pH on the transplacental equilibrium of bupivacaine. Anesthesiology, *51:*50, 1979.
223. Kennedy, R.L., Miller, R.P., Bell, J.U., *et al.*: Uptake and distribution of bupivacaine in fetal lambs. Anesthesiology, *65:*247, 1986.
224. Kennedy, W.F., Everett, G.B., Cobb, L.A., and Allen, G.D.: Simultaneous systemic and hepatic hemodynamic measurements during high peridural anesthesia in normal men. Anesth. Analg. (Cleve.), *50:*1069, 1971.
225. King, H.K., Xiao, C.S., and Wooten, D.J.: Prolongation of epidural bupivacaine analgesia with glycerine. Can. J. Anaesth. *40:*431, 1993.
226. Kishikawa, K., Namiki, I., Miyashita, K., and Saitoh, K.: Effects of famotidine and cimetidine on plasma levels of epidurally administered lignocaine. Anaesthesia, *45:*719, 1990.
227. Kitahara, T., Jun, S., and Yoshida, J.: The spread of drugs used for spinal anesthesia. Anesthesiology, *17:*295, 1956.
228. Klein, J.A.: Tumescent technique for regional anesthesia permits lidocaine doses of 35mg/kg for liposuction. J. Dermatol. Surg. Oncol., *16:*248, 1990.
229. Klingenstrom, P., Nylen, B., and Westermark, L.: A clinical comparison between adrenaline and octapressin as vasoconstrictors in local anaesthesia. Acta Anaesthesiol. Scand., *11:*35, 1967.
230. Kloss, M.W., Rosen, G.M., and Rauckman, E.J.: Cocaine-mediated hepatotoxicity. Biochem. Pharmacol., *33:*169, 1984.
231. Kopacz, D.J., Carpenter, R.L., and Mackey, D.C.: Effect of ropivacaine on cutaneous capillary blood flow in pigs. Anesthesiology, *71:*69, 1989.
232. Koster, H., Shapiro, A., and Leikensohn, A.: Procaine concentration changes at the site of injection in subarachnoid anesthesia. Am. J. Surg., *33:*245, 1936.
233. Kraus, E., Polnaszek, C.F., Scheeler, D.A., *et al.*: Interaction between human serum albumin and alpha$_1$-acid glycoprotein in the binding of lidocaine to purified protein fractions and sera. J. Pharmacol. Exp. Ther. *239:*754, 1986.
234. Kristoffersen, E., Sloth, E., Husted, J.C., Bach, A.B., Husegaard, H.C., and Zulow, I.: Spinal anaesthesia with plain 0.5% bupivacaine at 19 degrees C and 37 degrees C. Br. J. Anaesth., *65:*504, 1990.
235. Krogh, K., and Jellum, E.: Urinary metabolites of chloroprocaine. Anesthesiology, *56:*483, 1982.
236. Kuhnert, B.R., Knapp, D.R., Kuhnert, P.M., and Prochaska, A.L.: Maternal, fetal, and neonatal metabolism of lidocaine. Clin. Pharmacol. Ther. *26:*213, 1979.
237. Kuhnert, B.R., Kuhnert, P.M., Philipson, E.H., *et al.*: The half-life of 2-chloroprocaine. Anesth. Analg. (Cleve.), *65:*273, 1986.
238. Kuhnert, B.R., Kuhnert, P.M., Prochaska, A.L., and Gross, T.L.: Plasma levels of 2-chloroprocaine in obstetric patients and their neonates after epidural anesthesia. Anesthesiology, *53:*21, 1980.
239. Kuhnert, P.M., Kuhnert, B.R., Stitts, J.M., and Gross, T.L.: The use of a selected ion monitoring technique to study the disposition of bupivacaine in mother, fetus, and neonate following epidural anesthesia for Cesarian section. Anesthesiology, *55:*611, 1981.
240. Kuhnert, B.R., Zuspan, K.J., Kuhnert, P.M., *et al.*: Lack of influence of cimetidine on bupivacaine levels during parturition. Anesth. Analg. (Cleve.), *66:*986, 1987.
241. Labedzki, L., Scavone, J.M., Ochs, H.R., and Greenblatt, D.J.: Reduced systemic absorption of intrabronchial lidocaine by high frequency nebulization. J. Clin. Pharmacol., *30:*795, 1990.
242. Lalka, D., Vicuna, N., Burrow, S.R., *et al.*: Bupivacaine and other amide local anesthetics inhibit hydrolysis of chloroprocaine by human serum. Anesth. Analg. (Cleve.), *57:*534, 1978.

243. Langerman, L., Basinath, M., and Grant, G.J.: The partition coefficient as a predictor of local anesthetic potency for spinal anesthesia: evaluation of five local anesthetics in a mouse model. Anesth. Analg., *79:*490, 1994.
244. Langerman, L., Grant, G.J., Zakowski, M., Ramanathan, S., and Turndorf, H.: Prolongation of spinal anesthesia. Spinal action of a lipid drug carrier on tetracaine, lidocaine and procaine. Anesthesiology, *77:*475, 1992.
245. Laurito, C.E., Kirz, L.J., VadeBoncouer, T.R., *et al.*: Continuous infusion of interpleural bupivacaine maintains effective analgesia after cholecystectomy. Anesth. Analg. (Cleve.), *72:*516, 1991.
246. Lauven, P.M., Witow, R., Lussi, C., and Luhr, H.G.: Blutspiegel und pharmakokinetisches modell von prilocain bei der kontinuerlichen plexus-brachialis-blockade. Reg. Anesth. *13:*189, 1990.
247. Le Corre, P., Estebe, J.P., Chevanne, Y., Malledant, Y., and Le Verge, R.: Spinal controlled delivery of bupivacaine from DL-lactic acid oligomer microspheres. J. Pharm. Sci., *84:*75, 1995.
248. Lee-Son, S., Wang, G.K., Concus, A., Crill, E., and Strichartz, G.: Stereoselective inhibition of neuronal sodium channels by local anesthetics. Evidence for two sites of action? Anesthesiology, *77:*324, 1992.
249. Legros, F., Luo, H., Bourgeois, P., Lafont, N., and Boogaerts, J.: Influence of different liposomal formulations on pharmacokinetics of encapsulated bupivacaine. Anesthesiology, *73:*A851, 1990.
250. Lennard, M.S., Tucker, G.T., and Woods, H.F.: Time-dependent kinetics of lignocaine in the isolated perfused rat liver. J. Pharmacokinet. Biopharm., *11:*165, 1983.
251. Leor, R., Feinstein, M., Hod, H., Rabinowitz, B., and Kaplinsky, E.: The influence of pH on the intravenous delivery of lidocaine solutions. Eur. J. Clin. Pharmacol., *39:*521, 1990.
252. Lerman, J., Strong, A., LeDez, K.M., Swartz, J., Rieder, M.J., and Burrows, F.A.: Effects of age on the serum concentration of α_1-acid glycoprotein and the binding of lidocaine in pediatric patients. Clin. Pharmacol. Ther., *46:*219, 1989.
253. Lofstrom, B.: Blocking characteristics of etidocaine (Duranest). Acta. Anaesthesiol. Scand. *60:*21, 1975.
254. Lofstrom, B.: Tissue distribution of local anesthetics with special reference to the lung. Int. Anesthesiol. Clin., *16:*53, 1978.
255. Luduena, F.P.: Duration of local anesthesia. Annu. Rev. Pharmacol., *9:*503, 1969.
256. Lund, P.C., Bush, D.F., and Covino, B.G.: Determinants of etidocaine concentration in the blood. Anesthesiology, *42:*497, 1975.
257. McClure, J.H., and Scott, D.B.: Comparison of bupivacaine hydrochloride and carbonated bupivacaine in brachial plexus block interscalene technique. Br. J. Anaesth., *53:*523, 1981.
258. McEllistrem, R.F., Bennington, R.G., and Roth, S.H.: *In vitro* determination of permeability to opioids and local anaesthetics. Can. J. Anaesth., *40:*165, 1993.
259. Maclean, D., Chambers, W.A., Tucker, G.T., and Wildsmith, J.A.W.: Plasma prilocaine concentrations after three techniques of brachial plexus blockade. Br. J. Anaesth. *60:*136, 1988.
260. McLean, S., Starmer, G.A., and Thomas, J.: Methaemoglobin formation by aromatic amines. J. Pharm. Pharmacol., *21:*441, 1969.
261. McNamara, P.J., Slaughter, R.L., Pieper, J.A., *et al.*: Factors influencing serum protein binding of lidocaine in humans. Anesth. Analg. (Cleve.), *60:*395, 1981.
262. McNamara, P.J., Slaughter, R.L., Visco, J.P., *et al.*: Effect of smoking on binding of lidocaine to human serum proteins. J. Pharm. Sci., *69:*749, 1980.
263. Marathe, P.H., Shen, D.D., Artru, A.A., and Bowdle, A.: Effect of serum protein binding on the entry of lidocaine into brain and cerebrospinal fluid in dogs. Anesthesiology, *75:*804, 1991.
264. Martin, R., Lamarche, Y., and Tetreault, L.: Comparison of the clinical effectiveness of lidocaine hydrocarbonate and lidocaine hydrocloride with and without epinephrine in epidural anaesthesia. Can. Anaesth. Soc. J., *28:*217, 1981.
265. Mashimo, T., Uchida, I., Pak, M., *et al.*: Prolongation of canine epidural anesthesia by liposome encapsulation of lidocaine. Anesth. Analg. (Cleve.), *74:*827, 1992.
266. Mather, L.E.: Tachyphylaxis in regional anaesthesia: Can we reconcile clinical observation and laboratory measurements? Anaesth. Intenzivemed., *176:*3, 1986.
267. Mather, L.E.: Disposition of mepivacaine and bupivacaine enantiomers in sheep. Br. J. Anaesth., *67:*239, 1991.
268. Mather, L.E., and Cousins, M.J.: Local anaesthetics and their current clinical use. Drugs, *18:*185, 1979.
269. Mather, L.E., Long, G.J., and Thomas, J.: The binding of bupivacaine to maternal and foetal plasma proteins. J. Pharm. Pharmacol., *23:*359, 1971.
270. Mather, L.E., McCall, P., and McNicol, P.L.: Bupivacaine enantiomer pharmacokinetics after intercostal neural blockade in liver transplant patients. Anesth. Analg. (Cleve.), *80:*328, 1995.
271. Mather, L.E., Runciman, W.B., Carapetis, R.J., *et al.*: Hepatic and renal clearances of lidocaine in conscious and anesthetized sheep. Anesth. Analg. (Cleve.), *65:*943, 1986.
272. Mather, L.E., and Rutten, A.J.: Stereochemistry and its relevance in anaesthesiology. Curr. Opin. Anaesthesiol., *4:*473, 1991.
273. Mather, L.E., Rutten, A.J., and Plummer, J.L.: Pharmacokinetics of bupivacaine enantiomers in sheep: influence of dosage regimen and study design. J. Pharmacokinet. Biopharm., *22:*481, 1994.
274. Mather, L.E., and Thomas, J.: Bupivacaine binding to plasma protein fractions. J. Pharm. Pharmacol., *30:*653, 1978.
275. Mather, L.E., Tucker, G.T., Murphy, T.M., *et al.*: Haemodynamic drug interactions: Peridural lignocaine and intravenous ephedrine. Acta Anaesthesiol. Scand., *20:*207, 1976.
276. Mayumi, T., Dohi, S., and Takahashi, T.: Plasma concentrations of lidocaine associated with cervical, thoracic, and lumbar epidural anesthesia. Anesth. Analg. (Cleve.), *62:*578, 1983.
277. Mazoit, J.X., Boico, O., and Samii, K.: Myocardial uptake of bupivacaine: II. Pharmacokinetics and pharmacodynamics of bupivacaine enantiomers in the isolated perfused rabbit heart. Anesth. Analg. (Cleve.), *77:*477, 1993.
278. Mazoit, J.X., Denson, D.D., and Samii, K.: Pharmacokinetics of bupivacaine following caudal anesthesia in infants. Anesthesiology, *68:*387, 1988.
279. Mazoit, J.X., Lambert, C., Berdeaux, A., Gerard, J.-L., and Froideveaux, R.: Pharmacokinetics of bupivacaine after short and prolonged infusions in conscious dogs. Anesth. Analg. (Cleve.), *67:*961, 1988.
280. Mazumdar, B., Tomlinson, A.A., and Faulder, G.C.: Preliminary study to assay plasma amethocaine concentrations after topical application of a new local anaesthetic cream containing amethocaine. Br. J. Anaesth., *67:*432, 1991.
281. Merry, A.F., Cross, J.A., Mayadeo, S.V., and Wild, C.J.: Posture and spread of extradural analgesia in labour. Br. J. Anaesth., *55:*303, 1983.
282. Mets, B., Hickman, R., Allin, R., Van Dyk, J., and Lotz, Z.: Effect of hypoxia on the hepatic metabolism of lidocaine in the isolated perfused pig liver. Hepatology, *17:*668, 1993.
283. Meyer, J., and Nolte, H.: Liquorkonzentrationen zur bupivacain nach subduraler applikation. Anaesthesist, *29:*38, 1978.
284. Mogensen, T., Hojgaard, L., Scott, N.B., Henriksen, J.H., and Kehlet, H.: Epidural blood flow and regression of sensory analgesia during continuous postoperative epidural infusion of bupivacaine. Anesth. Analg. (Cleve.), *67:*809, 1988.
285. Mogensen, T., Simonsen, L., Scott, N.B., Henriksen, J.H., and Kehlet, H.: Tachyphylaxis associated with repeated epidural injections of lidocaine is not related to changes in distribution or the rate of elimination from the epidural space. Anesth. Analg. (Cleve.), *69:*180, 1989.
286. Monson, D.H.: A double blind comparison of carbonated lidocaine and lidocaine hydrochloride in epidural anaesthesia. Can. Anaesth. Soc. J., *28:*387, 1981.
287. Moore, D.C.: Intercostal nerve block: Spread of India ink injected to the rib's costal groove. Br. J. Anaesth., *53:*325, 1981.
288. Moore, D.C.: The pH of local anesthetic solutions. Anesth. Analg. (Cleve.), *60:*833, 1981.
289. Moore, D.C., Bridenbaugh, L.D., Van Ackeren, E.G., *et al.*: Spread of radio-opaque solutions in the epidural space of the human adult corpse. Anesthesiology, *19:*377, 1957.
290. Moore, D.C., Bush, W.H., and Burnett, L.L.: Celiac plexus block: A roentgenographic, anatomic study of technique and spread of solution in patients and corpses. Anesth. Analg. (Cleve.), *60:*369, 1981.
291. Moore, D.C., Bush, W.H., and Scurlock, J.E.: Intercostal nerve block: A roentgenographic anatomic study of technique and absorption in humans. Anesth. Analg. (Cleve.), *59:*815, 1980.
292. Moore, D.C., Mather, L.E., Bridenbaugh, P.O., *et al.*: Arterial and venous plasma levels of bupivacaine following peripheral nerve blocks. Anesth. Analg. (Cleve.), *55:*763, 1976.
293. Moore, D.C., Mather, L.E., Bridenbaugh, L.D., *et al.*: Arterial and venous plasma levels of bupivacaine (Marcaine) following epidural and intercostal nerve blocks. Anesthesiology, *45:*39, 1976.

294. Moore, R.A., Bullingham, R.E.S., McQuay, H.J., *et al.*: Dural permeability to narcotics: *In vitro* determination and application to extradural administration. Br. J. Anaesth., *54:*1117, 1982.
295. Moorthy, S.S., Dierdorf, S.F., and Yaw, P.B.: Influence of volume on the spread of local anesthetic-methylene blue solution after injection for intercostal block. Anesth. Analg. (Cleve.), *75:*389, 1992.
296. Morgan, D.J., Smyth, M.P., Thomas, J., and Vine, J.: Cyclic metabolites of etidocaine in humans. Xenobiotica, *7:*365, 1977.
297. Morikawa, K.I., Bonica, J.J., Tucker, G.T., and Murphy, T.M.: Effect of acute hypovolaemia on lignocaine absorption and cardiovascular response following epidural block in dogs. Br. J. Anaesth., *46:*631, 1974.
298. Morrison, L.M.M., Emanuelsson, B.M., McClure, J.H., *et al.*: Efficacy and kinetics of extradural ropivacaine: comparison with bupivacaine. Br. J. Anaesth., *72:*164, 1994.
299. Murphy, D.: Interpleural analgesia. Br. J. Anaesth., *71:*426–434, 1993.
300. Murphy, T.M., Mather, L.E., Stanton-Hicks, M.A., *et al.*: Effects of adding adrenaline to etidocaine and lignocaine in extradural anaesthesia. I: Block characteristics and cardiovascular effects. Br. J. Anaesth., *48:*893, 1976.
301. Nakazono, T., Murakami, T., Higashi, Y., and Yata, N.: Study on brain uptake of local anesthetics in rats. J. Pharmacobiodyn., *14:*605, 1991.
302. Nancarrow, C., Runciman, W.B., Mather, L.E., Upton, R.N., and Plummer, J.L.: The influence of acidosis on the distribution of lidocaine and bupivacaine into the myocardium and brain of the sheep. Anesth. Analg. (Cleve.), *66:*925, 1987.
303. Nancarrow, C., Rutten, A.J., Runciman, W.B., *et al.*: Myocardial and cerebral drug concentrations and the mechanisms of death after fatal intravenous doses of lidocaine, bupivacaine, and ropivacaine in the sheep. Anesth. Analg. (Cleve.), *69:*276, 1989.
304. Nation, R.L., Triggs, E.J., and Selig, M.: Lignocaine kinetics in cardiac patients and aged subjects. Br. J. Clin. Pharmacol., *4:*439, 1977.
305. Nayak, P.K., Misra, A.Z., and Mule, S.J.: Physiological disposition and biotransformation of ^{3}H-cocaine in acutely and chronically treated rats. J. Pharmacol. Exp. Ther., *196:*556, 1976.
306. Nicol, M.E., and Holdcroft, A.: Density of intrathecal agents. Br. J. Anaesth., *68:*60, 1992.
307. Nishikawa, T., Goyagi, T., Kimura, T., Dai, M., and Naito, H.: Oral clonidine preanesthetic medication does not alter plasma lidocaine elimination during epidural anesthesia in lightly anesthetized patients. Can. J. Anaesth., *39:*521, 1992.
308. Nishikawa, T. Inomata, S., Igarishi, M., Goyagi, T., and Naito, H.: Plasma lidocaine concentrations during epidural blockade with isoflurane or halothane anesthesia. Anesth. Analg. (Cleve.), *75:*885, 1992.
309. Nishimura, N., Kitahara, T., and Kusakabo, T.: The spread of lidocaine and I-131 solution in the epidural space. Anesthesiology, *20:*785, 1959.
310. Nishimura, N., and Ogura S.: The effect of the posture in the spread of epidural anesthesia. Masui *40:*350, 1991.
311. Nitescu, P., Hultman, E., Appelgren, L., Linder, L.E., and Curelaru, I.: Bacteriology, drug stability and exchange of percutaneous delivery systems and antibacterial filters in long term intrathecal infusion of opioid drugs and bupivacaine in "refractory" pain. Clin. J. Pain., *8:*324, 1992.
312. Noble, D.W., Smith, K.J., and Dundas, C.R.: The effects of H2-antagonists on the elimination of bupivacaine. Br. J. Anaesth., *59:*735, 1987.
313. Nordqvist, P.: The occurrence of procaine esterase in peripheral nerve and its influence on procaine block. Acta Pharmacol. Toxicol. (Kbh.), *8:*217, 1952.
314. Nunn, J.E., and Slavin, G.: Posterior intercostal nerve block for pain relief after cholecystectomy. Br. J. Anaesth., *52:*253, 1980.
315. Nydahl, P.-A., Philipson, L., Axelsson, K., and Johansson, J.-E.: Epidural anesthesia with 0.5% bupivacaine: Influence of age on sensory and motor blockade. Anesth. Analg. (Cleve.), *73:*780, 1991.
316. O'Brien, J.E., Abbey, V., Hinsvark, O., *et al.*: Metabolism and measurement of chloroprocaine, an ester-type local anesthetic. J. Pharm. Sci., *68:*75, 1979.
317. O'Bryan, S., Barry, M.G., Collins, W.C.J., *et al.*: Plasma protein binding of lidocaine and warfarin in insulin-dependent and non-insulin-dependent diabetes mellitus. Clin. Pharmacokinet., *24:*183, 1993.
318. O'Sullivan, G.M., Smith, M., Morgan, B., Brighouse, D., and Reynolds, F.: H2-antagonists and bupivacaine clearance. Anaesthesia, *43:*93, 1988.
319. Oda, Y., Furuichi, K., Tanaka, K., *et al.*: Metabolism of a new local anesthetic, ropivacaine, by human hepatic cytochrome P450. Anesthesiology, *82:*214, 1995.
320. Ohmura, S., Yamamoto, K., Kobayashi, T., and Murakami, S.: Displacement of lidocaine from the lung after bolus injection of bupivacaine. Can. J. Anaesth., *40:*676, 1993.
321. Ohno, H., Watanabe, M., Saitoh, J.Y., *et al.*: Effect of epinephrine concentration on lidocaine disposition during epidural anesthesia. Anesthesiology, *68:*625, 1988.
322. Palazzo, M.G.A., Kalso, E.A., Argiras, E., Madgwick, R., and Sear, J.W.: First-pass lung uptake of bupivacaine: effect of acidosis in an intact rabbit lung model. Br. J. Anaesth., *67:*759, 1991.
323. Palmer, S.K., Bosnjak, Z.J., Hopp, F., *et al.*: Lidocaine and bupivacaine differential blockade of isolated canine nerves. Anesth. Analg. (Cleve.), *62:*754, 1983.
324. Park, W.Y., Hagins, E.M., Massengale, M.D., and MacNamara, T.E.: The sitting position and anesthetic spread in the epidural space. Anesth. Analg. (Cleve.), *63:*863, 1984.
325. Park, W.Y., Hagins, F.M., Rivat, E.L., and MacNamara, T.E.: Age and epidural dose response in adult men. Anesthesiology, *56:*318, 1982.
326. Park, W.Y., Massengale, M., Kin, S.-I., *et al.*: Age and the spread of local anesthetic solutions in the epidural space. Anesth. Analg. (Cleve.), *59:*768, 1980.
327. Partridge, B.L., Katz, J., and Benirschke, K.: Functional anatomy of the brachial plexus sheath: implications for anesthesia. Anesthesiology, *66:*743–7, 1987.
328. Peeyush, M., Ravishankar, M., Adithan, C., and Sashindran, C.H.: Altered pharmacokinetics of lignocaine after epidural injection in Type II diabetics. Eur. J. Clin. Pharmacol., *43:*269, 1992.
329. Pere, P., Tuominen, M., and Rosenberg, P.H.: Cumulation of bupivacaine, desbutylbupivacaine and 4-hydroxybupivacaine during and after continuous interscalene brachial plexus block. Acta Anaesthesiol. Scand., *35:*647, 1991.
330. Perucca, E., and Richens, A.: Reduction of oral bioavailability of lignocaine by induction of first-pass metabolism in epileptic patients. Br. J. Clin. Pharmacol., *8:*21, 1979.
331. Petersen, M.C., Moore, R.G., Nation, R.L., McMeniman, W.: Relationship between the transplacental gradients of bupivacaine and alpha$_1$-acid glycoprotein. Br. J. Clin. Pharmacol., *12:*859, 1981.
332. Piafsky, K.M., and Knoppert, D.: Binding of local anesthetics to alpha$_1$-acid glycoprotein. Clin. Res., *26:*836A, 1979.
333. Piafsky, K.M., and Woolner, E.A.: The binding of basic drugs to alpha$_1$-acid glycoprotein in cord serum. J. Pediatr., *5:*820, 1982.
334. Pihlajamaki, K.K.: Inverse correlation between the peak venous serum concentration of bupivacaine and the weight of the patient during interscalene brachial plexus block. Br. J. Anaesth., *67:*621, 1991.
335. Pihlajamaki, K.K., Kanto, J., Lindberg, R., Karanko, M., and Kiilholma, P.: Extradural administration of bupivacaine: pharmacokinetics and metabolism in pregnant and non-pregnant women. Br. J. Anaesth., *64:*556, 1990.
336. Planas, M.E., Gonzalez, P., Rodriguez, L., Sanchez, S., and Cevc, G.: Noninvasive percutaneous induction of topical analgesia by a new type of drug carrier, and prolongation of local pain insensitivity by anesthetic liposomes. Anesth. Analg. (Cleve.), *75:*615, 1992.
337. Post, C., Andersson, R.G.G., Ryrfeldt, A., and Nilsson, E.: Physicochemical modification of lidocaine uptake in rat lung tissue. Acta Pharmacol. Toxicol., *44:*103, 1979.
338. Post, C., and Eriksdotter-Behm, K.: Dependence of lung uptake of lidocaine in vivo on blood pH. Acta Pharmacol. Toxicol., *51:*136, 1982.
339. Post, C., and Freedman, J.: A new method for studying the distribution of drugs in spinal cord after intrathecal injection. Acta Pharmacol. Toxicol., *54:*253, 1984.
340. Powell, M.F.: Stability of lidocaine in aqueous solution: effect of temperature, pH, buffer, and metal ions on amide hydrolysis. Pharm. Res., *4:*42, 1987.
341. Prengel, A.W., Lindner, K.H., Hahnel, J.H., and Georgieff, M.: Pharmacokinetics and technique of endotracheal and deep endobronchial lidocaine administration. Anesth. Analg. (Cleve.), *77:*985, 1993.
342. Quimby, C.W.: Influence of blood loss on the duration of regional anesthesia. Anesth. Analg. (Cleve.), *44:*387, 1965.
343. Quinlan, J.J., Oleksey, K., and Murphy, F.L.: Alkalinization of mepivacaine for axillary block. Anesth. Analg., *74:*371, 1992.

344. Radtke, H., Nolte, H., Fruhstorfer, H., and Zenz, M.: A comparative study between etidocaine and bupivacaine in ulnar nerve block. Acta Anaesthesiol. Scand., *60:*17, 1975.
345. Raj, P.P., Ohlweiler, D., Hitt, B.A., and Denson, D.D.: Kinetics of local anesthetic esters and effects of adjuvant drugs on 2-chloroprocaine hydrolysis. Anesthesiology, *53:*307, 1980.
346. Ramanathan, J., Bottorf, M., Jeter, J.N., Khalil, M., and Sibai, B.M.: The pharmacokinetics and maternal and neonatal effects of epidural lidocaine in preeclampsia. Anesth. Analg. (Cleve.), *65:*120, 1986.
347. Reidenberg, M.M., James, M., and Dring, L.G.: The rate of procaine hydrolysis in serum of normal subjects and diseased patients. Clin. Pharmacol. Ther., *13:*279, 1972.
348. Rice, A.S.C., Pither, C.E., and Tucker, G.T.: Plasma concentrations of bupivacaine after supraclavicular brachial plexus blockade in patients with chronic renal failure. Anaesthesia, *46:*354, 1991.
349. Richter, O., Klein, K., Abel, J., *et al.*: The kinetics of bupivacaine (Carbostesin) plasma concentrations during epidural anesthesia following intraoperative bolus injection and subsequent continuous infusion. Int. J. Clin. Pharmacol. Ther. Toxicol., *22:*611, 1984.
350. Rigler, M.L., and Drasner, K.: Distribution of catheter-injected local anesthetic in a model of the subarachnoid space. Anesthesiology, *75:*684, 1991.
351. Roberts, S.M., Harbison, R.D., and James, R.C.: Human microsomal N-oxidative metabolism of cocaine. Drug Metab. Disp., *19:*1046, 1991.
352. Robson, R.A., Wing, L.M.H., Miners, J.O., *et al.*: The effect of ranitidine on the disposition of lignocaine. Br. J. Clin. Pharmacol., *20:*170, 1985.
353. Rosen, M.A., Thigpen, J.W., Shnider, S.M., *et al.*: Bupivacaine-induced cardiotoxicity in hypoxic and acidotic sheep. Anesth. Analg. (Cleve.), *64:*1089, 1985.
354. Rosenberg, P.H., and Heavner, J.E.: Acute cardiovascular and central nervous system toxicity of bupivacaine and desbutylbupivacaine in the rat. Acta Anaesthesiol. Scand., *36:*138, 1992.
355. Rosenberg, P.H., and Heinonen, E.: Differential sensitivity of A and C nerve fibres to long-acting amide local anaesthetics. Br. J. Anaesth., *55:*143, 1983.
356. Rosenberg, P.H., Kytta, J., and Alila, A.: Uptake of bupivacaine, etidocaine, lignocaine and ropivacaine in n-heptane, rat sciatic nerve and human epidural and subcutaneous fat. Br. J. Anaesth., *58:*310, 1986.
357. Rosenberg, P.H., Pere, P., Hekali, R., and Tuominen, M.: Plasma concentrations of bupivacaine and two of its metabolites during continuous interscalene brachial plexus block. Br. J. Anaesth., *66:*25, 1991.
358. Rosenberg, P.H., Saramies, L., and Alila, A.: Lumbar epidural anaesthesia with bupivacaine in old patients: Effect of speed and direction of injection. Acta Anaesthesiol. Scand., *25:*270, 1981.
359. Ross, B.K., Coda, B., and Heath, C.H.: Local anesthetic distribution in a spinal model: a possible mechanism of neurologic injury after continuous spinal anesthesia. Reg. Anesth., *17:*69, 1992.
360. Ross, R.A., Clarke, J.E., and Armitage, E.N.: Postoperative pain prevention by continuous epidural infusion. Anaesthesia, *35:*663, 1980.
361. Rothstein, P., Arthur, G.R., Feldman, H., Kopf, G., and Covino, B.G.: Bupivacaine for intercostal nerve blocks in children: blood concentrations and pharmacokinetics. Anesth. Analg. (Cleve.), *65:*625, 1986.
362. Rothstein, P., Arthur, G.R., and Feldman, H., *et al.*: Pharmacokinetics of bupivacaine in children following intercostal block. Anesthesiology, *57:*A426, 1981.
363. Rothstein, P., Cole, J.S., and Pitt, B.R.: Pulmonary extraction of (3H) bupivacaine: modification by dose, propranolol and interaction with (14C) 5-hydroxytryptamine. J. Pharmacol. Exp. Ther., *240:*410, 1987.
364. Routledge, P.A., Barchowsky, A., Bjornsson, T.D., *et al.*: Lidocaine plasma protein binding. Clin. Pharmacol. Ther., *27:*347, 1980.
365. Routledge, P.A., Stargel, W.W., Finn, A.L., *et al.*: Lignocaine disposition in blood in epilepsy. Br. J. Clin. Pharmacol., *12:*663, 1981.
366. Rowland, M., Thomson, P., Guichard, A., and Melmon, K.L.: Disposition kinetics of lidocaine in normal subjects. Ann. N.Y. Acad. Sci., *179:*383, 1971.
367. Rowland, M.: Local anesthetic absorption, distribution and elimination. *In* Eger E. II (ed.): Anesthetic Uptake and Action. pp. 332–366. Baltimore, Williams & Wilkins, 1974.
368. Runciman, W.B., Mather, L.E., Ilsley, A.H., *et al.*: A sheep preparation for studying interactions between blood flow and drug disposition. III: Effects of general and spinal anaesthesia on regional blood flow and oxygen tensions. Br. J. Anaesth., *56:*247, 1984.
369. Runciman, W.B., Myburgh, J.A., Upton, R.N., and Mather, L.E.: Effects of anaesthesia on drug disposition. *In* Feldman, S.A., Scurr, C.F., and Paton, W. (eds.): Mechanisms of Action of Drugs in Anaesthetic Practice. 2nd ed. pp. 93–128. London, Edward Arnold, 1994.
370. Rutten, A.J., Mather, L.E., and McLean, C.F.: Cardiovascular effects and regional clearances of i.v. bupivacaine in sheep: enantiomeric analysis. Br. J. Anaesth., *67:*247, 1991.
371. Rutten, A.J., Mather, L.E., McLean, C.F., and Nancarrow, C.: Tissue distribution of bupivacaine enantiomers in sheep. Chirality, *5:*485, 1993.
372. Rutten, A.J., Mather, L.E., Nancarrow, C., Sloan, P.A., and McLean, C.F.: Cardiovascular effects and regional clearances of intravenous ropivacaine in sheep. Anesth. Analg., *70:*577, 1990.
373. Rutten, A.J., Mather, L.E., Plummer, J.L., and Henning, E.C.: Postoperative course of plasma protein binding of lignocaine, ropivacaine and bupivacaine in sheep. J. Pharm. Pharmacol., *44:*355, 1992.
374. Safran, D., Kuhlman, G., Orhant, E.E., Castelain, M.H., and Journois, D.: Continuous intercostal blockade with lidocaine after thoracic surgery. Clinical and pharmacokinetic study. Anesth. Analg. (Cleve.), *70:*345, 1990.
375. Sallie, R.W., Tredger, J.M., and Williams, R.: Extrahepatic production of the lignocaine metabolite monoethylglycinexylidide (MEGX). Biopharm. Drug. Disp., *13:*555, 1992.
376. Sanchez, V., Arthur, G.R., and Strichartz, G.R.: Fundamental properties of local anesthetics. I. The dependance of lidocaine's ionization and octanol:buffer partitioning on solvent and temperature. Anesth. Analg. (Cleve.), *66:*159, 1987.
377. Santos, A.C., Pedersen, H., Morishima, H.O., *et al.*: Pharmacokinetics of lidocaine in nonpregnant and pregnant ewes. Anesth. Analg. (Cleve.), *67:*1154, 1988.
378. Santos, A.C., Pedersen, H., Sallusto, J.A., *et al.*: Pharmacokinetics of ropivacaine in nonpregnant and pregnant ewes. Anesth. Analg. (Cleve.), *70:*262, 1990.
379. Sato, S., Baba, Y., Tajima, K., *et al.*: Prolongation of epidural anesthesia in the rabbit with the use of a biodegradable copolymer paste containing lidocaine. Anesth. Analg. (Cleve.), *80:*97, 1995.
380. Schenker, S., Yang, Y., Johnson, R.F., *et al.*: The transfer of cocaine and its metabolites across the term human placenta. Clin. Pharmacol. Ther., *53:*329, 1993.
381. Schug, S.A., Payne, J.P., Baker, P., and Holford, N.H.G.: Non-stationary pharmacokinetics of bupivacaine during continuous interpleural infusion. The International Monitor on Regional Anaesthesia, April 1994, p. 33; Abstracts XII Eur. Soc. Reg. Anaesth. Congr., Barcelona, May 1994.
382. Scott, D.B., Jebson, P.J.R., Braid, D.P., *et al.*: Factors affecting plasma levels of lignocaine and prilocaine. Br. J. Anaesth., *44:*1040, 1972.
382a Scott, D.B., Lee, A., Fagan, D., *et al.*: Acute toxicity of ropivacaine compared with that of bupivacaine. Anesth. Analg. (Cleve.) *69:*563, 1989.
383. Scott, D.B., Littlewood, D.G., Covino, B.G., and Drum, G.B.: Plasma lignocaine concentrations following endotracheal spraying with an aerosol. Br. J. Anaesth., *48:*899, 1976.
384. Seifen, A.B., Ferrari, A.A., Seifen, A.A., *et al.*: Pharmacokinetics of intravenous procaine infusion in humans. Anesth. Analg. (Cleve.), *58:*382, 1979.
385. Selander, D.: Axillary plexus block: paresthetic or perivascular. Anesthesiology, *66:*726, 1987.
386. Seow, L.T., Lips, F.J., and Cousins, M.J.: Effect of lateral posture on epidural blockade for surgery. Anaesth. Intensive Care, *11:*97, 1983.
387. Seow, L.T., Lips, F.J., Cousins, M.J., and Mather, L.E.: Lidocaine and bupivacaine mixtures for epidural blockade. Anesthesiology, *56:*177, 1982.
388. Sharrock, N.E.: Epidural anesthetic dose responses in patients 20 to 80 years old. Anesthesiology, *49:*425, 1978.
389. Sharrock, N.E., Go, G., and Mineo, R.: Effect of IV low-dose adrenaline and phenylephrine infusions on plasma concentrations of bupivacaine after lumbar extradural anaesthesia in elderly patients. Br. J. Anaesth. *67:*694, 1991.
390. Sharrock, N.E., Mineo, R., Stanton, J., Ennis, W.J., Urmey, W.F., and Arthur, G.R.: Single versus staged epidural injections of 0.75% bupivacaine: Pharmacokinetic and pharmacodynamic effects. Anesth. Analg. (Cleve.), *79:*307, 1994.
391. Shiroff, R.A., Schneck, D.W., Pritchard, J.F., *et al.*: Effects of acute blood pressure reduction by sodium nitroprusside on serum lidocaine levels. Fed. Proc., *36:*958, 1977.

392. Siler, J.N., and Rosenberg, H.: Lidocaine hydrochloride versus lidocaine bicarbonate for epidural anesthesia in outpatients undergoing arthroscopic surgery. J. Clin. Anesth., *2:*296, 1990.
393. Simon, R.P., Benowitz, N.L., and Culala, S.: Motor paralysis increases brain uptake of lidocaine during status epilepticus. Neurology, *34:*384, 1984.
394. Sinclair, C.J., Scott, D.B., and Edstrom, H.H.: Effect of the Trendelenburg position on spinal anaesthesia with hyperbaric bupivacaine. Br. J. Anaesth., *54:*497, 1982.
395. Skou, J.C.: Local anaesthetics: III. Distribution of local anaesthetics between the solid phase/aqueous phase of peripheral nerves. Acta Pharmacol. Toxicol. (Kbh.), *10:*297, 1954.
396. Skromstag, K.E., Hauge, O., and Steen, P.A.: Distribution of local anesthetics injected into the interpleural space, studied by computerized tomography. Acta Anaesthesiol. Scand., *34:*323, 1990.
397. Skromstag, K.E., Minor, B., and Steen, P.A.: Side effects and complications related to interpleural analgesia: an update. Acta Anesthiol. Scand., *34:*473, 1990.
398. Stanton-Hicks, Md' A., Berges, P.U., and Bonica, J.J.: Circulatory effects of peridural block: IV. Comparison of the effects of epinephrine and phenylephrine. Anesthesiology, *39:*308, 1973.
399. Starke, P., and Nolte, H.: pH des liquor spinalis wahrend subduraler blockade. Anaesthesist, *27:*41, 1978.
400. Stewart, D.J., Inaba, T., Lucassen, M., and Kalow, W.: Cocaine metabolism: Cocaine and norcocaine hydrolysis by liver and serum esterases. Clin. Pharmacol. Ther., *25:*464, 1979.
401. Stewart, D.J., Inaba, T., Tang, B.K., and Kalow, W.: Hydrolysis of cocaine in human plasma by cholinesterase. Life Sci., *20:*1557, 1977.
402. Stienstra, R., Gielen, M., Kroon, J.W., and Van Poorten, F.: The influence of temperature and speed of injection on the distribution of a solution containing bupivacaine and methylene blue in a spinal canal model. Reg. Anesth., *15:*6, 1990.
403. Stienstra, R., and Van Poorten, F.: Speed of injection does not affect subarachnoid distribution of plain bupivacaine 0.5%. Reg. Anesth., *15:*208, 1990.
404. Strichartz, G.R., Sanchez, V., Arthur, G.R., Chafetz, R., and Martin, D.: Fundamental properties of local anesthetics. II. Measured octanol:buffer partition coefficients and pKa values of clinically used drugs. Anesth. Analg., *71:*158, 1990.
405. Sukhani, R., Garcia, C.J., Munhall, R.J., Winnie, A.P., and Rodvold, K.A.: Lidocaine disposition following intravenous regional anesthesia with different tourniquet deflation technics. Anesth. Analg. (Cleve.), *68:*633, 1989.
406. Sundnes, K.O., Vaagenes, P., Skretting, P., *et al.*: Spinal analgesia with hyperbaric bupivacaine: Effects of volume of solution. Br. J. Anaesth., *54:*69, 1982.
407. Takasaki, M.: Blood concentrations of lidocaine, mepivacaine and bupivacaine during caudal analgesia in children. Acta Anaesthesiol. Scand., *28:*211, 1984.
408. Takasaki, M., and Kajitani, H.: Plasma lidocaine concentrations during continuous epidural infusion of lidocaine with and without epinephrine. Can. J. Anaesth., *37:*166, 1990.
409. Takman, B.: The chemistry of local anaesthetic agents. Br. J. Anaesth., *47:*183, 1975.
410. Tam, Y.K., Ke, J., Coutts, R.T., Wyse, D.G., and Gray, M.R.: Quantification of three lidocaine metabolites and their conjugates. Pharm. Res., *7:*504, 1990.
411. Tam, Y.K., Yau, M., Berzins, R., Montgomery, P.R., and Gray, M.R.: Mechanism of lidocaine kinetics in the isolated perfused rat liver. I. Effects of continuous infusion. Drug. Metab. Dispos., *15:*12, 1987.
412. Tanaka, K., Oda, Y., Asada, A., Fujimori, M., and Funae, Y.: Metabolism of lidocaine by rat pulmonary cytochrome P450. Biochem. Pharmacol., *47:*1061, 1994.
413. Tarkilla, P., Huhtala, J., and Tuominen, M.: Transient radicular irritation after spinal anaesthesia with hyperbaric 5% lignocaine. Br. J. Anaesth., *74:*328, 1995.
414. Terasaki, T., Pardridge, W.M., and Denson, D.D.: Differential effect of plasma protein binding of bupivacaine on its in vivo transfer into the brain and salivary gland of rats. J. Pharmacol. Exp. Ther., *239:*724, 1986.
415. Tetzlaff, J.E., and Rothstein, L.: Alkalinization of mepivacaine does not alter onset of caudal anesthesia. J. Clin. Anesth., *4:*301, 1992.
416. Tetzlaff, J.E., Yoon, H.J., O'Hara, J., *et al.*: Alkalinization of mepivacaine accelerates onset of interscalene block for shoulder surgery. Reg. Anesth., *15:*242, 1990.
417. Thomas, J., Long, G., Moore, G., and Morgan D.: Plasma protein binding and placental transfer of bupivacaine. Clin. Pharmacol. Ther., *19:*426, 1976.
418. Thompson, G.E.: This fight isn't fair. Anesth. Analg. (Cleve.), *79:*3, 1994.
419. Thompson, G.E., and Rowe, D.H.: Functional anatomy of the brachial plexus sheaths. Anesthesiology, *59:*117, 1983.
420. Thompson, P., Melmon, K.L., Richardson, J.A., and Rowland, M.: Lidocaine pharmacokinetics in advanced heart failure, liver disease and renal failure in humans. Ann. Intern. Med., *78:*499, 1973.
421. Truant, A.P., and Takman, B.: Differential physical-chemical and neuropharmacologic properties of local anesthetic agents. Anesth. Analg. (Cleve.), *38:*478, 1959.
422. Tu, Y.H., Stiles, M.L., Allen, L.V. Jr.: Stability of fentanyl citrate and bupivacaine hydrochloride in portable pump reservoirs. Am. J. Hosp. Pharm., *47:*2037, 1990.
423. Tucker, G.T.: Plasma binding and disposition of local anesthetics. Int. Anesthesiol. Clin., *13:*33, 1975.
424. Tucker, G.T.: Absorption and disposition of local anaesthetics in relation to regional blood flow changes. *In* Van Kleef, J.W., Burm, A.G.L., and Spierdijk, J. (eds.): Current Concepts in Regional Anaesthesia pp. 192–202. Boston and The Hague, Martinus Nijhof, 1984.
425. Tucker, G.T.: Pharmacokinetics of local anaesthetics. Br. J. Anaesth., *58:*717, 1986.
426. Tucker, G.T.: Safety in numbers: The role of pharmacokinetics in local anesthetic toxicity. Reg. Anesth., *19:*155, 1994.
427. Tucker, G.T., Bax, N.D.S., Lennard, M.S., *et al.*: Effects of beta-adrenoceptor antagonists on the pharmacokinetics of lignocaine. Br. J. Clin. Pharmacol., *17:*21S, 1984.
428. Tucker, G.T., and Boas, R.A.: Pharmacokinetic aspects of intravenous regional anesthesia. Anesthesiology, *34:*538, 1971.
429. Tucker, G.T., Boyes, R.N., Bridenbaugh, P.O., and Moore, D.C.: Binding of anilide-type local anesthetics in human plasma. I: Relationships between binding, physicochemical properties and anesthetic activity. Anesthesiology, *33:*287, 1970.
430. Tucker, G.T., Boyes, R.N., Bridenbaugh, P.O., and Moore, D.C.: Binding of anilide-type local anesthetics in human plasma. II: Implications in vivo with special reference to transplacental distribution. Anesthesiology, *33:*304, 1970.
431. Tucker, G.T., Cooper, S., Littlewood, D., *et al.*: Observed and predicted accumulation of local anaesthetic agent during continuous extradural analgesia. Br. J. Anaesth., *49:*237, 1977.
432. Tucker, G.T., and Lennard, M.S.: Enantiomer specific pharmacokinetics. Pharmacol. Ther., *49:*305, 1989.
433. Tucker, G.T., and Mather, L.E.: Pharmacokinetics of local anaesthetic agents. Br. J. Anaesth., *47:*213, 1975.
434. Tucker, G.T., and Mather, L.E.: Plasma protein binding of bupivacaine and its interaction with other drugs in man. Br. J. Anaesth., *47:*1029, 1975.
435. Tucker, G.T., and Mather, L.E.: Clinical pharmacokinetics of local anaesthetic agents. Clin. Pharmacokinet. *4:*241, 1979.
436. Tucker, G.T., and Mather, L.E.: Physicochemical properties, absorption and disposition of local anesthetic agents. *In* Cousins, M.J., and Bridenbaugh, P.O. (eds.): Neural Blockade in Clinical Anesthesia and Management of Pain, 2nd ed. pp. 47–110. Philadelphia, J.B. Lippincott, 1988.
437. Tucker, G.T., Mather, L.E., Lennard, M.S., and Gregory, A.: Plasma concentrations of the stereoisomers of prilocaine after administration of the racemate: implications for toxicity? Br. J. Anaesth., *65:*333, 1990.
438. Tucker, G.T., Moore, D.C., Bridenbaugh, P.O., *et al.*: Systemic absorption of mepivacaine in commonly used regional block procedures. Anesthesiology, *37:*277, 1972.
439. Tucker, G.T., Wiklund, L., Berlin, A., and Mather, L.E.: Hepatic clearance of local anesthetics in man. J. Pharmacokinet. Biopharm., *5:*111, 1977.
440. Tuominen, M., Pitkanen, M., and Rosenberg, P.H.: Effect of speed of injection of 0.5% plain bupivacaine on the spread of spinal anaesthesia. Br. J. Anaesth., *69:*148, 1992.
441. Turner, D., Williams, S., and Heavner, J.: Pleural permeability to local anesthetics—the influence of concentration, pH, and local anesthetic combinations. Reg. Anesth., *14:*128, 1989.
442. Ueda, J., Katsuji, O., and Arakawa, K.: True oil/water partition coefficients of procaine and lidocaine and estimation of their dissociation constants in organic solvents. Anesth. Analg. (Cleve.), *61:*56, 1982.

443. Ueda, W., Hirakawa, M., and Mon, K.: Inhibition of epinephrine absorption by dextran. Anesthesiology, *62:*72, 1985.
444. Upton, R.N., Mather, L.E., and Runciman, W.B.: The influence of drug sorption on pharmacokinetic studies of chlormethiazole and lignocaine. J. Pharm. Pharmacol., *39:*485, 1987.
445. Upton, R.N., Runciman, W.B., and Mather, L.E.: The relationship between some physiochemical properties of ionisable drugs and their sorption into medical plastics. Aust. J. Hosp. Pharm., *17:*267, 1987.
446. Urban, B.J.: Clinical observations suggesting a changing site of action during induction and recession of spinal and epidural anesthesia. Anesthesiology, *39:*496, 1973.
447. Vanhoutte, F., Vereecke, J., Verbeke, N., and Carmeliet, E.: Stereoselective effects of the enantiomers of bupivacaine on the electrophysiological properties of the guinea-pig papillary muscle. Br. J. Pharmacol., *103:*1275, 1991.
448. Van Kleef, J.W., Burm, A.G.L., and Vletter, A.A.: Single-dose interpleural versus intercostal blockade: nerve block characteristics and plasma concentration profiles after administration of 0.5% bupivacaine with epinephrine. Anesth. Analg. (Cleve.), *70:*484, 1990.
449. Van Kleef, J.W., Logeman, E.A., Burm, A.G.L., *et al.*: Continuous interpleural infusion of bupivacaine for postoperative analgesia after surgery with flank incisions: A double-blind comparison of 0.25% and 0.5% solutions. Anesth. Analg. (Cleve.), *75:*268, 1992.
450. Veering, B.T., Burm, A.G.L., Van Kleef, J.W., Hennis, P.J., and Spierdijk, J.: Epidural anesthesia with bupivacaine: Effects of age on neural blockade and pharmacokinetics. Anesth. Analg. (Cleve.), *66:*589, 1987.
451. Veering, B.T., Burm, A.G., Vletter, A.A., *et al.*: The effect of age on the systemic absorption, disposition and pharmacodynamics of bupivacaine after epidural administration. Clin. Pharmacokinet., *22:*75, 1992.
452. Veering, B.T., Burm, A.G.L., Vletter, A.A., van den Hoeven, R.A.M., and Spierdijk, J.: The effect of age on systemic absorption and systemic disposition of bupivacaine after subarachnoid administration. Anesthesiology, *74:*250, 1991.
453. Vester-Andersen, T., Christiansen, C., Hansen, A., *et al.*: Interscalene brachial plexus block: Area of analgesia, complications and blood concentrations of local anesthetics. Acta Anaesthesiol. Scand., *25:*81, 1981.
454. Vester-Andersen, T., Husum, B., Lindeburg, T., *et al.*: Perivascular axillary block. V: Blockade following 60 ml of mepivacaine 1% injected as a bolus or as 30 + 30 ml with a 20-min interval. Acta Anaesthesiol. Scand., *28:*612, 1984.
455. Vree, T.B., Beurner, E.M.C., Lagerwerf, A.J., Simon, M.A.M., and Gielen, M.J.M.: Clinical pharmacokinetics of R(+)- and S(−)-mepivacaine after high doses of racemic mepivacaine with epinephrine in the combined psoas compartment/sciatic nerve block. Anesth. Analg. (Cleve.), *75:*75, 1992.
456. Wang, B.C., Spielholz, N.I., Hillman, D.E., and Turndorf, H.: Reversal of tetracaine spinal block by exogenous subarachnoid cholinesterase. Anesthesiology, *59:*A209, 1983.
457. Wennberg, E., Haljamae, H., Edwall, G., and Dhuner, K.-G.: Effects of commercial (pH 3.5) and freshly prepared (pH 6.5) lidocaine-adrenaline solutions on tissue pH. Acta Anaesthesiol. Scand., *26:*524, 1982.
458. Wiklund, L., Tucker, G.T., and Engberg, G.: Influence of intravenously administered epinephrine on splanchnic haemodynamics and clearance of lidocaine. Acta Anaesthesiol. Scand., *21:*275, 1977.
459. Wildsmith, J.A.W., Brown, P.D., and Johnson, S.: Structure activity relationships in differential nerve block at high and low frequency stimulation. Br. J. Anaesth., *63:*444, 1989.
460. Wildsmith, J.A.W., Gissen, A.J., Gregus, J., and Covino, B.G.: Differential nerve blocking ability of amino-ester local anaesthetics. Br. J. Anaesth., *57:*612, 1985.
461. Wildsmith, J.A.W., Gissen, A.J., Takman, B., and Covino, B.G.: Differential nerve block: esters v amides and the influence of pKa. Br. J. Anaesth., *59:*379, 1987.
462. Wildsmith, J.A.W., McClure, J.H., Brown, D.T., and Scott, D.B.: Effects of posture on the spread of isobaric and hyperbaric amethocaine. Br. J. Anaesth., *53:*273, 1981.
463. Wildsmith, J.A.W., Tucker, G.T., Cooper, S., *et al.*: Plasma concentrations of local anaesthetics after interscalene brachial plexus block. Br. J. Anaesth., *49:*461, 1977.
464. Wilkinson, G.R., and Lund, P.C.: Bupivacaine levels in plasma and cerebrospinal fluid following peridural administration. Anesthesiology, *33:*482, 1970.
465. Williams, R., Blaschke, T.F., Meffin, P.J., *et al.*: Influence of viral hepatitis on the disposition of two compounds with high hepatic clearance: Lidocaine and indocyanine green. Clin. Pharmacol. Ther., *20:*290, 1976.
466. Wilson, T.D., and Forde, M.D.I.T.: Stability of milrinone and epinephrine, atropine sulfate, lidocaine hydrochloride, or morphine sulfate injection. Am. J. Hosp. Pharm., *47:*2504, 1990.
467. Wing, L.M.H., Miners, J.O., Birkett, D.J., *et al.*: Lidocaine disposition—Sex differences and effects of cimetidine. Clin. Pharmacol. Ther., *35:*695, 1984.
468. Winnie, A.P., Lavallee, D.A., Sosa, B.P., and Masud, K.Z.: Clinical pharmacokinetics of local anaesthetics. Can. Anaesth. Soc. J., *24:*252, 1977.
469. Winnie, A.P., Radonjic, R., Akkineni, S.R., and Durrani, Z.: Factors influencing distribution of local anesthetic injected into the brachial plexus sheath. Anesth. Analg. (Cleve.), *58:*225, 1979.
470. Winnie, A.P., Tay, C.-H., Patel, K.P., *et al.*: Pharmacokinetics of local anesthetics during plexus blocks. Anesth. Analg. (Cleve.), *56:*852, 1977.
471. Wood, M., and Wood, A.J.J.: Changes in plasma drug binding and alpha$_1$-acid glycoprotein in mother and newborn infant. Clin. Pharmacol. Ther., *29:*522, 1981.
472. Wulf, H., Munstedt, P., and Maier, C.H.: Plasma protein binding of bupivacaine in pregnant women at term. Acta Anaesthesiol. Scand., *35:*129, 1991.

Neural Blockade in Clinical Anesthesia and Management of Pain, Third Edition,
edited by M.J. Cousins and P.O. Bridenbaugh.
Lippincott–Raven Publishers, Philadelphia © 1998.

CHAPTER 4

Clinical Pharmacology of Local Anesthetic Agents

Benjamin G. Covino and John A. W. Wildsmith

A review of the physiological and pharmacological factors that underlie the clinical use of local anesthetic agents must consider the factors that influence the usefulness and toxicity of the drugs as a group, and of the specific agents. The clinical usefulness of a local anesthetic is determined by its inherent anesthetic potency, the rate of onset, and the duration of effect. Toxicity may include effects on the central nervous and cardiovascular systems, local irritant actions, allergic responses, and miscellaneous agent-specific reactions such as methemoglobinemia and addiction. A large number of local anesthetics are available commercially and they differ markedly in both clinical profiles and potential for toxicity. Knowledge of the clinical pharmacology of these various drugs is essential if the appropriate agent is to be selected for a specific clinical situation.

Most clinically useful local anesthetic agents belong to one of two chemically distinct groups. Amino-esters possess an ester link between the aromatic and amine portions of the molecule and include procaine, chloroprocaine, and tetracaine. Amino-amides have an amide linkage and include lidocaine, mepivacaine, prilocaine, ropivacaine, bupivacaine, and etidocaine. The chemical structures of the various agents, and the basic pharmacological differences between the ester and amide compounds, are presented in Table 3-1 (See Chapter 3). The clinical profiles of the commonly available agents are summarized in Table 4-1.

B. G. Covino: Department of Anesthesia, Harvard Medical School, Brigham and Women's Hospital, Boston, Massachusetts 02115. (*Deceased*)

J. A. W. Wildsmith: University Department of Anaesthesia, Ninewells Hospital and Medical School, Dundee DD1 9SY United Kingdom.

PHARMACOLOGIC FACTORS AFFECTING ANESTHETIC ACTIVITY

In humans, the potency, onset, and duration of anesthesia are primarily determined by the physicochemical properties of the various agents and their inherent vasodilator activity. In addition, onset, duration, and depth of anesthesia may be altered by such factors as dosage, addition of vasoconstrictors to the local anesthetic solution, and the site of injection. Attempts have been made to alter the onset and duration of anesthesia by using mixtures of various agents, carbonating local anesthetic solutions, and adding potassium and dextran to local anesthetic solutions.

Physicochemical Properties

The physicochemical properties that influence local anesthetic activity are primarily lipid solubility, protein binding, and pKa. The relative values for lipid solubility, protein binding, and pKa of the various local anesthetic agents are shown in Table 3-1 (Chapter 3).

Lipid solubility appears to be the primary determinant of intrinsic anesthetic potency (Fig. 4-1). Procaine and chloroprocaine, for example, represent agents of low lipid solubility, which have partition coefficients less than 1. These drugs must be administered in relatively high concentrations, that is, 2% to 3%, to attain effective conduction blockade in humans. On the other hand, tetracaine, bupivacaine, and etidocaine are compounds of high lipid solubility with partition coefficients varying from 4 to 140. These agents produce effective anesthesia at relatively low concentrations of 0.25% to 0.5%. Lidocaine, mepivacaine, and prilocaine are intermediate both in terms of lipid solubility (partition coefficients of about 1-3) and their anesthetic potency *in vivo* (effective anesthetic concentration of 1%–2%). A rather precise

TABLE 4-1. *Clinical profile of local anesthetic agents*

Agent	Concentration (%)	Clinical use	Onset	Usual duration (h)	Recommended maximum single dose[a] (mg)	pH of plain solutions[b]	Comments
Amides							
Lidocaine	0.5–1.0	Infiltration	Fast	1.0–2.0	300	6.5	Most versatile agent
	0.25–0.5	IV regional			500 + epinephrine		
	1.0–1.5	Peripheral nerve blocks	Fast	1.0–3.0	500 + epinephrine		
	1.5–2.0	Epidural	Fast	1.0–2.0	500 + epinephrine		
	4	Topical	Moderate	0.5–1.0	500 + epinephrine		
	5	Spinal	Fast	0.5–1.5	100		
Prilocaine	0.5–1.0	Infiltration	Fast	1.0–2.0	600	4.5	Least toxic amide agent
	0.25–0.5	IV regional			600		
	1.5–2.0	Peripheral nerve blocks	Fast	1.5–3.0	600		Methemoglobinemia occurs usually above 600 mg
	2.0–3.0	Epidural	Fast	1.0–3.0			
Mepivacaine	0.5–1.0	Infiltration	Fast	1.5–3.0	400 500 + epinephrine	4.5	Duration of plain solutions longer than lidocaine without epinephrine. Useful when epinephrine is contraindicated.
	1.0–1.5	Peripheral nerve blocks	Fast	2.0–3.0			
	1.5–2.0	Epidural	Fast	1.5–3.0			
	4.0	Spinal	Fast	1.0–1.5	100		
Bupivacaine	0.25	Infiltration	Fast	2.0–4.0	175 225 + epinephrine	4.5–6	Lower concentrations provide differential sensory/motor block. Ventricular arrhythmias and sudden cardiovascular collapse reported following rapid IV injection.
	0.25–0.5	Peripheral nerve blocks	Slow	4.0–12.0	225 + epinephrine		
	0.25–0.5	Obstetrical epidural	Moderate	2.0–4.0	225 + epinephrine		
	0.5–0.75	Surgical epidural	Moderate	2.0–5.0	225 + epinephrine		
	0.5–0.75	Spinal	Fast	2.0–4.0	20		
Ropivacaine	0.2	Infiltration	Fast	2.0–4.0			New drug in 1996 *S* enantiomer of homologue of bupivacaine; probably less toxic to myocardium than bupivacaine
	0.2–0.5	Peripheral nerve blocks	Slow	4.0–12.0			
	0.2	Postoperative analgesia (epidural)	–	–			
	0.2	Obstetrical epidural analgesia	–	–			
	0.75–1.0	Surgical epidural	Moderate	2.0–4.0			
Etidocaine	0.5	Infiltration	Fast	2.0–4.0	300 400 + epinephrine	4.5	Profound motor block useful for surgical anesthesia but not for obstetrical analgesia.
	0.5–1.0	Peripheral	Fast	3.0–12.0	400 + epinephrine		
	1.0–1.5	Surgical epidural	Fast	2.0–4.0	400 + epinephrine		
Dibucaine	0.25–0.5 hyperbaric	Spinal	Fast	2.0–4.0	10		Recommended only for spinal and topical use
	0.00067 hypobaric 1.0	Spinal	Fast	2.0–4.0	10		

(continued)

correlation exists between lipid solubility and anesthetic potency as determined on an isolated nerve; however, in humans the correlation between lipid solubility and anesthetic effectiveness is less precise owing to other biological considerations that exist *in vivo* but not in an *in vitro* preparation. In general, potency increases as a function of lipid solubility until a partition coefficient of about 4 is achieved. Further increases in lipid solubility do not appear to cause a further enhancement of anesthetic potency (Fig. 4-1).

The pKa of a chemical compound, which is essentially the pH at which the ionized and nonionized forms are present in equal amounts, will influence the onset of anesthesia because the uncharged form of the local anesthetic agent is primarily responsible for diffusion across the nerve sheath and

TABLE 4-1. *Continued*

Agent	Concentration (%)	Clinical use	Onset	Usual duration (h)	Recommended maximum single dose[a] (mg)	pH of plain solutions[b]	Comments
Esters	1.0	Topical	Slow	30–60	50		
Procaine						5–6.5	Used mainly for infiltration and differential spinal blocks. Allergic potential after repeated use
	1.0	Infiltration	Fast	30–60	1000		
	1.0–2.0	Peripheral nerve blocks	Slow	30–60	1000		
	2.0	Epidural	Slow	30–60	1000		
	10.0	Spinal	Moderate	30–60	200		
Chloroprocaine	1.0				800	2.7–4	Lowest systemic toxicity of all local anesthetics
		Infiltration	Fast	30–60	1000 + epinephrine		
	2.0				1000 + epinephrine		Intrathecal injection may be associated with sensory/motor deficits.
		Peripheral nerve block	Fast	30–60			
	2.0–3.0				1000 + epinephrine		
		Epidural	Fast	30–60			
Tetracaine	0.5					4.5–6.5	Use is primarily limited to spinal and topical anesthesia.
	2.0	Spinal	Fast	2.0–4.0	20		
		Topical	Slow	30–60	20		
Cocaine	4.0–10.0						Topical use only. Addictive, causes vasoconstriction. CNS toxicity initially features marked excitation ("fight and flight" response). May cause cardiac arrhythmias owing to sympathetic stimulation.
		Topical	Slow	30–60	150		
Benzocaine	Up to 20						Useful only for topical anesthesia.
		Topical	Slow	30–60	200		

[a] The recommended maximum single doses quoted are generally those in manufacturers' data sheets. Increasingly, it is recognized that the concept of maximum recommended doses is flawed.[129] The systemic kinetics of local anesthetics are influenced by the site of injection and the general physical status of the individual patient. Recommendations about "maximum doses" should be taken as guidance and adapted in the light of knowledge of the individual block procedure and the particular patient's general condition.

[b] Epinephrine-containing solutions have a pH 1 to 1.5 units lower than plain solutions.

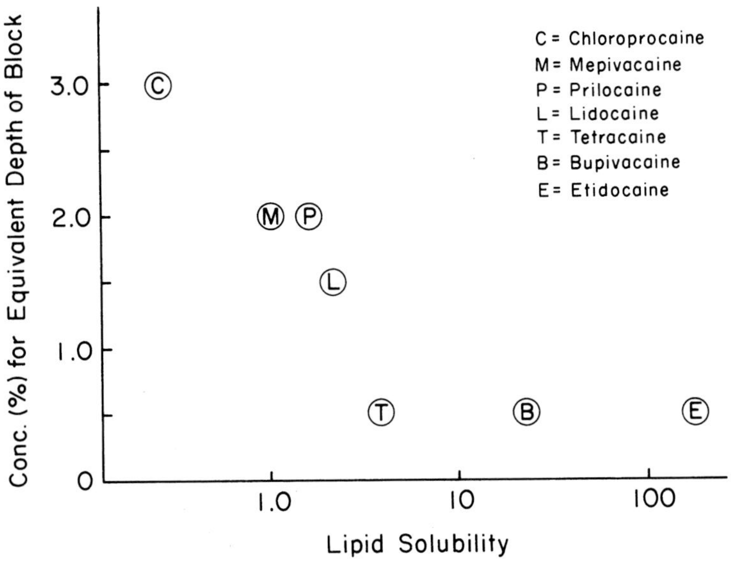

FIG. 4-1. Relation between lipid solubility and inherent potency of local anesthetic agents.

nerve membrane.[119] The onset of action will be directly related to the amount of drug that exists in the base form. The percentage of a specific local anesthetic that is present in the base form when injected into tissue, the pH of which is 7.4, is inversely proportional to the pKa of that agent. Mepivacaine, lidocaine, prilocaine, and etidocaine, for example, possess a pKa of about 7.7. When these agents are injected into tissue at a pH of 7.4, about 65% of these drugs exist in the ionized form and 35% in the nonionized base form. On the other hand, tetracaine possesses a pKa of 8.6, which means that only 5% is present in the nonionized form at a tissue pH of 7.4, whereas 95% exists in the charged cationic form. In humans, a correlation does exist between onset of conduction blockade and the pKa of the various local anesthetic agents (Fig. 4-2).[15,97] For example, the agents with relatively low pKa's, namely, lidocaine, mepivacaine, prilocaine, and etidocaine, have a fairly rapid onset of action. On the other hand, tetracaine and procaine, which have high pKa's, have a rather slow onset of action. Bupivacaine is intermediate, both in terms of pKa and onset of action. One exception to this rule appears to be chloroprocaine, which has a high pKa and a rapid onset of action in humans; however, if one considers that chloroprocaine generally is used at higher concentrations and larger dosages than other local anesthetics, the more rapid onset of action may be related simply to the larger number of molecules of this agent that are administered in order to achieve effective anesthesia.

Finally, the relative protein binding of various local anesthetics will influence the duration of anesthesia of the various agents (Fig. 4-2). If, indeed, a local anesthetic receptor site exists in the protein sodium channel in nerve membrane, then agents that possess a greater affinity for protein should remain at the receptor site for a longer time and therefore cause a longer duration of action. Thus, bupivacaine and etidocaine, which are about 95% protein bound, do demonstrate long durations of anesthesia. On the other hand, procaine, which is only 6% protein bound, has a relatively short duration of action. Prilocaine, mepivacaine, and lidocaine, which are intermediate in terms of protein binding (55%–75%), are also intermediate in terms of anesthetic duration.

Vasodilator Properties

The clinical activity of the various local anesthetics is also modified by factors not related to the physicochemical properties of the different drugs. In particular, the effect of local anesthetics on vascular smooth muscle will indirectly influence the apparent potency and duration of action of these agents. Local anesthetics are absorbed into the vascular compartment from the region of their injection. The rate of vascular absorption will determine the number of molecules of local anesthetic available for diffusion to the receptor site of the nerve membrane, which in turn will influence their *in vivo* potency and duration of action. All local anesthetics except cocaine exhibit a biphasic effect on vascular smooth muscle.[11,78] At extremely low concentrations they cause enhanced activity of vascular smooth muscle, leading to vasoconstriction. At concentrations commonly used for regional anesthesia, however, local anesthetics tend to be vasodilators. Differences in the relative degree of vasodilation produced by local anesthetics will influence their anesthetic profile. For example, *in vitro* studies have shown that lidocaine is significantly more potent than mepivacaine on an isolated nerve, whereas duration of conduction block is similar.[40] Studies in humans, however, have indicated that little difference exists in the relative anesthetic potency between these two agents and the duration of action of mepivacaine is somewhat longer than that of lidocaine.[97] These differences

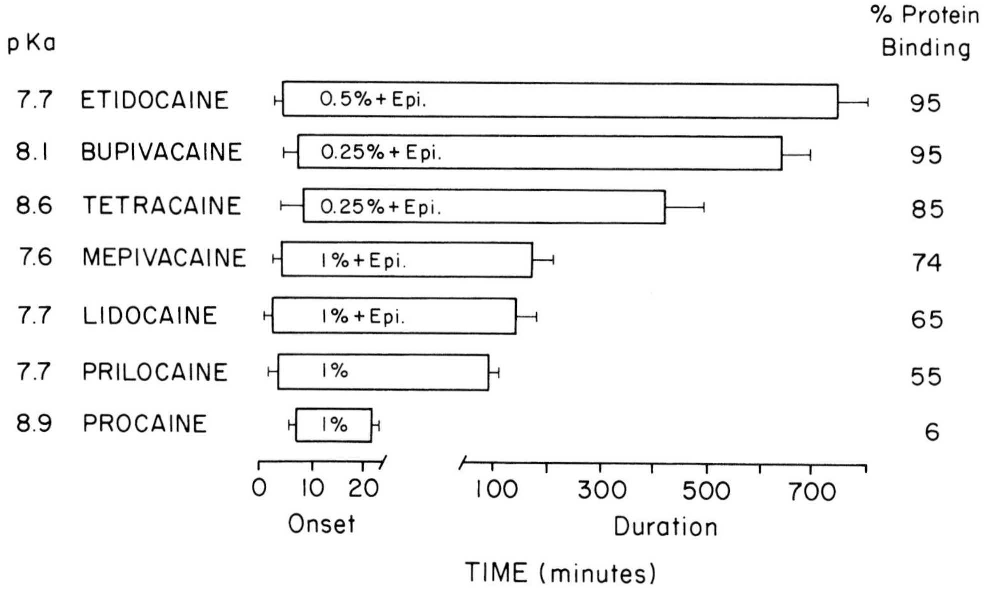

FIG. 4-2. Relation between pKa and onset of anesthesia (*left side* of figure) and relation between protein binding and duration of anesthesia (*right side* of figure).

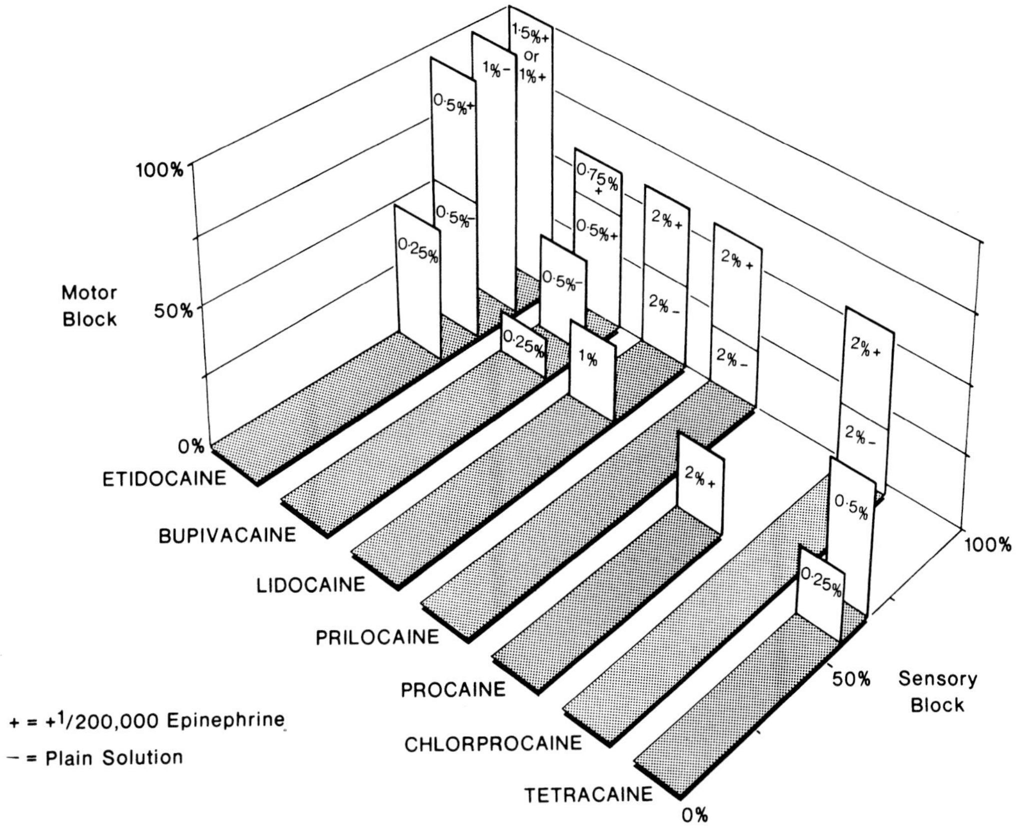

FIG. 4-3. Comparison of agents in epidural block. The percentage of motor blockade and the percentage of success of sensory blockade are illustrated for each agent. This illustration is based on subjective clinical data, and thus only approximate comparisons can be drawn.

are probably related to the greater degree of vasodilation induced by lidocaine. The addition of epinephrine to solutions of lidocaine and mepivacaine will essentially eliminate the difference in vasodilator activity produced by the two compounds. Under such conditions little difference in the duration of action is observed in humans when epinephrine-containing solutions of lidocaine and mepivacaine are used.[97]

In summary, the clinically important properties of local anesthetic agents include potency, onset, and duration of action. The clinical profile of the various agents is related primarily to their physicochemical properties. *In vivo*, however, the clinical activity of these drugs may be altered by other actions, such as their relative effects on vascular smooth muscle. On the basis of their anesthetic profile in humans, the various local anesthetics may be classified as follows:

1. Agents of low anesthetic potency and short duration of action, that is, procaine and chloroprocaine
2. Agents of intermediate anesthetic potency and duration of action, that is, lidocaine, mepivacaine, and prilocaine
3. Agents of high anesthetic potency and prolonged duration of action, that is, tetracaine, bupivacaine, ropivacaine, and etidocaine

In terms of onset, chloroprocaine, lidocaine, mepivacaine, prilocaine, and etidocaine possess a relatively rapid onset of action. Procaine and tetracaine have a long latency period except when used for spinal anesthesia, and bupivacaine is intermediate in terms of onset of anesthesia.

In addition to the anesthetic properties described above, one other important clinical consideration is the ability of local anesthetic agents to cause a differential blockade of sensory and motor fibers (Fig. 4-3). Although differential conduction blockade has been used for many years by altering the concentration of procaine administered intrathecally, this technique is useful primarily for the diagnosis of certain pain states. The introduction of bupivacaine into clinical practice provided anesthesiologists with the first agent that showed a relative specificity for sensory fibers such that adequate sensory analgesia without profound inhibition of motor fibers could be achieved for surgical, obstetric, and acute and chronic pain therapy.[21] Bupivacaine and etidocaine, two local anesthetic agents introduced into clinical practice at the same time, provide an interesting contrast in terms of their differential sensory/motor blocking activity, although they are both potent long-acting anesthetic agents. Bupivacaine, for example, is widely used epidurally for surgical and obstetric procedures and relief of pain postoperatively because of its ability to provide adequate sensory analgesia with minimal blockade of motor fibers, particularly when used as a 0.25% or 0.5% solution. Thus, the woman in labor can be rendered pain-free and still be able to move her legs, which is one of the primary reasons why this agent has enjoyed popularity for continuous epidural blockade during labor. Increasing the concentration of bupivacaine to 0.75% will increase the depth of both sensory and motor blockade while also shortening latency and producing a more prolonged duration of anesthesia.[131] Etidocaine, on the other hand, shows little separation between sensory and motor blockade. To achieve adequate epidural sensory anesthesia, 1.5% concentrations of etidocaine are usually required. At these concentrations, etidocaine has an extremely rapid onset of action and a prolonged duration of anesthesia; however, sensory anesthesia is associated with a profound degree of motor blockade. Thus etidocaine is a valuable agent, particularly for epidural blockade in surgical situations in which optimum muscle relaxation is desirable, because it combines a rapid onset, prolonged duration, and satisfactory quality of anesthesia with profound motor blockade. This marked effect on motor function renders etidocaine of limited value, however, for obstetric analgesia and postoperative pain relief.

NONPHARMACOLOGIC FACTORS INFLUENCING ANESTHETIC ACTIVITY

Although the inherent pharmacologic properties of the various local anesthetic agents will basically determine their anesthetic profile, other factors may influence the quality of regional anesthesia, including (i) dosage of local anesthetic administered; (ii) addition of a vasoconstrictor to the local anesthetic solution; (iii) site of administration; (iv) use of additives; and (v) mixtures of local anesthetic solutions.

Dosage of Local Anesthetic Solutions

The mass of drug administered will influence the onset, potency, and duration of anesthesia (Table 4-2).[21] As the dose of local anesthetic is increased, the frequency of satisfactory anesthesia and the duration of anesthesia will increase and the time for onset of anesthesia will decrease. In general, the dosage of local anesthetic administered can be increased by administering a larger volume of a less concentrated solution or a smaller volume of a more concentrated solution. In clinical practice, however, an increase in dosage is usually achieved by using a more concentrated solution of the specific agent. For example, a dose-response study involving the use of bupivacaine for epidural analgesia in women in labor showed that increasing the concentration from 0.125% to 0.5% while maintaining the same volume of injectate (10 ml) resulted in a decreased latency, improved incidence of satisfactory analgesia, and an increased duration of sensory analgesia.[92] A similar study involving the use of bupivacaine for surgical anesthesia also demonstrated that increasing the concentration from 0.5% to 0.75% with a concomitant increase in dosage from about 100 mg to 150 mg produced a more rapid onset and prolonged duration of sensory anesthesia.[131] In addition, the frequency of satisfactory sensory anesthesia was increased and the depth of motor blockade enhanced. The relative influence of volume, concentration, and dosage was demonstrated in a study in which prilocaine (600 mg) administered epidurally either as 30 ml of a 2% solution or 20 ml of 3% solution was evaluated.[41] No difference in onset, adequacy, or duration of anesthesia and onset, depth, and duration of motor blockade was observed despite differences in volume and concentration of anesthetic solution used, since the dosage was maintained constant. The volume of anesthetic solution administered may influence the spread of anesthesia; for example, 30 ml of 1% lidocaine administered into the epidural space was shown to produce a level of anesthesia that was 4.3 dermatomes higher than that achieved when 10 ml of 3% lidocaine was used.[52] Thus, except for the possible effect on the spread of anesthesia, the primary qualities of regional anesthesia, namely, onset, depth, and duration of blockade, are related to the mass of drug injected, that is, the product of volume times concentration.

TABLE 4-2. *Effects of dose and epinephrine on local anesthetic properties*

	Increased dose (concentration or volume)	Addition of epinephrine
Onset time	↓	↓[a]
Degree of motor blockade	↑	↑
Degree of sensory blockade	↑	↑
Duration of blockade	↑	↑
Area of blockade	↑	↑
Peak plasma concentration	↑	↓

[a] Minimal effect for etidocaine.

Addition of a Vasoconstrictor to Local Anesthetic Solutions

Vasoconstrictors, particularly epinephrine, are frequently added to local anesthetic solutions. The decrease in the rate of vascular absorption that results from adding epinephrine will allow more anesthetic molecules to reach the nerve membrane, thereby improving the depth and duration of anesthesia (Table 4-2). Local anesthetic solutions usually contain a 1:200,000 (5 μg/ml) concentration of epinephrine, a concentration that has been reported to provide an optimal degree of vasoconstriction when used with lidocaine for epidural or intercostal use.[13] Little information is available on the optimum concentration of epinephrine when used with other local anesthetic agents. Other vasoconstrictor agents such as norepinephrine and phenylephrine have been used as additives to solutions of local anesthetics. Regional blood flow studies indicate that epinephrine is more effective as a vasoconstrictor than norepinephrine when combined with local anesthetic agents.[46] Phenylephrine has been re-

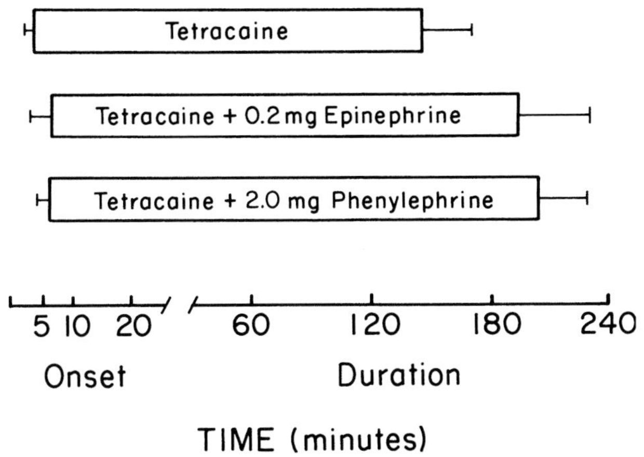

FIG. 4-4. Comparative effect of epinephrine and phenylephrine on the duration of spinal anesthesia produced by tetracaine. (Data derived from Concepcion, M., Maddi, R., Francis, D., *et al.*: Vasoconstrictors in spinal anesthesia with tetracaine. A comparison of epinephrine and phenylephrine. Anesth. Analg., *63*:134, 1984.)

ported to produce the greatest prolongation of spinal anesthesia when combined with tetracaine[102]; however, more recent studies conducted under double-blind conditions indicated that at equipotent doses no differences existed between the ability of epinephrine and phenylephrine to prolong the duration of spinal anesthesia produced by tetracaine (Fig. 4-4).[37]

Differences exist in terms of the effect of epinephrine in prolonging the duration of action of various local anesthetic agents. Procaine, lidocaine, and mepivacaine, for example, benefit greatly from the addition of epinephrine in terms of prolonging the duration of infiltration anesthesia, peripheral nerve blocks, and epidural blockade.[2,19,64,141] The duration of action of prilocaine, bupivacaine, and etidocaine is also prolonged by adding epinephrine when these agents are used for infiltration and peripheral nerve blocks.[2,97,141] The duration of action of these agents is not, however, markedly affected by epinephrine following epidural blockade.[19,26,83] The decreased vasodilator action of prilocaine compared to that of lidocaine is believed responsible for the reduced effect of added epinephrine to solutions of prilocaine. With bupivacaine and etidocaine, the high lipid solubility of these agents may be responsible for the diminished effect of epinephrine. These agents are taken up substantially by epidural fat and then slowly released, which contributes to their prolonged duration of action; however, the interaction of epinephrine and the long-acting agents, such as bupivacaine, is dependent on the concentration of drug used. In epidural blockade for labor, for example, the frequency and the duration of adequate analgesia were improved when epinephrine 1:200,000 was added to 0.125% and 0.25% bupivacaine[92]; however, the addition of epinephrine to 0.5% and 0.75% bupivacaine was not associated with a significant improvement in the frequency of satisfactory epidural blockade in obstetric or surgical patients.[92,134] The degree of motor blockade is enhanced following the epidural administration of epinephrine-containing solutions of bupivacaine and etidocaine.[134] The differential effect of epinephrine in terms of prolonging the duration of action of local anesthetic agents is most apparent in the subarachnoid space. Epinephrine significantly extends the duration of spinal anesthesia when combined with tetracaine.[7,37] The duration of effective surgical anesthesia is not, however, markedly enhanced when solutions of lidocaine or bupivacaine with epinephrine are administered intrathecally.[31,32]

Site of Injection

The site of administration of local anesthetic agents will influence their anesthetic profile. Although local anesthetics are frequently classified as agents of short, moderate, or long duration with a slow or rapid onset of action, these general properties are influenced by the type of anesthetic procedure performed. Tetracaine, for example, is usually considered an agent of slow onset and long duration, but its onset of action is quite rapid (about 3 min) when administered intrathecally, whereas the duration of spinal anesthesia with tetracaine is only 2 to 3 hours.[37] In terms of latency, the most rapid onset of action occurs after the intrathecal or subcutaneous administration of local anesthetics, whereas the slowest onset times are observed during the performance of brachial plexus blocks.[40] With regard to the duration of anesthesia, an agent such as bupivacaine possesses a duration of surgical anesthesia of about 4 hours when administered into the epidural space (Fig. 4-5). When bupivacaine is administered for brachial plexus blockade, however, the duration of anesthesia averages 10 hours. Differences in the onset and the duration of anesthesia depending on the site of injection are partly due to the particular anatomy of the area of injection, the variation in the rate of vascular absorption, and the amount of drug used for various types of regional anesthesia. In the case of spinal anesthesia, the lack of a nerve sheath around the spinal cord and the deposition of the local anesthetic solution in the immediate vicinity of the spinal cord are responsible for the rapid onset of action. On the other hand, the relatively small amount of drug used for spinal anesthesia probably accounts for the relatively short duration of action associated with this particular technique. With brachial plexus blockade, the onset of anesthesia is slow due to the anesthetic agent usually being deposited at some distance from the nerve roots, and therefore time for diffusion to the nerve membrane is required before signs of anesthesia are apparent. The long duration of brachial plexus blockade observed with most local anesthetics but, in particular, with the longer-acting agents is probably related to the decreased rate of vascular absorption from that site, and also the larger doses of drug commonly used for this regional anesthetic technique.

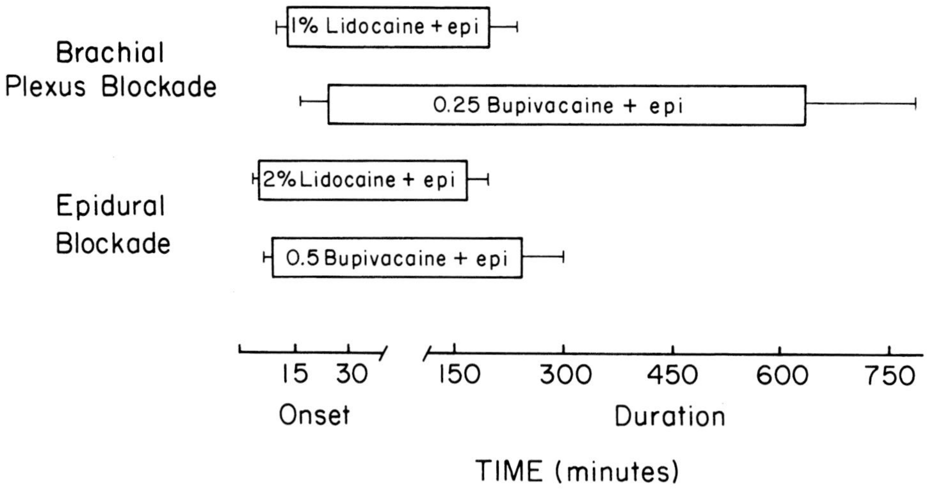

FIG. 4-5. Comparative onset and duration of anesthesia of lidocaine and bupivacaine following epidural and brachial plexus blockade.

Use of Additives with Local Anesthetic Solutions

Attempts have been made to modify local anesthetic solutions in a number of ways in order to improve the onset of action or prolong the duration of anesthesia. Carbonation of local anesthetic solutions has been attempted to reduce the onset of action of various local anesthetics (Fig. 4-6). It has been clearly shown in isolated nerve preparations that carbon dioxide will enhance the diffusion of local anesthetics through nerve sheaths and produce a more rapid onset of conduction block.[29,62] The mechanism is believed to be related to the diffusion of carbon dioxide through the nerve membrane resulting in a decrease in intracellular pH. The lower pH will increase the intracellular concentration of the cationic form of the local anesthetic, which represents the active form that binds to a receptor in the sodium channel. In

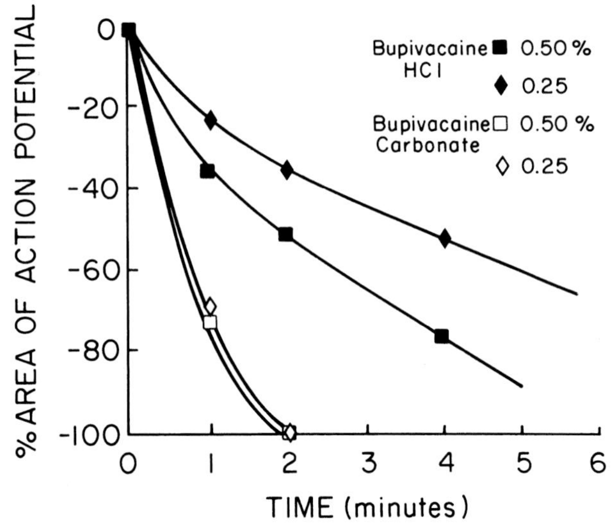

FIG. 4-6. Effect of CO_2 on the onset of conduction block in the isolated frog sciatic nerve.

addition, the local anesthetic cation does not readily diffuse through membranes such that the drug remains entrapped within the axoplasm, a situation referred to as ion trapping. The enhanced formation of the local anesthetic cation and the process of ion trapping are believed responsible for the more rapid onset and more profound degree of conduction block. A number of clinical studies have been carried out with carbonated solutions of lidocaine. Initial investigations in humans found that lidocaine carbonate solutions had a more rapid onset of brachial plexus and epidural blockade compared to lidocaine hydrochloride solutions.[18,20] More recent double-blind studies, however, have failed to demonstrate a significantly more rapid onset of action when lidocaine carbonate was compared with lidocaine hydrochloride for epidural blockade.[107] In theory an agent such as bupivacaine that has a relatively slow onset of action should benefit greatly from the use of a carbonated solution, and it has been reported that bupivacaine–carbon dioxide is associated with a more rapid onset of action in humans[47]; however, double-blind studies in which bupivacaine carbonate was compared with bupivacaine hydrochloride for brachial plexus or epidural blockade have failed to confirm these earlier reports of a significantly shorter onset of action of the carbonated solution.[25,100] Thus, at present, it is not certain whether carbonation of local anesthetic solutions imparts any advantage to the various local anesthetic agents in terms of onset of block when used under clinical conditions, although the depth of anesthesia may be improved.

The discrepancy between *in vitro* and *in vivo* studies suggests that the injected carbon dioxide is rapidly buffered *in vivo* such that the intracellular pH is not sufficiently altered and significantly increased levels of the cationic form of the local anesthetic are not achieved to produce a more rapid onset of anesthesia.

Attempts have been made to improve the onset of conduction blockade by adding sodium bicarbonate to local

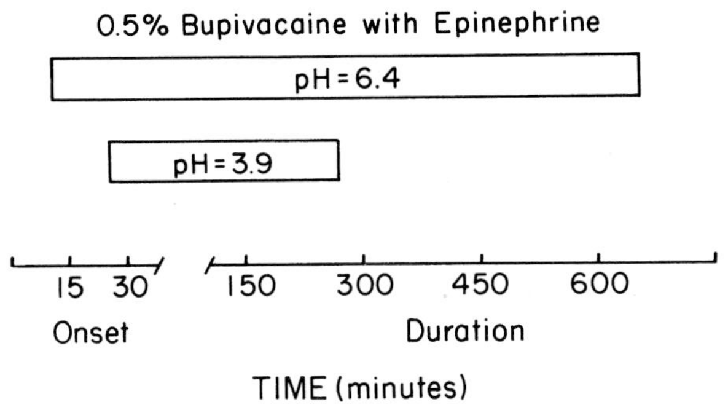

FIG. 4-7. Effect of pH on the onset and duration of brachial plexus blockade. (Data derived from Hilgier, M.: Alkalinization of bupivacaine for brachial plexus block. Reg. Anesth., *10*:59, 1985.)

anesthetic solutions immediately before injection.[59,74] Theoretically, sodium bicarbonate will increase the pH of the local anesthetic solution, which in turn will increase the amount of drug in the uncharged base form. Thus the rate of diffusion across the nerve sheath and nerve membrane should be enhanced, resulting in a more rapid onset of anesthesia. Several clinical studies have been performed in which the addition of sodium bicarbonate to solutions of bupivacaine did appear to produce a significant decrease in the latency of brachial plexus blockade.[59,74] Moreover, it has been reported that the duration of anesthesia was prolonged by increasing the pH of the local anesthetic solution (Fig. 4-7).[74]

Potassium has also been added to local anesthetic solutions in an attempt to improve the quality of anesthesia. Addition of 1% KCl to lidocaine was found to shorten the latency of spread and intensify the quality of sensory block in the epidural space.[22] In a subsequent study, the duration of digital and ulnar blocks with lidocaine was prolonged by the addition of KCl, but the onset of anesthesia was unaffected.[4]

Various attempts have been made to prolong the duration of anesthesia by incorporating dextran into local anesthetic solutions.[96,122] Discrepancies exist in studies of the effectiveness of dextran in prolonging the duration of regional anesthesia. In one controlled clinical study, prolonged durations of anesthesia were observed in some patients, but the mean duration of intercostal nerve blockade was not significantly altered when solutions of bupivacaine with and without dextran were compared.[14]

Rosenblatt and Fung have suggested that the difference in results obtained by various investigators may be related to the pH of the dextran solution used.[123] These authors have reported that dextran solutions with a pH of 8.0 significantly prolong the duration of bupivacaine-induced coccygeal nerve blocks in rats, whereas the duration of block is not altered when dextran with a pH of 4.5 to 5.5 is added to bupivacaine.[123] These results indicate that alkalinization of the anesthetic solution may be responsible for prolonged conduction blockade rather than the dextran itself.

Mixtures of Local Anesthetics

The use of mixtures of local anesthetics for regional anesthesia has become relatively popular in recent years. The basis for this practice is to compensate for the short duration of action of certain agents such as chloroprocaine or lidocaine and the long latency of other agents such as tetracaine and bupivacaine. The combination of lidocaine or mepivacaine and tetracaine was commonly used in some centers before the advent of bupivacaine and etidocaine as long-duration anesthetics. Because the slow onset of tetracaine for peripheral nerve blocks and epidural anesthesia was clinically unacceptable, the addition of lidocaine or mepivacaine provided a local anesthetic solution that afforded a relatively rapid onset of action and prolonged duration of anesthesia. Further, mixtures of chloroprocaine and bupivacaine have been used to produce a local anesthetic solution with a rapid onset and long duration of action. The low systemic toxicity of chloroprocaine afforded an additional advantage to such a mixture; however, the use of a chloroprocaine-bupivacaine mixture has produced contradictory results. Cunningham and Kaplan originally reported that a mixture of chloroprocaine and bupivacaine did result in a short latency and prolonged duration of brachial plexus blockade.[42] On the other hand, Cohen and Thurlow found that the duration of epidural anesthesia produced by a mixture of chloroprocaine and bupivacaine was significantly shorter than that obtained with solutions of bupivacaine alone.[35] This reduced duration has been attributed in part to a decrease in pH, since chloroprocaine solutions have a pH of about 3.0.[60] Reduction in pH will decrease the amount of bupivacaine available in the uncharged base form, which may reduce the number of molecules able to penetrate the nerve sheath. In addition, data from isolated nerve studies suggest that a metabolite of chloroprocaine may inhibit the binding of bupivacaine to membrane receptor sites.[38] In a randomized prospective study of mixtures of various concentrations of lidocaine and bupivacaine, no difference in onset of blockade was observed among the solutions tested. Duration of blockade with a 50:50 mixture of lidocaine/bupivacaine was only marginally greater than that for lidocaine alone.[132] At present there do not appear to be any clinically significant advantages to using mixtures of local anesthetic agents. Etidocaine and bupivacaine provide clinically acceptable onsets of action and prolonged durations of anesthesia. In addition, the use of catheter techniques for epidural anesthesia and for brachial plexus blockade makes it possible to administer repeated injections of rapidly acting agents such as chloroprocaine or lidocaine, which will provide an anesthetic duration of indefinite length.

TOXICITY OF LOCAL ANESTHETICS

Various types of toxic reactions have been reported in humans in association with the use of local anesthetic agents. The adverse reactions observed include systemic toxicity involving primarily the central nervous system (CNS) and the cardiovascular system, localized neural and skeletal muscle irritation, and specific side effects such as methemoglobinemia, allergy, and addiction. Cardiovascular and CNS toxicity and skeletal muscle irritation are toxicologic properties of all local anesthetic agents. The remaining adverse effects are associated with the use of certain specific drugs. If one considers the large number of local anesthetic administrations, the frequency of toxic reactions is extremely low. Moreover, most untoward effects are due to the inappropriate use of this class of drugs, such as accidental intravascular or intrathecal injections or administration of an excessive dosage.

Systemic Toxicity

Most toxic reactions to local anesthetics in humans involve the CNS. Local anesthetic-induced cardiovascular depression occurs less frequently but tends to be more serious and more difficult to manage.

Local anesthetics vary considerably in terms of their potential for causing systemic toxic reactions. The relative toxicity of the commonly used agents is depicted in Figure 4-8.

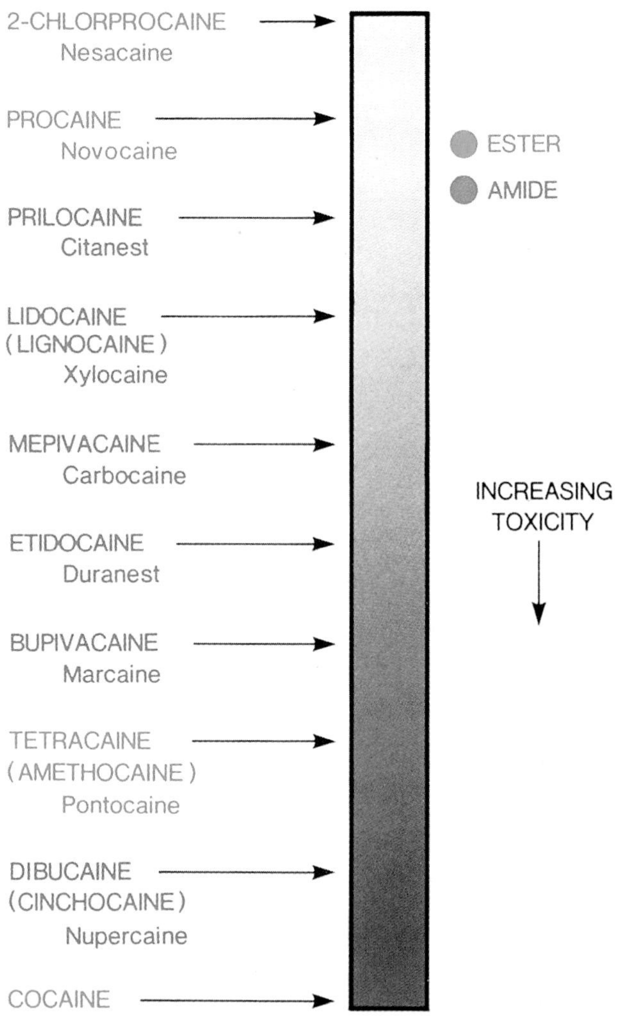

FIG. 4-8. Spectrum of local anesthetic agents. Agents are arranged in approximate order of increasing toxicity; it should be noted, however, that comparisons of all of the agents at "equi-effect" concentration, under the same conditions, have not yet been made in humans.

Central Nervous System Toxicity

The signs and symptoms of local anesthetic–induced CNS toxicity are shown in Figure 4-9. Human volunteers receiving intravenous infusions of local anesthetics describe feelings of lightheadedness and dizziness followed frequently by visual and auditory disturbances such as difficulty in focusing and tinnitus. Other subjective CNS symptoms include disorientation and occasional feelings of drowsiness. Objective signs of CNS toxicity are usually excitatory in nature and include shivering, muscular twitching, and tremors initially involving muscles of the face and distal parts of the extremities. Ultimately, generalized convulsions of a tonic-clonic nature occur. If a sufficiently large dose of a local anesthetic agent is administered systemically, the initial signs of CNS excitation are followed rapidly by a state of generalized CNS depression. Seizure activity ceases and respiratory depression and ultimately respiratory arrest occur. Occasionally in some patients CNS depression may occur without a preceding excitatory phase, particularly if other CNS depressant drugs have been used concomitantly.

The mechanism by which local anesthetic agents produce an initial state of CNS excitation involves the selective blockade of inhibitory pathways in the cerebral cortex.[44,76,142] The initial inhibition of inhibitory pathways by local anesthetic agents would allow facilitatory neurons to function in an unopposed fashion, which would result in an increase in excitatory activity, leading to convulsions. After an increase in the dose of local anesthetic administered, these agents would tend to inhibit both inhibitory and facilitatory pathways, resulting in a generalized state of CNS depression.

The potential CNS toxicity of various local anesthetic agents appears to be primarily related to their intrinsic anesthetic potency. In cats, for example, a dose of about 35 mg/kg of procaine was required to cause convulsions compared to a mean convulsive dose of 5 mg/kg of bupivacaine.[50] Lidocaine, mepivacaine, and prilocaine were intermediate with regard to the dose required to induce convulsions. A comparison of the intrinsic anesthetic potency and toxicity of these local anesthetics indicates that bupivacaine is about eight times more potent than procaine when used for production of regional anesthesia and about seven times more toxic than procaine with regard to the dose required to produce convulsive activity in cats. In a similar study in dogs a dose of about 20 mg/kg of lidocaine was required to produce convulsions compared to doses of 8 mg/kg for etidocaine and 5 mg/kg of bupivacaine.[95] Thus the relative CNS toxicity of bupivacaine, etidocaine, and lidocaine is about 4:2:1, which is similar to the relative anesthetic potency of these agents in humans. Intravenous infusion studies in human volunteers have also demonstrated a relationship between the intrinsic anesthetic potency of various local

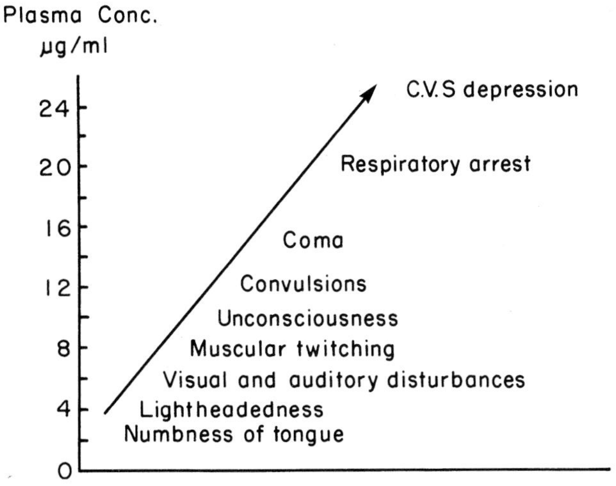

FIG. 4-9. Relationship of signs and symptoms of local anesthetic toxicity to plasma concentrations of lidocaine.

anesthetics and the dosage required to induce signs of CNS toxicity.[57,127,128]

A correlation also exists between the convulsive blood level of various local anesthetic agents and their relative anesthetic potencies. In monkeys, bupivacaine produced convulsions at a blood level of about 4.5 μg/ml, whereas lidocaine-induced convulsions were observed at a mean blood level of 25 μg/ml.[108] In humans, convulsions have been reported at venous blood levels of approximately 2 to 4 μg/ml of bupivacaine and etidocaine, whereas concentrations in excess of 10 μg/ml are usually required for production of convulsive activity when a less potent agent such as lidocaine is administered.

Although a general relationship exists between anesthetic potency and CNS toxicity, the rate of injection and rapidity with which a particular blood level is achieved will influence the toxicity of local anesthetic agents (Fig. 4-10). Scott, for

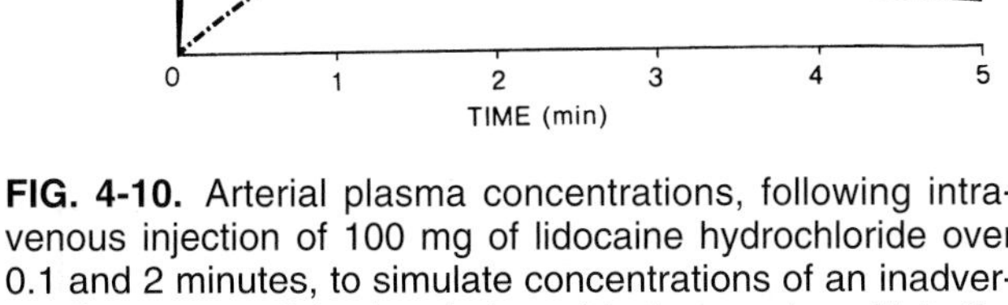

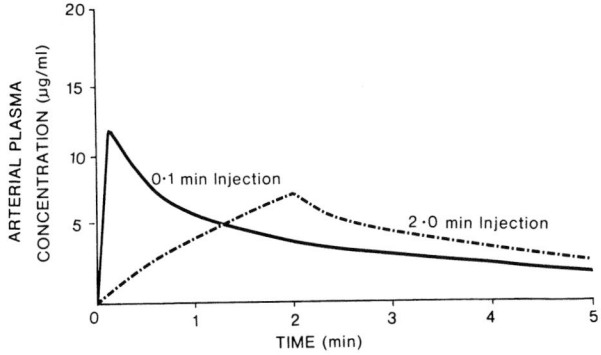

FIG. 4-10. Arterial plasma concentrations, following intravenous injection of 100 mg of lidocaine hydrochloride over 0.1 and 2 minutes, to simulate concentrations of an inadvertent intravenous injection during a block procedure. Note the reduction in peak concentrations brought about by prolonging injection time. (Data from Tucker, G.T., and Boas, R.A.: Pharmacokinetic aspects of intravenous regional anesthesia. Anesthesiology, *34*:538, 1971.)

TABLE 4-3. *Effect of P_{CO_2} on the convulsive threshold (CD_{100}) of various local anesthetic in cats*

Agent	CD (mg/kg) P_{CO_2} 25–40 mm Hg	CD (mg/kg) P_{CO_2} 65–81 mm Hg	Change in CD_{100}
Procaine	35	17	51
Mepivacaine	18	10	44
Prilocaine	22	12	45
Lidocaine	15	7	53
Bupivacaine	5	2.5	50

(Data derived from Englesson, S.: The influence of acid-base changes on central nervous system toxicity of local anesthetic agents. I. An experimental study in cats. Acta Anesthesiol. Scand., *18*:79, 1974.)

example, has shown that human volunteers could tolerate an average dose of 236 mg of etidocaine and a venous blood level of 3.0 μg/ml before the onset of CNS symptoms when etidocaine was infused at the rate of 10 mg/min.[126] When the infusion rate was increased to 20 mg/min, however, the volunteers could only tolerate an average of 161 mg of etidocaine, which produced a venous plasma level of about 2 μg/ml.

The acid-base status of animals and patients can markedly affect the CNS activity of local anesthetic agents.[50] Studies in cats have shown that the convulsive threshold of various local anesthetics is inversely related to the arterial P_{CO_2} level (Table 4-3). The convulsive threshold dose of various local anesthetics was decreased by about 50% when the P_{CO_2} was elevated from 25–40 mm Hg to 65–81 mm Hg. A decrease in arterial pH is also associated with a decrease in the convulsive threshold of these agents. The relationship between P_{CO_2}, pH, and the CNS activity of local anesthetic agents has been evaluated by Englesson and Grevsten.[51] Respiratory acidosis with a resultant increase in P_{CO_2} and a decrease in arterial pH will consistently decrease the convulsant threshold of local anesthetic agents; however, an elevated P_{CO_2} and pH, as may occur during metabolic alkalosis, exert less of an effect on the convulsive threshold of local anesthetic agents, suggesting that pH is primarily responsible for the changes in CNS toxicity. Acidosis may alter the convulsive threshold in several ways. An elevation of P_{CO_2} will enhance cerebral blood flow so that more anesthetic agent is delivered to the brain. A decrease in intracellular pH will enhance the conversion of the base form of local anesthetic agents to the cationic form, which is responsible for the effect of these drugs on nerve membranes. The cationic form does not diffuse well, which will increase the intracellular concentration. Hypercarbia or acidosis, or both, will also decrease the plasma protein binding of local anesthetic agents.[28] Therefore, an elevation in P_{CO_2} or decrease in pH will increase the portion of free drug available for diffusion into the brain. On the other hand, acidosis will increase the cationic form of the local anesthetic, which will decrease the rate of diffusion.

In summary, local anesthetic agents can produce marked effects on the central nervous system. In general, signs of CNS excitation leading to frank convulsions are the most common manifestation of systemic local anesthetic toxicity. Excessive doses of these drugs may also lead to CNS depression and respiratory arrest. In general the potential CNS toxicity of local anesthetics correlates with the inherent anesthetic potency of the various agents.

Cardiovascular System Toxicity

Local anesthetic agents can exert a direct action both on cardiac muscle and on peripheral vascular smooth muscle.

Cardiac Effects

Detailed electrophysiologic studies on cardiac muscle have been carried out with various local anesthetics, but particularly with lidocaine because this agent is used for treating ventricular arrhythmias. Lidocaine decreases the maximum rate of depolarization without altering the resting membrane potential of cardiac muscle.[61] Action potential duration and the effective refractory period are decreased by lidocaine; however, the ratio of effective refractory period to action potential duration is increased both in Purkinje fibers and in ventricular muscle (see Chapter 2, Fig. 2-18).

Considerable interest exists in the cardiac electrophysiologic effects of bupivacaine because of the observation that this agent may precipitate cardiac arrhythmias in various animal species, including man. Bupivacaine markedly depresses the rapid phase of depolarization (V_{max}) in isolated guinea pig papillary muscle preparations.[6,34] In addition, rate of recovery from a steady-state block was much slower in bupivacaine-treated papillary muscles as compared to lidocaine. This slow rate of recovery resulted in an incomplete restoration of V_{max} between action potentials when heart rate exceeded 100 beats/min. In contrast, recovery from lidocaine was complete, even at rapid heart rates. A decrease in rate of depolarization and action potential duration leading to conduction block and electrical inexcitability was also observed in canine Purkinje fibers.[49] These results suggest that bupivacaine may produce unidirectional block and a reentrant type of cardiac arrhythmia.

Electrophysiologic studies in intact dogs and in humans essentially reflect the findings observed in isolated cardiac tissue.[91,140] As the dose and blood levels of lidocaine are increased, a prolongation of conduction time through various parts of the heart occurs that is reflected in the electrocardiogram as an increase in the PR interval and QRS duration. Extremely high concentrations of local anesthetics will depress spontaneous pacemaker activity in the sinus node, resulting in sinus bradycardia and sinus arrest. A similar depression at the atrioventricular (AV) node also occurs, resulting in prolonged PR intervals and partial and complete AV dissociation.

Because depolarization in the heart and nerve is related to the influx of sodium ions, local anesthetics are believed to act primarily at the sodium channels to inhibit sodium conductance (see Fig. 2-18). In cardiac tissue the depolarization phase of the action potential is related to the influx of sodium ions through so-called fast channels and to the influx of calcium ions through slow channels (see Fig. 2-18). The slow calcium channels are responsible for the spontaneous depolarization observed in the region of the sino-atrial (SA) node. Most investigators believe that local anesthetics have little effect on the slow inward calcium currents. Josephson and Sperelakis have reported, however, that high concentrations of lidocaine, procaine, and tetracaine can block slow calcium channels in the myocardial sarcolemma (see Chapter 2).[80]

Local anesthetic agents also exert profound effects on the mechanical activity of cardiac muscle. Studies on isolated guinea pig atria and isolated whole rabbit hearts have shown that all local anesthetics exert a dose-dependent negative inotropic action.[12,55] The more potent local anesthetic agents tend to depress cardiac contractility at lower doses and concentrations than do the less potent local anesthetic agents[6] (Table 4-4).

Studies in dogs in which a strain gauge arch was sutured to the right ventricle revealed that a relationship exists between the local anesthetic potency of various agents and their ability to decrease myocardial contractility (Fig. 4-11).[139] Tetracaine, for example, which is about eight to ten times more potent than procaine as a local anesthetic, was found to be about eight times more depressant than procaine in intact dogs. The hemodynamic effects of the various clin-

TABLE 4-4. *Comparative effect of various local anesthetic agents on cardiac contractility*

Agent	Relative anesthetic potency	Local anesthetic concentrations (μg/ml) to produce 25–50% decrease in cardiac contractility: Isolated rabbit heart (25% ↓)[a]	Isolated guinea pig atria (50% ↓)[b]
Procaine	1	—	277
Chloroprocaine	1	—	102
Cocaine	2	—	56
Lidocaine	2	16.4	67
Prilocaine	2	11.7	42
Mepivacaine	2	9.9	55
Etidocaine	6	1.3	—
Bupivacaine	8	1.4	6
Tetracaine	8	0.9	6

[a] Data derived from Block, A., and Covino, B.G.: Effect of local anesthetic agents on cardiac conduction and contractility. Reg. Anesth., *6*:55, 1982.

[b] Data derived from Feldman, H.S., Covino, B.M., and Sage, D.J.: Direct chronotropic and inotropic effects of local anesthetic agents in isolated guinea pig atria. Reg. Anesth., *7*:149, 1982.

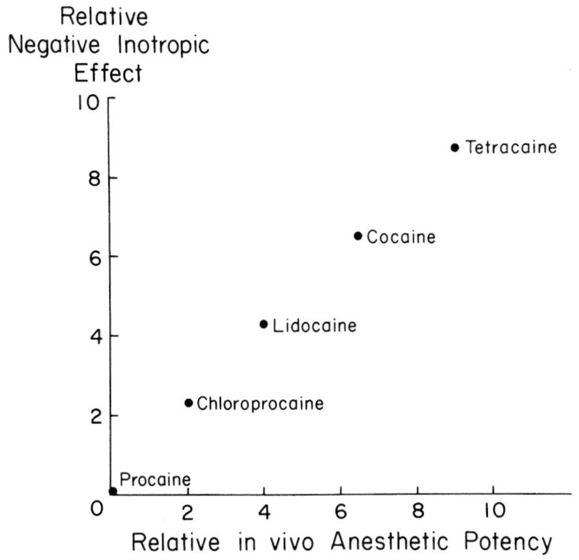

FIG. 4-11. Relation between anesthetic potency and negative inotropic effect of various local anesthetics. (Data derived from Stewart, D.M., Rogers, W.P., Mahaffrey, J.E., *et al.*: Effect of local anesthetics on the cardiovascular system in the dog. Anesthesiology, *24*:620, 1963.)

ically useful ester and amide local anesthetics were compared in closed-chest anesthetized dogs.[94,100] Again, a relationship existed between the anesthetic potency of the various agents and their depressant effect on heart rate, blood pressure, and cardiac output. The direct effect of lidocaine on myocardial contractility in patients under general anesthesia was evaluated by Harrison and colleagues during thoracic surgical procedures.[71] A strain gauge sutured to the right ventricle revealed that the intravenous administration of 2 to 4 mg/kg of lidocaine caused minimal changes in right ventricular contractile force.

The mechanism by which local anesthetics depress myocardial contractility is not precisely known. Both procaine and tetracaine can increase the release of calcium from isolated skeletal muscle preparations.[87] A similar displacement of calcium from cardiac muscle would result in a decrease in myocardial contractility; however, studies in the isolated guinea pig heart have shown that an increase in the extracellular concentration of calcium failed to reverse the negative inotropic action of bupivacaine or lidocaine.[143]

Over the years several case reports have appeared in the literature in which bupivacaine and etidocaine were associated with rapid and profound cardiovascular depression.[3,48,113] These cases differed from the usual cardiovascular depression seen with local anesthetics. The onset of cardiovascular depression occurred relatively early. In some cases, severe cardiac arrhythmias were observed, and the cardiac depression appeared resistant to various therapeutic modalities.

Insight into these clinical problems has been obtained in nonanesthetized sheep preparation with chronic vascular catheters.[109] After nonconvulsion-producing graded bolus doses of both lidocaine and bupivacaine, dose-dependent reductions in left ventricular *dp/dt* max occurred (as an index of myocardial contractility), as did increases in left ventricular end diastolic pressure (LVEDP) (Fig. 4-12A). Both of these parameters returned to control values within 3 minutes in keeping with negative inotropic drug effects. In addition, within seconds of drug administration into the inferior vena cava, dose-dependent increases in pulmonary artery pressure were noted, suggesting a direct pulmonary vasoconstrictive effect (Fig. 4-12B). These effects were of similar magnitude when lidocaine and bupivacaine were administered in doses considered to be of equal potency, that is, lidocaine:bupivacaine = 4:1.

With convulsion-producing doses (CD_{100} = 3.3 mg/kg for lidocaine, 1.5 mg/kg for bupivacaine), the initial transient depression in the indices of myocardial contractility was rapidly reversed, presumably by autonomic responses to the convulsion. During convulsions, elevations in LVEDP were marked for both drugs, but without significant changes in intrathoracic pressure, suggesting decreased myocardial compliance as a possible causative factor.

The cardiotoxicity of the more potent agents such as bupivacaine appears to differ from that of lidocaine in the following manner: (i) The ratio of the dosage required for irreversible cardiovascular collapse (CC) and the dosage that will produce CNS toxicity (convulsions), that is, the CC/CNS ratio, is lower for bupivacaine and etidocaine than for lidocaine; (ii) ventricular arrhythmias and fatal ventricular fibrillation may occur after the rapid intravenous administration of a large dose of bupivacaine (Fig. 4-12C) but not lidocaine; (iii) the pregnant animal or patient may be more sensitive to the cardiotoxic effects of bupivacaine than the nonpregnant animal or patient; (iv) cardiac resuscitation is more difficult after bupivacaine-induced cardiovascular collapse; and (v) acidosis and hypoxia markedly potentiate the cardiotoxicity of bupivacaine.

CC/CNS Ratio. Studies in adult sheep in which a continuous intravenous infusion of local anesthetic was administered have shown that a CC/CNS dose ratio of 7.1 ± 1.1 existed for lidocaine, indicating that seven times as much drug was required to induce irreversible cardiovascular collapse as was needed for the production of convulsions.[105,106] In comparison, the CC/CNS ratio for bupivacaine was 3.7 ± 0.5 and for etidocaine 4.4 ± 0.9. In terms of blood levels associated with CNS and cardiovascular collapse, lidocaine showed a CC/CNS blood level ratio of 3.6 ± 0.3 compared to values of 1.6 to 1.7 for bupivacaine and etidocaine (Fig. 4-13). Tissue levels of the various local anesthetics that were determined at the time of cardiovascular collapse indicate a greater uptake of bupivacaine and etidocaine by the myocardium compared to lidocaine (Fig. 4-13).

Ventricular Arrhythmias. deJong and colleagues initially reported that bupivacaine caused cardiac arrhythmias in awake, but paralyzed cats, whereas no such changes were observed with lidocaine.[45] Studies in unanesthetized sheep confirmed that severe cardiac arrhythmias occur after the

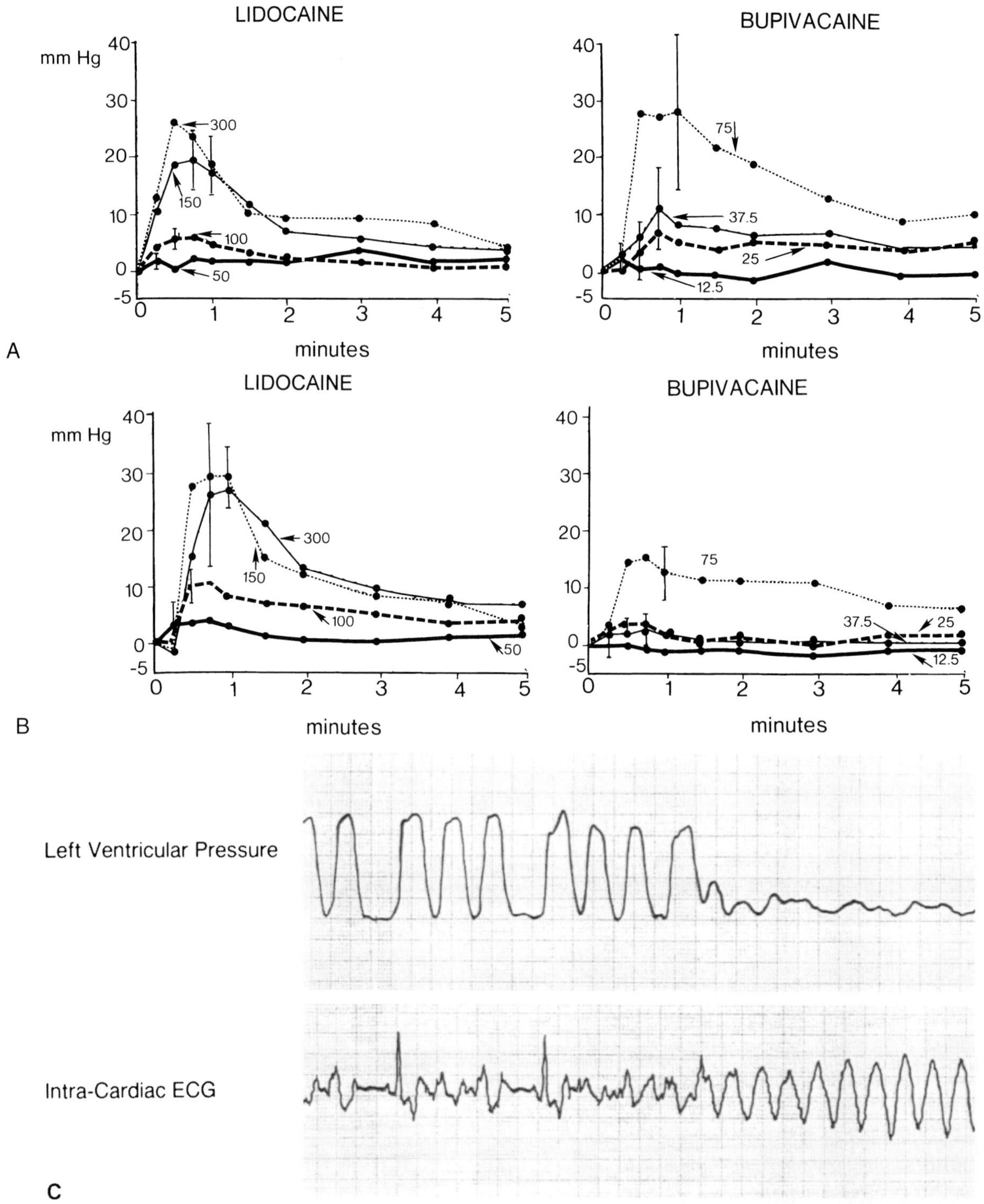

FIG. 4-12. Cardiovascular effects of local anesthetics in nonanesthetized sheep. **A:** Change in left ventricular end diastolic pressure (LVEDP) at increasing doses of lidocaine (lignocaine) and bupivacaine. **B:** Change in pulmonary artery pressure at the same doses of both drugs. The four doses (mg) were chosen for each drug to approximate equivalent clinical doses (lidocaine:bupivacaine = 4:1) (see text). **C:** Cardiac toxicity of bupivacaine. A rapid intravenous bolus of 150 mg of bupivacaine resulted in a fatal rapid decrease in left ventricular pressure (catheter tip transducer). Also ECG changed from a normal intracardiac quadripolar ECG pattern to that of ventricular tachycardia and subsequent ventricular fibrillation. (Reproduced with permission from Nancarrow, C. Acute Toxicity of Lignocaine and Bupivacaine. Ph.D. thesis, Flinders University of Southern Australia, 1986.)

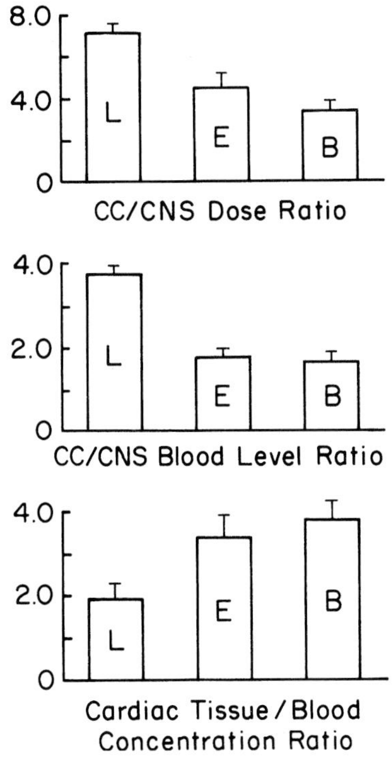

FIG. 4-13. Comparative CC/CNS toxicity dose ratio, CC/CNS toxicity blood level ratio, and myocardial tissue levels at time of cardiovascular collapse of lidocaine *(L),* bupivacaine *(B),* and etidocaine *(E).* (Data derived from Morishima, H.O., Peterson, H., Finster, M., *et al.*: Is bupivacaine more cardiotoxic than lidocaine? Anesthesiology, *59:*A409, 1983; and Etidocaine toxicity in the adult, newborn, and fetal sheep. Anesthesiology, *58:*342, 1983.)

were observed in awake paralyzed cats following the administration of etidocaine, although the frequency was less than that associated with the use of bupivacaine.[45] In addition, ventricular fibrillation was also observed in one of three dogs in which supraconvulsant doses of etidocaine were injected.[49] The results suggest that the occurrence of ventricular fibrillation is not related to the basic piperidine ring structure of bupivacaine because mepivacaine, which contains the piperidine moiety, failed to cause these cardiac abnormalities. Thus it appears that it is the bupivacaine molecule *per se* that is responsible for the actions on the heart.

The theory that ventricular arrhythmias are related to the degree of lipid solubility and protein binding may not be valid because etidocaine, which is more highly lipid soluble than bupivacaine and equally protein bound, appears to be associated with a lower incidence of ventricular fibrillation than is bupivacaine. In sheep, Nancarrow and colleagues found that mean values of maximum arterial drug concentrations during fatal experiments were 165 mg/liter (SD-22) for lidocaine-treated animals and 20.9 mg/liter (SD-7.9) after bupivacaine.[109] For both drugs, similar percentages of the initial dose (3% for lidocaine, 3.7% for bupivacaine) were found in the heart after analysis of tissue homogenate obtained postmortem.

Cardiac arrhythmias associated with bupivacaine do not appear related to the intensity of convulsive activity, although pentobarbital-treated dogs that did not convulse did not demonstrate these electrocardiographic abnormalities. Isolated guinea pig hearts perfused with a bupivacaine solution revealed evidence of conduction block and bigeminy and trigeminy, but did not when perfused with lidocaine.[143]

rapid intravenous administration of bupivacaine, whereas no cardiac irregularities were observed when lidocaine was injected intravenously.[86] Although no cardiac arrhythmias were observed in the canine toxicity studies conducted by Liu and co-workers, these dogs were anesthetized with pentobarbital.[93,94] Subsequent studies in unanesthetized dogs demonstrated the occurrence of ventricular tachycardia and ventricular fibrillation in some animals receiving intravenous bupivacaine.[95,124] No arrhythmias occurred when the same dogs were given intravenous lidocaine. The incidence of ventricular fibrillation has been ascertained in ropivacaine studies in awake dogs in which convulsant and supraconvulsant doses of lidocaine, mepivacaine, bupivacaine, and etidocaine were administered intravenously[54] (Table 4-5). Although the number of animals studied is relatively small in each group, it appears that ventricular fibrillation may occur in about 50% of dogs after the rapid intravenous injection of a convulsant or supraconvulsant dose of bupivacaine. Ventricular fibrillation was not observed in the lidocaine, etidocaine, or mepivacaine treated dogs. Ventricular arrhythmias

TABLE 4-5. *Frequency of ventricular fibrillation (VF) following the IV administration of convulsant or supraconvulsant doses of various local anesthetics in unanesthetized dogs*

Drug	Number of dogs	Dose (mg/kg)	Frequency of VR
Lidocaine	10	11–33	0
Mepivacaine	5	13–26	0
Etidocaine	8	4.6–9.2	13
Bupivacaine	16	3.4–13.6	44

(Data derived from Eicholzer, A.W., and Feldman, H.S.: Acute toxicity of etidocaine following various routes of administration in the dog. Toxicol. Appl. Pharmacol., *37:*13, 1976; Feldman, H.S., Arthur, G.R., Norway, S.B., *et al.*: Cardiovascular effects of mepivacaine and etidocaine in the awake dog. Anesthesiology, *61:*A229, 1984; and Sage, D., Feldman, H., Arthur, G.R., and Covino, B.G.: Cardiovascular effects of lidocaine and bupivacaine in the awake dog. Anesthesiology, *59:*A210, 1983.)

In addition, Reiz has observed the development of ventricular fibrillation in intact pigs in which bupivacaine was injected directly into the left anterior descending coronary artery (S. Reiz, personal communication). Thus these ventricular arrhythmias apparently are not related to the occurrence of convulsive activity.

The etiology of bupivacaine-associated ventricular arrhythmias is not known. As mentioned previously, electrophysiologic studies have shown that bupivacaine can markedly depress the rapid phase of depolarization (V_{max}) of the cardiac action potential and prolong the recovery phase, leading to conduction block and electrical inexcitability. These data suggest possible unidirectional blockade of conducting pathways, which may cause a re-entrant type of arrhythmia (see also Chapter 2).[34,149]

Enhanced Cardiotoxicity in Pregnancy. Many of the cardiotoxic reactions reported after the use of bupivacaine have occurred in pregnant patients. As a result, the 0.75% solution is no longer recommended for use in obstetric anesthesia in the United States. It is not certain whether the pregnant patient is more susceptible to the toxic effects of local anesthetics. Studies in sheep have shown that the CC/CNS dosage ratio of bupivacaine decreased from 3.7 ± 0.5 in nonpregnant sheep to 2.7 ± 0.4 in pregnant sheep.[104] Little difference was observed, however, in the CC/CNS blood level ratio, which varied from 1.6 ± 0.1 in nonpregnant sheep to 1.4 ± 0.1 in pregnant ones. The myocardial uptake of bupivacaine in pregnant sheep at the time of cardiovascular collapse did not differ from that in nonpregnant sheep. Additional studies are clearly warranted to determine the relative cardiotoxicity of bupivacaine and other local anesthetics in pregnant and nonpregnant animals.

Cardiac Resuscitation. Cardiopulmonary resuscitation is apparently extremely difficult in patients in whom cardiotoxicity has occurred following the administration of a toxic dose of bupivacaine. Studies in acidotic and hypoxic sheep have also indicated that cardiac resuscitation following bupivacaine-induced toxicity is difficult.[144] Recent studies in hypoxic dogs rendered toxic with bupivacaine indicate that resuscitation is possible if massive doses of epinephrine and atropine are used.[81] Studies in several animal species,[6,109] and man,[130] indicate that ropivacaine is less cardiotoxic than bupivacaine, but more toxic than lidocaine.

Effect of Acidosis and Hypoxia. Changes in acid-base status will alter the potential cardiovascular toxicity of local anesthetic agents. Studies on isolated atrial tissues have shown that hypercarbia, acidosis, and hypoxia will tend to potentiate the negative chronotropic and inotropic action of lidocaine and bupivacaine.[125] In particular, the combination of hypoxia and acidosis appears to markedly potentiate the cardiodepressant effects of bupivacaine. Studies in intact sheep have also demonstrated that hypoxia and acidosis markedly increase the cardiotoxicity of bupivacaine.[144] This enhanced toxicity is not related to a greater myocardial tissue uptake of local anesthetic, since investigations in rabbits demonstrated a decreased cardiac concentration of bupivacaine in the presence of acidosis.[69] Marked hypercarbia, acidosis, and hypoxia occur very rapidly in some patients after seizure activity caused by the rapid accidental intravascular injection of local anesthetic agents.[102] Thus it has been postulated that the cardiovascular depression observed with the more potent agents such as bupivacaine may in part be related to the severe acid-base changes that occur following the administration of toxic doses of these agents (see also Chapter 3).

Peripheral Vascular Effects

Local anesthetics exert a biphasic action on smooth muscle of peripheral blood vessels.[11] For example, exposure of arterioles in the cremaster muscle of rats to concentrations of lidocaine of 10 to 10^3 μg/ml produced a dose-related state of vasoconstriction varying from 88% to 60% of the control vascular diameter.[78] An increase in the concentration of lidocaine to 10^4 μg/ml produced approximately a 27% increase in arteriolar diameter, indicating a significant degree of vasodilation. Other studies using an isolated rat portal vein preparation have also demonstrated that local anesthetic drugs stimulate spontaneous myogenic contractions and augment basal tone at low concentrations and inhibit myogenic activity at higher concentrations.[11]

In vivo studies have also confirmed the biphasic effect of local anesthetic on the peripheral vasculature. The intra-arterial administration of mepivacaine in human volunteers resulted in a decrease in forearm blood flow without any change in arterial pressure, which suggests that mepivacaine caused vasoconstriction, which increases peripheral vascular resistance.[79] Similar studies with lidocaine also showed an increased tone in capacitance vessels, with less consistent effect on resistance vessels. As the dose of local anesthetic agent is increased, the stimulatory or vasoconstrictor action of these agents changes to one of inhibition and vasodilation.

Cocaine is the only agent that produces a state of vasoconstriction at most doses. Direct blood flow studies in dogs have shown that the initial effect of cocaine is one of vasodilation, but this is followed by a long period of vasoconstriction regardless of the dose of cocaine administered.[110] This unique property of cocaine is not related to a direct effect of cocaine itself on vascular smooth muscle but is basically an indirect action of this agent. Cocaine has been shown to inhibit the uptake of norepinephrine by tissue binding sites. Thus, after the release of norepinephrine from postganglionic sympathetic fibers, the decrease in the reuptake of norepinephrine by tissue binding sites will result in an excess amount of free norepinephrine, which will lead to a prolonged, profound state of vasoconstriction. This property of cocaine to inhibit the reuptake of norepinephrine has not been demonstrated to occur with other local anesthetics.

In summary, the sequence of cardiovascular events that usually occurs after the systemic administration of local anesthetic agents is as follows: At relatively nontoxic blood levels of these agents, either no change in blood pressure or a slight increase in blood pressure may be observed. Concentrations of local anesthetics that produce CNS toxicity will result in a marked increase in heart rate, blood pressure, and cardiac output that is directly related to the degree and duration of convulsive activity.[124] A further increase in dosage and blood level of local anesthetic leads to cardiovascular depression. The initial fall in blood pressure is primarily related to a decrease in cardiac output that is transient in nature and spontaneously reversible in most patients. If the amount of local anesthetic administered is excessive, however, a profound state of cardiovascular depression occurs that is related to the negative inotropic and peripheral vasodilator action of these agents. Ultimately, the combined peripheral vasodilation, decreased myocardial contractility, and depressant effect on cardiac rate and conductivity will lead to cardiac arrest and circulatory collapse. In addition, certain agents such as bupivacaine, and less so ropivacaine, may precipitate potentially fatal ventricular fibrillation.

Miscellaneous Systemic Effects

Other systemic actions have been ascribed to local anesthetic drugs, most of which are related to the generalized membrane stabilizing property of this class of drugs. For example, local anesthetics have been reported to possess neuromuscular blocking, ganglionic blocking, and anticholinergic activity. There is little evidence to suggest that any of these miscellaneous effects is clinically significant under normal conditions (However, see Chapter 27).

A unique systemic side effect is the formation of methemoglobinemia following the administration of large doses of prilocaine.[75,98] A dose–response relationship exists between the amount of prilocaine administered and the degree of methemoglobinemia. In general, doses of prilocaine of approximately 600 mg are required before the development of clinically significant levels of methemoglobinemia. The formation of methemoglobinemia is believed to be related to the degradation of prilocaine in the liver to O-toluidine, which is actually responsible for the oxidation of hemoglobin to methemoglobin.[75] Although methemoglobinemia is of little clinical significance in most patients with normal oxygen carrying capacity, it has limited the use of this potentially valuable drug, since prilocaine is the least toxic of the amide local anesthetics in terms of CNS toxicity. The methemoglobinemia associated with the use of prilocaine is spontaneously reversible or may be treated by the intravenous administration of methylene blue.

Allergic Effects

Reports of allergic reactions, hypersensitivity, or anaphylactic responses to local anesthetic agents appear periodically.[24,75,118] Unfortunately, systemic toxic reactions to local anesthetic agents are frequently misdiagnosed as representing allergic- or hypersensitivity-type reactions.[56] The aminoester agents such as procaine have been shown to produce allergic-type reactions. Because these agents are derivatives of *para*-aminobenzoic acid, which is known to be allergenic in nature, it is not unusual that a certain percentage of the population will demonstrate allergic reactions to this class of local anesthetics. The advent of the amino amide local anesthetics, that are not derivatives of *para*-aminobenzoic acid, markedly changed the incidence of allergic-type reactions to local anesthetic drugs. Reactions of an allergic type to the amino amides are extremely rare, although several cases have been reported in the literature over the years which suggest that this class of agents can on rare occasions produce an allergic-type phenomenon.[24,56,118] It should be remembered that solutions of amino amide agents from multiple-dose containers may contain a preservative, methylparaben, whose chemical structure is similar to that of *para*-aminobenzoic acid. It has been shown that patients in whom methylparaben was administered intradermally demonstrated a positive skin reaction.[5] Also some patients are allergic to metabisulfite, which is present in epinephrine-containing local anesthetic solutions. Cross-sensitivity reactions are possible because many other drugs, foods, and beverages contain preservatives such as metabisulfite and hydroxybenzoate. Two patients suspected of having allergic reactions to local anesthetics were confirmed by challenge testing to have allergies to benzoate and metabisulfite.

Progressive challenge with dilute (1:1000) and then undiluted intradermal injection of local anesthetics has been successfully used to diagnose adverse responses to local anesthetics. It is important to use local anesthetic solutions without additives in such testing, and also for neural blockade in patients with a history of allergy to preservatives in foods and drugs.[56]

Local Tissue Toxicity

Local anesthetic agents used clinically rarely produce localized nerve damage.[135] However, in 1980 some concern had been expressed regarding the potential neurotoxicity of chloroprocaine. Prolonged sensory motor deficits were reported in four patients after the epidural or subarachnoid injection of large doses of this particular drug.[115,117] Subsequently, Moore reported signs of neural damage in five additional patients in whom chloroprocaine had been used.[103] Studies in animals have proved somewhat contradictory regarding the potential neurotoxicity of chloroprocaine (Table 4-6). Barsa and associates, using an isolated

TABLE 4-6. *Summary of neurotoxicity studies involving chloroprocaine*

		Signs of neurotoxicity			
Reference	Type of study	2-CP	Lidocaine	Bupivacaine	$NaHSO_3$
8	Isolated rabbit vagus nerve	+ + +	0	–	–
64	Isolated rabbit vagus nerve	+ + +	–	0	+ + +
113	Intact rabbit sciatic nerve	0	0	–	–
117	Dog—total spinal	+ + +	–	0	–
148	Rabbit—spinal	+ + +	–	–	+ + +
122	Sheep—total spinal	+	+	0	–
122	Monkey—total spinal	+	–	+	–

0, no effect; +, mild toxicity; + + +, severe toxicity; –, not studied; 2-CP, commercial 2-chloroprocaine solution; $NaHSO_3$, sodium bisulfite.

rabbit vagus nerve preparation, reported that chloroprocaine was associated with signs of neural irritation, whereas the use of lidocaine under similar conditions failed to cause local toxic effects.[8] Histologic examination of rabbit sciatic nerves exposed to chloroprocaine for 6 hours did not, however, reveal any signs of nerve damage.[112] Doses of chloroprocaine sufficient to cause total spinal anesthesia in dogs produced paralysis in about 30% of the animals, whereas dogs treated with bupivacaine did not show evidence of permanent neurologic sequelae.[116] Studies of a similar nature in sheep and monkeys failed to show any difference in neurotoxicity between chloroprocaine and other local anesthetics or control solutions.[121] Paralysis observed in rabbits in which chloroprocaine solutions were administered intrathecally was believed to be related to sodium bisulfite, which is used as an antioxidant in chloroprocaine solutions.[147] The use of pure solutions of chloroprocaine without sodium bisulfite did not cause paralysis, whereas sodium bisulfite alone was associated with paralysis. A detailed series of studies has been conducted on the isolated rabbit vagus nerve to investigate the neurotoxicity of the various components of commercial chloroprocaine solutions (Table 4-7).[63] Commercial solutions of 3% chloroprocaine contain the local anesthetic agent itself, 0.2% sodium bisulfite, and hydrogen ions, which yield a pH of approximately 3.0. Application of commercial 3% chloroprocaine to isolated vagus nerves for 30 minutes resulted in irreversible conduction blockade. The use of 3% chloroprocaine with sodium bisulfite solution buffered to a pH of 7.3 caused reversible conduction block. A 3% chloroprocaine solution with a pH of 3.2 but without sodium bisulfite also resulted in reversible blockade. Application of a 0.2% sodium bisulfite solution at a pH of 3.3 resulted in irreversible conduction block, whereas the use of a 0.2% sodium bisulfite solution with a pH of 7.0 caused no conduction block. The results of these studies suggest that the combination of a low pH and the presence of sodium bisulfite may be responsible for the neurotoxic reactions observed following the use of large amounts of chloroprocaine solution. Chloroprocaine, itself, does not appear to be neurotoxic. The tolerance of peripheral nerves to bisulfite seems to be much higher than that of spinal nerve roots. Ford and colleagues (personal communication) injected 10% bisulfite at pH 4.8 near the saphenous nerve of the cat, and no damage was detected; however, at pH 2.8 moderate damage occurred (see also Chapter 30).

TABLE 4-7. *Effect of chloroprocaine, pH, and bisulfite on A- and C-fiber conduction in the isolated rabbit vagus nerve*

			Recovery time (min)	
Local anesthetic	pH	Bisulfite (%)	A	C
3% chloroprocaine	3.0	0.2	α	α
3% chloroprocaine	7.2	—	60	120
3% chloroprocaine	3.2	—	60	120
3% chloroprocaine	7.3	0.2	60	120
—	7.0	0.2	—	—
—	3.3	0.2	α	α

—, no block; α, irreversible block.

Skeletal muscle appears to be more sensitive to the local irritant properties of local anesthetic agents than other tissues. Skeletal muscle changes have been observed with most of the clinically used local anesthetic agents.[40,90] In general, the more potent longer-acting agents such as bupivacaine and etidocaine appear to cause a greater degree of localized skeletal muscle damage than the less potent, shorter-acting agents such as lidocaine and prilocaine. This effect on skeletal muscle is reversible, and muscle regeneration occurs rapidly and is complete within 2 weeks after injection of local anesthetic agents. These changes in skeletal muscle have not been correlated with any overt clinical signs of local irritation.

FACTORS INFLUENCING SYSTEMIC LOCAL ANESTHETIC ACTIVITY

The CNS and cardiovascular toxicity of local anesthetics is clearly related to the blood level of these agents, which in turn will influence the concentration in the brain and heart. The blood levels of local anesthetics that are achieved following the use of appropriate dosages and appropriate regional anesthetic techniques rarely cause adverse systemic reactions; however, toxic blood levels can occur, usually caused by an accidental intravascular injection or the extravascular administration of an excessive dose.

Extremely high blood levels of local anesthetics are achieved following rapid intravascular injection. Under these conditions toxicity is primarily related to the intrinsic anesthetic potency of the specific agents. The concentration of a drug in blood following an extravascular injection is determined by the rate of absorption, tissue redistribution, and metabolism and excretion. Thus, following an extravascular injection, the blood level and the toxicity of local anesthetics are in part related to the intrinsic potency of the agent, but also to the pharmacokinetic profile of the drug. The pharmacokinetics of the various local anesthetic agents have been described in Chapter 3.

Absorption of local anesthetics is related to site of injection, choice of drug, dosage, and addition of vasoconstrictors.

Site of Injection

Absorption from any site depends on the blood supply to that site, with richly supplied areas favoring rapid absorption.[13] Figure 4-14 shows mean plasma concentration curves following the injection of 400 mg of lidocaine at four different sites. The highest concentrations occurred after intercostal block and the lowest after subcutaneous abdominal infiltration. These results agree with the relative blood supplies of the four anatomic areas.

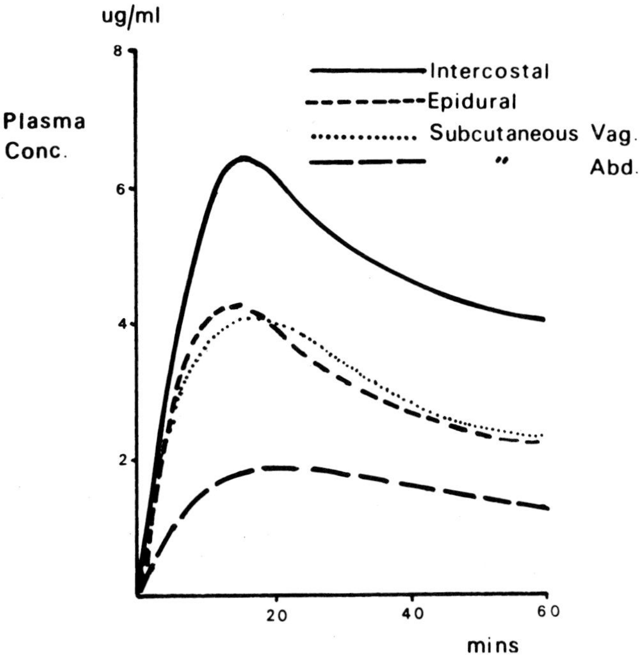

FIG. 4-14. Plasma concentrations of lidocaine following injection of 400 mg at four different sites.

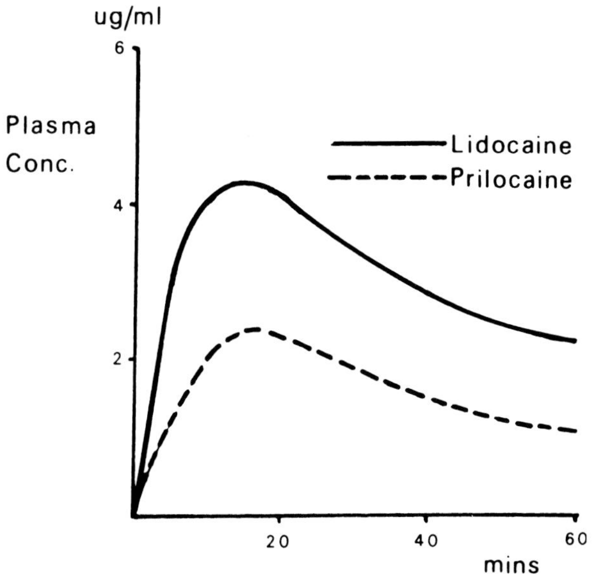

FIG. 4-15. Plasma concentrations of lidocaine and prilocaine following the epidural injection of 400 mg of each agent.

Choice of Drug

Figure 4-15 shows the plasma concentrations after epidural block, using the same dose of lidocaine or prilocaine. As can be seen, prilocaine yields lower plasma concentrations than does lidocaine. These differences may indicate a slower absorption for prilocaine, but it is more likely that they result from more rapid metabolism and a larger volume of distribution than for lidocaine. They explain the fact that intravenous prilocaine causes less toxicity, and for a shorter time, than does the same dose of lidocaine.[53] Similarly, etidocaine blood levels are lower than those of bupivacaine when equal doses are administered. This difference in blood levels allows the use of higher concentrations and dosages of etidocaine needed to achieve the same depth of anesthesia as buipvacaine. The epidural administration of 300 mg of etidocaine (20 ml of 1.5%) and 150 mg of bupivacaine (20 ml of 0.75%) produces similar depths and duration of anesthesia and similar blood levels.

Dosage

Within the clinical range of dosages for most local anesthetics, the relation between dosage and maximum plasma concentration appears reasonably linear (Fig. 4-16).

Addition of Epinephrine

The efficacy of epinephrine in reducing the absorption of local anesthetics depends on the sensitivity of the vasculature at the site of injection and the local anesthetic drug itself (Figs. 4-17, 4-18).

The rate of tissue redistribution, metabolism, and excre-

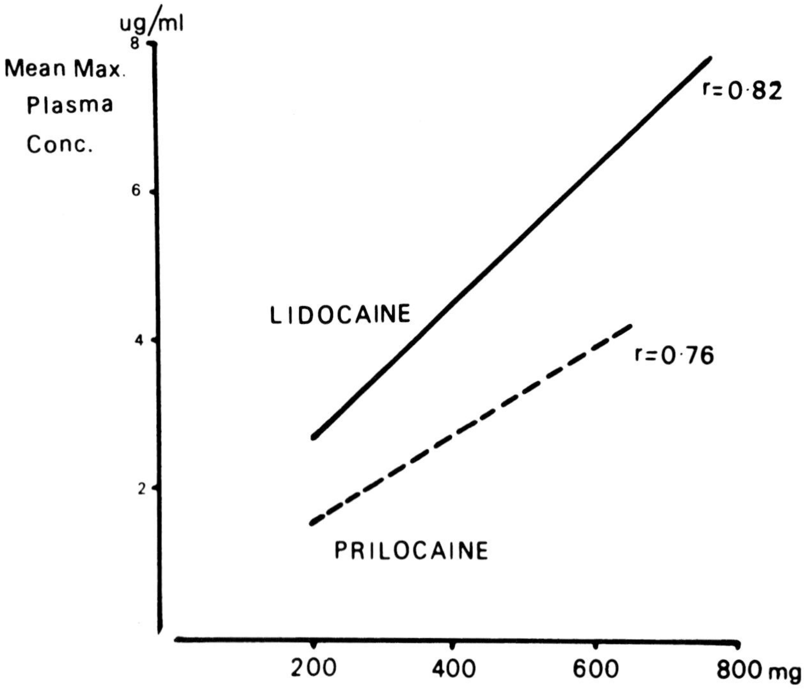

FIG. 4-16. Regression lines of mean maximum plasma concentration for lidocaine and prilocaine following epidural injection.

tion varies considerably among different local anesthetics. Among the amino amides prilocaine has the shortest distribution half-life ($t_{1/2}\alpha$), whereas the rates of tissue redistribution of the other amide agents are similar. The elimination half-life ($t_{1/2}\beta$) is also lower for prilocaine than for the other amide drugs because of its rapid rate of hepatic metabolism and possible metabolism by extrahepatic organs. The elimination half-lives of lidocaine, mepivacaine, and etidocaine are similar, whereas bupivacaine possesses the longest $t_{1/2}\beta$ value, which is indicative of a relatively slow rate of hepatic degradation. These differences in the pharmacokinetic and metabolic properties are responsible for the relatively low potential for systemic toxicity of prilocaine and the relatively high potential of bupivacaine.

Among the amino ester agents, chloroprocaine is hydrolyzed most rapidly, followed in order by procaine and tetracaine. The rate of hydrolysis of the ester agents is correlated with their relative potential for producing systemic tox-

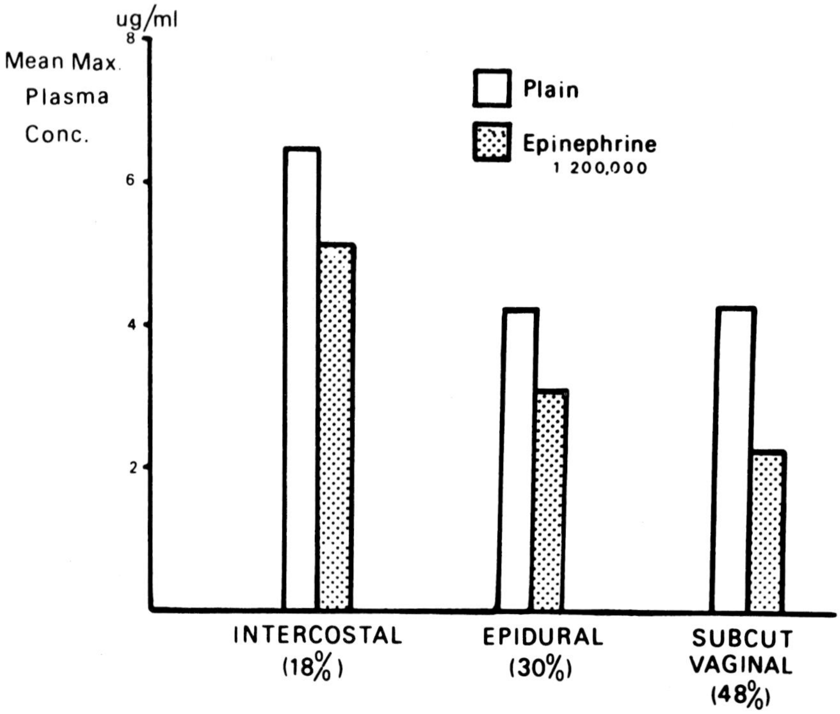

FIG. 4-17. Mean maximum concentrations of lidocaine with and without epinephrine, 1:200,000 given at three different sites. The most marked reduction caused by epinephrine occurs with the subcutaneous injection (48%), compared to 30% for epidural and 18% for intercostal (see also Fig. 3-14).

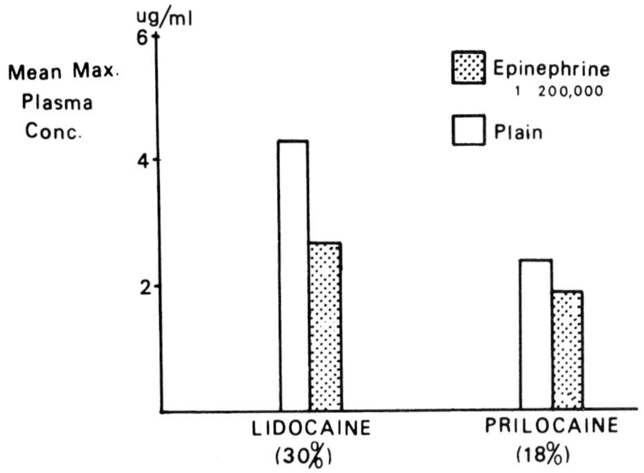

FIG. 4-18. Mean maximum concentration of lidocaine and prilocaine with and without epinephrine. 1:200,000, given epidurally. Epinephrine gives a larger reduction in plasma concentrations with lidocaine than with prilocaine (30% and 18%, respectively).

icity; thus chloroprocaine tends to be least toxic, whereas tetracaine is the most toxic and procaine is intermediate in terms of its toxic potential.

The clinical status of the patient will influence the pharmacokinetic properties and toxic potential of the various local anesthetics. The half-life of amide local anesthetics is prolonged in patients with a low cardiac output.[145] In such cases, an intravenous bolus injection results in a much higher blood concentration that persists for a longer period of time such that the proportion of drug reaching the brain and myocardium will be higher (Fig. 4-19).

Low cardiac output states are, in addition, often associated with a considerable reduction in liver blood flow.[70] Because the liver is responsible for detoxifying amide local anesthetics, reducing the liver blood flow will reduce the amount of drug available for degradation. This may produce very high blood concentrations during continuous intravenous infusion.[114] Hepatocellular disease could likewise reduce the speed of degradation and must be considered if high or repeated doses of local anesthetic are contemplated.

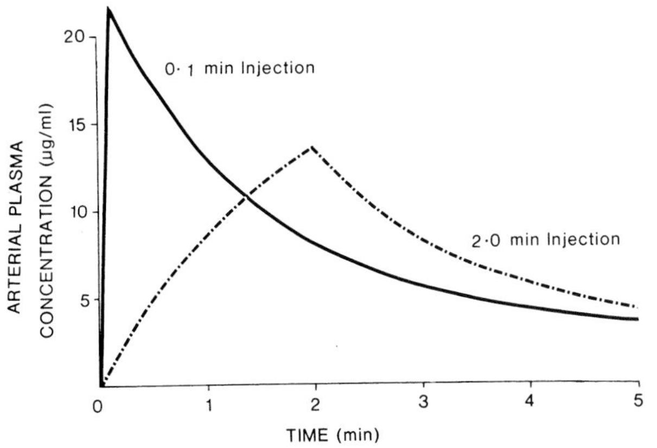

FIG. 4-19. Simulated arterial plasma concentrations of lidocaine, as described in Figure 4-10, show the likely outcome in patients with cardiac output reduced to about 50% of normal. (Data from Thomson, S.P.: Lidocaine pharmacokinetics in advanced heart failure, liver disease, and renal failure in humans. Ann. Intern. Med., *78*:499, 1973.)

DIAGNOSIS, PREVENTION, AND TREATMENT OF TOXIC REACTIONS

The differential diagnosis of systemic local anesthetic reactions is described in Table 4-8. Most toxic effects are preventable by the careful performance of regional anesthetic procedures, selection of the appropriate agent and dose, and a knowledge of the factors that affect absorption, distribution, and elimination of local anesthetics.

Prevention

As indicated previously, most toxic reactions are due to an accidental intravascular injection. This can often be avoided by careful technique and by allowing sufficient time for reflux of the blood down the needle or catheter used for injection (see also Table 4-9). Very gentle syringe aspiration before and during injection is also useful, although a negative result may be due to collapse of the vessel wall against the needle orifice rather than correct placement extravascularly. The use of a short bevel needle with a clear plastic hub allows easier recognition of vascular entry when performing nerve blocks such as brachial plexus blockade. Injections should be made slowly or by use of a fractionated dose technique. For example, during the performance of an epidural block, 3 to 4 ml of the anesthetic may be administered through the needle, followed by an additional 3 to 4 ml of solution after insertion of an epidural catheter. Once the catheter is taped in place and the patient properly positioned, additional increments of 3 to 4 ml of solution can be injected at 3- to 5-minute intervals as needed for attainment of a satisfactory level of anesthesia. The patient should be questioned during the injection of the local anesthetic to determine the presence of early numbness or any warning signs of toxicity such as circumoral numbness and tinnitus. In addition, monitoring of heart rate, blood pressure, and an electrocardiogram (ECG) should be performed before, during, and after the administration of any local anesthetic.

The use of a test dose is frequently helpful to detect an accidental intravascular or intrathecal injection. Three milliliters to 5 ml of anesthetic solution usually is required for an appropriate test dose. If there is no medical contraindication to the use of epinephrine, an epinephrine-containing solution is of value because a sudden increase in heart rate and blood pressure is usually diagnostic of an intravascular injection unless the patient has been taking β-adrenergic blockers. A period of 3 to 5 minutes is usually required after an epidural test dose in order to elicit signs of subarachnoid block.

TABLE 4-8. *Differential diagnosis of local anesthetic reactions*

Etiology	Major clinical features	Comments
Local anesthetic toxicity		
Intravascular injection	Immediate convulsion and/or cardiac toxicity	Injection into vertebral or a carotid artery may cause convulsion after administration of small dose.
Relative overdose	Onset in 5 to 15 minutes of irritability, progressing to convulsions	
Reaction to vasoconstrictor	Tachycardia, hypertension, headache, apprehension	May vary with vasopressor used
Vasovagal reaction	Rapid onset Bradycardia Hypotension Pallor, faintness	Rapidly reversible with elevation of legs
Allergy		
Immediate	Anaphylaxis (↓ BP, bronchospasm, edema)	Allergy to amides extremely rare
Delayed	Urticaria	Cross-allergy possible, for example, with preservatives in local anesthetics and food
High spinal or epidural block	Gradual onset Bradycardia[a] Hypotension Possible respiratory arrest	May lose consciousness with total spinal block and onset of cardiorespiratory effects more rapid than with high epidural or with subdural block.
Concurrent medical episode (e.g., asthma attack, myocardial infarct)	May mimic local anesthetic reaction	Medical history important

[a] Sympathetic block above T4 adds cardioaccelerator nerve blockade to the vasodilation seen with blockade below T4; total spinal block may have rapid onset.
BP, blood pressure.

TABLE 4-9. *Measures to prevent toxicity from neural blockade*[a]

PATIENT EVALUATION

Identification of significant systemic disease, age, and other factors, to permit individualization of local anesthetic dose

PREMEDICATION

Diazepam or other appropriate CNS depressant in moderate dosage

PREPARATION

Resuscitative drugs
- Midazolam or thiopentone, succinylcholine, atropine, vasopressor

Equipment
- Oxygen administration and suction equipment
- Airway (oropharyngeal airway, laryngoscope, endotracheal tube)

Ensure adequate IV available
Discard any cloudy solutions or those containing crystals
Physically separate neural blockade tray from any other drugs

PREVENTION

Personally check dose of local anesthetic and vasoconstrictor
Use test dose, 5–10% of total dose
Aspirate frequently and discard solution colored by blood
Monitor cardiovascular signs (rapid ↑ heart rate if epinephrine injected intravenously)
Constant verbal contact with patient past time of peak plasma concentration

[a] Local anesthetic toxicity may result in convulsions; however, with rapid and appropriate treatment, these should never be fatal in themselves. See also cardiac effects of bupivacaine in text.
CNS, central nervous system; IV, intravenous.

TABLE 4-10. *Treatment of acute local anesthetic toxicity*

AIRWAY

Establish clear airway; suction, if required

BREATHING

Oxygen with face mask
Encourage adequate ventilation (prevent cycle of acidosis, increased uptake of local anesthetic into CNS, and lowered seizure threshold)
Artificial ventilation, if required

CIRCULATION

Elevate legs
Increase IV fluids if ↓ blood pressure
CVS support drug if ↓ blood pressure persists (see below) or ↓ heart rate
Cardioversion if ventricular arrhythmias occur

DRUGS

CNS depressant
- Diazepam 5–10 mg, IV, Midazolam 2–5 mg
- Thiopental 50 mg, IV, incremental doses until seizures cease

Muscle relaxant
- Succinylcholine 1 mg/kg, if inadequate control of ventilation with above measures (requires artificial ventilation and may necessitate intubation)

CVS support
- Atropine 0.6 mg, IV, if ↓ heart rate
- Ephedrine, 12.5–25 mg, IV, to restore adequate blood pressure
- Epinephrine for profound cardiovascular collapse

CNS, central nervous system; CVS, cardiovascular system; IV, intravenous.

Treatment

Other than cessation of injection, it is seldom necessary to treat the minor signs and symptoms of toxicity (see Table 4-10) provided adequate respiration and cardiovascular function are maintained. Nevertheless, early signs of toxicity warrant constant verbal contact, cardiovascular monitoring, administration of oxygen, and encouragement to breathe at a normal minute volume.

Convulsions

If convulsions occur, the aim of treatment is to stop them and treat any respiratory or cardiovascular depression before cerebral hypoxia occurs. Currently, three pharmacologic approaches to controlling convulsions are available (see following). The simple nonpharmacologic measures should be carried out before any drug treatment is begun. The prevention of hypoxia and acidosis is the single most important feature of treatment (see also Chapter 6).

Intravenous Barbiturates

Thiopental (50–100 mg) can rapidly abort a convulsive episode. This agent has the great advantage of being familiar and usually readily available to the anesthesiologist. The possibility of enhanced respiratory and cardiovascular depression should be minimal and transient considering the small dosage required. Respiration must be carefully observed and a clear airway obtained, if necessary, by endotracheal intubation. If respiratory depression or apnea occurs, artificial ventilation with oxygen is required.

Diazepam/Midazolam

Diazepam may be administered intravenously in doses of 5 to 10 mg to control convulsions. Its onset may be somewhat slower than that of thiopental and its duration of action is longer. Respiration must be maintained and supported in the same fashion as described above. Although both thiopental and diazepam should abort the convulsions, they will not prevent the possibility of respiratory and cardiovascular depression. Midazolam (mg boluses) has a rapid onset.

Succinylcholine

Succinylcholine, a neuromuscular blocking agent, will also stop convulsions when administered intravenously. A dose of 50 mg is usually adequate, but administration is accompanied by paralysis and cessation of respiration. The patient should be immediately intubated and ventilated with oxygen. This agent should be used only by persons skilled in the art of endotracheal intubation. Of note, succinylcholine will inhibit muscular convulsive activity but not the convulsive process in the brain which might increase the oxygen demand of the brain; however, if respiration is controlled with oxygen and cardiovascular function is adequate, no deleterious CNS sequelae are likely.

Cardiovascular Depression

Hypotension should be treated by correction of hypoxia, elevation of legs, increased rate of infusion of intravenous fluids, and, if necessary, intravenous administration of a vasopressor agent. Because hypotension usually is due to a combination of myocardial depression and vasodilation, it is preferable to use an agent that stimulates both α- and β-adrenergic receptors such as ephedrine (15–30 mg or incremental doses of 5 mg until a positive response is obtained). Atropine (0.4 mg) can also be used to reverse a state of bradycardia.

Profound cardiovascular depression requires the immediate institution of cardiopulmonary resuscitation. Ventricular tachycardia or fibrillation should be treated by electrical cardioversion, which may require the use of higher than normal electrical energy. It has been reported that the use of large doses of epinephrine and atropine can reverse the cardiovascular collapse produced by bupivacaine in dogs. It may be necessary to continue cardiopulmonary resuscitative efforts for an hour or longer in situations of profound circulatory collapse. All other treatment modalities should be carried out, such as controlled ventilation with oxygen and administration of sodium bicarbonate to treat acidosis.

Respiratory and cardiovascular depression caused by a total spinal block should be treated in the same manner as described above. Assisted or controlled ventilation with oxygen and endotracheal intubation, if deemed necessary, should be instituted promptly to prevent hypoxia and acidosis. Rapid infusion of intravenous fluids, vasopressors, and anticholinergic agents should be given to treat hypotension and bradycardia (see also Chapter 8). Aspiration of 10 to 20 ml of cerebrospinal fluid (CSF) and replacement with saline may be useful for prevention of possible neural damage, particularly if solutions of chloroprocaine have been administered intrathecally.

Proper monitoring and immediate availability of resuscitative equipment are equally important when performing a regional or general anesthetic technique (see Chapter 6).

CLINICAL USE OF LOCAL ANESTHETICS

Amino Ester Agents

Procaine

Procaine is rarely used at present for peripheral nerve or extradural blocks because of its low potency, slow onset, and relatively short duration of action. Although the potential for systemic toxic reactions is quite small with procaine, this agent can cause allergic-type reactions. Currently procaine is used mainly for infiltration anesthesia and differential spinal blocks in chronic pain patients.

Chloroprocaine

Chloroprocaine became very popular in the United States because of its rapid onset of action and low systemic toxicity. Although the potency of the agent is relatively low, it can be used for epidural anesthesia in large volumes in a 3% solution because of its low systemic toxicity, and the large dose enhances its effect. The duration of action is between 30 and 60 minutes and the agent has enjoyed its greatest popularity for epidural analgesia and anesthesia in obstetrics because of the rapid onset and low systemic toxicity in both mother and fetus. However, frequent injections are needed to provide adequate pain relief in labor and it is more usual to establish analgesia with chloroprocaine and then change to a longer-acting agent such as bupivacaine (see Chapter 18).

Subsequently, the use of chloroprocaine declined because of reports of prolonged neurological deficit following accidental subarachnoid injection. As has been discussed previosly, this toxicity was ascribed to the bisulfite then included in the commercial preparation as a preservative. Because of this, the formulation was changed to eliminate bisulfite, and disodium ethylenediaminetetraacetic acid (EDTA) was used instead. However, since then, a number of reports[1,77,89,111,136] of back pain (sometimes severe enough to require opioid analgesia) have appeared. While the precise cause of the problem has yet to be elucidated, a number of factors have been implicated including the EDTA preservative, the use of very large volumes of the agent, the low pH of the solution, and irritation of the perispinous tissues during preparatory infiltration. A comparative study found that the use of very large volumes (greater than 40 ml) of chloroprocaine resulted in a significant incidence of the problem, but that 25 ml or less produced no greater incidence of back pain than did other anesthetic agents.[137]

Chloroprocaine has also proved of value for peripheral nerve blocks and epidural anesthesia when the duration of surgery is not expected to exceed 30 to 60 minutes. Thus this drug is useful for ambulatory surgical procedures performed under regional anesthesia. Chloroprocaine has also been mixed with other agents such as bupivacaine or tetracaine in order to provide a rapid onset and prolonged duration of anesthesia; however, as discussed previously, such mixtures may not result in the long duration of anesthesia usually associated with bupivacaine.

Tetracaine

Tetracaine remains a very popular drug for spinal anesthesia in the United States. Tetracaine may be used as an isobaric, hypobaric, or hyperbaric solution for spinal blockade, although hyperbaric solutions of tetracaine are probably used most commonly. Tetracaine provides a relatively rapid onset of spinal anesthesia—about 3 to 5 minutes—a profound depth of anesthesia, and a duration of 2 to 3 hours. The addition of epinephrine can extend the duration of anesthesia to 4 to 6 hours (see Chapter 7).

Tetracaine is rarely used for other forms of regional anesthesia because of its extremely slow onset of action and the potential for systemic toxic reactions when the larger doses required for other types of regional blockade are used. Before the introduction of bupivacaine and etidocaine, mixtures of tetracaine and other local anesthetics with a more rapid onset such as lidocaine or mepivacaine were used for various regional anesthetic procedures.

Tetracaine does possess excellent topical anesthetic properties, and solutions of this agent were commonly used for endotracheal surface anesthesia. The absorption of tetracaine from the tracheobronchial area is, however, extremely rapid, and several fatalities have been reported following the use of an endotracheal aerosol of tetracaine.

Cocaine

The original local anesthetic, cocaine, is still used clinically for its topical anesthetic and vasoconstrictor properties. Cocaine solutions are frequently used to anesthetize the nasal mucosa before nasotracheal intubation.

Amino Amide Agents

Lidocaine

Lidocaine was the first drug of the amino amide type to be introduced into clinical practice. This agent remains the most versatile and most commonly used local anesthetic because of its inherent potency, rapid onset, moderate duration of action, and topical anesthetic activity. Solutions of 0.5%, 1.0%, 1.5%, and 2.0% lidocaine are available for infiltration, peripheral nerve blocks, and epidural anesthesia. In addition, 5% lidocaine with 7.5% glucose is widely used for spinal anesthesia of 30 to 60 minutes' duration. (However, see Chapters 2 and 7 regarding concerns about possible neurotoxicity of 5% lidocaine when used for continuous spinal anesthesia.) Lidocaine is also used in ointment, jelly, and viscous and aerosol preparations for a variety of topical anesthetic procedures.

Although the duration of action of lidocaine is about 1 to 3 hours for various regional anesthetic procedures, the addition of epinephrine will significantly prolong the duration of this agent. Moreover, epinephrine will decrease the rate of absorption of lidocaine, which will significantly decrease its blood levels and potential for producing systemic toxic reactions (see Chapter 3).

Lidocaine also possesses a number of nonanesthetic uses. It is widely used as an intravenous antiarrhythmic agent in patients with ventricular arrhythmias. In addition, it has proved useful as an antiepileptic and intravenous analgesic agent. The systemic analgesic properties of lidocaine have proved to be of value in the treatment of certain chronic pain syndromes (see Chapter 27). In addition, the combination of intravenous lidocaine and CNS depressants such as barbiturates and general anesthetics has been used to provide a state of balanced analgesia and anesthesia. This systemic analgesic activity of lidocaine is apparently due to an action in CNS and is not related to its effect on peripheral nerves.

Mepivacaine

Mepivacaine is similar to lidocaine in terms of its anesthetic profile. Mepivacaine can produce a profound depth of anesthesia with a relatively rapid onset and a moderate duration of action. This agent may be used for infiltration, peripheral nerve blocks, and epidural anesthesia in concentrations varying from 0.5% to 2.0%. In some countries 4% hyperbaric solutions of mepivacaine are also available for spinal anesthesia.

Differences do exist between mepivacaine and lidocaine. Mepivacaine is not effective as a topical anesthetic agent and thus is less versatile than lidocaine. In addition, the metabolism of mepivacaine is markedly prolonged in the fetus and newborn such that this agent is not usually used for obstetric anesthesia. In adults, however, mepivacaine appears to be somewhat less toxic than lidocaine. Moreover, the vasodilator activity of mepivacaine is less than that of lidocaine. Thus mepivacaine provides a somewhat longer duration of anesthesia than lidocaine when the two agents are used without epinephrine. The duration of action of mepivacaine can be significantly prolonged by the addition of a vasoconstrictor such as epinephrine (see Chapter 3).

A 3% solution of mepivacaine is available specifically for dental anesthesia. A 2% solution of mepivacaine with the vasoconstrictor levonordefrin (NeoCobefrin) is also prepared specifically for the dental field.

Prilocaine

The clinical profile of prilocaine is also similar to that of lidocaine. Prilocaine has a relatively rapid onset of action while providing a moderate duration of anesthesia and a profound depth of conduction blockade. This agent causes significantly less vasodilation than lidocaine and thus can be used without epinephrine. In general, the duration of prilocaine without epinephrine is similar to that of lidocaine with epinephrine (see Chapter 3). Thus prilocaine is particularly useful in patients in whom epinephrine may be contraindicated. Prilocaine is useful for infiltration, peripheral nerve blockade, and epidural anesthesia. Although prilocaine possesses topical anesthetic activity and can induce spinal anesthesia of short duration, no specific formulations of this agent are available for topical or spinal anesthesia.

The primary advantage of prilocaine compared to lidocaine is its significantly decreased potential for producing systemic toxic reactions. Studies in animals and human volunteers indicate that prilocaine is approximately 40% less toxic than lidocaine. Prilocaine is the least toxic of the amino amide local anesthetics. Thus this agent is particularly useful for intravenous regional anesthesia because CNS toxic effects are rarely seen after tourniquet deflation, even when early accidental release of the tourniquet may occur. Forty milliliters of 0.5% prilocaine (200 mg) provides effective anesthesia for hand surgery using the intravenous regional anesthetic technique (see Chapter 12).

The major deterrent to the use of prilocaine is related to the formation of methemoglobinemia with this drug. This unusual side effect of prilocaine has essentially eliminated the use of this drug in obstetrics, although prilocaine has not been reported to cause any significant adverse effects in mother, fetus, or newborn; however, the cyanotic appearance of newborns delivered of mothers who have received prilocaine for epidural anesthesia during labor results in sufficient confusion concerning the etiology of the cyanosis such that the obstetric use of this potentially valuable drug has been virtually abandoned.

EMLA

This *E*utectic *M*ixture of *L*ocal *A*nesthetics (EMLA) lidocaine (25 mg/ml) and prilocaine (25 mg/ml) is available in an oily cream or as a 20-cm^2 "patch" with a central portion of 10 cm^2 containing the EMLA (25 mg of both drugs in 1 g of cream). *Eutectic* means equal proportions of solid crystals of prilocaine and lidocaine. The eutectic mixture takes on the convenient property of becoming a liquid at room temperature; in comparison the melting points of lidocaine and prilocaine are 67° and 37°C, respectively. The eutectic mixture is already an oil and requires only the addition of an emulsifier (arlatone) and a thickener (carbopol) to give it good consistency as a paste for application.[27,58]

In the EMLA, 80% of each droplet is local anesthetic compared to a standard emulsion where only 20% is local anesthetic. Thus there is a high *concentration* of drug in contact with the skin. This overcomes prior problems with local anesthetic creams which penetrate the epidermis of the skin with difficulty. The pH of the EMLA is relatively high (9.4) and thus a high percentage of the local anesthetic is in un-ionized base form. This facilitates passage of the drug across the diffusion barrier of the epidermis penetrating approximately 5 mm to the A-delta and C fibers in the dermis.[10,58]

The increased *efficacy* is accompanied by enhanced *safety* since the dose of drugs is small and plasma concentrations are well below toxic levels. Also because of the small dose of prilocaine, methemoglobinemia has not been a problem. However, in small children below 3 years of age, there is a small potential for systemic toxicity. Also, the biphasic vascular effects of prilocaine, in particular, may result in initial blanching of the skin followed by vasodilation.[27,58,138]

EMLA requires application at least 60 to 90 minutes prior to a procedure, and analgesia is still present 1 hour after removal. Local anesthetic uptake continues for several hours during application, thus application 2 hours or more beforehand is practical and desirable.[27]

The efficacy of EMLA has been documented for painful superficial procedures such as venipuncture and arterial cannulation, application prior to neural blockade, skin graft harvesting, arteriovenous shunt procedures, lumbar puncture, and as a method of anesthetizing gums prior to local anesthetic blocks for dentistry.[27,33,138]

The availability of EMLA patches[33] over the counter in some countries introduces the "patient control" concept to local anesthesia. Patients, or parents of children, appropriately instructed, can apply the patch prior to a painful procedure; this permits a sense of control, may reduce anxiety, and may increase patient satisfaction with the procedure. The "regional block" anesthesiologist can also apply EMLA, or instruct the patient to do so, prior to a neural blockade technique, thus preparing the area for a more comfortable start to the procedure.

Bupivacaine

Bupivacaine has probably had the greatest influence on the practice of regional anesthesia since the introduction of lidocaine. Bupivacaine was the first local anesthetic that combined the properties of an acceptable onset, long duration of action, profound conduction blockade, and significant separation of sensory anesthesia and motor blockade. This agent is used in concentrations of 0.125%, 0.25%, 0.5%, and 0.75% for various regional anesthetic procedures, including infiltration, peripheral nerve blocks, and epidural and spinal anesthesia. Bupivacaine has not been used for topical anesthesia. The average duration of surgical anesthesia of bupivacaine varies from about 3 to 10 hours. Its longest duration of action occurs when major peripheral nerve blocks such as brachial plexus blockade are performed. In these situations, average durations of effective surgical anesthesia of 10 to 12 hours have been reported. In some patients, durations of brachial plexus block of 24 hours or more have been observed with complete recovery of sensation. The vascular absorption of bupivacaine is influenced to a variable extent by epinephrine, but less so than for lidocaine.

The major advantage of bupivacaine appears to be in the area of obstetric analgesia for labor. In this situation, bupivacaine administered epidurally in concentrations varying from 0.125% to 0.5% provides satisfactory pain relief for 2 to 3 hours, which significantly decreases the need for repeated injections in the pregnant woman. More importantly, adequate analgesia is usually achieved without significant motor blockade such that the woman in labor is able to move her legs. This differential blockade of sensory and motor fibers is also the basis for the widespread use of bupivacaine for postoperative epidural analgesia and for certain chronic pain states (see Chapters 18, 26, 29).

Unfortunately the obstetric use of bupivacaine has been tempered somewhat in the mid 1980s because of reports of sudden cardiovascular collapse following the accidental rapid intravenous administration of this agent. The cardiotoxicity of bupivacaine, which has been discussed previously, has occurred primarily in the United States in obstetric patients. As a result, the 0.75% solution of bupivacaine is no longer recommended for obstetric anesthesia in the United States.

Bupivacaine had become relatively popular for intravenous regional anesthesia. The advantage of bupivacaine for intravenous (IV) regional anesthesia is related to the suggestion that there was an extended duration of anesthesia that occurred after tourniquet deflation. Several reports of sudden cardiovascular collapse after accidental early cuff deflation have resulted, however, in a recommendation in the United States that bupivacaine not be used for IV regional anesthesia (see Chapter 12).

In recent years, bupivacaine has been used extensively for spinal anesthesia. Isobaric and hyperbaric solutions of 0.5% to 0.75% bupivacaine have been investigated for various surgical procedures performed under subarachnoid blockade. Onset of spinal anesthesia with bupivacaine usually occurs within 5 minutes, whereas the duration of surgical anesthesia persists for 3 to 4 hours. Comparative studies of bupivacaine and tetracaine suggest little difference between the two agents in terms of onset, spread, and duration of spinal blockade. Several investigations have suggested that the frequency of satisfactory anesthesia may be greater with bupivacaine than with tetracaine. In addition, less hypotension is apparent after the intrathecal administration of bupivacaine, even in patients with an exaggerated spread of sensory anesthesia. The degree of motor blockade is greater when isobaric solutions of bupivacaine are used as opposed to hyperbaric formulations (see Chapter 7).

Ropivacaine

The concern about the potential of bupivacaine to produce cardiotoxicity after accidental intravenous injection, described earlier, has led to a search for an alternative long-acting local anesthetic drug. Ropivacaine has undergone considerable laboratory and clinical evaluation and has recently become approved for clinical use by the regulatory process in many parts of the world; it is not yet commercially available in any country. It belongs to the same chemical series as mepivacaine and bupivacaine, being intermediate in structure between the two agents (Chapter 3, Fig. 3-6). All the compounds in this series contain an asymmetric carbon atom which means that they may exist (and are usually presented) as a racemic mixture of two, optically active isomers.[99]

However, ropivacaine is unique in that it was marketed as an almost pure solution of the *S* isomer. This isomer was chosen because it is the longer acting of the two when used for nerve blockade in animals. Subsequent work has shown that the *S* isomer is also less cardiotoxic than the *R* isomer[147] so there is a double advantage (see also Chapter 3). Intravenous infusion studies in man have shown that ropivacaine can be administered in larger doses than bupivacaine before early features of both cardiovascular and CNS toxicity are apparent.[88,130] The implication is that the higher concentrations of ropivacaine (e.g., 0.75 or 1.0%) may be used with less risk of severe toxicity than is the case with bupivacaine.[99]

Early clinical studies have suggested that ropivacaine has a block profile very similar to bupivacaine (but with a marginally shorter duration) when used for major peripheral[72,73] and epidural[17,23,36,82] block. In addition, the epidural studies also suggest that the degree of motor block produced by ropivacaine is less than that produced by bupivacaine so it may be possible to produce a greater separation between sensory and motor block when the agent is used for pain relief in the postoperative period or during labor[99] (see also Chapter 8).

Ropivacaine has already undergone significant evaluation in these latter fields (although the work is not yet published), and it is likely to be the first agent to be marketed in most countries in a dilute formulation for constant infusion. Like other local anesthetics, ropivacaine has a biphasic effect on blood flow,[30] but the vasoconstrictor action is present at clinically used concentrations, the agent having been shown to reduce epidural blood flow.[43] Thus it is unlikely to be marketed in preparations containing epinephrine.[99]

Etidocaine

Etidocaine, which is chemically related to lidocaine, is one of the more recent local anesthetics introduced for clinical use. This agent is characterized by very rapid onset, prolonged duration of action, and profound sensory and motor blockade. Etidocaine may be used for infiltration, peripheral nerve blockade, and epidural anesthesia. Although etidocaine and bupivacaine provide prolonged durations of anesthesia, significant differences exist with regard to the anesthetic profile of these two local anesthetics. Etidocaine has a significantly more rapid onset of action than bupivacaine. In addition, the concentrations of etidocaine required for adequate sensory anesthesia produce profound motor blockade. As a result, etidocaine is primarily useful as an anesthetic for surgical procedures in which muscle relaxation is required. Thus this agent is of limited use for obstetric epidural analgesia and for postoperative pain relief because it does not provide a differential blockade of sensory and motor fibers. It is possible to take advantage of the different pharmacologic profiles of etidocaine and bupivacaine in certain clinical situations. For example, it is possible to initiate epidural blockade with 1.5% etidocaine for lower limb orthopedic procedures, such as total hip replacements, and for abdominal surgical procedures. Under these conditions etidocaine will provide a rapid onset of action and a profound depth of anesthesia and muscle relaxation. Supplemental intraoperative and postoperative anesthesia is then provided by 0.5% bupivacaine, which produces excellent sensory anesthesia with minimal motor blockade. Effects of epinephrine on vascular absorption of etidocaine are summarized in Chapter 3.

Agents Currently Undergoing Evaluation

Articaine

Articaine is an agent that has been used in dental practice in some European countries for nearly 20 years. It belongs to the anilide group of local anesthetics, but differs from drugs such as lidocaine in that it has a thiophene ring instead of a benzene ring in its structure.[149] It has been claimed that this agent has a faster onset and better spreading properties than lidocaine when used in dental blocks and this has resulted in its reevaluation for wider use. However, comparison with prilocaine in dental blocks has not demonstrated any difference[68] and comparison with lidocaine in epidural use also failed to show any significant differences.[16] Thus it seems unlikely that this agent will become much more widely available.

Butamben

Butyl aminobenzoate (BAB) is an amino ester local anesthetic patented in 1923 and originally used as a topical preparation, Butesin Picrate (Abbott Laboratories, North Chicago, IL). BAB is an ester of *para*-aminobenzoic acid and butyl alcohol, with a molecular weight of 193.24. An extraordinarily low pKa of 2.3 results in minimal ionization to the hydrophilic cation, and thus BAB is at the extreme low end of local anesthetic water solubility.[65]

BAB also has poor dural permeability, and these properties, together with its rapid hydrolysis, were previously thought to make it unattractive for epidural use. However, in the late 1980s, Shulman in the United States and Korsten in the Netherlands contemporaneously formulated suspension preparations of BAB, which produced long-lasting sensory blockade when given epidurally to cancer patients.[84,133] Subsequently Abbott Laboratories overcame substantial theoretical and technical difficulties to prepare a reproducible aqueous *suspension* of 5% butamben composed as follows: Each milliliter of BAB suspension contains 50 mg BAB; 0.25 mg polysorbate-80 (Tween-80) and 25 mg polyethylene glycol (PEG-3350) as suspending agents; and 9 mg sodium chloride for tonicity adjustment. The suspension has a pH of approximately 6.0 and a mean particle size of about 40 μm. Since 1 g of BAB dissolves in about 7 liters of water, very little of the BAB in the *suspension* is present in aqueous *solution* and thus the majority of BAB is present in a solid form which acts as a depot for very slow dissolution. In this respect the BAB suspension is like "slow-release" morphine preparations, where it is not the drug *per se* that is long-acting but the slow and *continuous* release of the drug. This explains the extraordinarily long duration (weeks to months) of pain relief associated with epidural butamben *suspension* administration in patients with cancer pain[84,133];

in contrast, BAB administered as a *solution* epidurally in rats had a shorter duration of action than a solution of bupivacaine.[67]

Another valuable attribute of BAB suspension administered epidurally is an apparent *selectivity* for A-delta and C fibers, with clear evidence in cancer patients of a lack of motor blockade and a sparing of bladder and bowel function, suggesting sparing of larger sensory fibers.[84,133] This selectivity is not seen after BAB *solution* administration epidurally in rats, again suggesting that it is the physicochemical properties of the suspension that result in apparent selectivity of BAB.[67] Postmortem studies in dogs[85] and humans[84] reveal semisolid BAB suspension material distributed only in the posterior epidural space close to the dorsal roots in a metameric pattern, in keeping with cryomicrotome studies of epidural space (see Chapter 8). It has been proposed that the short length of spinal nerve root in epidural space may permit neural blockade of a sufficient number of nodes of Ranvier (three) of A-delta and C fibers but *not* of larger motor and sensory fibers.[84] The poor dural penetration and rapid hydrolysis in CSF of BAB also may result in CSF concentrations too low to produce significant motor or sensory block due to BAB in CSF.

BAB solution is also unusual in its mode of action compared to other currently used local anesthetics (see Chapter 2), suggesting that some contribution to its unusual effects is possibly due to the inherent properties of BAB. *In vitro* studies reported that BAB selectively affects inactivation of fast sodium currents in cultured rat sensory neurons, thus producing a substantial reduction in membrane excitability due to a "hyperpolarization" type of block.[146] This is similar to that produced by another ester local anesthetic, benzocaine, and to the typical fast sodium channel blocker tetrodotoxin (TTX).[146] It is interesting that TTX was investigated as a local anesthetic and discarded. Also TTX has minimal effect on axonal transport, compared to substantial effects with amino amides such as lidocaine. Preservation of axonal transport is important when local anesthetics are used for long-duration blockade, since it may be associated with lower neurotoxicity.

The suspension formulation is not effective in achieving long-duration, selective local anesthesia without neurotoxicity when conventional local anesthetics are used. A lidocaine suspension, similar to that of BAB, produced only short-duration nonselective epidural blockade, which was associated with more significant neuropathological changes than those observed with BAB suspension.[66] Thus the physicochemical properties of the local anesthetic, that is, low pKa, lower water solubility, and a high octanol:water distribution coefficient, appear to be as important as the suspension formulation in achieving long-duration, selective neural blockade.

Thus, the promising pharmacodynamic properties of BAB in animals and in a small number of cancer patients clearly warrant further study of the efficacy and safety of BAB suspension.

DRUGS USED WITH LOCAL ANESTHETICS

Vasoconstrictors

Epinephrine is, of course, the active agent of the adrenal medulla. It is a powerful vasoconstrictor and has effects on both α- and β-adrenergic receptors.

On exposure to air or light, epinephrine may rapidly lose potency as a result of degradation. For this reason, stabilizing agents, such as sodium metabisulfite, are used. They slow the breakdown of the drug to as little as 2% per year. These agents also allow epinephrine-containing solutions to be autoclaved once without appreciable loss of activity. Epinephrine-containing solutions cannot, however, be reautoclaved. Epinephrine-containing solutions have a lower pH (3-4.5) than untreated solutions because of the added antioxidant.

When epinephrine is used with local anesthetic solutions, it must be in a concentration and dose to produce the desired vasoconstriction without leading to epinephrine overdose. Although the optimal concentration has been controversial, most authorities now agree on 1:200,000. More dilute solutions are of doubtful value; increasing the concentration does not achieve a correspondingly more effective vasoconstriction and increases the likelihood of toxicity. Even with 1:200,000, a total dose of 200 μg should not be exceeded.

The principal side effects of epinephrine are hypertension, bradycardia or tachycardia, and cardiac arrhythmias. Such reactions are likely to occur if the local anesthetic solution is accidentally injected intravenously. Animal experiments have shown that epinephrine increases the toxicity of local anesthetics when given directly into the circulation. The favorable cardiovascular effects of slowly absorbed 1:200,000 epinephrine are similar to those observed during recently developed "low-dose" constant infusion of epinephrine in intensive therapy; this differs markedly from the adverse effects of a relatively large bolus dose rapidly injected directly into the circulation. It is wise to avoid the use of epinephrine in patients sensitive to catecholamines (e.g., patients with hypertension, thyrotoxicosis).

Epinephrine also has local side effects, the most important being vasoconstriction of terminal arteries, leading to gangrene, for example, in the digits if the drug is used in a local anesthetic for ring blocks.

Phenylephrine (Neosynephrine) is a sympathomimetic drug with predominately alpha-receptor activity. It has been extensively used in spinal anesthesia.

Felypressin (Octapressin) is a synthetic drug similar to the naturally occurring vasopressin but without the antidiuretic and coronary vasoconstrictor effects of vasopressin. It has been shown to increase the intensity and duration of dental nerve blocks, and it is used in local anesthesia for this purpose in a concentration of 0.03 U/ml. It is a useful alternative in patients who are sensitive to catecholamines.

Ornipressin (POR-8) is another octapeptide related to vasopressin. It is supplied in ampules of 5 IU in 1 ml. A dose of 5 IU in 50 ml of 2% lidocaine has been used for plastic surgery. It is claimed to have a direct effect on the peripheral vasculature with minimal or no direct cardiac effects. Animal studies have revealed teratogenicity in high, subcutaneous doses considerably in excess of the maximum clinical level.

Levonordefrin (NeoCobefrin) is an alpha-receptor stimulator used with mepivacaine in dental blocks in a 1:20,000 concentration.

Antioxidants

Most of the commonly used local anesthetics, especially of the amide type, are extremely stable compounds and will remain unchanged in solution indefinitely. Thus solutions do not require additives if they are stored in ampules. If epinephrine is included in the preparation, however, antioxidants must be added to prevent breakdown of the vasoconstrictor.

The agent used for this purpose is sodium metabisulfite in a concentration of 0.1%. Epinephrine-containing solutions will retain their potency for 2 years with this agent and will withstand single autoclaving.

Studies discussed above indicate that bisulfite in the presence of low pH (below 3) may cause neurotoxicity. Thus spinal and epidural local anesthetic solutions should contain only low concentrations of bisulfite (0.1%) and pH should be buffered to be above 4.5 (see above).

Antimicrobials

Except for minor infiltration, local anesthetic solutions should not contain antimicrobials. Thus the ideal presentation is in a single-use, rubber-capped vial or ampule. Vials are preferred because their caps are easily removed, whereas glass fragments may contaminate solutions when ampules are opened.

In multiple-dose vials, methylparaben (1%) is often the antimicrobial included in the solution. Methylparaben is effective against gram-positive organisms and fungi but less so against gram-negative bacteria. It may be responsible for some of the allergic reactions attributed to local anesthetics—in theory, it should be considerably more antigenic than the local anesthetics. Chlorocresol has been used as an antibacterial agent and is more effective than methylparaben, but, like phenol, it is neurotoxic and should not be used in spinal, IV, or plexus blocks or extradural injections.

SUMMARY

The clinical pharmacologic properties of local anesthetic agents affect both the anesthetic profile and potential toxicity of the various drugs in current clinical use. The most important anesthetic properties are potency, onset, duration of action, and relative blockade of sensory and motor fibers. These qualities are related to the physicochemical properties of the various compounds. The toxicity of local anesthetics involves the central nervous system and the cardiovascular system. The toxicity of the different drugs is generally correlated with their inherent anesthetic potency but can be modified by the pharmacokinetic and metabolic properties of the specific agents. In general, the local anesthetics for infiltration, peripheral nerve blockade, and epidural anesthesia can be divided into three groups: (i) agents of short duration, that is, procaine and chloroprocaine; (ii) agents of moderate duration, that is, lidocaine, mepivacaine, and prilocaine; and (iii) agents of long duration, that is, tetracaine, bupivacaine, ropivacaine, and etidocaine. These local anesthetics also vary in terms of onset: Chloroprocaine, lidocaine, mepivacaine, prilocaine, and etidocaine have a rapid onset, whereas procaine, tetracaine, ropivacaine, and bupivacaine are characterized by a longer latency period.

The agents specifically formulated for intrathecal use include lidocaine, mepivacaine, and procaine, which have a short duration of action, and tetracaine, dibucaine, and bupivacaine, which provide a prolonged duration of spinal anesthesia.

Agents used in topical anesthetic preparations include lidocaine, EMLA, and tetracaine. Cocaine solutions are also used for topical anesthesia of the nasal mucosa.

With regard to the relative systemic toxicity of the various agents, chloroprocaine is the least toxic of the amino esters, whereas tetracaine is most toxic. Among the amino amides, prilocaine is least toxic, followed in order of increasing toxicity by mepivacaine, lidocaine, etidocaine, ropivacaine, and bupivacaine.

An appreciation of the pharmacologic and toxicologic profile of the various local anesthetics should make it possible to match a specific agent to a particular clinical situation.

REFERENCES

1. Ackerman, W.E.: Correspondence: Back pain after epidural Nesacaine MPF. Anesth. Analg., *70:*224, 1990.
2. Albert, J., and Lofstrom, B.: Bilateral ulnar nerve blocks for the evaluation of local anaesthetic agents. Acta Anaesthesiol. Scand., *9:*203, 1965.
3. Albright, G.A.: Cardiac arrest following regional anesthesia with etidocaine or bupivacaine. Anesthesiology, *51:*285, 1979.
4. Aldrete, J.A., Barnes, D.R., Sidon, M.A., and McMullen, R.B.: Studies on effects of addition of potassium chloride to lidocaine. Anesth. Analg., *48:*269, 1969.
5. Aldrete, J.A., and Johnson, D.A.: Evaluation of intracutaneous testing for investigation of allergy to local anesthetic agents. Anesth. Analg., *49:*173, 1970.
6. Arlock, P.: Actions of three local anaesthetics, lidocaine, bupivacaine, and ropivacaine on guinea pig papillary muscle sodium channels (V_{max}). Pharmacol. Toxicol., *63:*96, 1988.
7. Armstrong, I.R., Littlewood, D.G., and Chambers, W.A.: Spinal anesthesia with tetracaine—effect of added vasoconstrictor. Anesth. Analg., *62:*793, 1983.
8. Barsa, J.E., Batra, M., Fink, B.R., and Sumi, S.M.: Prolonged neural blockade following regional analgesia with 2-chloroprocaine. Anesth. Analg., *61:*961, 1982.
9. Benoit, P.W., and Belt, W.D.: Some effects of local anesthetic agents on skeletal muscle. Exp. Neurol., *34:*264, 1972.
10. Bjerring, P., and Arendt-Nielsen, L.: Depth and duration of skin analgesia to needle insertion after topical application of EMLA cream. Br. J. Anaesth., *64:*173, 1990.
11. Blair, M.R.: Cardiovascular pharmacology of local anaesthetics. Br. J. Anaesth., *47:*247, 1975.
12. Block, A., and Covino, B.G.: Effect of local anesthetic agents on cardiac conduction and contractility. Reg. Anaesth., *6:*55, 1982.

13. Braid, D.P., and Scott, D.B.: The systemic absorption of local analgesic drugs. Br. J. Anaesth., *37:*394, 1965.
14. Bridenbaugh, L.D.: Does the addition of low molecular weight dextran prolong the duration of action of bupivacaine? Reg. Anaesth., *3:*6, 1978.
15. Bridenbaugh, P.O.: Intercostal nerve blockade for the evaluation of local anaesthetic agents. Br. J. Anaesth., *47:*306, 1975.
16. Brinklov, M.: Clinical effects of Carticaine, a new local anaesthetic. Acta Anaesth. Scand., *21:*5, 1977.
17. Brockway, M.S., Bannister, J., McClure, J.H., McKeown, D., and Wildsmith, J.A.W.: Comparison of extradural ropivacaine and bupivacaine. Br. J. Anaesth., *66:*31, 1991.
18. Bromage, P.R.: A comparison of the hydrochloride and carbon dioxide salts of lidocaine and prilocaine in epidural analgesia. Acta Anaesthesiol. Scand. Suppl., *16:*55, 1965.
19. Bromage, P.R.: A comparison of the hydrochloride salts of lignocaine and prilocaine for epidural analgesia. Br. J. Anaesth., *37:*753, 1965.
20. Bromage, P.R.: An evaluation of two new local anesthetics for major conduction blockade. Can. Anaesth. Soc. J., *17:*557, 1970.
21. Bromage, P.R.: Mechanism of action of extradural analgesia. Br. J. Anaesth., *47:*199, 1975.
22. Bromage, P.R., and Burfort, M.D.: Quality of epidural blockade. II. Influence of physico-chemical factors: Hyaluronidase and potassium. Br. J. Anaesth., *38:*857, 1966.
23. Brown, D.L., Carpenter, R.L., and Thompson, G.E.: Comparison of 0.5% ropivacaine and 0.5% bupivacaine for epidural anesthesia in patients undergoing lower-extremity surgery. Anesthesiology, *72:*633, 1990.
24. Brown, D.T., Beamish, D., Wildsmith, J.A.W.: Allergic reaction to an amide local anaesthetic. Br. J. Anaesth., *53:*435, 1981.
25. Brown, D.T., Morrison, D.H., Covino, B.G., and Scott, D.B.: Comparison of carbonated bupivacaine and bupivacaine hydrochloride for extradural anaesthesia. Br. J. Anaesth., *52:*419, 1980.
26. Buckley, F.P., Littlewood, D.G., Covino, B.G., and Scott, D.B.: Effects of adrenaline and the concentration of solution on extradural block with etidocaine. Br. J. Anaesth., *50:*171, 1978.
27. Buckley, M.M., and Benfield, P.: Eutectic lidocaine/prilocaine cream: A review of the topical anesthetic/analgesic efficacy of a eutectic mixture of local anesthetics (EMLA). Drugs, *46*(1):126, 1993.
28. Burney, R.G., DiFazio, C.A., and Foster, J.A.: Effects of pH on protein binding of lidocaine. Anesth. Analg., *57:*478, 1978.
29. Catchlove, R.F.H.: The influence of CO_2 and pH on local anesthetic action. J. Pharmacol. Exp. Ther., *181:*291, 1972.
30. Cederholme, I., Evers, H., and Lofstrom, J.B.: Skin blood flow after intradermal injection of ropivacaine in various concentrations with and without epinephrine evaluated by laser doppler flowmetry. Reg. Anesth., *17:*322, 1992.
31. Chambers, W.A., Littlewood, D.G., Logan, M.R., and Scott, D.B.: Effect of added epinephrine on spinal anesthesia with lidocaine. Anesth. Analg., *60:*417, 1981.
32. Chambers, W.A., Littlewood, D.G., and Scott, D.B.: Spinal anesthesia with hyperbaric bupivacaine: Effect of added vasoconstrictors. Anesth. Analg., *61:*49, 1982.
33. Chang, P.C., Goresky, G.V., O'Connor, G., *et al.*: A multicentre randomised study of single-unit dose package of EMLA patch vs EMLA 5% cream for venipuncture in children. Can. J. Anaesth., *41:*59, 1994.
34. Clarkson, C.W., and Hondegheim, L.: Mechanisms for bupivacaine depression of cardiac conduction: Fast block of sodium channels during the action potential, with slow recovery from block during diastole. Anesthesiology, *62:*396, 1985.
35. Cohen, S.E., and Thurlow, A.: Comparison of a chloroprocaine-bupivacaine mixture with chloroprocaine and bupivacaine used individually for obstetric epidural analgesia. Anesthesiology, *51:*288, 1979.
36. Concepcion, M., Arthur, G.R., Steele, S.M., Bader, A.M., and Covino, B.G.: A new local anesthetic, ropivacaine—its epidural effects in humans. Anesth. Analg. *70:*80, 1990.
37. Concepcion, M., Maddi, R., Francis, D., *et al.*: Vasoconstrictors in spinal anesthesia with tetracaine. A comparison of epinephrine and phenylephrine. Anesth. Analg., *63:*134, 1984.
38. Corke, B.G., Carlson, C.G., and Dettbam, W.D.: The influence of 2-chloroprocaine on the subsequent analgesic potency of bupivacaine. Anesthesiology, *60:*25, 1984.
39. Covino, B.G., and Bush, D.F.: Clinical evaluation of local anesthetic agents. Br. J. Anaesth., *47:*289, 1975.
40. Covino, B.G., and Vassallo, H.G.: Local Anesthetics. Mechanisms of Action and Clinical Use: New York, Grune & Stratton, 1976.
41. Crawford, O.B.: Comparative evaluation in peridural anesthesia of lidocaine, mepivacaine, and L-67, a new local anesthetic agent. Anesthesiology, *25:*321, 1964.
42. Cunningham, N.L., and Kaplan, J.A.: A rapid onset long acting regional anesthetic technique. Anesthesiology, *41:*509, 1974.
43. Dahl, J.B., Simonsen, L., Morgensen, T., Henriksen, J.H., and Kehlet, H.: The effect of 0.5% ropivacaine on epidural blood flow. Acta Anaesth. Scand., *34:*308, 1990.
44. DeJong, R.H., Robles, R., and Corbin, R.W.: Central actions of lidocaine—Synaptic transmission. Anesthesiology, *30:*19, 1969.
45. DeJong, R.H., Ronfeld, R.A., and DeRosa, R.A.: Cardiovascular effects of convulsant and supraconvulsant doses of amide local anesthetics. Anesth. Analg., *61:*3, 1982.
46. Dhuner, K.G., and Lewis, D.: Effect of local anaesthetics and vasoconstrictors upon regional blood flow. Acta Anaesthesiol. Scand., *23:*347, 1966.
47. Eckstein, K.L., Vincente-Eckstein, A., Steiner, R., and Missler, V.: Klinische erprobung von bupivacaine CO_2. Anaesthesist, *27:*1, 1978.
48. Edde, R.R., and Deutsch, S.: Cardiac arrest after interscalene brachial plexus block. Anesth. Analg., *55:*446, 1977.
49. Eicholzer, A.W., and Feldman, H.S.: Acute toxicity of etidocaine following various routes of administration in the dog. Toxicol. Appl. Pharmacol., *37:*13, 1976.
50. Englesson, S.: The influence of acid-base changes on central nervous system toxicity of local anesthetic agents. I. An experimental study in cats. Acta Anaesthesiol. Scand., *18:*79, 1974.
51. Englesson, S., and Grevsten, S.: The influence of acid-base changes on central nervous system toxicity of local anaesthetic agents: II. Acta Anaesthesiol. Scand., *18:*88, 1974.
52. Erdimir, H.A., Soper, L.E., and Sweet, R.B.: Studies of factors affecting peridural anesthesia. Anesth. Analg., *44:*400, 1965.
53. Eriksson, E., Engelsson, S., Wahlquist, S., and Ortengren, B.: Study of the intravenous toxicity in man and some *in vitro* studies on the distribution and absorbability. Acta Chir. Scand., *358*(Suppl.):25, 1966.
54. Feldman, H.S., Arthur, G.R., and Covino, B.G.: Comparative systemic toxicity of convulsant and supraconvulsant doses of intravenous ropivacaine, bupivacaine and lidocaine in the conscious dog. Anesth. Analg., *69:*794, 1989.
55. Feldman, H.S., Covino, B.M., and Sage, D.J.: Direct chronotropic and inotropic effects of local anesthetic agents in isolated guinea pig atria. Reg. Anaesth., *7:*149, 1982.
56. Fisher, M.Mc.D., and Graham, R.: Adverse responses to local anaesthetics. Anaesth. Intensive Care, *12:*325, 1984.
57. Foldes, F.F., Davidson, G.M., Duncalf, D., and Kuwabara, J.: The intravenous toxicity of local anesthetic agents in man. Clin. Pharmacol. Ther., *6:*328, 1965.
58. Freeman, J.A., Doyle, E., Ng, T. I., and Morton, N.S.: Topical anaesthesia of the skin: A review. Paediatr. Anaesth., *3:*129, 1993.
59. Galindo, A., Schou, M., and Witcher, T.: pH adjusted local anesthetics. Proceedings of the American Society of Regional Anesthesia., pp. 50, 1981.
60. Galindo, A., and Witcher, T.: Mixtures of local anesthetics: Bupivacaine-chloroprocaine. Anesth. Analg., *59:*683, 1980.
61. Gettes, L.S.: Physiology and pharmacology of antiarrhythmic drugs. Hosp. Pract., *16:*89, 1981.
62. Gissen, A.J., Covino, B.G., and Gregus, J.: Differential sensitivity of fast and slow fibers in mammalian nerve. IV. Effect of carbonation of local anesthetics. Reg. Anaesth., *10:*68, 1985.
63. Gissen, A.J., Datta, S., and Lambert, D.: The chloroprocaine controversy II. Is chloroprocaine neurotoxic? Reg. Anaesth., *9:*135, 1984.
64. Grambling, Z.W., Ellis, R.G., and Valpitto, P.P.: Clinical experiences with mepivacaine (Carbocaine). J. Med. Assoc. Georgia, *53:*16, 1964.
65. Grouls, R., Ackerman, E., Machielsen, E., and Korsten, H.: Butyl-p-aminobenzoate. Preparation, characterisation and quality control of a suspension injection for epidural administration. Pharm. Wkbl, Sci. Ed., *12:*13, 1991.
66. Grouls, R.J.E., Hellebrekers, L.J., Noort R. van, *et al.*: Pharmacokinetics and effects of a lidocaine-base suspension in dogs following epidural administration. Anesthesiology, (In press).
67. Grouls, R.J.E., Meert, T.F., Korsten, H.H.M., Hellebrekers, L.J., and Breimer, D.D.: Epidural and intrathecal n-butyl-p-aminobenzoate solution in the rat: Comparison with bupivacaine. Anesthesiology, *86:*181, 1997.
68. Haas, D., Harper, D., Saso, M., and Young, E.: Comparison of articaine and prilocaine anesthesia by infiltration in maxillary and mandibular arches. Anesth. Prog., *37:*230, 1990.

69. Halpern, S.H., Eisler, E.A., Shnider, S.M., *et al.*: Myocardial tissue uptake of bupivacaine and lidocaine after intravenous injection in normal and acidotic rabbits. Anesthesiology, *61:*A208, 1984.
70. Harrison, D.C., and Alderman, E.L.: Relation of blood levels to clinical effectiveness of lidocaine. *In* Scott, D.B., and Julian, D.C. (eds.): Lidocaine in the Treatment of Ventricular Arrhythmias. pp. 178–188. Edinburgh, E & S Livingston, 1971.
71. Harrison, D.C., Sprouse, J.H., and Morrow, A.G.: The antiarrhythmic properties of lidocaine and procaine amide; clinical and physiologic studies of their cardiovascular effects in man. Circulation, *28:*486, 1963.
72. Hickey, R., Hoffman, J., and Ramamurthy, S.: A comparison of ropivacaine 0.5% and bupivacaine 0.5% for brachial plexus block. Anesthesiology, *74:*639, 1991.
73. Hickey, R., Rowley, C.L., Candido, K.D., Hoffman, J., Ramamurthy, S., and Winnie, A.P.: A comparative study of 0.25% ropivacaine and 0.25% bupivacaine for brachial plexus block. Anesth. Analg. *75:*602, 1992.
74. Hilgier, M.: Alkalinization of bupivacaine for brachial plexus block. Reg. Anaesth., *10:*59, 1985.
75. Hjelm, M., and Holmdahl, M.H.: Biochemical effects of aromatic amines II. Cyanosis, methemoglobinemia and Heinz-body formation induced by a local anaesthetic agent (prilocaine). Acta Anaesthesiol. Scand., *2:*99, 1965.
76. Huffman, R.D., and Yim, G.K.W.: Effects of diphenylaminoethanol and lidocaine on central inhibition. Int. J. Neuropharmacol., *8:*217, 1969.
77. Hynson, J.M., Sessler, D.I., and Glosten, B.: Back pain in volunteers after epidural anesthesia with chloroprocaine. Anesth. Analg., *72:*253, 1991.
78. Johns, R.A., DiFazio, C.A., and Longnecker, D.E.: Lidocaine constricts or dilates rat arterioles in a dose dependent manner. Anesthesiology, *61:*A204, 1984.
79. Jorfeldt, L., Lofstrom, B., Pernow, B., and Wahren, J.: The effect of mepivacaine and lidocaine on forearm resistance and capacitance vessels in man. Acta Anaesthesiol. Scand., *14:*183, 1970.
80. Josephson, I., and Sperelakis, N.: Local anesthetic blockade of Ca^{2+}-mediated action potentials in cardiac muscle. Eur. J. Pharmacol., *40:*201, 1976.
81. Kasten, G.W., and Martin, S.T.: Successful resuscitation after massive intravenous bupivacaine overdose in the hypoxic dog. Anesthesiology, *61:*A206, 1984.
82. Katz, J.A., Knarr, D., and Bridenbaugh, P.O.: A double-blind comparison of 0.5% bupivacaine and 0.75% ropivacaine administered epidurally in humans. Reg. Anesth., *15:*250, 1990.
83. Keir, L.: Continuous epidural analgesia in prostatectomy: comparison of bupivacaine with and without adrenaline. Acta Anaesthesiol. Scand., *18:*1, 1974.
84. Korsten, H.H.M., Ackerman, E.W., Grouls, R.J.E., *et al.*: Long-lasting epidural sensory blockade by n-butyl-p-aminobenzoate in the terminally ill intractable cancer pain patient. Anesthesiology, *75:*950, 1991.
85. Korsten, H.H.M., Hellebrekers, L.J., Grouls, R.J.E., *et al.*: Long-lasting sensory blockade by n-butyl-p-aminobenzoate in the dog. Neurotoxic or local anaesthetic effect? Anesthesiology, *73:*491, 1990.
86. Kotelko, D.M., Shnider, S.M., Dailey, P.A., *et al.*: Bupivacaine-induced cardiac arrhythmias in sheep. Anesthesiology, *60:*10, 1984.
87. Kuperman, A.S., Altura, B.T., and Chezar, J.A.: Action of procaine on calcium efflux from frog nerve and muscle. Nature, *217:*673, 1968.
88. Lee, A., Fagan, D., Lamont, M., Tucker, G.T., Halldin, M., and Scott, D.B.: Disposition kinetics of ropivacaine in humans. Anesth. Analg., *69:*736, 1989.
89. Levy, L., Randel, G.I., and Pandit, S.K.: Correspondence: Does chloroprocaine (Nesacaine MPF) for epidural anesthesia increase the incidence of backache? Anesthesiology, *71:*476, 1989.
90. Libelius, R., Sonesson, B., Stamenovic, B.A., and Thesleff, S.: Denervation-like changes in skeletal muscle after treatment with a local anesthetic (Marcaine). J. Anat., *106:*297, 1970.
91. Lieberman, N.A., Harris, R.S., Katz, R.I., *et al.*: The effects of lidocaine on the electrical and mechanical activity of the heart. Am. J. Cardiol., *22:*375, 1968.
92. Littlewood, D.G., Buckley, P., Covino, B.G., *et al.*: Comparative study of various local anesthetic solutions in extradural block in labour. Br. J. Anaesth., *51:*47, 1979.
93. Liu, P.L., Feldman, H.S., Covino, B.M., *et al.*: Acute cardiovascular toxicity of procaine, chloroprocaine and tetracaine in anesthetized ventilated dogs. Reg. Anaesth., *7:*14, 1982.
94. Liu, P.L., Feldman, H.S., Covino, B.M., *et al.*: Acute cardiovascular toxicity of intravenous amide local anesthetics in anesthetized ventilated dogs. Anesth. Analg., *61:*317, 1982.
95. Liu, P.L., Feldman, H.S., Giasi, R., *et al.*: Comparative CNS toxicity of lidocaine, etidocaine, bupivacaine and tetracaine in awake dogs following rapid IV administration. Anesth. Analg., *62:*375, 1983.
96. Loder, R.E.: A local anesthetic solution with longer action. Lancet, *2:*346, 1960.
97. Lofstrom, J.B.: Ulnar nerve blockade for the evaluation of local anaesthetic agents. Br. J. Anaesth., *47:*297, 1975.
98. Lund, P.C., and Cwik, J.C.: Propitocaine (Citanest) and methemoglobinemia. Anesthesiology, *26:*569–571, 1965.
99. McClure, J.H.: Ropivacaine [Review]. Br. J. Anaesth., *76:*300, 1996.
100. McClure, J.H., and Scott, D.B.: Comparison of bupivicaine hydrochloride and carbonated bupivacaine in brachial plexus block by the inter-scalene technique. Br. J. Anaesth., *53:*523, 1981.
101. Meagher, R.P., Moore, D.C., and DeVries, J.C.: The most effective potentiator of tetracaine spinal anesthesia. Anesth. Analg., *45:*134, 1966.
102. Moore, D.C., Crawford, R.D., and Scurlock, J.E.: Severe hypoxia and acidosis following local anesthetic-induced convulsions. Anesthesiology, *53:*259, 1980.
103. Moore, D.C., Spierdijk, J., VanKleef, J.D., *et al.*: Chloroprocaine neurotoxicity: Four additional cases. Anesth. Analg., *61:*155, 1982.
104. Morishima, H.O., Pederson, H., Finster, M., *et al.*: Bupivacaine toxicity in pregnant and nonpregnant ewes. Anesthesiology, *63:*134, 1985.
105. Morishima, H.O., Peterson, H., Finster, M., *et al.*: Is bupivacaine more cardiotoxic than lidocaine? Anesthesiology, *59:*A409, 1983.
106. Morishima, H.O., Pedersen, H., Finster, M., *et al.*: Etidocaine toxicity in the adult, newborn and fetal sheep. Anesthesiology, *58:*342, 1983.
107. Morrison, D.H.: A double-blind comparison of carbonated lidocaine and lidocaine hydrochloride in epidural anaesthesia. Can. Anaesth. Soc. J., *28:*387, 1981.
108. Munson, E.S., Tucker, W.K., Ausinsch, B., and Malagodi, H.: Etidocaine, bupivacaine, and lidocaine seizure thresholds in monkey. Anesthesiology, *42:*471, 1975.
109. Nancarrow, C. *et al.*: Myocardial and cerebral drug concentrations and mechanisms of death after fatal intravenous doses of lidocaine, bupivacaine and ropivacaine in the sheep. Anesth. Analg., *69:*276, 1989.
110. Nishimura, N., Morioka, T., Sato, S., and Kuba, T.: Effects of local anesthetic agents on the peripheral vascular system. Anesth. Analg., *44:*135, 1965.
111. Orkin, F.K., and Bogetz, M.S.: Back pain following uncomplicated epidural anaesthesia with chloroprocaine (Abstract). Anesthesiology, *71:*A716, 1989.
112. Pizzalato, D., and Reneger, O.J.: Histopathologic effects of long exposure to local anesthetics on peripheral nerves. Anesth. Analg., *38:*138, 1959.
113. Prentiss, J.E.: Cardiac arrest following caudal anesthesia. Anesthesiology, *50:*51, 1979.
114. Prescott, L.F., and Nimmo, J.: Plasma lidocaine concentrations during and after prolonged infusions in patients with myocardial infarction. *In* Scott, D.B., and Julian, D.C. (eds.): Lidocaine in the Treatment of Ventricular Arrhythmias. pp. 178–188. Edinburgh, E & S Livingston, 1971.
115. Ravindran, R.S., Bond, V.K., Tasch, M.D., *et al.*: Prolonged neural blockade following regional analgesia with 2-chloroprocaine. Anesth. Analg., *58:*447, 1980.
116. Ravindran, R.S., Turner, M.S., and Muller, T.: Neurological effects of subarachnoid administration of 2-chloroprocaine-CE, bupivacaine and low pH normal saline in dogs. Anesth. Analg., *61:*279, 1982.
117. Reisner, L.S., Hochman, B.N., and Plumer, M.H.: Persistent neuralgia deficit and adhesive arachnoiditis following intrathecal 2-chloroprocaine injection. Anesth. Analg., *58:*452, 1980.
118. Reynolds, F.: Allergy reaction to an amide local anaesthetic. Br. J. Anaesth., *53:*901, 1981.
119. Ritchie, J.M., Ritchie, B., and Greengard, P.: The active structure of local anesthetics. J. Pharmacol. Exp. Ther., *150:*152, 1965.
120. Rocco, A.G., Francis, D.M., Wark, J.A., *et al.*: A clinical double-blind study of dibucaine and tetracaine in spinal anesthesia. Anesth. Analg., *61:*133, 1982.
121. Rosen, M.A., Baysinger, C.L., Shnider, S.M., *et al.*: Evaluation of

neurotoxicity of local anesthetics following subarachnoid injection. Anesthesiology, *57:*A196, 1982.
122. Rosenblatt, R.M., and Fung, D.L.: Optional ratio of bupivacaine and dextran for regional anaesthesia. Reg. Anaesth., *4:*2, 1979.
123. Rosenblatt, R.M., and Fung, D.L.: Mechanism of action of dextran prolonging regional anesthesia. Reg. Anaesth., *5:*3, 1980.
124. Sage, D., Feldman, H., Arthur, G.R., and Covino, B.G.: Cardiovascular effects of lidocaine and bupivacaine in the awake dog. Anesthesiology, *59:*A210, 1983.
125. Sage, D.J., Feldman, H.S., Arthur, G.R., *et al.*: Influence of lidocaine and bupivacaine on isolated guinea pig atria in the presence of acidosis and hypoxia. Anesth. Analg., *63:*1, 1983.
126. Scott, D.B.: Evaluation of clinical tolerance of local anesthetic agents. Br. J. Anaesth., *47:*328, 1975.
127. Scott, D.B.: Evaluation of the toxicity of local anaesthetic agents in man. Br. J. Anaesth., *47:*56, 1975.
128. Scott, D.B.: Toxicity caused by local anaesthetic drugs. Br. J. Anaesth., *53:*553, 1981.
129. Scott, D.B.: Editorial: "Maximum recommended doses" of local anaesthetic drugs. Br. J. Anaesth., *63:*373, 1989.
130. Scott, D.B., Lee, A. Fagin, D. Bowler, G.M.R., Bloomfield, P., and Lund, H.R.: Acute toxicity of ropivacaine compared with that of bupivacaine. Anesth. Analg., *69:*563, 1989.
131. Scott, D.B., McClure, J.H., Giasi, R.M., *et al.*: Effects of concentration of local anaesthetic drugs in extradural block. Br. J. Anaesth., *52:*1033, 1980.
132. Seow, L.T., Lips, F.J., Cousins, M.J., and Mather, L.E.: Lidocaine and bupivacaine mixtures for epidural blockade. Anesthesiology, *56:*177, 1982.
133. Shulman, M.: Treatment of cancer pain with epidural butyl-aminobenzoate suspension. Reg. Anesth., *12:*1, 1987.
134. Sinclair, C.J., and Scott, D.B.: Comparison of bupivacaine and etidocaine in extradural blockade. Br. J. Anaesth., *56:*147, 1984.
135. Skou, J.C.: Local anesthetics. II. The toxic potencies of some local anesthetics and of butyl alcohol, determined on peripheral nerve. Acta Pharmacol. Toxicol., *10:*292, 1954.
136. Stevens, R.A., Chester, W.L., Artuso, J.D., Bray, J.G., and Mellestein, J.A.: Back pain after epidural anesthesia in volunteers: A preliminary report. Reg. Anesth., *16:*199, 1991.
137. Stevens, R.A., Urmey, W.F., Urquhart, B.L., and Kao, T.C.: Back pain after epidural anesthesia with chloroprocaine. Anesthesiology, *78:*492, 1993.
138. Steward, D.J.: Management of childhood pain: New approaches to procedure-related pain. Proceedings of a roundtable discussion held Jan. 9, 1993. J. Pediatr., 122(No. 5, Pt. 2):S2, 1993.
139. Stewart, D.M., Rogers, W.P., Mahaffrey, J.E., *et al.*: Effect of local anesthetics on the cardiovascular system in the dog. Anesthesiology, *24:*620, 1963.
140. Sugimoto, T., Schaal, S.F., Dunn, N.M., and Wallace, A.G.: Electrophysiological effects of lidocaine in awake dogs. J. Pharmacol. Exp. Ther., *166:*146, 1969.
141. Swerdlow, M., and Jones, R.: The duration of action of bupivacaine, prilocaine, and lignocaine. Br. J. Anaesth., *42:*335, 1970.
142. Tanaka, K., and Yamasaki, M.: Blocking of cortical inhibitory synapses by intravenous lidocaine. Nature, *209:*207, 1966.
143. Tanz, R.D., Heskett, T., Loehning, R.W., and Fairfax, C.A.: Comparative cardiotoxicity of bupivacaine and lidocaine in the isolated perfused mammalian heart. Anesth. Analg., *63:*549, 1984.
144. Thigpen, J.W., Kotelko, D.M., Shnider, S.M., *et al.*: Bupivacaine cardiotoxicity in hypoxic-acidotic sheep. Anesthesiology, *59:*A204, 1983.
145. Thomson, S.P.: Lidocaine pharmacokinetics in advanced heart failure, liver disease, and renal failure in humans. Ann. Intern. Med., *78:*499, 1973.
146. Van den Berg, R.J., van Soest, P.F., Wang, Z., Grouls, R.J. and Korsten, H.H.: The local anaesthetic n-butyl-p-aminobenzoate selectively affects inactivation of fast sodium currents in cultured rat sensory neurons. Anesthesiology, *82:*1463, 1995.
147. Vanhoutte, F., Vereecke, J., Verbeke, N., and Carmeliete.: Stereoselective effects of the enantiomers of bupivacaine on the electrophysiological properties of the guinea-pig papillary muscle. Br. J. Pharmacol., *103:*1275, 1991.
148. Wang, B.C., Hillman, D.E., Spiedholz, N.I., and Turndorf, H.: Chronic neurological deficits and Nesacaine-CE—an effect of the anesthetic, 2-chloroprocaine, or the antioxidant, sodium bisulfite? Anesth. Analg., *63:*445, 1984.
149. Winther, J., and Patirupanusara, B.: Evaluation of carticaine—A new local analgesic. Int. J. Oral Surg., *3:*422, 1974.
150. Wojtczak, J.A., Pratilas, V., Griffin, R.M., and Kaplan, J.A.: Cellular mechanisms of cardiac arrhythmias induced by bupivacaine. Anesthesiology, *61:*A37, 1984.

Neural Blockade in Clinical Anesthesia and Management of Pain, Third Edition,
edited by M.J. Cousins and P.O. Bridenbaugh.
Lippincott–Raven Publishers, Philadelphia © 1998.

CHAPTER 5

Modification of Responses to Surgery by Neural Blockade

Clinical Implications

Henrik Kehlet

Surgical trauma is an injury that may range from complications from minor elective procedures to a massive insult following major procedures complicated by sepsis. The body reacts to the noxious stimulus both locally and generally. The inflammatory reaction constitutes the local response and is considered to be important for healing and defense against infection. The general response is in the form of an endocrine metabolic activation leading to hypermetabolism with an acceleration of most biochemical reactions, including substrate mobilization. The general response is highly dependent on the severity of the injury and represents a stereotyped neurophysiologic reflex response. From a teleological viewpoint the stress response probably has evolved to provide a maximum chance of survival because of the resulting fluid preservation and supply of the increased demands for energy-generating substrates. If prolonged, however, the stress response may have a detrimental effect because of the resulting devastating nutritional consequences leading to depletion of several essential components of the body (For neural response to injury see Chapter 23.1).

During the past few decades there has been a tremendous increase of knowledge within anesthesia and surgery, allowing even major procedures to be performed in patients with severe complicating disease, previously contraindicating surgery. A key factor in the development of safe convalescence has been the development of surgical biology, because the proper treatment of surgical trauma requires knowledge of its biochemical effects. Thus a favorable postoperative outcome will most probably occur through a collaboration between anesthesiologists and surgeons taking advantage of the knowledge of precipitating factors of the stress response and applying modulatory therapeutic methods, thereby minimizing profound changes in fluid and electrolyte balances, nutritional metabolism, and host defense mechanisms.

This chapter updates the developments in the understanding of the release mechanisms involved in the stress response to surgical procedures and in the techniques that can modulate these responses. A review of the literature will be presented on the modulating effect of neural blockade on the stress response to surgical procedures, and the implications for anesthetic practice will be delineated based on a review of controlled studies on the effect of neural blockade on postoperative morbidity.

GENERAL STRESS RESPONSE TO SURGERY

The response to surgical trauma may be divided into two phases: The initial acute "ebb" or "shock" phase is characterized by a hypodynamic state, a reduction in metabolic rate, and depression of most physiologic processes. With surgical trauma this phase is either absent or very transient during the postoperative period. The second phase is the hyperdynamic "flow" phase, which may last for a few days or weeks depending on the magnitude of the surgical insult or occurrence of complications. Characteristically, metabolic rate and cardiac output are elevated. A summary of the endocrine and metabolic responses to surgical trauma is given in Table 5-1. There is a change in the endocrine milieu whereby plasma concentrations of the catabolic active hormones are elevated while those of the anabolic active hormones are lowered. Posttraumatic changes in the biological activity of thyroid hormone have not been clarified but are

H. Kehlet: Department of Surgical Gastroenterology, Hvidovre University Hospital, DK-2650 Hvidovre, Denmark.

TABLE 5-1. *Neuroendocrine and metabolic responses to surgery*

Endocrine	
Catabolic	
Due to increase in:	ACTH, cortisol, ADH, GH, catecholamines, renin, angiotensin-II, aldosterone, glucagon, IL-1, TNF, IL-6
Anabolic	
Due to decrease in:	Insulin, testosterone
Metabolic	
Carbohydrate	**Hyperglycemia, glucose intolerance, insulin resistance**
Due to increase in:	Hepatic glycogenolysis (epinephrine, glucagon), gluconeogenesis (cortisol, glucagon, GH, epinephrine, free fatty acids)
Due to decrease in:	Insulin secretion/action
Protein	**Muscle protein catabolism, increased synthesis of acute-phase proteins**
Due to increase in:	Cortisol, epinephrine, glucagon, IL-1, IL-6, TNF
Fat	**Increased lipolysis and oxidation**
Due to increase in:	catecholamines, cortisol, glucagon, GH
Water and Electrolyte Flux	**Retention of H_2O and Na^+, increased excretion of K^+, decreased functional extracellular fluid with shifts to intracellular compartments**
Due to increase in:	Catecholamines, aldosterone, ADH, cortisol, angiotensin-II, prostaglandins, and other factors

ACTH, adrenocorticotropic hormone; ADH, antidiuretic hormone; GH, growth hormone; IL, interleukin; TNF, tumor necrosis factor.

not reflected by changes in circulating levels of triiodothyronine (T_3) and thyroxine (T_4). The influence of surgery on insulin secretion is biphasic, with an impaired insulin response to glucose during the initial phase followed by an increased insulin response but with a concomitant increased peripheral insulin resistance (postreceptor defect). Hepatic glucose production is stepped up due to increased gluconeogenesis and initially increased glycogenolysis, and total body glucose utilization is elevated. Lipid turnover and oxidation are enhanced and protein turnover is increased, probably with a reduction in protein synthesis and a slight increase in breakdown during elective surgery. During major trauma, however, the increased protein breakdown exceeds synthesis. Synthesis of some specific proteins, that is, acute-phase proteins, is increased. Concomitantly, fluid and electrolyte balance shows a shift toward water and sodium retention, while urinary potassium excretion is increased. Vascular permeability to albumin is increased. Peripheral blood neutrophils increase whereas lymphocytes decrease, and most parameters of specific as well as nonspecific immunofunction show a deterioration. Coagulation is activated and fibrinolysis inhibited except for an initial transient activation.

Although the metabolic response to surgery is a net effect of responses to injury and (semi-) starvation, the changes in energy metabolism and substrate flow are predominantly determined by the injury response. The intensity of the stress response to surgery is directly related to the degree of tissue trauma,[226] that is, diagnostic procedures of short duration, procedures on the body surface, ear surgery, and superficial eye surgery evoke only a very slight, transient response, whereas procedures involving the thorax and abdominal cavity elicit a more pronounced response in which the flow phase may last up to several days or weeks if complications eventuate. Intracranial procedures lead to an intermediate, rather small, and short-lived response. A detailed description of the endocrine metabolic response to surgery and trauma has been given in recent reviews.[52,70,116,126,223,227]

RELEASE MECHANISMS OF THE STRESS RESPONSE

In contrast to our detailed knowledge of the changes in various hormonal and metabolic compartments of the stress response, information on the exact nature and relative role of the various signals that may initiate and potentiate the response is limited and not fully understood (Fig. 5-1).

Afferent Neural Stimuli

Much evidence has accumulated to demonstrate that the peripheral and central nervous systems represent a major common pathway mediating the stress response.[222] The nociceptive signals to the central nervous system are transmitted primarily by small myelinated (A-δ) and unmyelinated (C) sensory afferent fibers to the substantia gelatinosa in the dorsal horn, with further rostrad spread to the ventral-posterior nucleus of the thalamus.[225] Modulation of pain may occur at many levels, including midbrain, medulla, and spinal cord, by means of powerful descending inhibitory systems, as shown in Figure 5-2 (see also Chapters 23 and 24). The relative role of the various nociceptive stimuli (pressure, chemical, thermal) in arousing the stress response remains to be ascertained, as is the case for the peripheral substrates (transmitters) involved; however, local synthesis in the traumatized area of histamine, bradykinin, serotonin, kinins, prostaglandins, and substance P has been shown to facilitate the initiation of afferent neural stimuli. Afferent stimuli conducted through somatosensory and sympathetic pathways play a predominant role in precipitating the response to abdominal surgery compared to the vagal afferent pathway.

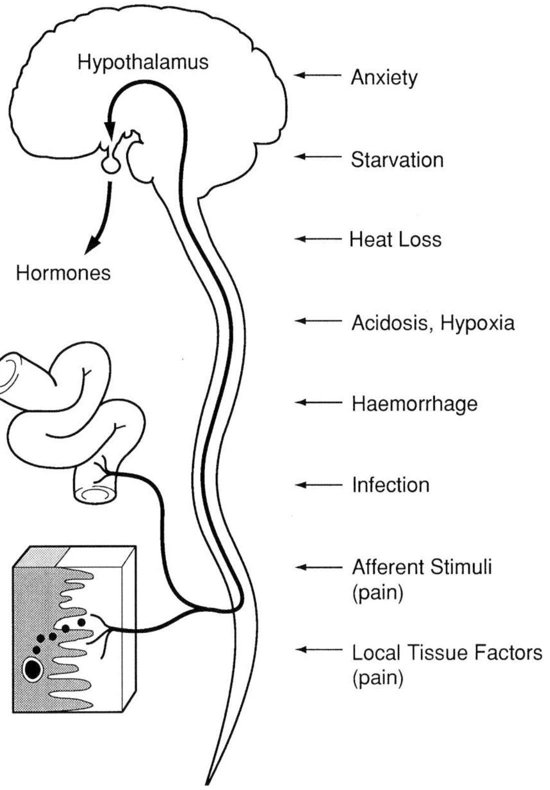

FIG. 5-1. Release mechanisms of the endocrine metabolic response to surgery. The principal mechanisms are afferent neural stimuli (*arrows on right*) due to noxious surgical/trauma stimuli and local tissue factors released at the trauma site; both of these categories of stimuli may be associated with pain. Interleukin-1 is released from circulating macrophages and forms part of the "inflammatory soup" that sensitizes nociceptors (see also Fig. 5-3). Secondary amplifiers of the response are psychological factors (e.g., anxiety), starvation, heat loss, acidosis, hypoxia, hemorrhage, and infection. Noxious stimuli from viscera (e.g., gut) travel via visceral nociceptive afferents (via sympathetic ganglia) and contribute to the trauma stimuli, and local tissue factors are also involved. Central responses to afferent stimuli involve hypothalamus and other central nervous system areas mediating the efferent humoral and neural components of the endocrine-metabolic response.

The role of the afferent parasympathetic pathways through the pelvic nerves has not been evaluated. The influence of efferent neural stimuli in raising the stress response is discussed below. The importance of afferent neural stimuli versus other stimuli (see Fig. 5-1) in mediating the trauma response has been evaluated in clinical studies using different techniques of neural blockade (see following). These studies have demonstrated that during relatively minor, clean surgery the neural pathway is the main release mechanism of most of the classic endocrine metabolic responses (see Table 5-1), but not of postoperative changes in various protein systems (acute-phase proteins), parameters of immunofunction (cytokines, cascade systems, etc.), and the coagulation and fibrinolytic systems. During major procedures, however, these other stimuli (see Fig. 5-1) may potentiate the response.

Local and Systemic Tissue Factors

The observation that severe injury to a denervated limb elicited an adrenocortical response during various experimental settings has emphasized that factors other than afferent neural stimuli may contribute to the response during a major insult. The nature of such substances, presumably released at the trauma site, has been studied extensively during recent years,[124,227] but a clear picture has not yet emerged. Important factors may involve the coagulation and fibrinolysis cascade systems, the plasma contact activation system, cytokines (predominantly tumor necrosis factor [TNF], interleukin-1 [IL-1], IL-6), adhesion molecules following neutrophil and macrophage activation, platelet activating factor, (PAF) and activation of the L-arginine–nitric oxide pathway.[39,14,228,229] Further, most nociceptive stimuli lead to a local release of histamine, serotonin, prostaglandins, leukotrienes, substance P, and other neurokinins,[225] but the exact role of these substrates in mediating the stress response, apart from facilitating the afferent neural stimuli, remains to be determined (Fig. 5-3). It is unlikely that one factor is responsible for most nociceptive and inflammatory changes and most probably it is a concerted action with several mediators involved.[124,230] A key question for further understanding of the release mechanisms of the injury response, in order to develop rational strategies for modification of injury-induced organ damage, is knowledge of the time course of release of the individual mediators. However, this has so far not been established. Some humoral mediators (histamine, oxygen radicals, etc.) and the neural mediated responses (hormones) represent fast, protein synthesis–independent responses that occur within minutes, while some protein synthesis–dependent mediators (adhesion molecules, cytokines, acute phase proteins, etc.) may take a longer time (hours).

In order to evaluate the relative role of neural factors (catabolic hormones) versus inflammatory mediators, the effects of combined hormonal infusions with epinephrine, norepinephrine, cortisol, and glucagon have been investigated. Such studies have demonstrated that the classical catabolic hormones may only be responsible for some of the metabolic responses observed after surgery.[11,71] Thus, hyperthermia, the acute-phase protein response, and the magnitude of the metabolic changes during major surgery could not be effected by hormonal infusion, while induction of "inflammation" with intramuscular administration of etiocholanolone resulted in fever, acute-phase protein synthesis, and hypoferremia, but not hypermetabolism or stress hormone release.[231] A combination of multihormonal infusion together with etiocholanolone, however, did reproduce a multicomponent stress response as seen in surgical procedures,[231] although the magnitude was lower. It is therefore likely that both inflammatory (tissue factors) and endocrine

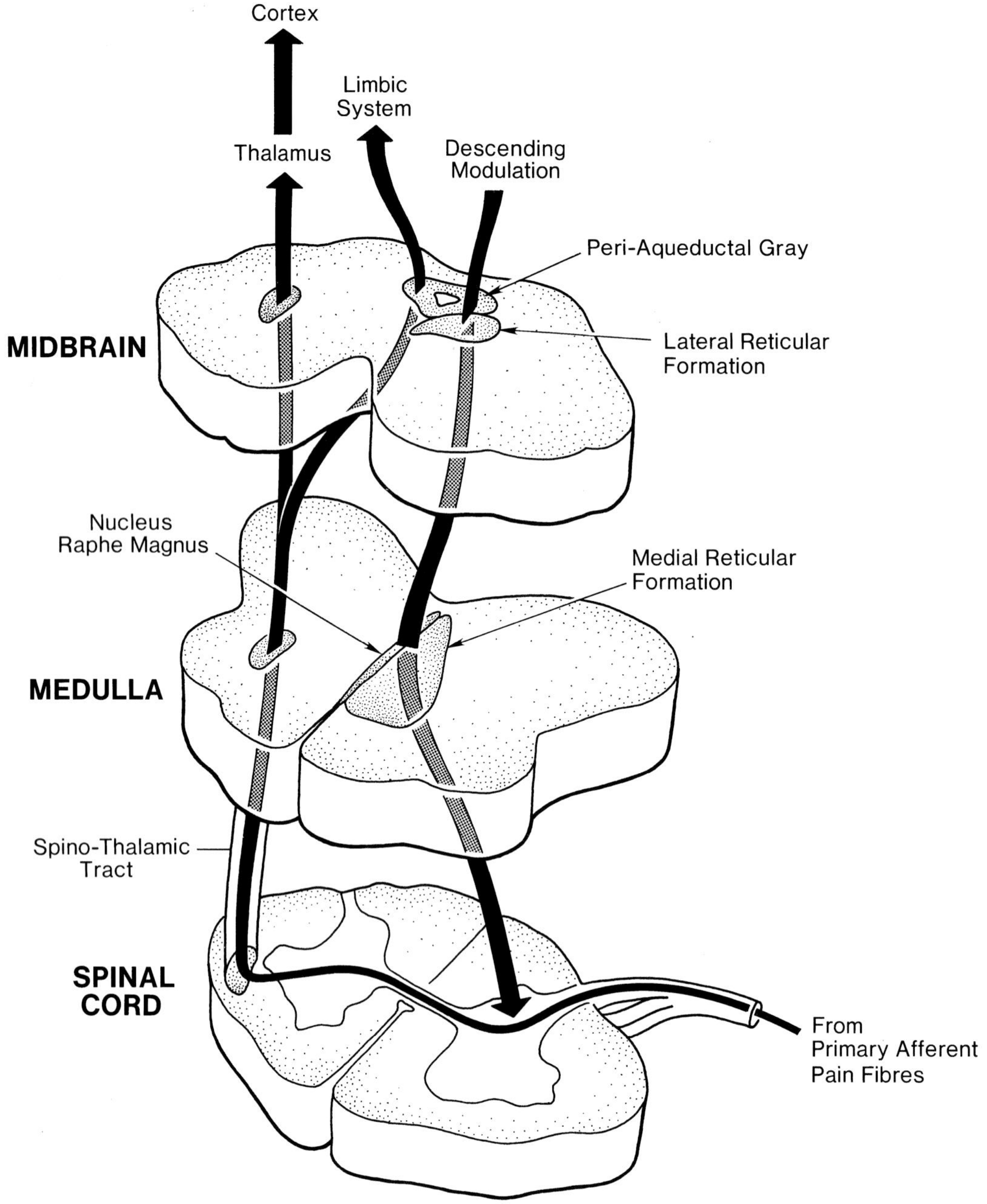

FIG. 5-2. Pain transmission and modulation. Primary afferent fibers are shown entering dorsal horn of spinal cord and crossing over to spinothalamic tract. Note descending modulation initiated in midbrain and medulla, impinging on primary afferent pathway in dorsal horn. Modulation also occurs more centrally (see Chapters 24 and 25), probably partly involving the limbic system. [Reproduced with permission from Phillips, G.D., and Cousins, M.J.: Neurological mechanisms of pain and the relationship of pain, anxiety, and sleep. *In* Cousins, M.J., and Phillips, G.D. (eds.): Acute Pain Management. London, Churchill Livingstone, 1986.]

mediators are necessary for the complete manifestation of host responses to surgical injury and critical illness.

Altered Set Point of Endocrine Metabolic Feedback Systems

In our effort to find a rational explanation for the necessity of the stress response, we hypothesized that trauma leads to a change in the set point of various endocrine and substrate feedback systems because of an extra need for substrate during the hypermetabolic state and in healing tissues. In several studies, however, the administration of hormones (cortisol), substrates (glucose, fat, various proteins), and fluids could not be demonstrated to prevent the trauma-induced increase in cortisol secretion, gluconeogenesis, various protein systems, antidiuretic hormone, or aldosterone.[111,113] These

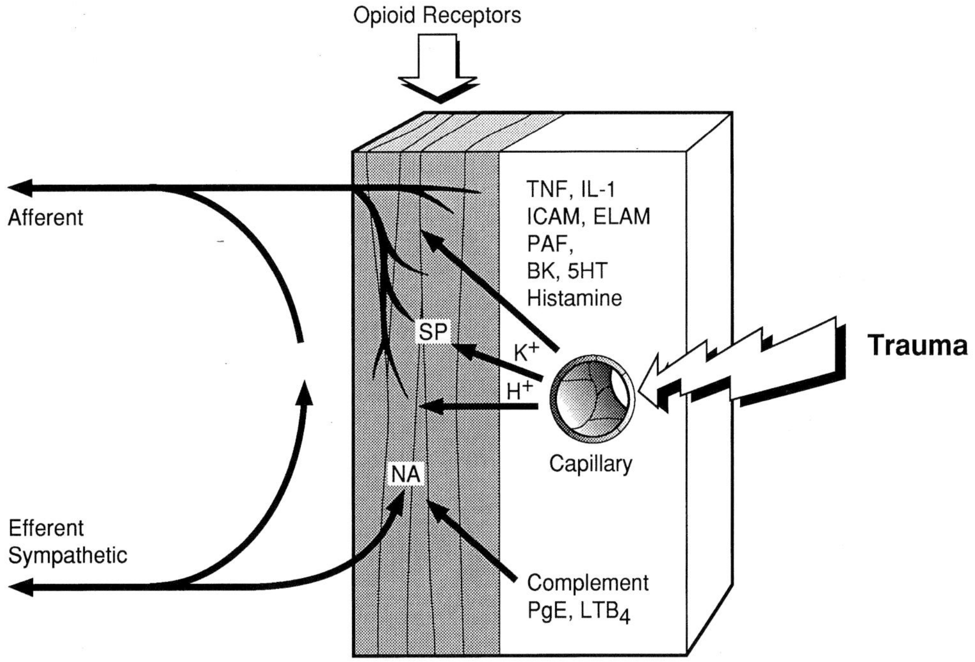

FIG. 5-3. Local tissue factors and peripheral pain receptors. The physical stimuli of "trauma," the chemical environment (e.g., H+), algesic substances (e.g., serotonin [5-HT], bradykinin [BK]), and microcirculatory changes may all modify peripheral receptor activity. Substance P released by the axon reflex is an important peripheral pain transmitter. Efferent sympathetic activity may increase the sensitivity of receptors by means of norepinephrine (NA) release. Histamine, complement, and arachidonic cascade metabolites (e.g., PGE_2, LTB_4) may all contribute to inflammation and increase the sensitivity of peripheral nociceptors, together with cytokines (e.g., TNF and IL-1), adhesion molecules (e.g., ICAM, ELAM), and PAF. Following injury there is an increased concentration of opioid receptors on the peripheral nerve terminals, where endogenous opioids may reduce sensitivity of nociceptive receptors. [Modified with permission from Phillips, G.D., and Cousins, M.J.: Neurological mechanisms of pain and the relationship of pain, anxiety, and sleep. *In* Cousins, M.J., and Phillips, G.D. (eds.): Acute Pain Management. London, Churchill Livingstone, 1986.]

findings may suggest that the classical catabolic endocrine stress response be considered as a reflex response[222] rather than as a response elicited because of a primarily increased need for hormones or substrates, or both. Similar data from humoral mediator administration are not available.

Other Factors

It is well documented that hemorrhage, even of small magnitude and not accompanied by hypotension, may activate atrial receptors and lead to an endocrine metabolic response. Similarly, acidosis and hypoxia may activate the response, and, if infection is superimposed on the surgical trauma, an exaggerated stress response will eventuate. All these factors, however, may not be considered as basic release mechanisms of the response but rather as amplifying factors.[111] Correspondingly, psychological factors *per se* may precipitate endocrine metabolic changes, but from a quantitative viewpoint these are negligible compared to the trauma-induced changes.

Heat loss, caused by the semi-nude condition of the patient and low ambient temperature of the operating room, may be an additional stimulus for increased metabolism in surgical patients. Heat loss is not, however, the causative factor of the stress response to surgery, but may act as an amplifying factor, since prevention of heat loss by various methods has not been demonstrated to prevent the responses.[111,113]

MODIFYING FACTORS OF THE STRESS RESPONSE

The stress response to surgery and other injuries has usually been considered to be a homeostatic defense mechanism important for healing of tissue and adaptation to the noxious insult of injury. It has also been believed to enhance resistance to stress. In modern anesthesia and surgery, however, the biochemical changes after injury need not be considered as a homeostatic response important for survival and restitution, since physiologic disturbances may be prevented or repeatedly treated and substrates, blood, and other fluids are readily available. Concern about detrimental effects of surgery such as increased demands on various organs, myocardial infarction, pulmonary complications, thromboembolism, pain and convalescence with fatigue, and inability to work—all of which may not be results of imperfections in surgical technique but rather sequelae to the stress responses—has therefore led to studies of an eventual modulation of the trauma response. Thus, with the availability of current therapy, the stress response may have become maladaptive, and instead the hypothesis has been proposed that the above-mentioned morbidity in high-risk surgical patients may be reduced by inhibiting the surgically induced endocrine response, hypermetabolism, and resulting increased demands on body mass and physiologic reserve.[111,113]

At present a variety of methods are available to modify the stress response to surgery (Fig. 5-4).[39,70,111,113,223,232]

General Anesthesia

Although the use of general anesthesia may limit the perception of the injury, a vast amount of data have indicated that this may not necessarily be followed by a concomitant interference with the processing of the noxious stimuli to the hypothalamus and thereby an altered stress response. Generally, almost all intravenous agents and volatile anesthetics in normal "low" doses have only a quantitatively minor influence on endocrine metabolic function *per se* and on endocrine metabolic changes induced by surgical trauma.[22,109,111,161] In circumstances in which a slight inhibitory or stimulatory effect of an anesthetic has been demonstrated intraoperatively, the endocrine metabolic changes in the recovery period and late convalescence were not different from the usual pattern.

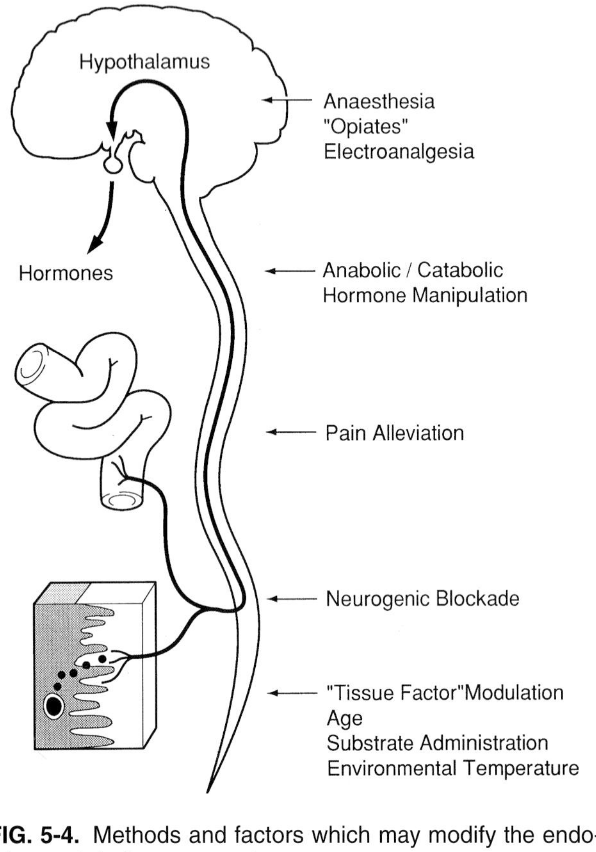

FIG. 5-4. Methods and factors which may modify the endocrine-metabolic response to surgery.

Exceptions to the general rule that general anesthetics are relatively inert as modifiers of the trauma response are ether and cyclopropane, both of which exert a stimulatory effect of the sympathetic nervous system and the adrenal cortex, and etomidate and high-dose opiate anesthesia, which have an inhibitory effect. Several studies have demonstrated that the hypnomimetic agent etomidate selectively inhibits the adrenocortical response to surgery through an inhibition of two enzymes in cortisol synthesis[68,213] but without influence on other responses. Much concern has arisen about the use of etomidate for anesthesia or intensive care[128] since uncontrolled observations have suggested an increased mortality among intensive care patients receiving long-term sedation with etomidate. Further data are needed, however, before implications can be settled for the use of etomidate in low doses as an adjuvant to anesthesia for surgical procedures. No severe side effects have been observed to the transient, selective inhibition of the cortisol response to surgical procedures by etomidate.

The use of high-dose opiate anesthesia has become popular especially during cardiovascular procedures, and it is well documented that this anesthetic principle may lead to a complete suppression of most endocrine and metabolic responses.[22,109,111] Most studies have been performed in patients undergoing open heart surgery, and the results have been rather uniform in demonstrating that morphine (2–4 mg/kg), fentanyl (50–200 μg/kg), and other synthetic opiates may either prevent or inhibit the initial endocrine metabolic response. This applies to the usual increase in plasma concentrations of cortisol, aldosterone, renin, vasopressin, growth hormone, epinephrine, and norepinephrine, glucose, and lactate. In most of these studies, however, the modifying effect disappeared during the cardiopulmonary bypass procedure, and no influence on flow-phase responses in the later postoperative period has been demonstrated. The effect of high-dose opioid anesthesia on postoperative endocrine metabolic function after abdominal procedures is probably not important although more data are needed before final conclusions can be made.[153,179,332] No differences have been demonstrated among the various synthetic opiates with regard to their inhibitory effect on the surgical stress response.

In summary, high-dose opiate anesthesia has only a transient inhibitory effect on the stress response as long as high concentrations are maintained in the blood and tissues, but prolonged postoperative metabolic effects do not eventuate. The use of this technique for a sustained reduction of the stress response is therefore limited because of the concomitant depression of the respiratory system. Further, fentanyl (50 μg/kg) could not reverse the established metabolic and cortisol response to pelvic surgery when administered 60 minutes after skin incision.[233] The use of high-dose opiate administration in the postoperative period needs further evaluation as a continuous intravenous infusion to prolong rewarming time and minimize shivering, heat loss, and metabolic demands and heart work.

Anabolic/Catabolic Hormone Modulation

Because the endocrine response to surgery is characterized by increased secretion of catabolic active hormones (catecholamines, cortisol, glucagon) and impaired secretion or effect of anabolic active hormones (insulin, testosterone), the catabolic postoperative state may be transformed to anabolism either by antagonizing the action of catecholamines by adrenergic blockade or by administration of anabolic hormones.[111,113]

It is well documented that some aspects of the metabolic response to surgery may be modified by adrenergic blockade, and in this context β-adrenergic blockade is more effective than α-adrenergic blockade.[111,113] No information is available, however, on eventual modulation of postoperative metabolism by adrenergic blockade. Administration of insulin has also been demonstrated to reduce posttraumatic protein breakdown.[232] Administration of growth hormone may improve nitrogen balance in traumatized patients[234,232] and several studies have shown anabolic steroids to be effective in improving postoperative nitrogen balance.[111,113]

Thus, endocrine manipulations may partly attenuate different metabolic responses after surgical trauma.[232] A major reduction of the stress response will probably not be achieved, however, unless a multicomponent regimen is used, and this may still be without effect on certain hormones (thyroid), various neural transmitters, and cytokines, among others. Furthermore, additional treatment of pain is necessary.

Pain Alleviation

During recent years, basic research on the mechanisms by which nociceptive stimuli are processed in the central nervous system has led to an improved understanding of pain and treatment of pain (see Chapters 23 and 24). The influence of pain relief on the stress response to surgery by the methods available (Fig. 5-5) will be reviewed in detail as it affects neural blockade by spinal and epidural analgesia with

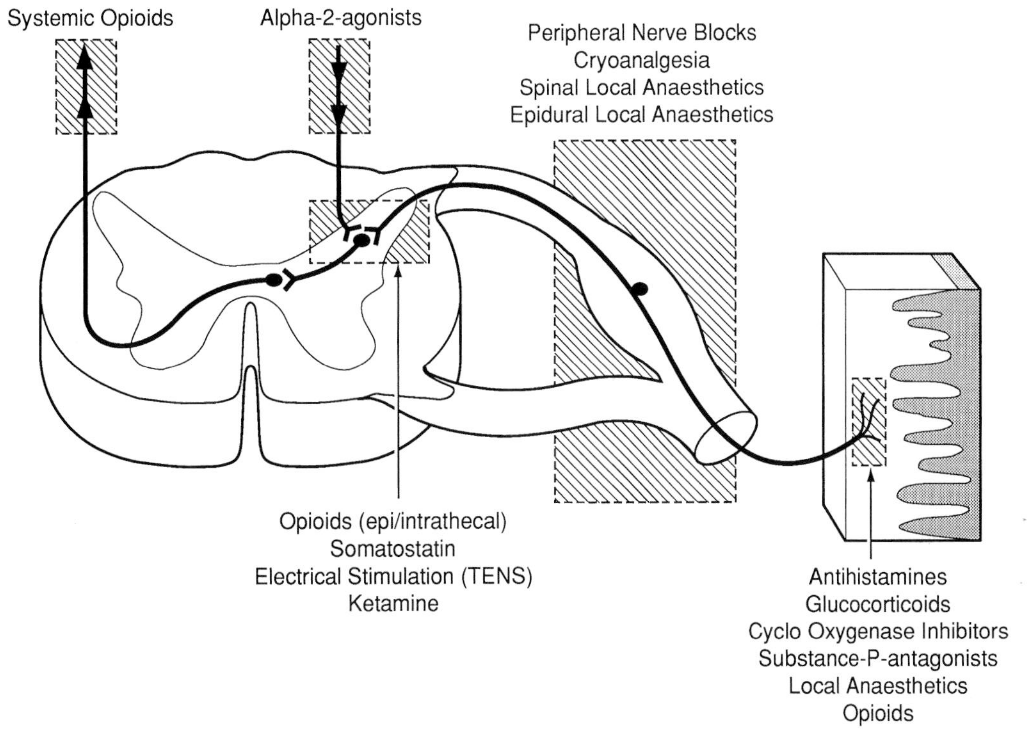

FIG. 5-5. Various techniques that may provide pain relief in surgical patients and thereby eventually modify the endocrine metabolic response. Peripheral treatment of pain with local anesthetics may suppress the stress response. The effect of peripheral treatment with opioids, substance P antagonists, serotonin antagonists, and antihistamines on the stress response has not been evaluated. Treatment with NSAIDs may slightly attenuate some endocrine metabolic responses. Preoperative glucocorticoids attenuate hyperthermia and acute-phase responses. Central neural blockade with local anesthetics inhibits a major part of the stress response. No data are available on cryo-analgesia. Pain relief with epidural intrathecal opioids or alpha-2-agonists (clonidine) is less efficient than local anesthetics in reducing the stress response, despite pain relief. TENS has no important effect on the stress response. Administration of systemic opioids in usual low doses has no consistent influence on the stress response.

local anesthetic agents and epidural/intrathecal administration of opiates and other analgesics. The influence of other pain treatment modalities will be briefly reviewed.

Influence of Pain Relief by Antagonizing Peripheral Mediators of Pain

Since the arachidonic cascade metabolites are involved in several steps of the responses to injury, perioperative nonsteroidal anti-inflammatory drug (NSAID) treatment may be expected to modify important parameters of the surgical stress response, and thereby organ dysfunction and outcome. Experimental studies have suggested that treatment with NSAIDs has favorable effects on posttraumatic immunosuppression and pulmonary dysfunction,[245] improves protein catabolism,[241,242] and reduces edema and wound-induced hypermetabolism in a burn model.[243,244] In clinical studies NSAIDs may attenuate the endocrine metabolic response to endotoxin but not to hypoglycemia.[239,240] In surgical studies NSAIDs had no important effects on the classical stress hormones[248,250,253] or on acute-phase proteins or leukcocytosis.[250–252,273] Hyperthermia may be reduced,[247,248,273] while the effect on nitrogen loss and net protein catabolism is debatable.[248,249] Although NSAIDs may improve some parameters of posttraumatic immunosuppression[246] there is no clinical evidence of less (or more) infectious complications after NSAID treatment.[247] Summarizing, perioperative use of NSAIDs may result in a slight modification of the surgical stress response and immunosuppression, but the clinical implications hereof are unknown.

There are no data on the potential effects of substance P antagonists, antihistamines, or serotonin antagonists on the surgical stress response, but preliminary data from multimodal regimens do not suggest an important effect.[112,249]

The effect of peripheral pain treatment with locally applied opioids[235] on the surgical stress response has not been evaluated.

Glucocorticoids may have some pain-alleviating effect and may alter several of the humorally mediated responses such as hyperthermia and acute-phase protein responses.[236–238] The clinical implications of a modified surgical stress response from high-dose glucocorticoids remain uncertain, except that the usual postoperative impairment in pulmonary function may be improved.[236]

Peripheral application of local anesthetics in the wound may reduce both pain and the pituitary response to surgery,[264] probably due to a direct neural as well as an anti-inflammatory effect of the local anesthetic.[265,266,397,473] The combination of incisional local anesthetic plus local hypothermia could not modify the systemic leukocyte, temperature, and transferrin response to herniotomy, despite no increase in plasma cortisol and glucose.[273] Other studies using peripheral instillation of local anesthetics intraperitoneally[269–271,275] or intrapleurally[267,268] have not been successful in reducing the surgical stress response. A combination of large doses of local anesthetics into an abdominal wound combined with continuous celiac plexus blockade with bupivacaine led to a slight reduction in the plasma glucose and cortisol response, but had no effect on the IL-6 response.[274]

Intravenous administration of local anesthetics has no important effect on postoperative pain or endocrine metabolic responses.[178,314]

Pain Relief by Stimulation of Inhibitory Descending Pathways and Alpha-2-Agonists

In experimental settings stimulation of the descending inhibitory pathways (see Fig. 5-2) from the brain stem using electrical stimulation or administration of the final transmitters (serotonin, alpha-2-agonists, and enkephalins) has analgesic effects. Correspondingly, clinical data have confirmed analgesia following systemic and epidural/intrathecal administration of alpha-2-agonists (predominantly clonidine).[254,255]

Systemic or epidural clonidine may reduce postoperative adrenergic responses, vasopression concentrations, plasma cortisol, and beta-endorphin.[256–260] The modifying effect on the surgical stress response is only moderate and similar to epidural morphine.[256]

Transcutaneous Electrical Nervous Stimulation (TENS)

Several controlled studies have demonstrated TENS to have only a slight to moderate analgesic effect following different operative procedures.[205,261] TENS has probably no or only very minor and clinically unimportant effects on intra- and postoperative endocrine and metabolic changes.[261–263]

Systemic Opiate Administration

Despite the widespread use of intermittent or continuous administration of various opiates for pain alleviation in surgical patients, very little information is available on subsequent mitigation of endocrine metabolic changes. The data suggest, however, that either no or only minor reductions will be obtained unless very high doses are used.[112] The recent use of systemic infusion of opiates by a demand technique has been shown to be an effective technique for postoperative pain relief, but without significant effects on plasma catecholamines, cortisol, and glucose.[306]

Age

It has been suggested that elderly patients might undergo surgical procedures at an increased risk because of abnormal endocrine and metabolic responses, but few studies have focused on this problem with appropriate matched control groups.

The limited data suggest that elderly patients elicit an increased cortisol response, whereas other responses may be similar to those of younger patients.[111,307] One study in lower extremity revascularization showed higher resting plasma norepinephrine levels preoperatively in older patients, but an increased intraoperative response in younger patients.[308]

Substrate Administration

It may be hypothesized that if trauma leads to increased requirements for certain substrates, then administration of such substrates should attenuate or prevent the stress response. As a general conclusion, however, provision of substrates may to some degree improve single aspects of postoperative catabolism, but the fundamental characteristics of the trauma response are not prevented. This also applies to administration of various specific substrates such as branched chain amino acids and ketones. Such considerations, however, obviously should not be an argument against nutritional support *per se*, but rather serve to emphasize that the basic mechanism of the stress response is not a lack of or an increased need for substrates.

Reduction of Heat Loss

Because injury leads to increased heat production and a rise in body temperature, it has been suggested that the stimulus to the stress response is a change in the set point of thermal neutrality at the hypothalamic level caused by the need for a higher core temperature. A logical approach to attenuate the responses would therefore be to raise environmental temperature. This principle is further argued by the usual increased heat loss in surgical patients owing to the semi-nude state and relatively low temperature in the operating rooms and wards. As mentioned above, recent observations suggest that the increased heat production and rise in body temperature are mediated by a synergistic effect of cortisol, catecholamines, and glucagon with a superimposed influence of IL-1.

One of the problems associated with surgical procedures is increased intra- and postoperative heat loss, leading to hypothermia which may be an additional stress on the body.[309] Recent studies suggest that there may be several physiological and metabolic advantages of providing thermal neutrality during and following surgical injury by reducing heat loss through the use of space blankets or by active warming. Thus, warming reduced urinary excretion of nitrogen and 3-methylhistidine, and the usual decrease in muscle glutamine concentration,[310,311] as well as plasma catecholamine responses and oxygen consumption were reduced, but without effects on acute-phase protein responses.[312] Also, postoperative nursing in a thermoneutral environment reduced urinary nitrogen, epinephrine and cortisol secretion, and leucine oxidation.[313]

METABOLIC FUNCTION BY NEURAL BLOCKADE MODIFICATION OF ENDOCRINE

The central role of the peripheral and central nervous system in mediating the response to surgical injury has stimulated research on the effects of blockade of nociceptive stimuli by peripheral or central nerve blocks on the injury response. Thus in 1910 George Crile launched the hypothesis of anociassociation,[50] suggesting that disruption of nociceptive stimuli by neural blockade might favorably affect posttraumatic outcome. In contrast, Walter Cannon demonstrated the importance of the sympathetic nervous system in maintaining homeostasis in response to a variety of stresses, such as fluid deprivation, hemorrhage, and cold[31]; however, the theory of anociassociation was supported in experimental studies, demonstrating that spinal anesthesia before injury reduced mortality due to blunt hind limb trauma.[160] Following the classic studies of Hume and Egdahl,[100] who demonstrated the importance of the peripheral and central nervous system in mediating the adrenocortical response to trauma, a vast amount of data has appeared during the last decades on the influence of neural blockade on various aspects of the responses to surgical injury. In the following sections these data are reviewed and the strength and limitations of these findings are discussed, aiming to identify issues relevant to future progress in our understanding of the surgical stress response. Finally, directions for future research are suggested.

Influence of Neural Blockade per se on Endocrine Metabolic Function

The effects of neural blockade by spinal or epidural analgesia with local anesthetic agents have predominantly been studied within the 20- to 30-minute interval between initiation of anesthesia and start of surgery. It appears that neural blockade per se has only a limited influence on endocrine metabolic function, except for the effect on catecholamines and pancreatic islet function. The data suggest that epidural analgesia has no important effect on resting plasma cortisol and growth hormone (GH) levels,[74,77,162,171] whereas minor decreases in plasma prolactin, luteinizing hormone (LH), and follicle-stimulating hormone (FSH) have been observed.[77] In metabolic parameters, no significant changes have been noted in blood glucose, lactate, alanine, free fatty acids, glycerol, and ketones during 20 to 30 minutes of epidural analgesia (T4–S5).[108]

In contrast, plasma epinephrine and norepinephrine decreased in relation to a higher rostrad spread of sensory analgesia during spinal anesthesia with tetracaine (Fig. 5-6).[156] Other studies have found the same relation between changes in plasma catecholamines and sensory level of analgesia during spinal anesthesia with hyperbaric tetracaine and bupivacaine, although less significant.[14]

On average, no significant changes in plasma catecholamines are to be expected during blockade, including

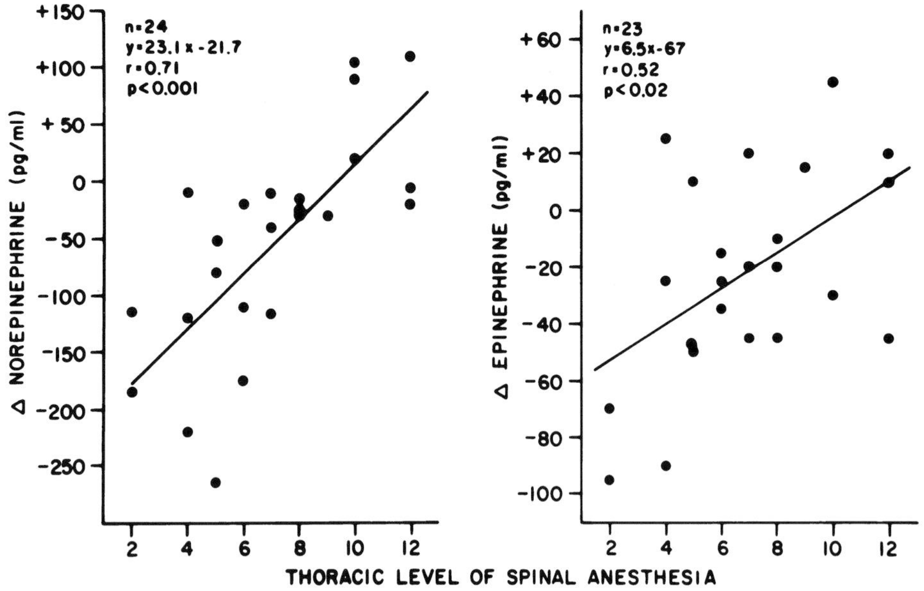

FIG. 5-6. Effect of spinal local anesthetic block *per se* on plasma catecholamines. Changes in plasma norepinephrine and epinephrine from pre-anesthesia to 30 minutes after subarachnoid injection of tetracaine. Regression analysis shows a significant correlation between thoracic level of anesthesia with both norepinephrine and epinephrine. (Reproduced with permission from Pflug, A.E., and Halter, J.B.: Effect of spinal anesthesia on adrenergic tone and the neuroendocrine responses to surgical stress in humans. Anesthesiology, *55:*120, 1981.)

lower (T9–T10) thoracic levels,[81,165] whereas decreased concentrations usually are seen during higher (T2–T6) dermatome blockade.[64,81,165,315] Plasma norepinephrine, but not epinephrine, decreased during epidural analgesia extending to between T4 and T10, whereas plasma renin activity and vasopressin were unchanged.[59] During subsequent tilt, epidural analgesia did not modulate plasma catecholamines and renin, whereas vasopressin increased compared to tilt without epidural analgesia.[59]

The acute insulin response to hyperglycemia is inhibited by a high thoracic (T2–T6) dermatome blockade, whereas a low (T9–T10) blockade has no influence on insulin secretion, suggesting that a baseline adrenergic input is important for maintenance of normal pancreatic islet function.[81] Plasma glucagon responses to a glucose load may be augmented by a high dermatome blockade.[81]

Epidural analgesia with local anesthetics may interfere with the normal counterregulatory mechanisms during hypoxemia and hypotension. Thus, epidural analgesia inhibits the renin response to hypotension but increases the vasopressin concentration,[316] thereby modifying the usual effects of vasopressin and the renin-angiotensin system to maintain blood pressure.[317] In experimental studies epidural analgesia blocks the catecholamine response to hypoventilation[318] and the cardiovascular response to hypoxemia, although the vasopressin response was enhanced.[319] Finally, an extensive epidural analgesia reduced cardiovascular and catecholamine responses to hypercapnia in dogs.[320] Thus, the studies in animals and nonsurgical patients have demonstrated that sympathetic blockade by epidural local anesthetics interfere with normal regulatory functions of the sympathetic pituitary and adrenal systems in various stress states, emphasizing the need for physiological support in surgical patients when such physiological disturbances occur.

There are no systematic studies on a possible differential effect of spinal versus epidural analgesia or of different local anesthetic agents on endocrine metabolic function. In a study in volunteers, cardiovascular and catecholamine responses to a cold pressor test were reduced during lidocaine epidural anesthesia compared to bupivacaine and 2-chloroprocaine,[321] but interpretation is difficult since it is unknown whether the doses administered represent equianesthetic doses.

The influence of circulating levels of local anesthetics on endocrine metabolic function is debatable; initial studies with intravenous infusion of lidocaine, bupivacaine, and etidocaine, in amounts resulting in plasma concentrations at the same levels observed during administration in epidural analgesia, showed epinephrine-like responses such as increased splanchnic uptake of glycerol and lactate and release of 3-hydroxybutyrate.[220] Recent controlled studies, however, did not observe any changes in plasma cortisol, catecholamines and various metabolites during infusion of bupivacaine or lidocaine unless plasma bupivacaine levels exceeded 3 to 4 μg/liter.[82,125]

INFLUENCE OF NEURAL BLOCKADE ON THE RESPONSE TO SURGICAL PROCEDURES

Lower Abdominal (Gynecologic) Procedures and Operations on the Lower Extremities

The modifying effects of neural blockade on intraoperative and postoperative endocrine and metabolic responses are summarized in Tables 5-2 and 5-3. Most studies have been performed during hysterectomy,[9,15,17,23,25,26,30,43,63,129,152,322,324] vaginal surgery,[166] inguinal herniotomy and minor orthopedic procedures,[6,81,105,155,165,323,325] prostatectomy,[66] and hip replacement.[37,94,177,193]

Pituitary Hormones

The normal increase in plasma prolactin during surgery is prevented by neural blockade,[9,23,77] but this effect is caused both by afferent neural blockade and by the omission of general anesthesia, since many general anesthetics in themselves exert a stimulatory effect on prolactin secretion. Thus during surgery performed under combined general anesthesia and epidural analgesia, plasma prolactin levels may be elevated already before skin incision.[23]

TABLE 5-2. *Influence of neural blockade (spinal/epidural) on the endocrine response to lower abdominal (gynecological) surgery or to procedures on the lower extremities*

Hormone level in plasma (supporting references)	Intraoperative response	Postoperative response[a]
Prolactin (9,23,77)	↓	↓
Growth hormone (15, 23,77,155,165,322, 330)	↓	↓
ACTH (155,325,328)	↓	?
ADH (17,166)	↓	↓
TSH (324)	↓	↓
FSH (77)	→	↘
LH (77)	→	↘
Beta-endorphin (66,325, 327)	↓	?
Cortisol (6,23,30,43, 63,74,77,94,105, 108,129,152,165, 171,177,322, 325–330,332)	↓	↓
Aldosterone (28,76, 325)	↓	↓
Dehydroepiandrosterone (325)	↓	↓
Renin (28,76)	↓	↓
Epinephrine (64,165, 308)	↓	↓
Norepinephrine (64,165, 308)	↓	↓
Insulin (6,26,30,105, 325)	↘	↘
C-peptide (6,26)	↘	↘
Glucagon (6,23)	→	→
T3 (24,25,324)	→	→
T4 (24,25,324)	→	→
Testosterone	?	?
Estradiol	?	?
Gastrointestinal hormones	?	?
Calcitonin gene-related peptide (322)	→	→
Serotonin (332)	↓	→
Substance P (327)	→	→

[a] Continuous epidural analgesia only. ?, no data; ↓, inhibition of response; →, no effect on response, ↘, slight inhibition.
ACTH, adrenocorticotropic hormone; ADH, antidiuretic hormone; FSH, follicle-stimulating hormone; LH, luteinizing hormone; TSH, thyroid-stimulating hormone.

TABLE 5-3. *Influence of neural blockade (spinal/epidural) on the metabolic response to lower abdominal (gynecological) surgery or to procedures on the lower extremities*

Metabolic response (supporting references)	Intraoperative response	Postoperative response[a]
Plasma-glucose (6,23,26, 30,63,108,152,171,177, 322,324–326,329–331)	↓	↓
Glucose tolerance (6,30, 99,105,323)	↑	→
Insulin clearance and action (323)	↓	?
Free fatty acid and glycerol (41,78, 108,324)	↓	→
Plasma-ketones (6,108)	↓	↗
Plasma-cAMP (157)	↓	↓
Plasma-lactate (108,193)	↓	→
Liver glycogen (7)	↓	?
Muscle amino acids (37)	?	↓
Nitrogen balance (27,331)	?	↑
Plasma-creatinine phosphokinase (173)	?	↘
Plasma-amino acids (37,108)	→	→↘
Plasma-acute-phase proteins (172,329–331)	→	→
IL-6 (330)	→	→
Oxygen consumption (67,175,331)	?	↘

[a] Continuous epidural analgesia only; ?, No data; ↑, improvement or normalization (nitrogen balance, glucose tolerance); ↘, slight inhibition of response; ↓, inhibition of response; →, no effect on response; ↗, slight increase.
cAMP, cyclic adenosine monophosphate; IL, interleukin.

Neural blockade also inhibits the growth hormone and adrenocorticotropic hormone (ACTH) response to surgery.[15,23,77,155,165,323,330] Similarly, the usual increase in antidiuretic hormone (ADH) is reduced by neural blockade.[17,166] Neural blockade accelerated the minor postoperative decrease in plasma FSH and LH in female patients.[77] The thyroid-stimulating hormone (TSH) increase is blocked.[324] The usual increase in beta-endorphin is prevented.[66,325,327]

Cortisol

Several studies have demonstrated that neural blockade with spinal or epidural analgesia may abolish or inhibit the cortisol response to surgery (Fig. 5-7).[6,23,30,36,43,63,74,77,94,105,108,129,165,171,177,322,325–330] In some of these studies, however, the influence was only marginal despite evidence that

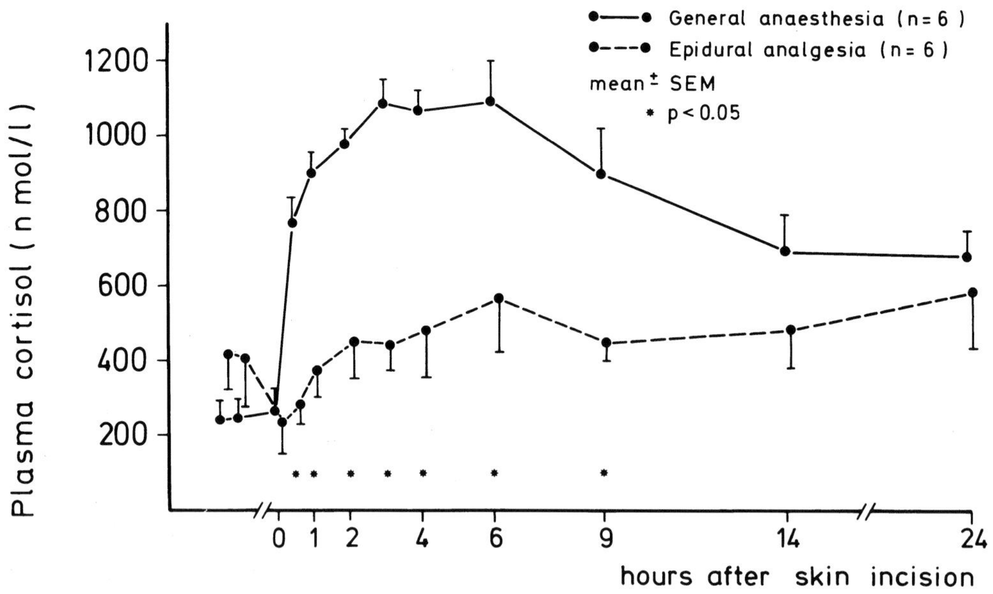

FIG. 5-7. Plasma cortisol: Comparison of intraoperative and postoperative changes in patients undergoing abdominal hysterectomy during general anesthesia (halothane) or continuous epidural analgesia with intermittent injections of plain bupivacaine 0.5%. Sensory level of analgesia was maintained from T4 to S5 during the 24-hour postoperative period. Plasma cortisol increased at all times after skin incision in patients operated on under general anesthesia, whereas no changes were observed in patients receiving continuous epidural analgesia. (Reproduced with permission from Brandt, M.R., Fernandes, A., Mordhorst, R., and Kehlet, H.: Epidural analgesia improves postoperative nitrogen balance. Br. Med. J., *1*:1106, 1978.)

these patients had sufficient alleviation of pain. The variable success in inhibiting the cortisol response to surgery in these studies may be explained by insufficient afferent neural blockade (see following).

Aldosterone and Renin

The limited data on the influence of neural blockade on plasma aldosterone and renin changes suggest that these responses are reduced both intraoperatively and postoperatively during hysterectomy and hip surgery.[28,76,325]

Catecholamines

Neural blockade leads to an abolished epinephrine response to surgery[64,165] in accordance with the inhibited cyclic adenosine monophosphate (cAMP) response.[157] Intraoperative and postoperative changes in plasma norepinephrine are probably also reduced[64,165,308]; looking at the data from major (upper) abdominal procedures, however, an abolished norepinephrine response is most likely (see below).

Thyroid Hormones

Neural blockade has no major influence on plasma T_4[24,25,324] but during combined general anesthesia and neural blockade an intraoperative and early postoperative increase in T_4 may be observed because several general anesthetic agents lead to hepatic release of T_4. Neural blockade alone or in combination with general anesthesia has no influence on the normal rapid decrease in plasma T_3 during hysterectomy or on the usual postoperative decrease in binding of thyroid hormones to plasma proteins.[24,25]

Insulin and Glucagon

Plasma insulin (and C-peptide) levels are unchanged during surgery under general anesthesia but may decrease during neural blockade (Fig. 5-8).[6,26] This is probably caused by blockade of resting adrenergic tone to the pancreatic islets, since baseline adrenergic input is important for normal islet function.[81] Plasma glucagon did not change during abdominal hysterectomy[23] or knee surgery[6] performed during general anesthesia or during combined general anesthesia and epidural analgesia[23] or epidural analgesia alone.[6]

Sex Hormones

No information is available on the influence of neural blockade on changes in plasma testosterone and estradiol.

Gastrointestinal Hormones and Neurotransmitters

P-calcitonin gene-related peptide does not change whether the operation is performed during general or epidu-

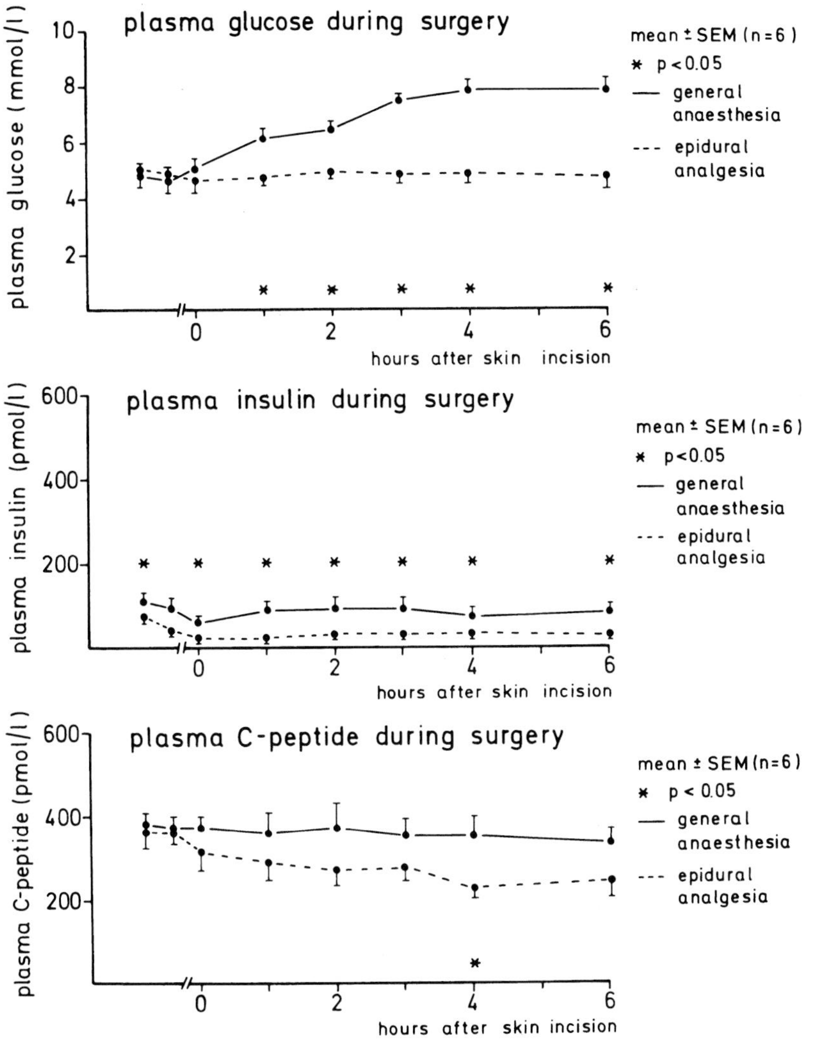

FIG. 5-8. Plasma glucose, insulin, and C-peptide: Comparison of changes in patients undergoing abdominal hysterectomy during general anaesthesia with halothane or enflurane or continuous epidural analgesia with intermittent injections of plain bupivacaine 0.5%. Sensory level of analgesia extended from T4 to S5 throughout the study. During general anaesthesia plasma glucose increased after skin incision despite unchanged levels in insulin and C-peptide. In contrast, patients receiving epidural analgesia showed no changes in plasma glucose, probably because of concomitant inhibition of plasma catecholamines and cortisol. Insulin and C-peptide decreased after epidural analgesia because of blockade of adrenergic tone to pancreatic islets. (Reproduced with permission from Brandt, M.R., Kehlet, H., Faber, O., and Binder, C.: C-peptide and insulin during blockade on the hyperglycemic response to surgery by epidural analgesia. Clin. Endocrinol., *6*:167, 1977.)

ral analgesia.[322] The usual decrease in plasma substance P is not modified by spinal anesthesia.[327]

Glucose Metabolism

The usual hyperglycemic response to surgery is reduced or blocked by neural blockade (Fig. 5-8).[23,26,30,63,108,152,171,177,322,324–326,329,330] This effect is not mediated through an increased insulin secretion, but probably by inhibition of hepatic glycogenolytic response to surgery.[7] The inhibitory effect of neural blockade on the glycogenetic response to surgery is caused by the abolished epinephrine response[64,185] or blockade of efferent sympathetic neural pathways to the liver,[102,123] or both. Probably both efferent sympathetic nerves to the liver and the adrenals must be deactivated to block the glucose response to surgery.[123]

Lower glucose concentrations in patients operated on during neural blockade have also been demonstrated in skeletal muscle biopsies.[193] No differences, however, in muscle content of creatinine phosphate, adenosine triphosphate, lactate, or glucose-6-phosphate were found between patients operated on under epidural analgesia or neuroleptanesthesia.[193] An intravenous glucose tolerance test carried out during inguinal herniotomy[105] or hysterectomy[99] performed under neural blockade was normal, in contrast to the impaired glucose tolerance observed during surgery under general anesthesia. This effect of neural blockade on intraoperative glucose tolerance is probably caused by several factors. First, inhibition of hepatic glucose output may be important. Second, inhibition of the cortisol and epinephrine response to surgery may be of importance because both hormones inhibit peripheral glucose clearance.[11] Third, preservation of normal insulin response to glucose during neural blockade[79,80,99] may be a causative factor, although this could not be demonstrated in one study.[105] Insulin clearance and action was kept normal when herniotomy was performed during epidural analgesia.[323] Also, omission of general anesthesia may be important because halothane has been shown to inhibit the acute insulin response to glucose independent of adrenergic mechanisms.[79,80] In two studies in which tests were performed 8 and 24 hours after surgery, glucose tolerance was found to be abnormal and similar to that of patients operated on under general anesthesia,[6,30] but in one of these the cortisol response was incompletely inhibited, suggesting insufficient afferent neural blockade.[30]

Altogether, the mechanisms involved in the modifying effect of neural blockade on glucose homeostasis, glucose tolerance, and insulin response to a glucose load are very complex. This is further emphasized by the demonstration that a high thoracic block (T2–T6) inhibits resting efferent sympathetic tonic activity to the pancreatic islets, thereby leading to an impaired insulin response to glucose.[81] This may be a contributing mechanism to the impaired glucose tolerance and insulin response to glucose during the late postoperative period in patients having continuous epidural analgesia who are normoglycemic prior to glucose "challenge."[30] Further investigations using either a glucose clamp technique or labeled glucose for glucose clearance studies are needed to clarify the underlying mechanisms to the modifying effect of neural blockade on perioperative glucose homeostasis (see Tables 5-2 and 5-3).

Fat Metabolism

Neural blockade probably inhibits intraoperative lipolysis as indicated by reduced levels of plasma free fatty acids and glycerol during lower abdominal surgery.[41,108,324] Postoperatively, levels return to control values despite continuous epidural analgesia (see Table 5-3).[108]

Spinal anesthesia (T10–L1) did not inhibit the increase in free fatty acids and glycerol during inguinal herniotomy unless the extent of analgesia was increased to high thoracic levels (T1–T3).[78]

Although a reduction of postoperative lipolysis by neural blockade is to be expected because of the concomitant sympathetic blockade, further studies are needed using radioactive techniques to assess lipid turnover and oxidation.

Lactate and Ketones

The normal perioperative increase in blood lactate, which is partly caused by the general anesthetics, may be reduced by neural blockade.[108,193] The intraoperative increase in 3-hydroxybutyrate is reduced by neural blockade during hysterectomy,[106] whereas late postoperative levels tend to increase compared to those in patients undergoing hysterectomy or knee surgery under general anesthesia.[6,108]

Amino Acids and Nitrogen Balance

No influence of neural blockade could be demonstrated in the first 24-hour postoperative blood alanine profile,[108] but the 5-day cumulative postoperative nitrogen balance was significantly less negative (about 50%) in patients undergoing abdominal hysterectomy during epidural analgesia for 24 hours compared to general anesthesia (Fig. 5-9).[27] Correspondingly, continuous 24-hour postoperative epidural analgesia following hip replacement prevented the usual postoperative shifts in amino acid composition in muscle.[37] There are no data on 3-methylhistidine excretion.

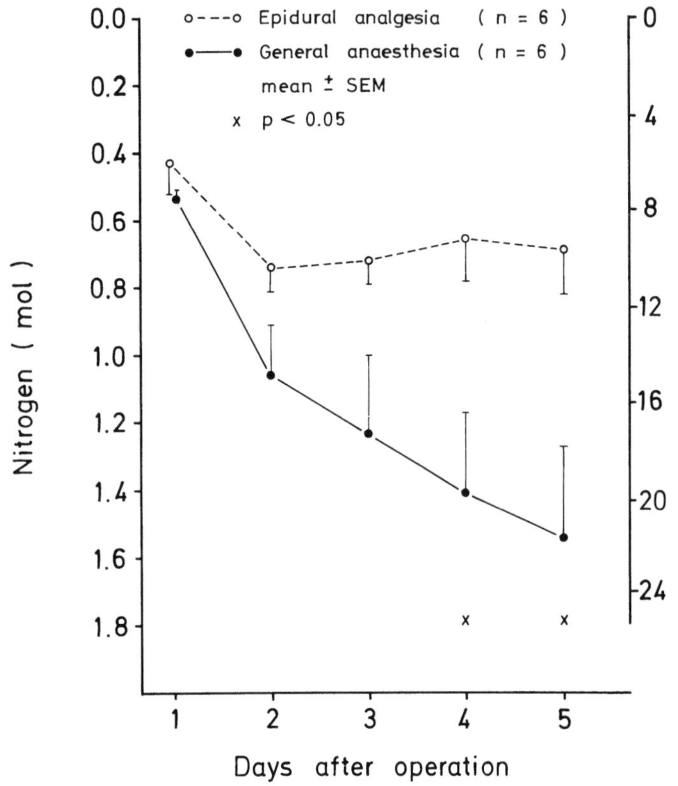

FIG. 5-9. Nitrogen balance: Comparison of urinary nitrogen excretion during the initial 5 days after abdominal hysterectomy in patients under general anesthesia with halothane or continuous epidural analgesia for 24 hours with intermittent injections of plain bupivacaine 0.5%. Sensory level of analgesia was held from T4 to S5. During the 5-day postoperative period, both groups received a hypocaloric oral intake amounting to 20 g of nitrogen and about 2900 calories. Patients receiving epidural analgesia had no intraoperative and postoperative increase in plasma cortisol and glucose, and concomitantly urinary nitrogen excretion was significantly reduced. (Reproduced with permission from Brandt, M.R., Fernandes, A., Mordhorst, R., and Kehlet, H.: Epidural analgesia improves postoperative nitrogen balance. Br. Med. J., *1*:1106, 1978.)

TABLE 5-4. *Effect of epidural or intrathecal analgesia on postoperative nitrogen economy*

	Surgery	Comment	Author
Lumbar epidural local anesthetic	Hysterectomy	24-h block with inhibition of cortisol and glucose response and improvement in nitrogen balance	Brandt[27]
	Colonic	44-h block. Postoperative nitrogen balance improved and 3-methylhistidine excretion reduced	Vedrinne[334]
	Hip surgery	No effect of single-dose epidural bupivacaine on urinary nitrogen and 3-methylhistidine excretion	Carli[333]
	Hip surgery	24-h block with reduction of cortisol and glucose response as well as usual 72-h postoperative shifts in amino acid composition in skeletal muscle	Christensen[37]
Thoracic epidural local anesthetic	Colonic	24-h block with reduction of urinary excretion of catecholamines, but not cortisol. Urinary nitrogen excretion and whole body protein turnover (leucin oxidation) reduced	Carli[335]
	Gastric	48-h block with reduced plasma cortisol and glucagon response and decreased urinary catecholamine excretion; urinary nitrogen excretion reduced compared to pain relief with systemic opioids and epidural opioids	Tsuji[336]
	Aortic	24-h block with reduced plasma cortisol and urinary catecholamine excretion; no effect on urinary nitrogen and cortisol excretion ($n = 2 \times 5$)	Smeets[337]
	Abdominal	Single-dose postoperative block (~ 6 h duration) with slightly reduced plasma catecholamines, glucagon, and cortisol levels; isotope study with decrease in glucose and urea turnover rates	Shaw[338]
	Abdominal and thoracic	24-h block with no influence on plasma glucose, free fatty acids, and lactate except at the end of operation, and no effects on postoperative nitrogen urea or 3-methylhistidine excretion	Seeling[187]
	Abdominal	Single-dose epidural analgesia; no effect on plasma cortisol, glucose prolactin, or nitrogen balance	De Lalande[54]
	Abdominal	24-h block, but without effects on plasma cortisol, glucose, or prolactin, but improved nitrogen balance	De Lalande[54]
Lumbar epidural opioid	Colonic	48-h treatment (epi.meperidine); no effect on nitrogen and 3-methylhistidine excretion	Vedrinne[334]
Lumbar or thoracic local anesthetic + opioid	Gastric	Intraoperative epidural local anesthetic + 72-h postoperative epidural morphine; Reduced plasma cortisol and glucagon and urinary excretion of catecholamines and nitrogen	Tsuji[336]
	Abdominal	24-h intermittent local anesthetic and 72-h epidural morphine with insignificant reduction in urinary catecholamines and cortisol, but unchanged 4-day nitrogen excretion	Hjortsø[91]
	Hysterectomy	24-h block with improved glucose homeostasis and insignificant reduction in urinary nitrogen excretion	Licker[331]

In contrast, a single-dose intraoperative epidural blockade had no effects on urinary excretion of nitrogen and 3-methylhistidine.[333]

The data on the effect of epidural analgesic techniques on postoperative nitrogen economy in lower and upper body procedures are shown in Table 5-4. In accordance with the pronounced reduction of the endocrine catabolic response by epidural local anesthetics in lower body procedures, a positive effect is observed on nitrogen economy in such procedures. However, in major (upper) abdominal procedures the effect is variable, probably explained by the insufficient afferent blockade and thereby less reduction of the catabolic endocrine response in those procedures (see following).

Renal Function, Water, and Electrolyte Balance

Renal function and urinary excretion of water and electrolytes may be profoundly altered in connection with anesthesia and surgery,[46] and neural blockade may influence this response by several mechanisms: (i) changes in glomerular filtration rate (GFR), second to universal hemodynamic effects of sympathetic blockade; (ii) effects mediated through an altered endocrine response to surgery by neural blockade; (iii) direct renal effects owing to blockade of efferent neural pathways or interruption of neural renal reflexes (afferent/efferent), or both. Renal innervation originates from T10–L1.[16] The influence of neural blockade on central and peripheral hemodynamics (see Chapters 7 and 8) may also affect renal hemodynamics and decrease effective renal blood flow.[212,417] GFR has been found to decrease during epidural analgesia parallel to the decrease in systemic blood pressure.[104] The influence of neural blockade on the endocrine response to surgery has been described (Table 5-2). Since most of the hormones (cortisol, catecholamines, aldosterone, renin, ADH) that may affect kidney function[58] are modified by neural blockade, a major influence should be expected on kidney function. Further, experimental studies have shown efferent sympathetic nervous activity to be important for kidney function, since denervation leads to an increase in sodium excretion and urine flow.[75,150] Also, neural blockade may interfere with reflexes recognized to influence efferent renal nerve activity and thereby tubular transport rates, although conclusive evidence has yet to be demonstrated.[150]

Despite the increased knowledge from both experimental and clinical studies on various mechanisms by which neural blockade may influence kidney function in the perioperative period, no final conclusion has emerged on the modifying effect of neural blockade on fluid and electrolyte balance in surgical patients. Thus the available data are very discordant (Table 5-5), and unfortunately the explanation hereto is not clear. A major problem hindering interpretation of these studies is that surgical procedures, the extent and duration of neural blockade, fluid administration, and duration of the studies are not similar. The observation in experimental studies that neural blockade may reverse posttraumatic anuria[42] has not been elucidated in clinical settings. Epidural analgesia does not alter hemodynamics during cross-clamping in aortic surgery.[340]

Further studies on this important aspect of the injury response and its eventual modulation by neural blockade are needed.

Hepatic Function and Serum Enzymes

It is well documented that surgical trauma may lead to changes in various serum enzymes considered to be of hepatic origin and to increases in hepatic microsomal enzyme activity.[127] This may contribute to accelerated drug pharmokinetics in the postoperative period.[61] These changes are predominantly observed within the first postoperative week and differ from results obtained intraoperatively where changes may be absent.[159] Although changes in hepatic functions and various serum enzymes probably are correlated to the intensity of the surgical trauma, the role of the general anesthetic agents in modifying hepatic function should not be overlooked. Thus, in experimental studies thiopentone anesthesia alone without surgery consistently decreased hepatic flow and extraction of test drugs, whereas these changes in hepatic function were not observed after high spinal anesthesia.[133,350] The effects of general anesthesia could be demonstrated up to 24 hours after application[133] and therefore should be reinvestigated in clinical settings.

The effect of neural blockade on the surgically induced changes in hepatic function has not been fully evaluated. Studies performed during spinal anesthesia with assessments either during surgery[159,341,342] or within the initial postoperative 3 weeks[127] have shown no difference in hepatic microsomal enzyme activity measured by the aminopyrine breath test or by antipyrine clearance, compared to changes in patients operated on under general anesthesia. That a single-dose spinal anesthesia has no effect on late postoperative hepative function is not, however, unexpected because studies on endocrine metabolic changes have shown only a transient (2–5 hours) inhibition (see following). In studies from patients operated on during continuous epidural analgesia no influence could be demonstrated on the normal postoperative changes in serum bilirubin, alkaline phosphatase, amino transferase, or aspartate amino transferase,[87,173] whereas the postoperative increase in serum lactate dehydrogenase and creatinine kinase was reduced.[173]

Oxygen Consumption, Thermoregulation, and Shivering

Epidural analgesia has been reported to reduce, although not normalize, the usual postoperative increase in oxygen consumption following prostatectomy,[175] colonic surgery,[312] and major vascular surgery.[67] However, no effect could be demonstrated following cholecystectomy[101] and hysterectomy.[331] Some reduction by neural blockade of the postoperative increase in oxygen consumption would be expected because the postoperative elevation in catabolic hormones (see Table 5-2) is attenuated, thereby reducing general metabolism.[11]

Neural blockade may, however, have a dual effect on oxygen consumption because vasodilation due to extensive neural blockade may predispose to hypothermia if vasodilated areas of the patient are left exposed in a cold environment. Most, but not all, studies have shown a more pronounced decrease in central temperature following neural blockade and a prolonged rewarming period.[86,92,103,210,345–347] When changes in mean skin temperature were combined with

TABLE 5-5. *Influence of neural blockade on perioperative fluid and electrolyte balance*

Surgery	Reference	Urinary H_2O excretion	Urinary Na^+ excretion	Urinary K^+ excretion
Hysterectomy	28,331	→	→	↓
Herniotomy	21	↑	↑	→
Hip replacement	17	→	–	–
Cholecystectomy	141		→	–
Vagotomy/pyloroplasty	339	→	↑	↓
Abdominal/thoracic	187	→	→	→
Prostatectomy	281	→	–	–

–, no influence; ↑, increased excretion; ↓, decreased excretion.

changes in core temperature to provide an estimate for changes in total body heat, however, no differences were observed between epidural or spinal analgesia and general anesthesia.[92,343] A single-dose spinal or epidural analgesia or a continuous low-dose epidural analgesia has no effect on the later hyperthermic response to surgery.[117,281,343]

Another factor that may counteract the reducing effect of neural blockade on postoperative oxygen consumption is shivering, which may represent an inappropriately programmed thermal response to raise the body temperature by increasing metabolism. Observations on the occurrence of postoperative shivering in patients receiving neural blockade are not uniform, although most studies have found an increased incidence.[86,92,210,344,345] The occurrence of postoperative shivering was not correlated to changes in central core temperature.[86] Efforts to minimize shivering by using warm solutions of the local anesthetics have been negative,[214,344] but a combination of warmed local anesthetics and parenteral fluids did reduce shivering following epidural analgesia in obstetrics.[139]

Epidural anesthesia changes thermal perception since a decrease in central temperature is poorly perceived,[344,348] and the sweating threshold is lower during epidural anesthesia alone compared to combined general/epidural anesthesia.[349]

Further studies are needed on the effect of neural blockade on posttraumatic oxygen consumption and thermoregulation to determine how to reduce postoperative demands. Prevention of heat loss during anesthesia and postoperative recovery is important, as these measures have been demonstrated to reduce postoperative nitrogen excretion[32,310,311] and oxygen consumption.[312,313]

Coagulation and Fibrinolysis

Surgical trauma initiates profound changes in both the coagulatory and fibrinolytic system.[356] Thus, the ability to coagulate is increased and changes in fibrinolysis are characterized by an initial, intraoperatively enhanced fibrinolytic function and decreased fibrinolysis in the postoperative period. As representing one of the factors of the triad of Virchow, these postoperative changes in coagulation and fibrinolysis may contribute to development of thromboembolic complications.

Modulation of the surgically induced changes in coagulation or fibrinolysis by neural blockade may be due to effects of the neural afferent/efferent blockade or to effects of the local anesthetics themselves (Table 5-6). Most studies have considered the effect of continuous epidural analgesia on coagulation and fibrinolysis, since a single-dose regional anesthesia probably will not lead to prolonged effects in the postoperative period,[352,353] in agreement with data on other stress responses.

Neural blockade has no effect on postoperative blood platelet count.[83,174,352,354] The usual increase in platelet aggregation may be inhibited,[332,351] although some studies have shown no effect.[361] Neural blockade does not modulate postoperative changes in plasma fibrinogen,[83,174,353,354,358,360]

TABLE 5-6. *Influence of neural blockade on perioperative changes in coagulation and fibrinolysis*

Parameter	Change (reference)
Coagulation	
Platelet count	No effect (83,174,352,354)
Platelet aggregation	Inhibition (351,332,359), no effect (361)
Plasma-fibrinogen	No effect (83,174,353,354,358,360)
Prothrombin time	No effect (83,174,351,353)
Partial thromboplastin time	No effect (83,352,353)
Plasma-antithrombin III	No effect (174,224,351–354,358)
Plasma-factor VIII capacity	Inhibition of response (174,352,354)
Factor VIII capacity	Inhibition of response (148,354), no effect (352,358)
von Willebrand factor	No effect (353), inhibition (354)
Thromboelastography	Inhibition of response (357)
Fibrinolysis	
Clot lysis time	No major effect (62,174,190,352)
Serum-fibrinogen degradation products	No effect (174,190,360)
Plasma-plasminogen	No effect (174,224,351,353,354,358)
alpha$_1$-antitrypsin	
alpha$_2$-macroglobin	
Serum-fibrinolysis inhibition activity	Inhibition of response (148)
Plasma-plasminogen activators and release after venous occlusion	Increased (148)
Tissue plasminogen activator (tPA)	No effect (353)
Plasminogen activator inhibitor-1 (PAI-1)	Inhibition of response (360)
Effects of local anesthetics per se	
Platelet aggregation	Inhibition (18), no effect (355)
Prothrombin time, partial thromboplastin time, antithrombin-III, platelets and aggregation, clot lysis time	No effect (40)
Endothelial structure and leukocyte adherence	Preserving/inhibition (194)

prothrombin time[83,174,351,353] partial thromboplastin time,[83,352,353] P-antithrombin-III,[174,224,351–358] and P-factor-VIII-antigen response,[174,352,354] while changes in factor-VIII capacity and von Willebrand factor may be inhibited[148,354] or unmodified.[352,353,358] Increased coagulation measured by thromboelastography may be inhibited by continuous epidural analgesia.[357]

The influence of neural blockade on the fibrinolytic response to surgery is debatable although some studies have shown an advantageous effect. No major effects have been observed in intra- and postoperative clot lysis time,[62,174,190,352] fibrin degradation products,[174,190,360] or changes in plasma plasminogen, alpha-1-antitrypsin, and alpha-2-macroglobin.[174,224,351,353,354,358] Continuous epidural anesthesia was found, however, to inhibit fibrinolysis inhibition activity in serum in patients undergoing hip surgery (Fig. 5-10)[148] and to reduce plasminogen activator inhibitor-1 (PAI-1) response,[360] as well as plasminogen activation and release after venous occlusion.[148] No effect has been demonstrated on tissue plasminogen activator (tPA).[353]

The explanation for the discordant results in the various investigations is not clear, but may be due to different techniques to assess coagulatory and fibrinolytic functions, and to differences in amount of blood loss and blood transfused between patients operated under general anesthesia and neural blockade as well as to differences in surgical procedures and type and duration of regional anesthesia. However, although the overall influence of neural blockade on unfavorable changes in postoperative coagulation and fibrinolysis are rather small, those observed may be one of several explanations for the reduced risk of postoperative thromboembolic complications after regional anesthesia (see following).

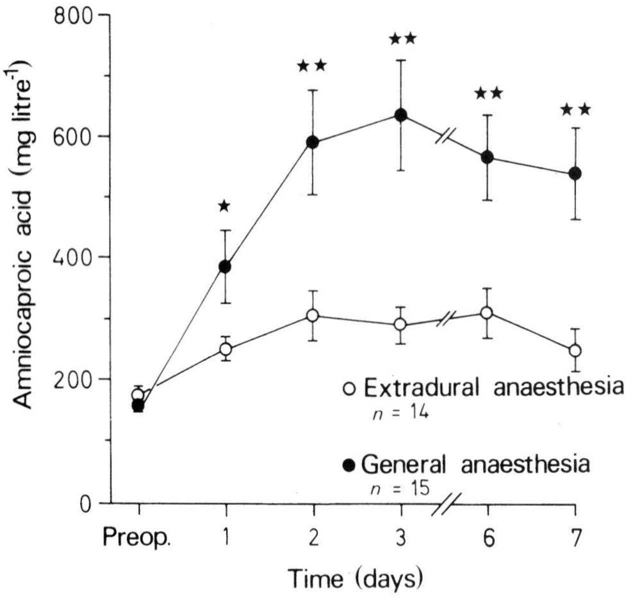

FIG. 5-10. Fibrinolysis inhibition activity expressed in dilution of aminocaproic acid in patients undergoing hip replacement under general anesthesia with nitrous oxide/oxygen and fentanyl or continuous epidural analgesia with intermittent injections of 0.5% bupivacaine with adrenaline for 24 hours. The results show that the increase in fibrinolysis inhibition activity in serum was avoided by epidural analgesia. At the same time the patients receiving epidural analgesia also showed higher concentrations of plasminogen activators and increased capacity for release of plasminogen activators; the capacity for activation of factor VIII was significantly reduced. Thus fibrinolytic function was improved by epidural analgesia. (Reproduced with permission from Modig, J., Borg, T., Bagge, L., and Saldeen, T.: Role of extradural and of general anaesthesia in fibrinolysis and coagulation after total hip replacement. Br. J. Anaesth., *55*:625, 1983.)

Besides the effects mediated through the afferent/efferent neural blockade on the trauma response, neural blockade *per se* or the local anesthetics themselves may influence coagulation and fibrinolysis. The effect of spinal or epidural analgesia *per se* on fibrinolysis and coagulation is not well defined, but during eye surgery no changes or differences in factor-II and factor-X, antithrombin-III, plasminogen, or alpha-2-antiplasmin were found between patients operated on under general and those under regional anesthesia.[176]

In order to elucidate the mechanisms for regional anesthesia–induced alterations in coagulatory and fibrinolytic responses for surgery, the effect of combined infusion of catabolic hormones (cortisol, epinephrine, and glucagon) has been studied.[362] Compared to saline infusion, platelet aggregation and Plasma-fibrinogen concentration increased after stress hormone administration; tPA activity increased, but without effects on tPA antigen levels or PAI-1 activity or antigen levels or α_2-AP-plasminogen.[362] Thus, differences in neuroendocrine response between general and regional anesthesia may explain some of the postoperative changes in platelet function, while factors other than the classical stress hormones are responsible for the demonstrated differences in fibrinolysis.

In *in vitro* studies lidocaine, bupivacaine, and tocainide caused an inhibition of ADP-induced platelet aggregation,[18] but this has not been confirmed in clinical studies using systemic administration of local anesthetics.[353] Intravenous infusion of lidocaine (2 mg/min) for 6 days after hip surgery did not modulate various tests of coagulation and fibrinolytic function.[40] Local anesthetics may exert an antithrombotic effect by blocking leukocyte locomotion and by preventing the cells from adhering to and invading venous walls, thus preserving endothelial structure (Fig. 5-11).[194]

The use of epinephrine or phenylephrine infusion to increase hemodynamic stability during continuous epidural analgesia and increase leg blood flow has no further effects on the fibrinolytic response to hip surgery.[363]

The clinical effects of neural blockade on thromboembolic complications is discussed later in this chapter.

Immunocompetence and Acute-Phase Proteins

Infectious complications continue to be one of the major factors leading to postoperative morbidity. Determinants of infection are host defense mechanisms, the environment

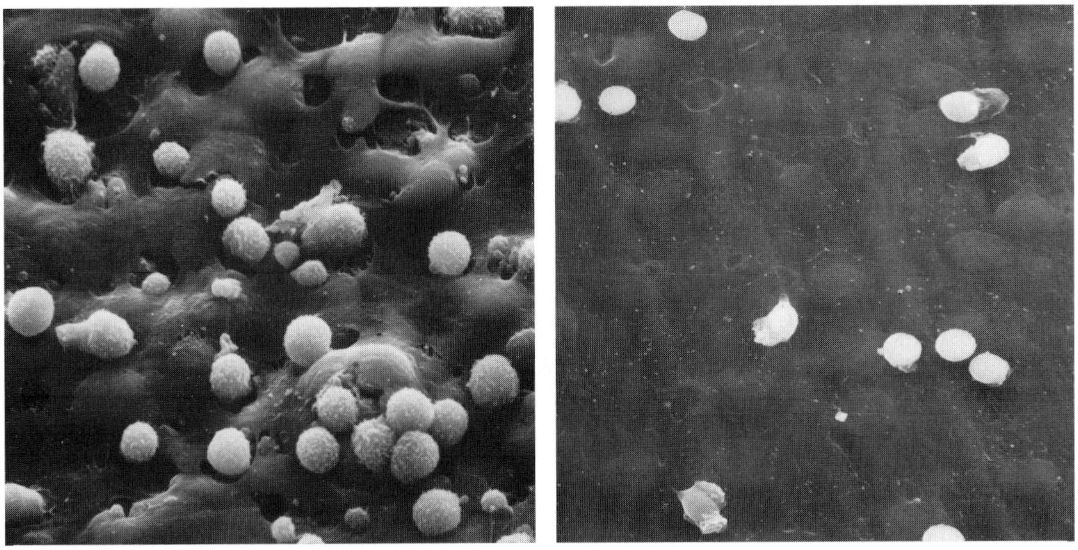

A B

FIG. 5-11. Luminal surface of jugular vein taken for bypass grafting from canine model (scanning electron micrograph × 1000). Vein was exposed and occluded briefly before local perfusion and fixation. **A:** Control: Endothelium is extensively damaged by leukocytes that had adhered and forced their way across junctions between endothelium and basement membrane. **B:** Lidocaine (load dose 1.25 mg/kg, then 0.125 mg/kg/min), 15 to 30 minutes before and during vein dissection and removal. Endothelial damage is greatly reduced, and leukocyte adherence and migration are essentially eliminated. (Reproduced with permission from Stewart, G.J.: Antithrombotic activity of local anesthetics in several canine models. Reg. Anaesth., *7*:S89, 1982.)

where the infection takes place, and the microorganisms producing the infection. Studies performed during different degrees of surgical trauma combined with general anesthesia have concluded that changes in immunocompetence are predominantly correlated to the magnitude of trauma and that the general anesthesia *per se* has only a minor role in this context.[110,364,365] Immunocompetence is a multicomponent mechanism by which the body protects itself against foreign organisms or substances and involves either nonspecific or specific immune mechanisms. In the following sections the influence of neural blockade and local anesthetic agents on nonspecific and specific immune mechanisms is reviewed; the influence of general anesthesia and different surgical procedures on immunocompetence has been discussed elsewhere.[110,364,365]

The influence of neural blockade on immunocompetence is probably negligible. Thus, no influence on peripheral blood neutrophils and lymphocytes was found[171,192] and the chemotactic response of neutrophils was not altered by epidural analgesia or spinal anesthesia, except for a slight depression when epinephrine was added to epidural analgesia.[192]

Neural blockade may alter some aspects of the surgically induced changes in *nonspecific immunity*. Thus, postoperative granulocytosis may be reduced by continuous epidural analgesia,[171,330,370,371] but not following a single-dose spinal or epidural anesthesia.[60,215,372–374] Late postoperative changes in leukocyte migration are not modified by a single-dose epidural analgesia.[60] Complement is probably not modified by regional anesthesia,[224,374,375] and no effect is observed on plasma fibronectin changes[376] or acute-phase protein responses[172,330] (Table 5-3; Fig. 5-12). In contrast, epidural analgesia led to an improved monocyte function (spreading and lysis) during hip surgery.[94] This effect was not due to omission of general anesthesia because the same observations were made during combined epidural and general anesthesia.[97] Caudal analgesia improved late postoperative leukocyte microbicidal activity,[377] and circulating neutrophils removed from patients undergoing hip arthroplasty during epidural analgesia also showed enhanced neutrophil microbicidal activity,[378] as well as improved neutrophil motility during chemotaxis.[373]

Neural blockade may also influence perioperative changes in *specific immunity* because the normal lymphopenic response may be obtunded.[171,215,330,370,371] Continuous epidural analgesia or spinal anesthesia has no influence on postoperative changes in immunoglobulins.[172,372] A slight decrease in the number of T cells following hip surgery was not modulated by epidural analgesia, and the ratio between T-suppressor (T8) cells and T-helper (T4) cells was unaffected.[98] A number of studies have considered the influence of neural blockade on the lymphoproliferative response of circulating lymphocytes to various immune stimuli, "mitogens," in the perioperative period. In several of these studies, however, interpretation of the results is impeded by the lack of appropriate control groups.[51,115,183] In other studies neural blockade by epidural analgesia[95] or spinal anesthesia[215] improved the normal decrease in blastogenic response of circulating lymphocytes to nonspecific and specific mitogens during hip surgery[95,372] and during

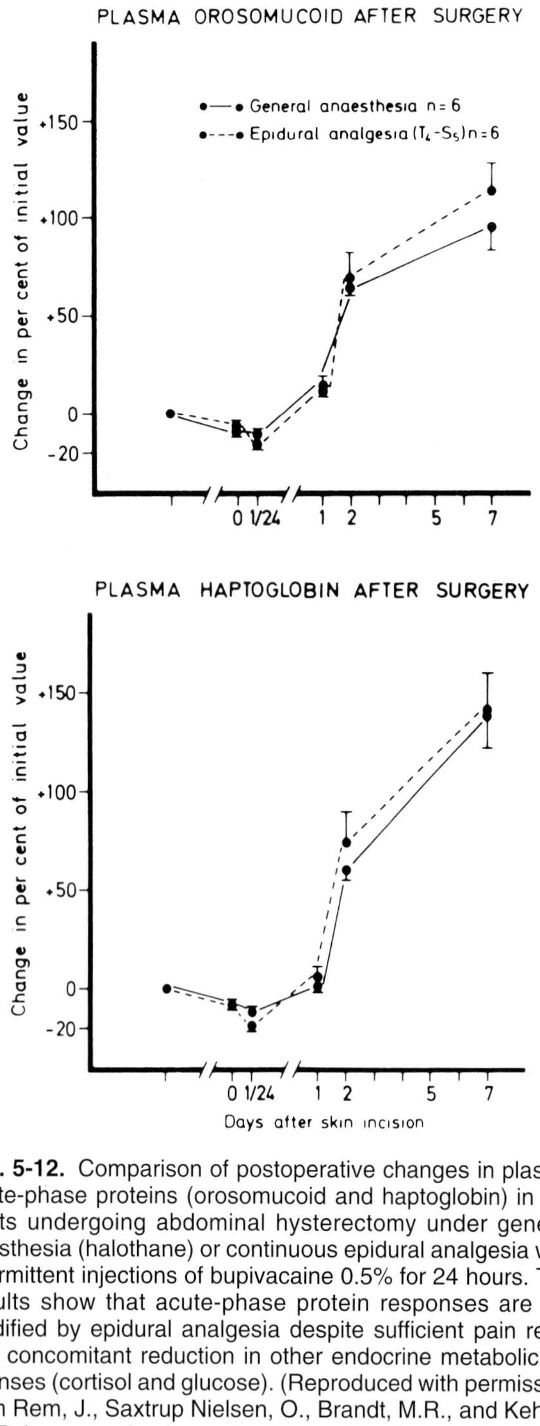

FIG. 5-12. Comparison of postoperative changes in plasma acute-phase proteins (orosomucoid and haptoglobin) in patients undergoing abdominal hysterectomy under general anesthesia (halothane) or continuous epidural analgesia with intermittent injections of bupivacaine 0.5% for 24 hours. The results show that acute-phase protein responses are not modified by epidural analgesia despite sufficient pain relief and concomitant reduction in other endocrine metabolic responses (cortisol and glucose). (Reproduced with permission from Rem, J., Saxtrup Nielsen, O., Brandt, M.R., and Kehlet, H.: Release mechanisms of postoperative changes in various acute phase protein and immunoglobulins. Acta Chir. Scand., *502*:51, 1980.)

prostatectomy.[215] In contrast, the usual intraoperative increase and postoperative decrease in natural killer (NK) cell activity were not modified by epidural analgesia during major upper abdominal surgery despite inhibition of some aspects of the endocrine response.[206] However, continuous epidural analgesia almost normalized changes in lymphocyte subpopulations and improved NK cell activity, concomitant with a reduction in cortisol and catecholamine responses after hysterectomy.[371] These results are supported by experimental data to demonstrate pronounced redistribution of lymphocytes to lymphatic tissue after laparotomy and hormone activation.[379] A single-dose epidural analgesia had no effect on late postoperative changes in lymphocyte response to phytohemagglutinin (PHA) and pokeweed mitogen stimulation.[60] In contrast, a single-dose spinal anesthesia improved PHA-induced lymphocyte response, but otherwise had no effect on lymphocyte subtype NK cell activity or immunoglobulins.[372] Epidural analgesia with combined administration of local anesthetics and morphine did not modify postoperative impairment in delayed hypersensitivity in patients undergoing major abdominal surgery,[89] but this regimen also failed to significantly alter the endocrine metabolic stress response.

Local anesthetic agents stabilize cell membrane function and may therefore influence neutrophil and lymphocyte function. Thus, *in vitro* studies have demonstrated that lidocaine and bupivacaine reduce the blastogenic lymphocyte response to PHA stimulation,[168] and that lidocaine[211] and procaine[195] reduce NK cell activity. No effect was seen on immunoglobulin synthesis.[369] Also ropivacaine, bupivacaine, prilocaine, lidocaine, and mepivacaine reduced chemoluminescence.[367] Lidocaine 0.2% and 0.5% inhibits leukocyte metabolism and motility.[368] In most of these studies, however, pharmacologic doses of local anesthetics were used, and extrapolation to the clinical situation is difficult. In other *in vitro* studies using local anesthetics in concentrations observed during epidural analgesia, no effect of lidocaine was observed on microbicidal oxidative function (neutrophil chemoluminescence)[217] or of bupivacaine on monocyte function (spreading and lysis) and lymphocyte blastogenic response to mitogens.[96] In experimental studies in rabbits, intravenous infusion of lidocaine (0.3 mg/kg) inhibited granulocyte adherence and suppressed delivery to inflammatory sites.[134] In a rat wound model, incisional lidocaine reduced leukocyte appearance and metabolic function.[397] Also, in a rat peritonitis model local application of lidocaine, but not bupivacaine, inhibited the inflammatory reaction and plasma extravasation.[366]

In summary, neural blockade may positively influence some aspects of the surgically induced impairment in various aspects of immunocompetence. The mechanism hereto has not been completely elucidated but may partly be explained by the concomitant inhibition of various endocrine metabolic responses.[96] The clinical relevance and implications for anesthetic practice have not, however, been settled. Nevertheless, the data on neural blockade and perioperative immunocompetence are extremely interesting and of potential value because posttraumatic immunodepression has been difficult to modulate by other therapeutic measures.

Major (Upper) Abdominal, Major Vascular, and Thoracic Surgery

The influence of neural blockade with local anesthesics on the endocrine metabolic response to major abdominal, vas-

TABLE 5-7. *Effect of epidural local anesthetic analgesia on the intraoperative and postoperative stress responses to major surgery*

ACTH	↓	
	↘	471
	→	189,328
Prolactin	↓	
	↘	
	→	54,206[a]
ADH/vasopressin	↓	19
	↘	
	→	38,457,471
Growth hormone	↓	
	↘	457
	→	480[a]
Cortisol	↓	29,204,479[a],481[a]
	↘	8,141,180,189,336,337,475,476,480[a]
	→	121,200[a],54,88,206[a],90,328,335,361[a],432,471
Aldosterone	↓	481[a]
	↘	141
	→	
Renin	↓	
	↘	
	→	
	↑	141
Glucagon	↓	
	↘	336
	→	121
Insulin	↓	200[a],481[a]
	↘	8
	→	121
Epinephrine	↓	180,312,335,336,476,481[a],482[a]
	↘	202,206[a],337,475,478[a],480
	→	90,457
Norepinephrine	↓	180,202,206[a],312,335,336,475,476,480,[a]482[a]
	↘	90,337,457
	→	
Thyroid hormones	↓	
	↘	
	→	181,189
TNF/endotoxin	↓	
	↘	
	→	328
Glucose	↓	29,200[a],8,101,189,204,479[a]
	↘	121,187,432,476,480[a]
	→	54,88,141,361,471,481[a]
Glucose tolerance/turnover	↓	
	↘	338,475
	→	187
Glycerol/FFA	↓	101,204
	↘	8,101
	→	187,200[a],481[a]
Lactate	↓	
	↘	101
	→	8,200[a],476,480[a]
cAMP	↓	
	↘	
	→	361[a]
O_2 consumption	↓	73,312,481[a]
	↘	
	→	101,477[a]

[a] *intra*operative epidural local anesthetics only, with or without postoperative assessments; all other data from continuous *post*operative regimens; for effects of epidural local anesthetics on nitrogen balance, see Table 5-4; for data from continuous spinal, combined epidural opioid–local anesthetic regimens, and other combined regimens, see text; endocrine metabolic parameters assessed by analysis of blood concentrations or urinary excretion.

↓, pronounced inhibition of response; ↘, slight inhibition of response; →, no effect on response; ↑, amplification of response.

ACTH, adrenocorticotropic hormone; ADH, antidiuretic hormone; cAMP, cyclic adenosine monophosphate; FFA,; TNF, tumor necrosis factor.

cular, and thoracic procedures is summarized in Table 5-7. In most studies plain 0.5% bupivacaine has been used intraoperatively and a continuous technique with intermittent injections or continuous infusion of lower concentrations of bupivacaine postoperatively. Although the surgical procedures and the technique of epidural analgesia (volume and concentration of local anesthetic) have varied, the results of these studies are reasonably consistent in that pronounced inhibitory effects such as seen during epidural analgesia in procedures in the lower part of the abdomen (see Tables 5-2 and 5-3) were not observed. However, a variable degree of inhibition was reported in many studies and predominantly in parameters such as changes in blood glucose and blood and urinary catecholamines (Table 5-7). The explanation of the varying results between the reported studies is not clearly related to the epidural regimen,[483] and probably several factors are involved: (i) The extents of sensory analgesia have varied and in some studies have not been defined; duration of neural blockade also differed; (ii) The technique of epidural analgesia and administration of local anesthetics varied and only in very few studies were data presented to document that the claimed area of analgesia was maintained throughout the study period by repeated assessments; (iii) The surgical procedures differed, and a combination of thoracic and abdominal operations in some studies may impede interpretation[19,29,187]; (iv) In some studies perioperative administration of fluids, glucose, or other substrates was not defined, also impeding interpretation. However, despite these flaws in methodology, the conclusion seems valid that neural blockade with local anesthetics is less efficient in reducing the surgical stress response to thoracic, major vascular, and upper abdominal procedures than the response to operations performed in the lower part of the body.

Several explanations may be given for the less pronounced effect of neural blockade in reducing the stress response to major abdominal, vascular, and thoracic procedures compared to other operations (Fig. 5-13). Thus, the unblocked *vagal afferent pathway* has been hypothesized to be of importance in this context,[29] but experimental studies in dogs with vagotomy, ventrolateral cordotomy, or combined vagotomy plus cordotomy failed to demonstrate an importance of the vagal pathway in the ADH response to surgery[207]; however, a concomitant neural blockade of sympathetic and somatic afferents was not performed. Correspondingly, clinical studies using infiltration of the vagal nerve with local anesthetics immediately after opening the abdomen[200] or preliminary surgical vagotomy or vagal blockade[203] failed to modify the stress response. The role of *unblocked phrenic afferents* is unknown. An *insufficient afferent sympathetic block* may be of importance because an additional celiac plexus block was found to further reduce the stress response when combined with epidural analgesia.[204] This was further confirmed by the demonstration of pronounced inhibition of plasma cortisol, glucose, free fatty acids, and urinary epinephrine excretion in patients undergoing gastrectomy during general anesthesia and intraoperative

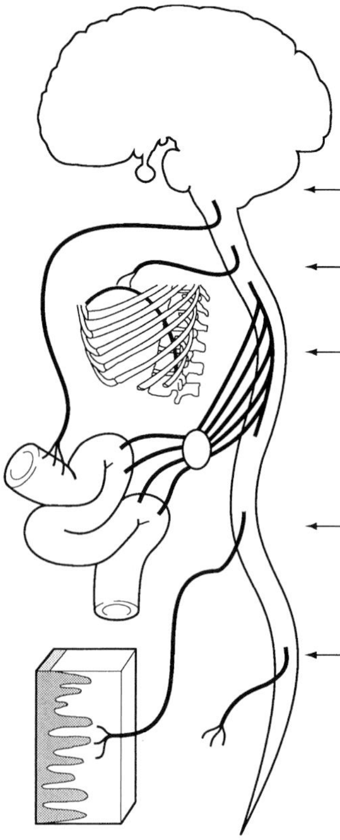

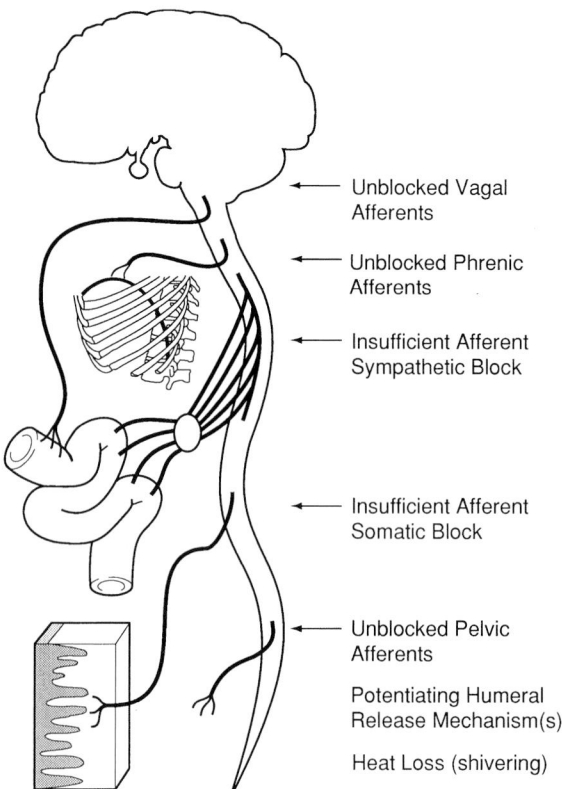

FIG. 5-13. Factors that may explain the demonstrated reduced inhibition of the surgical stress response by epidural analgesia during major (upper) abdominal procedures compared to procedures in the lower abdomen and lower extremities. Existent data suggest that the main cause is an insufficient afferent somatic and sympathetic block, whereas unblocked parasympathetic afferents probably are of minor importance. The role of potentiating humoral release mechanisms (local tissue factors and interleukin-1) and increased metabolism by shivering due to heat loss have not been fully evaluated.

splanchnic nerve blockade, when compared to general anesthesia alone or intraoperative local anesthetic and postoperative morphine.[451] According to previous observations, neural blockade as assessed by sensory level of analgesia extending to T4 may also lead to an autonomic blockade of the sympathetic plexuses in the abdomen,[16] but studies assessing sympathetic blockade by skin conductance and skin blood flow and temperature suggest that the level of sympathetic blockade in spinal anesthesia may be lower than that of sensory blockade.[10,130] Thus, the relative inefficiency of epidural analgesia in reducing the stress response to upper abdominal procedures may, at least in part, be due to inadequate inhibition of sympathetic afferent activity. The role of an *insufficient afferent somatic block* is difficult to assess because no consistent evaluation of the sensory blockade was reported in the various studies. However, studies with somatosensory evoked potentials to assess the depth of neural blockade have demonstrated that thoracic epidural techniques do not provide a total afferent blockade,[450,484,485] even with high concentrations of local anesthetics. In contrast, more pronounced reductions of evoked potentials are observed with lumbar epidural local anesthetic techniques[185,486] or intrathecal local anesthetics,[487] although a "chemical transsection" of the spinal cord was not observed. Use of high doses of 1.5% etidocaine in lumbar epidural analgesia, however, abolished somatosensory evoked potentials after dermatomal stimulation.[488] A correlation between inhibition of the cortisol response to cholecystectomy and reduction in somatosensory evoked potentials was observed in some, but not all dermatomal segments,[450] suggesting that insufficient somatic afferent blockade is an important factor to explain the smaller effect of thoracic epidural local anesthetic techniques in blocking the surgical stress response compared to lumbar epidural local anesthetic techniques. Furthermore, a pronounced variation in both proximal/distal and contralateral extent of analgesia has been demonstrated during continuous epidural analgesia with intermittent injections of identical doses of bupivacaine,[13] which may also explain the variable results shown in Table 5-7. The role of potentially *unblocked pelvic parasympathetic afferents* is unknown, but may be of importance because in most studies blocks extending from T4 to L1 to L2 were used. Finally, potentiating humoral release mechanisms (see above) may also be more important during major procedures than during minor procedures.[328] *Heat loss* and *shivering*, which are more pronounced after major than minor procedures, are additional factors that may reduce the inhibitory effect of neural blockade on the surgical stress response, but quantitative assessments have not been performed.

In an effort to increase the depth of the afferent blockade, a continuous spinal local anesthetic technique has been used and demonstrated to lead to a more pronounced reduction of the cortisol and glucose responses.[453,454] This is in accordance with the more efficient afferent blockade during continuous spinal anesthesia, especially in combination with epidural local anesthetics, as assessed by electrical sensory thresholds.[489] Also, the combination of a thoracic epidural local anesthetic to block catecholamines, etomidate to block cortisol, and somatostatin to block glucagon was very effective since the usual postoperative increase in amino acid clearance and urea synthesis was abolished.[490]

Combined Epidural Local Anesthetic–Opioid Analgesia

Combinations of analgesics in a multimodal or balanced analgesia regimen[472] improve pain relief and may therefore be expected to further reduce the surgical stress responses. In hip replacement addition of 2.5 mg morphine to a single-dose intrathecal cinchocaine led to a more pronounced inhibition of plasma cortisol than cinchocaine alone.[149] Similar results were found in a meniscectomy study.[491] However, during upper abdominal surgery or thoracotomy the combined use of epidural local anesthetic and morphine did not block the cortisol response.[492,493,495] A very effective analgesic regimen with combined epidural bupivacaine and morphine in relatively high doses and with systemic indomethacin eliminated pain during open cholecystectomy, but not changes in cortisol, glucose, acute-phase proteins, or the hyperthermic response.[440] Combined perioperative epidural bupivacaine and morphine together with systemic ibuprofen and incisional bupivacaine did not prevent the glucose and cortisol response to minilaparotomy cholecystectomy, compared to surgery with general anesthesia, incisional bupivacaine, and systemic ibuprofen and morphine postoperatively.[497]

In laparoscopic cholecystectomy thoracic epidural local anesthetics did not block the plasma cortisol or glucose response to surgery.[496]

The use of *intra*operative epidural local anesthetics and *post*operative epidural morphine did reduce urinary cortisol excretion in one study,[435] but had no effect on nitrogen balance, urinary catecholamines and cortisol,[90] or oxygen consumption[477] in other studies.

Improvement in postoperative analgesia by combined systemic prednisolone and epidural local anesthetic–opioid treatment further reduced the hyperthermic response as well as prostaglandin and acute-phase protein responses.[236,494]

In conclusion, the available data have clearly demonstrated neural blockade to be less efficient in reducing the surgical stress response to upper abdominal and thoracic procedures than the response to operations in the lower part of the body.

MECHANISM OF MODIFYING EFFECTS OF NEURAL BLOCKADE ON THE STRESS RESPONSE

The basic mechanism of the blocking effect of neural blockade on the stress response to surgery is the prevention of the nociceptive signal from the surgical area from reaching the central nervous system. Although small myelinated (A-delta) and unmyelinated (C) sensory fibers are primarily involved in the transmission of these stimuli, the ascending pathways have not been fully evaluated.[225] This also applies to the relative role of somatic versus autonomic afferent pathways (see above). Thus further data are needed on the role of pain stimuli versus other neural stimuli, and the role of afferent neural blockade versus blockade of efferent pathways to various organs. It is hoped that such data will clarify the reported discrepancies in the efficacy of neural blockade in altering the stress response to surgery and also point toward better techniques to obtain a more sufficient blockade of nociceptive stimuli and the stress response.

Role of Pain Stimuli versus Other Neural Stimuli

Although pain *per se* will elicit an endocrine metabolic response, the inhibitory effect of neural blockade on the endocrine metabolic response to surgery is mediated not only through alleviation of pain. Thus a definite adrenocortical response to hysterectomy was observed in patients receiving epidural analgesia with sufficient pain alleviation.[41,63,129]

Further, postoperative analgesia by epidural administration of a combination of local anesthetics and morphine[90,440] or morphine alone did not result in a pronounced inhibition of the stress response to various procedures.

Afferent versus Efferent Neural Blockade

The neural release mechanisms of the endocrine and metabolic response to surgery may involve both afferent and efferent pathways but differ among the individual endocrine glands. Thus predominantly afferent pathways are involved in the release of the pituitary hormone responses, whereas release of individual adrenocortical responses is more complex. In the experimental setting a pituitary-adrenal stress response may be observed after thermal injury without brain-pituitary connections,[448] indicating that factors other than neural stimuli may release pituitary-adrenal responses. Such factors include IL-1 and other immune mediators.[449]

The cortisol response is triggered by a dual mechanism involving an efferent neural limb to the pituitary and the humoral efferent limb to the adrenal cortex by ACTH. The aldosterone response may be mediated partly by the ACTH response, but afferent and efferent neural pathways are also involved in releasing the renin and angiotensin response. The epinephrine response is mediated by afferent neural pathways combined with efferent sympathetic pathways to the adrenal medulla. Further, afferent/efferent neural reflexes may directly affect various organs (e.g., liver, kidney) independent of endocrine changes.[123,150]

The literature is conflicting with regard to the influence of neural blockade on the cortisol response to surgery, probably because of an insufficient afferent block in most studies (see Tables 5-2 and 5-7). Thus systematic studies on the influence of the extent of sensory analgesia on the cortisol response to lower abdominal surgery have shown that an extensive blockade from T4 to S5 must be achieved to prevent the cortisol response (Fig. 5-14).[63] These findings have been confirmed in other studies during hysterectomy under spinal anesthesia, where plasma cortisol did not increase intraoperatively in patients in whom analgesia did not regress below T4, whereas a progressive increase was observed with waning analgesia (Fig. 5-15).[152] Afferent sensory blockade to T8 has no effect on the cortisol response to hysterectomy,[30,63] indicating that efferent pathways to the adrenal glands (T11–L1) are unimportant in this context. Also, a neural blockade from T3 to L1 has no influence on ACTH-stimulated cortisol secretion.[188]

The intensity of the afferent blockade on the modifying effect of neural blockade on the surgical stress response is obviously important, but little information is available with

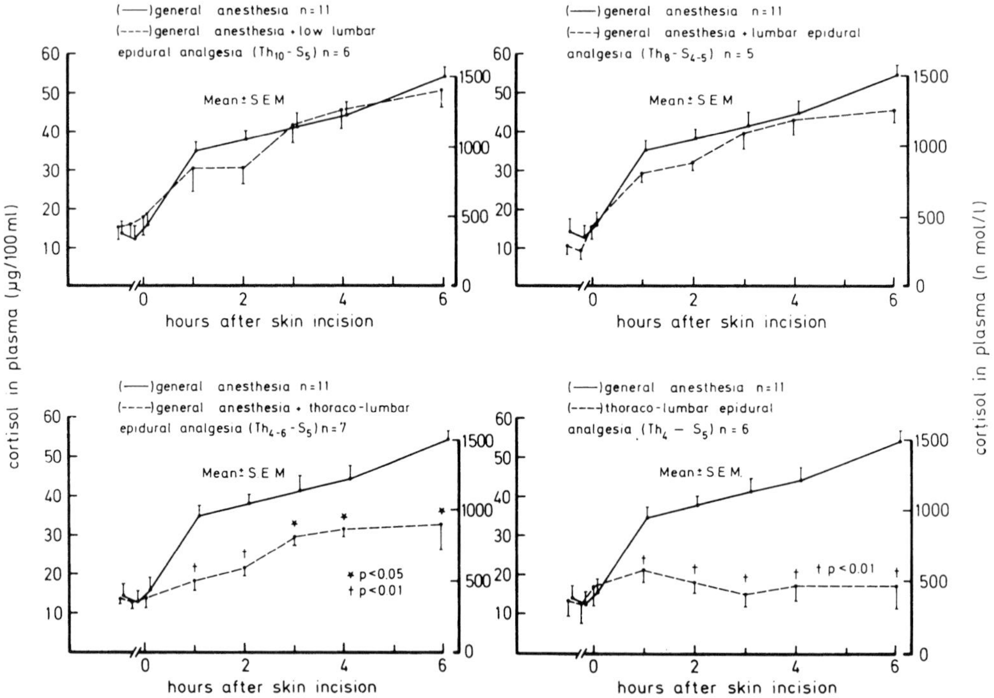

FIG. 5-14. Influence of varying sensory levels of analgesia during epidural analgesia with 0.5% plain bupivacaine in patients undergoing abdominal hysterectomies. Control patients received general anesthesia with halothane or enflurane. The results show that analgesia extending to T10 or T8 has no effect on the plasma cortisol response to surgery despite postoperative pain relief. Further extension of levels of analgesia leads to a reduction in plasma cortisol during and after surgery, and when the fourth thoracic segment is included the response is blocked. Similar results were found in changes in plasma glucose. (Reproduced with permission from Engquist, A., Brandt, M.R., Fernandes, A., and Kehlet, H.: The blocking effect of epidural analgesia on the adrenocortical and hyperglycemic response to surgery. Acta Anesthesiol. Scand., *21*:330, 1977.)

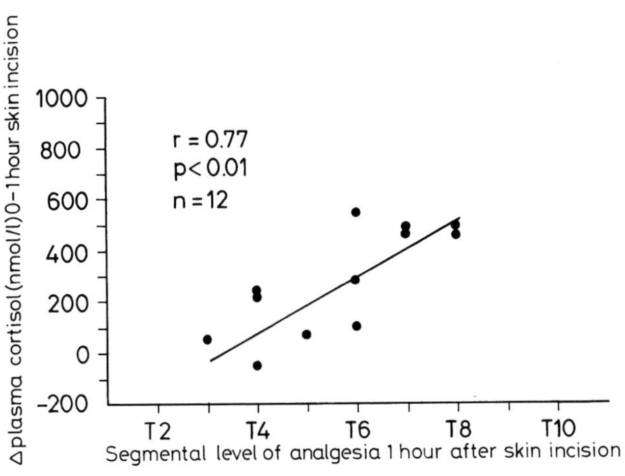

FIG. 5-15. Comparison between changes in analgesic level and plasma cortisol 1 hour after skin incision in patients undergoing abdominal hysterectomies under spinal anesthesia with 0.5% hyperbaric tetracaine or neuroleptanesthesia. Preoperative sensory level of analgesia to pinprick extended to at least T4. The results show unchanged plasma cortisol levels with maintenance of analgesic level at T4, while regression of analgesia leads to a progressive increase in plasma cortisol, in accordance with systematic studies on the influence of sensory levels of analgesia during epidural analgesia on the adrenocortical and hyperglycemic response to hysterectomy (see Fig. 5–12). (Reproduced with permission from Møller, I.W., Hjortsø, E., Krantz, T., *et al.*: The modifying effect of spinal anesthesia in intra- and postoperative adrenocortical and hyperglycemic response to surgery. Acta Anesthesiol. Scand., *28*:266, 84.)

concomitant objective assessment of the depth of neural blockade as well as stress responses. In one study during cholecystectomy the reduction of the cortisol response after epidural etidocaine 1.5% did correlate to reduction of somatosensory evoked potentals at the T10 level, but not to modification of potentials at the T6 and L1 segments.[450]

The role of sympathetic and parasympathetic stimulation in initiating the endocrine metabolic responses has been discussed above, and it appears that sympathetic blockade may be more effective than parasympathetic blockade in reducing the response. The relative efficacy of somatosensory blockade versus sympathetic blockade has not been definitely assessed, although the inhibitory effect of a splanchnic nerve blockade on plasma cortisol, glucose, and free fatty acids and urinary epinephrine excretion was almost as pronounced as found with high epidural blockade, and significantly reduced compared to general anesthesia alone.[451] However, other studies on celiac plexus block suggest that a pure sympathetic block has only a minor modulating effect on the surgical stress response,[33,219] whereas a combination of sympathetic and somatic neural blockade by celiac plexus and epidural blockade was most effective.[204] A combination of continuous wound infiltration with bupivacaine and continuous celiac plexus blockade significantly reduced the cortisol and glucose responses to upper abdominal surgery,[452] and more effectively than seen with many epidural low-dose bupivacaine studies in upper abdominal surgery (Table 5-7), although no specific comparison to epidural analgesia was performed.[452]

In contrast to most changes in adrenocortical function, the adrenal medullary and hyperglycemic responses to surgery apparently are released through both afferent and efferent neural pathways, and these responses generally are more easily inhibited. Thus several studies have shown that a neural blockade including efferent pathways to the adrenal glands (T11–L1) leads to an inhibition of the hyperglycemic response to lower abdominal surgery[30,63] and upper abdominal procedures[29,101,189,200] despite an unmodulated cortisol response. An additional factor in the reduction of the hyperglycemic response may be concomitant blockade of efferent sympathetic pathways to the liver.[102,123,463]

Spinal Analgesia versus Epidural Analgesia

Few systematic studies have been performed comparing endocrine metabolic responses to similar surgical procedures performed during either spinal (intrathecal) or epidural analgesia, except during hysterectomy, where no additional metabolic effect could be obtained by the more efficient blockade of efferent pathways with motor blockade during spinal analgesia.[63,152] In contrast, studies in major abdominal (colonic) surgery showed continuous spinal anesthesia[453] or a combined continuous spinal and epidural regimen[454] to be more effective in reducing the cortisol and glucose responses than epidural local anesthetic techniques.

Peripheral Blocks

Plasma catecholamine, glucose, and cortisol and cardiovascular responses to cataract surgery are blocked by a retrobulbar block compared to surgery during general anesthesia.[455,456] A pure somatic blockade with intercostal local anesthetic has no important effect on the surgical stress response in abdominal or thoracic procedures.[457,458] A paravertebral block did reduce classical catecholamine, cortisol, and glucose responses to cholecystectomy compared to general anesthesia alone.[459]

Influence of Duration of Neural Blockade

A single-dose neural blockade by spinal analgesia[152,184] or epidural analgesia[74] has only a short-lasting (2–5 hours) inhibitory effect on the stress response (Fig. 5-16). There is a lack of data on the effect of an intermediate blockade (6–12 hours) on later postoperative responses, but in studies with maintenance of epidural analgesia for 24 hours a prolonged effect could be demonstrated as a reduction of nitrogen loss[27] and in plasma creatinine phosphokinase[173] during the following 4 postoperative days, and the usual late postoperative changes in muscle amino acid pattern were blunted.[37] Further data are needed before any conclusion can be made on the optimal duration of the neural block to inhibit the stress response.

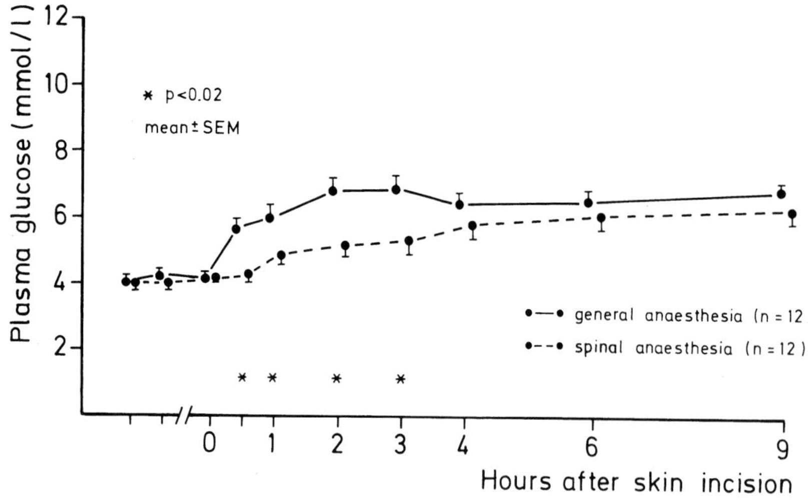

FIG. 5-16. Comparison between the hyperglycemic response to abdominal hysterectomy in patients operated on under neuroleptanesthesia or spinal anesthesia with 0.5% hyperbaric tetracaine. Sensory level of analgesia extended to at least T4 before skin incision. The results show a transient inhibition of the glucose response to surgery by spinal anesthesia, but parallel to regression of analgesia plasma glucose increased and attained levels as in the general anesthesia group 4 to 6 hours after skin incision. (Reproduced with permission from Møller, I.W., Hjortsø, E., Krantz T., *et al.*: The modifying effect of spinal anesthesia on intra-and postoperative adrenocortical and hyperglycemic response to surgery. Acta Anesthesiol. Scand., *28*:266, 1984.)

Differential Modifying Effect of Local Anesthetics

An increasing number of studies have demonstrated that the different local anesthetics may preferentially block some fibers (see Chapters 2 and 4), but no data have shown whether any single agent or a mixture of local anesthetics provides a more complete block, and thereby a more pronounced reduction of the stress response. A study in volunteers showed more pronounced reduction of cardiovascular and catecholamine responses by epidural lidocaine than by bupivacaine and 2-chloroprocaine during a cold pressor test,[321] but it is unknown if the doses given were equianesthetic.

Influence of Posttraumatic Neural Blockade

In contrast to the vast amount of data on the influence of neural blockade in abating endocrine and metabolic changes to a subsequent surgical trauma, there is a paucity of data on the influence of posttraumatic application of neural blockade. Initiation of continuous epidural analgesia 30 minutes after skin incision during abdominal hysterectomy prevented further amplification of the stress response to surgery as measured by changes in plasma cortisol and glucose, but preoperative levels in these stress parameters were not attained (Fig. 5-17).[151] Another hysterectomy study showed no differences between late (>6 hours) plasma glucose and corti-

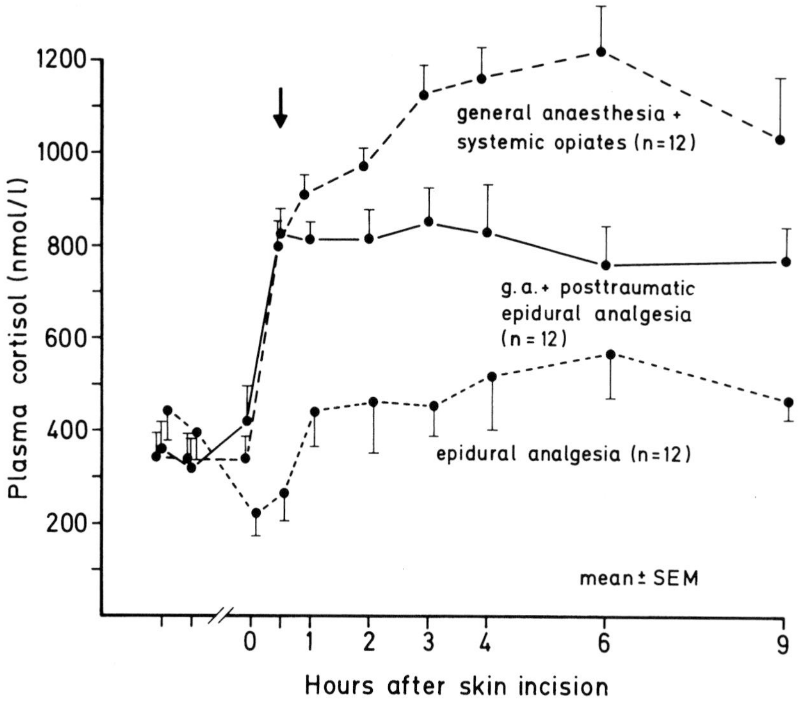

FIG. 5-17. Comparison of plasma cortisol response to abdominal hysterectomy in patients receiving general anesthesia (halothane) and systemic opiates for postoperative pain relief, and in patients receiving continuous epidural analgesia (T4 to S5) with intermittent injections of 0.5% plain bupivacaine. The third group was anesthetized with halothane but had an epidural catheter inserted before surgery; 30 minutes after skin incision an identical dose of bupivacaine (35 ml) was administered (indicated by ↓) as in the epidural group. The results show that epidural analgesia inhibits the plasma cortisol response to surgery. If administered postinjury, epidural analgesia prevented further amplification of the cortisol response, but levels did not attain preoperative levels within the 9-hour study period. Similar results were obtained by plasma glucose measurements. (Reproduced with permission from Møller, I.W., Rem, J., Brandt, M.R., and Kehlet, H.: Effect of posttraumatic epidural analgesia on the cortisol and hyperglycemic response to surgery. Acta Anesthesiol. Scand., *26*:56, 1982.)

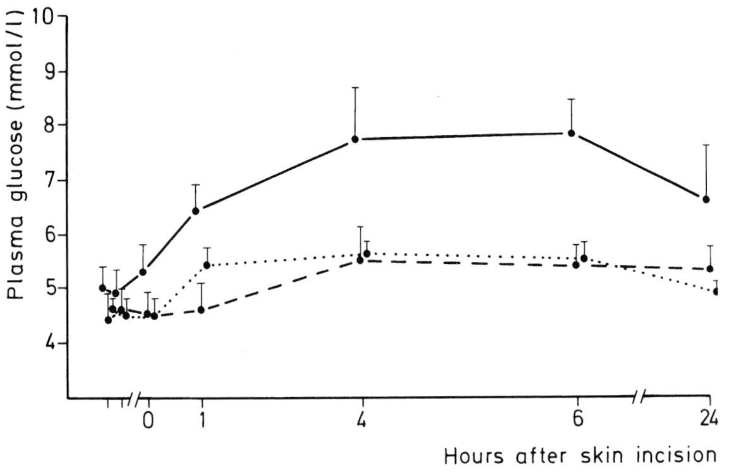

FIG. 5-18. Comparison of changes in plasma glucose in patients undergoing hip replacement who received general anesthesia (enflurane) (*unbroken line*, n = 10), general anesthesia plus epidural analgesia (T8) with intermittent injections of 0.5% plain bupivacaine for 24 hours (*broken line*, n = 10), or epidural analgesia alone (*dotted line*, n = 10) (all values mean ± SEM). The results show that usual hyperglycemic response to hip replacement is abolished by neural blockade with epidural analgesia. This reduction of the hyperglycemic response (and adrenocortical, results not shown) is independent of concomitant administration of general anesthesia. (Reproduced with permission from Riis, J., Lomholt, B., Haxholdt, O., *et al.*: Immediate and long term mental recovery from general vs epidural anesthesia in elderly patients. Acta Anaesthesiol. Scand., *27*:44, 1983.)

sol values whether a single-dose epidural bupivacaine was given before versus 30 minutes after incision.[447]

The influence of neural blockade on the stress response to accidental trauma and burn injury has not been clarified. Spinal anesthesia had no influence on the increased energy consumption in one burn patient.[221]

Modulating Effect of Combined Neural Blockade and General Anesthesia

Although neural blockade alone was used in most of the above-mentioned studies, the concomitant administration of general anesthesia has no additional inhibitory or stimulatory effects on endocrine metabolic function. Thus a pronounced inhibition of both the cortisol and hyperglycemic response to hip replacement was observed in patients receiving epidural analgesia alone or combined epidural analgesia and general anesthesia (Fig. 5-18).[177] Similarly, the intraoperative impairment in monocyte and lymphocyte function observed during general anesthesia was avoided by operating on patients during both epidural analgesia and combined epidural analgesia and general anesthesia.[95,97]

INFLUENCE OF EPIDURAL OR INTRATHECAL OPIATES ON THE STRESS RESPONSE

It is well documented that epidural or intrathecal opiate administration provides good postoperative pain relief. The modifying effect of this analgesic regimen on the stress response is less pronounced, however, compared to local anesthetics despite similar analgesia at rest with the two techniques. Thus epidural morphine or diamorphine administration had no influence on the intraoperative response in cortisol and glucose[36] and either little or no effect on postoperative responses in cortisol, glucose, and fluid and electrolyte balance following hysterectomy[36,48,106] thoracotomy[457] or abdominal surgery.[464,470,471] In abdominal aorta surgery epidural morphine (6 mg) resulted in marked reduction in plasma norepinephrine levels and hemodynamic responses, but with no effect on plasma epinephrine or arginine vasopressin levels.[428] Similarly, epidural morphine administration 4 mg twice daily for 3 days after major abdominal procedures did not reduce urinary excretion of cortisol, catecholamines, or nitrogen to any major extent, despite superior pain relief compared to intermittent systemic morphine administration.[90] These results are in contrast to other findings that epidural morphine 4 mg every 12 hours significantly reduced urinary excretion of cortisol and catecholamines, although less than following epidural local anesthetics.[336]

In a comprehensive comparison of the effect of epidural morphine versus bupivacaine and intermittent systemic morphine on the endocrine and metabolic changes following cholecystectomy, epidural morphine was less effective in reducing the stress response compared to bupivacaine, despite a similar degree of pain relief (Fig. 5-19).[101,180] Similar results were found comparing epidural bupivacaine with epidural morphine after hysterectomy[289] and gastrectomy.[336] The effect of epidural opioid on nitrogen balance is summarized in Table 5-4, and is less than observed with epidural local anesthetic.

The influence of epidural opiates on plasma ADH response to surgery is debatable because in one study fentanyl apparently reduced postoperative ADH concentrations,[19,20] while another study suggested that morphine increased ADH secretion.[120] In the latter study, however, patient groups were not comparable with regard to duration of surgery.[120]

Intrathecal diamorphine 0.5 mg/10 kg reduced plasma cortisol but not the glucose response to colonic surgery,[34] and similar results were found after intrathecal morphine 0.8 mg after upper abdominal surgery.[465]

Comparison of epidural versus systemic administration of fentanyl or alfentanil showed either no difference in plasma cortisol and catecholamine responses[466] or a more pronounced reduction in beta-endorphin, cortisol, and hyperglycemia, but not ACTH, GH, and prolactin,[467] by the epidural administration.

At present, no conclusion can be made as to a possible dif-

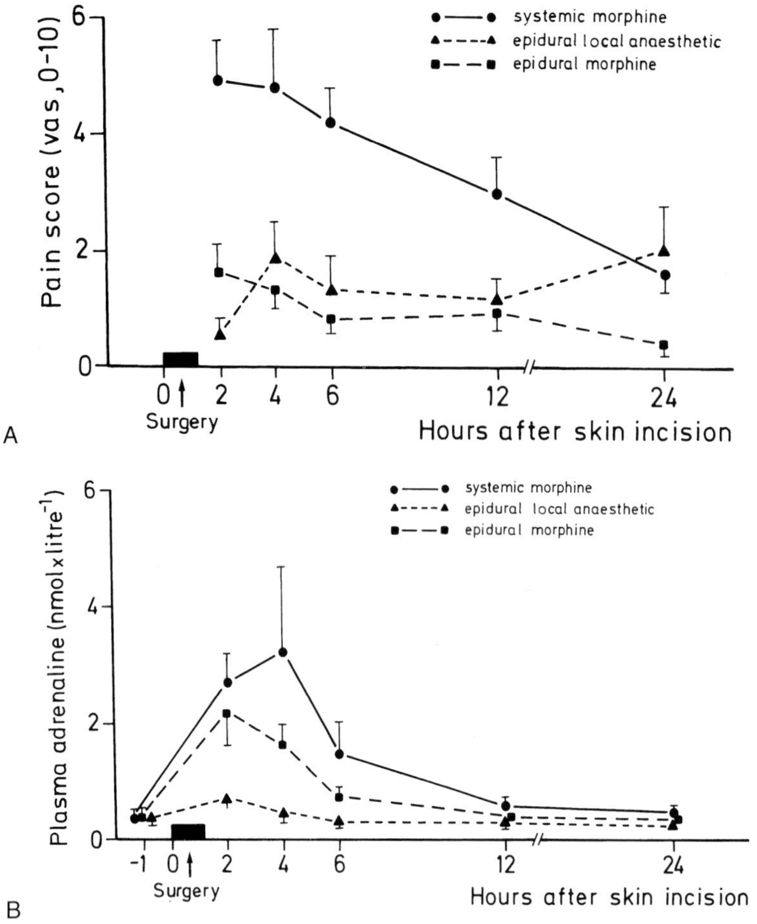

FIG. 5-19. Comparison of pain relief **(A)** and changes in plasma epinephrine **(B)** following cholecystectomy in patients receiving general anesthesia with nitrous oxide/oxygen, diazepam, and fentanyl and systemic opiates for postoperative pain relief (n = 8), general anesthesia plus epidural analgesia with 0.5% plain bupivacaine effective before surgery (T4 to L3) and continued with intermittent injections (0.25 − 0.375% bupivacaine for 24 hours) (n = 8), or general anesthesia plus epidural morphine 4 mg 1 hour before surgery and repeated every 10 hours (n = 8). The results show an improved postoperative pain relief by the two epidural regimens without differences between epidural local anesthetics and epidural morphine. Similar results were found in changes in plasma norepinephrine and in various metabolic responses (see Håkansson, E., Rutberg, H., Jorfeldt, L., and Mårtensson, J.: Effects of extradural administration of morphine or bupivacaine on the metabolic response to upper abdominal surgery. Br. J. Anesth. *57*:394, 1985). Thus epidural analgesia with morphine is less efficient in reducing the surgical stress response than are epidural local anesthetics despite similar pain relief. (Reproduced with permission from Rutberg, H., Håkansson, E., Anderberg, B., *et al.*: Effects of the extradural administration of morphine, or bupivacaine, on the endocrine response to upper abdominal surgery. Br. J. Anaesth., *56*:233, 1984.)

ferential effect of the different opiates in reducing the stress response following epidural/intrathecal administration (see also Chapter 28).

In a study comparing diamorphine with epidural somatostatin or general anesthesia alone, epidural diamorphine slightly reduced glucose responses but without effects on plasma glucagon, GH, insulin, or cortisol, while epidural somatostatin only reduced plasma GH and insulin responses compared to general anesthesia.[470]

Addition of intravenous naloxone 1 μg/kg/h reduced analgesia; also plasma cortisol and glucose concentrations were slightly reduced compared to intrathecal diamorphine without naloxone.[469]

In conclusion, epidural/intrathecal opiate administration is less efficient in reducing the surgical stress response than neural blockade techniques with local anesthetics. This is in accordance with the lack of effect of intrathecal morphine on sympathetic nerve activity, assessed by direct intraneural recordings, compared to the pronounced sympathetic blockade during spinal anesthesia with local anesthetics.[468]

Influence of Neural Blockade on Perioperative Morbidity

Despite an improved understanding of the physiologic changes resulting from anesthesia and surgery, major operative procedures may still be beset with morbidity such as myocardial infarction, pulmonary complications, thromboembolic complications, mental disturbances, and prolonged convalescence with fatigue and inability to work. It has been hypothesized that the occurrence of such complications may not necessarily be related to imperfections in surgical technique but rather to increased demands caused by the endocrine metabolic response to surgical trauma.[111] Neural blockade, which reduces the surgical stress response, may therefore be expected to mitigate some aspects of perioperative morbidity. The following sections review information available from controlled studies on the effect of neural blockade on various parameters of perioperative morbidity.

Mortality

Mortality is a well-defined end point parameter of postoperative morbidity, but the incidence of this complication is usually too low in modern anesthesia and surgery to allow any conclusion on the effect of a therapeutic regimen unless a very large number of patients are investigated. Accordingly, there is no conclusive evidence that neural blockade with local anesthetics reduces postoperative mortality following elective surgical procedures, although it certainly may be a contributing factor to reduced mortality.[426] So far, no meta-analysis on mortality has been performed in elective procedures.

In contrast, a fair amount of data has been collected from

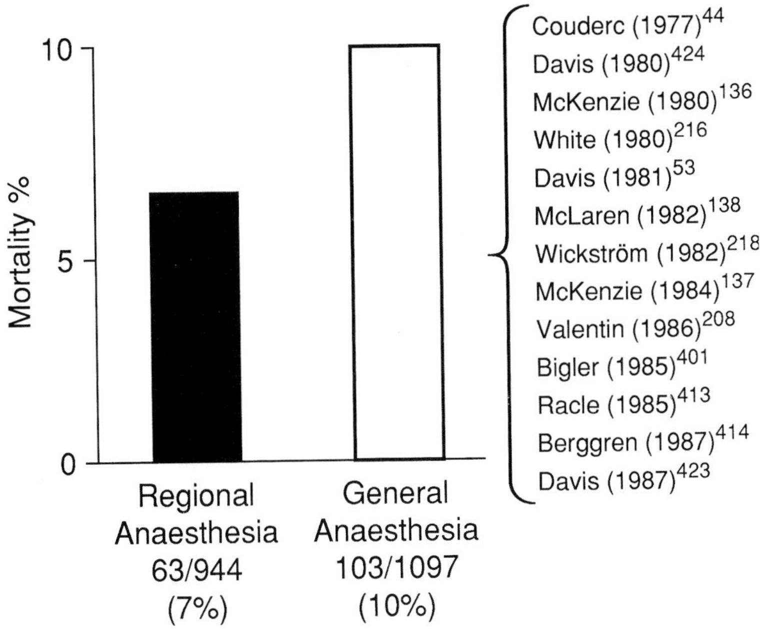

FIG. 5-20. Studies of mortality following acute hip surgery for fracture. Meta-analysis shows marginal statistically significant advantage for regional anesthesia compared to general anesthesia (see text).

patients undergoing acute hip surgery for fracture (Fig. 5-20). Although the compiled data suggest a significant reduction of mortality following surgery during regional anesthesia, a proper meta-analysis shows the advantage to be only of marginal statistical significance, and probably not clinically significant.[425] The data suggest that spinal anesthesia may be more effective than epidural analgesia, but no final conclusion can be drawn because of an inadequate number of studies using epidural anesthesia.[425]

Another reservation should be made however with regard to the influence of neural blockade on mortality following surgery for hip fracture, because follow-up in two studies[137,208] for 2 to 4 months postoperatively showed that the initial difference in mortality between neural blockade and general anesthesia disappeared (Fig. 5-21). The explanation for the identical survival rate during long-term postoperative follow-up,[137,208] despite an apparent initial reduction in mortality in patients operated on under neural blockade, is not clear. Analysis of causes of death in the reported studies is not complete, but pulmonary complications accounted for most fatalities. Retention of the potential early benefit of spinal/epidural block may depend on a vigorous program of activity/nutrition in the early postoperative phase. A large but nonrandomized study does not indicate that mortality is reduced by regional anesthesia after acute hip surgery.[460]

In summary, the only meta-analysis suggests a limited beneficial effect of regional anesthesia compared to general anesthesia on early postoperative mortality following acute surgery for hip fracture, while no similar meta-analysis data or other cumulative data are available for other procedures. These results are not unexpected since mortality depends on factors other than those influenced by regional anesthesia. Thus, further studies are needed focusing on continuous effective intra- and postoperative analgesia with neural blockade techniques combined with enforced postoperative mobilization and nutrition (see following).

Blood Loss

It is well documented that intraoperative blood loss is reduced by about 30% during elective hip replacement (Fig. 5-22). Accordingly, the need for blood transfusions was also

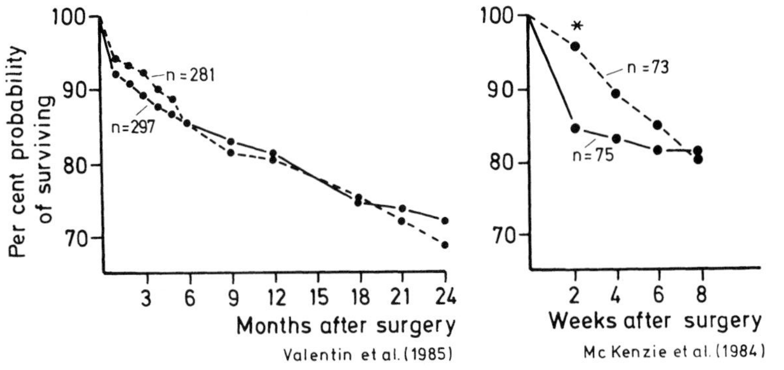

FIG. 5-21. Long-term survival in patients undergoing acute surgery for hip fracture who received spinal anesthesia or general anesthesia (controlled studies). Despite an initial reduction in early postoperative mortality (see also Table 5-7), no influence of spinal anesthesia was observed on long-term survival. (Reproduced with permission from Valentin, N., Lomholt, B., Jensen, J.S., *et al.*: Spinal or general anesthesia for surgery of the fractured hip? A prospective study of mortality in 578 patients. Br. J. Anaesth., *58*:284, 1986; and McKenzie, P.J., Wishart, H.Y., and Smith, G.: Long term outcome after repair of fractured neck of femur. Comparison of subarachnoid and general anesthesia. Br. J. Anaesth., *56*:581, 1984.)

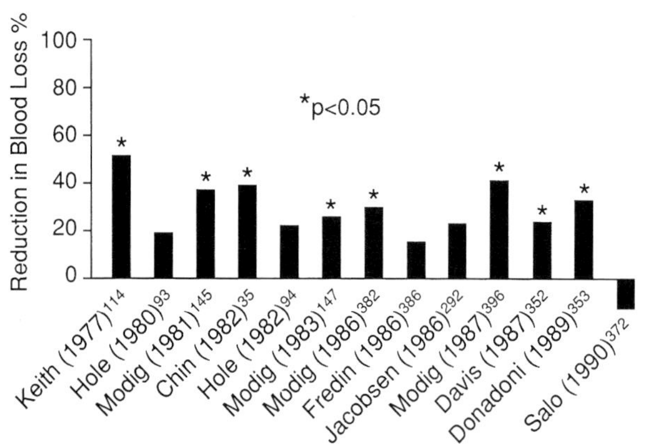

FIG. 5-22. Blood loss during elective hip replacement. Meta-analysis reveals a significant reduction in blood loss of close to 30% in patients receiving epidural analgesia.

reduced. The data are less consistent during acute surgery for hip fracture[44,53,137,208,216,425] probably because of the lower amount of blood loss during this procedure.

Neural blockade also reduced blood loss in four prostatectomy studies.[84,135,351,418]

Results from differing abdominal, gynecological, and vascular procedures are less consistent, probably because of inclusion of a variety of surgical procedures.

The mechanism of the apparent reduction in intraoperative bleeding during neural blockade is debatable.[57,419] However, hypotension is an important factor,[419–421] as well as reduction of peripheral venous pressure leading to diminished venous oozing.[419,420] During hypotensive epidural analgesia changes in cardiac output following epinephrine or phenylephrine, but with similar mean arterial pressure, did not influence intraoperative blood loss.[422] Intraoperative blood loss during hip replacement under spinal anesthesia did not increase in patients receiving epinephrine to maintain systolic arterial pressure at or above 100 mm Hg.[198] Induced hypotensive anesthesia with halothane or nitroprusside, but without regional anesthesia, also led to a similar reduction in intraoperative blood loss during hip replacement.[167,197]

Finally, continuous epidural analgesia has been reported to reduce postoperative blood loss through drains.[420]

In summary, a fair amount of data suggests that intraoperative blood loss is reduced about 30% during operations in the lower part of the body, whereas no such advantage has been demonstrated during major (upper) abdominal or thoracic procedures.

Thromboembolic Complications

The influence of neural blockade with local anesthetics on thromboembolic complications has been investigated in 13 controlled studies (Fig. 5-23). Thromboembolic complications have been verified by phlebography or ^{125}I-fibrinogen scan. In the two vascular studies,[357,380] clinical graft thrombosis was used as an indicator of thrombosis, and in two studies[147,382] additional assessments with ventilatory perfusion lung scan were done to verify pulmonary embolism. In most studies (Fig. 5-23) the control group did not receive prophylactic antithrombotic treatment, although in one of the vascular studies[380] an unknown number of patients received postoperative heparin. The results are uniform in that all six controlled studies[53,145,147,381–383] during hip surgery showed about 50% reduction in thromboembolic complications, including the risk of pulmonary embolism. Similar results were obtained during prostatectomy[84] and knee replacement.[384] In the two vascular studies,[357,380] a pronounced reduction in postoperative graft thrombosis was demonstrated in patients operated under regional anesthesia. In contrast, all three studies of abdominal surgery failed to show any effect of regional anesthesia on thromboembolic complications.[85,91,140] However, two of these studies[85,140] used thoracic epidural analgesia, and the third study[91] using an extensive intraoperative neural blockade was compared with a control group receiving prophylactic antithrombotic treatment. The relatively few studies on the influence of regional anesthesia on thromboembolic complications in different surgical operations do not resolve the issue of whether a single-dose neural blockade is inferior to a continuous epidural analgesia technique, although the latter was used in most studies. The pronounced reduction of thromboembolic complications in the two vascular studies[357,380] was observed despite the use of epidural fentanyl after the intraoperative lo-

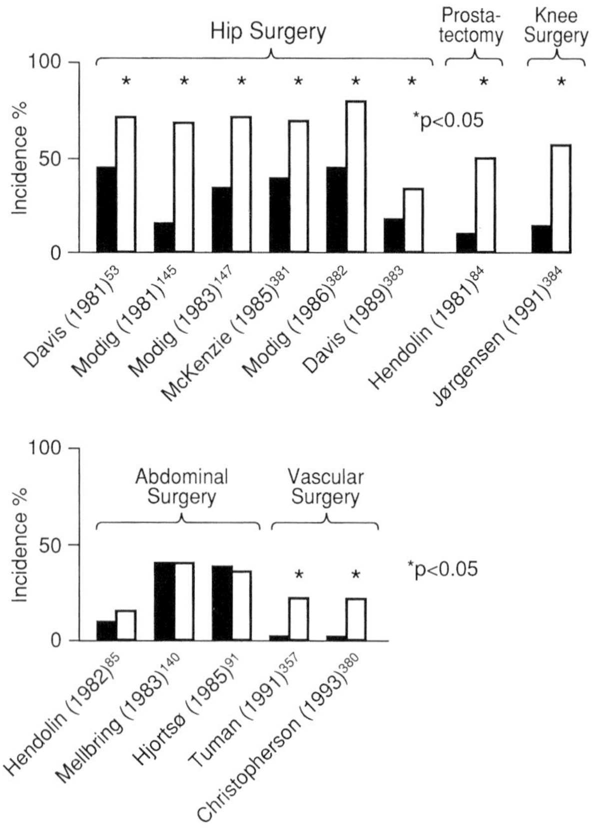

FIG. 5-23. Influence of neural blockade with local anesthetics on thromboembolic complications. Meta-analysis of 13 controlled studies (see text).

cal anesthetic blockade,[380] while the third study[357] used continuous epidural bupivacaine–morphine. From the data available, it therefore seems plausible that the intraoperative blockade, together with intraoperative anesthetic and surgical management,[474] is most important, but more data are needed on the relative influence of postoperative local anesthetics versus opioids on thromboembolic complications.

A meta-analysis from controlled studies in patients undergoing acute surgery for hip fracture showed a significant reduction of thromboembolic complications in patients operated during neural blockade compared with general anesthesia.[425]

The importance of combining regional anesthesia with other antithrombotic techniques has been poorly evaluated. No difference was observed in thromboembolism whether intraoperative epidural analgesia was combined with dextran of heparin plus dihydroergotamine[385] or whether intraoperative epidural analgesia plus stockings were combined with heparin plus dihydroergotamine versus placebo.[387] In contrast, addition of heparin to combined intraoperative epidural analgesia with stockings and aspirin reduced thromboembolism from 24% to 8%.[388] In a study of hip patients who received dextran, there was no difference in thromboembolic complications whether patients were operated on under epidural analgesia or general anesthesia.[386] Finally, additional use of pneumatic compression boots did not further reduce the low incidence of thromboembolic complications after hypotensive epidural anesthesia and aspirin.[389] Therefore, additional studies are needed to elucidate whether multiple combinations of antithrombotic prophylaxis combined with epidural techniques may further reduce or even eliminate thromboembolic complications.

The mechanism of the observed reduction in thromboembolism by neural blockade is probably a modulation of several of the factors of the triad of Virchow (see above). In addition to the mentioned favorable changes on coagulation and fibrinolysis, a pronounced increase in blood flow to the lower extremities has been demonstrated after sympathetic blockade by neural blockade with local anesthetics.[45,144,390–461,462] The effect is extended into the early postoperative period even after single-dose regional anesthesia. Also venous emptying rate and venous capacity were improved by continuous epidural analgesia.[144] A possible effect caused by a change in blood rheology[395] cannot be excluded, but the pronounced reduction in thromboembolism in lower extremities and lungs was observed without any differences in hematocrit between patients receiving neural blockade and those receiving general anesthesia.[147] Finally, experimental and *in vitro* studies have suggested that local anesthetics *per se* may influence endothelial structure (see Fig. 5-11).

Intravenous administration of lidocaine (2 mg/min) for 6 days after hip surgery has been reported to reduce thromboembolism[40] whereas administration of an oral analogue of lidocaine (tocainide) did not reduce thromboembolism after hip replacement.[146]

In summary, the favorable effects of regional anesthesia on pathogenic mechanisms of postoperative thromboembolic complications also result in a clinically important reduction in these complications.

Pulmonary Complications

It is well documented that neural blockade with local anesthetics or local anesthetic–opioid mixtures may improve several parameters of pulmonary function postoperatively (see Chapter 8). Epidural opioids alone may have a less advantageous effect compared to local anesthetics. Continuous postoperative epidural analgesia is apparently more effective than a single-dose blockade (see also Chapter 26).

There are limited data on the influence of neural blockade techniques on postoperative pulmonary (infective) complications from controlled clinical trials. In *lower* body operations such as prostatectomy,[83,199] hip replacement,[93,164] lower limb amputation,[131] and lower limb vascular surgery,[380,412] the data suggest that a reduction in pulmonary complications may be achieved by neural blockade, but a significant advantageous effect was only demonstrated in one study.[412] Obviously these preliminary data in a relatively small number of patients in a variety of surgical procedures should be further explored, since existing data are positive.

In *major* surgical procedures preliminary data from small-sized studies are inconclusive.[2,143,164,191] The compiled data from larger controlled studies do not allow a firm conclusion as to whether continuous epidural analgesia may reduce clinically relevant postoperative pulmonary complications (Table 5-8). However, the studies are relatively small and they use a variety of epidural analgesic techniques, a variable duration of analgesia, and a variety of surgical procedures. The data do not allow separation as to whether one epidural technique (i.e., local anesthetic vs. opioid) may be more effective in reducing pulmonary complications.

The use of intercostal or infiltration local anesthetic techniques may reduce the incidence of postoperative atelectasis and pulmonary complications, but the data are so far statistically inconclusive.[49,55,163,436–438] The data do not allow an analysis of whether continuous or repeated intercostal nerve block[436,438] may be more effective than single dose techniques.

In conclusion, the published data on postoperative pulmonary infective complications are insufficient to allow any conclusions as to whether neural blockade techniques may reduce this complication. However, the data from lower body procedures are most promising, which together with the well-documented improvement in postoperative pulmonary function by neural blockade emphasizes the need for further well-designed large-sized controlled clinical studies. In such studies it is important to use optimal epidural analgesic techniques with local anesthetics, and such studies should include a postoperative rehabilitation program in order to demonstrate the potential advantageous effect of ag-

TABLE 5-8. *Effect of continuous epidural analgesia on pulmonary infection after major abdominal/vascular/thoracic surgery*[a]

	Postoperative analgesic technique	Epidural analgesia	Systemic opioid
Rawal (1983)[169]	○		
Hjortsø (1985)[91]	○●		
Cuschieri (1985)[56]	●		
Yeager (1987)[435]	○	116 complications	146 complications
Hendolin (1987)[432]	●	in 545 patients	in 549 patients
Jayr (1988)[439]	○		
Seeling (1990)[295]	○●		
Tuman (1991)[357]	○●	21%	25%
Ryan (1992)[303]	●		
Kilbride (1992)[441]	○		
Davies (1993)[434]	●		
Jayr (1993)[296]	○●		$p > 0.05$

[a] Compiled data from controlled studies including more than 30 patients.
●, epidural local anesthetic; ○, epidural opioid.

gressive intra- and postoperative analgesia with neural blockade on pulmonary morbidity (see following).[305,442]

Cardiac Complications

The data on the influence of neural blockade on cardiovascular function in the perioperative period suggest that the normally increased demands are reduced (see Chap. 8), probably because of the concomitant inhibition of the sympathetic response to surgery. It might therefore be expected that neural blockade, and in particular continuous epidural analgesia with local anesthetics or mixtures of local anesthetics and opioids, may favorably affect postoperative cardiac complications, especially in high-risk patients. Unfortunately, the published studies do not allow any final conclusion on this important point.

The hypothesis that analgesia may reduce sympathetic cardiac stimulation and demands is attractive, and both systemic[427] and epidural[428,429] morphine may reduce the incidence of myocardial ischemia[427,429] and hemodynamic instability,[428] but without significant effects on clinically relevant cardiac outcome parameters (see also Chapter 8).

Single-dose epidural analgesia in high-risk surgical patients did not improve clinical cardiac outcome,[170,430,431] although intraoperative cardiovascular dysfunction was improved[170,199,431] (Fig. 5-24). The use of continuous epidural local anesthetics in low-risk patients undergoing open cholecystectomy did not reduce cardiac morbidity,[432] and intraoperative local anesthetics with continuous postoperative epidural fentanyl did not reduce cardiac morbidity in high-risk patients undergoing lower extremity vascular surgery,[380] although peripheral graft thromboembolic complications were reduced. In patients undergoing coronary artery bypass grafting, continuous epidural analgesia with local anesthetics and opioids reduced tachycardia and myocardial ischemia, but without significant positive effects on clinically relevant cardiac outcome parameters.[433]

The results from controlled studies on the effect of continuous epidural analgesic techniques on cardiac complications after major abdominal/vascular/thoracic surgery are

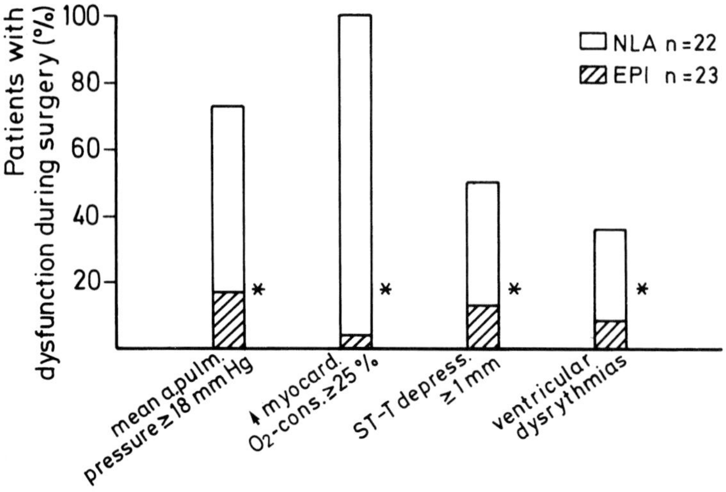

FIG. 5-24. Cardiac effects of thoracic epidural analgesia (0.5% plain bupivacaine) plus light balanced anesthesia or neuroleptanesthesia alone in patients undergoing major abdominal surgery. All patients had had a recent (less than 3 months) myocardial infarction. The results show a significant reduction in intraoperative hemodynamic, metabolic, and ECG changes in patients receiving epidural analgesia. Measurements were not performed in the postoperative period. Reinfarction rate was 1 of 23 in the epidural group and 5 of 22 in the neuroleptanesthesia group. (Modified from data by Reiz, S., Bålfors, E., Sørensen, M.B., *et al.*: Coronary hemodynamic effects of general anesthesia and surgery: Modification by epidural analgesia in patients with ischemic heart disease. Reg. Anaesth., *7*:S8, 1982.)

TABLE 5-9. *Effect of continuous epidural analgesia on cardiac complications after major abdominal/vascular/thoracic surgery*[a]

	Postoperative epidural analgesic technique	Epidural analgesia	Systemic opioid
Hjortsø (1985)[91]	●○	72 complications in 289 patients	81 complications in 307 patients
Yeager (1987)[435]	○		
Seeling (1990)[295]	●○		
Tuman (1991)[357]	●○		
Davies (1993)[434]	●		
Beattie (1993)[429]	○	25%	26%

[a] Compiled data from controlled studies including more than 30 patients.
●, epidural local anesthetic; ○, epidural opioid.

summarized in Table 5-9. It appears that the improved analgesia does not result in improved cardiac outcome based on the overall results and no positive effect was found in studies with different epidural analgesic techniques.

In summary, the well-established positive effects on cardiovascular hemodynamics of epidural analgesic techniques have so far not translated into a documented positive effect on clinically relevant cardiac outcome parameters (myocardial infarction, severe arrhythmias, death, etc.). The explanation for this is most probably that a variety of epidural techniques in a variety of surgical procedures are used. More data are needed from studies with prolonged effective epidural techniques continued into the late postoperative period in well-defined, high-risk patient groups undergoing similar types of surgery and well-defined treatment regimens for fluid replacement, oxygenation, etc.

Cerebral Complications

Postoperative impairment of mental function is a well-recognized phenomenon. The underlying mechanisms have not been completely evaluated, although old age, self-reported alcohol abuse, poor cognitive and functional status, electrolyte disturbances, hypoxemia, and psychoactive medications are most important.[142,398,399] The use of neural blockade might theoretically influence postoperative mental function by several mechanisms: (i) omission of general anesthetics may be advantageous because of their potential direct toxic effect on the cerebral cortex; and (ii) neural blockade may lower metabolic demands concomitant to inhibition of the endocrine metabolic response to surgery. Contrarily, the use of neural blockade may also adversely affect cerebral function, particularly in hypertensive patients with a blunted cerebrovascular autoregulation, although cerebral blood flow is not modified by a high spinal anesthesia in normotensive subjects.[118]

In superficial procedures with no significant surgical stress response such as eye surgery, no differences in postoperative mental dysfunction could be demonstrated between patients operated under general anesthesia and those operated under topical regional anesthesia.[102,411]

For other larger surgical procedures, predominantly major orthopedic surgery in elderly patients, much data are available from clinical randomized trials comparing cerebral outcome in patients operated on under general anesthesia and those operated on under regional anesthesia (Table 5-10). Overall, no difference has been demonstrated in cerebral outcome parameters in the reported studies. However, most of the studies have used a single dose of regional anesthesia, which may not be expected to have prolonged metabolic effects into the postoperative period. Furthermore, other pathogenic factors in postoperative cerebral dysfunction may be more important than the short-lasting metabolic effects of a single-dose regional anesthesia and the omission of general anesthesia.

In a randomized study of 60 patients undergoing bilateral knee replacement under epidural analgesia there was no difference in the incidence of postoperative delirium between patients receiving continuous combined epidural bupivacaine and fentanyl and those receiving continuous intravenous infusion of fentanyl.[416]

In conclusion, the available data do not suggest that neural blockade favorably influences postoperative mental function, but further data are needed from continuous epidural

TABLE 5-10. *Effect of regional versus general anesthesia on postoperative mental dysfunction (controlled studies)*

Improved function ($p < 0.05$)	No effect	Deteriorated function ($p < 0.05$)
Maurette (1988)[407a]	Williams-Russo (1995)[415]	Jones (1990)[409a]
Chung (1987)[402]	Crul (1992)[408]	Hughes (1988)[400a]
Racle (1986)[413]	Haan (1991)[410]	
Hole (1980)[93]	Nielson (1990)[406]	
	Asbjørn (1989)[405]	
	Chung (1989)[404]	
	Ghoneim (1988)[403]	
	Berggren (1987)[414]	
	Cook (1986)[412]	
	Bigler (1985)[401]	
	Mann (1983)[131]	
	Riis (1983)[177]	

[a] Denotes difference in one or few of the parameters studied.

techniques providing sufficient analgesia to allow restoration of various organ functions (see following).

Gastrointestinal Function

Postoperative adynamic ileus is a well-recognized problem which most often occurs after operations within the abdomen, but may also be seen after operations remote from the intestines.[5] Paralytic ileus is predominantly confined to the stomach and the colon, while the motility of the small intestine usually returns within a few hours postoperatively.[5,69] The mechanism of paralytic ileus is complex, but involves spinal sympathetic and parasympathetic afferents and inhibitory sympathetic and vagal efferents.[5,69] Assessment of postoperative gastrointestinal motility can be done by means of radiopaque markers,[275] water-soluble contrast with serial abdominal radiographs, acetaminophen absorption to assess gastric emptying, and measurements of end expiratory hydrogen concentration to assess orocecal transit time.[276,277] The time for the first passage of feces will primarily represent return of left colonic motility, which is the last to recover. The treatment of postoperative paralytic ileus by means other than neural blockade techniques has so far had very limited success.[5,154]

In studies in volunteers, epidural local anesthetics did not influence gastric emptying[276,277] or orocecal transit time.[277] In contrast, epidural morphine delays gastric emptying[276,278] as well as orocecal transit time.[278] In another study in volunteers, epidural bupivacaine had no detrimental effect on gastroduodenal motility, while epidural morphine reduced gastric emptying and orocecal transit time during fasting and after food intake.[285]

Peripheral Blocks

Neural blockade with an ileo-inguinal field block and wound infiltration has been reported to hasten postoperative oral intake after herniotomy[196] and following spinal anesthesia for lower limb amputation[131] compared with surgery under general anesthesia. Also celiac plexus blockade may reduce gastric paralysis in neurosurgical intensive care patients.[279] In contrast, a single-dose mesenteric root infiltration with bupivacaine did not improve ileus after open cholecystectomy.[280]

Epidural Opioids

The postoperative use of intrathecal or epidural opioids is expected to reduce gastrointestinal motility, but in a comparative study in adipose patients undergoing gastroplasty, epidural morphine increased the amount of gastric aspirate and reduced the time until first passage of flatus and feces.[159] In a study after cholecystectomy, gastric emptying was not different between patients receiving intrathecal morphine 0.8 mg and those receiving intramuscular papaveretum 10 mg.[183] These findings are in contrast to experimental studies which demonstrate that epidural fentanyl reduces inhibitory gastrointestinal reflexes responsible for postoperative paralytic ileus.[125] In a comparative study of epidural fentanyl given at the thoracic or lumbar level, postthoracotomy ileus was reduced by administration at the thoracic level.[184] The effect of epidural opioid administration on bile duct pressures is controversial.[209]

Based on these studies, pain relief with epidural or intrathecal opioids cannot be expected to have positive effects on postoperative ileus, while the administration of local anesthetics to inhibit gastrointestinal inhibitory reflexes may be of advantage, continuous techniques appear to be most rational. In a single-dose postcholecystectomy study, epidural morphine delayed gastric emptying in contrast to no detrimental effects after epidural bupivacaine.[298] These findings are in accordance with other studies showing enhanced postoperative gastric emptying rate following epidural bupivacaine compared to systemic opioid.[156]

Epidural Local Anesthetics

In experimental studies, epidural anesthesia has been demonstrated to accelerate recovery of postischemic bowel motility.[286]

In clinical studies, epidural local anesthetics may improve intestinal motility as assessed by an increased electrical activity over the stomach and intestines.[72] Intra-abdominal bupivacaine instillation[178] and intravenous lidocaine infusion[181] have also been reported to improve ileus after abdominal surgery.

Following radical prostatectomy there was no difference in intestinal ileus symptoms among patients receiving intraoperative epidural local anesthetics, general anesthesia with isoflurane, or combined epidural and general anesthesia, when all three groups received continuous patient-controlled epidural analgesia with a fentanyl–bupivacaine combination.[281]

The effect of continuous epidural analgesia techniques on *postlaparotomy* gastrointestinal motility has been evaluated in several controlled studies (Fig. 5-25). Thus, continuous epidural bupivacaine infusion for between 24 and 76 hours reduced gastrointestinal paralysis in five of six studies.[3,287,288,290–292] The only study[287] which showed a nonsignificant improvement in motility also was the only study to use short-term (24 hours) epidural bupivacaine. In studies comparing epidural bupivacaine versus epidural opioid or versus epidural mixtures of bupivacaine and opioid, epidural bupivacaine again shortened gastrointestinal paralysis (Fig. 5-25).[288,289,293] In studies comparing low-dose mixtures of epidural bupivacaine and opioid with epidural opioid or systemic opioid, there was either no effect on gastrointestinal paralysis or a slight improvement (Fig. 5-25).[91,293–296] It is therefore likely that addition of a small-dose opioid to a continuous epidural bupivacaine regimen may reduce some of the positive effects of the local anesthetic regimen on gastrointestinal ileus. However, uncontrolled observations with

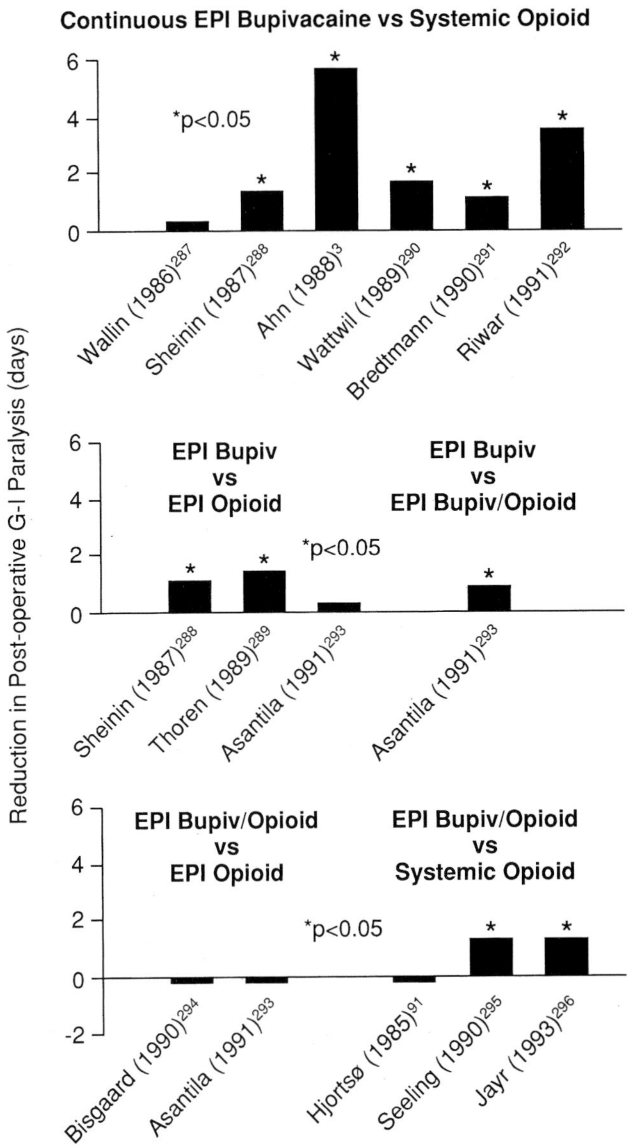

FIG. 5-25. Gastrointestinal paralysis and the effects of various epidural and systemic analgesic regimes (see text).

enforced oral nutrition during a low-dose epidural local anesthetic–morphine regimen suggest that early normalization of gastrointestinal function after colonic surgery may be attained despite the use of small amounts of epidural morphine.[297]

The effect of regional anesthetic techniques, including epidural analgesia, on postoperative nausea and vomiting has not been clarified, mostly due to the fact that the pathogenesis of postoperative nausea and vomiting is multifactorial,[65] and because most controlled studies of continuous epidural analgesia have included a limited number of patients. There are not enough well-performed controlled studies to demonstrate the preference of one opioid to another to reduce nausea and vomiting in continuous postoperative epidural regimens.

In addition to the effect on gastrointestinal motility, epidural local anesthetics may increase colonic and rectal activity and pressure with a further increase during neostigmine administration after pretreatment with atropine.[1] In experimental studies, epidural local anesthetics caused mesenteric venodilation,[299] and spinal anesthesia decreased colonic vascular resistance and increased colonic blood flow.[4] This has been confirmed in clinical studies,[132] although one study showed a decrease in superior mesenteric artery blood flow following epidural local anesthetics in patients undergoing aortofemoral reconstruction for obliterative vascular disease.[300]

It has been argued that the increased intestinal motility may be a risk factor for anastomotic breakdown, although the increase in intestinal blood flow should have a favorable effect on colonic anastomoses. Experimental studies have not shown detrimental effects on colonic blood flow, anastomotic bursting pressure, or hydroxyproline content after continuous epidural analgesia.[301] However, three cases of very early, immediate postoperative presentation of a disruption in colonic anastomosis have been reported.[12,201] These reports hardly justify the recommendation that surgery on the colon should be considered to be a relative contraindication to epidural analgesia,[201] since it is unlikely that the resulting sympatheticoly sis *per se* may trigger anastomotic breakdown. Rather, it may lead to an earlier presentation of a disruption already present and caused by failure of the surgical technique or other factors. Thus, four controlled trials after single-dose spinal anesthesia[302] or continuous epidural bupivacaine for 48 to 72 hours[291,292,303] have not demonstrated a significant risk for anastomotic dehiscence. Nevertheless, the cumulative incidence of anastomotic breakdown in the three continuous epidural bupivacaine studies[291,292,303] was 10 of 126 patients receiving epidural bupivacaine versus six of 118 patients receiving general anesthesia and systemic opioid postoperatively. Therefore, more data are needed from larger series before final conclusions can be made.

In conclusion, the available data clearly demonstrate that continuous epidural analgesia with local anesthetics improves postoperative gastrointestinal paralysis compared with pain relief with systemic opioids or epidural opioids. The limited data available suggest that a combination of epidural bupivacaine and small doses of opioid may reduce some of this advantageous effect. The enhanced normalization of postoperative gastrointestinal motility with regimens including epidural local anesthetics may facilitate early oral feeding, which otherwise has been demonstrated to reduce the risk of septic complications.[304] Continuous epidural analgesia with local anesthetics with or without additional opioids may therefore be an important method to enhance postoperative recovery of organ functions and to reduce fatigue.[305]

Convalescence, Fatigue, and Hospital Stay

Postoperative convalescence factors including hospital stay are determined by several factors independent of pain relief, neural blockade, and its potential advantageous effect on postoperative morbidity. It is therefore not unexpected that the available data from controlled clinical studies have shown inconclusive results on these parameters. Thus, intercostal blocks did not change overall hospital stay following renal surgery,[49,158] hysterectomy,[289,290] prostatectomy,[83,135,199,281] or lower limb vascular surgery.[380] Ambulation was improved by an inguinal field block in herniotomy,[196] while the data from continuous epidural analgesia in hip or knee replacement are discordant.[164,122] Small-sized abdominal surgery studies have not shown any significant effects of neural blockade techniques on hospital stay.[143,163,164] In major abdominal, vascular, or thoracic surgery, the relatively large-sized controlled studies have not demonstrated any significant advantages on hospital stay whatever the technique of epidural analgesia (Table 5-11).

The effect of neural blockade techniques on postoperative fatigue[47] is also questionable since effective epidural techniques have not been able to demonstrate significant reduction in postoperative fatigue.[91,122,182,440]

In summary, there is a need for a reconsideration of the effect of neural blockade techniques on postoperative fatigue and hospital stay; excellent perioperative care regimens with effective rehabilitation should utilize the excellent pain relief for increased activity, rather (see following) than just provide neural blockade *per se*.

Integration of Neural Blockade and Pain Relief with Postoperative Rehabilitation: A New Concept

It has generally been assumed that postoperative pain relief may reduce pulmonary, cardiovascular, thromboembolic, and other complications and may reduce hospital stay. However, as it appears from the above-mentioned review of available data from controlled clinical studies, it has not been possible to demonstrate overall important positive effects on outcome using patient-controlled analgesia, NSAIDs, epidural opioids, epidural local anesthetics, or epidural opioid–local anesthetic combinations or other neural blockade techniques. Exceptions are the positive effects of epidural or spinal local anesthetic techniques on postoperative thromboembolic complications, intraoperative blood loss in lower body procedures, and gastrointestinal ileus in abdominal procedures. The explanation for the relatively disappointing findings in major abdominal, thoracic, vascular, and other procedures during effective analgesic regimens is most probably that the provided pain relief and modification of physiological responses to surgery by neural blockade have not been used to enhance mobilization and intake of oral nutrition, that is integrated into an active rehabilitation program. Thus, the relative immobilization, which often occurs in postoperative patients despite good pain relief,[122] may enhance loss of muscle function and lead to fatigue, representing an overall hazard of hospitalization, especially in the elderly.[443] Also a conservative approach with gastrointestinal tubes and restrictions on oral intake is common clinical practice, despite the evidence that tubes have no advantages[444] and that early enteral nutrition is beneficial.[304] A significant improvement of outcome therefore requires a *combined* approach with effective pain relief and the reduction of perioperative stress responses and organ dysfunction together with active mobilization and nutrition.[498] This approach is similar to the concept of balanced or multimodal analgesia which is more effective on postoperative pain than single-modality treatment.[472]

In the future,[498] an integrated approach with intensified preoperative information, provision of effective pain relief allowing normal function, and stress reduction with neural blockade techniques will be necessary (Fig. 5-26). Together with the enforced mobilization and exercise and feeding, there may also be a place for administration of growth factors (GH or other anabolic agents) or specific nutrients (glutamine, arginine, etc.) to promote anabolism and enhanced healing in certain high-risk patients.[498] Such a strategy may seem obvious, but involves a change in several surgical and nurse traditions, as well as a change in the architecture or function of the general surgical ward, shifting from a bed-

TABLE 5-11. *Effect of continuous epidural analgesia on postoperative hospital stay (days) after major abdominal/vascular/thoracic surgery*[a]

	Epidural analgesia	Systemic opioid
Rawal (1984)[169], Yeager (1987)[435], Seeling (1990)[295], Bredtman (1990)[291], Tuman (1991)[357], Ryan (1992)[303], Davies (1993)[434], Jayr (1993)[296]	15 days	16 days
	$p > 0.05$	

[a] Mean values of compiled data from controlled studies including more than 30 patients.

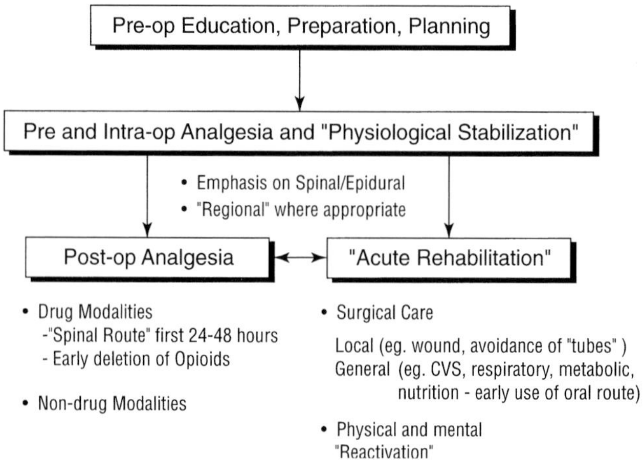

FIG. 5-26. The concept of "acute pain treatment and acute rehabilitation." The diagram emphasizes the need for an integrated approach to pain relief and acute rehabilitation, in order to return patients to normal activity as soon as possible.[498]

oriented ward to an activity-oriented ward. This approach represents an expansion of the conventional "acute-pain service" in order to draw advantages from the pain-free state achieved by neural blockade techniques, and requires an intensified collaboration between the patient, surgical nurse, surgeon, and anesthesiologist, probably within the setting of a "postoperative rehabilitation unit." So far, there are no data from controlled studies of such an approach, but preliminary data have suggested a considerable improvement in postoperative convalescence and reduction in hospital stay following hip replacement[445] and open colonic surgery[297] when a combined approach comprising optimal pain relief, enforced postoperative mobilization, and early enteral nutrition is used. A further step toward reduction of hospital stay and prevention of surgery-induced organ dysfunction is the combination of minimally invasive (laparoscopic) surgery with epidural local anesthetic blockade, enforced oral nutrition and mobilization, and avoidance of opioids to further reduce nausea, vomiting, and ileus.[498] Preliminary data in high-risk patients undergoing colonic cancer surgery suggest such an approach to be of major clinical importance, since gastrointestinal function was reestablished within 48 hours and hospital stay was reduced to 2 days, with normal convalescence and no increase in fatigue after discharge.[446]

There is a major need for further results from larger patient series in individual operations and from different institutions in order to define the role and the advantageous effects of neural blockade techniques and pain relief on outcome in such "accelerated surgical stay programs."[498]

CONCLUSIONS

In summary, this review has revealed that neural blockade with local anesthetics may diminish a predominant part of the physiological responses to surgical procedures in the lower part of the abdomen and to procedures on the lower extremities. The inhibitory effect is less pronounced during major (upper) abdominal, vascular, and thoracic procedures, probably because of insufficient afferent neural blockade by the currently available techniques. To obtain a pronounced reduction of the surgical stress response, a continuous postoperative epidural technique should be used, and probably with a continuous spinal or combined spinal/epidural technique intraoperatively in major procedures. Pain relief by epidural/intrathecal opioid administration is less efficient in reducing the stress response. On the basis of controlled studies, there is increasing evidence that neural blockade may mitigate various aspects of postoperative morbidity. However, the evidence is only convincing with regard to reduction in blood loss and thromboembolism in lower body procedures and gastrointestinal paralysis in abdominal procedures. The data from other procedures are inconclusive or show an insignificant reduction of morbidity. The studies on the effect of epidural/intrathecal opioid administration on postoperative morbidity compared to epidural local anesthetics do not allow any conclusion, but the effects will probably be less because of less modification of stress responses and organ dysfunction. Combined analgesia with epidural local anesthetic and opioids seems rational, but its superiority with regard to morbidity reduction has not been demonstrated.

Future studies should focus on an evaluation of humoral mediators on the stress response and their release and inhibitory mechanisms; an evaluation of a more selective and sufficient nociceptive blockade; and on an evaluation of the optimal duration of nociceptive blockade, in order to obtain a pronounced reduction in the surgical stress response. Studies should also focus on the effect of neural blockade on the stress response in traumatized patients.

Finally, there is a need for more controlled studies on clinical morbidity parameters where efficient analgesic techniques have been used in large patient series in well-defined surgical procedures. Such studies should also integrate the given neural blockade technique into an active rehabilitation program with enforced mobilization and nutrition in order to demonstrate potential improvement in outcome; these studies should also evaluate patients at risk for perioperative neural blockade.

REFERENCES

1. Carlstedt, A., Nordgren, S., Fasth, S., *et al.*: Epidural anesthesia and postoperative colorectal motility—A possible hazard to a colorectal anastomosis. Int. J. Colorect. Dis., *4:*144, 1989.
2. Addison, N.V., Brear, F.A., Budd, K., and Whittaker, M.: Epidural analgesia following cholecystectomy. Br. J. Surg., *61:*860, 1974.
3. Ahn, H., Andaker, L., Bronge, A., *et al.*: Effect of continuous epidural analgesia on gastrointestinal motility. Br. J. Surg., *75:*1176, 1988.
4. Aitkenhead, A.R., Gilmour, D.G., Hothersull, A.P., and Ledingham, I.M.A.: Effects of subarachnoid nerve block and arterial P_{CO_2} on colon blood flow in dog. Br. J. Anaesth., *52:*1071, 1980.
5. Livingston, E.H., and Passaro, E.P.: Postoperative ileus. Dig. Dis. Sci., *35:*121, 1990.
6. Altemeyer, K.-H., Seeling, W., Breuking, E., *et al.*: Untersuchungen zur stressreaktion bei knieoperationen unter kontinuerlicher periduralanaesthesie im vergleich zur neuroleptanalgesie. Anaesthesist, *32:*219, 1983.
7. Annamunthodo, H., Keating, V.J. and Patrick, S.J.: Liver glycogen alterations in anaesthesia. Anaesthesia, *131:*429, 1958.
8. Asoh, T., Tsuji, H., Shirasaka, C., and Takeuchi, Y.: Effect of epidural analgesia on metabolic response to major upper abdominal surgery. Acta Anaesthesiol. Scand, *27:*233, 1983.
9. Bellmann, O., and Stoeckel, H.: The influence of anaesthesia on prolactin secretion in man. *In* Stoeckel, H., and Oyama, T. (eds.): Endocrinology in Anaesthesia and Surgery, pp. 101. New York, Springer Verlag, 1980.
10. Bengtsson, M.: Changes in skin blood flow and temperature during spinal analgesia evaluated by laser Doppler flow-metry and infrared thermography. Acta Anaesthesiol. Scand., *281:*625, 1984.
11. Bessey, P.Q., Watters, J.M., Aoki, T.T., and Wilmore, D.W.: Combined hormonal infusion simulates the metabolic response to injury. Ann. Surg., *200:*264, 1984.
12. Bigler, D., Hjortsø, N.-C., and Kehlet, H.: A case of disruption of colonic anastomosis two hours postoperatively during continuous epidural analgesia. Anaesthesia, *40:*278, 1985.
13. Bigler, D., Hjortsø, N.-C., and Kehlet, H.: Variation in spread of sensory and temperature analgesia during intermittent postoperative epidural bupivacaine administration. Acta Anaesthesiol. Scand., *301:*289, 1986.
14. Bigler, D., Hjortsø, N.-C., Edstrøm, H., *et al.*: Comparative effects of intrathecal hyperbaric bupivacaine and tetracaine on sensory and cold analgesia, and cardiovascular and plasma catecholamine responses. Acta Anaesthesiol. Scand., *30:*199, 1986.

15. Blunnie, W.P., McIlroy, P.D.A., Merrett, J.D., and Dundee, J.W.: Cardiovascular and biochemical evidence of stress during major surgery associated with different techniques of anaesthesia. Br. J. Anaesth., *55:*611, 1983.
16. Bonica, J.J.: Autonomic innervation of the viscera in relation to nerve block. Anesthesiology, *29:*793, 1968.
17. Bonnet, F., Harari, A., Thibonnier, M., and Viars, P.: Suppression of antidiuretic hormone hypersecretion during surgery by extradural anaesthesia. Br. J. Anaesth., *54:*29, 1982.
18. Borg, T., and Modig, J.: Potential anti-thrombotic effects of local anaesthetics due to their inhibition of platelet aggregation. Acta Anaesthesiol. Scand., *29:*739, 1985.
19. von Bormann, B., Weidler, B., Dennhardt, R., and Hempelmann, G.: Anaesthesieverfahren und postoperative ADH-secretion. Anaesthesist, *321:*177, 1983.
20. von Bormann, B., Weidler, B., Dennhardt, R., *et al.*: Influence of fentanyl on stress-induced elevation of plasma vasopressin (ADH) after surgery. Anesth. Analg., *62:*727, 1983.
21. Boskovski, N.: The effects of epidural versus general anesthesia on perioperative water and electrolyte excretion. Reg. Anaesth., *9:*165, 1984.
22. Desborough, J.P., and Hall, G.M.: Modification of the hormonal and metabolic response to surgery by narcotics and general anaesthesia. Clin. Anaesthesiol. *3:*317, 1989.
23. Brandt, M.R., Kehlet, H., Binder, C., *et al.*: Effect of epidural analgesia on the glucoregulatory endocrine response to surgery. Clin. Endocrinol., *5:*107, 1976.
24. Brandt, M.R., Kehlet, H., Hansen, J.M., and Skovsted, L.: Serum triiodothyronine and surgery. Lancet, *1:*491, 1976.
25. Brandt, M.R., Kehlet, H., Skovsted, L., and Hansen, J.M.: Rapid decrease in plasma triiodothyronine during surgery and epidural analgesia independent of afferent neurogenic stimuli and of cortisol. Lancet, *2:*1333, 1976.
26. Brandt, M.R., Kehlet, H., Faber, O., and Binder, C.: C-peptide and insulin during blockade of the hyperglycemic response to surgery by epidural analgesia. Clin. Endocrinol., *6:*167, 1977.
27. Brandt, M.R., Fernandes, A., Mordhorst, R., and Kehlet, H.: Epidural analgesia improves postoperative nitrogen balance. Br. Med. J., *1:*1106, 1978.
28. Brandt, M.R., Ølgaard, K., and Kehlet, H.: Epidural analgesia inhibits the renin and aldosterone response to surgery. Acta Anaesthesiol. Scand., *23:*267, 1979.
29. Bromage, P.R., Shibata, H.R., and Willoughby, H.W.: Influence of prolonged epidural blockade on blood sugar and cortisol responses to operations upon the upper part of the abdomen and the thorax. Surg. Gynecol. Obstet., *132:*1051, 1971.
30. Buckley, F.P., Kehlet, H. Brown, N.S., and Scott, D.B.: Postoperative glucose tolerance during epidural analgesia. Br. J. Anaesth., *54:*325, 1982.
31. Cannon, W.B.: The Wisdom of the Body. New York, Norton, 1939.
32. Carli, F., Clark, M.M., and Wollen, J.W.: Investigation of the relationship between heat loss and nitrogen excretion in elderly patients undergoing major abdominal surgery under general anaesthesia. Br. J. Anaesth., *54:*1023, 1982.
33. Chari, P., Katariya, R.N., Dash, R.J., and Phanindranath, T.S.N.: Effect of coeliac plexus block on plasma cortisol in major abdominal surgery. Indian J. Surg., *42:*384, 1980.
34. Child, C.S., and Kaufman, L.: Effect of intrathecal diamorphine on the adrenocortical, hyperglycemic and cardiovascular responses to major colonic surgery. Br. J. Anaesth., *57:*389, 1985.
35. Chin, S.P., Abou-Madi, M.N., Eurin, B., *et al.*: Blood loss in total hip replacement. Extradural v. phenorperidine analgesia. Br. J. Anaesth., *541:*491, 1982.
36. Christensen, P., Brandt, M.R., Rem, J., and Kehlet, H.: Influence of extradural morphine on the adrenocortical and hyperglycaemic response to surgery. Br. J. Anaesth., *54:*24, 1982.
37. Christensen, T., Waaben, J., Lindeburg, T., *et al.*: Effect of epidural analgesia on plasma and muscle amino acid pattern after surgery. Acta Chir. Scand., *152:*407, 1986.
38. Cochrane, J.P.S., Forsling, M.L., Menzies Gow, N., and Le Quesne, L.P.: Arginine vasopressin release following surgical operations. Br. J. Surg., *68:*209, 1981.
39. Fong, U., and Lowry, S.F.: Cytokines and the cellular response to injury and infection. *In* Wilmore, D.W., Brennan, M.F., Harken, A.H., Holcroft, J.W., and Meakins, J.L. (eds.): Care of the Surgical Patient. New York, Scientific American, Inc., 1994.
40. Cooke, E.D., Bowcock, S.A., Lloyd, M.J., and Pilcher, M.F.: Intravenous lignocaine in prevention of deep venous thrombosis after elective hip surgery. Lancet, *2:*797, 1977.
41. Cooper, G.M., Holdcroft, A., Hall, G.M., and Alaghband-Zadeh, J.: Epidural analgesia and the metabolic response to surgery. Can. Anaesth. Soc. J., *26:*381, 1979.
42. Cort, J.H.: Relief of posttraumatic anuria. Am. J. Physiol., *164:*686, 1951.
43. Cosgrove, D.P., and Jenkins, J.S.: The effect of epidural anaesthesia on the pituitary-adrenal response to surgery. Clin. Sci. Mol. Med., *46:*403, 1974.
44. Couderc, E., Mauge, F., Duwaldstein, P., and Desmonts, J.-M.: Résultats comparatifs de l'anesthésia générale et peridurale chez le grand veillard dans lachirurgie de la hance. Anesth. Analg. Réanim., *34:*987, 1977.
45. Cousins, M.J., and Wright, C.J.: Graft, muscle and skin blood flow after epidural block in vascular surgical procedures. Surg. Gynecol. Obstet., *133:*59, 1971.
46. Cousins, M.J., and Mazze, R.I.: Anaesthesia, surgery and renal function. Anaesth. Intensive Care, *114:*355, 1973.
47. Christensen, T., and Kehlet, H.: Postoperative fatigue. World J. Surg., *17:*220, 1993.
48. Cowen, M.J., Bullingham, R.E.S., Paterson, G.M.C., *et al.*: A controlled comparison of the effects of extradural diamorphine and bupivacaine on plasma glucose and plasma cortisol in postoperative patients. Anesth. Analg., *61:*15, 1982.
49. Crawford, E.D., and Skinner, D.G.: Intercostal nerve block with thoracoabdominal and flank incision. Urology, *14:*25, 1982.
50. Crile, G.W.: Phylogenetic association in relation to certain medical problems. Boston Med. Surg. J., *631:*893, 1910.
51. Cullen, B.F., and von Belle, G.: Lymphocyte transformation and changes in leukocyte count: Effects of anesthesia and operation. Anesthesiology, *43:*563, 1975.
52. Douglas, R.G., and Shaw, J.H.F.: Metabolic response to sepsis and trauma. Br. J. Surg., *76:*115, 1989.
53. Davis, F.M., and Laurenson, V.G.: Spinal anaesthesia or general anaesthesia for emergency hip surgery in elderly patients. Anaesth. Intensive Care, *9:*352, 1981.
54. De Lalande, J.P., Le Page, J.L., Perramant, M., *et al.*: Influence of epidural analgesia on protein sparing in major visceral surgery. Ann. Fr. Anesth. Réanim., *3:*16, 1984.
55. Delilkan, A.E., Lee, C.K., Yong, N.K., *et al.*: Postoperative local analgesia for thoracotomy with direct bupivacaine intercostal blocks. Anesthesia, *281:*561, 1973.
56. Cuschieri, R.J., Morran, C.G., Howie, J.C., and McArdle, C.S.: Postoperative pain and pulmonary complications: Comparison of three analgesic regimens. Br. J. Surg., *721:*495, 1985.
57. Donald, J.R.: Induced hypotension and blood loss during surgery. J. Roy. Soc. Med., *75:*149, 1982.
58. Dworkin, L.D., Ischikawa, I., and Brenner, D.M.: Hormonal modulation of glomerular function. Am. J. Physiol., *244:*F95, 1983.
59. Ecoffey, C., Edouard, A., Pruszczynski, W., *et al.*: Effects of epidural anesthesia on catecholamines, renin activity and vasopressin changes induced by tilt in elderly men. Anesthesiology, *62:*294, 1985.
60. Edwards, A.E., Gemmel, L.W., Mankin, P.P., *et al.*: The effects of three differing anaesthetics on the immune response. Anaesthesia, *39:*1071, 1984.
61. Elfstrom, J.: Drug pharmacokinetics in the postoperative period. Clin. Pharmacokinet., *4:*16, 1979.
62. Engquist, A., Askgaard, B., and Funding, J.: Impairment of blood fibrinolytic activity during major surgical stress under combined extradural blockade and general anaesthesia. Br. J. Anaesth., *48:*903, 1976.
63. Engquist, A., Brandt, M.R., Fernandes, A., and Kehlet, H.: The blocking effect of epidural analgesia on the adrenocortical and hyperglycemic response to surgery. Acta Anaesthesiol. Scand., *21:*330, 1977.
64. Engquist, A., Fog-Møller, F., Christiansen, C., *et al.*: Influence of epidural analgesia on the catecholamine and cyclic AMP responses to surgery. Acta Anaesthesiol. Scand., *24:*17, 1980.
65. Watcha, M.F., and White, P.F.: Postoperative nausea and vomiting. Anesthesiology, *177:*162, 1992.

66. Finley, J.H., Cork, R.S., Hameroff, S.R., and Scherer, K.: Comparison of plasma beta-endorphine levels during spinal versus general anesthesia. Anesthesiology, *57:*A191, 1982.
67. Fournell, A., Wilhelmy, B., Falke, K., *et al.*: Kontinuerliche Messung der Sauerstofaufnahme bei postoperativer Periduralanalgesie. *In* Wüst, H.J., and Zindler, M. (eds.): Neue Aspekte in der Regionalanaesthesie 1. pp. 54. Berlin, Springer Verlag, 1980.
68. Fragen, R.J., Shanks, C.A., Molteni, A., and Avram, M.J.: Effects of etomidate on hormonal responses to surgical stress. Anesthesiology, *61:*652, 1984.
69. Furness, J.B., and Costa, M.: Adynamic ileus, its pathogenesis and treatment. Med. Biol., *52:*82, 1974.
70. Bessey, P.Q.: Metabolic response to critical illness. *In* Wilmore, D.W., Brennan, M.F., Harken, A.H., Holcroft, J.W., and Meakins, J.L. (eds.): Care of the Surgical Patient. New York, Scientific American, Inc., 1994.
71. Gelfand, R.A., Matthews, D.E., Bier, D.M., and Sherwin, R.S.: Role of counterregulatory hormones in the catabolic response to stress. J. Clin. Invest., *74:*2238, 1984.
72. Gelman, S., Feigenberg, Z., Dintzman, M., and Levy, E.: Electroenterography after cholecystectomy—The role of high epidural analgesia. Arch. Surg., *112:*580, 1977.
73. Gelman, S., Laws, H.L., Potzick, J., *et al.*: Thoracic epidural vs. balanced anesthesia in morbid obesity. An intraoperative and postoperative hemodynamic study. Anesth. Analg., *59:*902, 1980.
74. Gordon, N.H., Scott, D.B., and Percy Robb, I.W.: Modification of plasma corticosteroid concentrations during and after surgery by epidural blockade. Br. Med. J., *1:*581, 1973.
75. Güllner, H.-G.: Regulation of sodium and water excretion by catecholamines. Life Sci., *32:*921, 1983.
76. Hack, G., Marx, M., Witassek, F., and Vetter, H.: Zum Einfluss von Periduralanästhesie und Operation auf das Renin-Angiotensin-Aldosteron-System. *In* Wüst, H.J., and Zindler, M. (eds.): Neue Aspekte in der Regional-Anaesthesie, 1st ed. pp. 119. Berlin, Springer Verlag, 1980.
77. Hagen, C., Brandt, M.R., and Kehlet, H.: Prolactin, LH, FSH, GH and cortisol response to surgery and the effect of epidural analgesia. Acta Endocrinol., *94:*151, 1980.
78. Hallberg, D., and Orö, L.: Free fatty acids of plasma during spinal anaesthesia in man. Acta Med. Scand., *178:*281, 1965.
79. Halter, J.B., and Pfug, A.E.: Relationship of impaired insulin secretion during surgical stress to anesthesia and catecholamine release. J. Clin. Endocrinol., *51:*1093, 1980.
80. Halter, J.B., and Pflug, A.E.: Effects of anesthesia and surgical stress on insulin secretion in man. Metabolism, *29:*1124, 1980.
81. Halter, J.B., and Pflug, A.E.: Effect of sympathetic blockade by spinal anesthesia on pancreatic islet function in man. Am. J. Physiol., *239:*E151, 1980.
82. Hasselstrøm, L., Mogensen, T., Kehlet, H., and Christensen, N.J.: Effect of intravenous bupivacaine on cardiovascular function and plasma catecholamines in humans. Anesth. Analg., *63:*1053, 1984.
83. Hendolin, H.: The influence of continuous epidural analgesia and general anaesthesia on the peri- and postoperative course of patients subjected to retropubic prostatectomy. Thesis, University of Kuopio, Finland, 1980.
84. Hendolin, H., Mattila, M.A.K., and Poikolainen, E.: The effect of lumbar epidural analgesia on the development of deep vein thrombosis of the legs after open prostatectomy. Acta Chir. Scand., *147:*425, 1981.
85. Hendolin, H., Tuppurainen, T., and Lahtinen, J.: Thoracic epidural analgesia and deep vein thrombosis in cholecystectomized patients. Acta Chir. Scand., *148:*405, 1982.
86. Hendolin, H., and Länsimies, E.: Skin and central temperatures during continuous epidural analgesia and general anaesthesia in patients subjected to prostatectomy. Ann. Clin. Res., *14:*181, 1982.
87. Hendolin, H., and Penttila, I.M.: Liver enzymes after retropubic prostatectomy in patients receiving continuous lumbar epidural analgesia or general anaesthesia. Ann. Clin. Res., *14:*1, 1982.
88. Hennek, K., and Sydow, F.W.: Die thorakale Periduralanaesthesie zur intra- und postoperativen Analgesie bei Lungenresektionen. Reg. Anaesth., *7:*115, 1984.
89. Hjortsø, N.C., Andersen, T., Frøsig, F., *et al.*: Failure of epidural analgesia to modify postoperative depression of delayed hypersensitivity. Acta Anaesthesiol. Scand., *28:*128, 1984.
90. Hjortsø, N.C., Christensen, N.J., Andersen, T., and Kehlet, H.: Effects of the extradural administration of local anaesthetic agents and morphine on the urinary excretion of cortisol, catecholamines and nitrogen following abdominal surgery. Br. J. Anaesth., *57:*400, 1985.
91. Hjortsø, N.C., Andersen, T., Frøsig, F., *et al.*: Influence of epidural analgesia with local anaesthetics and morphine on morbidity after abdominal surgery. Acta Anaesthesiol. Scand., *29:*790, 1985.
92. Holdcroft, A., Hall, G.M., and Cooper, G.M.: Redistribution of body heat during anaesthesia. Anaesthesia, *34:*758, 1979.
93. Hole, A., Terjesen, T., and Breivik, H.: Epidural versus general anaesthesia for total hip arthroplasty in elderly patients. Acta Anaesthesiol. Scand., *24:*279, 1980.
94. Hole, A., Unsgaard, G., and Breivik, H.: Monocyte functions are depressed during and after surgery under general anaesthesia but not under epidural anaesthesia. Acta Anaesthesiol. Scand., *26:*301, 1982.
95. Hole, A., and Unsgaard, G.: The effect of epidural and general anaesthesia on lymphocyte functions during and after major orthopaedic surgery. Acta Anaesthesiol. Scand., *27:*135, 1983.
96. Hole, A.: Depression of monocytes and lymphocytes by stress-related humoral factors and anaesthetic-related drugs. Acta Anaesthesiol. Scand., *281:*280, 1984.
97. Hole, A.: Per- and postoperative monocyte and lymphocyte functions. Effects of combined epidural and general anaesthesia. Acta Anaesthesiol. Scand., *28:*367, 1984.
98. Hole, A., and Bakke, O.: T-lymphocytes and the subpopulations of T-helper and T-suppressor cells measured by monoclonal antibodies (T_{11}, T_4 and T_8) in relation to surgery under epidural and general anaesthesia. Acta Anaesthesiol. Scand., *28:*296, 1984.
99. Houghton, A., Hickey, J.B., Ross, S.A., and Dupre, J.: Glucose tolerance during anaesthesia and surgery. Comparison of general and extradural anaesthesia. Br. J. Anaesth., *50:*495, 1978.
100. Hume, D.M., and Egdahl, R.H.: The importance of the brain in the endocrine response to injury. Ann Surg., *150:*697, 1959.
101. Håkansson, E., Rutberg, H., Jorfeldt, L., and Martensson, J.: Effects of extradural administration of morphine or bupivacaine on the metabolic response to upper abdominal surgery. Br. J. Anaesth., *57:*394, 1985.
102. Järhult, J., Falck, B., Ingemansson, S., and Nobin, A.: The functional importance of sympathetic nerves to the liver and endocrine pancreas. Ann. Surg., *189:*96, 1979.
103. Jenkins, J., Fox, J., and Sharwood-Smith, G.: Changes in body heat during transvesical prostatectomy. Anaesthesia, *38:*748, 1983.
104. Jensen, B.H., Berthelsen, P., and Bröchner-Mortensen, J.: Glomerular filtration rate during halothane anaesthesia and epidural analgesia in combination with halothane anaesthesia. Acta Anaesthesiol. Scand., *21:*395, 1977.
105. Jensen, C.H., Berthelsen, P., Kühl, C., and Kehlet, H.: Effect of epidural analgesia on glucose tolerance during surgery. Acta Anaesthesiol. Scand., *24:*472, 1980.
106. Jørgensen, B.C., Andersen, H.B., and Engquist, A.: Influence of epidural morphine on postoperative pain, endocrine-metabolic, and renal responses to surgery: A controlled study. Acta Anaesthesiol. Scand., *26:*63, 1982.
107. Karhunen, U., and Jönn, G.: A comparison of memory function following local and general anaesthesia for extraction of senile cataract. Acta Anaesthesiol. Scand., *26:*291, 1982.
108. Kehlet, H., Brandt, M.R., Prange Hansen, A., and Alberti, K.G.M.M.: Effect of epidural analgesia on metabolic profiles during and after surgery. Br. J. Surg., *66:*543, 1979.
109. Kehlet, H.: The modifying effect of general and regional anesthesia on the endocrine-metabolic response to surgery. Reg. Anaesth., *7:*S38, 1982.
110. Kehlet, H., Wandall, J., and Hjortsø, N.C.: Influence of anesthesia and surgery on immunocompetence. Reg. Anaesth., *7:*S68, 1982.
111. Kehlet, H.: The stress response to anaesthesia and surgery: Release mechanisms and modifying factors. Clin. Anaesth., *21:*315, 1984.
112. Schulze, S., Drenck, N.E., Hjortsø, E., and Kehlet, H.: Influence of combined neural blockade, H_1 and H_2-receptor and serotonine-2 receptor blockade, indomethacin and tranexamic acid on leucocyte, temperature and acute phase protein response to surgery. Acta Chir. Scand., *154:*329, 1988.
113. Kehlet, H., and Schulze, S.: Modification of the general response to injury—Pharmacological and clinical aspects. *In* Little, R.A., and Frayn, K.N. (eds.): The Scientific Basis of Care of the Critically Ill. Manchester, Manchester University Press, 1986.

114. Keith, I.: Anaesthesia and blood loss in total hip replacement. Anaesthesia, *32:*444, 1977.
115. Kent, J.R., and Geist, S.: Lymphocyte transformation during operations with spinal anesthesia. Anesthesiology, *42:*505, 1975.
116. Deitch, E.A.: Multiple organ failure. Pathophysiology and potential future therapy. Ann. Surg., *216:*117, 1992.
117. Kirkeby, O.J., and Risöe, C.: Influence of neural pathways on the pyrexial response to surgical trauma. Acta Chir. Scand., *151:*7, 1985.
118. Kleinerman, J., Sancetta, S.M., and Hackel, D.B.: Effects of high spinal anesthesia on cerebral circulation and metabolism in man. J. Clin. Invest., *37:*285, 1958.
119. Klinck, J.R., and Lindop, M.J.: Epidural morphine in the elderly. A controlled trial after upper abdominal surgery. Anaesthesia, *37:*907, 1982.
120. Korinek, A.M., Languille, M., Bonnet, F., *et al.*: Effect of postoperative extradural morphine on ADH secretion. Br. J. Anaesth., *57:*407, 1985.
121. Kossman, B., Völk, E., and Spilker, E.D.: Influence of thoracic epidural analgesia on glucose, cortisol, insulin, and glucagon responses to surgery. Reg. Anaesth., *7:*107, 1982.
122. Møiniche, S., Hjortsø, N.-C., Hansen, B.L., *et al.*: The effect of balanced analgesia on early convalescence after major orthopedic surgery. Acta Anaesthesiol. Scand., *38:*328, 1994.
123. Lautt, W.W.: Afferent and efferent neural roles in liver function. Prog. Neurobiol., *21:*323, 1983.
124. Lamu, M., and Thijs, L.G. (eds.): Mediators of Sepsis. Update in Intensive Care and Emergency Medicine. Berlin, Springer Verlag, 1992.
125. Birch, K., Jørgensen, J., Jørgensen, B.C., and Kehlet, H.: Effect of IV lidocaine on postoperative pain and endocrine response. Br. J. Anaesth. *59:*721, 1987.
126. Weissman, C.: The metabolic response to stress: an overview and update. Anesthesiology, *73:*308, 1990.
127. Loft, S., Boel, J., Kyst, A., *et al.*: Increased hepatic microsomal enzyme activity after surgery under halothane or spinal anaesthesia. Anesthesiology, *62:*11, 1985.
128. Longnecker, D.E.: Stress free: To be or not to be? Anesthesiology, *51:*643, 1984.
129. Lush, D., Thorpe, J.N., Richardson, D.J., and Bowen, D.J.: The effect of epidural analgesia on the adrenocortical response to surgery. Br. J. Anaesth., *44:*1169, 1972.
130. Löfström, J.B., Malmquist, L.-Å., and Bengtsson, M.: Can the "sympathogalvanic reflex" (skin conductance response) be used to evaluate the height of the sympathetic block in spinal analgesia? Acta Anaesthesiol. Scand., *28:*578, 1984.
131. Mann, R.A.M., and Bisset, W.I.K.: Anaesthesia for lower limb amputation. Anaesthesia, *38:*1185, 1983.
132. Johansson, K., Ahn, H., Lindhagen, J., and Tryselius, U.: Effect of epidural anaesthesia on intestinal blood flow. Br. J. Surg., *75:*73, 1988.
133. Mather, L.E., Runciman, W.B., and Ilsley, A.H.: Anesthesia-induced changes in regional blood flow. Reg. Anaesth., *7:*S24, 1982.
134. MacGregor, R.R., Thorner, R.E., and Wright, D.M.: Lidocaine inhibits granulocyte adherence and prevents granulocyte delivery to inflammatory sites. Blood, *56:*203, 1980.
135. McGowan, S.W., and Smith, G.F.N.: Anaesthesia for transurethral prostatectomy. Anaesthesia, *35:*847, 1980.
136. McKenzie, P.J., Wishart, H.Y., Dewar, K.M.S., *et al.*: Comparison of the effects of spinal anesthesia and general anaesthesia on postoperative oxygenation and perioperative mortality. Br. J. Anaesth., *52:*49, 1980.
137. McKenzie, P.J., Wishart, H.Y., and Smith, G.: Long-term outcome after repair of fractured neck of femur. Br. J. Anaesth., *56:*581, 1984.
138. McLaren, A.D.: Mortality studies. A review. Reg. Anaesth., *7:*S172, 1982.
139. Mehta, P., Theriot, E., Mehrotra, D., *et al.*: Shivering following epidural anesthesia in obstetrics. Reg. Anaesth., *9:*83, 1984.
140. Mellbring, G., Dahlgren, S., Reiz, S., and Sunnegårdh, O.: Thromboembolic complications after major abdominal surgery: Effect of thoracic epidural analgesia. Acta. Chir. Scand., *149:*263, 1983.
141. Menzies Gow, N., and Cochrane, J.P.S.: The effect of epidural analgesia on postoperative sodium balance. Br. J. Surg., *66:*864, 1979.
142. Marcantonio, E.R., Goldman, L., Mangione, C.M., *et al.*: A clinical prediction rule for delirium after elective noncardiac surgery. J.A.M.A. *271:*134, 1994.
143. Miller, L., Gertel, M., Fox, G.S., and MacLean, L.D.: Comparison of effect of narcotic and epidural analgesia on postoperative respiratory function. Am. J. Surg., *131:*291, 1976.
144. Modig, J., Malmberg, P., and Karlström, G.: Effect of epidural versus general anaesthesia on calf blood flow. Acta Anaesthesiol. Scand., *24:*305, 1980.
145. Modig, J., Hjelmstedt, Å., Sahlstedt, B., and Maripuu, E.: Comparative influences of epidural and general anaesthesia on deep venous thrombosis and pulmonary embolism after total hip replacement. Acta Chir. Scand., *147:*125, 1981.
146. Modig, J., Borg, T., Karlström, G., *et al.*: Effects of tocainide, an oral analogue of lidocaine, on thromboembolism after total hip replacement. Ups. J. Med. Sci., *86:*269, 1981.
147. Modig, J., Borg, T., Karlström, G., *et al.*: Thromboembolism after total hip replacement. Role of epidural and general anesthesia. Anesth. Analg., *62:*174, 1983.
148. Modig, J., Borg, T., Bagge, L., and Saldeen, T.: Role of extradural and of general anaesthesia in fibrinolysis and coagulation after total hip replacement. Br. J. Anaesth., *55:*625, 1983.
149. Moore, R.A., Paterson, G.M.C., Bullingham, R.E.S., *et al.*: Controlled comparison of intrathecal cinchocaine with intrathecal cinchocaine and morphine. Br. J. Anaesth., *56:*837, 1984.
150. Moss, N.G.: Renal function of renal afferent and efferent nerve activity. Am. J. Physiol., *243:*F425, 1982.
151. Møller, I.W., Rem, J., Brandt, M.R., and Kehlet, H.: Effect of posttraumatic epidural analgesia on the cortisol and hyperglycaemic response to surgery. Acta Anaesthesiol. Scand., *26:*56, 1982.
152. Møller, I.W., Hjortsø, E., Krantz, T., *et al.*: The modifying effect of spinal anaesthesia on intra- and postoperative adrenocortical and hyperglycemic response to surgery. Acta Anaesthesiol. Scand., *28:*266, 1984.
153. Møller, I.W., Krantz, T., Wandall, E., and Kehlet, H.: Effect of alfentanil anaesthesia on the adrenocortical and hyperglycemic response to surgery. Br. J. Anaesth., *57:*591, 1985.
154. Neely, J., and Catchpole, B.: Ileus: The restoration of alimentary-tract motility by pharmacological means. Br. J. Surg., *58:*21, 1971.
155. Newsome, H.H., and Rose, J.C.: The response of human adrenocorticotropic hormone and growth hormone to surgical stress. J. Clin. Endocrinol. Metab., *33:*481, 1971.
156. Nimmo, W.S., Littlewood, D.G., Scott, D.B., and Prescott, L.F.: Gastric emptying following hysterectomy with extradural analgesia. Br. J. Anaesth., *50:*559, 1978.
157. Nistrup Madsen, S., Brandt, M.R., Engquist, A., *et al.*: Inhibition of plasma cyclic AMP, glucose and cortisol response to surgery by epidural analgesia. Br. J. Surg., *64:*669, 1977.
158. Noller, D.W., Gillenwater, J.Y., Howards, S.S., and Vaughan, E.D.: Intercostal nerve block with flank incision. J. Urol., *117:*759, 1977.
159. Oikkonen, M., Rosemberg, P.H., and Nwuvonen, P.J.: Hepatic metabolic ability during anaesthesia. Anaesthesia, *39:*660, 1984.
160. O'Shaughnessey, L., and Slome, D.: Etiology of traumatic shock. Br. J. Surg., *22:*589, 1934.
161. Oyama, T.: Influence of anaesthesia on the endocrine system. *In* Stoeckel, H., and Oyama, T. (eds.): Endocrinology in Anaesthesia and Surgery. pp. 39. Heidelberg, Springer Verlag, 1980.
162. Oyama, T., and Matsuki, A.: Plasma cortisol level during epidural anaesthesia and surgery in man. Anaesthesist, *20:*140, 1971.
163. Patel, J.M., Lanzafame, R.J., Williams, J.S., *et al.*: The effect of incisional infiltration of bupivacaine hydrochloride upon pulmonary functions, atelectasis and narcotic need following elective cholecystectomy. Surg. Gynecol. Obstet., *157:*338, 1983.
164. Pflug, A.E., Murphy, T.M., Butler, S.H., and Tucker, G.T.: The effects of postoperative peridural analgesia on pulmonary therapy and pulmonary complications. Anesthesiology, *41:*8, 1974.
165. Pflug, A.E., and Halter, J.B.: Effect of spinal anesthesia on adrenergic tone and the neuroendocrine response to surgical stress in humans. Anesthesiology, *55:*120, 1981.
166. Punnonen, R., and Viinamäki, O.: Vasopressin release following operation upon the vagina performed under general anesthesia or epidural analgesis. Surg. Gynecol. Obstet., *156:*781, 1983.
167. Qvist, T.F., Skovsted, P., and Bredgaard Sørensen, M.: Moderate hypotensive anaesthesia for reduction of blood loss during total hip replacement. Acta Anaesthesiol. Scand., *26:*351, 1982.
168. Ramus, G.V., Cesano, L., and Barbalonga, A.: Different concentrations of local anaesthetics have different modes of action on human lymphocytes. Agents Actions, *13:*333, 1983.

169. Rawal, N., Sjöstrand, U., Christoffersson, E., *et al.*: Comparison of intramuscular and epidural morphine for postoperative analgesia in the grossly obese. Anaesth. Analg., *63:*583, 1984.
170. Reiz, S., Bålfors, E., Bredgaard Sørensen, M., *et al.*: Coronary hemodynamic effects of general anesthesia and surgery. Reg. Anaesth., *7:*S8, 1982.
171. Rem, J., Kehlet, H., and Brandt, M.R.: Prevention of postoperative lymphopenia and granulocytosis by epidural analgesia. Lancet, *1:*283, 1980.
172. Rem, J., Saxtrup Nielsen, O., Brandt, M.R., and Kehlet, H.: Release mechanisms of postoperative changes in various acute phase proteins and immunoglobulins. Acta Chir. Scand. (Suppl.) *502:*51, 1980.
173. Rem, J., Møller, I.W., Brandt, M.R., and Kehlet, H.: Influence of epidural analgesia on postoperative changes in various serum enzyme patterns and serum bilirubin. Acta Anaesthesiol. Scand., *25:*142, 1981.
174. Rem, J., Feddersen, C., Brandt, M.R., and Kehlet H.: Postoperative changes in coagulation and fibrinolysis independent of neurogenic stimuli and adrenal hormones. Br. J. Surg., *68:*229, 1981.
175. Renck, H.: The elderly patient after anaesthesia and surgery. Acta Anaesthesiol. Scand., *34:*44, 1969.
176. Richard, L.C., Büller, H.R., Bovill, J., and Ten Cate, J.W.: Influence of anaesthesia on coagulation and fibrinolytic proteins. Br. J. Anaesth., *55:*869, 1983.
177. Riis, J., Lomholt, B., Haxholdt, O., *et al.*: Immediate and long-term mental recovery from general versus epidural anesthesia in elderly patients. Acta Anaesthesiol. Scand., *27:*44, 1983.
178. Rimbäck, G., Cassuto, J., Fax'en, A., *et al.*: The effect of intra-abdominal bupivacaine instillation on postoperative colonic motility. Gut, *27:*170, 1986.
179. Giesecke, K., Klingstedt, C., Ljungqvist, O., and Hagenfeld, L.: The modifying influence of anaesthesia on postoperative protein catabolism. Br. J. Anaesth., *72:*697, 1994.
180. Rutberg, H., Håkansson, E., Anderberg, B., *et al.*: Effects of extradural morphine and local anaesthetics on the endocrine response to upper abdominal surgery. Br. J. Anaesth., *56:*223, 1984.
181. Rutberg, H., Anderberg, B., Håkansson, E., *et al.*: Influence of extradural blockade on serum thyroid hormone concentrations. Acta Chir. Scand., *151:*97, 1985.
182. Zeiderman, M.R., Welchew, E.A., and Clark, R.G.: Influence of epidural analgesia upon postoperative fatigue. Br. J. Surg., *78:*1457, 1991.
183. Ryhänen, P.: Effects of anesthesia and operative surgery on the immune response of patients of different ages. Thesis, University of Oulu, Finland, 1977.
184. Sandberg, A.A., Eik-Nes, K., Samuels, L.T., and Tyler, F.H.: The effects of surgery on the blood levels and metabolism of 17-hydroxycorticosteroids in man. J. Clin. Invest., *33:*1507, 1954.
185. Saugbjerg, P., Asoh, T., Lund, C., *et al.*: Effects of epidural analgesia on scalp recorded somatosensory evoked potentials to posterior tibial nerve stimulation. Acta Anaesthesiol Scand., *30:*400, 1986.
186. Scheinin, B., and Rosenberg, P.H.: Effect of prophylactic epidural morphine or bupivacaine on postoperative pain after upper abdominal surgery. Acta Anaesthesiol. Scand., *26:*474, 1982.
187. Seeling, W., Altemeyer, K.-H., Berg, S., *et al.*: Die kontinuerliche thorakale periduralanaesthesie zur intra- und postoperativer analgesie. Anaesthesist, *31:*439, 1982.
188. Seeling, W., and Fehm, H.L.: Eine thorakale PDA mit 0,75%-igen bupivacain hat keinen einfluss auf die ACTH-stimulierte cortisolsekretion. Reg. Anaesth., *7:*11, 1984.
189. Seeling, W., Altemeyer, K.-H., Butters, M., *et al.*: Glukose ACTH, kortisol, T_4, T_3 und rT_3 in plasma nach cholecystektomie. Reg Anaesth., *7:*1, 1984.
190. Simpson, P.J., Radford, S.G., Forster, S.J., *et al.*: The fibrinolytic effects of anaesthesia. Anaesthesia, *37:*3, 1982.
191. Spence, A.A., and Smith, G.: Postoperative analgesia and lung function: A comparison of morphine with extradural block. Br. J. Anaesth., *43:*144, 1971.
192. Stanley, T.H., Hill, G.E., and Hill, H.R.: The influence of spinal and epidural anesthesia on neutrophil chemotaxis in man. Anesth. Analg., *57:*567, 1978.
193. Stefansson, T., Wickström, I., and Haljamäe, H.: Effects of neuroleptic and epidural analgesia on cardiovascular function and tissue metabolism in the geriatric patient. Acta Anaesthesiol. Scand., *261:*386, 1982.
194. Stewart, G.J.: Antithrombotic activity of local anesthetics in several canine models. Reg. Anaesth., *7:*S89, 1982.
195. Takagi, S., Kitagawa, S., Oshimi, K., *et al.*: Effect of local anaesthetics on human natural killer cell activity. Clin. Exp. Immunol., *53:*477, 1983.
196. Teasdale, C., McCrum, A., Williams, N.B., and Horton, R.E.: A randomized controlled trial to compare local with general anaesthesia for short-stay inguinal hernia repair. Ann. R. Coll. Surg. Engl., *64:*238, 1982.
197. Thompson, G.E., Miller, R.D., Stevens, W.C., and Murray, W.R.: Hypotensive anesthesia for total hip arthroplasty: A study of blood loss and organ function (brain, heart, liver and kidney). Anesthesiology, *48:*91, 1978.
198. Thorburn, J.: Subarachnoid blockade and total hip replacement; effect of epinephrine on intraoperative blood loss. Br. J. Anaesth., *57:*290, 1985.
199. Tolksdorf, W., Raiss, G., Stribel, J.-P., and Lutz, H.: Intra- und postoperative kardiopulmonale Komplikationen bei transurethralen Prostataresektionen in Intubationsnarkose und rückenmarksnaher leitungsanästhesie. *In* Wüst, H.J., and Zindler, M. (eds.). Neue Aspekte in der Regional-Anästhesie. I. pp. 146. Berlin, Springer Verlag, 1980.
200. Traynor, C., Paterson, J.L., Ward, I.D., and Hall, G.M.: Effects of extradural analgesia and vagal blockade on the metabolic and endocrine response to upper abdominal surgery. Br. J. Anaesth., *54:*319, 1982.
201. Treissmann, D.A.: Disruption of colonic anastomosis associated with epidural anesthesia. Reg. Anaesth., *5:*22, 1980.
202. Tsuji, H., and Shirasaka, C.: Inhibition of adrenergic response to upper abdominal surgery with prolonged epidural blockade. Jap. J. Surg., *12:*343, 1982.
203. Tsuji, H., Asoh, T., Takeuchi, Y., and Shirasaka, C.: Attenuation of adrenocortical response to upper abdominal surgery with epidural blockade. Br. J. Surg., *70:*122, 1983a.
204. Tsuji, H., Shirasaka, C., Asoh, T., and Takeuchi, Y.: Influences of splanchnic nerve blockade on endocrine-metabolic responses to upper abdominal surgery. Br. J. Surg., *70:*437, 1983b.
205. Tyler, E., Caldwell, C., and Ghia, J.N.: Transcutaneous electrical nerve stimulation: An alternative approach to the management of postoperative pain. Anesth. Analg., *61:*449, 1982.
206. Tönnesen, E., Hüttel, M.S., Christensen, N.J., and Schmitz, O.: Natural killer cell activity in patients undergoing upper abdominal surgery. Relationship to the endocrine stress response. Acta Anaesthesiol. Scand., *28:*654, 1984.
207. Ukai, M., Moran, W.H., and Zimmerman, B.: The role of visceral afferent pathways on vasopressin secretion and urinary excretory patterns during surgical stress. Ann. Surg., *168:*16, 1968.
208. Valentin, N., Lomholt, B., Jensen, J.S., *et al.*: Spinal or general anaesthesia for surgery of the fractured hip? Br. J. Anaesth., *58:*284, 1986.
209. Vatashsky, E., Beilin, B., and Aronson, H.B.: Common bile duct pressure in dogs after opiate injections—Epidural versus intravenous route. Can. Anaesth. Soc. J., *31:*650, 1984.
210. Vaugham, M.S., Vaugham, R.W., and Cork, R.C.: Postoperative hypothermia in adults. Relationship of age, anesthesia and shivering to rewarming. Anesth. Analg., *60:*746, 1981.
211. Verhoef, J., and Sharmu, S.D.: Inhibition of human natural killer activity by lysosomotropic agents. J. Immunol., *131:*125, 1983.
212. Wagenknecht, L.V., Zamora, M., and Madsen, P.O.: Continuous recording of renal clearance by external monitoring during epidural anesthesia. Invest. Urol., *8:*540, 1971.
213. Wagner, R.L., and White, P.F.: Etomidate inhibits adrenocortical function in surgical patients. Anesthesiology, *61:*647, 1984.
214. Webb, P.J., James, F.M., and Wheeler, A.S.: Shivering during epidural analgesia in women during labour. Anesthesiology, *55:*706, 1981.
215. Whelan, P., and Morris, P.J.: Immunological responsiveness after transurethral resection of the prostate: General versus spinal anaesthetic. Clin. Exp. Immunol., *48:*611, 1982.
216. White, I.W.C., and Chapell, W.A.: Anaesthesia for surgical correction of fractured femoral neck. A comparison of three techniques. Anaesthesia, *35:*1107, 1980.
217. White, I.W.C., Gelb, A.W., Wexler, H.R., *et al.*: The effects of intravenous anaesthetic agents on human neutrophil chemiluminescence. Can. Anaesth. Soc. J., *30:*506, 1983.
218. Wickström, I., Holmberg, I., and Stefansson, T.: Survival of female geriatric patients after hip fracture surgery. A comparison of 5 anaesthetic methods. Acta Anaesthesiol. Scand., *26:*607, 1982.

219. Wiklund, L.: Splanchnic oxygen uptake in relation to systemic oxygen uptake during postoperative splanchnic blockade and postoperative fentanyl analgesia. Acta Anaesthesiol. Scand., *19:*29, 1975.
220. Wiklund, L., and Jorfeldt, L.: Splanchnic turn-over of some energy metabolites and acid-base balance during intravenous infusion of lidocaine, bupivacaine, or etidocaine. Acta Anaesthesiol. Scand., *25:*200, 1981.
221. Wilmore, D.W.: Hormonal responses and their effect on metabolism. Surg. Clin. North Am., *56:*999, 1976.
222. Wilmore, D.W., Long, J.M., Mason, A.D., and Pruitt, B.A.: Stress in surgical patients as a neurophysiologic reflex response. Surg. Gynecol. Obstet., *142:*257, 1976.
223. Wilmore, D.E.: Catabolic illness. Strategies for enhancing recovery. N. Engl. J. Med., *325:*695, 1991.
224. Wüst, H.J., Fiedler, H.W., Trobisch, H., and Richter, O.: Fibrinolyse und Komplementsystem frofile während aortofemoraler bypassimplantation. Anaesthesist, *31:*564, 1982.
225. Yaksh, T.L., and Hammond, D.L.: Peripheral and central substrates involved in the rostrad transmission of nociceptive information. Pain, *13:*1, 1982.
226. Chernow, B., Alexander, H.R., Smallridge, R.C., *et al.*: Hormonal responses to graded surgical stress. Arch. Intern. Med., *147:*1273, 1987.
227. Beal, A.L., and Cerra, F.B.: Multiple organ failure syndrome in the 1990s. Systemic inflammatory response and organ dysfunction. J.A.M.A., *271:*226, 1994.
228. Benton, L.D., Khan, M., and Greco, R.S.: Integrins, adhesion molecules and surgical research. Surg. Gynecol. Obstet., *177:*311, 1993.
229. Moncada, S., and Higgs, A.: The L-arginine-nitric oxide pathway. N. Engl. J. Med., *329:*2002, 1993.
230. Dray, A., and Bevan, S.: Inflammation and hyperalgesia: highlighting the team effort. TiPS, *14:*287, 1993.
231. Watters, J.M., Bessey, P.Q., Dinarello, C.A., *et al.*: Both inflammatory and endocrine mediators stimulate host responses to sepsis. Arch. Surg., *121:*179, 1986.
232. Ziegler, T.R., Gatzen, C., and Willmore, D.W.: Strategies for attenuating protein-catabolic responses in the critically ill. Annu. Rev. Med., *45:*459, 1994.
233. Bent, J.M., Paterson, J.L., Machiter, K., and Hall, G.M.: Effect of high-dose fentanyl anaesthesia on the established metabolic and endocrine response to surgery. Anaesthesia, *39:*19, 1984.
234. Byrne, T.A., Morrissey, T.B., Gatzen, C., *et al.*: Anabolic therapy with growth hormone accelerates protein gain in surgical patients requiring nutritional rehabilitation. Ann. Surg., *218:*400, 1993.
235. Stein, C.: Peripheral mechanisms of opioid analgesia. Anesth. Analg., *76:*182, 1993.
236. Schulze, S., Sommer, P., Bigler, D., *et al.*: Effect of combined prednisolone, epidural analgesia and indomethacin on the systemic response after colonic surgery. Arch. Surg., *27:*325, 1992.
237. Rock, C.S., Coyle, S.M., Keogh, C.V., *et al.*: Influence of hypercortisolemia on the acute phase protein response after endotoxin in humans. Surgery, *112:*467, 1992.
238. Santos, A.A., Browning, J.L., Sheltinga, M.R., *et al.*: Are events after endotoxaemia related to circulating phospholipase-A_2? Ann. Surg., *219:*183, 1994.
239. Revhaug, A., Michie, H.R., Manson, J.M., *et al.*: Inhibition of cyclooxygenase attenuates the metabolic response to endotoxin in humans. Arch. Surg., *123:*162, 1988.
240. Michie, H.R., Majzoub, J.A., O'Dwyer, S.T., *et al.*: Both cyclooxygenase dependent and cyclooxygenase independent pathways mediate the neuroendocrine response in humans. Surgery, *108:*254, 1990.
241. Hulton, N.R., Johnson, D.J., Evans, A., *et al.*: Inhibition of prostaglandin synthesis improves postoperative nitrogen balance. Clin. Nutr., *7:*81, 1988.
242. Heindorff, H., Almdal, T., and Vilstrup, H.: Indomethacin prevents the increase in urea synthesis capacity and the weight loss after hysterectomy in rats. Clin. Nutr., *9:*103, 1990.
243. Demling, R.H., and Lalonde, C.: Tropical ibuprofen decreases early postburn edema. Surgery, *102:*857, 1987.
244. Lalonde, C., Knox, J., Daryani, R., *et al.*: Tropical flurbiprofen decreases burn wound induced hypermetabolism and systemic lipid peroxidation. Surgery, *109:*645, 1991.
245. Rockwell, W.B., and Ehrlich, H.P.: Ibuprofen in acute care therapy. Ann. Surg., *211:*78, 1990.
246. Faist, E., Ertel, W., Cohnert, T., *et al.*: Immunoprotective effects of cyclooxygenase inhibition in patients with major surgical trauma. Trauma, *30:*8, 1990.
247. Haupt, M.T., Jastremski, M.S., Clemmer, T.P., *et al.*: Effect of ibuprofen in patients with severe sepsis: A randomized double-blind multicenter study. Crit. Care Med., *19:*1339, 1991.
248. Asoh, T., Shirasaka, C., Uchida, I., and Tsuji, H.: Effects of indomethacin on endocrine responses and nitrogen loss after surgery. Ann. Surg., *206:*770, 1987.
249. Shaw, J.H.F., and Woolfe, R.R.: Metabolic intervention in surgical patients. Ann. Surg., *207:*274, 1988.
250. Engel, C., Kristensen, S.S., Axel, C., *et al.*: Indomethacin and the stress response to hysterectomy. Acta Anaesthesiol. Scand., *33:*540, 1989.
251. Jensen, A.G., Jensen, V.J., Gregersen, B., *et al.*: Influence of a single dose of indomethacin on some biochemical changes and on postoperative intestinal paralysis following minor surgery. A prospective randomized double-blind study. Acta Anaesthesiol. Scand., *34:*624, 1990.
252. Claeys, M.A., Camu, F., and Maes, V.: Prophylactic diclofenac infusions in major orthopedic surgery: effects of analgesia and acute phase proteins. Acta Anaesthesiol. Scand., *36:*270, 1992.
253. Varrassi, G., Panella, L., Piroli, A., *et al.*: The effects of perioperative ketorolac infusion on postoperative pain and endocrine metabolic response. Anesth. Analg., *78:*514, 1994.
254. Aanta, R., and Scheinin, M.: Alpha$_2$-adrenergic agents in anaesthesia. Acta Anaesthesiol. Scand., *37:*433, 1993.
255. Maze, M., and Tranquilli, W.: Alpha-2 adrenoceptor agonists: Defining the role in clinical anesthesia. Anaesthesiology, *74:*581, 1991.
256. Lund, C., Qvitzau, S., Greulich, A., *et al.*: Comparison of the effects of extradural clonidine with those of morphine on postoperative pain, stress responses, cardiopulmonary function and motor and sensory block. Br. J. Anaesth., *63:*516, 1989.
257. Aho, M., Scheinin, M., Lehtinen, A.-M., *et al.*: Intramuscularly administered dexmedetomidine attenuates hemodynamic and stress hormone responses to gynecologic laparoscopy. Anesth. Analg., *75:*932, 1992.
258. Eisenach, J.C., Lysak, S.Z., and Viscomi, C.M.: Epidural clonidine analgesia following surgery: Phase I. Anesthesiology, *71:*640, 1989.
259. Quintin, L., Roudot, F., Roux, C., *et al.*: Effect of clonidine on the circulation and vasoactive hormones after aortic surgery. Br. J. Anaesth., *66:*108, 1991.
260. Bernard, J.M., Bourréli, B., Homméril, J.L., and Pinaud, M.: Effects of oral clonidine premedication and postoperative i.v. infusion on haemodynamic and adrenergic responses during recovery from anaesthesia. Acta Anaesthesiol. Scand., *35:*54, 1991.
261. Leong, R.J., and Chernow, B.: The effects of acupuncture on operative pain and the hormonal responses to stress. Int. Anesthesiol. Clin., *26:*213, 1988.
262. Kho, H.G., van Egmond, J., Eijk, R.J.R., and Kapteyns, W.M.M.J.: Lack of influence of acupuncture and transcutaneous stimulation on the immunoglobulin levels and leucocyte counts following upper-abdominal surgery. Eur. J. Anaesthesiol., *8:*39, 1991.
263. Kho, H.G., Kloppenborg, P.W.C., and van Egmond, J.: Effects of acupuncture and transcutaneous stimulation analgesia on plasma hormone levels during and after major abdominal surgery. Eur. J. Anaesthesiol., *101:*197, 1993.
264. Sinclair, R., Cassuto, J., Högström, M., *et al.*: Topical anesthesia with lidocaine aerosol in the control of postoperative pain. Anesthesiology, *68:*895, 1988.
265. Rimbäck, G., Cassuto, J., Wallin, G., and Westlander, G.: Inhibition of peritonitis by amide local anesthetics. Anesthesiology, *69:*881, 1988.
266. Cassuto, J., Nellgård, P., Stage, L., and Jönsson, A.: Amide local anesthetics reduce albumin extravasation in burn injuries. Anesthesiology, *72:*302, 1990.
267. Rademaker, B.M.P., Sih, I.L., Kalkman, C.J., *et al.*: Effects of interpleurally administered bupivacaine 0.5% on opioid analgesic requirements and endocrine response during and after cholecystectomy: a randomized double-blind controlled study. Acta Anaesthesiol. Scand., *35:*108, 1991.
268. Scott, N.B., Mogensen, T., Bigler, D., and Kehlet, H.: Comparison of the effects of continuous intrapleural vs epidural administration of 0,5% bupivacaine on pain, metabolic response and pulmonary func-

tion following cholecystectomy. Acta Anaesthesiol. Scand., *33:*535, 1989.
269. Scott, N.B., Mogensen, T., Greulich, A., *et al.*: No effect of continuous i.p. infusion of bupivacaine on postoperative analgesia, pulmonary function and the stress response to surgery. Br. J. Anaesth., *61:*165, 1988.
270. Wallin, G.J.C., Högström, S., and Hedner, T.: Influence of intraperitoneal anaesthesia on pain and the sympathoadrenal response to abdominal surgery. Acta Anaesthesiol. Scand., *32:*553, 1988.
271. Rademaker, B.M.P., Kalkman, C.J., Odoom, J.A., *et al.*: Intraperitoneal local anaesthetics after laparoscopic cholecystectomy: effects on postoperative pain, metabolic responses and lung function. Br. J. Anaesth., *72:*263, 1994.
272. Schulze, S., Schierbeck, J., Sparsø, B.H., *et al.*: Influence of neural blockade and indomethacin on leucocyte, temperature, and acute-phase protein response to surgery. Acta Chir. Scand., *153:*255, 1987.
273. Schulze, S., Rye, B., Møller, I.W., and Kehlet, H.: Influence of local anaesthesia and local hypothermia on leucocyte, temperature and acute phase protein response to surgery. Dan. Med. Bull., *39:*86, 1992.
274. Hamid, S.K., Scott, N.B., Sutcliffe, N.P., *et al.*: Continuous coeliac plexus blockade plus intermittent wound infiltration with bupivacaine following upper abdominal surgery: a double-blind randomised study. Acta Anaesthesiol. Scand., *36:*534, 1992.
275. Tollesson, P.O., Cassuto, J., Faxén, A., and Björk, L.: A radiologic method for the study of postoperative colonic motility in humans. Scand. J. Gastroenterol., *26:*887, 1991.
276. Thorén, T., and Wattwil, M.: Effects on gastric emptying of thoracic epidural analgesia with morphine or bupivacaine. Anesth. Analg., *67:*687, 1988.
277. Thorén, T., and Wattwil, M., Järnerot, G., and Tanghöj, H.: Epidural and spinal anesthesia do not influence gastric emptying and small intestinal transit in volunteers. Reg. Anesth., *14:*35, 1989.
278. Thorén, T., Tanghöj, H., Wattwil, M., and Järnerot, G.: Epidural morphine delays gastric emptying and small intestinal transit in volunteers. Acta Anaesthesiol. Scand., *33:*174, 1989.
279. Weinstabl, C., Porges, P., Plainer, B., *et al.*: Coeliac plexus block with bupivacaine reduces intestinal dysfunction in neurosurgical ICU patients. Anaesthesia., *48:*162, 1993.
280. Carcía-Caballero, M., and Vara-Thorbeck, C.: The evolution of postoperative ileus after laparoscopic cholecystectomy. Surg. Endoscopy, *7:*416, 1993.
281. Shir, Y., Frank, S.M., Brendler, C.B., and Raja, S.N.: Postoperative morbidity is similar in patients anesthetized with epidural and general anesthesia for radical prostatectomy. Urology, *44:*232, 1994.
282. Rimbäck, G., Cassuto, J., and Tollesson, P.-O.: Treatment of postoperative paralytic ileus by intravenous lidocaine infusion. Anesth. Analg., *70:*414, 1990.
283. England, D.W., Davis, I.J., Timmins, A.E., *et al.*: Gastric emptying: a study to compare the effects of intrathecal morphine and i.m. papaveretum analgesia. Br. J. Anaesth., *59:*1403, 1987.
284. Guinard, J.-P., Mavrocordatos, P., Chiolero, R., and Carpenter, R.L.: A randomized comparison of intravenous versus lumbar and thoracic epidural fentanyl for analgesia after thoracotomy. Anesthesiology, *77:*1108, 1992.
285. Thörn, E.-E., Wattwil, M., and Källander, A.: Effects of epidural morphine and epidural bupivacaine on gastroduodenal motility during the fasted state and after food intake. Acta Anaesthesiol. Scand., *38:*57, 1994.
286. Uddasin, R., Eimerl, D., Schiffman, J., and Haskel, Y.: Epidural anesthesia accelerates the recovery of postischemic bowel motility in the rat. Anesthesiology, *80:*832, 1994.
287. Wallin, G., Cassuto, J., Högström, S., *et al.*: Failure of epidural anesthesia to prevent postoperative paralytic ileus. Anesthesiology, *65:*292, 1986.
288. Sheinin, B., Asantila, R., and Orko, R.: The effect of bupivacaine and morphine on pain and bowel function after colonic surgery. Acta Anaesthesiol. Scand., *31:*161, 1987.
289. Thorén, T., Wattwil, M., Garvill, J.-E., and Jürgensen, U.: Effects of epidural bupivacaine and morphine on bowel function and pain after hysterectomy. Acta Anaesthesiol. Scand., *33:*1181, 1989.
290. Wattwil, M., Torén, T., Hennerdal, S., and Garvill, J.-E.: Epidural analgesia with bupivacaine reduces postoperative paralytic ileus after hysterectomy. Anaesth. Analg., *68:*353, 1989.
291. Bredtman, R.D., Herden, H.N., Teichmann, W., *et al.*: Epidural analgesia in colonic surgery: results of a randomized prospective study. Br. J. Surg., *77:*638, 1990.
292. Riwar, A., Schär, B., and Grötzinger, U.: Effekt der kontinuerlichen postoperativen analgesie mit bupivacain peridural auf die darmmotilität nach kolorektalen resektionen. Helv. Chir. Acta, *58:*729, 1991.
293. Asantila, R., Eklund, P., and Rosenberg, P.H.: Continuous epidural infusion of bupivacaine and morphine for postoperative analgesia after hysterectomy. Acta Anaesthesiol. Scand., *35:*513, 1991.
294. Bisgaard, C., Mouridsen, P., and Dahl, J.B.: Continuous lumbar epidural bupivacaine plus morphine versus epidural morphine after major abdominal surgery. Eur. J Anaesthesiol., *7:*219, 1990.
295. Seeling, W., Bruckmooser, K.-P., Hüfner, C., *et al.*: Keine verminderung postoperativer Komplikationen durch Katheterepiduralanalgesie nach grossen abdominellen Eingriffen. Anaesthesis, *39:*33, 1990.
296. Jayr, C., Thomas, H., Rey, A., *et al.*: Postoperative pulmonary complications. Anesthesiology, *78:*666, 1993.
297. Møiniche, S., Bülow, S., Hesselfeldt, P., *et al.*: Convalescence and hospital stay after colonic surgery during balanced analgesia, enforced oral feeding and mobilization. Eur. J. Surg., *161:*283, 1995.
298. Thörn, S.-E., Wattwil, M., and Näslund, I.: Postoperative epidural morphine, but not epidural bupivacaine, delays gastric emptying on the first day after cholecystectomy. Reg. Anesth., *17:*91, 1992.
299. Hogan, Q.H., Stadnicka, A., Stekiel, T.A., *et al.*: Mechanism of mesenteric venodilation after epidural lidocaine in rabbits. Anesthesiology, *81:*939, 1994.
300. Lundberg, J., Lundberg, D., Norgren, L., *et al.*: Intestinal hemodynamics during laparotomy: effects of thoracic epidural anesthesia and dopamine in humans. Anesth. Analg., *71:*9, 1990.
301. Schnitzler, M., Kilbride, M.J., and Senagore, A.: Effect of epidural analgesia on colorectal anastomotic healing and colonic motility. Reg. Anesth., *17:*143, 1992.
302. Worsley, M.H., Wishart, H.Y., Peebles Brown, D.A., and Aitkenhead, A.R.: High spinal nerve block for large bowel anastomosis. Br. J. Anaesth., *60:*836, 1988.
303. Ryan, P., Schweitzer, S.A., and Woods, R.J.: Effect of epidural and general anaesthesia compared with general anaesthesia alone in large bowel anastomoses. Eur. J. Surg., *158:*45, 1992.
304. Moore, F.A., Feliciano, D.V., Andrassy, R.J., *et al.*: Early enteral feeding, compared with parenteral, reduces postoperative septic complications. The results of a meta-analysis. Ann. Surg., *216:*172, 1992.
305. Kehlet, H.: Postoperative pain relief. A look from the other side. Reg. Anesth., *19:*369, 1994.
306. Møller, I.W., Dinesen, K., Søndergaard, S., *et al.*: Effect of patient controlled analgesia on plasma catecholamines, cortisol and glucose concentration after cholecystectomy. Br. J. Anaest., *61:*160, 1988.
307. Håkansson, I., Rutberg, H., Jorfeldt, L., and Wiklund, L.: Endocrine and metabolic responses after standardized moderate surgical trauma: Influence of age and sex. Clin. Physiol., *4:*461, 1994.
308. Breslow, M.J., Parker, S.D., Frank, S.M., *et al.*: Determinants of catecholamine and cortisol responses to lower extremity revascularization. Anesthesiology, *79:*1202, 1993.
309. Carli, F.: Metabolic disturbances of hypothermia. Clin. Anaesthesiol., *3:*405, 1989.
310. Carli, F., Emery, P.W., and Freemantle, C.A.J.: Effect of perioperative normothermia on postoperative protein metabolism in elderly patients undergoing hip arthroplasty. Br. J. Anaesth., *63:*276, 1989.
311. Carli, F., and Itiaba, K.: Effect of heat conservation during and after major abdominal surgery on muscle protein breakdown in elderly patients. Br. J. Anaesth., *58:*502, 1986.
312. Carli, F., Webster, J., Nandi, P., *et al.*: Thermogenesis after surgery: effect of perioperative heat conservation and epidural anesthesia. Am. J. Physiol., *263:*E441, 1992.
313. Carli, F., Webster, J., Pearson, M., *et al.*: Postoperative protein metabolism: Effect of nursing elderly patients for 24 h after abdominal surgery in a thermoneutral environment. Br. J. Anaesth., *66:*292, 1991.
314. Wallin, G., Cassuto, J., Högström, S., *et al.*: Effects of lidocaine infusion on the sympathetic response to abdominal surgery. Anesth. Analg., *66:*1008, 1987.
315. Stevens, R.A., Artuso, J.D., Kao, T.-C., *et al.*: Changes in human plasma catecholamine concentrations during epidural anesthesia depend on the level of block. Anesthesiology, *74:*1029, 1991.
316. Hopf, H.-B., Schlaghecke, R., and Peters, J.: Sympathetic neural blockade by thoracic epidural anesthesia suppresses renin release in response to arterial hypotension. Anesthesiology, *80:*992, 1994.

317. Carp, H., Vadhera, R., Jayaram, A., and Garvey, D.: Endogenous vasopressin and renin-angiotensin systems support blood pressure after epidural block in humans. Anesthesiology, *80:*1000, 1994.
318. Stevens, R.A., Lindeberry, P.J., Arcario, T.J., *et al.*: Epidural anaesthesia attenuates the catecholamine response to hypoventilation. Can. J. Anaesth., *37:*867, 1990.
319. Peters, J., Kutkuhn, B., Merdert, H.A., *et al.*: Sympathetic blockade by epidural anesthesia attenuates the cardiovascular response to severe hypoxemia. Anesthesiology, *72:*134, 1990.
320. Shibata, K., Futagami, A., Taki, Y., and Kobayashi, T.: Epidural anesthesia modifies the cardiovascular response to marked hypercapnia in dogs. Anesthesiology, *81:*1454, 1994.
321. Stevens, R.A., Beardsley, D., White, J.L., *et al.*: Does the choice of local anesthetic affect the catecholamine response to stress during epidural anesthesia? Anesthesiology, *79:*1219, 1993.
322. Bythell, V.E., Lacoumenta, S., Breimer, L.H., *et al.*: Effects of epidural analgesia on plasma calcitonin gene-related peptide. Acta Anaesthesiol. Scand., *33:*666, 1989.
323. Magnüsson, J., Nybell-Lindahl, G., and Tranberg, K.-G.: Clearance and action of insulin during general or epidural anaesthesia. Clin. Nutr., *51:*159, 1986.
324. Noreng, M.F., Jensen, P., and Tjelldén, N.U.: Per- and postoperative changes in the concentration of serum thyreotropin under general anaesthesia, compared to general anaesthesia with epidural analgesia. Acta Anaesthesiol. Scand., *31:*292, 1987.
325. Seitz, W., Luebbe, N., Bechstein, W., *et al.*: A comparison of two types of anaesthesia on the endocrine and metabolic responses to anaesthesia and surgery. Eur. J. Anaesthesiol., *3:*283, 1986.
326. Davies, F.M., Laurenson, V.G., Lewis, J., and Wells, J.E.: Metabolic response to total hip arthroplasty under hypobaric subarachnoid or general anaesthesia. Br. J. Anaesth., *59:*725, 1987.
327. Janicki, P.K., Erskine, R., and van der Watt, M.L.: Plasma concentrations of immunoreactive beta-endorphin and substance P in patients undergoing surgery under general vs. spinal anaesthesia. Horm. Metab. Res., *25:*131, 1993.
328. Naito, Y., Tamai, S., Shingu, K., *et al.*: Responses of plasma adrenocorticotropic hormone, cortisol and cytokines during and after upper abdominal surgery. Anesthesiology, *77:*426, 1992.
329. Murat, I., Walker, J., Esteve, C., *et al.*: Effect of lumbar epidural anaesthesia on plasma cortisol levels in children. Can. J. Anaesth., *35:*20, 1988.
330. Moore, C.M., Desborough, J.P., Powell, H., *et al.*: Effects of extradural anaesthesia on interleukin-6 and acute phase response to surgery. Br. J. Anaesth., *72:*272, 1994.
331. Licker, M., Suter, P.M., Krauer, F., and Rifat, N.K.: Metabolic response to lower abdominal surgery: Analgesia by epidural blockade compared with intravenous opiate infusion. Eur. J. Anaesthesiol., *111:*193, 1994.
332. Anand, K.J., and Hickey, P.R.: Halothane—morphine compared with high-dose sufentanil for anaesthesia and postoperative analgesia in neonatal cardiac surgery. N. Engl. J. Med., *326:*1, 1992.
333. Carli, F., and Emmery, P.W.: Intraoperative epidural blockade with local anesthetics and postoperative protein breakdown associated with hip surgery in elderly patients. Acta Anaesthesiol. Scand., *34:*263, 1990.
334. Vedrinne, C., Vedrinne, J.M., Guiraud, M., *et al.*: Nitrogen sparing effect of epidural administration of local anesthetics in colon surgery. Anesth. Analg., *69:*354, 1989.
335. Carli, F., Webster, J., Pearson, M., *et al.*: Protein metabolism after abdominal surgery: effect of 24-h extradural block with local anaesthetic. Br. J. Anaesth., *69:*729, 1991.
336. Tsuji, H., Shirasaka, C., Asoh, T., and Uchida, I.: Effects of epidural administration of local anesthetics and morphine on postoperative nitrogen loss and catabolic hormones. Br. J. Surg., *74:*421, 1987.
337. Smeets, H.J., Kievit, J., Dulfer, F.T., and van Kleef, J.W.: Endocrine metabolic response to abdominal aortic surgery: A randomised trial of general anesthesia versus general plus epidural anesthesia. World J. Surg., *17:*601, 1993.
338. Shaw, J.H.F., Galler, L., Holdaway, I.M., and Holdaway, C.M.: The effect of extradural blockade upon glucose and urea kinetics in surgical patients. Surg. Gynecol. Obstet., *165:*260, 1987.
339. Bevan, D.R.: Modification of the metabolic response to trauma under extradural analgesia. Anaesthesia, *26:*188, 1971.
340. Gamulin, Z., Forster, A., Simonet, F., *et al.*: Effects of renal sympathetic blockade on renal hemodynamics in patients undergoing major aortic abdominal surgery. Anesthesiology, *65:*688, 1986.
341. Nancarrow, C., Plummer, J.L., Ilsley, A.H., *et al.*: Effects of combined extradural blockade and general anaesthesia on indocyanine green clearance and halothane metabolism. Br. J. Anaesth., *58:*29:1986.
342. Darling, J.R., Murray, J.M., Hainsworth, A.M., and Trinick, T.R.: The effect of isoflurane or spinal anesthesia on indocyanine green disappearance rate in the elderly. Anesth. Analg., *78:*706, 1994.
343. Bredahl, C., Hindsholm, K.B., and Frandsen, P.C.: Changes in body heat during hip fracture surgery: a comparison of spinal analgesia and general anaesthesia. Acta Anaesthesiol. Scand., *35:*548, 1991.
344. Sessler, D.I., and Ponte, J.: Shivering during epidural anesthesia. Anesthesiology, *72:*816, 1990.
345. Hynson, J.M., Sessler, D.I., Glosten, B., and McGuire, J.: Thermal balance and tremor patterns during epidural anesthesia. Anesthesiology, *74:*680, 1991.
346. Joris, J., Ozaki, M., Seesler, D.I., *et al.*: Epidural anesthesia impairs both central and peripheral thermoregulatory control during general anesthesia. Anesthesiology, *80:*268, 1994.
347. Frank, S.M., Beattie, C., Christopherson, R., *et al.*: Epidural versus general anesthesia, ambient operating room temperature, and patient age as predictors of inadvertent hypothermia. Anesthesiology, *77:*252, 1992.
348. Glosten, B., Sessler, D.I., Faure, E.A.M., *et al.*: Central temperature changes are poorly perceived during epidural anesthesia. Anesthesiology, *77:*10, 1992.
349. Lopez, M., Ozaki, M., Sessler, D.I., and Valdes, M.: Physiologic responses to hyperthermia during epidural anesthesia and combined epidural/enflurane anesthesia in women. Anesthesiology, *78:*1046, 1993.
350. Whelan, E., Wood, A.J.J., Shay, S., *et al.*: Lack of effect of spinal anesthesia on drug metabolism. Anesth. Analg., *69:*307, 1989.
351. Henny, C.P., Odoom, J.A., ten Cate, H., *et al.*: Effects of extradural bupivacaine on the haemostatic system. Br. J. Anaesth., *58:*301, 1986.
352. Davis, F.M., McDermott, E., Hickton, C., and Wells, E.: Influence of spinal and general anaesthesia on haemostasis during total hip arthroplasty. Br. J. Anaesth., *59:*561, 1987.
353. Donadoni, R., Baele, G., Devulder, J., and Rolly, G.: Coagulation and fibrinolytic parameters in patients undergoing total hip replacement: Influence of the anaesthesia technique. Acta Anaesthesiol. Scand., *33:*588, 1989.
354. Bredbacka, S., Blombäck, M., Hägnevik, K., and Irestedt, L.: Per- and postoperative changes in coagulation and fibrinolytic variables during abdominal hysterectomy under epidural or general anaesthesia. Acta Anaesthesiol. Scand., *30:*204, 1986.
355. Berntsen, R.F., Simonsen, T., Sager, G., and Olsen, H.: Therapeutic lidocaine concentrations have no effect on blood platelet function and plasma catecholamine levels. Eur. J. Clin. Pharmacol., *43:*109, 1992.
356. Murphy, W.G., Davies, M.J., and Eduardo, A.: The haemostatic response to surgery and trauma. Br. J. Anaesth., *70:*205, 1993.
357. Tuman, K.J., McCarthy, R.J., March, R.J., *et al.*: Effects of epidural anesthesia and analgesia on coagulation and outcome after major vascular surgery. Anesth. Analg., *73:*696, 1991.
358. Gibbs, N.M., Wrawford, G.P.M., and Michalopoulos, N.: The effect of epidural blockade on postoperative hypercoagulability following abdominal aortic bypass surgery. Anesth. Intensive Care, *201:*487, 1992.
359. Naesh, O., Hindberg, I., Friis, J., and Christiansen, C.: General versus regional anaesthesia and platelet aggregation in minor surgery. Eur. J. Anaesthesiol., *11:*169, 1994.
360. Rosenfeld, B.A., Beattie, C., Christopherson, R., *et al.*: The effect of different anesthetic regimens on fibrinolysis and the development of postoperative arterial thrombosis. Anesthesiology, *79:*435, 1993.
361. Naesh, O., Hindberg, I., Friis, J., *et al.*: Platelet activation in major surgical stress: influence of combined epidural and general anaesthesia. Acta Anaesthesiol. Scand., *38:*820, 1994.
362. Rosenfeld, B.A., Faraday, N., Campbell, D., *et al.*: Hemostatic effects of stress hormone infusion. Anesthesiology, *81:*1116, 1994.
363. Sharrock, N.E., Go, G., Mineo, R., and Harpel, P.C.: The hemodynamic and fibrinolytic response to low dose epinephrine and phenylephrine infusions during total hip replacement under epidural anesthesia. Thromb. Haemost., *68:*436, 1992.
364. Salo, M.: Effects of anaesthesia and surgery on the immune response. Acta Anaesthesiol. Scand., *36:*201, 1992.

365. Stevenson, G.W., Hall, S.C., Rudnick, S., *et al.*: The effect of anesthetic agents on the human immune response. Anesthesiology, *72:*542, 1990.
366. Rimbäck, G., Cassuto, J., Wallin, G., and Westlander, G.: Inhibition of peritonitis by amide local anesthetics. Anesthesiology, *69:*881, 1988.
367. Cederholm, I., Briheim, G., Rutberg, H., and Dahlgren, C.: Effects of five amino-amide local anaesthetic agents on human polymorphonuclear leukocytes measured by chemiluminescence. Acta Anaesthesiol. Scand., *38:*704, 1994.
368. Hammer, R., Dahlgren, C., and Stendahl, O.: Inhibition of human leukocyte metabolism and random mobility by local anaesthesia. Acta Anaesthesiol. Scand., *29:*520, 1985.
369. Salo, M.: Effects of lignocaine and bupivacaine on immunoglobulin synthesis *in vitro*. Eur. J. Anaesthesiol., *7:*133, 1990.
370. Jakobsen, B.W., Pedersen, J., and Egeberg, B.B.: Postoperative lymphocytopenia and leucocytosis after epidural and general anaesthesia. Acta Anaesthesiol. Scand., *30:*668, 1986.
371. Tønnesen, E., and Wahlgreen, C.: Influence of extradural and general anaesthesia on natural killer cell activity and lymphocyte subpopulations in patients undergoing hysterectomy. Br. J. Anaesth., *60:*500, 1988.
372. Salo, M., and Nissilä, M.: Cell-mediated and humoral immune responses to total hip replacement under spinal or general anaesthesia. Acta Anaesthesiol. Scand., *34:*241, 1990.
373. Erskine, R., Janicki, P.K., Ellis, P., and James, M.F.M.: Neutrophils from patients undergoing hip surgery exhibit enhanced movement under spinal anaesthesia compared with general anaesthesia. Can. J. Anaesth., *39:*905, 1992.
374. Wanscher, M., Antonsen, S., Toft, P., *et al.*: Attenuation of intraoperative surgical stress response has no influence on postoperative degranulation of polymorphonuclear granulocytes. Eur. J. Anaesthesiol., *8:*393, 1991.
375. Bengtson, A., Lannsjö, W., and Heideman, M.: Complement and anaphylatoxin responses to cross-clamping of the aorta. Br. J. Anaesth., *59:*1093, 1987.
376. Hesselvik, F., Brodin, B., Haåkanson, E., *et al.*: Influence of epidural blockade on postoperative plasma fibronectin concentrations. Scand. J. Clin. Invest., *47:*435, 1987.
377. Busoni, P., Sarti, A., De Martino, M., *et al.*: The effect of general and regional anesthesia on oxygen-dependent microbicidal mechanisms of polymorphonuclear leukocytes in children. Anesth. Analg., *67:*453, 1988.
378. Erskine, R., Janicki, P.K., Neil, G., and James, M.F.M.: Spinal anaesthesia but not general anaesthesia enhances neutrophil biocidal activity in hip arthroplasty patients. Can. J. Anaesth., *41:*632, 1994.
379. Toft, P., Svendsen, P., Tønnesen, E., *et al.*: Redistribution of lymphocytes after major surgical stress. Acta Anaesthesiol. Scand., *37:*245, 1993.
380. Christopherson, R., Beattie, C., Frank, S.M., *et al.*: Perioperative morbidity in patients randomized to epidural or general anesthesia for lower extremity vascular surgery. Anesthesiology, *79:*422, 1993.
381. McKenzie, P.J., Wishart, H.Y., Gray, I., and Smith, G.: Effects of anaesthetic technique on deep vein thrombosis. Br. J. Anaesth., *57:*853, 1985.
382. Modig, J., Maripuu, E., and Sahlstedt, B.: Thromboembolism following total hip replacement. A prospective investigation of 94 patients with emphasis on the efficacy of lumbar epidural anesthesia in prophylaxis. Reg. Anesth., *11:*72–79, 1986.
383. Davis, F.M., Laurenson, V.G., Gillespie, W.J., *et al.*: Deep vein thrombosis after total hip replacement. J. Bone Joint Surg., *71B:*181, 1989.
384. Jørgensen, L.N., Rasmussen, L.S., Nielsen, P.T., and Leffers, A.: Antithrombotic efficacy of continuous extradural analgesia after knee replacement. Br. J. Anaesth., *66:*8–12, 1991.
385. Fredin, H.O., Rosberg, B., Arborelius, M., and Nylander, G.: On thromboembolism after total hip replacement in epidural analgesia: A controlled study of dextran 70 and low-dose heparin combined with dihydroergotamine. Br. J. Surg., *71:*58–60, 1984.
386. Fredin, H., and Rosberg, B.: Anaesthetic techniques and thromboembolism in total hip arthroplasty. Eur. J. Anaesth., *3:*273, 1986.
387. Christensen, S.W., Wille-Jørgensen, P., Bjerg-Nielsen, A., and Kjaer, L.: Prevention of deep venous thrombosis following total hip replacement, using epidural analgesia. Acta Orthoped Belg., *55:*58, 1989.
388. Sharrock, N.E., Brien, W.W., Salvati, E.A., *et al.*: The effect of intravenous fixed-dose heparin during total hip arthroplasty on the incidence of deep-vein thrombosis. J. Bone Joint Surg., *72A:*1456, 1990.
389. Lieberman, J.R., Huo, M.M., Hanway, J., *et al.*: The prevalence of deep venous thrombosis after total hip arthroplasty with hypotensive epidural anesthesia. J Bone Joint Surg., *76A:*341, 1994.
390. Poikolainen, E., and Hendolin, E.: Effects of lumbar epidural analgesia and general anaesthesia on flow velocity in the femoral vein and postoperative deep vein thrombosis. Acta Chir. Scand., *149:*361, 1983.
391. Bowler, G.M.R., Lamont, M.C., and Scott, D.B.: Effect of extradural bupivacaine or i.v. diamorphine on calf blood flow in patients after surgery. Br. J. Anaesth., *59:*1412, 1987.
392. Perhoniemi, V., and Linko, K.: Effect of spinal versus epidural anaesthesia with 0.5% bupivacaine on lower limb blood flow. Acta Anaesthesiol. Scand., *31:*117, 1987.
393. Haljamäe, H., Frid, I., Holm, J., and Åkerström, G.: Epidural vs general anaesthesia and leg blood flow in patients with occlusive atherosclerotic disease. Eur. J. Vasc. Surg., *2:*395, 1988.
394. Davis, F.M., Laurenson, V.G., Gillespie, W.J., *et al.*: Leg blood flow during total hip replacement under spinal or general anaesthesia. Anaesth. Intensive Care, *17:*136, 1989.
395. Odoom, J.A., Bovill, J.G., Hardeman, M.R., and Oosting, J.: Effects of epidural and spinal anesthesia on blood rheology. Anesth. Analg., *74:*835, 1992.
396. Modig, J., and Karlström, G.: Intra- and postoperative blood loss and hemodynamics in total hip replacement when performed under lumbar epidural vs general anaesthesia. Eur. J. Anaesth., *4:*345, 1987.
397. Eriksson, A.S., Sinclair, R., Cassuto, J., and Thomsen, P.: Influence of lidocaine on leukocyte function in the surgical wound. Anesthesiology, *77:*74, 1992.
398. Marcantonio, E.R., Juarez, G., Goldman, L., *et al.*: The relationship of postoperative delirium with psychoactive medications. J.A.M.A., *272:*1518, 1994.
399. O'Keefe, S.T., and Chonchubhair, A.N.: Postoperative delirium in the elderly. Br. J. Anaesth., *73:*673, 1994.
400. Hughes, D., Bowes, J.B., and Brown, M.W.: Changes in memory following general or spinal anaesthesia for hip arthroplasty. Anaesthesia, *43:*114, 1988.
401. Bigler, D., Adelhøj, B., Petring, O.U., and Pedersen, N.O.: Mental function and morbidity after acute hip surgery during spinal and general anaesthesia. Anaesthesia, *40:*676, 1985.
402. Chung, F., Meier, R., Lautenschlager, E., *et al.*: General or spinal anesthesia: which is better in the elderly? Anesthesiology, *67:*422, 1987.
403. Ghoneim, M.M., Hinrichs, J.V., O'Hara, M.W., and Mehta, M.P.: Comparison of psychologic and cognitive functions after general or regional anesthesia. Anesthesiology, *69:*507, 1988.
404. Chung, F.F., Chung, A., Meier, R.H., and Lautenschlaeger, E.: Comparison of perioperative mental function after general anaesthesia and spinal anaesthesia with intravenous sedation. Can. J. Anaesth., *36:*382, 1989.
405. Asbjørn, A., Jakobsen, B.W., Pilegaard, H.K., and Blom, L.: Mental function in elderly men after surgery during epidural analgesia. Acta Anaesthesiol. Scand., *33:*369, 1989.
406. Nielson, W.R., Gelb, A.W., Casey, J.E., *et al.*: Long-term cognitive and social sequelae of general versus regional anesthesia during arthroplasty in the elderly. Anesthesiology, *73:*1103, 1990.
407. Maurette, P., Castagnera, L., Vivier, C., and Erny, P.: Répercussions comparées de l'anesthésie générale et de la rachianesthésie sur le fonctions psychiques du sujet âgé. Ann. Fr. Anesth. Réanim., *7:*305, 1988.
408. Crul, B.J., Hulstijn, W., and Burger, I.C.: Influence of the type of anaesthesia on postoperative subjective physical well-being and mental function in elderly patients. Acta Anaesthesiol. Scand., *36:*615, 1992.
409. Jones, M.J.T., Piggott, S.E., Vaughan, R.S., *et al.*: Cognitive and functional competence after anaesthesia in patients aged over 60: controlled trial of general and regional anaesthesia for elective hip or knee replacement. Br. Med. J., *300:*1683, 1990.
410. Haan, J., van Kleef, J.W., Bloem, B.R., *et al.*: Cognitive function after spinal or general anesthesia for transurethral prostatectomy in elderly men. J. Am. Geriatr. Soc., *39:*596, 1991.
411. Campbell, D.N.C., Lim, M., Muir, M.K., *et al.*: A prospective randomised study of local versus general anaesthesia for cataract surgery. Anaesthesia, *48:*422, 1993.

412. Cook, P.T., Davies, M.J., Cronin, K.D., and Moran, P.: A prospective randomised trial comparing spinal anaesthesia using hyperbaric cinchocaine with general anaesthesia for lower limb vascular surgery. Anaesth. Intensive Care, *14:*373, 1986.
413. Racle, J.P., Benkhadra, A., Poy, J.Y., Glezial, B., and Gaudray, A.: Etude comparative de l'anesthésie générale et de la rachianesthésie chez la femme âgée dans la chirurgie de la hance. Ann. Fr. Anesth. Réanim., *5:*24, 1986.
414. Berggren, D., Gustafson, Y., Eriksson, B., *et al.*: Postoperative confusion after anesthesia in elderly patients with femoral neck fractures. Anesth. Analg., *66:*497, 1987.
415. Williams-Russo, P., Sharrock, N.E., Mattis, S., *et al.*: A randomized trial of epidural versus general anesthesia for non-cardiac surgery in older adults: General anesthesia carries no additional risk for cognitive complications. J. Am. Med. Assc., *274:*44, 1995.
416. Williams-Russo, P., Urquart, B.L., Sharrock, N.E., and Charlson, M.E.: Post-operative delirium: Predictors and prognosis in elderly orthopedic patients. J. Am. Geriatr. Soc., *40:*759, 1992.
417. Zayas, V.M., Blumenfeld, J.D., Bading, B., *et al.*: Adrenergic regulation of renin secretion and renal hemodynamics during deliberate hypotension in humans. Am. J. Physiol., *265:*F686, 1993.
418. Nielsen, K.K., Andersen, K., Asbjørn, J., *et al.*: Blood loss in transurethral prostatectomy: epidural versus general anaesthesia. Int. Urol. Nephrol., *19:*287, 1987.
419. Modig, J.: Regional anaesthesia and blood loss. Acta Anaesthesiol Scand., *32* (Suppl. 89):44, 1988.
420. Modig, J., and Karlström, G.: Intra- and postoperative blood loss and haemodynamics in total hip replacement when performed under lumbar epidural versus general anaesthesia. Eur. J. Anaesthesiol., *4:*345, 1987.
421. Sharrock, N.E., Mineo, R., Urquhart, B., and Salvati, E.A.: The effect of two levels of hypotension on intraoperative blood loss during total hip arthroplasty performed under lumbar epidural anesthesia. Anesth. Analg., *76:*580, 1993.
422. Sharrock, N.E., Mineo, R., and George, B.S.: The effect of cardiac output on intraoperative blood loss during total hip arthroplasty. Reg. Anesth., *18:*24, 1993.
423. Davies, F.M., Woolner, D.F., Frampton, C., *et al.*: Prospective, multicenter trial of mortality following general or spinal anesthesia for hip fracture in elderly. Br. J. Anaesth., *59:*280, 1987.
424. Davies, F.M., Quince, M., and Laurenson, W.G.: Deep vein thrombosis and anaesthetic technique in emergency hip surgery. Br. Med. J., *281:*1528, 1980.
425. Sorenson, R.M., and Nathan, L.P.: Anesthetic techniques during surgical repair of femoral neck fractures. Anesthesiology, *77:*1095, 1992.
426. Sharrock, N.E., Cazan, M.G., Hargett, M.J.L., *et al.*: Changes in mortality after total hip and knee arthroplasty over a ten-year period. Anesth. Analg., *80:*242, 1995.
427. Mangano, D.T., Siliciano, D., Hollenberg, M., *et al.*: Postoperative myocardial ischemia. Anesthesiology, *76:*342, 1992.
428. Breslow, M.J., Jordan, D.A., Christopherson, R., *et al.*: Epidural morphine decreases postoperative hypertension by attenuating sympathetic nervous system hyperactivity. J.A.M.A., *261:*3577, 1989.
429. Beattie, W.S., Normal, D., and Forrest, J.B.: Epidural morphine reduces the risk of postoperative myocardial ischaemia in patients with cardiac risk factors. Can. J. Anaesth., *40*,532,1993.
430. Baron, J-F., Bertrand, M., Barré, E., *et al.*: Combined epidural and general anesthesia versus general anesthesia for abdominal aortic surgery. Anesthesiology, *75:*611, 1991.
431. Reinhart, K., Foehring, U., Kasting, T., *et al.*: Effects of thoracic epidural anesthesia on systemic haemodynamic function and systemic oxygen supply–demand relationship. Anaesth. Analg., *69:*360, 1989.
432. Hendolin, H., Lahtinen, J., Länsimies, E., and Tuppurainen, T.: The effect of thoracic epidural analgesia on postoperative stress and morbidity. Ann. Chir. Gynaecol., *76:*234, 1987.
433. Liem, T.H., Hasenbos, M.A.W.M., Booij, L.H.D.J., and Gielen, M.J.M.: Coronary artery bypass grafting using two different anesthetic techniques: Part 2: Postoperative outcome. J. Cardiothorac. Vasc. Anesth., *6:*156, 1992.
434. Davies, M.J., Silbert, B.S., Mooney, P.J., *et al.*: Combined epidural and general anaesthesia versus general anaesthesia for abdominal aortic surgery: A prospective randomised trial. Anaesth. Intensive Care, *21:*790, 1993.
435. Yeager, M.P., Glass, D., Neff, R.K., and Brinck-Johnsen, T.: Epidural anesthesia and analgesia in high-risk surgical patients. Anesthesiology, *66:*729, 1987.
436. Engberg, G., and Wiklund, L.: Pulmonary complications after upper abdominal surgery: their prevention with intercostal blocks. Acta Anaesthesiol. Scand., *32:*1, 1989.
437. Ross, W.B., Tweedie, J.H., Leong, Y.P., and Wyman, A.: Does intercostal blockade improve patient comfort after cholecystectomy? Br. J. Surg., *74:*63, 1987.
438. Sabanathan, S., Mearns, A.J., Bickford Smith, P.J., *et al.*: Efficacy of continuous extrapleural intercostal nerve block on post-thoracotomy pain and pulmonary mechanics. Br. J. Surg., *77:*221, 1990.
439. Jayr, C., Mollié, A., Bourgain, J.L., *et al.*: Postoperative pulmonary complications: General anesthesia with postoperative parenteral morphine compared with epidural analgesia. Surgery, *104:*57, 1988.
440. Schulze S., Roikjaer, O., Hasselstrøm, L., *et al.*: Epidural bupivacaine and morphine plus systemic indomethacin eliminates pain but not systemic response and convalescence after cholecystectomy. Surgery, *103:*321, 1988.
441. Kilbride, M.J., Senagore, A.J., Mazier, W.P., *et al.*: Epidural analgesia. Surg. Gynecol. Obstetr., *174:*137, 1992.
442. Simpson, T., Wahl, G., DeTraglia, M., *et al.*: The effects of epidural versus parenteral opioid analgesia on postoperative pain and pulmonary function in adults who have undergone thoracic and abdominal surgery: A critique of research. Heart Lung, *21:*125, 1992.
443. Creditor, M.C.: Hazards of hospitalization in the elderly. Ann. Intern Med., *118:*219, 1993.
444. Sagar, P.M., Kruegener, G., and MacFie, J.: Nasogastric intubation and elective abdominal surgery. Br. J. Surg., *79:*1127, 1992.
445. Møniche, S., Hansen, B.N., Christensen, S.E., *et al.*: Activity of patients and duration of hospitalization following hip replacement with balanced treatment of pain and early mobilization. Ugeskr. Laeger., *154:*1495, 1992.
446. Bardram, L., Funch-Jensen, P., Jensen, P., *et al.*: Recovery after laparoscopic colonic surgery with epidural analgesia, enforced oral nutrition and mobilization. Lancet, *345:*763, 1995.
447. Katz, J., Clarioux, M., Kavanagh, B.P., *et al.*: Pre-emptive lumbar epidural anaesthesia reduces postoperative pain and patient-controlled morphine consumption after lower abdominal surgery. Pain, *59:*395, 1994.
448. Carr, D.B., Ballantyne, J.C., Osgood, P.F., *et al.*: Pituitary-adrenal stress response in the absence of brain-pituitary connections. Anesth. Analg., *69:*197, 1989.
449. Lilly, M.P., and Gann, D.S.: The hypothalamic-pituitary-adrenal-immune axis. A critical assessment. Arch. Surg., *127:*1463, 1992.
450. Dahl, J.B., Rosenberg, J., and Kehlet, H.: Effect of thoracic epidural etidocaine 1.5% on somatosensory evoked potentials, cortisol and glucose during cholecystectomy. Acta Anaesthesiol. Scand., *36:*378, 1992.
451. Shirasaka, C., Tsuji, H., Asoh, T., and Takeuchi, Y.: Role of the splanchnic nerves in endocrine and metabolic response to abdominal surgery. Br. J. Surg., *73:*142, 1986.
452. Hamid, S.K., Scott, N.B., Sutcliffe, N.P., *et al.*: Continuous coeliac plexus blockade plus intermittent wound infiltration with bupivacaine following upper abdominal surgery: A double-blind randomised study. Acta Anaesthesiol. Scand., *36:*534, 1992.
453. Webster, J., Barnard, M., and Carli, F.: Metabolic response to colonic surgery: extradural vs continuous spinal. Br. J. Anaesth., *67:*467, 1991.
454. Dahl, J.B., Rosenberg, J., Dirkes, W.E., *et al.*: Prevention of postoperative pain by balanced analgesia. Br. J. Anaesth., *64:*518, 1990.
455. Barker, J.P., Robinson, P.N., Vafidis, G.C., *et al.*: Local analgesia prevents the cortisol and glycaemic responses to cataract surgery. Br. J. Anaesth., *64:*442, 1990.
456. Barker, J.P., Vafidis, G.C., Nobinson, P.N., and Hall, G.M.: Plasma catecholamine response to cataract surgery: a comparison between general and local anaesthesia. Anaesthesia, *46:*642, 1991.
457. Scheinin, B., Scheinin, M., Asantila, R., *et al.*: Sympatho-adrenal and pituitary hormone responses during and immediately after thoracic surgery—modulation by four different pain treatments. Acta Anaesthesiol. Scan., *31:*762, 1987.
458. Pither, C.E., Birdenbaugh, L.D., and Reynolds, F.: Preoperative intercostal nerve block: effect on the endocrine metabolic response to surgery. Br. J. Anaesth., *60:*730, 1988.
459. Giesecke, K., Hamberger, B., Järnberg, P.-O., and Klingstedt, C.: Par-

avertebral block during cholecystectomy: effects on circulatory and hormonal responses. Br. J. Anaesth., *61:*652, 1988.
460. Sutcliffe, A.J.: Mortality after spinal and general anaesthesia for surgical fixation of hip fractures. Anaesthesia, *49:*237, 1994.
461. Rørdam, P., Jensen, L.P., Schroeder, T., *et al.*: Intra-arterial papaverine and leg vascular resistance during in situ bypass surgery with high or low epidural anaesthesia. Acta Anaesthesiol. Scand., *37:*97, 1993.
462. Bading, B., Blank, S.G., Sculco, T.P., *et al.*: Augmentation of calf blood flow by epinephrine infusion during lumbar epidural anesthesia. Anesth. Analg., *78:*1119, 1994.
463. Niijima, A. Nervous regulation of metabolism. Prog. Neurobiol., *33:*135, 1989.
464. Normandale, J.P., Schmulian, C., Paterson, J.L., *et al.*: Epidural diamorphine and the metabolic response to upper abdominal surgery. Anaesthesia, *40:*748, 1985.
465. Downing, R., Davis, I., Black, J., and Windsor, C.W.O.: Effect of intrathecal morphine on the adrenocortical and hyperglycaemic responses to upper abdominal surgery. Br. J. Anaesth., *58:*858, 1986.
466. Camu, F., and Debucquoy, F.: Alfentanil infusion for postoperative pain: a comparison of epidural and intravenous routes. Anesthesiology, *75:*171, 1991.
467. Salomäki, T.E., Leppäluoto, J., Laitinen, J.O., *et al.*: Epidural versus intravenous fentanyl for reducing hormonal, metabolic and physiologic responses after thoracotomy. Anesthesiology, *79:*672, 1993.
468. Kirnö, K., Lundin, S., and Elam, M.: Effects of intrathecal morphine and spinal anaesthesia on sympathetic nerve activity in humans. Acta Anaesthesiol. Scand., *37:*54, 1993.
469. Wright, P.M.C., O'Toole, D.P.O., and Barron, D.W.: The influence of naloxone infusion on the action of intrathecal diamorphine: low-dose naloxone and neuroendocrine responses. Acta Anaesthesiol. Scand., *36:*230, 1992.
470. Desborough, J.P., Edlin, S.A., Burrin, J.M., *et al.*: Hormonal and metabolic responses to cholecystectomy: comparison of extradural somatostatin and diamorphine. Br. J. Anaesth., *63:*508, 1989.
471. Wiedemann, B., Leibe, S., Kätzel, R., *et al.*: The influence of epidural combination anesthesia on stress reaction, pain reaction, and respiration in upper abdominal surgery. Anaesthesist, *40:*608, 1991.
472. Kehlet, H., and Dahl, J.B.: The value of "multimodal" or "balanced analgesia" in postoperative pain treatment. Anesth. Analg., *77:*1048, 1993.
473. Sinclair, R., Eriksson, A.S., Greetzer, C., *et al.*: Inhibitory effects of amide local anaesthetics on stimulus-induced human leukocyte metabolic activation, LTB_4 release and IL-1 secretion *in vitro*. Acta Anaesthesiol. Scand., *37:*159, 1993.
474. Sharrock, N.E., Ranawat, C.S., Urquhart, B., and Peterson, M.: Factors influencing deep vein thrombosis following total hip arthroplasty under epidural anesthesia. Anesth. Analg., *76:*765, 1993.
475. Uchida, I., Asoh, T., Shirasaka, C., and Tsuji, H.: Effect of epidural analgesia on postoperative insulin resistance as evaluated by insulin clamp technique. Br. J. Surg., *75:*557, 1988.
476. Stenseth, R., Bjella, L., Berg, E.M., *et al.*: Thoracic epidural analgesia in aortocoronary bypass surgery II: Effects on the endocrine metabolic response. Acta Anaesthesiol. Scand., *38:*834, 1994.
477. Watters, J.M., March, R.J., Desai, D., *et al.*: Epidural anaesthesia and analgesia do not affect energy expenditure after major abdominal surgery. Can. J. Anaesth., *40:*314, 1992.
478. Kirnö, K., Friberg, P., Grzegorczyk, A., *et al.*: Thoracic epidural anesthesia during coronary artery bypass surgery: Effects on cardiac sympathetic activity, myocardial blood flow and metabolism, and central hemodynamics. Anesth. Analg., *79:*1075, 1994.
479. Stelzner, J., Reinhart, K., Föhring, U., and Henneberg, M.: Die Auswirkungen der thorakalen periduralanalgesie auf die kortisol- und glukoseantwort bei operationen an der abdominellen aorta. Reg. Anaesth., *11:*16, 1988.
480. Lund, J., Stjernström, H., Jorfeldt, L., and Wiklund, L.: Effect of extradural analgesia on glucose metabolism and gluconeogenesis. Br. J. Anaesth., *58:*851, 1986.
481. Hosoda, R., Hattori, M., Shimada, Y., *et al.*: Favorable effects of epidural analgesia on hemodynamics, oxygenation and metabolic variables in the immediate postanesthetic period. Acta Anaesthesiol. Scand., *37:*469, 1993.
482. Gold, M.S., DeCrosta, D., Rizzuto, C., *et al.*: The effect of lumbar epidural and general anesthesia on plasma catecholamines and hemodynamics during abdominal aortic aneurysm repair. Anesth. Analg., *78:*225, 1994.
483. Kehlet, H.: Modification of responses to surgery and anesthesia by neural blockade: Clinical implications. *In* Cousins, M.J., and Bridenbaugh, P.O. (eds.): Neural Blockade in Clinical Anesthesia and Management of Pain. pp. 145. Philadelphia, J.B. Lippincott, 1987.
484. Dahl, J.B., Rosenberg, J., Lund, C., and Kehlet, H.: Effect of thoracic epidural bupivacaine 0.75% on somatosensory evoked potentials after dermatomal stimulation. Reg. Anesth., *15:*73, 1990.
485. Lund, C., Hansen, O.B., Mogensen, T., and Kehlet, H.: Effect of thoracic epidural bupivacaine on somatosensory evoked potentials after dermatomal stimulation. Anesth. Analg., *66:*731, 1987.
486. Lund, C., Selmar, P., Hansen, O.B., Hjortsø, N.-C., and Kehlet, H.: Effect of epidural bupivacaine on somatosensory evoked potentials after dermatomal stimulation. Anesth. Analg., *66:*34, 1987.
487. Lund, C., Selmar, P., Hansen, O.B., and Kehlet, H.: Effect of intrathecal bupivacaine on somatosensory evoked potentials following dermatomal stimulation. Anesth. Analg., *66:*809, 1987.
488. Lund, C., Hansen, O.B., Kehlet, H., *et al.*: Effects of etidocaine administered epidurally on changes in somatosensory evoked potentials after dermatomal stimulation. Reg. Anesth., *16:*38, 1991.
489. Dirkes, W.E., Rosenberg, J., Lund, C., and Kehlet, H.: The effect of subarachnoid lidocaine and combined subarachnoid lidocaine and epidural bupivacaine on electrical sensory thresholds. Reg. Anesth., *16:*262, 1991.
490. Heindorff, H., Schulze, S., Mogensen, T., *et al.*: Hormonal and neural blockade prevents the postoperative increase in amino acid clearance and urea synthesis. Surgery, *111:*543, 1992.
491. Nielsen, T.H., Nielsen, H.K., Husted, S.E., *et al.*: Stress response and platelet function in minor surgery during epidural bupivacaine and general anaesthesia: effect of epidural morphine addition. Eur. J. Anaesthesiol., *6:*409, 1989.
492. Zwarts, S.J., Hasenbos, M.A.M.W., Gielen, M.J.M., and Kho, H-G.: The effect of continuous epidural analgesia with sufentanil and bupivacaine during and after thoracic surgery on the plasma cortisol concentration and pain relief. Reg. Anesth., *14:*183, 1989.
493. Scott, N.B., Mogensen, T., Bigler, D., *et al.*: Continuous thoracic extradural 0.5% bupivacaine with or without morphine: effect on quality of blockade, lung function and the surgical stress response. Br. J. Anaesth., *62:*253, 1989.
494. Schulze, S., Møller, I.W., Bang, U., *et al.*: Effect of combined prednisolone, epidural analgesia and indomethacin on pain, systemic response and convalescence after cholecystectomy. Acta Chir. Scand., *156:*203, 1990.
495. Liem, T.H., Booij, L.H.D.J., Gielen, M.J.M., *et al.*: Coronary artery bypass grafting using two different anesthetic techniques: part 3: adrenergic responses. J. Cardiothorac Vasc. Anesth., *6:*162, 1992.
496. Rademaker, B.M., Ringers, J., Odoom, J.A., *et al.*: Pulmonary function and stress response after laparoscopic cholecystectomy: comparison with subcostal incision and influence of thoracic epidural analgesia. Anesth. Analg., *75:*381, 1992.
497. Dahl, J.B., Hjortsø, N.-C., Stage, J.G., *et al.*: Effects of combined perioperative epidural bupivacaine and morphine, ibuprofen, and incisional bupivacaine on postoperative pain, pulmonary, and endocrine-metabolic function after minilaparotomy cholecystectomy. Reg. Anesth., *19:*199, 1994.
498. Kehlet, H.: Multimodal approach to contro postoperative pathophysiology and rehabilitation. Br. J Anaesth. *78:*606, 1997.

PART II

Techniques of Neural Blockade

Neural Blockade in Clinical Anesthesia and Management of Pain, Third Edition,
edited by M.J. Cousins and P.O. Bridenbaugh.
Lippincott–Raven Publishers, Philadelphia © 1998.

CHAPTER 6

Perioperative Management of Patients for Neural Blockade

Phillip O. Bridenbaugh and James C. Crews

Without regard to which nerve block technique might be considered or which local anesthetic agent may be used, the principles applied to a general anesthetic are just as essential for a successful regional anesthetic outcome. These basic principles include, of course, a well-trained physician working in a well-equipped anesthetizing location. There are, however, additional requirements for the successful practice of the subspecialty of regional anesthesia. The anesthetist must be skilled, not just in the technical aspects of how to accomplish a selected technique, but also in its indications, contraindications, and proper intraoperative management. Presumably, these skills and knowledge are taught early in the anesthesia training period by experts in the subspecialty. From this beginning, the anesthetist who has a sincere interest in neural blockade and who is convinced of its efficacy will continue to employ and polish his or her technical skills until they become an essential part of the anesthetic armamentarium.

A thorough knowledge of the pertinent anatomy, obtained from textbooks and atlases, should be reinforced through the study of cadavers and surgical specimens. In addition, one should be familiar with the physiology of neural blockade, pharmacology of the local anesthetic agents themselves, and the physiologic effects and potential complications associated with the various regional anesthetic techniques. One can, therefore, anticipate changes in the patient's status and not only determine the suitability of a given technique for a specific patient and procedure, but also be prepared to institute appropriate therapy if and when these changes occur.

Finally, this thorough knowledge of the requirements for successful neural blockade also requires that the anesthetist undertake these activities in a suitable location well equipped with not only suitable block equipment, but also with all other appropriate monitors, resuscitation drugs, and equipment. Under all but the most unusual circumstances, an assistant to the anesthetist is essential for optimal patient care. This applies to regional anesthesia as well as general anesthesia.

P. O. Bridenbaugh: and J. C. Crews: Department of Anesthesia, University of Cincinnati College of Medicine, Cincinnati, Ohio 45267-0531.

PRE-ANESTHETIC MANAGEMENT

Almost every anesthetic encounter begins when the anesthetist consults an operative schedule and notes the procedure to be done, the patient's name, (sometimes age), and the operating surgeon. Based on the procedure alone, the anesthetic planning begins by considering appropriate techniques, general or regional, and then some specific choices. Knowledge of the surgeon's personality and technical skills will also play a role in selecting not only a specific block technique but also the drug (i.e., duration) and considerations of supplementary drugs. With that degree of advanced planning one can then approach the patient assessment for final selection.

The advent of ambulatory surgery has somewhat complicated the selection process because the anesthetist usually does not have access to the patients or their medical records until 1 or 2 hours before the actual procedure. If the anesthetic choices being considered require any degree of advance planning it is highly recommended that the anesthetist discuss these concerns with the surgeon and, if helpful, telephone or personally visit the patient to ensure proper planning and preparation for the proposed procedure.

PATIENT SELECTION

The most important determinant in the selection of a regional anesthetic technique is the suitability of that technique to that specific patient for the specific procedure. Unless thorough and careful consideration is given to the patient, all else will likely fail. Patient factors to be considered include anatomy, pathophysiology, and psychological state.

Because nearly all regional anesthetic techniques are based on the identification and utilization of anatomic landmarks, both surface and bony, it is essential that the patient display those landmarks. Examples of anatomic impediments to the conduct of a successful nerve block technique include morbid obesity, deforming arthritis, and other physical deformities that would limit accurate patient positioning or palpation of local landmarks at the site of the block.

Pathophysiologic considerations may be either local or systemic. Local conditions such as infection, abnormalities, trauma, burns, or dressings could all preclude the opportunity to perform a satisfactory block technique. More subtle, and often more important, are the systemic problems of the patient. Clearly, a severely hypovolemic patient should not be considered for a technique that involves major sympathetic neural blockade unless appropriate prophylaxis is accomplished beforehand. Patients with neurologic disease, coagulopathies, or severe cardiovascular disease all need to have thorough pre-anesthetic medical and laboratory evaluation of their pathology. It may turn out that one type of block technique will be contraindicated whereas another might be perfectly acceptable. It must be remembered that the anesthetic choice involves not only the selection of a block technique but also consideration of the risks and benefits of all anesthetic options tailored for the individual patient for the best possible outcome. Coincident with the assessment of the patient's pathophysiology is the consideration of the drug therapy the patient has been receiving. Of special concern for selection of central neuraxial blocks (spinal or epidural) is the patient's use of vasoactive drugs such as antihypertensive, alpha- and beta-adrenergic receptor blocking agents, and calcium channel blocking drugs. These agents, in combination with a major sympathetic nerve block can result in precipitous blood pressure changes and cardiac problems intraoperatively.

The use of neural blockade techniques for patients with a large variety of disease processes is a very subjective choice. The literature does not contain absolute documentation of when it is safe or unsafe, indicated or contraindicated, preferable or optional to use any given anesthetic technique or agent. The decision is multifactorial but ultimately becomes the responsibility of the attending anesthetist. Controversial issues in the use of neural blockade include coagulopathies or presence of anticoagulants, preexisting peripheral neurologic disease of a variety of causes, and medicolegal concerns. In view of the fact that the choice considers all that has been previously noted here it is probably inappropriate for a textbook to provide a list of diseases or circumstances when regional anesthesia should or should not be used. See Chapter 21 for a review of complications and side effects of regional anesthesia. This should be consulted when anticipating the risks of a given technique.

Finally, the mental attitude or psychological makeup of the patient will play a major role in determining the advisability of selecting a regional anesthetic technique. This is highly specific to the surgical procedure and the anesthetic options being presented. For example, the patient who would accept a single venipuncture for a 45-minute intravenous regional arm block might become hysterical at the thought of a spinal anesthetic for amputation of the leg. Such conditions may impose major management problems intraoperatively.

Equally difficult to manage is the disoriented patient. Mental disorientation, whether senile, pathologic, or pharmacologic (including social drugs) may not prevent the actual accomplishment of a successful block technique but will likely commit the anesthetist to very deep to unconscious levels of sedation throughout the operative period. Uncooperative patients nearly always must be put to sleep without regard to the depth of the regional anesthetic. Clearly, nerve blocks that require patient cooperation with positioning or identification of paresthesias are difficult to accomplish (and may be dangerous) in uncooperative, psychologically disturbed patients. Parenthetically, it may be noted that somnolent or unconscious patients may be ideal candidates for nerve block techniques that can be accomplished with a peripheral nerve stimulator, rendering patient participation unnecessary.

The anesthetist must also undertake other elements of a pre-anesthetic evaluation, including a complete history and physical examination. The usual elements of systemic disease, current medications, past operations and anesthetics, allergies, dental status, and family history of anesthetic problems must be recorded. Laboratory studies essential for the conduct of a general anesthetic must also be recorded. Patients must first be evaluated as candidates for general anesthesia and then evaluated for suitability for regional anesthesia.

It is a rare regional anesthetic (or an anesthetist) that can be guaranteed as 100% satisfactory with zero chance of needing additional medication, anesthetic, or resuscitation.

PATIENT INTERVIEW

Once the anesthetist has decided upon the anesthetic plan, the patient should be so informed. A broad but useful definition of informed consent is the obligation to explain to the patient the risks and benefits of the selected anesthetic plan, as opposed to the risks and benefits of an alternate plan. Clearly, the anesthetist must first be personally convinced that the recommended technique is the preferred choice or it will be difficult to provide the patient with the necessary assurance.

A significant number of patients refuse a regional anesthetic because "they don't want to be awake during the operation." It is essential, therefore, that the anesthetist describe in chronological detail the events that will occur from arrival in the surgical/anesthesia area through admission to the recovery area. Patients should be assured that as soon as an intravenous infusion is established, systemic sedatives will be given to make the patient comfortable prior to the anesthetic. Patients also need to be told, early in the interview, that they will be provided with additional systemic drugs throughout the operation to produce a state of sedation up to unconsciousness as needed for their comfort. When available, the use of headphones with music, visual screens, and other distracting techniques should be discussed.

The anesthetist should describe in detail the performance of the block and the patient's role in that process. This description should include start of the intravenous (IV) infusion, position, identification of paresthesias (if likely), signs and symptoms of normal onset of neural blockade, and systemic toxicity. If the patient knows what to expect and has the anesthetist's assurance that incremental sedation or analgesia will be administered as desired, most patients will consent to a regional anesthetic.

Informing the patient about the rationale for neural blockade will further motivate patients toward acceptance. Factors such as a reduced likelihood of side effects from general anesthetics, muscle relaxants, and endotracheal intubation should be noted. The increased public awareness of postoperative pain relief facilitates patient acceptance of regional anesthesia. The painless emergence from operative sedation in the recovery unit with a plan for earlier discharge with fewer risks of opioid analgesic side effects should also be discussed. The amount of information given will vary for each patient; however, such discussions invariably increase the confidence of the patient and may positively affect the recovery. All that remains, then, is for the anesthetist to write on the patient's medical record that a selected anesthetic plan (including a regional anesthetic technique) has been discussed with the patient, questions answered, and that the patient agrees.

PREMEDICATION OF PATIENTS FOR NEURAL BLOCKADE TECHNIQUE

Just as the principles applied to selection of a regional anesthetic technique are primarily those used for general anesthesia, so too are the basic tenets similar in the administration of the anesthetic orders and medications.

Pre-anesthesia Fasting

In the past, *all* patients scheduled to receive any type of anesthetic were restricted from all oral intake for a minimum of 6 hours and preferably from midnight the day before surgery. The efficacy of this practice was reexamined in the early 1990s. Because unconsciousness may be a required or desired part of any regional anesthetic procedure it is important that the rationale for pre-anesthetic fasting be the same for all healthy patients. There are many individual circumstances, especially in pediatric procedures, where these practices will be modified, but some general guidelines are helpful.

Phillips et al.[37] prospectively compared the effect of allowing unrestricted clear fluids until the time of oral medication (2 hours prior to surgery). Patients otherwise underwent conventional fasting. The residual volume and pH of gastric contents after induction of anesthesia were measured in 100 elective surgical patients allocated randomly to a group allowed unrestricted fluids or to a control group who fasted for 6 hours (mean = 388 ml vs. 0 ml). There was no significant difference in mean residual gastric volume (22 ml vs. 19 ml) or pH (2.64 vs. 2.26) between the study group and the control group. Problems with aspiration were not encountered. The authors concluded that elective surgical patients could be allowed to drink clear fluids until 2 hours before anesthesia to enhance patient comfort without compromising safety. This paper was accompanied by an editorial in the British Journal of Anaesthesia[45] which stated: "Returning to elective operations which concern the vast majority of patients requiring an anaesthetic, it is clear that 'nil by mouth after midnight' should be abandoned. In its place, there should be agreement by anaesthetists, surgeons, and nurses on guidelines that both day-case and inpatients may take, if they wish, clear fluids by mouth up to 3 hours before surgery." The list of clear fluids excluded alcoholic drinks and those containing milk or sugar but it did include orange juice and apple juice.

To further endorse the liberalization of clear liquid intake from the empirical 6-hour rule, the Canadian Anaesthetists' Society revised its 1987 *Guidelines to the Practice of Anaesthesia* which suggested a minimum of 5 hours from the last oral intake until the induction of anaesthesia. It went on to note, "consideration should be given to the same guidelines when elective regional anesthesia is undertaken." Because of the results of reliable clinical studies, the Canadian Anaesthetists' Society revised its guidelines to state, "Recognizing that there is currently no fixed period of fasting recommended before all procedures, departments must establish policies concerning patients' oral intake before elective induction of anaesthesia."[29]

In 1995, the American Society of Anesthesiologists released its Practice Parameters entitled, *Guidelines for Sedation and Analgesia by Non-Anesthesiologists*; they made the following recommendations[20] for pre-anesthesia fasting (Table 6-1):

> Patients undergoing sedation/analgesia for elective procedures should not drink fluids or eat solid foods for a sufficient period of time to allow for gastric emptying prior to their procedure ... In urgent, emergent, or other situations where gastric emptying is impaired, the potential for pulmonary aspiration of gastric contents must be considered in determining the timing of the intervention and the degree of sedation/analgesia.

Pre-anesthetic Medications

The advent of ambulatory surgery and the current practice that most patients are seen for the first time by their anesthesiologist a few hours before surgery has changed the ratio-

TABLE 6-1. *Example of fasting protocol for sedation and analgesia for elective procedures[a]*

Patient group	Solids and nonclear liquids[b]	Clear liquids
Adults	6–8 hours or none after 12 A.M.[c]	2–3 hours
Children >36 months old	6–8 hours	2–3 hours
Children 6–36 months old	6 hours	2–3 hours
Children <6 months old	4–6 hours	2 hours

[a] Gastric emptying may be influenced by many factors including anxiety, pain, abnormal autonomic function (e.g., diabetes), pregnancy, and mechanical obstruction. Therefore, the suggestions below do not guarantee that complete gastric emptying has occurred. Unless contraindicated, pediatric patients should be offered clear liquids until 2 to 3 hours before sedation to minimize the risk of dehydration.

[b] This includes milk, formula, and breast milk. (High fat content may delay gastric emptying.)

[c] There are no data to establish whether a 6- to 8-hour fast is equivalent to an overnight fast prior to sedation/analgesia.

(Reprinted with permission from Guidelines for Sedation and Analgesia by Non-Anesthesiologists. American Society of Anesthesiologists, 1995.)

nale and types of drugs used for premedication. Although inpatients for elective procedures may be seen and sedated the evening before surgery; by very nature of being in-house suggests they are too sick or at too great a risk to be done as same-day cases. Premedication has as its goals the rapid onset of amnesia and analgesia with very short duration of action and a minimum of postoperative sequelae (i.e., nausea, vomiting, pain, etc.). In considering the timing of premedication, it is essential that all pre-anesthetic and presurgical discussions and consents be obtained and documented prior to administration. As many as 20% of same-day surgery cases are canceled for a variety of reasons. Patients may fail to arrive for the procedure, they may have a full stomach or abnormal laboratory values, electrocardiogram (ECG), or chest x-ray, or they may have had an interim illness since the last office visit which requires surgical reevaluation with postponement or cancellation. Thus, the anesthetist must be sure that a scheduled procedure will take place before administering premedications to a patient.

Anticholinergics

Most practitioners of regional anesthesia have abandoned the routine use of anticholinergic drugs unless they plan to combine their technique with an inhalation anesthetic. Those abandoning the preoperative use of these drugs considered their action as primarily antisialagogue. Anticholinergic drugs in adult, premedication doses do not alter gastric fluid pH or volume.[44] A published review of postoperative nausea and vomiting states that "the incidence of nausea and vomiting during spinal anesthesia is decreased by the intravenous administration of atropine." However, the quoted references date to the late 1950s and raise the question of whether such conclusions are still valid.[49] In summary, the pre-anesthetic use of this class of drugs is limited to a knowledge of their various clinical actions and the application of that action to specific needs of a select patient (Table 6-2). Routine use of anticholinergics as premedications for regional anesthesia is not recommended.

Antiemetics

One of the inducements anesthesiologists offer to patients when comparing regional and general anesthesia is the reduced likelihood of postoperative nausea and/or vomiting with regional anesthesia. Actually, that cause and effect relationship has not been proven in the scientific literature. Nonetheless, nausea and vomiting have been a major cause of postanesthesia morbidity since the days of ether anesthesia. In the current climate of cost-effective health care, early discharge of ambulatory surgical patients has become a major focus. Included in a study of strategies to decrease post anesthesia care unit (PACU) costs was the role of nausea and vomiting.[12] They determined that if nausea and vomiting could have been eliminated in each patient, without causing sedation, the total time to discharge would have been decreased by less than 5%. The authors' conclusion was that anesthesiologists cannot control PACU economics via the choice of anesthetic drugs or techniques.

Cost alone should not be the determining factor, however.

TABLE 6-2. *Comparative effects of anticholinergic drugs*

	Sedation	Antisialagogue	Increase heart rate	Relax smooth muscle	Mydriasis cycloplegia	Prevent motion sickness	Decrease gastric hydrogen ion secretion	Alter fetal heart rate
Atropine	+	+	+ + +	+ +	+	+	∓	0
Scopolamine	+ + +	+ + +	+	+	+ + +	+ + +	±	?
Glycopyrrolate	0	+ +	+ +	+ +	0	0	±	0

0, none; +, mild; + +, moderate; + + +, marked, ±, variable effects (may or may not).

(Reprinted with permission from Stoelting, R.K.: Pharmacology and Physiology in Anesthetic Practice, 2nd ed. pp. 244. Philadelphia, J.B. Lippincott, 1991.)

In the eyes of many patients, postoperative nausea and vomiting is perceived as a failure of anesthesia rather than an unavoidable consequence of the perioperative experience. Many patients complain about the distress they felt due to nausea and vomiting from a previous operation and beg to be spared that experience again.[21] Although regional anesthesia has been considered an attractive alternative to general anesthesia, the confusion arises from the practice of most anesthesiologists using concomitant intravenous sedatives and opioids during regional anesthesia to provide anxiolysis and analgesia for position discomfort. Thus it is difficult to separate the emetic effects of the sedative/analgesic medications from those associated with neural blockade.

The incidence of emesis associated with central neuraxial block is greater than with peripheral nerve block because of the side effects of the resultant sympathetic nervous system blockade (i.e., hypotension and perhaps central hypoxemia). Studies of the actual benefit, if any, of central neuraxial block in reducing emesis are conflicting. Even studies with local anesthesia and monitored anesthesia care fail to document conclusively that neural blockade is better. Clearly the multifactorial causes of perioperative nausea and vomiting are influenced more by total patient management than the use of any single drug or technique. An extensive review of postoperative nausea and vomiting clearly illustrates this point.[49] In summary, the authors note "that factors clearly associated with an increased risk of postoperative emesis include age, gender (menses), obesity, previous history of motion sickness or postoperative vomiting, anxiety, gastroparesis, and type of surgery (especially, laparoscopy, strabismus, and middle ear procedures) ... Although anesthesiologists have little, if any, control over these factors, they do have control over the emesis-related risk factors of pre-anesthetic medication, anesthetic drugs, and techniques, and postoperative pain management." The authors conclude: "Although routine antiemetic prophylaxis is clearly unjustified, patients at high risk for postoperative emesis should receive special considerations with respect to the prophylactic use of antiemetic drugs."

Analgesics

There is a popular belief among many anesthesiologists that induction of anesthesia is not painful and thus does not require administration of an analgesic agent in the pre-anesthetic period. However, practitioners of regional anesthesia or other potentially painful invasive procedures should give strong consideration to their use. Furthermore, the regional anesthetic renders only portions of the patient's anatomy analgesic. An analgesic will enhance total body comfort and likely reduce the dosage of supplementary sedation.

Recently, there has been much interest in the phenomenon of preemptive analgesia (see Chapter 23). Woolf et al.[53] described peripheral and central sensitization of nociceptive receptors and neurons to tissue injury. Together these result in the postoperative/postinjury pain state. The observation that sensory signals during surgery can trigger this prolonged hypersensitivity encouraged clinical trials to determine if *pre*operative regional anesthesia or systemic opioid *pre*medication could "preempt" postoperative pain by preventing establishment of central sensitization. A number of clinical studies have been undertaken to determine the role of opioid premedication in reducing postoperative pain, but, to date, results are inconclusive.

Two major determinants for the inclusion of an opioid pre-anesthetic are the type of nerve block and the mental attitude of the patient. Nerve blocks that require paresthesias or multiple insertions, especially paravertebral, are painful and analgesia is beneficial. Similarly, the more apprehensive or excitable the patient the greater the need for both analgesia and sedation. Excitable patients heavily medicated with sedatives may tend to be drowsy and relaxed until painfully stimulated, when they are likely to overreact or react inappropriately and uncooperatively during an invasive procedure.

Selection of a specific opioid as a pre-anesthetic analgesic must be made with a consideration of the patient's analgesic requirements during the ensuing procedure and recovery period. For a brief period of painful stimulus in an outpatient setting, (e.g., diagnostic nerve block), a short-acting opioid with a fast onset is best. On the other hand, if one uses pre-anesthetic opioids for placement of a thoracic epidural prior to pulmonary surgery that uses endotracheal general anesthesia, then a long-acting opioid may be preferable (see Chapter 26). The preferred route of administration for all premedication is, obviously, intravenous through a continuous infusion line. Fentanyl is probably the pre-anesthetic opioid of choice for analgesia during nerve block procedures because its analgesic effects at 50 to 150 μg doses produce few to no side effects and provide a cooperative patient with a relatively clear sensorium. Once satisfactory neural blockade is achieved or if longer procedures are undertaken, one may choose to consider a longer-acting opioid analgesic.

Sedatives and Hypnotics

Early practitioners of regional anesthesia combined short-acting barbiturates with opioids as their premedication of choice. Usually, atropine or scopolamine accompanied that combination. As noted earlier in this chapter, most anesthesia practices today are for same-day patients, most of whom will leave the hospital or surgical facility 1 to 3 hours after their procedure. In addition to the desirable analgesia prior to regional anesthesia, most patients prefer to be sedated and usually amnestic during presurgical procedures. Just as the selection of an analgesic considered the needs and duration of the procedure, so too does the selection of a sedative. The chosen drug is usually continued into the operative management of the patient as well.

The benzodiazepines, principally midazolam, are commonly used as sedative agents because of their wide spectrum of central nervous system (CNS) depressant activity, low incidence of side effects, and wide margin of safety. All benzodiazepines possess the same properties of anxiolysis, amnesia, and sedation to varying degrees. Diazepam was the early favorite for premedication and supplementation for regional anesthesia and could be given orally or parenterally. Its prolonged duration was finally recognized with the advent of ambulatory surgery, where although the patient appeared to be awake, impairment of memory, cognitive, and motor skills was noted to persist for several hours. A secondary benefit of using benzodiazepines as premedication for regional anesthesia techniques is their anticonvulsant properties. deJong[11] first reported the superiority of diazepam over barbiturates in preventing seizures from local anesthesia overdose in animals (see Chapter 2). As a result of those studies, diazepam enjoyed widespread use as a prophylactic against local anesthetic seizures as well as for its sedative properties. A serious criticism must be given, however, against the use of diazepam as a prophylactic to permit the use of larger than recommended safe doses of local anesthetic. Many factors contribute to a given patient's toxicity threshold to local anesthetics. It is important, therefore, that the selected dose of a local anesthetic be at or below that recommended dose. Giving a large dose of diazepam will not necessarily prevent a seizure in the event of a local anesthetic overdose.

For those patients in whom prolonged amnesia is desired, other benzodiazepines may be considered (lorazepam, flunitrazepam, and midazolam). Currently, midazolam is the most frequently used benzodiazepine for pre-anesthetic sedation. Because it is water-soluble, it causes significantly less pain on injection than diazepam.[11,14] Midazolam has a rapid onset of action and a short elimination half-life (2–4 hours) and is significantly more potent than diazepam (Fig. 6-1). Failure to recognize its potency led to some early overdoses and resulted in the current recommendation of dose titration to the desired sedative level. Midazolam also produces more amnesia and sedation than diazepam, making it highly suitable for use with regional anesthesia. The other benzodiazepines, lorazepam and oxazepam, are potent amnestic agents but have such a prolonged duration of action that they are less suitable as premedication or supplements to most regional anesthesia procedures.[13,27]

Other drugs have been used as pre-anesthetic adjuvants prior to administration of regional anesthesia. The tranquilizing drugs (phenothiazines and butyrophenones) were popular earlier but their hypotensive effects in conjunction with sympathetic blocks resulting from regional anesthesia led to some major complications. The perceived advantage of the butyrophenones is their ability to produce a state of mental calm and indifference with little hypnotic effect. It was discovered, however, that larger doses, especially without analgesic or sedative drugs already present, could produce hallucinations, restlessness, and even extrapyramidal dyskinesia.[47] Droperidol is still useful, however, in lower doses (0.625–2.5 mg), as a potent antiemetic. Excess sedation and delayed discharge time are likely only after doses of droperidol greater than 2.5 mg.[44]

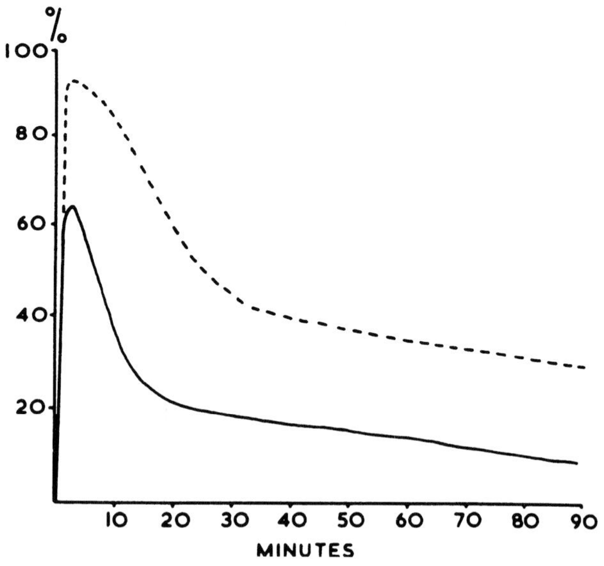

FIG. 6-1. Incidence of complete amnesia (—) and partial amnesia (----) following midazolam 6 mg. (Dundee, J.W., Samuel, I.O., Toner, W., and Howard, P.J.: Midazolam: A water-soluble benzodiazepine. Anaesthesia, *35*:460, 1980.)

Although not truly in the category of pre-anesthetic medication, the need for a rapid-acting sedative to alleviate the anxiety during the performance of a regional block technique can be effectively met with thiopental, methohexital, or propofol. (These agents will be discussed later in this chapter). During a regional blockade procedure, small intravenous bolus doses may be given by an assistant who also monitors the patient's airway, vital signs, and level of consciousness. Alternatively, some use a continuous intravenous infusion of dilute solutions of methohexital to achieve the same purpose. The advantage of the use of low doses of these drugs is the rapid recovery of sensorium immediately after the block technique is completed. This allows for accurate patient response to onset and level of sensory and motor blockade. The disadvantage of using these drugs lies primarily in their extreme potency and potential for relative overdose resulting in significant respiratory depression (or apnea) which may require ventilatory support. Both the barbiturates and propofol are nonanalgesic, or hyperalgesic, so repeat or high doses may be required during induction of painful and/or difficult neural block techniques.

EQUIPMENT, SUPPLIES, LOCATION, AND PATIENT POSITIONING

Prior to performing any neural blockade procedure, the anesthesiologist should locate and insure the proper functioning of the necessary monitoring and resuscitation equipment and drugs. Minimal basic resuscitation drugs and equipment for airway management (airways, suction equipment, laryngoscope, endotracheal tubes, muscle relaxants), support of cardiorespiratory function (oxygen, mask and reservoir bag, epinephrine, anticholinergic drugs, inotropic and/or vasopressor drugs), and sedative/induction agents (benzodiazepines, barbiturates) should be immediately available in case of adverse patient reaction associated with the procedure or the anesthetic agents administered (Fig. 6-2). Monitoring should include, at a minimum, the application of a pulse oximeter to monitor pulse rate, peripheral perfusion, and oxygen saturation.[3] For all but the least invasive, least complicated procedures, one should consider electrocardiograph and blood pressure monitoring as well. Peripheral temperature monitoring may be helpful if monitoring for effects of sympathetic blockade (see Chapter 4, Tables 4-9, 4-10).

The location most appropriate for performance of neural blockade procedures will vary according to the type of procedure and practice setting. Local anesthetic infiltration and minor neural blockade procedures may be safely performed in outpatient locations such as physicians' offices and emergency departments. More complex neural blockade procedures should be carried out in an otherwise suitable anesthetizing location such as the pre-induction area, operating room, PACU, or an appropriately equipped special procedure area (radiological procedure area, pain management unit, etc.). Regardless of the location, an area of sufficient size, with proper lighting and equipment to safely and efficiently perform the procedure is required. Neural blockade procedures for surgical patients may be more conveniently and efficiently performed in pre-induction areas, where the block can be performed while a preceding operative procedure is being completed or while the operating room is being prepared for the patient.

Considerations for patient positioning for neural blockade procedures should insure patient safety and comfort and optimize the successful performance of the anesthetic procedure. Some neural blockade procedures may require the enlistment of an assistant to help maintain patient safety and comfort.

Equipment Specific to Neural Blockade

The necessary equipment for a neural blockade procedure will again vary according to the anesthetic procedure being performed. Nonetheless, suggestions regarding basic equipment may be useful to most and can be modified to the needs of the specific procedure, patient, and practitioner.

Block Trays

Basically, three types of neural blockade procedures are most frequently performed by the anesthesiologist: (i) spinal (subarachnoid) neural blockade; (ii) epidural or caudal neural blockade; and (iii) peripheral neural blockade. Because the specific equipment required for each of these three types of blockade procedures is sufficiently different, most anes-

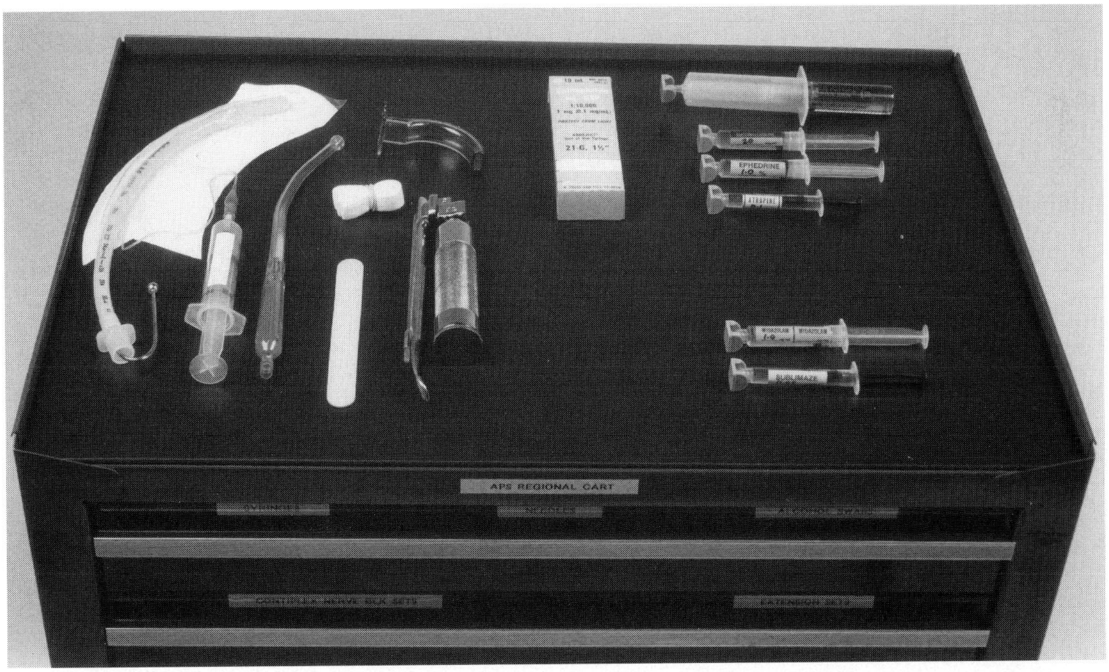

FIG. 6-2. Equipment for patient resuscitation and treatment of adverse reactions for neural blockade procedures. (*Left to right*) Endotracheal tube with stylet and cuff syringe; Yankauer suction; tongue-depressor; endotracheal tube tape; oropharyngeal airway; laryngoscope and blade; prefilled syringe containing epinephrine (0.1 mg/ml); labeled syringes containing (*front to back*) fentanyl, midazolam, atropine, succinylcholine, ephedrine, and thiopental. (*Not pictured*) Oxygen source, bag and mask, suction source.

thesia departments find it most efficient to have separate block trays for each procedure. (In some situations, a fourth tray for other, major neural blockade procedures may be indicated for celiac plexus block, hypogastric plexus block, or lumbar sympathetic block.) The specific requirements for needles, syringes, and ancillary equipment are discussed in the chapters that describe the various neural blockade techniques.

Apart from the needles, syringes, local anesthetic agents, adjuvant drugs, and ancillary equipment specific to the procedure, some basic supplies are required for all neural blockade procedures including (i) a container for a skin preparation solution; (ii) sponges or other applicators for skin preparation solution application; (iii) sterile drapes; and (iv) gauze sponges for wiping the skin during the procedure. These supplies may be assembled from individual sterile packages at the time of the procedure or be supplied as components of either a preassembled nerve block pack or a commercially prepared, disposable nerve block tray.

Anesthesiologists have witnessed a progressive improvement in the quality and reliability of disposable, commercially prepared nerve block trays. In many higher volume centers, commercially produced "custom trays" tailored to the specific needs and preferences of the department are frequently used. The convenience of the prepackaged tray, improvements in the quality of disposable needles and other equipment components, and the desirability of single-use equipment from the standpoint of sterility and patient safety have virtually eliminated the use of internally prepared nerve block trays (Fig. 6-3). While most major centers in the United States currently use disposable, commercially produced trays, the choice of these trays versus internally prepared reusable nerve block trays or packs is still subjective and is based on cost, convenience, reliability, number of procedures performed, type of procedures performed, and locale. High-quality, single-use, disposable needles are probably here to stay, but in this era of environmental consciousness and cost containment, a "hybrid tray" consisting of some reusable supplies (skin preparation solution container, drapes, tray) and disposable needles, syringes, and sponges may offer advantages for some types of procedures in some practice situations. Convenience, efficiency, and flexibility in the practice of regional anesthesia may be further enhanced through the use of a specially equipped regional anesthesia cart (Fig. 6-4).

Special Equipment

To improve the success rate of neural blockade or to make it possible in very difficult cases or extreme circumstances, special devices, needles, and pieces of equipment have been advocated or introduced. Various needles and modifications of the technique of identification of the epidural space have been described (see Chapter 7). Radiological localization of needle placement using fluoroscopy or computed tomography guidance may be indicated for certain more difficult neural blockade procedures. The use of Doppler or ultrasound guidance to locate nerves or associated vascular structures has also been described. Although these more sophisticated adjuncts can be recommended for difficult procedures or for the placement of neurolytic solutions, they may be too expensive and time-consuming to become routine for the daily practice of neural blockade.

Peripheral Nerve Stimulators

The use of a nerve stimulator to assist in the location of peripheral nerves with motor fiber components has been advo-

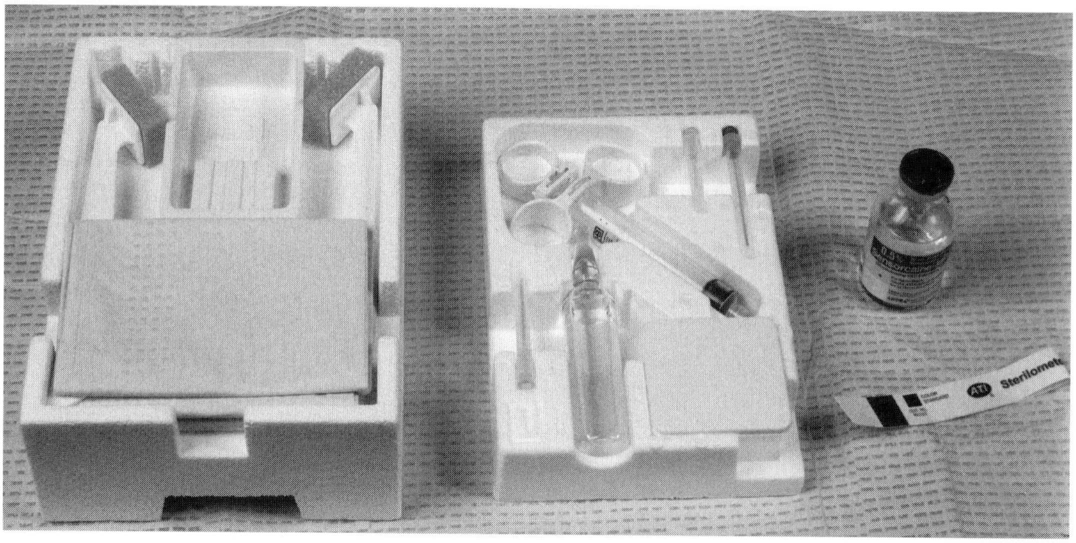

FIG. 6-3. Sterile disposable tray for peripheral neural blockade procedures. Pictured are separate trays for skin preparation and neural blockade supplies: skin prep solution container, prep sponges, paper drapes, gauze sponges, local anesthetic for skin infiltration, local anesthetic solution cup, plastic disposable three-ring syringe, 18-gauge, 22-gauge, and 25-gauge disposable needles. Gas sterilized bottle of local anesthetic solution is also shown.

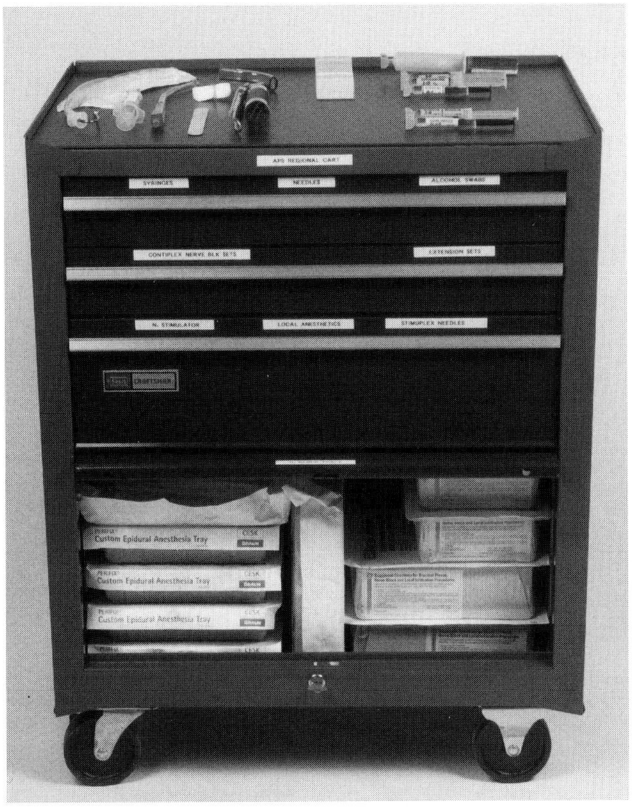

FIG. 6-4. Regional anesthesia procedure cart. The *top shelf* is the work surface for resuscitation drugs and equipment or block tray. The *drawers* contain syringes, needles, skin preparation solutions, dressing supplies, peripheral nerve stimulator and insulated needles, plastic extension sets, local anesthetic solutions. The *bottom shelf* has sterile disposable trays for minor peripheral neural blockade, major peripheral neural blockade, spinal, and epidural neural blockade procedures.

cated for peripheral neural blockade procedures on the basis of efficacy, efficiency, and patient safety.[6,8,10,26,38,43,54] The peripheral nerve stimulator allows for localization of a peripheral nerve without the need for elicitation of a paresthesia; thus peripheral neural blockade can be performed in patients who are sedated, unconscious, or otherwise unable to understand or cooperate, or in circumstances where the nerve is difficult to localize due to anatomic variability.

The technique of peripheral nerve stimulation was originally described in 1912.[48] The stimulating current was transmitted to the nerve using a pure nickel needle insulated with lacquer down to the tip. Needle localization of nerves with motor responses using electrical stimulation with an insulated needle was described in 1955.[35] In 1962 the construction and use of a portable needle nerve stimulator-locator as an instrument to assist in the locating of nerves for neural blockade procedures was reported.[22] This relatively small transistorized stimulator provided variable, pulsed output of between 0.3 and 30 V and utilized a plastic coating as insulation of all but the tip of the needle.

In 1973, the use of a nerve stimulator with standard, unsheathed (uninsulated) needles commonly used for neural blockade procedures was reported.[32] The nerve stimulator output was attached to the stimulating needle with a standard alligator clamp. The reported advantages of the use of uninsulated needles included better feel of the tissue planes, fewer complications resulting from problems with the insulating materials, and less dependence on special equipment. While the use of uninsulated needles may result in stimulation of the nerve due to proximity of the nerve and segments of the needle other than the tip, experimental investigation demonstrated greater current density at the tip of unsheathed hypodermic needles than at the shaft.

In a comparative investigation of sheathed and unsheathed needles in the cat, sheathed (insulated) needles were reported to be more precise in locating the peripheral nerve.[16] In this study it was reported that unsheathed (uninsulated) needles were capable of displaying the "least stimulating current" when the tip of the needle was beyond the nerve by as much as 0.8 cm. In a study of the electrical characteristics of peripheral nerve stimulators that contributed to the localization of peripheral nerves,[17] the following characteristics were found to be important:

1. A *linear output*, that is, a plot of percent output versus percentage of meter scale gives a straight line passing through zero and with 100% of the meter scale corresponding to 100% output.
2. *High and low output ranges* which allow the use of higher output when the needle is distant from the nerve and a wide range of low output control when the needle is close to the nerve. Stimulators developed for monitoring neuromuscular blockade may not have the required control in the low output range, making them unsuitable for use in the location of peripheral nerves for neural blockade.
3. *Clearly marked polarity of the output* extending to the ends of the connecting cables. It is important to attach the cathode (−) to the stimulating needle and the anode (+) to the surface of the patient. On some stimulators, it is difficult to determine which is the cathode (−) by color in that on some models the anode (+) is red, and on others the cathode (−) is red.
4. *Constant current output,* that is, current output remains the same regardless of different resistance applied to the output. In contrast, a constant voltage output instrument will decrease current output as resistance increases.
5. *A short stimulation pulse.* The shorter the stimulation pulse, the greater the ratio of the current required to stimulate the nerve when the needle is 1 cm away from the nerve compared to when the needle is on the nerve. For example, for a pulse width of 40 μsec, this ratio is 11, whereas for a pulse width of 1000 μsec the ratio is only 5.
6. *Design features*, including a large, easily turned current output dial, a digital current output meter, and a battery check.

Several sophisticated peripheral nerve stimulators and a variety of prepackaged, sterile, single-use, insulated needle

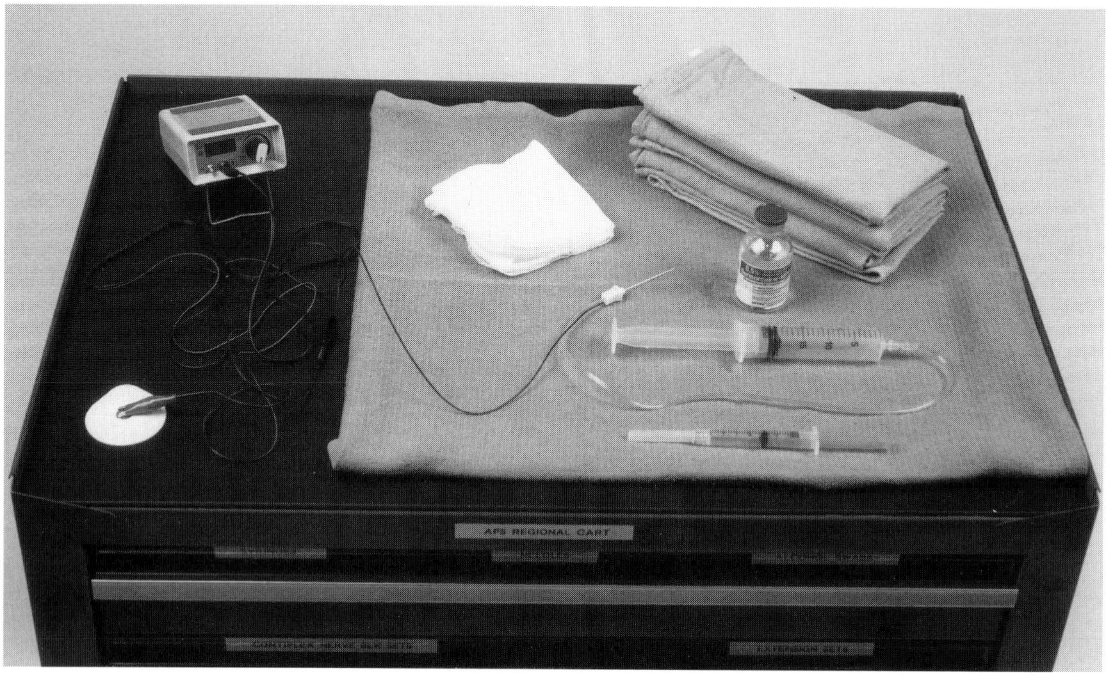

FIG. 6-5. Peripheral nerve stimulator apparatus. (*Right to left*) Peripheral nerve stimulator with low output variable intensity control, connecting cables with ground electrode, sterile disposable insulated block needle with extension set, 20-ml syringe containing local anesthetic solution for neural blockade procedure (attached), 3-ml syringe containing local anesthetic with 25-gauge needle for skin infiltration, gauze sponges, gas sterilized bottle of local anesthetic solution, and sterile drapes.

systems are currently commercially available incorporating the design features outlined above (Fig. 6-5).

Polarity of the stimulating needle when using a peripheral nerve stimulator affects the current required for nerve stimulation during neural blockade procedures.[46] In a study of patients undergoing axillary brachial plexus blockade, as much as two to three times the current output of the nerve stimulator was required to obtain nerve stimulation when the stimulating needle was attached to the positive terminal (anode) compared to when the stimulating needle was attached to the negative terminal (cathode). For this reason, it is imperative that the stimulating needle be connected to the negative output terminal (cathode) of the nerve stimulator and the patient be connected via the positive terminal (anode) to allow nerve stimulation detection at the lowest possible current output.

Technical Considerations

1. The anode (+) terminal of the stimulator is connected to an electrode on the patient's skin clear of the prepped site of the block.
2. The cathode (−) terminal of the stimulator is connected to the stimulating needle. The needle is inserted and advanced near the nerve. The stimulator is set to an output of 1 to 2 mA. Local muscle contraction should be minimal at this setting.
3. Stimulation of the nerve to be blocked should be measured by observing or feeling for muscle contractions within the motor distribution of the nerve. When using an insulated (sheathed) needle, stimulation will increase as the needle tip approaches the nerve and then decrease as the needle tip passes the nerve. The current output of the stimulator is decreased, as the needle approaches the nerve, to the lowest output which results in nerve stimulation and muscle contraction (usually less than 0.5 mA). At the point of maximum stimulation with the minimum stimulator output the needle tip should be proximate to the nerve and the local anesthetic solution may be injected. When using an uninsulated (unsheathed) needle, the same techniques are utilized, but care must be taken to determine that the nerve stimulation is resulting from proximity of the needle tip to the nerve rather than from the needle shaft. This may be determined by systematically advancing and withdrawing the needle to the point of maximum nerve stimulation with minimum stimulator output.
4. Injection of 1 to 2 ml of local anesthetic will immediately abolish nerve stimulation and muscle contraction if the tip of the needle is at the site of the nerve. If this does not occur the needle should be withdrawn slightly and the process repeated. A further test is to increase the output of the stimulator after the test dose. It should still be

possible to elicit some muscle response at the higher output. After a successful test dose, the full dose of local anesthetic required for the nerve block may be injected.

Future Considerations

The peripheral nerve stimulator has traditionally been used to locate nerves with motor fiber components as described above. However, the use of a peripheral nerve stimulator to determine the location of a peripheral nerve with purely sensory fiber components has been described recently.[42] Peripheral surface stimulation of peripheral nerves and proximal location of nerve trunks using detection of mixed nerve action potentials has also been reported as a method to facilitate peripheral neural blockade.[50] Potential advantages of this method of nerve location include avoidance of direct local muscle stimulation and avoidance of the pain which may be produced by muscle contraction at a peripheral site of injury. Potential application of this methodology to clinical practice awaits the development of a simple stimulation and detection apparatus.

Syringes, Needles, and Drugs

The major variation in what otherwise might be an "all purpose" block tray is the numbers and kinds of syringes, needles, and drugs that would be included. Other than the personal preferences for size, glass versus plastic, or three ringed versus plain syringes, there is little to choose among syringes.

Interest in needles has focused primarily on patient safety and comfort, speed of injection, angle of bevel, and the role of needle size in nerve trauma and association with the incidence of postdural puncture headache. Commensurate with the ability to aspirate blood as an indication of possible intravascular injection, generally one should consider using the smallest needle possible. Because most practitioners must do multiple needle insertions to accomplish a successful block, all patients deserve skin and subcutaneous infiltration with a 25-gauge or smaller needle. The use of a needle with a security bead at its proximal shaft has been advocated to preclude loss of broken needles.[33] The use of high-quality disposable needles makes this practice unnecessary and expensive. The role of the needle, its size, and angle of bevel (i.e., sharp point) in producing nerve injury has been studied.[41] In a study comparing the "paresthesia" approach with the "trans-arterial" approach in axillary brachial plexus blockade among 433 patients, a 2.8% incidence of neurologic symptoms was reported after paresthesias and only 0.8% in the transarterial group (Table 6-3). To separate drug effects from needle trauma, the neural damage resulting from a sharp, 14° needle bevel and a blunt, 45° needle bevel was also compared in the isolated rat sciatic nerve model.[40] The 45° needle reportedly produced significantly less damage than did the sharper needle (Table 6-4).

TABLE 6-3. *Number of patients with symptoms of postanesthetic nerve lesion*

	Patients	Patients with nerve lesion	%
Paresthesia group	290	8	2.8
Artery group	243	2	0.8
Total	533	10	1.9

(Selander, D., Edshage, S., and Wolff, T.: Paresthesiae or no paresthesiae? Acta Anesthesiol. Scand., *23*:29, 1979.)

An additional word of caution needs to be mentioned with the use of long-bevel disposable needles. The metal with which these needles are made is relatively soft. After such a needle point strikes a bony surface (rib or spine), it may develop a hook or barb at its tip (Fig. 6-6). This barb can cause significant damage as it passes through nerves, vessels, and tissue. Frequent observation for development of deformities at the needle tip or wiping of the tip of the needle across sterile cotton or gauze will allow recognition of this problem. Needles that are bent or otherwise deformed during the performance of a neural blockade procedure should be discarded and a new needle should be used.

Drugs packaged in commercially prepared, disposable trays have been sterilized, usually with ethylene oxide. Bridenbaugh[9] demonstrated that it was not only safe but beneficial to autoclave the drugs to be used in neural blockade. In the past this was done by adding drugs to the hospital-prepared trays, so that all drugs and equipment were sterilized together. Ampules and vials of drugs may be individually wrapped and autoclaved to be added to an opened sterile tray at the time of use, much the same as extra needles and syringes are added. This not only ensures sterile drug within the container, but also allows the anesthetist freedom to handle the sterile outer container without benefit of an assistant. All local anesthetic drugs used for neural blockade may be safely steam-autoclaved. Dextrose-containing solutions will often acquire a brownish discoloration if autoclaved more than once; if this occurs, the drug should be discarded.

TABLE 6-4. *Fascicular injury after intraneural injections with nerve in situ*

	Long Bevel		Short Bevel	
	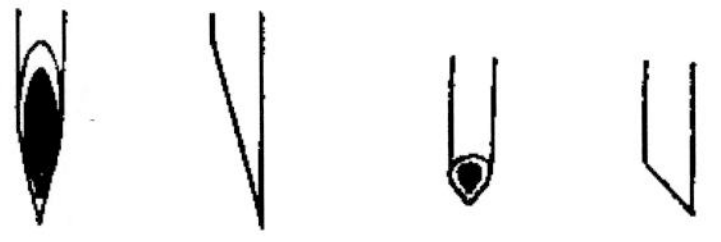			
n	15	15	15	15
Fascicular injury	9	5	0	3

(Selander, D., Dhuner, K.-G., and Lundborg, G.: Peripheral nerve injury due to injection needles used for regional anesthesia. Acta Anesthesiol. Scand., *21*:186, 1977.)

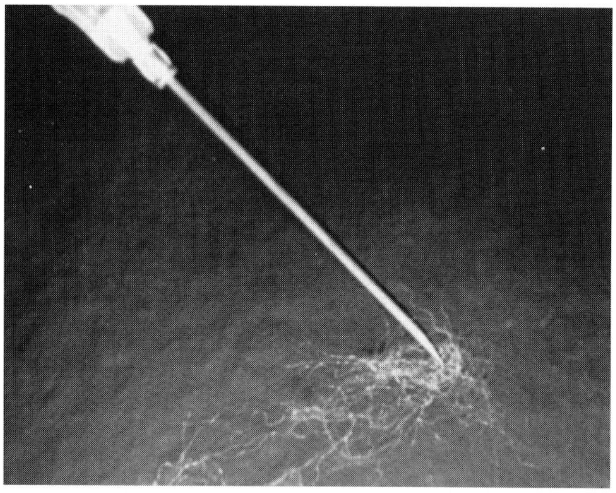

FIG. 6-6. Needle with barb or "fish hook."

In an effort to determine the safety of subjecting these drugs to gas autoclaving with ethylene oxide, Abram[1] studied both ampules and vials of local anesthetic agents, some of which had intentionally been "pre-cracked." There was no evidence of ethylene oxide metabolites, that is, ethylene glycol, in any of the intact ampules. However, some of the drugs in vials with rubber stoppers or in pre-cracked ampules had detectable ethylene glycol. In a separate animal study of the neurologic effect of ethylene glycol, Abram found no effect in doses several times greater than that found in the "cracked ampules." His conclusion was that it was safe to sterilize local anesthetic agents with ethylene oxide, especially those in snap-top ampules. It is important, however, that 24 to 72 hours be allowed for the extrusion of ethylene oxide if it is used to sterilize the entire block tray. Without regard to how hospital-prepared trays are sterilized, there should be indicator tape or tags to assure the anesthetist that the equipment has, in fact, been sterilized.

PERFORMANCE OF NEURAL BLOCKADE

Appropriately selected and premedicated patients should arrive at a well-equipped anesthetizing area adequately prepared for performance of the selected regional block technique. Hyperbaric or hypobaric spinals should be performed on a surface that allows easy manipulation of patient position, sitting, lateral, prone, or supine (head up or head down). Other neural blockade procedures not affected by the patient's position can usually be done with the patient on a stretcher or bed, as long as it allows for appropriate resuscitation efforts, should they be necessary.

Before starting the regional anesthetic procedure, the anesthetist should check the patient's record to determine if and when the patient received the prescribed premedication and if the premedication has—or has had time to have—the desired effect. Only then should a judgment be made of the need for sedative or analgesic supplementation during the block procedure.

The use of supplemental sedative or analgesic agents during the administration of regional anesthesia is actually a continuation of the philosophy of the pre-anesthetic indications previously discussed. The goal of the anesthetist is to provide the patient with a pleasant anesthetic experience throughout the entire perioperative period. The amount of additional supplemental medication required depends not only on the specific requirements of the patient, but also on the degree of painful stimulation associated with the performance of the selected block technique. Most patients require little additional supplementation for the simple, single-injection procedures such as spinal, epidural, and axillary block. In fact, patients often are more easily positioned and responsive to paresthesias if they are not heavily medicated. Conversely, procedures such as deep paravertebral blocks (celiac plexus and sympathetic blocks) or multiple intercostal nerve blocks are quite painful and will likely require additional parenteral sedation and/or analgesics. Nervous or hypersensitive patients may also benefit from additional parenteral supplementation.

As discussed earlier, the selection of sedative or analgesic drugs for administration during performance of a neural blockade procedure is as individual as the choice of premedication. The common goal, however, is to either retain the patient's consciousness (albeit depressed) or have it restored very soon after the procedure has been completed. Excessive sedation incurs the risks of airway obstruction or circulation collapse and will also mask the early warnings of complications of the block, such as an unintentional high spinal or epidural block or an intravascular injection. Excessive doses of some of the psychotropic or dissociative drugs may also render a previously cooperative patient excitable or unmanageable. Short-acting intravenous drugs given in small doses or by a continuous infusion can be carefully titrated to produce the desired level of sedation and analgesia and still ensure a rapid recovery at the conclusion of the block.

Any time supplemental intravenous agents are being used, it is especially important that the anesthetist have an assistant to monitor the patient's vital signs and level of consciousness and ensure maintenance of proper patient positioning for the procedure. Minimum monitoring standards for patients undergoing neural blockade procedures should include pulse oximetry monitoring of pulse rate and oxygen saturation.[3] ECG and blood pressure monitoring should be immediately available. For patients receiving supplemental sedative-hypnotic or opioid analgesic drugs, supplemental oxygen administration should be considered. Following the administration of supplemental sedative or analgesic drugs or performance of the neural blockade procedure, the patient should not be left alone for at least 30 minutes. Regular verbal contact should be maintained to insure consciousness and comfort until the patient has recovered from the effects and the potential side effects of all drugs administered and until delayed systemic toxicity from the local anesthetics is ruled out.

INTRAOPERATIVE MANAGEMENT OF PATIENTS FOR NEURAL BLOCKADE

The most important, and often most challenging, aspect of the successful practice of regional anesthesia is the intraoperative management of the patient. A major concern of patients when discussing regional anesthesia for their surgery is that they will have to remain awake. This all too common approach to the management of patients with nerve blockade may be traced back to the earliest days of surgery when there were no, or too few, anesthetists. Surgeons performed all of the nerve blocks first, and then left their patients wide awake and unmonitored while they proceeded with the surgical procedure. It is not surprising, then, that early anesthetists were expected only to provide general anesthesia to those patients and/or procedures not suitable for a nerve block administered by the surgeon.

It has taken decades for surgeons and anesthetists to accept the fact that it is not a sign of failure if a patient who has had a nerve block, capable of providing 100% of the surgical anesthesia, received enough supplemental sedation to sleep lightly during the operative period.

Gaston Labat,[25] a surgeon and the "Father of Regional Anesthesia," acknowledged in his early writings the importance of sedative supplementation of regional anesthesia. Even more important are his comments relating to excessive noise in the operating room, unnecessary conversation that might be misinterpreted by the patient, and avoidance of the surgeon querying the patients about their level of sedation or comfort. Many patients would be content with little or no sedation if the operating room environment were quiet and nonthreatening.

At present, more anesthetists and surgeons accept the philosophy that every surgical patient deserves the same anesthetic goals of anesthesia care (amnesia, analgesia, etc.) without regard to which drugs are used and how, when, or where they are administered. If one adopts the attitude of patient-oriented total anesthesia care, then the intraoperative administration of supplemental drugs in addition to the neural blockade may be a single anesthetic plan based on the needs of the patient, the surgeon, and the anesthetist.

Patient Considerations

Often, the compelling indication for a regional block technique rather than a general anesthetic is the patient who should *not* be rendered unconscious. This may be due to a full stomach, difficult airway, or high risk (poor physical status), all factors that impose serious risks under general anesthesia. Clearly, these patients should be awake or sedated just enough to provide anxiolysis and a cooperative attitude. Specific pharmacologic agents will be discussed later, but this is a situation in which "vocal anesthesia" (reassuring conversation) or music via headphones can be very helpful.

The antithesis of the high-risk, slightly sedated patient is the pediatric or otherwise overly anxious patient who will likely become uncooperative or agitated intraoperatively. Although these patients may need to be asleep during surgery, it does not preclude their receiving a regional anesthetic for surgical anesthesia prior to induction of unconscious sedation. Supplementation of regional anesthesia thus covers the extremes of patient needs. It is a rare patient, however, who must be denied any kind of supplementation just as a matter of principle. Our armamentarium of drugs and techniques no longer makes this argument valid.

Surgical Considerations

Frequently, the determinant of supplemental drugs and techniques is the location or anticipated duration of the surgical procedure, or both. In general, the closer the surgical procedure is to the head and neck, the more complex the anesthetic management. Patients tend to be more apprehensive about operations in these areas. The proximity of darkening and smothering surgical drapes, retractors, and surgical manipulation around the eyes and the airway may further add to the patient's apprehension and feelings of claustrophobia. For these reasons one would tend toward heavy sedation. Unfortunately, as the surgical team occupies the area at the head of the patient, the anesthetist as protector of the airway is likely dislocated to areas more distant, creating anxiety and caution in balancing sedation with safety. In these surgical procedures, the anesthetist must never render patients unconscious without first securing the airway.

The duration of the surgical procedure affects the complete range of supplemental pharmacology. Extremely short procedures may require no supplemental drugs, whereas lengthy procedures will likely require both sedation and analgesia. Depending on surgical position, most patients will become progressively more uncomfortable from lying still on an operating table. Although high sensory levels of spinal or epidural anesthesia supply their own analgesia, low levels of block and peripheral nerve blocks have limited areas of analgesia. Remember, "all of the body wants to be comfortable." One must review if and what drugs were given in the pre-block period because many are of short duration and will wear off soon after surgery starts. There must be a continuum of necessary sedation and analgesia throughout the perioperative period.

Anesthesiologists who work with otolaryngologists, ophthalmologists, oral surgeons, and plastic surgeons providing monitored anesthesia care (MAC) are especially vulnerable to the aforementioned balance of "conscious airways" in comfortable and cooperative patients. Adding to the situation is the variable expertise of the operating surgeon with the required local and peripheral nerve block techniques. Anesthetists tend to be more forgiving when they supplement their own failed or inadequate blocks than they are when the surgeon has the same results. It is wise and good practice to remember that very light levels of endotracheal inhalation agents provide the same clinical effect as intravenously administered sedatives or analgesics.

Anesthetic Considerations

There are at least three features of regional anesthesia that are primary indications for supplementation. First is a thorough knowledge of the neural elements involved in the surgical procedure and of the regional block to be performed. Will the nerve block provide anesthesia for all of the anticipated surgical stimuli? For example, the use of an intercostal nerve block is extremely beneficial as the anesthetic technique for placement of a gastrostomy feeding tube. One must appreciate, however, that the intercostal nerve block provides only somatic sensory blockade of that portion of the abdominal wall. When the surgeon enters the abdomen, visceral pain will be noted by the patient since the viscera are innervated via the unblocked autonomic fibers. Obviously, some degree of supplemental analgesia will be required.

Second is the possibility that the block is inadequate due to missed or partially blocked neural elements. This could result from poor technique or improper choice of local anesthetic drug, concentration, or volume. On occasion, the operation extends beyond the area of neural blockade. In these cases, supplementary analgesia and sedation in the amount and duration necessary to provide completely satisfactory anesthesia must be rapidly instituted. Withholding or delaying adequate anesthesia is a disservice to the patient. Conversely, it is equally inappropriate to have a 90% satisfactory regional anesthetic converted to a 100% general anesthetic because the patient responded. One should supplement only to the degree and duration necessary to restore the contribution of the regional technique to overall anesthetic satisfaction.

A final factor overlooked by anesthesiologists and surgeons alike is total comfort for the patient. The patient may have a totally numb and paralyzed extremity only to subsequently suffer progressive back and body aches and pains from lying immobilized on a hard operating surface. A ready solution to this problem for healthy patients receiving epidural or spinal anesthesia is to produce a higher level of sensory blockade. For example, a T11 spinal anesthetic would be sufficient for lower extremity surgery. However, if no significant adverse physiologic effects are anticipated, then a T6 level would provide patient comfort up to the mid-thorax without use of large doses of systemic analgesics. All too many "perfect block techniques" have had to be abandoned because of poor management of the patient's total anesthetic needs.

Drugs and Techniques

Specific agents or techniques for intraoperative supplementation of regional anesthesia include the entire gamut of anesthesia practice. For a variety of surgical, anesthetic, and patient factors, every regional anesthetic could potentially require induction of a general anesthetic at a moment's notice, and the anesthetic preparations should be made accordingly. With that in mind, supplementation methods will be discussed from the least to the most intrusive since that is actually the recommended practice, that is, to give no more or do no more than is required to provide a satisfactory anesthetic.

Nonpharmacologic Techniques

A surprising number of patients will request a regional anesthetic because they are actually afraid of being rendered unconscious. Other patients are ambivalent about the need for or desirability of sedation and defer to the anesthetist. A thorough explanation to the patient of the anesthetic and surgical happenings will be helpful in their decision. Reassurance that the anesthetist will be in constant attendance and able to increase levels of supplementation as required or desired is essential. It is important that patients be unaware of the actual events of the procedure, that is, they should be psychologically or pharmacologically distracted from the operative procedures.

Techniques for distraction vary, but are designed to prevent anticipation of pain and fear by the patient. Office practitioners of local and/or nerve block anesthesia become adept at these techniques of "vocal anesthesia." It is equally important that all operating room personnel project the same professional reassurance to the patient.

Music has been a part of the surgical experience for nearly a century, beginning with live performances in dental and operating theaters.[34] Music exerts a calming or distracting influence on patients both in the preoperative holding area and during the surgical procedure.

Since "live" music performances are impractical in this day of cost-effective medicine, simpler techniques must be used. This varies from a simple radio with headsets turned to a music station of the patient's choice to portable tape and CD players with headphones and a sufficient music library to provide music of the patient's choice. Commercially available headphones can be wired into induction operating and recovery rooms as well. Many recovery units now provide closed-circuit or commercial television viewing for patients awaiting discharge home.

Intravenous Techniques

The most common method of administering sedative and analgesic drugs intraoperatively is intravenously. With improved technology the single or combined uses of bolus, continuous drip, continuous infusion, and even patient-controlled administration are now available. The selection of methods should be tailored to the circumstances of patient and procedure. Nearly all the pre-anesthesia and preoperative medications are given as single bolus into the IV line. An exception to this is a propofol or methohexital drip during the administration of prolonged neural blockade such as intercostal nerve block or a celiac plexus block using radiographic needle placement. Intraoperative administration of ongoing sedation in a stable surgical procedure can be accomplished using any of a variety of continuous infusion devices. In circumstances where the patient with satisfactory surgical anesthesia is provided with regional anesthesia and wants to be conscious, a patient-controlled sedation device may be used. In a study in Japan, patients having total abdominal hysterectomy under epidural anesthesia received either self-administered or anesthesiologist-administered bolus doses of midazolam (1.0–1.5 mg) until desired sedation was obtained. The total amount of midazolam in the anesthesiologist-administered group was 12.15 mg ± 3.9 mg (mean ± SD). By comparison, the total amount in the self-administered group was 7.43 mg ± 1.81 mg (mean ± SD). The level of sedation showed wider variation in the patient-controlled series than in the anesthesiologist-sedated group. This suggests that lower doses of sedatives may be used when patients under regional anesthesia are allowed to self-administer the medication to a desired level of comfort.

A very early study[19] provided evidence of the advantage of administering a premedication dose of sedative with the continuing administration of intraoperative supplementation. The 229 outpatients receiving regional anesthesia for surgery were divided into either a placebo group or a diazepam group to determine whether a small IV dose of diazepam confers any benefit to the patient in terms of sedation and/or acceptance of the surgery under local anesthesia. Forty of the patients received no premedication; the remainder received atropine and a phenothiazine. Of the non-premedicated patients who also received placebo intraoperatively, 50% needed additional sedation within the first 15 minutes of the procedure. In contrast, only 1 of 13 unmedicated patients who received intraoperative diazepam needed additional sedative (Table 6-5). In the larger premedicated group, 36% of placebo patients required additional sedation and 37% of the diazepam patients required sedation (Table 6-6). Although the patients who received diazepam had the same need for additional sedation as the placebo group, the level of sedation in the diazepam-treated patients was deeper. It was concluded that "while the use of intravenous diazepam reduces the need for premedications yet the premedication does assist in producing an improved level of sedation." Major disadvantages have led to the decline in the use of diazepam as an intraoperative supplement. These include significant pain with injection, increased risk of venous thrombophlebitis (up to 48%), and long-lasting residual effects. The terminal half-life of diazepam may extend 30 to 50 hours. Kortilla[24] reported impairment of driving skills up to 10 hours after doses of 0.3 to 0.45 mg/kg.

TABLE 6-5. *Distribution of numbers of patients requiring additional sedation*

	Diazepam	Placebo	
Unpremedicated			
Additional sedation	1	13	p = 0.0125
No additional sedation	14	12	
Premedicated			
Additional sedation	13	30	p = 2.005
No additional sedation	83	63	

(Gjessing, J., and Tomlin, P. I.: Intravenous sedation and regional analgesia. Anaesthesia, *32*:66, 1977.)

TABLE 6-6. *Value of premedication*

	Reduced need for additional sedation	
	Additional sedation	No additional sedation
Diazepam group		
Unpremedicated	1	14
Premedicated	13	83
Total	14	97
p = 0.35 (not significant)		
Placebo group		
Unpremedicated	13	12
Premedicated	30	63
Total	43	75
p = 0.025 (very significant)		
	Deepened level of sedation (time only 15 minutes)	
	Unpremedicated	Premedicated
Diazepam group		
Asleep	1	41
Drowsy	6	17
Relaxed	7	18
Total	14	76
p = 0.005 (very significant)		

(Gjessing, J., and Tomlin, P. I.: Intravenous sedation and regional analgesia. Anaesthesia, *32*:66, 1977.)

In addition to midazolam and diazepam, other benzodiazepines have been studied to find an agent that produces better amnesia with less venous irritation and that has a shorter biologic half-life. Although all benzodiazepines can be used effectively as supplements during regional anesthesia, none has proven more efficacious than midazolam (Table 6-7).

Analgesics

Opioids

Use of low-dose opioids alone to supplement regional anesthesia is of limited value. Although their use will address the additional analgesic needs of the patient, most opioids have little effect on the production of amnesia and on levels of consciousness. Mather studied intramuscular meperidine[30] and the subjective effects it produced. They included dryness of the mouth, drowsiness without tranquility,

TABLE 6-7. *Pharmacokinetic parameters of diazepam, lorazepam, midazolam, and flunitrazepam*

	$t_{1/2\alpha}$ (min)	V_1 (liters/kg)	$t_{1/2\beta}$ (h)	Vd_β (liters/kg)	Cl (ml/min)
Diazepam	9–130	0.31–0.41	31.3–46.6	0.9–1.2	26–35
Lorazepam	3–10	0.30–0.72	14.3–14.6	1.14–1.30	1.05–1.10 (ml/min/kg)
Midazolam	3–38	0.17–0.44	2.1–2.4	0.8–1.14	202–324
Flunitrazepam	15 ± 8	0.61 ± 0.36	25 ± 11	3.6 ± 1.3	94 ± 37

$t_{1/2\alpha}$, half-life of distribution; V_1, volume of the central compartment; $t_{1/2\beta}$, elimination half-life; Vd_β, apparent volume of distribution; Cl, total plasma clearance.

(Kanto, J., and Klotz, U.: Intravenous benzodiazepines as anaesthetic agents. Acta Anesthesiol. Scand., *26*:555, 1982.)

visual disturbances, and loss of concentration and ability to keep track of time. It is advantageous intraoperatively if patients do lose track of time. In Mather's study, volunteers believed only 10 minutes had passed when, in fact, 45 to 60 minutes had elapsed.

The addition of an analgesic to benzodiazepine sedation has been shown to reduce the requirements of the latter. Combinations of midazolam and alfentanil and propofol and fentanyl provided highly satisfactory intraoperative conditions during extra corporeal shock wave lithotripsy compared with a pure epidural technique.[31] Caution and careful monitoring are important when combining opioid and benzodiazepine sedation for long procedures and/or in poor-risk patients. Respiratory depression is clearly the most dangerous of the opioid side effects. In a study of volunteers receiving fentanyl 2μg/kg, 50% developed hypoxemia as defined by oxygen saturation (SaO_2) of less than 90%.[5] Although midazolam alone (0.05 mg/kg) produced no adverse respiratory events, the combination of those doses of fentanyl and midazolam produced hypoxemia in 92% of the patients and apnea lasting more than 15 seconds in 50%. The use of supplemental oxygen and adequate monitoring of respiratory function and hemoglobin oxygen saturation are essential for all regional anesthesia techniques in which sedation and analgesia, alone or in combination, are used.

The implementation of continuous infusion techniques for intraoperative supplementation has led to the use of very potent, short-acting agents. In the opioid class of drugs, remifentanil, a fentanyl derivative, has attracted interest. It is rapidly metabolized by tissue esterases with an elimination half-life of 8 to 10 minutes. Its brief duration of action is said to be independent of the duration of administration so it provides no postoperative analgesia. However, with a satisfactory regional block this is less important. Further studies are required to clarify remifentanil's interaction with midazolam and propofol for continuous infusion supplementation, however. Alfentanil is also a short-acting opioid suitable for continuous infusions. Its redistribution half-life is 11.6 minutes. Its elimination half-life of 94 minutes is significantly longer than remifentanil's. When compared to fentanyl, alfentanil is said to be one-fourth as potent and with a duration of action one-third as long.[36]

Ketamine

Ketamine is a potent analgesic that provides amnesia and a state of "dissociative anesthesia." Although it has been used in conjunction with other intravenous agents such as propofol and midazolam to provide total intravenous anesthesia, the reported uses as a supplement to local or regional anesthesia are limited.

A very early study[4] compared low-dose ketamine and diazepam using intermittent doses as supplements to spinal analgesia in elderly patients and noted equivalent benefits. Ketamine (0.25–0.75 mg/kg) given intravenously produced satisfactory analgesia during the subcutaneous infiltration of large volumes of dilute local anesthetic in patients premedicated with midazolam. The analgesia resulting from this dose of ketamine may also prove beneficial in the event of an incomplete local anesthetic block.[52] Even in low doses, ketamine may produce, as part of the dissociative state, varying degrees of muscle rigidity and purposeful skeletal movements independent of surgical stimulation. A study compared alfentanil and ketamine infusions in combination with midazolam for outpatient lithotripsy in patients not deemed to require regional anesthesia. All patients received 4 to 10 mg midazolam prior to starting the treatment. The ketamine group received a loading dose of 0.4 mg/kg and continued with an infusion of 25 μg/kg/min. Ketamine provided superior intraoperative cardiorespiratory stability; however, it was associated with more disruptive movements and dreaming during the procedure. Postoperatively, confusion also occurred more frequently in the ketamine group (31% vs. 5%).[31] The analgesic benefits of ketamine may be used to advantage as a supplement to epidural analgesia for cesarean section. Although its analgesia is greater for somatic than visceral pain it is often helpful to alleviate the pain of delivery of the infant and may be used without associated depression of the neonate.[2]

Nonsteroidal Anti-inflammatory Drugs

The respiratory depressant side effects of the sedative and analgesic drugs frequently used (e.g., barbiturates, opioids, midazolam, and propofol) can be a real problem especially when used in combination for long operative procedures. For that reason, there has been significant interest in determining the efficacy of some of the more potent nonsteroidal anti-inflammatory drugs (NSAIDS) as supplements to regional anesthesia.

The most commonly administered of these drugs are ketorolac and diclofenac. They are more often given intravenously preoperatively to decrease the dosage requirements for opioids when more profound analgesic supplement may be anticipated. One report of ketorolac (1 mg/kg intravenously) intraoperatively noted a similar degree of intraoperative and postoperative analgesia to fentanyl (3μ/kg) when each agent was used as the sole supplement to local anesthesia during minor operations.[7] In addition, substitution of ketorolac for fentanyl prevented pruritus and significantly decreased the incidence of postoperative nausea and vomiting. Because ketorolac produces no sedation, its use intraoperatively may result in less postoperative sedation and thus shorten the time for discharge from the hospital or office. Adverse effects of ketorolac include occasional prolonged bleeding time, gastric irritation, and renal dysfunction.

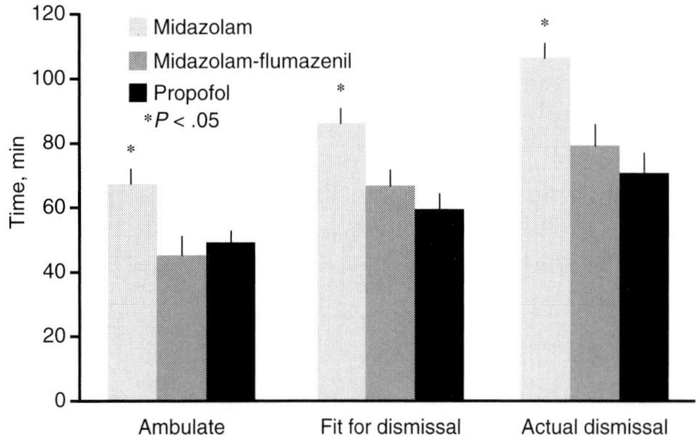

FIG. 6-7. Recovery times after operation during local anesthesia in patients receiving midazolam, midazolam–flumazenil, or propofol for sedation. Mean values ± standard error of the mean; $^*P < .05$ compared with other groups. (Data from Ghouri A.F., Ramirez-Ruiz, M.A., and White, P.E.: Effect of flumazenil on recovery after midazolam and propofol sedation. Anesthesiology, *81*:333–339, 1994) (Reprinted with permission from Brown, D.L.: Regional Anesthesia and Analgesia. pp. 182. Philadelphia, W.B. Saunders, 1996.)

Antagonist Drugs

Now that effective antagonists are available to reverse the actions of benzodiazepines (flumazenil) and opioids (naloxone), there is the risk that clinicians may oversedate or overmedicate patients intraoperatively with the attitude that it is easy to use an antagonist postoperatively. A knowledge of the efficacy and side effects of these antagonists is essential if one is to avoid significant complications.

Flumazenil

Flumazenil is a specific benzodiazepine receptor antagonist that can rapidly reverse the amnestic and sedative properties of the benzodiazepines without incurring a rebound effect of *increased* anxiety after reversal.[51] After 0.1 to 0.2 mg/min of midazolam given intravenously (average of 10 mg over 60–70 min) during minor operations with local anesthesia, flumazenil (1 mg intravenously) improved recovery and permitted patients to be dismissed more than 20 minutes earlier than a placebo control group (Fig. 6-7). Flumazenil was effective for decreasing the duration of postoperative amnesia but had no effect on amnesia during the operation.[18] Of note was the fact that patients receiving the midazolam-flumazenil combination, as opposed to propofol-based sedation, were more likely to report an increase in their level of sedation after their return home. This resedation was likely due to the fact that the half-life of flumazenil is significantly shorter than that of midazolam, allowing sedation to recur 1 to 2 hours after flumazenil was administered.

Naloxone

Naloxone is a pure opioid receptor antagonist with no intrinsic analgesic properties. In low doses, naloxone has been used to antagonize adverse side effects of the opioids while preserving their analgesic effects. Clinically, there seems little doubt that low doses of naloxone will reverse the severity, if not the occurrence, of the nausea, vomiting, and itching that often accompany clinical doses of opioids. Interestingly, the doses of opioids used to premedicate or intraoperatively supplement regional anesthesia seldom result in these troublesome side effects. Furthermore, use of naloxone to reverse side effects of these low doses would very likely reverse their analgesic activities. Naloxone, like flumazenil, has a considerably shorter half-life than most of the opioids. Caution is necessary to prevent a recurrence of the opioid-related side effects. More important is the need to ensure that patients given naloxone will not experience pain in the recovery period. If caregivers are unaware that naloxone was given they will order more opioids for the patient at discharge. Then the risk of opioid overdose after naloxone clearance may be significant. In the future, continuous infusions of short-acting opioids intraoperatively should avoid the need for naloxone reversal.

Inhalation Techniques

There are three major reasons for combining inhalation techniques with a regional anesthetic technique. First, there are operative positions and procedures about the head, neck, thorax, and upper abdomen that require endotracheal tube protection of the airway against obstruction or aspiration. Although patients in critical care units tolerate indwelling endotracheal tubes with little or no sedation, most surgical patients need to be anesthetized if the endotracheal tube is to be tolerated during surgical manipulation. Second, procedures of very long duration can be performed with regional anesthesia using continuous catheter techniques or long-acting local anesthetics such as bupivacaine or ropivacaine. However, the cumulative doses of the parenteral sedatives and opioids can become very high over several hours of administration, leading to a prolonged postoperative recovery time. In these instances, once significant basal sedation is achieved with sedatives and opioids, it may be desirable to switch to low concentrations of inhaled agents. Third, there is always the possibility that the regional anesthetic technique, even with significant sedative supplementation, will not meet all of the needs of the patient or the surgeon. At that point, it is essential to proceed to an inhalation anesthetic technique. Anesthesiologists must always remember that the goal is to provide the patient with the very best anesthetic possible from start to finish. The numbers and types of drugs required or their routes of administration (i.e., regional, intravenous, or inhalation) are not as important as the outcome.

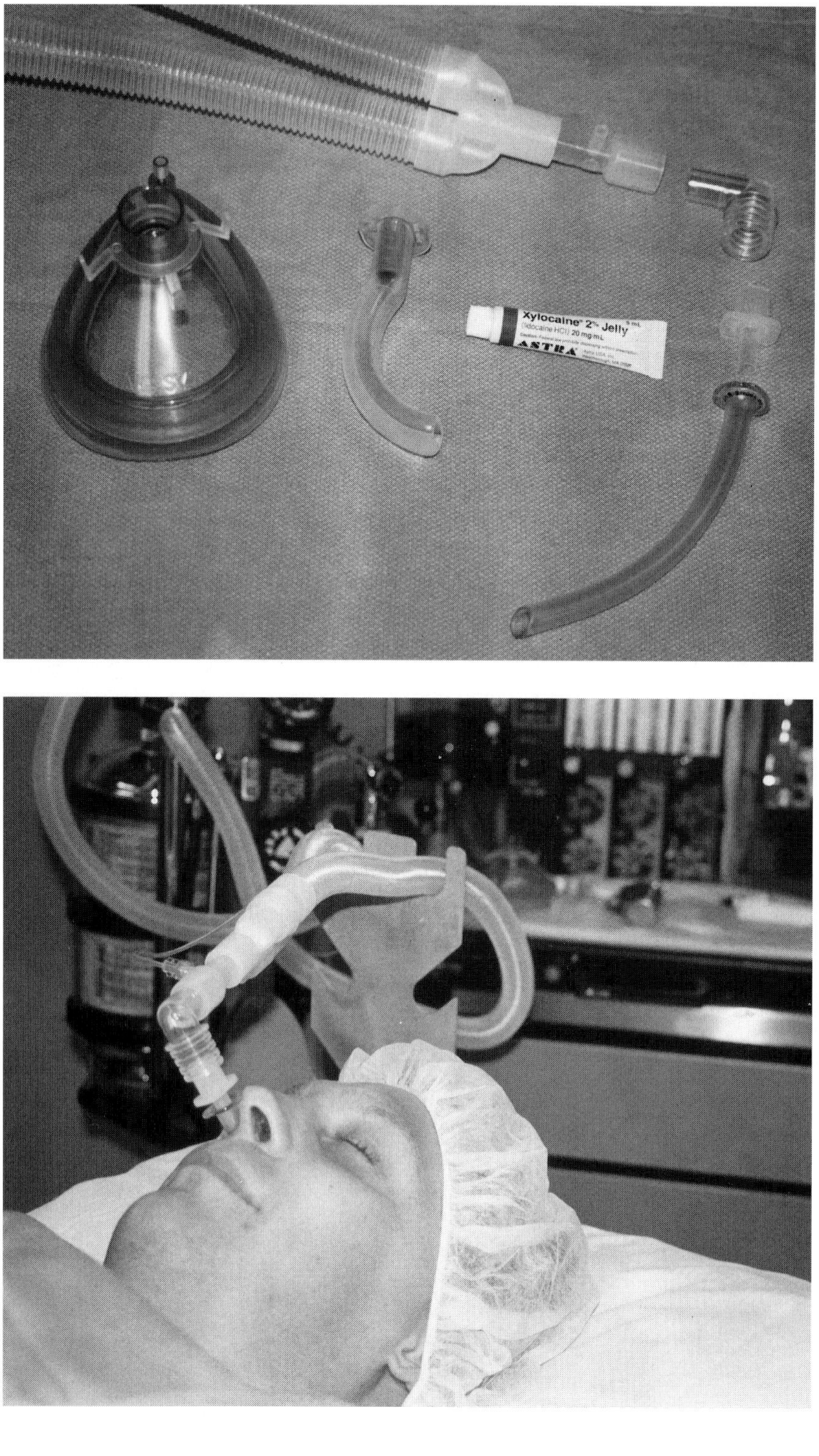

A

B

FIG. 6-8. (A) Equipment used for inhalation supplement of neural blockade using the anesthesia system. The plastic mask with or without oral airway may be used. Alternatively, the plastic nasal airway plus a standard 15-mm fitting may be adapted to the circle system. **(B)** Demonstration of the use of the plastic nasal airway and circle system used for inhalation anesthesia supplement of neural blockade.

For situations in which an endotracheal tube is not required for protection of the airway, there is greater opportunity of using very light concentrations of inhaled drugs as another means of continuously administered sedation or analgesia in a spontaneously breathing patient. This can be administered by mask, nasal airway, or laryngeal mask airway (LMA). For patients who dislike or resist the claustrophobic feeling of head straps and face mask, a nasal airway connected to the circle breathing circuit of an anesthetic machine is a very satisfactory alternative. After gentle insertion of the lubricated airway into the anesthetized nasal passage, an endotracheal tube connector is inserted into the proximal end of the airway and the breathing circuit of the anesthesia machine attached (see Fig. 6-8a,b)

The use of inhaled agents for supplemental sedation is very common in dental practice. Because intravenous injections are not required, this technique is of benefit to pediatric patients. More importantly, inhalation agents are rapidly eliminated through the lungs so recovery may be faster than that following administration of intravenous drugs.

Nitrous oxide is the most popular of the supplemental inhalation agents because of its significant analgesic properties and its low potency, providing a wide margin of safety. Recommended concentrations of nitrous oxide for "inhalation sedation" are 25% to 50%. An early study[15] reported on 394 patients who received 1005 outpatient dental treatments with the usual local anesthetic techniques plus a fixed concentration of 25% nitrous oxide via a nasal mask. Ninety-nine percent of their patients received adequate analgesia without loss of consciousness. More important, the change in anxiety level on subsequent treatments declined from the initial 86% who were "very anxious" to less than 10% on the fourth visit (Fig. 6-9). Generally, these results apply to the proper management of most regional anesthetic procedures. The patient who is pain-free and sedated will be less anxious and more compliant toward future regional anesthetics. Kortilla and co-workers[23] studied the time course of the effects of 30% nitrous oxide on selective cognitive and psychomotor tasks, clearly, a function of importance for outpatient anesthesia. They concluded that "the distinct impairment in hand-eye coordination 12 minutes after cessation of the (45-min test period) administration of the nitrous oxide suggests that even in healthy young subjects, total recovery is not instantaneous and that outpatients need supervision for at least 20 to 30 minutes after administration." However, this evidence does seem to indicate that recovery from nitrous oxide may be faster than after similar doses of most intravenous drugs.

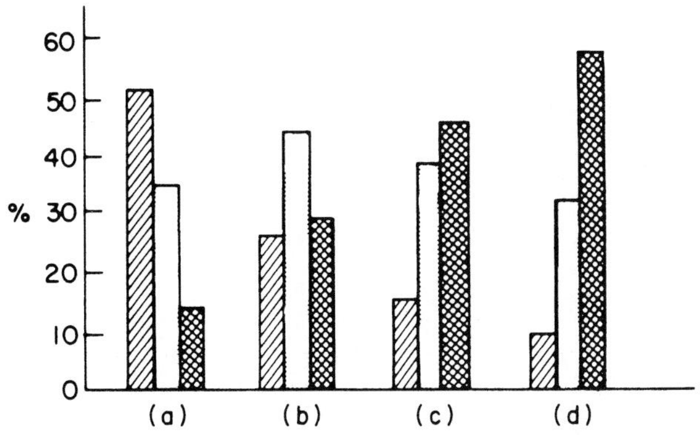

FIG. 6-9. Change in anxiety level as course of treatment proceeds, excluding patients who attended only once. ▨, extremely anxious; □, very anxious; ▩, slightly or not anxious. *(a)* First visit, n = 197; *(b)* second visit, n = 197; *(c)* third visit, n = 135; *(d)* fourth visit, n = 97. (Edmunds, D.H., and Rosen, M.: Inhalation sedation with 25% nitrous oxide. Anaesthesia, *39:*140, 1984.)

Low concentrations of volatile anesthetics may also be used to provide intraoperative sedation and analgesia. In a crossover study of patients in labor, inhalation of 0.75% isoflurane provided analgesia superior to 50% nitrous oxide. Patients receiving isoflurane also had more drowsiness.[28] Another study in dental patients compared inhalation of 0.5% isoflurane with 33% nitrous oxide. Patients breathing isoflurane were more relaxed, had marginally more rapid recovery and, in spite of a slightly unpleasant odor, would prefer isoflurane again.[39] Because of the extensive potency of isoflurane, especially if administered in conjunction with other sedatives and opioids, extreme vigilance and careful monitoring of SaO_2 and other vital signs must be done. Supplemental oxygen should be administered to all patients receiving significant doses of sedative and analgesic drugs without regard to route of administration. All practitioners of local and regional anesthesia must know the fundamentals of administering and monitoring conscious sedation whether it is done by anesthesiologists or other operating room personnel. The practice guidelines of the American Society of Anesthesiologists are excellent basic principles that all should follow.[20]

SUMMARY

The use of sedative and analgesic adjuncts during local and regional anesthesia can enhance patient comfort and improve operative conditions. In turn, this can expand the range of procedures that can safely and comfortably be performed without a major general anesthetic.

There are two basic principles to be derived from the preceding discussion of perioperative management of patients undergoing neural blockade. First, neural blockade is just one technique in the total armamentarium of the anesthesiologist. The anesthesiologist must be intellectually, psychologically, and technically prepared to perform inhalation or intravenous anesthesia techniques, as well as regional anesthesia techniques. The successful outcome of regional as well as general anesthesia practices requires provision of adequate space, equipment, and assistance. Finally, and most important, one should not feel that regional anesthesia techniques are failures if additional drugs and techniques are required for complete patient or surgical satisfaction. To exploit each drug and technique, alone or in combination, to the maximum benefit is the ultimate consultant practice of anesthesiology.

Second, it follows that the use of regional anesthesia techniques is only a part of the total anesthetic care of the patient. The anesthesiologist must deal with the whole patient from the pre-anesthetic visit through the discharge from the facility. The goal of correct premedication and supplementation of regional anesthesia is to maximize the benefits of what was, presumably, the appropriately selected and well-administered regional anesthetic technique. Empirical or premature overmedication carries the risk of respiratory and cardiovascular complications. This will also discourage anesthesiologists and surgeons from using regional anesthesia because "they take too long to accomplish and they all have to be put to sleep anyway." Conversely, refusing to supplement when and to the degree necessary will only incur the ill will of the patient and surgeon. The appropriate use of analgesics and sedatives as premedication and for intraoperative supplementation is the key to an ever-increasing acceptance of the practice of regional anesthesia.

REFERENCES

1. Abram, S.E., Ho, K.C., and Doumas, B.T.: Ethylene oxide sterilization of local anesthetics a potential hazard? Reg. Anesth., *4:*2, 1979.
2. Akamatsu, T.J., Bonica, J.J., and Rehmet, R.: Experiences with the use of ketamine for parturition. Anesth. Analg., *53:*284, 1974.
3. American Society of Anesthesiologists, House of Delegates: Standards for Basic Intraoperative Monitoring. Park Ridge, IL, ASA, October 21, 1986, amended October 13, 1993.
4. Austin, T.R.: Low dose ketamine and diazepam during spinal analgesia. Anaesthesia, *35:*391, 1980.
5. Bailey, P.L., Pace, N.L., Ashburn, M.A., *et al.*: Frequent hypoxemia and apnea after sedation with midazolam and fentanyl. Anesthesiology, *73:*826, 1990.
6. Baranowski, A.P., and Pither, C.E.: A comparison of three methods of axillary brachial plexus anaesthesia. Anaesthesia, *45:*362, 1990.
7. Basek, V., Smith, D.B., and Cox, C.: Keterolac or fentanyl to supplement local anesthesia? J. Clin. Anesth., *4:*480, 1992.
8. Bosenberg, A.T.: Lower limb nerve blocks in children using unsheathed needles and a nerve stimulator. Anaesthesia *50:*206, 1995.
9. Bridenbaugh, L.D., and Moore, D.C.: Does repeated heat sterilization of local anesthetic drugs affect potency? Anesthesiology, *25:*372, 1964.
10. Davies, M.J., and McGlade, D.P.: One hundred sciatic nerve blocks: A comparison of localisation techniques. Anaesth. Intensive Care, *21:*76, 1993.
11. deJong, R.H., and Heavner, J.E.: Diazepam prevents local anesthetic seizures. Anesthesiology, *34:*523, 1971.
12. Dexter, F., and Tinker, J.H.: Analysis of strategies to decrease post anesthesia care unit costs. Anesthesiology, *82:*94, 1995.
13. Dundee, J.W., Lilburn, J.K., Toner, W., and Howard, P.J.: Plasma lorazepam levels. A study following single dose administration of 2 and 4 mg by different routes. Anaesthesia, *33:*15, 1978.
14. Dundee, J.W., and Wilson, D.B.: Amnesic action of midazolam. Anaesthesia, *35:*459, 1980.
15. Edmunds, D.H., and Rosen, M.: Inhalation sedation with 25% nitrous oxide. Anaesthesia, *39:*183, 1984.
16. Ford, D.J., Pither, C., and Raj, P.P.: Comparison of insulated and uninsulated needles for locating peripheral nerves with a peripheral nerve stimulator. Anesth. Analg., *63:*925, 1984.
17. Ford, D.J., Pither, C.E., and Raj, P.P.: Electrical characteristics of peripheral nerve stimulators: Implications for nerve localization. Reg. Anaesth., *9:*73, 1984.
18. Ghouri, A.F., Ramirez-Ruiz, M.A., and White, P.F.: Effect of flumazenil on recovery after midazolam and propofol sedation. Anesthesiology, *81:*333, 1994.
19. Gjessing, J., and Tomlin, P.I.: Intravenous sedation and regional analgesia. Anaesthesia, *32:*63, 1977.
20. Guidelines for Sedation and Analgesia by Non-Anesthesiologists. American Society of Anesthesiologists, 1995.
21. Kapur, P.A.: The big little problem [Editorial]. Anesth. Analg., *73:*243, 1991.
22. Koons, R.A.: The use of the Block-Aid monitor and plastic intravenous cannulas for nerve blocks. Anesthesiology, *31:*290, 1962.
23. Kortilla, K., Ehoneim, M.M., Jacobs, L., Mewaldt, S.P., and Petersen, R.C.: Time course of mental and psychomotor effects of thirty percent nitrous oxide during inhalation and recovery. Anesthesiology, *54:*220, 1981.
24. Kortilla, K., and Linnoula, M.: Recovery and skills related to driving after intravenous sedations: Dose-response relationship with diazepam. Br. J. Anaesth., *47:*457, 1975.
25. Labat, G.: Regional Anesthesia. Philadelphia, W.B. Saunders, 1922.
26. Lavoie, J., Martin, R. Tetrault, J.-P., Cote, D.J., and Colas, M.J.: Axillary plexus block using a peripheral nerve stimulator: Single or multiple injections. Can. J. Anaesth., *39:*538, 1992.
27. McKay, A.C., and Dundee, J.W.: Effect of oral benzodiazepines on memory. Br. J. Anaesth., *52:*1247, 1980.
28. McLead, D.D., Ramayya, G.P., and Tunstall, M.E.: Self-administered isoflurane in labour. A comparative study with entonox. Anaesthesia, *40:*424, 1985.
29. Maltby, J.R.: The shortened fluid fast and the Canadian Anaesthetists' Society's new guidelines for fasting in elective/emergency patients. Can. J. Anaesth., *37:*905, 1990.
30. Mather, L.E., Lindop, M.J., Tucker, G.T., and Pflug, A.E.: Pethidine revisited: Plasma concentrations and effects after intramuscular injection. Br. J. Anaesth., *47:*1269, 1975.
31. Monk, T.G., Boure, B., White, P.F., *et al.*: Comparison of intravenous sedative-analgesic techniques for outpatient immersion lithotripsy. Anesth. Analg., *72:*616, 1991.
32. Montgomery, S.J., Raj, P.P., Nettles, D., and Jenkins, M.T.: The use of the nerve stimulator with standard unsheathed needles in nerve blockade. Anesth. Analg., *52:*827, 1973.
33. Moore, D.C.: Regional Block, 4th ed. Springfield, IL, Charles C. Thomas Publishers, 1965.
34. Neal, J.J., and McMahon, D.J.: Equipment. *In* Brown, D.B. (ed): Regional Anesthesia and Analgesia, 1st ed. p. 162. Philadelphia, Saunders, 1996.
35. Pearson, R.B.: Nerve block in rehabilitation: A technique of needle localization. Arch. Phys. Med. Rehab., *36:*631, 1955.
36. Philip, B.K.: Supplemental medication for ambulatory procedures under regional anesthesia. Anesth. Analg., *64:*1117, 1985.
37. Phillips, S., Hutchinson, S., and Davidson, T.: Preoperative drinking does not affect gastric contents. Br. J. Anaesth., *70:*6, 1993.
38. Riegler, F.X.: Brachial plexus block with the nerve stimulator: Motor response characteristics at three sites. Reg. Anaesth., *17:*295, 1992.
39. Rodrigo, M.R., and Rosenquist, J.B.: Isoflurane for conscious sedation. Anaesthesia, *43:*369, 1988.
40. Selander, D., Dhuner, K.G., and Lundborg, G.: Peripheral nerve injury due to injection needles used for regional anesthesia. Acta Anaesthesiol. Scand., *21:*182, 1977.
41. Selander, D., Edshage, S., and Wolff, T.: Paresthesiae or no paresthesiae? Acta Anaesthesiol. Scand., *23:*27, 1979.
42. Shannon, J., Lang, S.A., Yip, R.W., and Gerard, M.: Lateral femoral cutaneous nerve block revisited. Reg. Anesth., *20:*100, 1995.
43. Smith, B.L.: Efficacy of a nerve stimulator in regional analgesia; experience in a resident training program. Anaesthesia, *31:*778, 1976.
44. Stoelting, R.K.: Responses to atropine, glycopyrrolate, and Riopan of gastric fluid pH and volume in adult patients. Anesthesiology, *48:*367, 1978.
45. Strunin, L.: How long should patients fast before surgery? Time for new guidelines [Editorial]. Br. J. Anaesth., *70:*1993.
46. Tulchinsky, A., Weller, R.W., Rosenblum, M., and Gross, J.B.: Nerve stimulator polarity and brachial plexus block. Anesth. Analg., *77:*100, 1993.
47. Vickers, M.D., Wood-Smith, F.G., and Stewart, H.C.: Central nervous system depressants. *In* Drugs in Anaesthetic Practice, 5th ed. pp. 66. London, Butterworth & Co., 1978.

48. vonPerthes, G.: Uker leitungsanasthesie unter zuhilfenahme elektrischer reizung. Med. Wschr., *47:*2545, 1912.
49. Watcha, M.F., and White, P.F.: Postoperative nausea and vomiting, its etiology, treatment and prevention. Anesthesiology, *77:*162, 1992.
50. Wee, M.Y.K., Geeurickx, A., and Wimalaratna, S.: A method to facilitate regional anaesthesia by detection of mixed nerve action potentials. Br. J. Anaesth., *69:*411, 1992.
51. White, P.F., Shafer, A., Boyle, W.A., *et al.*: Benzodiazepine antagonism does not provoke a stress response. Anesthesiology, *70:*636, 1989.
52. White, P.F., Vasconez, L.O., Mathes, S.A., *et al.*: Comparison of midazolam and diazepam for sedation during plastic surgery. Plas. Reconstr. Surg., *81:*703, 1988.
53. Woolf, C.J., and Chang, M.S.: Preemptive analgesia—Treating postoperative pain by preventing the establishment of central sensitization. Anesth. Analg., *77:*362, 1993.
54. Zahari, D.T., Englund, K., and Girolamo, M.: Peripheral nerve block with use of nerve stimulator. J. Foot Surg., *29:*162, 1990.

A

Central Neural Blockade

Neural Blockade in Clinical Anesthesia and Management of Pain, Third Edition,
edited by M.J. Cousins and P.O. Bridenbaugh.
Lippincott–Raven Publishers, Philadelphia © 1998.

CHAPTER 7

Spinal (Subarachnoid) Neural Blockade

Phillip O. Bridenbaugh, Nicholas M. Greene, and Sorin J. Brull

Spinal anesthesia consists of the temporary interruption of nerve transmission within the subarachnoid space produced by injection of a local anesthetic solution into cerebrospinal fluid. Used widely, safely, and successfully for almost 100 years, spinal anesthesia has many potential advantages over general anesthesia, especially for operations involving the lower abdomen, the perineum, and the lower extremities.

In this chapter we review the techniques of spinal anesthesia and its advantages and disadvantages based on anatomic, pharmacologic, and physiologic principles. Spinal anesthesia for diagnostic and therapeutic purposes, including differential spinal anesthesia, is discussed in Chapter 27. Intrathecal injection of opioids is discussed in Chapter 29.

Many terms have been used to describe the injection of local anesthetics into the subarachnoid space, including *spinal anesthesia*, *spinal* or *subarachnoid analgesia*, *spinal* or *subarachnoid block*, and *subarachnoid anesthesia*. *Subarachnoid* is semantically correct: The injection is made into the subarachnoid space, and that is where the neural response occurs. Subarachnoid is certainly clear and unambiguous to physicians. Subarachnoid is not equally clear to any but the patient with the most sophisticated knowledge of anatomy. In communicating with patients, *subarachnoid* is best avoided if truly informed consent is to be obtained for the type of anesthesia to be used. The term *block*, as in *spinal* or *subarachnoid block*, is incorrect. To neurologists, neurosurgeons, and other nonanesthesiologists, spinal block means obstruction to the flow of cerebrospinal fluid (CSF) within the spinal subarachnoid space. *Analgesia* is also not entirely correct. Injection of local anesthetics (not local "analgesics") into CSF produces anesthesia, not analgesia, in the operative field. All sensation is lost, not just the ability to feel pain. It is suggested that *spinal anesthesia*, the term used in this chapter, is preferable. It is accurate. It is unambiguous.

P. O. Bridenbaugh: Department of Anesthesia, University of Cincinnati College of Medicine, Cincinnati, Ohio 45267-0531.

N. M. Greene: Department of Anesthesiology, Yale University School of Medicine, New Haven, Connecticut 06520-8051.

S. J. Brull: Department of Anesthesiology, Yale University School of Medicine; and Section of General Anesthesia, Yale-New Haven Hospital, New Haven, Connecticut 06510.

HISTORY

The history of anesthesia is not the story of random events. It was logical, almost predictable in fact, that anesthesia would be first introduced about 1846 and that, when introduced, the first anesthetic would be an inhalation agent of rather simple chemical structure.[56] It was equally logical, almost inevitable, that the next type of anesthesia to be introduced would be local, not intravenous, anesthesia. But other things had to take place before local anesthesia could be introduced. The needle and syringe had to be invented. The industrial revolution had to develop to the point where needles and syringes could be mass produced with accuracy great enough to ensure a perfect match between barrels and plungers of the syringes. Above all, the germ theory of disease had to be introduced, and, after that, the ability to avoid infection by asepsis had to be proved. Invasive anesthetic techniques using needles were impossible until the fear of creating infection was resolved.

The prerequisites necessary for the introduction of local anesthesia were all realized by the 1880s, and in 1884 Koller reported that the topical application of cocaine to the eye produced anesthesia of the cornea and conjunctiva.[72] Again, there is a sense of inevitability about what Koller did, not only in its timing but also in the fact that cocaine was the first local anesthetic. The first local anesthetic almost had to be a naturally occurring compound. Industrial chemistry had not advanced in the 1880s to the point where compounds as chemically complex as local anesthetics could be synthesized. Also, doctors of the time had to know about and be acquainted with the first local anesthetic in the same way they had to be already familiar with the first inhalation anesthetic, ether.[56] Cocaine, identified in 1855 and isolated in 1860, was a naturally occurring alkaloid that, by the 1880s, had been purified and medically used for nonanesthetic purposes (see Chapter 1).

Within months of publication of Koller's paper, cocaine was being injected to produce regional anesthesia, not just topical anesthesia. In the same year, 1885, Halsted used cocaine to block the brachial plexus, and Corning, a neurologist in New York, injected cocaine intervertebrally in dogs and in patients.[34] As a neurologist, Corning's objective was to relieve chronic pain in his patients, not to produce operative anesthesia. Indeed, whether his injections were made into the subarachnoid or the epidural space is not clear. Corning thus cannot be considered as the one who introduced operative spinal anesthesia. In fact, spinal anesthesia could not become an acceptable means for use of cocaine until a safe, predictable means for performing lumbar punctures was described. Quincke did this in 1891, but even so it was not until 1899 that August Bier used Quincke's technique to inject cocaine in order to produce operative anesthesia in six patients, the first real spinal anesthesia[9] (Table 7-1). Bier's report of his success with spinal anesthesia was rapidly seized upon by others. In the same year Matas in New Orleans and Tuffier in France also reported on the use of cocaine spinal anesthesia,[88,129] as did Tait and Caglieri in San Francisco in 1900.[126] In 1901, there were no less than 27 papers published on cocaine spinal anesthesia.[5] In 1902, Morton, in New York,[96] reported a series of cocaine spinal anesthetics for operations on all portions of the body, including the head and neck.

TABLE 7-1. *History of spinal anesthesia*

1885	J.L. Corning (New York Neurologist):? epidural;? spinal; cocaine for pain relief
1891	Quincke (Germany): lumbar puncture
1899	August Bier (Germany): first cocaine spinal anesthesia in six patients
1899	Matas (New Orleans), Tuffier (France), Tait and Caglieri (San Francisco): cocaine spinal anesthesia
1905	H. Braun (Germany): procaine spinal anesthesia
1907	Barker (United Kingdom): hyperbaric procaine (glucose); hypobaric procaine (alcohol)
1930	Jones (United Kingdom): dibucaine spinal anesthesia
1935	Sise (USA): tetracaine spinal anesthesia
1940	Lemmon (USA): continuous spinal anesthesia
1945	Tuohy (USA): continuous spinal anesthesia
1945	Prickett (USA): report on neurologic safety of intrathecal epinephrine to prolong spinal anesthesia
1954	Wooly and Roe (United Kingdom): report of paraplegia in association with spinal anesthesia
1954	Dripps and Vandam (USA): study demonstrating absence of neurologic sequelae
1965	Re-emergence of use of spinal anesthesia

The first phase in the history of spinal anesthesia, from 1899 to 1905, was characterized by the use of only cocaine for spinal anesthesia. However, the popularity of cocaine spinal anesthesia in the year following 1899 was limited principally to a relatively few enthusiasts who, despite their almost evangelical fervor, were unsuccessful in convincing others of the advantages of their new-found technique. They were unable to do so mainly because of the high frequency of conspicuous central nervous system side effects, including tremors, hyperreflexia, severe headaches, and muscle spasms and pains. By the turn of the century, however, the German chemical and pharmaceutical industry had advanced to the point where new and totally synthetic drugs were being developed. Among these was procaine, first synthesized by Einhorn in 1904. In 1905, Heinrich Braun, a German surgeon, reported the use of procaine for operative spinal anesthesia.[17] With the introduction of procaine, spinal anesthesia entered a new phase, an era of development, refinement, and widespread popularity. Procaine for spinal anesthesia initiated this new era because it was the first neurologically safe local anesthetic. Within an astonishingly brief time, spinal anesthesia became widely used, even though still not universally accepted as a safe, convenient, and effective anesthetic technique. It was, in the eyes of many, vastly superior to general anesthesia with ether or chloroform. It was also simpler than other more complex types of regional anesthesia. Equally important, thanks to the remarkably astute observations of clinicians like Babcock, Koster, Labat, and Pitkin,[4,73,77,108] came understanding of the causes of hypotension during spinal anesthesia and how to manage it. So, too, came refinements in the techniques of spinal anesthesia, including means for controlling levels of anesthesia by making procaine solutions hyperbaric by adding glucose, first reported by Barker in 1907,[6] or hypobaric, initially by adding alcohol. The popularity of spinal anesthesia was further advanced by the synthesis of tetracaine in 1931 and its introduction into clinical practice by Sise in 1935, as well as by the synthesis of dibucaine and its introduction into clinical practice by Jones in 1930.[66,118] These new local anesthetics provided longer duration of spinal anesthesia than did procaine. Duration of spinal anesthesia was further extended by the use of continuous spinal anesthesia by Lemmon in 1940 and Tuohy in 1945.[80,130] In 1945, Prickett and associates published their report on the neurologic safety of intrathecal epinephrine to prolong the duration of spinal anesthesia,[110] a practice introduced as early as 1903 by Braun[16] but never widely accepted because of the fear of neurologic complications.

By the mid-1940s spinal anesthesia had reached a peak of its popularity, a popularity soon followed by almost equally widespread avoidance and neglect. The era of neglect of spinal anesthesia was brought about by a combination of circumstances, including the fear of neurologic complications, a fear based on widely publicized legal decisions, especially in the United Kingdom, and scientifically unsound but widely publicized articles on extraordinarily high incidences of neurologic sequelae (see Chapter 1). The demise of spinal anesthesia was further contributed to by the introduction and popularization of intravenous anesthetics, neuromuscular relaxants, and, somewhat later, modern halogenated inhalation anesthetics. The pharmacologic explosion in anesthesia between 1945 and 1965 made spinal anesthesia appear unnecessarily demanding, inconvenient, and tedious, as well as, at least medicolegally, unsafe. To all of this was added the introduction of ever increasingly radical operations, the magnitude and duration of which were incompatible with spinal anesthesia.

Around 1965, spinal anesthesia began a recovery that has persisted and even accelerated over the last 30 years. One factor in this renaissance was the epidemiologically impeccable studies of Dripps and Vandam demonstrating that, when properly performed, spinal anesthesia is neurologically safe.[44] Another factor was the introduction of new amide-type local anesthetics. Finally, there was gradual acceptance of the fact that general anesthesia, too, has risks and hazards, a concept to which the halothane hepatitis controversy of the 1960s and 1970s also contributed.

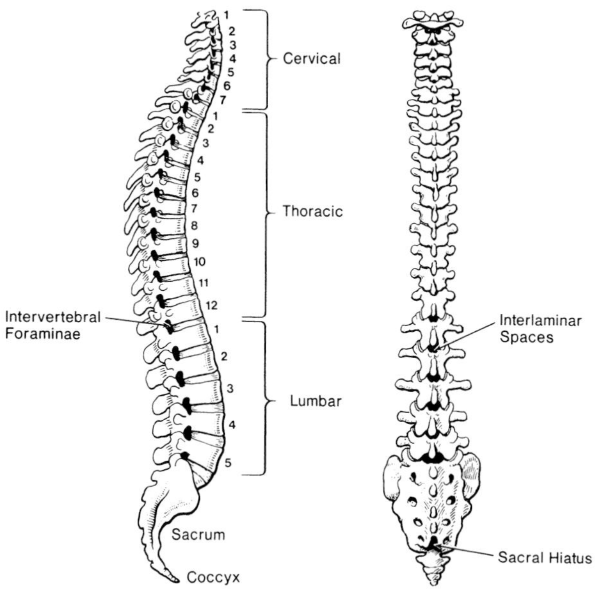

FIG. 7-1. Vertebral column, lateral (*left*) and posterior (*right*) views, illustrating curvatures and interlaminar spaces.

ANATOMY

Intimate knowledge of the anatomy of the vertebral column and its contents is the keystone to successful, safe spinal anesthesia, not only in terms of the performance of lumbar puncture but also in terms of the spread of local anesthetics in CSF and the level of anesthesia achieved.

Vertebral Column

The vertebral column, comprising 33 vertebrae (7 cervical, 12 thoracic, 5 lumbar, 5 fused sacral, and 4 coccygeal), has four curves (Fig. 7-1). The cervical and lumbar curves are convex anteriorly, whereas the thoracic and sacral curves are convex posteriorly. The curves of the vertebral column have a significant influence on the spread of local anesthetics in the subarachnoid space. In the supine position, the high points of the cervical and lumbar curves are at C5 and L5; the low points of the thoracic and sacral curves are at T5 and S2, respectively. The vertebral column is bound together by several ligaments, which give it stability and elasticity (Fig. 7-2).

Supraspinous Ligament. This strong fibrous cord connects the apices of the spinous processes from the sacrum to C7, where it is continued upward to the external occipital protuberance as the ligamentum nuchae. It is thickest and broadest in the lumbar region and varies with patient age, sex, and body build.

Interspinous Ligament. This thin, membranous ligament connects the spinous processes, blending anteriorly with the ligamentum flavum and posteriorly with the supraspinous ligaments. Like the supraspinous ligaments, the interspinous ligaments are broadest and thickest in the lumbar region.

Ligamentum Flavum. Also known as the "yellow ligament," this ligament comprises yellow elastic fibers and connects adjacent laminae that run from the caudal edge of the vertebra above to the cephalad edge of the lamina below. Laterally, this ligament begins at the roots of the articular processes and extends posteriorly and medially to the point where the laminae join to form the spinous process. Here the two components of the ligaments are united, thus covering the interlaminar space.

Longitudinal Ligaments. The anterior and posterior longitudinal ligaments bind the vertebral bodies together.

Epidural Space. This space surrounds the spinal meninges and extends from the foramen magnum, where the dura is fused to the base of the skull, to the sacral hiatus, which is covered by the sacrococcygeal ligament (see Chapter 8). It is bounded anteriorly by the posterior longitudinal ligament, laterally by the pedicles and the intervertebral foramina, and posteriorly by the ligamentum flavum and the

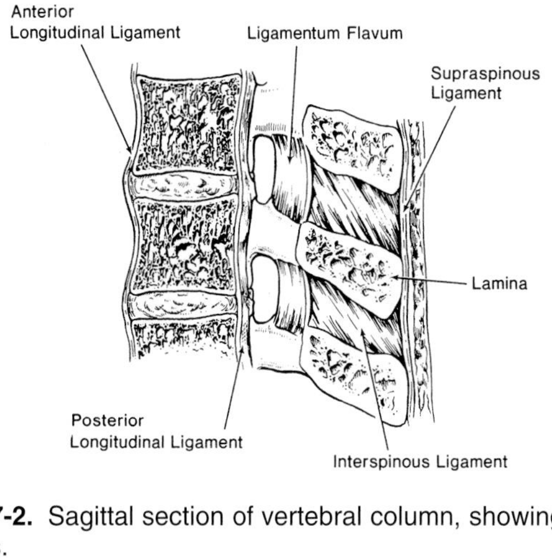

FIG. 7-2. Sagittal section of vertebral column, showing ligaments.

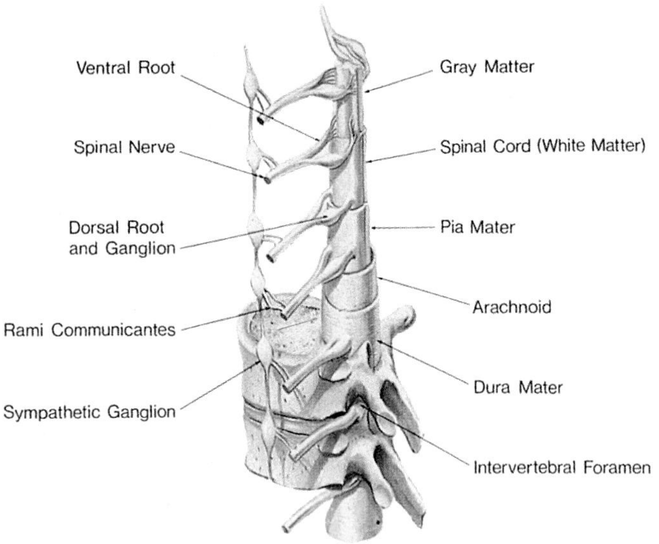

FIG. 7-3. The spinal cord and its related structures.

anterior surface of the lamina. The anterior epidural space is very narrow because of the proximity of the dura and the anterior surface of the vertebral canal. The epidural space is widest posteriorly and varies with the vertebral level, ranging from 1 to 1.5 mm at C5 to 2.5 to 3 mm at T6 to its widest point 5 to 6 mm at the level of L2. In addition to nerve roots that traverse the epidural space, the contents of the epidural space are fat, areolar tissue, lymphatics, arteries, and the extensive internal vertebral venous plexus of Batson.[7]

Spinal Meninges. The spinal cord is protected by both the bony vertebral column and three connective tissue coverings, the meninges (Fig. 7-3; Table 7-2).

Dura mater, the outermost membrane, is a tough, fibroelastic tube the fibers of which run longitudinally. Although continuous, it can be described in two parts: the *cranial* and the *spinal*. The cranial dura consists of an outer layer (endosteal), which lines the skull, and an inner layer (meningeal), which invests the brain and folds inward to form the falx cerebri. The two layers are closely united except where they enclose the great venous sinuses that drain the blood from the brain (Fig. 7-4).

At the spinal level, the outer (endosteal) layer continues down the vertebral canal as periosteal lining. The inner (meningeal) layer continues caudad as the spinal dura, or *theca*. Superiorly, it is firmly attached to the circumference of the foramen magnum of the occipital bone. Inferiorly, or caudally, the dural sac ends at the lower border of S2, where it is pierced by the filum terminale. The filum terminale is the terminal thread of the pia mater, which extends from the tip of the spinal cord to blend with the periosteum on the back of the coccyx. The filum terminale anchors the cord and spinal dura, the latter being further steadied in the lower end of the vertebral column by a few fibrous strips from the posterior longitudinal ligament. The spinal dura also provides a thin cover for the spinal nerve roots, becoming progressively thinner near the intervertebral foramina, where it continues as epineural and perineural connective tissue of the peripheral nerves (Fig. 7-5).

TABLE 7-2. *Applied anatomy: spinal anesthesia*

Ligaments attached to spine	Ligamentum nuchae (cervical) → supraspinous (thickest lumbar region) → sacrum Interspinous, ligamentum flavum, anterior/posterior longitudinal
Epidural space	(see Chapter 8)
Dura	Spinal dura = brain meningeal dura Spinal periosteum = brain endosteal dura Ends at lower S2, pierced by filum terminale
Arachnoid	Attached to dura, but capillary space between the two = subdural space Subdural space—wider laterally and in cervical area
Pia mater	Delicate vascular membrane investing spinal cord
Subarachnoid space	Space between arachnoid and pia Contains arachnoid trabeculae and also CSF Extends from brain to cord to spinal roots
Denticulate ligaments	Lateral projections of pia, anchor spinal cord to dura
Vertebrae	7 cervical, 12 thoracic, 5 lumbar, 5 fused sacral, 4 coccygeal
Spinal nerves	8 cervical, 12 thoracic, 5 lumbar, 5 sacral, 1 coccygeal **Cervical above C7;** exit *above* vertebral level **C8** exits below C7 **Thoracic/lumbar:** exit *below* vertebral level L5 exits between L5 and sacrum **Sacral:** exit via anterior/posterior foramina

Arachnoid mater is the middle of the three coverings of the brain and spinal cord. It is a delicate nonvascular membrane closely attached to the dura and, with it, ends at the

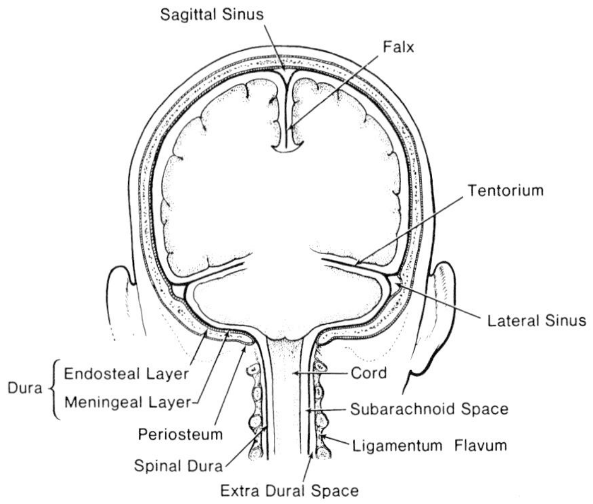

FIG. 7-4. Meningeal coverings of brain and proximal cord.

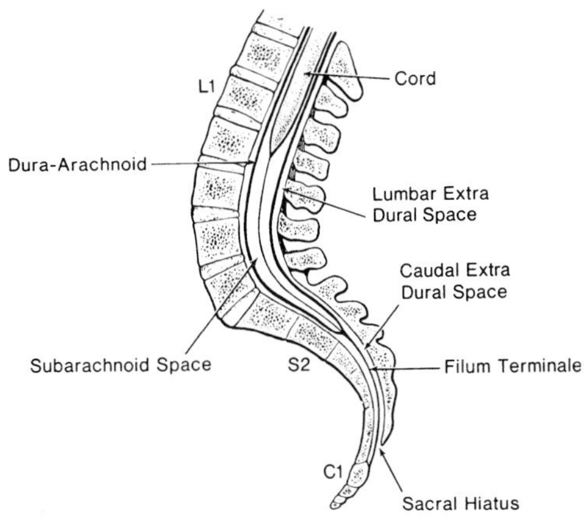

FIG. 7-5. Lumbosacral portion of vertebral column, showing terminal spinal cord and its coverings.

lower border of S2. There is a capillary interval or potential cavity between the dura and arachnoid mater called the *subdural space*, which contains a minute quantity of serous fluid that moistens the smooth surfaces of the opposed membranes. It does not communicate directly with the subarachnoid space but extends laterally over the nerve roots and ganglia. The subdural space is wider in the cervical region and more accessible than elsewhere in the spinal column. It is also wider laterally adjacent to the nerve roots, which can be shown after injection of radioactive dye (Fig. 7-6). In this situation, the injected solution curves downward between the arachnoid and dura to lymph spaces within root ganglia.[92] Analgesic solutions introduced into this space are said to ascend, but only very slowly in the cranial cavity with which this space communicates.

Although most subdural injections of local anesthetics are unintentional, Mehta[90] describes the technique for intentional entry into the space with x-ray control. He notes that if the needle enters the subarachnoid space with flow of CSF, one withdraws the needle until the flow stops, and at this point the bevel of the needle is likely to rest in the subdural space. This could also allow CSF to flow into the subdural space. The subdural space has long been recognized by radiologists during the performance of a myelogram. If dye leaks through the needle puncture into the subdural space, it obscures the radiologic field for weeks, which may account for a few, but clearly not all, of the failed spinals despite aspiration of "some" spinal fluid. The case reports of subdural injection indicate unilateral or inordinately high levels of anesthesia, but usually after volumes of local anesthetic intended for epidural anesthesia.[87,105] This occasional phenomenon explains why the term "subdural block" is incorrect when referring to spinal anesthesia and explains the rare case of spinal subdural hematoma (see Chapter 21).

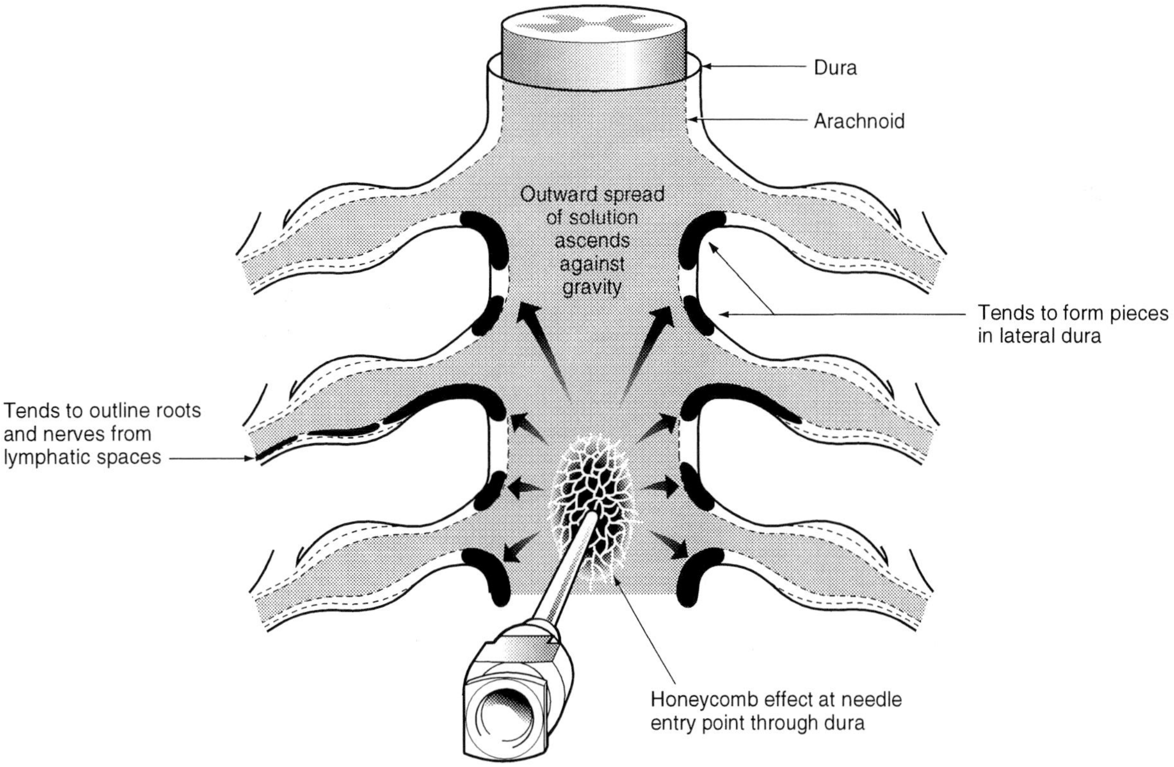

FIG. 7-6. Diagrammatic representation of the spread of radiopaque contrast medium injected into the cervical subdural space. The initial honeycomb effect at the injection site is replaced by the collection on either side of small pools or pieces in the lateral dura owing to outward spread of the solution. (Redrawn with permission from Mehta, M., and Maher, R.: Injection into the extra-arachnoid subdural space. Anaesthesia, *32*:761, 1977.)

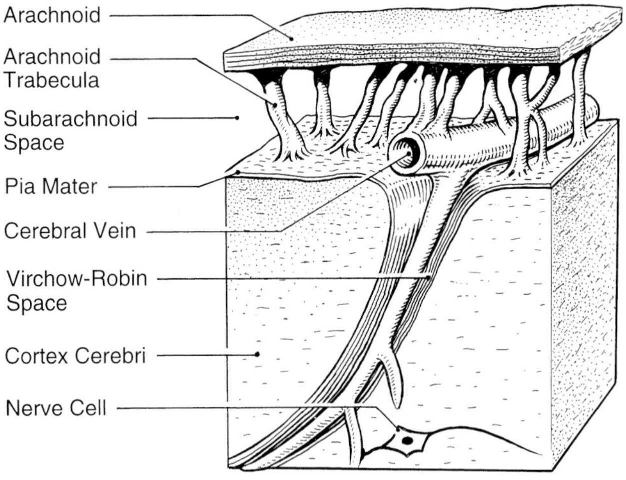

FIG. 7-7. Diagram of subarachnoid space showing blood vessels and arachnoid trabecula. (Redrawn after Strong, O.S., and Elwyn, A.: Human Neuroanatomy. Baltimore, Williams & Wilkins, 1959.)

Pia mater is a delicate, highly vascular membrane closely investing the spinal cord and brain. It clings to the surface of both throughout their entire course. The space between the arachnoid and the pia is thus called the *subarachnoid space* (see Table 7-2). A large number of cobweb-like trabeculae run between these two membranes, and, of course, the space contains the spinal nerves and the CSF as well. The many blood vessels that supply the spinal cord are also found in this space (Fig. 7-7). Lateral projections of the pia, the denticulate ligaments, are attached to the dura and aid in supporting the spinal cord.

Spinal Cord. The spinal cord, which is continuous above with the medulla oblongata, begins at the level of the foramen magnum and ends below as the conus medullaris. At birth, the cord ends at the level of L3 but rises to end in adult life at the lower border of L1 (Fig. 7-8).

Spinal Nerves. There are 31 pairs of symmetrically arranged spinal nerves, which are attached to the spinal cord by two roots (see Table 7-2). Both the anterior and posterior roots arise from the cord as several filaments, or rootlets. The lumbar and sacral nerve roots extending beyond the termination of the spinal cord at the lower border of L1 form the cauda equina. The greater surface area of nerves in the cauda equina as they traverse the subarachnoid space from their point of origin in the cord to their point of exit through the dura, together with the fact that they are covered by only a thin layer of pia, means that lumbar and sacral nerve roots are especially sensitive to the effects of local anesthetics in the CSF by which they are bathed.

Subarachnoid Space. Bounded internally by the pia and externally by the arachnoid, this space is filled with cerebrospinal fluid and contains numerous arachnoid trabeculae, which form a delicate, spongelike mass. This space has three divisions: cranial (surrounding the brain), spinal (surrounding the spinal cord), and root (surrounding the dorsal and ventral spinal nerve roots). All of these components are in "free communication" with each other. Again, as the dorsal and ventral nerve roots leave the spinal cord, they are covered only by pia and bathed in CSF (see Fig. 7-3). As these spinal nerve roots pass beyond the spinal dura and traverse the epidural space, they carry with them all three meningeal layers and have distinct epidural, subdural, subarachnoid, and subpial spaces. As indicated above, as the dura extends further out toward the intervertebral foramen, it becomes much thinner. The subarachnoid space extends separately along both the dorsal and ventral roots to the level of the dorsal root ganglion, where the arachnoid and the pia continue as the perineural epithelium of the peripheral nerve. The spinal nerve root arachnoid contains proliferations of arachnoid cells, or villi, which have been identified in humans and other animals, along with dorsal and ventral roots.[114] These proliferations are of many shapes and sizes and may protrude into adjacent subdural spaces (see Chapter 8).

Cerebrospinal Fluid. This is an ultrafiltrate of the blood plasma, with which it is in hydrostatic and osmotic equilibrium (Table 7-3). It is a clear, colorless fluid found in the spinal and cranial subarachnoid spaces and in the ventricles of the brain. At 37°C, the specific gravity ranges from 1.003 to 1.009, with a mean of 1.006. The total volume of CSF in the average adult ranges from 120 to 150 ml, of which 25 to 35 ml is in the spinal subarachnoid space. The majority of the spinal subarachnoid volume lies distal to the cord in the area of the cauda equina. In the horizontal position, the pressure of CSF ranges from 60 to 80 mm H_2O.

Acid-Base. In normal subjects, the pH of CSF is slightly lower than that of the arterial blood (7.32). The Pco_2 is higher (48 mm Hg) and the bicarbonate level about the same in both fluids (23 mEq/liter). Cisternal and lumbar CSF samples obtained at the same time in steady-state have very similar pH, Pco_2 and bicarbonate levels; however, during rapidly changing conditions, as in respiratory alkalosis or acidosis, the lumbar CSF is slow to respond, whereas cisternal values reflect changes in systemic acid-base parameters.[49]

TABLE 7-3. *Composition of cerebrospinal fluid*

Specific gravity	1.006 (1.003–1.009) (at 37°C)
Volume	120–150 ml (25–35 ml spinal space)
CSF pressure (lumbar)	60–80 mm H_2O (in horizontal position)
pH	7.32 (7.27–7.37) (cisternal pH follows blood; lumbar pH lags behind)
Pco_2	48 mm Hg
Hco^{3-}	23 mEq/L
Sodium	133–145 mEq/L
Calcium	2–3 mEq/L
Phosphorus	1.6 mg/dl
Magnesium	2.0–2.5 mEq/L
Chloride	15–20 mEq/L
Proteins (lumbar)	23–38 mg/dl (↑ permeability to protein in lumbar area)

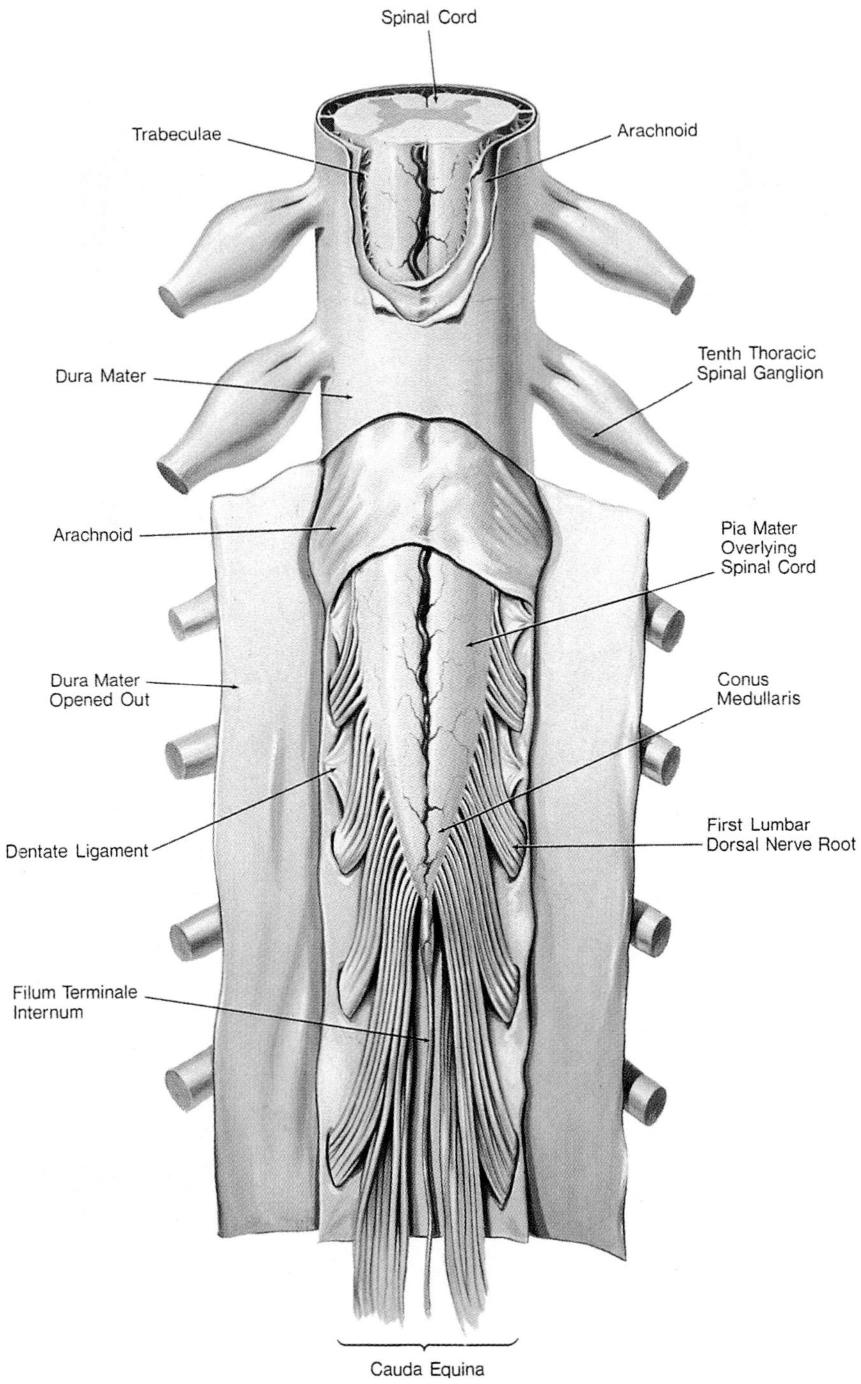

FIG. 7-8. Terminal spinal cord and cauda equina, showing relationship of overlying structures.

Electrolytes. The concentrations of electrolytes in CSF are similar to, but vary from, those in serum. The sodium ion is the major cation present in plasma and CSF. Whereas the normal concentration range in both fluids is similar, varying between 133 and 145 mEq/liter, the absolute concentration is slightly greater in plasma. The CSF calcium levels vary between 2 and 3 mEq/liter and the total serum levels between 4 and 5 mEq/liter. Not only is CSF calcium not affected by diseases of the nervous system, but also it is even maintained postmortem. Thus there seems little basis for measuring CSF calcium in clinical practice. Similar stability occurs with CSF phosphorus (largely phosphate). The normal CSF level is about 60% of the serum level (1.6 mg/dl compared with 4.0 mg/dl). There has been more interest in the magnesium levels in CSF because magnesium is the sole cation in which the concentration in CSF is substantially greater (30%) than that in serum. The CSF level lies between 2.0 and 2.5 mEq/liter and the serum level between 1.5 and 2.0 mEq/liter.

Interest in the CSF chloride results from its role as the major anion of CSF and the fact that its concentration exceeds the plasma level. CSF chloride level is normally 15 to 20 mEq/liter higher than the serum level. It is slightly reduced in the presence of a very elevated CSF protein level and otherwise follows serum level, but absolute changes are less than those in serum. There seems to be no indication for measurement of CSF chloride in clinical practice.[49]

Proteins. In normal children and adults, there is a concentration gradient of protein from a low level in the ventricles (6–15 mg/dl) to an intermediate level in the cisterna magna (15–25 mg/dl) to the highest level in the lumbar sac (20–50 mg/dl). This gradient is best explained by the relatively increased permeability of the blood–CSF barrier to proteins in the spinal subarachnoid space. Normal values reported for the lumbar CSF total protein have varied. Normal patients and volunteers have mean values ranging from 23 to 28 mg/dl. Since the reported upper and lower limits vary from 9 to 58 mg/dl, it is essential that clinicians know the range of normal values for the laboratory performing the test.

Cerebrospinal fluid is formed by either secretion or ultrafiltration from the choroid arterial plexuses of the lateral, third, and fourth ventricles. The choroid plexus comprises invaginations of capillaries from the subarachnoid space (Fig. 7-9). These capillaries are supported in a flimsy connective tissue framework of pia mater, which, in turn, is in intimate contact with the ependyma, a single-layered epithelium lining the ventricle. It is presumed that these ependymal cells are primarily responsible for the secretion of CSF. Although it is possible, experimentally, to induce both increased and decreased rates of CSF formation, there is a great tendency for it to be maintained at a constant rate.[50] Cardiac glycosides in usual clinical doses probably have no measurable effect, whereas systemic administration to animals of acetazolamide, a carbonic anhydrase inhibitor, reduces the rate of CSF formation by as much as 50%.

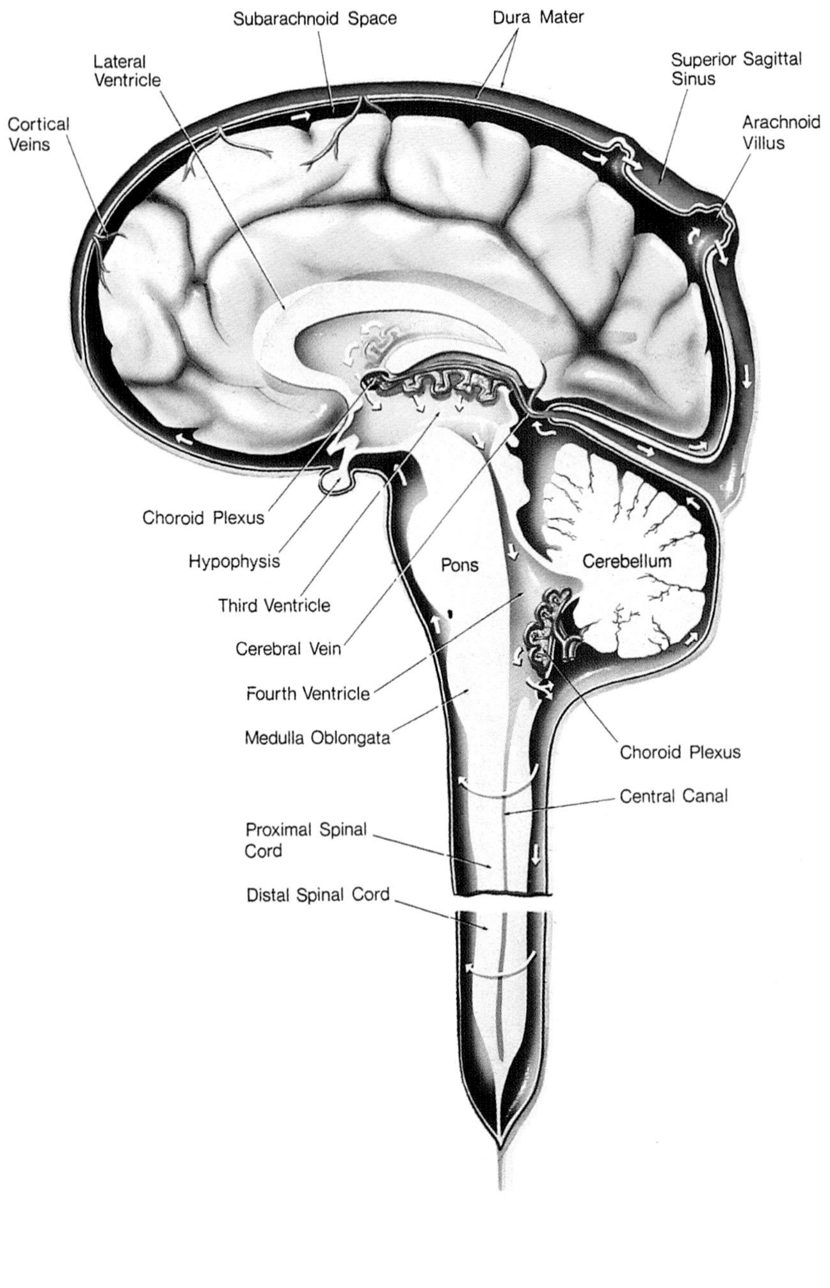

FIG. 7-9. Production, circulation, and resorption of cerebrospinal fluid.

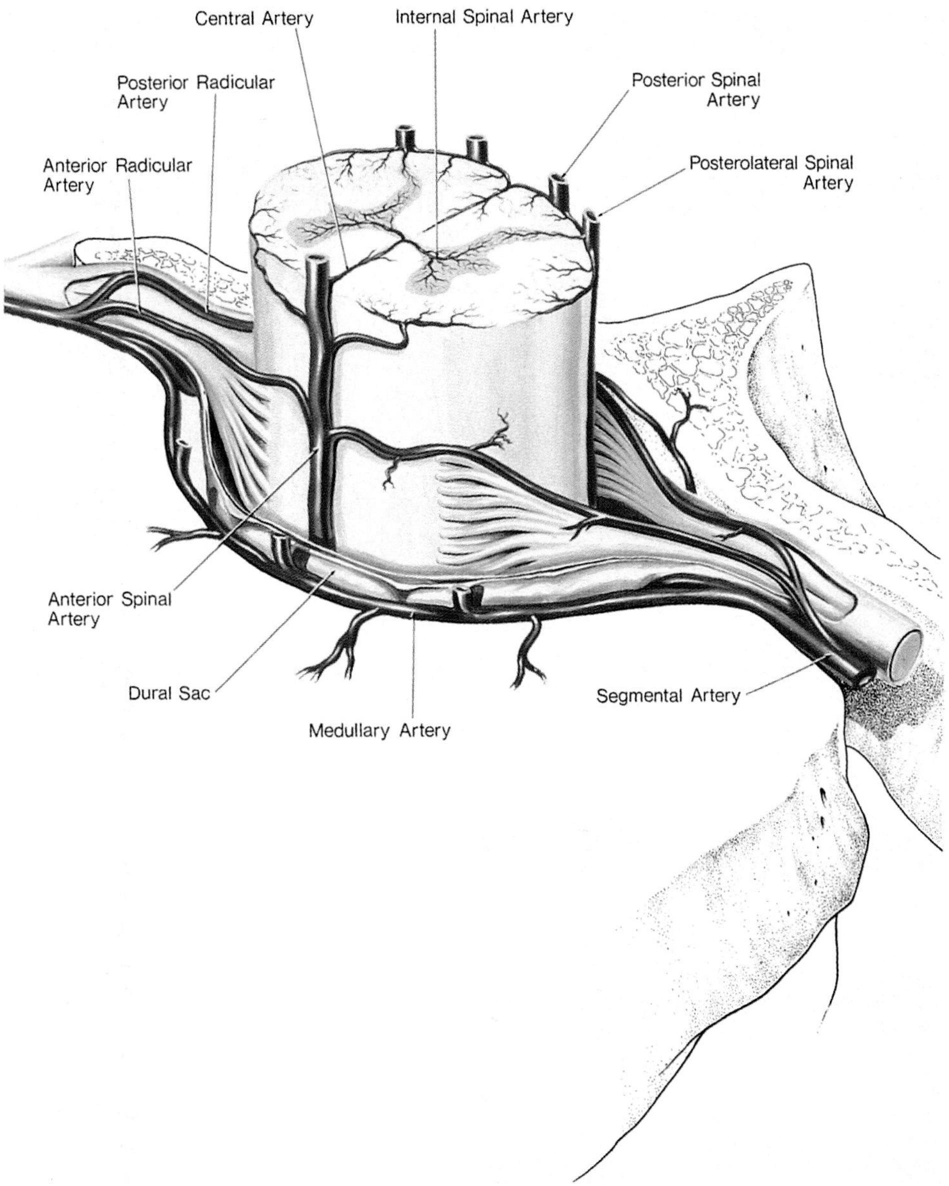

FIG. 7-10. Arterial supply of the spinal cord.

Furosemide, in large doses, may reduce the rate of CSF formation, whereas steroids have an inconsistent effect. Drugs such as norepinephrine, insulin, chlorothiazide, neostigmine, and phenytoin, among several others less used, have no or an insignificant effect on CSF formation. Studies of the effect of hydrostatic pressure showed that CSF formation declines as intraventricular pressure increases to a sufficient degree and duration. CSF formation is reduced when serum osmolality increases, and increases when serum is made hypotonic. The relationship is approximately linear, with a 1% change in serum osmolality causing a 6.7% change in CSF formation. During equilibrium, the rate of absorption of CSF equals its rate of formation. These rates are about 0.35 ml/min or 500 ml/day.

Spinal arteries. The spinal cord receives its blood supply from arteries of the brain above, and from spinal branches of the subclavian, aorta, and iliac arteries below. These last-mentioned spinal arteries enter the intervertebral foramina, cross the epidural space, and enter the subarachnoid space in the region of the dural cuff of the spinal nerve roots to gain access to the spinal cord (Fig. 7-10). Although the major purpose of these branches is to serve as blood supply to the spinal nerve roots, only a few feed into the anterior spinal artery. It has been shown, however, that these "nonfeeder" arteries do actually penetrate into the spinal cord and contribute to the segmental nature of the blood supply to the cord.[35]

The paired posterior arteries arise from the posterior inferior cerebellar arteries and descend medially to the posterior nerve roots, sending penetrating vessels to the posterior white columns and the remainder of the posterior gray column. These arteries are fed by 25 to 40 radicular arteries.

The anterior spinal artery is a single, midline artery formed between the pyramids of the medulla oblongata by the union of a branch from the terminal part of each vertebral artery. It descends in front of the anterior longitudinal sulcus of the spinal cord and the corresponding vein to the filum terminale. It gives off numerous circumferential vessels that supply the periphery of the cord and send some 200 branches into the sulcus toward the center of the cord, while also sending radiating twigs into the anterior and lateral gray and white columns and into the anterior part of the posterior gray column. As previously noted, these three longitudinal vessels (two posterior arteries and a single anterior artery) are "fed" by only a few of the spinal branches of the vertebral, deep cervical, ascending cervical, posterior intercostal, lumbar, and lateral sacral arteries. Only about 6 or 7 of these arteries make a significant contribution to the anterior artery,

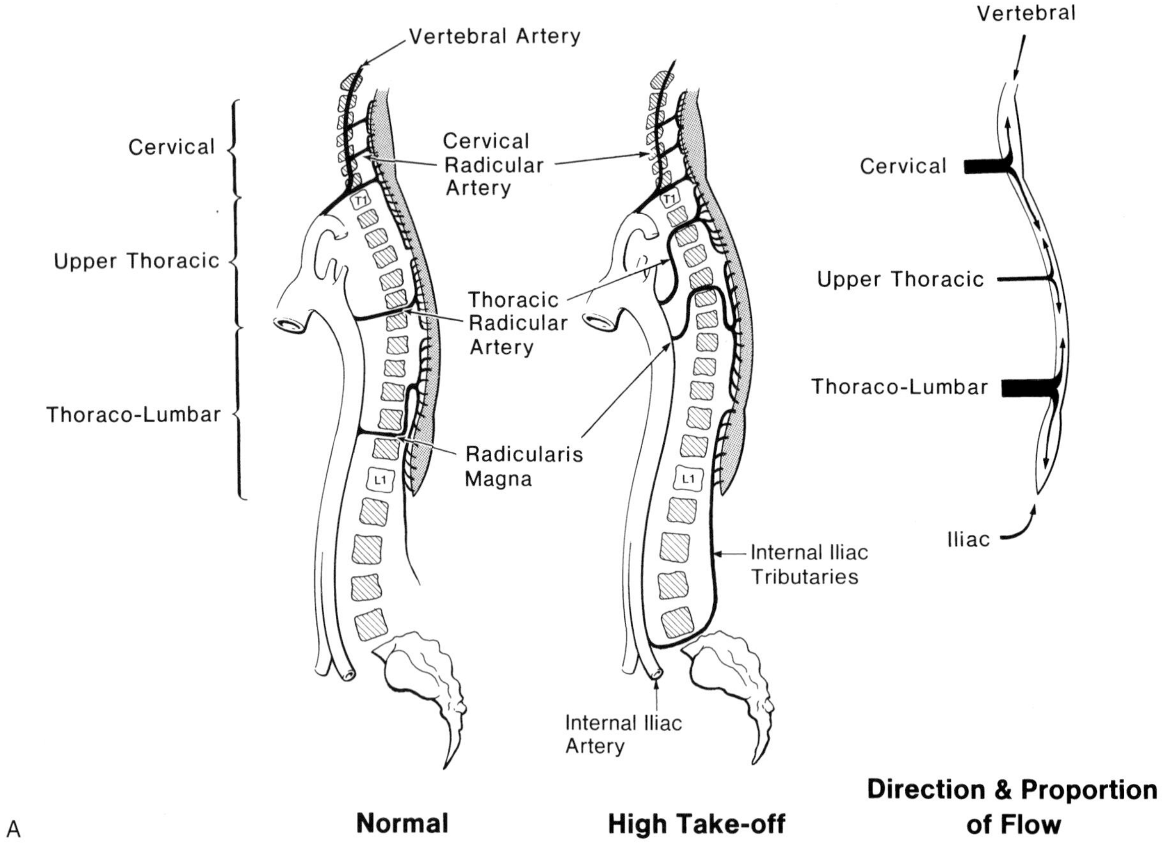

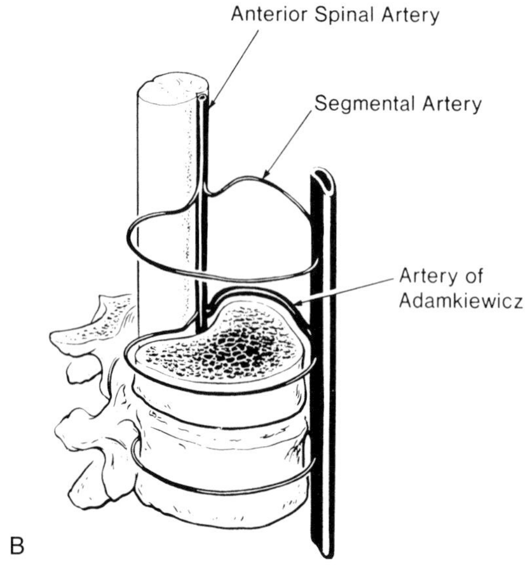

FIG. 7-11. A: Blood supply of spinal cord, vertical distribution; functional concept. *In "normal" situations*, note the following: relatively discrete vertical areas with little anastomosis; direction of flow dependent on relationship of area to major "feeder" artery; proportion of flow greatest from radicularis magna "feeder" artery (artery of Adamkiewicz) to thoracolumbar region. *In abnormal situations* (e.g., "high take-off"), note the following: The iliac artery branch may supply the lower thoracolumbar region of cord entering by way of the intervertebral foramen in the vicinity of L4-L5. **B: Blood supply of spinal cord; anatomic description.** This highlights recent demonstration of "segmental" anatomic distribution of spinal arteries; however, note that although all spinal arteries reach the spinal cord, many are extremely small and offer only a minimal contribution to nutritive blood flow. (Modified from data of Crock, H.V., and Yoshizawa, H.: The Blood Supply of the Vertebral Column and Spinal Cord in Man. New York, Springer-Verlag, 1977).

and a similar number make a contribution to the posterior arteries, but not at the same level. These feeders are broken into series of short lengths freely anastomosing posterior to anterior across the midline, providing adequate cord blood flow over three large and relatively discreet segments of spinal cord (Fig. 7-11).

The largest of the feeder arteries is the *radicularis magna* (artery of Adamkiewicz), which supplies the anterior spinal artery in the area of the lumbar enlargement of the cord. It enters by way of a single intervertebral foramen (78% of the time on the left) between the T8 and L3 foramina. Damage to this artery by needle trauma or other means could result in ischemia in the lumbar area of the cord. This is possible because there is poor vertical anastomosis between cervical, thoracic, and lumbar segments of the anterior spinal artery. Anterior spinal artery ischemia results in a predominantly motor lesion, since the anterior two thirds of the spinal cord, including the anterior horn cells, is supplied almost exclusively by the anterior spinal artery. In a small percentage of cases (15%), the artery of Adamkiewicz takes off high (T5), and the usually slender contribution of iliac tributaries to the conus medullaris and lumbar cord enlarges; under these circumstances, iliac tributaries may feed the anterior spinal artery by means of vessels passing through low lumbar intervertebral foramina. Ligation of these iliac tributaries during pelvic surgery or trauma during epidural anesthesia may result in a lesion in the region of the conus medullaris.

In the midthoracic region, relatively small feeder arteries reach the anterior spinal artery by way of intervertebral foramina between T4 and T9. In the cervical and upper thoracic regions, the anterior spinal artery begins with a contribution descending from both vertebral arteries and then receives feeder branches, through intervertebral foramina, from the subclavian artery to help maintain anterior spinal artery blood flow in the upper thoracic region, although this is reduced near T4. The T4 region appears to be the most tenuously supplied, since blood flow from the midthoracic region becomes sluggish near T4.

PHARMACOLOGY

The versatility of spinal anesthesia is afforded by a wide range of local anesthetics and additives that allow control over the level, the time of onset, and the duration of spinal anesthesia. A brief discussion of some of the more common local anesthetics used for spinal anesthesia (see Chapter 4) is followed by consideration of factors governing the distribution of local anesthetic solutions in CSF (i.e., the level of anesthesia), the uptake of local anesthetics by neural elements within the subarachnoid space (i.e., the types of nerves blocked), and the elimination of local anesthetics from the subarachnoid space (i.e., duration of action).

Drugs

Procaine produces spinal anesthesia with an onset of effect in about 3 to 5 minutes and a duration of 50 to 60 minutes. In the United States, procaine for spinal anesthesia is marketed in 2-ml ampules of 10% aqueous solution. The 10% solution, when diluted with an equal volume of CSF, produces a 5% solution of procaine that weighs about the same as CSF and, when mixed with an equal volume of 10% glucose, produces a 5% solution of procaine that is heavier than CSF. Aqueous solutions of 2.5% procaine, lighter than CSF, are used principally for differential or diagnostic rather than operative spinal anesthesia. Procaine should not be injected in concentrations exceeding 5%. The suggested dosage ranges from 50 to 100 mg for perineal and lower extremity surgery to 150 to 200 mg for upper abdominal surgery (Table 7-4).

Lidocaine also provides onset of anesthesia in 3 to 5 minutes and lasts slightly longer than procaine, 60 to 90 minutes. Lidocaine for spinal anesthesia is available as a commercial solution of 5% lidocaine in 7.5% glucose. It is also packaged in the United States as a 2-ml ampule of 1.5% concentration in 7.5% glucose for spinal anesthesia in obstetrics. Usual doses range from 25 to 50 mg for perineal surgery and sad-

TABLE 7-4. *Drugs for spinal anesthesia*

Drug and concentration	Dose (mg)			Duration (min)[a]	
	To L4	To T10	To T4	Plain	With 0.2 mg epinephrine
Procaine (5%)	50–75	100–150	150–200	40–55	60–75
Lidocaine (5%)	25–50	50–75	75–100	60–70	60–70
Tetracaine (0.5%)	4–6	6–10	12–16	60–90	120–180
Bupivacaine (0.75%)[b]	4–8	8–12	14–20	90–110	90–110

[a] For a given local anesthetic in spinal anesthesia the larger mg dose, the longer the duration of surgical anesthesia (e.g., a 16 mg dose of tetracaine will have a duration of two- to three times longer than a 4 mg dose, either plain or with epinephrine.

[b] Bupivacaine 0.5% is available as an isobaric solution that is ideal for surgery below the level of T10, such as hip surgery. Motor block with this solution is profound and long lasting in the legs. Doses are 10 to 15 mg for the L4 level and 15 to 20 mg for the T10 level. A heavy solution of bupivacaine 0.5% is also available and is suitable for abdominal surgery. Doses and effects are similar to those obtained with the bupivacaine 0.75% solution.

dle block anesthesia to 75 to 100 mg for upper abdominal surgery (see Table 7-4).

Tetracaine (amethocaine) provides anesthesia with time to onset of 3 to 6 minutes but with a considerably longer duration of action (210–240 minutes) than procaine or lidocaine. Tetracaine is marked both in ampules that contain 20 mg of crystals and in ampules that contain 2 ml of a 1% aqueous solution of tetracaine. Solutions of 1% tetracaine diluted to 0.1% to 0.33% by the addition of distilled water are lighter than CSF. The 1% solution, when mixed with equal volumes of 10% glucose (0.5% tetracaine in 5% glucose), is widely used as a spinal anesthetic solution that is heavier than CSF. The suggested dosages for tetracaine spinal anesthesia range from 5 mg for perineal and lower extremity surgery to 15 mg for abdominal surgery (see Table 7-4).

Bupivacaine produces onset of anesthesia in 5 to 8 minutes. Anesthesia lasts about as long as that produced by tetracaine.[74] Bupivacaine for spinal anesthesia is commercially available in the United States in a 2-ml ampule containing 0.75% bupivacaine in 8.5% glucose. Elsewhere, 0.5% concentrations, plain or with glucose, are used for spinal anesthesia. The plain solutions of bupivacaine are slightly lighter than CSF but can be treated as isobaric solutions. Recommended dosages of bupivacaine for spinal anesthesia range from 8 to 10 mg for perineal and lower extremity surgery and from 15 to 20 mg for abdominal surgery (see Table 7-4).

Vasoconstrictors

Vasoconstrictors have been used for more than 80 years to prolong the duration of spinal anesthesia. Initially, there was concern that vasoconstrictors might produce ischemia of the spinal cord sufficient to cause postoperative neurologic complications. This fear has been proved to be groundless. Although none of several carefully controlled clinical studies[44,84,110] of spinal anesthesia with and without vasoconstrictors has shown that vasoconstrictors are associated with neurologic complications, there are conflicting animal data on the effect of vasoconstrictors on spinal cord blood flow. Studies using unmedicated dogs showed a dose-response reduction in spinal cord blood flow with the subarachnoid administration of phenylephrine.[43] Conversely, measurement of spinal cord blood flow in anesthetized cats after subarachnoid injection of lidocaine, mepivacaine, and tetracaine, with and without epinephrine, showed no changes.[109]

Epinephrine and phenylephrine are the vasoconstrictors most widely used to prolong the duration of spinal anesthesia. Dosages of epinephrine vary from 0.2 to 0.5 mg (0.2–0.5 ml of 1:1000 epinephrine). Dosages of phenylephrine range from 0.5 to 5 mg (0.05–0.5 ml of a 1% solution). Despite the wide range of doses, there is no discernible relationship in published reports between dose of vasoconstrictor and the extent to which duration of anesthesia is prolonged. When, for example, the dose of epinephrine is kept constant at 0.2 mg, the duration of hyperbaric tetracaine spinal anesthesia has been variously reported as being increased by 12%,[47] by 25%,[94] and by 53%.[104] Furthermore, although 0.5 mg of epinephrine has been reported to increase the duration of tetracaine spinal anesthesia by only 27%,[47] 0.2 mg has been found to prolong tetracaine spinal anesthesia by 25%[94] to 53%[104] (Table 7-5).

Failure to establish a clear relation between dose of epinephrine added and the magnitude of prolongation of spinal anesthesia can be ascribed to two factors: (i) failure to control other determinants of duration of spinal anesthesia, including age of the patient, the amount of local anesthetic injected, and the area over which the anesthetic is distributed within the subarachnoid space (i.e., level of anesthesia),[57] and (ii) failure of past reports to use a clear, consistent, and logical definition of the duration of anesthesia.

Rigidly controlled double-blind clinical studies have recently evaluated the extent to which epinephrine and phenylephrine prolong spinal anesthesia while keeping constant the age of patients studied, the dose of local anesthetic used, and the level of anesthesia. Duration of anesthesia was defined as the time required for the maximum level of sensory anesthesia to decrease by a certain number of spinal segments. These clinical studies, subsequently confirmed by pharmacokinetic studies (see "Elimination" following), indicate that the effect of epinephrine or phenylephrine on duration of spinal anesthesia depends on the local anesthetic used. The addition of epinephrine or phenylephrine to lidocaine or bupivacaine, for example, produces no *clinically meaningful* prolongation of spinal anesthesia as determined by two-segment regression.[28,29,121] If, on the other hand, one compares duration of anesthesia in lumbar and sacral segments, as would be clinically relevant for perineal and lower extremity surgery, one sees longer anesthesia time with the epinephrine-containing solutions. As previously mentioned, it is important to note the measured end point when making judgments about the role of vasoconstrictors in prolonging clinical anesthesia. The time required for four-segment regression of lidocaine spinal anesthesia averaged 109 minutes without epinephrine and 100 minutes with 0.3 mg of epinephrine.[28] On the other hand, in equally well-controlled studies of tetracaine spinal anesthesia, both epinephrine and phenylephrine produced prolongation of duration of spinal anesthesia that was both clinically and statistically significant.[2,24,32] The time to regression of the sensory level to L1 following 12 mg of hyperbaric tetracaine, for example, averaged 171 minutes without epinephrine, 383 minutes with 0.3 mg of epinephrine, and 357 minutes with 1.0 mg of phenyle-

TABLE 7-5. *Vasoconstrictors and spinal anesthesia: 0.3 mg epinephrine or 1 mg phenylephrine*

Added to lidocaine or bupivacaine
No clinically significant ↑ duration (determined by 2 segment regression)
Anesthesia in lumbosacral segments is longer lasting
Added to tetracaine
↑ Duration (2 segment regression) 171 min (plain); 383 min (epinephrine)

phrine.[32] Epinephrine and phenylephrine prolong the duration of tetracaine spinal anesthesia and do so equally well when equipotent doses are used. Indeed, one of these studies was so rigidly controlled that a dose-response effect of epinephrine could be seen: The time to regression to L1 when 0.2 mg of epinephrine was added (272 minutes) was significantly less than when 0.3 mg was used (383 minutes).[32] However, there was no significant difference between the time to regression to L1 when 1.0 mg of phenylephrine was used (357 minutes) and when 2.0 mg of phenylephrine was added (324 minutes) (see Table 7-5).

Why vasoconstrictors prolong tetracaine spinal anesthetics consistently and markedly, while having substantially less, if any, effect on the duration of lidocaine and bupivacaine anesthetics, remains unclear.

Distribution

Distribution of local anesthetic solutions within the subarachnoid space determines the extent of the neural blockade produced by spinal anesthesia.

At one extreme, the distribution of a local anesthetic solution injected at the L3–L4 interspace may be limited to sacral roots only. At the other extreme, the local anesthetic solution may spread to produce blockade of sacral, lumbar, thoracic, and even cervical roots, even though injected at the same L3–L4 interspace. In either case, the local anesthetic injected at L3–L4 is not homogeneously distributed in CSF. Instead, the concentration of local anesthetic in CSF decreases as a function, not of distance from the site of injection, but of distance from the epicenter at which the concentration of local anesthetic is greatest. A spinal anesthetic solution injected at the L3–L4 interspace may have an epicenter of greatest concentration in the sacral area, at the site of injection, or in the high thoracic area depending on where the solution has spread and been distributed after injection. Determinants of where the epicenter of concentration lies are to be discussed later, but the existence of a decrease in concentration of anesthetic in CSF on either side of the point of maximum concentration means that uptake of local anesthetic by neural elements within the subarachnoid space, a function of concentration of anesthetic in CSF, varies at different levels of the cord. The result is the existence of clinically important zones of differential block, as discussed in the following section on uptake.

At least 23 factors have been invoked as being involved in determining where and how far local anesthetic solutions spread in CSF (Table 7-6A & B). However, not all are of demonstrable clinical importance. When all other factors that affect distribution are kept constant, factors that have **no demonstrable significant effects** on distribution include patient weight, composition of CSF, concentration of local anesthetic in the solution injected, diffusion of local anesthetics in CSF independent of the effects of baricity, addition of vasoconstrictors to the local anesthetic solution, and circulation of CSF[58,122] (Table 7-6A).

TABLE 7-6A. *Distribution of L.A. in CSF: factors with no proven effects*

Patient weight
CSF composition
Circulation of CSF
Concentration of L.A. in solution injected
Diffusion in CSF, independent of baricity
Addition of vasoconstrictors (see Table 7-4)
Direction of needle bevel during injection
Rate of injection
Turbulence in CSF, e.g., by "barbotage"
Coughing to increase CSF pressure
Age (small or no effect)
Gender

CSF, cerebrospinal fluid; L.A., local anesthetic

TABLE 7-6B. *Distribution of L.A. in CSF: factors with proven effects*

Site of injection
Anatomic configuration of spinal column
Patient height (only at extremes)
Angulation of needle, e.g., angled cephalad → ↑ cephalad spread hyperbaric solutions injected in lateral position
Volume of CSF, e.g., ↓ CSF volume with ↑ intra-abdominal pressure (pregnancy and other situations)
Characteristics of L.A. solution
Density of L.A. solution (L.A. weight vs. CSF weight)
Specific gravity (density L.A./density water)
Baricity (density L.A./density CSF)
Dose of L.A.
Volume of L.A. solution (minor effect if hyperbaric L.A.)
Position of patient during injection
Position of patient after injection

CSF, cerebrospinal fluid; L.A., local anesthetic

The direction in which the bevel of the needle is facing during injection also plays no role in determining where the anesthetic solution goes. Nor, clinical impression to the contrary, does turbulence within CSF during injection affect distribution, except locally at the site of injection. That turbulence has no significant effect on distribution is shown by the fact that, under controlled conditions, differing the rate of injection of a spinal anesthetic solution through needles of the same size has no effect on the level of anesthesia achieved.[89,98] Not even deliberate production of considerable turbulence at the site of injection by barbotage affects distribution.[81,100] Sudden increases in CSF pressure produced by coughing or straining fail to affect spread of local anesthetic solutions in CSF.[45] Age has little[107] or no[134] effect on the level of isobaric spinal anesthesia (see Table 7-6A).

Ten of the 23 factors in Table 7-6 do, nevertheless, influence how far and in what direction a spinal anesthetic solution spreads during and after injection into CSF.[58] The site of injection, especially if at a level other than lumbar intervertebral spaces is, of course, a determinant of spread. So, too, is anatomic configuration of the spinal column, particularly when pronounced, as in kyphosis. The normal lordotic curve will, when the patient is in the supine horizontal position, cause a hyperbaric anesthetic solution to move to the apex of the lumbosacral area and upward to the thoracic area. Elimination of the lordotic curve by flexion of the thighs on the abdomen has been reported to decrease slightly the cephalad spread.[120] Another study[82] found, however, creation of a bimodal distribution of levels of anesthesia, but no significant change in cephalad spread with flexion. Placing patients in the lithotomy position immediately after injection of hyperbaric tetracaine results in a level of anesthesia similar to that observed when patients are left in the supine horizontal position for 10 minutes after injection before being placed in the lithotomy horizontal position.[113]

How tall an adult patient may be has in general no clinically significant effect on the level of spinal anesthesia achieved when evaluated under suitably controlled conditions.[101,102] This is because of the relatively restricted range in height observed in most adults. In a patient 210 cm tall, however, the number of spinal segments blocked when a given amount and volume of local anesthetic is injected at L3–L4 will be less than if the same amount and volume of anesthetic solution were injected at L3–L4 in a patient 130 cm tall. This becomes even more apparent when spinal anesthetics are used in pediatric patients.

The direction in which the needle is pointing during injection of the anesthetic solution also plays a role in distribution of the anesthetic.[124] If the long axis of the needle is pointing in a cephalad direction, distribution of hyperbaric solutions injected with the patient in the horizontal lateral position will be slightly more cephalad than if the long axis of the needle is at right angles to the spinal column.

The volume of CSF also affects distribution significantly. Increased intra-abdominal pressure, as in term pregnancy or in patients with ascites or large intra-abdominal tumors, may often be associated with the development of collateral venous channels that pass through the lumbar epidural space because of obstruction of blood flow through the inferior vena cava. If chronic, epidural venous engorgement causes the dura to impinge upon the subarachnoid space with a consequent reduction in volume of CSF in the lumbar subarachnoid space. The decrease in lumbar CSF volume may explain why otherwise normal doses of spinal anesthetics produce unexpectedly high levels of anesthesia in term parturients.

The **most important factors in determining the spread** of spinal anesthetic solutions and the factors most susceptible to manipulation in order to achieve predictable levels of spinal anesthesia are the weight of the anesthetic solution injected in relation to the weight of CSF, the dosage and volume of anesthetic solution injected, and the position of the patient during and immediately after injection (Table 7-6B).

The weights of spinal anesthetic solutions are expressed in terms of density. Density is the weight in grams of 1 ml of a liquid. The specific gravity of a solution is a ratio: the density of the solution divided by that of water. The baricity of a spinal anesthetic solution is also a ratio: the density of the anesthetic solution divided by that of CSF. Because density is inversely related to temperature, when it is involved in the calculation of specific gravity or baricity, it must be measured at the same temperature, preferably 37°C, if data are to be clinically meaningful. Baricity is the most useful index for determining how spinal anesthetic solutions distribute themselves when added to CSF. Being the ratio between density of the anesthetic solution and density of CSF, baricity is a more direct and simpler index than are calculations based on specific gravities that depend upon the ratio between two ratios, each of which has water as a common denominator. If the baricity of a solution is 1.0, it is by definition isobaric; if greater than 1.0 it is hyperbaric; if less than 1.0 it is hypobaric. The density of normal CSF varies, however, by 0.0003 (two standard deviations) above and below the mean value of 1.0003. For spinal anesthetic solutions to be predictably hypobaric or hyperbaric in all patients requires, therefore, that their baricities be, respectively, less than 0.9990 and greater than 1.0010. Representative densities, specific gravities, and baricities of solutions of importance are given in Table 7-7.

Hypobaric Solutions. Tetracaine is the local anesthetic most frequently used for hypobaric spinal anesthesia. Solutions of 0.1% to 0.33% tetracaine in water are reliably hypobaric in all patients (Table 7-7). Because of the high anesthetic potency and lipid solubility of tetracaine, even solutions of 0.1% to 0.33% in water provide good sensory anesthesia and motor relaxation for up to 2 hours. Such solutions are readily prepared by diluting commercially available 1% tetracaine for spinal anesthesia with sterile distilled

TABLE 7-7. *Physical characteristics of spinal anesthetic solutions at 37°C[a]*

	Density	Specific Gravity	Baricity
Water	0.9934	1.0000	0.9931
CSF	1.0003	1.0069	1.0000
Tetracaine			
0.33% in water (*hypobaric*)	0.9980	1.0046	0.9977
1.0% in water	1.0003	1.0007	1.0000
0.5% in 50% CSF	0.9998	1.0064	0.9995
0.5% in half normal saline	1.0000	1.0066	0.9997
0.5% in 5% dextrose (*hyperbaric*)	1.0136	1.0203	1.0133
Bupivacaine			
0.5% in water (*isobaric*)	0.9993	1.0059	0.9990
0.5% in 8% dextrose (*hyperbaric*)	1.0210	1.0278	1.0207
Procaine			
2.5% in water (*hypobaric*)	0.9983	1.0052	0.9983
Lidocaine			
2% in water (*isobaric*)	1.0003	1.0066	1.0003
5% in 7.5% dextrose (*hyperbaric*)	1.0265	1.0333	1.0265

[a] Mean values. (Reproduced with permission from Greene, N.M.: Distribution of local anesthetic solutions within the subarachnoid space. Anesth. Analg., *64*:715, 1985.)
CSF, cerebrospinal fluid.

water without preservatives or other additives. Hypobaric solutions of bupivacaine with baricities substantially less than 0.9990 would also be expected to be equally effective but have not been studied extensively to date. Hypobaric solutions of procaine, lidocaine, and other local anesthetics with relatively low anesthetic potencies are generally unsuitable for operative hypobaric spinal anesthesia. When diluted in distilled water sufficiently to produce hypobaric solutions, they approach the minimum effective concentrations. When further diluted by CSF after intrathecal injection, their concentrations decrease to the point that muscle relaxation is usually incomplete and sensory anesthesia becomes too brief for many procedures.

The position of the patient during and for the first few minutes after intrathecal injection of hypobaric solutions determines spread in CSF. If the patient is in the head-up position during and after injection, the anesthetic ascends in a cephalad direction; if in the head-down position, the anesthetic solution spreads caudad. Hypobaric solutions are particularly useful for perineal and rectal operations performed in the prone, jack-knife position. In such cases, anesthesia is induced in the same position as that required for surgery, thus avoiding the need to change the position of the patient after induction of anesthesia. Hypobaric solutions are also useful for low unilateral anesthesia, especially operations on a lower extremity. However, hypobaric solutions are not recommended for intra-abdominal procedures. The head-up position required to achieve high enough levels of anesthesia may be dangerous in the presence of extensive sympathetic denervation, and arterial hypotension may be severe in such a situation.

Isobaric Solutions. Isobaric solutions of tetracaine are readily prepared by mixing equal volumes of the commercial 1% tetracaine solution and either CSF or half normal saline (see Table 7-7). The 1% tetracaine solution is itself isobaric but is too concentrated to allow wide enough distribution in CSF to produce levels of anesthesia sufficient for most procedures. Bupivacaine 0.5% in water is slightly hypobaric (see Table 7-7), but so slightly hypobaric that it has been widely and successfully used as an isobaric solution. The slight hypobaricity of 0.5% aqueous solutions of bupivacaine is demonstrated by the fact that lumbar injection of 0.5% bupivacaine in patients in the seated position who remain seated for the next 2.5 minutes results in sensory levels of anesthesia about one to two segments higher than levels produced in patients in whom the same amount of the same solution is injected with the patients in the lateral horizontal position who are then immediately placed in the supine horizontal position.[27,67,131] Isobaric solutions of lidocaine or procaine (see Table 7-7) are easily prepared but are of limited value in operative spinal anesthesia for the same reasons as those mentioned previously for hypobaric solutions.

A major clinical advantage of isobaric spinal anesthetics is that position of the patient during and after injection has no effect on distribution of the anesthetic and thus no effect on the levels of anesthesia. Injection can be made with the patient in any position, and the patient can then be placed in the operative position without affecting the level of anesthesia. Isobaric spinals are particularly useful when levels of anesthesia to T10 or below are required. Isobaric solutions, to produce midthoracic or high thoracic levels of anesthesia, will require larger doses and volumes and are used less frequently.

Hyperbaric Solutions. The easiest, safest, and most widely used way to render spinal anesthetic solutions hyperbaric is by adding glucose. Commercially marketed hyperbaric solutions of bupivacaine and lidocaine contain 5% to 8% glucose. Commercial solutions of 1% tetracaine are usually made hyperbaric by mixing with equal volumes of 10% glucose to produce a 5% glucose solution to be injected intrathecally. Five percent to 8% glucose solutions have densities far in excess of those required to render them hyperbaric (see Table 7-7). Once enough glucose has been added to increase the baricity of the solution above 1.0010, the concentration of glucose has no effect on distribution.[3,27,36]

Distribution of hyperbaric solutions is governed by position of the patient during injection and for the next 20 to 30 minutes. After that, distribution should no longer be significantly affected by position; however, sensory level should be monitored an additional 10 to 20 minutes, since occasional higher levels have been reported. The seated position during and after injection restricts distribution to lower lumbar and sacral roots. The head-down position results in thoracic levels of anesthesia, depending on the degree and duration of head-down position.[19,27,36,79,91,92,123,138]

Concentration and Dose

Concentration and *dose* of local anesthetic injected, together with *volume* of injectate, have all been said to affect distribution. Separation of the individual effects on distribution of each of these three variables is difficult because changing one of the three affects either or both of the other two variables. However, this problem has been resolved in a double-blind study by Shesky and colleagues, in which age, height, position, and other factors that affect distribution[115] were controlled. The 72 patients given isobaric glucose-free bupivacaine in this study were divided into six groups of 12 patients each with concentrations of bupivacaine, volumes (ml) of injectate, and amounts (mg) of bupivacaine being systematically altered as shown in Table 7-8. Levels of anesthesia were significantly higher (T2–T4) in patients given 15 or 20 mg of bupivacaine (groups II, III, V, and VI) than they were in patients given 10 mg (T5–T8; groups I and IV). Further, levels of anesthesia were similar in patients given the same dose of bupivacaine (groups I and IV) even though the concentration of bupivacaine and the volume injected differed. Also, patients given the same volume of anesthetic solution (2 ml) had levels of anesthesia significantly higher when 0.75% bupivacaine was injected (group V) than when 0.5% was used (group I). The authors concluded that "total dosage of bupivacaine is more important than volume or

TABLE 7-8. *Concentration and dose of glucose-free bupivacaine and volume of solution used in the six groups studied by Shesky and co-workers*[a]

Group	Concentration (%)	Volume (ml)	Dose (mg)
I	0.5	2.0	10
II	0.5	3.0	15
III	0.5	4.0	20
IV	0.75	1.3	10
V	0.75	2.0	15
VI	0.75	2.7	20

[a] n = 12 patients each.

(From Sheskey, M.C., Rocco, A.G., Bezzari-Schmid, M., *et al.*: A dose-response study of bupivacaine for spinal anesthesia. Anesth. Analg., *62*:931, 1983.)

concentration of anesthetic solution" in determining spread of local anesthetic solution in CSF. These results with isobaric solutions of bupivacaine have been confirmed by others[10,83,98,133] but may not be directly applicable to solutions that are clearly hypobaric or strongly hyperbaric. These data demonstrate, nevertheless, that dosage significantly affects distribution independently of concurrent changes in concentration and volume. There is no evidence that concentration of the injectate *per se* has any influence on clinical spinal anesthesia. Once the selected dose of local anesthetic is injected into the CSF, it takes on a new concentration dependent upon the other factors of drug distribution within the CSF. The concentration of the drug in the injecting syringe has no relevance to any of these other factors. The adjective "more" in the conclusion that dosage is more important than volume is most appropriate. It does not preclude the possibility that volume is also a determinant of distribution, although probably of secondary importance compared to dosage.

Uptake

Uptake of local anesthetics into neuronal tissues within the subarachnoid space during spinal anesthesia depends on four factors: concentration of local anesthetic in CSF; surface area of nerve tissue exposed to CSF; lipid content of nerve tissue; and blood flow to nerve tissue (Table 7-9).

Uptake of local anesthetics is greatest where the concentration of local anesthetic in CSF is greatest. Since concentration of local anesthetic in CSF decreases as a function of distance above and below the site of highest concentration, so too does uptake by neuronal tissue.

The surface area of nerve roots and their uptake of local anesthetics in CSF is considerable as they cross the subarachnoid space from the cord to their points of exit through the dura.[31] The spinal cord also takes up local anesthetics. This involves two processes. One is diffusion of local anesthetic down a concentration gradient from CSF through the pia mater directly into the cord. This is a slow process affecting only the most superficial portions of the cord. The other process involves extensions of the subarachnoid space, known as the spaces of Virchow-Robin, which accompany blood vessels penetrating the spinal cord from the pia mater. Through the spaces of Virchow-Robin, local anesthetics in CSF have access to deeper structures in the cord (see Fig. 7-7). If accessibility were the only factor governing tissue levels of local anesthetics, concentrations in the spinal cord might be expected to be lower than those present in nerve roots traversing the subarachnoid space. This is not the case; concentrations of local anesthetics are greater in the spinal cord than in nerve roots[31] because of the role played by lipid content in determining uptake of local anesthetics.

Since local anesthetics are more soluble in lipids than in water, heavily myelinated tissues within the subarachnoid space, which have high lipid contents, would be expected to have high concentrations of local anesthetics. This is borne out by the observations of Cohen,[31] who found not only higher concentrations of local anesthetics in tracts within the spinal cord than in nerve roots, but also a correlation between concentrations of local anesthetics in spinal cord tracts and the degree of myelination of fibers within spinal cord tracts.

Tissue blood flow governs tissue concentrations of local anesthetics within subarachnoid nerve tissues because blood flow determines the rate at which local anesthetics are removed from tissue. Highly perfused areas of the cord may thus not always have high concentrations of local anesthetics even though they may contain more lipid and more spaces of Virchow-Robin, and thus greater accessibility to CSF than more poorly perfused areas.[57]

TABLE 7-9. *Uptake and elimination of local anesthetics (L.A.) from CSF*

Uptake of L.A. into neural tissue
- Concentration of L.A. in CSF
- Surface area of neural tissue exposed to CSF
- Lipid content of nerve
- Blood flow to nerve

Spinal nerve rootlets
- Large surface area → *rapid* onset of block (also DRG, sympathetic fibers)

Spinal cord
- *Slow* diffusion via subarachnoid extensions accompanying blood vessels into cord (Virchow-Robin spaces)
- High lipid in cord → high cord L.A. concentrations

Elimination of L.A. from CSF
- By vascular absorption via subarachnoid and epidural blood vessels
- No significant metabolism of L.A. in CSF

General order of uptake by fiber size (see also Chapter 2)

Motor ←	Touch ←	Pinprick ←	Sympathetic block (B)
$A\alpha$ 1 seg	$A\beta$? 1 seg	? $A\delta$? 2 segs	cold sense (C)

DRG, dorsal root ganglion; CSF, cerebrospinal fluid.

During spinal anesthesia, local anesthetics are found both in nerve roots and within the substance of the spinal cord[31] (Table 7-9). However, the major cause of loss of sensation and muscle relaxation during spinal anesthesia is the presence of local anesthetics in spinal nerve roots and in dorsal root ganglia, not within the spinal cord. The concentration of local anesthetics in nerve roots is, as mentioned above, a function of distance from the site of highest concentration of local anesthetic in CSF. This, combined with the fact that different types of nerve fibers differ in their sensitivities to the blocking effects of local anesthetics, gives rise to zones of differential blockade of great clinical and physiologic importance. These zones of differential blockade are most apparent and most readily measured above, that is, cephalad to, the site of highest concentration of local anesthetic in CSF. During hyperbaric tetracaine spinal anesthesia, for example, the concentration of tetracaine in CSF decreases in cephalad direction until it becomes so low that it is sufficient to block only those nerve fibers in the subarachnoid space that are most sensitive to local anesthetics. These are the preganglionic sympathetic nerves. This decrease in local anesthetic concentration gives rise to a *zone of differential sympathetic denervation* as measured by loss of cold temperature discrimination (C fiber) during spinal anesthesia that averages *two* spinal segments above the level of pinprick sensory blockade (A-delta fiber). Because the most cephalad preganglionic sympathetic fiber comes off the spinal cord at the level of T1, the two-segment zone of differential sympathetic block means that a sensory level at T3 is associated with total preganglionic sympathetic (B fibers) denervation. This zone of differential blockade remains constant in extent during maintenance and regression of the level of spinal anesthesia as the anesthesia wears off from above downward.[22] The extent of the zone of differential sympathetic blockade is the same with tetracaine and bupivacaine and, presumably, with other local anesthetics. Furthermore, the spinal segmental level at which the cutaneous sense of cold is lost lies about two segments above the level of pinprick anesthesia, which in turn lies about one segment above the level of anesthesia to light touch.[22,138] Therefore, testing for the level of loss of the sensation of light touch would be the best sensory modality to test for the level of block adequate for surgery. To test level of sympathetic denervation and thus the potential for changes in cardiovascular function during spinal anesthesia, in theory one should test for the level of loss of temperature discrimination (see Table 7-9). Another study, using laser Doppler technique, suggested that spinal sympathetic block was less than sensory blockade in intensity, level, and duration.[8] Thus, the subject of zones of "differential block" is complex, as discussed in Chapter 2.

Somatic sensory afferent fibers are in general also more sensitive to local anesthesia than are somatic motor fibers. This creates another zone of differential blockade during spinal anesthesia, a level of somatic motor blockade that lies below the level of somatic sensory blockade. This zone of differential blockade also averages two spinal segments below pinprick level[51,136] (see Table 7-9). It determines the extent of surgical relaxation of the anterior abdominal wall as well as the effect of spinal anesthesia on the respiratory muscles, neither of which is the same as the level of surgical anesthesia or the extent of sympathetic denervation and thus the extent of physiologic trespass during spinal anesthesia.

The functional significance of the presence of local anesthetics within the spinal cord during spinal anesthesia remains unproven. The result is certainly not chemical transection of the cord. Some neural elements within the cord fail to absorb appreciable amounts of local anesthetics. The concentrations of local anesthetics in neural elements that do absorb local anesthetics vary widely.[31] That the spinal cord is itself relatively unaffected during spinal anesthesia is nevertheless indicated by the observation in patients that while stimuli applied to the posterior tibial nerve no longer elicit cortical evoked responses during high diagnostic spinal anesthesia to T2–T3, direct stimulation of the cord at T8–T9 still elicits cortical evoked responses during high spinal anesthesia that differ only slightly from evoked responses measured before induction of spinal anesthesia.[78]

Clinically, the functional integrity of the spinal cord is maintained during spinal anesthesia, at least in terms of transmission of somatic sensory afferent impulses, by the relatively frequent development of segmental spinal anesthesia. In the presence of profound blockade of midthoracic sensory and motor fibers during operative spinal anesthesia, it is often possible to detect, in lumbar and sacral areas, normal or nearly normal motor function, as well as transmission of pain sensation in these same lumbar and sacral regions.

The uptake of local anesthetics by neuronal tissues and blood vessels within the subarachnoid space results in a decrease in concentration of local anesthetic in CSF. Figure 7-12 shows the decrease in CSF concentration of four solutions of lidocaine as a function of time after injection. The lowest concentration 5 minutes after injection occurred with an isobaric hypo-osmotic solution. After 10 minutes, however, disappearance curves of lidocaine from CSF became parallel for all solutions for the next 50 minutes and were not significantly different.[39] The initial sharp decline in concentration of local anesthetic in CSF is primarily the result of distribution of lidocaine away from the site of injection with consequent dilution in a larger volume of CSF. It is secondarily the result of uptake of lidocaine into intrathecal tissue. This initial rapid decline in concentration is followed by a more gradual decrease due mainly to elimination of local anesthetic from the subarachnoid space. As the concentration of local anesthetic (and glucose injected with it) decreases, a point is reached where the solution, previously hyperbaric, approaches isobaricity. When this point is reached (about 30–35 minutes with lidocaine), changes in position of patients given hyperbaric spinal anesthetic solutions no longer influence distribution of the anesthetic solution in CSF. The level of anesthesia becomes "fixed." The position

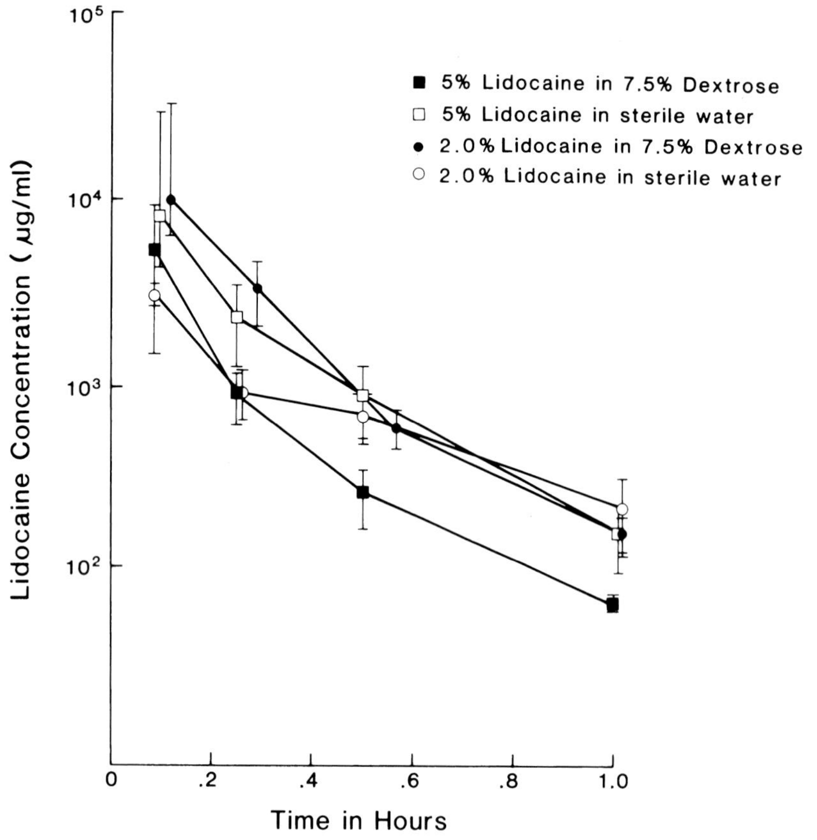

FIG. 7-12. Cerebrospinal fluid lidocaine concentrations as a function of time after injection of lidocaine solutions of different osmolalities and baricities. Data are presented as mean ± SD for the four animals in the Latin square study. (From Denson, D.D., Bridenbaugh, P.O., Turner, P.A., and Phero, J.C.: Comparison of neural blockade and pharmacokinetics after subarachnoid lidocaine in the rhesus monkey: II. Effects of volume, osmolality, and baricity. Anesth. Analg., *62*:995, 1983).

of the patient can be changed without changing the level of anesthesia[39] (see previous section on Hyperbaric Solutions).

Elimination

The rate at which local anesthetics are removed or eliminated from the subarachnoid space determines the duration of spinal anesthesia. Elimination does not involve metabolism of local anesthetics within the subarachnoid space (see Table 7-9). Elimination is entirely by vascular absorption and is reflected by systemic blood levels of intrathecally injected local anesthetics.[23,39–41,52,111]

Elimination by vascular absorption occurs in two areas: the epidural space and the subarachnoid space. Just as local anesthetics pass through the dura into CSF after injection into the epidural space, so, too, do local anesthetics in CSF cross the dura as they move down the concentration gradient between CSF and the epidural space.[57] Movement of drugs across the dura is related to neither lipid solubility nor degree of ionization (and thus not to pKa).[95] Once in the epidural space, local anesthetics originally injected into CSF are again susceptible to vascular absorption. The blood supply in the epidural space is, in terms of ml blood flow/g/min, greater than in the subarachnoid space. Therefore, vascular absorption of local anesthetics from the epidural space represents as important a route of elimination of local anesthetics from CSF as does vascular reabsorption from the subarachnoid space. Vascular absorption within the subarachnoid space is accomplished principally by vessels in the pia mater on the surface of the cord and by vessels within the cord. Because vascular perfusion of the cord varies in different areas, the rate of elimination, and thus the concentration of local anesthetics in the cord, also varies from one area to another.

The rate at which a given dose of local anesthetic is eliminated from the subarachnoid space in part depends on the vascular absorptive surface area to which that dose is exposed. For example, spinal anesthesia with 10 mg of tetracaine to a level of T12 lasts longer than with a sensory level of T3. It lasts longer because the absorptive surface to which the 10 mg of tetracaine is exposed is greater with T3 than with T12 levels. Differences in rate of vascular absorption as a function of differences in absorptive surface have yet to be pharmacokinetically proved. However, Burm and colleagues made the interesting observation that times to peak plasma levels of bupivacaine are significantly shorter with 15 mg of hyperbaric bupivacaine than with 15 mg of isobaric bupivacaine, even though peak levels show no significant difference.[23] By contrast, primate studies of lidocaine spinal solutions of varying baricity show significantly faster rates of absorption of lidocaine in sterile water than do the corresponding dextrose solutions, suggesting that rate of absorption from CSF increases with decreasing baricity. There were no differences in height of block or time to two-segment regression among the test solutions.[39]

Lipid solubility would also be expected to determine the

rate of elimination of intrathecal local anesthetics. Lipid solubility of local anesthetics is directly related to their duration of action. The more tightly a local anesthetic is bound to lipids, the less susceptible it is to vascular absorption, and the less susceptible it is to removal from its site of action. The rate of vascular absorption, and therefore plasma levels of long-acting, highly lipid-soluble local anesthetics, should be expected to differ from plasma levels of less lipid-soluble, shorter-acting local anesthetics injected intrathecally, but this has not been quantitated. Indeed, Burm and co-workers found that times to peak plasma levels of intrathecal hyperbaric lidocaine and bupivacaine were similar as were, dose for dose, the peak levels themselves[23,134] despite the greater lipid solubility of bupivacaine.

Decreases in spinal cord blood flow would be expected to decrease the rate of elimination of local anesthetic from the subarachnoid space and so prolong the duration of spinal anesthesia. This has been proposed as an explanation for the greater duration of spinal anesthesia in older patients, as quantitated by Veering et al.[134] in a study that also showed that age had no effect on either time to peak plasma levels or terminal half-life of intrathecal bupivacaine.[134]

Prolongation of spinal anesthesia by the addition of vasoconstrictors such as epinephrine and phenylephrine has also been ascribed to decreased rates of elimination of intrathecal local anesthetic as a consequence of intrathecal vasoconstriction. However, Kozody and colleagues found that neither 0.2 mg of epinephrine nor 5 mg of phenylephrine decreased spinal blood flow in dogs.[75] Pharmacokinetically more meaningful are data on plasma levels of lidocaine following the intrathecal injection of lidocaine with or without added epinephrine or phenylephrine in experimental animals.[39–41,46] In all of these studies, times to peak levels and peak levels of plasma lidocaine were similar with or without epinephrine or phenylephrine added to the injectate. The disparity between the lack of effect of vasoconstrictors on peak plasma levels of local anesthetics injected into CSF and conflicting reports on their clinical effects needs further study. It appears that local anesthetics placed into CSF are simultaneously and quickly being deposited into neural and vascular tissue. The rate and amount absorbed into the vascular bed are apparently unaffected by vasoconstrictors, but there still remains significant amounts of local anesthetic bound to neural tissue in equilibrium with CSF which must be eliminated therefrom by continued vascular absorption. Here, apparently, factors such as total dose of drug, baricity, vasoconstrictors, cord blood flow, and lipid solubility may play a role in the intensity and duration of neural blockade.

PHYSIOLOGIC RESPONSES

The injection of local anesthetic solutions into the subarachnoid space produces important and often widespread physiologic responses. Understanding the etiology and significance of these physiologic effects is the key to the safe management of patients during spinal anesthesia and to understanding the indications and contraindications of spinal anesthesia.

Cardiovascular

The most important physiologic responses to spinal anesthesia involve the cardiovascular system.[60] They are mediated by the combined effects of autonomic denervation and, with higher levels of neural blockade, the added effects of vagal nerve innervation. The cardiovascular effects of spinal anesthesia are not due to the presence of local anesthetics in ventricular CSF in concentrations sufficient to produce direct depression of medullary vasomotor centers. The concentration of local anesthetics in cisternal CSF during even cervical levels of anesthesia is below the concentration required to produce effects on medullary vasomotor centers when applied directly to the brain stem.[60] Similarly, plasma levels of local anesthetics during spinal anesthesia are below those required to produce direct effects on the myocardium or on peripheral vascular smooth muscles.[52] Vasoconstrictors that are injected into the subarachnoid space along with local anesthetics in order to prolong the clinical duration of anesthesia do not have direct effects on the myocardium or the peripheral vascular smooth muscles. The alpha-2 agonist clonidine, however, when administered in small doses intrathecally during tetracaine spinal anesthesia, has resulted in a decrease of diastolic blood pressure in some,[14] although not all,[15] reports. Therefore, despite the need for clarification under clinical conditions of the effects of spinally administered clonidine,* the generalization that local anesthetics and vasoactive substances administered in small doses intrathecally lack direct cardiovascular effect remains accurate. Because of the importance of sympathetic denervation in the genesis of cardiovascular changes during spinal anesthesia, the effect of spinal anesthesia on the sympathetic nervous system warrants discussion before consideration of the cardiovascular responses themselves (see Chapter 8).

Sympathetic Denervation. Because the level of sympathetic denervation determines the magnitude of cardiovascular responses to spinal anesthesia, it might be anticipated that the higher the level of neural blockade, the greater would be the change in cardio-circulatory parameters. The relationship is neither predictable nor precise. In the presence of partial sympathetic blockade, a reflex increase in sympathetic activity occurs in sympathetically intact areas. The result is vasoconstriction that tends to compensate for the peripheral vasodilation taking place in the sympathetically denervated areas. This can be seen in the changes in arterial pulse wave contours and in cutaneous blood flow in the upper extremities in the presence of low or midthoracic sensory levels of spinal anesthesia.[18] Of even greater importance is the fact that the most cephalad preganglionic sympathetic fibers exit the spinal cord at the level of T1. Existence of a zone of dif-

*Doses of clonidine of the order of 20 to 100 micrograms intrathecally are associated with dose-related hypotension.

TABLE 7-10. *Some aspects of cardiovascular (CV) effects of spinal anesthesia*

CV effects with C4 sensory block = T3 sensory block
Both → total sympathetic block
Arterial vasodilatation but local compensation
Only 15–18% ↓ total vascular resistance
Mean arterial pressure only ↓ 15–18% even with high block *provided* cardiac output maintained
Venodilatation may be maximal
May be venous pooling with changes in posture
Pooling effects → ↓ preload → ↓ cardiac output
Cardiac output
Determined by preload
May be normal—*if* normovolemia
—*if* legs above heart level
Heart rate (HR)
↓ if T1–T4 block
? ↓ if RA pressure ↓↓
Usually HR ↓ 10%–15% unless T1 block or ↓↓ RA pressure
Mean arterial blood pressure (MAP)
↓ 10–15% even with high block, *unless* ↓↓ RA pressure
Myocardial oxygenation
↓ MAP → ↓ Coronary blood flow
→ ↓ Myocardial O_2 delivery (approx. 48% ↓)
↓ Myocardial O_2 consumption (approx. 48% ↓)
↓ Myocardial O_2 consumption, due to:
↓ Afterload (↓ LV minute work)
↓ Preload (↓ work of LV and RV)
↓ HR (↓ frequency of contraction)
Cerebral blood flow (CBF)
Autoregulation maintains CBF (↓ cerebral vascular resistance,
Over MAP range 90–60 mm Hg CBF is constant, except if essential hypertension

RA, right atrial.

ferential sympathetic denervation means that the level of sympathetic denervation is even higher than the level of sensory anesthesia.[22,26] Since sympathetic denervation is complete at the T1 level, cardiovascular changes are no greater with midcervical sensory levels of anesthesia than they are with T1 levels (Table 7-10). Finally, as will be seen below, with proper intraoperative management, vascular hypotension may be modest or even absent in the presence of total sympathetic denervation. The correlation of spinal levels of anesthesia and changes in blood pressure is weak indeed. Sympathetic denervation is similar following epidural and subarachnoid anesthesia to similar levels of sensory blockade.[125]

Arterial Circulation. Sympathetic denervation produces arterial and, physiologically more important, arteriolar vasodilation, although vasodilation is not maximal. Vascular smooth muscle on the arterial side of the circulation retains a significant degree of autonomous tone following acute, pharmacologically induced, sympathetic denervation. As a result, total peripheral vascular resistance (TPVR) decreases only modestly, about 15% to 18% in normal subjects even in the presence of total sympathetic denervation, provided cardiac output, the other determinant of blood pressure, is kept normal.[60] Because TPVR decreases only 15% to 18%, mean arterial pressure decreases only 15% to 18% in the presence of a normal cardiac output (Table 7-10).

Venous Circulation. Veins and venules, with only few smooth muscles in their walls, retain no significant residual tone following acute pharmacologic denervation, and so they can vasodilate maximally. Whether they do so or not is determined by intraluminal hydrostatic pressure. Intraluminal hydrostatic pressure on the venous side of the circulation depends on gravity. If denervated veins lie below the level of the right atrium, gravity causes peripheral pooling of blood in these capacitance vessels. If the denervated veins lie above the level of the right atrium, gravity causes the blood to flow back to the heart. Preload, that is, venous return to the heart, therefore depends on the position of the patient during spinal anesthesia, especially during high spinal anesthesia (Table 7-10).

Cardiac Output. Preload is an important determinant of cardiac output. During levels of spinal anesthesia high enough to produce total sympathetic denervation, cardiac output remains unchanged in normovolemic subjects as long as they are positioned with the legs elevated above the level of the heart. The head-up (legs-down) position, on the other hand, leads to severe decreases in venous return to the heart, and thus to significant decreases in cardiac output.

Heart Rate. Heart rate characteristically decreases during spinal anesthesia in the absence of autonomically active drugs and medications. The bradycardia is due in part to blockade of preganglionic cardiac accelerator fibers arising from T1–T4 during high (i.e., T3–T4) levels of anesthesia.[137] The bradycardia is also mediated by significant decreases in right atrial pressure and pressure in the great veins as they enter the right atrium. This can be seen during fixed levels of high spinal anesthesia. Placing the patient in the modest head-down position (or with legs elevated) increases venous return, which in turn increases right atrial pressure and thus heart rate at a time when blockade of cardiac accelerator fibers remains constant. The slight head-up position, on the other hand, further decreases venous return, right atrial pressure, and heart rate. The direct relationship between right atrial pressure and heart rate during high spinal anesthesia is mediated by intrinsic chronotropic stretch receptors located in the right atrium and adjacent great veins (see Chapter 8). The extent to which heart rate decreased in response to total sympathetic denervation (during spinal anesthesia) has been found to be, on the average, only moderate (10%-15%).[59,103] However, severe bradycardia[62] and even asystole[76] have been reported in normal patients during otherwise uneventful spinal anesthesia. The mechanism responsible for such extreme cardiovascular responses has been described as the Bezold-Jarisch reflex.[86]

Hypotension. The preceding indicates that slight decreases in arterial pressure in the range of 15% or so during high spinal anesthesia in normovolemic patients can be ascribed to decreases in afterload, that is, decreases in TPVR.

Severe hypotension, however, can be due only to decreases in cardiac output secondary to decreases in preload associated with peripheral pooling of blood in vasodilated capacitance vessels or to hypovolemia, or both.

The indications for treatment of arterial hypotension during spinal anesthesia and the methods to be used are best considered in light of what arterial hypotension caused by sympathetic denervation means in terms of oxygenation of the myocardium and the central nervous system (the organs most susceptible to hypoxia). The following discussion applies only to hypotension during spinal anesthesia in normovolemic subjects. Hypovolemic subjects are highly susceptible to the hypotensive effects of spinal anesthesia because, in the presence of hypovolemia, maintenance of cardiovascular function depends on compensatory reflex increases in sympathetic activity. Elimination of these compensatory reflexes by sympathetic denervation during spinal anesthesia can result in such catastrophic hypotension (due to decreases in TPVR and venous return to the heart) that spinal anesthesia is contraindicated in the presence of hypovolemia (Fig. 7-13) (see Chapter 8).

Myocardial Oxygenation. A major determinant of coronary blood flow, and thus myocardial oxygen supply, is the perfusing pressure in the coronary vasculature. A decrease in mean arterial pressure during spinal anesthesia is therefore associated with a decrease in coronary blood flow. In normal subjects, Hackel and colleagues found that as mean arterial pressure decreased from 119.5 mm Hg before to 67.20 mm Hg during spinal anesthesia, coronary flow decreased from 153.2 ml/100 g/min to 73.6 ml/100 g/min. The 48% decrease in myocardial oxygen supply was associated with a parallel 53% decrease in myocardial oxygen requirements; myocardial oxygen consumption averaged 16.1 ml/100 g/min before, and 7.5 ml/100 g/min during, spinal anesthesia.[63] Similar data have also been reported in experimental animals.[46,119] Myocardial oxygen demands decrease during hypotension associated with spinal anesthesia for three reasons: (i) afterload decreases; the resistance against which the left ventricle ejects blood during systole is diminished, and therefore left ventricular work decreases; (ii) preload decreases; as venous return and cardiac output decrease, so too does the work load of both ventricles because the amount of blood to be ejected per unit of time is lessened; (iii) heart rate decreases; ventricular work load is diminished as the frequency of contraction diminishes (Table 7-10). Recognition of the fact that myocardial work and oxygen requirements diminish to essentially the same extent as does myocardial oxygen supply during moderate levels of arterial hypotension in normal subjects has altered past concepts of when and how hypotension should be treated during spinal anesthesia (see following).

Cerebral Blood Flow. Cerebrovascular autoregulatory mechanisms maintain cerebral blood flow in humans at constant levels even in the presence of wide fluctuations in mean arterial pressure. Not until mean arterial pressure decreases below about 55 mm Hg does cerebral blood flow become pressure dependent. Cerebrovascular autoregulation is independent of the sympathetic nervous system.

Cerebral blood flow remains unaffected in normal persons, therefore, even when mean arterial pressure decreases from control levels of 93 mm Hg to levels of 63 mm Hg during spinal anesthesia, because cerebrovascular resistance decreases proportionately (from 2.1 to 1.5 units).[71] Cerebrovascular autoregulatory mechanisms are blunted, however, in patients with essential hypertension (Table 7-10). In hypertensive subjects, a 50% decrease in mean arterial pressure (from 158 mm Hg before to 79 mm Hg during spinal anesthesia) is associated with a 17% decrease in cerebral flow, from 47 ml/100 g/min to 38 ml/100 g/min.[70,71] The level of blood pressure during spinal anesthesia that requires initiation of corrective measures is accordingly higher in hypertensive than in normotensive patients, both in absolute terms and in terms of percent decrease in pressure from preanesthetic control levels. In neither normotensive nor hypertensive patients need arterial pressure be maintained exactly at preoperative control levels during spinal anesthesia in order to ensure maintenance of adequate cerebral perfusion.

Regional Blood Flow. In addition to the effects of spinal anesthesia on cardiac and cerebral blood flow, it is of interest to know whether blood flow to other organs, such as kidney and liver, is affected and whether the changes are of clinical importance. In awake, unrestrained sheep, the effects of five drugs with flow-limited characteristics on regional blood flow and organ oxygen tensions were compared with the effects induced by spinal anesthesia.[112] Aside from a 10% decrease in hepatic blood flow, there were no significant changes in any hemodynamic variable or in any of the arterial or venous oxygen tensions induced by spinal anesthesia. The intravenous infusion of adequate volumes of saline at the time of the spinal blockade probably contributed to the maintenance of the normal variables.

Under general anesthesia (1.5% end tidal halothane), cardiac output and hepatic blood flow were decreased to 70% and renal blood flow to 50% of control values. Heart rate was unchanged and mean arterial pressure decreased by an average of 10%. Hepatic and renal oxygen tensions decreased significantly. If these findings are confirmed in humans, it would suggest that well-controlled spinal anesthesia may be preferred to general anesthesia with halothane, especially in patients with hepatic or renal disease (Fig. 7-14 A, B).[112]

Management of Hypotension. Oxygenation of the two most critical organs, the brain and the myocardium, is now recognized as being maintained in normal subjects in the presence of moderate levels of hypotension during spinal anesthesia. It is thus no longer considered necessary or desirable to maintain blood pressure at "normal" levels during spinal anesthesia. There comes a point, nevertheless, at which hypotension becomes so great that decreases in cerebrovascular resistance and decreases in myocardial oxygen

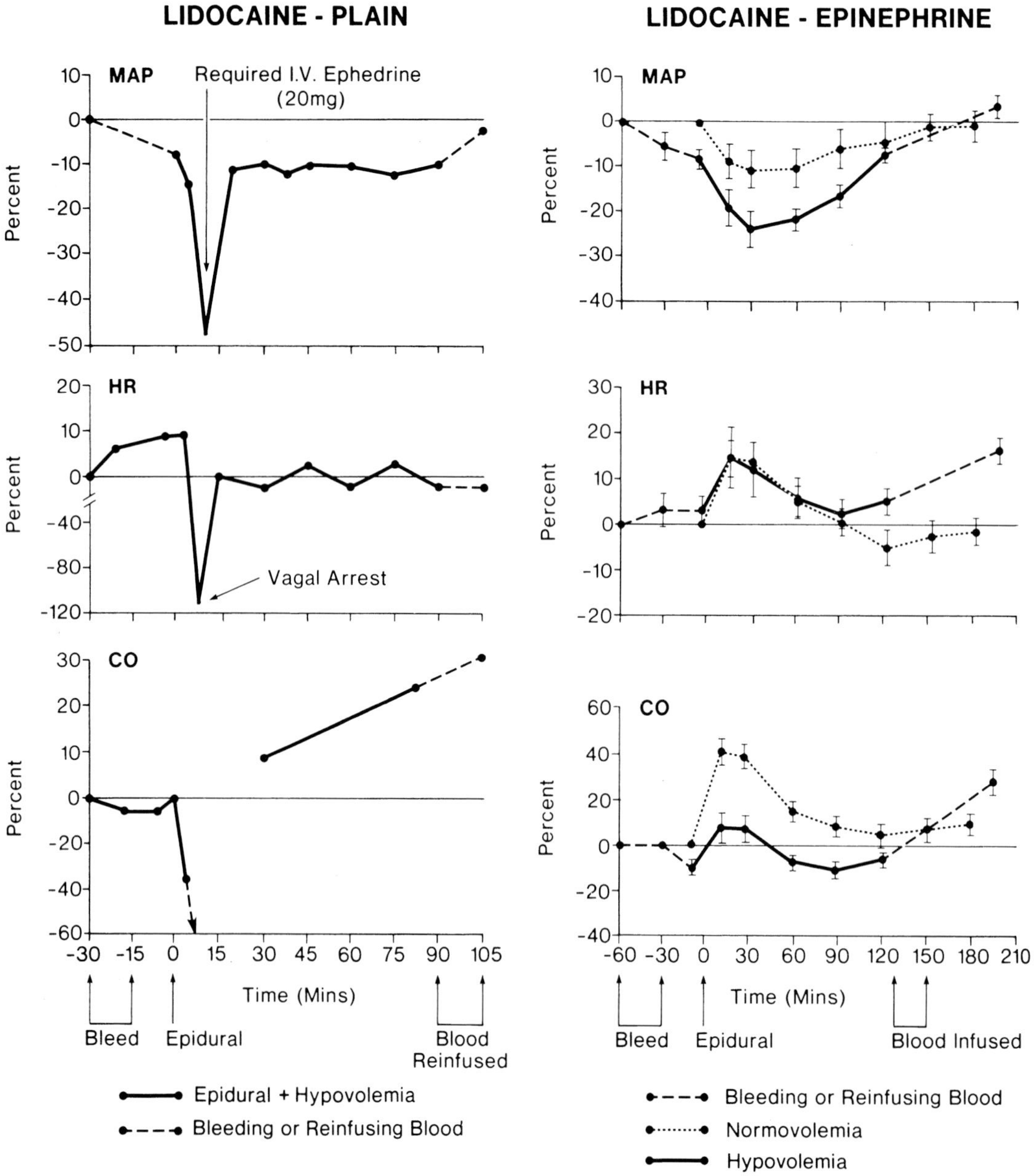

FIG. 7-13. Cardiovascular effects of epidural block, effect of hypovolemia in conscious volunteers; epidural block to T5 with plain and epinephrine-containing solutions. The mean percent changes are shown for each variable. Lidocaine-epinephrine (*right*). The cardiovascular changes after lidocaine-epinephrine in the presence of normovolemia are compared with hypovolemia (−13%). During normovolemia, note the marked increase in heart rate and cardiac output, lasting about 60 minutes. During hypovolemia, mean arterial pressure is significantly lower (−23%), but cardiac output remains close to control levels as a result of an elevated heart rate. Lidocaine plain (*left*). A representation of a typical response is shown. Severe bradycardia is associated with extreme hypotension, and in two subjects, vagal arrest occurred that required rapid resuscitation with ephedrine and oxygen. In only one subject was hypotension associated with increased heart rate, and this prevented the extreme hypotension seen in the other five subjects. (Modified from data of Bonica, J.J., Berges, P.U., and Morikawa, K.: Circulatory effects of peridural block. I. Effects of level of analgesia and dose of lidocaine. Anesthesiology, 33:619, 1970; Bonica, J.J., Akamatsu, T.J., Berges, P.U., Morikawa, K., and Kennedy, W.F., Jr.: Circulatory effects of peridural block. II. Effects of epinephrine. Anesthesiology, 34:514, and Bonica, J.J., Kennedy, W.F., Akamatsu, T.J., and Gerbershagen, H.U.: Circulatory effects of peridural block: III. Effects of acute blood loss. Anesthesiology, *36*:219, 1972.)

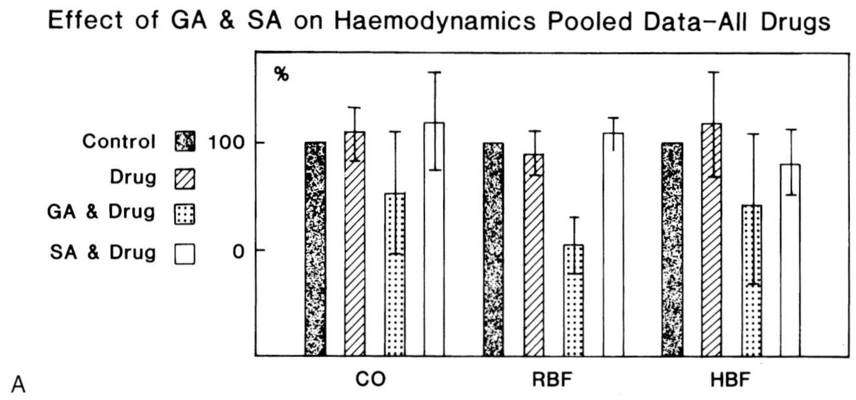

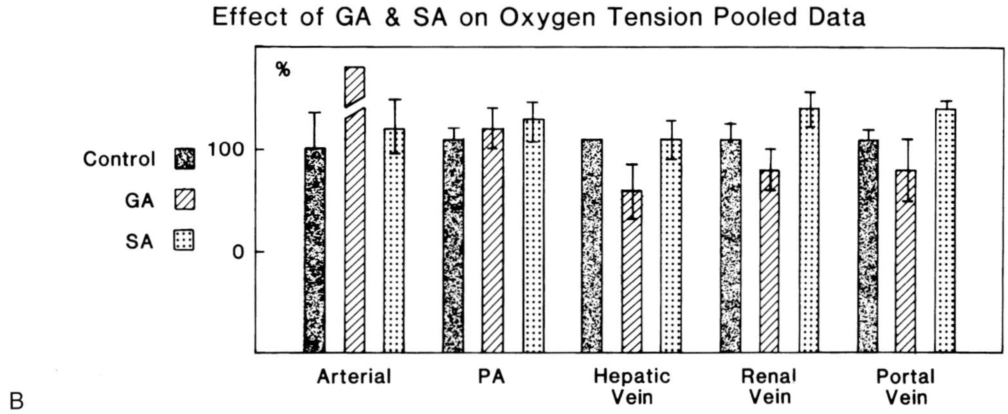

FIG. 7-14. Summary of blood flow **(A)** and oxygen tension data **(B)**. The mean value of each variable during control-drug, general anesthesia, or subarachnoid anesthesia studies has been expressed as a percentage of the mean value of the corresponding variable during the control preinfusion period on the same day. The mean and SD of these percentages for all five drugs studied are shown. Drug, control-drug study; GA & Drug, general anesthesia study; SA & Drug, subarachnoid anesthesia study; CO, cardiac output; RBF, renal blood flow; HBF, hepatic blood flow; PA, pulmonary artery. (Modified from Runciman, W.B., Mather, L.E., Ilsley, A.H., Carapetis, R.J., and Upton, R.N.: A sheep preparation for studying interactions between blood flow and drug disposition. III: Effects of general and spinal anaesthesia on regional blood flow and oxygen tensions. Br. J. Anaesth., *56*:1247, 1984).

requirements are no longer able to compensate for decreases in cerebral and coronary artery perfusing pressures. Exactly what this critical pressure is has not yet been defined. Pragmatically, however, decreases in systolic blood pressure to levels 33% below resting control levels (preferably as measured before the patient gets out of bed in the morning) need not be treated during spinal anesthesia in healthy, asymptomatic patients (Table 7-11). Although also not quantitated, similar levels of hypotension may be tolerated in patients with coronary arterial disease. Such statements are based on equivalent decreases in arterial blood pressure being deliberately induced in coronary care units by use of nitroprusside or nitroglycerin as a means of favorably affecting the ratio between myocardial oxygen supply and demand, even in patients with demonstrable myocardial ischemia. Physiologic responses to nitroprusside or nitroglycerin are quite similar to those associated with spinal anesthesia. Pragmatically, in patients with essential hypertension it would appear prudent to initiate corrective measures when systolic blood pressure decreases to more than 25% below the resting control levels. Clearly, appropriate monitors to detect significant blood pressure and ST-segment changes as well as delivery of supplemental oxygen *are to be recommended.*

Vasopressors are no longer routinely relied on in the management of hypotension during spinal anesthesia. Alpha-adrenoceptor agonists, such as methoxamine and phenylephrine, may so increase after load that increases in left ventricular oxygen demand because of increased work load may exceed the increase in myocardial oxygen supply brought about by the increase in coronary perfusing pressure (see Table 7-11). Also, of course, the cause of hypotension significant enough to require treatment during spinal anesthesia is not a decrease in TPVR, which alpha-adrenoceptor agonists would correct, but rather decreases in preload and cardiac output, neither of which is favorably affected by alpha-adrenoceptor agonists. Proportionately greater increases in myocardial oxygen requirements than in myocardial oxygen supply may also result when positive chronotropic drugs, including atropine, are used to elevate blood pressure by increasing heart rate and thus cardiac output.

Positive inotropic agents that increase cardiac output by increasing myocardial contractility may not be effective ei-

TABLE 7-11. *Treatment of hypotension associated with spinal anesthesia*

In "normal" patients *treat* if systolic BP ↓ by 30%
In "essential hypertension" *treat* if systolic BP ↓ by 20%
However, monitor CVS and CNS function

Principles of use of vasopressors

? Peripherally acting vasoconstrictors, e.g. α-agonists phenylephrine, methoxamine, not ideal because of: ↑ afterload, ↑ LV work, ↑ O_2 consumption, whereas the problem is ↓ preload and ↓ CO

Ideal is pure venoconstrictor (+ mild vasoconstrictor): → ↑ preload → ↑ CO; no such drugs exist

Treatment steps

1. ∴ → Use ephedrine or mephentermine
 → ↑ preload → ↑ CO
 → ↑ CO
2.[a] Elevate legs or Trendelenburg, but not 20° (→ ↑ internal jugular venous pressure → ↑ CBF)
3.[a] Administer oxygen
4.[a] ↑ IV fluids but:
 If normovolemia ephedrine more effective
 IV fluid "preloading" not very effective

[a] Often steps 2–4 will be used prior to step 1.
BP, blood pressure; CBF, cerebral blood flow; CNS, central nervous system; CVS, cardiovascular system; LV, left ventricle.

ther. Myocardial contractility is not impaired by spinal anesthesia. Increasing ventricular contractility when end diastolic filling volumes are decreased because of decreased preload may be misguided. The ideal vasopressor for treatment of hypotension during spinal anesthesia would be one that acts selectively to produce venoconstriction without affecting afterload, heart rate, or myocardial contractility. Such an ideal vasopressor would selectively remedy the cause of severe hypotension during spinal anesthesia, decreased preload. Such an ideal vasopressor, however, is not available. The best means for treating hypotension during spinal anesthesia is thus physiologic, not pharmacologic. In instances in which physiologic measures (see following) need to be supplemented by vasopressors, the most useful are ephedrine and mephentermine. Both have at least some venoconstrictive properties without major undesirable effects on the ratio between myocardial oxygen supply and demand (Table 7-11).

Physiologic treatment of hypotension during spinal anesthesia consists of restoration of preload by increasing venous return to the heart, and thus restoring cardiac output. This is most simply and most effectively done by providing the patient with an internal autotransfusion: merely placing the patient in the slight head-down or legs-up position. By doing so, the venous return and cardiac output improve, and in normovolemic patients, blood pressure returns to near normal levels.[117] The remaining minor decrease in blood pressure represents the decrease in afterload secondary to arterial and arteriolar vasodilatation. The head-down position need not, and should not, exceed about 20°. Extreme Trendelenburg position may be counterproductive by increasing internal jugular venous pressure to such an extent that effective cerebral perfusion pressure and cerebral blood flow are diminished. Use of the head-down position to maintain blood pressure or to correct hypotension during hyperbaric spinal anesthesia may result in unnecessarily high levels of anesthesia if used before the level of anesthesia becomes fixed. This can be avoided by elevating the lower body above the level of the heart at the same time the upper thorax and cervical area are elevated at about the T4 level by placing a pillow or other support under the patient's shoulders. This arrests the rising spinal at the T4 level at the same time that venous return is being maximized. This technique also reduces the chance of producing significant respiratory depression.

Another means for restoration of venous return, preload, and cardiac output during spinal anesthesia consists of the rapid intravenous infusion of large volumes of electrolyte solutions. Restoration of blood pressure alone, however, is not the sole objective in treating hypotension during spinal anesthesia. The objective is restoration of tissue oxygenation, especially myocardial oxygenation. Vasoconstrictors also restore blood pressure, as discussed above, but their adverse effects on the balance between myocardial oxygen supply and demand are so well recognized that they should be used infrequently today. The rapid intravenous infusion of a relatively large volume of fluids (1.0–1.5 L/70 kg) within 10 to 15 minutes for treatment of arterial hypotension during spinal anesthesia has been reported.[30,135] In one such study, Venn and colleagues concluded that the fluid preload was only of benefit in reducing the extent of the hypotension induced by spinal anesthesia, and even then, only in those patients in whom the sympathetic block extended above the T6 dermatome. By contrast, a vasopressor such as ephedrine was much more effective in treating hypotension, even when fluid administration (1 L or more) was ineffective. In another study, Coe and Revanäs compared the incidence of hypotension induced by spinal anesthesia in patients who received no intravascular volume preload, with the incidence of hypotension in patients given 8 ml or 16 ml of intravascular fluid (Ringer's acetate solution) per kg body weight. The authors found that the incidence of hypotension was a function of the level of sympathetic denervation, occurring in 60% of patients with a T7 sympathectomy, and in 100% of patients with a T4 or higher level of sympathectomy. However, the overall incidence of hypotension (27%) was similar in the three groups of patients, regardless of the intravenous fluid preload. Even when the intravenous fluid administration was guided by objective criteria such as central venous pressure monitoring, fluid preloading failed to prevent significant blood pressure decreases in 35% of patients[117] (see Table 7-11). It is apparent, then, that intravenous fluid preloading is relatively ineffective in the prophylaxis or treatment of hypotension induced by clinical spinal anesthesia in patients with normal circulating blood volume (fluid preloading and management in the gravid patient undergoing spinal anesthesia are discussed in Chapter 18).

In addition to being relatively ineffective, other considerations are to be borne in mind when large amounts of intravenous fluids are administered to patients undergoing spinal anesthesia. Although intravenous crystalloids may increase peripheral blood flow by decreasing viscosity and improving blood rheology, the oxygen content is decreased because of hemodilution. Thus, the decreased oxygen delivery to the tissues may exceed the benefits of increased tissue perfusion. Relatively large amounts of intravenous fluids also may be poorly tolerated by patients with myocardial dysfunction or those with valvular heart disease. Excess intravenous fluids also increase the need for postoperative urinary bladder catheterization, because the duration of parasympathetic nervous system denervation induced by spinal anesthesia far outlasts the duration of sensory denervation. These patients (and especially the elderly males with some degree of prostatism) are much more likely to develop urinary retention and some of the complications associated with catheterization, such as urinary bladder infection. Finally, intravenous crystalloid administration may counteract the salutary effects of spinal anesthesia on the coagulation system; according to one study, intravenous crystalloids increased coagulability and the incidence of deep venous thrombosis.[65]

Ventilatory

Arterial blood gas tensions are unaffected during high spinal anesthesia in patients spontaneously breathing room air.[60] Resting tidal volume, maximum inspiratory volume, and negative intrapleural pressure during maximal inhalation are similarly unaffected.[47,51] They remain unaltered despite the intercostal paralysis associated with high thoracic sensory levels of spinal anesthesia because diaphragmatic activity is unimpaired. Maximum breathing capacity and maximum expiratory volumes, on the other hand, are significantly diminished during high thoracic levels of anesthesia, as are maximum intrapleural pressures during forced exhalation, including coughing. Pulmonary mechanics during exhalation are impaired because the muscles involved in forced exhalation, especially the anterior abdominal muscles, are denervated by high thoracic levels of spinal anesthesia. The effects of high spinal anesthesia on forced exhalation are of clinical importance in patients with tracheal or bronchial secretions in whom the ability to maintain clear airways depends on their ability to cough.

The phrenic nerves are unaffected by even midcervical levels of sensory anesthesia because the level of motor blockade is usually below the level of sensory anesthesia, as discussed previously. Respiratory arrest owing to phrenic paralysis secondary to excessively high or "total" spinal is relatively rare. Nor is respiratory arrest caused by the presence of local anesthetics in ventricular CSF in concentrations adequate to produce direct depression of medullary respiratory neurons. Even the concentration of local anesthetic in cisternal CSF during high spinal anesthesia, greater than that in ventricular CSF, is below the threshold concentration of local anesthetic required to produce depression of central respiratory neurons when applied directly to the medulla. The most likely cause of transient respiratory arrest during high spinal anesthesia is ischemia of medullary respiratory neurons secondary to decreases in blood pressure and cardiac output severe enough to impair cerebral blood flow. Medullary ischemia as the cause of apnea during high spinal anesthesia is evidenced by the fact that respiratory arrest rarely occurs in the absence of hypotension severe enough to be associated with impending loss of consciousness. Further, restoration of blood pressure and cardiac output in cases of respiratory arrest during spinal anesthesia, if done promptly, is associated with immediate return of spontaneous respirations. This would not happen if the respiratory arrest were caused by pharmacologic block of the phrenic nerves or central respiratory neurons.

The character of spontaneous respirations serves as a valuable indication of the adequacy of medullary blood flow during high spinal anesthesia. It is therefore advisable to let patients breathe spontaneously during high spinal anesthesia rather than to control ventilation. Elimination of the negative intrapleural pressure of spontaneous inhalation by positive pressure ventilation not only removes a valuable indication of the adequacy of cerebral blood flow, but also may further decrease venous return, cardiac output, and arterial blood pressure.

The frequency and the type of postoperative respiratory complications have been reported to be similar after spinal anesthesia, local infiltration anesthesia, and general anesthesia in normal patients, as well as in patients with pre-existing respiratory disease, provided all other factors involved in determining the incidence of postoperative respiratory complications are kept constant.[68] These other factors include the site and type of operation; age, sex, obesity, and smoking history of the patient; and frequency with which narcotics are administered for relief of postoperative pain. In studies of spinal anesthesia, no special advantage has been reported in the respiratory cripple. There may be an advantage, however, in using saddle block or low spinal anesthesia for perineal, urologic, and other surgery in order to avoid general anesthesia and possible artificial ventilation in patients on the brink of respiratory failure, with severe bronchospasm, excessive amounts of sputum, or a difficult airway. Data are lacking to document these theoretic advantages.

Hepatic

Hepatic blood flow decreases during spinal anesthesia to the extent that arterial blood pressure decreases.[69,85,97] The decrease in hepatic blood flow is associated with an increase in the difference between systemic arterial and hepatic venous oxygen content. This reflects an increase in hepatic oxygen extraction, not hepatic hypoxia. The frequency and the magnitude of postoperative hepatic dysfunction are the same following spinal anesthesia in normal patients, as well as in patients with pre-existing hepatic disease, as they are when similar operations are performed under general anesthesia. This is true not only when blood pressure is maintained at normal levels during spinal anesthesia but also when severe hypotension is intentionally produced, as with hypotensive spinal anesthesia.[61] Spinal anesthesia has not been proven to represent either an advantage or a disadvantage in patients with pre-existing liver disease. Further data are needed. Spinal anesthesia, when possible, could avoid hepatotoxicity caused by halogenated anesthetics if susceptible patients were able to be identified preoperatively. Recent data from a sheep model with chronic vascular catheters indicate that spinal anesthesia to T4 is associated with minimal changes in hepatic blood flow, oxygenation, and drug metabolism. In contrast, general anesthesia with halothane resulted in reduced hepatic blood flow, decreased hepatic vein oxygen content, and decreased intrinsic clearance of drugs metabolized by the liver.

Renal

Renal blood flow, much like cerebral blood flow, is maintained by autoregulatory mechanisms through a wide range of changes in arterial perfusing pressure. In the absence of vasoconstriction, renal blood flow does not decrease until mean arterial pressure decreases below about 50 mm Hg. In the absence of severe hypotension, renal blood flow, and therefore urinary output, thus remain unaffected during spinal anesthesia. When spinal anesthesia is associated with mean arterial pressures below about 50 mm Hg, transient decreases in renal blood flow and urinary output occur. Even during severe, prolonged periods of hypotension, blood flow remains adequate to provide oxygenation of renal tissues so that renal function returns to normal as the blood pressure returns to normal in the postoperative period.[61]

Endocrine and Metabolic

Spinal anesthesia blocks hormonal and metabolic responses to nociceptive stimuli arising from the operative site to a degree not observed with general anesthesia.[60] The effect is only transient, however. Soon after the spinal anesthesia wears off, metabolic and hormonal responses in patients having had spinal anesthesia for their operation become indistinguishable from those having had general anesthesia for the same operation. The value of temporary inhibition of these responses on ultimate outcome remains to be defined (see also Chapter 5).

Gastrointestinal

Preganglionic fibers from T5 to L1 are inhibitory to the gut. The small intestine therefore contracts during midthoracic levels of spinal anesthesia owing to the relatively unopposed activity of the vagus nerve. Sphincters are relaxed, and peristalsis is normally active. The combination of a contracted gut and complete relaxation of the abdominal muscles provides exceptionally fine operating conditions for intra-abdominal procedures.

Obstetric

The physiology of spinal anesthesia in mother, fetus, and neonate is discussed in Chapter 18.

TECHNIQUE

Equipment

The preference of the anesthesiologist can dictate whether disposable, commercially prepared, or reusable department-prepared spinal anesthesia trays are used. Reusable department-prepared trays must be meticulously prepared by conscientious, well-trained personnel, with care being taken to prevent chemical and bacterial contamination. Because the manufacturers of disposable trays have been able to duplicate almost completely the traditional reusable tray for spinal anesthesia, it appears that disposable spinal trays will eventually replace the traditional reusable tray (see Chapter 6).

Needles for Spinal Anesthesia. A needle with a close-fitting, removable stylet is essential. This will prevent coring of the skin and the rare, though possible, occurrence of epidermoid spinal cord tumors from the introduction of pieces of epidermis into the subarachnoid space. Over the years, a large number of spinal needles of various diameters with numerous types of points have been developed. In general, in order to keep the incidence of postpuncture headache to a minimum, needles either of small bore or with a rounded, noncutting bevel (Greene, or Whitacre, or Sprotte) should be used.

A description of a few of the more popular spinal needles follows (Fig. 7-15). The Quincke-Babcock spinal needle, the so-called standard spinal needle, has a sharp point with a medium-length cutting bevel. The Pitkin spinal needle has a sharp point but short bevel with cutting edges and a rounded heel. Despite Pitkin's original claims, the incidence of postpuncture headache with this needle is relatively high. The Greene spinal needle has a rounded point and a rounded noncutting bevel of medium length.

The Whitacre and Sprotte needles (the pencil-point needles) have a completely rounded, noncutting bevel with a solid tip, the opening of the needle being on the side, 2 to 4 mm proximal to the tip of the needle.[48] The Huber point Tuohy needle has a curved tip for introducing catheters into the subarachnoid space. For the inexperienced, the use of either a 22-gauge Greene needle or a 22-gauge Whitacre needle is recommended because the characteristic "feel" of the various structures can more readily be learned than with smaller-bore spinal needles, while simultaneously keeping the incidence of postpuncture headache low (2%–7%).

Combination, or double-needle, sets are available. One such set is composed of the standard 5-cm, 21-gauge Quincke-Babcock spinal needle with a stylet and a 9-cm, 26-

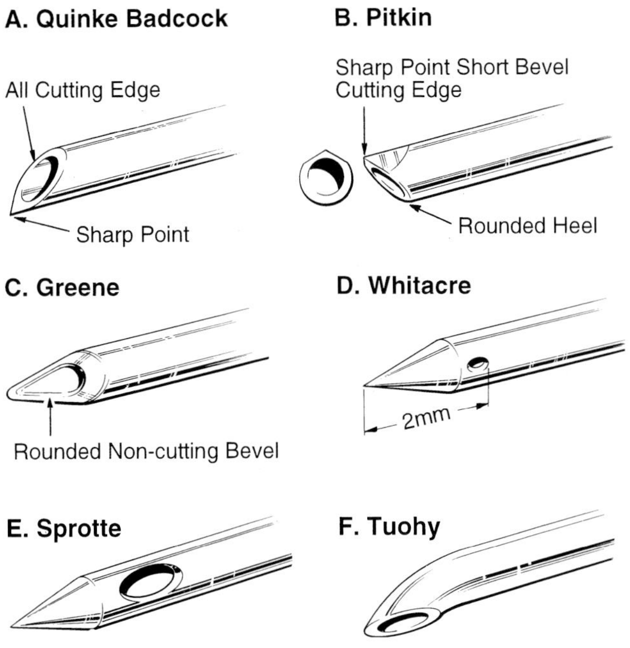

FIG. 7-15. Spinal needles.

gauge Quincke-Babcock needle with a close-fitting stylet. The 21-gauge introducer is inserted into either the ligamentum flavum or the epidural space, and puncture of the dura arachnoid is made with the fine 26-gauge needle. *Combined spinal-epidural sets* are becoming increasingly popular (see Chapters 8 and 18). Although manufacturers have slight modifications, all sets provide a Tuohy needle for introduction of an epidural catheter and a slightly longer spinal needle for subarachnoid injection of local anesthetics or narcotics. Some of the Tuohy needles have a double lumen, one that serves as a guide for the spinal needle and the other an additional aperture on the curved side for passage of the spinal needle without bending around the Huber tip (see Fig. 8-31).

Regardless of the size of the needle used, care must be taken so that the dural fibers that run longitudinally are separated rather than transected. With that in mind, the opening bevel is always on the side of the notch on the hub of the needle; the notch is then arranged so that the needle bevel is parallel to the longitudinal dural fibers.

Introducers. Various introducers have been developed both to facilitate the introduction of small-bore spinal needles, which are not easily directed, and to prevent contact of the spinal needle with the skin, hence reducing the incidence of coring and the introduction of pieces of epidermis or bacteria into the subarachnoid space. As an alternative, a disposable 18-gauge needle may be used. The use of an introducer is particularly helpful with 25-gauge or 26-gauge needles (Fig. 7-16).

Preparation and Monitoring of the Patient

Inasmuch as all conduction anesthetics may potentially become general anesthetics, the preparation for spinal anesthesia should be the same as that for general anesthesia. This includes a functional intravenous line, blood pressure and heart rate monitor, pulse oximeter, and appropriate equipment for airway management and oxygen administration. Emergency drugs also must be prepared (see Chapter 6). As in the management of any technique, the spinal anesthesia should be administered to a cooperative patient who is lying on a table that can be tipped upward or downward. The primary advantage of spinal over epidural anesthesia is the ability to control the spread of the anesthetic by manipulation of the specific gravity of the solution and the position of the patient. Except when using isobaric solutions, failure to use a movable table will lead to a higher incidence of both unsatisfactory anesthesia and complications. Similarly, the anesthesiologist must be able to assess the spread if it is to be controlled. The spread in overly sedated or anesthetized patients is virtually impossible to assess, and again this will lead to a greater degree of failure or complications.

Position of the Patient

Lateral decubitus position is undoubtedly the most popular position for the performance of spinal anesthesia because of the comparative comfort it affords the patient (Fig. 7-17). The patient should be placed on the very edge of the table closest to the anesthesiologist. The vertebral column is then flexed to widen the interlaminar spaces, which is accomplished by drawing the knees up to the chest and putting the chin down on the chest, the head supported by a pillow. (Care must be taken so that the vertebral column remains parallel with the edge of the table and the iliac crest and shoulders perpendicular to the table.) An assistant must stand in front of the patient to help the patient maintain the correct position. If the anesthesiologist is right-handed, the left lateral decubitus position should be used with the spinal

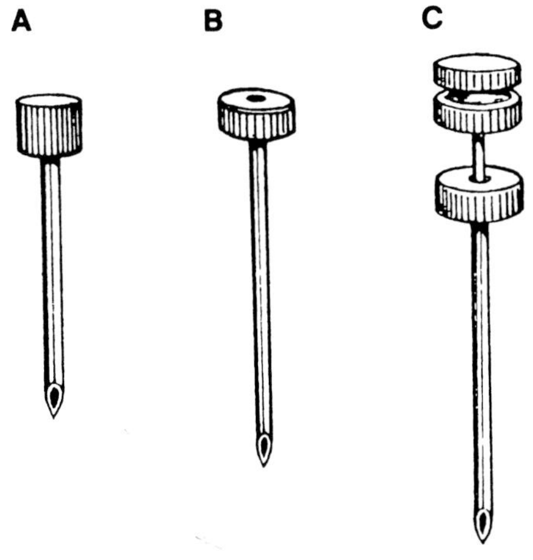

FIG. 7-16. Spinal needle guides and introducers. **A.** Pitkin guide. **B.** Sise introducer for 20-gauge or smaller spinal needles. **C.** Lund modification of Sise with locking stylet. (Lund, P.C.: Principles and Practice of Spinal Anesthesia. Springfield, IL, Charles C. Thomas, 1971).

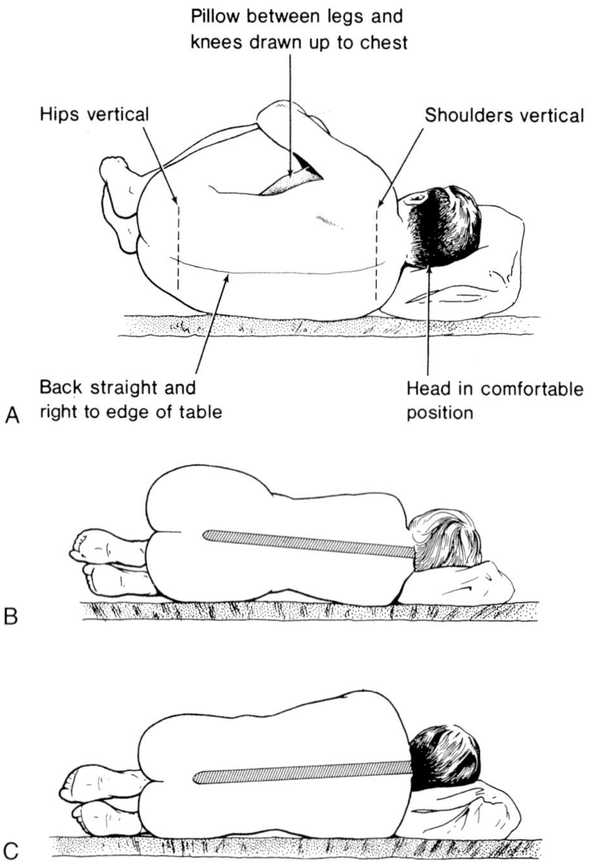

FIG. 7-17. A–C: Lateral decubitus position for spinal anesthesia. Note skeletal differences of female **(B)** and male **(C)** on level of subarachnoid space.

anesthesia tray to the right of the anesthesiologist. If the patient is to be positioned prone or supine at the conclusion of administering the spinal anesthetic, the location of the operative site is irrelevant. If, on the other hand, unilateral or hypobaric techniques are being used, then position of the operative site appropriate to the relative baricity of solution is essential.

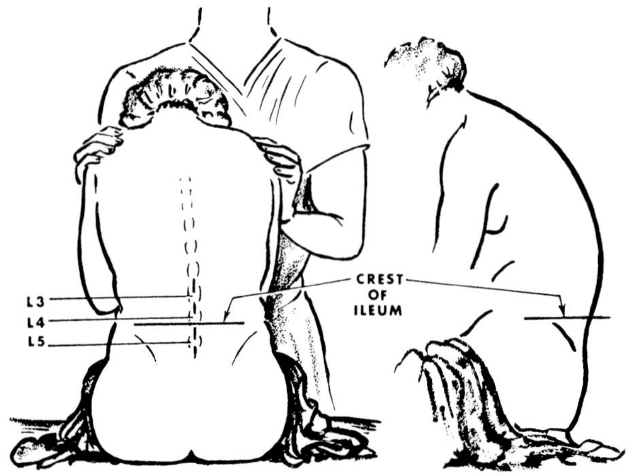

FIG. 7-18. Sitting position correctly demonstrated for spinal anesthesia. (Lund, P.C.: Principles and Practice of Spinal Anesthesia. Springfield, IL, Charles C. Thomas, 1971).

Sitting position is used less frequently than lateral decubitus, with the exceptions of low spinal anesthesia in obstetrics, certain gynecologic and urologic procedures, and certain hypobaric (and hyperbaric) techniques. The sitting position also facilitates lumbar puncture in obese patients (Fig. 7-18). Precautions must be taken against hypotension when patients who have received moderate to heavy premedication or are subject to fainting are in the sitting position. The patient sits on the table as close to the anesthesiologist as possible, the feet supported by a stool. The patient's neck and back are flexed again to provide maximum opening of the interspinous spaces. An assistant must stand in front of the patient at all times both to support and to maintain the correct position of the patient.

Prone position is used primarily for the hypobaric technique for procedures on rectum, sacrum, and lower vertebral column. Preferably, the patient is placed on his abdomen on the operating table to avoid repositioning after induction of spinal anesthesia. The technique is most easily accomplished if the lumbar curve is extended by flexion of the table or by placing a pillow under the patient's abdomen. The spinal fluid pressure is low in this position, and therefore aspiration may be necessary to obtain a free flow of spinal fluid. Flow of spinal fluid may be facilitated by elevating the head of the table. If this is to be done and the technique is hypobaric, it is critical that the table be repositioned before injection of the anesthetic so that the highest portion of the vertebral column is at the desired level of anesthesia.

TECHNIQUE OF LUMBAR PUNCTURE

Preparation of Equipment and Puncture Site. A previously prepared tray (hospital or commercial) should then be opened, and its sterility noted by checking the sterilization indicator. All subsequent activity should be performed using careful aseptic technique. The patient's back is then widely prepared with an antiseptic solution and sterile drapes applied. After discarding the preparation solution, one should prepare the anesthetic drugs, being careful at all times to prevent contamination of drugs or equipment with the preparation solution.

A line between the upper border of the iliac crest passes through either the spinous process of L4 or the interspace between L4 and L5 (see Fig. 7-18). The anesthesiologist should be positioned with the tray on the right (if right-handed) and the patient as nearly at eye level as possible. One may sit or stand as desired. Before any injection, the spinal needle should be inspected to ascertain that the stylet fits properly and that there are no barbs or foreign material on the tip of the needle. Care is taken to avoid handling the plunger of the syringe, which contains the spinal anesthetic solution, or touching the shaft of the spinal needle, which will subsequently be introduced into the subarachnoid space.

Depending on the interspace and approach selected, an intracutaneous skin wheal is made at the puncture site with a 25- to 27-gauge, 1-cm needle attached to a 2- to 5-ml syringe. One milliliter to 2 ml of 1% lidocaine is the usual dosage and drug for skin wheals. After this, subcutaneous infiltration of additional local anesthetic may be accomplished with a 2- to 3-cm, 22-gauge needle. The patient is then ready for the spinal needle to be introduced.

Midline Approach. Traditionally, the midline approach with the patient in the lateral position is the most popular approach (Fig. 7-19). If an introducer is being used, it is inserted through the skin wheal firmly into the interspinous ligament. Then the spinal needle is held like a dart (i.e., the hub is held between the thumb and index finger with the third finger along the proximal part of the shaft of the needle). If no introducer is used, the skin and soft tissues are fixed against the bony landmark by the second and third fingers of the left hand, which straddle the interspace.

The spinal needle is inserted through the same hole in the skin that was used to perform the intracutaneous wheal and subcutaneous infiltration. The bevel of the spinal needle should be directed laterally so that the dural fibers that run longitudinally are spread rather than transected. After traversing the skin and subcutaneous tissues, the needle is advanced in a slightly cephalad direction (100° to 105° on the cephalad side) with the long axis of the vertebral column (see Fig. 7-19), care again being taken to stay absolutely in the midline. (Even in the lumbar area, where the spinous processes of the lumbar vertebrae are relatively straight, the interlaminar space is slightly cephalad to the interspinous space). There is a characteristic change in resistance as the needle traverses the ligamentum flavum and the dura arachnoid, a change that becomes quite recognizable as experience is gained with this technique. The stylet is removed and CSF allowed to appear at the hub of the needle. If proper flow of spinal fluid does not occur, the needle is rotated in 90° increments until good flow is achieved. Occasionally, with patients in the prone position or if a small-bore spinal needle is being used, free flow of CSF will not be apparent. Gentle aspiration with a small, sterile syringe may then be used to obtain fluid.

With the hub of the spinal needle held firmly between the thumb and index finger of the left hand—the back of the left hand against the patient's back to prevent either withdrawal or advance of the spinal needle—the syringe containing the local anesthetic solution is firmly attached to the needle. Aspiration of spinal fluid is then performed, and if there is free flow, the local anesthetic solution is injected. Before removing the spinal needle, one again performs aspiration and reinjection of a small amount of fluid to reconfirm that the tip of the needle is still in the subarachnoid space. The patient is then placed in the desired position; cardiovascular and respiratory functions are monitored frequently; and the analgesic level to pinprick or temperature level with alcohol is checked at 5-minute intervals until the desired level is achieved. The patient should be repositioned as necessary, according to the baricity of the injected solution, to achieve this desired level; however, this must be accomplished within the "fixing time" of about 20 to 30 minutes for the local anesthetic.

Paramedian (Lateral) Approach. Many variations of the paramedian (lateral) approach avoid traversing the sometimes narrowed or calcified interspinous space. This approach is especially useful when degenerative changes are

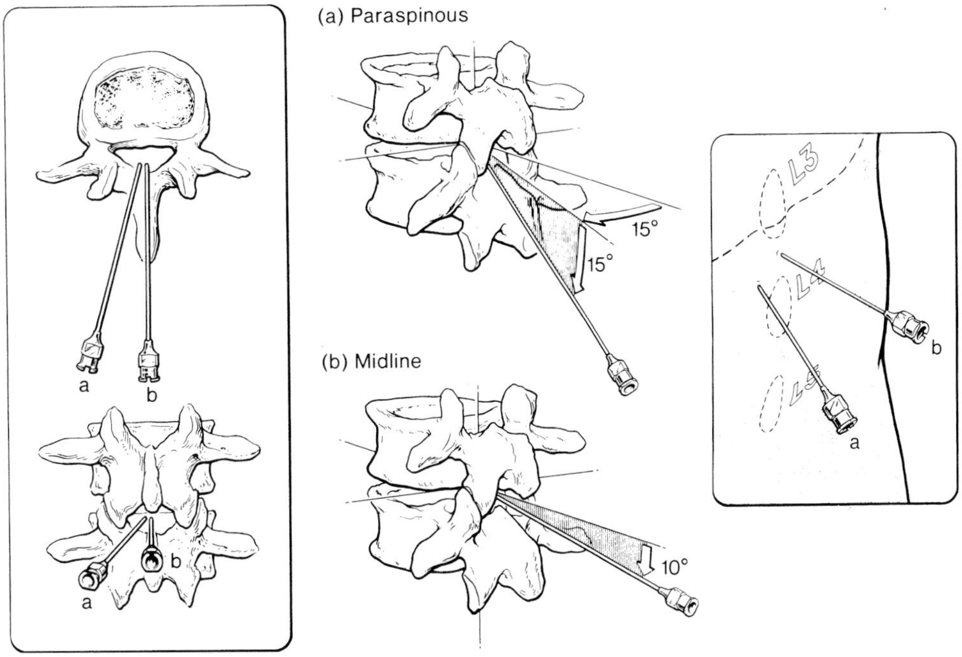

FIG. 7-19. Two common techniques of lumbar puncture for spinal anesthesia. **(a):** Paraspinous, paramedian, or lateral approach. **(b):** Midline.

encountered in the interspinous structures (e.g., in elderly patients) and when ideal positioning of the patient cannot be achieved, owing to pain (e.g., fractures, and dislocations involving the hips and lower extremities).

The patient is placed in the flexed lateral decubitus position, and a skin wheal is raised 1.5 cm lateral to the midline directly opposite the cephalad tip of the spinous process below the selected interspace. The direction of the spinal needle is at an angle of about 15° to 20° with the midline and slightly cephalad, 100° to 105° on the cephalad side (see Fig. 7-19). As with the midline approach, there is a characteristic "feel" encountered as the needle passes through the ligamentum flavum and dura arachnoid. At this point, the advance is stopped and the stylet withdrawn to allow spinal fluid to appear in the hub of the needle. If periosteum rather than the subarachnoid space is encountered, the needle should be redirected slightly cephalad, thus walked off the laminae into the interspace. Anesthesiologists should remember that the interlaminar space is created by the failure of the laminae to unite in the midline. If the needle is walked off the laminae, it must enter the interlaminar space and go into the subarachnoid space. Once the tip of the needle lies within the subarachnoid space, the remainder of the technique for administering spinal anesthesia is identical to that described previously for the midline approach.

The Taylor Approach. This is a special paramedian approach to enter the L5 interspace (the largest interlaminar space). It was originally described for urologic procedures but was subsequently used for other operations in the pelvis and perineum.[128] The patient is placed in the flexed lateral decubitus position, and a 12-cm spinal needle is inserted through a skin wheal made 1 cm medial and 1 cm caudad to the lowest part of the posterior-superior iliac spine. The needle is directed medially and cephalad at an angle of 55° into the subarachnoid space. Again, if periosteum is encountered, the needle is withdrawn and redirected slightly cephalad or walked into the correct location. Once the needle has been placed in the subarachnoid space, the remaining steps are identical to those described for the midline approach (Fig. 7-20).

Continuous Catheter Technique. This technique for spinal anesthesia uses a standard midline approach with a Tuohy-tip needle, which will allow passage of a plastic catheter through its lumen. The bevel of the needle is most advantageously directed cephalad during the advancement of the needle through the interspinous ligament. Once the needle is in, or just through, the ligamentum flavum, the bevel is rotated 90° to be parallel to the dural fibers before entry into the subarachnoid space. Once free flow of CSF is observed, the needle should be advanced another 1 to 2 mm to ensure that the entire tip of the needle is within the subarachnoid space; otherwise, the catheter will impinge on the dura as it emerges from the tip of the needle. The threading and fixation of the catheter are identical to the technique used for epidural anesthesia (see Chapter 8).

Because stimulation of the nerve roots by the catheter tip is painful and the catheter could conceivably enter a subarachnoid vessel, it is preferable to thread it only 2 to 4 cm beyond the tip of the needle. Once free flow of CSF through the catheter has been demonstrated, local anesthetic may be injected. The use of a Millipore filter placed at the injection end of the catheter is recommended for all subsequent local anesthetic injections.

There is obviously no advantage to adding epinephrine to agents being injected through the catheter because the duration is limitless anyway. Subsequent doses through the catheter may be reduced by 30% to 50% from the original dose.

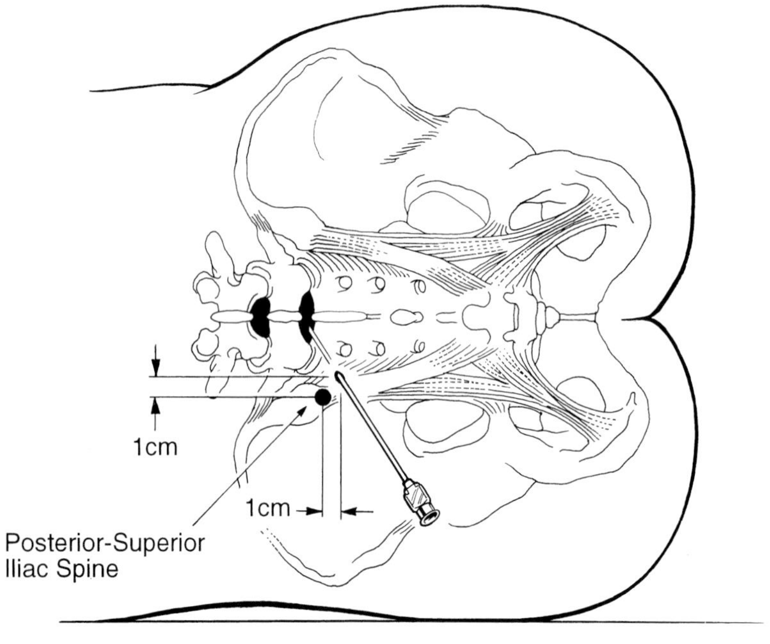

FIG. 7-20. Taylor approach to spinal anesthesia. (Redrawn with permission from Lund, P.C.: Principles and Practice of Spinal Anesthesia. Springfield, IL, Charles C. Thomas, 1971).

INTRAOPERATIVE AND POSTOPERATIVE MANAGEMENT

The first 5 to 10 minutes after administration of the spinal anesthetic are the most critical in adjusting the level of anesthesia when hyperbaric or hypobaric solutions are used. Levels of spinal anesthesia required for common surgical procedures are shown in Table 7-12. The first 10 to 20 minutes are also the most critical in assessing the cardiovascular responses to spinal anesthesia. Frequent measurements of blood pressure and heart rate will allow early recognition of any degree of hypotension. Indications and methods for treatment of hypotension have been previously described in this chapter (see Hypotension). Patient monitoring, as described in Chapter 6, should include pulse oximetry and electrocardiogram.

After surgical anesthesia levels and cardiovascular stability have been achieved, the anesthesiologist may determine whether supplemental drugs should be administered to make the patient comfortable. Not all patients will need intravenous medications during the course of surgery under spinal anesthesia. Many need only reassurance by a caring, empathetic anesthesiologist. When drugs are required to allay apprehension or discomfort arising from the unanesthetized upper extremities and trunk, benzodiazepines, which have both sedative and anxiolytic properties, are most useful. Particularly useful is midazolam, with its relatively short duration of action. The object of intraoperative medication during spinal anesthesia is to render the patient free of fear, anxiety, and discomfort. The object is not to induce light general anesthesia unless the patient or surgical circumstances require it. Midazolam, for example, should be administered in low doses, and its effects should be assessed frequently, especially in the elderly; once the desired effect is achieved, maintenance of sedation should be accomplished with additional low doses at increasingly longer intervals. Opioids during spinal anesthesia are best reserved for management of discomfort or slight pain from the operative site and for discomfort that occurs in the unanesthetized upper part of the body when patients lie immobile on the operating table for long periods. The low doses of opioids required for this type of analgesia will have minimal depressant effects on respiration. The amount of opioids given to produce satisfactory intraoperative analgesia during spinal anesthesia can be greatly decreased by administration of 50% nitrous oxide in oxygen by mask or by insufflation through a nasopharyngeal catheter (see Chapter 6). If pain is severe because the level of spinal anesthesia is inadequate, induction of light general anesthesia is preferred instead of reliance upon large doses of opioids.

TABLE 7-12. *Level of spinal anesthesia required for common surgical procedures*

Level	Surgical procedure
T4–T5 (nipple)	Upper abdominal surgery
T6–T8 (xiphoid)	Intestinal surgery (including appendectomy)[a], gynecologic pelvic surgery, and ureter and renal pelvic surgery
T10 (umbilicus)	Transurethral resection, obstetric vaginal delivery, and hip surgery
L1 (inguinal ligament)	Transurethral resection, if no bladder distension; thigh surgery; lower limb amputations
L2–L3 (knee and below)	Foot surgery
S2–S5 (perineal)	Perineal surgery, hemorrhoidectomy, anal dilation

[a] Blockade to T10 is not adequate for appendectomy because of splanchnic nerve supply to peritoneum (T6–L1).

Although supplemental oxygen by mask or by nasopharyngeal insufflation is usually not necessary in normal patients with low levels of spinal anesthesia, it is often used in patients with high thoracic levels or if the patient's respirations are depressed by hypnotics, tranquilizers, or opioids. The anesthesiologist should bear in mind that supplemental oxygen given to a hypoventilating patient may improve arterial oxygenation, but it will not relieve the accompanying increase in arterial carbon dioxide tension and may even aggravate it (see Chapter 6).

The anesthesiologist's role postoperatively can be divided into two periods. The first is actually a continued monitoring of the anesthetized patient in the recovery unit until complete cessation of the spinal anesthesia has occurred. Concerns during this period start with the careful movement and transport of the patient from the operating room to the unit. It is not uncommon for such activities to precipitate some degree of hypotension owing to redistribution of blood volume with movement; thus careful monitoring of the blood pressure is essential. If the patient does not have an indwelling urinary catheter, recovery room personnel should be alert for a distended bladder. The voiding mechanism is mediated through sacral autonomic fibers, which are the last to regain function after spinal anesthesia. Even after patients are able to move their extremities and respond to sensory stimuli, they may have some residual autonomic blockade, and thus may not only be unable to void but may also become hypotensive in the sitting or standing position. Postspinal headache is not related, either in severity or in incidence, to the patient's position while spinal anesthesia is wearing off and during the immediate postoperative period. Patients are kept flat in bed after spinal anesthesia only if necessary to avoid hypotension, not postoperative headaches. The role of the anesthesiologist in the postoperative period becomes surveillance with special attention to the possible development of postanesthetic complications, which are discussed in Chapter 21. Equally as important as the detection of bona fide complications is good rapport with the patient, which will permit the explanation of postsurgical aches and pains and the appropriate dismissal of them when clearly not caused by spinal anesthesia.

INDICATIONS AND ADVANTAGES

Indications for spinal anesthesia are much the same as they are for any type of regional anesthesia. These may include, for example, the presence of a full stomach, but only if a "low" spinal is used and full precautions for a full stomach are taken. However, vomiting and aspiration can occur during spinal anesthesia, especially in overly sedated patients, but their occurrence is less likely with spinal anesthesia. Anatomic distortions of the upper airway that might make maintenance of a clear airway difficult under general anesthesia also may, in certain circumstances, indicate use of spinal anesthesia. Certain types of operations are also relative, although not usually absolute, indications for spinal anesthesia. A spinal anesthetic technique is particularly preferable in operations such as rectal procedures. The area in which anesthesia and muscle relaxation are required is so circumscribed in rectal operations that the physiologic trespass associated with a small, discrete area of regional anesthesia is substantially less than that associated with general anesthesia. Operations such as transurethral resection of the prostate are also often relative indications for epidural or spinal anesthesia; not only is the physiologic trespass in geriatric patients having this procedure under spinal anesthesia less than that associated with general anesthesia, but complications associated with this operation, including perforation of the bladder and hypervolemia with congestive heart failure secondary to vascular absorption of irrigating fluid, can be more rapidly recognized during spinal anesthesia than during general anesthesia. As a general principle, however, the greater the extent of anesthesia required, the fewer are the indications for regional anesthesia.

Although cholecystectomies and gastrectomies can be, and in past years have been, successfully performed under spinal anesthesia, upper abdominal operations require T4 levels of sensory anesthesia. The physiologic trespass associated with such high levels of anesthesia is greater than that associated with use of modern general anesthetic techniques. Spinal anesthesia by itself is infrequently strongly indicated for operations above the level of the umbilicus. It may be valuable however, as part of a "balanced" technique.

Indications for major regional anesthesia are especially frequent in obstetrics. The role of regional anesthesia in obstetrics is fully discussed in Chapter 18 but some of the advantages, and thus indications, deserve emphasis. They include resolution of the problem associated with the fact that the mother almost invariably has a full stomach. Spinal anesthesia is also free of significant blood concentrations of drugs that can cross the placenta and affect the fetus. Early bonding between mother and neonate is not impaired by spinal anesthesia.

The advantages of spinal anesthesia over major nerve blocks are most evident in operations involving the lower extremities. Either spinal anesthesia or nerve blocks can be used for operations below the knee, but spinal anesthesia has the advantage of being simpler, more rapidly induced, and optimal for bilateral lower limb procedures. For operations involving the knee and upper leg, these advantages become even more evident. The number and the complexity of nerve blocks needed for operations on the knees, the thigh, and the hip are so great that spinal anesthesia is usually the preferred technique.

A new and special advantage of spinal anesthesia, as well as other forms of regional anesthesia, is their ability to decrease the intensity and duration of postoperative pain by the production of intraoperative deafferentation of the operative site.[37,68,116,132] Failure to block afferent stimuli arising from peripheral traumatized sites establishes a state of central nervous system hyperexcitability that increases pain to a clinical significant degree above that seen when nerve blocks prevent nociceptive impulses from entering the spinal cord. However, in order to maintain the advantage obtained with spinal anesthesia, it may be helpful to add a small dose of opioid to the spinal local anesthesia, thus providing a continuum of analgesia as the local anesthetic wears off. Subsequently, analgesia can be maintained by *prearranged* use of patient-controlled analgesia (PCA), which usually will maintain pain relief with lower than expressed doses, as a result of the pre-emptive spinal analgesia (see Chapter 26).

Continuous catheter spinal anesthesia has advantages over single injection spinal anesthesia that may specifically indicate its use.[33] The advantages include the ability to control the duration of spinal anesthesia, shortening it by using short-acting local anesthetics or prolonging it for hours, if necessary, by repetitive injection of local anesthetic solutions through the catheter. Equally important advantages include the ability to decrease or increase the level of anesthesia intraoperatively and to decrease the hypotension seen in elderly patients given a single-injection spinal anesthesia. Also, continuous spinal anesthesia to midthoracic levels needs only about 10% of the local anesthetic that epidural anesthesia would require. Placing the catheter preoperatively facilitates the operating schedule and allows the patient to be positioned for surgery before induction of anesthesia, thereby decreasing the risk of cardiovascular instability. Finally, the presence of the catheter allows the intrathecal injection of an opioid postoperatively for prolonged relief of postoperative pain.

CONTRAINDICATIONS

Contraindications to spinal anesthesia can be either usual or relative. Usual *contraindications* include the following:

1. Infections at the site of injection.
2. Dermatologic conditions (e.g., psoriasis) that preclude aseptic preparation of the skin at the site of injection.
3. Septicemia or bacteremia.
4. Shock or severe hypovolemia.
5. Pre-existing disease involving the spinal cord. This contraindication is based on the untested and untestable hypothesis that abnormal nervous tissue is more suscepti-

ble to the neurotoxicity of local anesthetics than is normal nervous tissue. Although there are no objective data to support this hypothesis, common sense and medicolegal considerations make it prudent to avoid spinal anesthesia in patients with progressive disease involving the cord lest the progression be blamed on the spinal anesthetic. Traumatic paraplegia and carcinoma of the prostate with metastases to lumbar vertebrae, however, are not necessarily absolute contraindications to spinal anesthesia when neurologic status is stable.

6. Increased intracranial pressure is a contraindication because of the risk of herniation of the medullary vasomotor and respiratory centers. Intracranial diseases without increased intracranial pressure (e.g., cerebral arteriosclerosis) are, on the other hand, often indications for spinal anesthesia.
7. Gross abnormality of blood clotting mechanisms (see also minor abnormalities of blood clotting mechanisms under relative contraindications). (See also Chapter 21.)
8. Patient refusal or patients who are psychologically or psychiatrically unsuited.
9. Lack of skill in, and experience with, spinal anesthesia. Spinal anesthesia is not for the unsupervised novice, nor is it for the anesthesiologist who, although skilled in general anesthesia, gives spinal anesthesia only rarely.
10. For the operating surgeon who cannot predictably complete the proposed operation in the time provided by spinal anesthesia or the surgeon who is unaccustomed to operating (especially intra-abdominally) under regional anesthesia.
11. Uncertainty about the extent or duration of the proposed operation, for example, "Exploratory laparotomy;? Whipple."

Relative contraindications to spinal anesthesia include the following:

1. Major surgical procedures above the umbilicus, using spinal anesthesia as the sole technique.
2. Deformities of the spinal column, including severe arthritis, severe kyphoscoliosis, and fusion of lumbar vertebrae at several levels.
3. Chronic severe headache or backache.
4. Blood in the CSF that fails to clear after 5 to 10 ml of CSF have been aspirated.
5. Inability to achieve a spinal tap after three attempts; after unsuccessful attempts, one should either abandon spinal anesthesia or obtain the help of a more experienced anesthesiologist.
6. Failure to obtain free flow of CSF through the lumbar puncture needle achieving satisfactory spinal anesthesia in this situation is not impossible, but the chances of doing so are significantly diminished.
7. Minor abnormalities of blood clotting, including "mini" doses of heparin administered up to the time of surgery.

Cardiac disease, whether myocardial, valvular, or ischemic, is best considered a major contraindication to spinal anesthesia if sensory levels to T6 or above are required. On the other hand, spinal anesthesia is often indicated in patients with even severe cardiac disease if only perineal levels of anesthesia are required.

COMPLICATIONS

Side effects and complications during spinal anesthesia involving respiration and the cardiovascular system were previously discussed in this chapter and also in Chapter 21. Another complication is complete failure of anesthesia to develop despite apparently correct injection of the local anesthetic solution into CSF. This is probably most frequently due to movement of the needle during injection but may occasionally be a result of subdural instead of subarachnoid injection (see Chapter 21). Although often attributed to injection of pharmacologically inert local anesthetic solutions (*i.e.*, the failure is blamed on the drug manufacturer), this is rarely the case. If the anesthesiologist routinely retains a portion of the uninjected local anesthetic and performs a bioassay of its anesthetic potency by placing a drop or two of the solution on the tongue or by making an intracutaneous wheal with it, only rarely, if ever, will the commercially supplied preparation be found to be devoid of local anesthetic activity when apparent injection of local anesthetic solution into CSF has produced no anesthesia.

Backache. Back pain is a frequent postoperative complaint after spinal anesthesia. Lund, in reviewing the literature, found an incidence of backache varying from 2% to 25%.[84] Although it is remotely possible that needle puncture of an intervertebral disk might result in postanesthetic backache, the more likely and more understandable cause is the flattening of the normal lordotic lumbar curve secondary to relaxation of the muscles and ligaments of the back. Presumably, this results in stretching of joint capsules, ligaments, and muscles beyond their normal "self-protective" range and results in pain. To this extent, it seems just as likely that a patient who receives paralyzing doses of muscle relaxants would suffer the same problem and that the lithotomy position might even exaggerate the condition. A study by Brown and Elman found the incidence of postoperative backache to be similar following general and spinal anesthesia.[20] A more recent clinical report recorded the incidence of transient (14%) and prolonged (3%) backache in 2046 patients receiving either epidural or spinal lumbar spine puncture in the usual way. They claimed that paraspinous infiltration of local anesthetic agent at the puncture site blocked the recurrent spinal nerves innervating the interspinous ligaments and muscles. In the succeeding 322 patients, the incidence of backache was reduced to 5.6% and to 0 for prolonged backache.[106]

Headache. The next most common complication of spinal anesthesia postoperatively is headache. This is more appropriately called postdural-puncture headache rather than spinal headache (see also Chapter 18).

The incidence of postdural-puncture headaches over the years has varied from 0.2% to 24%.[53,54,64,127] They are more frequent in women and in younger patients. The highest incidence is in obstetric patients. Also, the larger the size of the needle, the more frequent and severe are the postdural-puncture headaches. Although headaches after spinal anesthesia can be a postspinal-anesthetic problem, diagnostic lumbar punctures and myelography are associated with an even higher incidence of headaches. Further, postoperative headaches occur after general anesthesia. Not all headaches after spinal anesthesia are due to the dural puncture. It is important, therefore, to be conversant with the diagnostic features that are unique to this complication.

Clinical features. Although a history of dural puncture is helpful, the clinical features of postdural puncture headache are still diagnostic. First, the onset of headache occurs a minimum of several hours after the puncture but usually in the first or second day postpuncture. A recent controlled study showed that bed rest did not prevent, but merely postponed, the onset of headache.[25] The headache has been described[21] as invariably bifrontal and occipital, frequently involving the neck and upper shoulders. Severity varies from mild to incapacitating and may be aggravated, especially by the upright position and also by coughing and straining. The headache usually subsides completely when the patient is lying down. Associated symptoms are related to the severity of the headache and may include nausea and loss of appetite, photophobia, changes in hearing acuity and tinnitus, and depression. Patients whose headache persists for any period of time feel miserable, tearful, bedridden, and dependent. In more severe cases, diplopia and cranial nerve palsies have been attributed to traction on those cranial nerves (Fig. 7-21).

Once the diagnosis of postdural-puncture headache has been established, prompt treatment is essential. Until the past few years, treatment was conservative to the point that therapeutic efficacy could not be separated from the self-limiting nature of the process itself. The earliest measure was prophylactic in the form of enforced flat bed rest for 24 to 48 hours. This, of course, became therapeutic once the headache had occurred. Symptomatic treatment with analgesics or sedatives is just that, and probably has no beneficial effect in reversing the process. The most popular current concept of the pathophysiology is loss of CSF through the puncture site with resultant intracranial tension on meningeal vessels and nerves. Therapeutic modalities therefore have been directed at restoring the pressure relationships in the epidural and subarachnoid spaces. This has included measures such as abdominal binders to force more venous blood through epidural plexus; injection of saline in large volumes into the epidural space; overhydration of the patient, orally or intravenously, to stimulate production of CSF; and antidiuresis. In practical terms, many mild headaches may be resolved with forced fluid intake of 3

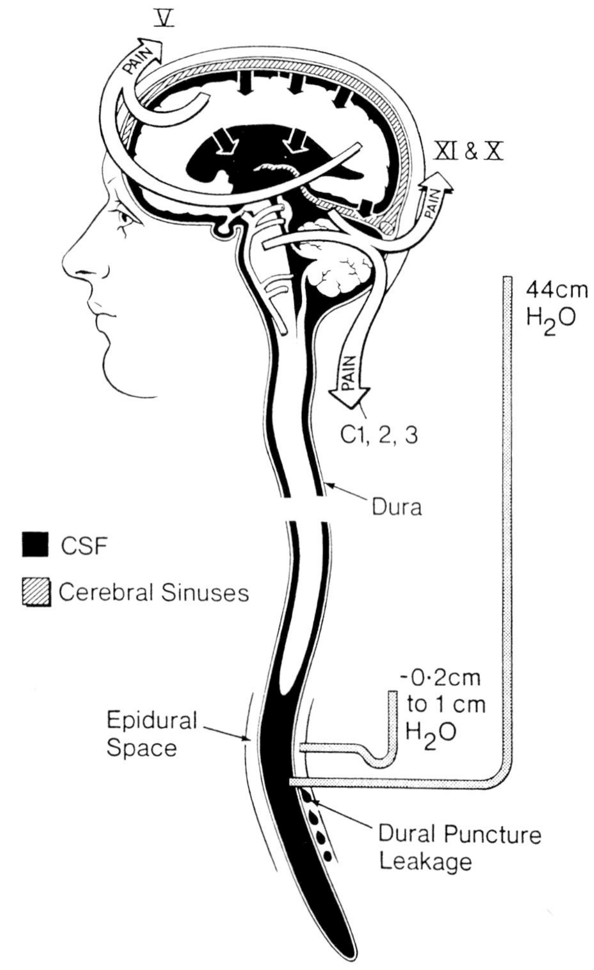

FIG. 7-21. Pathophysiology of post-dural puncture headache. Barometric figures are those to be expected in the subarachnoid and epidural spaces in the upright position at the site of lumbar puncture. The pressure differential favors CSF leakage. Note that CSF pressure is approximately atmospheric at the base of the brain. CSF leakage leads to descent of the brain in the upright position (*dark arrows*) on pain-sensitive intracranial vessels and the tentorium. Pain is referred (*open arrows*) above the tentorium via the trigeminal nerve (*V*) to the frontal region, and below the tentorium via the glossopharyngeal and vagal nerves (*IX, X*) to the occiput and via the upper cervical nerves (*C1, 2, 3*) to the neck and shoulders. (Brownridge, P.: The management of headache following accidental dural puncture in obstetric patients. Anaesth. Intensive Care, *11*:9, 1983.)

liters/day or more, plus the use of a tight abdominal binder when the patient is sitting or standing.

In 1970, DiGiovanni reported on 50 patients who received epidural injections of autologous blood as treatment for postlumbar-puncture headache.[42] Subsequently, and despite fears of infection and neurologic sequelae, the procedure has become an important therapy, employed progressively earlier. Abouleish summarized 524 cases reported by 11 centers.[1] He also reported a prospective study of an additional 118 patients. The technique of autologous blood patch is simply the insertion of a needle in the epidural space by the usual methods, followed by the injection of 5 to 15 ml of blood drawn aseptically from the patient's own anticubital vein. If patients are at all volume depleted, it is desirable to simultaneously infuse 1000 ml of intravenous fluid. Subsequent to the injection, the patient remains supine for 30 to 60 minutes. The success rate after the first injection varies from 89% to 95%. The procedure may be repeated 24 hours later and will provide equivalent success. Reported complications are few and mild but include backache (35%), neckache (0.9%), and transient temperature elevation (5%) of 24 to 48 hours' duration. It appears, then, that this is a worthwhile procedure with known minor risk that should be considered if early conservative measures fail.

Neurologic Sequelae. The remaining complications of postspinal anesthesia fall into the category of neurologic sequelae (see Chapters 8 and 21). Although these are the most feared and most serious of all complications, they are extremely rare.[44,93] Lund tabulated the major series of spinal anesthesia reported between 1948 and 1958.[84] Of these 582,190 cases of spinal anesthesia, he stated that "no incidence of permanent motor paralysis [was] reported," (see Table 7-5). Nonetheless, cases have been reported. It is obviously important to both patient and anesthetist alike that every postanesthetic complication be examined critically with reference to prevention of similar complications. This is especially important with neurologic sequelae after spinal anesthesia.

Nowhere in the foregoing has any of these neurologic complications been identified as being caused by spinal anesthesia. This is not to say that it is not possible, but rather that not all postspinal-anesthetic neurologic complications are directly related to the anesthetic; perhaps they are not even indirectly related to the anesthetic and, even more perplexing, may never have a proven etiology. Much of the negative image of spinal anesthesia has been a result of "speculative etiology by association."

It is important to keep the perspective that determination of etiology should not be fault-motivated but rather therapy-oriented. To that end, the important first step in any neurologic complication is early detection, diagnosis, and treatment. The degree of irreversibility of many of these complications is time related. Since most anesthesiologists are not trained neurologists, an early neurologic consultation is mandatory.

Anatomically, injuries may be categorized as peripheral nerve, cauda equina, spinal cord, and intracranial. Peripheral nerves usually have multiple nerve root origins. A complication in a unilateral peripheral nerve distribution (e.g., hypoesthesia or weakness) is likely to be secondary to trauma to the nerve, secondary to positioning, or secondary to operative trauma rather than being due to spinal anesthesia. The precise localization, by a neurologist, of the neural distribution of the lesion is essential in arriving at an appropriate differential diagnosis and treatment. In contrast, bilateral involvement, whether cauda equina or higher up the spinal cord, would be more indicative of an epidural or subarachnoid injury with totally different therapeutic and prognostic implications. Anesthesiologists and surgeons alike should realize that patients who have complications are not interested in fault if they are assured that everyone is working together for an early diagnosis and treatment (see also Chapter 21).

From the prophylactic viewpoint, strict attention must be paid to the cleansing of the patient, particularly the locally or systemically infected patient. Care should be exercised to eliminate introduction of detergents or chemicals into the subarachnoid space, and extreme caution is necessary to ensure use of the correct drugs and vasopressors in the correct concentrations. Traumatic complications can usually be avoided by careful and cooperative positioning of the patient by the surgeon and the anesthesiologist with awareness of the vulnerability of peripheral nerves for the particular surgical procedure. Certainly, the anesthesiologist always endeavors to use an atraumatic spinal technique but should be sensitive to early abandonment rather than perseverance in technically extremely difficult cases.

Despite their rarity, unequivocal cases of *cauda equina syndrome* have been reported in recent years. Although most of these cases have been associated with the simultaneous reintroduction and popularization of continuous spinal anesthesia, the suggestion by de Jong that 5% lidocaine in 7.5% dextrose may be inherently neurotoxic, even when used correctly as a single-dose technique, deserves further consideration.[38] To date, most of the reports of cauda equina syndrome following spinal anesthesia have been associated with use of plastic microcatheters.[33] The most likely explanation for these unfortunate instances of cauda equina paralysis is that the anesthesia was carried out in such a way that neurotoxically high concentrations of local anesthetics were created in the area of the cauda equina. These high concentrations were most frequently caused by repeated injections of hyperbaric local anesthetic solutions through a microcatheter, the tip of which lay in the area of the cauda equina. The combination of using a hyperbaric solution with malpositioning of the patient or catheter so that the anesthetic solution never migrated out of the sacrolumbar area to the thoracic level of the spinal cord probably resulted in pooling of neurotoxic concentrations of local anesthetic in the sacrolumbar area.

Regardless of whether *hyper*baric solutions of local anesthetic are injected into the subarachnoid space through a needle, microcatheter or macrocatheter, the desired level of neural blockade is obtained partly by dose, but to a major degree by changing the position of the table (head-down for cephalad spread). It has never been recommended that hyperbaric solutions of any local anesthetic be repeatedly administered to neurotoxic levels as the sole means to achieve the desired level. The Trendelenburg position achieves the maximum result with the maximum safety. In some countries, clinicians are now avoiding hyperbaric 5% "spinal" lidocaine for continuous *or* single-shot spinal anesthesia. Since it is the *dose* of local anesthetic that contributes to level of blockade, the 2% lidocaine isobaric solution, in appropriate dose, seems a logical alternative to the controversial 5% lidocaine. Whether catheters of 30 gauge and smaller add to the risk of inducing toxicity is debatable, as are the roles of speed of injection and number of openings at the tip of the catheter in CSF. Catheters of a size used for continuous epidural anesthesia also may be used for continuous spinal anesthesia, even though they may by associated with an increase in the incidence of postpuncture headaches.

COMPARISON OF SPINAL AND EPIDURAL

Although spinal and epidural anesthesia are major regional anesthetic techniques, there are significant differences between them. Efforts to compare the upper levels of sensory and sympathetic block after epidural have not been done as carefully as with spinal anesthesia (see Chapter 8 for factors influencing level and degree of sympathetic blockade with epidural)[8]; however, obstetric anesthesiologists have the distinct clinical impression that the speed of onset of sympathetic block and therefore the adverse cardiovascular side-effects occur more rapidly with spinal than with epidural anesthesia. Some anesthesiologists regard the slower onset of side-effects, which allows more time to initiate treatment, as a reason for preferring epidural over spinal for cesarean section.

An offsetting disadvantage of epidural anesthesia is the requirement for larger volumes and doses of local anesthetic agents, which result in pharmacologically active plasma concentrations of local anesthetics. Equivalent levels of sensory analgesia with spinal anesthesia are accompanied by plasma levels of local anesthetics too low to have direct systemic effects (see Chapter 3). By acting directly on the myocardium and on peripheral vascular smooth muscles, epidurally injected local anesthetics, with their varying systemic effects, produce cardiovascular changes that are often additive to those produced by high sympathetic blockade (see Chapter 8).

An additional problem with epidural anesthesia is that many of the local anesthetics have contained additives such as methylparaben and bisulfite, which, when unintentionally placed into the subarachnoid space, have produced major complications (see Chapter 8). These same drugs in low doses and without additives or low pH have been used safely for spinal anesthesia. The effect of higher plasma levels of local anesthetics during epidural anesthesia also becomes important when comparing epidural and spinal anesthesia for obstetrics because local anesthetics pass from the maternal to the fetal circulation (see Chapter 18).

One major advantage of epidural anesthesia is that continuous epidural catheter techniques can extend the duration of anesthesia beyond that usually possible with spinal anesthesia. This difference is especially useful when continuous epidural analgesia is used for control of pain during labor. This difference is also particularly appreciated by those who are hesitant to use either intrathecal vasoconstrictors with spinal anesthesia or continuous spinal catheter techniques.

Many anesthesiologists believe that more predictable levels of anesthesia can be achieved with single injection spinal than with single injection epidural anesthesia. This advantage of spinal over epidural is lost when continuous epidural catheter techniques are used that allow one to increase or decrease the levels of epidural anesthesia when short-acting local anesthetics are applied. The potential benefit of epidural over spinal as regards avoidance of postdural-puncture headaches is not always fully realized under clinical conditions. Even in the hands of experts, dural punctures do occur during planned epidural anesthesia. Given the size of epidural needles, especially those used for insertion of catheters, when this happens the likelihood of a postdural-puncture headache may be considerable.

Anesthesiologists equally well trained in epidural and spinal anesthesia realize that both techniques have advantages and both have disadvantages. Neither should be used to the exclusion of the other. Both should be used and the choice based upon advantages for individual patients. "Combined" spinal-epidural technique is discussed in Chapter 8.

REFERENCES

1. Abouleish, E., Vega, S., Blendinger, I., and Tio, T.O.: Long-term follow-up of epidural blood patch. Anesth. Analg., *54:*459, 1975.
2. Armstrong, I.A., Littlewood, D.G., and Chambers, W.A.: Spinal anesthesia with tetracaine—the effect of added vasoconstrictors. Anesth. Analg., *62:*793, 1983.
3. Axelsson, K., and Widman, B.: Clinical significance of specific gravity of spinal anaesthetic agents. Two double-blind studies with hyperbaric 5% lidocaine. Acta Anaesthesiol. Scand., *23:*427, 1979.
4. Babcock, W.W.: Spinal anaesthesia: A clinical study of 658 administrations. N.Y. Med. J., *98:*897, 1913.
5. Bibliographia Medica II. Cocaine spinal anesthesia. pp. 855, Paris 1901.
6. Barker, A.E.: Clinical experiences with spinal analgesia in 100 cases. Br. Med. J., *1:*665, 1907.
7. Batson, O.V.: The function of the vertebral veins and their role in the spread of metastases. Ann. Surg., *112:*138, 1940.
8. Bengtsson, M., Lofstrom, J.B., and Malmquist, L.A.: Skin conductance responses during spinal analgesia. Acta Anaesthesiol Scand., *29:*67, 1985.
9. Bier, A.: Versuche über Kokainisierung des Rückenmarks. Dtsch. Z. Chir., *51:*361, 1899.
10. Blomquist, H., Nilsson, A., and Arwestrom, E.: Spinal anesthesia with 15 mg bupivacaine 0.25% and 0.5%. Reg. Anesth., *13:*165, 1988.
11. Bonica, J.J., Akamatsu, T.J., Berges, P.U., Morikawa, K., and Kennedy, W.F., Jr. Circulatory effects of peridural block. II. Effects of epinephrine. Anesthesiology, *34:*514, 1971.
12. Bonica, J.J., Berges, P.U., and Morikawa, K.: Circulatory effects of peridural block. I. Effects of level of analgesia and dose of lidocaine. Anesthesiology, *33:*619, 1970.
13. Bonica, J.J., Kennedy, W.F., Akamatsu, T.J., and Gerbershagen, H.U.: Circulatory effects of peridural block. III. Effects of acute blood loss. Anesthesiology, *36:*219, 1972.
14. Bonnet, F., Brun-Buisson, V., Saada, M., *et al.*: Dose-related prolongation of hyperbaric tetracaine spinal anesthesia by clonidine in humans. Anesth. Analg., *68:*619, 1989.
15. Bonnet, F., Diallo, A., Saada, M., *et al.*: Prevention of tourniquet pain

by spinal isobaric bupivacaine with clonidine. Br. J. Anaesth., *63:*93, 1989.

16. Braun, H.: Über den Einfluss der Vitalität der Gewebe auf die örtlichen und allgemeinen Gifturkungen localanästhesirender Mittel und über die Bedeutung des Adrenalins für die Localanästhesis. Arch. F. Klin. Chir., *19:*541, 1903.
17. Braun, H.: Über einige neue örtliche Anästhetica (Stovain, Alypine, Novokain). Dtsch. Med. Wochenschr. *31:*1667, 1905.
18. Bridenbaugh, P.O., Moore, D.C., and Bridenbaugh, L.: Capillary Po_2 as a measure of sympathetic blockade. Anesth. Analg., *50:*26, 1971.
19. Brown, D.T., Wildsmith, J.A.W., Covino, B.G., and Scott, D.B.: Effect of baricity on spinal anaesthesia with amethocaine. Br. J. Anaesth., *52:*589, 1980.
20. Brown, E.M., and Elman, D.S.: Postoperative backache. Anesth. Analg., *40:*683, 1961.
21. Brownridge, P.: Management of headache following dural puncture in obstetric patients. Anaesth. Intensive Care, *11:*4, 1983.
22. Brull, S.J., and Greene, N.M.: Time courses of zones of differential spinal anesthesia with hyperbaric tetracaine or bupivacaine. Anesth. Analg., *69:*342, 1989.
23. Burm, A.G., van Kleef, J.W., Gladines, M.P., Spierdijk, J., and Breimer, D.D.: Plasma concentrations of lidocaine and bupivacaine after subarachnoid administration. Anesthesiology, *59:*191, 1983.
24. Caldwell, C., Nielsen, C., Baltz, T., *et al.*: Comparison of high-dose epinephrine and phenylephrine in spinal anesthesia with tetracaine. Anesthesiology, *62:*804, 1985.
25. Carbaat, P.A.T., and Van Crevel, H.: Lumbar puncture headache: Controlled study of the preventive effect of 24 hours bedrest. Lancet, *2:*1133, 1982.
26. Chamberlain, D.P., and Chamberlain, B.D.L.: Changes in skin temperature of the trunk and their relationship to sympathetic blockade during spinal anesthesia. Anesthesiology, *65:*139, 1986.
27. Chambers, W.A., Edstrom, H.H., and Scott, D.B.: Effect of baricity on spinal anaesthesia with bupivacaine. Br. J. Anaesth., *53:*279, 1981.
28. Chambers, W.A., Littlewood, D.G., Logan, M.R., and Scott, D.B.: Effect of added epinephrine on spinal anesthesia with lidocaine. Anesth. Analg., *60:*417, 1981.
29. Chambers, W.A., Littlewood, D.G., and Scott, D.B.: Spinal anesthesia with bupivacaine: Effect of added vasoconstrictors. Anesth. Analg., *61:*49, 1982.
30. Coe, A.J., and Revanäs, B.: Forum: Is crystalloid preloading useful in spinal anaesthesia in the elderly? Anaesthesia, *45:*241, 1990.
31. Cohen, E.N.: Distribution of local anesthetic agents in the neuraxis of the dog. Anesthesiology, *29:*1002, 1968.
32. Concepcion, M., Maddi, R., Francis, D., *et al.*: Vasoconstrictors in spinal anesthesia with tetracaine—A comparison of epinephrine and phenylephrine. Anesth. Analg., *63:*134, 1984.
33. Continuous Spinal Anesthesia Symposium. Reg. Anesth., 18, Nov-Dec. Supplement, 1993.
34. Corning, J.L.: Spinal anesthesia and local medication of the cord. N.Y. State J. Med., *42:*483, 1885.
35. Crock, H.V., and Yoshizawa, H.: The Blood Supply of the Vertebral Column and Spinal Cord in Man. New York, Springer-Verlag, 1979.
36. Cummings, G.C., Bamber, D.B., Edstrom, H.H., and Rubin, A.P.: Subarachnoid blockade with bupivacaine: A comparison with cinchocaine. Br. J. Anaesth., *56:*573, 1984.
37. Dahl, J.B., and Kehlet, H.: The value of pre-emptive analgesia in the treatment of postoperative pain. Br. J. Anaesth., *70:*434, 1993.
38. De Jong, R.H.: Last round for a "heavyweight"? Anesth. Analg., *78:*3, 1994.
39. Denson, D.D., Bridenbaugh, P.O., Turner, P.A., and Phero, J.C.: Comparison of neural blockade and pharmacokinetics after subarachnoid lidocaine in the rhesus monkey. II. Effects of volume, osmolality, and baricity. Anesth. Analg., *62:*995, 1983.
40. Denson, D.D., Bridenbaugh, P.O, Turner, P.A., Phero, J.C., and Raj, P.P.: Neural blockade and pharmacokinetics following subarachnoid lidocaine in the rhesus monkey. I. Effects of epinephrine. Anesth. Analg., *61:*746, 1982.
41. Denson, D.D., Turner, P.A., Bridenbaugh, P.O., and Thompson, G.A.: Pharmacokinetics and neural blockade after subarachnoid lidocaine in the rhesus monkey. III. Effects of phenylephrine. Anesth. Analg., *63:*129, 1984.
42. DiGiovanni, A.J., and Dunbar, B.S.: Epidural injections of autologous blood for postlumbar puncture headache. Anesth. Analg., *49:*268, 1970.
43. Dohi, S., Matsumiya, N., Takeshima, R., and Naito, H.: Effects of subarachnoid lidocaine and phenylephrine on spinal cord and cerebral blood flow in dogs. Anesthesiology, *61:*238, 1984.
44. Dripps, R.D., and Vandam, L.D.: Long-term follow-up of patients who received 10,098 spinal anesthetics. I. Failure to discover major neurological sequelae. J.A.M.A., *156:*1486, 1954.
45. Dubelman, A.M., and Forbes, A.R.: Does cough increase the spread of subarachnoid anesthesia? Anesth. Analg., *58:*306, 1979.
46. Eckenhoff, J.E., Hafkenschiel, J.H., Foltz, E.L., and Driver, R.L.: Influence of hypotension on coronary blood flow, cardiac work, and cardiac efficiency. Am. J. Physiol., *152:*545, 1948.
47. Egbert, L.D., and Deas, T.C.: Effect of epinephrine on the duration of spinal anesthesia. Anesthesiology, *21:*345, 1960.
48. Etherington-Wilson, W.: Intrathecal nerve root block: Some contributions and a new technique. Proc. R. Soc. Med. (Anaesth.), *27:*323, 1937.
49. Fishman, R.A.: Cerebrospinal Fluid in Diseases of the Nervous System. pp. 168. Philadelphia, W.B. Saunders, 1980.
50. Fishman, R.A.: Cerebrospinal Fluid in Diseases of the Nervous System. p. 15. Philadelphia. W.B. Saunders, 1980.
51. Freund, F.G., Bonica, J.J., Ward, R.J., Akamatsu, T.J., and Kennedy, W.F., Jr.: Ventilatory reserve and level of motor block during high spinal and epidural anesthesia. Anesthesiology, *28:*834, 1967.
52. Giasi, R.M., D'Agostino, E., and Covino, B.G.: Absorption of lidocaine following subarachnoid and epidural administration. Anesth. Analg., *58:*360, 1979.
53. Greene, B.A.: A 26-gauge lumbar puncture needle: Its value in the prophylaxis of headache following spinal analgesia for vaginal delivery. Anesthesiology, *11:*464, 1950.
54. Greene, H.M.: A technique to reduce the incidence of headache following lumbar puncture in ambulatory patients with a plea for more frequent examination of cerebrospinal fluids. Northwest Med., *22:*240, 1923.
55. Greene, N.M.: The area of differential block during spinal anesthesia with hyperbaric tetracaine. Anesthesiology, *19:*45, 1958.
56. Greene, N.M.: A consideration of factors involved in the discovery of anesthesia and their effect on subsequent development of anesthesia. Anesthesiology, *35:*515, 1971.
57. Greene, N.M.: Uptake and elimination of local anesthetics during spinal anesthesia. Anesth. Analg., *62:*1013, 1983.
58. Greene, N.M.: Distribution of local anesthetic solutions within the subarachnoid space. Anesth. Analg., *64:*715, 1985.
59. Greene, N.M., and Bachand, R.G.: Vagal component of the chronotropic response to baroreceptor stimulation in man. Am. Heart J., *82:*22, 1971.
60. Greene, N.M., and Brull, S.J.: Physiology of Spinal Anesthesia. 4th ed. Baltimore, Williams & Wilkins, 1981.
61. Greene, N.M., Bunker, J.P., Kerr, W.S., *et al.*: Hypotensive spinal anesthesia: Respiratory, metabolic, hepatic, renal and cerebral effects. Ann. Surg., *140:*641, 1954.
62. Gregoretti, S.: Paroxysmal atrioventricular heart block during spinal anesthesia. Reg. Anesth., *10:*149, 1985.
63. Hackel, D.B., Sancetta, S.M., and Kleinerman, J.: Effect of hypotension due to spinal anesthesia on coronary blood flow and myocardial metabolism in man. Circulation, *13:*92, 1956.
64. Hart, J.R., and Whitacre, J.J.: Pencil-point needle in prevention of postspinal headache. J.A.M.A., *147:*657, 1951.
65. Janvrin, S.B., Davies, G., and Greenhalgh, R.M.: Postoperative deep vein thrombosis caused by intravenous fluids during surgery. Br. J. Surg., *67:*690, 1980.
66. Jones, W.H.: Spinal analgesia: A new method and a new drug. Br. J. Anaesth., *7:*99, 1930.
67. Kalso, E., Tuominen, M., and Rosenberg, P.H.: Effect of posture and some CSF characteristics on spinal anaesthesia with isobaric 0.5% bupivacaine. Br. J. Anaesth., *54:*1179, 1982.
68. Katz, J., Kavanagh, B.P., Sandler, A.N., *et al.*: Pre-emptive analgesia: Clinical evidence of neuroplasticity contributing to postoperative pain. Anesthesiology, *77:*439, 1992.
69. Kennedy, W.F. Jr., Everett, G.B., Cobb, L.A., and Allen, G.D.: Simultaneous systemic and hepatic hemodynamic measurements during high spinal anesthesia in normal man. Anesth. Analg., *49:*1016, 1970.
70. Kety, S.S., King, B.D., Horvath, S.M., Jeffers, W.A., and Hafkenschiel, J.H.: The effects of acute reduction in blood pressure by means of differential spinal sympathetic block on the cerebral circulation of hypertensive patients. J. Clin. Invest., *29:*402, 1950.

71. Kleinerman, J., Sancetta, S.M., and Hackel, D.B.: Effects of high spinal anesthesia on cerebral circulation and metabolism in man. J. Clin. Invest., *37:*285, 1958.
72. Koller, C.: Uber Verwendung des Kokains zur Anasthesierung am Auge. Wien. Med. Wochenschr., *43:*46, 1884.
73. Koster, H.: Spinal analgesia with special reference to its use in surgery of the head, neck and thorax. Am. J. Surg., *5:*554, 1928.
74. Koster, H., Shapiro, A., and Leikensohn, A.: Spinal anesthesia: Procaine concentration changes at site of injection in subarachnoid anesthesia. Am. J. Surg., *33:*245, 1936.
75. Kozody, R., Palahniuk, R.J., Wade, J.G., and Cumming, M.O.: The effect of subarachnoid epinephrine and phenylephrine on spinal cord blood flow. Can. Anaesth. Soc. J., *31:*503, 1984.
76. Kreutz, J.M., and Mazuzan, J.E.: Sudden asystole in a marathon runner: The athletic heart syndrome and its anesthetic implications. Anesthesiology, *73:*1266, 1990.
77. Labat, G.: Regional Anesthesia: Its Technique and Clinical Application. Philadelphia, W.B. Saunders, 1922.
78. Lang, E., Krainick, J.U., and Gerbershagen, H.U.: Spinal cord transmission during high spinal anesthesia as measured by cortical evoked potentials. Anesth. Analg., *69:*15, 1989.
79. Lee, A., Ray, D., Littlewood, D.G., and Wildsmith, J.A.W.: Effect of dextrose concentration on the intrathecal spread of amethocaine. Br. J. Anaesth., *61:*135, 1988.
80. Lemmon, W.T.: A method of continuous spinal anaesthesia. Ann. Surg., *111:*140, 1940.
81. Levin, E., Muravchick, S., and Gold, M.I.: Isobaric tetracaine spinal anesthesia and the lithotomy position. Anesth. Analg., *60:*810, 1981.
82. Logan, M.R., and Drummond, G.B.: Spinal anesthesia and lumbar lordosis. Anesth. Analg., *67:*338, 1988.
83. Logan, M.R., McClure, J.H., and Wildsmith, J.A.W.: Plain bupivacaine: An unpredictable spinal anesthetic agent. Br. J. Anaesth., *58:*292, 1986.
84. Lund, P.C.: Principles and Practice of Spinal Anesthesia. Springfield, IL, Charles C. Thomas, 1971.
85. Lynn, R.B., Sancetta, S.M., Simeone, F.A., and Scott, R.W.: Observations on the circulation during high spinal anesthesia. Surgery, *32:*195, 1952.
86. Mackey, D.C., Carpenter, R.L., Thompson, G.E., Brown, D.L., and Bodily, M.N.: Bradycardia and asystole during spinal anesthesia: A report of three cases without morbidity. Anesthesiology, *70:*866, 1989.
87. Manchanda, V.N., Murad, S.H., Shilyansky, G., and Mehringer, M.: Unusual clinical course of accidental subdural local anesthetic injection. Anesth. Analg., *62:*1124, 1983.
88. Matas, R.: Report of successful spinal anesthesia. Medical News. J.A.M.A., *33:*1659, 1899.
89. McClure, J.H., Brown, D.T., and Wildsmith, J.A.W.: Effect of injected volume and speed of injection on the spread of spinal anaesthesia with isobaric amethocaine. Br. J. Anaesth., *54:*917, 1982.
90. Mehta, M., and Maher, R.: Injection into the extra-arachnoid subdural space. Anaesthesia, *32:*760, 1977.
91. Mitchell, R.W.D., Bowler, G.M.R., Scott, D.B., and Edström, H.H.: Effects of posture and baricity on spinal anaesthesia with 0.5% bupivacaine 5 ml. Br. J. Anaesth., *61:*139, 1988.
92. Moller, I.W., Fernandes, A., and Edstrom, H.H.: Subarachnoid anaesthesia with 0.5% bupivacaine: effects of density. Br. J. Anaesth., *56:*1191, 1984.
93. Moore, D.C.: Complications of Regional Anesthesia. Springfield, IL, Charles C. Thomas, 1955.
94. Moore, D.C.: Spinal anesthesia: Bupivacaine compared with tetracaine. Anesth. Analg., *59:*743, 1980.
95. Moore, R.A., Bullingham, R.E.S., McQuay, H.J., et al.: Dural permeability to narcotics: *In vitro* determination and application to extradural administration. Br. J. Anaesth., *54:*1117, 1982.
96. Morton, A.W.: The subarachnoid injection of cocaine for operations on the upper part of the body. J.A.M.A., *39:*1162, 1902.
97. Mueller, R.P., Lynn, R.B., and Sancetta, S.M.: Studies of hemodynamic changes in humans following induction of low and high spinal anesthesia. II. The changes in splanchnic blood flow, oxygen extraction and consumption and splanchnic vascular resistance in humans not undergoing surgery. Circulation, *6:*894, 1952.
98. Mukkada, T.A., Bridenbaugh, P.O., Singh, P, and Edstrom, H.H.: Effects of dose, volume and concentration of glucose-free bupivacaine in spinal anesthesia. Reg. Anesth., *11:*98, 1986.
99. Neigh, J.L., Kane, P.B., and Smith, T.C.: Effects of speed and direction of injection on the level and duration of spinal anesthesia. Anesth. Analg., *49:*912, 1970.
100. Nightingale, P.J.: Barbotage and spinal anaesthesia. Anaesthesia, *38:*7, 1983.
101. Norris, M.C.: Height, weight, and the spread of subarachnoid hyperbaric bupivacaine in the term parturient. Anesth. Analg., *67:*555, 1988.
102. Norris, M.C.: Patient variables and the subarachnoid spread of hyperbaric bupivacaine in the term parturient. Anesthesiology, *72:*478, 1990.
103. O'Rourke, G.W., and Greene, N.M.: Autonomic blockade and the resting heart rate in man. Am. Heart J., *80:*469, 1970.
104. Park, W.Y., Balingot, P.E., and McNamara, T.E.: Effects of patient age, pH of cerebrospinal fluid and vasopressor on onset and duration of spinal anesthesia. Anesth. Analg., *54:*455, 1975.
105. Pearson, A.: A rare complication of extradural analgesia. Anaesthesia, *39:*460, 1984.
106. Peng, A.T., Behar, S., and Blancato, L.S.: Reduction of postlumbar puncture backache by the use of field block anesthesia prior to lumbar puncture. Anesthesiology, *63:*227, 1985.
107. Pitkanen, M., Haapaniemi, L., Tuominen, M., and Rosenberg, P.H.: Influence of age on spinal anaesthesia with isobaric 0.5% bupivacaine. Br. J. Anaesth., *56:*279, 1984.
108. Pitkin, G.P.: Controllable spinal anesthesia. Am. J. Surg., *5:*537, 1928.
109. Porter, S.S., Albin, M.S., Watson, W.A., Bunogin, L., and Pantoja, G.: Spinal cord and cerebral blood flow responses to subarachnoid injection of local anesthetics with and without epinephrine. Acta Anaesthesiol. Scand., *29:*330, 1985.
110. Prickett, M.D., Gross, E.G., and Cullen, S.C.: Spinal anesthesia with solutions of procaine and epinephrine: preliminary report of 108 cases. Anesthesiology, *6:*469, 1945.
111. Ravindran, R.S., Viegas, O.J., Pantazis, K.L., and Baldwin, S.J.: Serum lidocaine levels following spinal anesthesia with lidocaine and epinephrine in dogs. Reg. Anesth., *8:*6, 1983.
112. Runciman, W.B., Mather, L.E., Ilsley, A.H., Carapetis, R.J., and Upton, R.N.: A sheep preparation for studying interactions between blood flow and drug disposition. III: Effects of general and spinal anaesthesia on regional blood flow and oxygen tensions. Br. J. Anaesth., *56:*1247, 1984.
113. Schmidt, K.A., and Snyder, S.A.: Effect of horizontal lithotripsy position on hyperbaric tetracaine spinal anesthesia. Anesth. Analg., *67:*894, 1988.
114. Shantha, T.R., and Evans, J.A.: The relationship of epidural anesthesia to neural membranes and arachnoid villi. Anesthesiology, *37:*543, 1972.
115. Sheskey, M.C., Rocco, A.G., Bizzarri-Schmid, M., *et al.*: A dose-response study of bupivacaine for spinal anesthesia. Anesth. Analg., *62:*931, 1983.
116. Shir, Y., Raja, S.N., and Frank, S.M.: The effect of epidural vs. general anesthesia on postoperative pain and analgesia requirements in patients undergoing radical prostatectomy. Anesthesiology, *80:*49, 1994.
117. Sidi, A., Pollak, D., Floman, Y., and Davidson, J.T.: Hypobaric spinal anesthesia in the operative management of orthopedic emergencies in geriatric patients. Isr. J. Med. Sci., *20:*589, 1984.
118. Sise, L.F.: Pontocaine-glucose solution for spinal anesthesia. Surg. Clin. North Am., *124:*1501, 1935.
119. Sivarajan, M., Amory, D.W., Lindbloom, L.E., and Schwettman, R.S.: Systemic and regional blood-flow changes during spinal anesthesia in the Rhesus monkey. Anesthesiology, *43:*78, 1975.
120. Smith, T.C.: The lumbar spinal and subarachnoid block. Anesthesiology, *29:*60, 1968.
121. Spivey, D.L.: Epinephrine does not prolong lidocaine spinal anesthesia in term parturients. Anesth. Analg., *64:*468, 1985.
122. Steinstra, R., and Greene, N.M.: Factors affecting the subarachnoid spread of local anesthetic solutions. Reg. Anesth., *16:*1, 1991.
123. Stienstra, R., and Van Poorten, J.F.: Plain or hyperbaric bupivacaine for spinal anesthesia. Anesth. Analg., *66:*171, 1987.
124. Stienstra, R., van Poorten, F., and Kroon, J.W.: Needle direction affects the sensory level of spinal anesthesia. Anesth. Analg., *68:*497, 1989.
125. Stevens, R.A., Beardsley, D., White, L., *et al.*: Does spinal anesthesia result in more complete sympathetic block than that from epidural anesthesia? Anesthesiology, *82:*877, 1995.

126. Tait, D., and Caglieri, G.: Experimental and clinical notes on the subarachnoid space. Trans. Med. Soc. Calif., *30:*266, 1900.
127. Tarrow, A.B.: Solution to spinal headaches. Int. Anesthesiol. Clin., *1:*877, 1963.
128. Taylor, J.A.: Lumbosacral subarachnoid tap. J. Urol., *43:*561, 1940.
129. Tuffier, *et al.*: Analgesie chirurgicale per l'injection sous-arachnoidienne lombaire de cocaine. C.R. Soc. Bull. (Paris), *51:*882, 1899.
130. Tuohy, E.B.: Continuous spinal anesthesia: Its usefulness and technic involved. Anesthesiology, *5:*142, 1944.
131. Tuominen, M., Kalso, E., and Rosenberg, P.H.: The effects of posture in the spread of spinal anaesthesia with isobaric 0.75% or 0.5% bupivacaine. Br. J. Anaesth., *54:*313, 1982.
132. Tverskoy, M., Cozacov, C., Ayache, M., Bradley, E.L., and Kissin, I.: Postoperative pain after inguinal herniorrhaphy with different types of anesthesia. Anesth. Analg., *70:*29, 1990.
133. Van Zundert, A.A., and De Wolf, A.M.: Extent of anesthesia and hemodynamic effects of subarachnoid administration of bupivacaine with epinephrine. Anesth. Analg., *67:*784, 1988.
134. Veering, B.T., Burm, A.G.L., Van Kleef, J.W., *et al.*: Spinal anesthesia with glucose-free bupivacaine: effects of age on neural blockade and pharmacokinetics. Anesth. Analg., *66:*965, 1987.
135. Venn, P.J.H., Simpson, D.A., Rubin, A.P., and Edstrom, H.H.: Effect of fluid preloading on cardiovascular variables after spinal anaesthesia with glucose-free 0.75% bupivacaine. Br. J. Anaesth., *63:*682, 1989.
136. Walts, L.F., Koepke, T., and Margules, R.: Determination of sensory and motor levels after spinal anesthesia with tetracaine. Anesthesiology, *25:*634, 1964.
137. Ward, R.J., Bonica, J.J., Freud, F.G., and Akamatsu, T.: Epidural and subarachnoid anesthesia: Cardiovascular and respiratory effects. J.A.M.A., *191:*275, 1965.
138. Wildsmith, J.A.W., McClure, J.H., Brown, D.T., and Scott, D.B.: Effects of posture on the spread of isobaric and hyperbaric amethocaine. Br. J. Anaesth., *53:*273, 1981.

Neural Blockade in Clinical Anesthesia and Management of Pain, Third Edition,
edited by M.J. Cousins and P.O. Bridenbaugh.
Lippincott–Raven Publishers, Philadelphia © 1998.

CHAPTER 8

Epidural Neural Blockade

Michael J. Cousins and Bernadette T. Veering

Although techniques of epidural anesthesia do not offer the economy of drug dosage or degrees of blockade of spinal anesthesia, they are currently more versatile and better studied. No other neural blockade techniques are used as extensively in each of the fields of surgical anesthesia, obstetric anesthesia, and diagnosis and management of acute and chronic pain. Epidural blockade is also unique because of special features of the anatomic site of injection and the resultant diverse sites of action of the local anesthetic solution (see following).

The most practical and widely used continuous method of neural blockade is spinal epidural blockade; pharmacokinetic data have helped to increase the efficacy and safety of epidural infusion techniques (see Chapter 26). Continuous caudal blockade has useful but limited applications, and continuous spinal anesthesia is beginning to be used more frequently (see Chapter 7). As indicated in Chapters 24 and 29, new developments in the understanding of pain conduction have extended the use of continuous epidural blockade to the administration of drugs that selectively block pain conduction, while leaving sensation, motor power, and sympathetic function essentially unchanged. The safety and the reliability of spinal epidural catheter techniques, with the addition of bacterial filters, have permitted relief of acute pain (see Chapters 18 and 26) and chronic pain (see Chapters 27 to 29) for many days, often with patients remaining ambulatory. This has heralded an even more vigorous and fruitful era of investigation and clinical application of epidural blockade than did the unprecedented development of the past 20 years.

APPLIED ANATOMY OF EPIDURAL BLOCKADE

The reader should review the description of the anatomy of bony spine, ligaments, meninges, cerebrospinal fluid (CSF), and spinal arteries in Chapter 7, since this is directly applicable to epidural blockade.

The epidural space is not as voluminous as the subarachnoid space. Nevertheless, it extends from the base of the skull to the sacrococcygeal membrane and has complicated direct communications with the paravertebral space and indirect communications with the CSF. It also leads directly to the vascular system by way of its large epidural veins, which have no valves and connect with the basivertebral venous plexus, intracranial veins, and the azygos vein (see Fig. 8-15); this is a potential direct route to the brain and heart for drugs, air, or other material inadvertently injected into an epidural vein. Within the cranium, there is no epidural space, as the meningeal dura and endosteal dura are closely adherent, except where they separate to form the venous sinuses. At the foramen magnum, these two layers separate: the former becomes the spinal dura, and the latter becomes the periosteum of the spinal canal (Figs. 8-1 to 8-3). Thus, although local anesthetics cannot enter between the endosteal and meningeal layer of the cerebral dura, they can diffuse across the spinal dura at the base of the brain into the CSF and, thence, to the brain (Fig. 8-3). Between the spinal dura and the spinal periosteum lies the epidural space. The ligamentum flavum completes the posterior wall in direct continuity with the periosteum of the spinal canal (Figs. 8-1, 8-4 to 8-6). Because the spinal canal is approximately triangular in cross section and the articular processes indent the triangle (Fig. 8-4), the epidural space narrows posterolaterally and then widens again laterally toward the intervertebral foramina (Fig. 8-5). Thus, the safest point of entry into the epidural space is in the midline.

The Posterior Epidural Space

During recent years new techniques have been used to investigate the anatomy of the epidural space, in particular the lumbar region. These developments include endoscopic examination, computed tomography, magnetic resonance and cryomicrotome section.[31,32,190,193,334,407]

M. J. Cousins: Department of Anaesthesia and Pain Management, Royal North Shore Hospital, University of Sydney, St. Leonards, New South Wales 2065 Australia.

B. T. Veering: Department of Anesthesiology, University Hospital Leiden, 2300 RC Leiden, The Netherlands.

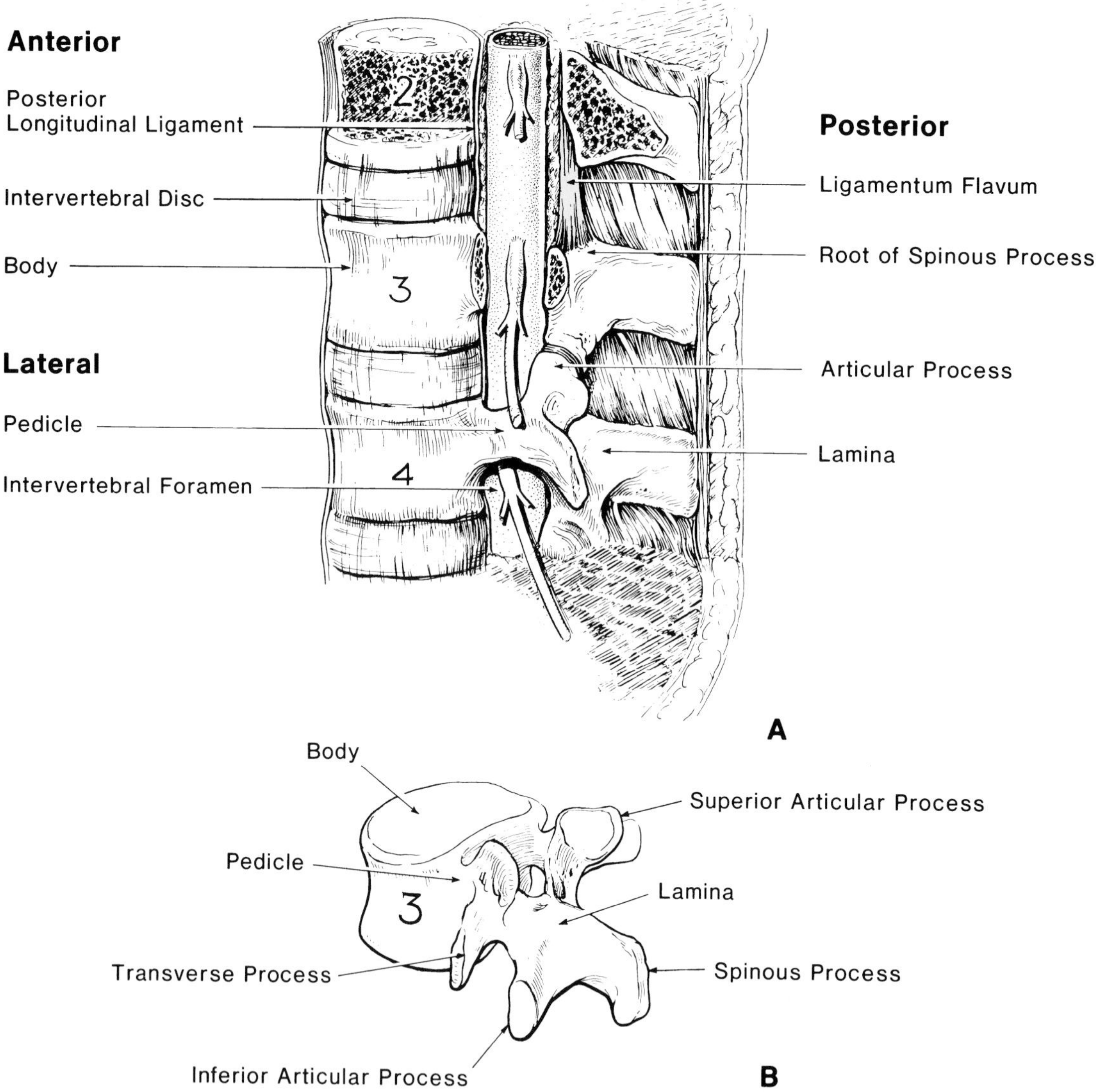

FIG. 8-1. A: Boundaries of the epidural space. Note the superior portion of ligamentum flavum, hidden from posterior view because of attachment to the anterior aspect of the lamina, and the inferior attachment of the ligamentum flavum to the posterior aspect of the lamina (see also Fig. 8-11). **B:** Lumbar vertebra. (Macintosh, R.R.: Lumbar Puncture and Spinal Analgesia. Edinburgh, E. & S. Livingstone, 1957.)

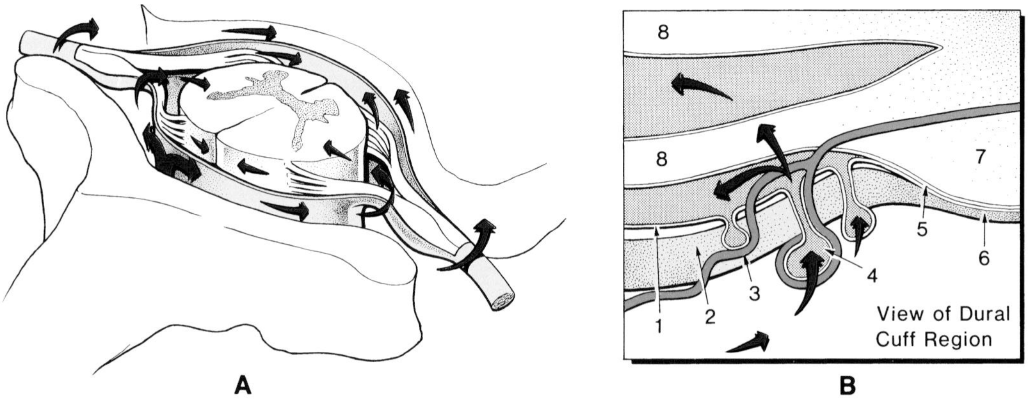

FIG. 8-2. A: Schematic representation of horizontal spread of local anesthetic in epidural space. Major spread posteriorly to the region of "dural cuff" (root sleeve) region is shown, with subsequent entry to cerebrospinal fluid (CSF) and spinal cord. Minor spread into anterior epidural space is also shown. **B:** Enlarged view of dural cuff region shows rapid entry of local anesthetic into CSF by way of arachnoid granulations: *1,* arachnoid membrane; *2,* dura; *3,* epidural vein; *4,* arachnoid "granulation" protruding through dura and contacting epidural vein; *5,* perineural epithelium of spinal nerve in continuity with arachnoid; *6,* epineurium of spinal nerve in continuity with dura; *7,* dorsal root ganglion; *8,* intradural spinal nerve roots. *Note:* This figure does not depict the anatomical shape of the epidural space, which is shown in Fig. 8-7.

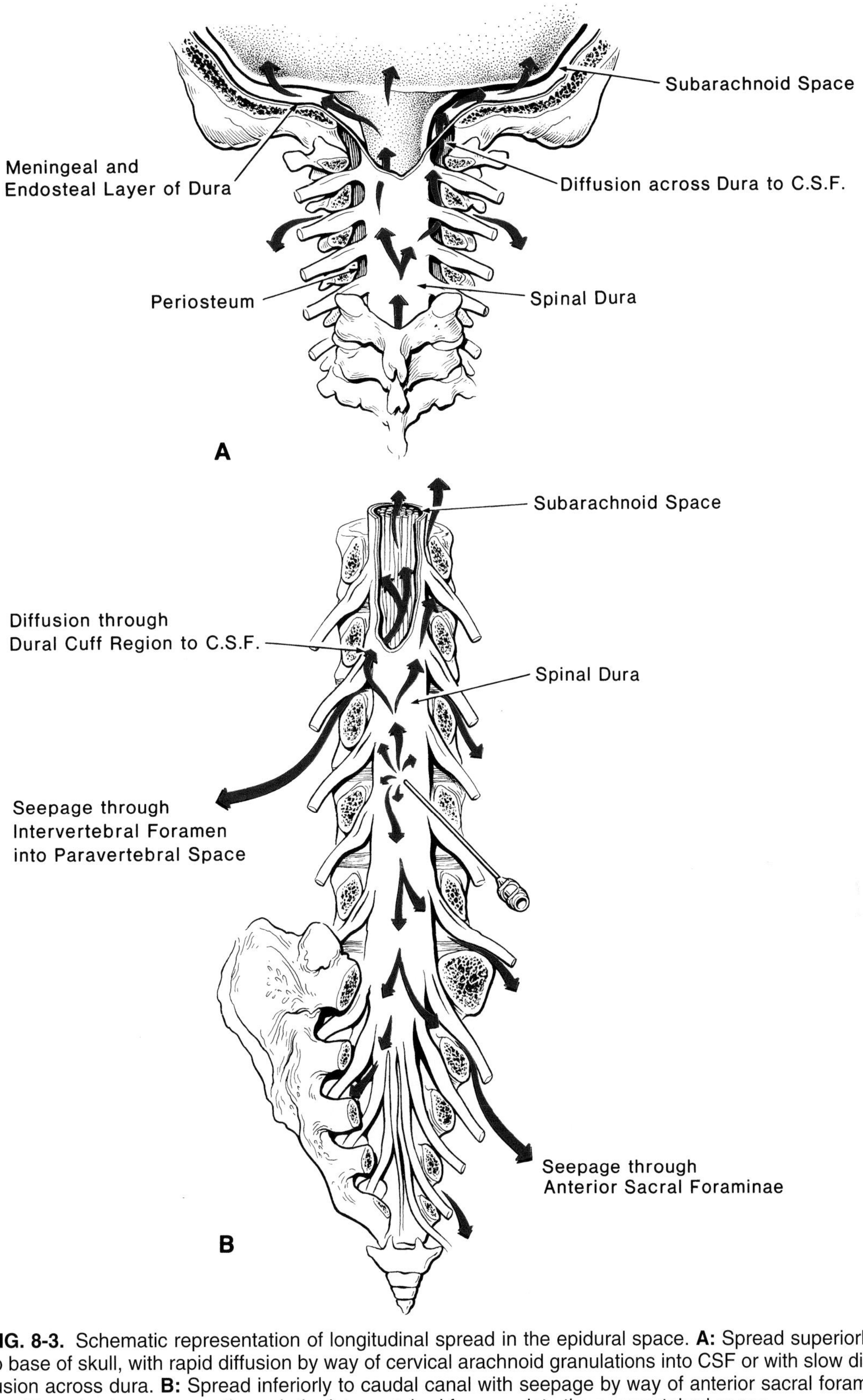

FIG. 8-3. Schematic representation of longitudinal spread in the epidural space. **A:** Spread superiorly to base of skull, with rapid diffusion by way of cervical arachnoid granulations into CSF or with slow diffusion across dura. **B:** Spread inferiorly to caudal canal with seepage by way of anterior sacral foramina. There is also seepage through the intervertebral foramen into the paravertebral space.

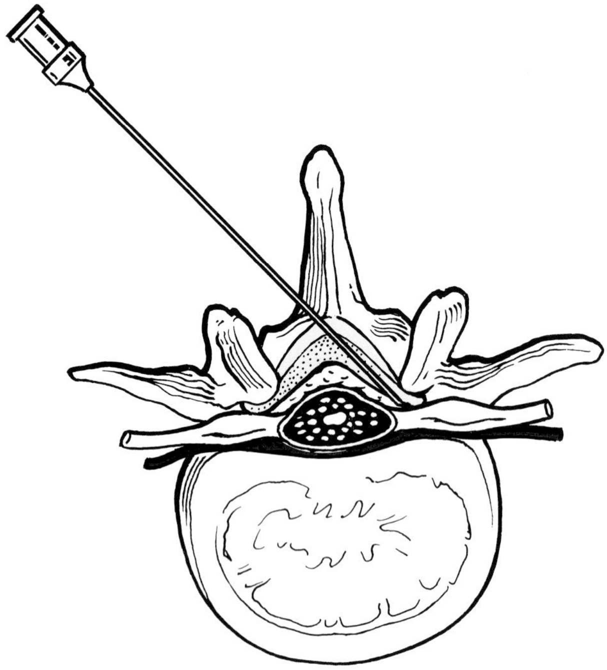

FIG. 8-4. Ligamentum flavum, cross-sectional view. The triangular shape of each half of the ligament is apparent. They narrow toward the articular processes, as does the underlying epidural space. Also, incorrect extreme lateral angulation of a needle is shown. Oblique penetration of the ligamentum flavum results, with continued resistance for several millimeters and eventual loss of resistance in the dural cuff region, where there are two main hazards: The epidural space is very narrow and the dura is thin (see also Fig. 8-2); the needle is close to spinal nerve and vessels. (Macintosh, R.R.: Lumbar Puncture and Spinal Analgesia. Edinburgh, E. & S. Livingstone, 1957.)

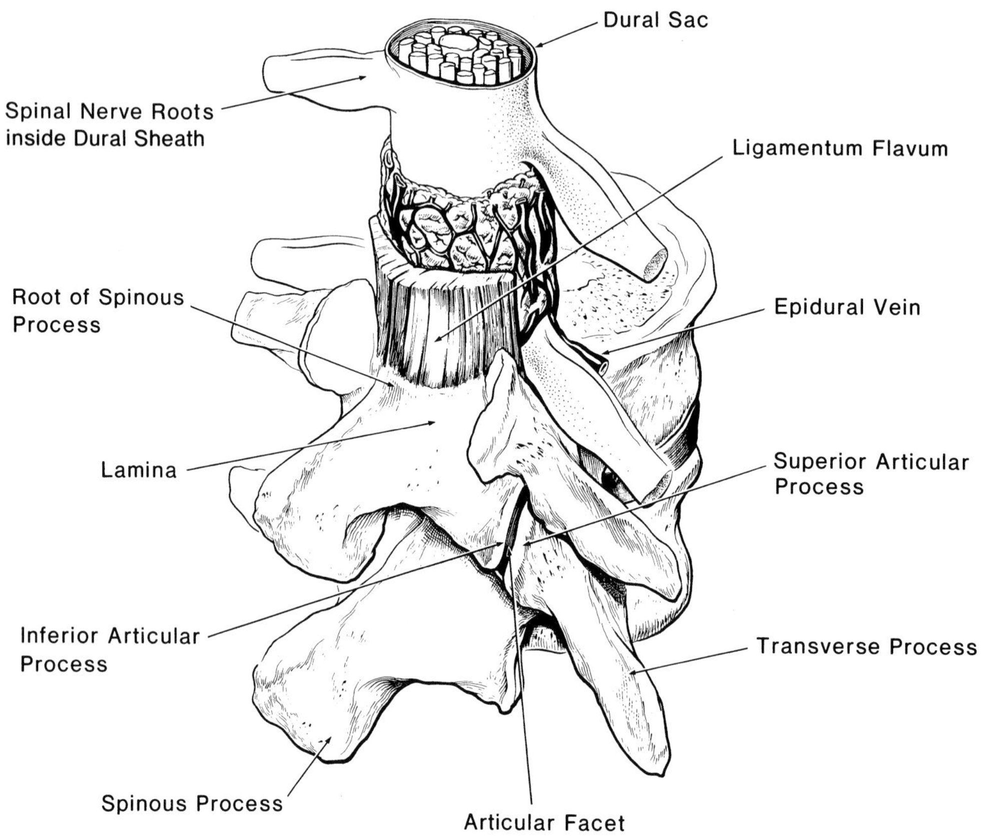

FIG. 8-5. Epidural space, relationships from the posterior view. Note the increased prevalence of epidural veins lateral to the midline; narrowing of the ligamentum flavum and epidural space laterally; slight downward slope of spinous processes; proximity of articular facets at lateral aspect of lamina (see also Fig. 8-12B). (Macintosh, R.R.: Lumbar Puncture and Spinal Analgesia. Edinburgh, E. & S. Livingstone, 1957.)

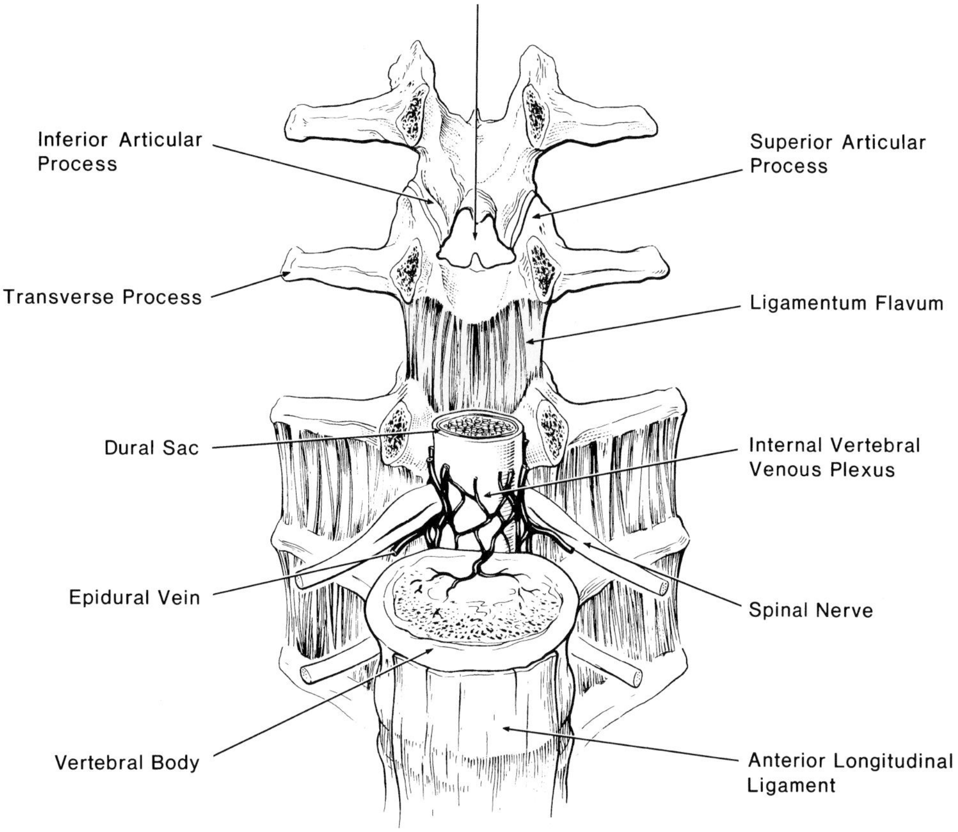

FIG. 8-6. Epidural space, relationships from anterior view. Note "interlaminar space" at one level and covered by ligamentum flavum at the level below. Epidural veins are in continuity with veins draining vertebral body ("internal vertebral venous plexus"). (Macintosh, R.R.: Lumbar Puncture and Spinal Analgesia. Edinburgh, E. & S. Livingstone, 1957.)

Cryomicrotome sectioning of cadavers, in which the spine is frozen *in situ*, allows examination of the epidural anatomy less distorted by artefact.[193] Using this technique, segmentally distributed compartments in the epidural space were observed posteriorly, laterally, and anteriorly, being partly occupied with nerves, fat, and fibrous tissue. Fat appeared to be the principal epidural tissue. Basically posterior and lateral compartments were found to be discontinuous circumferentially, with a repeated metameric segmentation of the epidural contents in the longitudinal axis (Fig. 8-7). Posterior compartments were formed between the middle of one lamina and the cranial edge of the next lower lamina, limited dorsally by the flaval ligaments. These posterior compartments were separated by areas where the dura is attached directly to the cranial part of the vertebral lamina and the vertebral arches. The contents of the posterior epidural compartment are separated from the lateral contents by an intervening area where the dura is against the lamina with no tissue between. In normal conditions the respective subcompartments usually show a mutually free communication as can be demonstrated on epidurograms (canalograms).[247] In-

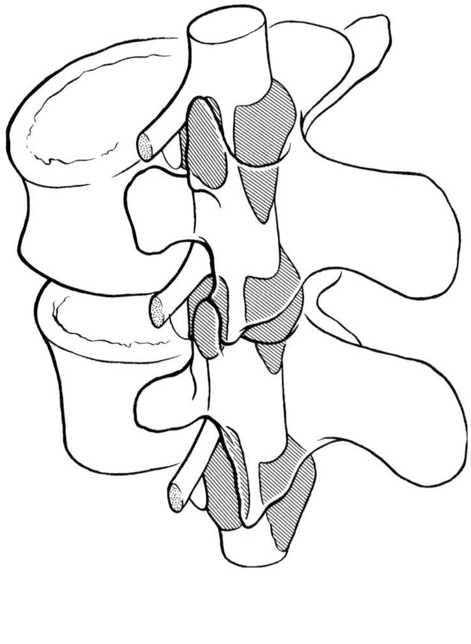

FIG. 8-7. A drawing of the compartments of the epidural space (stippled) as seen in cryomicrotomy. The epidural contents are discontinuous circumferentially and repeat metamerically. Where no contents are represented, the dura is in contact with the spinal canal wall. The pedicles are concealed behind the transverse processes. (Hogan, G.H.: Lumbar epidural anatomy. A new look by cryomicrotome section. Anesthesiology, *75*:767, 1991).

jected solutions can pass from compartment to compartment, since the dura is not adherent to the canal wall. The compartmentization of the epidural space is supported by observations using computed tomographic and magnetic resonance imaging.[190,334,407] Various studies have demonstrated a fold in the posterior dura along the midline.[31,32,246] This fold has been termed the *plica mediana dorsalis* and is formed as the dura is prevented from collapsing by fibrous strands going from the ligamentum flavum to the medial portion of the dura (Fig. 8-8). This is the matter that is demonstrated when a considerable quantity of air or fluid is injected in the lumbosacral epidural space, compressing the dural sac and distorting the anatomy. During epiduroscopy Blomberg (1986) observed in cadavers a dorsomedian connective tissue band between the dura and the flaval ligaments, which fixed the dura and caused a dorsomedian fold.[31] However, conclusions derived from examination of cadavers should be applied with care to the situation of clinical epidural anesthesia. The pressure of the cerebrospinal space in cadavers is low or completely equalized with atmospheric pressure, causing the dura to collapse. The observed dorsomedian fold is thereby accentuated. In living humans a dorsomedian connective tissue band causing a dorsomedian fold of the dura mater was also seen by epiduroscopy, but not as prominent as that seen in cadavers.[32] In this study, the epidural space was found to be present as a potential space, which opened up only temporarily as small increments of air were injected. A distinction should be made, however, between the substantial fold of the dura mater itself and the dorsomedian ligamentous strands connecting the lumbar sac to the ventral side of the vertebrae.[204]

The clinical relevance of the dorsomedian connective tissue band connected to the dura mater has been related to the possibility of developing unilateral epidural blockade.[260] Probably it is not the dorsomedian tissue band that causes problems but the technique used. Most likely other factors, such as the position of the catheter and injection of small volumes of local anesthetic solution, are more frequently responsible for the development of an unilateral block. This subject will be covered in the section: problems in epidural block.

Surface Anatomy

The key anatomy for safe placement of a needle in the epidural space is summarized in Tables 8-1 to 8-3. However, before considering deep structures, the anesthesiologist should be certain of the level and direction of insertion of the needle; thus, surface anatomy is important. Because the easiest and safest point of entry into the epidural space is in the midlumbar region, a reliable surface marking for this level is important: The line drawn between the highest point of the

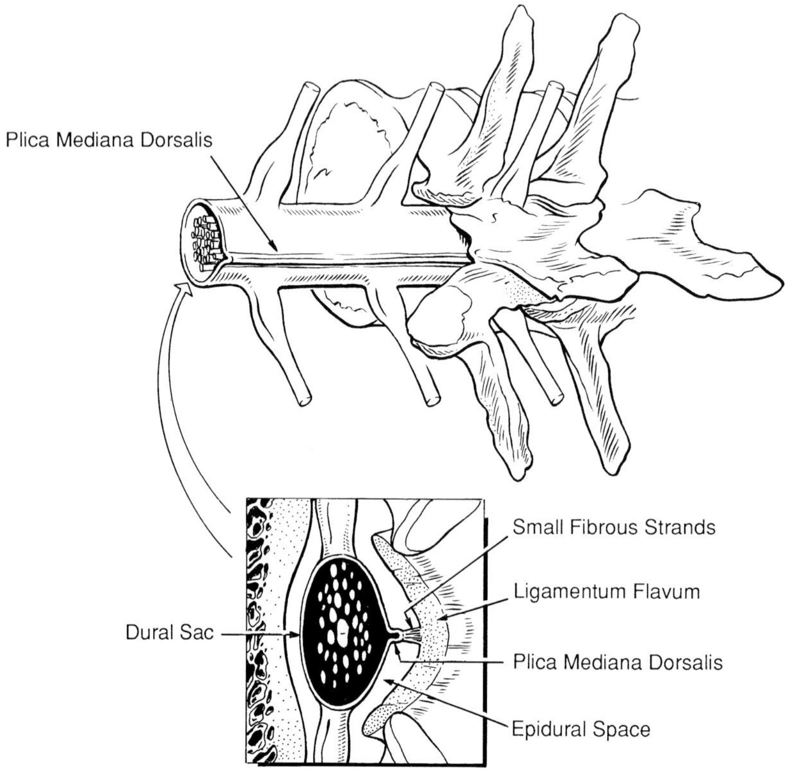

FIG. 8-8. The dural sac after removal of an arch of a vertebra. The dorsal plica mediana is seen as a dural fold. Enlarged view shows median fibrous strands going from the ligamentum flavum to the median portion of the dura. Consequently these strands will give rise to a dorsomedian fold of the dura mater, i.e., the plica mediana dorsalis.

TABLE 8-1. *Key anatomic features for administration of lumbar epidural anesthesia*

Spine and ligaments	Relationships of epidural space
Spinous process – Widest in midlumbar region – Only slight downward angulation (see Fig. 8-1) – Inferior border opposite widest point of interlaminar space (see Fig. 8-14B) – Superior border over upward-sloping lamina (see Fig. 8-14B) – Narrower superiorly. Needle inserted beside spinous process guided into midline by lateral aspect of spinous process (see Fig. 8-30A) Interspinous ligament – Well defined above L4. Below L4 narrower and loose—may offer less resistance Lamina – Posterior surface slopes down and back – Needle may strike lamina superficially at inferior aspect of slope or deep at superior aspect of slope (see Fig. 8-5) Interlaminar space – Increased by flexing lumbar spine – Larger "target" area in midline and in midlumbar region – Smaller target laterally (see Fig. 8-14B) Articular facets – Needle directed past lateral aspect of interlaminar space may impinge on articular facets, causing severe radiating pain and muscle spasm (see Fig. 8-14B) Ligamentum flavum – Thickest in midlumbar region in midline (see Fig. 8-10) – Attached to anteroinferior aspects of lamina above and posterosuperior aspects of lamina below; thus, needle entering at inferior aspect may be held up by lamina (see Fig. 8-11)	Epidural space – Widest in midlumbar region in midline (5–6 mm), narrower next to articular processes where ligamentum flavum and dura almost touch (see Fig. 8-4) – Widens laterally where spinal nerve surrounded by dural cuff (see Fig. 8-2A) – Communicates with paravertebral space by way of intervertebral foramen (see Fig. 8-1); therefore, epidural catheter may stimulate spinal nerve—unisegmental paresthesia Spinal nerve – Needle inserted past depth of lamina with lateral angulation on *same* side may penetrate past spinous process to spinal nerve (Fig. 8-5) – Needle angled across midline to *opposite* side may run in substance of ligamentum flavum laterally to reach spinal nerve and/or dural cuff (see Fig. 8-4) Arterial supply of spinal cord (see Figs. 7-10 and 7-11) – Only one anterior spinal artery – In thoracolumbar region fed mainly by "radicularis magna," which usually enters by way of an intervertebral foramen on left side at T11–T12 (may be at other interspaces T8–L3) – Supply to anterior thoracolumbar cord is discontinuous with higher levels – Sharp demarcation between anterior and posterior spinal artery territory Epidural veins – Prominent in lateral portion of epidural space (see Fig. 8-5) – Drain to azygos vein and connect to pelvic veins, providing an alternative route from pelvis to right heart. Therefore, they become distended when inferior vena cava is obstructed (see Fig. 8-15) – Also connect to cerebral venous sinuses by way of basivertebral veins (see Fig. 29-13)

TABLE 8-2. *Key anatomic features for administration of midthoracic epidural anesthesia*

- Spinous process
  - Extreme downward slope, inferior border opposite midpoint of lamina below
  - Small posterior surface, processes close together and difficult to identify
  - Therefore, the paraspinous (paramedian) technique is easier (see Fig. 8-30B)
- Interspinous ligament
  - Difficult to identify because spinous processes close to one another
- Lamina
  - Broader than lumbar laminae, but shorter in vertical dimension
  - Large area available for location of depth of ligamentum flavum with less fear of accidental puncture of dura
- Ligamentum flavum
  - Thick but less so than midlumbar
- Epidural space
  - In midline 3–5 mm, narrow laterally

TABLE 8-3. *Key anatomic features for administration of cervicothoracic epidural anesthesia*

- Spinous process
  - At C7 (vertebra prominens) and T1, direction is almost horizontal
  - Inferior border C7 opposite widest point of C7–T1 interlaminar space
- Lamina
  - Shaped like narrow rectangle
- Interlaminar space
  - Accessible with midline puncture if neck flexed
- Ligamentum flavum
  - Thinner than at any other level
- Epidural space
  - Width at first thoracic interspace is 3 to 4 mm (note width at C3–C6 is 2 mm)
  - Increased width if neck flexed
  - Usually marked negative pressure (increased if sitting)

two iliac crests usually passes through the spinous process of the fourth lumbar vertebra (Fig. 8-9). The interspinous space above this spinous process (L3–L4) or one higher (L2–L3) is the standard site of needle insertion for epidural block in adults, since the spinal cord usually ends at the lower border of vertebra L1. As noted in Chapter 20, this is not the case in children and is one reason why the caudal route of entry is preferred to the lumbar route in young children. Also, the dural sac terminates at the level of S2 in adults (S3 in small children): A line through the posterior superior iliac spines crosses this level. As noted in Table 8-1, puncture below L4 increases the difficulty of "midline" epidural block because of the ill-defined interspinous ligament; also, puncture above L2 increases the risk of damage to the conus medullaris, so that the interspaces of L2–L3 and L3–L4 are both the safest and the easiest; identification of L4 reassures that an easy entry may be achieved. Identification of L1 acts as a double check and confirms that the point of entry is safely below the conus medullaris. There is no difference in the potential danger of damaging the cord if one chooses the T12–L1 interspace or the C7–T1 interspace, both of which can often be technically easy; however, the spinal cord lies directly beneath the epidural space in both instances. Thus, only anesthesiologists experienced with epidural techniques require the anatomic landmarks above L1: the inferior angle of scapula (T7), the root of the spine of the scapula (T3), and the vertebra prominens (C7).

Because of the extreme angulation of the spinous pro-

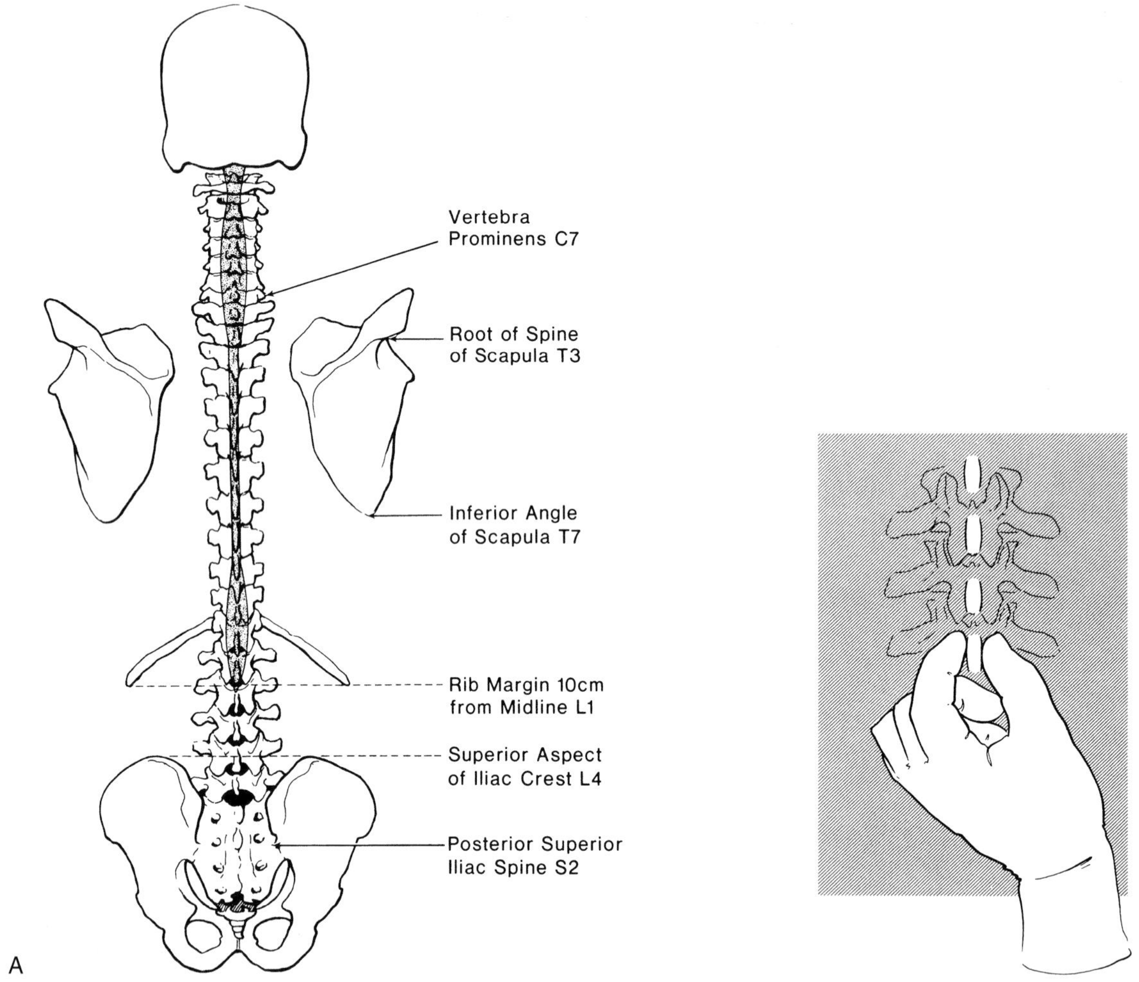

FIG. 8-9. A: Surface anatomy and landmarks for epidural blockade. The spinous process (vertebra prominens) at C7 is the most prominent spinous process when the neck is flexed. The spinous process at T3 lies opposite the root of the spine of the scapula (arm by side). The spinous process at T7 lies opposite the inferior angle of the scapula (arm by side). For puncture between C7 and T1 there is direct access to the interlaminal space, but there are other hazards (see text). Puncture below T3 and above T7 is difficult because of angled spinous processes. Puncture below T7 becomes progressively similar to L2–L3. Other hazards are the same as those for high puncture (see text). The spinous process at L1 (*lower border*) is noted by a line meeting the costal margin 10 cm from the midline. The spinous process at L4 (*center*) lies at the top of the iliac crests. S2 is noted by the posterior superior iliac spines. Puncture is safest and easiest in the lumbar region. L2–L3 and L3–4 are the preferred levels. **B: Method of checking midline**. Labat's method of checking center of spinous processes uses the thumb and forefinger to grasp the spinous processes above and below the site of the needle puncture.

TABLE 8-4. *Key levels of dermatomal blockade*

Cutaneous landmark	Segmental level	Significance
Little finger	C8	All cardioaccelerator fibers (T1–T4) blocked
Inner aspect of arm and forearm	T1 and T2	Some degree of cardio-accelerator blockade
Apex of axilla	T3	Easily remembered landmark
Nipple line (midway sternal notch and xiphisternum)	T4–T5	Possibility of cardioaccelerator blockade
Tip of xiphoid	T7	Splanchnics (T5–L1) may become blocked
Umbilicus	T10	Sympathetic blockade limited to lower limbs
Inguinal ligament	T12	
Outer side of foot	S1	No lumbar sympathetic blockade Most difficult nerve root to block

cesses in the midthoracic region, midline puncture is difficult, and the paraspinous (paramedian) approach is preferable. In contrast, there is excellent access to the interlaminar space in the midline at C7–T1 and T1–T2; the same applies in the low thoracic region. However, it should be noted that anatomic differences, such as a narrower epidural space (Tables 8-2 and 8-3), require greater technical skill at these levels and a technique somewhat different from that usually used for lumbar epidural block.

In the lumbar region, correct needle insertion takes full advantage of the fact that it is both easier and safer to insert the needle at the L2–L3 or L3–L4 interspace, with the needle entering the epidural space in the midline. The latter does not necessarily imply that the needle must start in the midline, although in most cases that is an easy approach. As shown in Figures 8-1 and 8-14B, the inferior aspects of the spinous processes, in the midlumbar region, lie opposite the line across the widest lateral extent of the interlaminar space. Thus, needle insertion should be close to the superior spinous process, since the upper border of the inferior spine lies over the lamina of its underlying vertebral body. A needle inserted with due regard to this requires very slight upward angulation to give an unobstructed approach to the interlaminar space (see Fig. 8-30). A surface anatomic aid that is often neglected involves checking that the needle is inserted in the center of a line running through the middle of the superior and inferior aspects of the spinous processes, that is, in the center of the supraspinous ligament. This is best achieved by grasping the spinous processes adjacent to the site of puncture between thumb and forefinger while the needle is inserted through skin and subcutaneous tissue into the supraspinous ligament (Fig. 8-9B). If this is done, the needle should sit firmly in the supraspinous ligament without angulation to one side. Obese subjects may require additional maneuvers (see section on Technique).

Segmental Levels

In assessing the level of epidural blockade, it is important for the anesthesiologist to have a method of using simple surface landmarks to indicate level of dermatomal blockade and thus segmental spinal nerve (and sympathetic blockade). Table 8-4 lists the key levels (see Fig. 8-35).

There is no point in testing for blockade of T1–T2 by testing above the nipple line, since this area has double innervation from T1–T2 and C3–C4, so that normal sensation remains even when T1–T2 are blocked. Thus, residual activity in the important cardiac sympathetics T1 and T2 is checked by testing skin sensation on the inside of the arm above the elbow (T2) and below the elbow (T1). Residual motor activity in T1 can also be checked by testing the ability of the patient to hold a sheet of paper between the outstretched fingers (interossei C8, T1). In a lightly anesthetized patient, spinal reflexes may be useful for testing level of blockade: epigastric (T7–T8); abdominal (T9, T12), cremasteric (L1, L2), plantar (S1, S2), knee-jerk (L2–L4), ankle-jerk (S1, S2).

Structures Encountered During Midline Insertion of Epidural Needle

If correct use of surface anatomy described above is observed and prior skin puncture is made with a larger needle (or scalpel blade), an epidural needle should encounter no resistance in the skin and subcutaneous tissue, but should then penetrate the tough supraspinous ligament (Figs. 8-10 and 8-11), which will support it at right angles to the skin in all di-

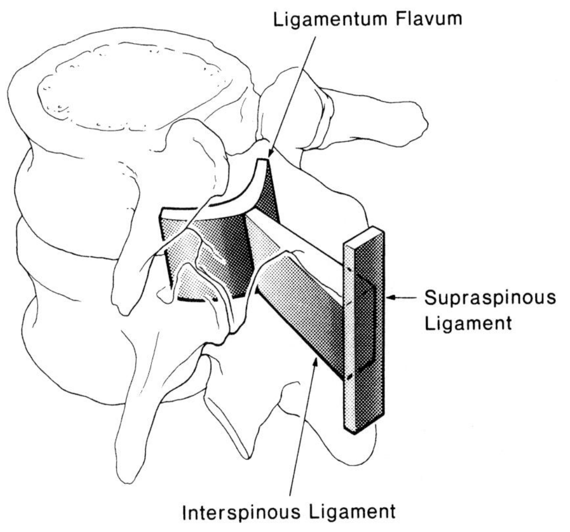

FIG. 8-10. Ligaments encountered during a midline puncture.

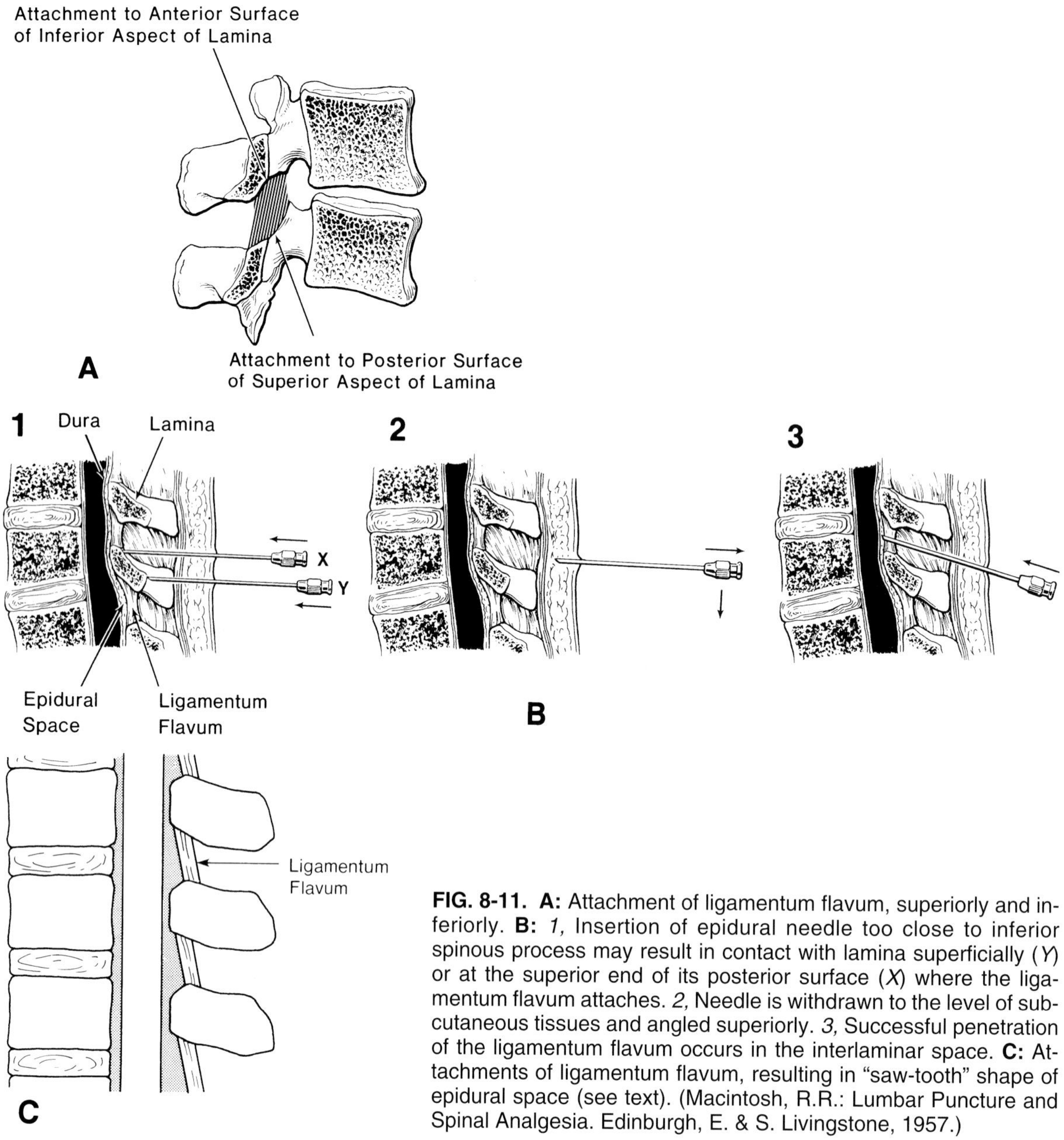

FIG. 8-11. **A:** Attachment of ligamentum flavum, superiorly and inferiorly. **B:** *1,* Insertion of epidural needle too close to inferior spinous process may result in contact with lamina superficially (*Y*) or at the superior end of its posterior surface (*X*) where the ligamentum flavum attaches. *2,* Needle is withdrawn to the level of subcutaneous tissues and angled superiorly. *3,* Successful penetration of the ligamentum flavum occurs in the interlaminar space. **C:** Attachments of ligamentum flavum, resulting in "saw-tooth" shape of epidural space (see text). (Macintosh, R.R.: Lumbar Puncture and Spinal Analgesia. Edinburgh, E. & S. Livingstone, 1957.)

rections. The interspinous ligament then offers continued resistance to advancing the needle. An increase in resistance to advancement of the needle signals that the needle tip has entered the thick, elastic ligamentum flavum; after only a few millimeters of advancement, a sudden loss of all resistance occurs as the needle tip enters the epidural space.

The distance of the epidural space from the skin varies widely. It is most commonly 4 cm (50%) and is 4 to 6 cm in 80% of the population according to detailed records of 3200 cases[176] and other recent studies.[296,322] In obese patients, however, this distance may be greater than 8 cm but is less than 3 cm in thin patients.

Incorrect procedure (Tables 8-5 and 8-6), or sometimes inadvertent aberrant needle placement owing to anatomic difficulties, may result in quite a different sequence of events than that described earlier and contact with different anatomic structures. Failure to clearly define the midline results in needle entry beside the supraspinous ligament. If the anesthesiologist persists with this unsatisfactory start, it is likely that the needle will next enter the interspinous ligament obliquely, resulting in only a transient resistance, followed by loss of resistance; or, it may miss the ligament completely, resulting immediately in a feeling of no resistance, in the paravertebral muscles. Both of these situations may be interpreted as rapid entry into the epidural space. However, injection of local anesthetic is followed by marked "drip back," and subsequent attempts to thread an epidural catheter will be met with considerable resistance. If the needle is inserted too close to the spinous process (or during any attempt at midline puncture in the midthoracic region), it is

TABLE 8-5. *Structures encountered during epidural block*

Structure	Comment
With Correct Procedure (Midline Technique)	
Skin	Prior puncture with 19-gauge needle should ensure no "drag" on epidural needle
Supraspinous ligament	Needle sits *firmly* in midline
Interspinous ligament	Clear-cut resistance to syringe plunger (above L4) ? Poorly defined resistance (below L4, or sometimes at other levels, ? choose another interspace)
Ligamentum flavum	Increase in resistance to syringe plunger, with marked "elastic" quality Increased resistance to advancing needle
Epidural space	*Controlled* and well-defined loss of resistance No resistance to injected solution No, or minimal, "drip back" of injected solution Catheter passes easily
Incorrect Procedure or Unintentional Misplacement of Needle	
Skin	Lack of prior puncture causes marked "drag" on epidural needle
Supraspinous ligament	Entered to one side, causes needle to angle laterally Missed completely, causes needle to flop to one side and appear to have no support
Interspinous ligament	Entered obliquely, results in transient resistance, then loss of resistance, which is interpreted as entrance to epidural space; however, there is marked run back of injected solution, and catheter will not thread Missed completely, results in low resistance—needle in paravertebral muscles
Spinous process	Very superficial contact: interspace not marked ?; spine flexed? (see Fig. 8-14B) Deep contact: needle angled much too acutely?
Lamina	Posterior end of slope: superficial obstruction to needle advancement Anterior end of slope: deep obstruction (see Fig. 8-11)
Articular processes	Sudden pain in back Muscle spasm on one side of back
Ligamentum flavum (LF)	
LF pierced midline but with poor control of entry	Needle "overshoots" through epidural space and punctures dura (see Table 8-6)
LF pierced to side of midline where dura close and veins prominent	Dural puncture ± CSF flow; or cannulation of epidural vein, +/− bleeding
Failure to identify LF with subsequent entry into subdural space	No CSF aspirated Some resistance to injected solution and "drip back," which is local anesthetic Catheter passes with difficulty Small dose of local anesthetic results in widespread block with bizarre distribution
Needle enters lateral aspect from opposite side and continues within ligament to region of spinal nerve (see Fig. 8-4)	Continued "elastic resistance" for several millimeters and then sudden unisegmental paresthesia May be followed by CSF flow if dural cuff entered
Epidural space	
Entry uncontrolled, needle against dura, no solution injected to expand epidural space	Catheter threads with difficulty or sudden loss of resistance—CSF in catheter
Entry to side of midline into epidural vein or CSF	Blood or CSF via needle or bleeding as catheter threaded—clot in catheter unless flushed with saline
Entry at extreme inferior aspect of ligamentum flavum at attachment to lamina of lower vertebra	Loss of resistance to syringe plunger but needle progress halted by upper edge of lamina and catheter will not thread
Entry at extreme superior aspect with only tip of needle piercing ligament	Loss of resistance to syringe plunger but some resistance to injected solution and catheter will not thread Further progress of needle easy
Entry at lateral aspect	Catheter may impinge on spinal nerve

CSF, cerebrospinal fluid

TABLE 8-6. *Suspected dural puncture*

Sign	Cause	Management
Second loss of resistance and fluid flows from needle	Dural puncture	Convert to spinal anesthetic or move to higher interspace for epidural
Second loss of resistance after identifying ligamentum flavum and no fluid flows from needle, but injected solution → some "drip back"	? Entry into subdural space ? Dural puncture	Test "drip back" on arm: Cold = L.A.; warm = CSF Drip into container[a] With glucose test tape: CSF → color change If drip back only L.A. withdraw needle and reidentify epidural space If drip back = CSF ± L.A., move to a rostrad[b] interspace or convert to spinal anesthetic
One loss of resistance only; however, "drip back" at: A shallow level	Interspinous ligament pierced and needle in paravertebral muscle	Reinsert needle in midline
A deeper level	Low compliance of epidural fat Needle only partially through ligamentum flavum Needle in CSF	Test as above, if drip back only L.A.: Attempt to pass catheter → easy passage Attempt to pass catheter → does not pass: Superiorly needle can be advanced and then catheter threaded Inferiorly needle will not advance Test for CSF, if positive move to rostrad interspace or convert to spinal

[a] Few drops of CSF in thiopental will form a precipitate; however local anesthetic will also form a precipitate with thiopental.[4]

[b] Do not attempt to withdraw needle into epidural space at the same level, as this may result in subdural cannulation.[365]

L.A., local anesthetic; CSF, cerebrospinal fluid.

not uncommon for the needle to contact the spinous process. Perhaps the most common obstruction to the needle is the lamina of the vertebral body. Because the posterior surface of the lamina slopes gently down and back from its anterior end to its posterior end (see Fig. 8-5), an epidural needle inserted too far laterally may encounter lamina either at a superficial depth or deeper, close to its junction with the ligamentum flavum (see Fig. 8-11). Even more extreme lateral insertion or lateral angulation of the needle may result in the needle point contacting the superior or inferior articular processes or the joint space (see Fig. 8-14B), where their articular facets meet. The latter can be particularly painful, since the articular facets have a rich nerve supply, and needle trauma may result in sudden severe localized pain on one side of the back with accompanying paravertebral muscle spasm on that side. This pain is not dissimilar to that caused by direct contact with a nerve root: "radicular pain." Both may result in pain that radiates into the leg. Radicular pain is usually more discreet with only one area involved (e.g. the inside of the knee for L3 or inside of the leg for L4). Facet pain may radiate but is somewhat more diffuse.

Ligamentum Flavum. The ligamentum flavum should be entered in the center of the interlaminar gap, regardless of where the needle enters the skin (midline or paraspinous). Even with midline puncture, failure to control the penetration of the ligament results in a second loss of resistance, signalling dural puncture. Entry at the lateral aspect of the interlaminar gap may also result in dural puncture, since the epidural space is narrow at this point (see Figs. 8-4 and 8-7); there is also an increased risk of puncturing an epidural vein with return of blood from the epidural needle.

Epidural Space. This space should permit easy injection of solution and easy threading of an epidural catheter, if it is entered in the midline in a controlled manner. Uncontrolled entry or failure to fix the needle securely during subsequent injections or catheter insertions may result in pushing the needle tip forward until it touches the dura. This results in some resistance to injected local anesthetic and may cause the epidural catheter to puncture the dura if undue force is used when catheter insertion becomes difficult. Many textbooks fail to explain why catheter insertion is impossible, and why further progress of the needle is obstructed immediately after an otherwise impeccably correct loss of resistance through the ligamentum flavum. The explanation lies in the anatomy of the lamina and ligamentum flavum; the latter attaches to the anteroinferior aspects of the lamina below (see Figs. 8-1, 8-6, and 8-7). Thus, a needle piercing the ligamentum flavum at its extreme inferior aspect may be held up by the upper edge of the sloping lamina (see also Fig. 8-11). Usually reinsertion of the needle, more to the center of the interlaminar space, is then necessary. Less commonly, a needle angled sharply upward may undergo a clear-cut loss of resistance as its tip penetrates the ligamentum flavum, but attempts to pass a catheter meet with bony resistance. In this case, the recurved tip of an epidural needle still lies partially in the ligamentum flavum immediately adjacent to its attachment to the lamina above. If the epidural needle can be advanced without further resistance, and the catheter then threads easily without aspiration of CSF, this confirms a high entry through the interlaminar gap. More rarely, but of great importance, a needle angled acutely laterally may penetrate the ligamentum flavum close to a spinal nerve. Subsequent attempts to pass a catheter may lead to resistance and the immediate report of a unisegmental paresthesia. This calls for repositioning of the needle, since persistence may lead to spinal nerve trauma.

It is unusual not to obtain a jet of CSF back through an 18-gauge (or larger) needle if it enters the subarachnoid space. Thus, the syringe should always be disconnected as soon as the loss of resistance through the ligamentum flavum is obtained, or if a subsequent second loss of resistance is noted. The width of the posterior epidural space, beneath the ligamentum flavum, varies considerably, depending on the level of the bony spine at which it is approached and the horizontal point of needle entry (see Tables 8-1, 8-2, and 8-3); it is widest in the midline in the midlumbar region (5-6 mm) but narrows next to the articular processes (see Figs. 8-4 and 8-7). In the midthoracic region, it is 3 to 5 mm in the midline and very narrow laterally. In the lower cervical region, the distance between ligamentum flavum and dura is only 1.5 to 2 mm in the midline; however, this increases below C7 to 3 to 4 mm, particularly if the neck is flexed.

Epidural Veins. These veins are most prominent along the lateral walls of the spinal canal in the lateral portion of the epidural space (see Fig. 8-5).

Spinal Arteries. These arteries reach the spinal cord by way of the intervertebral foramina and enter the epidural space to reach spinal nerve roots in the region of the dural cuffs (see Chapter 7, Figs. 7-10, 7-11, and Fig. 8-4). It is thus possible to cause spinal cord ischemia if a spinal artery is traumatized by a needle inserted toward a spinal nerve root. The spinal cord territory supplied by the anterior spinal artery is most vulnerable, since there is only one anterior artery (Fig. 8-12) and since the major feeder to this artery usually enters unilaterally (on the left in 75%) by way of a single intervertebral foramen, between T5 and L3 (see Chapter 7, Fig. 7-11). This further supports the practice of ensuring that the needle enters the epidural space in the midline and suggests that the L3–L4 interspace is the best choice for beginners.

Aspects of Individual Anatomic Structures with Relevance to Epidural Block

The description given of applied anatomy of epidural puncture highlights relevant aspects of the anatomy of the bony spine, ligaments, meninges, spinal nerves, and blood vessels. Anesthesiologists are strongly advised to study the detailed anatomy of the individual lumbar vertebrae, as well as the articulated skeleton, with the aid of an atlas of anatomy.

Only by direct handling of the bony spine and its articulations will the reader fully appreciate the important relationships discussed (see Tables 8-1 to 8-3).

Vertebrae and Vertebral Column. These structures hold the key to both spinal subarachnoid and epidural blockade (see Figs. 8-1, 8-5, 8-6, 8-9, 8-13, 8-14, and 8-30). These are

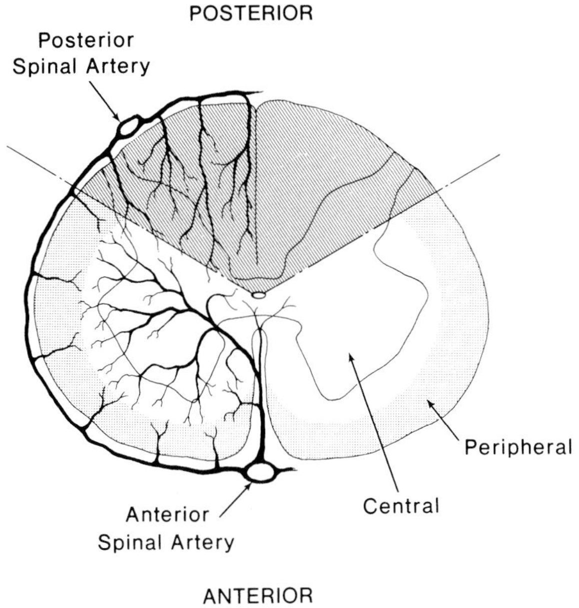

FIG. 8-12. Blood supply of spinal cord, horizontal distribution. The "central" area, supplied only by anterior spinal artery, is predominantly a motor area (see text).

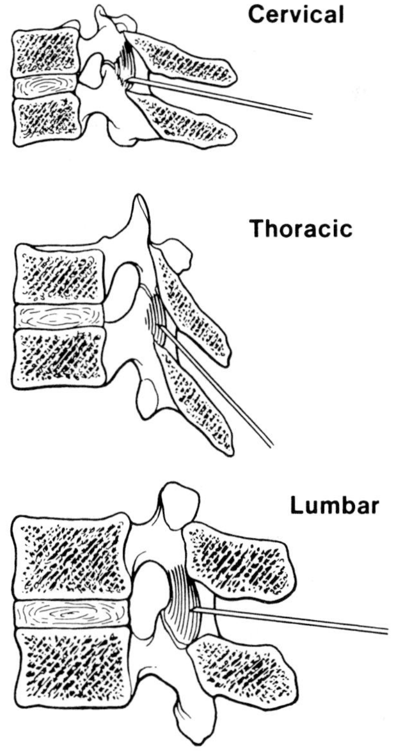

FIG. 8-13. Ligamentum flavum in cervical, thoracic, and lumbar regions.

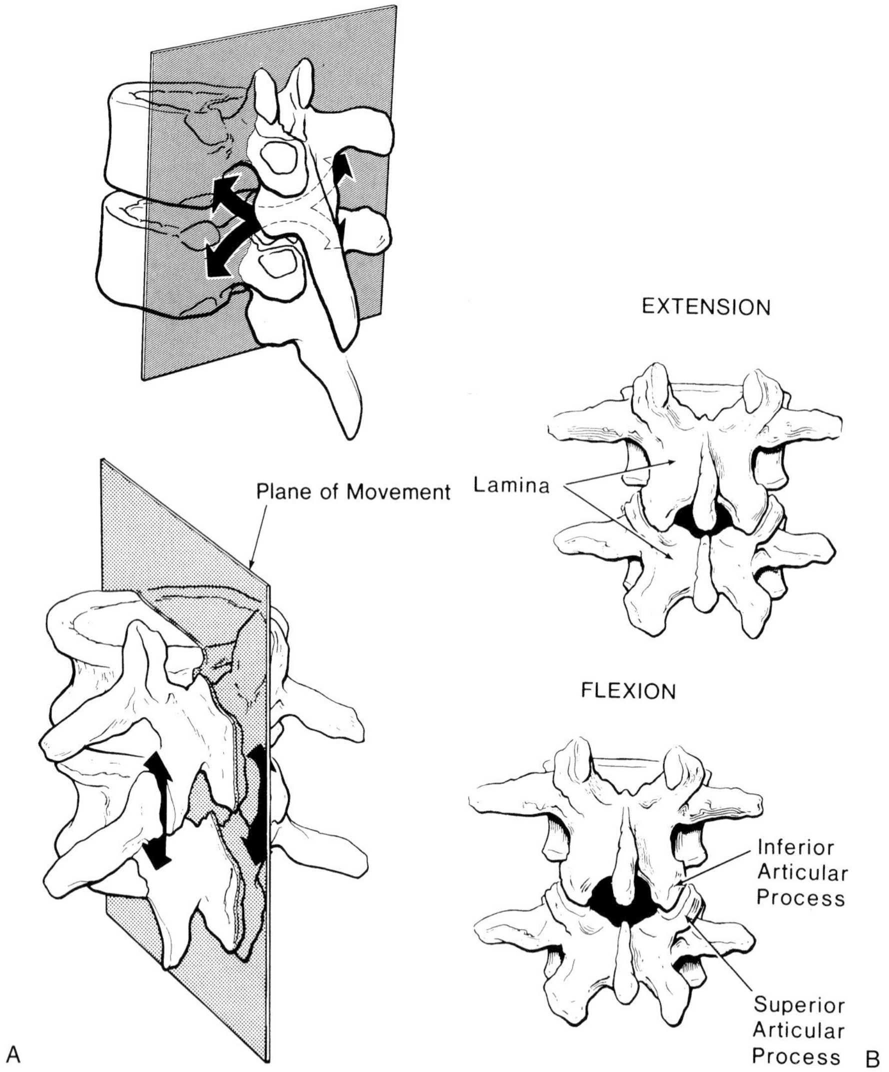

FIG. 8-14. A: Articular facets, plane of rotation. In the **thoracic** region, the plane through the facets is the coronal plane (at right angles to median plane) so that lateral rotation can occur. In the **lumbar** region, the plane through the facets is the median plane (bisecting the body into right and left halves), so that lateral rotation cannot occur and the only possible movement is flexion and extension. (*Arrows* indicate direction of movement.) **B: Interlaminar space, lumbar region**, in extension and flexion. In extension, the boundaries are roots of spinous processes and laminae. With flexion, articular processes form the lateral boundary, and articular facets are exposed at the lateral extremity of the interlaminar space. (Part **B** modified from Macintosh, R.R.: Lumbar Puncture and Spinal Analgesia. Edinburgh, E. & S. Livingstone, 1957.)

also discussed in Chapter 7. However, the following are of particular importance to epidural blockade. The spinous processes are widest in the midlumbar region and have only slight angulation, making insertion of the 16- to 18-gauge Tuohy needle into the center of the supraspinous ligament relatively easy compared with elsewhere in the spine. The inferior border of the spinous process lies over the widest part of the interlaminar space (Fig. 8-14). The process becomes somewhat narrower superiorly, so that a needle can be guided by the lateral aspect of the spinous process to enter the midpoint of the ligamentum flavum. In the midthoracic region, the spinous processes are much narrower, closer together, and angulated sharply downward, thus obscuring the interlaminar space (see Chapter 7, Fig. 7-1). The inferior border of spinous processes in this region lies opposite the lamina of the vertebral body below. Insertion of an epidural needle may necessitate a paraspinous (paramedian) approach. If the needle is inserted beside the lower border of the spinous process and angled upward at 130°, the lateral aspect of the process can once again be used to guide the needle inward 15° toward the center of the ligamentum flavum (see Fig. 8-30). In the cervical region, the spinous processes widen and become bifid with a wide supraspinous ligament. They are almost horizontal in the lower cervical region and permit easy access to the interlaminar space (see Fig. 8-13).

Supraspinous Ligament. This ligament runs vertically between the apices of the spinous processes of lumbar and thoracic vertebrae and continues above as ligamentum nuchae. It varies in width directly with the width of the spinous process; in the lumbar region, it may be as much as 1 cm wide (see Fig. 8-10). In persons who engage in heavy physical activity and in laborers and the aged, the ligament may become ossified, making midline puncture impossible.

Interspinous Ligament. This ligament runs obliquely between the spinous processes and is continuous anteriorly with the ligamentum flavum and posteriorly with the supraspinous ligament. As indicated in Tables 8-1 through 8-3, its thickness is greatest above L4 in the lumbar region. Although it is a thin ligament, its fibers are attached along the entire superior and inferior surfaces of the spinous processes; thus, in the lumbar region, the ligament is rectangular and provides an identifiable resistance to injected air or solution (see Fig. 8-10).

Laminae and Articular Processes. These form the boundaries of the interlaminar foramen. In the lumbar region, the foramen is triangular when the lumbar spine is extended, with the base being formed by the upper borders of the laminae of the lower vertebra, and the sides by the medial aspects of the inferior articular processes of the vertebra above. However, if the lumbar spine is flexed, the inferior articular processes glide upward by means of the synovial joints between facets of articular processes, thus enlarging the interlaminar foramen to a diamond shape (Fig. 8-14B); borders of the superior articular process of the vertebra below now form the lower part of the lateral boundaries of the foramen. It is worth noting that, in the lumbar region, the facets of the articular processes articulate in a plane at right angles to the lamina, so that rotation cannot take place; by contrast, in the thoracic region, the facets articulate in the same plane as the lamina, so that lateral rotation readily occurs.[249] This further indicates the potential increased difficulty of puncture in the thoracic compared with the lumbar region (Fig. 8-14A).

The *lamina* itself slopes down and back on its posterior surface, so that it may be contacted by a needle either superficially or deep (see Figs. 8-5 and 8-11B). As indicated above, the lamina forms only the wide base of the interlaminar space. The remaining boundaries are formed laterally and superiorly by the articular processes (see Fig. 8-6).

Ligamentum Flavum. Composed almost entirely of elastic fibers, this ligament is aptly named since it is indeed yellow. Because of its tough elasticity and its thickness of several millimeters in the lumbar region, the ligament imparts a characteristic "springy" resistance, particularly to a large-bore needle with an upturned end (Tuohy needle). The ligament runs from the anterior and inferior aspects of the lamina above to the posterior and superior aspects of the lamina below. Laterally, the ligament narrows as it blends with the capsule of the joint between the articular processes (see Figs. 8-4 to 8-6). Because developmentally two laminae fuse at each level to form the root of the spinous process, two ligamenta flava meet in the median plane and here become continuous with the deep fibers of the interspinous ligament (see Fig. 8-10). Thus, an epidural needle advancing in the midline encounters continuing resistance that increases immediately as the needle passes into the ligamentum flavum. New information about the anatomy of ligamentum flavum is contained in the foregoing section on posterior epidural space.

Pedicles. These join the laminae to the vertebral bodies and complete the bony spinal canal that protects the dural sac. Each pedicle is notched, so that pedicles of adjacent vertebral bodies form the intervertebral foramen. The inferior pedicle of each foramen is notched more deeply. The intervertebral foramina are completed posteriorly by the capsule surrounding the articular processes of adjoining vertebrae and anteriorly by an intervertebral disk and the lower part of the body above it (see Fig. 8-1). Because the epidural space is continuous with the paravertebral space, it is possible to produce an epidural block by injection close to an intervertebral foramen (see Chapter 10), or to penetrate the dura at the dural cuff region if a needle is inserted into an intervertebral foramen. The degree of patency of intervertebral foramina is thought to influence the spread of local anesthetics and contrast media injected into the epidural space[352]; it has been shown that extensive "leakage" of local anesthetic occurs through intervertebral foramina.[250] There are a total of 58 foramina, so the potential for "leakage" is considerable. However, the density of areolar tissue around the foramina varies considerably, and with advancing age it may form a recognizable "operculum" that effectively blocks off foramina. This may play a part in the declining dose requirements with advancing age,[62,352,392,393] although a declining neural population may also contribute.[100] Similar mechanisms probably result in reduction in dose requirements that may occur in atherosclerosis.[60]

Contents of the Epidural Space. These are also discussed in Chapter 7. However, several aspects deserve further comment with relation to epidural block.

Epidural fat. This semifluid lobulated areolar tissue extends throughout the spinal and caudal epidural space. It is most abundant posteriorly, diminishes adjacent to the articular processes, and then increases laterally around the spinal nerve roots, where it is continuous with the fat surrounding the spinal nerves in the intervertebral foramina and thence with the fat in the paravertebral space. Anteriorly, it is sparse, and thus the dura may lie close to the posterior longitudinal ligament. Overall, the amount of fat in the epidural space tends to vary in direct relation to that present elsewhere in the body, so that obese patients may have epidural spaces that are occupied by generous amounts of fat. Mostly, the epidural fat lies free in the epidural space except near the nerve roots, where connective tissue tends to tether the fat in the intervertebral foramina. The epidural fat is surprisingly vascular, with small capillaries that form a rich network in its substance. The fat itself has a great affinity for drugs with high lipid solubility, such as bupivacaine and etidocaine, which may remain in epidural fat for long periods (see Chapter 3); uptake of local anesthetic into epidural fat competes with vascular and neural uptake. The compliance of the epidural fat varies considerably between persons and with increasing age.[386,387] In children and young adults, it offers little resistance to injection, but in some adults, a low compliance may result in considerable "drip back" of injected local anesthetic. A fiberoptic endoscopy study of 48 cadavers reported a dorsomedian connective tissue band, of varying thickness, in every case[31] (see Epidural Space).

Epidural veins. The large valveless epidural veins are part of the internal vertebral venous plexus,[19] which drains the neural tissue of spinal cord, the CSF, and the bony spinal canal. The major portion of this plexus lies in the anterolateral part of the epidural space,[45] out of reach of a correctly placed epidural needle (see Figs. 8-5 and 8-6). The plexus has rich segmental connections at all levels within intervertebral foramina and epidural space, and within the body of the vertebrae (the basivertebral veins). Superiorly, the plexus communicates with the occipital, sigmoid, and basilar venous sinuses within the cranium. Inferiorly, anastomoses by way of the sacral venous plexus link the vertebral plexus to uterine and iliac veins. By way of the intervertebral foramina at each level, the vertebral plexus communicates with thoracic and abdominal veins, so that pressure changes in these cavities are transmitted to the epidural veins but not to the supporting bony elements of the neural arch and the vertebral bodies. Thus, marked increases in intra-abdominal pressure may compress the inferior vena cava while distending the epidural veins and increasing flow up the vertebrobasilar plexus. This increased flow is accommodated mostly by means of the azygos vein, which ascends in the right chest over the root of the right lung into the superior vena cava (Fig. 8-15). However, it is also possible for a small dose of local anesthetic injected rapidly into an epidural vein to be channeled directly up the basivertebral system to a cerebral venous sinus; this is most likely to occur in a pregnant woman in the supine position when the inferior vena cava is obstructed, and intrathoracic pressure rises during active bearing down, so that the azygos flow is temporarily increased. Clearly, local anesthetic should not be injected into

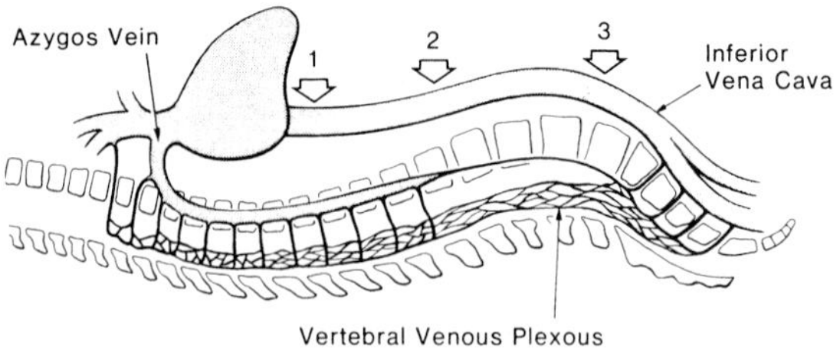

FIG. 8-15. Epidural veins (vertebral venous plexus) and their connections with inferior vena cava (IVC) and azygos vein. Epidural veins are protected from compression by the vertebral canal; thus, obstruction to IVC results in rerouting of venous return by way of epidural veins, and thence to the azygos vein above the level of obstruction. Some common sites of IVC obstruction are shown: *(1)* below the liver (e.g., severe ascites); *(2)* thoracolumbar junction (e.g., abdominal pressure) in prone position; *(3)* pelvic brim (e.g., pregnancy). (Modified from Bromage, P.R.: Epidural Analgesia. Philadelphia, W.B. Saunders, 1978.)

the epidural space under such conditions. More likely, distention of epidural veins, owing to direct inferior vena caval obstruction (e.g., by the uterus) or owing to increased thoracoabdominal pressure, will also diminish the effective volume of the epidural space, with the result that injected local anesthetics spread more widely up and down the epidural space. In addition, the potential absorptive area of venules and capillaries is increased, with increased drug reaching the heart by way of the azygos vein. The impressive size of the epidural veins on the lateral wall of the spinal canal (see Figs. 8-5 and 8-6) can be confirmed by epidural phlebography during a Valsalva maneuver.[157] Three important aspects of safety emerge:

1. The epidural needle should pierce the ligamentum flavum in the midline to avoid the large laterally placed epidural veins.
2. Insertion of epidural needles or catheters or injection of local anesthetic should be avoided during episodes of marked increase in size of epidural veins, such as that which occurs with increased thoracoabdominal pressure during straining.
3. The presence of vena caval obstruction calls for a reduction in dose, a decreased rate of injection, and increased care in aspirating for blood (see following) before epidural injection.

An intriguing feature of the epidural veins is of importance in draining CSF and in the transfer of local anesthetic to the CSF. In the region of the dural cuffs, bulbs of arachnoid mater protrude through the dura into the epidural space, where they often invaginate the walls of epidural veins that drain the spinal cord and nerve root area.[352] Although the primary function of these arachnoid granulations is to drain CSF[127] and remove debris from the CSF into the vascular system,[203] they also provide a favorable site for transfer of local anesthetic into the spinal fluid (see Fig. 8-2).

Spinal arteries. The spinal cord receives its blood supply from arteries on the surface of the brain above or from arteries that enter the intervertebral foramina and then gain access to the spinal cord by way of the spinal nerve roots (see Chapter 7, Figs. 7-10 and 7-11).

It is of significance to epidural block that the spinal branches of the subclavian, aortic, and iliac arteries cross the epidural space and enter the subarachnoid space in the region of the dural cuffs (see Chapter 7, Fig. 7-10). The anterior spinal artery territory supplying the anterior horn or motor area of the spinal cord is most vulnerable[162] (see Fig. 8-12). Details of spinal arterial supply are given in Figure 7-11 and adjacent text in Chapter 7.

Epidural lymphatics. The dural cuff region is supplied with a rich lymphatic network that rapidly conveys debris from arachnoid villi out through intervertebral foramina to reach lymph channels in front of the vertebral bodies.[51] It is reassuring that foreign material can be carried away rapidly by an efficient system that runs in a direction away from spinal fluid and the spinal cord.

Dural sac. Containing dura, arachnoid, spinal fluid, pia, spinal nerves, and spinal cord, the dural sac is, strictly speaking, contained within the annular epidural space. A detailed description of the meninges and CSF is given in Chapter 7. For the purposes of this chapter, it is important to examine some aspects of the anatomy of the dura, arachnoid, and spinal nerves in the region adjacent to the intervertebral foramina, the so-called dural cuff region.

The Dura. This can be considered as a protective tube that is pierced by and gives a short "cuff" to each pair of spinal nerves; at this point, the dura becomes markedly thinner and is closely adherent to the dorsal surfaces of the dorsal root ganglia as far as the point where anterior and posterior roots fuse to form the spinal nerve. Within these dural cuffs, there is a small blind pocket of CSF, which is separated from the epidural space only by the greatly thinned dura (see Fig. 8-2). Here, the dura is pierced by veins, arteries, and lymphatics, running to and from the underlying subarachnoid space. Also, the arachnoid membrane pushes small "granulations"[352] through the dura; these may either indent epidural veins or come into contact with epidural lymphatics, to facilitate drainage of CSF and elimination of foreign material.[51] This region also provides a ready route for passage of local anesthetics into the spinal fluid. Although the dura and arachnoid are usually in close apposition, they are easily separated, and it is possible to inadvertently insert an epidural catheter into the subdural space[46,345] (see Chapter 7, Fig. 7-6).

Arachnoid Membrane. It is now known that the arachnoid membrane is metabolically active[397] and is capable of forming giant vacuoles, which may temporarily communicate with the subdural space or, in the dural cuff region, directly with the epidural space. This probably provides a system for rapid drainage of CSF and clearance of debris from the CSF.[375]

Spinal Nerves. Some advances in neuroanatomy have helped to explain the segmental onset of epidural blockade. Studies of the size of dorsal roots indicate a considerable variation in size, with large roots at C8 and S1 and a "valley" between these two peak sizes in the thoracic region.[154] Studies of the number of myelinated and nonmyelinated fibers in ventral roots also reveal a peak at S1 and in the lower cervical region at C5–C8.[90] This is in keeping with the relative resistance of the lower cervical region and S1 to neural blockade. Anatomic studies suggested that the pia of the spinal cord and spinal nerve roots is continuous with the perineurium of the spinal nerves. Because the epineurium of spinal nerves is continuous with the dura, this raises the possibility of continuity between the subarachnoid space and a subepineurial space.[351] This would explain reports of transverse myelitis after injection of neurolytic agents directly beneath spinal nerve epineurium. All that is required for rapid spread of injected solution from spinal nerve to CSF is accurate needle placement beneath the spinal nerve epineurium (see Fig. 8-2).

Spinal Cord. It is known that local anesthetics, injected into the epidural space, can subsequently be detected in spinal nerve roots and the peripheral areas of the spinal cord[67] in concentrations sufficient to block nerve conduction. However, even the combination of nerve root and spinal cord effects of local anesthetics may not abolish afferent "traffic" in spinal cord due to noxious input (see section on somatosensory evoked potentials). Blockade may be more difficult in situations such as severe nociceptive input or neuropathy resulting in "central sensitization"; this is associated with enhanced spinal cord neural responses which are much longer, more long-lasting, and excite a much more extensive area of the spinal cord (see Chapter 24).

Epidural Pressures. The epidural space is identified traditionally by the negative pressure in the space believed to be created by tenting of the dura by the advancing needle.[56,139,209,384] Blunt needles with side openings produce the greatest negative pressures; they produce a good "coning" effect of the dura without puncturing it and transmit the negative pressure well because of their side opening.

By using a manometer attached to the advancing needle, Usubiaga[386] found negative epidural entry pressures measured at cervical, thoracic, lumbar and sacral levels. Also, a relationship was demonstrated between the pressure generated at injection into the epidural space and the extent of block that developed. However, in these early reports only the instantaneous epidural entry pressures were obtained. Using a closed measurement system, which permitted continuous measurement of positive and negative pressure, Telford and Hollway[369] studied the pressures generated during deliberate dural puncture with a Tuohy needle. Such a closed measurement system facilitates the development of large transdural pressure gradients because of the inability of the epidural space pressure to equilibrate with subatmospheric pressure. Epidural space pressures were always positive with the needle stationary in the epidural space, except when the subarachnoid space was to be entered (Fig. 8-16). The negative pressure that then developed was stated to be artificial and caused by tenting of the dura by the blunt Tuohy needle. The authors reported that spontaneous respiration with its associated negative interpleural pressure would be insufficient to cause negative lumbar epidural pressure. A similar device was used to measure thoracic epidural pressure continuously at the time of insertion a Tuohy needle at the T7–T8 intervertebral level using a loss of resistance technique.[289] High negative epidural pressures up to −60 mm Hg were only observed at the moment of epidural puncture, equilibrating to a positive value within 90 seconds in both expiratory and inspiratory phases. This suggests that subsequent adaptation of the surrounding tissue results in restoration of the normal positive epidural pressure.

Shah[349] demonstrated with Macintosh balloon indicators attached to Tuohy needles that the lumbar epidural pressure increased with stimuli known to increase CSF pressure like jugular venous compression, ventilation with carbon dioxide, and positive end expiratory pressure. The increase in epidural pressure produced by jugular venous compression agreed with those of Usubiaga.[386] This suggests that the lum-

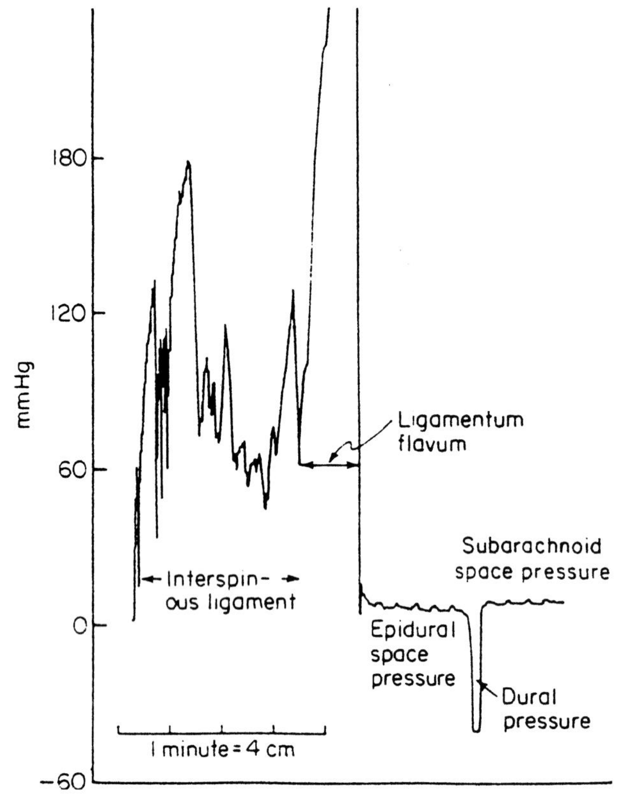

FIG. 8-16. A typical pressure, compared with time recording. Note the increasing pressure during passage through the interspinous ligaments, the high pressure generated during passage through the ligamentum flavum and the precipitous decrease in pressure on entering the epidural space. The pressure is only negative on entry into the subarachnoid space. (Telford, R.J., and Holbway, T.E.: Observations on deliberate dural puncture with a Tuohy needle: Pressure measurement. Anaesthesia, *46*:725, 1991.)

bar epidural pressure is in equilibrium with the prevailing spinal CSF pressure.

Paul and Wildsmith[301] investigated the influence of the pressure generated by low lumbar epidural injection of two different volumes of bupivacaine upon epidural pressure and showed that the epidural pressure stabilized within 60 seconds, irrespective of the pressure applied by the local anesthetic injection. The same plateau pressure in both groups at the upper limit of normal for CSF pressure suggests a pressure-limiting feature in the epidural space; displacement of CSF may be the main safety valve limiting epidural pressure. In addition, no significant correlation was found between the individual level of analgesia and the epidural pressure at any time or with patient characteristics. The authors suggest that a relationship might exist between the height of the pressure and an increase in the escape of injected fluid from the space through the intervertebral foramina to the paravertebral space.

Studies by Usubiaga et al. (1967) have helped to explain why successful entry into the epidural space is sometimes followed by "drip back" when local anesthetic is subsequently injected; classic pressure-volume compliance studies showed that compliance decreased with increasing age and that residual pressure after injection of 10 ml of solution at a standard rate had a positive correlation with age.[387] Thus, some patients with a low compliance in the epidural space will be unable to accommodate a large volume of solution if it is injected rapidly; "drip back" will be less common in young patients and if injection is made slowly because, although there was a transient increase in epidural pressure in young patients, Usubiaga found that pressure was essentially back to baseline in 30 seconds. If one routinely uses a negative pressure test for epidural puncture, it is important to be aware of factors that result in marked changes in epidural pressure.

In severe lung diseases such as emphysema, epidural negative pressure may be abolished, particularly if the patient is lying down.[150] Any factor that increases abdominal pressure and/or occlusion of the inferior vena cava may distend the epidural veins (see earlier) and increase pressure in the lumbar epidural space. This results in only slight changes in the thoracic epidural space, particularly if the patient is sitting.[386]

During labor, baseline lumbar epidural pressures are higher in women in the supine position compared with those in the lateral position. As labor progresses, baseline pressures increase to as high as +10 cm H_2O at full dilatation.[153] Also, there are peaks of epidural pressure during each uterine contraction, with increases of 8 to 15 cm H_2O.[58]

Coughing or a Valsalva maneuver increases both intrathoracic and intra-abdominal pressure, so that pressure in thoracic and lumbar epidural space increases,[386] resulting in high positive pressures being recorded throughout the epidural space.

Comparison of patients having prior lumbar surgery to those who did not revealed a higher baseline lumbar epidural space in patients with previous lumbar surgery.[371] However, additional pressure from epidural injections decays at a rate similar to that in patients who did not undergo operations. This suggests that the alteration induced by surgery is one of different initial condition, rather than a change in distensibility. On the other hand, the resistance to fluid injection in the epidural space was higher in patients with a diseased space as the result of epiduroarachnoiditis compared with that of the normal space.[318] Therefore one should be careful with the injection of fluid into parts of the epidural space that do not communicate freely with the surroundings.

PHYSIOLOGIC EFFECTS OF EPIDURAL BLOCKADE

With currently available local anesthetic agents, spinal epidural neural blockade implies sympathetic blockade accompanied by somatic blockade, which may involve sensory and motor blockade alone or in combination. Although it is possible to avoid blockade of "peripheral" lumbar sympathetic fibers if only sacral segments are blocked by a caudal approach to the epidural space, spinal epidural blockade almost invariably results in some degree of sympathetic block-

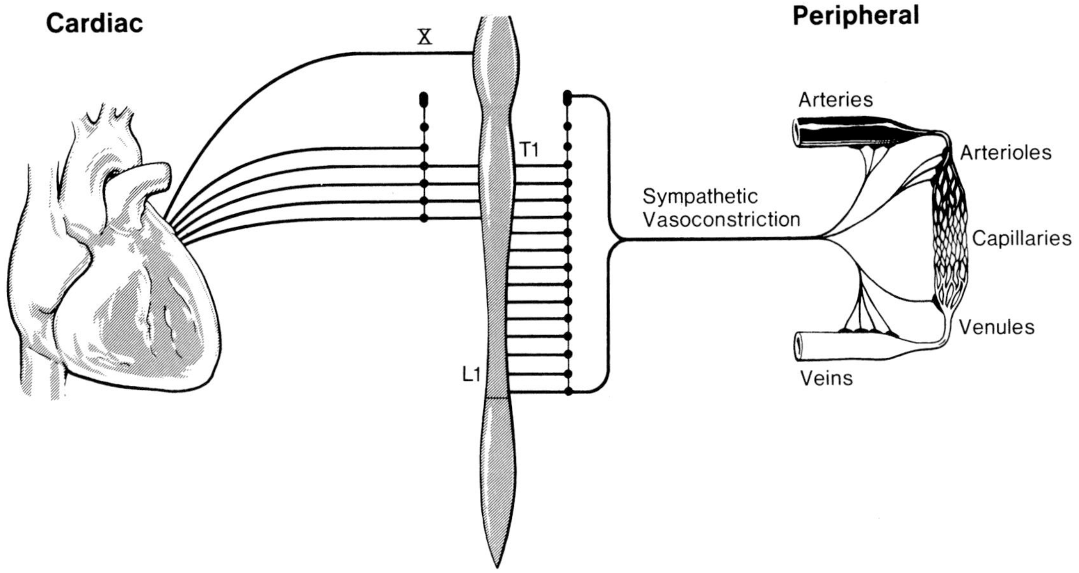

FIG. 8-17. Sympathetic blockade: "central" (cardiac) and "peripheral" components. These consist of T1–T4 cardiac sympathetic fibers and T1–L2 "peripheral" sympathetic fibers. Note important innervation of veins and venules. Vagal cardiac fibers are also shown.

ade. Some of the most important (but not all) of the physiologic effects of epidural blockade can be discussed in relation to either sympathetic blockade only of vasoconstrictor fibers (below T4) and/or of cardiac sympathetic fibers (T1–T4; Fig. 8-17). Many clinicians prefer to have a wide margin of safety if they are intent on avoiding major sympathetic blockade. Thus, they aim to restrict the level of analgesia to T10. Studies discussed in Chapter 13, however, indicate that the level of sympathetic block with epidural anesthesia may be lower than the level of sensory block and more incomplete in terms of the quality of block.[22] This concept of sympathetic blockade is still a practical approach in considering the physiologic effects of epidural blockade because inguinal, perineal, urologic, and lower limb surgical procedures can be carried out with blockade to T10 or lower, which at most will produce only a "peripheral" sympathetic blockade. However, lower abdominal surgery (such as appendectomy, gynecologic surgery, and cesarean section) necessitates blockade to T4. Thus, the most frequent use of epidural block will be to either T4 or T10 level. Occasionally, a T1 level is needed for chest injury or thoracotomy. We will consider the cardiovascular effects of epidural block with respect to the degree of sympathetic block (and its effects) with sensory blockade to T1, T4, or T10.

Subtler and somewhat more indirect is the reduced input to the central nervous system (CNS), which accompanies various levels of sensory blockade. This "deafferentation" has long been thought capable of exerting a "protective" effect that reduces the efferent neurohumoral response to surgical stimulation or trauma. Objective data have now become available to support this hypothesis (see Chapter 5).

Finally, it is important to remember that extensive epidural blockade often requires large doses of local anesthetic (with or without epinephrine). Large doses themselves may cause physiologic changes as a result of the direct pharmacologic effects of circulating blood concentrations. These are an inevitable outcome of vascular absorption from the epidural space. Because of the unique epidural venous system (see earlier), direct intravascular injection may result in the rapid attainment of high concentrations of local anesthetic in the brain and/or heart with the potential for convulsions and/or sudden depression of cardiac output (see Chapters 2 to 4). Also, important changes in vagal tone accompany sympathetic block (see Fig. 8-21). The various mechanisms for physiologic effects of epidural block are summarized in Table 8-7.

Cardiovascular Effects of Epidural Blockade

In order to understand the cardiovascular effects of epidural blockade, a sound knowledge of the autonomic control of circulation is required (see Chapter 13).[237,257] Although it has been claimed that epidural block results in a lesser degree of sympathetic block and much greater cardiovascular stability than subarachnoid block,[128] there are no controlled data to support this. In general, cardiovascular depression may occur with both epidural and subarachnoid blockade (Fig. 8-18) and is at least partly related to the level of sympathetic blockade (see Figs. 8-17 and 8-19; see also Chapter 7).[41,43,224,225] While the potential for cardiovascular changes owing to sympathetic block is present for epidural and subarachnoid blockade,[a] vascular absorption of local anesthetic and vasoconstrictor may result in significant hemodynamic changes after epidural but not after subarachnoid blockade;

[a] Level of sympathetic block is the same as (or lower than) sensory with epidural blockade. In comparison, sympathetic block is two to three segments higher than sensory level with subarachnoid block.

TABLE 8-7. *Mechanisms for physiologic effects of epidural analgesia*

By way of vascular absorption of local anesthetic (L.A.) or Epinephrine (EPI)	By way of direct neural blocking effects or indirect results of blockade
Receptor	Spinal nerves (roots and trunks) by axonal blockade
β-stimulation by EPI	*Sympathetic*
α-stimulation by EPI or phenylephrine	Efferent blockade
Smooth muscle	Peripheral (T1–L2) vasoconstrictor
Blood vessels, L.A. or EPI	"Adrenal" (T6–L1)
Heart, L.A. or EPI	"Central" (T1–T4) cardiac sympathetic
Other organs, L.A. or EPI	*Sensory*
Cardiac muscle	Afferent blockade
By L.A. or EPI	Reduced peripheral sensation
Neural tissue	Blockade of visceral pain fibers
CNS, by L.A.	Reduced efferent neurohumoral response to surgical or other stimulus within the blocked area
Conducting system of heart, by L.A.	
Miscellaneous	*Motor*
Neuromuscular junction by L.A.	Efferent blockade
	Varying degrees of motor paralysis
	Reflex muscle relaxation without paralysis (deafferentation)
	Spinal cord
	Axons
	Superficial, sensory tracts blocked (e.g., bupivacaine, lidocaine, and etidocaine)
	Deep motor paths blocked (e.g., etidocaine)
	Dorsal horn modulation of pain transmission (? axons, ?cells)
	Possibility of "antianalgesic" effect owing to block of inhibitory paths
	Cell Bodies: "selective" blockade, by opioids (see Chapter 29)
	Secondary changes in parasympathetic activity
	Sympathetic block to T5 + ↓ venous return may → ↑↑ vagus
	Sympathetic block to T1 → unopposed vagus (see Fig. 8-21)
	Secondary changes in vasoactive hormones
	Sympathetic block to T1 → blockade of ↑ renin but not ↑ vasopressin, that usually helps maintain BP in response to ↓ BP challenge (see Fig. 8-22)

BP, blood pressure; CNS, central nervous system

the reason for this lies predominantly in the much larger doses of drugs used in epidural blockade and in the proximity of the large epidural veins, which, owing to their anatomy, have considerable potential for rapid transport of drug to the heart (Table 8-8) and CNS. The more gradual onset of sympathetic blockade after epidural analgesia compared with subarachnoid block may provide a mechanism for initial responses that are less severe for epidural block.[356] When used for epidural block, lidocaine, chlorprocaine, and etidocaine have a rapid onset of sympathetic block (especially etidocaine). This is even more evident if epinephrine-containing solutions are used. In comparison, onset of sympathetic block is slower with bupivacaine and there is a lesser tendency for rapid development of hypotension; indeed, sympathetic block may take 25 to 30 minutes to develop and even then may be only a "partial" block (see Chapter 13). Animal studies have shown that autoregulation at the level of the precapillary sphincters develops within 30 minutes of complete ablation of neural activity.[170]

Although controlled studies are not available, experience with large series of thoracic epidural blocks administered in intensive care units by continuous catheter techniques further supports the allowance of adequate time for autoregulation. A common management protocol for "topping up" thoracic epidural blockade for chest trauma involves keeping the patient supine during, and for 20 to 30 minutes after, "top-up." When this procedure is used, serious hypotension is uncommon, whereas topping up in the semirecumbent position or allowing inadequate time in the supine position after blockade may result in large reductions in blood pressure (see Chapter 26). A more practical alternative is to use a continuous infusion, which usually permits patients to remain semirecumbent after an initial period of stabilization in the supine position.

Blockade Below T4

Epidural blockade that is restricted to the level of the low thoracic and lumbar region (T5–L4) results in a "peripheral" sympathetic blockade with vascular dilatation in the pelvis and lower limbs; if all splanchnic fibers are blocked (T6–L1), then pooling of blood in the gut and abdominal viscera also may occur. This "peripheral" blockade has been demonstrated by measurements of large increases in lower limb blood flow owing to arteriolar vasodilation[41,112,358] and "pooling" of blood in the venous capacitance vessels.[356] Be-

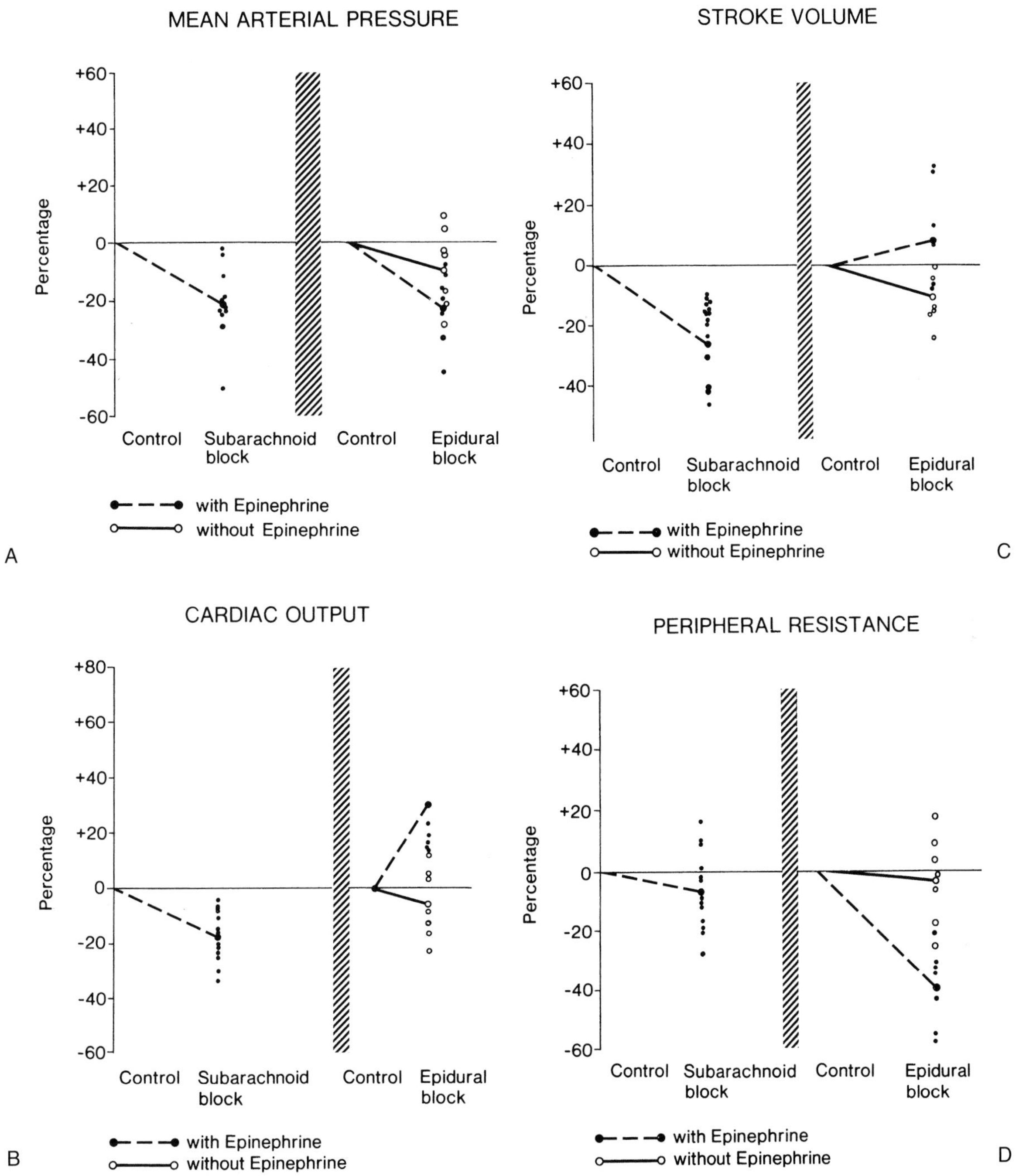

FIG. 8-18. Cardiovascular effects of epidural block to T5 level, with and without epinephrine. **A:** Mean arterial pressure. **B:** Cardiac output. **C:** Stroke volume. **D:** Peripheral resistance. Percentage changes for each variable are shown after epidural block, with a comparison given for a similar level of subarachnoid block. (Ward, R.J., *et al.*: Epidural and subarachnoid anesthesia. Cardiovascular and respiratory effects. J.A.M.A., *25*:275, 1965. Copyright © 1965, American Medical Association.)

cause the latter contain 80% of blood volume, venodilatation has a potential for dramatic changes in venous return, reduction in right atrial pressure, and reduced cardiac output. The decrease in venous return has been shown to result in increased cardiac vagal tone. This explains why heart rate remains unchanged or decreased despite hypotension and activation of cardiac sympathetic accelerator fibers.[18] A precise quantitative measurement of increased venous capacitance requires venous occlusion plethysmography of the calf (see Chapter 13).

Distribution of blood to the splanchnic area was studied by Arndt and co-workers in healthy young volunteers after injection of 20 ml of plain 2% lidocaine in the lumbar region.[12] Sympathetic block was not assessed independently;

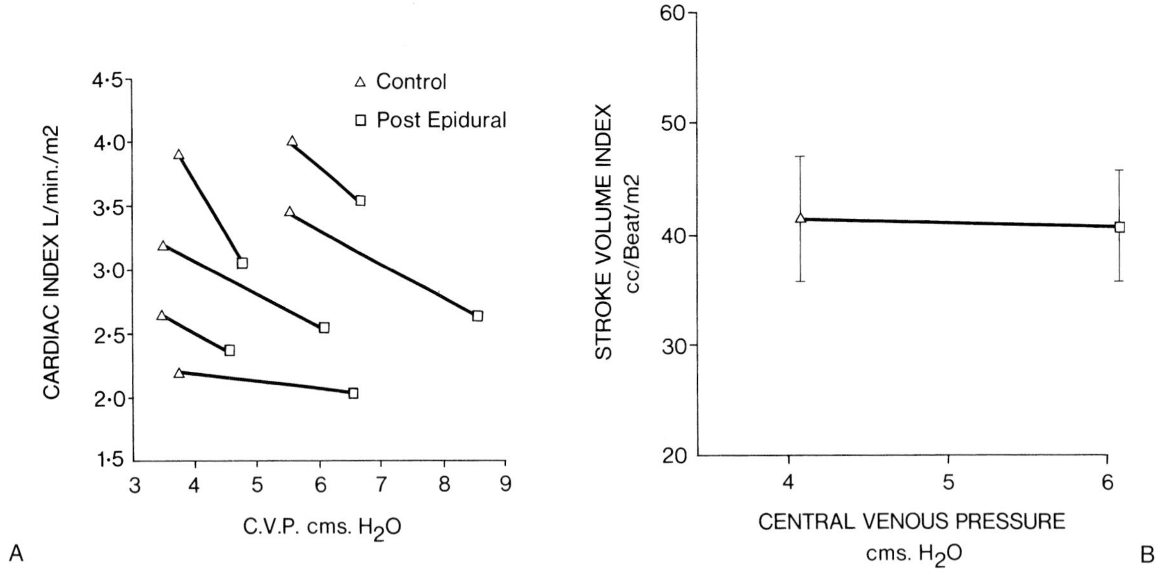

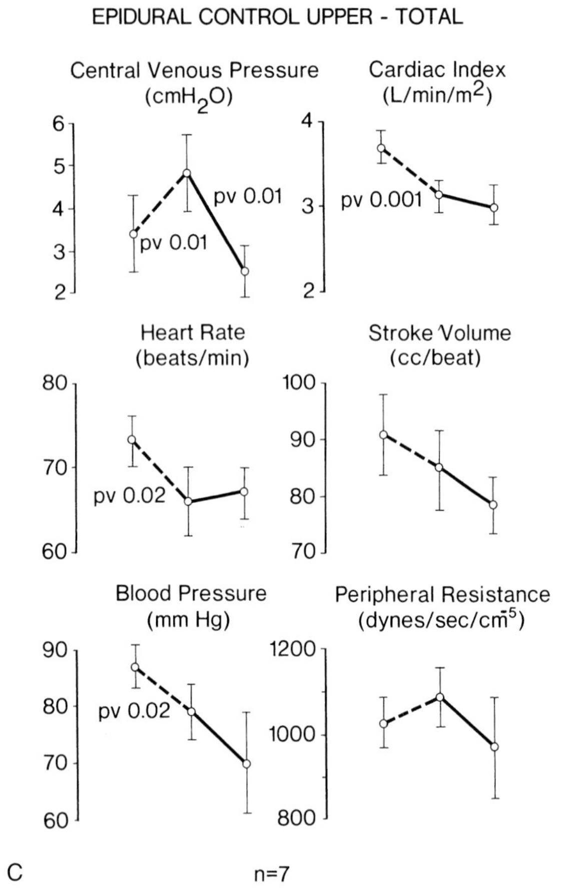

FIG. 8-19. Cardiovascular effects of epidural block. **A, B:** Blockade of T1–T4 alone compared with control measurements (control). **C:** Blockade of T1–T4 alone (upper) is compared with total blockade of T1–S5 (total) and control measurements (control). *Note:* Block of T1–T4 alone results in reductions in blood pressure, heart rate, and cardiac index, accompanied by a rise in central venous pressure. Extension of block to T1–S5 results in a further fall in CVP and cardiac index. (Parts **A** and **B** from Otton, P.E., and Wilson, E.J.: The cardiocirculatory effects of upper thoracic epidural analgesia. Can. Anaesth. Soc. J., *13:*541, 1966; Part **C** from McLean, A.P.H., Mulligan, G.W., Otton, P., and MacLean, L.D.: Hemodynamic alterations associated with epidural anesthesia. Surgery, *62:*79, 1967.)

however, it is unlikely that it spread much higher than the lower thoracic segments[22] (see Chapter 13). In all eight subjects except two, splanchnic blood volume decreased as assessed by distribution of radiolabeled red cells. Radioactivity also decreased in thorax and upper limbs, indicating compensatory vasoconstriction.[12] It is possible that the two subjects with increased splanchnic region blood volume did achieve blockade of the T6–L1 splanchnic sympathetic fibers.

Compensatory Mechanisms. Peripheral sympathetic activity. Even without intravenous "rehydration," healthy subjects in the supine position compensate for a decrease in mean arterial pressure with a reflex increase in efferent sympathetic vasoconstriction above the level of the block. Thus,

TABLE 8-8. *Cardiovascular effects of epidural blockade*

Mechanism	Effect
Neural effects	
"Peripheral" sympathetic block (T10–L2)	
Blockade of vasoconstrictor fibers to lower limbs	Arteriolar dilatation. Increased venous capacitance and pooling of blood in lower limbs → decreased venous return → ↓ CO
Reflex increase in vasoconstrictor fiber activity in upper limbs via baroreceptors	Increased vasomotor tone in upper limbs → ↑ venous return → ↑ CO
Reflex increase in cardioaccelerator nerve activity	↑ HR ↑ CO
Reduced right atrial pressure, due to ↓ venous return[a]	? ↓ HR (Note ↓↓ RA pressure → ↓↓ HR[a]; see Fig. 8-21)
Adrenal medullary sympathetic block (T6–L1)	
(Blockade of splanchnic nerves)	
Vasoconstrictor fibers to abdominal viscera	Pooling of blood in gut → decreased venous return
Adrenal medullary catecholamine secretion	Decreased levels of circulating catecholamines → ↓ HR ↓ CO
"Central" sympathetic block (T1–T4)	
Blockade of	
Cardiac sympathetic outflow from vasomotor center	↓ HR ↓ CO
Cardiac sympathetic reflexes at segmental level	
Vasoconstrictor fibers to head, neck, and arms	Vasodilatation in upper limbs. Blockade of compensatory lower limb vasoconstriction if T5–L1 is also blocked
Vagal predominance	"Inappropriate bradycardia"; "sudden bradycardia"; vagal arrest (see Fig. 8-21 and Table 8-11)
Effects of drug absorption	
Absorbed local anesthetic	Usually no measurable effects on HR, CO, MAP, or TPR even in patients with vascular disease
Moderate blood levels	Lidocaine may → ↑ CO, which is balanced ↓ TPR, so that MAP is unchanged
Antiarrhythmic	
Maintenance of normal CO	
Minimal reduction in vascular tone	
High blood levels (toxic)	↓ CO ↓ HR
Decreased contractility	↓ MAP
If convulsions occur hypoxia results in further reduction in CO	
Cardiac conducting tissue,? unidirectional blockade	Bupivacaine (very high levels) may → VT, VF, and cardiac arrest
Vascular dilatation	↓ TPR
Absorbed epinephrine	↑ CO ↑ HR ↓ TPR
β-stimulation	MAP may be unchanged or slightly reduced Antagonism of reflex vasoconstriction above level of blockade because of β-effects on muscle vasculature (→ ↓ TPR)

CO, Cardiac output; HR, heart rate; MAP, mean arterial pressure; TPR, total peripheral resistance; VT, ventricular tachycardia; VF, ventricular fibrillation.

[a] Decreased venous return was associated with increased vagal activity in one study. This may offset any increases in sympathetic activity.[18]

blood flow and venous capacitance are reduced in the head, neck, and upper limbs.[41,356,358] This increased efferent sympathetic activity is mediated predominantly (by means of the baroreceptors) by those sympathetic vasoconstrictor nerves (T1–T5) that remain unblocked and by circulating catecholamines released from the adrenal medulla owing to increased activity in any unblocked fibers in the splanchnic nerves (T6–L1). Although blood vessels in some viscera, such as the kidney, appear to be more responsive to direct neural stimuli,[2] in other vascular beds both neural and hormonal influences have major effects, although at different levels of the vasculature. Major arterioles respond mostly to neural stimuli, whereas small arterioles and venules near the capillary bed respond predominantly to circulating catecholamines. Thus, while any splanchnic fibers remain unblocked, there is a potential for vasoconstrictor activity below (as well as above) the level of blockade, by release of catecholamines from the adrenal medulla. Finally, the ability of precapillary sphincters to achieve autoregulation within a short time of cessation of neural activity[170] provides a further mechanism for regaining vascular tone and minimizing vascular pooling below the level of blockade.

Increased activity in cardiac sympathetic fibers (T1–T4). This increased activity may result in increased cardiac contractility and increased heart rate; similar effects are produced by increased levels of circulating catecholamines. Evidence that the latter are important in maintaining homeostasis in some clinical situations is provided by the surprisingly small changes in heart rate and cardiac output (−16%) with blockade of C5–T4, but with splanchnic fibers to the adrenal medulla (T6–L1) intact (Fig. 8-19).[291] Although quite large compensatory cardiac effects may be observed in unmedicated volunteers (*e.g.*, a 20% increase in heart rate and cardiac output[41]), these changes are not seen in premedicated patients (Table 8-9).[161] In premedicated patients, despite decreased peripheral resistance, an unchanged heart rate, and cardiac output, mean arterial pressure was reduced by only 10%, since changes in total vascular resistances were held to only a 25% reduction by increased sympathetic activity in unblocked areas.

The studies by Germann and colleagues[161] and Sjögren and Wright[358] report changes that are close to those that the anesthesiologist may anticipate in clinical practice, although patients in the latter study were not rehydrated. The practice of preblock "rehydration" with intravenous balanced salt solution is capable of maintaining mean arterial blood pressure close to preblock levels in healthy patients, including parturients, provided the level of blockade is below T4 and inferior vena caval obstruction is avoided.[41]

Is There Any Reason To Believe That Blockade To T10 Is Any Safer Than Extending Up To T5? Data available from studies in healthy volunteers[41] and healthy patients[161,358] indicate that, even with block to T5, changes are minimal, provided bradycardia is avoided. There are, however, several inescapable differences if blockade is extended right up to T5: (i) A larger number of vasoconstrictor fibers are blocked; (ii) the level of blockade is close to the cardiac sympathetics, so that any "overshoot" with initial or "top up" doses will pro-

TABLE 8-9. *Cardiovascular effects of epidural blockade by level of blockade with plain solutions*

		Change from control value (%)										
Extent of block	Dose of local anesthetic	CPP	Cardiac output	HR	MAP	SV	CVP	TPR	dp/dt	Arm flow	Leg flow	Reference
	Lower abdominal block											
T10–S5	20–25 ml 1.5% lidocaine				−6[a]							132
T10–S5	10 ml 2% lidocaine		0	+5	0	0	0	0	−25	+300	+300	41
	Upper abdominal block											
T4/5–S5	20–25 ml 1.5% lidocaine				−21[a]							132
T4/7–S5	30 ml 1.5% lidocaine		0	0	−16	0		0		0	+64	356
T5–S5	25–40 ml 2% lidocaine		−5	+7	−9		−10	−3				402
T3–S5	20–35 ml 2% lidocaine[b]		+21	+22	+5	+1	+13	−17	+23	−51	+287	41
T4–L4	15 ml 2% lidocaine		+7	+3	−1	+6	+6	−13		−35	+510	358
T7–S5	15–20 ml 1.5% lidocaine		0	0	−20	0		−24				161
	High thoracic block											
C5–T4	6–8 ml 1% mepivacaine		−17	−17	−8	0	+45	+8				291
C8–S5	30–40 ml 2% lidocaine[b]		+2	+6	−17	−3	+26	−21	−12	+91	+177	41
C5–S5	24–32 ml 1% mepivacaine		−19	−8	−20	−13	−27	−6				262
T1–T5	2–5 ml 0.5% bupivacaine[c]	+2	0	−9	−1	+4	−35	0				35
T2–T12	8 ml 2% lidocaine		−1	−7	−12	+10	−3	−3		+47	+21	358
T3–?	20–25 ml 1.5% lidocaine				−23[a]							132

[a] Systolic pressure
[b] Incremental doses
[c] Patients with coronary artery disease
CCP, coronary perfusion pressure; CVP, central venous pressure; HR, heart rate; MAP, mean arterial pressure; SV, stroke volume; TPR, total peripheral resistance

TABLE 8-10. *Danger signals: cardiovascular effects of epidural block*

Signal	Mechanisms and potential sequelae	Treatment
↑ HR ↓ BP in supine parturient with sensory level T11–L4 or ↓ HR ↓ BP—a more dangerous sign	Inferior vena caval occlusion venodilatation in lower limbs → ↓ Venous return, ↓ CO, ↓ organ perfusion (incl. fetus) → Epidural vein engorgement → ↓ spinal cord perfusion → "spinal stroke" → ↑ Sympathetic → ↑ HR (baroreceptors) vasoconstriction activity (above level of block) in upper limbs → ↓ RA pressure → ↓ HR (↑ vagal tone) (Note ↓↓ RV pressure may → ↓↓ HR; see Table 8-11 and Fig. 8-21)	Lateral position IV fluids, oxygen until MAP normal May require atropine and/or ephedrine if above measures fail
Gradual ↓ HR ↓ BP with level above T4	Venodilatation (as above) ↓ cardiac sympathetic activity → ↓ CO ↓ HR ↓ MAP → ↓ Cardiac sympathetic activity initially accompanied by ↓ parasympathetic (see also Fig. 8-21). → However, ↓↓ venous return → ↑ vagal activity Therefore, ↓↓ HR may occur before blockade of all T1-T4	IV fluids. Elevate legs. Atropine. Oxygen until MAP normal. Vasopressor (ephedrine) if required
"Sudden bradycardia" in either condition above	↓↓ Venous return may result in sudden ↑ parasympathetic tone ("faint response"); see Table 8-11; Fig. 8-21) ↓↓ HR → cardiac arrest	As above, but emphasis on sequence: elevate legs, oxygen, IV atropine, IV fluids—ephedrine rapidly if no response to above. May need epinephrine[a]
"Inappropriate" bradycardia (i.e., "normal" HR in face of ↓ MAP with sensory level T3–T4)	Peripheral vasodilatation should evoke an ↑ HR. But ↓ venous return → ↑ vagal tone, so HR remains at preblock rate but is "inappropriately" slow	IV atropine if MAP does not respond to fluids and elevation of legs, and relief of venous obstruction
Reduced blood volume or known obstruction of inferior vena cava	Hemorrhage Increased intra-abdominal pressure (see Fig. 8-15)	Restore blood volume, Relieve vena caval obstruction } Before epidural block
↓ HR with visceral traction in presence of blockade to T1	Total sympathetic block Unopposed vagus Changes in vagal tone → profound changes in HR; may → transient asystole (see Table 8-11 and Fig. 8-21)	IV atropine(?) Local infiltration to block vagal stimulus Ensure venous return adequate + arterial P_{O_2} adequate since ↑ HR (atropine) → ↑ myocardial oxygen demand

[a] Sudden bradycardia and hypotension may also result from cardiac toxicity of local anesthetics. This may require rapid resuscitative measures, including large doses of epinephrine.

BP, blood pressure; CO, cardiac output; HR, heart rate; IV, intravenous; MAP, mean arterial pressure; RA, right atrial; RV, right ventricular.

duce changes similar to those shown for blockade to T1 in Figure 8-19; and (iii) the splanchnic nerves T6–L1 may be blocked; thus varying degrees of blockade of visceral pain are provided, but also blockade of adrenal medullary activity and splanchnic vasoconstrictor fibers may be produced.

The combination of (i) and (iii) may become important if a patient's state of hydration has been wrongly assessed, if blood volume is reduced[42] owing to occult blood loss or disease states, or if compensatory mechanisms are for any other reason impaired. It is to be expected that the cardiovascular effects of other sedative and narcotic drugs will be additive. Such effects are mild if anesthesia is light and patients are healthy; however, the additional cardiovascular depression can be clearly documented even in healthy patients[161,364] and may be much greater in ill patients (Tables 8-9 and 8-10). It seems wise, then, to be most cautious about the level of blockade and the dose of sedative/narcotic in patients with any compromise of compensatory mechanisms.

The role of the splanchnic blood vessels in hypotension after epidural blockade has not been clearly defined. It is well known that blockade of the celiac plexus may produce marked pooling of blood in the splanchnic region, which receives 25% of cardiac output (splanchnicectomy faint), although this pooling is no greater than in the limbs; the potential for hypotension owing to both these mechanisms is markedly accentuated in patients with hypovolemia.

In a study of blood volume distribution after epidural block, two subjects with increases in splanchnic blood volume had substantial decreases in thoracic blood volume and arterial blood pressure. In one subject this was accompanied by a low heart rate and incipient faint reaction.[12] This is in keeping with the evidence of increased vagal tone in response to reduced venous return (see earlier).[18]

Blockade Above T4 (High Thoracic Block)

Total Sympathetic Blockade (T1–L4). It has been thought that control of cardiac rate (chronotropy) and force of contraction (inotropy) resided in the vasomotor center and was mediated by means of the cardiovascular sympathetic fibers (T1–T4). Although this is substantially true, it now appears that changes of cardiovascular sympathetic activity of approximately 20%[253] can be accomplished at a spinal cord level by reflex activity in the upper four or five thoracic segments (particularly T1), without vasomotor center control[26,99,359]; this can still be overridden by changes in parasympathetic activity.[237] Thus, epidural blockade of T1–T5 segments has the following effects on cardiac sympathetic activity: blockade of segmental cardiac reflexes in segments T1–T4; blockade of outflow from vasomotor center to cardiac sympathetic fibers (T1–T4); vasoconstrictor nerve blockade in head, neck, and upper limbs.

If, as is often the case, blockade extends from T1 to L4, the following effects will be added to the above: splanchnic nerve blockade (T6–L1) with resultant blockade of adrenal medullary secretion of catecholamines and blockade of splanchnic vasoconstrictor fibers; blockade of vasoconstrictor fibers in the lower part of the body, most important the capacitance vessels of the lower limbs (see Table 8-8).

The magnitude of cardiovascular changes has been documented in unmedicated volunteers[40,41] and in unmedicated patients[351,358] (see Fig. 8-19). In general, the mean arterial blood pressure was reduced approximately 20%, with a similar reduction in total peripheral resistance. Although Bonica and colleagues found that cardiac output was increased slightly or unchanged, McLean and colleagues found a 15% to 20% reduction.[262] Bonica and colleagues found that central venous pressure was markedly raised (26%).[40,41] Because only the studies of McLean and Bonica achieved blockade above T1, their results are more indicative of the effects of complete cardiac sympathetic block. Most surprising was the minimal change in heart rate observed despite blockade of C5–S5, that is, complete blockade of cardio-accelerator fibers and adrenal medullary catecholamine secretion. Because changes in cardiac rate are known to be controlled chiefly by the balance of sympathetic and parasympathetic tone at any moment, it must be assumed that parasympathetic tone was reduced to almost the same degree as sympathetic tone to maintain heart rate at a normal or near normal level (see Table 8-11). This small change in heart rate gives a deceptive picture of cardiac sympathetic activity, since Otton and Wilson have shown that blockade of T1–T4 alone produced an increase in central venous pres-

TABLE 8-11. *Vagal and sympathetic activity: effects on heart rate*

	Venous return "sensors" in great veins, atria, ventricles	Arterial pressure "sensors" in carotid sinus and aortic arch
Afferent path	Vagus	Vagus, glossopharyngeal
Efferent path	Vagus	Sympathetic
Effect of increased venous return + ↑ BP	↑ Venous return ↘ ↓ Vagal activity → ↑ HR	↑ BP ↘ ↓ sympathetic activity → ↓ HR
Effect of decreased venous return + ↓ BP		
Mild ↓: (? ↓ atrial volume)	↑ Vagal activity → ↓ HR ↓ HR (vagus) balanced by ↑ HR (sympathetic).: HR unchanged	↑ sympathetic activity → ↑ HR
Severe ⇊: (? ↓ ventricular pressure)	⇈ Vagal activity → ⇊ HR	⇈ Sympathetic activity ? Accentuates activation of vagal receptors in ventricle[a]
	If cardiac sympathetics blocked, vagus is unopposed, and with sensitized vagal receptors (serum catecholamines) → ⇊ HR and possible cardiac arrest	

[a] ⇊ BP also → ↓ carotid body oxygen supply. This initiates a "hypoxic" response and further increases vagal efferent activity.

BP, blood pressure; HR, heart rate

sure (CVP) without an increase in stroke volume output of the heart (see Fig. 8-18).[291] That is, the heart did not empty as well as before blockade—a reduced response of the Frank-Starling mechanism. Because the other major determinant of stroke volume is catecholamine stimulation determining the level of Frank-Starling response, the patient with blockade extending from T1 to L2 potentially has both mechanisms obtunded. Thus, one may view the rise in CVP in Bonica's study[41] as a warning sign that the myocardium has exhausted its compensatory mechanisms. Although the associated changes in mean arterial pressure and cardiac output were surprisingly small in the studies of T1 blockade (see Table 8-9), the cardiovascular system has essentially no further mechanisms to respond if called on to do so. In this situation, the anesthesiologist has "assumed control of the circulation" and must be prepared to make rapid adjustments in body position, blood volume, vascular tone, cardiac rate, and cardiac contractile state; this may require administration of various combinations of crystalloids, colloids, atropine, ephedrine, and catecholamines. Although such control can be (see Table 8-17) and has been accomplished, it is by no means easy to mimic the subtle balance of responses achieved by the vasomotor center.

Effects of Thoracic Epidural Blockade on the Ischemic Heart[a]

During experimentally induced myocardial ischemia in anesthetized dogs it has been shown that thoracic epidural anesthesia (TEA) with a selective blockade of cardiac sympathetic segments favorably alters the myocardial oxygen supply/demand ratio.[126,226] Furthermore, during coronary occlusion TEA improved the transmural distribution of regional myocardial blood flow by increasing the endocardial-to-epicardial blood flow ratio, with maintenance of the coronary perfusion pressure.[226] The altered distribution of myocardial blood flow is most likely to occur by the decreased inotropy, heart rate, and impedance to left ventricular injection. Using a similar model, Davis et al. (1986) confirmed this observation.[126] The authors discovered that not only did thoracic sympathetic blockade enhance regional myocardial blood flow, but it also reduced the anatomic extent of the experimentally induced infarction. The most likely mechanism for this reduction in tissue injury was the pronounced reduction of heart rate and inotropy with little effect on coronary perfusion pressure observed in dogs with high TEA compared to control animals. In addition, the incidence of ischemia-induced malignant arrhythmias in anesthetized rats was reduced by high TEA.[33] Thus high TEA exerts a cardioprotective effect during experimental myocardial ischemia by improving the myocardial oxygen supply/demand ratio.

The influence of high thoracic epidural anesthesia with a plain solution of bupivacaine on central hemodynamics has been studied in patients with severe coronary artery disease and unstable angina pectoris.[34,36] During basal conditions, i.e., during rest without ischemic pain, high TEA did not change the central hemodynamic variables. However, TEA achieved during ischemic chest pain, was associated with significantly reduced indices of myocardial oxygen demand, such as systolic arterial blood pressure, heart rate, and pulmonary capillary wedge pressure, accompanied in some patients by less pronounced ST segment depression. The main variable regulating myocardial oxygen availability, coronary perfusion pressure, remained unchanged, as well as stroke volume, cardiac output, and systemic vascular resistance. Significant arterial hypotension did not occur, possibly due to limited spread of the small volumes of bupivacaine injected. On the other hand, a more extended TEA (from T1 to T12) caused pronounced arterial hypotension to the detriment of coronary perfusion in similar patients.[315] High TEA in association with physical stress also reduced ischemic chest pain and decreased heart rate in patients with unstable angina pectoris, in spite of maximal β-adrenergic blockade, to a greater degree than in patients with β-adrenergic blockers at rest.[34] Thus depending on the prevailing cardiac sympathetic tone, high TEA may cause a greater or lesser number of changes in central hemodynamics in patients with coronary artery disease (CAD) who are being treated with β-adrenergic blockers. Furthermore it has been reported that high TEA improves ischemia-induced left ventricular global and regional wall motion abnormalities, while diminishing associated changes in ST segments in patients with CAD during physical stress.[228] This is probably related to the decrease in left ventricular afterload *per se,* improving regional wall motion (see also Chapter 5, Table 5-9).

Regional cardiac sympathetic blockade with high TEA has been shown to increase the diameter of the lumina of diseased portions of epicardial coronary arteries in patients with severe coronary artery disease treated with beta-blockers.[35] However, the diameter of nonstenotic epicardial coronary artery segments remained unchanged. These results indicate that there is a resting cardiac sympathetic alpha constrictor tone of the atherosclerotic epicardial coronary arteries.

Regional cardiac sympathetic blockade caused no changes in coronary perfusion pressure, myocardial blood flow, or coronary venous oxygen content, indicating a lack of effect on coronary resistance vessels. High TEA had probably no influence upon the autoregulation of coronary resistance vessels; it should therefore not adversely affect regional blood flow distribution in patients with coronary artery disease with a pattern that provides a basis for coronary steal (i.e., maldistribution of coronary blood flow).[75,183]

Absorbed Local Anesthetics

Plain Solutions. Pharmacokinetic studies (see Chapter 3) have provided a precise picture of the blood concentration profile resulting from absorption of local anesthetics from the epidural space. This formed the basis for determining

[a] See also Meigner, A., *et al.*: Thoracic epidural anesthesia and the patient with heart disease. Anesth. Analg., *85*:1,1997.

systemic effects after intravenous infusion of local anesthetics to achieve blood concentrations similar to those occurring with epidural block. Early observations came from intravenous use of lidocaine in the treatment of cardiac arrhythmias.[181] At blood concentrations of lidocaine similar to those resulting from epidural blockade (3–5 μg/ml), Harrison reported excellent cardiovascular stability, even in patients with severe myocardial disease. Subsequent studies in healthy patients reported minimal changes in cardiovascular function with blood concentrations of lidocaine of 4 to 8 μg/ml.[212] Indeed, there was even some evidence of cardiovascular stimulation. The latter was postulated as the cause of surprising increases in cardiac output, cardiac rate, and mean arterial pressure associated with thoracic epidural block accomplished with large incremental doses of lidocaine (1500 mg). Because these changes were not reported by other studies of thoracic blockade, Bonica and colleagues postulated that the high blood concentrations of lidocaine (4–7 μg/ml) resulted in stimulatory effects on the circulation.[41] Such stimulation was thought to be caused by a central effect of lidocaine enhancing sympathetic activity by means of remaining cardiac sympathetic fibers. An alternative peripheral mechanism would have to invoke potentiation of peripheral sympathetic activity. Although local anesthetics can exert a biphasic effect on vascular smooth muscle (see Chapter 3), it seems unlikely that a peripheral mechanism is responsible for the changes observed by Bonica and colleagues.[41]

Epinephrine-Containing Solutions. The preceding discussion has focused on studies using plain solutions of local anesthetic. Vascular absorption of added epinephrine does result in systemic actions on β-adrenergic receptors. It is now well established that the cardiovascular effects of low-dose epinephrine are quite different from its traditional picture of tachycardia, hypertension, and peripheral ischemia. Systemic effects of doses of epinephrine in the range of 80 to 130 μg, as used in epidural block, are a moderate increase in heart rate, increased cardiac output, decreased peripheral resistance, and decreased mean arterial pressure. Bonica and colleagues[40] attribute these effects solely to β-adrenergic stimulation. In order to investigate this hypothesis, they administered epinephrine epidurally without local anesthetic in doses similar to those usually incorporated in local anesthetic solutions (80–130 μg). The epinephrine *per se* produced changes similar to those seen with epinephrine-containing local anesthetics, except that the changes were of lesser magnitude and shorter lived. Also, Bromage[65] has postulated that the epinephrine-containing solutions result in more profound sympathetic neural blockade, in a manner similar to the increase in intensity of motor blockade that results from epinephrine-containing solutions.[66] There is direct evidence that epidural and subarachnoid local anesthetic blockade may produce a variable degree of sympathetic blockade. Using the skin conductance response and laser Doppler flowmetry, sympathetic blockade was much lower in segmental level, and of briefer duration, than sensory block[22] (see Chapter 13). Indirect support is provided by Bonica's observation that two out of ten of his subjects failed to develop evidence of sympathetic blockade despite sensory analgesia to T1.[41] Furthermore, Cousins and Wright[112] observed that, in patients with postoperative pain, abolition of vasoconstrictor responses sometimes did not occur with 1% plain lidocaine but appeared more satisfactory with 2% plain lidocaine. They attributed this effect to more profound sensory blockade with better "deafferentation" of the operative site and prevention of adrenal medullary release of catecholamines; level of blockade was only from T7 to T10 in these studies (i.e., incomplete denervation of adrenal medulla). However, it is entirely possible that the stronger solution produced more effective sympathetic nerve penetration over the same number of segments or over a more extensive area. The latter may be important, since there is ample evidence of large individual variations in extent of sympathetic innervation of upper and lower limbs.[148]

The most likely explanations for the more pronounced cardiovascular effects of epinephrine-containing local anesthetic solutions appear to be as follows:

1. Systemic absorption of epinephrine: β-adrenergic effects on the heart, resulting in increased heart rate and cardiac output; peripheral vascular β-adrenergic effects, resulting in further vasodilatation within the area of sympathetic block and antagonism of compensatory vasoconstrictor responses outside the area of blockade. Thus, total peripheral resistance falls, and mean arterial blood pressure is reduced to a degree comparable to that seen with equivalent levels of subarachnoid blockade (Fig. 8-18).
2. More intense neural penetration or more extensive spread of neural blockade, resulting in more reliable sympathetic block.

Hypovolemia and Epidural Block

It has long been said that subarachnoid or epidural neural blockade may result in dangerously accentuated cardiovascular depression in the presence of uncorrected hypovolemia. However, this was largely anecdotal until the studies of Bonica and colleagues. Healthy volunteers received epidural block to T5 with and without epinephrine. Subjects were normovolemic or had undergone withdrawal of 13% of blood volume.[40–42] In comparison to the mild cardiovascular changes at normovolemia, major reductions in heart rate, cardiac output, and mean arterial pressure occurred in the presence of hypovolemia; in five of seven patients who had received plain solutions of lidocaine, vigorous resuscitation, including ephedrine administration, was required. Cardiovascular homeostasis was better maintained with epinephrine-lidocaine blockade. However, marked reductions in mean arterial blood pressure still occurred (Fig. 8-20). Because cardiac sympathetic fibers were thought not to be blocked in these patients, an explanation was sought for the large reductions in heart rate and cardiac output. Morikawa and colleagues repeated the same studies of plain

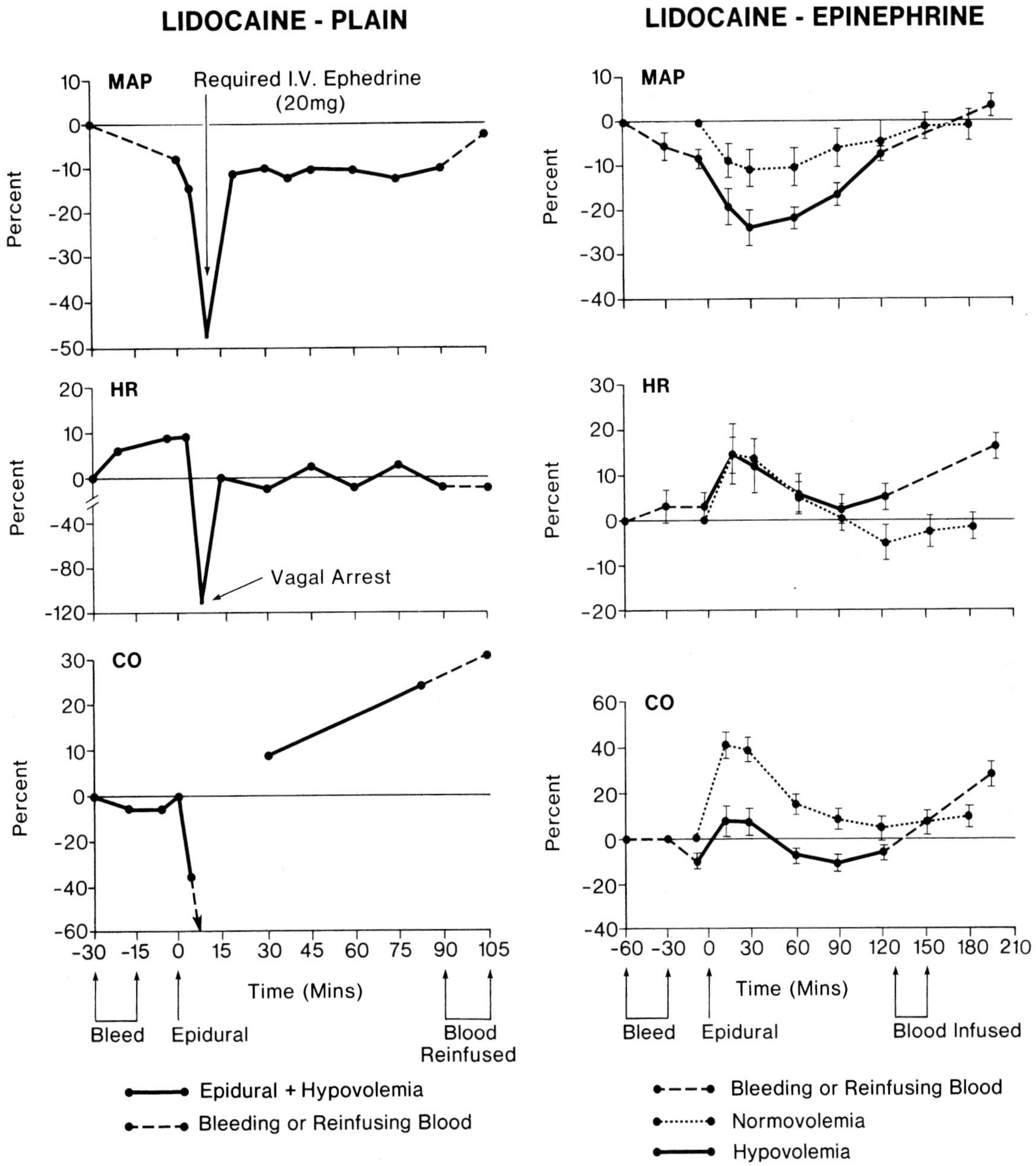

FIG. 8-20. Cardiovascular effects of epidural block, effect of hypovolemia in conscious volunteers; epidural block to T5 with plain and epinephrine-containing solutions. The mean percentage of change is shown for each variable. **Right:** Lidocaine–epinephrine. The cardiovascular changes after lidocaine-epinephrine in the presence of normovolemia are compared with hypovolemia (−13%). During normovolemia, note the marked increase in heart rate and cardiac output, lasting about 60 minutes. During hypovolemia, mean arterial pressure is significantly lower (−23%), but cardiac output remains close to control levels as a result of an elevated heart rate. **Left:** Lidocaine plain. A representation of a typical response is shown. Severe bradycardia is associated with extreme hypotension, and in two subjects, vagal arrest occurred that required rapid resuscitation with ephedrine and oxygen. In only one subject was hypotension associated with increased heart rate, and this prevented the extreme hypotension seen in the other five subjects. (Modified from data of Bonica, J.J., Berges, P.U., and Morikawa, K.: Circulatory effects of epidural block: I. Effects of levels of analgesia and dose of lidocaine. Anesthesiology, *33*:1619, 1970; Bonica, J.J., Akamatsu, T.J., Berges, P.U., Morikawa, K., *et al.*: Circulatory effects of epidural block: II. Effects of epinephrine. Anesthesiology, *34*:514, 1971 and Bonica, J.J., *et al.*: Anesthesiology, *36*:219, 1972.)

lidocaine in anesthetized dogs.[271] Although they recorded large reductions in mean arterial pressure and cardiac output, heart rate was not reduced and cardiovascular collapse did not occur in the presence of withdrawal of 13% of blood volume. It thus seemed likely that the sudden bradycardia resulting in cardiovascular collapse in human subjects may have been due to parasympathetic activity similar to that seen in the "faint" response to decreased venous return.[52] This sudden increase in parasympathetic activity is a vagal response to marked reductions in venous return[18] (Tables 8-10 and 8-11; Fig. 8-21). Usually this response occurs only in conscious humans (and in no other species) and is abolished by general anesthesia. It is worth emphasizing that severe reductions in venous return, such as those observed in Bonica's study,[42] result in a sudden large increase in vagal activity[283–286] (Fig. 8-21). Thus, a patient's condition may suddenly deteriorate to the point of loss of consciousness and perhaps asystole. This situation may be confused with "cardiac toxicity" if bupivacaine is the local anesthetic used. However, "cardiac toxicity" usually occurs soon after injection of the local anesthetic, whereas there is a time lag for the response described above.

What factors were responsible for the somewhat less pronounced cardiovascular depression in hypovolemic subjects receiving epidural block with lidocaine-epinephrine? It has already been noted that absorbed lidocaine-epinephrine results in increased heart rate and cardiac output, but a lower mean arterial pressure, owing to decreased peripheral resistance, compared with plain lidocaine; however, the higher cardiac rate may protect the heart from increases in vagal ac-

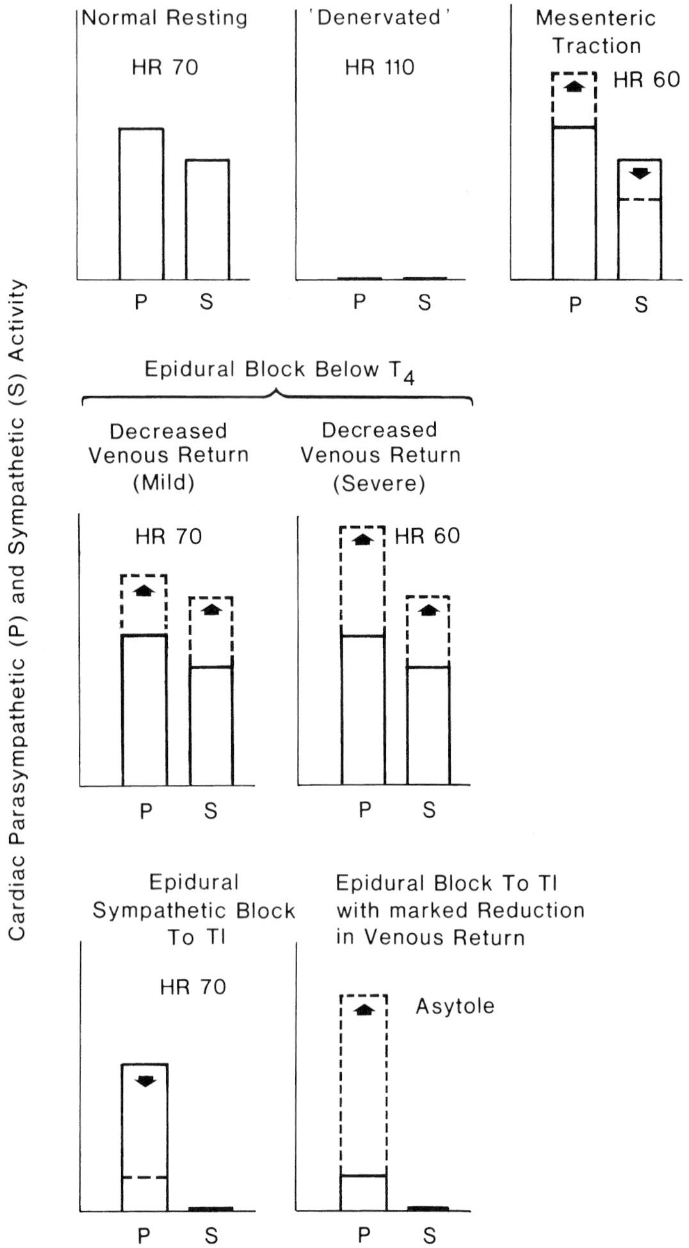

FIG. 8-21. Vagal effects of epidural block. **Top, left:** The balance of cardiac parasympathetic *(P)* activity and sympathetic *(S)* activity is shown with a normal resting heart rate of 70. **Top, middle**: The presence of a heart rate of 110 following complete "denervation" of the heart emphasizes the dominant action of the vagus. **Top, right:** Autonomic reflexes such as mesenteric traction usually result in bradycardia by an opposite change in P and S. **Center:** Epidural block to T4. **Center, left:** A mild reduction in venous return results in increased vagal tone,[18] which may offset the increase in sympathetic tone (arterial baroreceptors) so that heart rate is unchanged or slightly decreased. **Center, right:** Marked reduction in venous return stimulates a marked increase in P, and S increases in an attempt to minimize the bradycardia. **Bottom:** Epidural block to T1. **Bottom, left:** Usual situation, in which P has diminished to compensate for a blocked S. A heart rate of 70 is the result of the same dominance of P over S that exists at rest; however, P is now completely unopposed. **Bottom, right:** Marked reduction in venous return (or other stimulus to P) results in unopposed increase in P, which may lead to asystole. Such responses are much more likely in the conscious patient.

tivity, although it has been noted that a high level of sympathetic activity may accentuate cholinergic effects in patients with poor venous return.[286] It is also possible that peak arterial blood concentrations of lidocaine were higher after plain lidocaine in patients with hypovolemia, owing to decreased cardiac output and thus a smaller volume of distribution (see Chapter 3, Table 3-12). In this situation, the myocardium receives a larger percentage of cardiac output and thus is potentially exposed to higher concentrations of local anesthetics (see Chapter 4, Fig. 4-19). Any coexistent hypercapnia or acidosis would tend to accentuate the depressant effects of local anesthetic on the myocardium (see Chapter 3). The moral of Bonica's study is clear[43]: Epidural block should be avoided or used with great care in patients with uncorrected hypovolemia or in any other patient in whom venous return is markedly impaired (e.g., patients with large intra-abdominal masses in whom the pressure of the mass on the vena cava cannot be relieved before blockade; see Fig. 8-15).

Thoracic-Epidural Anesthesia and General Anesthesia

TEA associated with light general anesthesia is increasingly used for upper abdominal surgery and for major vascular surgery. Light general anesthesia with mechanical ventilation added to thoracic epidural anesthesia may induce substantial hypotension. Such hypotension arises mainly from a decrease in venous return and is also due to attenuation of the compensatory vasoconstriction of nonanesthetized sympathetic tone via central depressant effects on vasomotor center. Thus a combined technique of TEA plus light general anesthesia may alter hemodynamics, principally by a decrease in the loading conditions of the heart and by a negative inotropic effect resulting from both the cardiac sympathetic blockade and the direct myocardial depressant effect of general anesthesia.[314,405]

Obviously the greatest concern for the consequences of hypotension is in patients with coronary artery disease. Coronary artery disease is common in patients undergoing major vascular surgery. Therefore these patients are prone to develop cardiac complications.[377] Several studies have demonstrated a beneficial effect of TEA on the heart and coronary circulation in patients with coronary artery disease (see Effects of Thoracic Epidural Blockade on the Ischemic Heart).[34–36,228] However, this beneficial effect cannot be extrapolated to patients receiving TEA combined with light general anesthesia. The fall in blood pressure induced by such a technique may compromise coronary blood flow and so myocardial oxygen supply, despite a decrease in myocardial oxygen consumption. In this context, Saada et al. (1992) examined the effect of TEA, induced during light general anesthesia, on segmental ventricular wall motion (SWM) as monitored by transesophageal echocardiography.[328] In patients with coronary artery disease scheduled for major vascular surgery, 12.5 ml of lidocaine 2% was injected through an epidural catheter placed at T6–T7 or T7–T8 30 minutes after induction of general anesthesia. TEA induced a decrease in heart rate, mean arterial pressure, cardiac index, and estimated coronary perfusion pressure due to sympathetic blockade. Pulmonary occlusion pressure remained constant owing to colloid infusion. Despite these reductions, TEA plus light general anesthesia did not worsen (or improve) ventricular wall motion or induce myocardial ischemia, suggesting that myocardial oxygen balance was maintained. In an earlier almost identical study by the same group it was shown that lumbar epidural anesthesia may cause impairment of SWM, indicating myocardial ischemia.[329] In comparing these two studies it would seem that block of the efferent sympathetic innervation to the heart that occurs with TEA but not with lumbar epidural blockade has beneficial effects.

Despite prophylactic intravenous hydration, TEA plus general anesthesia may cause hypotension requiring vasopressor therapy. In clinical practice ephedrine and phenylephrine are the two agents that are commonly recommended to treat hypotension during epidural anesthesia associated with general anesthesia.[411] Ideally the vasopressor agent should restore blood pressure without increasing heart rate or impairing left ventricular function. Ephedrine and phenylephrine may differently affect left ventricular (LV) function in high-risk patients. Accordingly, Samain et al. (1989) determined the effects of ephedrine versus phenylephrine on LV function in high-risk patients who developed arterial hypotension during high thoracic epidural anesthesia combined with general anesthesia.[332] Level of analgesia extended to T3 in these patients who received epidural block before general anesthesia. LV function was assessed by transesophageal echocardiography. Both cardiac index and ejection fraction area were significantly compromised when phenylephrine was given. This is consistent with the results of Goertz (1993), who determined the effect of phenylephrine bolus administration on LV function during TEA combined with general anesthesia in patients with cardiovascular disease.[169] When ephedrine was given, no acceleration of heart rate was noted. In addition, the rise in blood pressure did not compromise LV emptying. Thus ephedrine appears to be the drug of choice to restore blood pressure under TEA associated with general anesthesia.

Lumbar Epidural Block and General Anesthesia

Lumbar epidural anesthesia combined with general anesthesia is commonly used for prolonged major lower abdominal and pelvic surgery. Combined epidural and general anesthesia offers the advantage of a rapid and less painful recovery. This combination technique may result in a greater degree of hypotension than with each technique alone. However, the cardiovascular effects of combined lumbar epidural and general anesthesia have received relatively little attention in the literature to date.

Stephen and colleagues[364] studied the combination of lumbar epidural block administered approximately 20 minutes after the induction of light anesthesia consisting of thiopentone, nitrous oxide and oxygen. Unfortunately, the level of blockade could not be recorded in this study, although it was likely to be in the region of T5, considering the dose of local anesthetic used (30 ml of 2% plain lidocaine). This combination produced large reductions in arterial blood pressure up to 30%. Elevation of legs (to simulate a head-down tilt) resulted in increased mean arterial pressure, central venous pressure, and peripheral resistance, but no change in cardiac output, whereas intravenous bolus administration of ephedrine (10 mg) increased both cardiac output and mean arterial pressure. Further reductions in arterial pressure were observed when epinephrine was added to the epidurally administered local anesthetic solution.[343] The absorbed epinephrine stimulates β-adrenergic receptors in peripheral vascular beds, leading to vasodilatation and hypotension.

Germann and colleagues demonstrated that there were no significant differences between the hemodynamic effects of placing lumbar epidural catheter with a dose of plain lidocaine before or after the induction of anesthesia, consisting of thiopentone, nitrous oxide, oxygen, and succinylcholine.[161] The level of analgesia extended to T6 (± two segments) in patients who received epidural block before general anesthesia, and it was assumed that similar levels were achieved in those who had epidural block induced before general anesthesia. Mean arterial blood pressure decreased to 35% below control values. Head-down tilt did not affect the hemodynamic variables during established epidural block and general anesthesia. In contrast, subsequent administrations of 0.6 mg intravenous atropine resulted in a return of arterial pressure to essentially baseline values. Decreased venous return associated with this level of analgesia will result in increased vagal activity[18] (see Fig. 8-21 and Table 8-10).

Nancarrow and associates compared the cardiovascular effects of epidural block to T5 level, given before nitrous oxide-halothane (0.35% end-tidal) general anesthesia, with the same general anesthesia minus epidural block.[276] Decreases in mean arterial pressure were significantly greater (up to 58%) in the epidural group, whereas no changes were observed in the general anesthesia group. However, decreases in liver blood flow and reductive metabolism of halothane were similar in both groups, despite the occurrence of significant decreases in arterial pressure.[276]

Wright and Fee (1992) examined the effect of prophylactic treatment with intravenous fluid, 1000 ml, and ephedrine or methoxamine on cardiovascular responses to combined lumbar epidural anesthesia and isoflurane general anesthesia.[411] Systolic arterial pressure was significantly greater after ephedrine than after preloading or methoxamine. The reduction in arterial blood pressure after induction of general anesthesia was associated with a decrease in vascular resistance after methoxamine. A decrease in venous return, resulting mostly in hypotension during epidural block, is less likely to occur following prophylactic administration of ephedrine, since the systemic vascular resistance is maintained at preblock values. Goertz et al. (1993) demonstrated that administration of phenylephrine boluses effectively restored mean arterial pressure in patients who were moderately hypotensive during lumbar epidural anesthesia combined with general anesthesia.[169] The range of the level of analgesia was T8–T11. In addition, the left ventricular function assessed by transesophageal echocardiography was unaltered.

In summary, it appears that light general anesthesia can be safely combined with epidural block to the level of T5 in healthy patients. Use of a slight head-down tilt to maintain venous return and small incremental doses of atropine to maintain heart rate of approximately 90 beats per minute are recommended to treat moderate hypotension during combined lumbar epidural and general anesthesia. If additional cardiovascular support is required, ephedrine should be used depending on each patient's cardiovascular status.

Important Aspects of Venous Return and Epidural Blockade

As indicated in Tables 8-10 and 8-11 and in Figure 8-21, reduced venous return may play a dominant role in initiating sudden reductions in cardiac rate, which should be viewed as a danger signal that venous return is markedly reduced and oxygenation of the myocardium is at risk. There is no doubt that obstruction to venous return, by whatever means, must be avoided in patients being given epidural block. If postural changes are added to obstruction in the presence of the increased venous capacitance of epidural block, serious impairment of venous return will follow. In addition, pressure in epidural veins will rise owing to channeling of blood from the pelvis by way of the alternative route of the vertebral venous plexus and azygos vein to the right atrium; this has important consequences for increased spread of segmental analgesia and may impair arterial blood flow to the spinal cord.[357] Partial occlusion of the inferior vena cava in dogs has been reported to markedly decrease cardiac output and increase the resuscitation time for cardiac toxicity resulting from intravascular injection of bupivacaine. Also, much larger doses of epinephrine and bicarbonate were required for resuscitation.[216] Although not measured, presumably peak arterial concentrations of bupivacaine were much higher in animals with inferior vena cava occlusion.

Situations in which venous return may be compromised may be summarized (see Fig. 8-15):

Supine hypotensive syndrome in pregnancy resulting from uterine compression of the vena cava is accentuated by increased venous capacitance owing to sympathetic block of epidural analgesia and postural changes favoring pooling of blood in the lower limbs.[339,340]

Uterine contraction during labor in supine position may cause compression. Mean brachial arterial pressure may be maintained at deceptively normal levels because of simultaneous compression of vena cava and aorta (Poseiro effect). However, mean femoral arterial pressure drops precipitously, as does uterine blood flow.[29] These effects are accentuated by epidural block if the patient is allowed to remain supine.

Intestinal obstruction, ascites, and large intra-abdominal tumors may compress the vena cava at three main sites: (i) *below the liver*, owing to abdominal distention, by intestinal obstruction,[21] or by ascites[310] (this site is also commonly occluded by overenthusiastic retraction or by abdominal packs during upper abdominal surgery); (ii) *in the upper lumbar region*, by large intra-abdominal tumors (including the uterus); and (iii) *at the pelvic brim*, by stretching of the iliac vessels owing to extreme backward tilting of the pelvis. This is sometimes an accompaniment of later pregnancy and may also result from extreme lordotic posturing on the operating table. The "extended lordotic posture" may occlude the vena cava below the liver as well—with potential for venous congestion in the kidney and resultant proteinuria.[76]

The most common causes of vena caval obstruction in surgical applications of epidural block are poor positioning, heavy-handed retraction, and incorrect use of abdominal packs. Extreme positions, such as the jackknife prone, lateral "kidney," and hyperflexed lithotomy, should be avoided in association with any anesthetic and with epidural block in particular.[251,339] Whenever possible, caval obstruction should be relieved before epidural block or carefully avoided after epidural block. If it occurs and cannot be corrected for a period of time, venous return may be assisted by restoring venous capacitance to normal levels by using carefully titrated doses of ephedrine (5-10 mg) intravenously. In some patients with large abdominal tumors, both the aorta and the vena cava may be partially obstructed, but with maintenance of sufficient venous return to keep mean arterial pressure normal, with a partly occluded aorta. Sudden relief of the aortic obstruction as the tumor is removed may cause a precipitous fall in blood pressure owing to the reactive hyperemia below the level of obstruction. This situation may be avoided by ensuring adequate hydration and perhaps by using appropriate amounts of colloid before tumor removal. Also, one should be prepared to use small doses of ephedrine until reactive hyperemia subsides.

Epidural Blockade and Reduction of Blood Loss

Although initial emphasis on methods to reduce operative blood loss focused on reduction of arterial blood pressure,[142] it was also well known that position played an important part.[142]

There has been a gradual recognition of the importance of avoidance of venous obstruction and the use of position in combination with sympathetic blockade to aid venous pooling away from the operative site. Thus, although epidural blockade has been used to produce hypotension and, in turn, control operative blood loss,[381,382] others have found that blood loss can be reduced without the levels of hypotension commonly required if general anesthesia and hypotensive drugs are used.[222,374] Keith deliberately avoided arterial hypotension in a randomized prospective study of blood loss using epidural or general anesthesia for surgery for total hip replacement.[222] Blood loss intraoperatively was determined by a colorimetric technique and postoperatively by closed suction drains. Patients receiving epidural block had operative blood losses that were half those associated with general anesthesia. In contrast, there was no difference in postoperative blood losses between the two groups. Other studies reported a reduction in blood loss by 30% to 40% if epidural block is used for hip surgery.[267,362] Thus, it appears that epidural block may reduce operative blood loss by factors other than a mild reduction in arterial blood pressure, increased venous capacitance,[356] and the use of appropriate position. Additional factors may include the prevention of high venous pressure in response to sympathetic activity resulting from pain,[65] avoidance of "reactive arterial hypertension," and avoidance of increased airway pressure with resultant effects on venous pressure (see also Chapter 5, Fig. 5-22).

Function of Hollow Viscera After Epidural Blockade

The Bladder

One of the most commonly observed sequels of lumbar epidural block is temporary atonia of the bladder owing to blockade of sacral segments S2–S4. This is similar to lower motor neuron lesions in which bladder sensation is lost. Fortunately, this type of effect after epidural blockade is usually short-lived and causes no or minimal increases in postblock bladder dysfunction.[116]

When continuous epidural techniques are used, however, catheterization of the bladder may be necessary.[195] On the other hand, segmental thoracic epidural block (e.g., T5–L1) may spare the sacral segments and thus leave bladder sensation intact. In addition, relief of severe abdominal pain by epidural block from T5 to L1 may prevent reflex sympathetic activity (via T12–L1 spinal segments), which increases bladder sphincter tone and may predispose to acute retention.

The Gut

Epidural block extending from T6 to L1 effectively denervates the splanchnic sympathetic supply to the abdominal viscera (see Chapter 13, Figs. 13-1 and 13-2). The sympathetic blockade results in a small contracted gut owing to parasympathetic dominance. However, the question has been raised whether this predisposes to postoperative ileus.

Gelman et al. (1977) demonstrated that epidural anesthesia increased the electrical activity of the stomach and intestine after cholecystectomy.[160] Also, volunteer studies indicate that gastric emptying was not delayed during thoracic epidural anesthesia with local anesthetics.[372] Epidural morphine injected at the T4 level, however, delayed gastric emptying, as evidenced by slow absorption of acetaminophen. These results suggest that intraoperative and postoperative epidural anesthesia with local anesthetic agents may be useful in preventing and relieving postoperative ileus. Discrepancies exist, however, between studies that have examined the effect of epidural anesthesia on gastrointestinal motility. In patients undergoing cholecystectomy, propulsive colonic motility did not return faster in patients who had been given epidural anesthesia with local anesthetics than in those who had received parenteral opioids.[401] On the other hand, after gastrointestinal surgery the transit time of barium contrast and the time until the passing of flatus and feces were significantly shorter in patients who received postoperative epidural anesthesia with bupivacaine than in those who had been given opioid injection[6] or epidural morphine.[335] Thus there is evidence that compared with parenteral and epidural opioids, epidural anesthesia with local anesthetics shortens the duration of postoperative colonic ileus (see Chapter 5, Fig. 5-25).

Although there has been some concern about the effects of accelerated bowel motility on the integrity of gut anastomotic lines, this fear has never been supported by controlled studies. However, retrospective studies show that colorectal leak rate was lower with combined epidural and general anesthesia than with general anesthesia alone.[327] The lowest leak rate was reported in patients receiving combined epidural and general anesthesia intraoperatively and continuous epidural bupivacaine for postoperative pain relief. The highest wound dehiscence rate was observed when epidural morphine analgesia was given postoperatively. Blood flow in the intestine, as assessed by laser Doppler flowmetry, has been shown to increase in patients undergoing colon surgery under epidural anesthesia.[210] This increase may be beneficial and may contribute to the healing of the gut anastomoses if epidural local anesthetic agents are used for postoperative analgesia (see Chapter 5, pages 162–163).

Thus epidural anesthesia with local anesthetics seems to be the best method for relieving pain after gastrointestinal surgery because of its minimal effects on gastric emptying, stimulating effects on bowel motility, and possibly beneficial effects on the integrity of bowel anastomoses. Additional prospective studies are clearly indicated to investigate the role of epidural anesthesia in the postoperative gastrointestinal outcome.

Thermoregulation and Shivering

Hypothermia (a decrease in core temperature) is common in patients undergoing surgery with epidural anesthesia and is thought to result from heat loss to the cold environment due to sympathectomy-induced vasodilatation. The normal process by which thermoregulation usually minimizes intraoperative core temperature is prevented, since epidural anesthesia directly inhibits vasoconstriction in the analgesic dermatomes. However, recent studies investigating the thermal balance during epidural anesthesia demonstrated that hypothermia following epidural injection of local anesthetic solution may result in part from redistribution of heat from central to peripheral regions.[166,206,348] Sympathectomy-induced vasodilatation produced central hypothermia via net convection of heat from warmer central to cooler peripheral tissues. The net effect is an increase in peripheral tissue temperature at the expense of decreased central temperature. Warming the body via the skin for 2 hours before inducing epidural anesthesia raised the skin temperature (but not the core temperature) and helped prevent hypothermia during the induction of epidural anesthesia.[166] These results support the hypothesis that redistribution of heat within the body, not heat loss to the environment, is the most important etiology of hypothermia from epidural anesthesia.

Shivering-like tremors occur in approximately 30% of patients with epidural anesthesia. The relationship of shivering-like tremors to the hypothermia associated with epidural anesthesia is unclear, as the onset of tremor does not always coincide with the decrease in central temperature. In addition, those tremors are not always accompanied by a sensation of coldness.[167] The decrease in core temperature triggers thermoregulatory vasoconstriction and shivering above the level of epidural anesthesia.[206,348] Patients with uncontrollable tremor during epidural anesthesia do not necessarily feel cold, probably because epidural local anesthetics inhibit tonic cutaneous cold receptor input to hypothalamic thermoregulatory centers.[167] Therefore skin temperature is probably more important than decreased central temperature in determining thermal perception. Tremor is preceded by central hypothermia, and electromyographic (EMG) analyses of tremor pattern were quantatively similar to those produced by normal thermoregulatory shivering in cold-exposed volunteers.[206,348] Also, warming the body before inducing epidural anesthesia limited the occurrence of shiver-like tremor because of a smaller decrease in core temperature.[167] Therefore it is likely that most tremors during epidural anesthesia in nonpregnant subjects are primarily due to normal thermoregulatory shivering.

A direct effect of cold solutions injected into the epidural space upon thermosensitive structures within the spinal cord may cause shivering during epidural anesthesia. Two peripartum studies have demonstrated that tremors during epidural anesthesia were significantly more common after cold (4°) than warm (37°) bupivacaine administration.[306,402] Additionally, epidural injection of warm anesthetic stopped shivering, suggesting that pregnancy may enhance the contribution of spinal thermoregulatory input. However, an influence of epidural injectate temperature on tremor intensity in nonpregnant subjects could not be demonstrated.[348] Therefore the role of spinal or epidural thermoreceptors in initiating shivering during epidural anesthesia is likely to be minimal.

Proposed nonthermoregulatory etiologies include systemic absorption of epidurally administered local anesthetic and central transfer of epidural anesthetic in cerebrospinal fluid. Intravenous lidocaine in doses sufficient to approximate the plasma levels of lidocaine during epidural anesthesia did not affect core temperature, vasoconstriction, or shivering in response to cold and is therefore unlikely to contribute to tremor or shivering.[168]

Injection of either epidural meperidine (25 mg) or epidural fentanyl (50 μg) has been reported to abolish shivering during epidural local analgesia in a high percentage of patients in labor[72,355] and during cesarean section.[367]

In summary, tremor during epidural anesthesia is due to normal thermoregulatory shivering, which results largely from central hypothermia and is preceded by peripheral vasoconstriction above the level of sympathetic blockade.

Neuroendocrine Effects of Epidural Blockade

Surgical stress is associated with a variety of changes in endocrine and metabolic function, including protein metabolism, leading to a state of negative nitrogen balance in the postoperative period. Most of the surgically induced endocrine and metabolic changes (increased plasma concentrations of catecholamines, cortisol, glucose, antidiuretic hormone and growth hormone) are abolished by an appropriate level of sensory blockade produced by regional anesthesia. The mechanism by which epidural anesthesia may diminish endocrine changes and metabolic alterations during surgery is probably related to a blockade of either afferent or efferent pathways or both. The extent of the epidural blockade and the site of surgery will influence the degree of inhibitory effect on the stress response to surgical procedures.[220] If the level of anesthesia extends from T4 to S5 and if the epidural blockade is initiated before the onset of surgery, epidural anesthesia for lower abdominal procedures and operations on the lower extremities may completely abolish the hormonal and metabolic response. However epidural anesthesia is less efficient in decreasing the surgical stress response to major upper abdominal and thoracic procedures.[189] This is probably due to the inability of the epidural anesthetic to completely block all nociceptive afferent pathways.[220] The role of the open afferent vagal pathway is probably of minor importance in this context, based upon experimental and clinical studies (see Chapter 5). At present the most plausible explanation is incomplete afferent somatic and sympathetic blockade.[220] Also, there is evidence that the afferent neural impulses as well as humoral factors, such as cytokines, which are released from the site of action, may initiate the stress response in the hypothalamus during upper abdominal surgery.[275]

Epidural opioids are widely used in the management of postoperative pain relief. Despite providing complete pain relief, epidural opioids are less effective than local anesthetics in blocking the stress response, indicating that pain relief *per se* does not modify the stress response.[400] However, combinations of local anesthetics and opioids administered epidurally in the postoperative period provide more complete blunting of the neuroendocrine response than opioids.[108]

The important clinical question, whether the reduction in stress response may lead to an improvement in postoperative morbidity and mortality, has not been finally answered. Results are inconclusive to date, despite some improvements in a few indices such as thromboembolic complication, nitrogen balance, and reduced immunocompetence.[108] Further studies are clearly needed to answer that question. The metabolic alterations observed during surgery and the modifying effect of intra- and postoperative epidural anesthesia-analgesia on the metabolic stress response to surgery are discussed in detail in Chapter 5. However, the focus of postoperative pain relief has now shifted since it has been recognized that pain relief must be provided in a way that permits rapid return of physical and mental activity, as part of "acute rehabilitation"[108,221] (see Chapter 5, Fig. 5-26).

Vasoactive hormones

Current evidence suggests that the arginine-vasopressin (AVP) system and the renin-angiotensin system (RAS) play an important role in maintaining arterial blood pressure under conditions in which the sympathetic system is impaired.[48,308] Angiotensin, the most effective constrictor of resistance vessels, plays a dominant role in stabilization of arterial blood pressure, whereas vasopressin apparently comes into play as the last line of defense, when the filling of the heart is reduced to the extent that cardiac output can no longer be maintained.[308] Experimentally the role that RAS and AVP play in maintaining blood pressure can be studied by administering specific antagonists of these vasopressor systems and measuring the resultant effect on blood pressure.

Studies in awake sedated dogs demonstrated that high thoracic epidural anesthesia is associated with hemodynamically effective increases in vasopressin concentrations.[303] On the other hand, profound hypotension occurred during high thoracic epidural anesthesia when AVPA, a specific vasopressin V1-receptor antagonist, was administered, preventing vasopressin from acting.

Renin plasma concentrations did not change significantly despite the marked hypotension observed after combined sympathetic and vasopressin blockade. Therefore loss of neurogenic vasomotor control during high epidural anesthesia in dogs is most likely to be compensated for by an intact vasopressin system. In addition, vasopressin plasma concentrations, which increase considerably during epidural anesthesia alone, increase even more when epidural is combined with additional challenges such as severe hypoxemia.[303] The increase in vasopressin concentrations is most likely to compensate for decreased cardiac filling and/or arterial blood pressure when sympathoadrenal responses are impaired.

In contrast to the findings of Peters,[303] Carp et al. (1994) found that both renin and vasopressin support blood pressure and prevent severe hypotension following epidural anesthesia.[83] They studied healthy volunteers and administered lidocaine through a lumbar epidural catheter to obtain a sensory block to T2. Blood pressure did not change after T2-epidural anesthesia in subjects treated with the vasopressin antagonist AVPA; however, the plasma concentrations of renin increased.

Conversely when the angiotensin-converting enzyme inhibitor enalapril was administered, epidural anesthesia was not associated with hypotension, but the concentration of vasopressin increased. In contrast, combined treatment with both inhibitors resulted in a marked decrease in blood pressure by more than 30% after epidural anesthesia. In healthy humans, therefore, AVP and RAS both play an important role in maintaining blood pressure after epidural blockade. Differences between the study of Peters in dogs[303] and the study of Carp in humans[83] may be attributable to species differences in the hierarchy of blood pressure regulation.

Hopf et al. (1994) examined the relative importance of these systems in surgical patients exposed to a hypotensive challenge.[197] Nonpremedicated patients without cardiovascular disease, scheduled for elective upper abdominal surgery, received an intravenous infusion of sodium nitroprusside (SNP) to achieve a 25% reduction in mean arterial pressure. Thereafter epidural anesthesia was induced with bupivacaine to obtain a sensory block from T1–T11. After thoracic epidural anesthesia was fully established, the challenge with the SNP dose was adjusted to achieve the same mean arterial pressure as with the sympathetic system intact. Active renin and vasopressin concentrations were measured in response to SNP-induced arterial hypotension both before and during sympathetic blockade by epidural anesthesia. SNP-induced hypotension was associated with increased plasma renin concentrations with the sympathetic system intact, but not during sympathetic blockade by thoracic epidural anesthesia. Vasopressin plasma concentrations increased during SNP-induced hypotension in the presence of widespread epidural sympathetic blockade, but not with the sympathetic system intact (see Fig. 8-22B). With sympathetic innervation intact, SNP infusion increased heart rate and decreased mean arterial pressure. During sympathetic blockade by epidural anesthesia, the responses to the second hypotensive challenge were significantly different from the first: heart rate increased by less than the half of the increase following the first challenge (see Fig. 8-22A).

In summary, sympathetic blockade by thoracic epidural anesthesia abolished the increase in renin activity in response to arterial hypotension. This indicates in humans that the renal sympathetic system probably plays a key role in mediating renin release in response to hypotension. In addition, thoracic epidural anesthesia activates the vasopressin system in response to hypotension.

Understanding the role of these endogenous vasopressor systems in maintaining blood pressure after epidural blockade in healthy subjects may help to explain why certain high-risk patients become hypotensive during high thoracic epidural anesthesia.

Effects of Epidural Blockade on Respiration

Two important questions concerning respiration and epidural blockade require an answer: Does epidural block interfere with respiration? Is the ability to cough impaired?

The following aspects of epidural blockade may influence respiration:

Aspects of Epidural Blockade That May Influence Respiration
Sensory ("afferent") neural blockade reduces nociceptive afferent drive to respiratory center
Motor ("efferent") neural blockade of intercostal muscles, abdominal muscles, and diaphragm (rarely)
Sympathetic neural blockade with resultant changes in cardiac output and pulmonary blood flow
Vagal dominance in the presence of complete sympathetic blockade
Effects of systematically absorbed epinephrine and local anesthetic on:
Respiratory control center in midbrain and on chemoreceptors in medulla and carotid bodies
Myoneural junction
Metabolism of succinylcholine in serum

The potential for phrenic (C3–C5) palsy is extremely low with epidural block, since even blockade to T1 produces motor blockade to only the T4–T5 level. The only exception may be intentional epidural block at the cervical level or inadvertent epidural block during interscalene brachial plexus block (see Chapter 10).

Respiratory arrest during high epidural blockade is not usually the result of the effects of sensory or motor blockade, nor is it due to depressant effects of local anesthetic in the CSF; the concentrations attained in the brain by means of this route are insufficient to depress neuronal activity unless gross overdosage is administered.[67] The most common causes of the rare instances of respiratory arrest associated with epidural block are extensive sympathetic blockade, reduced cardiac output, and reduced oxygen delivery to the CNS. It cannot be overemphasized that meticulous attention to maintenance of organ perfusion, by means of the clinical measures described earlier, should ensure that respiratory arrest in association with epidural block occurs extremely seldom and that such an occurrence should be rapidly reversible, with proper management.

It has been claimed that extensive sensory blockade may result in loss of consciousness owing to lack of input to the reticular activating system. However, epidural block to T1 does not cause loss of consciousness. This requires complete afferent blockade, including blockade of cervical nerve roots and the cranial nerves.[65]

Many factors may contribute to the respiratory effects of epidural block. At present, our knowledge in this area is meager. However, the documented changes produced by epidural block *per se* appear to be mild. For example, a sensory level of T3, associated with a motor level of T8, may be expected to result in essentially no change in vital capacity (VC) and functional residual capacity (FRC) in normal patients, so that respiration and the ability to cough are not im-

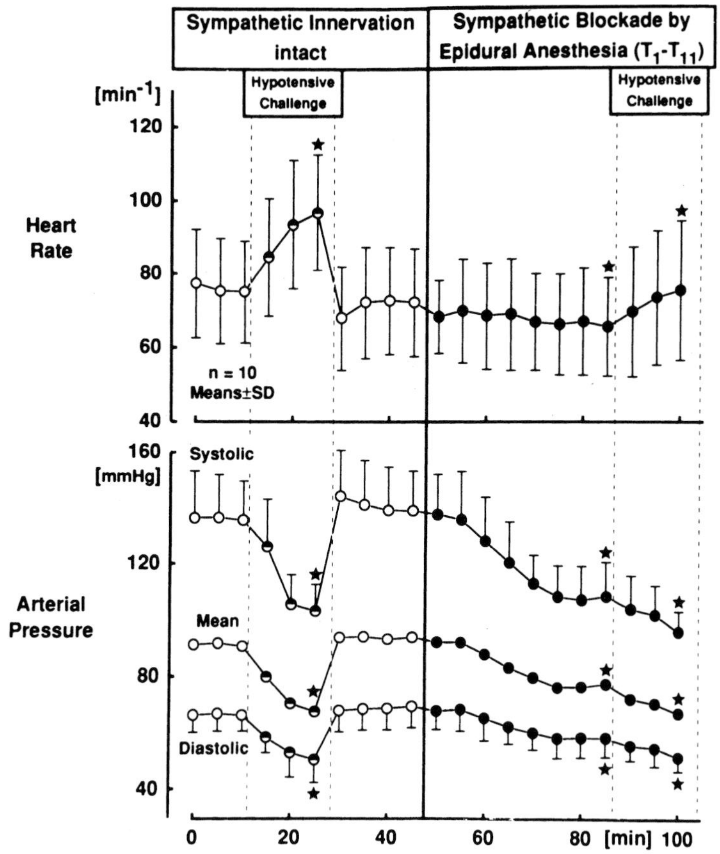

A

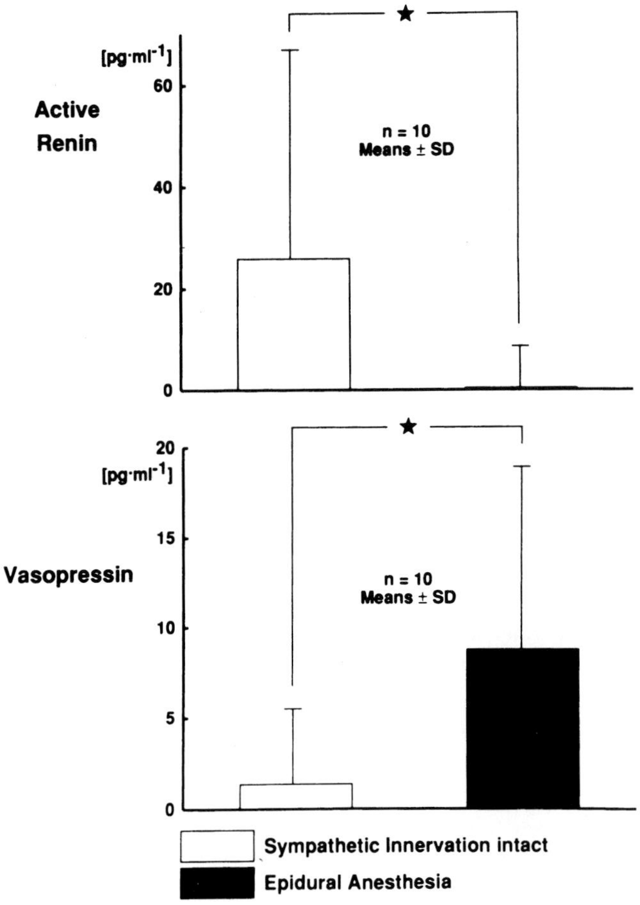

B

FIG. 8-22. **A**. Cardiovascular effects of sodium nitroprusside (SNP)-induced arterial hypotension (hypotensive challenge; vertical stippled lines) in awake nonsedated patients. Data points are mean values with standard deviations. **Left:** With the sympathetic innervation intact (o-o). Note the marked increase in heart rate and decrease in arterial blood pressure. **Right:** With sympathetic blockade by thoracic epidural blockade from T1 to T11 with plain bupivacaine (●-●). Heart rate increased albeit to a much smaller extent, whereas blood pressure decreased significantly. Sympathetic blockade by thoracic epidural anesthesia is usually (and here) associated with a decrease of both heart rate and blood pressure. **B:** Changes in plasma renin and vasopressin concentrations evoked by hypotensive challenge. SNP-induced hypotension was associated with increased renin plasma concentrations with the sympathetic system intact, but not during sympathetic block by epidural anesthesia. In contrast, vasopressin plasma concentrations remained unchanged with SNP-induced hypotension, but increased significantly during epidural anesthesia. (From Hopf, H.B., Schlaghecke, R., and Peters, J.: Sympathetic neural blockade by thoracic epidural anesthesia suppresses renin release in response to arterial hypotension. Anesthesiology, *80*:992, 1994.)

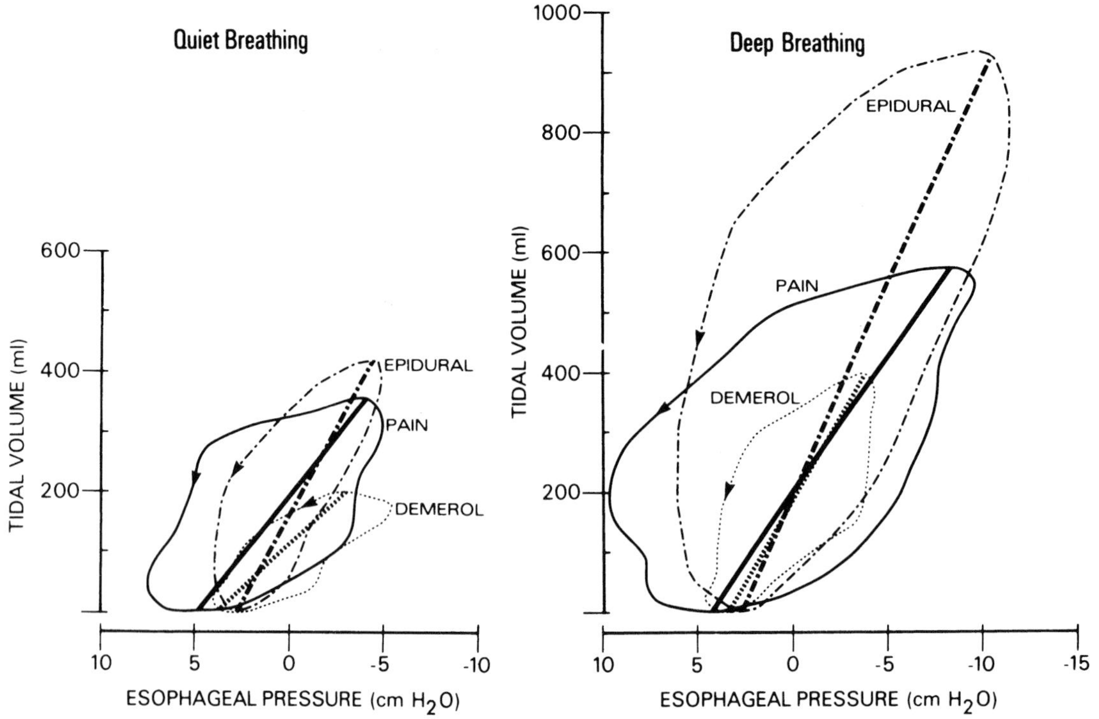

FIG. 8-23. Effect of pain and analgesia on thoracic pressure volume relationships. Pressure volume loops are shown 2 to 6 hours after cholecystectomy during quiet breathing **(left)** and deep breathing **(right)**. Pain is associated with decreased tidal volume, which is marked when deep breathing is attempted. During expiration there is high positive pressure, particularly during deep breathing. Such high pressure would be associated with glottic closure, abdominal splinting, and grunting type of respiration. Demerol decreases tidal volume but decreases the high pressure during expiration; thus grunting diminishes, an apparent and deceptive improvement. Epidural blockade increases tidal volume, particularly during deep breathing. This is achieved with much lower positive pressure during expiration and would be accompanied by elimination of grunting and abdominal splinting. A tidal volume of nearly 1000 ml would be associated with effective coughing. (Reproduced with permission from Bromage, P.R.: Epidural Analgesia. Philadelphia, W.B. Saunders, 1978.)

paired.[259,398] In patients with severe pain, epidural block probably improves VC and FRC as well as Pa_{O_2}, at least in the early postoperative period (see also Chapter 26); this may result in improved respiratory exchange and more effective coughing (Fig. 8-23).[65,195,266,358,399]

Effect of Thoracic Epidural Anesthesia on Respiration

Since epidural anesthesia induces segmental block of spinal nerves, an adequate extension of the block of motor nerves can selectively affect respiratory muscles in the rib cage. Therefore the effect of thoracic epidural anesthesia (TEA) on the performance of the parasternal intercostal muscles was investigated by measuring electromyographic activity and length changes of the parasternal muscles in anesthetized spontaneous breathing dogs.[366] TEA caused rib cage distortion by impaired contraction of the parasternals and conceivably other respiratory muscles in the rib cage as well. Extrapolation to the clinical situation is difficult. However, in healthy awake volunteers TEA caused a reduction of ventilatory response to CO_2 during spontaneous respiration principally because of decreased contribution of the rib cage to tidal breathing.[229] Mechanical impairment of rib cage movement can produce decreased ventilatory response to carbon dioxide, probably reflecting blockade of the efferent or afferent pathway (or both) of the intercostal nerve roots. These changes, however, are of an order unlikely to be of clinical relevance. Prevention of respiratory failure by blocking pain-related effects on ability to cough and breathe deeply usually outweighs any consideration of ventilatory impairment from the block itself, especially as diaphragmatic function may be improved.

Furthermore TEA does not impair the hypoxic drive, e.g., the ventilatory response to progressive isocapnic hypoxemia as has been shown in unpremedicated patients.[331] There appears to be no reason to avoid TEA in patients who are reliant on hypoxic drive, such as those with chronic airway disease.

Diaphragmatic dysfunction is a major determinant of the impaired respiratory function observed after upper abdominal and thoracic surgery. Mankikian et al. (1988) showed that thoracic epidural anesthesia increased postoperative esophageal and gastric pressure and diaphragmatic motion indices of diaphragm function after upper abdominal surgery in humans, suggesting a partial reversal of the diaphragmatic dysfunction.[255] These results, however, were based upon indirect measurements and may also reflect changes in abdominal muscle activity. Pansard et al. (1993) obtained direct diaphragmatic electromyogram recording from intramuscular electrodes that had been inserted into the costal and crural parts of the muscle during elective abdominal aorta surgery.[297] The electrical diaphragmatic activity was increased but was not associated with improved diaphragmatic contractility. It seems unlikely that diaphragmatic activity increased during thoracic epidural anesthesia as a compensation for reduction in parasternal muscle inspiratory activity produced by motor blockade, since rib cage motion did not change after thoracic epidural blockade. In an awake sheep model 24 hours after thoracotomy, there was a significant decrease of both costal and crural diaphragmatic shortening; following thoracic epidural administration of lidocaine, tidal volume increases were recorded, but there was markedly reduced rib cage expansion.[305] This finding may be due to a shift of the workload of breathing from the chest wall to the diaphragm, to explain the unexpected observation that rib cage function decreased in this animal model. By using the same study design in humans undergoing thoracic surgery, this group observed a marked impairment of active diaphragmatic shortening, which was not reversed by thoracic epidural anesthesia, despite improvement of other indices of respiratory function.[152] This probably suggests that diaphragmatic contraction could not overcome the increased external forces placed upon it by other respiratory muscles. Differences in outcome of both investigations may be species related (see also Chapter 5, Fig. 5-8).

In summary, the effects of epidural anesthesia on diaphragmatic function after upper abdominal and thoracic surgery are complex. The most likely explanation for the TEA-related increase in diaphragmatic activity seems to be the interruption of an inhibitory reflex of phrenic nerve motor drive, either related to direct deafferentation of visceral sensory pathways or related to a diaphragmatic load reduction due to increased abdominal compliance.

Epidural Block and Motor Function

Clinical Applications of Deliberate Preservation of Motor Function

With respect to respiratory function, it is clear from the previous section that the aim is to use the appropriate drug and regimen to preserve motor function, and thus to permit deep breathing and coughing. In postoperative patients, continuous infusion of bupivacaine has proved to be an attractive method of achieving this goal. This method is described in detail in Chapter 26. Preservation of motor function also permits ultra-early ambulation, since patients who are pain-free are able to ambulate soon after surgery.[65] It may be necessary to use vasopressors if epidural block is continued with only local anesthetic. Alternatives are to use dilute bupivacaine plus opioid (some risk of hypotension) or opioid alone (no risk of hypotension) as described in Chapter 26. Ultra-early ambulation probably decreases the risk of venous thrombosis and may decrease the hospitalization time.[65] More controlled data are required (see also Chapter 5).

Clinical Applications of Motor Function Depression

In abdominal and hip surgery, depression of motor function is necessary during surgery. In this situation, the powerful motor blockade of etidocaine or lidocaine may be used (see Fig. 8-25). Some of the motor effects are obtained by "deafferentiation," preventing reflex muscle contraction by blocking nociception before it reaches the spinal cord (see Fig. 8-23).

Factors determining motor effects of epidural block are as follows (see pharmacology section):

1. *The local anesthetic drug:* Bupivacaine has the least motor effects; etidocaine has the most potent effects.
2. *Dose of drug:* Degree of motor blockade is increased as dose of drug increases.
3. *Repeated doses of drug:* With "top-up" techniques, both motor and sensory blockade tend to become more intense with repeated doses; however, if dilute solutions of bupivacaine are used by controlled continuous infusion, motor blockade can be kept to a minimum.
4. *Epinephrine as an adjuvant* increases the degree of motor blockade.

Epidural Blockade and Pregnancy

The known and potential physiologic effects of epidural block on mother, placenta, and fetus must be viewed in the light of contemporary knowledge of the physiology and pathophysiology of pregnancy, fetal physiology, and pharmacology. The detailed implications for regional anesthesia are discussed further in Chapter 18 (see Figs. 18-3 through 18-7 and Fig. 18-12).

By recognizing the modifications in management that are predicted by the impact of the physiologic changes of pregnancy, one can administer epidural anesthesia to the gravid women with efficacy and safety.

PHARMACOLOGY OF EPIDURAL BLOCKADE

The essence of the clinical pharmacology of epidural block is the provision of safe and effective neural blockade. To safely institute an epidural block, a knowledge of the physiology of epidural block is necessary, as well as a revision of the pharmacokinetics of local anesthetics as related to their administration by means of the epidural route. The efficacy of epidural block depends on this and on the clinical effects of the local anesthetics used.

In considering the pharmacokinetics of local anesthetics, both the systemic absorption and systemic disposition are of importance. Systemic absorption of local anesthetics limits the duration of nerve blocks and is of concern in view of systemic toxicity. The general absorption and disposition characteristics of local anesthetics are discussed in detail in Chapter 3. The potential for systemic toxicity should also be considered when choosing a local anesthetic agent for epidural use. The pharmacokinetic characteristics of the local anesthetics currently used for epidural analgesia and the implications for the time course of neural blockade and systemic toxicity have been reviewed in detail by Burm.[77,391] Toxic effects of local anesthetics mainly involve the central nervous system and the cardiovascular system, depending on the rapidity of absorption from the epidural space and the total dose of the drug administered. This topic is covered in detail in Chapters 2, 3, and 4.

Thus, a thorough knowledge of the pharmacokinetics and toxicity of local anesthetics is a prerequisite to the safe use of epidural analgesia.

"Efficacy" of Epidural Block

Mechanisms and sites of action

Before discussing factors that influence the clinical efficacy of epidural blockade, it is helpful to summarize current data concerning the site(s) at which local anesthetics act after their injection into the epidural space. The anatomic spread, which is an important determinant of the pharmacologic response, is summarized in Figures 8-2 and 8-3. The possible sites of action of local anesthetic drugs administered into the epidural space include the nerve trunks in the paravertebral space, the dorsal root ganglia, the dorsal and ventral spinal roots, the spinal cord itself, and the brain[64] (see also Chapters 2 and 3).

Studies concerning tissue uptake of local anesthetics indicate that the intradural spinal roots show the highest concentration of local anesthetic agents following both subarachnoid and epidural injection.[67,92] However, the amount of the local anesthetic drug found in the dorsal root ganglia is very small, indicating a minor contribution of these ganglia to the epidural blockade. The initial segmental onset of epidural anesthesia is probably related to the conduction blockade of the spinal roots within the dural sleeves,[352] where high concentrations build up rapidly, as the dura is very thin in this region. Probably 40% of the dural root sleeves ("cuff") have arachnoid proliferations and villi, reducing the thinkness of the dura mater (Figure 8-2B). Subsequently, diffusion of local anesthetics from the epidural space through the dura mater into the cerebrospinal fluid occurs to the periphery of the spinal cord.[64,113] Likewise, opioids rapidly gain access to CSF (see also Chapter 29).[110,111]

In addition, vascular transport of local anesthetic via spinal radicular arteries may contribute to the distribution of local anesthetic from the epidural space to the spinal cord. The concentrations attained within the cord, however, are lower than those in the spinal roots.[92] Spinal cord involvement in epidural anesthesia is indicated by studies of lower limb reflex changes during midthoracic epidural anesthesia.[63] In addition, the regression of epidural anesthesia does not follow the classic segmental pattern seen during onset of analgesia, suggesting a spinal cord involvement.[380] Electrophysiologic studies in monkeys also confirmed involvement of the spinal cord.[121,122]

For highly lipid-soluble local anesthetic drugs, the diffusion across the dural cuff into the CSF and then the spinal cord may be rapid. The primary site of action of local anesthetics in the cord may vary with the differences in their physicochemical properties, resulting in differences in sensory and motor blockade between agents.[121,122]

Seepage through the intervertebral foramina occurs, which may result in multiple paravertebral blocks. However, this blockade of the multiple mixed spinal nerves is generally confined to young people and will play a minor role in the mechanism of epidural anesthesia.

Longitudinal Spread of Solutions in the Epidural Space

Studies using radiologic contrast media and radiolabeled solutions have mostly shown that these solutions tend to spread more in a cranial than a caudal direction.[78,279,387] However, radiologic contrast media cannot be expected to accurately reflect the spread of a local anesthetic drug; mixtures of local anesthetics and radioactive substances, such as ^{131}I, may result in different rates of diffusion of the local anesthetic and the radioactive substance. Because access to the CSF is important in determining clinical effects of local anesthetics, studies that determine only longitudinal spread in the epidural space may have limited value. More useful would be studies with labeled local anesthetics in which autoradiographs were taken at different levels to determine concentrations in epidural space, CSF, spinal roots, spinal cord, and so forth.

Clinical Considerations for the Efficacy of Epidural Blockade

There is no question now that epidural block can be effective in nearly all cases if attention is paid to the anatomy, physiology, and pharmacology of the technique. Yet there are still many major medical centers throughout the world that hold the belief that epidural blockade has a high failure rate compared with subarachnoid blockade. This merely serves to underline the relatively recent acquisition of relevant data on which to base the effective use of epidural block.

Assessment of Epidural Blockade

In defining important factors in effective epidural block, the development of standardized methods of assessment of epidural block has been essential:

Sensory Block. Sensory block is graphed by testing for loss and return of pinprick sensation (*partial sensory block*) in each dermatome on both sides of the body (Fig. 8-24). An

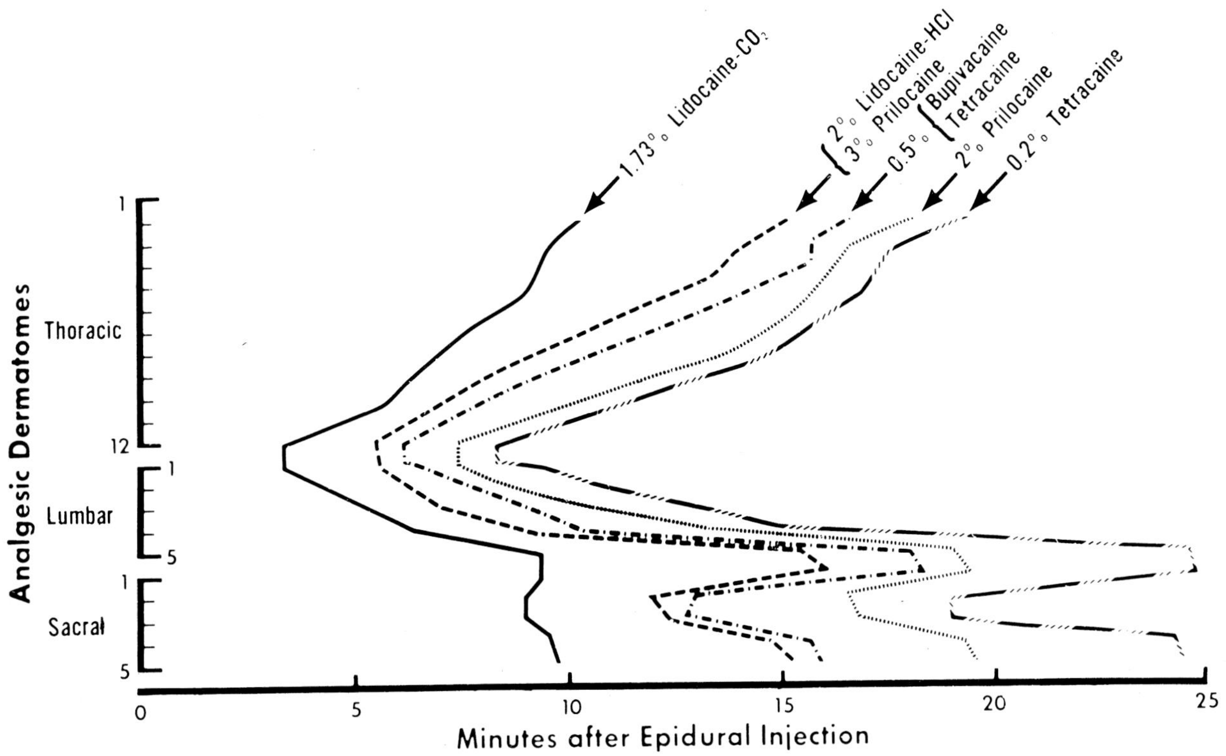

FIG. 8-24. *Sensory blockade.* Mean latency profile of 1.73% carbonated lidocaine contrasted with 2% lidocaine HCl, 2% and 3% prilocaine, 0.5% bupivacaine, and 0.2% tetracaine. All solutions contained 1:200,000 epinephrine. Injection was given at the second lumbar interspace. (Reproduced with permission from Bromage, P.R.: Epidural Analgesia. Philadelphia, W.B. Saunders, 1978.)

alternative method of testing initial onset is to use an alcohol swab to assess loss of temperature sensation, which is the most sensitive indicator of initial onset of sensory block (see Chapter 2, Table 2-1). Complete loss of touch sensation may also be charted.[109,346]

From a "time-segment" graph, the following can be obtained: time to initial onset and complete spread of analgesia; time to regression of two segments and complete regression of analgesia (Fig. 8-24); total number of segments blocked on both sides of the body; milliliters of local anesthetic per mean segmental spread (total segments R + L divided by two); and area of the segment-time diagram (segment minutes), which can be related to the dose of local anesthetic, in segment minutes per dose. The latter expression is used to assess the development of tachyphylaxis (see below).

Somatosensory evoked potentials (SEPs). Cortical derived somatosensory evoked potentials (SEPs) have been used in the qualitative assessment of the intensity of peripheral and central neural blockade.[24,124,134,242–244,254]

SEPs reflect the net results of neuronal activities coming from peripheral nerves through the spinal cord to the brain. SEPs are generated by repetitive stimulation of peripheral nerves and can be monitored at several points along the sensory pathway, including over the spinal cord, subcortical structures, and cerebral cortex. Intraoperative monitoring of SEPs is an accepted technique to assess the functional integrity of the sensory pathways, particularly during spinal and scoliosis surgery.[173]

Despite a clinically adequate block as assessed by pinprick, afferent impulses generating SEPs still passed through an expected blocked area following epidural administration of bupivacaine, mepivacaine, or etidocaine. This probably indicates that total afferent blockade often is not obtained. Abolishment of SEP has only been accomplished using 1.5% etidocaine.[242] This is possibly due to the ability of etidocaine to penetrate the white matter of the spinal cord more readily.[121]

Sympathetic Block. Sympathetic block is assessed by measuring skin temperature with a telethermometer (see Chapter 13, Fig. 13-17), thermography, or temperature-sensitive papers. Alternatively, a digital plethysmogram may be used (see Chapter 13, Fig. 13-6). Skin conductance can be measured in the clinical setting by use of the psychogalvanic response; reliable measurements are much more difficult than usually acknowledged. More precise, but of research application only, are the use of various sweat tests, such as cobalt blue and starch iodine, or the response of skin plethysmography to ice during venous occlusion plethysmography (see Chapter 13, Figs. 13-6 and 13-5). A full discussion of the clinical and laboratory tests of sympathetic block is given in Chapter 13.

Motor block. Motor block is usually assessed by use of the Bromage scale for motor blockade in the lower limbs.[65]

Bromage Scale

No block (0%)	Full flexion of knees and feet possible
Partial (33%)	Just able to flex knees, still full flexion of feet possible
Almost complete (66%)	Unable to flex knees. Still flexion of feet
Complete (100%)	Unable to move legs or feet

Motor blockade in the lower limbs can be assessed with reference to specific myotomes (e.g., L2 hip flexion).[346] A score of 0 is assigned for no block and 1 for complete block (no movement) at each joint on each side. Thus maximal motor block is present bilaterally with a score of 10:

	Right		Left
Hip flexion (L2)	1		1
Knee extension (L3)	1		1
Ankle dorsiflexion (L4)	1		1
Great toe dorsiflexion (L5)	1		1
Ankle plantar flexion (S1)	1		1
	5	+	5 = 10 (complete motor block)

This test removes some observer error because only a "move" (0) or "no move" (1) decision needs to be made at each joint.

An onset profile for motor blockade can be presented as a "myotome score/time" diagram. For research purposes, Axelsson reported an apparatus that measures maximal isometric strength by a force transducer at ankle, knee, and hip. This provides objective, reproducible measurements of muscle power.[13]

Abdominal muscle power may be assessed by the rectus abdominis muscle (RAM) test.[388] This is useful in abdominal surgery when abdominal muscle blockade is required rather than lower limb muscle blockade. On the other hand, the Bromage scale is useful for lower limb surgery. Both scales may be used when a comprehensive picture is required: RAM-test (T5–T12) and Bromage scale (L1–S2).

"RAM" Test of Abdominal Muscles

100%	Able to rise from supine to sitting position with hands behind head
80% power	Can sit only with arms extended
60% power	Can lift only head and scapulae off bed
40% power	Can lift only shoulders off bed
20%	An increase in abdominal muscle tension can be felt during effort; no other response

Testing of 100% and 80% power has limitations in patients with vasodilation; blood pressure and pulse rate must be carefully monitored if these tests are to be used.

A broad comparison of agents used for epidural block can be compiled based on their "success rate" in producing motor and sensory block. Because different methods of testing have been used in many studies, the comparisons are only qualitative (Fig. 8-25).

EMG. Few studies have used the more quantitative method of EMG, although this would provide more sensitive assessment.

Reflex Response. Under general anesthesia without muscle relaxation, sensation can still be crudely assessed by use of reflex response to pinch by a forceps at appropriate segmental levels. Alternatively, the tendon reflexes in the lower limbs give a gross index of both motor and sensory block, while reflexes such as those of the cremaster, anal, and abdominal may also be useful as a gross guide to adequacy of blockade.

Factors Affecting Epidural Blockade

Many factors may affect the efficacy, spread of blockade, fiber types blocked, and other aspects of epidural blockade. These are summarized in Table 8-12 and are discussed below.

Site of Injection and Nerve Root Size

It can readily be seen from the time-segment diagram in Figure 8-24 that blockade tends to be most intense and has the most rapid onset close to the site of injection. The subsequent spread of analgesia depends to some extent on whether the injection is made in thoracic or lumbar regions.

After *lumbar epidural* injection, analgesia spreads in the manner shown in Figure 8-24. There is a somewhat greater cranial than caudal spread and there may be a delay in the L5 and S1 segments. The delay in onset at these segments appears to be due to the large size of these nerve roots.[154]

After *midthoracic epidural* injection, analgesia spreads quite evenly from the site of injection. However, the upper thoracic and lower cervical segments are resistant to blockade because of the large size of the nerve roots and the large number of nerve fibers within them. Repeated doses by the midthoracic route eventually may cause analgesia to spread into lumbar and sacral segments, with the expected lag in onset at L5–S1. Careful control of dose in the thoracic region permits sparing of the lumbar segments and thus avoidance of sympathetic block in the lower limbs and maintenance of normal bladder function—that is, a true segmental block. Similarly, a small dose injected at L2–L3 for labor pain may block only T11 and L3–L4 segments, while it spares the sacral segments.

The profile of onset of caudal epidural block spreads upward from S5, and the S1 segment is the last to be blocked, as expected (see Chapter 9, Fig. 9-5).

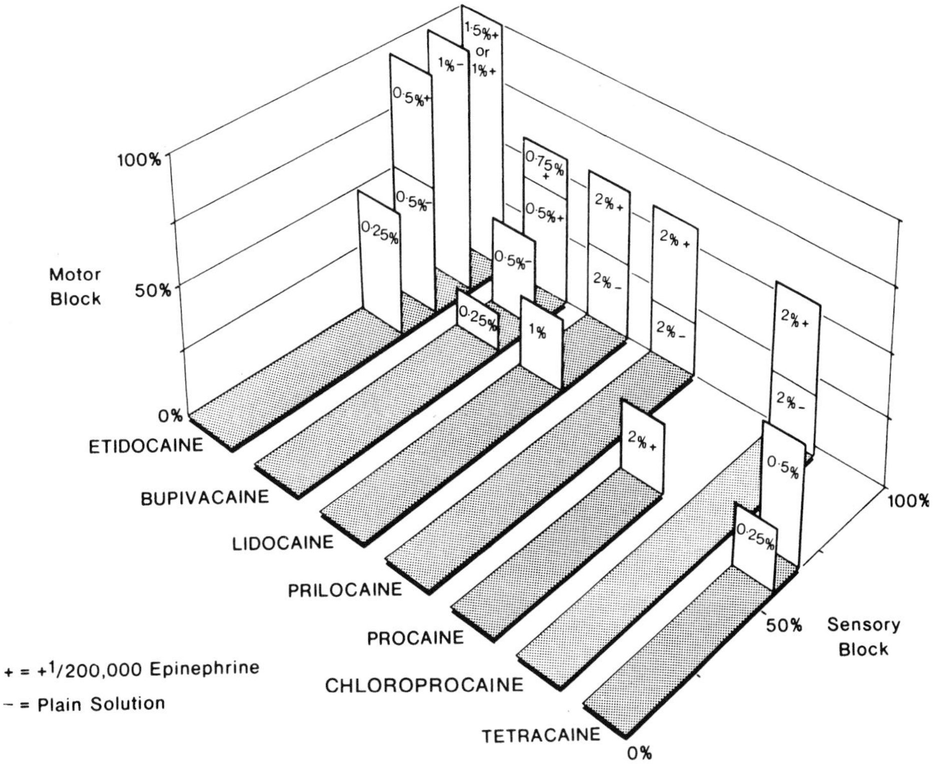

FIG. 8-25. Motor and sensory block percentage success rate. Comparison of agents, concentrations, and addition of epinephrine are based on subjective data, so that only approximate comparisons can be made.

Age

Over the past several years the anesthesiologist has been faced with a growing number of elderly patients presenting for surgery. Epidural anesthesia has enjoyed a resurgence of popularity for elderly patients undergoing surgery in areas amenable to conduction anesthesia. With advancing age, anatomic changes do occur in the epidural space.[64] In the young individual, the areolar tissue around the intervertebral foramina is soft and loose. In the elderly, this areolar tissue becomes dense and firm, partially sealing the intervertebral foramina.[65] With aging, the dura becomes more permeable to local anesthetic because of significant increase in the size of the arachnoid villi.[352]

Discrepancies exist between studies in which the influence of age on epidural anesthesia has been assessed. The classic study of Bromage regarding the influence of age on epidural spread reported a strong relationship between age and the epidural segmental dose requirement (ESDR); i.e. the amount (dose) of local anesthetic required to block one spinal segment.[62] Assuming a linear dose-relationship, Bromage demonstrated that with age the ESDR decreased in a linear way. In contrast to Bromage's assumption, others have found no direct linear relationship between volume and anesthetic spread.[174,300,354] The greater the total amount used, the greater the ESDR calculated. From this it can be concluded that the results of Bromage's study concerning the linear decrease of ESDR with age are questionable because he assumed a direct linear relationship between the amount (dose) of local anesthetic and extent of anesthesia and because he used variable total anesthetic amounts.[62]

Using a given dose (fixed volume and concentration) other investigators have found a significantly greater number of spinal segments blocked in older patients. However, the magnitude of this effect was small: only 1 to 3 segments more in the elderly patients compared to younger adult patients (Fig. 8-26).[174,281,299,300,324,393] When using different volumes, the dose-effect relationship varied with these volumes.[9,354]

Age has also been shown to be associated with a higher upper level of analgesia following thoracic epidural administration of a fixed dose; increased levels of analgesia with

TABLE 8-12. *Factors affecting epidural blockade*

Site of injection and nerve root size
Weight (? no), age, height
Position—sitting (? minimal)
—lateral (? yes)
Local anesthetic agent
Dose (? volume/concentration)
Addition of epinephrine
Carbon dioxide solutions
Number and frequency of injections
? Injection by needle compared with catheter

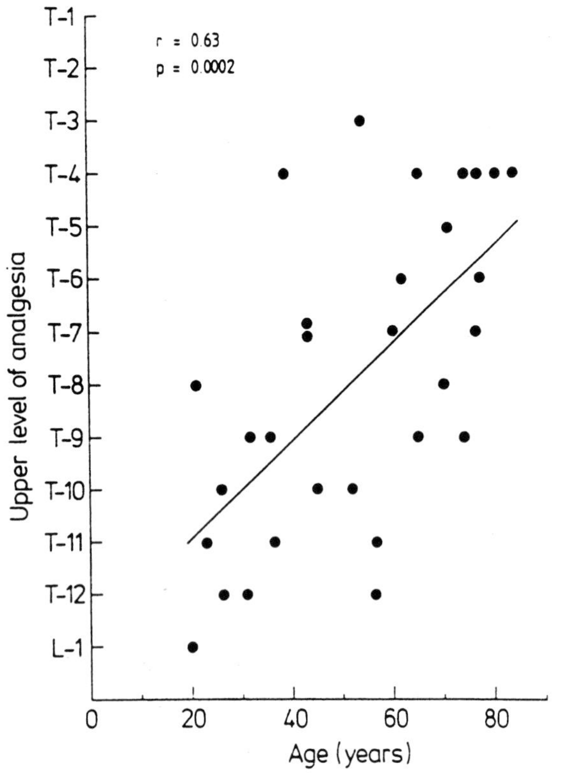

FIG. 8-26. Relationship between the upper level of analgesia and age after epidural administration of 0.5% bupivacaine. Segmental spread is increased with age (Veering, B.T., Burm, A.G.L., Van Kleef, J.W., Hennis, P.J., and Spierdÿk, J.: Epidural anesthesia with bupivacaine: Effects of age on neural blockade and pharmacokinetics. Anesth. Analg., *66:*589, 1987).

increasing age have been attributed to reduced leakage of local anesthetic solution because of progressive sclerotic closure of intervertebral foramina.[64,65] Also, the cephalad spread of radioactivity after epidural injection of iodine-131 mixed in 2% lidocaine was higher in patients older than 50 years than in younger ones.[279] Radiologic studies, however, have failed to show a relationship between age and spread in the epidural space.[78] It is possible that radiopaque material and local anesthetic do not spread in an identical manner. On the other hand, the increased permeability of the dura with aging, as described by Shantha and Evans,[352] may contribute to the higher levels of the analgesic spread in the elderly. Usubiaga[387] reported that older patients have a higher residual pressure and that there is a positive relationship between residual epidural pressure and the extent of analgesic spread. Also, increased epidural compliance and decreased epidural resistance with advancing age may contribute to this enhanced spread in the elderly.[188]

The onset time to maximal caudad spread has been reported to decrease with advancing age following epidural administration of bupivacaine, allowing surgery in areas innervated by these segments to be started sooner in older patients than in younger patients.[392,393] In addition, a more rapid onset and enhanced intensity of motor blockade has been shown in older patients.[393] With aging, the neural population declines steadily within the spinal cord, and peripheral nerves show a linear reduction in conduction velocity, especially in motor nerves.[136] This could make older patients more sensitive to local anesthetics, which is probably (partially) the cause of the shorter onset time of analgesia in the caudad segments and the altered motor block profile. Nydahl[281] reported a shorter duration of motor blockade, as assessed by electromyographic recordings, following epidural administration of epinephrine-containing bupivacaine solutions. This may be attributed to a stronger reaction of younger subjects to epinephrine.[395]

Epidural anesthesia carries some problems in elderly patients. The technique is technically more difficult, and so there is always a chance of a failure. This is partially attributed to the fact that the ligamentum flavum probably changes into a form that is easily ossified.[288] The more extensive spread of analgesia is likely to be accompanied by more extensive sympathetic blockade. Therefore, prevention of hypotension by intravenous administration of crystalloid fluids will be important in older patients. It should be emphasized, however, that rapid volume preloading constitutes a potential risk in elderly patients with poor cardiac function, in whom there is a risk of pulmonary edema and cardiac failure.

With epidural anesthesia there is a decline in the thermoregulatory response with age, as has been shown by the decrease in core temperature.[151] Consequently the postoperative rewarming process will occur more slowly in older patients. Lumbar epidural anesthesia with lidocaine did not affect the resting ventilation parameters, such as minute ventilation and tidal volume, in older patients and stimulated the ventilatory response to hypercapnia is to the same degree as in young patients.[331] Therefore lumbar epidural anesthesia appears to be a safe technique in elderly patients.

Important considerations for the use of epidural anesthesia in pediatric patients is covered in Chapter 20.

Position

Comparison of sitting and lateral positions for epidural block reveals no significant differences in cephalad spread.[298] An exception is the obese patient, who achieves a lower level of block when seated.[191] Caudad spread of block in seated patients is slightly favored by the sitting position.[59] From these studies it seems that the differences between sitting and lateral positions are small. The lateral position favors spread of analgesia to the dependent side in both pregnant and nonpregnant patients,[11,175,345] but the differences are small. In surgical patients, however, Seow and associates found that onset of sensory and motor block was significantly more rapid on the dependent side and had a longer duration (Fig. 8-27A). In addition to being more rapid in onset, motor blockade was greater on the dependent side at all time intervals tested out to 40 minutes after injection (Fig. 8-27B). Onset time for sympathetic block was not faster on the

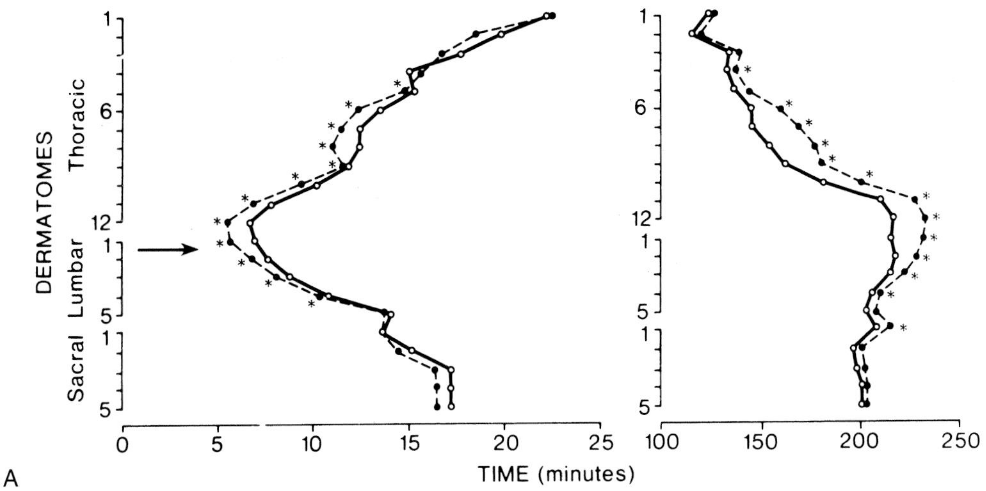

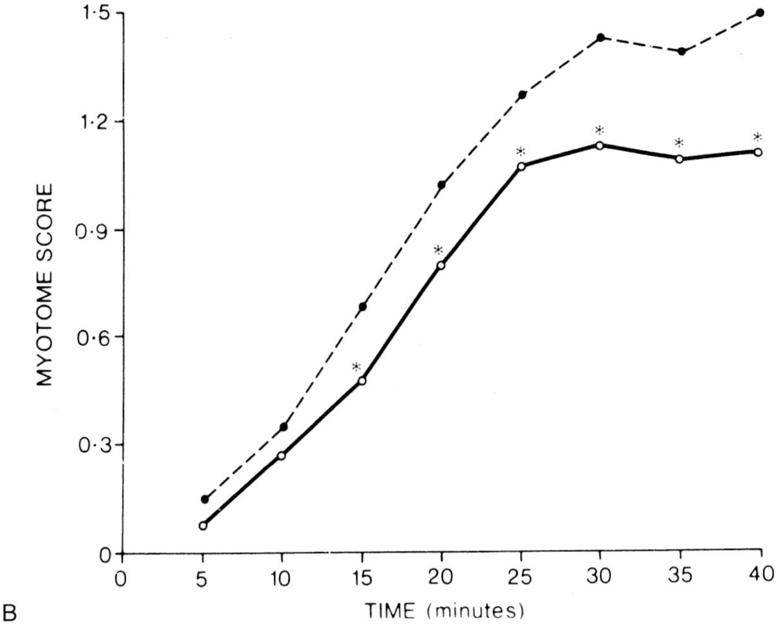

FIG. 8-27. A: Mean time-segment diagram for partial sensory blockade at each dermatome level. Data points plotted are mean values. → Site of injection of local anesthetic; *Denotes significant difference between the (●---●) dependent and (○—○) nondependent sides ($p < 0.05$). A similar time-segment diagram for complete sensory blockade was obtained, with significant difference between the two sides for dermatomes T8-L4 inclusive for onset profile and T8-L3 inclusive for sensory regression profile. **B:** Mean myotome score for total number of myotomes with complete motor blockade at each time interval after administration of epidural blockade (maximum possible number = 10 myotomes, that is, five for each right and left side). *Denotes significant difference between (●---●) dependent and nondependent (○—○) sides ($p<0.05$). (Reproduced with permission from Seow, L.T., Lips, F.J., and Cousins, M.J.: Effect of lateral posture on epidural blockade for surgery. Anaesth. Intensive Care, *11*:97, 1983.)

dependent side, but duration of maximum elevation of skin temperature was greater on the dependent side.[345] The differences in sensory and motor block are great enough to indicate an advantage in placing patients on the operative side during epidural block before lower limb surgery.[345]

There appears to be no correlation between spread of analgesia and weight and height in adults.[65]

Speed of Injection

Increasing the speed of injection has no effect on bulk flow of solutions in the epidural space.[78,279] Also, spread of analgesia is only minimally influenced. However, rapid injection of large volumes of solution may increase CSF pressure,[165] decrease spinal cord blood flow, increase intracranial pressure, and pose a risk of spinal or cerebral complications. In susceptible patients, sudden increases in CSF pressure may compromise spinal cord blood flow (see Chapter 30), and this may increase susceptibility to neurotoxicity[165] or, in atherosclerotics, may possibly cause "spinal stroke." There is evidence that nutritive vessels crossing the perineurium of nerves are subject to a pathologic "valve" mechanism initiated by perineurial edema.[241] This edema could be initiated by sudden increases in CSF pressure. Subsequent hypotension owing to sympathetic block may decrease spinal cord flow if CSF pressure and perineurial pressure remain high. A combination of these effects could result in neural damage (see also Chapter 30).

Sudden increases in intracerebral pressure may cause headache, cerebral hemorrhage, or isolated hemorrhage in a small vessel, such as a retinal vessel. Headache is commonly reported if epidural solutions are injected rapidly. Intraocular hemorrhage has been described after rapid epidural injection of 30 ml of solution of local anesthetic.[87] Thus, rapid injection is not only ineffective in "forcing solution up the epidural space," but also potentially dangerous. Local anesthetics should be injected into the epidural space slowly and preferably in incremental doses.

TABLE 8-13. *Choice of agent for epidural block*

Application and requirements	Agent(s)	Comment
Surgical analgesia (medium to long duration)		
Sensory + + + Motor + + +	2% Lidocaine (HCl or CO_2) +	Rapid onset, excellent analgesia and motor block, medium duration
	3% Chloroprocaine	For brief procedures only. Rapid onset
	1.5%–1% Etidocaine ±	Rapid onset, profound analgesia and motor block, long duration
	0.5%–0.75% Bupivacaine 0.75%–1% Ropivacaine[a]—	Slow onset, good analgesia, moderate motor block, long duration
	2% Mepivacaine	Similar to lidocaine. Can be used for medium duration if epinephrine is undesirable
	3% Prilocaine—	Single-shot techniques. Dose of <600 mg, low toxicity
Postoperative or post-trauma pain (long duration)	0.25% Bupivacaine—	Slow onset, long duration of sensory analgesia with little motor blockade (0.25%)
Sensory + + + Motor O	0.2% Ropivacaine[a]—	
Obstetric analgesia (long duration)	0.125%–0.5% Bupivacaine— 0.2% Ropivacaine[a]—	0.125%–0.25% may be brief duration
Sensory + + Motor O	1% Lidocaine–CO_2+	Useful for resistant "missed segments" Rapid onset, medium duration
Obstetric surgery or instrumental delivery (medium to long duration) Sensory + + + Motor + +	3% Chloroprocaine + 2% Lidocaine + 0.75% Ropivacaine[a]—	Considerations similar to surgical analgesia (*Note:* 0.25% bupivacaine is not potent enough and 0.5% bupivacaine provides inadequate analgesia in 5%–10% of patients. Bupivacaine 0.75% not recommended for obstetrics.)
Diagnostic and therapeutic neural blockade		
Range of blockade from sympathetic to motor	0.5%–2% Lidocaine	0.5%—sympathetic, 1%—sensory, 2%+ motor blockade, for diagnostic blockade
	0.25% Bupivacaine 0.2% Ropivacaine[a]—	May be useful for diagnostic blockade requiring long-duration sensory block with no motor block, also used for "therapeutic block" (see Chapter 27)

+ = with epinephrine; — = without epinephrine.
[a] Ropivacaine is labelled 2 mg/ml (0.2%), 7.5 mg/ml (0.75%), 10 mg/ml (1%).
Note: This table does not (and cannot) cover all the shades of difference between agents. See also Chapter 3, Table 3-1 and Chapter 4, Table 4-1.

Volume, Concentration, and Dose of Local Anesthetic

Extensive studies by Bromage indicated that the dose of drug (concentration × volume) determined the spread of analgesia,[64] at least between the concentrations of 2% and 5% lidocaine and 0.2% and 0.5% tetracaine. However, data were not obtained to compare 0.5% lidocaine with a range of 1% to 2%, which is a typical clinical range of concentrations. It did appear from Bromage's data that dose requirements diminished from about 30 mg per segment to 20 mg per segment when concentration was reduced from 2% to 1% lidocaine. Erdemir and colleagues have shown that 30 ml of 1% lidocaine produced a higher sensory level than 10 ml of a 3% solution.[145] Burn and colleagues showed that large volumes of contrast media (40 ml) were more likely to spread into cervical regions compared with higher concentrations and smaller volumes (20 ml).[78]

With regard to motor blockade, dosage becomes less important when dilute solutions are used. Below concentrations of 1% lidocaine, motor block is minimal regardless of dose, unless injections are repeated at intervals. Then intensity of sensory and motor block increases with each successive injection. This mechanism is important in obstetric analgesia when dilute solutions of 0.125% or 0.065% bupivacaine are used.

Increasing dosage results in a linear increase in degree of sensory block and duration of epidural block, whereas increasing concentration results in a reduction in onset time and intensity of motor blockade (see also Fig. 8-25). A general summary of the effects of local anesthetic dose and added epinephrine is given in Chapter 4, Table 4-2. However, it should be recognized that choice of drug influences these effects.

Choice of Local Anesthetic

The concept of a "spectrum" of local anesthetics depicted in Chapter 4, Figure 4-8 relates significantly to epidural block. The great flexibility of sensory and motor block that can be obtained by careful choice of drug is seen in Figure

8-25. For example, 0.25% bupivacaine may provide satisfactory analgesia for acute pain with close to zero motor block, whereas 0.25% etidocaine results in close to 50% motor block, but variable analgesia.

If more potent analgesia with minimal motor block is required, 0.5% bupivacaine or 2% plain lidocaine may be chosen, although the former is the best choice for continuous techniques. The requirements of profound sensory block and excellent muscle relaxation (e.g., for surgery or operative obstetrics) are best met by 2% lidocaine with epinephrine or 1.5% etidocaine[240] or 0.75% to 1.0% ropivacaine (if long duration is required).

Procaine, dibucaine, and tetracaine are not usually chosen for epidural block because of their rather inferior sensory and motor blocking properties. An exception may be the use of tetracaine if chloroprocaine is unavailable and amides are thought to be contraindicated.

Chloroprocaine has become an attractive alternative for short procedures and for obstetric analgesia; it is a safe drug because of its high rate of metabolism (however, see Chapter 4, Table 4-7).

Use of prilocaine for epidural block is worthy of consideration. It is still the safest amide agent when used in a dose of less than 600 mg and should be considered for single-shot epidural block, except in obstetrics. Of practical use, the 2% plain solution provides intense sensory block and minimal motor block; with 2% plain solutions levels are similar to those of the 2% epinephrine-containing solution, provided the dose is below 400 mg. This solution has appeal for outpatient caudal blocks or for single-shot epidural block for brief procedures. Alternatively, the 3% solution may be used if rapid onset is required, although a 20-ml dose produces some degree of motor block even with the plain solution (Table 8-13).

Ropivacaine. Ropivacaine is the S-enantiomer of a chain-shortened homologue of bupivacaine (propyl instead of butyl side chain).

In isolated nerve preparations ropivacaine produces a differential block, with less A-fiber action potential depression (motor blockade) than bupivacaine at equal degrees of suppression of C-fiber action potentials (sensory block).[15]

The dose causing convulsive activity in dogs is the same for ropivacaine as for bupivacaine,[146] but ropivacaine appears to be less arrhythmogenic and less potent than bupivacaine in depressing electrophysiologic variables.[268] Scott et al. (1989) compared the acute toxicity of ropivacaine with that of bupivacaine on both the CNS and the cardiovascular system (CVS) in human volunteers during intravenous infusion at a rate of 10 mg/min up to a maximal dose of 150 mg.[342] Ropivacaine caused fewer CNS symptoms and was at least 25% less toxic than bupivacaine in regard to the dose tolerated. Subtle changes in cardiac contractility and conductivity at subconvulsive plasma levels were seen with both drugs, although the changes were less frequent and less prominent with ropivacaine.

Studies to date have demonstrated ropivacaine to be an effective, long-lasting local anaesthetic when given epidurally[54,70,96,218] (see Tables 8-13 and 8-14). In one study there were no major differences regarding the characteristics of sensory and motor blockade between 0.5% ropivacaine and 0.5% bupivacaine.[70] In another study, however, it was shown that 0.5% ropivacaine was less potent in terms of producing motor block than 0.5% bupivacaine.[54] The intensity and duration of motor block are clearly dependent on the concentration of ropivacaine.[414] For surgical anesthesia, 0.75% or 0.1% ropivacaine will probably be more suitable.[218,272]

A difference between bupivacaine and ropivacaine, with regard to their disappearance from the area of injection in connection with epidural block, has been demonstrated by Dahl et al. (1990) using a clearance technique, indicating vasoconstrictive properties of ropivacaine in clinically tested concentrations.[125] However, prolongation of the duration of neural blockade did not occur when combining ropivacaine with a strong vasoconstrictor such as epinephrine.[85]

The distinct separation of sensory and motor fiber blockade with 0.5% ropivacaine may be advantageous for obstetric epidural anesthesia and postoperative epidural analgesia.

TABLE 8-14. *Clinical effects of local anesthetic solutions commonly used for epidural blockade*

Drug	Time spread to ± four segments ± 1 SD (min)	Approximate time to two-segment regression ± 2 SD[a] (min)	Recommended "top-up" time from initial dose[a] (min)
Lidocaine, 2%	15 ± 5	100 ± 40	60
Prilocaine, 2%–3%	15 ± 4	100 ± 40	60
Chloroprocaine, 2%–3%	12 ± 5	60 ± 15	45
Mepivacaine, 2%	15 ± 5	120 ± 150	60
Bupivacaine, 0.5%–0.75%	18 ± 10	200 ± 80	120
Ropivacaine, 0.75%–1%	20.5 ± 7.9	177 ± 49	120
Etidocaine, 1%–1.5%	10 ± 5	200 ± 80	120

[a] Note "top-up" time is based on duration minus 2 SD, which encompasses the likely duration in 95% of the population. In a conscious, cooperative patient, an alternative is to use frequent checks of segmental level to indicate need to "top up." All solutions contain 1:200,000 epinephrine, except ropivacaine. (Data from studies of Allen, P.R., and Johnson, R. W.[7]; Brown, D. T., et al.[70]; Cohen, S.E., and Thurlow, A.,[95]; Bromage, P.R.[65]; Cousins, M.J., et al.[109]; Murphy, T.M., et al.[273]; Seow, L.T., et al.[346]; Katz, J.A., et al.[218]; and Morrison, L.M.M., et al.[272]

Limited experience is available with ropivacaine in pregnancy; however, the first study comparing bupivacaine with ropivacaine showed no major differences regarding the characteristics of pain relief in labor.[261] Preliminary results show that postoperative epidural infusion of ropivacaine 0.2% provided good pain relief with minimal motor block in patients having major lower abdominal surgery and major orthopedic surgery.[16,337] Zaric et al. (1994) assessed motor blockade by a quantitative method (measurements of isometric muscle force) during continuous epidural infusion of ropivacaine 0.1%, 0.2%, or 0.3% in healthy volunteers.[415] The quality of sensory and motor blockade were clearly dependent on the concentration of ropivacaine. Ropivacaine 0.2% caused moderate motor blockade and provided the most satisfactory conditions for postoperative pain relief.[415]

Differential Block. The differential capabilities of local anesthetics to block sensory and motor fibers has been referred to as "sensory-motor dissociation" (see Fig. 8-25). The basis for this phenomenon is discussed in Chapters 2 and 3.

Local Anesthetic Mixtures. The basis of mixing (compounding) of local anesthetic agents is to obtain a rapid onset as well as a long duration of blockade. 2-chloroprocaine was used in combination with bupivacaine to have a faster onset as well as prolonged sensory block following epidural anesthesia in the obstetric setting.[95] Unfortunately, 2-chloroprocaine shortened the duration of bupivacaine's block. Isolated nerve studies suggest that a metabolite of chloroprocaine may inhibit the binding of bupivacaine to the membrane site of action.[101]

Currently, there does not appear to be any clinically significant advantage to the use of mixtures of local anesthetic agents if a catheter technique is to be used. The use of continuous techniques of administration of the shorter-acting agents has considerable advantages in that duration is not a problem and a rapid effect can be obtained with a single drug. Only when a single-dose (through the needle) technique is used does the 1:1 mixture of lidocaine-bupivacaine have some merit in achieving rapid onset of profound motor blockade, followed by some increases in duration of analgesia compared with lidocaine alone; however, the gains are small.[346]

Epinephrine

There is general agreement that addition of epinephrine reduces vascular absorption to a variable extent (see Chapter 4, Table 4-2, and Figs. 4-17 and 4-18) and enhances the efficacy of epidural blockade. However, with respect to efficacy, the following distinctions must be drawn: Enhancement of blockade is much less marked with the longer-acting agents bupivacaine and etidocaine; addition of fresh epinephrine in a concentration of 1:200,000 may enhance the intensity of motor block, quality of sensory blockade, and duration of blockade, at least for lidocaine and prilocaine.[66]

As indicated in Chapter 3, Table 3-4, the combination of local vasoconstriction (owing to epinephrine) and acidity (owing to antioxidants) in premixed epinephrine-containing solutions may lower tissue pH below 7 for more than 90 minutes. This theoretically would result in reduced release of local anesthetic base and reduced penetration of neural tissue. It has been proposed that this may be responsible for increased latency to onset of sensory blockade.[66]

Despite these considerations, addition of fresh epinephrine to local anesthetic, *at the time of injection*, does not prolong the onset of clinical epidural or subarachnoid neural blockade with lidocaine or bupivacaine. In fact, with lidocaine or etidocaine the opposite has been reported[50,273] (Fig. 8-28). A controlled study comparing commercially prepared epinephrine-containing solutions with solutions containing freshly added epinephrine is not available. However, reduced tissue pH results from epinephrine-containing solutions regardless of whether the solution has a pH of 3.5 or 6.5, so that adding epinephrine freshly may not have a great advantage. Another effect of epidurally administered

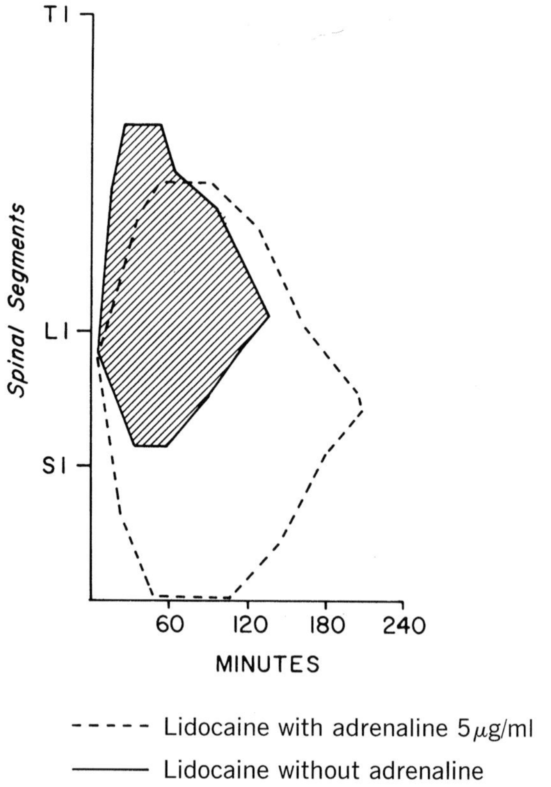

FIG. 8-28. Effect of epinephrine; segmental spread and duration of sensory blockade for lidocaine. Segmental spread and duration of analgesia are enhanced by addition of epinephrine. Caudad spread of analgesia is also markedly improved with epinephrine-containing solutions. *Broken line,* + epinephrine (5 μg/ml); *solid line,* plain solution. (Murphy, T.M., Mather, L.E., Stanton-Hicks, M.D.A., Bonica, J.J., *et al.*: Effects of adding adrenaline to etidocaine and Lignocaine in extradural anaesthesia: I. Block characteristics and cardiovascular effects. Br. J. Anaesth., *48*:893, 1976.)

epinephrine has become apparent: inhibitory receptors in the dorsal horn of the spinal cord are responsive to epidural or subarachnoid administration of α-agonists.[313] In one study in dogs, clonidine was as effective as epinephrine in prolonging duration of sensory blockade of subarachnoid tetracaine. Interestingly, clonidine was more effective in prolonging motor blockade.[20] Because clonidine does not produce vasoconstriction, it seems that at least part of the enhancement of analgesia seen with epinephrine is due to activation of dorsal horn inhibitory systems (see Chapter 29). For more detailed information on α-agonists, the reader is referred to Chapters 23, 24, and 29.

Carbon Dioxide Salts

Injection of carbonated local anesthetics instead of the regular hydrochloride salt solutions may influence the onset of blockade by a direct effect of carbon dioxide on axons, enhanced diffusion, and/or a decrease in intraneural pH, which enhances the fraction of active ionized drug in the axons. This effect appears to be more pronounced with epidurally administered lidocaine than with bupivacaine solutions.[263,278] Carbonated local anesthetics are used extensively in Canada, but are not marketed in other countries. This topic is covered in more detail in Chapter 2.

Number and Frequency of Local Anesthetic Injections

Whether augmentation or diminution of neural blockade occurs after repeated epidural injection of local anesthetics depends on the local anesthetic agent, the number of injections, and the timing between injections (Fig. 8-29).

A single "repeat" dose (20% of total dose) given approximately 20 minutes after the main dose of local anesthetic has been said to consolidate blockade within the level of blockade already established. Thus, "missed segments" may be "filled in," but the level of blockade may not be extended.[57]

A second dose of approximately 50% of initial dosage will maintain the initial segmental level of analgesia if given when the upper level of segmental analgesia has receded one to two dermatomes. On the other hand, administration of the same dose as given for induction of block will result in augmentation of level of blockade at this time. Clinical practice relies on either mean duration times (Table 8-14) or careful monitoring for signs of regression of blockade, to determine the need for a second or refill dose.

A "refill" dose given more than 10 minutes outside regression of analgesia (the "interanalgesic interval") may result in tachyphylaxis, that is, an *increase* in dosage is required to maintain a constant level of blockade. Tachyphylaxis increases with the length of interanalgesic interval up to 60 minutes, but then it remains constant; at 60 minutes there is a 30% to 40% decrease in effect of a repeated dose (see Fig. 8-29).[69]

Tachyphylaxis has been most clearly demonstrated in association with "continuous" epidural block in patients in whom repeated injections of the short-acting amides—lidocaine, prilocaine, or mepivacaine—are used. Because the interanalgesic interval seems so important, it is not surprising that tachyphylaxis has been much less a problem with the longer-acting agents, such as bupivacaine (see Fig. 8-29).

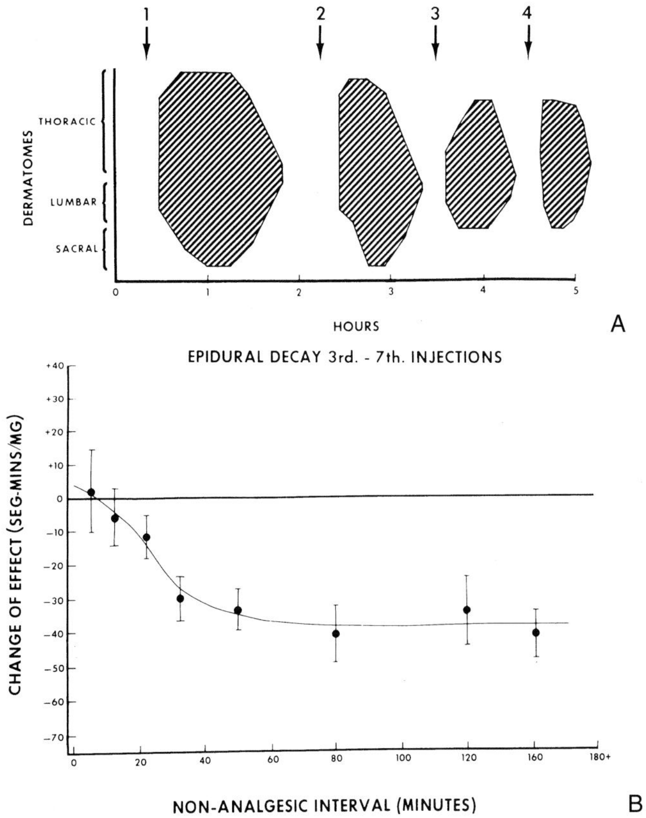

FIG. 8-29. Tachyphylaxis. **A:** Diminished segmental spread and duration of action of repeated epidural injections of the same dose of local anesthetic, injected at each arrow. Note reinjection has been made at least 30 minutes after analgesia has regressed two segments. **B:** "Nonanalgesic interval." As the time lag from loss of analgesia to reinjection exceeds 10 to 15 minutes, there is a progressive reduction in analgesic effect that reaches a maximum reduction of about 35% to 40% at 60 minutes. (Bromage, P.R., Pettigrew, R.T., and Crowell, D.E.: Tachyphylaxis in epidural analgesia: I. Augmentation and decay of local anesthesia. J. Clin. Pharmacol., *9*:30, 1969.)

Bromage found that tachyphylaxis increased with the number of injections administered. This again indicates the desirability of using long-acting agents. Finally, it should be recalled that bupivacaine and etidocaine have a lesser tendency to accumulate in the blood, whereas the short-acting agents are associated with gradually increasing blood concentrations with increased risks of toxicity (see Chapter 3, Fig. 3-12 and Table 3-7).

The mechanism of tachyphylaxis is not known. It may be partly explained by pH changes[82] in spinal fluid with repeated injections; however, this is not an adequate explanation on its own (see Chapters 2 and 3).

TECHNIQUE OF EPIDURAL BLOCKADE

Epidural Trays

There are now available a large number of commercially prepared disposable epidural trays that contain a variable number of the ideal components for epidural blockade. Individual preference plays a considerable part in choice of a tray. However, there are several desirable features:

Separation of a preparation section from the equipment section of the tray is desirable.

Glass syringes for testing loss of resistance should be of highest quality, with freely moving, snug-fitting plungers. High-quality plastic "loss of resistance" syringes are also available.

Disposable epidural needles should not have the "chisel" tip of the original Tuohy needle, since this increases the risk of dural puncture. Some disposable epidural needles are dangerously sharp (Fig. 8-30A).

Epidural needle stylets should fit the needle precisely, particularly at the needle tip.

Epidural catheters should be made of clear material so that aspirated blood can be clearly seen in the catheter. Also, catheters should be strong and flexible, should be inert, and should not have sharp tips capable of tearing blood vessels or puncturing dura. They should also be marked for roentgenographic detection.

Local anesthetics to be used in disposable trays should be packed in sterile protective covering on the tray or in individual sterile containers. Single-use vials are available with a "top hat"-shaped cap that can easily be grasped and pulled off without contaminating the solution with particles of glass or rubber, as may occur with ampuls and some types of vials.

Mixing cups should be free of any particulate matter.

Unfortunately, many disposable trays fall short of these ideals. However, sterility is guaranteed by the manufacturer, and needles and syringes should be free of imperfections.

Many anesthesiologists still prefer department-prepared trays, which contain all items decided on by that particular group. This works well in a practice in which all can agree on a "standard" tray and a dedicated and skilled staff prepare the trays to ensure sterility and exclusion of chemical materials that may be neurolytic. In smaller hospitals that use epidural trays infrequently, commercial trays may be a valuable insurance against chemical and bacterial contamination. Larger units may prefer to design their own trays and use carefully maintained, reusable, high-quality needles and syringes. The following "traps" should be avoided.

Syringe barrels and plungers should be kept together, since "odds" may not fit with the precision required for loss of resistance testing. Powder or other material on syringe plungers may result in sticking, which can be dangerous if entry into the epidural space is missed, particularly above the level of L1; plastic epidural "loss of resistance" syringes have special plungers that prevent this problem.

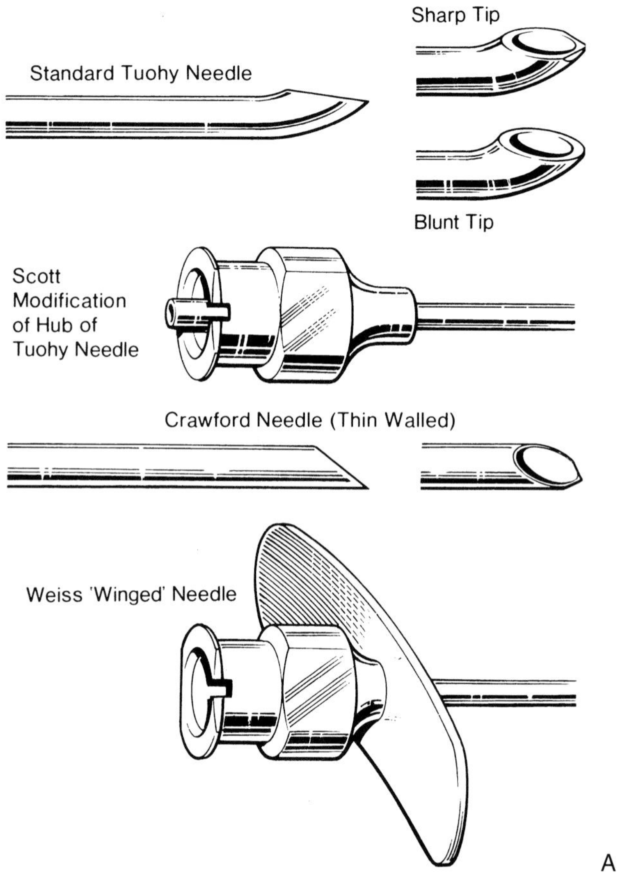

FIG. 8-30. A: *Epidural needles.*

Epidural needles should be skillfully machined and maintained, so that rough and sharp edges are avoided. Stylets must fit perfectly to avoid tissue damage or plugs in the end of the needle.

Epidural local anesthetics must be carefully sterilized, using a technique approved by a trained pharmacist, so that sterility, potency, and freedom from chemical contamination are ensured.

Hospital-prepared anesthetic trays should have the date of sterilization marked on the outside of the pack and a sterilization indicator included inside the pack.

Epidural Needles

As for spinal analgesia, a close-fitting removable stylet is essential for epidural anesthesia, to prevent plugging of the needle tip with skin and failure to recognize loss of resistance. The possibility of a large epidermal plug being carried into the epidural or subarachnoid space must also be avoided. The epidural space can also be identified by compression of a 10- to 20 ml air-filled syringe attached to a 22-gauge Greene or Whitacre spinal needle; this is a useful teaching aid while performing lumbar puncture and may also be an alternative technique for single-shot epidural block. The "standard" Tuohy needle has a gentle curve of the "Huber" tip, but with a rather sharp point at the end, and this is favored by some experienced epiduralists. For the novice, a

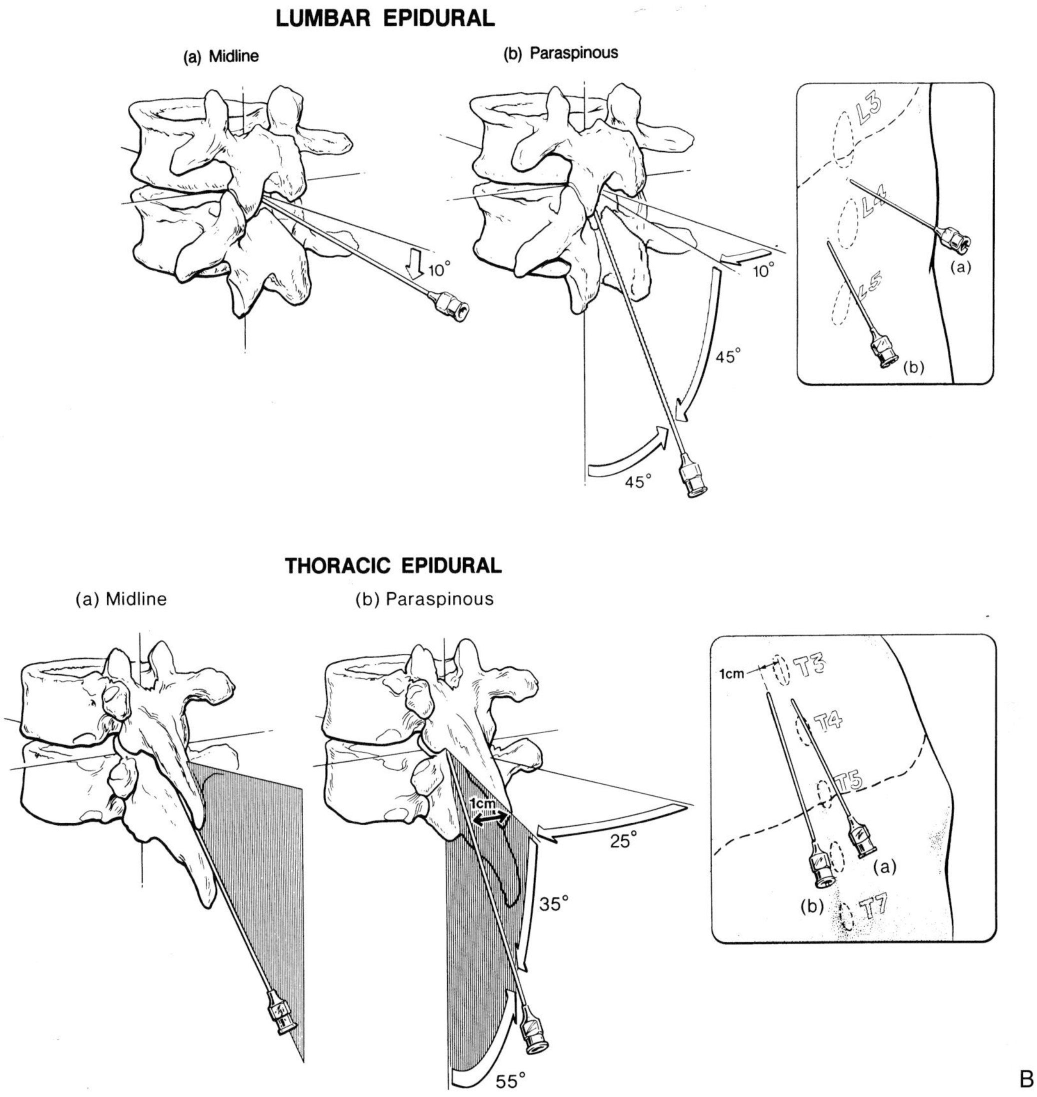

FIG. 8-30. *Continued.* **B:** *Epidural Block: Sites of needle insertion. Upper panel*: **Lumbar epidural**. *(a)* Midline. Note insertion closer to the superior spinous process and with a slight upward angulation; *(b)* paraspinous (paramedian). Note insertion beside caudad edge of "inferior" spinous process, with 45° angulation to long axis of spine below. *Lower panel*: **Thoracic epidural**. *(a)* Midline. Note extreme upward angulation required in midthoracic region. Therefore, a paraspinous approach may be easier: *(b)* paraspinous. Note needle insertion next to caudad tip of the spinous process above interspace of intended level of entry through ligamentum flavum. Upward angulation is 55° to long axis of spine below and inward angulation is 10° to 15°.

rounded blunt needle end of the Huber tip is less likely to puncture the dura[378] (Fig. 8-30A). This type of needle end also permits easier identification of the ligamentum flavum, sometimes requiring considerable force to penetrate the ligament. Some authorities like to teach with a 16-gauge needle and then let the novice "graduate" to an 18-gauge needle.

A useful refinement is the Scott needle, which has the shaft protruding from the hub.[110] This permits easier threading and advancement of epidural catheters, particularly with 18-gauge catheters, which sometimes kink and curl within the standard hub. Calibrated needles with centimeter markings also are available.[137,235]

The 18-gauge Crawford, thin-walled needle is often used for the paramedian, "paraspinous" (lateral) approach, since a catheter threads directly up the epidural space if the needle is angled at 45° to 60° upward. With a Tuohy needle, the catheter is sometimes difficult to thread with this approach, since the recurved needle tip is angled back against the ligamentum flavum or lamina. However, the Crawford needle with its "front end" orifice is more likely to penetrate the tissues, like an "apple corer," and to become plugged with tissue fragments than is the Tuohy needle with its recurred orifice. Other needles, such as the large Cheng[86] and Crawley needles[102] and the fine 22-gauge Wagner needle, are less commonly used, since they have little advantage over standard needles.

"Winged needles" are ideal for "hanging-drop" techniques, since the grip on the needle should be well away from the fluid drop on the hub of the needle. Many variants of the original Labat winged needle are available, and detachable wings made of plastic have also been designed[410] for use with standard Tuohy needles. Some anesthesiologists prefer more versatile and more solid "spool"-type needles with a Barker style of hub, (e.g., the Bromage needle).[58]

Epidural Catheters

Plastic epidural catheters have replaced those made of other materials. There are various plastic materials, and no systematic study has been made of the requirements for epidural catheters and the features of different plastic materials. Only sporadic information is available. For example, some Teflon catheters were found to kink, and this led to breakages in the wall. Bromage has summarized ideal characteristics: biochemical inertness, low coefficient of friction, high tensile strength, maneuverable rigidity, kink resistance, atraumatic tip, depth indicators, radiopacity. A stylet is not recommended, since it increases the risk of trauma to blood vessels, nerve roots, and so on. One catheter (the Racz catheter) has a stainless steel coil at the tip that makes the tip flexible.

Epidural Cannulas

In an attempt to overcome the risk of pulling a catheter back through a Tuohy needle and shearing it off, epidural "cannula-over-needle" equipment was developed, analogous to intravascular equipment. This includes the Winnie-Jelco cannula, the Henkin-Bard cannula, and others.[65] They all suffer from the need to connect the cannula to a catheter after it is advanced over the straight epidural needle. In our view this equipment is not an advantage over standard equipment.

Epidural equipment should be simple. A steady pair of hands with a highly trained feel for loss of resistance, a freely running glass syringe, and a high-quality epidural needle are far superior to the multitude of mechanical devices offered as aids to identify the epidural space.[129]

Required Equipment for Epidural Blockade

- A satisfactory preparation section of tray (sterilizing fluid cup, swabs, swab holder, sterile towels)
- 1 × 2.5 cm, 25-gauge needle for skin analgesia
- 1 × 4 cm, 22-gauge needle for deep infiltration
- 1 × 18 gauge needle for drawing up epidural solutions and then piercing skin[a] before inserting the epidural needle
- Epidural needle (Tuohy, Crawford)
- Epidural catheter
- 1 × 2 ml, glass syringe for infiltration, syringe mount
- 2 × 10 ml, all-glass syringes for loss of resistance tests[b] and drawing up local anesthetic
- Local anesthetic mixing cup
- Normal saline
- Local anesthetics
- Filters and caps for epidural catheter
- Sterility indicator

[a]Alternatively a small scalpel blade is used.
[b]Excellent plastic "testing syringes" are available.

Some practitioners prefer to have sterilized vials of local anesthetic on the tray and to draw them up into 10-ml glass syringes, rather than using a "mixing" container and exposing the solution to possible contamination. Although Millipore filters have not been conclusively shown to reduce the incidence of epidural infection, they may have other advantages. Particulate matter has been reported from mixing containers and "snap-neck" glass ampuls.[217] The Millipore filter offers some protection against this material reaching the epidural space. (see Chapter 6 for general information regarding equipment for neural blockade and preparation of the patient.)

Combined Spinal-epidural anesthesia

A combined spinal-epidural technique (CSE) can be used to reduce or eliminate some of the disadvantages of spinal and epidural anesthesia while preserving advantages of both. Spinal anesthesia offers rapid onset of action, reliable surgical anesthesia, and full muscle relaxation. On the other hand, an indwelling epidural catheter offers the advantage of adding local anesthetic top-up doses to extend the duration of the block, to improve inadequate spinal block, and to provide postoperative pain relief. This sequential technique has been shown to be particularly useful in patients undergoing cesarean section and major hip and knee surgery.[389] Controlled studies comparing a regular or epidural block with sequential CSE block for cesarean section showed that CSE technique proved to be as safe and effective as spinal and epidural anesthesia for cesarean section.[312] Initially an epidural needle was introduced at one lumbar interspace followed by a subarachnoid puncture at another interspace.[120] Brownridge[71] advocated this double-interspace technique for cesarean section (see Chapter 18).

Currently the most commonly used technique is the single-interspace spinal needle through the epidural needle method, as first described by Coates in 1982 (Fig. 8-31A).[89] A 16- or 18-gauge Tuohy needle is used to identify the epidural space, after which a long spinal needle is inserted through it to perforate the dura mater. Correct placement of the spinal needle in the subarachnoid space is confirmed by aspiration of cerebrospinal fluid. After the subarachnoid injection of a local anesthetic solution, the spinal needle is removed and the epidural catheter introduced into the epidural space in the usual manner.

Specially designed needle sets for the CSE have been produced. For example a modified Tuohy needle with a hole (back eye) in its curve has been manufactured, so that the

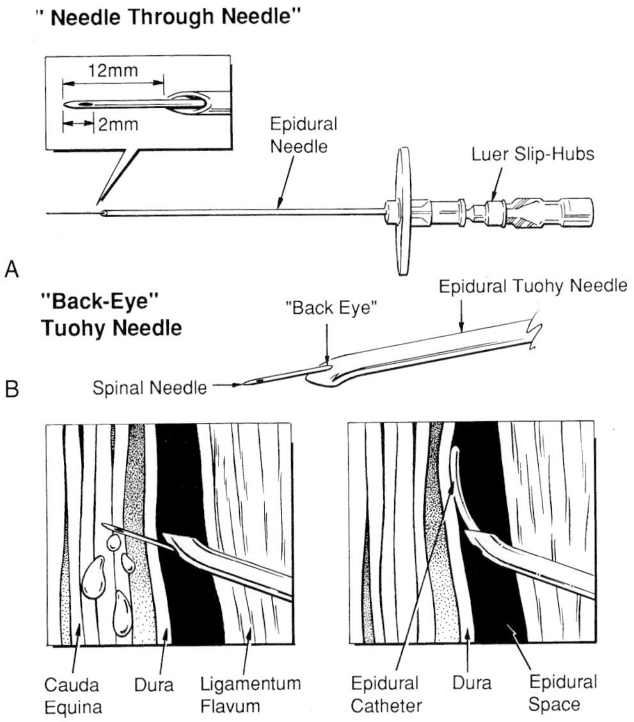

FIG. 8-31. **A:** Combined spinal and epidural needle. It shows a needle-through-needle technique. **B:** Tuohy needle with back eye. Left panel shows subarachnoid needle protruding through back eye of Tuohy needle into subarachnoid space, while the Tuohy needle remains in the epidural space. Right panel shows an epidural catheter subsequently threaded into the epidural space for continuous epidural analgesia.

spinal needle passes through the back eye directly into the subarachnoid space, instead of exiting from the end of the Tuohy needle (Fig. 8-31B). This back eye is only of interest in those Tuohy needles with a long distal curve, and has been developed in order to eliminate the need to thread the spinal needle through the distal opening of the Tuohy needle with all the supposed disadvantages. Very recently Joshi et al. (1994) evaluated the CSE technique using the standard 16-gauge Tuohy needle or the modified Tuohy needle with the back eye.[213] It was concluded that an improved needle set for the "needle-through-needle" technique would be one with a modified Tuohy needle having the back eye and a spinal needle protruding more than 13 mm beyond the Tuohy needle.

Concerns regarding the CSE technique include an accidental passage of the epidural catheter through the hole in the dura mater, the possibility of extensive subarachnoid effects from epidurally injected local anesthetics by passage through the hole in the dura, and failure to thread the epidural catheter after the intrathecal injection has been given. Routine precautions to avoid intravascular or intrathecal injection should be carried out, including aspiration and test dose administration. Spinal-epidural needle-through-needle technique may cause metallic fragments by friction between the spinal needle and the epidural bent tip inner surface.[141] Theoretically, the particles produced by the friction between the two needles can be pushed forward by the force extended into the epidural space. It is clear that this technique requires technical skills and therefore should be performed only by experienced anesthesiologists.

Patient Evaluation and Preparation

As in any preanesthetic evaluation, certain essential information should be obtained. Its implications must be considered before epidural blockade is selected as part of the anesthetic regimen. If epidural block seems appropriate, the necessary preoperative steps should be taken: The minimum entails adequate psychological preparation, adequate baseline data (e.g., blood sugar levels in a diabetic), and correction of reversible abnormalities, such as dehydration (Table 8-15). Informed consent is obtained.

TABLE 8-15. *Checklist: a safety procedure before spinal epidural blockade*

Patient evaluation
Psychological suitability
Physical suitability with emphasis on the following:
Obesity and/or bony spine abnormalities
Pre-existing neurologic disease
Cardiorespiratory function (e.g., ability to withstand sympathetic blockade)
Blood volume
Drug factors:
Anticoagulants, aspirin, and other antiplatelet drugs, sensitivity to local anesthetics, antihypertensive agents, monoamine oxidase inhibitors (and other drugs interferring with sympathetic function)
History of previous anesthetic and other drug administration
Family history of adverse drug effects
Patient preparation
Explanation of blockade procedure and its benefits (intraoperative and postoperative)
Inquiry as to patient's desire for sedation or full unconsciousness
Baseline information
Spine radiograph for undefined pathology, blood sugar level for diabetics
Correction of reversible abnormalities (e.g., dehydration)
Informed consent is obtained.
Record history and management plan in notes
Order
Changes (if any) in current medication
Premedication
Preoperative discussion
Operative details with surgeon to determine the following:
Level of blockade required
Appropriate supplementation
Necessity for intubation
Management plan with surgical staff: equipment and drug requirements
Timing for patient transport to operating room
Assistance from nursing staff

Preoperative Discussion with Medical Staff

A discussion with the medical staff should not be omitted just because the choice of anesthesia is considered the province of the anesthesiologist. Consultation with the surgeon is necessary to help determine the precise nature of operative approach and therefore the level of blockade required, the need for supplementation, and the necessity for intubation if exploration will markedly impinge on upper abdominal areas. Preoperative communication with nursing staff can be accomplished by a telephone call, to inform them beforehand of requirements for special equipment, timing of transportation of the patient to the operating room, and the need for assistance during positioning of the patient for a block (Table 8-15).

Planning for Technique of Block and Drug Dose

Choice of patient's position for puncture follows the same principles outlined in Chapter 7, Figures 7-17 and 7-18. Although the effect of gravity may be debatable, reliability of blockade of S1 is probably increased with the patient in the sitting position. Also, it is easier to enter the epidural space in obese patients if the sitting position is used. On the other hand, patients who have a history of fainting or who are heavily premedicated should have their block induced while in the lateral position. Site of puncture is usually at L2–L3 or L3–L4 (see Fig. 8-7A), unless the anesthesiologist is an experienced epiduralist; puncture at L5–S1 aids in ensuring blockade of the resistant S1 segment for ankle or knee surgery. At higher levels, experienced epiduralists may choose an interspace close to the center of the dermatomal segments required.[195] However, the degree of difficulty of needle insertion should also be considered. Thus, one may choose T9–T10 for a thoracic operation, even though the more difficult T5–T6 level may be closer to the center of the required dermatomes. Similarly, C7–T1 level may be chosen for an upper thoracic procedure rather than the more difficult T3–T4 level. We believe that the midline approach should be learned thoroughly before using the paraspinous (lateral) approach, since the chance of needle entry into the lateral aspects of the ligamentum flavum (see Fig. 8-4) may be greater if inexperienced attempts are made to "angle" the needle toward the midline. However, careful use of the spinous process to guide the needle for a paraspinous approach to a midline entry through the ligamentum flavum can be extremely reliable and easy in the hands of an experienced epiduralist (see Table 8-1), and this feature is helpful in the midthoracic region (see Table 8-2). In the cervical region, midline puncture becomes more reliable again, and it is best to choose the C7–T1 level, since the epidural space is wider than at higher cervical levels, and access between the spinous processes is easy if the neck if flexed (see Table 8-3).

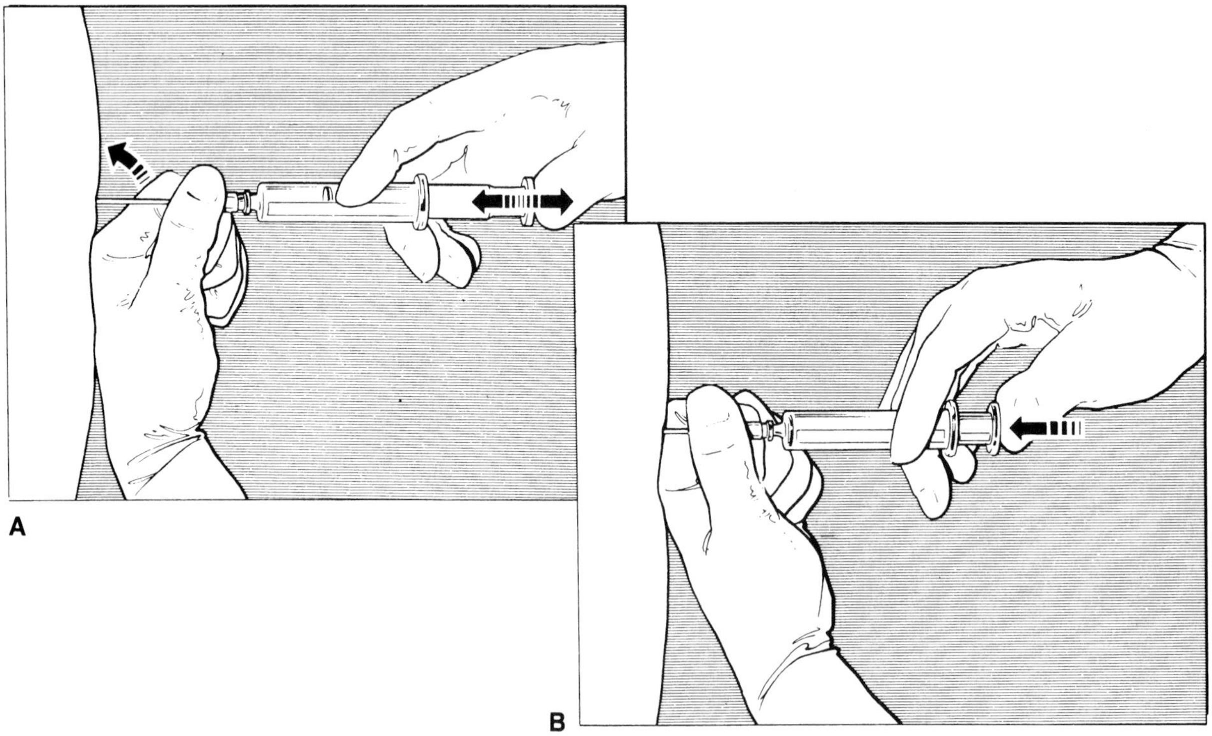

FIG. 8-32. "Bromage" grip for loss of resistance technique. **A:** Note the viselike grip of needle between thumb and *entire fist.* Metacarpal heads are braced against the back. The needle is advanced by rotation of the entire hand around the metacarpal heads; only a small, highly controlled movement is possible without repositioning the hand on the needle. There is continual compression of syringe plunger, with a "bouncing" movement. **B:** As soon as the ligamentum flavum is pierced, resistance to syringe plunger is lost, and the needle is immediately halted. (This sequence is seen from above.)

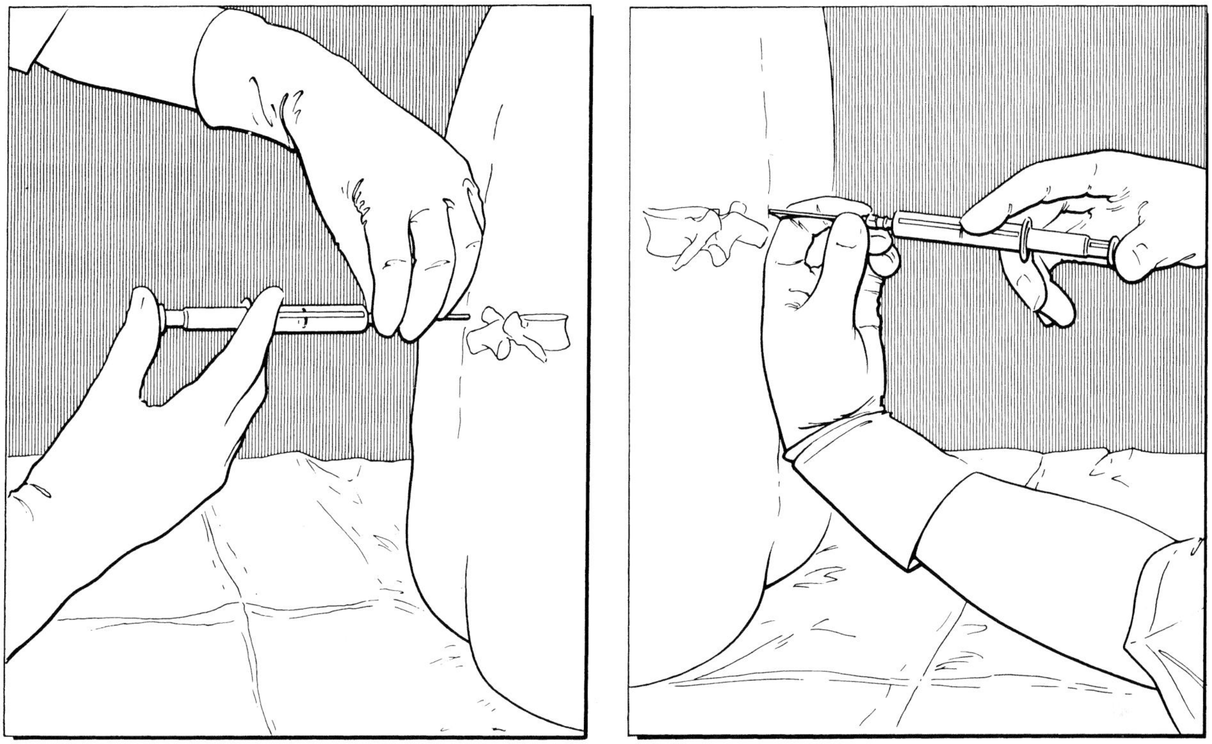

A B

FIG. 8-33. Alternative, less-controlled grips. **A:** Hand gripping needle from above. **B:** Hand gripping needle from below. Note that in both **A** and **B** the hand holding the needle is braced against the patient's back at all times, and the needle is advanced by forward movement of the forefinger and thumb.

The *technique chosen for identification of epidural space* depends largely on personal preference and familiarity with technique.[270] We prefer the technique of loss of resistance, using an air-filled syringe at all levels, provided the firm "Bromage" grip is used.[65] Certainly, the two-handed grip of the "hanging-drop" technique ensures excellent control; however, the slight risk that there may be a plug in the needle tip and the occurrence of low or no negative pressure tends to outweigh the benefits of the "hanging-drop," or "Gutierrez," technique. We prefer to use the midline approach (Fig. 8-30), with an air-filled syringe (Figs. 8-32 and 8-33) at lumbar, low-thoracic, and C7–T1 levels, unless midline entry proves difficult; then a paraspinous approach is used. In the midthoracic region, the paramedian, paraspinous (lateral) approach (see Fig. 8-30) is routinely used with an air-filled syringe.

A case for avoiding air-filled syringes could be made in patients presenting for ablation of renal stones by extracorporeal shock wave lithotripsy.[1] The focused shock waves set up turbulence and tissue damage at air-water or air-tissue interfaces, and so epidural or paravertebral bubbles of air might conceivably predispose to local neural damage if traversed by the shock beam. Thus, there are theoretic grounds for using saline-filled syringes for loss of resistance in such cases.[1] The chances of problems arising from epidural bubbles would seem to be extremely remote if puncture is made in the thoracic region and above the path of the shock beam.

It is desirable when puncture is made above the L2 level to routinely infiltrate down beside the spinous process and check the depth of the lamina as a guide to the depth of the interlaminar space. This avoids the danger of continuing to advance a needle with a plug in the end. Experience with the use of the Bromage grip develops a keen sense of resistance in the hand advancing the needle and the hand compressing the syringe plunger. Unfortunately, the "hanging-drop" is not under the anesthesiologist's control; it may impart a visual sign only on entry into the epidural space without premonitory sign of increased plunger resistance, which becomes highly developed during routine use of lumbar epidural block. Nevertheless, many anesthesiologists find that the two-handed grip of the "hanging-drop" technique gives them greater control. If this technique is used, the stylet must not be withdrawn until the needle is close to the ligamentum flavum. It should be reinserted if the needle contacts periosteum and requires repositioning. Also, it is preferable to advance the needle only during inspiration so that negative pressure in the epidural space is maximal.

The *choice of single-shot or catheter technique* depends on the patient and the type of operation. Catheter techniques are useful in debilitated and aged patients, since level of blockade can be gradually extended to the required level; this is also a wise approach in operative obstetrics. Prolonged surgery requires catheter techniques. Healthy patients undergoing brief procedures can be adequately managed with a single shot by the needle, even if it is planned to thread a catheter for "insurance." In this situation we prefer to inject the dose by way of the needle, since catheters may malfunction owing to transforaminal escape or superficial placement,[49] "curling up,"[333] or sometimes passage into the anterior epidural space.[384] Threading catheters only 3 to 4 cm into the epidural space reduces, but does not eliminate, malfunction.[350]

Dosage calculation and choice of agent depend on factors discussed on page 288. Single-shot techniques depend on a generous calculation of dose requirements, so that catheter techniques are preferable if it is essential to restrict dose and level of blockade. Considerations of the most appropriate drug and concentration, and addition of epinephrine are also discussed on page 289 and are outlined in Table 8-13.

Needle insertion under general anesthesia is certainly more comfortable for the patient. However, comfort is bought at the price of safety, since valuable signs of contact with neural tissue and of intravascular or subarachnoid injection may be lost, so that considerable experience or supervision by an experienced epiduralist is required.

Conduct of Epidural Blockade

Epidural neural blockade should be viewed as part of a complete anesthetic procedure (Table 8-16), which includes preparative steps, continuous surveillance, and appropriate responses (e.g., supplementation if indicated). It should be stressed that technical expertise in inserting an epidural needle is insufficient, by itself, to safely manage epidural block. Reports of anesthetic mortality committees[360] have drawn attention to

1. Deficiencies in knowledge of physiology and pharmacology of epidural blockade and treatment of altered physiology and of pharmacologic side effects;
2. Inadequate preparation (e.g., failure to restore blood volume);
3. Inadequate monitoring before, during, and after surgery;
4. Inadequate supplementation and general management (e.g., failure to use artificial ventilation in situations where it is required);
5. Slowness and inappropriate responses to sudden changes in physiology;
6. Lack of appropriate resuscitative skills.

All of the above have parallels in the safe administration of *general* anesthesia. Somehow some individuals attempting to use epidural block have failed to realize that the same level of knowledge, surveillance, and technical skill is required for epidural block and its management.

Initial steps in the operating room must always include preparation of drugs and equipment for life support, the means of supplementation, and provision of a contingency plan for general anesthesia, to provide complete coverage for the operative procedure if the epidural block is inadequate. There should be no delay in deciding whether epidural block can be counted on to provide analgesia and muscle relaxation (if required). Inadequate or patchy blockade should be swiftly covered by appropriate supplementation, and this should be done in a manner that is not discernible to the patient or the surgeon. This is extremely important in maintaining acceptability of the technique to patient, surgeon, and other medical staff. Also, emphasis is placed on erecting a screen as soon as the patient is placed on the operating table.

Supplementation agents are discussed in Chapter 6. Some practitioners have a preference for supplementation with low-dose opioid infusion (e.g., pethidine[363]) or with low-dose infusion of rapidly cleared drugs, such as methohexitone, hexobarbital, midazolam, low-dose ketamine, etomidate, propofol, or chlormethiazole (hemineurin).[258,338,347] The aim of "low-dose" sedative infusion is to produce "natural" sleep with maintenance of an unobstructed airway, even with the patient in the prone position. This technique permits patients to tolerate uncomfortable positions without the long-standing problems associated with induction of general anesthesia and an obstructed airway. Because such drugs are rapidly cleared from the body, cessation of infusion may result in a rapid recovery from sedation within a few minutes.[258]

Once the patient arrives in the operating room, all of the above should be ready, and activity should then concentrate on aspects relating directly to the patient (Table 8-16). For example, adequacy of sedation before needle insertion should be assessed. Any recent untoward events, such as severe angina during the night, should be elicited. The medical record should be checked. In particular, drug therapy should be scrutinized to determine whether prescribed drugs (e.g., insulin) have been given and undesired drugs (e.g., heparin) have been discontinued. The steps of the procedure should be reassuringly outlined for the patient, and any changes in patient requirements determined (e.g., a desire to be completely asleep rather than lightly sedated).

Although there are many approaches to *locating the desired interspace*, we prefer to make an indentation with the thumb nail in the chosen interspace, to leave a mark at the level of the anterior superior iliac crest with the skin preparation solution, and then finally to palpate the rib margin as a guide to location of L1 (see Fig. 8-9A). With this approach, the landmarks can be identified immediately before needle insertion. In contrast, marking with a skin "pen" is carried out before skin preparation, and the patient may move in the interim. Baseline blood pressure and heart rate should always be recorded on the anesthetic record before blockade.

Skin preparation and preparation of the neural block tray should require two separate steps. Also, it should be stressed that the neural block tray must be kept separate from all other drugs, since human error may result in injection of inappropriate agents into the epidural space with potentially disastrous sequelae.[383] It is preferable to complete the skin preparation before uncovering the epidural needles and drugs. In any event, splashing of preparatory solutions on neural block equipment must be avoided (Table 8-16).

TABLE 8-16. *Therapeutic procedures[a] for epidural block*

Initial steps in the operating room
Preparation
Resuscitative drugs and equipment (see Chapter 4, Table 4-9); monitoring equipment (see Chapter 6, Fig. 6-2)
Plastic oxygen mask and appropriate connection to anesthetic machine
Supplementation: drugs and equipment
Opioid, sedative requests from drug "safe"
Stereo headphones
Screen (to be erected as soon as patient is in operating room)
Contingency plan for general anesthesia if needed, equipment and drugs prepared
The patient
Inquire about adequacy of sedation and other problems
Insert IV line and rehydrate
Position correctly but comfortably
Reiterate step of procedure
Mark landmarks with skin marker or other means
Check blood pressure, heart rate; attach ECG electrodes; monitor ECG continuously
Skin preparation and preparation of neural block tray
Equipment physically separated from all other drugs (see Chapter 6, Figs. 6-3, 6-4)
Sterile tray
Sterile wrapped drugs
Check sterility control indicator
Skin preparation
Keep equipment and drugs covered and separated from cleansing solutions during skin preparation
Discard cleansing solution and equipment before uncovering block equipment
Discard entire block tray if cleansing solution splashed onto drugs/needles
Allow at least 3 minutes for solution to act (draw up drugs during this time)
Preparation of drugs and equipment
Discard drug solutions that are cloudy or have crystals
Double check identity of drugs
Check dose of local anesthetic (and vasoconstrictor)
Draw up solution for epidural block in 10-ml syringes (to facilitate aspiration)
Draw up infiltration solution
Check fit of stylet, tip of epidural needle, fit of catheter through needle, patency of catheter
Check that "loss of resistance" syringe operates without sticking
Insertion of needle (midline technique)
Infiltrate skin and interspinous region (then recheck epidural equipment)
Puncture skin with 18-gauge needle or scalpel blade
Check that epidural needle insertion is midline by "Labat" palpation of spinous process (see Fig. 8-9B)
Maintain constant pressure on "testing" syringe
Control needle advancement in vicelike grip with hand braced against patient at all times (see Fig. 8-32)
Halt needle immediately if resistance is lost or if there is any doubt about position (see Table 8-5)
Aspirate gently and then immediately inject "test dose," 4 ml of prepared solution, again with hand holding needle braced against back
Disconnect syringe and check temperature of any backflow solution on arm (? cold = L.A. ? warm = CSF)
Question patient about warmth or numbness in lower limbs
Maintain constant verbal contact; check heart rate, blood pressure, ECG, pulse oximeter
Single shot
Inject (<0.3 ml/sec) one-half the full dose, aspirate; then disconnect syringe, check as above, and inject remainder of dose if no adverse sequelae
Catheter technique
Insert catheter and inject 4-ml dose through catheter; wait 5 minutes; check level, blood pressure, heart rate, aspirate: then inject remainder of dose in 5 ml increments (use Millipore filters)
Caution: Reposition needle/catheter if the following occur:
Paresthesia during insertion in a conscious patient
Muscle twitching in segmental nerve distribution
Excessive force appears necessary
CSF or blood are aspirated
Onset of analgesia appears excessively prolonged
No resistance is felt in interspinous ligament (? below L4) Choose another interspace or use paraspinous approach to check depth of lamina and ligamentum flavum

(continued)

TABLE 8-16. *Continued*

Insertion of needle (paraspinous)
Infiltrate skin, 0.5–1 cm lateral to caudad edge of spinous process
Using 22-gauge "spinal needle," infiltrate at 90° to skin down to lamina; note depth
Insert epidural needle beside spinous process (see Fig. 8-30B) and angle toward midline 10°–15°
Lumbar epidural
Epidural needle angled at 45° to long axis of spine, caudad to point of insertion
Needle beside spinous process, caudad to intended level of entry
Thoracic epidural
Epidural needle angled at 55° to long axis of spine, caudad to point of insertion
Needle beside spinous process above intended level of entry
Further steps in techniques are same as those for midline, except that little resistance is encountered until ligamentum flavum is engaged
Epidural needle should enter epidural space in midline
Continuing management
Monitor
By constant verbal contact (if patient conscious). Continuous ECG, end tidal CO_2, and pulse oximetry are desirable additions
Cardiorespiratory systems for "danger signals" (see Table 8-10)
Level of blockade
Respond to altered physiology
(see Tables 8-7 through 8-11 and Figs. 8-17 through 8-21)
Diagnose and treat local anesthetic "reactions"
(see Chapter 4, Tables 4-8 and 4-10)
Supplement as needed
With additional opioid or sedative agents
By superimposed general anesthesia if operative or patient requirements warrant it
Maintain adequate epidural block
Check for "missed" segments
Top up at mean duration minus 2 SD (see Table 8-14) or when measured segmental level regresses two segments, or use continuous infusion (see Chapter 26)
Diagnose and treat problems such as tachyphylaxis, vascular cannulation, delayed dural puncture
Follow-up
Early
Arrange continuing postoperative epidural analgesia if needed
Prevent infection
Late
Check for any sequelae and, if present, participate in diagnosis and management

[a] The term "therapeutic procedure" is used to include the planning and preparation, the technical procedure, monitoring, and prompt responses to adverse effects.

CSF, cerebrospinal fluid; ECG, electrocardiogram; L.A., local anesthetic; SD, standard deviation.

Except for skin infiltration, complete preparation of neural block equipment should take place before the block is begun. The remaining steps are completed while skin analgesia ensues. It should be noted that the local anesthetic to be used for epidural block is drawn up and ready to inject and the catheter (if used) has been checked and is ready to thread. Care should be taken that glove powder or other material does not soil the barrel of the "loss of resistance" syringe, since this may result in dangerous sticking of the barrel.

Midline Technique

The essential anatomy of needle insertion in the midline is described in detail in the text accompanying Tables 8-1 to 8-3, 8-5, and 8-6 (see also Figs. 8-32 and 8-33). The anesthesiologist should constantly think of the structures the needle encounters. The practical steps are outlined in Table 8-16, and the following aspects should be emphasized: Needle insertion should be in the center of the interspace; deep infiltration with a 22-gauge needle is important to "explore" the anatomy and to make subsequent insertion of the epidural needle comfortable; the skin should be punctured with a large-bore (18- or 19-gauge) needle or scalpel blade to avoid "drag" on the epidural needle or carriage of an epidermal "plug" into the epidural space; if the midline approach is used, the spinous processes should be gripped, as shown in Figure 8-9B, to assist in identification of the midline; constant pressure on the testing syringe should be maintained (Fig. 8-32A), and the epidural needle should be held in a vice-like grip that permits only a small forward movement at a time; the hand holding the needle must be braced firmly against the patient at all times; even in the lumbar region, a slight upward angulation is required to reach the interlaminar space (see Figs. 8-9 to 8-11). If the "Bromage" grip shown in Figure 8-32 is used, it is possible to readily identify changes in resistance, transmitted by the hand holding the needle and the syringe plunger, as the needle enters supraspinous, interspinous, and ligamentum flavum (see Fig. 8-10). Constant pressure on the syringe plunger permits immediate recognition of loss of resistance as the needle tip enters the epidural space, and the vice-like grip on the needle permits immediate halting of needle progress (Table 8-16). Gentle aspiration or, preferably, mere disconnection of the syringe is carried out to check for flow of CSF or blood. If neither is present, 4 ml of solution is immediately injected to push the dura away from the needle tip. Two points require emphasis: The injected solution should meet no resistance and the hand holding the needle must remain braced against the patient's back; otherwise, the needle may be advanced as the solution is injected. The syringe is disconnected again and any drip back is tested as in Table 8-6 while the patient is questioned about warmth and numbness in lower limbs; a subarachnoid injection results in almost immediate onset of blockade of β fibers (Chapter 2, Table 2-1). If no evidence of onset of a subarachnoid block is present, one may proceed to inject the calculated epidural dose as follows:

Single-Shot Techniques. After gentle aspiration, a *test dose* of 5 ml (preferably epinephrine-containing) local anesthetic solution is injected at 10 ml min.$^{-1}$ The syringe is disconnected, and any drip back is tested (see Table 8-6). The patient is observed for increased heart rate owing to intravascular injection of epinephrine and is questioned about sudden onset of warmth or numbness in the legs. If the response to these is negative, further 5-ml increments are injected until the full dose has been given. It should be noted that a "negative" response to a test dose does not provide absolute proof of correct placement.

Catheter Techniques. The catheter is inserted 3 to 4 cm while the hand holding the needle is braced against the patient's back to ensure that the needle does not move. After removal of the needle and careful aspiration, a 5 ml test dose (see above) is then injected through the catheter. After 5 to 10 minutes, the level of blockade, heart rate, and blood pressure are checked; if satisfactory, a careful aspiration test is carried out, and then the remainder of the dose is injected. Alternatively, the remainder of the dose can be injected slowly in 5-ml increments. As noted in Table 8-16, needle or catheter insertion should be halted if undue force is required or if paresthesias or muscle twiches are elicited. If blood flows freely from an epidural needle, it may be necessary to move to an adjacent interspace and ensure that the subsequent entry through the ligamentum flavum is in the midline (see Figs. 8-5 and 8-6). If clear solution drips back or is aspirated from needle or catheter, the steps outlined in Table 8-6 must be taken to determine whether the fluid is local anesthetic or CSF.[84,158] Aspiration of blood from the epidural catheter may be overcome by withdrawing the catheter (*provided the catheter is not still in the epidural needle*) or by injecting some saline. The catheter must not be left with blood in it, since it may rapidly become occluded. If blood aspiration does not cease, the catheter should be reinserted at another level. Two further indications to reposition needles or catheters are important: If resistance is poorly defined at any level, it is helpful to either try another interspace or choose the paraspinous (lateral) approach, which permits checking of the depth of the lamina by an exploring needle; if onset of analgesia is excessively prolonged, it is likely that injection has not been made into the epidural space.

Paraspinous Techniques (Paramedian)

Paraspinous, paramedian (lateral) insertion is a useful alternative technique. The term *paraspinous* is favored for the following reasons:

The needle should be inserted close to the spinous process because in both lumbar and thoracic regions, the spinous process narrows superiorly and thus guides the needle to a midline entry through the ligamentum flavum.

Extreme lateral angulation of the needle should be avoided, since it may result in oblique penetration of the ligamentum flavum (see Fig. 8-4) and vascular or neural damage. In most instances, the needle need not be angulated and merely follows the spinous process; thus, "paraspinous" describes the essence of the technique.

Techniques with extreme angulation of the needle should be disregarded in favor of the safer paraspinous approach (see Fig. 8-30B).

In the lumbar region infiltration is made 1 to 1.5 cm lateral to the caudad tip of the inferior spinous process of the chosen interspace. A 9 to 10-cm, 22-gauge spinal needle is then used to infiltrate perpendicular to the skin beside the spinous process; this permits the depth of the lamina to be determined before the epidural needle is inserted. It is worth noting that the epidural space can be identified, for single-shot techniques, if an air-filled syringe is attached to the 22-gauge needle and constant pressure is applied to the plunger. However, in most patients an 18-gauge epidural needle is next inserted beside the spinous process and angled upward at 45° to the skin (Fig. 8-30B); often the spinous process carries the needle slightly inward 10° to 15° to the sagittal plane. This may not always be so, and the needle may pass directly to the ligamentum flavum without any necessity for inward angulation. With this technique, resistance to the advancing needle and syringe plunger is encountered only when the needle tip enters the ligamentum flavum. Thus, careful location of the depth of ligamentum flavum is essential; from this point the technique is identical to that at the midline.

In the thoracic region skin infiltration is made 1 to 1.5 cm lateral to the caudad tip of the spinous process, *cephalad to* the intended level of needle insertion (Fig. 8-30B). Infiltration down to the level of the lamina is carried out as described above. The epidural needle is inserted beside the spinous process and 55° to 60° to the skin (sagittal plane); this angulation should permit the needle to reach ligamentum flavum *caudad to* the chosen spinous process (Fig. 8-30B).

For both thoracic and lumbar paraspinous approaches, the Crawford 18-gauge thin-wall needle is an option for single-shot and catheter techniques. The angulation of the needle may permit easier threading of a catheter if a straight-tip Crawford needle is used rather than the Huber tip of the Tuohy needle.

Technique for Obese Subjects and Those with Impalpable Spinous Processes

If preoperative evaluation determines that the patient is obese or of a very "squat" stature, or if bony landmarks are impalpable for other reasons, additional maneuvers may be required. In this situation it may be helpful to plan to carry out the epidural block with the patient in the sitting position, since landmarks may be more readily palpable and epidural puncture is often easier than in the lateral position.

At the time of epidural block, absence of bony landmarks need not cause dismay, since they can be identified during gentle infiltration with local anesthetic. A 5-cm, 22-gauge needle is used to infiltrate the deeper tissues in the region where the spinous processes are judged to lie. The needle is used to probe gently for the underlying spine.[65] Each time the needle touches bone, the depth is noted and the needle is systematically redirected medially or laterally until bone is located at the most superficial depth (i.e., the spinous process).[b] At this stage it may be necessary to infiltrate a new "track" directly toward the spinous process. The epidural needle is then inserted as for the "midline technique" above. Alternatively, the lamina may also be located and the "paramedian" approach used as above.

TABLE 8-17. *Cardiovascular support—epidural block: cardioactive drugs (70-kg adult)*

Drugs of Choice	
Atropine	0.3 mg IV increments[161]
Ephedrine	5–10 mg IV increments[42,143,144,364,403]
Epinephrine	1 mg in 500 ml solution (2 μg/ml) Infuse at rate 2–4 μg/min Titrate against heart rate, mean arterial blood pressure, improved tissue perfusion At low rates of infusion mainly β-effects; at higher rates, increasing α-effects
Metaraminol	100 mg in 500 ml solution (0.5 μg/ml) Infuse at rate 30–60 μg/min Titrate as above Both α- and β-effects May be given as a bolus of 5–10 mg if a long-acting agent (1–2 h) of indirect activity is needed
Norepinephrine	1 mg in 500 ml solution (2 μg/ml) Infuse at rate 2–4 μg/min Titrate as above At <6 μg/min β- as well as α-effects, and thus perfusion (e.g., urine flow) not reduced 2–4 μg/min usually sufficient to maintain blood pressure in presence of total sympathetic block
Other Drugs	
Dopamine and dobutamine[10] are alternatives to epinephrine; however, dopaminergic receptors are blocked by butyrophenones and phenothiazines. Isuprel (β) is usually inadequate alone, since both α- and β-effects are needed.[264] Methoxamine produces mainly α-effects with reflex slowing of the heart and decreased cardiac output.	

IV, intravenous

Continuing Management

As indicated in Table 8-16, monitoring and response to altered physiology are important aspects of the conduct of epidural block. The management of sudden reactions to injection of local anesthetic requires a sound knowledge of the differential diagnosis of local anesthetic reactions (see Chapter 4, Table 4-8) and their treatment, as well as detailed knowledge of the cardiovascular effects of epidural block (Tables 8-7 through 8-11). Only with constant monitoring can the appropriate responses to physiologic changes be made (Table 8-17). Atropine is often used for situations of vagal dominance (see Table 8-10). Ephedrine is useful for cardiovascular support if it is desired to use bolus injections of a medium-duration drug. Ephedrine is not useful in patients with depleted norepinephrine in sympathetic nerve endings, such as some elderly and debilitated patients and those under treatment with drugs that chronically deplete norepinephrine stores. In this situation, direct-acting drugs, such as epinephrine and norepinephrine, are required (Table 8-17). Both of these drugs have a brief duration of action, and thus it is more rational to use them by intravenous infusion, with careful titration against response. Metaraminol by bolus injection is another alternative (Table 8-17). Surveillance also permits appropriate supplementation with sedative-opioid or anesthetic agents and also appropriately timed "top-up" doses for the epidural block.

Maintenance of effective epidural block may entail overcoming common deficiencies in blockade and problems in the management of epidural catheters.

Problems in Epidural Blockade

Blockade Too Low at Upper Level or Inadequate Blockade at Lower Level. Approximately half the initial dose is administered 30 minutes after the first dose. However, if the initial dose was small (e.g., 4-8 ml), it may be necessary to repeat the initial dose. This is particularly so in the region of L5–S1, which is difficult to block. If not already done, it may be helpful to add opioid to the local anesthetic solution, since this will speed onset of block and will also extend the number of segments blocked; rapid-acting opioids such as fen-

[b] It may be helpful to leave the infiltration needle *in situ* and to use this as a guide to the location of the spinous process, when the epidural needle is inserted by means of a separate "track."

tanyl and hydromorphone may be the best choices (see Chapter 29).

"Missed Segments." Manage missed segments as above, depending on the size of initial dose and size of nerve root of "missed segment(s)." If a segment is missed on one side, it is worthwhile turning the patient onto that side before injection.[345] Epinephrine-containing solutions are the most effective, particularly 2% lidocaine with 1:200,000 epinephrine, in dealing with missed segments or inadequate block. This is a useful practice even if another agent has been used for the initial injection. If available, 2% lidocaine–carbon dioxide is a good choice for such problems.

Inadequate Motor Block within The Segmental Area Blocked. This requires further injection, 30 minutes after the initial dose, of approximately half this dose, preferably as 2% lidocaine with epinephrine.

Level Too High but Inadequate Sacral Analgesia. Careful monitoring of the physiologic effects of the high block and appropriate treatment are essential. Approximately 30 to 60 minutes after the initial dose, a small dose of 8 to 10 ml may be injected by a separate single-shot caudal needle. Such a dose will reliably block sacral segments without extending the upper level of lumbar epidural block. If access to the sacral hiatus is impossible, it is preferable to wait as long as possible (approximately 60 minutes) and inject a small increment (e.g., 5-8 ml by the epidural catheter), since blockade tends to spread progressively into the sacral segments with each repeat injection. Careful monitoring is required for signs of total epidural block. Another alternative is a single-shot subarachnoid "saddle" block (see Chapter 7); the spinal needle can be inserted without discomfort since the lumbar segments are already blocked, also there is no need for time delay since the additional dose of local anesthetic is small.

"Visceral" Pain During Lower Abdominal Surgery. It is not commonly recognized that peritoneal stimulation during appendectomy and sometimes during a difficult herniorrhaphy may require blockade to the level of T5–T6. Thus, adequate provision should be made to block to this level or, alternatively, to "top-up" to this level if required. If there is a delay in onset of T5 block, intravenous or epidural opioid or light general anesthesia may be required.

Inability to Thread Epidural Catheter. This is often a confirmatory sign that a false loss of resistance has been encountered in a tissue space dorsal to the ligamentum flavum and that the needle has been halted superficial to the ligamentum flavum. Clearly injection of local anesthetic at this point will be ineffectual. The most prudent course is to withdraw the needle and catheter together, after noting the depth of the needle. The needle is then redirected in the midline and maintained in resistant ligamentous tissues until a convincing loss of resistance is achieved.

On the other hand, if the anesthetist is firmly convinced, by all the evidence available, that the needle is properly sited and if the planned operative procedure is likely to be accomplished within the duration of a long-acting local anesthetic, it may be reasonable to proceed with a "single-shot" injection through the needle, using bupivacaine or etidocaine. However, the latter course of action involves two assumptions: that the needle is properly sited and that the operation will not extend longer than expected. One or both of these assumptions may be wrong; thus this course is not recommended because of the unpredictability of outcome.

Dural Puncture. Often it is feasible to convert to a subarachnoid block merely by maintaining the needle in position and injecting the appropriate intrathecal dose of tetracaine, dibucaine, or bupivacaine. If the anesthesiologist wants to persevere with epidural block, another interspace should be chosen (preferably above) and a catheter should be threaded upward. Injection should be made entirely by the catheter and should be slow. A test dose is essential (see above).

Subarachnoid Cannulation. This may occur at the time of initial insertion of the needle or epidural catheter.[214] It has an incidence of 0.2% to 0.7%.[214] Failure to recognize malplacement of needle or catheter and injection of the usual epidural dose would result in a total spinal anesthesia (see Chapter 4, Table 4-8). Epidural catheters have also been found to penetrate the dura at the time of a "top-up" dose, having initially functioned as if normally placed in the epidural space.[304] Thus, a small test dose administered by an epidural catheter is always advisable.

Subdural Cannulation. This results from perforation of the dura without penetration of the underlying arachnoid membrane (see Chapter 21). This is a rare result of intended epidural cannulation.[46,365] It occurs frequently during myelography[91] and in spinal anesthesia, with an incidence of up to 1 in 100. Spread of analgesia is patchy, markedly asymmetric, and sometimes extensive.[46,365] Replacement of the epidural catheter at a more rostrad interspace level is required (see also Chapter 7, Fig. 7-6).

Cannulation of an Epidural Vein. This is a greater hazard, especially in pregnant women because of epidural venous distention during labor, particularly if the needle or catheter enters the epidural space other than in the midline (see Fig. 8-5). Usually the risk of epidural venous cannulation is small.[205] The best treatment is *prevention*, which depends on gentle insertion of catheters that do not have sharp ends, and avoidance of use of stylets; insertion of only 3 to 4 cm of the catheter length; aspiration before injection by way of an epidural catheter; use of a test dose, preferably with epinephrine (injected into an epidural vein results in a rapid increase in heart rate and blood pressure).

Injection of a small amount of saline and withdrawal of the catheter by 1 to 2 cm usually permits retrieval of the catheter from the vein; if not, the catheter should be reinserted at another level. Delayed entry of a catheter into a vein may occur at the time of a "top-up" dose, with resulting CNS toxicity.[326] Once again, the catheter must be withdrawn, or if it is inaccessible, epidural block must be discontinued.

Venous cannulation is less likely to occur if the catheter is inserted into a "wet" epidural space, expanded by prior injection of local anesthetic, rather than into a dry one.[394] The practice of injecting a "priming" dose of local anesthetic through the needle is therefore a logical precaution against venous cannulation. Expansion of the epidural space can be accomplished by using a test dose of 4 ml via the needle, before inserting the catheter.

Epidural Hematoma. Needle or catheter trauma to epidural veins may result in bleeding, but this is usually minimal and stops rapidly; it is rare for an epidural hematoma and neurologic symptoms to arise if coagulation is normal. Only one case is currently recorded.[236] However, patients on anticoagulant therapy may develop large epidural hematomas and, possibly, paraplegia if either an epidural needle or catheter is inserted[131,164] (see section below on anticoagulants).

In the majority of cases, alternative means of providing most of the beneficial effects of epidural block are now available if anticoagulation is believed to be essential. For example, epidural block increases graft blood flow in association with vascular procedures on the lower limb.[112] However, limb blood flow may also be increased by prior sympathetic blockade using long-acting local anesthetics or intravascular reserpine injected into the affected limb, or even surgical sympathectomy (see Chapter 13). It is also important to note that surgical procedures involving the abdominal aorta may cause paraplegia. This may be the result of prolonged clamping of the aorta[105] or sectioning of nutrient arteries to nerve plexuses and the spinal cord.[383] Thus, while in lower limb vascular surgery, anticoagulation or epidural block, or both, may lead to epidural hematoma and paraplegia; in aortic surgery, direct cord ischemia must be added to the differential diagnosis of postoperative paraplegia (however, see Anticoagulants and Epidural, page 306).

It is important to allow any sensory or motor deficits of a continuous epidural block to wear off for a long enough time to assess as soon as possible after the surgery. The use of low-dose bupivacaine and opioid infusion usually does not result in significant motor or sensory loss, so that neurologic function can be monitored, and it is usually readily apparent that there has been the sudden onset of new symptoms and signs in the form of sensorimotor disturbances and/or back pain. Failure to recover function fully and, in some cases, severe lumbar pain indicate the possibility of epidural hematoma. Anticoagulants should then be stopped and myelography and/or CT scan carried out immediately because most patients who have recovered from epidural hematoma have been decompressed within 12 hours of the onset of symptoms.[32] The variability in individual response to "low-dose" heparin therapy means that some patients may still develop epidural hematomas, and this risk will continue until rapid methods are available to measure plasma levels of heparin and to assess the effect of heparin therapy on coagulation[413] (see following). Patients with potential interference with normal hemostatic mechanisms include those with disease (e.g., severe pre-eclampsia, intrauterine death) or medication (e.g., heparinization or oral warfarin, aspirin and other nonsteroidal anti-inflammatory drugs). Epidural puncture should be avoided if the platelet count falls below 100,000/mm^3. However, aspirin-like drugs do not change platelet *count;* they alter platelet *function.* In patients with pre-eclampsia and other conditions likely to alter the coagulation cascade, a full range of clotting studies should be performed in consultation with a hematologist.

Management of Epidural Catheters

Accurate placement of a minimal length of catheter is described in the foregoing discussion as an essential aid to successful "continuous" catheter epidural blockade. The problems of patchy blockade, missed segments, intravascular cannulation, and subarachnoid and subdural cannulation can usually be effectively managed if the "correct procedure" is carefully followed and close monitoring is carried out (see Table 8-16). The long-term complications of catheter placement, owing to damage to neural tissue, should be avoidable if catheters are withdrawn at the first sign of pain or paraesthesias on insertion or on reinjection. The complications of epidural hematoma are mostly (but not always) avoidable.

Prevention of Infection

Perhaps the most important aspect of management of epidural catheters is the avoidance of infections:

A strict antiseptic routine should always be carried out during catheter insertion. Adequate time should be allowed for the skin preparation to exert its antibacterial effect, and great care should be taken not to contaminate the epidural catheter before insertion.

Multidose local anesthetic vials should not be used: Preservative-free, single-use local anesthetic solutions should be used, and any residuum should be discarded after injection.

Local anesthetics should not be aspirated through "rubber bungs" in tops of local anesthetic vials; the top should be removed and the vial discarded after single use.

Glass syringes should be used only once and then resterilized, since the outside of the plunger may be contaminated during use. Many hospitals now use plastic single-use syringes.

During "top-up," the syringe nozzle and epidural catheter connection must not be contaminated, and if they are touched directly, the appropriate components should be changed. Wiping with alcohol swabs is not advised, since it is possible that neurolytic alcohol solution may then be carried into the epidural space.

The use of micropore (Millipore) filters has been shown in one study to reduce catheter contamination.[208] Although other studies have not substantiated this finding,[3] it seems reasonable to recommend the use of such filters. They provide at least some protection against infection and reduce the chance of contamination with particulate matter.[217]

If reasonable precautions are taken, the risk of infection from contamination of epidural catheters or local anesthetic solution should be small (e.g., 30,000 epidurals without a single infection).[65] However, endogenous infection owing to blood-borne spread from a pre-existing focus of infection may be a hazard.[17] Also, patients with septicemia clearly pose a considerable risk of metastatic epidural infection, and insertion of an epidural catheter is best avoided in such patients. Infection in the pelvic region could possibly spread to the epidural space by way of the venous connections to epidural veins (see Fig. 8-15); thus, the use of epidural catheters should be avoided unless the pelvic infection has been treated adequately with antibiotics. The risk of metastatic infection is even further increased in diabetics and in patients with suppressed immune responses.[336] The diabetic patient has proved to be a problem with long-term epidural catheters in treatment of cancer pain. However, immunosuppressed patients with cancer have been safely managed with long-term totally implanted epidural systems (see Chapter 29).

More complex measures to combat contamination at reinjection include the enclosure of large-volume syringes in a sterile bag[65] and the use of continuous drips and syringe pumps.[344]

Procedure for "Top-Up" and Catheter Removal

In conscious and cooperative patients, careful monitoring for signs of segmental regression will indicate the need for "top-up." In other situations, it is most convenient to top-up at the approximate time of regression of analgesia (−2 SD) as determined in clinical studies (see Table 8-14), provided that this timing coincides with safe blood concentrations of local anesthetic (see Chapter 4, Fig. 4-14). The mean −2 SD predicts the duration in 95% of patients. In practice, injection of half the initial dose of lidocaine approximately every hour results in maintenance of blockade associated with a small but significant gradual increase in blood lidocaine concentration (see Chapter 3, Fig. 3-12). This is usually not of importance during surgery, when one to two top-ups are often sufficient. In contrast, for the long-acting agents bupivacaine and ropivacaine, topping up with half the initial dose every 2 hours maintains level of blockade without appreciable increase in blood concentration over many successive top-ups. Thus, for long-term catheter techniques, bupivacaine is preferable with respect to toxicity and because the generous margin between top-up and two-segment regression lessens the chance that tachyphylaxis may occur. It should be clearly understood that we are interested in duration of blockade from time of complete spread to regression of two segments, provided an appropriate level of blockade is achieved with the initial dose; duration to two-segment regression is considerably shorter than complete duration. If initial level of blockade is much too high, initial top-up should be appropriately delayed, and size of top-up dose should be reduced in proportion to the level of "overshoot." A routine for topping-up is important.

Topping-Up Routine

Check level if possible: pinprick or ice in conscious patients, reflexes, and presence or absence of bradycardia (? level above T2) in anesthetized patients. Do not top-up if a high level is suspected.

Aspirate for CSF or blood.

Inject a small test dose (3–4 ml) of epinephrine-containing solution and check heart rate and blood pressure: Intravascular injection results in rapid increase in heart rate and blood pressure; subarachnoid injection results in extensive blockade with hypotension and sometimes bradycardia.

Inject remainder of top-up dose slowly with frequent aspiration, only if no complications ensue after the step above.

Monitor closely for one-half hour after top-up. If the patient is conscious and mobile, he should lie flat during top-up and for one-half hour afterward. In any patient, be prepared to increase rate of intravenous infusion or to manage local anesthetic reactions or extensive sympathetic blockade (see Chapter 4, Table 4-8).

Routine for Catheter Removal

Durations of maintenance of epidural catheters for more than 2 weeks have been reported. Bromage advocates replacement of catheters at a different site every 72 hours,[65] and this is supported on the grounds that epidural catheters become walled off by fibrous tissue reaction after about 72 hours.[138] However, if a catheter is functioning satisfactorily with no sequela, it is reasonable for it to remain *in situ* for approximately 1 week (see also Chapter 29). Catheters should be removed gently, and the end of the catheter should be carefully checked for completeness. If difficulty is experienced in withdrawing the catheter, the spine should be flexed and gentle continuous traction exerted. There is a remote possibility that a knot may form in the catheter if excessively long lengths have been inserted; this is impossible if only 3 to 4 cm of catheter is inserted into the epidural space. There is an even more remote possibility that a catheter may loop around a spinal nerve if excess lengths are inserted; pain on removal of catheter should alert the anesthesiologist to this possibility. If subsequent radiographs, after injection of 0.3 ml of contrast media into the catheter, show that it is located in the region of a spinal nerve, removal by laminectomy may have to be considered. Sequestration of a small amount of catheter in the epidural space should be noted, and the patient must be carefully assessed over the ensuing weeks. However, it is usually not necessary to remove this foreign body, nor is it technically easy to locate it at laminectomy. Thus, in general, laminectomy is reserved for situations associated with symptoms or signs.

Anticoagulants and Epidural Anesthesia

Patients hospitalized for major vascular surgery, orthopedic procedures, and lower abdominal surgery frequently have prophylactic anticoagulation therapy to prevent thrombosis and embolism. The combination of anticoagulation therapy and epidural anesthesia remains a difficult choice for the anesthesiologist. Theoretically, there is a greater risk of hemorrhagic complications. Neurologic complications of epidural anesthesia due to compressing hematoma in the spinal canal are extremely rare. Case reports do exist, especially in connection with therapeutic doses of anticoagulation, although there are few, indicating that the fear of epidural hematoma should not be overemphasized. Moreover, it is important to know that such a hematoma may occur spontaneously in anticoagulated patients not undergoing epidural blockade.[361] It is not clear whether the incidence of epidural hematoma in the anticoagulated patient following epidural anesthesia is any greater than the spontaneous incidence of epidural hematoma. The infrequency of this specific complication makes it impossible to perform prospective randomized studies to solve the problem.[27]

The decision to perform epidural anesthesia on a patient receiving antiplatelet or anticoagulant medications should be made on an individual basis, weighing the risk of epidural hematoma and benefits from the use of epidural blockade and thrombo-prophylaxis for a specific patient[107] (see above).

Aspirin and NSAIDs

Low-dose aspirin (60–120 mg) has been proven to markedly reduce the incidence of pre-eclampsia and intrauterine growth retardation by selectively inhibiting the platelet-synthesized thromboxane.[23] Epidural anesthesia is frequently indicated for labor and cesarean section in this group of obstetric patients.

Low-dose aspirin has also been proven to be useful in the prevention of thrombotic complications of arterial diseases in patients with cardiovascular diseases. It is obvious that this patient population may need vascular surgery of the lower extremity. Epidural anesthesia offers the advantage of the associated sympathetic blockade, which enhances blood flow in the lower limbs. Thus the anesthetist is faced with a growing number of patients treated with low-dose aspirin or some other antiplatelet drugs, who may all potentially benefit from epidural anesthesia.

Orthopedic patients undergoing major joint surgery frequently use preoperative nonsteroidal anti-inflammatory drugs (NSAIDs) for pain treatment. These agents cause variable inhibition of platelet aggregation comparable to effects of aspirin.

It is unknown whether the use of aspirin and other antiplatelet agents elevates the risk of epidural bleeding.[292] Although a few cases of spontaneous or traumatic epidural hematomas have been reported in patients taking aspirin, the incidence of epidural hematoma in aspirin-treated patients is extremely low.

Two studies, one retrospective and one prospective, failed to demonstrate an increased incidence of epidural hematoma in orthopedic patients who underwent surgery under epidural anesthesia and were receiving preoperative NSAIDs therapy. In both studies, preoperative antiplatelet therapy was associated with a slightly higher incidence of minor hemorrhagic complications, such as aspiration of blood through the epidural needle.[199,200]

Trying to assess the risk by means of the routine use of a bleeding time of an individual is controversial, since this test is subject to wide observation variation and is known to lack sensitivity and specificity.[248,282] Although the bleeding time may return to normal within 72 hours after aspirin ingestion, it may take 7 to 10 days for *in vitro* platelet aggregation tests to return to normal.[185] At present, the bleeding time is the only feasible bedside test that gives information about the aggregating capabilities of the patient's platelets. It is unknown how much bleeding will occur in relation to prolongation of the bleeding time. If this bleeding time is below 8 minutes, an atraumatic and prudent epidural puncture may be performed. However, if bleeding time is prolonged beyond 10 minutes, the anesthetist must balance the advantages and disadvantages of siting the epidural in that particular patient. Thus with aspirin and antiplatelet therapy the risk of developing epidural hematoma is unknown but seems to be minimal. For safety reasons, however, postoperative neurologic monitoring should be undertaken in all aspirin-treated patients who have received epidural anesthesia. Careful prospective trials are still needed to determine whether the bleeding time can be a useful predictor of clinically significant bleeding.[140]

Low-Dose Heparin

The prophylactic administration of low-dose subcutaneous unfractionated heparin has been clearly shown to reduce the incidence of deep venous thrombosis and subsequent pulmonary thromboembolism. As far as standard low-dose subcutaneous heparin prophylaxis is concerned, only two cases of epidural hematoma formation have been reported.[265,390] Metzger et al.[265] reported one case of epidural hematoma; however, no information was given about the time interval between administration of heparin and epidural anesthesia.[390] It was concluded that with regard to the epidural hematoma and low-dose heparinization, the possible coincidence of spontaneous lumbar hematoma and lumbar epidural block should be taken into consideration. A recent national Danish survey reports that more than 60% of practicing Danish anesthesiologists use epidural anesthesia in patients on low-dose subcutaneous heparin.[409] Only one case of epidural hematoma was reported under these circumstances. A great deal of uncertainty about whether to administer epidural anesthesia after low-dose heparin relates to the unpredictability of the individual's coagulation response to heparin. Some patients develop therapeutic blood levels of heparin rather than prophylactic blood levels within 2 to 4 hours of subcutaneous administration.[97] Thus it would seem wise to avoid the institution of an epidural block or removal of a catheter within 4 to 6 hours of low-dose heparin administration, if possible.

At present, more and more patients are prophylactically treated with low-molecular-weight heparin (LMWH). The newer LMWHs have been shown to be at least as effective and safe and sometimes more effective than unfractionated heparin in the prevention of deep venous thrombosis.[25] The advantages with LMWH in low doses as compared with unfragmented low-dose heparin are: a higher and more predictable bioavailability after subcutaneous injection; a longer biologic half-life, which makes one injection daily sufficient and a smaller influence on platelet function and lipolysis.[8] In a recent review article concerning clinical trials of LMWHs, more than 9,000 patients were reported to have undergone spinal or epidural anesthesia without any neurologic complication.[25] Proper dosing of the LMWH and respecting a minimum time span between administration of the LMWH and insertion/removal of the epidural needle or catheter are crucial in the prevention of bleeding.[390] At least 2 hours should separate injection of LMWH and the epidural technique; a period of 8 to 12 hours is even better.

Anticoagulation and Epidural Catheterization

The timing of insertion and removal of an indwelling epidural catheter in an anticoagulated patient remains controversial. Several studies have documented the relative safety of intravenous or subcutaneous heparin in the presence of an indwelling catheter. Rao and El-Etr (1981) analyzed patients who received continuous epidural anesthesia with subsequent intraoperative heparinization.[311] If blood was freely aspirated during needle insertion, surgery was cancelled and rescheduled for the following day under general anesthesia. The epidural catheters were removed prior to the administration of the maintenance dose of heparin. There were no incidences of epidural hematomas. Odoom and coworkers (1983) performed continuous epidural anesthesia in patients undergoing vascular procedures and receiving oral anticoagulation therapy with an intraoperative bolus and a continuous intraoperative infusion of heparin.[287] Epidural catheters were removed 48 hours postoperatively. Despite this intensive therapy, no patient in this combined series of 4164 cases developed signs of epidural hematoma.[286,311] Both studies, however, analyzed patients whose management of the epidural complied with strict guidelines. Patients with blood dyscrasias, prior heparinization, aspirin therapy of long duration, or a Thrombo-test of below 10% were excluded from the study. Horlocker et al. (1994) evaluated retrospectively the risk of epidural hematoma in patients receiving postoperative epidural analgesia while receiving low-dose warfarin.[201] Epidural catheters were left indwelling for 4 days or less. There were no signs of epidural hematoma. It is recommended that an epidural catheter should be removed 4 to 6 hours after the last heparin dose to allow for normalization of the activated partial thromboplastin time and that subsequent anticoagulation should not to be initiated for at least 1 hour after the catheter is removed.[198] Patients who have an epidural catheter removed during or immediately before anticoagulation should have their neurologic status followed until adequate mechanisms of hemostasis exist. A high index of suspicion must be maintained to facilitate the early detection of complications.

If fibrinolytic agents (such as tissue plasminogen activator, urokinase, or streptokinase) are to be used, epidural anesthesia should be avoided. It seems reasonable to assume that dangerous hematoma formation is more likely in the case of full anticoagulation. One must weigh the real risk of hematoma against the risk of coexisting diseases, which may have greater potential for morbidity.

APPLICATIONS OF EPIDURAL BLOCKADE

A discussion of the "indications" and "contraindications" of epidural block is not the scope of this section. The preceding material in this chapter has provided a broad anatomic, technical, pharmacologic, and physiologic basis on which to answer two important questions: Does epidural blockade offer significant benefits to the *individual* patient under consideration for the proposed operative or other application? Do the benefits outweigh the risks, owing to factors peculiar to the patient and/or procedure?

When viewed in this context, lists of "indications" and "contraindications" can be misleading and dangerous, since they cannot take into consideration factors that vary in individual patients. The only absolute *contraindications* to epidural blockade are patient refusal, major coagulation defects, uncorrected hypovolemia, infection in the area of proposed needle insertion, or severe systemic infection. As with spinal anesthesia, the benefits of epidural blockade in patients with neurologic disease should be carefully weighed; it appears wise, although there is no clear supportive evidence, to avoid blockade in patients with unstable neurologic disease, particularly if the spinal cord is involved. However, if epidural block offers significant benefits in patients with stable "peripheral" neurologic disease, such as diabetic neuropathy, its use may be considered in light of individual patients and procedures. The use of epidural block in many thousands of patients with back pain and neurologic deficit after back surgery (see Chapter 28) attests to its safety in carefully selected patients with stable neurologic signs. Abnormalities of the bony spine may increase the difficulty of epidural block, although by no means do they make it impossible; this difficulty must be weighed against the skill of the anesthesiologist and the risk-benefit ratio for the patient and procedure; both anteroposterior and lateral radiographs of the lumbar spine may be useful in making such a decision.

Other anatomic, pharmacologic, and physiologic factors in individual patients may lead to a decision not to use epidural block. However, they cannot be merely "listed" here, since the balance of risk to benefit must be decided for each

TABLE 8-18. *Some applications of epidural blockade*

1. Surgery
   - Upper and lower abdominal surgery, urologic surgery, pelvic surgery, hip surgery, vascular surgery, surgery in the obese patient, thoracic surgery, surgery of the neck and upper limb, radical mastectomy
   - Surgery in patients with medical conditions (see Chapter 7), e.g., buccal pemphigus, malignant hyperthermia
   - Specialized surgical procedures
     - Pheochromocytoma
     - Surgery of spine
     - Bladder distention for bladder cancer
     - Extracorporeal shock wave lithotripsy
2. Postoperative and post-trauma pain relief
   - See Chapter 26.
3. Obstetrics (see also Chapter 18)
   - For patient comfort, to avoid incoordinate uterine action, to minimize fetal acidosis, to reduce use of "urgent" instrumental delivery or "painful delivery" needing general anesthesia, to relieve pain during labor for medical indications, pre-eclampsia, for cesarean section
4. Diagnosis and management of chronic pain
   - "Differential" epidural block (see Chapter 27)
   - "Diagnostic epidural opioid blockade" (see Chapter 27)
   - Epidurography with metrizamide
   - Neurolytic epidural block (see Chapter 31)
   - Pain due to vasospasm due to ergot poisoning, cold injuries of extremities, Raynaud's disease or phenomenon and other vasospastic problems, phantom limb pain and causalgia, post-herpetic neuralgia, pancreatitis, renal colic, acute priapism
5. New epidural techniques
   - Epidural electrical stimulation (see Chapter 32)
   - Epidural opiods (see Chapter 29)

patient. For example, a patient with a low fixed cardiac output owing to constrictive pericarditis may be better managed during a perineal procedure by a saddle-block spinal anesthetic rather than an epidural anesthetic. A patient with severe congestive cardiac failure may be safely managed by epidural block for lower abdominal surgery, provided incremental doses are used by a catheter and the "internal phlebotomy" owing to sympathetic block has a slow onset. In addition, the vasodilation must be carefully balanced by titrating a slow vasopressor infusion, as shown in Table 8-17, to prevent the blood pressure from falling more than 30% below the preblock mean. The vasopressor must be given with great caution, since hypertension is more harmful than a little hypotension in congestive cardiac failure. Indeed, mild hypotension may be beneficial.

The considerations above enable the anesthesiologists to determine which benefits epidural blockade offers to each patient in each clinical setting. The potential applications may include operative surgery; postoperative pain management; post-trauma pain management (see also Chapter 26); obstetric analgesia and operative obstetrics (see also Chapter 18); chronic and cancer pain diagnosis and management (see also Chapters 26–32); and special applications in the management of particular medical and surgical conditions (see Table 8-18).

COMPLICATIONS OF EPIDURAL BLOCKADE

The problems discussed on pages 302–304 may be considered minor complications. Any complication should be viewed in the light of a sound knowledge of the anatomy, pharmacology, and physiology of epidural block.

Complications Relating to Anatomic or Technical Problems

Several problems have been discussed elsewhere: inadvertent dural puncture and total spinal blockade; massive subdural spread; total epidural blockade; epidural venous injection; epidural hematoma; epidural abscess; anterior spinal artery syndrome; ligation of spinal cord blood supply during major vascular surgery; injection of local anesthetics contaminated with neurolytic agents; injection of the "wrong drug" (e.g., thiopental); broken epidural catheters; and local anesthetic toxicity.

Rigid adherence to a "therapeutic procedure," as outlined in Table 8-16, greatly reduces the risks of major complications.

The occurrence and management of postdural puncture headache are discussed in Chapter 7. Unfortunately, the incidence of headache is high (70%–80%) if the dura is punctured with a 16- to 18-gauge epidural needle.[114,115] Thus, routine prophylaxis is advisable if the dura is punctured with an epidural needle; this includes use of the supine posture, increased oral and intravenous fluid intake, use of abdominal binders, and systemic analgesics. If an epidural catheter has been inserted at another level, it should be left *in situ* and 1500 ml of saline should be infused over 24 hours.[114,115] The use of epidural blood patch is discussed in Chapter 7 (see also Fig. 7-21).

Backache is supposed to be more severe when large epidural needles (compared with spinal needles) are used. However, there are no data to support this contention.

Bladder dysfunction is a distinct possibility if blockade of the sacral segments continues into the postoperative period. As discussed in more detail in Chapter 26, it is important to attempt to restrict epidural block to the required segments, which often do not include S2–S5. Also, it is vital to ensure that the bladder does not become overdistended if epidural block extends into the sacral segments during surgery; this is particularly important in aged men with incipient prostatic obstruction. Careful management of level of blockade in obstetric patients results in a similar incidence of catheterization, whether or not epidural block is used.[115]

Major neurologic sequelae of epidural block are potentially the same as for spinal anesthesia (see Chapter 7). It was initially thought that these sequelae followed spinal anesthesia and not epidural block, but this has been disproved. In a major world review of the use of epidural blockade, Usubiaga uncovered a number of cases of neurologic sequelae that were purportedly caused by epidural block.[383] However, the retrospective nature of the documentation in many of these cases often makes it impossible to determine the relative contribution of pre-existing medical factors, the surgical procedure itself, and the epidural block. As with spinal anesthesia, several large epidural case series report no neurologic sequelae in major hospitals where a standard procedure is followed: Bromage reports more than 40,000 epidural blocks without major neurologic sequelae.[65] The majority of cases of serious neurologic sequelae occur in small hospitals or occur after epidural block by an inexperienced operator who violates some aspect of a reasonable therapeutic regimen. Even so, there is a *potential* for neurologic sequelae resulting from anatomic, technical, physiologic, and pharmacologic factors associated with epidural block (Fig. 8-34) and the surgery, obstetric delivery, or other procedure for which the epidural block is used (see also Chapter 21). A survey of the literature revealed only a small number of cases of neurologic deficit in association with epidural block.[215] Some of these have subsequently been shown to be due to inadvertent subarachnoid injection of large volumes of a preparation of chloroprocaine that had a low pH and contained bisulfite in a concentration now recognized as being higher than desirable (see Chapter 4, Tables 4-6 and 4-7). Many anesthesiologists were not aware of the precise composition of this preparation of the drug, and indeed it has been changed over the years as the manufacture of the drug changed hands. There is an important lesson in this story: Subtle changes in the formulation of local anesthetic solutions may have vital importance, *particularly* for spinal anesthesia and epidural anesthesia (see also Chapter 30). Unfortunately, history tends to repeat itself. In the 1930s, solutions of procaine were prepared with 15% ethanol and glycerine; cauda equina syndromes resulted and it was concluded that procaine was the causative factor, the other ingredients apparently being regarded as harmless.[215] The same situation arose with the use of amylocaine (Stovaine) and piperocaine, solutions containing neurolytic components.[215] Local anesthetic solutions for epidural block should, as far as possible, contain only local anesthetic with pH adjusted as close as possible to normal pH. The precise solution to be used clinically should be tested under the most extreme conditions that could be experienced clinically (see also Chapter 30). Changes in formulation should not occur without repeating this testing, approval by drug regulatory bodies, and full information of the medical community. Possible causes of neurologic sequelae are summarized in Tables 8-19 and 8-20, and in Figure 8-34.

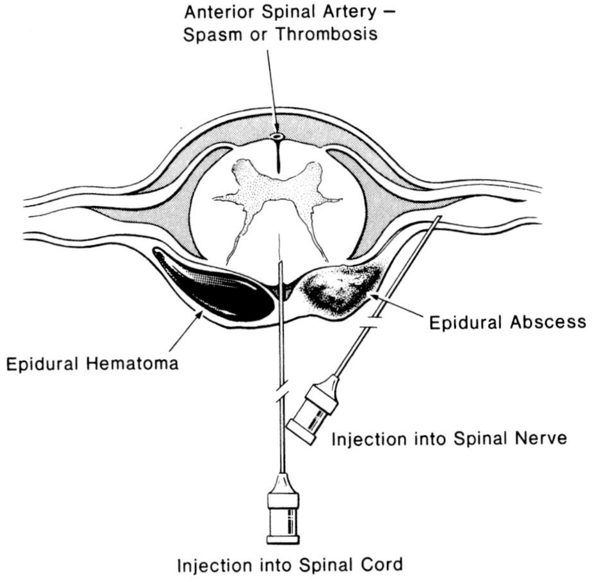

FIG. 8-34. Complications of epidural block (see text).

TABLE 8-19. *Possible factors in neurologic sequelae in patients receiving epidural block*

1. Direct trauma to spinal nerve roots, spinal cord
2. Compression of spinal cord or nerve roots
   - Epidural hematoma
   - Epidural abscess
   - Postpartum paresis owing to cephalopelvic disproportion (may also compress spinal cord "feeder" vessels)
3. Neurotoxicity
   - Low pH, high concentration of antioxidants (e.g., bisulfite) (see Chapter 4 and Chapter 30)
   - Neurotoxic additives (e.g., ethanol, benzyl alcohol, chlorocresol, methylparaben)[a]
   - Injection of "wrong drug" (i.e., not a local anesthetic)
4. Ischemia
5. Anterior spinal artery spasm or thrombosis
   - Trauma by needle
   - Spasm ? by epinephrine or other factors
   - Thrombosis owing to very low blood pressure (e.g., only in those with vascular disease)
   - ? Combination of hypotension and injection of large volume of local anesthetic raising CSF pressure (see Chapter 30)
6. Ischemia within spinal cord
   - ? "Neurotoxic" effects by way of reduced perineurial blood flow
   - —Only with neurotoxic additives and inappropriate use of local anesthetics (see Chapter 30).
7. Factors unrelated to epidural may frequently be found to be the causative factors e.g., pre-existing disease (see Table 8-20), surgical factors

[a] Such additives should never be used in epidural solutions (they have been in some multiple-use solutions in the past).

Direct trauma to the spinal cord can be eliminated if puncture is below L2. In all reported cases in which the patient was conscious, insertion of needle or catheter was followed by *severe lancinating pain* in dermatomes adjacent to or below the site of puncture.[65,196]

Epidural hematoma is discussed on page 304.[107,164] This complication can be prevented if the combination of coagulation defects or complete heparinization and epidural block is avoided. It is remotely possible for epidural hematoma to occur in patients without coagulation defects. Constant

TABLE 8-20. *Associated but unrelated neurologic sequelae in patients receiving epidural block[a]*

Anatomic abnormalities
"High take off" of artery radicularis magna and supply of lumbosacral area of cord by sacral branches of internal iliac artery (15% of population). Ligation or compression of this artery at surgery (? incidence 1:20,000)
Undiagnosed neurologic disease
AV abnormalities of spinal cord—1:15,000
Vertebral angioma—1:4–6,000
Atherosclerotic "spinal stroke"—1:20,000
Unrecognized prolapsed intervertebral disk— ? 1:6000
Unrecognized spinal metastases (≃5% of all cancer cases)
Unrecognized primary spinal cord tumor—? undiagnosed incidence
Damage to neuraxis during surgery
Compression of pelvic nerves (lumbosacral trunk) ? incidence 1:4000 (in labor related to duration and difficulty of labor)
Ligation or compression of spinal arteries during aortic surgery—? incidence
Compression of peripheral nerves by retraction, pressure on operating table
Stretching of peripheral nerves by extreme postures

[a] Incidence of condition is given where known (see also Chapter 21).
AV, arteriovenous

surveillance and early investigation are most important. In all reported cases, there is a rapid onset of signs of neurologic deficit or severe back pain, or both. These signs should always be rapidly investigated by myelography and/or computed tomography (CT) scan, and if necessary, laminectomy should be performed within a maximum of 12 hours, since recovery is unlikely if decompression is delayed beyond this time.[30] Note that uncommon arteriovenous abnormalities of the spinal cord may pose a risk of excessive bleeding into epidural or subarachnoid space either because of, or associated with, epidural block (see Table 8-20).

Epidural Abscess

In a series of 39 cases of epidural abscess, Baker and colleagues found that 38 cases were associated with endogenous infection.[17] In this series, an epidural abscess occurred in association with epidural block in only one case. Important diagnostic features present in all cases were severe back pain, local back tenderness, fever, leukocytosis, and abnormal myelogram with obstruction to flow of contrast medium. As for epidural hematoma, rapid investigation and laminectomy are essential for complete recovery. Because *Staphylococcus aureus* is the most common infecting organism,[178] antibiotic administration should include treatment for a staphylococcus infection if positive cultures are not available. A disturbing case of extensive epidural empyema has been reported after midthoracic epidural blockade.[147] It should be noted that epidural abscess may occur in association with general systemic infection,[251] which reinforces the view that epidural block should be avoided in this situation. Epidural corticosteroid administration may result in immune suppression. For example, epidural methylprednisolone, 80 mg, results in significant suppression of adrenal function for about 3 weeks.[207] Theoretically, this could pose a risk of epidural infection. To date, epidural abscess has not been reported in association with epidural steroids; however, meticulous care with sterility should be observed when epidural steroids are injected.

Subarachnoid infection has also been reported after epidural block, and contamination of equipment or drugs appears to be responsible.[47]

Trauma to Spinal Nerves or Blood Vessels in Dural Cuff Region

Oblique lateral entry into the ligamentum flavum may direct the needle into the dural cuff region (Fig. 8-34). This may result in direct trauma to a nerve root, with resultant unisegmental paresthesia; such a sign should warn the anesthesiologist not to persist with needle insertion in this position and not to attempt to thread a catheter. It is also possible that a major "feeder" artery to the anterior spinal artery may be damaged as it enters by way of an intervertebral foramen (see Chapter 7, Fig. 7-11), resulting in the so-called anterior spinal artery syndrome, or possibly in a large epidural hematoma (even in a patient with normal coagulation).

Unexplained Causes of Anterior Spinal Artery Syndrome

The most likely explanations for unexplained cases of anterior spinal artery syndrome are direct trauma and reduced perfusion pressure and/or venous congestion. The contribution of the small doses of epinephrine (1:200,000) in modern epidural local anesthetic solutions is doubtful, except perhaps in patients with severe arteriosclerosis if epidural block has been used in association with hypotension (see also Chapter 7). Studies of spinal cord blood flow, with concentrations of epinephrine in local anesthetic solutions, have not shown deleterious reductions in blood flow[230] (see also Chapter 7). Spinal cord ischemia and anterior spinal artery syndrome may result from low spinal cord perfusion unassociated with epidural block.[149] It is not known whether epidural block increases the risk of low spinal cord perfusion. However, it is certain that the same precautions should be taken, whether or not epidural block is used.

It should be noted that angiomas of vertebrae or the spinal cord are relatively common and may compress the spinal cord, particularly if intraspinal pressure is increased (e.g., during labor).[277] Once again, investigation by myelography and CT scan, and rapid exploration, if indicated, must be carried out if permanent sequelae are to be avoided.

Unexplained Arachnoiditis and Transverse Myelitis

Arachnoiditis and transverse myelitis are discussed in Chapter 7. Meticulous precautions must be taken to ensure that chemical agents capable of causing these lesions[227] are excluded from epidural block equipment and drugs (see Table 8-16). Only preservative-free local anesthetics from sterile single-use containers should be used for epidural block. The lack of neurotoxicity of any agent should be established before it is injected epidurally. Previous tragedies have occurred with the neurolytic carriers present in the so-called long-acting local anesthetic "efocaine."[87] As is the case with paraplegia after spinal anesthesia, it seems likely that reported cases of adhesive arachnoiditis after epidural blockade are due to chemical contamination.[65] However, the features of adhesive arachnoiditis may be produced by infection, trauma, and hemorrhage in the region of the arachnoid. Perhaps the best example of the latter is adhesive arachnoiditis after laminectomy or spinal fusion for "back pain." We have seen a number of these patients, who were neurologically normal before laminectomy, apart from symptoms of back pain; they developed classic signs of adhesive arachnoiditis after operation. Subsequent re-exploration revealed no infective process, but signs of extensive tissue trauma and classic features of adhesive arachnoiditis were present.

Partial or complete lesions of the cauda equina resulting in loss of bladder function, incontinence of feces, and sacral analgesia are sometimes attributed to epidural block. Although these lesions are possible, owing to abscess, hematoma, or chemical contamination, a more widespread neurologic deficit would be expected, considering the usual level of needle insertion. More likely causes are ligation of nutrient iliac vessels supplying the distal spinal cord in some patients or, alternatively, compression of sacral nerve roots or the pudendal nerve during pelvic surgery.

Complications Relating to Altered Physiology

The potential for complications owing to alteration in oxygen delivery to vital organs is outlined in detail in Tables 8-10 and 8-11. Thus, like general anesthesia, it is possible for epidural block to result in compromise of oxygen delivery to heart, brain, liver, or kidney, with sequelae that depend on the degree and duration of compromise. Full knowledge of pre-existing physical status and careful monitoring throughout the use of epidural block are essential to avoid such complications.

Complications of epidural block are given further consideration in Chapters 21 and 22.

DIFFERENTIAL DIAGNOSIS OF POSTOPERATIVE NEUROLOGIC SEQUELAE

It is all too easy to attribute a serious neurologic deficit after anesthesia and surgery to epidural block if the latter has been used as part of the anesthetic regimen. This is comforting for the surgical team, but it has no greater validity than does labeling all cases of postoperative jaundice as "halothane hepatitis." Factual evidence that links epidural blockade with neurologic sequelae is scarce: Local anesthetics in clinical concentrations do not cause neural damage or meningeal irritation; a properly placed epidural needle or catheter with no evidence of contact with nerve root during insertion does not damage spinal nerves or spinal cord, unless gross infection or epidural hematoma results, usually from associated medical or surgical problems; epinephrine used in a concentration of 1:200,000 almost certainly does not result in anterior spinal artery spasm.[230]

TABLE 8-21. *Investigative steps in the management of postoperative neurologic sequelae*

1. Thorough review of pre-existing medical problems and drug therapy (pre-existing signs and symptoms of a spinal cord tumor may be elicited or a family history of neurologic problems, or drug therapy capable of causing neurologic side effects)
2. Review of anesthetic management and surgical procedure (e.g., evidence of poor spinal cord perfusion; see physiology section): dangerous posturing during surgery? surgical section of nutrient vessels to spinal cord? surgical section or retraction of spinal nerves or peripheral nerves?
3. An attempt to anatomically localize the lesion (Fig. 8-35)
4. Consideration of most likely causes of a lesion located at such a level
5. Appropriate further investigations, such as blood culture, coagulation studies, myelography, CT scan, NMR scan, EMG
6. Careful surveillance for signs of progression of the lesion or associated medical problems
7. Rapid response to significant abnormalities (e.g., progressive neurologic deficit, back pain, pyrexia, and leukocytosis require myelogram to identify possible epidural abscess, and urgent laminectomy)
8. Follow-up documentation of outcome with appropriate investigation of progress of lesion (e.g., repeated EMG, serial cystometric measurements to document return or otherwise of bladder function)
9. Careful postmortem examination of nervous system by a skilled neuropathologist, if possible in conjunction with the anesthesiologist and surgeon involved. The pertinence of the pathologist's examination is greatly enhanced by firsthand information, and the education of medical staff is best served by direct participation in examining the morbid anatomy of such major complications
10. Precise reporting in the medical literature, avoiding misleading titles. For example, an excellent report by Usubiaga[385] provided clear evidence that paraplegia after vascular surgery under epidural block was due to ligation of nutrient vessels to the spinal cord during the surgery; unfortunately, the title of this article was "Neurological Complications of Prevertebral Surgery Under Regional Anesthesia." This implies that the regional anesthesia was to blame

CT, computed tomography; EMG, electromyography; NMR, nuclear magnetic resonance

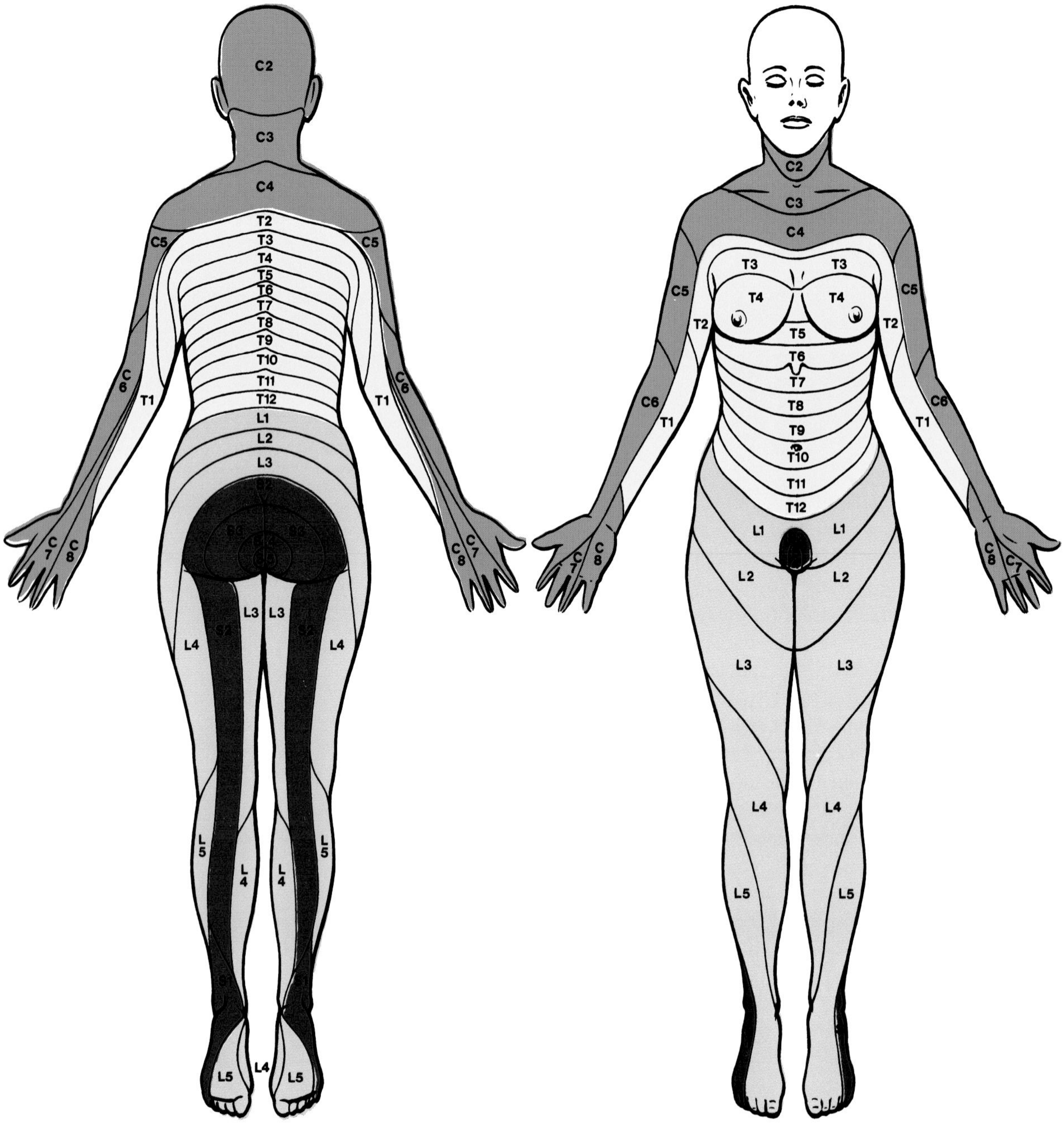

FIG. 8-35. Dermatomal chart. The segmental areas are illustrated to emphasize the most reliable cutaneous area to test for blockade of individual spinal cord segments.

There are a large number of common causes of neurologic deficit after anesthesia and surgery, just as there are common causes of postoperative jaundice. The medical team must consider a differential diagnosis with these common causes at the top of the list and must ensure that a readily treatable condition is not overlooked.

"Associated but unrelated" cases of spastic paraplegia may occur after childbirth in patients who received epidural block. This is strongly supported by the report of five cases of spastic paraplegia in parturients who did *not* have epidural block.[14] All were associated with spontaneous vertex deliveries, two of which were forceps deliveries.

The effective management of postoperative neurologic sequelae requires the collaboration of the anesthesiologist, the surgeon, and a neurologist. The assistance of a radiologist and neurosurgeon also may well be required. A frank discussion aimed at defining etiology rather than fault should take place after each physician has had an opportunity to examine the patient and history. The investigative steps are as listed in Table 8-21.

Anesthesiologists should have a thorough knowledge of the causes of postoperative neurologic sequelae that have been reported in patients who did not receive epidural block (see Table 8-20):

1. *Spinal cord lesions* resulting from ligation of nutrient spinal cord vessels during abdominal surgery[385] or during pelvic surgery (iliac vessels, see anatomy section and Chapter 7, Fig. 7-11); prolonged clamping of the aorta[105]; extreme posture and severe retraction causing epidural venous congestion, combined with low cardiac output and leading to "spinal stroke."

2. *Lesions of the cauda equina* or *spinal nerve roots.* "Adhesive arachnoiditis" has been found at re-exploration after major back surgery, and damage to spinal nerve roots has also resulted from surgery in the paravertebral region. Epidural hematoma associated with coagulation defects and systemic heparinization are discussed on page 304. Bladder dysfunction or complete loss of bladder and bowel control is a difficult diagnostic problem. Careful neurologic examination, including cystometry, EMG, and sometimes myelography, is required to determine etiology. Ligation of nutrient "iliac" supply to sacral segments of spinal cord may result in a clinical picture that mimics a cauda equina lesion. Severe retraction of sacral nerve roots during pelvic surgery may also result in such a lesion.

3. *Peripheral nerve lesions* are the most common neurologic sequelae[53] and should be carefully distinguished from more "central" causes on the basis of distribution of sensory, motor, and autonomic deficit and EMG to determine pattern of "muscle denervation" (if present) and timing of onset of denervation. This assists in determining whether spinal root(s) or peripheral nerves are involved and whether the lesion predates or postdates the operation or is consistent with an intraoperative episode.[256]

Such data alone, however, are not definitive and provide only a guide.[65] Knowledge of potential sites of peripheral nerve injury during surgery and a tendency for such lesions to be unilateral also serve as a basis for differentiation. Examples of sites of peripheral lesions are (i) *lumbosacral trunk* (L4–L5): compression on the ala of the sacrum during pregnancy, with resultant footdrop and weakness or analgesia[274] at L4–L5; (ii) *sacral nerves:* during delivery or pelvic surgery; (iii) *femoral nerve* (L2–L4): during pelvic surgery; (iv) *lateral femoral cutaneous nerve* (L2–L3): commonly damaged in the lithotomy position or because of direct pressure or retraction close to the inguinal ligament; (v) *lateral popliteal nerve* (L4–S2): pressure over the head of the fibula. It should be noted that patients with pre-existing neurologic disease, such as diabetic neuropathy, are at greater risk.[81]

CONCLUSION

Epidural neural blockade is capable of great diversity in terms of its range of neural blocking effects and the clinical applications of these effects. It is undoubtedly a most complex technique in terms of its anatomy, site of action, physiology, and pharmacology. Because of this, it is a technique for the specialist—the anesthesiologist. However, if used with due attention to the data presented in this chapter, it can be used with a high degree of safety and efficacy.

REFERENCES

1. Abbott, M.A., Samuel, J.R., and Webb, D.R.: Anaesthesia for extracorporeal shock wave lithotripsy. Anaesthesia, *40:*1065, 1985.
2. Abboud, F.M.: Control of the various components of the peripheral vasculature. Fed. Proc., *31:*1226, 1972.
3. Abouleish, E., Amortegui, A.J., and Taylor, F.H.: Are bacterial filters needed in continuous epidural analgesia for obstetrics? Anesthesiology, *46:*351, 1977.
4. Ackerman, W.E., Mustaque, Juneja, M.M., Kaczorowski, D.O.: The accuracy of using thiopental or test strips to detect dural puncture during continuous epidural analgesia. Reg. Anesth., *13:*169, 1988.
5. Adamkiewicz, A.: Die blutgefasse des menschlichen ruckenmarkes. II. Die gefasse der ruckenmarksoberflache. S.B. Heidelberg Akad. Wiss., *85:*101, 1882.
6. Ahn, H., Bronget, A., Johansson, K., Ygge, H., and Lindhagen, J.: Effect of continuous postoperative epidural analgesia on intestinal motility. Br. J. Surg., *75:*1176, 1988.
7. Allen, P.R., and Johnson, R.W.: Extradural analgesia in labor. A comparison of 2-chloroprocaine hydrochloride and bupivacaine hydrochloride. Anaesthesia, *34:*839, 1979.
8. Anderson, L.O.: Prevention and treatment of thrombosis by low-molecular-weight heparins. Drug Des. Discov., *5:*1, 1989.
9. Anderson, S., and Cold, G.E.: Dose response studies in elderly patients subjected to epidural analgesia. Acta Anaesthesiol. Scand., *25:*279, 1981.
10. Andy, J.J., *et al.*: Cardiovascular effects of dobutamide in severe congestive heart failure. Am. Heart J., *94:*175, 1977.
11. Apostolou, G.A., Zarmakoupis, P.K., and Mastrokostopoulos, G.T.: Spread of epidural anesthesia and the lateral position. Anesth. Analg. (Cleve.), *60:*584, 1981.
12. Arndt, J., Hock, A., Stanton-Hicks, M., and Stuhmeier, K.D.: Peridural anesthesia and the distribution of blood in supine humans. Anesthesiology, *63:*616, 1985.
13. Axelsson, K.H.: A double-blind study of motor blockade in the lower limbs. Studies during spinal anaesthesia with hyperbaric and glucose-free 0.5% bupivacaine. Br. J. Anaesth., *57:*960, 1985.
14. Bademosi, O.: Obstetric neuropraxia in the Nigerian African. Int. J. Gynaecol. Obstet., *17:*611, 1980.
15. Bader, A.M., Datta, S., Flanagan, H., and Covino, B.G.: Comparison of bupivacaine and ropivacaine induced conduction blockade in isolate rabbit vagus nerve. Anesth. Analg., *68:*724, 1989.
16. Badner, N.H., Sullivan, P., Ganapathy, S., *et al.*: Continuous epidural infusion of ropivacaine for the prevention of postoperative pain after major orthopedic surgery: A dose-finding study. Anesthesiology, *81:*A1017, 1994.
17. Baker, A.S., Ojemann, R.G., Swartz, M.N., and Richardson, E.P.: Spinal epidural abscess. N. Engl. J. Med., *293:*463, 1975.
18. Baron, J.F., Decaux-Jacolot, A., Edouard, A., *et al.*: Influence of venous return on baroreflex control of heart rate during lumbar epidural anesthesia in humans. Anesthesiology, *64:*188, 1986.
19. Batson, O.V.: The vertebral vein system. A. J. R., *128:*195, 1957.
20. Bedder, M.D., Kozody, R., Palahniuk, R.J., *et al.*: Clonidine prolongs tetracaine spinal anesthesia in dogs. Anesth. Analg., *65:*S14, 1986.
21. Bellis, C.J., and Wangensteen, O.H.: Venous circulatory change in the abdomen and lower extremities attending intestinal distention. Proc. Soc. Exp. Biol. Med., *41:*490, 1939.
22. Bengtsson, M.: Changes in skin blood flow and temperature during spinal analgesia evaluated by laser Doppler flowmetry and infra-red thermography. Acta Anaesthesiol. Scand., *28:*625, 1984.
23. Benigni, A., Greorini, G., Frusca, T., *et al.*: Effect of low-dose aspirin on fetal and maternal generation of thromboxane by platelets in women at risk for pregnancy-induced hypertension. N. Engl. J. Med., *321:*351, 1989.
24. Benzon, H.T., Toleikis, J.R., Shanks, C., Ramseur, A., and Slaon, T.: Somatosensory evoked potential quantification of ulnar nerve blockade. Anesth. Analg., *65:*843, 1986.
25. Bergqvist, D., Lindblad, B., and Matzsch, T.: Risk of combining low molecular weight heparin for thromboprophylaxis and epidural or spinal anesthesia. Semin. Thromb. Hemost., *19:*147, 1993.
26. Berne, R.M.: Haemodynamics and sodium excretion of denervated kidney in anaesthetized and unanaesthetized dog. Am. J. Physiol., *171:*148, 1952.
27. Berquist, E., Berquist, D., Bronge, A., Dahlgreen, S., and Lindquist,

B.: An evaluation of early thrombosis prophylaxis following fracture of the femoral neck. Acta Chir. Scand., *138:*689, 1972.

28. Bevan, D.R.: The sodium story: Effects of anaesthesia and surgery on intrarenal mechanisms concerned with sodium homeostasis. Proc. R. Soc. Med., *66:*1215, 1973.
29. Bieniarz, J., *et al.*: Aortocavial compression by the uterus in late human pregnancy. II: An arteriographic study. Am. J. Obstet. Gynecol., *100:*203, 1968.
30. Binnert, D., Thierry, A., Michiels, R., Soichot, P., and Perrin, M.: Presentation d'un nouveau cas d'hematome extradural rachidien spontane observe au cours d'un accouchement. J. Med. Lyon, *52:*1307, 1971.
31. Blomberg, R.: The dorsomedian connective tissue band in the lumbar epidural space of humans. Anesth. Analg., *65:*747, 1986.
32. Blomberg, R.G., and Olsson, S.S.: The lumbar epidural space in patients examined with epiduroscopy. Anesth. Analg., *68:*157, 1989.
33. Blomberg, S., and Ricksten, S.E.: Thoracic epidural anesthesia decreases the incidence of ventricular arrhythmias during acute myocardial ischemia in anaesthetised rats. Acta Anaesthesiol. Scand., *32:*173, 1988.
34. Blomberg, S., Curelaru, J., Emanuelsson, H., *et al.*: Thoracic epidural anaesthesia in patients with unstable angina pectoris. Eur. Heart J., *10:*437, 1989.
35. Blomberg, S., Emanuelsson, H., Kvist, H., *et al.*: Effects of thoracic epidural anesthesia on coronary arteries and arterioles in patients with coronary artery disease. Anesthesiology, *73:*840, 1990.
36. Blomberg, S., Emanuelsson, H., and Ricksten, S.E.: Thoracic epidural anesthesia and central hemodynamics in patients with unstable angina pectoris. Anesth. Analg., *69:*558, 1989.
37. Blomberg, S.C.: Long-term home self-treatment with high thoracic epidural anesthesia in patients with severe coronary artery disease. Anesth. Analg., *79:*413, 1994.
38. Bonica, J.J.: Principles and Practice of Obstetric Analgesia and Anesthesia. pp. 725, 745. Philadelphia, F.A. Davis, 1967.
39. Bonica, J.J., *et al.*: Peridural block: Analysis of 3637 cases and a review. Anesthesiology, *18:*723, 1957.
40. Bonica, J.J., Akamatsu, T.J., Berges, P.U., Morikawa, K., and Kennedy, W.F.: Circulatory effects of peridural block. II. Effects of epinephrine. Anesthesiology, *34:*514, 1971.
41. Bonica, J.J., Berges, P.U., and Morikawa, K.: Circulatory effects of peridural block. I. Effects of levels of analgesia and dose of lidocaine. Anesthesiology, *33:*619, 1970.
42. Bonica, J.J., Kennedy, W.F., Akamatsu, T.J., and Gerbershagen, H.U.: Circulatory effects of peridural block. III. Effects of acute blood loss. Anesthesiology, *36:*219, 1972.
43. Bonica, J.J., Kennedy, W.F., Ward, R.J., and Tolas, A.G.: A comparison of the effects of high subarachnoid and epidural anesthesia. Acta Anaesthesiol. Scand., *23* (Suppl.):429, 1966.
44. Bowdle, T.A., Freund, P.R., and Slattery, J.T.: Age-dependent lidocaine pharmacokinetics during lumbar peridural anesthesia with lidocaine hydrocarbonate or lidocaine hydrochloride. Reg. Anesth., *11:*123, 1986.
45. Bowsher, D.: A comparative study of the azygos venous system in man, monkey, dog, cat, rat and rabbit. J. Anat., *88:*400, 1954.
46. Boys, J.E., and Norman, P.F.: Accidental subdural analgesia. Br. J. Anaesth., *47:*1111, 1975.
47. Braham, J., and Saia, A.: Neurological complications of epidural anaesthesia. Br. Med. J., *2:*657, 1958.
48. Brand, P.H., Metting, P.J., and Britton, S.L.: Support of arterial blood pressure by major pressor systems in conscious dogs. Am. J. Physiol., *255:*H483, 1988.
49. Bridenbaugh, L.D., Moore, D.C., Bagdi, P., and Bridenbaugh, P.O.: The position of plastic tubing in continuous block techniques: An x-ray study of 552 patients. Anesthesiology, *29:*1047, 1968.
50. Bridenbaugh, P.O., *et al.*: Role of epinephrine in regional block anesthesia with etidocaine: A double-blind study. Anesth. Analg. (Cleve.), *53:*430, 1974.
51. Brierley, J.B., and Field, E.J.: The connections of the spinal sub-arachnoid space with the lymphatic system. J. Anat., *82:*153, 1948.
52. Brigden, W., Howarth, S., and Sharpey-Schafer, E.P.: Postural changes in the peripheral blood flow of normal subjects with observations on vasovagal fainting reactions as a result of tilting, the lordotic posture, pregnancy and spinal anaesthesia. Clin. Sci. Mol. Med., *9:*79, 1950.
53. Britt, B.A., and Gordon, R.A.: Peripheral nerve injuries associated with anaesthesia. Can. Anaesth. Soc. J., *11:*514, 1964.
54. Brockway, M.S., Bannister, J.P., McClure, J.H., McKeown, D., and Wildsmith, J.A.W.: Comparison of extradural ropivacaine and bupivacaine. Br. J. Anaesth, *66:*31, 1991.
55. Bromage, P.R.: Vascular hypotension in 150 cases of epidural analgesia. Anaesthesia, *6:*26, 1951.
56. Bromage, P.R.: The "hanging-drop" sign. Anaesthesia, *8:*237, 1953.
57. Bromage, P.R.: Spinal Epidural Analgesia. Edinburgh, E. & S. Livingstone, 1954.
58. Bromage, P.R.: Epidural needle. Anesthesiology, *22:*1018, 1961.
59. Bromage, P.R.: Spread of analgesic solutions in the epidural space and their site of action: A statistical study. Br. J. Anaesth., *34:*161, 1962.
60. Bromage, P.R.: Exaggerated spread of epidural analgesia in arteriosclerotic patients. Dosage in relation to biological and chronological ageing. Br. Med. J., *2:*1634, 1962.
61. Bromage, P.R.: A comparison of the hydrochloride salts of lignocaine and prilocaine for epidural analgesia. Br. J. Anaesth., *37:*753, 1965.
62. Bromage, P.R.: Ageing and epidural dose requirements. Segmental spread and predictability of epidural analgesia in youth and extreme age. Br. J. Anaesth., *41:*1016, 1969.
63. Bromage, P.R.: Lower limb reflex changes in segmental epidural analgesia. Br. J. Anaesth., *46:*504, 1974.
64. Bromage, P.R.: Mechanism of action of extradural analgesia. Br. J. Anaesth., *47:*199, 1975.
65. Bromage, P.R.: Epidural Analgesia. Philadelphia, W.B. Saunders, 1978.
66. Bromage, P.R., Burfoot, M.F., Crowell, D.F., and Pettigrew, R.T.: Quality of epidural blockade. I. Influence of physical factors. Br. J. Anaesth., *36:*342, 1964.
67. Bromage, P.R., Joyal, A.C., and Binney, J.C.: Local anesthetic drugs: Penetration from the spinal extradural space into the neuraxis. Science, *140:*392, 1963.
68. Bromage, P.R., and Millar, R.A.: Epidural blockade and circulating catecholamine levels in a child with phaeochromocytoma. Can. Anaesth. Soc. J., *5:*282, 1958.
69. Bromage, P.R., Pettigrew, R.T., and Crowell, D.E.: Tachyphylaxis in epidural analgesia. I. Augmentation and decay of local anesthesia. J. Clin. Pharmacol., *9:*30, 1969.
70. Brown, D.T., Carpenter, R.L., and Thompson, G.E.: Comparisons of 0.5% ropivacaine and 0.5% bupivacaine for epidural anesthesia in patients undergoing lower extremity surgery. Anesthesiology, *72:*633, 1990.
71. Brownridge, P.: Epidural and subarachnoid analgesia for elective cesarean section. Anaesthesia, *36:*70, 1981.
72. Brownridge, P.: Shivering related to epidural blockade in labor, and the influence of epidural pethidine. Anesth. Intens. Care, *14:*412, 1986.
73. Bryce-Smith, R.: Pressures in the extradural space. Anaesthesia, *5:*213, 1950.
74. Bryce-Smith, R., and Williams, E.O.: The treatment of eclampsia (imminent or actual) by continuous conduction analgesia. Lancet, *1:*1241, 1955.
75. Buffington, C.W., Davis, K.B., and Gillispie, S.: The prevalence of steal prone-coronary anatomy in patients with coronary artery disease: an analysis of the coronary artery surgery study registry. Anesthesiology, *69:*721, 1988.
76. Bull, G.M.: Postural proteinuria. Clin. Sci. Mol. Med., *7:*77, 1948.
77. Burm, A.G.L.: Clinical pharmacokinetics of epidural and spinal anaesthesia. Clin. Pharmacokinet., *16:*283, 1989.
78. Burn, J.M., Guyer, P.B., and Langdon, L.: The spread of solutions injected into the epidural space: A study using epidurograms in patients with the lumbosciatic syndrome. Br. J. Anaesth., *45:*338, 1973.
79. Calder, A.A., Moar, V.A., Qunsted, M.K., and Turnbull, A.C.: Increased bilirubin levels in neonates after induction of labour by intravenous prostaglandin E_2 or oxytocin. Lancet, *2:*1339, 1974.
80. Calnan, J.S., and Allenby, F.: The prevention of deep vein thrombosis after surgery. Br. J. Anaesth., *47:*151, 1975.
81. Calverley, J.R., and Mulder, D.W.: Femoral neuropathy. Neurology, *10:*963, 1960.
82. Campbell, H.H., and Walker, F.G.: Continuous epidural analgesia in the treatment of frostbite. A report of three cases. Can. Med. Assoc. J., *84:*87, 1961.
83. Carp, H., Vadherra, R., Jayaram, A., and Garvey, D.: Endogenous vasopressin and reninangiotension systems support blood pressure after epidural block in humans. Anesthesiology, *80:*1000, 1994.

84. Catterberg, J.: Local anesthetic vs. spinal fluid. Anesthesiology, *46:*309, 1977.
85. Cederholm, J., Anskar, S., and Bengtsson, M.: Sensory, motor, and sympathetic lock during epidural analgesia with 0.5% and 0.75% ropivacaine with and without epinephrine. Reg. Anesth., *19:*18, 1994.
86. Cheng, P.A.: Blunt-tip needle for epidural anesthesia. Anesthesiology, *19:*556, 1958.
87. Clarke, C.J., and Whitewell, J.: Intradural haemorrhage after epidural injection. Br. Med. J., *2:*1612, 1961.
88. Clarke, E., Momson, R., and Roberts, H.: Spinal cord damage by Efocaine. Lancet, *1:*896, 1955.
89. Coates, M.B.: Combined subarachnoid and epidural techniques. Anaesthesia, *37:*89, 1982.
90. Coggeshall, R.E., Coulter, J.D., and Willis, W.D.: Unmyelinated axons in the ventral roots of the cat lumbosacral enlargement. J. Comp. Neurol., *153:*39, 1974.
91. Cohen, C.A., and Kallos, T.: Failure of spinal anesthesia due to subdural catheter placement. Anesthesiology, *37:*352, 1972.
92. Cohen, E.N.: Distribution of local anesthetic agents in the neuraxis of the dog. Anesthesiology, *29:*1002, 1968.
93. Cohen, E.N., Levine, D.A., Colliss, J.E., and Gunther, R.E.: The role of pH in the development of tachyphylaxis to local anesthetic agents. Anesthesiology, *29:*994, 1968.
94. Cohen, S., Luykx, W.M., and Marx, G.F.: High versus low flow rates during lumbar epidural block. Reg. Anaesth., *9:*8, 1984.
95. Cohen, S.E., and Thurlow, A.: Comparison of a chloroprocaine-bupivacaine mixture with chloroprocaine and bupivacaine used individually for obstetric epidural analgesia. Anesthesiology, *51:*288, 1979.
96. Concepcion, M., Arthur, G.R., Steele, S.M., Bader, A.M., and Covino, B.G.: A new local anaesthetic ropivacaine. Its epidural effects in humans. Anesth. Analg., *70:*80, 1990.
97. Cooke, E.D., Lloyd, M.J., Bowcock, S.A., and Pilcher, M.D.: Monitoring during low-dose heparin prophylaxis. N. Engl. J. Med., *294:*1066, 1976.
98. Corbett, J.L., Frankel, H.L., and Harris, P.J.: Cardiovascular reflex responses to cutaneous and visceral stimuli in spinal man. J. Physiol. (Lond.), *215:*395, 1971.
99. Corbett, J.L., Frankel, H.L., and Harris, P.J.: Cardiovascular responses to tilting in tetraplegic man. J. Physiol. (Lond.), *215:*411, 1971.
100. Corbin, K.B., and Gardner, E.D.: Decrease in number of myelinated fibers in human spinal roots with age. Anat. Rec., *68:*63, 1937.
101. Corke, B.G., Carlson, C.G., and Dettbarn, W.D.: The influence of 2-chloroprocaine on the subsequent analgesic potency of bupivacaine. Anesthesiology, *60:*25, 1984.
102. Corning, J.L.: Spinal anaesthesia and local medication of the cord. N.Y. Med. J., *42:*483, 1885.
103. Cort, J.H.: Relief of post-traumatic anuria. Am. J. Physiol., *164:*686, 1951.
104. Cort, H.J.: Effect of nervous stimulation on the arterio-venous oxygen and carbon dioxide differences across the kidney. Nature, *171:*784, 1953.
105. Coupland, G.A.E., and Reeve, T.S.: Paraplegia: A complication of excision of abdominal aortic aneurysm. Surgery, *64:*878, 1968.
106. Cousins, M.J.: Vascular responses in arteriosclerotic patients. Anesthesiology, *35:*99, 1971.
107. Cousins, M.J.: Hematoma following epidural block. Anesthesiology, *37:*263, 1972.
108. Cousins, M.J.: Acute pain and the injury response: Immediate and prolonged effects. Reg. Anesth., *14:*162, 1989.
109. Cousins, M.J., *et al.*: Epidural block for abdominal surgery: Aspects of clinical pharmacology of etidocaine. Anaesth. Intens. Care, *6:*105, 1978.
110. Cousins, M.J., and Mather, L.E.: Intrathecal and epidural administration of opioids. Anesthesiology, *61:*276, 1984.
111. Cousins, M.J., Mather, L.E., Glynn, C.J., Wilson, P.R., and Graham, J.R.: Selective spinal analgesia. Lancet, *1:*1141, 1979.
112. Cousins, M.J., and Wright, C.J.: Graft, muscle, skin blood flow after epidural block in vascular surgical procedures. Surg. Gynecol. Obstet., *133:*59, 1971.
113. Covino, B.G., and Scott, D.B.: Handbook of Epidural Anaesthesia and Analgesia. Orlando, Grune & Stratton, 1985.
114. Craft, J.B., Epstein, B.S., and Coakley, C.S.: Prophylaxis of dural-puncture headache with epidural saline. Anesth. Analg. (Cleve.), *52:*228, 1973.
115. Crawford, J.S.: The prevention of headache consequent upon dural puncture. Br. J. Anaesth., *44:*598, 1972.
116. Crawford, J.S.: Principles and Practice of Obstetric Anaesthesia. 4th Ed. Oxford, Blackwell Scientific Publications, 1978.
117. Crawley, B.E.: Catheter sequestration. A complication of epidural analgesia. Anaesthesia, *23:*270, 1968.
118. Crock, H.V., and Yoshizawa, H.: The Blood Supply of the Vertebral Column and Spinal Cord in Man. New York, Springer-Verlag, 1977.
119. Cullen, M.L., Staren, E.D., El-Ganzouri, A., *et al.*: Continuous epidural infusion for analgesia after major abdominal operations: A randomized, prospective, double-blind study. Surgery, *98:*718, 1985.
120. Curelaru, I.: Long duration subarachnoid anesthesia with continuous epidural block. Prakt. Anaesth., *14:*71, 1979.
121. Cusick, J.F., Myklebust, J.B., and Abram, S.E.: Differential neural effects of epidural anesthetics. Anesthesiology, *53:*299, 1980.
122. Cusick, J.F., and Davidson, A.: Altered neural conduction with epidural bupivacaine. Anesthesiology, *57:*31, 1982.
123. Dahl, J.B., Rosenberg, J., and Kehlet, H.: Effect of thoracic epidural etidocaine 1.5% on somatosensory evoked potentials, cortisol and glucose during cholecystectomy. Acta Anesthesiol. Scand., *36:*378, 1992.
124. Dahl, J.B., Rosenberg, J., Lund, C., and Kehlet, H.: Effect of thoracic epidural bupivacaine 0.75% on somatosensory evoked potentials after dermatomal stimulation. Reg. Anesth., *15:*73, 1990.
125. Dahl, J.B., Simonsen, L., and Mogensen, T.: The effect of 0.5% ropivacaine on epidural blood flow. Acta Anaesthesiol. Scand., *34:*308, 1990.
126. Davis, R.F., DeBoer, W.V., and Maroko, P.R.: Thoracic epidural anesthesia reduces myocardial infarct size after coronary artery occlusion in dogs. Anesth. Analg., *65:*711, 1986.
127. Davson, H., Demer, F.R., and Hollingsworth, J.R.: The mechanism of drainage of the cerebrospinal fluid. Brain, *96:*329, 1973.
128. Dawkins, C.J.M.: Discussion on extradural spinal block. Proc. R. Soc. Med., *38:*299, 1945.
129. Dawkins, C.J.M.: The identification of the epidural space. A critical analysis of the various methods employed. Anaesthesia, *18:*66, 1963.
130. Dawkins, C.J.M.: The relief of pain in labour by mean of continuous-drip epidural block. Acta Anaesthesiol. Scand., *37* (Suppl.):248, 1970.
131. De Angelis, J.: Hazards of subdural and epidural anesthesia during anticoagulant therapy: A case report and review. Anesth. Analg. (Cleve.), *51:*676, 1972.
132. Defalque, R.J.: Compared effects of spinal and extradural anesthesia upon the blood pressure. Anesthesiology, *23:*627, 1962.
133. Dinnick, O.P.: Discussion on general anaesthesia for obstetrics: An evaluation of general and regional methods. Some aspects of general anaesthesia. Proc. R. Soc. Med., *50:*547, 1957.
134. Dirkes, W.E., Rosenberg, J., Lund, C., and Kehlet, H.: The effect of subarachnoid lidocaine and combined subarachnoid lidocaine and epidural bupivacaine on electrical sensory thresholds. Reg. Anesth., *16:*262, 1991.
135. Dogliotti, A.M.: Segmental peridural anesthesia. Am. J. Surg., *20:*107, 1933.
136. Dorfman, L.J., and Bosley, T.M.: Age-related changes in peripheral and central nerve conduction in man. Neurology, *29:*38, 1979.
137. Doughty, A.: A precise method of cannulating the lumbar evidural space. Anaesthesia, *29:*63, 1974.
138. Durant, P.A., and Yaksh, T.L.: Epidural injections of bupivacaine, morphine, fentanyl, lofentanil, and DADL in chronically implanted rats: a pharmacologic and pathologic study. Anesthesiology, *64:*43, 1986.
139. Eaton, L.M.: Observations on the negative pressure in the epidural space. Mayo Clin. Proc., *14:*566, 1939.
140. Editorial: A time to be born. Lancet, *2:*1183, 1974.
141. Eldor, J.: Metallic particles in the spinal-epidural needle technique. Letter to the Editor. Reg. Anesth., *19:*219, 1994.
142. Enderby, G.E.H.: Controlled circulation with hypotensive drugs and posture to reduce bleeding in surgery. Preliminary results with pentamethonium iodide. Lancet, *1:*1145, 1950.
143. Engberg, G., and Wiklund, L.: The use of ephedrine for prevention of arterial hypotension during epidural blockade. A study of the central circulation after subcutaneous premedication. Acta Anaesthesiol. Scand., *66* (Suppl.):1, 1978.
144. Engberg, G., and Wiklund, L.: The circulatory effects of intravenously administered ephedrine during epidural blockade. Acta Anaesthesiol. Scand., *66* (Suppl.):27, 1978.

145. Erdemir, H.A., Soper, L.E., and Sweet, R.B.: Studies of factors affecting peridural anesthesia. Anesth. Analg. (Cleve.), *44:*400, 1965.
146. Feldman, H.S., Arthur, G.R., and Covino, B.G.: Comparative systemic toxicity of convulsant and supraconvulsant doses of intravenous ropivacaine, bupivacaine and lidocaine in the conscious dog. Anesth. Analg., *69:*794, 1989.
147. Ferguson, J.F., and Kirsch, W.M.: Epidural empyema following thoracic extradural block. J. Neurosurg., *41:*762, 1974.
148. Folkow, B.: Nervous control of blood vessels. Physiol. Rev., *35:*629, 1955.
149. Forrester, A.C.: Mishaps in anaesthesia. Anaesthesia, *14:*388, 1959.
150. Frank, N.R., Mead, J., and Ferris, B.G.: The mechanical behaviour of the lungs in healthy elderly persons. J. Clin. Invest., *36:*1680, 1957.
151. Frank, S.M., Shir, Y., Raja, S.N., Fleisher, L.A., and Beattie, C.: Core hypothermia and skin surface temperature gradients. Epidural versus general anesthesia and the effects of age. Anesthesiology, *80:*502, 1994.
152. Fratacelli, M., Kimball, W.R., Wain, J.L., *et al.*: Diaphragmatic shortening after thoracic surgery in humans. Effects of mechanical ventilation and thoracic epidural anesthesia. Anesthesiology, *79:*654, 1993.
153. Galbert, M.W., and Marx, G.F.: Extradural pressures in the parturient patient. Anesthesiology, *40:*499, 1974.
154. Galindo, A., Hernandez, J., Benavides, O., *et al.*: Quality of spinal extradural anaesthesia: The influence of spinal nerve root diameter. Br. J. Anaesth., *47:*41, 1975.
155. Galindo, A., and Sprouse, J.H.: The influence of epidural anaesthesia on cardiac excitability in profound hypothermia. Can. Anaesth. Soc. J., *11:*614, 1964.
156. Galindo, A., and Witcher, T.: Mixtures of local anesthetics: bupivacaine-chloroprocaine. Anesth. Analg., *56:*683, 1980.
157. Gargano, F.P., Meyer, J.D., and Sheldon, J.J.: Transfemoral ascending lumbar catheterization of the epidural veins in lumbar disk disease. Radiology, *111:*329, 1974.
158. Gavin, R.: Continuous epidural analgesia, an unusual case of dural perforation during catheterisation of the epidural space. N.Z. Med. J., *64:*280, 1965.
159. Gavras, H., Hatzinikolaou, P., North, W.G., Bresnahan, M., and Gravas, I. Interaction of the sympathetic nervous system with vasopressin and renin in the maintenance of blood pressure. Hypertension, *4:*400, 1982.
160. Gelman, S., Feigenberg, Z., Dintzman, M., and Levy, E.: Electroenterography after cholecystectomy. The role of high epidural analgesia. Arch. Surg., *112:*580, 1977.
161. Germann, P.A.S., Roberts, J.G., and Prys-Roberts, C.: The combination of general anaesthesia and epidural block. I. The effects of sequence of induction on haemodynamic variables and blood gas measurements in healthy patients. Anaesth. Intens. Care, *7:*229, 1979.
162. Gillies, F.H., and Nag, D.: Vulnerability of human spinal cord in transient cardiac arrest. Neurology, *21:*833, 1971.
163. Gillies, I.D.S., and Morgan, M.: Accidental total spinal analgesia with bupivacaine. Anaesthesia, *28:*441, 1973.
164. Gingrich, T.F.: Spinal epidural hematoma following continuous epidural anesthesia. Anesthesiology, *29:*162, 1968.
165. Gissen, A.J., Datta, S., and Lambert, D.: The chloroprocaine controversy. Reg. Anesth., *9:*124, 1984.
166. Glosten, B., Hynson, J., Sessler, D.I., and McGuire, J.: Preanesthetic skin-surface warming reduces redistribution hypothermia caused by epidural block. Anesth. Analg., *77:*488, 1993.
167. Glosten, B., Sessler, D.I., Faure, A.M., Karl, L., and Thisted, R.A.: Central temperature changes are poorly perceived during epidural anesthesia. Anesthesiology, *77:*10, 1992.
168. Glosten, B., Sessler, D.I., Ostman, L.G., *et al.*: Intravenous lidocaine does not cause shivering-like tremor or alter thermoregulation. Reg. Anesth., *16:*218, 1991.
169. Goertz, A.W., Seeling, W., Heinriech, H., *et al.*: Effect of phenylephrine bolus administration on left ventricular function during high thoracic and lumbar epidural anesthesia combined with general anesthesia. Anesth. Analg., *76:*541, 1993.
170. Granger, H.J., and Guyton, A.C.: Autoregulation of the total systemic circulation following destruction of the central nervous system in the dog. Circ. Res., *25:*379, 1969.
171. Greene, N.M.: Area of differential block in spinal anesthesia with hyperbaric tetracaine. Anesthesiology, *19:*45, 1958.
172. Griffiths, D.P.G., Diamond, A.W., and Cameron, J.D.: Postoperative extradural analgesia following thoracic surgery: A feasibility study. Br. J. Anaesth., *47:*48, 1975.
173. Grundy, B.L., Heros, R.C., Tung, A.S., and Doyle, E.: Intraoperative loss of somatosensory evoked potentials predicts loss of spinal cord function. Anesthesiology, *57:*321, 1982.
174. Grundy, E.M., *et al.*: Extradural analgesia revisited. A statistical study. Br. J. Anaesth., *50:*805, 1978.
175. Grundy, E.M., Rao, L.N., and Winnie, A.P.: Epidural anesthesia and the lateral position. Anesth. Analg. (Cleve.), *57:*95, 1978.
176. Gutierrez, A.: Valor de la aspiracion liquida en el espacio peridural en la anestesia peridural. Rev. Circ. Buenos Aires, *12:*225, 1933.
177. Gutierrez, A.: Anesthesia extradural. Rev. Cirurg. Buenos Aires, 34, 1939.
178. Hancock, D.O.: A study of 49 patients with acute spinal extradural abscess. Paraplegia, *10:*285, 1973.
179. Hank, S.I., Raichle, M.E., and Reis, D.J.: Spontaneously remitting spinal epidural hematoma in a patient on anticoagulants. N. Engl. J. Med., *284:*1355, 1971.
180. Harper, A.M., Deshmukh, D., Rowan, J.O., and Jennett, W.B.: The influence of sympathetic nervous activity on cerebral blood flow. Arch. Neurol., *27:*1, 1972.
181. Harrison, D.C., Sprouse, J.H., and Morrow, A.G.: The antiarrhythmic properties of lidocaine and procaine amide. Clinical and physiologic studies of their cardiovascular effects in man. Circulation, *28:*486, 1963.
182. Heldt, J.H., and Moloney, J.C.: Negative pressure in the epidural space. Am. J. Med. Sci., *175:*371, 1928.
183. Heusch, G., Deussen, A., and Thamer, V.: Cardiac sympathetic nerve activity and progressive vasoconstriction distal to coronary stenosis: feedback aggravation of myocardial ischemia. J. Auton. Nerve Syst., *13:*311, 1985.
184. Hills, N.H.; Pflug, J.J., Jeyasingh, K., Boardman, L., and Calnan, J.S.: Prevention of deep vein thrombosis by intermittent pneumatic compression of calf. Br. Med. J., *1:*131, 1972.
185. Hindman, B.J., and Koka, B.V.: Usefulness of the post-aspirin bleeding time. Anesthesiology, *64:*368, 1986.
186. Hindmarsh, T.: Methiodal sodium and metrizamide in lumbar myelography. Acta Radiol. (Stockh.), *355*(Suppl.):359, 1973.
187. Hirabayashi, Y., and Shimozu, R.: Effect of age on extradural dose requirement in thoracic extradural anaesthesia. Br. J. Anaesth., *71:*445, 1993.
188. Hirabayashi, Y., Shimizu, R., Matsuda, I., and Inoue, S.: Effect of extradural compliance and resistance on spread of extradural analgesia. Br. J. Anaesth., *65:*508, 1990.
189. Hjorts, N.C., Neumann, P., Frsig, F., *et al.*: A controlled study on the effect of epidural analgesia with local anesthetics and morphine on morbidity after abdominal surgery. Acta Anaesthesiol. Scand., *29:*790, 1985.
190. Ho, P.S., Yu, S., Sether, L., *et al.*: Ligamentum flavum: Appearance on sagittal and coronal MR images. Radiology, *168:*469, 1988.
191. Hodgkinson, R., and Husain, F.J.: Obesity gravity and spread of epidural anesthesia. Anesth. Analg. (Cleve.), *60:*421, 1981.
192. Hoffman, J.I.E., and Buckberg, G.D.: Transmural variations in myocardial perfusion. *In* Yu, P., and Goodwin, J. (eds.): Progress in Cardiology. Vol. V. pp. 37–89, Philadelphia, Lea & Febiger, 1976.
193. Hogan, Q.H.: Lumbar epidural anatomy: A new look by cryomicrotome section. Anesthesiology, *75:*767, 1991.
194. Hollmen, A., and Saukkonen, J.: The effects of postoperative epidural analgesia versus centrally acting opiate on physiological shunt after upper abdominal operation. Acta Anaesthesiol. Scand., *16:*147, 1972.
195. Holmdahl, M.H., Sjorgren, S., Strom, G., and Wright, B.: Clinical aspects of continuous epidural blockade for postoperative pain relief. Ups. J. Med. Sci., *77:*47, 1972.
196. Honkomp, J.: Zur Begutachtung Bleibender Neurologischer Schaden nach Periduralanaesthesie. Der Anaesthesist, *15:*246, 1966.
197. Hopf, H.B., Schlaghecke, R., and Peters, J.: Sympathetic neural blockade by thoracic epidural anesthesia suppresses renin release in response to arterial hypotension. Anesthesiology, *80:*992, 1994.
198. Horlocker, T.T., and Wedel, D.J.: Anticoagulants, antiplatelet therapy and neuraxis blockade. Epidural and spinal analgesia and anesthesia: Contemporary issues. Anesth. Clin. North Am., 1992.
199. Horlocker, T.T., Wedel, D.J., and Offord, K.P.: Does preoperative antiplatelet therapy increase the risk of hemorrhagic complications associated with regional anesthesia. Anesth. Analg., *70:*631, 1990.
200. Horlocker, T.T., Wedel, D.J., Offord, K.P., *et al.*: Preoperative an-

tiplatelet drugs do not increase the risk of spinal hematoma associated with regional anesthesia. Reg. Anesth., *19*(2S):8, 1994.

201. Horlocker, T.T., Wedel, D.J., and Schlichting, J.L.: Postoperative epidural analgesia and oral anticoagulant therapy. Anesth. Analg., *79:*89, 1994.
202. Howarth, F.: Studies with a radioactive spinal anaesthetic. Br. J. Pharmacol., *4:*333, 1949.
203. Howarth, F.: Observations on the passage of a colloid from cerebrospinal fluid to blood and tissues. Br. J. Pharmacol., *7:*573, 1952.
204. Huson, A., Luyendyk, W., Tielbeek, A., and Van Zundert, A.: CT epidurography and the anatomy of the human epidural space. Anesthesiology, *69:*797, 1988.
205. Hylton, R.R., Eger, E.I., and Rovno, S.H.: Intravascular placement of epidural catheters. Anesth. Analg. (Cleve.), *43:*379, 1964.
206. Hynson, J.M., Sessler, D.I., Glosten, B., and McGuire, J.: Thermal balance and tremor patterns during epidural anesthesia. Anesthesiology, *74:*680, 1991.
207. Jacobs, S., Pullan, P.T., Potter, J.M., and Shenfield, G.M.: Adrenal suppression following extradural steroids. Anaesthesia, *38:*953, 1983.
208. James, F.M., George, R.H., Haiem, H., and White, G.J.: Bacteriologic aspects of epidural analgesia. Anesth. Analg. (Cleve.), *55:*187, 1976.
209. Janzen, E.: Der Negative Vorschlag bei Lumbalpunktion. Dtsch. Z. Nervenheilk., *94:*280, 1926.
210. Johansson, K., Ahn, H., Lindhagen, J., and Tryselius, U.: Effect of epidural anaesthesia on intestinal blood flow. Br. J. Surg., *75:*73, 1988.
211. Johnsson, S.R., Bygdeman, S., and Eliasson, R.: Effect of dextran on postoperative thrombosis. Acta Chir. Scand., *387:*(Suppl.):80, 1968.
212. Jorfeldt, L., *et al.*: The effect of local anaesthetics on the central circulation and respiration in man and dog. Acta Anaesthesiol. Scand., *12:*153, 1968.
213. Joshi, G.P., and McCarroll, S.M.: Evaluation of combined spinal-epidural anesthesia using two different techniques. Reg. Anesth., *19:*169, 1994.
214. Kalas, D.B., and Hehre, E.W.: Continuous lumbar peridural anesthesia in obstetrics. VIII. Further observations on inadvertent lumbar puncture. Anesth. Analg. (Cleve.), *51:*192, 1972.
215. Kane, R.F.: Neurologic deficits following epidural or spinal anesthesia. Anesth. Analg., *60:*150, 1981.
216. Kasten, G.W., and Martin, S.T.: Resuscitation from bupivacaine-induced cardiovascular toxicity during partial inferior vena cava occlusion. Anesth. Analg., *65:*341, 1986.
217. Katz, H., Borden, H., and Hirscher, D.: Glass-particle contamination of color-break ampules. Anesthesiology, *39:*354, 1973.
218. Katz, J.A., Knarr, D., and Bridenbaugh, P.O.: A double-blind comparison 0.5% bupivacaine and 0.75% ropivacaine administered epidurally in humans. Anesth. Analg., *15:*250, 1990.
219. Kehlet, H.: The stress response to anaesthesia and surgery: Release mechanisms and modifying factors. Clin. Anaesth., *2:*215, 1984.
220. Kehlet, H.: Surgical stress: the role of pain and analgesia. Br. J. Anaesth., *63:*189, 1989.
221. Kehlet, H.: Postoperative pain relief: A look from the other side. Reg. Anesth., *19:*369, 1994.
222. Keith, I.: Anaesthesia and blood loss in total hip replacement. Anaesthesia, *32:*444, 1977.
223. Kennedy, W.F., Jr.: Effects of spinal and peridural blocks on renal and hepatic functions. *In* Clinical Anesthesia Series. pp. 110–121. F.A. Davis, Philadelphia, 1969.
224. Kennedy, W.F., Everett, G.B., Cobb, L.A., and Allen, G.D.: Simultaneous systemic and hepatic hemodynamic measurements during high spinal anesthesia in normal man. Anesth. Analg., (Cleve.), *49:*1016, 1970.
225. Kennedy, W.F., Everett, G.B., Cobb, L.A., and Allen, G.D.: Simultaneous systemic and hepatic hemodynamic measurements during high peridural anesthesia in normal man. Anesth. Analg., (Cleve.), *49:*1016, 1970.
226. Klassen, G.A., Bramwell, R.S., Bromage, P.R., and Zborowska-Sluis, D.T.: The effect of acute sympathectomy by epidural anesthesia on the canine coronary circulation. Anesthesiology, *52:*8, 1980.
227. Kliemann, F.A.D.: Paraplegia and intercranial hypertension following epidural anesthesia. Report of four cases. Arq. Neuropsiquiatr., *33:*217, 1975.
228. Koch, M., Blomberg, S., Emanuelsson, H., *et al.*: Thoracic epidural anesthesia improves global and regional left ventricular function during stress induced myocardial ischemia in patients with coronary artery disease. Anesth. Analg., *71:*625, 1990.
229. Kochi, T., Sako, S., Nishino, T., and Mizuguchi, T.: Effect of high thoracic extradural anaesthesia on ventilatory response to hypercapnia in normal volunteers. Br. J. Anaesth., *62:*362, 1989.
230. Kosody, R., Palahniuk, R.J., Wade, J.G., and Cumming, M.O.: The effect of subarachnoid epinephrine and phenylephrine on spinal cord blood flow. Can. Anaesth. Soc. J., *31:*503, 1984.
231. Lahnborg, G., and Bengstrom, K.: Clinical and haemostatic parameters to thromboembolism and low-dose heparin prophylaxis in major surgery. Acta Chir. Scand., *141:*590, 1975.
232. Lassen, N.A.: Control of cerebral circulation in health and disease. Circ. Res., *34:*749, 1974.
233. Lazorthes, G., *et al.*: La vascularisation arterielle du renflement lombaire. Etude des variations et des suppleances. Rev. Neurol. (Paris), *114:*109, 1966.
234. Lazorthes, G., Poulhes, J., Bastide, G., Chancolle, A.R., and Zadeh, O.: Le vascularisation de la moelle epiniere (etude anatomique et physiologique). Rev. Neurol. (Paris), *106:*535, 1962.
235. Lee, J.A.: Specially marked needle to facilitate extradural block. Anaesthesia, *15:*186, 1960.
236. Lerner, S.M., Gutterman, P., and Jenkins, F.: Epidural hematoma and paraplegia after numerous lumbar punctures. Anesthesiology, *39:*550, 1973.
237. Levy, N.M.: Sympathetic-parasympathetic interactions in the heart. Circ. Res., *29:*437, 1971.
238. Li, T.-H., Shimosato, S., and Etsten, B.E.: Methoxamine and cardiac output in non-anesthetised man and during spinal analgesia. Anesthesiology, *26:*21, 1965.
239. Lock, R.F., Greiss, F.C., and Winston-Salem, N.C.: The anesthetic hazards in obstetrics. Am. J. Obstet. Gynecol., *70:*861, 1955.
240. Löfström, B.: Blocking characteristics of etidocaine (Duranest). Acta Anaesthesiol. Scand., *60* (Suppl.):21, 1975.
241. Low, P.A.: Endoneural fluid pressure and microenvironment of nerve. *In* Dyck, P.J., Thomas, P.K., Lambert, E.H., and Bunge, R. (eds.): Peripheral Neuropathy. pp. 599. Philadelphia, W.B. Saunders, 1984.
242. Lund, C., Hansen, O.B., Kehlet, H., Mogensen, T., and Qvitzau, S.: Effects of etidocaine administered epidurally on changes in somatosensory evoked potentials after dermatomal stimulation. Reg. Anesth., *16:*38, 1991.
243. Lund, C., Hansen, O.B., Mogensen, T., Hjortso, N.C., and Kehlet, H.: Effect of thoracic epidural bupivacaine on somatosensory evoked potentials after dermatomal stimulation. Anesth. Analg., *66:*731, 1987.
244. Lund, C., Selmar, P., Hansen, O.B., Hjortso, N.C., and Kehlet, H.: Effect of epidural bupivacaine on somatosensory evoked potentials after dermatomal stimulation. Anesth. Analg., *66:*34, 1987.
245. Lund, P.C.: Peridural Analgesia and Anesthesia. pp. 71,93. Springfield, Charles C. Thomas, 1966.
246. Luyendyk, W.: The plica mediana dorsalis of the dura mater and its relation to lumbar peridurography (canalography). Neuroradiology, *11:*147, 1976.
247. Luyendyk, W., and van Voorthuisen, A.E.: Contrast examination of the spinal epidural space. Acta Radiol., *5:*1051, 1966.
248. Macdonald, R.: Aspirin and extradural blocks. Br. J. Anaesth., *66:*1, 1991.
249. Macintosh, R.R.: Lumbar Puncture and Spinal Analgesia. Edinburgh, E. & S. Livingston, 1957.
250. Macintosh, R.R., and Mushin, W.W.: Observations on the epidural space. Anaesthesia, *2:*100, 1947.
251. Malatinsky, J., and Kadlic, T.: Inferior vena caval occlusion in the left lateral position. Br. J. Anaesth., *46:*165, 1974.
252. Male, C.G., and Martin, R.: Puerperal spinal epidural abscess. Lancet, *1:*608, 1973.
253. Malliani, A., Peterson, D.F., Bishop, V.S., and Brown, A.M.: Spinal sympathetic cardiocardiac reflexes. Circ. Res., *30:*158, 1972.
254. Malmquist, E.L-A., Berg, S., and Holmgren, H.: Effects of epidural bupivacaine or mepivacaine on somatosensory evoked potentials and skin resistance responses. Reg. Anesth., *17:*205, 1992.
255. Mankikian, B., Cantineau, J.P., Bertrand, M., *et al.*: Improvement of diaphragmatic function by a thoracic extradural block after upper abdominal surgery. Anesthesiology, *68:*379, 1988.
256. Marinacci, A.A.: Applied Electromyography. pp. 163–180. Philadelphia, Lea & Febiger, 1968.
257. Mason, D.T.: The autonomic nervous system and regulation of cardiovascular performance. Anesthesiology, *29:*670, 1968.
258. Mather, L.E., and Cousins, M.J.: Low-dose chlormethiazole infusion

as a supplement to epidural blockade: Blood concentrations and clinical effects. Anaesth. Intens. Care, *8:*421, 1980.
259. McCarthy, G.S.: The effect of thoracic extradural analgesia on pulmonary gas distribution. Functional residual capacity and airway closure. Br. J. Anaesth., *48:*243, 1976.
260. McCrae, A.F., Whitfield, A., and McClure, J.H.: Repeated unilateral epidural blockade. Anaesthesia, *47:*859, 1992.
261. McGrae, A.G., Jozwiak, H., and McClure, J.H.: Bupivacaine v ropivacaine in obstetric epidural analgesia. Reg. Anesth., *18:*64, 1993.
262. McLean, A.P.H., Mulligan, G.W., Otton, P., and McLean, L.D.: Hemodynamic alterations associated with epidural anesthesia. Surgery, *62:*79, 1967.
263. Mehta, P.M., Theriot, E., Mehrotra, D., Patel, K., and Kimbali, B.G.: A simple technique to make bupivacaine a rapid-acting epidural anesthetic. Reg. Anesth., *12:*135, 1987.
264. Mellander, S., and Johansson, B.: Control of resistance, exchange and capacitance functions in the peripheral circulation. Pharmacol. Rev., *20:*117, 1968.
265. Metzger, G., and Singbarl, G.: Spinal epidural hematoma following epidural anesthesia versus spontaneous spinal subdural hematoma. Two case reports. Acta Anaesthesiol. Scand., *35:*105, 1991.
266. Miller, L., Gertel, M., Fox, G.S., and MacLean, L.D.: Comparison of effect of narcotic and epidural analgesia on postoperative respiratory function. Am. J. Surg., *131:*291, 1976.
267. Modig, J., Borg, T., Karlstrom, G., Manpuu, E., and Sahltedt, B.: Thromboembolism after total hip replacement: Role of epidural and general anesthesia. Anesth. Analg., *62:*174, 1933.
268. Moller, R.A., and Covino, B.G.: Cardiac electrophisiologic properties of bupivacaine and lidocaine compared to those of ropivacaine, a new local anaesthetic. Anesthesiology, *72:*322, 1990.
269. Moloney, P.J., Elliott, G.B., and Johnson, H.W.: Experience with priapism. J. Urol., *114:*72, 1975.
270. Moore, D.C.: Regional Block. 4th Ed. Springfield, Charles C Thomas, 1976.
271. Morikawa, K.-I., Bonica, J.J., Tucker, G.T., and Murphy, T.M.: Effect of acute hypovolaemia on lignocaine absorption and cardiovascular response following epidural block in dogs. Br. J. Anaesth., *46:*631, 1974.
272. Morrison, L.M.M., Emanuelsson, B.M., McClure, J.H., *et al.*: Efficacy and kinetics of extradural ropivacaine: comparison with bupivacaine. Br. J. Anaesth., *72:*164, 1994.
273. Murphy, T.M., Mather, L.E., Stanton-Hicks, M.D'A., *et al.*: Effects of adding adrenaline to etidocaine and lignocaine in extradural anaesthesia. I. Block characteristics and cardiovascular effects. Br. J. Anaesth., *48:*893, 1976.
274. Murray, R.R.: Material obstetrical paralysis. Am. J. Obstet. Gynecol., *88:*399, 1964.
275. Naito, Y., Tamai, S., and Shingu, K.: Responses of plasma adrenocorticotropic hormone, cortisol and cytokines during and after upper abdominal surgery. Anesthesiology, *77:*426, 1992.
276. Nancarrow, C., Plummer, J.L., Ilsley, A.H., McLean, C.F., and Cousins, M.J.: Effects of combined extradural blockade and general anaesthesia on indocyanine green clearance and halothane metabolism. Br. J. Anaesth., *58:*29, 1986.
277. Nelson, D.A.: Spinal cord compression due to vertebral angiomas during pregnancy. Arch. Surg., *11:*408, 1964.
278. Nickel, P.M., Bromage, P.R., and Sherrill, D.L.: Comparison of hydrochloride and carbonated salts of lidocaine for epidural analgesia. Reg. Anaesth., *11:*62, 1986.
279. Nishimura, N., Kitahara, T., and Kusakabe, T.: The spread of lidocaine and 1–131 solution in the epidural space. Anesthesiology, *20:*785, 1959.
280. Noble, A.D., *et al.*: Continuous lumbar epidural analgesia using bupivacaine: A study of the fetus and newborn child. Br. J. Obstet. Gynaecol., *78:*559, 1971.
281. Nydahl, P.A., Philipson, L., Axelsson, K., and Johansson, J.E.: Epidural anesthesia with 0.5% bupivacaine: Influence of age on sensory and motor blockade. Anesth. Analg., *73:*780, 1991.
282. O'Kelly, Lawes, E.G., and Luntley, J.B.: Bleeding time: Is it a useful clinical tool. Br. J. Anaesth., *68:*313, 1992.
283. Oberg, B., and Thoren, P.: Studies on left ventricular receptors signalling in non-medullated vagal afferents. Acta Physiol. Scand., *85:*145, 1972.
284. Oberg, B., and Thoren, P.: Increased activity in left ventricular receptors during hemorrhage or occlusion of caval veins in the cat. A possible cause of vaso-vagal reaction. Acta Physiol. Scand., *85:*164, 1972.
285. Oberg, B., and White, S.: Circulatory effects of interruption and stimulation of cardiac vagal afferents. Acta Physiol. Scand., *80:*383, 1970.
286. Oberg, B., and White, S.: The role of vagal cardiac nerves and arterial baroreceptors in the circulatory adjustments to hemorrhage in the cat. Acta Physiol. Scand., *80:*395, 1970.
287. Odoom, J.A., and Sih, I.L.: Epidural analgesia and anticoagulant therapy. Experience with 1,000 cases of continuous epidurals. Anaesthesia, *38:*254, 1983.
288. Okada, A., Harata, S., Takeda, Y., *et al.*: Age-related changes in proteoglycans of human ligamentum flavum. Spine, *18:*2261, 1993.
289. Okutomi, T., Watanable, S., and Goto, F.: Time course in thoracic epidural pressure measurement. Can. J. Anaesth., *40:*1044, 1993.
290. Ottesen, S., Renck, H., and Jynge, P.: Cardiovascular effects of epidural analgesia. An experimental study in sheep of the effects on central circulation, regional perfusion and myocardial performance during normoxia, hypoxia and isoproterenol administration. Acta Anaesthesiol. Scand. *69* (Suppl.):1, 1978.
291. Otton, P.E., and Wilson, E.J.: The cardiocirculatory effects of upper thoracic epidural analgesia. Can. Anaesth. Soc. J., *13:*541, 1966.
292. Owens, E.L., Kasten, G.W., and Hessel, E.A.: Spinal subarachnoid hematoma after lumbar puncture and heparinization. Anesth. Analg., *65:*1201, 1986.
293. Oyama, T., and Matsuki, A.: Serum levels of thyroxine in man during epidural anesthesia and surgery. Der Anaesthetist, *19:*298, 1970.
294. Pages, F.: Anesthesia met America. Rev. Sanid. Mil. (Madr.), *11:*351, 1921.
295. Palmeiro, C., *et al.*: Denervation of the abdominal viscera for the treatment of shock. N. Engl. J. Med., *269:*709, 1963.
296. Palmer, S.H., Abram, S.E., Maitra, A.M., and Colditz, J.H.: Distance from the skin to the lumbar epidural space in an obstetric population. Anesth. Analg., *62:*944, 1983.
297. Pansard, J.L., Mankikian, B., Bertrand, M., *et al.*: Effects of thoracic extradural block on diaphragmatic electrical activity and contractility after upper abdominal surgery. Anesthesiology, *78:*63, 1993.
298. Park, W.Y., Hagins, F.M., Massengale, M.D., and MacNamara, Y.: The sitting positions and anesthetic spread in the epidural space. Anesth. Analg (Cleve.), *63:*863, 1984.
299. Park, W.Y., Hagins, F.M., Rivat, E.L., and MacNamara, T.E.: Age and epidural dose response in adult men. Anesthesiology, *56:*318, 1982.
300. Park, W.Y., Massengale, M., Kin, S.I., *et al.*: Age and the spread of local anesthetic solutions in the epidural space. Anesth. Analg (Cleve.), *59:*768, 1980.
301. Paul, D.L., and Wildsmith, J.A.W.: Extradural pressure following the injection of two volumes of bupivacaine. Br. J. Anaesth., *62:*368, 1989.
302. Peters, J., Kutkuhn, B., Medert, H.A., *et al.*: Sympathetic blockade by epidural anesthesia attenuates the cardiovascular response to severe hypoxemia. Anesthesiology, *72:*134, 1990.
303. Peters, J., Schlaghecke, R., Thouet, H., and Arndt, J.O.: Endogenous vasopressin supports blood pressure and prevents severe hypotension during epidural anesthesia in conscious dogs. Anesthesiology, *72:*694, 1990.
304. Philip, J.H., and Brown, W.U.: Total spinal anesthesia late in the course of obstetric bupivacaine epidural block. Anesthesiology, *44:*340, 1976.
305. Polaner, D.M., Kimball, W.R., Fratacci, M., Wain, J.C., and Zapol, W.: Thoracic epidural anesthesia increases diaphragmatic shortening after thoracotomy in the awake lamb. Anesthesiology, *79:*808, 1993.
306. Ponte, J., and Sessler, D.I.: Extradurals and shivering: Effects of cold and warm extradural saline injections in volunteers. Br. J. Anaesth., *64:*731, 1990.
307. Price, H.L., *et al.*: Can general anesthetics produce splanchnic visceral hypoxia by reducing regional blood flow? Anesthesiology, *27:*24, 1966.
308. Quail, A.W., Woods, R.L., and Korner, P.J.: Cardiac and arterial baroreceptor influences in release of vasopressin and renin during hemorrhage. Am. J. Physiol., *252:*H1120, 1987.
309. Ramsey, R., and Doppman, J.L.: The effects of epidural masses on spinal cord blood flow. An experimental study in monkeys. Radiology, *107:*99, 1973.
310. Rannigner, K., and Switz, D.M.: Local obstruction of the inferior vena cava by massive ascites. A. J. R., *93:*935, 1965.

311. Rao, T.L.K., and El-Etr, A.A.: Anticoagulation following placement of epidural and subarachnoid catheters: An evaluation of neurologic sequelae. Anesthesiology, *55:*618, 1981.
312. Rawal, N., Schollin, J., and Wesstrom, G.: Epidural versus combined spinal epidural block for caesarean section. Acta Anaesthesiol. Scand., *32:*61, 1988.
313. Reddy, S.V.R., and Yaksh, T.L.: Spinal noradrenergic terminal system mediates antinociception. Brain Res., *189:*391, 1980.
314. Reiz, S., Balfors, E., Sorensen, M.B., *et al.*: Coronary hemodynamic effects of general anesthesia and surgery: Modification by epidural analgesia in patients with ischemic heart disease. Reg. Anaesth. *7* (Suppl.):S8, 1982.
315. Reiz, S., Nath, S., and Rais, O.: Effects of thoracic block and prenalterol on coronary vascular resistance and myocardial metabolism in patients with coronary artery disease. Acta Anaesthesiol. Scand., *24:*11, 1980.
316. Roberts, V.C.: Fibrinogen uptake scanning for deep vein thrombosis: A plea for standardization. Br. Med. J., *3:*455, 1975.
317. Roberts, V.C., and Cotton, L.T.: Failure of low-dose heparin to improve efficacy of preoperative intermittent calf compression in preventing postoperative deep vein thrombosis. Br. Med. J., *3:*458, 1975.
318. Rocco, A.G., Scott, D.A., Boas, R.A., and Philip, J.H.: Epidural space behaves as a Starling resistor and inflow resistance is higher in spinal stenosis than in disc desease. Anesthesiology, *73:*A816, 1990.
319. Roizen, M.F., Horrigan, R.W., and Frazer, B.M.: Anaesthetic doses blocking adrenergic (stress) responses to incision-MacBar. Anesthesiology, *54:*390, 198.
320. Rooth, G., McBride, R., and Ivy, B.J.: Fetal and maternal pH measurements—a basis for common normal values. Acta Obstet. Gynecol. Scand., *52:*47, 1973.
321. Rosenbaum, S.H., and Barash, P.G.: Is anesthesia therapeutic. Editorial. Anesth. Analg., *69:*555, 1989.
322. Rosenberg, H., and Keyhak, M.M.: Distance to the epidural space in nonobese patients. Anesth. Analg., *63:*538, 1984.
323. Rosenberg, I.L., Evans, M., and Pollock, A.V.: Prophylaxis of postoperative leg vein thrombosis by low dose subcutaneous heparin or preoperative calf muscle stimulation: A controlled clinical trial. Br. Med. J., *1:*649, 1975.
324. Rosenberg, P.H., Saramies, L., and Alila, A.: Lumbar epidural anaesthetic with bupivacaine in old patients: Effect of speed and direction of injection. Acta Anaesth. Scand., *25:*270, 1981.
325. Runciman, W.B., Mather, L.E., Ilsley, A.H., *et al.*: A sheep preparation for studying interactions between blood flow and drug disposition. III. Effects of general and spinal anaesthesia on regional blood flows and oxygen tensions. Br. J. Anaesth., *56:*1247, 1984.
326. Ryan, D.W.: Accidental intravenous injection of bupivacaine: A complication of obstetrical epidural anaesthesia. Br. J. Anaesth., *45:*907, 1973.
327. Ryan, P., Schweitzer, S., Collopy, B., and Taylor, D.: Combined epidural and general anesthesia versus general anesthesia in patients having colon and rectal anastomoses. Acta Chir. Scand., *550*(Suppl.):146, 1988.
328. Saada, M., Catoire, P., Bonnet, F., *et al.*: Effects of thoracic epidural anesthesia with general anesthesia on segmental wall motion assessed by transesophageal echocardiography. Anesth. Analg., *75:*329, 1992.
329. Saada, M., Duval, A.M., Bonnet, F., *et al.*: Abnormalities in myocardial segmental wall motion during lumbar epidural anesthesia. Anesthesiology, *71:*26, 1989.
330. Sakura, S., Saito, Y., and Kosaka, Y.: Effect of extradural anaesthesia on the ventilatory response to hypoxaemia. Anaesthesia, *48:*205, 1993.
331. Sakura, S., Saito, Y., and Kosaka, Y.: Effect of lumbar epidural anesthesia on ventilatory response to hypercapnia in young and elderly patients. J. Clin. Anesth., *5:*109, 1993.
332. Samain, E., Coriat, P., Le Bret, F., *et al.*: Ephedrine vs phenylephrine for hypotension due to thoracic epidural anesthesia associated with general anesthesia: Effects on left ventricular function. Anesthesiology, *73:*A82, 1989.
333. Sanchez, R., Acuna, L., and Rocha, F.: An analysis of the radiological visualization of the catheters placed in the epidural space. Br. J. Anaesth., *39:*485, 1967.
334. Savolaine, E.R., Pandya, J.B., Greenblatt, S.H., and Conover, S.R.: Anatomy of the human lumbar epidural space: New insights using CT-epidurography. Anesthesiology, *68:*217, 1988.
335. Scheinin, B., Asantila, R., and Orko, R.: The effect of bupivacaine and morphine on pain and bowel function after colonic surgery. Acta Anaesthesiol. Scand., *31:*161, 1987.
336. Schreiner, E.J., Lipson, S.F., Bromage, P.R., and Camporesi, E.M.: Neurological complications following general anaesthesia. Anaesthesia, *38:*226, 1983.
337. Schug, S.A., Scott, D.A., Payne, J., Mooney, P., and Hagglof, B.: Epidural infusion of ropivacaine for postoperative analgesia following upper abdominal surgery: A dose-finding study. Anesthesiology, *81:*A977, 1994.
338. Schweitzer, S.A.: Chloremethiazole (Hemineurin) infusion as supplemental sedation during epidural block. Anaesth. Intens. Care, *6:*248, 1978.
339. Scott, D.B.: Inferior vena caval pressure. Changes occurring during anaesthesia. Anaesthesia, *18:*135, 1963.
340. Scott, D.B.: Inferior vena caval occlusion in late pregnancy. Clin. Anesth., *10:*37, 1973.
341. Scott, D.B., Jebson, P.J.R., and Boyes, R.N.: Pharmacokinetic study of the local anaesthetics bupivacaine (Marcaine) and etidocaine (Duranest) in man. Br. J. Anaesth., *45:*1010, 1973.
342. Scott, D.B., Lee, A., Fagan, D., *et al.*: Acute toxicity of ropivacaine compared with that of bupivacaine. Anesth. Analg., *69:*563, 1989.
343. Scott, D.B., Littlewood, D.G., Drummond, G.B., Buckley, P.F., and Covino, B.G.: Modification of the circulatory effects of extradural block combined with general anaesthesia by the addition of adrenaline to lignocaine solutions. Br. J. Anaesth., *49:*917, 1977.
344. Scott, D.B., and Walker, L.R.: Administration of continuous epidural analgesia. Anaesthesia, *18:*82, 1963.
345. Seow, L.T., Lips, F.J., and Cousins, M.J.: Effect of lateral posture on epidural blockade for surgery. Anaesth. Intens. Care, *11:*97, 1983.
346. Seow, L.T., Lips, F.J., Cousins, M.J., and Mather, L.E.: Lidocaine and bupivacaine mixtures for epidural blockade. Anesthesiology, *56:*177, 1982.
347. Seow, L.T., Mather, L.E., and Cousins, M.J.: Comparison of the efficacy of chlormethiazole and diazepam as I.V. sedatives for supplementation of extradural anaesthesia. Br. J. Anaesth., *57:*747, 1985.
348. Sessler, D.I., and Ponte, J.: Shivering during epidural anesthesia. Anesthesiology, *72:*816, 1990.
349. Shah, J.L.: Positive lumbar extradural space pressure. Br. J. Anaesth., *73:*309, 1994.
350. Shanks, C.A.: Four cases of unilateral analgesia. Br. J. Anaesth., *40:*999, 1968.
351. Shantaveerappa, T.R., and Bourne, G.H.: Perineural epithelium: A new concept of its role in the integrity of the peripheral nervous system. Science, *154:*1464, 1966.
352. Shantha, T.R., and Evans, J.A.: The relationship of epidural anesthesia to neural membranes and arachnoid villi. Anesthesiology, *37:*543, 1972.
353. Sharpey-Schafer, E.P.: Syncope. Br. Med. J., *1:*506, 1956.
354. Sharrock, N.E.: Epidural anesthetic dose responses in patients 20 to 80 years old. Anesthesiology, *49:*425, 1978.
355. Shehabi, Y., Gatt, S., Buckman, T., and Isert, P.: Effect of adrenaline, fentanyl and warming of injectate on shivering following extradural analgesia in labour. Anaesth. Intens. Care, *18:*31, 1990.
356. Shimosato, S., and Etsten, B.E.: The role of the venous system in cardiocirculatory dynamics during spinal and epidural anesthesia in man. Anesthesiology, *30:*619, 1969.
357. Silver, J.R., and Buxton, P.H.: Spinal stroke. Brain, *97:*539, 1974.
358. Sjogren, S., and Wright, B.: Circulation, respiration and lidocaine concentration during continuous epidural blockade. Acta Anaesthesiol. Scand., *16* (Suppl.):5, 1972.
359. Smith, O.A.: Reflex and central mechanisms involved in the control of the heart and circulation. Annu. Rev. Physiol., *36:*93, 1974.
360. South Australian Health Commission, 1985. Report of the Anaesthetics Mortality Committee. Anaesthetic Deaths in South Australia, 1974–1983.
361. Sreerama, V., Ivan, L.P., Dennery, J.M., and Richard, M.T.: Neurosurgical complications of anticoagulant therapy. Can. Med. Assoc. J., *108:*305, 1973.
362. Stanton-Hicks, M.D.'A.: A study using bupivacaine for continuous peridural analgesia in patients undergoing surgery of the hip. Acta Anaesthesiol. Scand., *15:*97, 1971.
363. Stapleton, J.V., Austin, K.L., and Mather, L.E.: A pharmacokinetic approach to postoperative pain: Continuous infusion of pethidine. Anaesth. Intens. Care, *7:*25, 1979.
364. Stephen, G.W., Lees, M.M., and Scott, D.B.: Cardiovascular effects of

epidural block combined with general anaesthesia. Br. J. Anaesth., *41:*933, 1969.
365. Stevens, R.A., and Stanton-Hicks, M.D.'A.: Subdural injection of local anesthetic: A complication of epidural anesthesia. Anesthesiology, *63:*323, 1985.
366. Sugimori, K., Kochi, T., Nishiro, T., Shinozuka, N., and Mizuguchi, T.: Thoracic epidural anesthesia causes rib cage distortion in anesthetised, spontaneously breathing dogs. Anesth. Analg., *77:*494, 1993.
367. Sutherland, J., Seaton, H., and Lowry, C.: The influence of epidural pethidine on shivering during lower segment caesarean section under epidural anaesthesia. Anaesth. Intens. Care, *19:*282, 1991.
368. Sutton, J.R., Cole, A., Gunning, J., Hickie, J.B., and Seldon, W.A.: Control of heart-rate in healthy young men. Lancet, *2:*1398, 1967.
369. Telford, R.J., and Hollway, T.E.: Observations on deliberate dural puncture with a Tuohy needle: Pressure measurement. Anaesthesia, *46:*725, 1991.
370. The bleeding time. Lancet, *337:*1447, 1991.
371. Thomas, P.S., Gerson, J.I., and Strong, G.: Analysis of human epidural pressures. Reg. Anesth., *17:*212, 1992.
372. Thoren, T., and Wattwil, M.: Effects on gastric emptying of thoracic epidural analgesia with morphine or bupivacaine. Anesth. Analg., *67:*607, 1988.
373. Thoren, T., Holmstrom, B., Rawal, N., *et al.*: Sequential combined spinal epidural block versus spinal block for cesarean section: Effects on maternal hypotension and neurobehavioral function of the newborn. Anesth. Analg., *78:*1087, 1994.
374. Thorud, T., Lund, I., and Holme, I.: The effect of anesthesia on intraoperative and postoperative bleeding during abdominal prostatectomies: A comparison of neurolept anesthesia, halothane anesthesia and epidural anesthesia. Acta Anaesthesiol. Scand., *57*(Suppl.):83, 1975.
375. Tripathi, B.J., and Tripathi, R.C.: Vacuolar transcellular channels as a drainage pathway for cerebrospinal fluid. J. Physiol., *239:*195, 1974.
376. Tsuji, H., Shirasaka, C., Asoh, T., and Takeuchi, Y.: Influences of splanchnic nerve blockade on endocrine metabolic responses to upper abdominal surgery. Br. J. Surg., *70:*437, 1983.
377. Tuman, K.J., McCarthy, R.J., March, R.J., *et al.*: Effects of epidural anesthesia and analgesia on coagulation and outcome after major vascular surgery. Anesth. Analg., *73:*696, 1991.
378. Tuohy, E.B.: Continuous spinal anesthesia: A new method of utilising a ureteral catheter. Surg. Clin. North Am., *25:*834, 1945.
379. Turnbull, I.M.: Blood supply of the spinal cord: Normal and pathological considerations. Clin. Neurosurg., *20:*56, 1973.
380. Urban, B.J.: Clinical observations suggesting a changing site of action during induction and recession of spinal and epidural anesthesia. Anesthesiology, *39:*496, 1973.
381. Urquhat-Hay, D., Marshall, N.G., and Marsland, J.M.: Comparison of epidural and hypotensive anaesthesia in open prostatectomy. Series 1. N.Z. Med. J., *69:*280, 1969.
382. Urquhat-Hay, D., Marshall, N.G., and Marsland, J.M.: Comparison of epidural and hypotensive anaesthesia in open prostatectomy. Series 2. N.Z. Med. J., *70:*223, 1969.
383. Usubiaga, J.E.: Neurological complications following epidural anesthesia. Int. Anaesthesiol. Clin., *13:*2, 1975.
384. Usubiaga, J.E., Dos Reis, A., and Usubiaga, L.E.: Epidural misplacement of catheters and mechanisms of unilateral blockade. Anesthesiology, *32:*158, 1970.
385. Usubiaga, J.E., Kolodny, J., and Usubiaga, L.E.: Neurological complications of prevertebral surgery under regional anesthesia. Surgery, *68:*304, 1970.
386. Usubiaga, J.E., Moya, F., and Usubiaga, L.E.: Effect of thoracic and abdominal pressure changes on the epidural space pressure. Br. J. Anaesth., *39:*612, 1967.
387. Usubiaga, J.E., Wikinski, J.A., and Usubiaga, L.E.: Epidural pressure and its relation to spread of anesthetic solutions in epidural space. Anesth. Analg. (Cleve.), *46:*440, 1967.
388. Van Zundert, A., Vaes, L., Van Der Aa, P., *et al.*: Motor blockade during epidural anesthesia. Anesth. Analg., (Cleve.), *65:*333, 1986.
389. Vandermeersch, E.: Combined spinal-epidural anaesthesia. *In* Van Aken, H. (ed.): New Developments in Epidural and Spinal Drugs Administration. pp. 691. London, Bailliere Tindall, 1993.
390. Vandermeulen, E.P.E., Vermylen, J., and Van Aken, H.: Epidural and spinal anaesthesia in patients receiving anticoagulant therapy. Balliere's Clin. Anaesthesiol., *7:*663, 1993.
391. Veering, B.T., and Burm, A.G.L.: Pharmacokinetics and pharmacodynamics of medullar agents. Balliere's Clin. Anaesthesiol., *7:*557, 1993.
392. Veering, B.T., Burm, A.G.L., Van Kleef, J.W., Hennis, P.J., and Spierdyk, J.: Epidural anesthesia with bupivacaine: Effects of age on neural blockade and pharmacokinetics. Anesth. Analg., *66:*589, 1987.
393. Veering, B.T., Burm, A.G.L., Vletter, A.A., *et al.*: The effect of age on the systemic absorption and systemic disposition of bupivacaine after epidural administration. Clin. Pharmacokinet., *22:*75, 1992.
394. Verniquet, A.J.W.: Vessel puncture with epidural catheters. Experience in obstetric patients. Anaesthesia, *35:*660, 1980.
395. Vestal, R.E., Wood, A.J.J., and Shand, D.G.: Reduced beta-adrenoceptor sensitivity in the elderly. Clin. Pharmacol. Ther., *26:*181, 1979.
396. Wagenknecht, L.V., Zamora, M., and Madsen, P.O.: Continuous recording of renal clearance by external monitoring during epidural anesthesia. Invest. Urol., *8:*540, 1971.
397. Waggener, J.D., and Beggs, J.: The membranous coverings of neural tissues: An electron microscopy study. J. Neuropathol. Exp. Neurol., *26:*412, 1967.
398. Wahba, W.M., Craig, D.B., Don, H.F., and Becklake, M.R.: The cardio-respiratory effects of thoracic epidural anaesthesia. Can. Anaesth. Soc. J., *19:*8, 1972.
399. Wahba, W.M., Don, H.F., and Craig, D.B.: Post-operative epidural analgesia: Effects on lung volumes. Can. Anaesth. Soc. J., *22:*519, 1975.
400. Waisick, J., Hurfor, W., Gelb, C., and Chernow, B.: Epidural opioid analgesia does not alter the neuro-endocrine response to thoracotomy. Anesth. Analg., *70:*S422, 1990.
401. Wallin, G., Cassuto, J., Hogstrom, S., *et al.*: Failure of epidural anesthesia to prevent postoperative paralytic ileus. Anesthesiology, *65:*292, 1986.
402. Walmsley, A.J., Giesecke, A.H., and Lipton, J.M.: Epidural temperature: A cause of shivering during epidural anesthesia. Anesth. Analg., *65:*S1, 1986.
403. Ward, R.J., *et al.*: Epidural and subarachnoid anesthesia. Cardiovascular and respiratory effects. J.A.M.A., *191:*275, 1965.
404. Ward, R.J., *et al.*: Experimental evaluation of atropine and vasopressors for the treatment of hypotension of high subarachnoid anesthesia. Anesth. Analg. (Cleve.), *45:*621, 1966.
405. Wattwil, M., Sundberg, A., Arvill, A., and Lennquist, C.: Circulatory changes during high thoracic epidural anesthesia—influence of sympathetic block and of systemic effect of the local anaesthetic. Acta Anaesthesiol. Scand., *29:*849, 1985.
406. Weil, J.V., McCullough, R.E., Kline, I.S., and Sodal, I.E.: Diminished ventilatory response to hypoxia and hypercapnia after morphine in normal man. N. Engl. J. Med., *292:*1103, 1975.
407. Werner, M.H., Hayes, D.F., Lucas, C.E., and Rosenberg, I.K.: Renal vasoconstriction in association with acute pancreatitis. Am. J. Surg., *127:*185, 1974.
408. Westbrook, J.L., Renowden, S.A., and Carrie, L.E.S.: Study of the anatomy of the extradural region using magnetic resonance imaging. Br. J. Anaesth., *71:*495, 1993.
409. Wille-Jorgensen, P., Jorgensen, L.N., and Rasmussen, L.S.: Lumbar regional anaesthesia and prophylactic anticoagulant therapy. Is the combination safe? Anaesthesia, *46:*624, 1991.
410. Winnie, A.P.: A grip to facilitate the insertion of epidural needles. Anesth. Analg. (Cleve.), *50:*23, 1971.
411. Wright, P.M.C., and Fee, J.P.H.: Cardiovascular support during combined extradural and general anaesthesia. Br. J. Anaesth., *68:*585, 1992.
412. Wugmeister, M., and Hehre, F.W.: The absence of differential blockade in peridural anaesthesia. Br. J. Anaesth., *39:*953, 1967.
413. Yin, E.I., Wessler, S., and Butler, J.V.: Plasma heparin: A unique, practical, submicrogram sensitive assay. J. Lab. Clin. Med., *81:*298, 1973.
414. Zaric, D., Axelsson, K., Nydahl, P.A., *et al.*: Sensory and motor blockade during epidural analgesia with 1%, 0.75% and 0.5% ropivacaine—a double-blind study. Anesth. Analg., *72:*509, 1991.
415. Zaric, D., Axelsson, K., Nydahl, P.A., Philipson, L., and Samuelsson, L.: Sensory and motor blockade during continuous epidural infusion of ropivacaine 0.1%, 0.2% and 0.3% in volunteers—a double-blind study. Reg. Anesth., *19:*60, 1994.

APPENDIX

Epidural Block—Future Developments

Review of the physiology of epidural block points to a number of areas in which basic information or further development of current data is indicated. A brief summary with some appropriate references is given in this appendix. References refer to studies of epidural block and relevant source information where no studies of epidural block have yet been reported. It is encouraging to note that many of the questions raised in this section of the Second Edition have been addressed and a number have been successfully answered.

Cardiovascular Physiology

??Does thoracic epidural block improve morbidity/mortality in patients with ischemic heart disease undergoing surgery?[34–37]

??Effects of thoracic epidural block on myocardial excitability.[42,155]

??Relative roles of vasopressin and renin in blood pressure support during thoracic epidural block.[83,197,303]

??Mechanism of sudden cardiac arrest in healthy patients who become mildly hypovolemic during epidural block. ?Sudden vagal activation. ?Loss of renin/vasopressin support. ?Contribution of responses triggered by hypoxia.[18,83,197,303]

Liver Blood Flow (LBF) and Liver Function

??Is sympathetic block by epidural techniques capable of protecting the liver from toxic injury[276] or shock?[223,295]

Renal Blood Flow (RBF) and Renal Function

??Sympathetic denervation by epidural block prevents renal changes associated with anesthesia.[26,325,396]

??Epidural block prevents renal failure after trauma[103] or medical conditions such as pancreatitis.[407]

Central Nervous System

Brain

??Do rapid reductions in cerebral perfusion pressure with epidural block initiate neurogenic cerebral vasoconstriction that initially overcomes local vasodilatory mechanisms?[180]

??Does "pre-emptive" epidural blockade need to aim to eliminate spinal neuronal activity in order to influence postoperative analgesia requirements?[123,134,242–244,254]

Gut

??Epidural local anesthetic increases gut blood flow and has a favorable effect on gut anastamoses after gut surgery?[6,210,327]

Hematologic Effects

??In reducing venous thrombosis as judged by fibrinogen scanning,[316] which treatment(s) are most effective or in combination: ?epidural block,[231,362] electric calf stimulation,[323] ?calf compression with a pump,[80,184,317] ?dextran, ?heparin.[27,210]

??Does preoperative use of NSAIDs increase the risk of epidural hematoma in patients receiving epidural block?[199,200,292]

??Does use of low-dose low-molecular-weight heparin (LMWH) increase the risk of epidural hematoma in association with epidural block?[25,390]

Respiratory Effects

??Thoracic epidural analgesia (TEA) is safe in patients reliant on hypoxic drive, since ventilatory response to hypoxia is not changed?[330]

??Reduced ventilatory response to CO_2 is only a minor effect of decreased rib cage contribution to tidal breathing.[229]

??TEA prevents noxious input from viscera, which initiate inhibitory phrenic reflexes, and also reduces diaphragm muscle load due to abdominal muscle relaxation.[152,255,297,305]

??The above favorable effects of TEA in patients with pain are responsible for improved diaphragmatic function, outweighing other effects of epidural block on intercostal muscles?

Neural Blockade in Clinical Anesthesia and Management of Pain, Third Edition, edited by M.J. Cousins and P.O. Bridenbaugh. Lippincott–Raven Publishers, Philadelphia © 1998.

CHAPTER 9

Caudal Epidural Blockade

Richard J. Willis

Local anesthetic injection into the sacral canal by way of the sacral hiatus, or caudal anesthesia as it is now known, was first introduced in 1901[23] and was used as the only available form of epidural anesthesia until the lumbar approach was described by Pages in Spain in 1921. Since that time, caudal epidural blockade has consistently suffered from comparison with central neural blockade induced at a higher level by both lumbar epidural and subarachnoid spinal techniques.

The reasons for these unfavorable comparisons are clear. First, there is considerable variation in the anatomy of the tissues near the sacral hiatus, in particular, in the bony sacrum. Frequently, the bony landmarks are obscured to a greater or lesser extent both by asymmetric bony overgrowth and by the overlying fibrous or fatty soft tissues. Attempts have been made to assess the incidence of sacral bony features that would make caudal blockade "impossible." One old study quoted an incidence of 7.7% of "absent hiatus."[8] This pessimistic figure takes no account of differences with advancing age, it being well accepted that distorted anatomy is less common in younger patients and quite rare in children. It is difficult to correlate this figure with some modern success rates of 94% and greater.[28,78] It remains conjectural whether this represents a difference in the age distribution of the population studied, or whether a modern study of bony abnormalities would reveal a lesser incidence of "impossible" anatomy. There is certainly no doubt that the failure rate with caudal blockade decreases markedly with greater experience. Another reason for the unfavorable comparison of caudal with lumbar block is also anatomic, relating to the dermatomal distribution of the nerve roots, the site of the entry hiatus at the exit of the most terminal roots, and the frequency of minor bony obstructions in the sacral canal. In the lumbar region, spread of anesthetic solution can occur both cephalad and caudad, giving rise to a wide dermatomal distribution of anesthesia. Clearly, with caudal entry to the epidural space, spread can only be cephalad and may be limited by minor bony obstructions, with the result such that the total number of segments blocked is bound to be less. To achieve a wide distribution of anesthesia predictably, with marked cephalad spread of solution, a large dose of local anesthetic drug must be used, with its inherent risk of drug toxicity and occasional excessive spread. Although single dose caudal anesthesia has been and still is used to block thoracic segments, it seems an inappropriate use of the technique and partly to blame for the block's poor reputation. When an indwelling catheter is inserted via the sacral hiatus and is freely introduced in the line of the canal so that the tip of the catheter lies closer to the lumbosacral junction, there is a greater likelihood of cephalad spread with a moderate dose. This is a worthwhile technique as long as the primary requirement for anesthesia is still in the lumbosacral distribution.

If one viewed the caudal approach merely as the lowest of segmental approaches to the epidural space, and restricted the block to the dermatomes supplied by lumbosacral roots, the technique would have a much lower failure rate, a lower incidence of complications, and, hence, a much greater popularity.

ANATOMY

The key to success in any regional anesthetic technique is a clear understanding of the normal anatomy of the region and an appreciation of variations of normality that may be encountered. This is possibly more relevant to the success of caudal blockade than to most other techniques. Wide variations of normality in the region can readily lead the unwary into needle misplacement, which, at best, results in failed block, and, at worst, may contribute to serious complications.

The Sacrum

The sacrum is a triangular bone, dorsally convex, that consists of the fused five sacral vertebrae. It articulates

R. J. Willis: Department of Anaesthesia and Intensive Care, Royal Adelaide Hospital, Adelaide, South Australia 5000 Australia.

cephalad with the fifth lumbar vertebra and caudad with the coccyx. Detailed descriptions of the sacrum can be found in standard textbooks of anatomy and should be studied by all trainees unfamiliar with the technique of caudal blockade. Only those features of the sacrum relevant to caudal blockade will be discussed in this chapter.

The concave anterior surface features four pairs of large anterior sacral foramina that provide passage from the midline sacral canal for the anterior rami of the upper four sacral nerves. In contrast with their posterior counterparts, the anterior foramina are unsealed and provide a ready passage for escape of local anesthetic solution injected into the sacral canal (Figs. 9-1, 9-2).

The anesthetically important dorsal surface of the sacrum is variably convex and irregular, with important prominences representing the fused elements of the sacral vertebrae. In the midline, there is a median crest with three or more, but commonly four, variably prominent tubercles, representing the sacral spinous processes. Lateral to this crest and medial to the four posterior sacral foramina is the intermediate sacral crest with a row of four tubercles, representing the upper four sacral articular processes. The posterior sacral foramina are smaller than their anterior counterparts and are sealed effectively by multifidus and sacrospinal muscles. The remnants of the S5 inferior articular processes are free and prominent, and flank the sacral hiatus. They constitute the sacral cornua, and, together with the adjacent coccygeal cornua, which they abut, are key landmarks for identification of the sacral hiatus and successful caudal blockade. The fused sacral transverse processes give rise to a variably raised lateral sacral crest with transverse tubercles, the most caudad of which occurs where the lateral border of the sacrum deviates more medially at the inferior lateral sacral angle. This is clinically important because it may be confused with one of the cornua (see Figs. 9-1 and 9-2).

The shape of the sacrum varies somewhat between sexes and between different races. In the female, the bone is shorter and wider, with the curvature being less in the upper part and more acute in the lower part. The anterior concave surface faces downward more than in the male. The angle of the sacral canal varies between the white and black populations in North America; in black patients there is a steeper

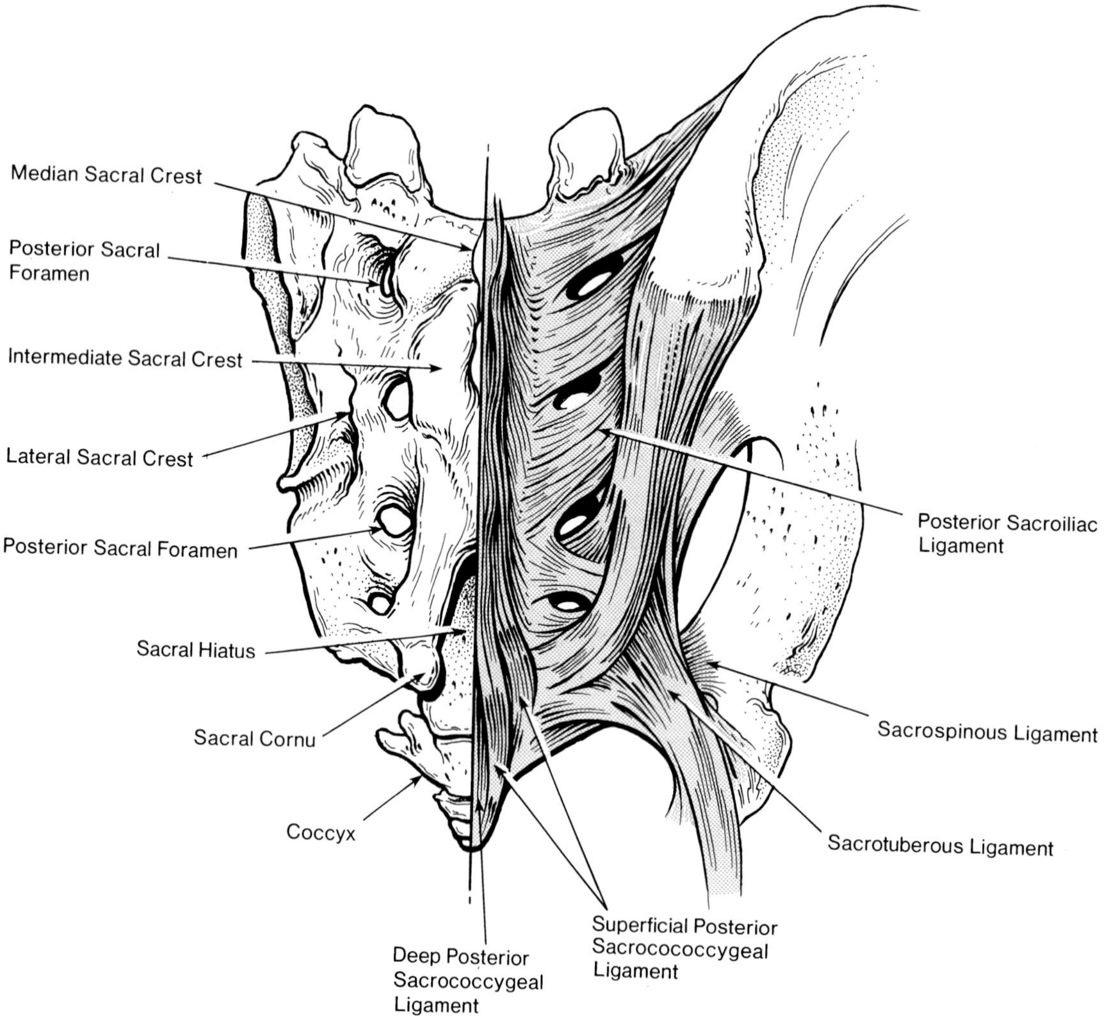

FIG. 9-1. The sacrum, dorsal aspect. Anatomy of bone structures and ligaments shown.

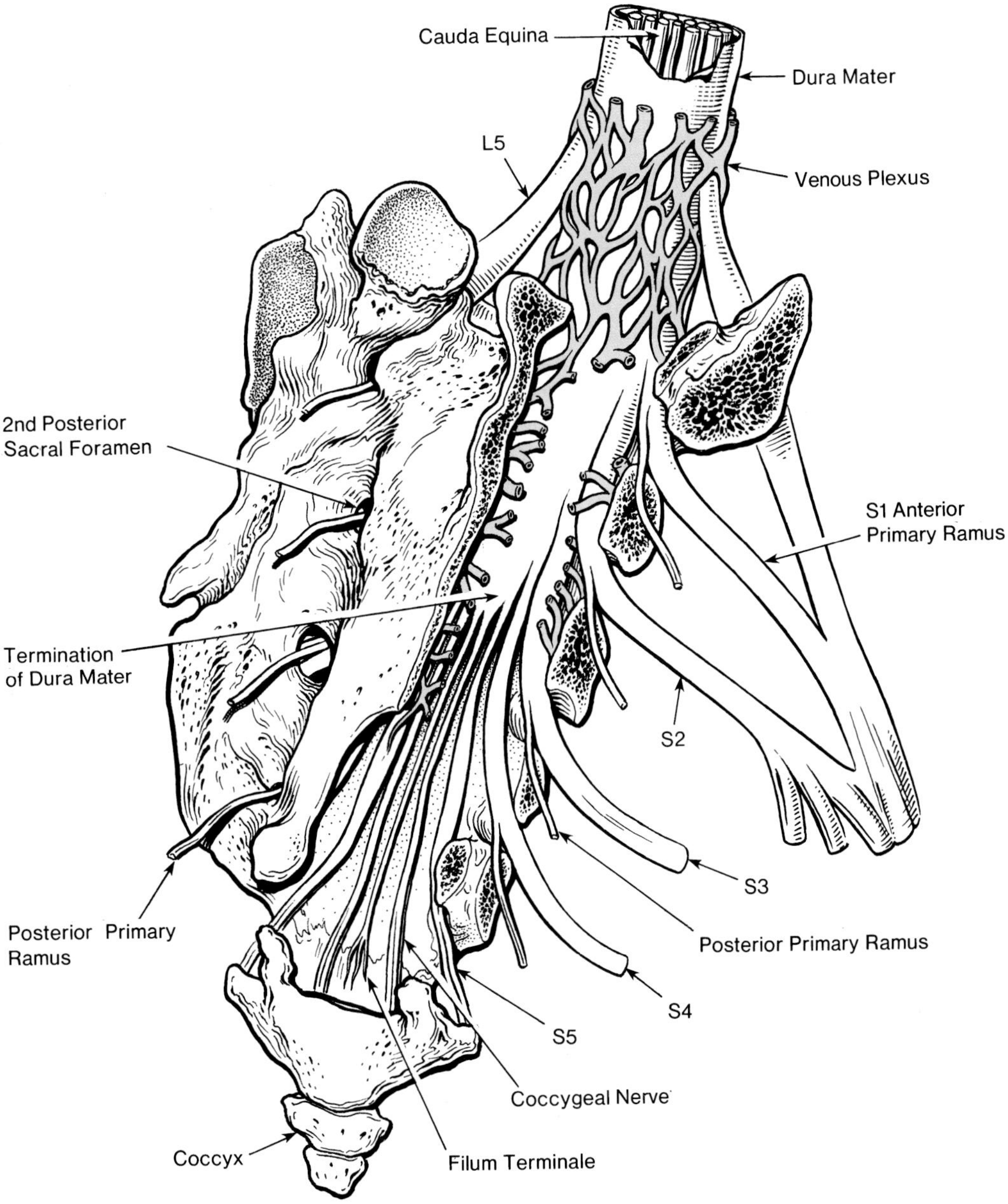

FIG. 9-2. Sacral canal, sacral nerves, and sacral venous plexus. The posterior wall of the sacral canal has been removed on the right side. *Note:* Posterior sacral foramina and small posterior primary rami; large anterior sacral foramina through which pass relatively large anterior primary rami; extensive venous plexus; termination of dural sac near S2 posterior sacral foramen; continuity of sacral epidural space with lumbar epidural space.

angle of needle insertion, which allows a slightly easier procedure.[88]

Coccyx

The coccyx is a small triangular bone consisting of three to five fused rudimentary vertebrae; it attaches by means of its upper articular surface to the lower articular surface of the sacrum. It has two prominent coccygeal cornua that abut their sacral counterparts. The bone tends to be angulated forward from the sacroccygeal junction, with its pelvic surface facing anteriorly and upward. This angulation can be quite marked, making palpation difficult, but the bone should be sought because its tip is a useful confirmatory landmark for the midline of the sacrum (see Figs. 9-1, 9-2, and 9-6).

Sacral Hiatus

The sacral hiatus is a defect in the lower part of the posterior wall of the sacrum, formed by the failure of the laminae of S5, and usually part of S4, to meet and fuse in the median plane. This leaves a space of variable dimension, often described as being like an inverted U or V, which is covered by the thick fibrous posterior sacrococcygeal ligament, part of a network of fibrous ligaments covering the sacroiliac and sacrococcygeal areas (Fig. 9-1). Penetration of this ligament by a needle yields direct access to the caudal limit of the epidural space in the sacral canal. It is in this area that there is considerable variation in "normal" anatomy.[111] Anatomic studies of sacra of mixed sex and race[8,69,116] have confirmed this variability (Fig. 9-3). Relevant findings are as follows:

1. The hiatus varies widely in size and shape from the "normal" inverted U (Fig. 9-3A) to longitudinal (Figs. 9-3B and 9-3G) or horizontal slits.
2. The apex of the hiatus lies higher than the lower one-third of S4 in about 50% of specimens (Figs. 9-3G, H, I).
3. The distance between the tip of the dural sac and the apex of the hiatus, obviously important in order to avoid dural puncture, is variable but almost always exceeds 20 mm and is usually closer to 45 mm.
4. In about 1% of specimens, however, there is total sacral spina bifida (Fig. 9-3I), and there is at least one recorded case of the dura directly underlying the hiatus at a distal level.
5. The hiatus is absent in up to 7.7% of specimens.
6. The anteroposterior diameter of the canal at the apex of the hiatus is less than 2 mm in 5% of specimens.

Some of these features of variable anatomy will make the procedure easier, rather than more difficult. It is really only item 5 that makes the block impossible, and reasons have already been given as to why the quoted incidence of 7.7% may be excessive.

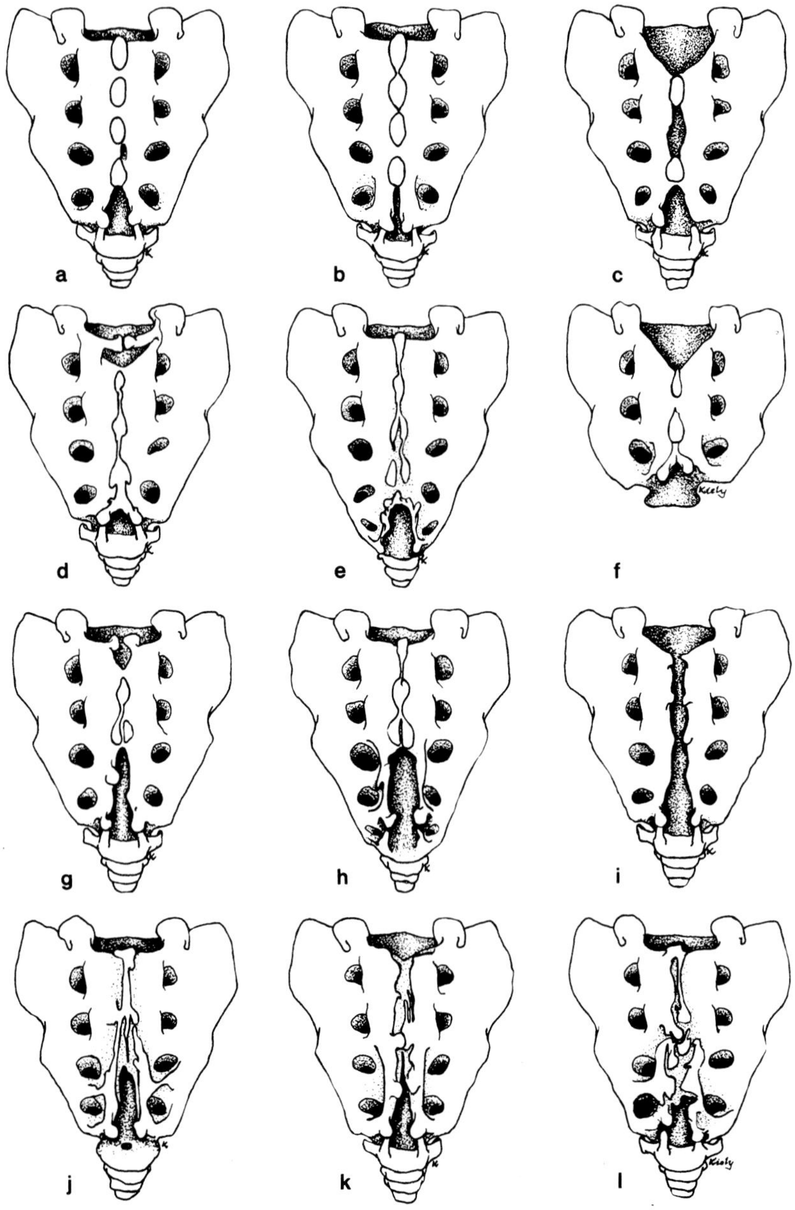

FIG. 9-3. Anatomic variants of dorsal wall of sacrum and sacral hiatus. **Dorsal Wall:** Despite its many structural variations, the sacral canal is open at the lower half of S5 and the hiatus is invariably in line with the median sacral crest (where present and palpable). **Sacral Hiatus: (a)** normal; **(b)** longitudinal slit-like hiatus; **(c)** second midline hiatus; **(d)** transverse hiatus; **(e)** large hiatus with absent cornua; **(f)** transverse hiatus with absent coccyx and two prominent cornua, with two proximal "decoy" hiatuses lateral to the cornua; **(g,h,i)** large midline defects in posterior sacral wall continuous with sacral hiatus; **(j,k,l)** enlarged longitudinal hiatuses, each with an overlying "decoy hiatus." In **(l)** the "decoy hiatus" is large and is surrounded by "cornua-like" structures, which could lead to needle insertion through posterior sacral ligaments but not into sacral canal. Also in **(l)** the sacral cornu is absent on the left side; this could lead to identification of the right S4 posterior sacral foramen as the sacral hiatus.

Sacral Canal and its Contents

The sacral canal is the continuation of the lumbar spinal canal. It communicates laterally with the anterior and posterior sacral foramina. Inferiorly, it terminates at the sacral hiatus. The volume of the sacral canal, including the sacral foraminal extensions, has been measured to vary between 12 and 65 ml, with a mean of about 30 to 34 ml.[115] These volumes were measured in dried specimen bones; they therefore are of little use in estimating *in vivo* dose requirement and serve only to underline its great variability.

The canal contains the terminal part of the dural sac, ending between S1 and S3, but generally at S2, on a line joining the posterior superior iliac spines. The five sacral nerve roots and the coccygeal nerve, which constitute the cauda equina, all transit the canal. The sacral epidural venous plexus, a part of the valveless internal vertebral venous plexus, generally ends at S4, but may extend throughout the canal. It tends to lie against the anterior wall of the canal, but this is an inconstant feature. It is very much at risk from needle or catheter puncture. Also found in the canal is the filum terminale, the non-nervous terminal filament of the spinal cord, which exits through the sacral hiatus to attach to the back of the coccyx (Fig. 9-2). The remainder of the canal is filled with epidural fat, the character of which changes from a loose texture in children to a more fibrous, close-meshed texture in adults. It has been suggested that this difference that gives rise to the predictability of caudal local anesthetic spread in children and its unpredictability in adults.[99]

Sacral and Coccygeal Nerves

The anterior and posterior primary rami of S1–S4 exit from the sacral canal by way of the anterior and posterior foramina, respectively. S5 and the minute coccygeal nerve exit laterally through the sacral hiatus and wind laterally around the sacrum and coccyx, respectively (see Fig. 9-2).

These roots give rise to the following nerves: posterior cutaneous nerve of the thigh (subdividing into gluteal, perineal, and terminal branches to the back of the thigh and leg), perforating cutaneous nerve (inconstant), pudendal nerve (subdividing into inferior rectal nerve, perineal nerve, scrotal or labial branches, nerve to urethral bulb, and dorsal nerve of penis or clitoris), anococcygeal nerves, pelvic splanchnic nerves, and various muscular branches. These nerves relay total sensory input from the vagina, anorectal region, floor of the perineum, anal and bladder sphincters, urethra, and scrotal skin. The vulva is sacrally innervated except for its most anterior margin (see Chapter 18, Fig. 18-2). It is the same with the penis, except that the base is not sacrally innervated. Sacral nerves also innervate a narrow band of skin extending from the posterior aspect of the gluteal region to the plantar and lateral surface of the foot.

In addition to these areas that have exclusive sacral innervation, several organs on the pelvic floor and perineum have multiple innervation through preaortic and sacrococcygeal nerve groups (see Chapter 18, Fig. 18-1), including the uterus, fallopian tubes, bladder, and possibly prostate. Although unsupplemented caudal blockade may not provide full pain control for operations on these structures, it can provide a major component of a combined anesthetic sequence (see also Chapter 18).

PHARMACOLOGY

Various studies have attested to safety of caudal anesthesia in terms of the local anesthetic blood levels attained. As would be expected, there are such wide variations between the doses, concentrations, and drugs used in the different studies that comparisons are difficult to make. In addition, some of these studies have measured the time of onset of the block and the duration. This information has been tabulated in Tables 9-1 and 9-2. The following generalizations can be made from this information:

1. Plasma levels for all local anesthetic drugs tend to be low after caudal administration.[22,36,37,43,82] Even very large doses in children have given plasma levels well below the accepted adult toxic levels.[110] Higher peak serum concentrations in infants under 12kg, and the presence of a greater free fraction, suggest that there should be greater caution with dose in this age group.[37,81] The addition of epinephrine 1:200,000 to bupivacaine solutions injected in children under 5 years of age provides a significantly longer duration of action than in adults, where epinephrine is of questionable value.[123]
2. Onset time or latent interval seems to be longer with caudal than with lumbar epidural anesthetic when similar drugs and doses are administered.[44]
3. The time to attainment of maximum spread is variable and takes longer than for lumbar epidural block. Ranges from 10 to 60 minutes have been reported with a mean of about 30 minutes.[19,37,81]
4. Block of the large diameter S1 root is less predictable than it is after lumbar epidural block when moderate doses are used.[44]
5. Concentrations of solution that are adequate to block sensory fibres are bupivacaine, 0.25%; etidocaine, 1%; mepivacaine, 1%; lidocaine, 1%; prilocaine, 1%; and chloroprocaine, 2%. Increased concentration will increase the degree of motor block and, possibly, will improve speed of onset. The addition of epinephrine will increase the degree of motor block, decrease the plasma levels, and increase the duration of the shorter-acting drugs (see also Chapter 3).

Dose and Spread

Through the years, many factors have been implicated in influencing the spread of a standard dose of local anesthetic solution injected into the caudal canal. Such factors as age, weight, height, dose (both volume and concentration of drug), speed of injection, and patient position, will be known

TABLE 9-1. *Pharmacokinetics and caudal block*

Study	Drug	Dose	Mean peak blood concentration and range	Mean time to peak blood concentration	Comments
Mazze, et al., 1966[82] Young adults	1.5% lidocaine with epinephrine 1:200,000	5.8–7.5 mg/kg mean 428 mg = 28.5 ml	1.4 μg/ml (0.5–2.9)	30 min	Lower blood levels with caudal than with lumbar epidural or IV regional
Cousins and Bromage, 1971[28] Adults	Lidocaine HCl and CO_2 lidocaine 1.75% base	About 17 ml	CO_2 lidocaine 3.1 μg/ml (2.6–3.8), lidocaine HCl 2.7 μg/ml (1.5–4.2)	CO_2 lidocaine 7 min, lidocaine HCl 12 min	
Moore, et al., 1968[84] Obstetric patients with caudal catheter	1.5% mepivacaine	300–450 mg = 20–30 ml	About 3.0 μg/ml	Not stated; 40 min for one patient	Blood levels rose after equivalent top-up doses to reach 7–9 μg/ml in four of five patients at delivery
Freund, et al., 1984[43] Young males <40 years compared with older males >55 years; caudal catheters inserted to 10 cm	2% lidocaine or 0.75% bupivacaine, both with epinephrine 1:200,000	Lidocaine 6 mg/kg, bupivacaine 2.2 mg/kg	Lidocaine <40y 2.47 μg/ml ± 0.23 lidocaine >55y 2.61 μg/ml ± 1.45 bupivacaine <40y 0.86 μg/ml ± 0.22 bupivacaine >50y 0.69 μg/ml ± 0.25	Lidocaine <40, 45 min, lidocaine >55, 25 min, bupivacaine <40, 30 min, bupivacaine >55, 20 min	No significant difference between peak plasma lidocaine or bupivacaine levels with age; no significant difference in dermatomal levels for the four groups
Eyres, et al., 1978[38] Children	1% lidocaine, 0.5% bupivacaine	Lidocaine 4 mg/kg, bupivacaine 2 mg/kg	Lidocaine 2 μg/ml, bupivacaine 0.7 μg/ml	Lidocaine 10–20 min, bupivacaine ?about 15 min	
Ecoffey, et al., 1984[36] Children	1% lidocaine	5 mg/kg	2.05 ± 0.08 μg/ml	28.2 ± 2.9 min	Long terminal half-life in children attributed to larger volume of distribution
Takasaki, 1984[109] Children	1.5% lidocaine, 1.5% mepivacaine, 0.5% bupivacaine, all with epinephrine	Lidocaine 11 mg/kg, mepivacaine 11 mg/kg, bupivacaine 3.7 mg/kg	Lidocaine 2.2 μg/ml, mepivacaine 2.53 μg/ml, bupivacaine 0.67 μg/ml	45 min 45 min 45 min	Low blood concentrations with slow decrease in concentrations

IV, intravenous; y = years of age.

or controllable. Their influences have been studied by a number of investigators. There are, however, a number of other factors in which the influences remain both unknown and uncontrollable, and which must inevitably give rise to the significant unpredictability of all epidural spread, but particularly in the sacral canal. These factors follow.[90]

1. The size of the caudal epidural space.
2. The size and patency of the sacral canal and the anterior sacral foramina.
3. The amount of bony distortion of the sacral canal.
4. The presence of septa in the epidural space.
5. The amount and nature of the soft tissues in the epidural space, especially fatty tissues.
6. The permeability of the neural tissue and dural cuffs to the drug.

Adults

The only factors that have been shown to affect caudal spread in adults are volume, speed of injection,[90] and patient posture.[127]

In another study, 30 ml of 1.5% lidocaine with epinephrine 1:200,000 injected over 1 minute gave a mean upper level of T6–T7 (L3–T1), whereas a similar volume injected over 2 minutes gave a mean upper level of T11 (S2–T2).[90] There was an 8% incidence of transient acute hypertension and tachycardia in the more rapid injection group. The lack of influence of age in adults is well shown in a study in which the dose of anesthetic per spinal segment is plotted against age for both lidocaine HCl and carbonated lidocaine[28] (Fig. 9-4). In the same study, there was also no correlation with height or weight. In another study, comparing spread with

TABLE 9-2. *Onset and duration of caudal block*

Study	Drug	Onset (min)	Spread (segments)	Two-segment regression (min)	Total regression (min)	Comments
Cousins and Bromage, 1971[28] Adult outpatients	2% lidocaine HCl, 17 ml	14.4 (3–32)	6.8 in 24.8 ± 6.4 min	At 67	At 87	Very rapid onset confirmed for carbonated lidocaine
	CO_2 lidocaine 1.75% base, 17 ml	3.2 (1–8)	9.6 in 12.8 ± 5.8 min	At 66	At 94	
Seow, et al., 1976[103] Adults	1% etidocaine with epinephrine 1:200,000, 25 ml	7.06 SD = 4.54	11.7 SD = 3.9	Not measured	Not measured	Rapid onset but persisting motor block noted with etidocaine
	1.5% lidocaine with epinephrine 1:200,000, 25 ml	12.44 SD = 6.14	12.7 SD = 5.8	Not measured	Not measured	
Park, et al., 1979[90]	30 ml 1.5% lidocaine with 1:200,000 epinephrine					Several instances of acute hypertension >200/100 in 1 min injection group
	Injection over 1 min	3.9 (2–15)	17 (8–22)		203 ± 5.3	
	Injection over 2 min	3.6 (2–12)	12 (3–21)	Not measured	192 ± 11	
Willis and Macintyre, 1986[128] Young female adults	2% lidocaine with 1:200,000 epinephrine					
	20 ml		9.5 (range 6.5–13)			
	10 ml		7 (4–13)			
	5 ml		4 (3–5)			
	0.5% bupivacaine with 1:200,000 epinephrine					
	20 ml		9 (4–12.5)			
	10 ml		6.5 (3–10)			
	5 ml		4 (3–5)			
			Block of S1 Root			
			Delay (min)	Failure (%)		
Galindo, et al., 1978[44]	1.5% chloroprocaine	4.8 (SD = 1.5)	20 (8.6)	20		All onset times are similar and very fast. The delay in the block of the large S1 root is very variable. Because individual doses range from 10–20 ml, it is difficult to assess the significance of these data.
	3% chloroprocaine	5.5 (0.7)	24.3 (6.7)	25		
	2% mepivacaine	5.9 (2.6)	27 (8.4)	23		
	0.75% bupivacaine	4.9 (2.0)	17.9 (5.6)	13		
	1% etidocaine	4.9 (1.4)	17.8 (3.5)	0		
	1.5% etidocaine	4.2 (2.5)	15 (3.8)	0		
	All with epinephrine 1:200,000—dose range, 10–20 ml					

both lidocaine and bupivacaine in a group of older and a group of younger adult males, there was no significant difference between any of the four groups.[43]

The effect of posture on the spread of caudal solutions was studied in patients in the horizontal position, 15° head-up on 15° head-down. Higher levels of analgesia were obtained in the head-up position.[127]

Children

In children, the situation is different: Schulte-Steinberg and Rahlfs in 1970 established that there was a high correlation between dose and age.[101] There were lesser degrees of correlation between dose and weight and dose and height in children. In 1977, the same authors produced a single regression line for three drugs (1% lidocaine, 1% mepivacaine, and 0.25% bupivacaine, all with epinephrine) showing in children the linear relation between age and spread (measured in ml/spinal segment).[102] Reference to this study shows that an adequate dosing schedule would be:

0.1 ml/segment/yr + 0.1 ml/segment (see Chapter 20)

There is strong agreement between this work and that done by Bromage with lumbar epidural anesthesia.[17]

Despite the academic appeal of the dosing schedule cited above, it has been challenged by a number of authors. This has given rise to a bewildering collection of formulae, some for specific purposes, and some for such vague indications as "routine surgical procedures." These are summarized in Table 9-3.

Three dosing schedules are worthy of further mention. The Armitage formula of 0.5 ml of 0.25% bupivacaine/kg

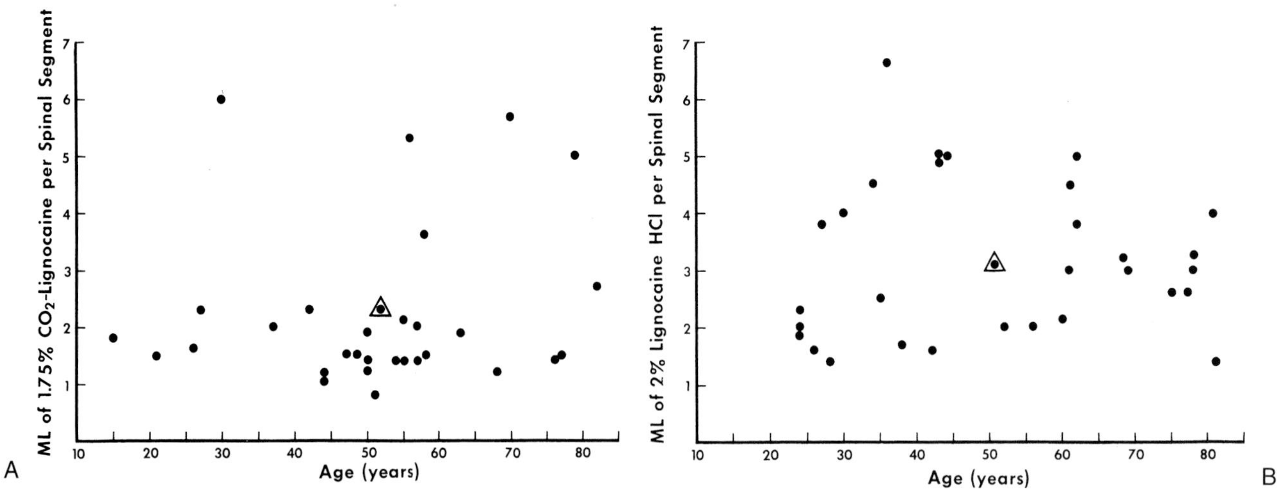

FIG. 9-4. Caudal blockade in adults: Segmental spread analgesia with advancing age. **A:** 1.75% lidocaine carbonate. **B:** 2% lidocaine hydrochloride. Dose requirements in milliliter per spinal segment are plotted against age, with the mean dose indicated by a dot in a triangle. There is no consistency in spread of analgesia at any age or any correlation between age and segmental spread. (Cousins, M.J., and Bromage, P.R.: Br. J. Anaesth., *43:*1149, 1971.)

for circumcision and anal surgery (low sacral) is easy to use, reliable, and safe, but requires much larger doses of drug.[5] The same author recommends 1 ml/kg of 0.25% bupivacaine to block the lower thoracic nerves and 1.25 ml/kg to block the midthoracic nerves (e.g., for orchidectomy or umbilical herniorrhaphy). This latter dose is high, but seems to have proven safe in children.

In the second study, Busoni and Andreuccetti[18] analysed 763 caudal blocks in children and produced two graphs. The first related spread of analgesia to dose and age, while the

TABLE 9-3. *Dose regimens for caudal block*

Study	Formula	Indication	Comments
Schulte-Steinberg and Rahlfs, 1977[102]	0.1 ml/segment/year + 0.1 ml/segment	Adapt to number of segments required	Gives rise to low doses
Armitage, 1979[5]	0.5 ml/kg 0.25% bupivacaine 1 ml/kg 1.25 ml/kg	For circumcision For inguinal herniotomy For umbilical herniorraphy or orchidopexy	
Kay, 1974[65]	0.5 ml 0.5% bupivacaine with epinephrine per year of age	Circumcision	Similar to Schulte-Steinberg and Rahlfs
Takasaki, et al., 1977[110]	ml/segment = 0.056 × weight (kg)	Adapt to number of segments required	Very slow speed of injection 0.15 ml/sec
Yeoman, et al., 1983[129]	1 ml 0.5% bupivacaine/year + 2 ml (max 20 ml)	Circumcision	
Lourey and McDonald, 1973[72]	3–4 mg 1% lidocaine/kg, 1.0 mg 0.5% bupivacaine/kg	Lower abdominal and urogenital operations	
McGown, 1982[78]	To S3: 0.55 ml/kg 1–2% lid. + epinephrine; to L2: 1.1 ml/kg 1–2% lid. + epinephrine; to T11: 1.7 ml/kg 1–2% lid. + epinephrine	Areas innervated by these nerve roots	Dose of 1.7 ml/kg is unacceptable even with 1% lidocaine with epinephrine
Spiegel, 1962[107]	$\text{Volume (ml)} = 4 + \frac{D - 15}{2}$ D = distance between C7 and sacral hiatus in cm	? upper abdominal surgery	
Satoyoshi and Kamiyama, 1984[97]	Volume (ml) = D − 13 (ml) D = distance between C7 and sacral hiatus in cm	Upper abdominal surgery, T4–T5	Excessive dose
Hassan, 1977[54]	7 mg/kg 1.5% lidocaine or mepivacaine	"Routine surgical procedures"	
Touloukian, et al., 1971[114]	2.7–7.6 mg/kg of 0.5–1% lidocaine	Neonatal surgery no higher than inguinal herniotomy	Seems satisfactory
Fortuna, 1967[41]	To T12: 10 mg/kg 0.5–2% lidocaine; to T10: 12.5 mg/kg 0.5–2% lidocaine; to T6: 15 mg/kg 0.5–2% lidocaine	Areas innervated by these nerve roots	High to excessive dose

lid., lidocaine.

second related spread of analgesia to dose and weight. Knowing the age and/or weight, the dose required for a given degree of spread can be determined. Weight proved to be a better predictor in infants, while age was better for older children (see also Chapter 20).

The third study[78] is notable for the extent of the detail presented. It states that with at least 97% confidence, 0.55 ml of 1% to 2% lidocaine/kg will produce a block to S3 or higher, 1.1 ml/kg will produce a block to L3 or higher, and 1.7 ml/kg will produce a block to T11 or higher. These doses gave rise to some excessively high blocks, and there was an alarmingly high incidence of respiratory or cardiac arrest (2.8%), or both, which one must deduce was at least contributed to by the very high doses of drug given. Such large doses should not be administered.

Dose by Means of Caudal Catheter

As previously stated, the tip of a caudal catheter may readily reach the L5–S1 level. The block then tends to behave more like a lumbar epidural. Estimation of dose can be done using the criteria that one uses for this latter block. "Top-up" doses should be scaled down, as with lumbar epidural "top-ups." Accumulation of mepivacaine during labor, with steadily rising blood levels and toxicity, has occurred, where caudal top-up doses have been the same as the initial dose.[84]

Onset and Duration

To understand and use rationally any regional anesthetic technique, it is important to know the following time intervals: the time to achieve maximum spread of block and the duration (usually measured for a central block as the time from onset to regression of two spinal segments). It is also useful to know the onset interval (latency) and the time to total regression of the block. Only limited data are available on this subject, the most notable feature of which is the great variability, particularly with regard to onset interval (see Table 9-2). This is probably due to use of different methods as criteria for "onset." In most studies, time of onset is the period from injection until the patient first notices loss of sensation to pinprick or other stimulus.

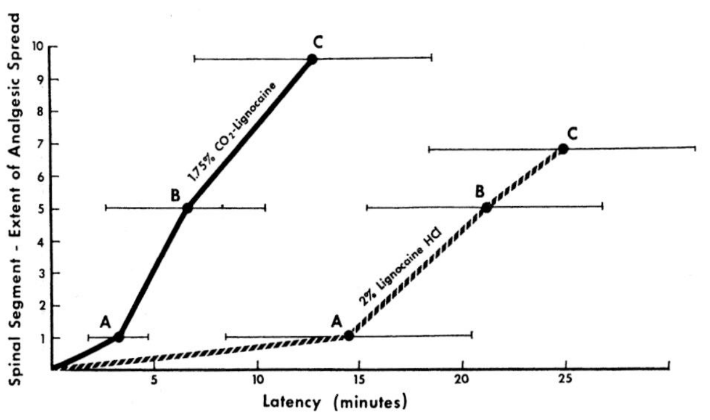

FIG. 9-5. Caudal blockade: Latency of onset and spread of complete blockade (i.e., "surgical" analgesia). Two percent lidocaine hydrochloride is compared to 1.75% lidocaine carbonate. Onset of blockade and complete loss of sensation are much more rapid with lidocaine carbonate. Even with the lidocaine carbonate solution, blockade of five segments may require nearly 10 minutes, whereas with the lidocaine hydrochloride solution it may require in excess of 20 minutes. (Cousins, M.J., and Bromage, P.R.: Br. J. Anaesth., *43:*1149, 1971.)

Probably the most useful clinical information comes from the study by Cousins and Bromage,[28] in which 1.75% carbonated lidocaine was compared with 2% lidocaine HCl. Although this study confirmed the usefulness of carbonated lidocaine, a drug not generally available, it also showed that the time to attain total sacral anesthesia with 2% lidocaine HCl was 21 minutes (mean), with some taking more that 30 minutes (Fig. 9-5). Two-segment regression took 67 minutes (mean), and total duration was 87 minutes (mean).

PHYSIOLOGICAL EFFECTS

The physiological changes associated with epidural anesthesia are well documented in Chapter 8. A limited sacral block from a caudal epidural would be expected to cause minimal physiological trespass.

Besides the sensory and motor block of the sacral roots, one could expect a degree of autonomic block. The sacral component of the parasympathetic craniosacral outflow (the pelvic splanchnic nerves) will be blocked, causing loss of visceromotor function in the bladder and bowel distally from the splenic flexure of the colon. There should, in theory, also be an increase in anal and bladder sphincter tone, but this is seldom seen in practice because of a coexistent sympathetic block, which is outlined below. Since the sympathetic outflow from the spinal cord ends at L1 level, a limited caudal block should theoretically avoid any sympathetic block. It would seem in practice, however, that this is not necessarily so. Vascular dilatation in the lower limb is often seen with a low level of caudal block. There seems no doubt that the level of sympathetic block is higher than that of sensory block, although there is very little "hard" evidence in the literature to confirm this (see Chapter 7). An often-quoted study[83] has shown evidence of sympathetic block of the eye in 17 of 20 consecutive obstetric patients having caudal analgesia. Although in this study the dose of drug and supine positioning of the patient have been rightly criticized, nevertheless the upper level of sensory block was significantly lower than T1 in all patients. It would seem, therefore, that the potential exists for a degree of unwanted sympathetic block. Pooling of blood in the denervated lower extremities, and reflex vasoconstriction in the innervated upper limbs, has been shown to occur.[92] Carotid flow was unchanged. Of course, if an extensive sensory block occurs (intentional or otherwise), inevitably a similarly extensive sympathetic block will occur, with all the consequences outlined in Chapter 8. Likewise, similar respiratory and neuroendocrine effects of high epidural anesthesia would be expected with an extensive caudal block.

Changes in adrenocorticotropic hormone (ACTH), immunoreactive beta-endorphin, antidiuretic hormone (ADH), cortisol, catecholamines, insulin, and growth hormone levels were measured in children undergoing surgery with either halothane anesthesia or caudal anesthesia. The normal rises in these hormone levels associated with general anesthesia and surgery in the perioperative period were blocked by caudal anesthesia.[45,86]

TECHNIQUE OF CAUDAL BLOCK

As in the preparation for any major regional anesthetic technique, all equipment must be assembled and checked, including block tray, resuscitation equipment, monitors, and suction. Secure intravenous access must be obtained (see Chapter 6).

The needles used for this procedure will depend to some extent on the clinical circumstances. For single-injection caudal block in a child, a 2 to 3 cm disposable 23- to 25-gauge needle should be used. In an adult, the slightly greater rigidity of a 22-gauge needle may make the procedure easier. The needles should be short-bevelled, because they give a better feel when different tissues are penetrated, they have less tendency to form barbs if bone is struck, the bevel is more likely to fully enter the canal when it is very shallow, and they may cause less trauma to blood vessels. If a catheter is to be inserted, a short 5 to 7 cm 18T-gauge Crawford-tip needle and a standard epidural catheter, are recommended. Some operators prefer to use a plastic intravenous cannula of small caliber.[89] Although this has some advantages, it has a tendency to kink and is less reliable. A large gauge IV needle can be used to insert a standard epidural catheter. The use of a Tuohy needle to insert a catheter is not recommended because the needle will lie in the long axis of the canal and the Tuohy tip will direct the catheter toward the wall, rather than into the axis of the canal, as would happen with a Crawford or an IV needle.

The patient can be positioned in one of three ways: The preferred position is the lateral Sims position (left-side down for a right-handed operator), with the lower leg only slightly flexed at the hip and the upper leg more flexed so that it lies over and above the lower leg and is also in contact with the bed. This maneuver tends to separate the buttocks. In contrast to lumbar epidural block, excess hip flexion is unnecessary and may on occasion stretch the skin to such an extent that palpation of the landmarks may become more difficult. This position has the advantages of comfort for the patient, a familiar working position for the anesthesiologist, and easy access to the airway if the patient is sedated, or in the event of an adverse reaction. Sagging of the gluteal cleft occasionally may cause some confusion in confirming landmarks in inexperienced hands, but can be readily corrected by an assistant, who holds the upper buttock to reposition the gluteal cleft in the median plane of the sacrum. This is in accordance with the general principle that skin creases are poor landmarks for regional anesthesia (Fig. 9-6A).

The prone position, with a pillow under the pelvis, is still popular with some anesthesiologists. Both legs are rotated so that the toes of both feet are facing medially. This again separates the buttocks. In this position, there is no distortion from movement of the gluteal cleft, but access to the mouth and airway is compromised.

The less popular knee-chest position may still be useful, particularly for the pregnant patient.

Skin preparation should be done over a large area so that all the landmarks can be palpated aseptically. If alcoholic solutions are used, a swab should be placed deep in the gluteal cleft, to prevent pain in the exposed sensitive perineal area.

Confirmation of bony landmarks is the key to success. In a thin, young patient, the protrusions of the sacral cornua can be seen without palpation, and the shallow depression over the sacral hiatus can be seen between them, Successful needle placement in these circumstances is exceedingly easy; however, the majority of patients have less obvious surface anatomy and require very careful palpation of all the bony landmarks. Needle penetration of a posterior sacral foramen may mimic the feel of entering the sacral hiatus. Often, closed bony depressions covered by fibrous ligament can also mimic the sacral hiatus, although injection is impossible (Fig. 9-7B). Only the most meticulous attention to the landmarks can prevent needle entry into these "decoy hiatuses."

It is important, initially, to identify the midline positively. This can be achieved by palpating the tip of the coccyx with the finger and moving cephalad, about 4 to 5 cm in an adult, until the fingertip lies over the sacral hiatus with the prominent sacral cornua palpable on each side by moving the fingertip from side to side (Fig. 9-6B). The use of excessive pressure while moving the finger in this latter manner can be painful. Considerable variability occurs in the prominence of the cornua, causing problems for the unwary. If one cornu is much less obvious than the other, there may be a tendency to palpate further laterally until a prominent tubercle of the lateral sacral crest at the inferior lateral sacral angle is felt. The importance of establishing the midline of the sacrum cannot be overemphasized. Palpation of the median sacral crest in a caudad direction can also lead to the sacral hiatus, but it is a less reliable method. The posterior superior iliac spines form an equilateral triangle with the sacral hiatus; this should be used as a confirmatory landmark for correct needle placement. Unfortunately, these spines are not always readily palpable. It is useful to remember that the line joining these spines is an approximate indication of the level of termination of the dural sac (S2 level). In patients in whom landmark palpation is difficult, digital examination, with one finger inserted into the rectum, may be performed to help select a point of needle entry. A useful alternative method of palpating the cornua and hiatus, using the thumb of each hand has been described.[74]

Once the area of the suspected hiatus has been found, one should keep the palpating hand in position until after the needle insertion, because the landmarks can be quickly obscured, especially in an obese patient. Because the canal has

A.

B.

C.

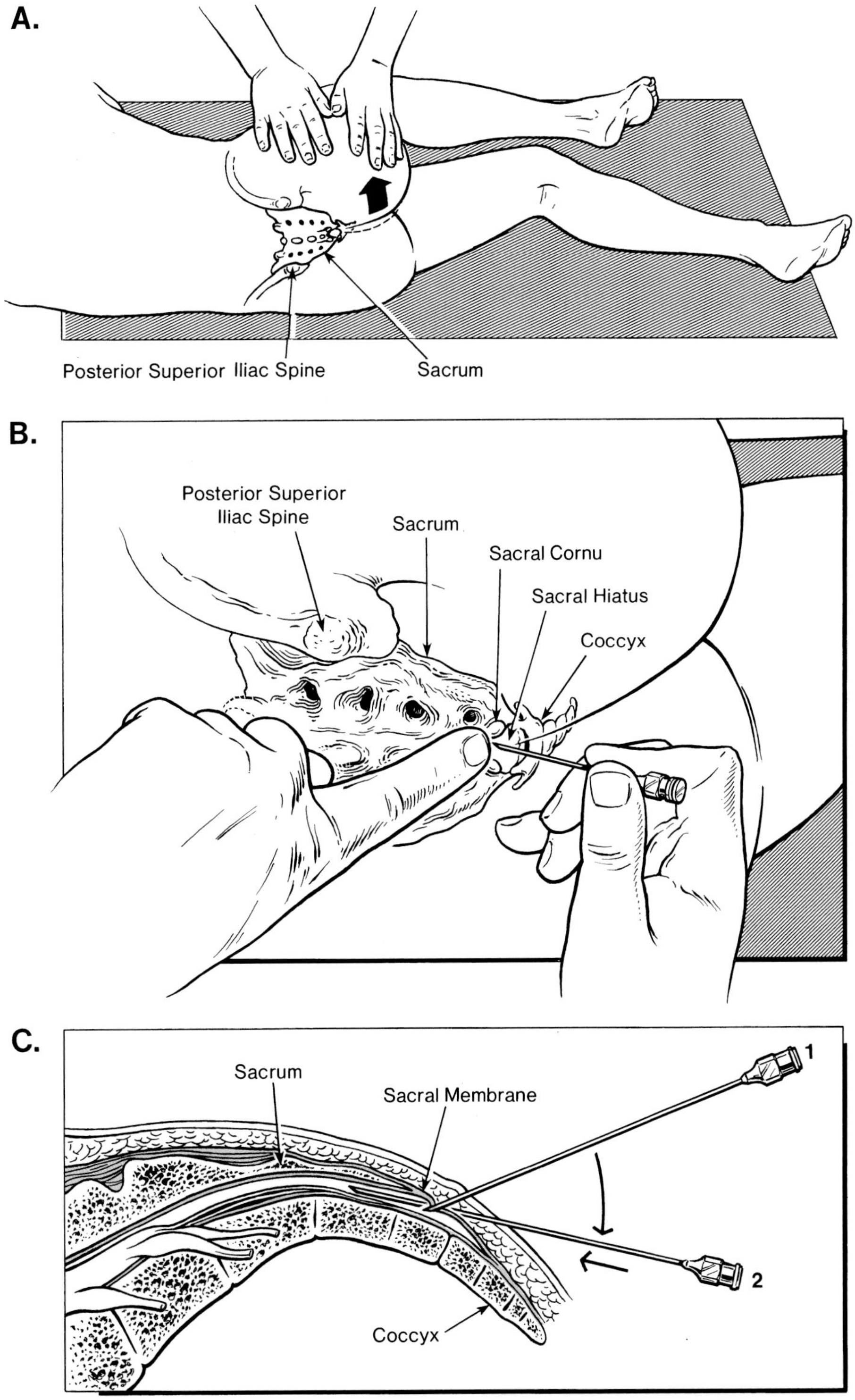

FIG. 9-6. Technique of caudal block (see text). **A:** Positioning for caudal block. **B:** Palpation of landmarks and needle insertion. **C:** Needle insertion through sacrococcygeal (sacral) membrane.

a tendency to become deeper as one progresses cephalad, canal entry is facilitated if a point of needle entry is chosen toward the upper end of the hiatus. The initial angle of needle insertion should be about 120° to the back (Fig. 9-6C). Penetration of the sacrococcygeal ligament has a characteristic feel to it. This "pop" can be learned only by practice. There is a feeling of nonresistance after penetration of the ligament, until the anterior sacral wall is contacted. This contact should not be sought deliberately. The needle, both hub and shank, should be depressed toward the skin to align the

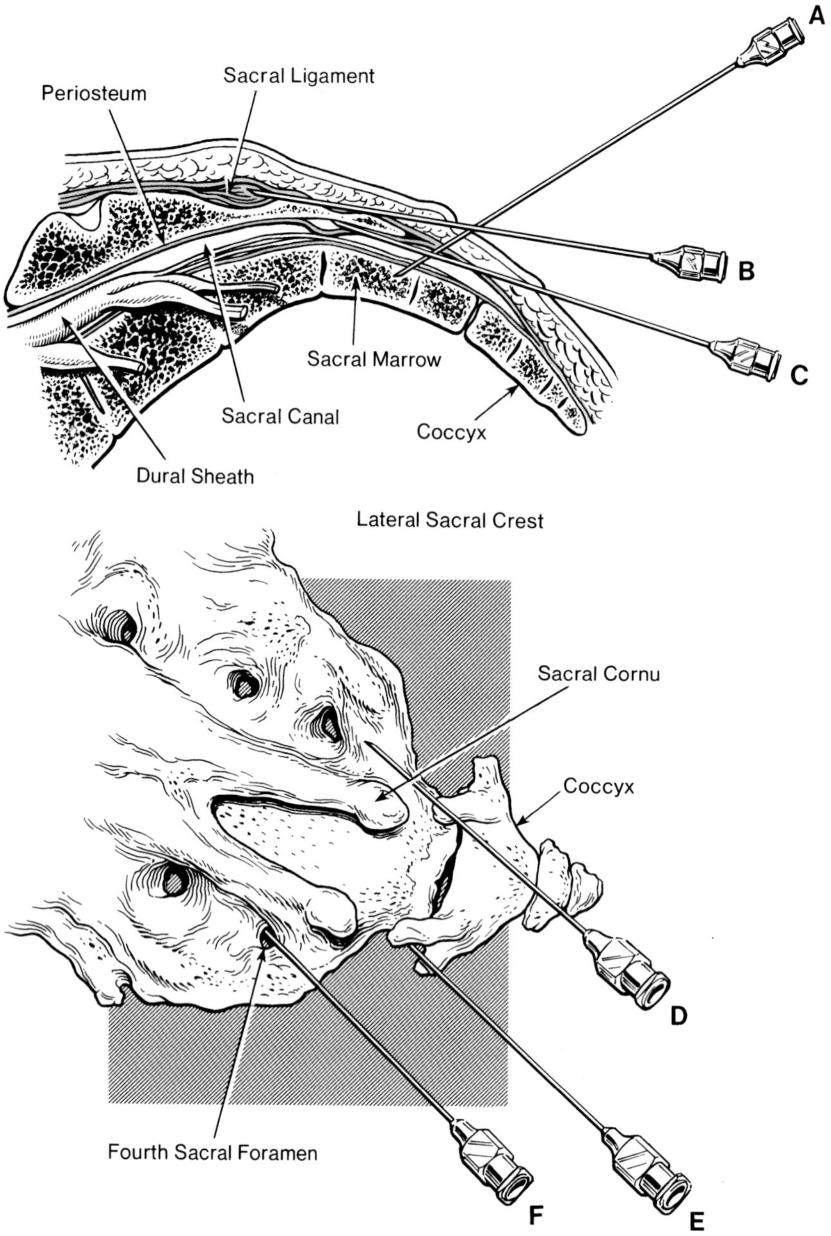

FIG. 9-7. Misplacement of needle during attempted caudal block. *Note:* injection into posterior sacral ligaments **(B)**; subperiosteal injection **(C)**; and injection into marrow **(A)**; lateral injection into a "decoy hiatus" **(D)** (see also Fig. 9-3); injection lateral to coccyx and toward anterior sacral wall **(E)**, with a risk of damaging intrapelvic structures (including a fetus); injection into 4th sacral foramen **(F)**, perhaps one of the most common causes of a unilateral limited block.

needle approximately in the long axis of the canal. It may then be inserted a further centimeter (Fig. 9-6C). On occasion, further needle insertion is not possible because of obstruction of some kind. This should be accepted. After both aspiration and a test of the local anesthetic drug are safely accomplished, the full dose of local anesthetic may be injected in 3–5 ml increments.

Signs of Correct Needle Placement

The following are the objective and subjective signs of accurate needle positioning, and those that appear appropriate should be elicited before completion of injection; the first four should be regarded as essential (modified from McCaul[74]).

1. Presence of sacral bone on each side of, in front of, and behind the needle at its point of insertion, does not exclude the possibility of entry into a decoy hiatus, but does protect against injection lateral to the sacral or coccygeal margins or into the presacral tissues or rectum.
2. The lack of cerebrospinal fluid (CSF), air, or blood on aspiration is important. Light blood staining is not uncommon and may indicate that entry into the sacral

canal has been achieved and that repeat aspiration should be attempted during the injection of solution.
3. There should be no subcutaneous bulge or superficial crepitus after rapid injection of 2 or 3 ml of anesthetic solution or air.
4. There should be no tissue resistance to injection; the force required to inject should not exceed that necessary to overcome syringe and needle resistances and should be constant throughout. Injection should feel like any other injection into the epidural space.
5. The so-called "whoosh" test can be used to predict successful needle placement.[9,70] This involves listening with a stethoscope over the midline lumbar spine for a characteristic "whoosh" sound on injection of 2 to 3 ml of air via the caudal needle. This test is more reliable than the "pop" of sacrococcygeal ligament penetration or "loss of resistance" tests.[24] Venous air embolism in an 11 kg child has been suggested following the use of 2.5 ml of air for this test.[49]
6. When correctly positioned, the needle should be able to move in the canal, pivoting at the point of penetration of the sacrococcygeal ligament. Eliciting the sign may, however, cause trauma to the tissues in the canal, particularly blood vessels, and usually is not necessary.
7. There should be no local pain during injection of solution; pain indicates misplacement of the needle, and injection should stop.
8. Paresthesia or a feeling of fullness that extends from the sacrum to the soles of the feet is common during injection, but ceases on completion and portends successful blockade.
9. The feeling of grating as the needle moves along the anterior wall of the sacral canal indicates accurate positioning but should not be purposefully elicited lest the sacral venous plexus be damaged.
10. An epidural catheter or other plastic cannula should enter the canal freely with the same or greater ease than in the lumbar epidural space.

It is recommended that one use a test dose containing epinephrine before the full dose is given. Because of the proximity of needle and catheter to venous plexuses, there is a risk of intravascular injection and a toxic reaction. Slow injection is also recommended in order to avoid rapid increases in spinal and intraepidural pressure.

Catheter Techniques

The epidural catheter should enter the canal without difficulty. Because of the angle of insertion, it will progress cephalad more predictably in all age groups[10,11,50,131] than will lumbar epidural catheters.

Fixation of the epidural catheter to prevent soiling is important. One secure method is to spray the area lightly with an adhesive such as tincture of benzoin compound and then apply a sterile adhesive plastic dressing initially into the previously separated gluteal cleft, and then directly over the site of insertion of the catheter. Because many of these patients will have surgery in the lithotomy position, the aim is to have a very adherent dressing in the gluteal cleft that will *not* form a pocket to collect fluids from the operative site, which may run down directly over the anus.

Monitoring

Despite the limited extent of block anticipated with caudal anesthesia, it is still mandatory to monitor the patient, including blood pressure (BP), electrocardiogram (ECG), and pulse oximetry. Intravenous or intraosseous misplacement of the caudal needle or excessive spread of block may give rise to unwanted effects. Maintaining verbal communication with the patient is the simplest, and in some ways the most reliable method of detecting adverse side effects. However, blood pressure and pulse should be measured frequently, and the progress of the block should be plotted.

INDICATIONS

Obstetric Anesthesia and Analgesia (see Chapter 18)

The widespread and safe use of epidural analgesia to control the pain of labor has been a major factor in increasing the popularity of regional anesthesia for elective and emergency surgery. Although the lumbar approach is now used as the technique of choice in most obstetric units, it should be remembered that it was the report in 1943 by Hingson and Edwards entitled *Continuous Caudal Analgesia: An Analysis of the First 10,000 Confinements Thus Managed with the Report of the Authors' First 1,000 Cases*,[59] that first popularized the method. The advantages were immediately obvious: high-quality analgesia with a low incidence of complications and a low failure rate for that time of only 7%.

In later years, clinical studies confirmed some of the advantages.[39,58] Most, but not all,[4] studies showed that caudal analgesia had essentially no effect on uterine activity during labor. Local anesthetic blood levels did not correlate with any measured changes in uterine activity.[117] Cardiac output increases during labor were decreased, and the tachycardia of the second stage and the early postpartum period was prevented by caudal analgesia.[53,118] One study demonstrated the prolongation of analgesia achieved by adding epinephrine to the caudal local anesthetic solution.[52] It also reported that epinephrine, 25 ml of 1:200,000 dilution, significantly prolonged labor; however, "top-up" doses of 15 to 20 ml were given in this study, and patients were supine; thus the epinephrine dose was large, and some supine hypotension may have occurred.

As regional anesthetic techniques became more refined, it became apparent that there were significant objections to the use of the caudal route for routine analgesia in labor. The pathways for the pain of first-stage labor are by way of T10–L1 (see Chapter 18). Thus a technique that initially and predominantly blocked sacral roots was less effective for early labor. Large doses of local anesthetic drug needed to be given. Admittedly, the caudal approach offered superb management of the sacrally mediated pain of second stage, but it did so for what could be a lengthy period of first stage, when it was not required. What was previously a tolerable failure rate of 7% became no longer acceptable. An unfortunate objection was the report of four cases in which local anesthetic drugs were injected into the fetus during attempted caudal injection.[40,105] For these reasons, continuous caudal analgesia in labor fell into disuse in most obstetric units, to an extent that facility in performing the technique has now been largely lost. There is still a place for continuous caudal analgesia in labor in those cases in which lumbar epidural analgesia is contraindicated because of anatomic abnormalities or localized infection. On occasions, sacral analgesia is required either early in labor or cannot be obtained via a lumbar catheter.

A two-catheter technique, one lumbar and one caudal, has been used in an effort to lower the total dose of local anesthetic drug.[1,27] This would seem to compound the likelihood of complications without a sufficiently significant positive advantage. The technique of using a lumbar catheter for first-stage analgesia, supplemented late in labor by single-injection caudal block, is popular in some centers.[74,91] Single-injection caudal is useful as an alternative to saddle-block spinal anesthesia for forceps delivery. In these circumstances, the proximity of the needle to the presenting part of the fetus must be remembered. The procedure is safe if bone of the sacrum and coccyx is palpable on all sides of the needle. Rectal examination is advised when there is any doubt. It has been stated that caudal block should not be performed if the presenting part is at the perineum.[74]

An excellent review of the use of caudal anesthesia in obstetrics is provided by Paull in a symposium on obstetric anesthesia.[91]

Pediatric Anesthesia (see Chapter 20)

Caudal block has been used successfully for anesthesia in children since about 1960,[107] with many studies attesting to its success. It is in this group of patients that the caudal technique has found its greatest application. In children, the sacral hiatus is usually very easy to palpate, making the procedure very simple, quick, and reliable.[31,78,122] Because of the ease of its performance in children, the block has been recommended for a wide variety of surgical procedures, both as the sole anesthetic and in combination with light general anesthesia. In summary, the surgical indications for the block divide into three groups: sacral block (e.g., circumcision, anal surgery), lower thoracic block (e.g., inguinal herniotomy), and upper thoracic block.

The significance of these three groups relates to the doses of local anesthetic drug required to consistently achieve the desired spread. This subject has been discussed at length in a previous section, but it should be reemphasized here that there is no justification for the use of doses of lidocaine in excess of 5 to 7 mg/kg, despite the allegations of safety by some authors. Midabdominal or upper abdominal surgery is not an indication for conventional caudal block. Thoracic epidural anesthesia in children has been achieved via a 24 g epidural catheter inserted through the sacral hiatus. The radiographically determined epidural catheter tip position was within two segments of the target position in 17 of 20 patients.[50]

For subumbilical surgery, caudal anesthesia is excellent. Since young children do not tolerate the frightening environment of the operating room, light general anesthesia seems to be the preferred technique for both induction of the caudal block and throughout the surgery. In those patients in whom sedation or general anesthesia is not desired or is contraindicated,[41,54,78] eutectic mixture of local anesthetics (EMLA) cream under adhesive plastic can be applied to the skin over the sacral hiatus an hour or so prior to the procedure.[46]

A modification of the standard caudal technique has been described by Busoni and Sarti for use in children.[19] This sacral intervertebral epidural block is based on the fact that fusion of the sacral segments is not complete until after the 25th year. The caudal needle is inserted into the S2-S3 space in the midline just below a line drawn between the posterior superior iliac spines. The epidural space was identified by loss of resistance to air. Successful block was achieved in 100% of 74 children aged between 2 months and 13 years.

Low-birth-weight and pre-term or former pre-term neonates constitute a high risk group of patients for whom the appropriate use of regional anesthesia can obviate the need for general anesthesia and minimize[124] the associated serious respiratory complications common to this group. The author's personal series, as well as several published studies, attest to the success and safety of single-shot or continuous caudal anesthesia for lower abdominal and perineal surgery in this challenging group of patients.[51,57,93,106,112,114,122]

A specific indication for caudal anesthesia in children is surgery in patients with congenital dystrophia myotonica. Regional anesthesia enables the anesthesiologist to avoid the respiratory depression associated with general anesthesia in these patients.[3,14]

Relief of pain in the early postoperative period is probably the major advantage of caudal anesthesia in children. Several studies have confirmed the benefit of caudal anesthesia for control of postoperative pain following circumcision.[65,73,79,80,130] It would seem to be better than intramuscular (IM) morphine, IM buprenorphine,[80] and IM dihydrocodeine,[13] and at least equivalent to penile block,[130] wound infiltration,[98] and ilioinguinal/iliohypogastric block, when appropriate[17] (see also Caudal Opioids). The following coexistent motor block has, however, been considered a disadvantage by some authors.[126,130] For postoperative pain management, bupivacaine 0.125% with epinephrine 1:200,000 is equianalgesic but has less motor block than 0.25% bupivacaine with epinephrine. Suggested safe infusion rates for caudal bupivacaine are 0.2–0.3 mg/kg/hr in infants and 0.2–0.5 mg/kg/hr in older children, with a limit of 48 hours. Higher infusion rates have given rise to toxicity.[75] Safe guidelines have been described by Berde.[6]

The duration of postoperative analgesia with caudal bupivacaine was significantly increased by the addition of 1 μg/kg of clonidine.[61] Caudal ketamine 0.5 mg/kg is equianalgesic with 0.25% bupivacaine.[85]

Adult Anesthesia

Caudal blockade can be used whenever the area of surgery is primarily innervated by the sacral and lumbar nerve roots. When the area is innervated from a higher level, lumbar epidural blockade and spinal subarachnoid block are preferable techniques. The following procedures are appropriate indications: anal surgery, especially hemorrhoidectomy and anal dilatation, surgery on the vulva and vagina, surgery on the scrotal skin and penis, and surgery of the lower limb. If a caudal catheter is used with its tip positioned higher in the canal, a higher level of anesthesia can be assured and more extensive surgery accommodated. Such procedures could include vaginal hysterectomy and inguinal herniorrhaphy. The use of caudal blockade for relief of postoperative pain following hemorrhoidectomy is well documented[7] and more recently has been recommended for pain relief following lower limb surgery.[76]

Chronic Pain Management

The caudal approach to the epidural space has been used for many years by pain physicians both to diagnose and to treat a variety of largely unspecified low back pain syndromes. In the main, the therapeutic techniques have involved injecting large volumes (up to 64 ml) of diluted procaine, lidocaine, or bupivacaine, with or without steroid, often at a fairly rapid rate.[30,48,87,104] Cure or improvement rates of more than 50% have been claimed[48,56] (see Chapter 28). Rapid injection of large volumes of any solution into the epidural space is not recommended. Such practice can result in large increase in spinal CSF pressure, with a risk of cerebral hemorrhage, visual disturbances, headache, or compromised spinal cord blood flow (spinal stroke). Central nervous system vascular catastrophies are particular hazards in patients with atherosclerosis.

Caudal Opioids

The caudal epidural route has been used for the administration of opioids, with varying claims of success.[12,62,63,95] With the exception of analgesia following hemorrhoidectomy, there is a paucity of studies of the use of caudal opioids in adults. However, in children there are numerous clinical studies comparing the postoperative pain relief obtained from caudal opioids with that obtained from a wide variety of regional anesthetic techniques and drugs given by other routes. From this large amount of literature, the following statements can be made:

1. Caudal morphine is effective and safe and has a prolonged duration of action for postoperative analgesia.[67,96,129]
2. An effective caudal analgesic dose of morphine is 50μg/kg, which gives rise to plasma levels lower than those generally required for systemic analgesia.[129]
3. Caudal morphine gives a significantly longer duration of analgesia than IM/IV morphine or caudal bupivacaine,[63,67,129] but is approximately equivalent to caudal buprenorphine.[47]
4. The addition of fentanyl to caudal solutions of bupivacaine[21] or lidocaine[64] does not prolong the duration of analgesia.
5. Single-shot caudal morphine can provide adequate postoperative analgesia following thoracic surgery.[96]
6. Despite the alleged safety of caudal opioids, respiratory depression is still possible,[66,108] particularly in infants.[119] All the usual precautionary measures must be taken.

In general, the side effects of caudal epidural opioids are similar to those from the more common lumbar epidural route. Certainly itching has been reported and claimed in a single report to be dose-related.[60]

COMPLICATIONS

The range of complications seen with caudal anesthesia is predictable and, in common with most other regional anesthetic procedures, decreases markedly with experience and with meticulous attention to technique (see Chapter 21).[33]

Improper Needle Placement

It is to be expected that in this region of renowned variability of anatomy, malpositioning of the caudal needle, particularly by novices, is not uncommon. There is no substitute for practical experience coupled with a sound knowledge of the possible anatomic variants. The possible consequences of improper needle placement follow.

Absent or Patchy Block

Particularly in an obese patient, the needle may come to lie in the soft tissues superficial to the sacrum. The experienced hand can often detect the absence of firm fixation of the needle that is present when the needle has correctly penetrated the sacrococcygeal ligament. Palpation over the needle tip during rapid injection of air or fluid will detect the appearance of a subcutaneous lump (Fig. 9-7B). With malplacement of the needle under periosteum, either outside the canal or inside the canal anteriorly or posteriorly, the needle will be "fixed," but there will be considerable resistance to injection (Fig. 9-7C).

If the needle is misplaced laterally, it may penetrate a posterior sacral foramen, or it may miss any hiatus and lie in the presacral soft tissues (Figs. 9-7E, 9-7F). In either case, injection may be easy, but absent or patchy block will result. Penetration of a ligament-covered sealed depression (decoy hiatus) may sometimes give the "correct feel," but injection will be impossible (Figs. 9-3I and 9-7D). With any malplacement where periosteum is needled or stretched, the awake patient will feel pain that can be severe. This pain may continue into the postoperative period and give rise to patient complaints. There is no place for persistent clumsy attempts to locate the correct hiatus.

Intravenous or Intraosseous Placement

Claims for a high incidence of local anesthetic toxic reactions during caudal anesthesia are not substantiated by studies.[32] Nevertheless, the potential exists for producing early-onset high blood levels of local anesthetic due either to intravenous or intraosseous injection.[94] The venous plexus of the caudal canal has already been described (Fig. 9-2). When a fine needle is used, free aspiration of blood on entering an epidural vein may not be obvious.

Several cases have been reported of cardiac arrhythmias associated with hemodynamic changes following caudal injection of bupivacaine with adrenaline in children.[31,42,78,121] Of particular interest were case reports of five infants who developed ST segment elevation and increased T-wave amplitude in association with a significant *decrease* in heart rate, but without seizures.[42] The importance of the test dose is again emphasized.

Of at least equal importance in toxicity potential is the possibility of intraosseous injection, produced by penetrating the thin layer of cortical bone of the anterior wall of the sacral canal, in those circumstances when the ligament penetration has not been felt (Fig. 9-7A). The feeling of bone penetration may be confused with that of ligament penetration, and then it is possible that the local anesthetic drug will be injected into the marrow. The result is similar to an intravenous injection with rapid attainment of a high blood level of local anesthetic; this, again, supports the need for use of a test dose. This complication was reported initially following aspiration of marrow cells during clinical caudal anesthesia[35,77] and was reproduced in animal studies.[35] A further, more recent, case has been reported.[125] Any suggestion of a feeling of "granularity" during needle insertion or during attempted aspiration should alert one to the possibility of this hazard; the test dose provides the only practical protection against this complication.

Dural Puncture

With the dural sac ending at S2 level, or approximately on a line joining the posterior-superior iliac spines, dural puncture should be exceedingly rare. An incidence of more than 1% has been quoted,[32] although the rate of consequent accidental spinal block was much lower, at 0.1%. Total spinal anesthesia has been reported following attempted caudal block in infants.[34] A knowledge of the variable distance from the tip of the sac to the apex of the sacral hiatus should warn of the possibility of dural puncture. Advancement of the needle, in adults, by more than 1–2 cm in the sacral canal should be avoided, while in children it should be correspondingly less.

Subdural Injection

As with epidural injection at any level, subdural injection is possible, though less likely, when the needle is inserted via the sacral hiatus. A slow onset but extensive block is highly suggestive of subdural injection.[20]

Injection into Fetus

There have been reports of fetal intoxication by local anesthetic drug injected into the fetal scalp during attempted caudal injection.[40,105] Two babies died. Unfortunately, these isolated reports have done much to discourage the use of caudal anesthesia during labor, despite the fact that the risk exists only when the presenting part has descended to the perineum and questionable techniques are used.

Excessive Spread

Unpredictability of spread of the local anesthetic solution, especially in adults,[28] has already been mentioned. Although *limited* cephalad spread is a more common problem with caudal, on rare occasions *excessive* spread may occur to a high thoracic level, even in the absence of a subarachnoid or subdural injection.[32] This extensive region of blockade is of itself no particular problem. After all, such levels are deliberately sought, with lumbar epidural anesthesia, for a variety of surgical procedures, and the physiologic changes that result are well controlled by simple standard measures. There is, however, a difference in the degree of expectation of these changes, often resulting in a lesser degree of vigilance by the anesthesiologist. One must not forget that the potential exists for a caudal to give rise to a somatic and sympathetic block at least as extensive as a lumbar epidural block, though it is less common. Secure intravenous access, adequate monitoring, and normal resuscitation equipment must be assured (see Chapter 8 for details of management of extensive epidural or total spinal block).

Catheter Problems

Problems from caudal epidural catheters are no different from those that occur with lumbar insertion. Catheter insertion when the needle is correctly placed is generally very easy, occurring more readily than with lumbar insertion. Early resistance to insertion is usually an indication that the needle is incorrectly placed. The catheter should never be withdrawn through the needle because of the risk of shearing it off. Shearing has also been reported when a properly placed needle was being withdrawn over the catheter in the accepted fashion.[26] This was caused by a barb directed toward the lumen, which had developed during a difficult insertion. Dural or venous puncture by the catheter is possible, particularly with older, more rigid catheters with sharper tips. There has also been a case report of a catheter knotting in the caudal canal, requiring neurosurgical exploration for its removal.[26]

Postoperative Problems

Pain

Pain at the injection site is the most common postoperative complaint. Ligament penetration without periosteal trauma will give rise to only minimal pain both during insertion and postoperatively. On the other hand, a periosteal hematoma may cause pain that lasts several weeks. There is no substitute for careful technique, using the information from all landmarks before needle insertion. It is worth remembering that coccygodynia resulting from the stress of childbirth may be erroneously blamed on the caudal block.

Urinary Retention

There seems little doubt that some increased risk of urinary retention occurs after epidural block of the sacral segments, especially when a long-acting local anesthetic drug is used.[15] The likelihood of retention may be greater in those patients who would normally be considered at risk, that is, elderly men, puerperal women, and those who will undergo ano-perineal surgery. These groups, of course, make up the bulk of the indications for adult caudal blockade. A single bladder catheterization should not cause significantly increased morbidity if proper technique is followed.[15]

Infection

Intuitively, one would think that the infection rate would be significantly higher with caudal block than with lumbar epidural block. In a bacteriologic comparison between simultaneous caudal and lumbar epidural catheters (two-catheter technique) during childbirth, cultures were taken from skin at the puncture site, catheter tip, catheter fluid, and catheter subcutaneously.[2] Specimens from the skin surface in the caudal area produced a significantly larger number of positive cultures than did those from the epidural area. This result was repeated when a more extensive skin preparation, including povidone-iodine ointment, was used in the caudal area; however, there were no clinical infections, and in fact all cultures in both areas taken from sites deep into the skin were negative. The study indicates that the risk of infection, although remote, does exist. Compromises in sterile technique have no place in regional anesthesia.

Neurological Complications

In common with lumbar epidural and subarachnoid anesthesia, caudal epidural anesthesia is inevitably associated with some slight risk of neurological damage. In his analysis of complications, Dawkins mentions one permanent lesion in nearly 23,000 cases, but the details are not specified.[32] Whatever the true incidence, it must be very small. Of greater significance is the likelihood that a coexistent neurologic lesion will be blamed on the block. Neurologic sequelae of traumatic vaginal delivery notoriously fall into this group. As anesthesiologists, we need to ensure that our medical colleagues maintain a balanced view of regional anesthetic techniques and that any neurologic lesions be thoroughly examined and investigated. In almost all cases, such investigations will reveal the coincident nature of the lesion (see Chapter 21).

CONCLUSION

Objective data obtained from randomized, prospective, controlled studies are still needed for many aspects of caudal blockade. Such data as are available indicate that caudal block can provide safe, effective analgesia of lumbosacral spinal segments.

The caudal route to the epidural space is particularly attractive in children (see Chapter 20) and in adults who require sacral block. In children, the technique is reliable, easy to perform, and has a consistent dose/spinal segment response relationship. In adults, there is an inevitable failure rate that is higher than that for lumbar epidural block, but with a knowledge of pertinent anatomy and with practical experience, failure rate can be reduced to an acceptable level.

REFERENCES

1. Abouleish, E.: Pain Control in Obstetrics, pp.285. Philadelphia, J.B. Lippincott, 1977.
2. Abouleish, E., Orig, T., and Amortegui, A.J.: Bacteriologic comparison between epidural and caudal techniques. Anesthesiology, *53:*511, 1980.
3. Alexander, C., Wolf, S., and Ghia, J.N.: Caudal anesthesia for early onset myotonic dystrophy. Anesthesiology, *55:*597, 1981.
4. Alexander, J.A., and Franklin, R.R.: Effects of caudal anesthesia on uterine activity. Obstet. Gynecol., *27:*436, 1966.
5. Armitage, E.N.: Caudal block in children. Anaesthesia, *34:*396, 1979.
6. Berde, C.B.: Convulsions associated with pediatric regional anesthesia. Anesth. Analg., *75:*164, 1992.
7. Berstock, D.A.: Haemorrhoidectomy without tears. Ann. R. Coll. Surg. Engl., *61:*51, 1979.
8. Black, M.G.: Anatomic reasons for caudal anesthesia failure. Anesth. Analg (Cleve.), *28:*33, 1949.
9. Bollinger, D., and Mayne, P.: The "whoosh" test in children (letter), Anaesthesia, *47:*1002, 1992.
10. Bonica, J.J.: Principles and Practice of Obstetric Analgesia and Anesthesia. Philadelphia, F.A. Davis, 1967.
11. Bosenberg, A.T., Bland, B.A., Schulte-Steinberg, O., and Downing, J.W.: Thoracic epidural anesthesia via caudal route in infants. Anesthesiology, *69:*265, 1988.
12. Boskovski, N., Lewinski, A., Xuereb, J., and Mercieca, V.: Caudal epidural morphine for postoperative pain relief. Anesthesia, *36:*67, 1981.
13. Bramwell, R.G., Bullen, C., and Radford, P.: Caudal block for postoperative analgesia in children. Anaesthesia, *37:*1024, 1982.
14. Bray, R.J., and Inkster, J.S.: Anaesthesia in babies with congenital dystrophia myotonica. Anaesthesia, *39:*1007, 1984.
15. Bridenbaugh, L.D.: Catheterization after long- and short-acting local

anesthetics for continuous caudal block for vaginal delivery. Anesthesiology, *46:*357, 1977.

16. Bromage, P.R.: Ageing and epidural dose requirements: Segmental spread and predictability of epidural analgesia in youth and extreme age. Br. J. Anaesth., *41:*1016, 1969.
17. Bromage, P.R.: Epidural Analgesia. Philadelphia, W.B. Saunders, 1978.
18. Busoni, P., and Andreuccetti, T.: The spread of caudal analgesia in children: A mathematical model. Anaesth. Intensive Care, *14:*140, 1986.
19. Busoni, P., and Sarti, A.: Sacral intervertebral epidural block. Anesthesiology, *67:*993, 1987.
20. Calder, T.M., and Harris, A.P.: Subdural block during attempted caudal epidural analgesia for labor. Anesthesiology, *76:*316, 1992.
21. Campbell, F.A., Yentis, S.M., Fear, D.W., and Bissonnette, B.: Analgesic efficacy and safety of a caudal bupivacaine–fentanyl mixture in children. Can. J. Anaesth., *39:*661, 1992.
22. Camboulives, J., Couvely, J.P., Alphonsi, R., and Unal, D.: Plasma determination of lidocaine and bupivacaine after caudal anesthesia in children. Ann. Fr. Anesth. Reanim., *5:*115, 1986.
23. Cathelin, M.F.: Une nouvelle voie d'injection rachidienne: Methôde des injections épidurales pas le procède du canal sacre. C.R. Soc. Biol. (Paris), *53:*452, 1901.
24. Chan, S.Y., Tay, H.B., and Thomas, E.: "Whoosh" test as a teaching aid in caudal block. Anaesth. Intensive Care, *21:*414, 1993.
25. Charlton, A.J., and Lindahl, S.G.E.: Ventilatory response during halothane and enflurane anaesthesia. Anaesthesia, *40:*18, 1985.
26. Chun, L., and Karp, M.: Unusual complications from placement of catheters in caudal canal in obstetrical anesthesia. Anesthesiology, *27:*96, 1966.
27. Cleland, J.G.P.: Continuous peridural and caudal analgesia in obstetrics. Anesth. Analg., *28:*61, 1949.
28. Cousins, M.J., and Bromage, P.R.: A comparison of the hydrochloride and carbonated salts of lignocaine for caudal analgesia in outpatients. Br. J. Anaesth., *43:*1149, 1971.
29. Cross, G.D., and Barrett, R.F.: Comparison of two regional techniques for postoperative analgesia in children following herniotomy and orchidopexy. Anaesthesia, *42:*845, 1987.
30. Cyriax, J.H.: Textbook of orthopaedic medicine. Diagnosis of soft tissue lesions. Vol 1., London, Bailliere Tindall, 1978.
31. Dalens, B., and Hasnaoui, A.: Caudal anesthesia in pediatric surgery: Success rate and adverse effects in 750 consecutive patients. Anesth. Analg., *68:*83, 1989.
32. Dawkins, C.J.M.: An analysis of the complications of extradural and caudal block. Anaesthesia, *24:*554, 1969.
33. DeJong, R.H.: Anesthetic complications during continuous caudal analgesia for obstetrics: Analysis of 826 cases. Anesth. Analg. (Cleve), *40:*384, 1961.
34. Desparmet, J.F.: Total spinal anesthesia after caudal anesthesia in an infant. Anesth. Analg., *70:*665, 1990.
35. DiGiovanni, A.J.: Inadvertent intraosseous injection—A hazard of caudal anesthesia. Anesthesiology, *34:*92, 1971.
36. Ecoffey, C., Desparmet, J., Berdeaux, A., and Maury, M., *et al.*: Pharmacokinetics of lignocaine in children following caudal anaesthesia. Br. J. Anaesth., *56:*1399, 1984.
37. Ecoffey, C., Desparmet, J., Maury, M., Berdeaux, A., *et al.*: Bupivacaine in children: Pharmacokinetics following caudal anesthesia. Anesthesiology, *63:*447, 1985.
38. Eyres, R.L., Kidd, J., Oppenheim, R., and Brown, T.C.K.: Local anaesthetic plasma levels in children. Anaesth. Intensive Care, *6:*243, 1978.
39. Fernandez-Sepulveda, R., and Gomez-Rogers, C.: Single dose caudal anesthesia: Its effect on uterine contractility. Am. J. Obstet. Gynecol., *98:*847, 1967.
40. Finster, M., Poppers, P.J., Sinclair, J.C., Morishima, H.O., *et al.*: Accidental intoxication of the fetus with local anesthetic drug during caudal anesthesia. Am. J. Obstet. Gynecol., *92:*922, 1965.
41. Fortuna, A.: Caudal analgesia: A simple and safe technique in paediatric surgery. Br. J. Anaesth., *39:*165, 1967.
42. Freid, E.B., Bailey, A.G., and Valley, R.D.: Electrocardiographic and haemodynamic changes associated with unintentional intravascular injection of bupivacaine with adrenaline in infants. Anesthesiology, *79:*394, 1993.
43. Freund, P.R., Bowdle, T.A., Slattery, J.T., and Bell, L.E.: Caudal anesthesia with lidocaine or bupivacaine: Plasma local anesthetic concentration and extent of sensory spread in old and young patients. Anesth. Analg., *63:*1017, 1984.
44. Galindo, A., Benavides, O., Ortega De Munos, S., Bonilla, O., *et al.*: Comparison of anesthetic solutions used in lumbar and caudal peridural anesthesia. Anesth. Analg., *57:*175, 1978.
45. Giaufre, E., Conte-Devolx, B., Morrison-Lacombe, G., Boudouresque, F., *et al.*: Caudal epidural anesthesia in children: Study of endocrine changes. Presse Med., *14:*201, 1985.
46. Giaufre, E., Le Gal, M., and Trinquet, F.: Clinical study of EMLA analgesic cream in pediatric regional anesthesia. Ann. Fr. Anesth. Reanim., *11:*384, 1992.
47. Girotra, S., Kumar, S., and Rajendran, K.M.: Comparison of caudal morphine and buprenorphine for postoperative analgesia in children. Eur. J. Anaesthesiol., *10:*309, 1993.
48. Gordon, J.: Caudal extradural injection for the treatment of low back pain. Anaesthesia, *35:*515, 1980.
49. Guinard, J.P., and Borboen, M.: Probable venous air embolism during caudal anesthesia in a child. Anesth. Analg., *76:*1134, 1993.
50. Gunter, J.B., and Eng, C.: Thoracic epidural anesthesia via the caudal approach in children. Anesthesiology, *76:*935, 1992.
51. Gunter, J.B., Watcha, M.F., Forestner, J.B., Hirshberg, G.E., *et al.*: Caudal epidural anesthesia in conscious premature and high-risk infants. J. Pediatr. Surg., *26:*9, 1991.
52. Gunther, R.E., and Bellville, J.W.: Obstetrical caudal anesthesia: II. A randomized study comparing 1 percent mepivacaine with 1 percent mepivacaine plus epinephrine. Anesthesiology, *37:*288, 1972.
53. Hansen, J.M., and Ueland, K.: The influence of caudal analgesia on cardiovascular dynamics during normal labour and delivery. Acta Anaesthesiol. Scand., *23* (Suppl):449, 1966.
54. Hassan, S.Z.: Caudal anesthesia in infants. Anesth. Analg., *56:*686, 1977.
55. Hatch, D.J., Hulse, M.G., and Lindahl, S.G.: Caudal analgesia in children: Influence on ventilatory efficiency during halothane anaesthesia. Anaesthesia *39:*873, 1984.
56. Hauswirth, R., and Michot, F.: Sacral epidural anesthesia in the treatment of lumbosacral backache. Schweiz Med. Wochenschr., *112:*222, 1982.
57. Henderson, K., Sethna, N.F., and Berde, C.B.: Continuous caudal anesthesia for inguinal hernia repair in former preterm infants. J. Clin. Anesth, *5:*129, 1993.
58. Hingson, R.A., Cull, W.A., and Benzinger, M.: Continuous caudal analgesia in obstetrics: Combined experience of a quarter of a century in clinics in New York, Philadelphia, Memphis, Baltimore, and Cleveland. Anesth. Analg. (Cleve.), *40:*119, 1961.
59. Hingson, R.A., and Edwards, W.B.: Continuous caudal analgesia: An analysis of the first ten thousand confinements thus managed with the report of the authors' first thousand cases. J.A.M.A., *123:*538, 1943.
60. Hirlekar, G.: Is itching after caudal epidural morphine dose related? Anaesthesia, *36:*68, 1981.
61. Jamali, S., Monin, S., Begon, C., Dubousset, A.M., *et al.*: Clonidine in pediatric caudal anesthesia. Anesth. Analg., *786:*633, 1994.
62. Jensen, B.H.: Caudal block for post-operative pain relief in children after genital operations: A comparison between bupivacaine and morphine. Acta Anaesthesiol. Scand., *25:*373, 1981.
63. Jensen, P.J., Siem-Jorgensen, P., Nielsen, T.B., Wichmand-Nielson, H.: Epidural morphine by the caudal route for postoperative pain relief. Acta Anaesthesiol. Scand., *26:*511, 1982.
64. Jones, R.D., Gunawardene, W.M., and Yeung, C.K.: A comparison of lignocaine 2% with adrenaline 1:200,000 and lignocaine 2% with adrenaline 1:200,000 plus fentanyl as agents for caudal anaesthesia in children undergoing circumcision. Anaesth. Intensive Care, *18:*194, 1990.
65. Kay, B.: Caudal block for postoperative pain relief in children. Anaesthesia, *29:*610, 1974.
66. Krane, E.J.: Delayed respiratory depression in a child after caudal epidural morphine. Anesth. Analg., *67:*79, 1988.
67. Krane, E.J., Jacobsen, L.E., Lynn, A.M., Parrot, C., *et al.*: Caudal morphine for postoperative analgesia in children: A comparison with caudal bupivacaine and intravenous morphine. Anesth. Analg., *66:*647, 1987.
68. Larsen, M.D., Sessler, D.I., Ozaki, M., McGuire, J., *et al.*: Pupillary assessment of sensory block level during combined epidural/general anesthesia. Anesthesiology, *79:*42, 1993.
69. Letterman, G.S., and Trotter, M.: Variations of the male sacrum: Their significance in caudal analgesia. Surg. Gynecol. Obstet., *78:*551, 1944.

70. Lewis, M.P., Thomas, P., Wilson, L.F., and Mulholland, R.C.: The "whoosh" test: A clinical test to confirm correct needle placement in caudal epidural injections. Anaesthesia, *47:*57, 1992.
71. Lim, E.T., Chong, K.Y., Singh, B., and Jong, W.: Use of warm local anaesthetic solution for caudal blocks. Anaesth. Intensive Care, *20:*453, 1992.
72. Loury, C.J., and McDonald, I.H.: Caudal anaesthesia in infants and children. Anaesth. Intensive Care, *1:*547, 1973.
73. Lunn, J.N.: Postoperative analgesia after circumcision: A randomized comparison between caudal analgesia and intramuscular morphine in boys. Anaesthesia, *34:*552, 1979.
74. McCaul, K.: Caudal blockade. *In* Cousins M.J., and Bridenbaugh, P.O. (eds.): Neural Blockade in Clinical Anesthesia and Management of Pain. 1st ed. pp. 275–293. Philadelphia, J.B. Lippincott, 1980.
75. McCloskey, J.J., Haun, S.E., and Deshpande, J.K.: Bupivacaine toxicity secondary to continuous caudal epidural infusion in children. Anesth. Analg., *75:*287, 1992.
76. McCrirrick, A., and Ramage, D.T.: Caudal blockade for postoperative analgesia: A useful adjunct to intramuscular opiates following emergency lower leg orthopaedic surgery. Anaesth. Intensive Care, *19:*551, 1991.
77. McGown, R.G.: Accidental marrow sampling during caudal anaesthesia. Br. J. Anaesth, *44:*613, 1972.
78. McGown, R.G.: Caudal analgesia in children. Anaesthesia, *37:*806, 1982.
79. Martin, L.V.: Postoperative analgesia after circumcision in children. Br. J. Anaesth., *54:*1263, 1982.
80. May, A.E., Wandless, J., and James, R.H.: Analgesia for circumcision in children. A comparison of caudal bupivacaine and intramuscular buprenorphine. Acta Anaesthesiol. Scand., *26:*331, 1982.
81. Mazoit, J.X., Denson, D.D., and Samii, K.: Pharmacokinetics of bupivacaine following caudal anesthesia in infants. Anesthesiology, *68:*387, 1988.
82. Mazze, R.I., and Dunbar, R.W.: Plasma lidocaine concentrations after caudal, lumbar epidural, axillary block, and intravenous regional anesthesia. Anesthesiology, *27:*574, 1966.
83. Mohan, J., and Potter, J.M.: Pupillary constriction and ptosis following caudal epidural analgesia. Anaesthesia, *30:*769, 1975.
84. Moore, D.C., Bridenbaugh, L.D., Bagdi, P.A., and Bridenbaugh, P.O.: Accumulation of mepivacaine hydrochloride during caudal block. Anesthesiology, *29:*585, 1968.
85. Naguib, M., Sharif, A.M., Seraj, M., el Gammal, M., *et al.*: Ketamine for caudal analgesia in children: Comparison with caudal bupivacaine. Br. J. Anaesth., *67:*559, 1991.
86. Nakamura, T., and Takasaki, M.: Metabolic and endocrine responses to surgery during caudal analgesia in children. Can. J. Anaesth., *38:*969, 1991.
87. Natelson, S.E., Gibson, C.E., and Gillespie, R.A.: Caudal block: Cost-effective primary treatment for back pain. South. Med. J., *73:*286, 1980.
88. Norenberg, A., Johanson, D.C., and Gravenstein, J.S.: Racial differences in sacral structure important in caudal anesthesia. Anesthesiology, *50:*549, 1979.
89. Owens, W.D., Slater, E.M., and Battit, G.E.: A new technique of caudal anesthesia. Anesthesiology, *39:*451, 1973.
90. Park, W.Y., Massengale, M., and MacNamara, T.E., Age, height, and speed of injection as factors determining caudal anesthetic level, and occurrence of severe hypertension. Anesthesiology, *51:*81, 1979.
91. Paull, J.D.: The place of caudal anaesthesia in obstetrics. Anaesth. Intensive Care, *18:*313, 1990.
92. Payen, D., Ecoffey, C., Carli, P., and Dubousset, A.M.: Pulsed Doppler ascending aortic, carotid, brachial and femoral artery blood flows during caudal anesthesia in infants. Anesthesiology, *67:*681, 1987.
93. Peutrell, J.M., and Hughes, D.G.: Epidural anaesthesia through caudal catheters for inguinal herniotomies in awake ex-premature babies. Anaesthesia, *48:*128, 1993.
94. Prentiss, J.E.: Cardiac arrest following caudal anesthesia. Anesthesiology, *50:*51, 1979.
95. Pybus, D.A., Dubras, B.E., Goulding, G., Liberman, H., *et al.*: Postoperative analgesia for haemorrhoid surgery. Anaesth. Intensive Care, *11:*27, 1983.
96. Rosen, K.R., and Rosen, D.A.: Caudal epidural morphine for control of pain following open heart surgery in children. Anesthesiology, *70:*418, 1989.
97. Satoyoshi, M., and Kamiyama, K.: Caudal anaesthesia for upper abdominal surgery in infants and children: A simple calculation of the volume of local anaesthetic. Acta Anaesthesiol. Scand. *28:*57, 1984.
98. Schindler, M., Swann, M., and Crawford, M.: A comparison of postoperative analgesia provided by wound infiltration or caudal anaesthesia. Anaesth. Intensive Care, *19:*46, 1991.
99. Schulte-Steinburg, O.: Spread of extradural analgesia following caudal injection in children. Br. J. Anaesth., *50:*973, 1978.
100. Schulte-Steinberg, O., and Rahlfs, V.W.: Caudal anesthesia in children. Anesthesiology, *49:*372, 1978.
101. Schulte-Steinberg, O., and Rahlfs, V.W.: Caudal anaesthesia in children and spread of 1 percent lignocaine: A statistical study. Br. J. Anaesth., *42:*1093, 1970.
102. Schulte-Steinberg, O., and Rahlfs, V.W.: Spread of extradural analgesia following caudal injection in children: A statistical study. Br. J. Anaesth., *49:*1027, 1977.
103. Seow, L.T., Chiu, H.H., and Tye, C.Y.: Clinical evaluation of etidocaine in continuous caudal analgesia for pelvic floor repair and postoperative pain relief. Anaesth. Intensive Care, *4:*239, 1976.
104. Sharma, P.K.: Indications, technique and results of caudal epidural injection for lumbar disc retropulsion. Postgrad. Med. J., *53:*1, 1977.
105. Sinclair, J.C., Fox, H.A., Lentz, J.F., Fuld, G.L., *et al.*: Intoxication of the fetus by a local anesthetic: A newly recognized complication of maternal caudal anesthesia. N. Engl. J. Med., *273:*1173, 1965.
106. Spear, R.M., Deshpande, J.K.M., and Maxwell, L.G.: Caudal anesthesia in the awake high-risk infant. Anesthesiology, *69:*407, 1988.
107. Spiegel, P.: Caudal anesthesia in pediatric surgery: A preliminary report. Anesth. Analg., *41:*218, 1962.
108. Steinstra, R., and Van Poorten, F.: Immediate respiratory arrest after caudal epidural sufentanil. Anesthesiology, *71:*993, 1989.
109. Takasaki, M.: Blood concentrations of lidocaine, mepivacaine and bupivacaine during caudal analgesia in children. Acta Anaesthesiol. Scand., *28:*211, 1984.
110. Takasaki, M., Dohi, S., Kawabata, Y., and Takahashi, T.: Dosage of lidocaine for caudal anesthesia in infants and children. Anesthesiology, *47:*527, 1977.
111. Thompson, J.E.: An anatomical and experimental study of sacral anaesthesia. Ann. Surg., *66:*718, 1917.
112. Tobias, J.D., Flannagan, J., Brock, J., and Brin, E.: Neonatal regional anesthesia: Alternative to general anesthesia for urologic surgery. Urology, *41:*362, 1993.
113. Tobias, J.D., Lowe, S., and O'Dell, N.: Continuous regional anaesthesia in infants. Can. J. Anaesth., *40:*1065, 1993.
114. Touloukian, R.J., Wugmeister, M., Pickett, L.K., and Hehre, F.W.: Caudal anesthesia for neonatal anoperineal and rectal operations. Anesth. Analg. (Cleve.), *50:*565, 1971.
115. Trotter, M.: Variations of the sacral canal: Their significance in the administration of caudal analgesia. Anesth. Analg., *26:*192, 1947.
116. Trotter, M., and Letterman, G.S.: Variations of the female sacrum: Their significance in continuous caudal anaesthesia. Surg. Gynecol. Obstet., *78:*419, 1944.
117. Tyack, A.G., Parsons, R.J., Millar, D.R., and Nicholas, A.D.G.: Uterine activity and plasma bupivacaine levels after caudal epidural analgesia. J. Obstet. Gynaecol. Br. Common W., *80:*896, 1973.
118. Ueland, K., and Hansen, J.M.: Maternal cardiovascular dynamics III: Labour and delivery under local and caudal analgesia. Am. J. Obstet. Gynecol., *103:*8, 1969.
119. Valley, R.D., and Bailey, R.G.: Caudal morphine for postoperative analgesia in infants: A report of 138 cases. Anesth. Analg., *72:*120, 1991.
120. Vater, M., and Wandless, J.: Caudal or dorsal nerve block? A comparison of two local anaesthetic techniques for postoperative analgesia following day case circumcision. Acta Anaesthesiol. Scand., *29:*175, 1985.
121. Ved, S.A., Pinosky, M., and Nicodemus, H.: Ventricular tachycardia and brief cardiovascular collapse in two infants after caudal anesthesia using a bupivacaine–epinephrine solution. Anesthesiology, *79:*1121, 1993.
122. Veyckemans, F., Van Obbergh, L.J., and Gouverneur, J.M.: Lessons from 1,100 pediatric caudal blocks in a teaching hospital. Reg. Anesth., *17:*119, 1992.
123. Warner, M.A., Kunkel, S.E., Offord, K.O.: The effects of age, epinephrine, and operative site on duration of caudal analgesia in pediatric patients. Anesth Analg., *66:*995, 1987.
124. Watcha, M.F., Thach, B.T., and Gunter, J.B.: Postoperative apnea af-

ter caudal anesthesia in an ex-premature infant. Anesthesiology, *71:*613, 1989.

125. Weber, S.: Caudal anesthesia complicated by intraosseous injection in a patient with ankylosing spondylitis. Anesthesiology, *63:*716, 1985.
126. White, J., Harrison, B., Richmond, P., Proctor, A., *et al.*: Postoperative analgesia for circumcision. Br. Med. J., *286:*1934, 1983.
127. Williams, N.E., Hardy, P.A., and Evans, A.F.: Spread of local anaesthetic solutions following sacral extradural (caudal) block: Influence of posture. J. Spinal Disord., *2:*249, 1989.
128. Willis, R.J., and Macintyre, P.E.: The effect of dose and drug on the spread of caudal anaesthesia. (Unpublished personal communication).
129. Wolf, A.R., Hughes, D., Hobbs, A.J., and Prys-Roberts, C.: Combined morphine–bupivacaine caudals for reconstructive penile surgery in children: Systemic absorption of morphine and postoperative analgesia. Anaesth. Intensive Care, *19:*17, 1991.
130. Yeoman, P.M., Cooke, R., and Hain, W.R.: Penile block for circumcision: A comparison with caudal blockade. Anaesthesia, *38:*862, 1983.
131. Zaaijman, J.D., and Slabber, C.F.: The position of epidural catheters in obstetric regional anaesthesia. S. Afr. Med. J., *55:*915, 1979.

B

Extremities

Neural Blockade in Clinical Anesthesia and Management of Pain, Third Edition,
edited by M.J. Cousins and P.O. Bridenbaugh.
Lippincott–Raven Publishers, Philadelphia © 1998.

CHAPTER 10

The Upper Extremity

Somatic Block

David L. Brown and L. Donald Bridenbaugh

All of the deep structures of the upper extremity and the skin distal to the middle of the upper arm are rendered insensitive by blocking the brachial plexus. The nerves of the plexus may be blocked anywhere along their course: from their emergence from intervertebral foramina and entrance into the sheath between the anterior and middle scalene muscles until they terminate in the specific nerves in the hand. Techniques for blocking of the plexus involve infiltration at one of five anatomic areas—that is, paravertebral (interscalene), supraclavicular, infraclavicular, in the axilla, and by blocking the specific terminal nerves. Thus, any surgical procedure on the arm—for example, reduction of fractures or dislocations, suturing of tendons, or repair of lacerations—is an indication for the use of this kind of anesthesia. In spite of the wide applicability of upper extremity somatic block, the fundamental issue for brachial plexus block or general anesthetic procedure frequently is the desire of the patient or the surgeon, or even the abilities of the anesthesiologist.

HISTORY

Brachial plexus nerve block was performed first by Halsted in 1884, when he "freed the cords and nerves of the brachial plexus, after blocking the roots in the neck with cocaine solution." In 1887, Crile disarticulated a shoulder joint after rendering a patient's arm insensitive by blocking the "brachial plexus by direct intraneural injection of each nerve trunk with 0.5 percent cocaine under direct vision."[18] In 1911, Hirschel and Kulenkampff, working independently, were the first to inject the brachial plexus percutaneously (blindly through the skin), without exposure of the nerves.[24,28] There have been many subsequent modifications of these original techniques, varying mostly according to site; they include the following: interscalene, supraclavicular, infraclavicular, axillary, and continuous techniques.[12,19,23,25,28,30,32,35,39,42,47–49,56–58,60,62,68,71–73] With the introduction of barbiturates and cyclopropane, the enthusiasm for block anesthesia waned in the early 1940s. In current years, however, the technique has had a resurgence, due in large part to increased understanding of neural plasticity and the possibility of minimizing hospital length-of-stay by effective use of regional block anesthesia.

Advantages

Brachial plexus block, like all other regional anesthetics, offers specific advantages to the patient, surgeon, anesthesiologist, and surgical facility, that may not be true for use of general anesthesia. These include the following:

1. *The anesthesia is limited to a restricted portion of the body on which the surgery will be performed*, leaving the other vital centers unaffected. The physiologic impact of the anesthesia on the patient may be less than with general anesthesia because metabolism of the rest of the body is undisturbed. This consideration is important in the poor-risk patient, who may not tolerate the stress imposed by general anesthesia. Patients who have complicating conditions, such as heart, renal, and pulmonary disease, chest injuries, diabetes, etc., are able to withstand surgery performed with brachial block anesthesia, without aggravation of the disease. This does not imply that the technique should be reserved only for poor-risk patients. On the contrary, nearly all patients who present themselves for surgery of the upper ex-

D. L. Brown: Department of Anesthesia, University of Iowa, Iowa City, Iowa 52242.
L. D. Bridenbaugh: Department of Anesthesiology, Virginia Mason Medical Center, Seattle, Washington 98111.

tremity can be afforded the benefits of this form of regional anesthesia.

2. *It is possible and desirable for the patient to remain ambulatory.* Outpatients may be sent home after procedures such as closed reduction of fractures or repair of lacerations. Brachial plexus block is also of benefit in aged patients, for whom early ambulation minimizes bed-rest related complications.
3. *The use of brachial block may minimize development of central nervous system hyperexcitability during a surgical procedure carried out during general anesthesia.* The use of brachial block may minimize the development of pathophysiologic neuropathic pain states, which occasionally follow even routine elective or emergent upper extremity operations. More specifically, patients who undergo upper extremity amputation may have a lower incidence of phantom limb pain than those who have the amputation carried out during general anesthesia.
4. *Whenever fluoroscopy is a necessary adjunct to the surgical procedure, brachial plexus block eliminates the potential general anesthetic dangers of explosions, respiratory depression, or airway obstruction in a darkened room* in which the patient cannot be readily observed. It also permits the patient to cooperate with the surgeon or the radiologist.
5. *Postanesthetic nausea, vomiting, and other side-effects of general anesthesia, such as atelectasis, hypotension, ileus, and dehydration, are reduced.* This allows the patients to advance their diets, and thus, to benefit from oral feeding earlier in the perioperative period.
6. *Prolonged operations on the upper extremity, if they are performed with general anesthesia, are sometimes followed by postoperative cardiovascular and CNS depression* because of the comparatively large doses of drugs required. Complex operations, such as tendon repairs and plastic procedures, can therefore have complications or side-effects out of proportion to the surgical procedure.
7. *Brachial plexus block anesthesia allows patients who fear losing consciousness ("control") to be awake.* If it is effectively performed, brachial plexus block provides a minimum degree of discomfort to the patient.
8. *Patients who present for surgery with an upper extremity at risk of vascular compromise may improve as soon as the pain has been relieved and vasodilation has been produced by the block.* The improved circulation resulting from the associated sympathetic blockade may be a positive factor in the prognosis of the traumatized upper extremity, which often has areas of severely compromised circulation and questionable tissue viability.
9. *Patients who arrive at surgery with full stomachs face less danger of aspiration if they vomit.* Aspiration remains one of the primary risks for patients emergently undergoing general anesthesia with a full stomach.
10. *Ideal operating conditions can be obtained to meet surgical requirements.* Complete motor relaxation can be accomplished. If it is desirable to have the patient move and cooperate—such as for surgical repair of tendons—this can also be accomplished by using a lower concentration of the local anesthetic.
11. *If an anesthesiologist is not continuously present, such as in rural regions, or during wartime, brachial block anesthesia permits the maximum utilization of special expertise.* The surgeon can perform the block and then perform the operation, or one anesthesiologist can furnish anesthesia for more than one patient.
12. *Post-anesthesia care unit (PACU) and ward nurses particularly appreciate the use of regional anesthesia.* Patients who return to the PACU, or to the wards, awake, without nausea or vomiting, and are able to help themselves immediately, allow nursing staff to direct their efforts to more dependent patients.

Anatomy

The brachial plexus supplies all of the motor and almost all of the sensory function of the upper extremity. The remaining area—the skin over the shoulder—is supplied by

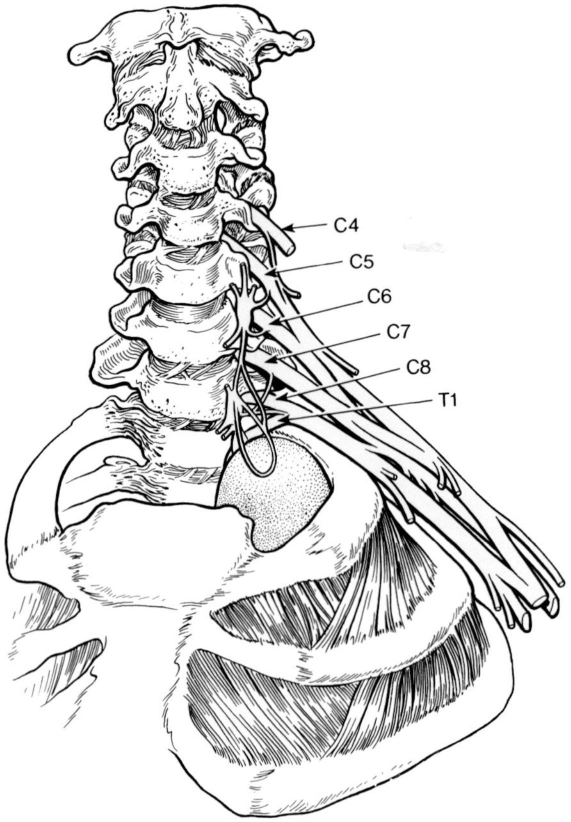

FIG. 10-1. Brachial plexus. Note the components of the plexus and the relationship to intervertebral foramina and "gutters" of transverse processes.

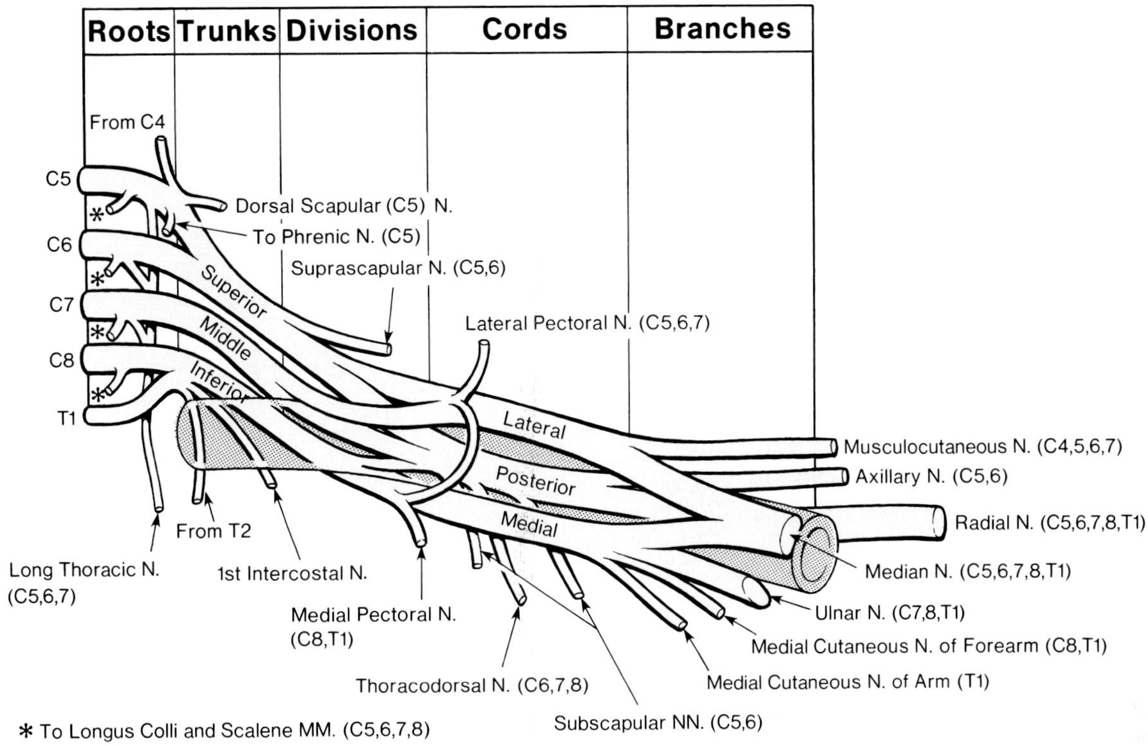

FIG. 10-2. Roots, trunks, divisions, cords, and branches of brachial plexus. Note also relationship to subclavian artery. Note that the intercostobrachial nerve is not shown in this diagram. N, nerve; M, muscle.

the caudad branches of the cervical plexus, and the posterior medial aspect of the arm, extending nearly to the elbow, is supplied by the medial cutaneous nerve of the arm and the intercostobrachial branch of the second intercostal nerve. The plexus is formed from the anterior primary rami of the fifth, sixth, seventh, and eighth cervical and the first thoracic nerves, and frequently receives small contributing branches from the fourth cervical and second thoracic nerve (Fig. 10-1).

After these nerves leave their respective intervertebral foramina, they proceed anterolaterally and caudally to occupy the interval between the anterior and middle scalene muscles, where they unite to form three trunks, thus initiating the formation of the plexus proper. These trunks emerge from the interscalene space at the lower border of these muscles and continue anterolaterally and inferiorly to converge toward the upper surface of the first rib, where they are closely grouped cephaloposterior to the subclavian artery. (It is to be noted that, as the newly formed trunks approach the first rib, they are arranged according to their designations as "superior," "middle," and "inferior"—i.e., one above the other, vertically, not next to the others, horizontally, as they are depicted in many texts). At the lateral edge of the rib, each trunk divides into an anterior and posterior division, each of which pass inferior to the midportion of the clavicle, to enter the axilla through its apex. These divisions, by which fibers of the trunk reassemble to innervate the ventral and dorsal aspects of the limb, reunite within the axilla to form three cords—the lateral, medial, and posterior—named because of their relationship with the second part of the axillary artery.

At the lateral border of the pectoralis minor, the three cords break up to give rise to the peripheral nerves of the upper extremity. The lateral cord gives off the lateral head of the median nerve and the musculocutaneous nerve; the medial cord gives off the medial head of the median nerve, the ulnar, the medial antebrachial, and the medial brachial cutaneous nerves; and the posterior cord terminates as the axillary and radial nerves (Fig. 10-2).

In its course, the brachial plexus is closely related to specific osseous and fascial structures, some of which serve as important landmarks during the injection of the anesthetic. In its position between the anterior and middle scalene muscles, the plexus lies superior and posterior to the second and third parts of the subclavian artery, which is also located between the two muscles. Anteromedial to the lower trunk and posteromedial to the artery lies the dome of the pleura.

Livingston and Werthein originally pointed out, and Winnie has refocused our attention on, the fascial barriers that surround these structures.[39,68,73] The prevertebral fascia divides to invest the anterior and middle scalene muscles and then fuses at the lateral margins to form an enclosed interscalene space. Therefore, as the nerve roots leave the trans-

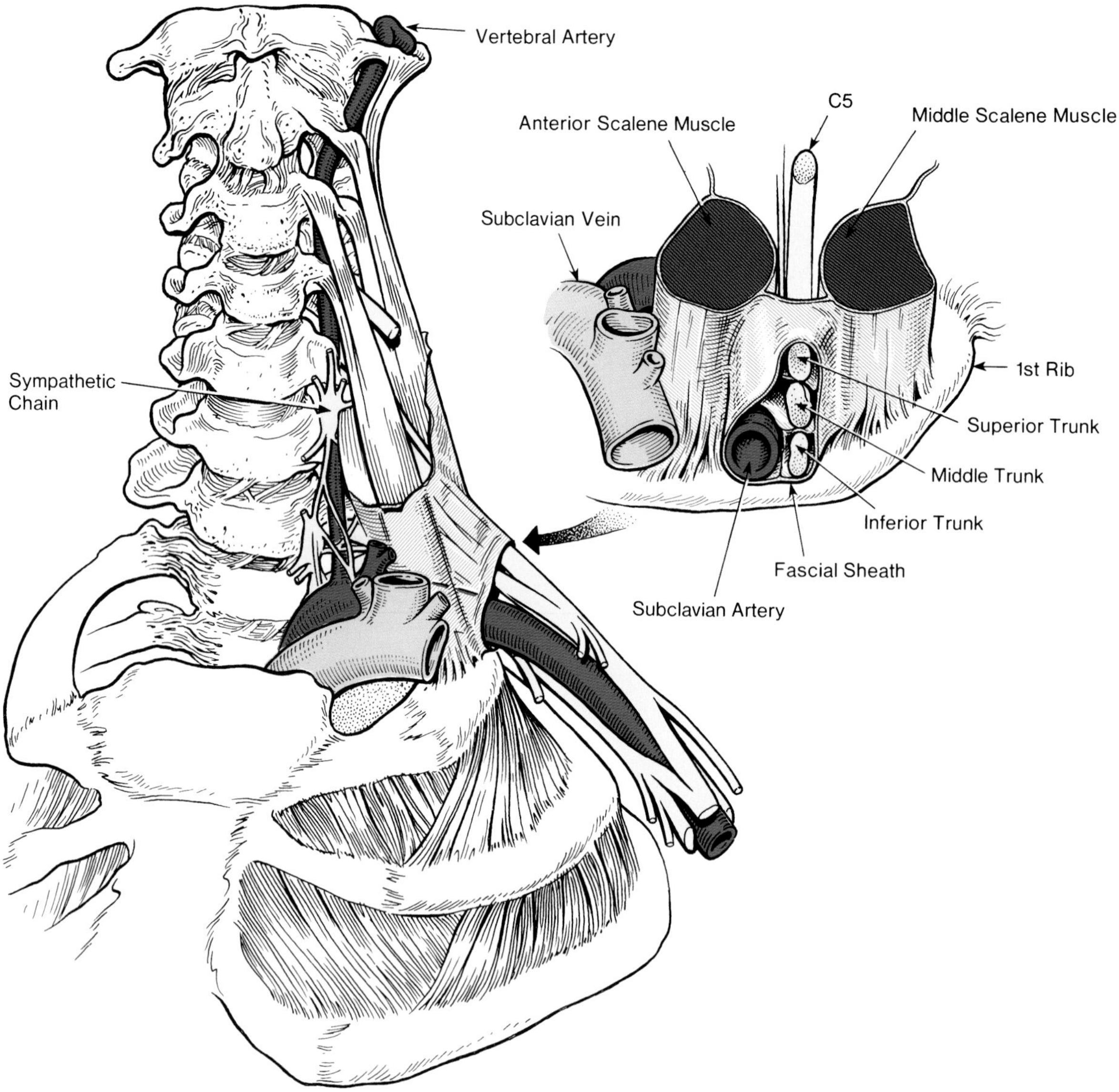

FIG. 10-3. Brachial plexus sheath and scalene muscles. Note brachial plexus "sandwiched" between anterior and middle scalene muscles, prevertebral fascia splitting to enclose scalenes and then forming a fascial sheath around the brachial plexus. Note also relationships to vertebral artery, subclavian artery, and sympathetic chain.

verse processes, they emerge between the fascia that covers the anterior and middle scalene muscles; and, in their descent toward the first rib to form the trunks of the plexus, the roots may be considered to be "sandwiched" between the anterior and middle scalene muscles, the fascia of which serves as a "sheath" of the plexus (Fig. 10-3). As the roots pass through this space, they converge to form the trunks of the brachial plexus and, together with the subclavian artery, invaginate the scalene fascia which forms a subclavian perivascular sheath. This, in turn, becomes the axillary sheath as it passes under the clavicle (Fig. 10-4). It is important for the anesthesiologist to recognize a continuous fascia-enclosed space, extending from the cervical transverse process to several centimeters beyond the axilla, and enclosing the entire brachial plexus, from the cervical roots to the great nerves of the upper arm. All the techniques for blocking the brachial plexus involve the location of the nerves and injection of the local anesthetic within the fascial sheath.

PATIENT CARE, DRUGS, AND EQUIPMENT

Premedication

Patients presenting for upper extremity block may be accident cases in whom opportunities for formal preparation and early premedication may not be possible. Accordingly,

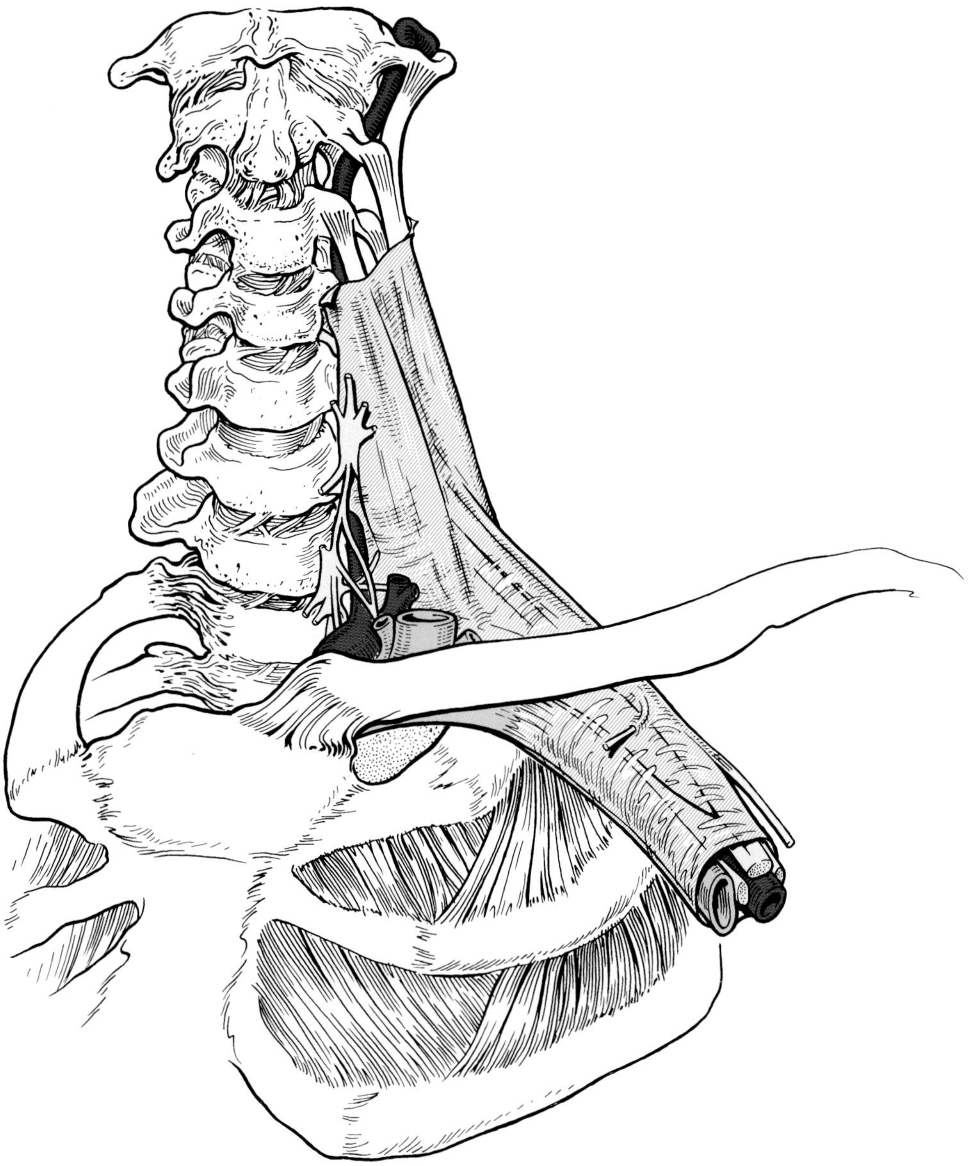

FIG. 10-4. Brachial plexus sheath extending from interscalene to subclavian and axillary regions. Note the brachial plexus enclosed in a vertical tube (the interscalene fascia or sheath), which is invaginated to form a horizontal tube (the subclavian and axillary sheath). An expanded view at the level of axillary block is shown in Fig. 10-8B.

the following points should be noted. First, the best way to achieve adequate pain relief is to provide neural blockade as quickly as possible. Second, patients who have sustained injuries to their hands are especially anxious about the outcome. Third, fractures are most common in children and the elderly. Fourth, many patients can be treated as outpatients; and last, because paresthesias are sought to facilitate many upper limb blocks, cooperation of the patient is required.

For both elective surgery and, where practicable, with emergencies, premedication is strongly recommended, preferably a narcotic (25 to 100 μg of fentanyl) combined with small doses of benzodiazepine (1.0 mg of midazolam) or another mild sedative. It is important that the patient be alert and cooperative enough for administration of the block procedure, but not distressed by it (see Chapter 6).

Intraoperative Analgesia and Sedation

Requirements for intraoperative analgesia and sedation depend on the patient's preference, the effects of premedication, the duration of the surgical procedure, additional stimuli such as a tourniquet, and the possibility of need for active tendon movement during stages of the operation. Even though complete analgesia is provided by nerve block, intraoperative sedation and additional analgesia may still be advisable, such as a combination of fentanyl and midazolam, a low-dose infusion of propofol, or even small, intermittent, doses of thiopental (see Chapter 6).

Postoperative Analgesia

Pain may not be prominent after surgery on the upper limb. It is usually relieved by simple oral analgesics and the release of compression dressings, if this is appropriate. Except in situations of extensive surgery and trauma, when stronger analgesics may be required for a short time, severe pain should be regarded as a sign of possible surgical complication. Because of this, the use of bupivacaine for nerve blocks may not be appropriate. However, many surgeons also believe that after hand surgery, the prolonged period of immobility, together with functional sympathectomy and good pain relief from a long-acting block, outweighs the potential disadvantage of minimizing the pain that might help identify complications. Further, the increasing application of brachial block to major total joint arthroplasty procedures on the upper extremity (shoulder, elbow, and wrist) identifies another group of patients in whom postoperative analgesia needs may be increased.

Posture of the Blocked Arm

Special care must be taken with the anesthetized limb. The arm must not be allowed to fall and strike the face; this may occur when patients attempt to move their half-paralyzed limbs. Second, it is important that the arm should not be put into a position that would stretch the brachial plexus (i.e., extended further than 90° or displaced posteriorly).[32] Third, the ulnar nerve at the elbow should be properly padded, particularly if the forearm is pronated. Finally the arm should be properly supported when the patient is moved, whether in transit from the operating table, or at all other times, until motor-power and sensation return. If patients are discharged to their homes with residual motor or sensory neural blockade, it is important that the blocked extremity be placed in a sling or other protective device. Patients also should be instructed to avoid sensory injury (burns, cuts, etc.) to the denervated extremity.

Local Anesthetic Drugs

At present, all upper extremity block techniques may be adequately performed with any of the local anesthetic drugs approved for peripheral nerve block (see Chapter 4). For emergency room use, practitioners may desire a short-acting drug with rapid onset, such as 2-chloroprocaine or lidocaine. A long-acting drug like bupivacaine or ropivacaine not only will provide anesthesia for long operative procedures, but will ensure a prolonged period of postoperative analgesia and sympathetic blockade. In general, a selection of a short-acting drug, a drug of intermediate action, or a long-acting drug, will suffice to meet the needs of most practitioners.

As in other peripheral nerve blocks, the use of solutions containing epinephrine depends generally on the agent to be used, the total dose of drug to be administered, and the duration of the block desired. Solutions containing epinephrine should not be used on the digital nerves of the hands.

Concentration of the drug required depends primarily on the size of the nerve trunk, the properties to be blocked (i.e., fiber size), and the disposition of these fibers within the nerve trunk (see Chapter 2). Muscle relaxation is important for shoulder surgery, particularly in the reduction of dislocations. Although the brachial plexus trunks are quite large, the actual nerve fibers that supply the shoulder are thought to be distributed in their periphery as "mantle fibers," so that they are blocked quickly and relatively easily. In contrast, hand surgery requires little muscle relaxation but a profound degree of sensory anesthesia. The nerves to the hand at the brachial plexus level are centrally situated within the nerve trunks, thus they are more difficult to block and may require a higher concentration of local anesthetic, despite relatively small fiber size (see Chapter 2, Fig. 2-17).

Equipment

In institutions where many regional blocks are performed and in which adequate preparation and sterilization can be assured, packs of appropriate syringes, needles, and other equipment can be assembled for various blocks. Commercially provided disposable block trays do not have the same variety of needles available, and their long bevels may "spur" if they come into contact with bony surfaces. For the nerve blocks described in this chapter, either 23-gauge, 32-mm or 25-gauge, 16-mm needles are suitable. Use of the smallest needle possible will help minimize effects of direct trauma to peripheral nerves (see Chapter 6).

INTERSCALENE BLOCK

The interscalene block was developed and later described as an alternative to the supraclavicular approach to the brachial sheath.[37,39,68] It provides excellent anesthesia of the caudad cervical plexus and cephalad portion of the brachial plexus.[37]

Advantages

Interscalene block is indicated when a proximal block is required, such as for shoulder surgery; it is often necessary to block the cervical plexus, as well. Another advantage of interscalene block is that it can be performed with the arm in virtually any position, and the risk of pneumothorax is small. Finally, the landmarks are more easily identified in obese patients.

Limitations and Problems

It is essential to elicit paresthesias.[a] Also, even with large volume injections (>40 mL), lower trunk anesthesia may be minimal; supplementary ulnar block may then be required. Uncommon, but potentially serious complications can occur. It is clear that the caudad portion of the brachial plexus (C8 or ulnar n.) is frequently not blocked with this technique.

Anatomy

The cervical nerves of the brachial plexus, after leaving their respective intervertebral formina, pass laterally in a deep groove or "gutter" in the superior surface of the transverse process of the cervical vertebrae. This groove separates the transverse process into anterior and posterior tubercles, which give origin to the scalenus anterior and scalenus medius muscles, respectively (see Fig. 10-3). The direction of the "gutters" in the lower cervical vertebrae is primarily lateral but also slightly anterior and almost 45° caudad, as if the transverse processes were drawn down by the scalene muscles. Although transverse processes in this region tend to overlap, it must be remembered that they are quite short and offer little protection to the intervertebral foramina from a horizontally directed needle. Before attempting this block, the anesthesiologist should examine closely the skeleton of the cervical vertebral column, with particular regard to the intervertebral foramina and the shape and direction of the transverse processes (see previous description of Anatomy).

Techniques

Position and Landmarks. The patient lies supine with the neck in the sagittal plane and the head turned slightly to the side opposite that to be blocked. The arm is placed by the side with the shoulder depressed. The head is temporarily lifted by the patient so that the posterior border of the tensed sternocleidomastoid muscle can be palpated. The interscalene groove is palpated by rolling the fingers posteriorly from the border of the sternocleidomastoid over the belly of the scalenus anterior to the groove, which is then marked. A line is extended directly laterally from the cricoid cartilage, to intersect the interscalene groove. The point of entry is at this intersection, which should be directly opposite the transverse process of C6. The external jugular vein may overlie this point (Fig. 10-5A,B).

Needle Insertion and Injection. After suitable aseptic preparation and the initiation of a skin wheal, the index and middle fingers of the left hand palpate the groove. A 23-gauge, 32-mm needle is inserted in a direction almost perpendicular to the floor of the "gutter" on the superior aspect of the transverse process, that is 45° caudad, posterior, and medial (Fig. 10-5B,C). The anesthesiologist should visualize the transverse process as being directed primarily laterally, but also caudad and slightly anterior.

The needle is advanced until paresthesias are elicited. If the paresthesias are not elicited on the first needle insertion, the palpating fingers are systematically rolled in an anterior-posterior direction, with needle insertion and reinsertion also carried out in a systematic fashion (Fig. 10-5E). Once a paresthesia is elicited, an injection of the full volume of solution in increments is performed. To avoid the problem of needle displacement, it should be held firmly by the hub during the period of injection. The transverse process is surprisingly superficial in the normal patient, no more than 1.5 to 2 cm beneath the skin. If bone is encountered at this depth, but no paresthesias, using a technique similar to the previously outlined anterior-posterior redirection of the interscalene needle, one should walk the needle across the transverse process, and thus across the path of the nerve. If bony contact is made only on deep insertion, it is likely that the transverse process has been missed and what has been reached is the vertebral body. If no bony contact is made near full depth of the needle, the vertebral column has been missed and needle redirection should be undertaken.[63] Anesthesiologists believe more interscalene blocks are missed posteriorly than anteriorly, because less experienced anesthesiologist mistake the groove between the middle and posterior scalene muscles for the groove between the anterior and middle scalene muscles.

In most cases superficial paresthesias are easily obtained. If a blunt bevel needle is used, the anesthesiologist may also appreciate the "pop" of the penetration of the fascia. Twenty to 40 ml of solution is injected, depending on the extent of the block required, as well as the condition and stature of the patient. Volume-to-anesthesia relationships have been studied with radiopaque contrast, and these suggest that 20 ml of solution will anesthetize the lower cervical nerves and most of the brachial plexus; however, with this volume the lower trunk is often spared.[67] Forty ml of solution optimizes blocking all of the cervical and the brachial plexuses, although even that dose does not guarantee block of C8–T1 (ulnar n.).

Comments

Anesthesia of the cervical plexus can be readily obtained by a single injection into the interscalene groove.[72] The C4 level can be identified by extending a line laterally from the upper border of the thyroid cartilage. Injection of 10 to 15 ml is made in identical fashion to that for interscalene brachial plexus block. Conversely, the superficial cervical plexus can be blocked at the mid-portion of the posterior border of the sternocleidomastoid muscle by injecting 10 to 15 ml of local anesthetic. This block can often be combined with an interscalene block for shoulder surgery (see Chapter 15, Fig. 15-9).

Complications

As with any paravertebral technique, unintentional epidural or spinal anesthesia is always possible and has been reported with this block.[36,52] Also, the vertebral artery is

[a]Paresthesias below the elbow are associated with a higher incidence of successful block.

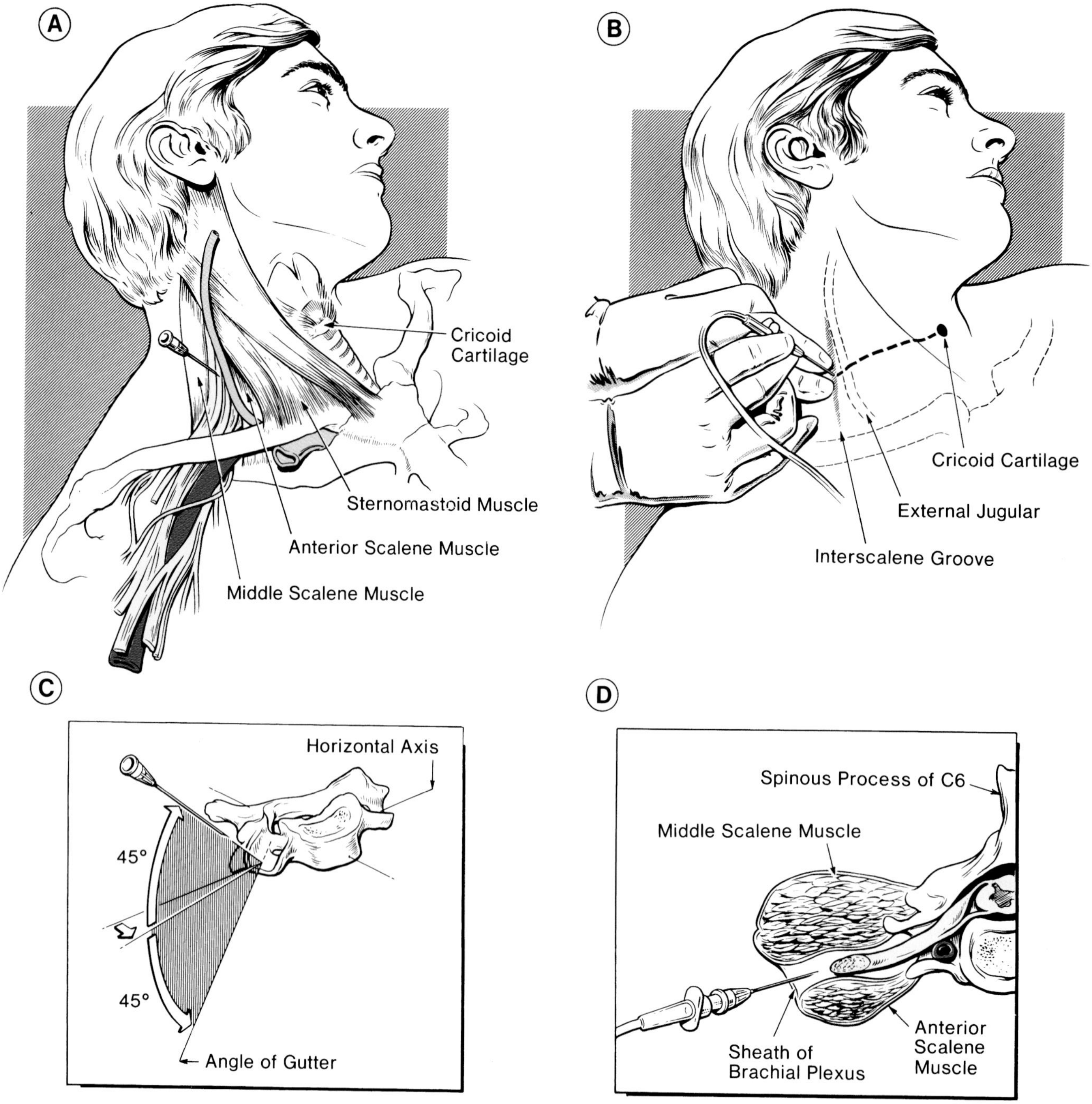

FIG. 10-5. A: Interscalene block. Anatomic landmarks. **B:** Interscalene block. Method of palpating interscalene groove and inserting needle. Note hand holding needle braced against clavicle. **C, D**: Interscalene block. Needle direction in relation to spine from anterolateral view **(C),** from above **(D).**

close to the point of even a correctly placed needle. The phrenic nerve is blocked almost uniformly either because of direct C4 root involvement or anterior spread to reach the anterior surface of the anterior scalene muscle, but this is seldom significant, at least in unilateral blocks.[48,61] Vagus, recurrent, laryngeal, and cervical sympathetic nerves are sometimes blocked, but these are of no significance except that it may be important to reassure the patient (see Chapter 21).

SUPRACLAVICULAR BLOCK

Advantages

There are several advantages to the use of the supraclavicular block. The brachial plexus is blocked where it is most compactly arranged—at the level of the three trunks. A low volume of solution is required and quick onset is achieved. Also, the technique can be performed with the arm in virtually any position. Block at this site provides the most homo-

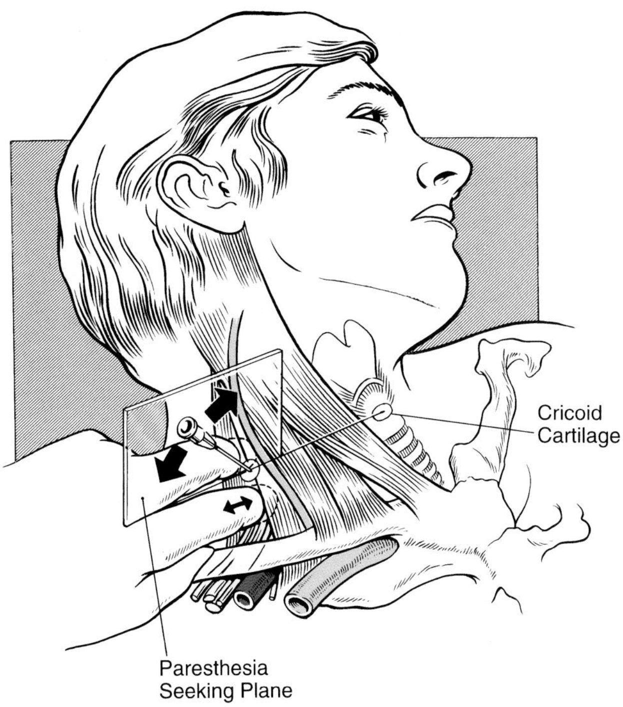

FIG. 10-5. *Continued.* **E:** Method of "rolling" finger anteroposterior across interscalene groove when seeking paresthesia.

geneous block of the brachial plexus.[38] There is minimal possibility of missing peripheral or proximal nerve branches because of failure of local anesthetic spread.

Limitations and Problems

Supraclavicular block has certain drawbacks. A reliable rapid onset block is achieved only if paresthesias are elicited. Furthermore, the classic technique is rather difficult to describe and teach. As a result of this difficulty with teaching the classic approach to supraclavicular block, a modification—the plumb-bob technique—has been designed to make the description and mastery of the technique more understandable. In any case, considerable experience is required to master it, and this is best accomplished by personal observation of an experienced anesthesiologist or by time spent in the postmortem room. The risk of pneumothorax is present with either of the two approaches to supraclavicular block.

Contraindications

This approach to the brachial plexus is best avoided in the following patients: those who are uncooperative, those of difficult stature in whom bony and muscular landmarks are not clear; or those with severe respiratory disease in whom pneumothorax or even phrenic nerve block would result in significant respiratory distress. Patients who require bilateral upper extremity block should not have them performed by either of the proximal techniques (interscalene or supraclavicular), to avoid the risk of bilateral phrenic nerve block, pneumothoraces, or a combination of the two. In addition, supraclavicular block should not be performed by a person who is unfamiliar with the technique or has not performed the block under the supervision of an experienced colleague.

Anatomy

The following are important points in the descriptive and topographic supraclavicular anatomy (Fig. 10-6A,B). First, the component parts of the plexus unite in a bundle that lies caudad and posterior to the clavicle at about its midpoint, cepahaloposterior to the subclavian artery. Second, the artery can often be palpated as a valuable landmark. Third, the first rib is an important landmark to prevent the needle from passing medially and piercing the lung. The rib is short, broad, and flat. It slopes caudally as it passes anteriorly. Although it is deeply curved, the small anterior-posterior-oriented portion is related to the subclavian artery and can be used as a backstop for needle insertion.

Technique: Classic Approach

The classic approach for supraclavicular block of the brachial plexus should be regarded as a combination of the early published techniques. It calls for a caudad, posterior, and medial direction for insertion of the needle from a point immediately posterior to the midpoint of the clavicle (Fig. 10-6C). This is generally satisfactory; however, strict interpretation may not always be appropriate. In some patients, beginning at a point just superior to the clavicle results in a posterior direction of the needle. A starting point 2 to 3 cm superior to the clavicle may make it easier to locate the interscalene groove and the nerve trunks cephalad to the first rib. If a point is taken immediately superior to the clavicle, it almost certainly will lie outside the lateral margin of the rib. Inward (medial) inclination of the needle easily penetrates the lung. The more lateral the starting point, and *the more medial the inclination*, the more likely it is that this will occur.

The pulsation of the subclavian artery against the palpating finger or needle is the surest guide to the brachial plexus. It may not be felt if the clavicle is raised, if the platysma muscle is tense, or if the patient is obese. An additional guide to locating the midpoint of the clavicle is finding the point where the straight portion of the external jugular vein, if continued, would cross the clavicle. Asking the patient to "blow out his cheeks" will frequently make the external jugular vein very prominent.

Rib-walking to achieve paresthesias, if they are not more simply obtained, is important for a satisfactory block. However, rib-seeking or further rib-walking after eliciting paresthesias is unnecessary and will only increase the risk of pneumothorax.

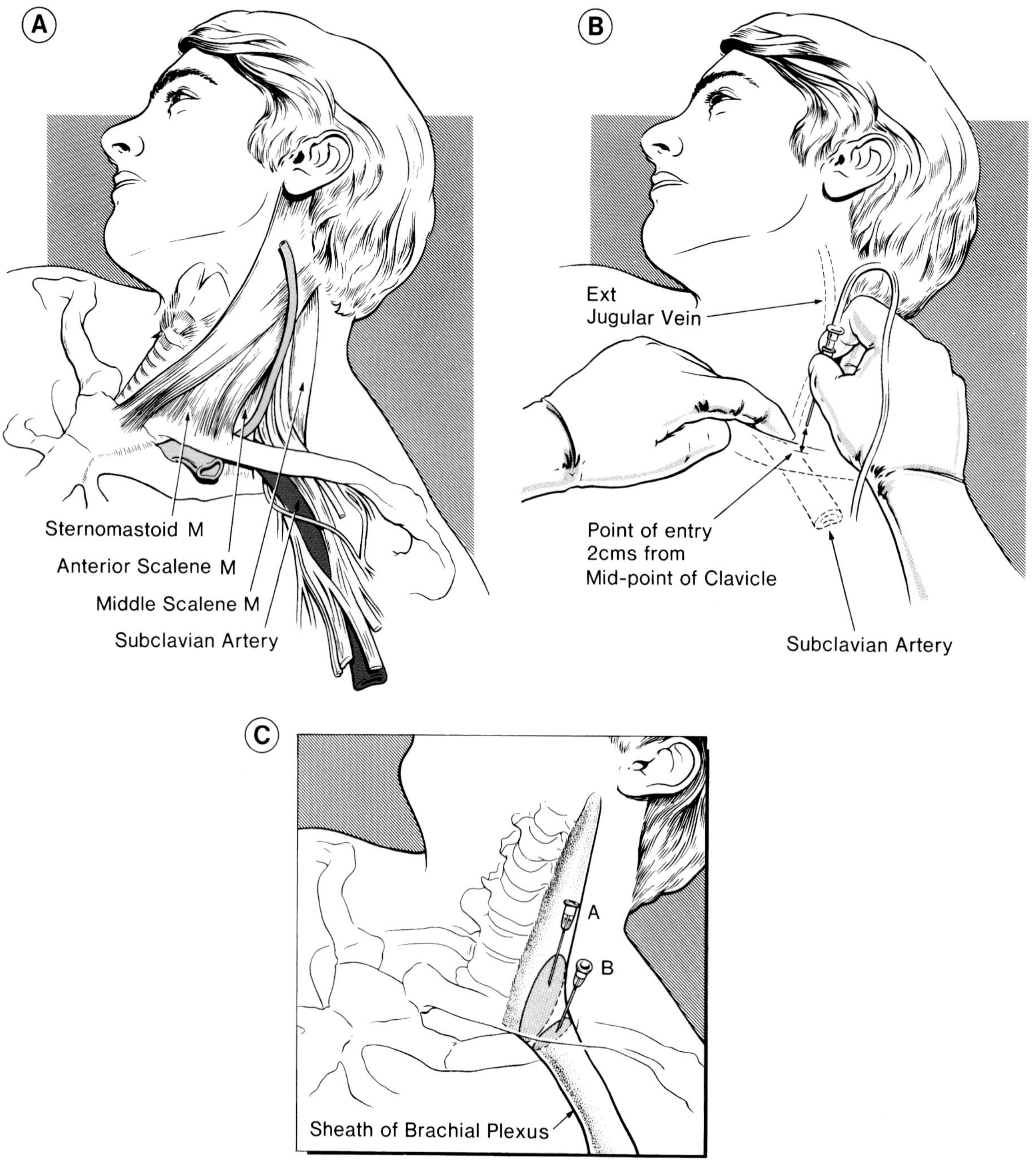

FIG. 10-6. **A:** Supraclavicular block. Classic approach. Anatomic landmarks. **B:** Supraclavicular block. Technique of needle insertion. **C:** Supraclavicular block. Note that the brachial plexus sheath becomes deeper as one moves medially and further back from the clavicle (*position A*) than it is at the lateral margin of the first rib immediately behind the clavicle (*position B*).

Positions and Landmarks

The patient should lie supine, without a pillow, arms at the side, and head turned slightly to the opposite side. The shoulder should be depressed caudad and posterior by gentle pressure on the relaxed shoulder, and by asking the patient to touch his or her knee. This posterior displacement of the shoulder can be exaggerated by molding the shoulders over a roll placed between the scapulae. The patient should then be instructed to raise his/her head approximately 20° from the table, putting strain on the neck muscles. This permits the clavicular head of the sternocleidomastoid muscle to be palpated and marked. The interscalene groove is palpated by rolling the finger back from the posterior border of the lower end of the identified sternocleidomastoid muscle and over the belly of the anterior scalene muscle. Because the brachial plexus makes its exit at the lateral border of the anterior scalene muscle, the skin is marked at this point, immediately above the clavicle. Usually this point lies approximately at the middle of the clavicle, 1.5 to 2 cm from the lateral border of the clavicular head of the sternocleidomastoid muscle. The subclavian artery often can be easily palpated in the supraclavicular fossa, because it also emerges from the caudad portion of the interscalene groove. This serves as a cross-check to the other landmarks.

Despite the multiple landmarks, this block is one of the simplest to perform if the subclavian artery can be palpated easily, because the needle is inserted immediately cephaloposterior to the pulsating artery. If neither the artery nor the interscalene groove can be felt clearly, a point is taken approximately 2 cm along a line marked superior to the midpoint of and perpendicular to the clavicle (Fig. 10-6B). In a patient with a protuberant clavicle, or in whom it is difficult to achieve adequate posterior displacement of the shoulder, this point should be taken nearer to 3 cm superior to the clavicle.

Procedure

The area should be aseptically prepared and draped. The anesthesiologist stands at the side of the patient to be blocked, facing the head of the table, since this position allows optimal needle control and observation of the patient's face. An intradermal wheal is raised at the previously determined point. If the anesthesiologist is right-handed, a filled 10-ml syringe with a 23-gauge, 32-mm needle attached, is held in the right hand and the patient is instructed to say "now" and *not* to move, as soon as he/she feels a "tingle" going down below his/her elbows. This initial technique varies slightly, depending on whether or not the subclavian artery is palpable. If the artery is palpable, the tip of the index finger is rested in the supraclavicular fossa, directly upon the arterial pulsation. The needle is inserted through the skin wheal and advanced slowly caudad, rolled slightly medially and posteriorly, so that the shaft of the needle and syringe are almost parallel to the patient's head (Fig. 10-6B,C). The index finger and thumb of the left hand firmly hold the hub of the needle and control the movement of the needle at all times (an assistant changes syringes).

Paresthesias usually will be elicited immediately. If so, the needle is fixed in position, and 15 to 25 ml of the local anesthetic drug is injected. If paresthesias are not elicited immediately, then one should proceed on to the rib, either depositing all the solution on or slightly superficial to the rib, in this position just posterior to the artery, or making further attempts to seek paresthesias by gentle reinsertions posteriorly, for an estimated 2 cm along the length (not breadth) of the rib. After the rib is encountered, the anesthesiologist, by gently tapping it with the point of the needle, walks the needle anteriorly along the rib for approximately 1.5 cm, maintaining the initial plane of direction of the needle, and seeking paresthesias. With each insertion of the needle, aspiration tests should be undertaken to see that the needle point is not in the subclavian artery. If it is, the anesthesiologist should not become alarmed, because a valuable landmark has been located. By withdrawing the needle and reinserting it posterolaterally to the subclavian artery, paresthesias usually will be elicited as the needle is slowly advanced. If no paresthesias are elicited, but the rib is contacted, a barrage of solution (40–50 ml) between the skin and the rib behind the artery can be used. This is the principle of the Patrick technique.[47]

If the artery is not palpable and has not been located, the previously located point 2 cm superior to the midpoint of the clavicle can be used and will be placed over the rib more certainly. The needle is inserted directly downward (caudad) until the paresthesias are elicited or the rib is contacted; and again, if necessary, the needle should be walked anteroposteriorly along the rib to seek the plexus. In a robust patient, it sometimes happens that the rib cannot be contacted at the full depth of this needle. Under these circumstances, the anesthesiologist should make a sweep with gentle reinsertions posteriorly as before, each time to the depth of the needle, in an attempt to elicit paresthesias superficial to the rib. If no paresthesias or rib are encountered at full depth of the needle, a needle 1 cm longer may be used, with caution. Alternatively, it may be advisable to choose another method. If the patient is properly positioned and all of the available landmarks are used and checked against one another, the need to change techniques will be rare.

Technique: Plumb-bob Approach

The development of the plumb-bob approach of supraclavicular block developed from efforts to simplify the anatomic projection necessary for the block.[11]

Positions and Landmarks

The patient should be positioned in a manner similar to that for the classic approach, lying supine without a pillow, with the head turned slightly away from the side to be blocked. The anesthesiologist should stand lateral to the patient, at the level of the patient's upper arm. This block involves inserting the needle and syringe assembly at approximately a 90° angle to the classic approach. The patient is asked to raise his or her head slightly off the block table, so that the lateral border of the sternocleidomastoid can be marked as it inserts onto the clavicle. From that point, a "mental" plane is created that runs parasagittally through that site (Fig. 10-7). The name "plumb-bob" was chosen for this block concept because if one suspends a plumb-bob over the entry site, as shown in Figure 10-7A, needle insertion through that point will result in contact with the brachial plexus in most patients. Figure 10-7B also illustrates a parasagittal section, obtained by MRI scanning, in the sagittal plane necessary to carry out this block. As illustrated, the brachial plexus at the level of the first rib lies posterior-cephalad to the subclavian artery.

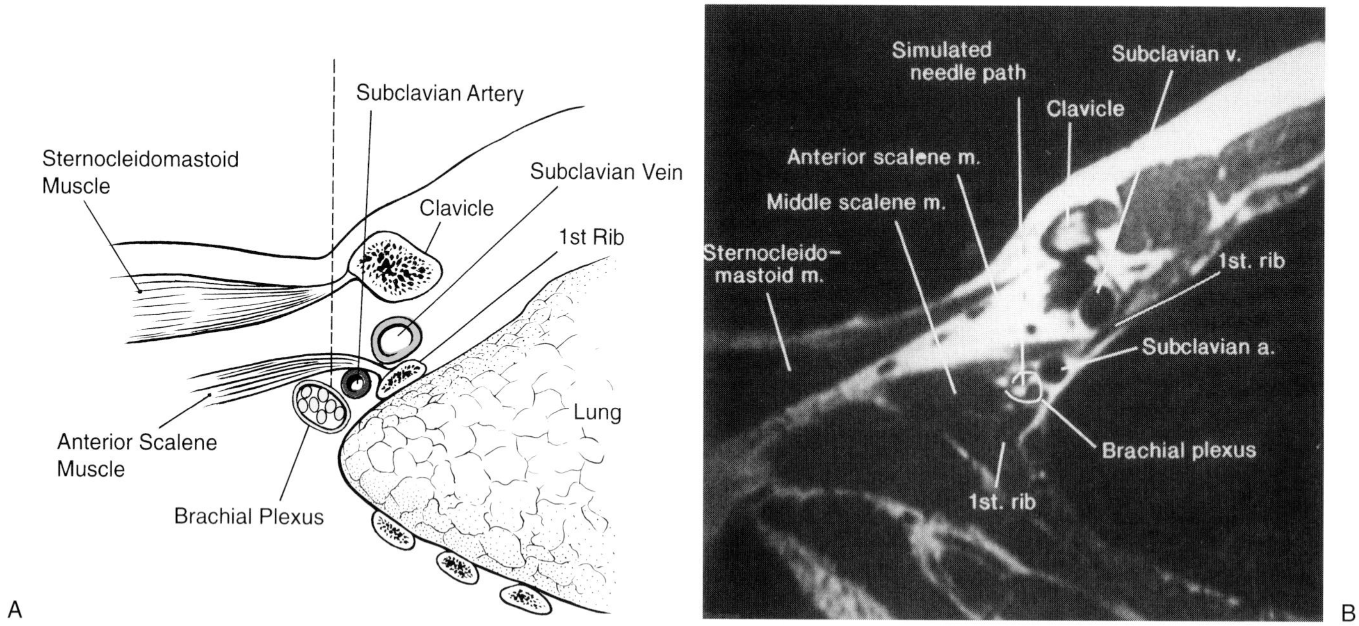

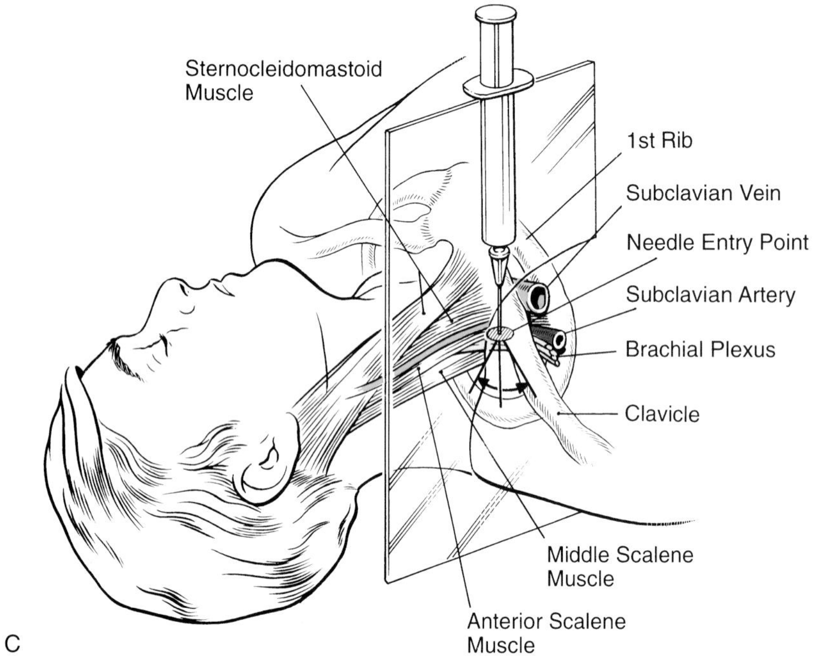

FIG. 10-7. Supraclavicular block—plumb-bob approach. **A:** Parasagittal anatomy. **B:** Magnetic resonance image of parasagittal anatomy. **C:** Technique of needle-syringe insertion for parasagittal plumb-bob technique. The plane of repositioning the needle is shown, with the *small arrows* indicating the limits (20°) of cephalad and caudad redirection.

Procedure

A skin wheal is placed immediately superior to the clavicle at the lateral border of the clavicular insertion of the sternocleidomastoid muscle. The needle is inserted in the parasagittal plane at a 90° angle to the table top. If a paresthesia is not elicited on the first pass, the needle and syringe are redirected cephalad in small steps through an arc of approximately 20°. If a paresthesia still has not been obtained, needle and syringe are reinserted at the starting position and then moved in small steps through an arc of approximately 20° in a caudad direction (Fig. 10-7C). Since the brachial plexus lies cephaloposterior to the artery as it crosses the first rib, a paresthesia often can be elicited prior to contacting the first rib. If that occurs, approximately 15 to 30 ml of local anesthetic are injected at this single site. If paresthesia is not elicited with these maneuvers, but the first rib is contacted, the block is carried out just like the classic approach—walking along the first rib until paresthesia is evoked. As with the classic approach, care should be taken not to allow the syringe and needle assembly to be medially directed toward the cupola of the lung.

Complications (see Chapter 21)

Pneumothorax. Serious complications seldom ensue. The most significant complication of the supraclavicular approach for blocking the brachial plexus is development of pneumothorax. The frequency of occurrence is between 0.5% and 6.0% and decreases as the anesthesiologist becomes more skilled.[19] Tall, thin patients, who characteristically have a high apical pleura, usually account for the greater number of these complications. Most likely the pneumothoraces are caused by the needle piercing the lung as exhalation occurs and a small bronchial-pleura opening is created by the needle point. The pneumothorax that results is then caused by air escaping from the lung. The risk of pneumothorax can be minimized by careful attention to detail, taking time, and being gentle; by the avoidance of multiple indiscriminate probings; and by the use of the shortest needles possible.

A pneumothorax must be suspected when there is dyspnea, cough, or pleuritic chest pain, but the diagnosis can be confirmed only by chest x-ray. It is important to realize, when assessing the size of the pneumothorax, that there is apparent exaggeration on a film taken in full expiration. A minority of the pneumothoraces become obvious within hours. These are usually extensive and accompanied by symptoms. The majority of pneumothoraces take up to 24 hours to develop, are usually small to moderate, and may or may not cause symptoms, so there is little point in taking x-rays routinely in the hours immediately after the block. It is also encouraging to note that it is most unusual for a "brachial block" pneumothorax to get any larger after 24 hours.

The treatment of pneumothorax depends on the extent and symptoms. In the early, more extensive, pneumothorax (i.e., greater than 50%), the patient should be admitted to the hospital and the air should be removed; this may be possible with a Heimlich valve positioned on a small catheter, rather than with the often-used larger thoracostomy cannula. Pneumothoraces that are asymptomatic and not extensive usually can be followed on an outpatient basis with suitable advice and warnings. Analgesics, such as codeine and aspirin, may be prescribed for pain and discomfort, if indicated. Serial films of the chest should be taken to assure that expansion of the lung is proceeding. However, there is no point to taking daily films, when it may take weeks for the air to be absorbed completely.

Other complications seen with supraclavicular brachial plexus blocks include the following:

Block of the Phrenic Nerve. This occurs in 40% to 60% of cases and usually causes no symptoms.[33] However, if a bilateral phrenic block occurs in a patient with underlying chest disease, dyspnea may result. Ordinarily, no treatment is necessary for the unilateral phrenic nerve block. Symptoms, if present, clear as the block dissipates. If dyspnea occurs, oxygen should be given by bag and mask or by other forms of oxygen therapy.

Horner Syndrome (Stellate Ganglion Block). This occurs in approximately 70% to 90% of the brachial plexus blocks when large volumes of local anesthetic drugs are injected. The symptoms clear as the block is dissipated, and no treatment is necessary. These symptoms of dysphagia and hoarseness should be explained to the patient, with the assurance that they will disappear as the local anesthetic wears off.

Nerve Damage or Neuritis. This is an uncommon but possible complication of all peripheral nerve blocks, including the supraclavicular technique for blocking the brachial plexus. When it occurs, immediate implication of the block technique itself should be avoided, since there are other, and perhaps more frequent, reasons for the development of neuropathy. Infrequently, needle trauma or faulty positioning of the anesthetized arm perioperatively may be the cause. Other remote causes include excessive tourniquet time, concentrated solutions with vasoconstrictors, and susceptible host tissues.[10,34] A neurologic consultation should be obtained to establish the level, extent, and treatment of the lesion, as well as to protect against legal action. Treatment usually consists of watchful waiting for spontaneous resolution. Physiotherapy and hone exercises are helpful in preventing muscle atrophy if motor nerves are involved. Complete restoration of normal function may take several weeks.

Systemic Toxic Reactions. The causes and treatment of toxic reactions to local anesthetic drugs are discussed in detail in Chapters 4 and 21. The most common reason for its occurrence in supraclavicular brachial plexus block is an unintentional intravascular injection of the local anesthetic drug or use of an excessive amount of solution. Properly treated, it should not be a serious complication.

Comments

It is strongly advised that paresthesias be obtained (preferably below the elbow), since they denote contact with the plexus, assuring a successful block with quicker onset. Promiscuous probing should be avoided. If, after five or six careful insertions, a paresthesia is not obtained, one of the other techniques should be used. Minor nerve injury after paresthesias has been reported (see Chapter 21).

One of the most certain causes of presumed failure of the block is to commence the operation before the selected local anesthetic has had time to become completely effective. This interval may be as brief as 5 minutes or as long as 30 minutes. The custom of prematurely using needle sticks to test the degree of anesthesia cannot be condemned too strongly. The patient's confidence in a successful anesthetic may be lost. Preferably, patients should be sedated for 15 minutes and the first tests for anesthesia made after the local anesthetic has had ample time, between 15 to 20 minutes, to become effective (see Chapter 6).

Because the trunks of the brachial plexus are so compact at the point of crossing the first rib, 25 ml of local anesthetic solution may be sufficient to produce a total brachial plexus block, even in the robust patient. If no paresthesias are obtained, larger volumes are required (e.g., 40–50 ml 1% lidocaine with epinephrine), and even then there may be a delay in onset and patchy anesthesia may occur.

Axillary Block

The perivascular axillary infiltration is the most popular technique for blocking the nerves of the arm. Needle insertion is carried out at a site distant from both the neuroaxis and the lung, avoiding complications to those areas.

Advantages

Axillary block provides excellent operating conditions for surgery of the forearm and hand, with less risk of major complications than is associated with alternative supraclavicular methods. This makes it suitable for emergency department

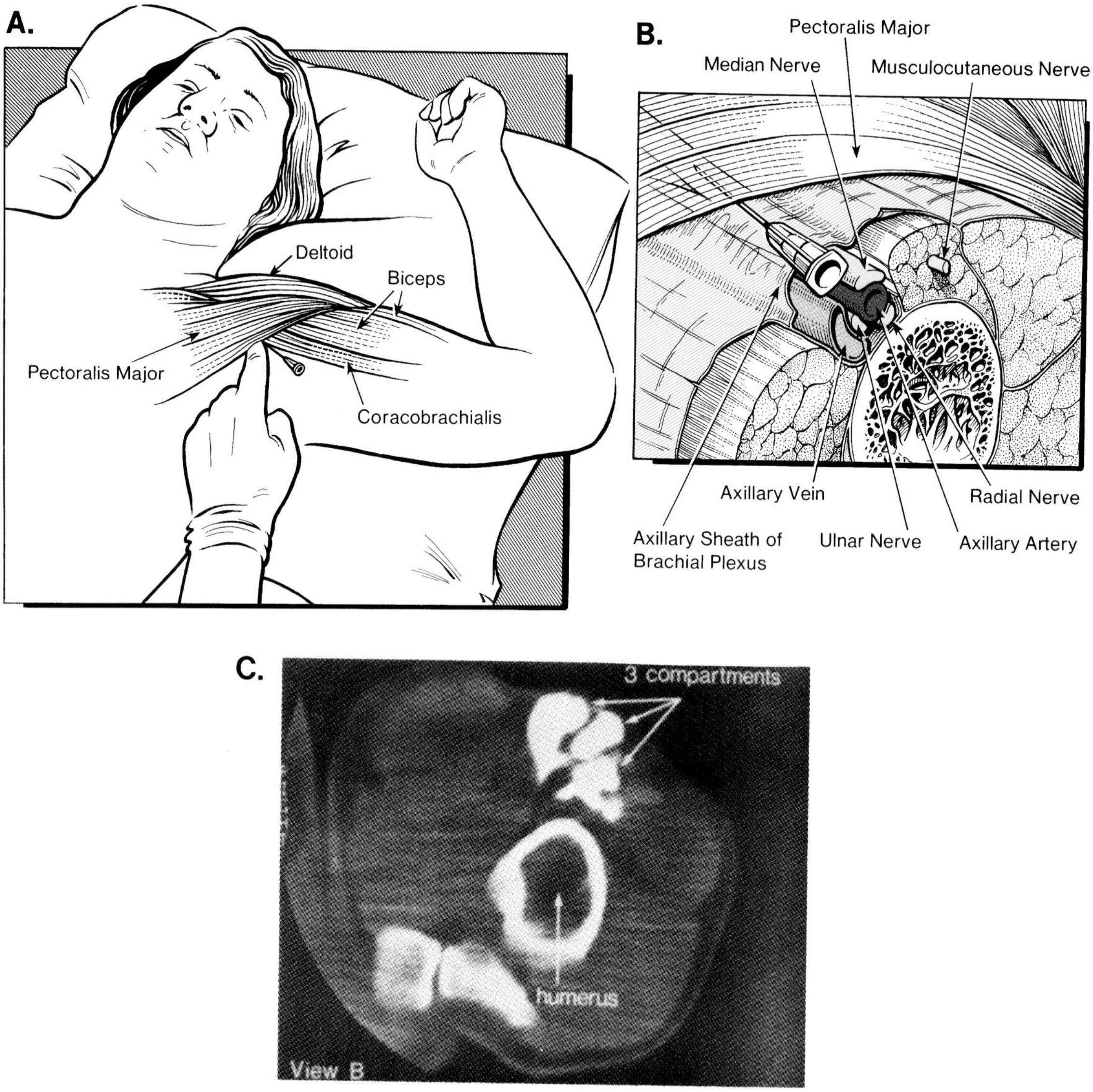

FIG. 10-8. Axillary block. **A, B:** Technique of needle insertion. **(A)** Note forefinger palpating axillary artery. Hand holding needle (not shown) should be braced against arm. Needle insertion is adjacent to coracobrachialis and pectoralis major muscles, immediately superior to tip of forefinger (see text). **(B)** Note direction of needle toward apex of axilla, in same direction as neurovascular bundle. Needle enters neurovascular sheath and may run inside sheath to a higher level. The medial head of triceps, lying between the neurovascular sheath and the humerus, has been compressed by the palpating finger and is not shown in this cross-section. **C:** Computer tomogram, after axillary block with bupivacaine 0.5% and iodothalamate. Separate injections of 10-ml solution were made after obtaining paresthesias in median and radial nerves and also on passing a needle through the axillary artery. Contrast medium apparently remained in three discrete compartments; it is not certain whether these relate to major branches of brachial plexus. Also local anesthetic may diffuse in a different manner to contrast medium. (Part **C** reproduced with permission from Thompson, G.E., and Rorie, D.H.: Functional anatomy of brachial plexus sheaths. Anesthesiology, *59*:117, 1983.)

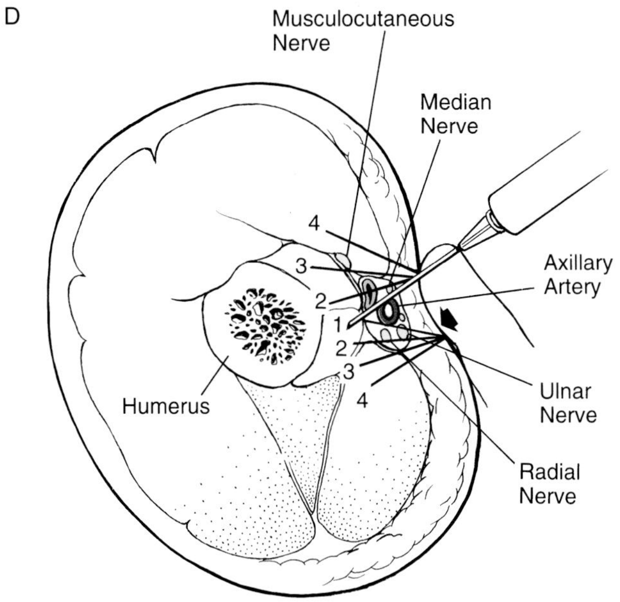

FIG. 10-8. *Continued.* **D:** Method of depositing local anesthetic in all quadrants surrounding the axillary artery.

and outpatient use. It is an easy technique to master, and probably the safest and most reliable for the patient of stout build. It is useful but not necessary to seek paresthesias, and fine needles are quite satisfactory. The block is, therefore, particularly useful in children (e.g., for the reduction of fractures).[15,27]

Limitations

The axillary approach does have certain limitations, the first of which is that the arm must be abducted in order to perform the block. The extent of anesthesia also is insufficient for shoulder and upper arm surgery. Sometimes anesthesia for elbow surgery may be inadequate even after using large volumes of local anesthetic solution. The circumflex and musculocutaneous nerves are sometimes missed because they leave the axillary sheath proximal to the point of injection. The musculocutaneous nerve is most important because of its extensive area of innervation on the radial side of the forearm, often extending onto the thenar eminence.

Anatomy

A cross section of the arm at the level of the anterior axillary fold demonstrates several anatomic points, including the compact, axillary neurovascular bundle (Fig. 10-8B).[45] On its medial (superficial) aspect, the axillary sheath is covered only by connective tissue, being posterior to the biceps/coracobrachialis and anterior to the triceps muscles. On its lateral or deep aspect, the sheath lies close to the neck of the humerus. At the level of axillary block, the median nerve tends to lie anterior to the axillary artery (as does the musculocutaneous nerve higher up the sheath), the ulnar nerve, medial and posterior to the artery, and the radial nerve, posterior and somewhat lateral to the artery. The medial antebrachial cutaneous nerve, and the medial brachial cutaneous nerves, are further medial to the artery. The axillary vein overlays the artery on its medial aspect. At this level, the musculocutaneous nerve has already left the sheath and is now in the body of the coracobrachialis muscle.

Technique

Position and Landmarks. The patient is placed in a supine position, with the head turned away from the side to be blocked. The arm is abducted to approximately 90° and the forearm flexed to 90° and externally rotated, so the dorsum of the hand lies on the table and the forearm lies parallel to the long axis of the patient's body. Although it is tempting to have the patient's hand under the head, it should not be done, because frequently the hyperabduction obliterates the brachial artery pulse.

The brachial artery is palpated and the pulse is followed proximally as far as possible, ideally to the pectoralis major muscle, if block of the musculocutaneous nerve is desired. If musculocutaneous block is not as important, needle insertion does not need to be performed in the proximal axilla and, in fact, needle insertion in the mid-to-lower portion of the axillary hair patch, or even more distal, is often effective.[9]

Point of Entry

The artery is fixed against the humerus by the index and middle fingers of the left hand, and a skin wheal is raised directly over the arterial pulse (Fig. 10-8).

Needle Insertion and Injection. A line should be imagined overlying the course of the axillary artery at the level of the mid-axilla; overlaying this line, the index and long fingers of the anesthesiologist's left hand are used to identify the artery and minimize the amount of subcutaneous tissue overlying the neurovascular bundle. In this manner, the anesthetist can develop a sense of the longitudinal course of the artery, which is essential for axillary blockade. With the index and long fingers still on the pulse of the axillary artery, a skin wheal is raised directly over the pulse (Fig. 10-8). A 25-gauge (20–25 mm) or 23-gauge (25 mm) needle is inserted as shown in Figure 10-8D. The needle may be "bare," or attached to a syringe or tubing.

During needle insertion, evidence of entering the axillary sheath may be identified by the feel of the "fascia click" as the needle penetrates the fascia; paresthesias, blood flowback, or oscillation of a free needle. If introducing a continuous catheter, the feeling penetrating the sheath is facilitated by the use of a short-bevel needle and the elimination of skin drag. Puncturing the skin first with a larger needle helps, but resistance can be reduced further by a needle-through-needle technique.[54]

Evoking paresthesias is encouraging and reliable evidence of correct position, but is not essential for a satisfactory block, and may be distressing to some patients. Selander[55] indicates that elicitation of paresthesia may carry a slight risk of postanesthetic neuropathy; there is no conclusive evidence of this theory. The use of the nerve stimulator (as described in Chapter 6) may obviate the need for soliciting paresthesias in uncooperative patients.

The flow or aspiration of arterial blood strongly suggests that the needle tip is within the sheath. The needle can either be withdrawn from the vessel, or pushed on through to the other side, before injection. Although it is not our preferred technique, it is the practice of some anesthesiologists to puncture the artery deliberately, as the means to identify the plexus.

Single-Injection Technique. After aspiration, which is particularly important in this site, the entire volume of local anesthetic may be injected. On the basis of sheath volume, and assuming equal proximal and distal spread, de Jong theorized that 42 ml of solution was needed to fill an adult's sheath in order to reach the coracoid process, at the approximate level where the musculocutaneous nerve leaves the sheath.[19] This kind of volume-to-anesthesia relationship has been confirmed with radiopaque contrast studies.[73] Studies by Vester-Andersen and others,[62] however, showed that increasing the volume of the injected local anesthetic drug above 40 ml did not improve spread to the musculocutaneous or radial nerve area.

Prevention of needle movement during injection may be a little awkward in the axilla, but is an important component of this technique. There are methods that can help: with a direct needle-syringe assembly, the anesthetist should fix the needle hub with the thumb and index finger of the left hand, or with the right hand, if using a needle attached to extension tubing. This "immobile needle" helps to prevent movement during syringe removal and reattachment.[67]

A few ml of solution are deposited in the subcutaneous tissue on withdrawal, to block the intercostobrachial nerve and its communications with the medial cutaneous nerve of the arm (Fig. 10-8B).

Double-Injection Technique. Nearly all early descriptions of axillary block have used the technique of injection on both sides of the artery.[12,19,25,43,64] Many anesthesiologists believe that if the first insertion is correct and the needle is not moved, the second injection should not be necessary, provided sufficient volume is used. Thompson and Rorie[59] and Partridge, et al.,[46] however, have demonstrated that the sheath may be divided into a fascial compartment created for each nerve, which functionally limits the circumferential spread of injected solutions of local anesthetic (Fig. 10-8C). Thompson and Rorie recommend a double- or multiple-injection technique.

There are some advantages to a double-injection technique. If the anesthesiologist is prepared to disregard the musculocutaneous nerve to block it separately, the volume of solution injected into the sheath may be reduced. Ten to 15 ml with each injection should be enough to block the nerves within the sheath.

The double-injection technique can be performed with one or two needles. With a single needle, half the total volume of local anesthetic solution is injected anterior to (above) the artery; the needle is then withdrawn from the fascia and redirected posterior (below) to the artery, and the remainder of the solution is injected. When two needles are used, they are inserted through the same skin wheal, but one is directed anterior and the other posterior to the artery before injecting through each needle.[30] With multiple injections, 10 ml of solution may be injected with each paresthesia or needle reposition. Usually 3 to 4 injections will suffice.

Promotion of Central Flow Within the Sheath. With the single-injection, large-volume technique, measures should be taken to promote proximal flow within the sheath. Digital pressure should be applied immediately distal to the needle, with the index and middle fingers, both during and immediately after injection. If these fingers are required for fixation of the needle hub, pressure on the distal sheath can be applied with the ulnar side of the hand. The application of a distal tourniquet frees the left hand but is of doubtful effectiveness and causes some discomfort.[26] Directing the needle toward the apex of the axilla has also been used in an effort to gain more proximal spread and higher block. Winnie has suggested the use of a 37-mm needle directed centrally at approximately 20° to the artery.[69] Hopcroft uses a 21-gauge, 50-mm needle directed centrally along the axis of the artery.[29] These techniques no doubt achieve the desired goal; but at some point, the pneumothorax problem must again arise. As soon as the injection is completed and while still applying some form of distal pressure, the arm should be adducted. This removes the effect of pressure on the humeral head, which may be a factor in limiting proximal spread.[70]

Comments

Axillary block is probably the most widely used technique for brachial plexus block today. More modifications, technical variations, and "tricks of the trade" are associated with this technique than with any other. Some actually decrease the effectiveness of the block.

In children particularly, a standard 25-gauge axillary block needle or scalp vein needles may be useful (see Chapter 20). Paresthesias can be an important part of this method, especially in a large arm with vague arterial pulsation or when there is difficulty in identifying the sheath. A nerve stimulator may be helpful in such circumstances, or for when patients are unresponsive or uncooperative.

Continuous Axillary Block

Continuous axillary block has been advocated as the anesthesia of choice for prolonged surgical procedures, such as reimplantations and postoperative pain relief.[2,53,54] Toxic reactions to local anesthetic drugs used in this manner are infrequent.[59] Pharmacokinetic data indicate that a continuous infusion of 0.25% bupivacaine at a rate of 20 to 30 mg/h (e.g., 10 ml) is effective and does not result in cumulative increases in blood concentration[21] (see Chapter 3). In practice, a standard bolus dose is given to establish the block (see above), and 15 to 60 minutes later the infusion is started.[21]

Complications and Contraindication

There are few complications or contraindications specific to this block, but the risk of intravascular injection must always be kept in mind, and the patient with a bleeding diathesis is probably at an increased risk of incurring a hematoma with this approach.

INFRACLAVICULAR BRACHIAL PLEXUS BLOCK

Several modifications of the original infraclavicular approach to the brachial plexus (Raj et al.,[50] Sims,[57] and Whiffler[66]) suggest that the perivascular sheath may be injected in this area as an alternative to other more popular approaches.

Advantages

While maintaining the advantage of the interscalene or axillary sheath blocks, injection of the local anesthetic drug in the sheath above the level where the musculocutaneous and axillary nerves are formed would block these nerves frequently missed on an axillary approach. Blocking lower than the first rib would eliminate the potential for pneumothorax or for missing the ulnar segment of the medial cord which occasionally is missed when the supraclavicular technique is used. It also blocks the intercostobrachial nerve, which is not blocked on any of the other approaches. It does not require positioning of the arm, as does the axillary block.

Limitations and Problems

The success of the infraclavicular approach may be enhanced by the use of a nerve stimulator to locate the plexus; however, a gentle paresthesia-seeking technique is also possible. Because the palpating finger cannot identify the arterial pulse in that area, the needle must be advanced blindly, increasing the likelihood of vascular puncture or of causing the patient more pain. If the ultimate needle point position is distal to the coracoid process (clinically frequent), most of the solution will move distally and the musculocutaneous and axillary nerves will be missed, as in the axillary approach.

Anatomy

Because this is essentially a sheath block of the plexus in the upper axilla from an infraclavicular approach, the axillary landmarks are (i) the outer border of the first four ribs, (ii) the posterior surface of the clavicle, (iii) the pectoralis major and minor anteriorly, and (iv) the subscapularis, teres major, and latissimus dorsi muscles posteriorly (Fig. 10-9). The contents of the axilla are the axillary vessels, the

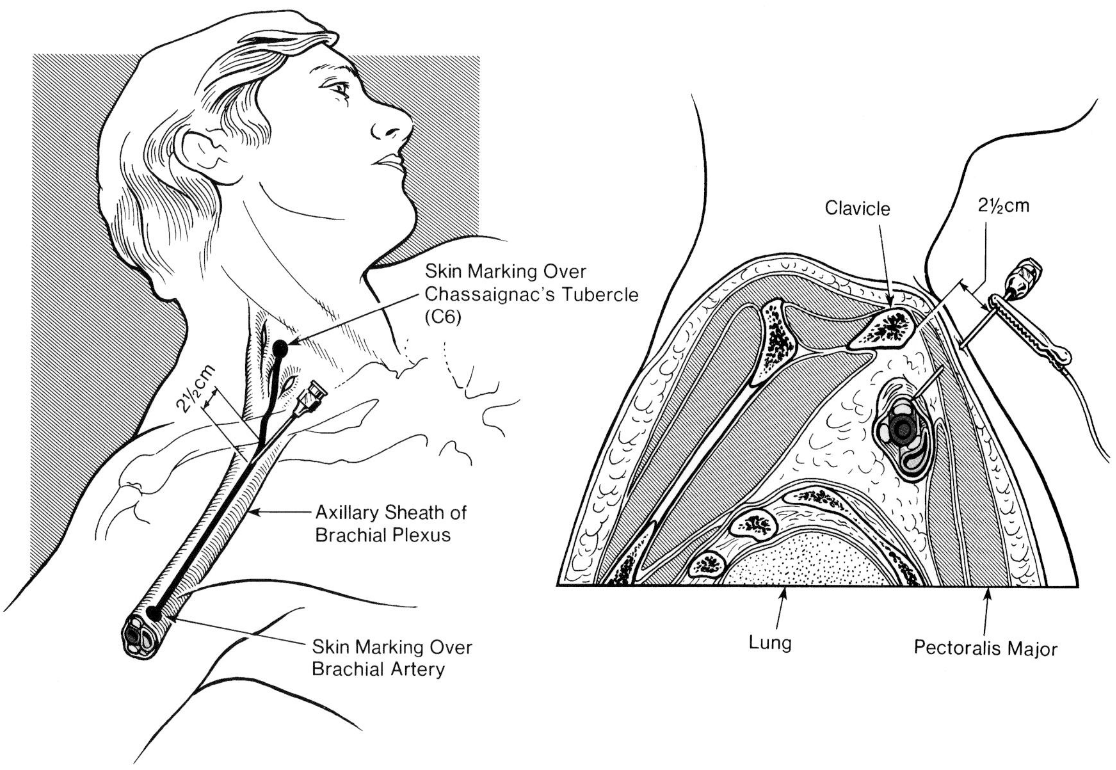

FIG. 10-9. Infraclavicular brachial plexus block (see text). Note position of arm abducted to 90° and supinated. Point of insertion is 2.5 cm below clavicle, along a line from C6 tubercle across clavicle to brachial artery. Note direction of needle laterally, inferiorly, and posteriorly toward brachial artery.

brachial plexus with its branches, some branches of the intercostal nerves, lymph glands and fat, and loose areolar tissue.

Technique

Position and Landmarks. Patients lie supine with their heads turned away from the arm to be blocked. If possible, the arm is abducted to 90° and allowed to rest comfortably. The physician stands on the opposite side from the arm to be blocked. The entire length of the clavicle is marked after palpation. The subclavian artery is palpated where it dips under the clavicle and then marked; it is usually at the midpoint of the clavicle. If the subclavian artery is not palpable, the midpoint of the clavicle is marked. The brachial artery is palpated in the arm and marked, and the C6 tubercle on the ipsilateral side is palpated and marked. A line is drawn from the C6 mark to the brachial artery in the arm. This line should go through the midpoint of the clavicle and is the surface marking of the brachial plexus (Fig. 10-9).

Needle Insertion and Injection. If a nerve stimulator is used the ground electrode of a peripheral nerve stimulator is attached to the opposite shoulder (see Chapter 6, Fig. 6-5). A skin wheal is raised 1 inch below the inferior border of the clavicle at its marked midpoint, or where the subclavian artery dips under the clavicle. A 22-gauge unsheathed standard 80-mm spinal needle is introduced through the skin wheal. The needle point is directed laterally toward the brachial artery (Fig. 10-9). Then the exploring electrode is attached either to the stem or to the hub of the needle, with a sterile alligator clip. The controls of the peripheral nerve stimulator are set to deliver 2 to 3 milliamperes (ma), and the needle is advanced at an angle of 45° to the skin. As the needle approaches the fibers of the brachial plexus, movement of the muscles supplied by those fibers will confirm that the needle point is in proximity to the nerve fibers of the brachial plexus. The current is decreased to 0.5 to 1 ma. The needle is then advanced. The muscle movements seen previously increase as the needle tip moves closer to the brachial plexus, and the needle is advanced until the muscle movements start to decrease. The needle is slowly withdrawn until the maximum muscle movements are observed again; the needle should be positioned so motor activity is still present with only 0.5 to 0.1 ma. Now the needle is held in that position while 2 ml of 2% lidocaine is injected through the needle with the one-impulse-per-second button on the nerve stimulator turned on. If the needle is located correctly, there is loss of the previously seen muscle movements within 30 seconds. If the needle is not located correctly, it may have been pushed past the nerve, and should be withdrawn and the process repeated. When the needle tip is properly located, 20 to 30 ml of local anesthetic drug is injected at that site. (The use of sheathed needles and other modifications on the use of the nerve stimulator are described in Chapter 6.) Conversely, a paresthesia-seeking technique simply demands that a logical and systematic "insertion and redirection" movement of the needle be carried out while the patient is asked to say "now" when a distal paresthesia is produced. As with the axillary block, digital pressure in the axilla distal to the injection site can theoretically increase the central flow of the local anesthetic drug.

Comments

Injection of local anesthetic drug into the perivascular spaces between the axilla and interscalene area, alternative to interscalene/supraclavicular and axillary block techniques that might preserve the advantages and overcome the disadvantages. This approach to the plexus is at a higher level than that of the axillary approach, assuring blockade of all the nerves derived from the plexus, but at a lower level than that of the supraclavicular approach, minimizing the risk of pleural injury. Although such an *infraclavicular* approach was originally suggested by Bazy and co-workers[5] in 1917, it did not gain much popularity because the available equipment and technology did not give anesthesia comparable to the classic Kulenkampff technique, and still resulted in pleural trauma. In 1977, Raj and associates[50] modified the infraclavicular technique by a lateral direction of the needle; thus avoiding the potential pneumothorax and using the nerve stimulator to make the technique of locating the plexus more acceptable to the patients. It is still not widely used, since most believe it requires the use of a nerve stimulator and a long needle able to penetrate both the pectoralis major and minor muscles, which can potentially cause greater patient discomfort than other perivascular techniques that block the plexus at more superficial points. It has recently gained favor for use with patients in whom the continuous block technique is desired, because maintaining an aseptic dressing at this site is more practical than at one in the axilla.

USE OF A NERVE STIMULATOR FOR ARM BLOCKS

The availability of high-quality insulated needles and stimulators designed for peripheral nerves provides a practical adjunct to plexus and peripheral nerve blocks in the arm and elsewhere in the body. It is important that the characteristics of the stimulator are suitable and that it is applied correctly, as described in Chapter 6 and Figure 6-5. It must be emphasized that use of a nerve stimulator as an adjunct to brachial plexus block is no substitute for anatomic knowledge and the use of appropriate landmarks, as described in the foregoing sections. The stimulator should not be turned on until the needle is approaching the "target," having first used standard technique. It is vital that a motor response be obtained at only minimal current output; otherwise, the tip of the needle may be still some distance from the nerve. Although uninsulated needles can be used at times successfully, it is now clear that accuracy increases with coated needles (see Chapter 6). It is important to be sure that the cathode (-) of the stimulator is attached to the needle; otherwise, 4 times as much current is needed to stimulate the nerve (see Chapter 6, Fig. 6-5); because current output is what stimulates the nerve; this is what the operator wants to be displayed (from 0.1 to 1.0 ma) on the stimulator. With precise needle placement, a motor response should be obtained with approximately 0.1 ma of current output. With a sheathed needle, muscle contraction will increase as the needle nears the nerve and then decrease as the needle moves past the nerve. The use of anatomic landmarks to position the needle close to the nerve or plexus obviates the need to turn on the stimulator with a superficially placed needle and high current output. Such a practice is to be condemned, since it produces confusing and painful local muscle contractions.

The major muscle responses obtained for a needle located close to radial, ulnar, median, and musculocutaneous nerves are shown in Figure 10-10.

Peripheral Blocks

With safe and reliable plexus anesthesia, and particularly with the more widespread use of axillary block, the need for distal nerve blocks has diminished; however, at times these can be of considerable value. Peripheral block can be useful when circumstances such as infection, difficult anatomy, bilateral surgery, or a physician's inexperience may preclude the use of more proximal plexus blocks. Also, it can be used for surgery on the hand that is of limited extent and duration, when it is on a part supplied by individual nerves, or as an alternative to digital, particularly multiple digital, blocks. With nerve block at the wrist, long flexor motor power is retained; this is of considerable value in certain kinds of hand procedures, such as tenolysis.[16,31] Peripheral block is always available to supplement patchy brachial plexus anesthesia. The peripheral ulnar nerve block is also the most reliable model for testing local anesthetic drugs.[40]

General Considerations

Tourniquet

A pneumatic tourniquet is often part of the surgical procedure of the arm. This has often been said to contraindicate peripheral blocks as the method of anesthesia. Up to 30 minutes of tourniquet time is well tolerated by most patients, even when they are unpremedicated, and this can easily be extended to an hour with suitable analgesic sedation.[24] A sterile Esmarch bandage should be available for the surgeon to apply *after* skin preparation and marking. The method of tourniquet application may also be a factor in patient tolerance.[17] Use of circumferential subcutaneous infiltration, although extensively used, would appear to be unnecessary and of doubtful value.[43]

Elbow or Wrist?

There may be little to be gained by blocking the nerves at the elbow as opposed to the wrist for surgical anesthesia. Only hand anesthesia can be achieved by blocking the three major nerve trunks at the elbow, because the forearm cutaneous nerves arise in the upper arm and are quite separate at this level. The wrist block is usually simpler to perform, but it is sometimes preferable to use a combination of the two levels (see Fig. 10-17 for areas of sensory supply of individual nerves of the arm). When caring for chronic pain patients, a block at the elbow can sometimes be an advantage, since a more discrete sensory block is produced: The effect of proximal injection does not preclude the possibility that the pain relief is from the local injection rather than from the specific nerve blocked.

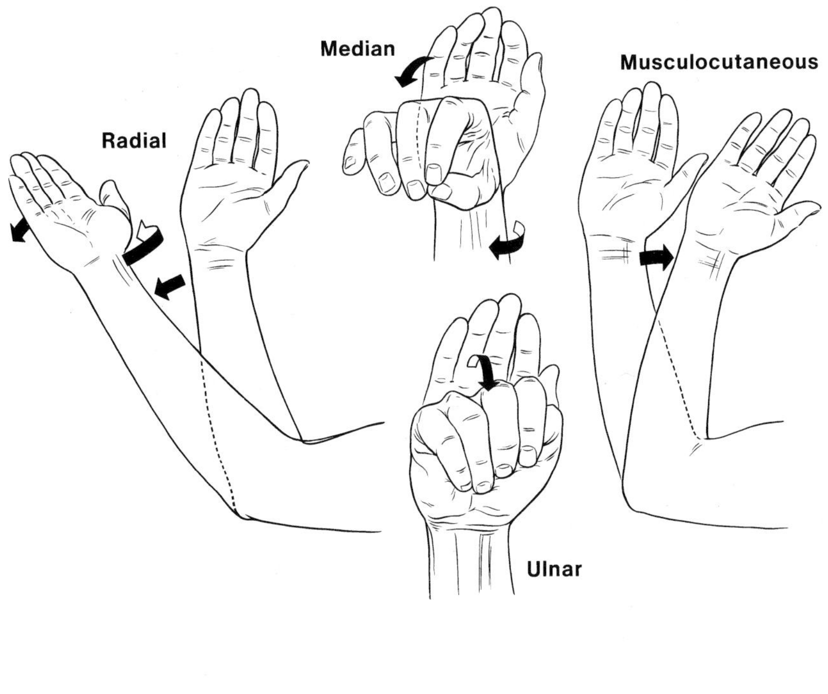

FIG. 10-10. Some characteristic movements of fingers, wrist, and elbow in response to nerve stimulation. *Radial*: Note extension at elbow, supination of arm, and extension at wrist and of fingers. *Median*: Note pronation of arm, flexion of wrist, opposition of middle, forefinger, and thumb, and flexion of lateral three fingers. *Ulnar*: Note flexion of wrist, adduction of all fingers (clenched together), and flexion and opposition of lateral two fingers toward thumb. *Musculocutaneous*: Note flexion at elbow. In general, it is not always possible to obtain stimulation of each major nerve or all components of that nerve. Thus motor responses vary considerably.

Paresthesias

As a general rule, anesthesia is quicker in onset and more reliable if paresthesias are sought when blocking the median and ulnar nerves at either elbow or wrist. Care should be taken, however, to avoid injecting the solution intraneurally. Intense paresthesias on injection of a small volume would tend to suggest intraneural placement, and the needle should be either advanced or withdrawn slightly (or both) as the injection is made. Another method of avoiding intraneural injection is to keep moving the needle in and out while injecting; this will deposit solution superficial and deep to the nerve but has the potential disadvantage of greater needle trauma.[44]

Paresthesias, if they are not elicited on initial insertion, are sought by gentle fanwise insertions across the path of the nerve. If no paresthesias are found, the anesthesiologist should retrace the fan and inject as the needle is moved gently in and out, the aim being to lay down a wall of solution over an area of approximately 2 cm^2 across the path of the nerves.

Median Nerve Block

Median nerve block is applicable for surgery on the radial side of the palm and 3½ digits, and for reduction of fractures, particularly the first metacarpal. It is usually combined with either ulnar or radial nerve blocks, depending on whether surgery extends to the ulnar side or to the dorsum of the hand. There is also occasional variation in innervation, which may necessitate multiple blocks.

Technique for Block at Elbow

The arm is abducted on a board with the elbow extended and the forearm supinated. One should stand alongside the radial aspect of the forearm. The intercondylar line between medial and lateral epicondyles of the humerus is drawn across the cubital fossa and the brachial artery is palpated and marked at this level (Fig. 10-11). A 25-gauge, 16-mm needle is inserted at a point just medial to the artery and directed perpendicular to the skin (Fig. 10-12). Three to 5 ml should be injected after eliciting paresthesias. If no paresthesias are obtained on initial insertion, the needle should be systematically redirected fanwise, medially from the artery, to inject local anesthetic near the path of the nerve.

Technique for Block at Wrist

The arm is abducted on a board with the elbow extended and the forearm supinated. One should sit beside the ulnar side of the hand for right arm block and the radial side for left arm block. The palmaris tendon should be made prominent by flexing the patient's wrist against resistance, with the fingers extended. The radial border of the tendon should be marked at a point approximately 2 cm proximal to the most distal wrist crease. If the tendon is absent, the point will be approximately 1 cm medial to the ulnar edge of the flexor carpi radialis tendon. With the wrist slightly extended, a 25-gauge, 16-mm needle is inserted perpendicular to the skin. The nerve is contacted on penetration of the deep fascia, usually at a depth of less than 1 cm (Fig. 10-14A). Three to 5 ml should be injected after eliciting paresthesias. If paresthesias

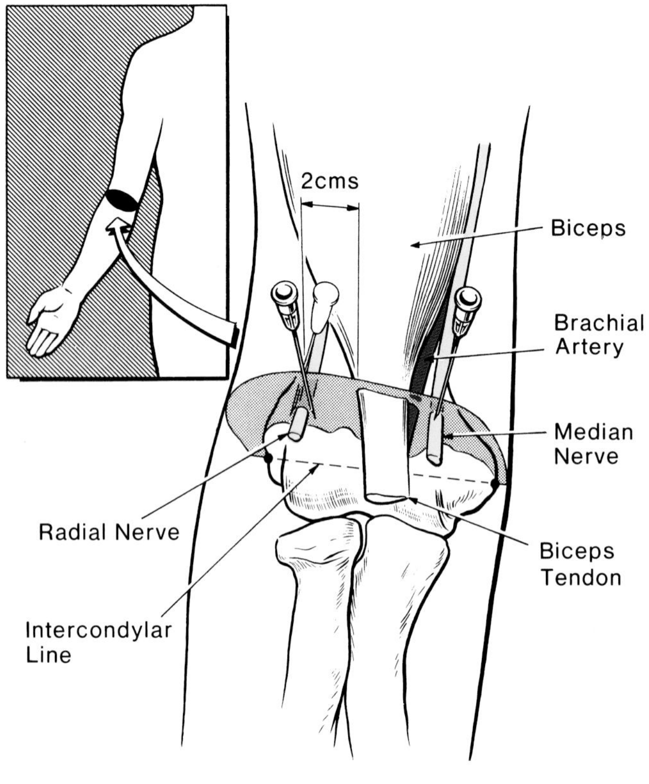

FIG. 10-11. Anatomic landmarks for median and radial nerve block at elbow.

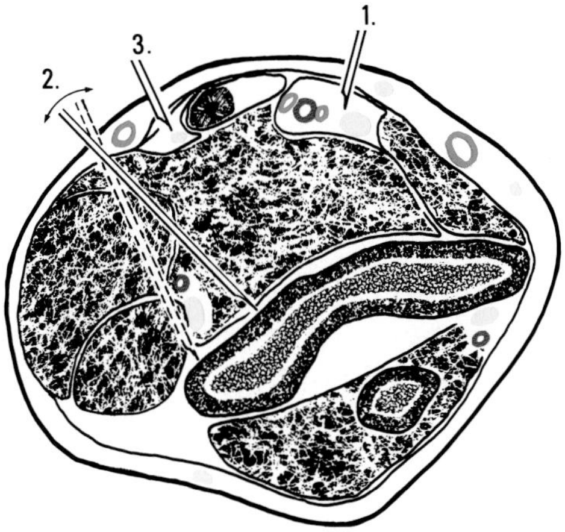

FIG. 10-12. Cross-section of arm at elbow. *(1)* Median nerve block. *(2)* Radial nerve block. *(3)* Lateral cutaneous nerve of forearm block. (Note nerve under deep fascia and close to biceps tendon.)

are not obtained on initial insertion, they should be sought in a more ulnar direction, under cover of the palmaris tendon. One ml of solution is deposited in the subcutaneous tissue on withdrawal to block the palmar cutaneous branch.

Ulnar Nerve Block

This anesthetic technique is applicable for surgery of the ulnar side of the hand and one and one-half (usually) digits and for reduction of fractures of the fifth digit, commonly the neck of the metacarpal. It is often used on its own, but may be combined with median and radial nerve blocks. Block of the ulnar nerve at the elbow is believed by some to lead to a significant incidence of residual ulnar neuritis. This is probably because where the nerve is palpable, it is well protected within a fibrous tunnel, and a high intraneural pressure may be generated. This approach is quite satisfactory, provided it is performed with a fine needle and only a small volume, such as 1 ml, is injected.[40] However, it may be preferable to block the nerve 2 to 3 cm proximal to the medial epicondyle, with 5 to 8 ml of solution.

Technique for Block at Elbow

With the patient lying supine, the elbow is flexed, with the forearm across the chest. One should stand beside the patient on the side of the arm to be blocked. The medial epicondyle and ulnar groove are palpated and a point taken 2 to 3 cm proximal and along the line of the nerve. A 25-gauge, 16-mm needle is introduced perpendicular to the skin and advanced gently, until a paresthesia is obtained or periosteum encountered (Fig. 10-13). Five to 8 ml should be injected after paresthesias. If no paresthesias are obtained on initial insertion, the needle should be moved fanwise across the path of the nerve until they are elicited. No paresthesias will probably result in a long delay or inadequate anesthesia.

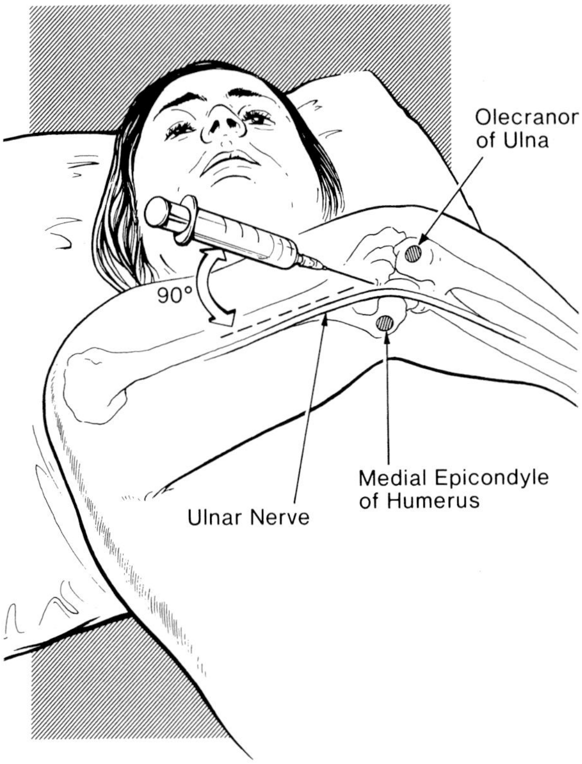

FIG. 10-13. Anatomic landmarks for ulnar nerve block at elbow. Note direction of needle at 90° to humerus.

Technique for Block at Wrist

Ulnar block at the wrist is more reliable and reportedly carries less risk of post-procedure neuritis than block of the ulnar nerve at the elbow. The arm is abducted on a board with the elbow extended and the forearm supinated. One should sit alongside the ulnar side of the hand.

At the wrist, the ulnar nerve is blocked where it lies under cover of the flexor carpi ulnaris tendon just proximal to the pisiform bone, before the nerve bifurcates into its terminal deep (motor) and the superficial (sensory) branches. At this point, the nerve lies on the ulnar side of, but deep to, the ulnar artery, and it has already given off its palmar cutaneous and dorsal branches (see Fig. 10-15).

The nerve may be approached either from the volar aspect of the wrist, with the needle directed dorsally from the radial side of the flexor carpi ulnaris tendon, or, preferably, from the ulnar side of the tendon with the needle directed radially for a distance of approximately 1.5 cm (see Fig. 10-14). A 25-gauge, 16-mm needle is again most suitable, and 3 to 5 ml is injected after paresthesias is elicited. It is important to seek paresthesias with this second approach, in case the needle comes into a plane anterior to the neurovascular bundle, and thus anterior to a thick fascial layer. The approach from the side of the wrist is preferred because it is possible to block the cutaneous branches from the same site of entry. Also, there is probably less chance of damaging the ulnar artery. If necessary, the two cutaneous branches may be blocked be-

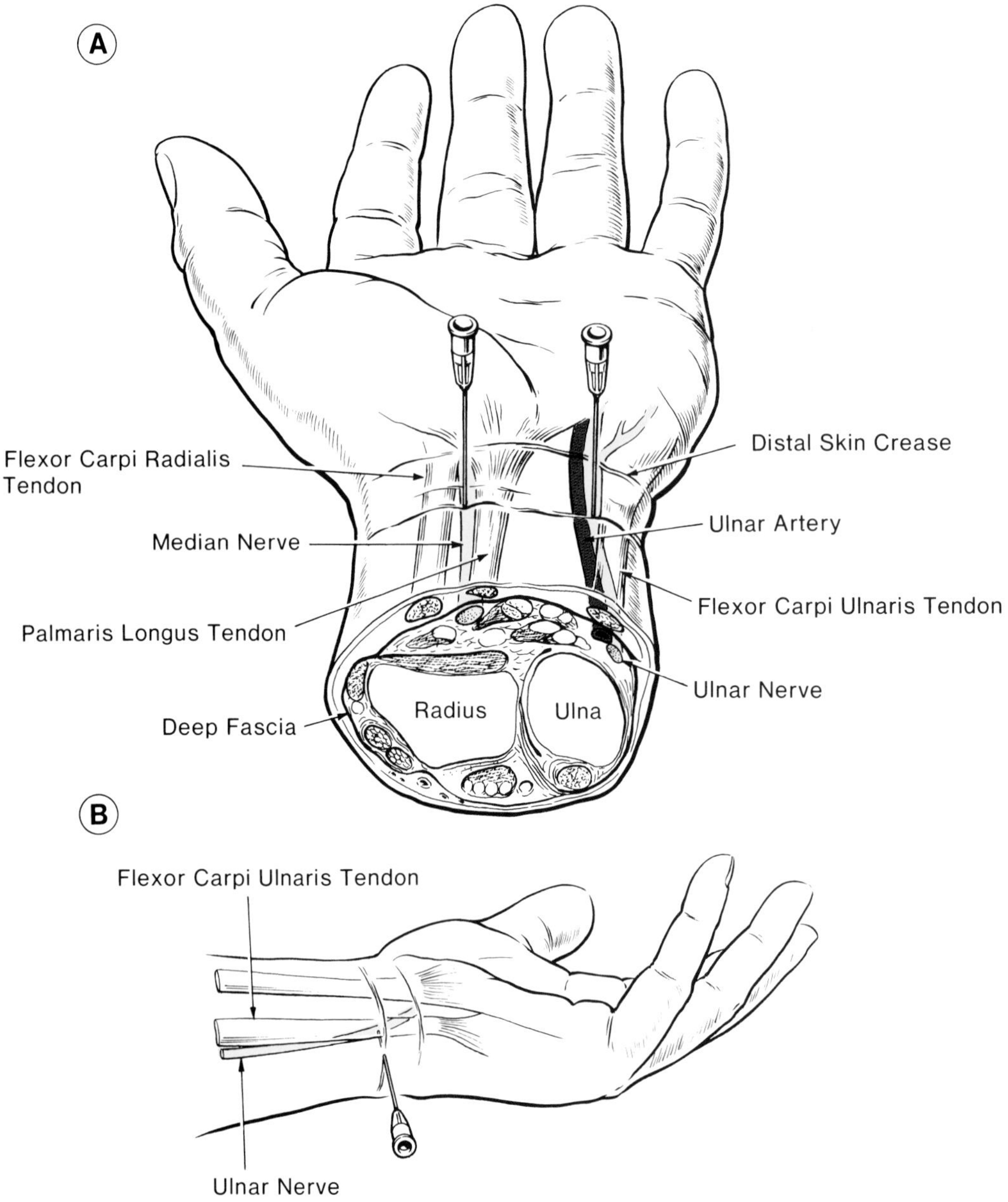

FIG. 10-14. A: Landmarks and technique of needle insertion for median and ulnar nerve block at wrist. **B:** Alternative method of ulnar nerve block, from ulnar side of wrist.

fore removing the needle completely: the dorsal branch by subcutaneous infiltration of 2 to 3 ml back along the ulnar border of the carpus and the palmar branch, by directing the needle onto the volar aspect of the wrist as far as the radial side of the flexor carpi ulnaris tendon, and then injecting 1 to 2 ml (see Fig. 10-15).

Radial Nerve Block

This is an easy and useful block at the wrist to interrupt the terminal cutaneous branches that supply the radial side of the dorsum of the hand and proximal dorsal parts of the radial 3½ (usually) digits. It is often combined with median nerve block.

Block at the elbow is more difficult and uncertain and has limited surgical applications. It may be combined with block of the lateral cutaneous nerve of the forearm for arteriovenous fistula surgery at the wrist, and it may be needed to supplement inadequate plexus block, particularly when fractures of the radius are involved. Conversely, performing a diagnostic radial nerve block at the elbow may allow more complete understanding of some chronic pain syndromes.

Technique for Block at Elbow

The radial nerve is blocked as it passes over the anterior aspect of the lateral epicondyle, close to the bone (see Fig.

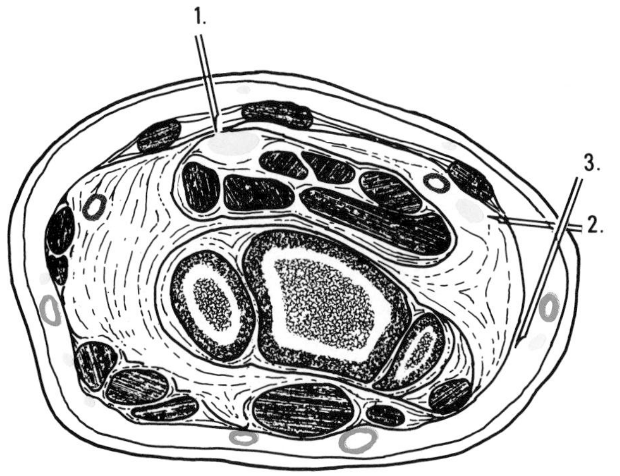

FIG. 10-15. Cross-section of forearm at wrist showing alternative method of ulnar nerve block *(2)* from ulnar side of flexor carpi ulnaris tendon. The dorsal cutaneous branch of the ulnar nerve can also be blocked by redirecting the needle superficially in a dorsal direction *(3)*. Median nerve block *(1)* is also shown. Note necessity to pierce the deep fascia; however, the median nerve lies less than 1 cm below the skin.

10-11). The arm is abducted on a board with the elbow extended and the forearm supinated. One should stand alongside the ulnar aspect of the arm for left arm block and the radial aspect for right arm block.

The intercondylar line is marked and the biceps tendon palpated at this level. From a point along the intercondylar line 2 cm lateral to the biceps tendon, a longer (4 to 5 cm) 23-gauge needle is inserted directly toward the humerus, that is, onto the bone of the lateral epicondyle toward its lateral margin (see Figs. 10-11, 10-12). The palpating index finger of the left hand on the posterior aspect of the epicondyle is used as a guide to direction. Two to 4 ml is injected as the needle is withdrawn 0.5 to 1 cm. The needle is withdrawn almost to the skin and redirected twice, slightly more medially each time but again onto bone, and further injections are made in the same fashion.

Technique for Block at Wrist

Radial nerve block at the wrist is a field block of the superficial terminal branches as they pass in a variable manner over the radial side of the carpus. The anatomic "snuffbox" is made prominent by extension of the thumb. The extensor pollicis longus and brevis tendons are both marked. A point is taken over the extensor longus tendon, opposite the base of the first metacarpal. A 25-gauge, 16-mm needle is directed proximally along the tendon as far as the dorsal radial tubercle as 2 ml is injected subcutaneously. The needle is withdrawn almost to the skin and redirected at a right angle across the snuffbox, to a point just past the brevis tendon, as a further 1 ml is injected (Fig. 10-16).

Musculocutaneous Nerve Block

Block of the musculocutaneous nerve usually is performed as a supplement to axillary plexus block, but it may be indicated as an independent procedure or in combination with block of the radial nerve.

First, it may be blocked as the main nerve trunk in the substance of the coracobrachialis muscle, from the same point of entry as in the axillary block procedure.[20] Second, it may be blocked 5 cm proximal to the elbow crease, where the terminal sensory *lateral cutaneous nerve of the forearm* is said to emerge from between the brachialis and biceps muscles.[20] Third, a technique has been described in which the block is performed just lateral to the tendon of the biceps muscle at the level of the intercondylar line. Olson has shown in 64 cadaver dissections that the nerve, rather than emerging from the brachialis biceps groove and running down over the cubital fossa superficially and somewhat lateral to the biceps tendon, stays deep to the fascia and close in under cover of

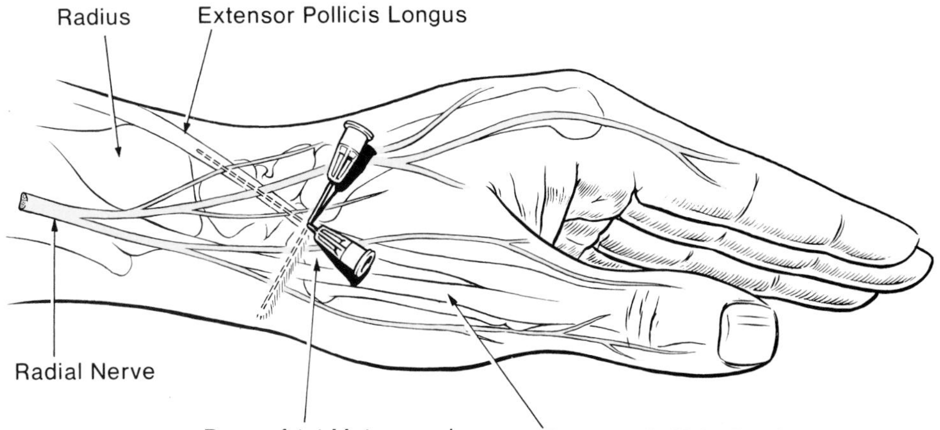

FIG. 10-16. Landmarks and method of needle insertion for radial nerve block at the wrist.

the lateral side of the tendon before it becomes superficial, at a variable distance distal to the elbow crease (Figs. 10-11, 10-12).[45] Last, the musculocutaneous nerve may be blocked as a subcutaneous field block.

Technique for Blocking Lateral to the Tendon of the Biceps Muscle. The arm is abducted on a board with the elbow extended and the forearm supinated; the intercondylar line and biceps tendon are marked. A 25-gauge, 16-mm needle is inserted at the point at which the intercondylar line crosses the lateral border of the biceps tendon, and 2 ml of anesthetic is injected deep to the fascia, just lateral to the tendon. Failures of block result from too deep an insertion (Figs. 10-11, 10-12).

This method is more definitive than block in the biceps brachialis groove, much less solution is required, and it can be performed in a few seconds.

Field Block of the Cutaneous Nerves of the Forearm

The *lateral cutaneous nerve* often does not pierce the deep fascia until it is distal to the elbow crease (see above). Subcutaneous infiltration should begin from a point 5 cm distal to the crease and in line with the biceps tendon, and then directed laterally for a distance of 3 to 4 cm.

The *medial cutaneous nerve of the forearm* arises from the medial cord of the brachial plexus in the axilla. It pierces the deep fascia in company with the basilic vein in the midarm and then bifurcates. Its anterior, or volar, branch passes down over the front of the cubital fossa medial to the biceps tendon to supply the anteromedial aspect of the forearm. The smaller posterior, or ulnar, branch passes downward, farther back, just in front of the medial epicondyle, to supply the posterior aspect (Fig. 10-17). Subcutaneous infiltration should extend from the biceps tendon to the medial epicondyle (see Figs. 10-11, 10-12).

The *posterior cutaneous nerve of the forearm* arises from the radial nerve and pierces the deep fascia above the elbow. It descends along the lateral side of the arm and then along the back of the forearm to the wrist. From a point directly over the lateral epicondyle of the humerus, with the elbow slightly flexed, subcutaneous infiltration should extend for 3 to 4 cm toward the olecranon.

Local Anesthetic Block of the Digital Nerves

Digital nerve block is a commonly used and effective method of anesthesia for a wide variety of minor outpatient surgical procedures on the digits. However, because of the uncommon but serious complications of ischemia and necrosis, it should not be undertaken lightly; alternatives such as nerve block at the wrist should be considered, particularly when more than one digit is involved. When digital nerve block is used, specific technical details must be strictly followed.

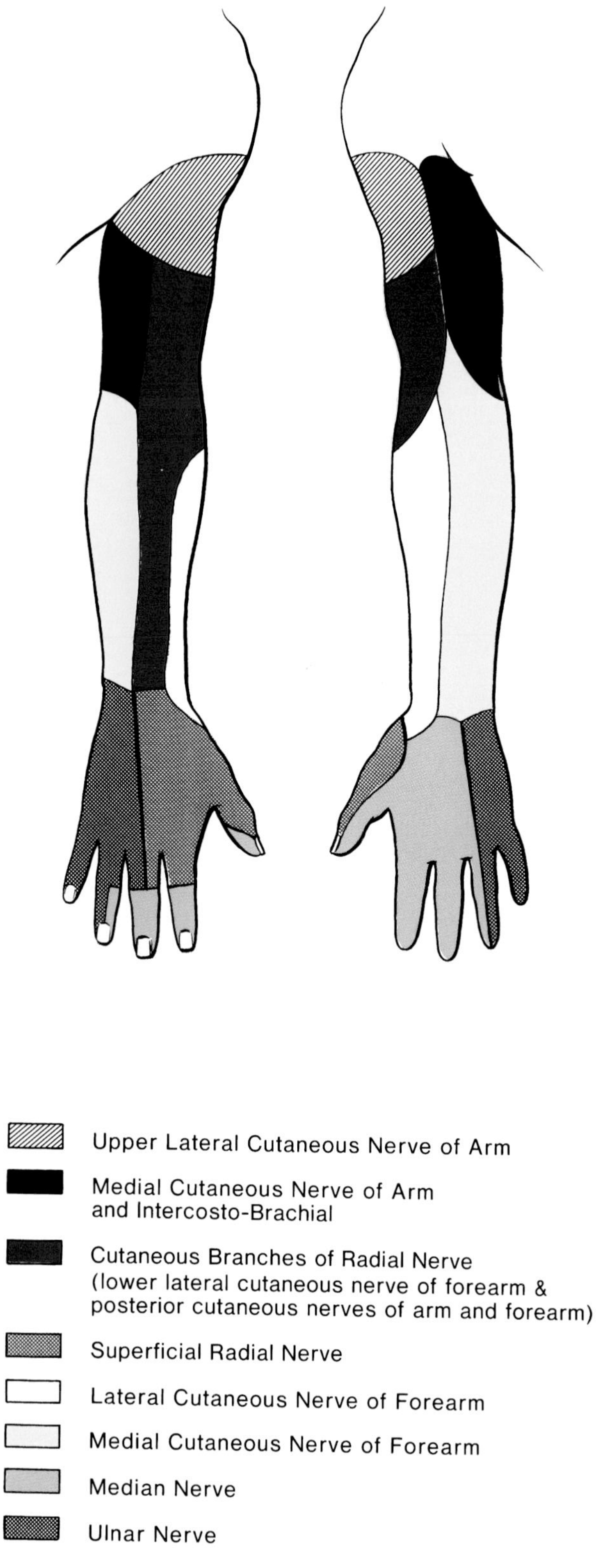

FIG. 10-17. Cutaneous nerve supply of upper limb.

Anatomy

The common digital nerves are derived from the median and ulnar nerves and divide in the distal palm into the volar digital nerves, to supply adjacent sides of the fingers, palmar aspect, tip, and nail bed area. These main digital nerves are accompanied by digital vessels and run on the ventrolateral aspect of the finger immediately lateral to the flexor tendon sheath. Small dorsal digital nerves supply the back of the fingers as far as the proximal (distal) joint. These run on the dorsolateral aspect of the finger.

Techniques

Block of Both Volar and Dorsal Digital Nerves at Each Side of the Base of the Finger. A 25-gauge, 16-mm needle is inserted at a point on the dorsolateral aspect of the base of the finger and directed anteriorly to slide past the base of the phalanx (Fig. 10-18A). The needle is advanced until the anesthesiologist feels the resistance of the palmar dermis, while observing for protrusion of palmor dermis directly opposite the needle path. One ml of solution is injected as the needle is withdrawn 2 to 3 mm to block the volar nerve, and

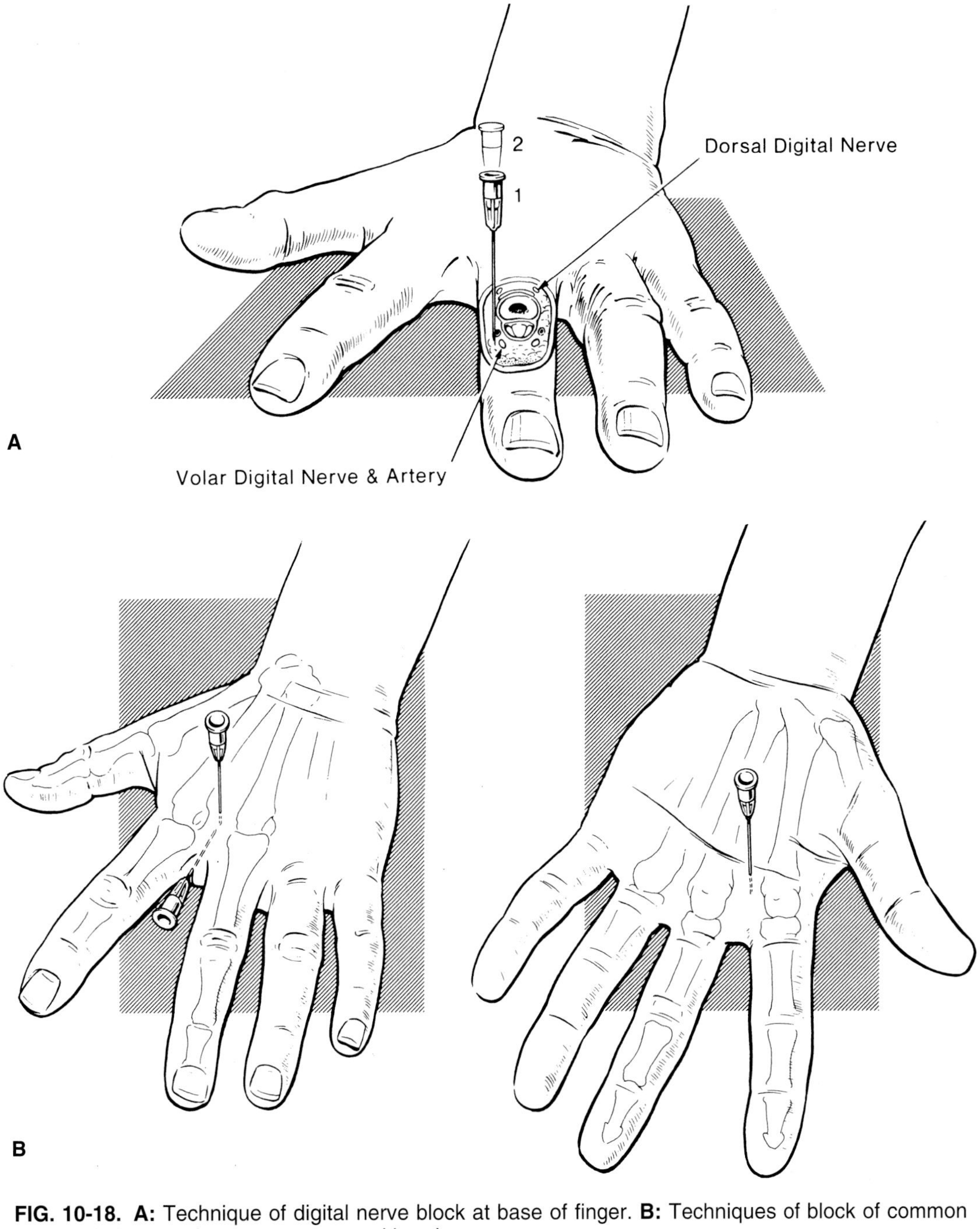

FIG. 10-18. A: Technique of digital nerve block at base of finger. **B:** Techniques of block of common volar digital nerves between metacarpal heads.

0.5 ml is injected just deep to the point of entry to block the dorsal nerve. The volar digital nerves can also be approached from the side of the finger.

Block of the Common Volar Digital Nerves near Their Bifurcation Between the Metacarpal Heads. With the fingers widely extended, a 25-gauge, 16-mm needle is inserted into the web 2 to 3 mm dorsal to the junction of the web and palmar skin. It is directed proximally toward the hand in line with the extended fingers, and 2 ml of solution is injected when the needle almost reaches the hub (Fig. 10-18B). Redirection from the same point of entry to the region of the dorsal nerves on each side can be performed easily, if necessary.

A metacarpal approach may also be performed, either from the dorsal aspect and inserting the needles between the bones almost as far as the palmar skin, or from the palmar aspect at the level of the distal crease, and inserting a short fine needle just through the palmar aponeurosis[13,14,51] (Fig. 10-18B). This second approach would seem to be unnecessarily painful. For those digital blocks, lower concentrations of local anesthetics are satisfactory and *must be used without vasoconstrictors.*

Thumb Block

The thumb is supplied by superficial branches of the radial nerve (see Fig. 10-16) and by digital branches of the median nerve (see Fig. 10-17). Thus, complete sensory block of the thumb is produced by median nerve block at the wrist (see Fig. 10-14A) and radial nerve block at the wrist (see Fig. 10-16). The thumb can also be blocked by circumferential infiltration at the base of the thumb ("ring block"), using a solution without epinephrine.

Infiltration of Fracture Sites

The principle of this technique is to render insensitive the periosteum in the region of the bony fracture. It has most commonly been applied in the treatment of Colles's fractures. The results with expert, careful, and patient technique, would appear to be satisfactory.[22]

Technique. Under very strict aseptic conditions, 10 to 15 ml (if it is a Colles's fracture) of 1% lidocaine or mepivacaine without epinephrine is injected into the periosteum at and around the fracture site from the dorsal aspect. At least 10 minutes must then elapse before the fracture is manipulated gently. This technique is not recommended for routine use, not only because of the risk of infection and the possibility of rapid uptake of the local anesthetic, but also because it often does not produce the satisfactory analgesia or muscle relaxation that is found after brachial plexus block.

Complications and Contraindications (see Chapter 21)

One specific complication of these peripheral blocks, apart from those already mentioned, is vascular insufficiency and gangrene after digital nerve block. This catastrophe is a result of digital artery occlusion, together with collateral circulation insufficiency, and often a series of causative factors must be involved to produce this problem.

Epinephrine-containing Solutions. Although not the only cause of gangrene, vasoconstrictor solutions used in this region undoubtedly have been responsible for such cases in the past and should never be used.

Volume of Solution. The mechanical pressure effects of injecting solution into a potentially confined space should always be borne in mind, particularly in blocks at the base of the digit. Maximum volumes of 2 ml on each side should not be exceeded.

Tourniquets. These are commonly applied to produce a bloodless field (and perhaps in the hope that they will both hasten and prolong anesthesia). Bradfield, in a report on 44 cases of gangrene, could not exonerate the tourniquet, but recommended that an upper limit of 15 minutes' duration could be set, and that it never be used in patients with Raynaud's phenomena.[8] Bunnell has condemned the use of rubber-band-type tourniquets at the base of the digit and has stated that whenever a tourniquet is needed, a proper upper arm tourniquet should be applied.[7]

Peripheral Vascular Disease. In patients with small vessel disease, perhaps an alternative method should be sought in addition to avoidance of digital tourniquet.

Direct Vascular Damage. Direct vascular damage caused by the needle may contribute to the complication. The incidence of digital gangrene is unknown. Even in reported cases, the duration of tourniquet use and other important facts often are not recorded. With the current level of knowledge, it would seem wise to avoid vasoconstrictors; avoid a digital tourniquet, or, certainly, limit its duration to 15 minutes; use small volumes of solution; avoid digital blocks in patients whose vessels may be suspect; and, as with all nerve blocks, be gentle and patient.

A source of infection proximate to the proposed site of injection is probably the main contraindication to nerve blocks on the upper limb.

REFERENCES

1. Accardo, N.J., and Adriani, J.A.: Brachial plexus block—A simplified technique using the axillary route. South Med. J. *42:*920, 1949.
2. Ang, E.T., Lassale, B., and Goldfarb, G.: Continuous axillary brachial plexus block—A clinical and anatomical study. Anesth. Analg. *63:*680–684, 1984.
3. Babitski, P.: A new method of anesthetizing the brachial plexus. Zentralbl Chir, *45:*215, 1918.
4. Bazy, L., and Blondin, S.: L'anesthésie du plexus brachial. Anesth. Anal. (Paris), *1:*190, 1935.
5. Bazy, L., Pouchet, V., Sourdat, P., and Laboure, J.: Anesthesie Regionale. pp. 222–225. Philadelphia, W.B. Saunders, 1917.
6. Bonica, J.J., Moore, D.C., and Orlov, M.: Brachial plexus block anesthesia. Am. J. Surg., *65*, 1949.
7. Boyes, J.H.: Bunnell's Surgery of the Hand, 5th ed. Philadelphia, J.B. Lippincott, 1970.
8. Bradfield, W.J.D.: Digital block anesthesia and its complications. Br. J. Surg., *50:*495, 1962.
9. Brown, D.L.: Atlas of Regional Anesthesia, Philadelphia, W.B. Saunders Co. 1992.

10. Brown, D.L.: Neurologic complications of anesthesia. *In:* Aminoff, M.J., (ed.): Neurology and General Medicine, 2nd Ed., New York, Churchill-Livingstone, 1994.
11. Brown, D.L., Cahill, D.R., and Bridenbaugh, L.D.: Supraclavicular nerve block: Anatomic analysis of a method to prevent pneumothorax. Anesth. Analg. *76:*530, 1993.
12. Burnham, P.J.: Simple regional nerve block for surgery of the hand and forearm. J.A.M.A., *169:*109, 1959.
13. Burnham, P.J.: Regional block anaesthesia for surgery of the fingers and thumb. Ind. Med. Surg., *27:*67, 1958.
14. Chase, R.A.: Atlas of Hand Surgery. Philadelphia, W.B. Saunders, 1973.
15. Clayton, M.L., and Turner, D.A.: Upper arm block anesthesia in children with fractures. J.A.M.A., *169:*99, 1959.
16. Conolly, W.B., and Berry, F.R.: Selective peripheral nerve blocks for reconstructive hand surgery. Med. J. Aust., *2:*94, 1974.
17. Crews, J. C., Hilgenhurst, G., Leavitt, B., *et al.*: Tourniquet pain: The response to the maintenance of tourniquet inflation on the upper extremity of volunteers. Reg. Anesth. *16:*314, 1991.
18. Crile, G.W.: Anesthesia of nerve roots with cocaine. Cleve. Med. J., *2:*355, 1897.
19. de Jong, R.H.: Axillary block of the brachial plexus. Anesthesiology, *22:*215, 1961.
20. de Jong, R.H.: Modified axillary block. Anesthesiology, *26:*615, 1965.
21. Denson, D.D., Raj, P.P., and Saldahna, F., *et al.*: Continuous perineural infusion of bupivacaine for prolonged analgesia: Pharmacokinetic considerations. Int. J. Clin. Pharmacol. Ther. Toxicol., *21:*591, 1983.
22. Dinley, R.J., and Michelinakis, E.: Local anaesthesia in the reduction of Colles' fracture. Injury, *4:*345, 1972–1973.
23. Dogliotti, A.M.: Anesthesia: Narcosis, Local, Regional, and Spinal. (Authorized English translation by Scuderi, C.S.) Chicago, S.B. Debour, 1939.
24. Dupont, C., *et al.*: Hand surgery under wrist block and local infiltration anesthesia using an upper arm tourniquet. Plast. Reconstr. Surg., *50:*532, 1972.
25. Eather, K.F.: Axillary brachial plexus block. Anesthesiology, *19:*683, 1958.
26. Erikkson, E.: A simplified method of axillary block. Nord. Med., 681325, 1962.
27. Erikkson, E.: Axillary brachial plexus anaesthesia in children with Citanest. Acta Anaesthesiol. Scand., *16* (Suppl):291, 1965.
28. Hirschel, G: Die Anasthesierung des Plexus Brachialis fur die Operataionen an der oberen Extremitat. Munch. Med. Wochenschr., *58:*1555, 1911.
29. Hopcroft, S.C.: The axillary approach to brachial plexus anaesthesia. Anaesth. Intensive Care, *1:*232, 1973.
30. Hudon, F., and Jacques, A.: Block of the brachial plexus by the axillary route. Can. Anaesth. Soc. J., *6:*400, 1959.
31. Hunter, J.M., *et al.*: A dynamic approach to problems of hand function. Clin. Orthop., *104:*112, 1974.
32. Jackson, L., and Keats, A.S.: Mechanism of brachial plexus palsy following anesthesia. Anesthesiology, *26:*190, 1965.
33. Knoblanche, G.E.: The incidence and aetiology of phrenic nerve blockade associated with supraclavicular bronchial plexus block. Anesth. Intens. Care, *7:*36, 1979.
34. Kroll, D.A., Caplan, R.A., Posner, K., Ward, R.J., and Cheney, F.W.: Nerve injury associated with anesthesia. Anesthesiology, *73:*202, 1990.
35. Kulenkampff, D.: Die anasthesierung des Plexus Brachialis. Zentralbl. Chir., *38:*1337, 1911.
36. Kumar, A., *et al.*: Bilateral cervical and thoracic epidural blockade complicating interscalene brachial plexus block. Anesthesiology, *35:*650, 1971.
37. Labat, G.: Brachial plexus block: Details of technique with lantern slides. Br. J. Anaesth., *4:*174, 1926–1927.
38. Lanz, E., Theiss, D., Jankovic, D.: The extent of brachial blockade following various techniques of brachial plexus block. Anesth. Analg. *62:*55, 1984.
39. Livingston, E.M., and Werthein, H.: Brachial plexus block: Its clinical application. J.A.M.A., *88:*1464, 1927.
40. Lofstrom, J.B.: Ulnar nerve blockade for the evaluation of local anaesthetic agents. Br. J. Anaesth., *47:*297, 1975.
41. Lofstrom, J.B., *et al.*: Late disturbance in nerve function after block with local anaesthetic agents. Acta Anaesthesiol. Scand., *10:*111, 1966.
42. Macintosh, R.R., and Mushin, W.W.: Local Anesthesia: Brachial Plexus. Oxford, Blackwell Scientific Publishers, 1944.
43. Moir, D.D.: Axillary block to the brachial plexus. Anaesthesia, *17:*274, 1962.
44. Neuhof, H.: Supraclavicular anesthetization of the brachial plexus. J.A.M.A., *62:*1629, 1914.
45. Olson, I.A.: The origin of the lateral cutaneous nerve of the forearm and its anesthesia for modified brachial plexus block. J. Anat., *105:*381, 1969.
46. Partridge, B.L., and Benirschke, K.: Functional anatomy of the brachial plexus sheath: Implications for anesthesia. Anesthesiology *66:*743, 1987.
47. Patrick, J.: The technique of brachial plexus block anesthesia. Br. J. Surg., *27:*734, 1939–1940.
48. Pere, P., Pitkanen, M., Rosenberg, P.H., *et al.*: Effects of continuous interscalene brachial plexus block on diaphragm motion and on ventilatory function. Acta Anaesthesiol. Scand. *36:*53, 1992.
49. Pitkin, W.M., Southworth, J.L., and Hingson, R.A.: Conduction Anesthesia. Philadelphia, J.B. Lippincott, 1953.
50. Raj, P.P., Montgomery, S.J., Nettles, D., and Jenkins, M.T.: Infraclavicular brachial plexus block—A new approach. Anesth. Analg., *52:*897, 1973.
51. Rank, B.K., Wakefield, A.R., and Hueston, J.T.: Surgery of Repair as Applied to Hand Injuries, 4th ed., pp. 88. Edinburgh, E. & S. Livingstone, 1973.
52. Ross, S., and Scarborough, C.D.: Total spinal anesthesia following brachial plexus block. Anesthesiology, *39:*458, 1973.
53. Sada, T., Kobbayashi, T., and Murakami, S.: Continuous axillary brachial plexus block. Can. Anaesth. Soc. J. *30:*201, 1983.
54. Selander, D.: Catheter technique in axillary plexus block. Acta Anaesthesiol. Scand., *21:*324, 1977.
55. Selander, D., Edshage, S., and Wolff., T.: Paresthesiae or no paresthesiae? Nerve lesions after axillary block. Acta Anaesthesiol. Scand., *23:*27, 1979.
56. Sherwood-Dunn, B.: Reg. Anesth., pp. 242. Philadelphia, F.A. Davis, 1920.
57. Sims, J.K.: A modification of landmarks for infraclavicular approach to brachial plexus block. Anesth. Analg., *56:*554, 1977.
58. Strachauer, A.C.: Brachial plexus anesthesia: A complete local anesthesia of upper extremities permitting all major surgical procedures. Lancet, *34:*301, 1914.
59. Thompson, G.E., and Rorie, D.H.: Functional anatomy of the brachial plexus sheaths. Anesthesiology, *59:*117, 1983.
60. Tuominen, M., Rosenberg, P., and Kalso, E.: Blood levels of bupivacaine after single dose, supplementary dose, and continuous infusion in axillary plexus block. Acta Anaesthesiol. Scand., *27:*303, 1983.
61. Urmey, W.F., and McDonald, M.: Hemidiaphragmatic paresis during interscalene brachial plexus block: Effects on pulmonary function and chest wall mechanics. Anesth. Analg., *74:*352, 1992.
62. Vester-Andersen, T., Christiansen, C., Sorensen, M., *et al.*: Perivascular axillary block: II. Influence of injected volume of local anaesthetic on neural blockade. Acta Anaesthesiol. Scand., *27:*95, 1983.
63. Ward, M.E.: The interscalene approach to the brachial plexus. Anaesthesia, *29:*147, 1974.
64. Webling, D.D.: Anaesthesia of the upper limb for casualty procedures. Med. J. Aust., *2:*496, 1960.
65. Wen-Hsien, W.U.: Brachial plexus block. J.A.M.A., *215:*1953, 1971.
66. Whiffler, K.: Coracoid block—A safe and easy technique. Br. J. Anaesth., *53:*845, 1981.
67. Winnie, A.P.: An "immobile" needle for nerve blocks. Anesthesiology, *31:*577, 1969.
68. Winnie, A.P.: Interscalene brachial plexus block. Anesth. Analg., (Cleve.), *49:*455, 1970.
69. Winnie, A.P.: The perivascular techniques of brachial plexus anaesthesia. ASA Refresher Courses in Anesthesiology, *2:*151, 1974.
70. Winnie, A.P.: Recent developments in anesthesia. Surg. Clin. North Am., *55:*878, 1975.
71. Winnie, A.P.: Plexus anesthesia: I. Perivascular Techniques of Brachial Plexus Block. Philadelphia, W.B. Saunders, 1983.
72. Winnie, A.P., *et al.*: Interscalene cervical plexus block. Anesth. Analg. (Cleve.), *54:*370, 1975.
73. Winnie, A.P., and Collins, V.J.: The subclavian perivascular technique to brachial plexus anaesthesia. Anesthesiology, *25:*353, 1964.

Neural Blockade in Clinical Anesthesia and Management of Pain, Third Edition,
edited by M.J. Cousins and P.O. Bridenbaugh.
Lippincott–Raven Publishers, Philadelphia © 1998.

CHAPTER 11

The Lower Extremity

Somatic Blockade

Phillip O. Bridenbaugh and Denise J. Wedel

Although there are many anatomic similarities between the innervation and bony landmarks of the upper and lower extremities, there are fewer techniques for peripheral neural blockade of the lower extremity than for the upper extremity, and the enthusiasm for performing them is not as great. It is very probable that peridural or subarachnoid anesthesia, which provides rapid, complete, safe anesthesia of the lower extremities, is more easily accomplished by anesthesiologists than is lower extremity peripheral neural blockade. Further, although it is possible to accomplish complete anesthesia of the upper extremity with a single injection, that is still not the case with the lower extremity. Nonetheless, peripheral neural blockade of the lower extremity is easily accomplished with a minimum of side-effects and should have a place in the armamentarium of anesthesiologists who use regional anesthesia as part of their overall practice.

Like other forms of neural blockade, lower extremity techniques are not new. Braun mentions that blockade of the lateral cutaneous femoral nerve was described by Nystrom in 1909.[4] Laewen expanded on this by describing the additional blockade of the anterior crural nerve, and Keppler improved both techniques by advocating the elicitation of paresthesias. Earlier than all of this—around 1887—Crile performed amputations by exposing the sciatic nerve in the gluteal fold and the femoral nerve in the inguinal fold, and injecting cocaine intraneurally. Subsequently, no fewer than six others advocated percutaneous approaches to the sciatic nerve alone. Some of these same authors wrote about blockade of other nerves of the leg as well (see Chapter 1).

Not only is this old concept still valid today, but many of the techniques are nearly identical to the original descriptions. This emphasizes remarks made by Labat that: "Anatomy is the foundation upon which the entire concept of regional anesthesia is built;" that "Landmarks are anatomic guideposts of the body which are used to locate the nerves;" that "Superficial landmarks are distinguishing features of the surface of the body which can be easily recognized and identified by sight or palpation. Bones and their prominences, blood vessels and tendons serve as deep landmarks. Deep landmarks can be defined only by the point of the needle. They are the only reliable guide for advancing the needle in attempting to reach the vicinity of the nerve;" and that "The anesthetist should attempt to visualize the anatomic structures traversed by the needle and utilize the tactile senses to determine the impulses transmitted by the point of the needle as it approaches a deep landmark (e.g., bone)."[31]

The importance of anatomic landmarks is illustrated by the many approaches proposed for blockade of the sciatic nerve. The course of the nerve through the pelvis and medial to the femoral head provides a plethora of bony landmarks, all at some time in the past 100 years having been advocated as essential to an author's favorite technique.

NERVE SUPPLY

The nerve supply to the lower extremity is composed of the lumbar and sacral plexuses. The lumbar plexus is formed in the psoas muscle by the anterior rami of the first four lumbar nerves, including, frequently, a branch from the 12th thoracic nerve and occasionally one from the 5th lumbar nerve. The sacral plexus is derived from the anterior rami of the 4th and 5th lumbar and the first two or three sacral nerves.

While the lumbosacral plexus as a whole contributes to the nerve supply of the lower extremities, the upper part of the lumbar division supplies the iliohypogastric and ilioin-

P. O. Bridenbaugh: Department of Anesthesia, University of Cincinnati College of Medicine, Cincinnati, Ohio 45267-0531.

D. J. Wedel: Department of Anesthesiology, Mayo Clinic, Rochester, Minnesota 55905.

guinal nerves, which are in series with the thoracic nerves and innervate the trunk above the level of the extremity (see Chapter 14). Specifically, the iliohypogastric nerve provides cutaneous innervation to the skin of the buttock and the muscles of the abdominal wall. The ilioinguinal nerve supplies the skin of the perineum and adjoining portion of the inner thigh. A third nerve, the genitofemoral, arises from the first and second lumbar nerves. It supplies filaments to the genital area and adjacent parts of the thigh. It also gives off a lumboinguinal branch, which supplies the skin over the area of the femoral artery and femoral triangle (see Chapter 14, Fig. 14-11).

Caudad to these nerves are the five major nerves that supply all of the lower extremity. The *lateral femoral cutaneous nerve*, the *femoral nerve* (sometimes called the *anterior crural nerve*), and the *obturator nerve* are derived from the lumbar plexus, along with minor contributions from the iliohypogastric, ilioinguinal, and genitofemoral nerves. The two remaining nerves are the *posterior cutaneous nerve of the thigh* and the *sciatic nerve* (see Fig. 11-5B). The posterior cutaneous nerve has sometimes been referred to as the "small sciatic" nerve. It derives from the first, second, and third sacral nerves, as does the larger sciatic nerve, which also receives branches of the anterior rami of the fourth and fifth lumbar nerves. Inasmuch as the two nerves course through the pelvis together and out through the greater sciatic foramen, they are considered together when techniques for blocking the sciatic nerve are discussed.

The sciatic nerve is really an association of two major nerve trunks. The first is the tibial, derived from the ventral branches of the anterior rami of the fourth and fifth lumbar and first, second, and third sacral nerves. The second is the common peroneal, derived from the dorsal branches of the anterior rami of the same five nerves. These two major nerve trunks pass as the sciatic to the proximal angle of the popliteal fossa, where they separate, with the tibial portion passing medially and the common peroneal (lateral popliteal) laterally. This division can occur more cephalad or caudad to the popliteal fossa.

The smaller branches of these nerves, which provide distal innervation of the lower extremity, are discussed in detail in conjunction with techniques for nerve block at the knee and ankle.

LUMBAR SOMATIC NERVE BLOCK

Anatomy

In considering neural blockade of the lower extremity at the lumbar level, the bony, muscular, and fascial relation-

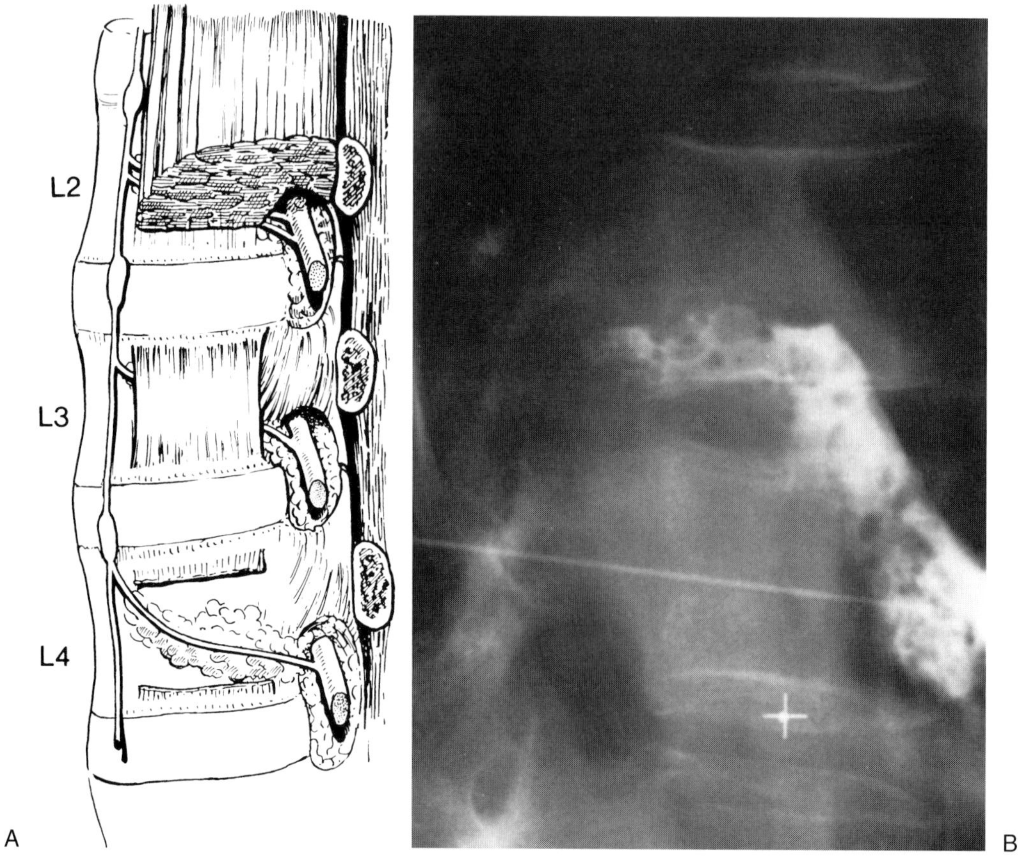

FIG. 11-1. Relationship of lumbar somatic nerve roots to sympathetic chain. Note the separation of somatic and sympathetic nerves by the psoas major muscle; however, there is also a potential path of communication via the fibrous arch illustrated at the L4 level (see also Chapter 13, Fig. 13-22).

ships to the emerging nerves must be recalled. The spinal nerve that leaves the spinal cord at each level is formed by the union of a ventral motor root with a dorsal sensory root. This mixed spinal nerve gives off a dorsal ramus, a ventral ramus, and a ramus communicans; the latter contributes to the formation of the sympathetic ganglion and trunk. The lumbar plexus, as previously noted, is formed by the anterior (ventral) divisions of the first, second, third, and fourth lumbar nerves, with about 50% inclusion of a branch from the 12th thoracic nerve and occasionally from the 5th lumbar nerve. The lumbar plexus is formed in front of the transverse processes of the lumbar vertebrae into a series of oblique loops that lie deep in the substance of the psoas major muscle and at the medial border of the quadratus lumborum muscle. From here, the individual nerves form and course in the direction of their terminal innervation.

The relation of the lumbar somatic plexus to the sympathetic chain should be remembered, since each may be blocked separately, but with a similar approach. The first and second lumbar spinal nerves, frequently the third, and sometimes the fourth, send communicating rami to form the lumbar portion of the sympathetic trunk. The sympathetic trunk lies on the ventrolateral surface of the lumbar and sacral bodies medial to the anterior foramina. It is apparent, therefore, that although these two nerve systems are separated by distance, muscle, and tissue planes, they have considerable intercommunication (Fig. 11-1).

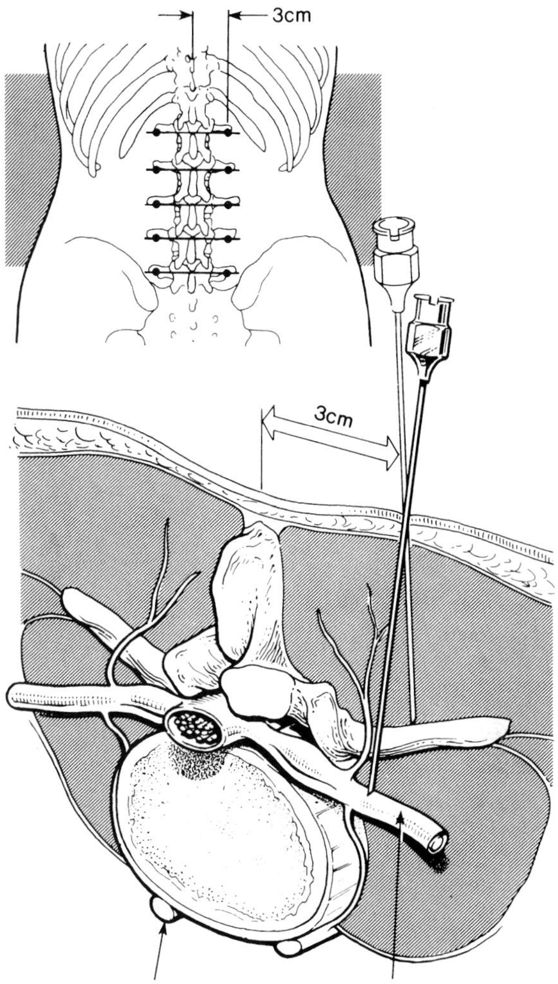

FIG. 11-2. Paravertebral lumbar somatic nerve block. **Upper Panel:** Skin markings are made by drawing lines across the cephalad aspect of spinous processes and then drawing vertical lines 3 cm from the midline. **Lower Panel:** A needle inserted perpendicular to the skin will contact the cephalad edge of a spinous process. Angulation of the needle in a cephalad direction to slide superior to the transverse process will reach the spinal nerve 2 to 3 cm deeper than the transverse process.

Technique

The standard approach to blockade of the lumbar somatic nerves is paravertebral (see also Chapter 14). The original writings of Labat and Pitkin advocate having the patient lie on the side opposite the one to be blocked. A soft roll placed between the iliac crest and the costal margin will minimize the lateral spinal curvature. A preferred position, in a healthy patient, is that of having the patient lie prone over a soft pillow, which will flatten (or elevate) the lumbar curve. Regardless of position, the landmarks used are the spinous processes of the lumbar vertebrae. Skin wheals are raised opposite the cephalad aspect of the spinous processes, on a line 3 to 4 cm laterally from, and parallel to, the midline of the back (Fig. 11-2). Depending on the size of the patient, an 8- or 10-cm needle is inserted through each of the skin wheals and advanced perpendicular to the surface of the skin until its tip comes into contact with the transverse process of the vertebral body, usually at a depth of 4 to 5 cm. The needle is then partially withdrawn and reintroduced slightly more cephalad and medially, making an angle of about 25° with the sagittal plane of the body. This should allow the needle to pass just tangential to the superior aspect of the transverse process and to be advanced an additional 2 to 3 cm. Paresthesias may frequently be elicited and a nerve stimulator can aid in accurate needle placement. If so, 8 to 10 ml of the selected local anesthetic solution should be injected. If no paresthesias are elicited, the solution is distributed in front of the transverse process.

It should be remembered that, unlike the thoracic spines, the spinous processes of the lumbar vertebrae do not slope downward, their upper and lower borders being more nearly horizontal. Their average thickness is from 0.5 to 1 cm. The distance between the tip of the lumbar spinous process and its attachment to the vertebral lamina is approximately 3 to 4 cm. A horizontal line drawn tangential to the superior aspect of the spine will overlie the transverse process of that vertebrae. The transverse processes of the lumbar vertebrae are short, accounting for the paravertebral skin wheal being only 2 to 3 cm from the midline. The average depth of the transverse process to the skin is 5 cm, which varies with the size of the patient and the paraspinous musculature. The transverse processes of L4 and L5 are more deeply situated than are those of the vertebrae above. When the needle passes superior to the transverse process, it is in proximity to the somatic nerve of the preceding segment (e.g., the needle passing over the transverse process of L1 injects the T12 nerve root). The L5 root is blocked through the same skin wheal as L4, by redirecting the needle in a caudad direction until it passes from the lower border of the L4 transverse process and by injecting the nerve root in a manner similar to the technique used in other roots (Fig. 11-2).

Inguinal Paravascular Block

A more peripheral approach to the major branches of the lumbar plexus that supply the leg has been described by Winnie.[62] His *inguinal paravascular* technique of lumbar plexus block utilizes the fascial envelope around the femoral nerve as a conduit, which carries injected anesthetic superiorly to the level where the lumbar plexus forms (Fig. 11-3).

As previously noted, the lumbar plexus lies between the quadratus lumborum muscle posteriorly and the psoas major muscle anteriorly, being invested, therefore, by the fasciae of those two muscles. Although the other nerves to the leg take divergent courses through the pelvis, the femoral nerve descends from under the psoas muscle and remains in the groove between the psoas and iliacus muscle. Proximal to the inguinal ligament, the femoral nerve is then in a fascial sheath, with the anterior covering being provided by the transversalis fascia (fascia iliaca over iliacus).

Technique

The technique for inguinal paravascular block is very similar to that for femoral nerve block. The patient lies supine with the anesthesiologist standing next to the side that is to be blocked. After careful palpation, a skin wheal is raised just lateral to the femoral artery, where it emerges distal to the inguinal ligament. A short-bevel 22-gauge needle, connected to a syringe filled with anesthetic, is inserted just over the tip of the palpating finger in a cephalad direction. A paresthesia of the femoral nerve or stimulation of the motor response must be produced as an indication that the tip of the needle is within the fascial sheath. The needle is then fixed and the desired volume of local anesthetic injected, while firm digital pressure is applied just distal to the needle in an attempt to force the flow of local anesthetic proximally into the area of the lumbar plexus. A volume of 25 to 30 ml of local anesthetic should be injected.

Indication

The lumbar plexus and its somatic nerves supply the cutaneous nerves not only to the upper thigh but also to the lower abdominal area. (Analgesia for the abdomen is covered more completely in Chapter 14.) Lumbar somatic block is indicated in cases where a unilateral block is desirable, or where

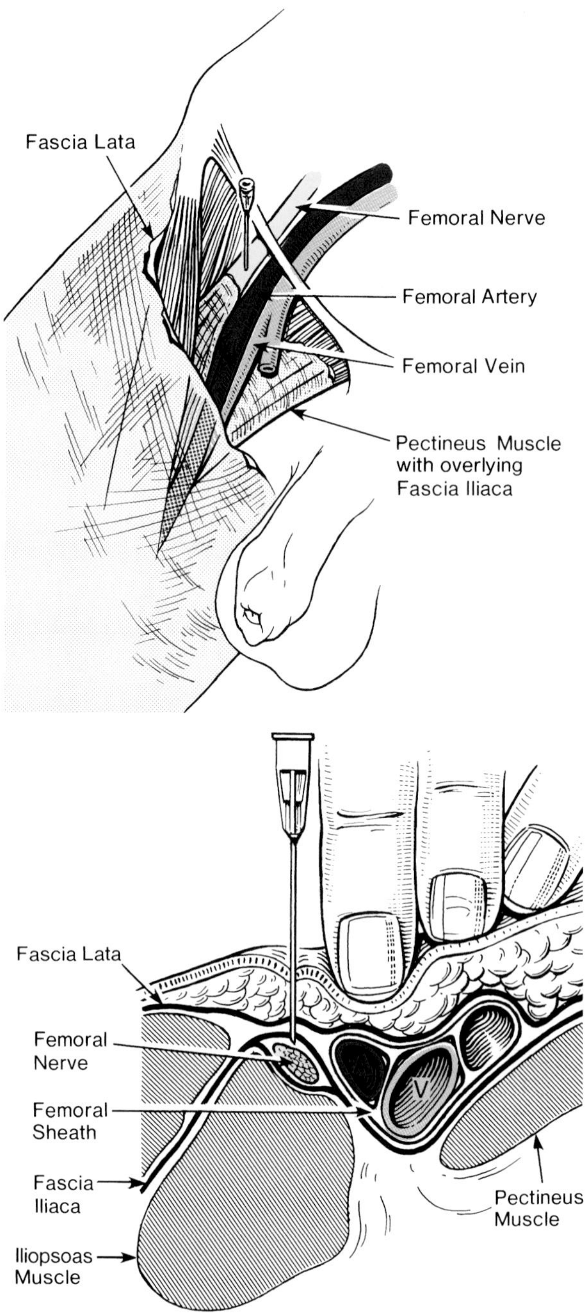

FIG. 11-3. Inguinal structures showing fascial envelope around femoral nerve and relationships for inguinal paravascular femoral nerve block techniques. Note that both the facia lata and facia iliaca must be penetrated.

for some reason a spinal or epidural anesthetic is contraindicated for operations of the hip, thigh, or upper leg.

Branches of the first three lumbar nerves provide cutaneous distribution to the inner and outer aspects of the thigh and the anterior gluteal region, along with adjacent perineal and suprapubic areas. With lumbar plexus block, it is possible to block these fibers. If the five major peripheral nerve blocks are performed, however, and procedures proximal to the midthigh are anticipated, then paravertebral blockade of the appropriate nerves is indicated. In contrast, lumbar somatic blockade alone will not be sufficient for complete anesthesia of the lower extremity, because it cannot achieve blockade of the sacral roots that supply the sciatic nerve.

Side Effects and Complications

For purposes of clarification, side effects, as used here, are physiologic occurrences that result from a particular technique or local anesthetic agent, which may not be desirable in a particular patient. The classic example is sympathetic nerve blockade. In theory, a carefully performed paravertebral lumbar somatic nerve block should not give rise to blockade of the lumbar sympathetic fibers. Nonetheless, in clinical practice, local anesthetic may reach the sympathetic chain, and the anesthesiologist should watch for such side effects, especially in the hypovolemic patient in whom the magnitude of response (usually hypotension) may be exaggerated.

Persistent paresthesias are uncommon and usually self-limited, resolving within several weeks. A rare complication of the paravertebral approach to neural blockade is that of epidural or subarachnoid injection. In a large patient, with considerable soft tissue overlaying the paraspinous area, a needle introduced at a slight medial angle can pass quite easily through the interspace and accomplish a paramedian approach to the epidural or subarachnoid space (see Chapter 7).

Finally, anterior to the vertebral column are major blood vessels. If caution is not observed in recalling or marking the depth of the transverse process when the anesthesiologist is advancing the needle to the level of the lumbar plexus, the needle may be inserted too deeply and these vessels entered. Careful aspiration before injection of local anesthetic solutions and use of a test dose containing epinephrine should prevent the serious complication of direct intravascular injection, with a likely systemic toxic reaction. Mere needle entry into a normal blood vessel without injection of drug is usually of no consequence. The most frequently encountered vessel with the right paravertebral approach is the inferior vena cava–and on the left, of course, is the aorta.

SACRAL PLEXUS NERVE BLOCK

Since the derivation of the sciatic nerve comes in part from spinal roots S1–S3, it is apparent that blockade of these roots must be combined with the aforementioned lumbar somatic block if complete anesthesia of the lower extremity is to be obtained by paravertebral blockade.

Anatomy

The sacral plexus is formed by the union of the first three sacral nerves and the fourth and fifth lumbar nerves. It also connects with the ascending division of the fourth sacral nerve. The sacral plexus is located on the anterior surface of the sacrum and is separated from the sacrum by the piriformis muscle. It is covered by the parietal portion of the pelvic fascia. In front of it lie the ureter, the pelvic colon, part of the rectum, and the iliac artery and vein. The plexus gives off two sets of branches: the collateral and the terminal. The collateral branches (anterior and posterior) supply the pudendal plexus, the hip joint, the gluteal structures, and the adductor and hamstring muscles. More pertinent to this discussion is that the terminal branches supply the greater and lesser sciatic nerves.

The sacrum is the wedge-shaped, fused, lower five sacral vertebrae attached by joints and ligaments to the iliac bones. On its posterior surface are two rows of openings—the posterior sacral foramina, present on each side of the fused spinous processes (see Chapter 9, Fig. 9-1). The posterior divisions of the sacral nerves pass through these foramina to the soft tissues of the sacral region at the back. Although these rows of foramina are not exactly parallel, angling toward the midline, they are not as steeply angulated as the edges of the sacrum. This is an important point to remember when surface landmarks are plotted (Fig. 11-4).

Another important anatomic relationship is that of the anterior sacral foramina to the homologous posterior foramina, which constitute the transsacral canal. The depth of the canal varies from 2.5 cm at the level of S1 to 0.5 cm at S4 (see Chapter 9, Fig. 9-7). It is important to have these figures in mind when blocking the sacral nerves by the trans-sacral method; otherwise, the needle may be introduced into the pelvis.

Technique

For trans-sacral block, the patient is prone over a pillow placed under the hips. The posterior superior iliac spine and the sacral cornu are palpated and marked bilaterally. A skin wheal is raised immediately lateral to and above the sacral cornu, and another placed 1 cm medial to and below the posterior superior iliac spine of the side to be blocked. The distance between the wheals is bisected, and an additional

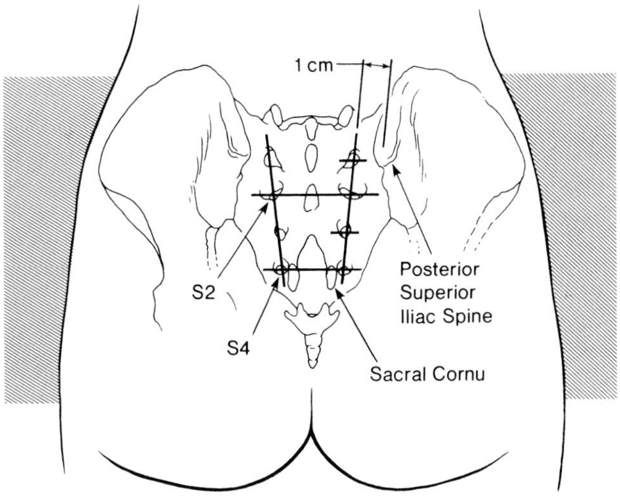

FIG. 11-4. Landmarks for sacral plexus nerve block.

wheal is raised at this site. Those three wheals thus identify the second, third, and fourth sacral foramina. The first sacral foramen is found by placing a wheal 1 to 2 cm above the second and on the same line as the others. There is no fifth sacral foramen. The fifth sacral nerves lie 1 to 2 cm caudad to the fourth foramen on the lines marked. The thickness of the soft tissues overlying the sacrum is greater superiorly—and, therefore, requires longer needles—than the lower segments. An 8- to 10-cm, 22-gauge needle is satisfactory for S1 and S2 and a 5-cm needle for the lower segments. The second foramen is often easiest to locate and thus usually attempted first. This helps in locating the others. The needle is inserted toward the posterior aspect of the sacrum, inclined slightly medially until striking bone. The needle is then withdrawn and reintroduced until it enters the respective transsacral canal. The needle is advanced approximately 2 to 2.5 cm into the first sacral canal and in 0.5-cm decrements for each succeeding canal moving caudad. Similarly, 5 to 7 ml of solution should be injected into the first sacral foramen, the volume being reduced by 1 to 1.5 ml for each subsequent injection. The precision of this block is aided by use of a peripheral nerve stimulator.

Side Effects and Complications

Since the sacral nerves represent the parasympathetic portion of the autonomic nervous system, sympathetic blockade and its potential for hypotension are not seen with transsacral block unless excessive volumes of solution spread proximally to the lumbar sympathetic fibers. Loss of parasympathetic function to bowel, bladder, and sphincters may occur, however. Injection of local anesthetic through misdirected needles into the subarachnoid or vascular compartments is a remote risk. Classically, the dural sac is said to terminate at the lower border of S2; however, there are enough clinical reports of subarachnoid puncture with a 6- to 7-cm caudal needle to suggest individual variations below this "classic" location. Finally, an appreciation of the pelvic contents, especially colon, rectum, and bladder, is important; should a deeply inserted needle enter the colon or rectum and not be noticed, it could result in seeding fecal material into the sacral canals.

Indications

The combined lumbosacral paravertebral approach to neural blockade of the lower extremity conserves neither the number of needle insertions nor the total volume of solution used, compared to the more traditional "four-nerve block" approach to be described. It does offer the benefit of anesthesia over the upper thigh, hip, and perineum, which the peripheral nerve blocks do not. It may thus be used for high amputations and for the relief of sciatic pain. It is also useful when immediate access to the individual nerves is not possible; for example, owing to trauma or infection.

SCIATIC NERVE BLOCK

Anatomy

The largest of the four major nerves supplying the leg is the sciatic nerve (L4–L5, S1–S3). The sciatic nerve, as previously noted, arises from the sacral plexus, where it is nearly 2 cm in width as it leaves the pelvis in company with the posterior cutaneous nerve of the thigh. It passes from the pelvis through the sacrosciatic foramen beneath the lower margin of the piriformis muscle, and between the tuberosity of the ischium and the greater trochanter of the femur. The nerve becomes superficial at the lower border of the gluteus maximus muscle. From there, it courses down the posterior aspect of the thigh to the popliteal fossa, where it divides into the tibial and common peroneal nerves. Branches supplying the posterior thigh are given off during the descent of the nerve to the popliteal space. The sciatic nerve supplies sensory innervation to the posterior thigh and entire leg and foot from just below the knee.

Technique

Several approaches to blockade of the sciatic nerve have been proposed, primarily to avoid positioning problems that are difficult for trauma patients and the elderly.

Classic Approach of Labat. The classic approach to the sciatic nerve block is with the patient lying on the side opposite the one to be blocked, rolled forward onto the flexed knee, with the heel in opposition to the knee of the outstretched dependent leg (Fig. 11–5A).

After careful palpation, a line is drawn between points made over the upper aspect of the greater trochanter of the femur and the posterior superior iliac spine. This line should coincide with the upper border of the piriformis muscle and also the upper border of the sacrosciatic foramen (sciatic notch). A line perpendicular and bisecting this is then drawn downward 3 cm and represents the point for injection. A second verification of this point may be made by projecting a line from the greater trochanter to a point 1 to 2 cm below the sacral cornua. This line crosses the perpendicular at about 3 cm and also represents a point overlying the sciatic nerve where it exits from the pelvis.[61]

A 10- to 12-cm needle is inserted through a wheal made at this point in a direction perpendicular to the skin until it strikes bone. Usually this will occur at 6 to 8 cm in a patient of average stature. Occasionally, the needle will pass into the sciatic notch when it is first introduced. If this occurs, it should be withdrawn nearly to the skin and the tip redirected more cephalad along the perpendicular line, until bone is contacted. Determination of the depth of the bony pelvis assists in the correct evaluation of paresthesias, which must be elicited in the leg below the level of the thigh. A geometric-grid approach in searching the notch for sciatic paresthesias also will ensure greater success, compared to random thrusts up and down through the notch. Some also advocate the use of a nerve stimulator (see Chapter 6).

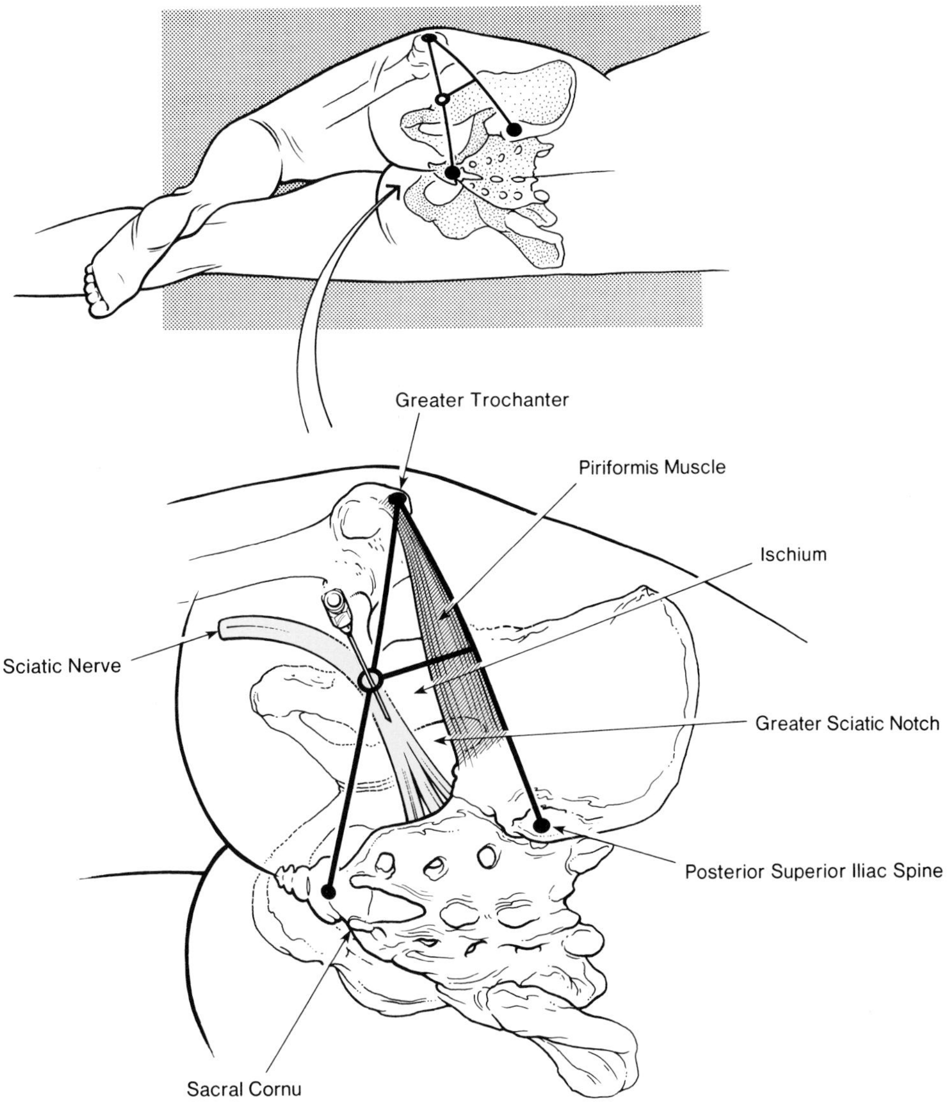

FIG. 11-5. A: Landmark anatomy of sciatic nerve components.

Although successful blockade may be accomplished by injecting 10 ml of local anesthetic solution after one paresthesia, the sciatic is a large nerve, and it is often helpful to seek additional paresthesias and inject a total volume of 20 to 30 ml of solution. Conceivably, a single paresthesia at the edge of the nerve and injection there would not provide complete anesthesia over the entire nerve. This was demonstrated in a recent study, comparing single to double-injection techniques, using a nerve stimulator to locate the sciatic nerve in 50 patients. The double-injection technique had a faster onset of blockade and higher efficacy with no increase in complications.[1]

Surface landmarks can be difficult to identify accurately in sciatic nerve blockade, due to the variable amount of subcutaneous tissue overlying the bony landmarks. Two recent techniques describe approaches which rely on more consistent landmarks. The superior gluteal artery, the largest branch of the internal iliac artery, passes between L5 and S1 and emerges from the upper border of the piriformis muscle at the upper aspect of the sciatic notch. A pencil probe doppler was used to locate this structure in 20 patients, followed by localization of the sciatic nerve with a stimulator. The artery was located 1 to 2 cm medial to Labat's line and usually slightly cephalad to Labat's point, with the nerve slightly inferior and lateral to the artery. The authors reported a 70% success rate with 1 or 2 needle passes, and only one failure, in a diabetic patient.[22]

The ischial spine can be palpated readily rectally, and is a reliable bony landmark for locating the sciatic nerve. In a study of 40 patients, comparing the Winnie modification of the Labat technique to localization of the nerve, using rectal palpation of the ischial spine as a landmark and crossing over to the alternate technique if unsuccessful after two tries, the success rate was 87.5% overall (52% with the classic technique and 76% with the alternative). Though this difference was not statistically significant, when crossover occurred it

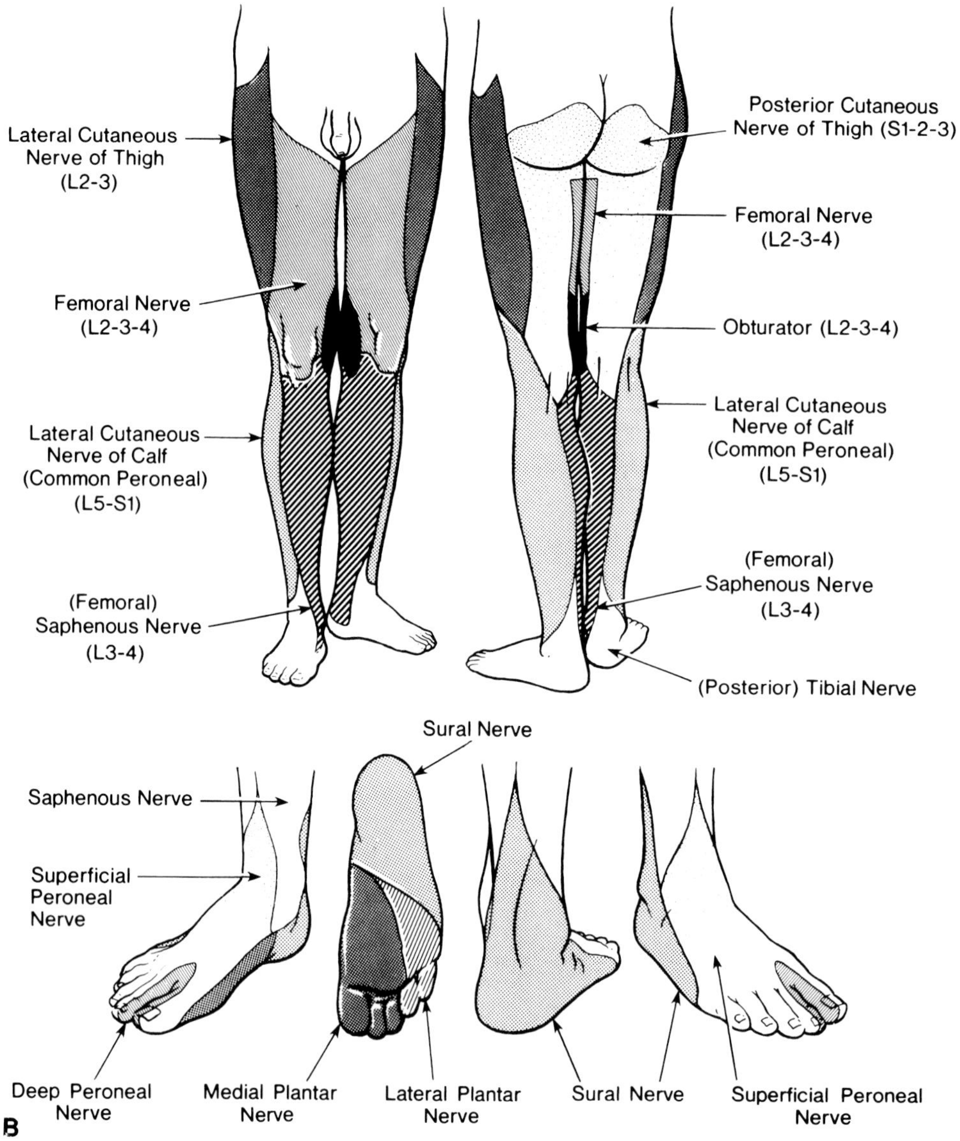

FIG. 11-5. Continued. B: Cutaneous nerve distribution of the lower limb.

was more likely from the classic to the alternative technique. The primary advantage of the alternative technique was the avoidance of surface landmarks as the sole anatomical markers for nerve location.[9]

A technique of continuous sciatic nerve block has been described to relieve pain from ischemic gangrene of the foot. This was subsequently combined with a continuous inguinal paravascular block (described later in this chapter) to provide regional anesthesia for the operative procedure and for postoperative pain relief for the first few postoperative days.[57]

The standard posterior approach was used, except that the sciatic nerve was identified with a nerve stimulator attached to a standard 16-gauge intravenous infusion cannula. An epidural-type catheter was passed through the cannula and advanced about 6 cm into the neurovascular space. Correct catheter placement was verified with radiologic contrast medium. Continuous infusion of a local anesthetic agent, with the use of a continuous infusion device connected to the well-anchored catheter, should then provide continuous analgesia.

Other Approaches. Labat also described an anterior approach to the sciatic nerve. The nerve passes from the lower border of the gluteus maximus where it is bounded medially by the hamstring muscles. It runs down the thigh, lying on the medial surface of the femur. The posterior femoral cutaneous nerve sometimes branches away from the greater sciatic nerve above the level of blockade, and may be missed with this approach.

The patient is placed supine with the lower extremity in a neutral position. A line that represents the inguinal ligament is trisected, and a perpendicular line from the junction of the middle and medial thirds of this line is extended downward and laterally on the anterior aspect of the thigh. The greater trochanter is located by palpation and a line extended from its tuberosity medially across the anterior surface of the thigh, parallel to the inguinal ligament. The point of intersection of this line and the perpendicular line from the inguinal ligament represents the point of injection (Fig. 11-6). A 10- to 12.5-cm needle is inserted through a wheal at this point and directed slightly laterally from a plane perpendicular to the skin. The needle is advanced until bone is contacted, then withdrawn and redirected medially and more perpendicularly to pass 5 cm beyond the femur, where it should be resting slightly posterior and medial to the femur within the neurovascular compartment (containing the sciatic nerve). After aspiration, a small test dose should be injected to determine ease of injection, indicating whether the needle lies in a muscle bundle or fascial space. The former offers firm resistance to injection, and the needle should be advanced until minimal resistance to injection indicates correct placement. Paresthesias, although not sought, would be helpful. The use of a nerve stimulator would also assist in locating the nerve in this approach. A modification of the anterior approach has been described to aid in locating the neurovascular compartment in children.[37] In adults, the average distance from the femoral surface to the sciatic neurovascular compartment varies little from 4.5 to 6 cm. In pediatric practice, the depth varies with the age and size of the child. A "loss of resistance" technique similar to that used for identifying the epidural space proved helpful in achieving correct needle placement. The metal needle removed from a standard 16-gauge intravenous catheter was attached to a 10-ml syringe without regard to the volume of solution intended for injection. The needle with syringe attached was inserted through the skin wheal in the traditional manner, until it struck the surface of the femur. It was then walked off the medial edge of the femur until it entered the thigh muscles. Continuous pressure was applied to the plunger of the syringe and the needle advanced through the muscle mass. At the point where the needle entered the neurovascular compartment, a sudden loss of resistance occurred, similar to that encountered when performing an epidural block. Following aspiration to exclude an intravascular injection, the predetermined amount of solution (15 to 30 ml of local anesthetic solution) was injected and the needle removed. It should be noted that smaller-bore needles may have too much internal resistance to clearly reflect loss of resistance upon entry into the neurovascular compartment. Once mastered, the success rate with this technique was said to be 95.2%.[37]

A more recent pediatric study compared the posterior, anterior, and lateral approaches to the sciatic nerve in 180 patients undergoing surgery below the knee. During light general anesthesia, the nerve was localized using either a nerve stimulator or (if no twitch) the loss of resistance technique. Of the 154 cases where twitches were elicited, all but 1 had a block. Twenty-six patients had atypical twitches (8) or no twitch (16), with only 50% resulting in blockade. The success rate overall was greater than 90%. The authors reported that the needle depth was least in the posterior approach, the first attempt success rate with the nerve stimulator was lower in the anterior group, and that there were three arterial punctures in the anterior group. They recommended the posterior approach in children.[11] Serious complications of the anterior approach to the sciatic nerve are rare. However, theoretical concerns regarding muscle trauma and puncture of a variety of vascular structures, including the femoral and profunda vessels, must be considered. The lithotomy position has also been advocated to facilitate approaching the sciatic nerve.[46] The anatomy is nearly identical to that in the aforementioned anterior approach. After the sciatic nerve passes between the ischial tuberosity and the greater trochanter, it lies just anterior to the gluteus maximus muscle. The nerve is accompanied at this point by the sciatic artery and the inferior gluteal veins, but they are relatively small vessels and add little risk to the procedure.

The patient is placed supine, and the extremity to be blocked is flexed at the hip as far as possible (90°–120°). The extremity may be supported by stirrups, mechanical devices, or by an assistant. In this position, the gluteus maximus muscle is flattened and the sciatic nerve relatively more superficial, lying in the readily palpable hollow between the semitendinosus and biceps femoris muscles. A line is drawn between the ischial tuberosity and the greater trochanter and a wheal raised at its midpoint. A 12- to 15-cm needle is inserted perpendicular to the skin and advanced until a paresthesia is elicited. (A peripheral nerve stimulator has been advocated but is seldom necessary unless the patient is unable to respond to paresthesias.) Twenty to 25 ml of a local anesthetic solution are then injected.

A lateral approach to the sciatic nerve has also been described.[17] The sciatic nerve is approached from the lateral thigh with the patient lying supine. The earliest report of a lateral approach was by Ichiyanaghi in 1959; it was thought by many to be "extremely difficult."[23] The quadratus femoris is the lowermost of the short rotators of the hip crossed by the sciatic nerve on its way to the posterior compartment of the thigh. The subgluteal space, within which the sciatic nerve lies as it crosses this muscle, can be identified in relation to the femur and the ischial tuberosity.

The block is performed with a 15-cm needle and uses the nerve stimulator (see Chapter 6). The patient lies supine with the whole limb exposed and with the hip held in the natural position. After appropriate skin preparation and drape, the needle is inserted through a skin wheal made 3 cm distal to the point of maximum lateral prominence of the trochanter, along the posterior profile of the femur (Fig. 11-7). Upon striking the bone of the femoral shaft, the needle is redirected to slide under the femur and is advanced to a total depth of 8 to 12 cm to reach the sciatic nerve. The nerve stimulator may elicit responses from any of the three motor components of the sciatic. After correct identification of the nerve, a minimum of 20 ml of local anesthetic is injected.

Side Effects and Complications

Sciatic nerve block is primarily a somatic nerve block. It does carry some sympathetic fibers to the extremity, however, and may therefore allow pooling of small quantities of blood—usually insufficient to cause significant hypotension. On some occasions, such as limb reimplantations and sympathetically mediated pain conditions, this sympathetic block may be therapeutically exploited. The effect of compensatory vasoconstriction on the opposite extremity should, however, be considered. There is some evidence that tissue oxygenation may be further reduced during this period of compensation, although it is unlikely that this is of clinical significance.[5]

No significant complications secondary to this block have been documented. Residual dysesthesias for periods of 1 to 3 days are reported by some patients, but are usually self-remitting.[53] It is reported that these minor problems may result from the use of long-bevel needles, producing damage to nerve fascicles.

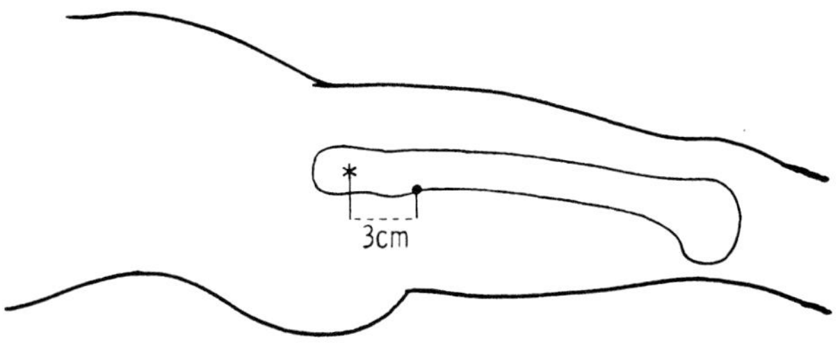

FIG. 11-7. Landmarks for insertion of the needle for lateral approach to sciatic nerve. (Guardini, R., Waldron, B.A., and Wallace, W.A.: Sciatic nerve block: A new lateral approach. Acta Anaesthiol. Scand., *29*:515, 1985.)

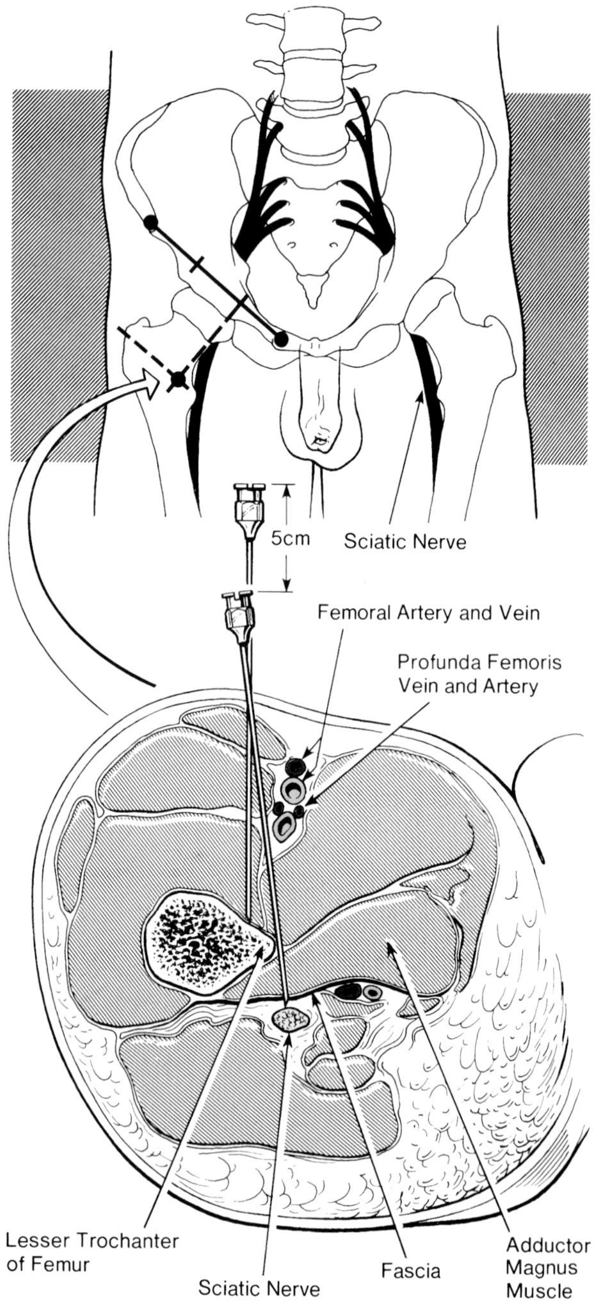

FIG. 11-6. Anterior approach to sciatic nerve block (see text). Cross-section of the leg at the level of the lesser trochanter to show the relationship between the sciatic nerve and the femur, and the fascia separating it from adductor magnus.

Indications

As one considers the sensory and cutaneous distribution of the sciatic nerve, it is not surprising that few surgical procedures could be accomplished using sciatic nerve block as the sole anesthetic (perhaps operations on the sole of the foot and the digits). More frequently, however, it is combined with one or more of the nerve blocks yet to be described, to provide a significantly larger field of surgical anesthesia.

In recent times, with increasing emphasis on pain relief, sciatic nerve block has been advocated for children for postoperative pain relief.[11,37] Although blocks were done before surgery but after induction of anesthesia, general anesthesia was maintained during surgery and the effectiveness of the block evaluated in providing postoperative pain relief. In a series of 82 patients, the analgesic success rate was 95.2%. The use of sciatic block, either single-injection or with the continuous infusion technique, for treatment of long-term pain, acute or chronic, secondary to ischemia, or sympathetically mediated pain, has also been reported.[17,57] Certainly when there are contraindications to epidural or lumbar paravertebral blocks in the treatment of these pain syndromes, one should consider the use of sciatic nerve blocks.

FEMORAL NERVE BLOCK

The femoral nerve (L2–L4) proceeds from the lumbar plexus in the groove between the psoas major and iliac muscles, where it enters the thigh by passing deep to the inguinal ligament. At the level of the inguinal ligament, the femoral nerve lies anterior to the iliopsoas muscle and slightly lateral to the femoral artery (see Fig. 11-3). It is important to remember that at, or even above, the level of the inguinal ligament, the femoral nerve divides into an anterior and posterior bundle. The anterior branches innervate the skin that covers the anterior surface of the thigh along with the sartorius muscle; the posterior branches innervate the quadriceps muscles, the knee joint, and its medial ligament, and give rise to the saphenous nerve, which descends over the medial side of the calf to supply the skin down to the medial malleolus. Another classification of the divided femoral nerve is into superficial and deep, which correspond to the aforementioned anterior and posterior. It may be helpful to recall that, in general, the deep branches are chiefly motor in function with articular branches to the hip and knee joints. The superficial branches are chiefly sensory and cutaneous in their distribution. They supply the anterior, anteromedial, and medial aspects of the thigh, the knee, and the upper portion of the leg.

Technique

Classic Approach of Labat. The patient lies supine and may be sedated, since paresthesias are helpful but not essential to this particular method. The femoral artery is palpated immediately below the inguinal ligament, and a wheal raised immediately lateral to the artery. A line drawn from the anterior superior iliac spine to the symphysis pubis will approximate the inguinal ligament, with the wheal adjacent to the femoral artery being approximately 1 to 2 cm below this line (see Fig. 11-3). A 3- to 4-cm needle, without syringe, is advanced perpendicular to the skin until a paresthesia is elicited or the needle undergoes maximum lateral pulsation from its position adjacent to and slightly deep to the artery. It should be repositioned until one of these two indicators has been achieved. If paresthesias occur, 10 to 20 ml of local anesthetic solution should be injected, after careful aspiration, to ensure against intravascular injection. If no paresthesias occur, 7 to 10 ml of local anesthetic is deposited fanwise lateral to the artery. The needle should then be carefully repositioned adjacent to the artery and the injection repeated. The fanwise injection is an important aspect of this technique since the nerve is not contained within the same fascial plane as the artery, and therefore a single injection adjacent to the vessel may be inadequate.

An alternate technique uses a single needle placement similar to the paravascular inguinal technique previously described.[27] This technique is based on the fact that two fascial layers can be identified by the use of a short-beveled needle. Recall that the femoral triangle is covered by the fascia lata; however, in contrast to the femoral vessels that are in a plane between the fascia lata and the underlying fascia iliaca, the femoral nerve lies deep to both.

The fundamental technique is the same as the others previously described; however, the advancing needle is felt to "pop" through the two layers of fascia, that is, a sudden loss of resistance upon passing through each fascial layer. Paresthesias need not be elicited. The needle is aspirated and 20 to 30 ml of local anesthetic solution is injected.

Paravascular Approach. An alternate technique for femoral nerve block has been noted in conjunction with blockade of the lumbar plexus (see Fig. 11-3).[62] This paravascular technique requires elicitation of paresthesias and a cooperative patient or, failing that, a nerve stimulator.

Side Effects and Complications

As with the sciatic nerve block, some of the sympathetic fibers to the lower extremity are blocked with the femoral procedure; however, with femoral block this is more likely to be advantageous to blood flow without being of a magnitude likely to produce systemic hypotension. Inasmuch as the site of blockade is adjacent to the major artery and vein, hematoma at the site is a possibility. Although this probably occurs, it is seldom if ever a complication of clinical significance. With the advent of vascular surgery, the anesthesiologist should be alert to the presence of vascular grafts of the femoral artery, which would be a relative contraindication for elective femoral nerve block.

Residual nerve involvement—dysesthesias or paresis—is remotely possible, but trauma to the nerve from these techniques is minimal, and such a complication therefore highly unlikely.

Indications

Surgical use of femoral nerve block includes operations of the anterior portion of the thigh, both superficial and deep. As with sciatic nerve block, the femoral nerve block is usually part of the combined block approach, incorporating not only sciatic but also lateral femoral cutaneous and obturator nerves.

Recently, additional uses for femoral nerve block have been recommended. Femoral nerve block combined with lateral femoral cutaneous nerve block was used successfully in 103 patients suspected of malignant hyperthermia, ranging in age from 4 to 76 years, undergoing muscle biopsy as the diagnostic test for the suspected trait.[2]

The analgesic role of femoral nerve block was noted to be effective in patients with a fractured shaft of the femur[3,20] and has now been expanded to the total perioperative period. Orthopedic surgeons evaluating acute knee injuries in outpatients used a combination of sciatic and femoral nerve blocks to examine patients in whom clinical examination under local infiltration was considered totally unreliable secondary to severe pain. They achieved a 96% successful examination rate and suggested its potential for outpatient arthroscopy.[50] It is not surprising, then, that a report has appeared comparing the paravascular inguinal technique, alone and in combination with the lateral femoral cutaneous nerve block, with traditional general anesthesia for outpatient knee arthroscopy.[44] Both regional techniques were deemed better than general anesthesia, but inclusion of the lateral femoral cutaneous nerve block improved analgesia on the lateral side of the knee. Recovery time for general anesthesia was significantly longer than with either regional technique.

Femoral nerve blocks alone have also been shown to be an effective adjunct to general anesthesia for knee joint surgery.[48] It was also noted that blocks performed before surgery were more effective than those done after surgery. Postoperative opiate administration was reduced by 80% in the recovery room and by 40% in the first 24 hours postoperatively in patients receiving nerve blocks. In a similar study comparing continuous 3-in-1 blocks with postoperative infusions to general anesthesia and opiates in patients undergoing total knee arthroplasty, the femoral nerve block afforded better pain relief and lower opioid doses.[15]

Although these studies were done in adults, similar work has been performed in a group of 50 children undergoing procedures on the lower limbs who would require postoperative narcotic analgesia.[38] After induction of general anesthesia, a combination of femoral and lateral femoral cutaneous nerve block was performed. There was a 96% success rate with a significant reduction in postoperative narcotic analgesia.

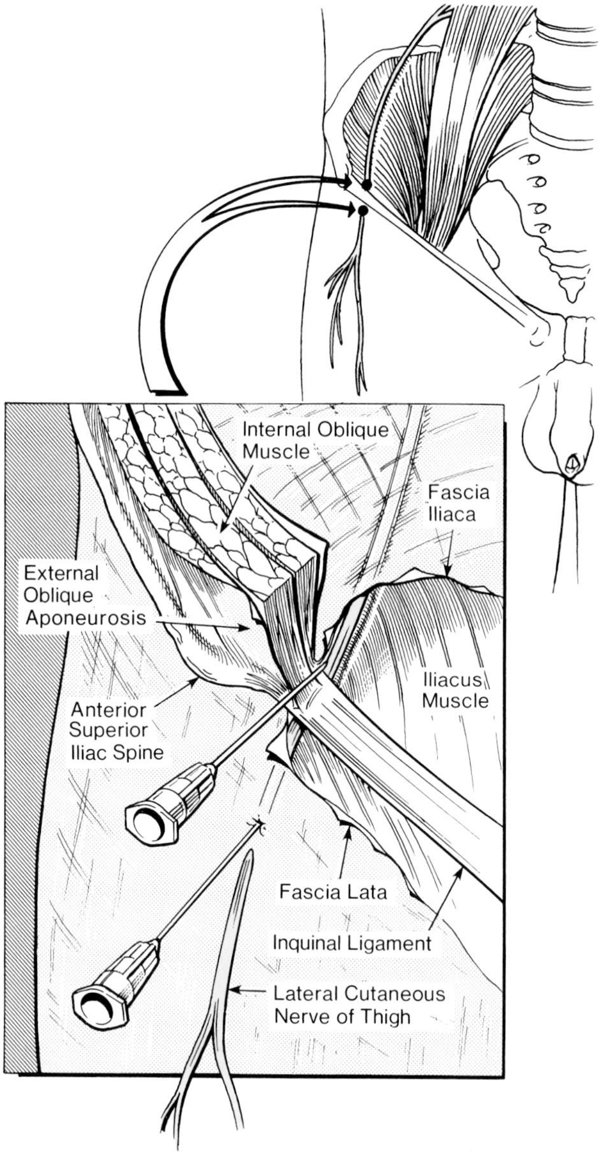

FIG. 11-8. Lateral cutaneous nerve block (see text). The lateral cutaneous nerve of the thigh passes inferiorly on iliacus muscle covered by iliacus fascia. Just medial to the anterior superior iliac spine it turns anteriorly to pass just below the inguinal ligament and runs deep to the fascia lata until it emerges subcutaneously. The lateral cutaneous nerve can be blocked just medially to the anterior superior iliac spine or 1 to 2 cm below it.

LATERAL FEMORAL CUTANEOUS NERVE BLOCK

The lateral femoral cutaneous nerve (L2–L3) emerges at the lateral border of the psoas muscle at a level lower than the ilioinguinal nerve. It passes obliquely under the iliac fascia and across the iliac muscle to enter the thigh deep to the inguinal ligament, at a point approximately 1 to 2 cm medial to the anterior superior iliac spine. It then crosses or passes through the tendinous origin of the sartorius muscle, and courses downward beneath the fascia lata. It emerges from the fascia lata at a point 7 to 10 cm below the anterior superior iliac spine, where it branches into anterior and posterior branches. The anterior branch supplies the skin over the anterolateral aspect of the thigh as low as the knee. The posterior branch pierces the fascia lata and passes backward to supply the skin on the lateral side of the thigh from just below the greater trochanter to about the middle of the thigh (Fig. 11-8).

Technique

The patient is placed in the supine position. After palpation of the anterior superior iliac spine, a skin wheal is placed 2 to 3 cm inferior and 2 to 3 cm medial to it. A 3- to 4-cm needle with syringe attached is then inserted through the wheal and perpendicular to the skin surface. Soon after passing through the skin, the firm fascia lata is felt and then a sudden release as the needle passes through. Ten mls of a local anesthetic solution should be deposited fanwise as the needle is moved upward and downward, depositing solution both above and below the fascia; most of it should be deposited below (Fig. 11-8).

An alternate technique is to direct the needle through the skin wheal in a slightly lateral and cephalad direction to strike the iliac bone, just medial and below the anterior superior iliac spine. Since the nerve emerges here, the deposition of 10 ml of local anesthetic solution in a medial fanwise fashion will also accomplish satisfactory blockade of the nerve. If the volume of the solution is of no concern to the total dose of drug administered, then the nerve can be blocked in both places on the same patient to double the chance of success.

Another modification of this technique attempts to locate the fascial canal in which the nerve lies as it passes under the inguinal canal. Reportedly, this allows a single injection of a lesser volume of local anesthetic, an important consideration in nerve blocks for children.[8] A short-beveled needle is inserted just medial to the anterior superior iliac spine and advanced until the loss of resistance ("pop") is felt as the needle passes through the external oblique aponeurosis. With syringe attached, the needle is advanced through the second loss of resistance of the internal oblique muscle and the underlying fascia iliacus. At this point, the 5- to 10-ml volume of local anesthetic should be injected easily (Fig. 11-8). If a paresthesia is elicited during needle placement, injection of the local anesthetic will result in a high success rate.

Side Effects and Complications

With the exception of a remotely possible dysesthesia or hypoesthesia, there are no known risks to this nerve block technique.

Indications

Lateral femoral cutaneous nerve block by itself is extremely suitable for anesthetizing the donor site before the removal of small skin grafts. Its primary indication as a supplement to the femoral and sciatic nerve blocks for operations on the lower extremity is the provision of analgesia for tourniquet pain. Since one of the terminal anterior branches forms part of the patellar plexus, it must be included with the other nerve blocks for operations on the knee, with or without tourniquet.

OBTURATOR NERVE BLOCK

The obturator nerve (L2–L4) derives its major source from L3–L4—the portion coming from L2 is very small and sometimes even lacking. The nerve appears at the medial border of the psoas muscle, covered anteriorly by the external iliac vessels, and passes downward in the pelvis. It continues with the obturator vessels along the obturator groove and passes through the obturator foramen into the thigh. As the nerve passes through the obturator canal, it divides into posterior and anterior branches. The anterior branch supplies an articular branch to the hip joint, the anterior adductor muscles, and cutaneous branches to the lower inner thigh. The size or existence of this cutaneous innervation is small and variable depending on which anatomic reference material is quoted. The posterior branch innervates the deep adductor muscles and frequently sends an articular branch to the knee joint, which may be important in providing analgesia for knee surgery.

Some anatomy books describe an accessory obturator nerve that leaves the medial border of the psoas muscle in company with the obturator nerve. It has been said to be incorrectly named, having much more in common with the femoral nerve.[32] Like the femoral nerve, it passes over, not under, the pubic ramus where it supplies the pectineus muscle. It is present in about one third of individuals.

Technique

The patient is placed supine with the leg to be blocked in slight abduction. Caution should be taken to protect the skin of the genitalia from irritating antiseptic solutions used in preparing the area. It should not be necessary to shave the pubic area.

The pubic tubercle is palpated and a skin wheal raised 1 to 2 cm below and 1 to 2 cm lateral to it. A 7- to 8-cm needle, without syringe attached, is introduced through the wheal in a slight medial direction to strike the horizontal ramus of the pubis. It is then withdrawn and redirected approximately 45% in a cephalad direction, to identify the superior bony portion of the obturator canal. The depth at which the needle strikes bone in each direction should be noted. The needle is withdrawn again and the point redirected slightly laterally and inferiorly until it passes into the obturator canal. It should be advanced 2 to 3 cm beyond the previously noted depth of bone, where, after careful aspiration to ensure the obturator vessels have not been entered, 10 to 15 ml of local anesthetic are injected. Only by identifying the bony wall of the canal can the anesthesiologist be certain that the needle has passed into the canal rather than into the soft tissues (e.g., bladder or vagina) medially or superiorly (Fig. 11-9). The presence of successful obturator nerve block is determined by demonstrating paresis of the adductor muscles, since the cutaneous distribution is small and inconstant.

A modification of this technique advocates searching for paresthesias to the area of the inner thigh.[43] If paresthesias are not elicited, then it is suggested that a fan-like wall of anesthesia be deposited. The major difference in the two techniques lies in a greater attempt to palpate the tendon on the adductor longus muscle, which constitutes the upper medial aspect of the obturator foramen. With gentle, deep palpation, one may be able to palpate the entire foramen and, placing the skin wheal inferior to the midpoint of the superior pubic ramus, gain a more precise location of the obturator nerve.

A recent modification advocated in treatment of patients with severe spasticity described the insertion of the needle behind the upper end of the adductor longus muscle to reach the obturator canal. The needle was directed laterally, and slightly upward and posterior with the correct position, identified by use of a nerve stimulator. This modified technique had a higher success (80% vs. 60%), fewer needle passes, greater overall patient satisfaction, less discomfort during the block, and better relief of symptoms than with the tradi-

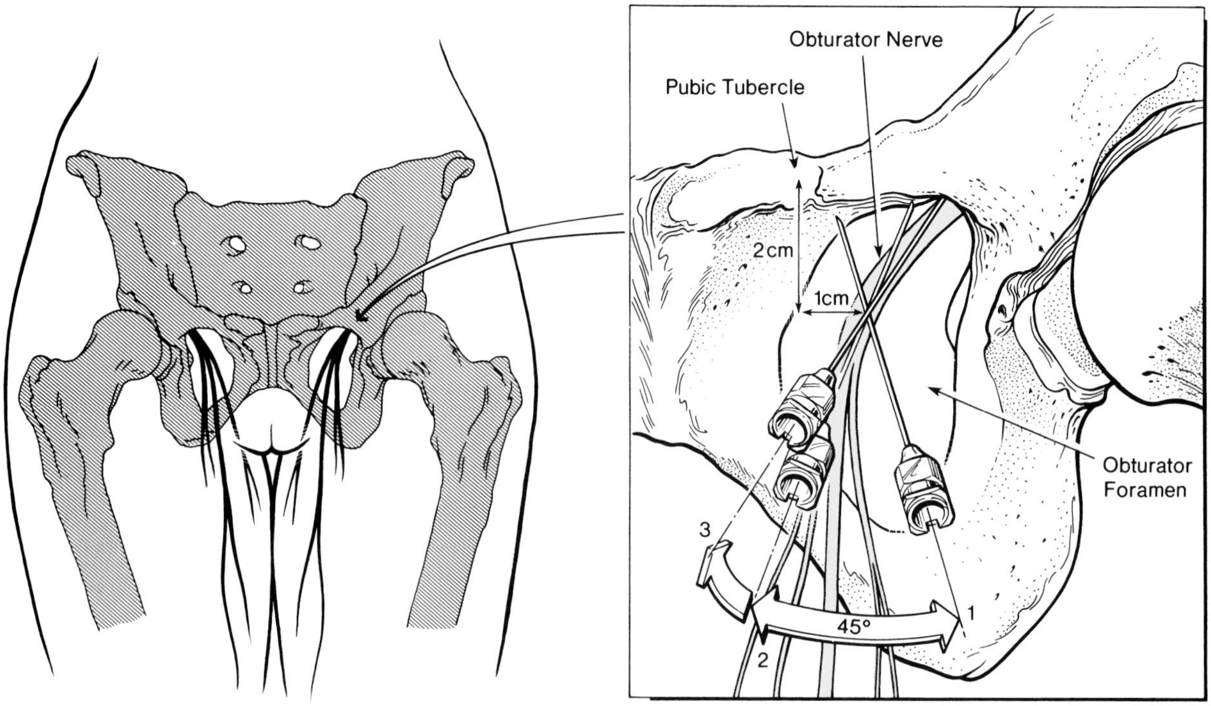

FIG. 11-9. Anatomy of obturator nerve, showing bony landmarks used in nerve block technique (see text).

tional method. The success of this method may be due to better alignment of the needle with the obturator canal.[59]

Side Effects and Complications

Obturator nerve block has vascular and neural complications and side effects nearly identical to those of the femoral nerve. Similarly, these represent remote possibilities rather than clinically important considerations.

Indications

Obturator nerve block is a valuable technique in diagnosing painful conditions of the hip and in the relief of adductor spasm of the hip. It is also necessary as a supplement to sciatic, femoral, and lateral femoral cutaneous nerve blocks, for surgery on or above the knee.

NERVE BLOCKS AROUND THE KNEE

Three major nerve trunks can be blocked at the level of the knee: the saphenous, the common peroneal, and the tibial.

Anatomy

The saphenous nerve is the cutaneous and terminal extension of the femoral nerve. It supplies the skin over the medial, anteromedial, and posteromedial aspects of the leg, extending from above the knee as far distal as the ball of the great toe.

The common peroneal and tibial nerves are divisions of the sciatic nerve. The tibial nerve often arises at the upper end of the popliteal fossa, though the sciatic nerve can bifurcate more superiorly. The tibial nerve is the larger of the two terminal branches of the sciatic nerve and has both a muscular branch to the back of the leg and cutaneous branches in the popliteal fossa and down the back of the leg to the ankle. The common peroneal nerve is about one half the size of the tibial nerve, being the other portion of the sciatic nerve when it bifurcates. It contains articular branches to the knee joint and cutaneous nerves to the lateral side of the leg, heel, and ankle (see Figs. 11-5B and 11-10).

Technique

One of the unexplained phenomena of regional blockade is the uniform lack of enthusiasm for, and even less advocacy of, blockade of individual nerves at the level of the knee, by any of the authors of studies on regional anesthesia (Braun, Labat, Pitkin, Sherwood-Dunn, Eriksson, and Moore). Some have reluctantly recommended circular infiltration at the thigh, and Löfström advocates only a block of the saphenous nerve, stating that ". . . tibial nerve block is difficult to perform and peroneal nerve block, though simple to carry out where the nerve winds round the head of the fibula, may carry a considerable risk of postanesthetic neuritis."[34] Documentation of these criticisms, however, seems lacking in the literature. It is important, therefore, that the anesthesiologist wishing to pursue nerve blocks of the knee undertake a careful review of the associated anatomy. More recently, there have been reports in the literature, advocating nerve blocks in this area, with documentation of both efficacy and safety.[26,29,30,51,56]

The popliteal fossa is a diamond-shaped area bounded inferiorly by the medial and lateral heads of the gastrocnemius muscles and superiorly by the long head of the biceps femoris laterally and the superimposed tendons of the semitendinosus and semimembranosus medially. As the sciatic nerve bifurcates, the larger tibial nerve goes medially and the common peroneal nerve laterally. Because the popliteal fossa is filled with fat, diffusion of injected local anesthetics may be impaired and administration requires that the needle tip be as close as possible to the nerve before injection. This is usually achieved by the use of paresthesias or the nerve stimulator. It is particularly important to know that the nerves are superficial to the popliteal vessels and are located about midway between the skin and the posterior surface of the femur. The distance from skin to nerve in the average adult is 1.5 to 2.0 cm.[51]

The patient, in the prone position, is asked to flex (lift) the leg, which allows the upper borders of the popliteal fossa to become more palpable. Once outlined, the popliteal fossa is divided into equal medial and lateral triangles, with the base of the two triangles being the skin crease behind the knee joint (Fig. 11-10). A skin wheal 5 cm superior to the skin crease and 1 cm lateral to the midline of the triangles should lie over the tibial and common peroneal nerves. Insert a 6- to 7.5-cm, 22-gauge needle at an angle of 45° to 60° to the skin with the tip in an anterior and superior direction. The needle is advanced until a paresthesia is obtained and 35 to 40 ml of local anesthetic solution are injected. The saphenous nerve block is performed by injecting 5 to 10 ml of local anesthetic solution deeply subcutaneous in a 5-cm area just below the medial surface of the tibial condyle.[51]

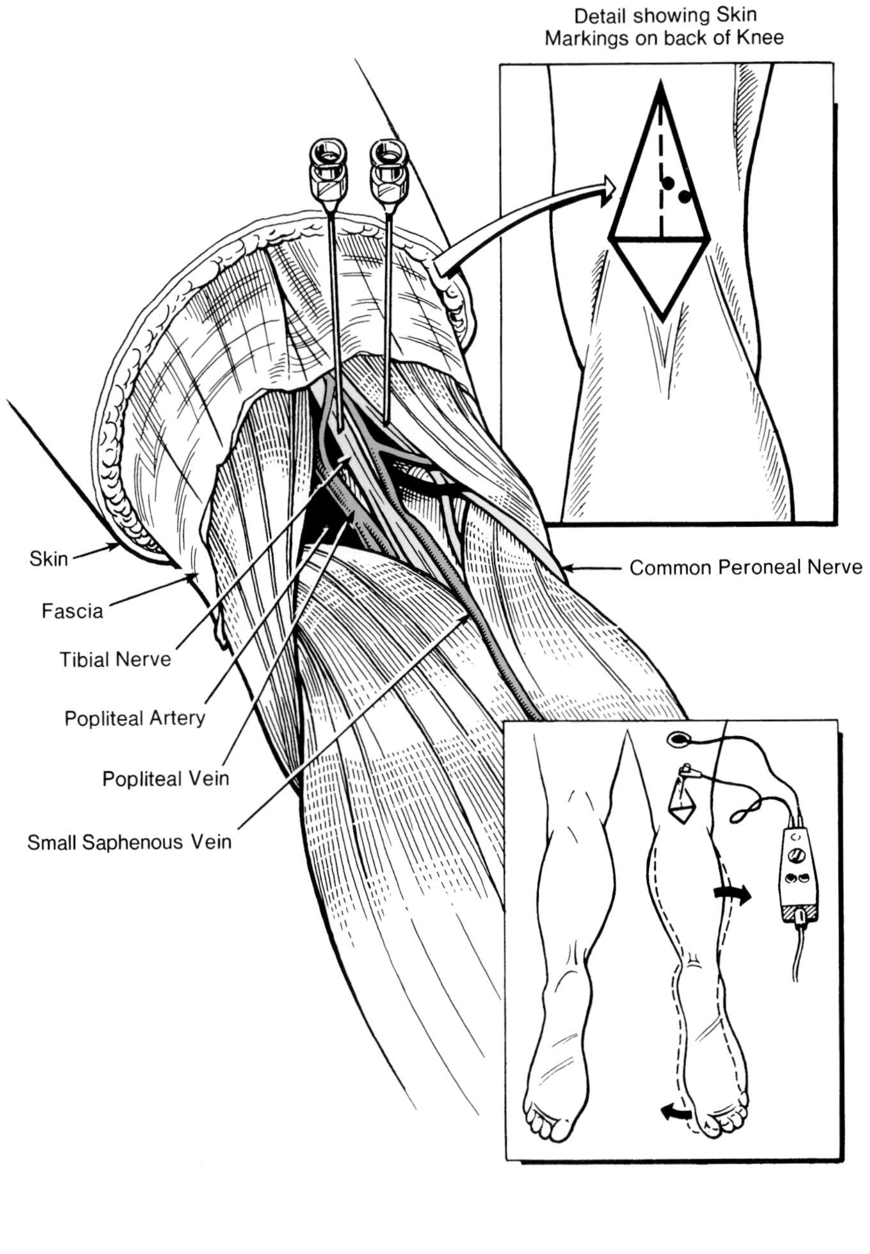

FIG. 11-10. Tibial and common peroneal nerve block. The tibial and common peroneal (lateral popliteal) nerves diverge in the popliteal fossa, which is bounded by biceps femoris muscle laterally and semimembranosus muscle medially. They can be blocked as they pass through the triangle formed by these muscles and a line drawn between the femoral condyles. As the needle is inserted, a loss of resistance should be felt as the needle penetrates the fascia overlying the popliteal fossa.

Indications

The paucity of reports on nerve blocks at the knee may be due to the relative narrow area of analgesia provided when compared to the more proximal nerve blocks previously described, or to blockade of nerves at the ankles. Even so, lack of access to these nerves proximally and reduced dose of local anesthetic drugs in blocks at the knee justify familiarity with these techniques. Kofoed[30] reported 284 outpatients receiving peripheral nerve blocks at the knee and ankle for a variety of operations such as hallux valgus, suture of ligaments and tendons, removal of soft tissue and bony tumors, synovectomy of metatarsal joints, and toe amputations. Singelyn[56] reported 625 blocks in 507 patients with a 92% success rate. The authors used a midline approach to avoid muscle trauma and inserted the needle 10 cm above the popliteal crease. This relatively cephalad needle position was felt to be more successful in blocking the nerve prior to its division. In contrast to these positive reports, Kilpatrick[29] reported a lower success rate and patient comfort when comparing the popliteal approach to the classic Labat technique for sciatic nerve block. Kempthorne and Brown[26] noted the benefit of these blocks in children as an adjunct to surgical anesthesia as well as for postoperative analgesia. Block of the tibial nerve has also been used as a diagnostic block in a child with myotonia and as an adjunct to physiotherapy for treatment of severe equinus deformity in children.

Complications and Efficacy

The satisfactory response to these blocks is similar to other peripheral nerve blocks and likely reflects appropriate management of the patient and satisfactory performance of the block (see Chapter 6). Rorie and associates[51] reported 82% success in 130 patients, with 6.2% requiring general anesthesia. Four patients reported postoperative symptoms similar to dysesthesias, all spontaneously remitting in less than 1 month. Kofoed[30] and Singelyn[56] reported 95% and 92% success rates without any complications, whereas Kempthorne[26] did not quote a success rate but noted no complications after 50 nerve blocks at the knee.

NERVE BLOCKS AT THE ANKLE

Five branches of the principal nerve trunks supply the ankle and foot: posterior tibial, sural, superficial peroneal (musculocutaneous), saphenous, and deep peroneal (anterior tibial).[36] These nerves are relatively easy to block at the ankle (Fig. 11-11).

Tibial Nerve Block

The tibial nerve (L4–L5, S1–S3), the larger of the two branches of the sciatic nerve, reaches the distal part of the leg from the medial side of the Achilles tendon, where it lies behind the posterior tibial artery. The nerve then gives off the medial calcaneal branch to the inside of the heel, after which it divides at the back of the medial malleolus into the medial and lateral plantar nerves, both under the abductor hallucis running to the sole of the foot. The medial branch supplies the medial two-thirds of the sole and plantar portion of the medial 3½ toes up to the nail. The lateral branch supplies the lateral one-third of the sole and plantar portion of the lateral one-and-one-half toes.

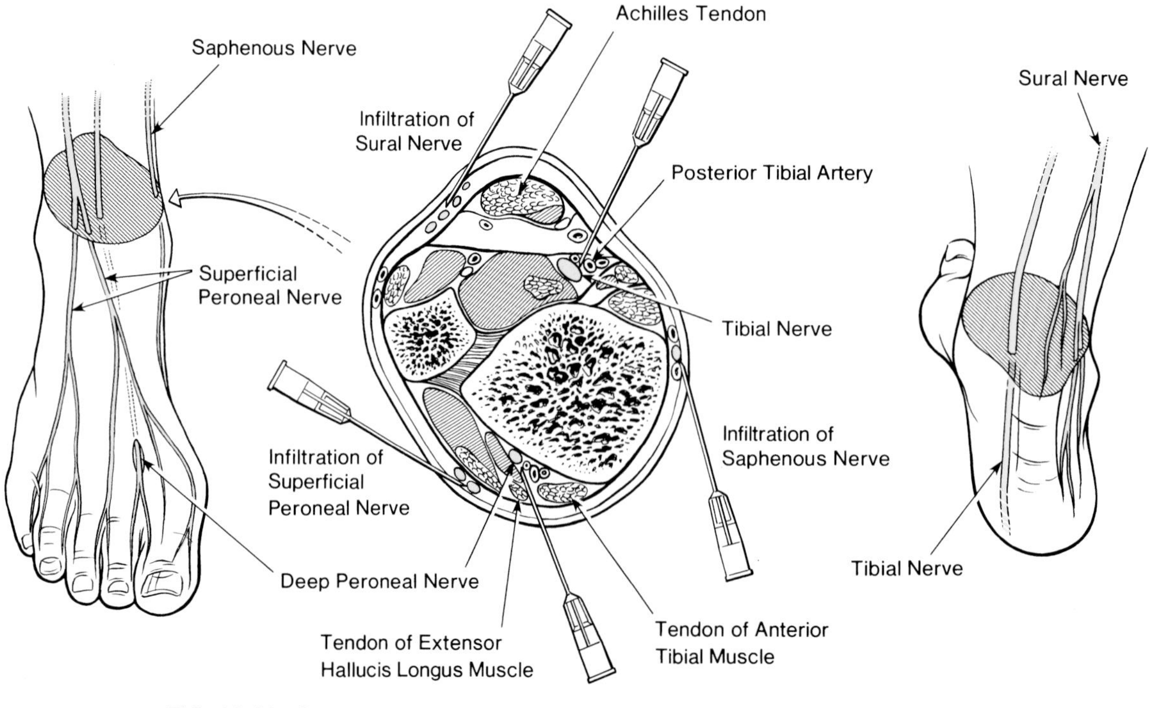

FIG. 11-11. Anatomy and technique of neural blockade for nerves at the ankle.

The patient lies prone or supine with the ankle supported by a pillow or foot rest. A skin wheal is raised lateral to the posterior tibial artery, if the artery is palpable. If the artery is not palpable, then the wheal is placed to the medial side of the Achilles tendon, level with the upper border of the medial malleolus. A 1- to 3-cm needle is advanced through the wheal at a right angle to the posterior aspect of the tibia, lateral to the artery. Shifting the needle in a mediolateral position may elicit a paresthesia, and then 3 to 5 ml of local anesthetic solution should be injected. If paresthesias are not obtained, 5 to 7 ml of local anesthetic solution is injected against the posterior aspect of the tibia, while the needle is withdrawn 1 cm.

Sural Nerve Block

The sural nerve is a cutaneous nerve that arises through the union of a branch from the tibial nerve and one from the common peroneal nerve. It becomes subcutaneous somewhat distal to the middle of the leg and proceeds along with the short saphenous vein behind and below the lateral malleolus to supply the lower posterolateral surface of the leg, the lateral side of the foot, and the lateral part of the fifth toe (Fig. 11-11).

With the patient in the same position as for tibial nerve block, a skin wheal is raised lateral to the Achilles tendon at the level of the lateral malleolus. A 1- to 3-cm needle is inserted through the wheal approximately 1 cm and angled toward the fibula, where paresthesias may be sought. If no paresthesias occur, infiltration is accomplished from the Achilles tendon to the outer border of the lateral malleolus. Three to 5 ml of local anesthetic solution injected fanwise are usually sufficient to produce analgesia. Often the tibial and sural nerves are blocked at the same time with the same needles and equipment.

Superficial Peroneal Nerve Block

The superficial peroneal nerve (L4–L5, S1–S2) perforates the deep fascia on the anterior aspect of the distal two-thirds of the leg and runs subcutaneously to supply the dorsum of the foot and toes, except for the contiguous surfaces of the great and second toes.

The superficial peroneal nerve is blocked immediately above and medial to the lateral malleolus. A subcutaneous infiltration of 5 to 10 ml of local anesthetic solution is spread from the anterior border of the tibia to the superior aspect of the lateral malleolus (Fig. 11-11).

Deep Peroneal Nerve Block

The deep peroneal nerve (L4–L5, S1–S2) courses down the anterior aspect of the interosseus membrane of the leg and continues midway between the malleoli onto the dorsum of the foot. Here, it innervates the short extensors of the toes, as well as the skin on the adjacent areas of the first and second toes. At the level of the foot, the anterior tibial artery lies medial to the nerve, as does the tendon of extensor hallucis longus muscle.

The deep peroneal nerve is blocked in the lower portion of the leg by placing a wheal between the tendons of the anterior tibial and extensor hallucis longus muscles, at a level just superior to the malleoli. Often the anterior tibial artery may be palpated. If this is possible, the skin wheal and nerve should be just lateral to the artery. The needle is advanced toward the tibia, and 3 to 5 ml of local anesthetic solution are injected (Fig. 11-11).

Saphenous Nerve Block

The saphenous nerve, which is the sensory terminal branch of the femoral nerve, becomes subcutaneous at the lateral side of the knee joint. It then follows the great saphenous vein to the medial malleolus and supplies the cutaneous area over the medial side of the lower leg, anterior to the medial malleolus and the medial part of the foot, as far forward as the midportion. Occasionally, its innervation extends to the metatarsophalangeal joint.

To block the saphenous nerve, a skin wheal is raised immediately above and anterior to the medial malleolus, and 3 to 5 ml of local anesthetic solution is infiltrated subcutaneously around the great saphenous vein (Fig. 11-11).

Ankle Block for Foot Anesthesia

All five nerve blocks at the ankle, undertaken simultaneously, would produce a ring of infiltration around the ankle at the level of the malleoli. Such an approach has, in fact, been advocated by more than one textbook of regional anesthesia; it is possible and usually successful at the distal extremes of all extremities and digits. Nonetheless, with circular infiltration, there is the hazard of vascular occlusion if large volumes of anesthetic solutions are injected, especially if they contain epinephrine. In general, block to a specific nerve, such as one of these just described, with smaller quantities of non-epinephrine-containing solutions of local anesthetic agents has a higher success rate with less risk.

A technique has been reported for a "midtarsal" approach to nerve block of the forefoot.[54] Injections are made immediately distal to the ankle joint where the nerves are accessible without having to reposition the patient.

Posterior Tibial Nerve. With the patient in the supine position, the leg is rotated externally. The posterior tibial artery is palpated where it passes behind the medial malleolus. Three to 5 ml of local anesthesia is injected on either side of the artery. If no pulse is palpable, local anesthesia is still injected at this point and deep to the fascia (Fig. 11-11).

Deep Peroneal Nerve. The patient, lying supine, is asked to extend the great toe to facilitate palpation of the extensor hallucis longus tendon. The dorsalis pedis artery is usually palpable several millimeters lateral to the tendon. Two or 3 ml of local anesthesia is injected deep to the fascia and on either side of the artery and distal to the extensor retinaculum (Fig. 11-11).

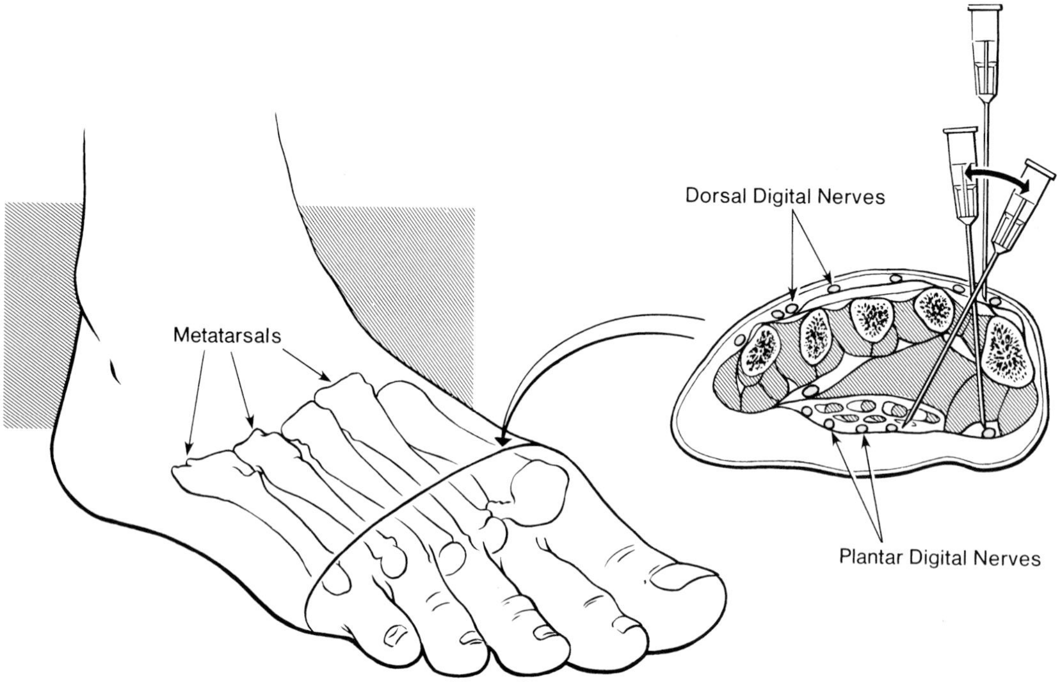

FIG. 11-12. Anatomic relationships and needle placement for metatarsal nerve block.

Saphenous, Superficial Peroneal, and Sural Nerves. The technique for these nerves is the same as previously described. A total of 15 ml of local anesthetic per foot is acceptable; however, this can be reduced to 10 ml for bilateral foot procedures once the necessary skills are obtained.

Still another modification of nerve block at the ankle has been proposed while leaving the patient in the supine position.[52] The foot is extended to 90° relative to the leg and propped up on sheets or some other lift for easier access. Flexing and supporting the knee also improve access to the posterior tibial nerve. This nerve can also be blocked at a more proximal site—two fingerbreadths proximal to the medial malleolus, with the needle inserted tangential to the medial border of the Achilles tendon and perpendicular to the tibia. The remainder of the nerves are approached as previously noted.

Indications and Complications

Ankle block is indicated in nearly all surgical procedures of the foot. In the two series previously noted, these include such procedures as Morton's neuroma, operations on the great toe, including bunionectomy and amputation, amputation of midfoot and toes for peripheral vascular disease, metatarsal osteotomy, incision, drainage, and debridement procedures. Chronic edema may obscure landmarks, but in the absence of draining infected lesions, needle insertion is not contraindicated.

No major complications have been reported. In one series, patients did not even complain significantly of tourniquet pain.[54] One patient complained of dysesthesias for 3 to 4 weeks. A simple alternative to a calf or upper leg tourniquet is the midfoot Esmarch bandage tourniquet. Following routine exsanguination of the foot, the elastic bandage is left tightly wound around the midfoot, serving as a sterile tourniquet within the anesthetized area.

METATARSAL AND DIGITAL NERVE BLOCK

The relationship of the terminal nerves to the metatarsal bones and the toes is very similar to that of the structures of the hand, with the nerve fibers passing through the intermetatarsal space and alongside each toe, where they become the digital nerves.

Nerve block in the intermetatarsal space is very similar to the metacarpal block. Skin wheals are raised on the dorsum of the foot over the proximal aspect of each metatarsal space that bounds the toes to be blocked. Local anesthetic solutions are then infiltrated in a fanwise direction between the two wheals, taking care not to pierce the sole of the foot. Solution should be injected carefully around the plantar surface of the metatarsal bone as well. Digital block alone can be accomplished by injecting through the wheals at the webs of the toes, depositing 2 to 3 ml of local anesthetic solution along either side of the toes to be blocked. Use of epinephrine in the anesthetic solutions and excessive volumes should be avoided in these blocks (Fig. 11-12).

INTRAVENOUS REGIONAL ANESTHESIA

Although intravenous regional anesthesia in the upper extremity is a widely used technique,[19] it has not been reported extensively for use in the lower limbs (see Chapter 12). When a tourniquet is applied to the thigh, a large dose of local anesthetic agent is required, with resultant failures and occasional reports of toxicity. The tourniquet may be placed either proximally on the thigh or at the ankle.

One prospective study of 58 consecutive unselected patients requiring anesthesia of the lower extremity employed placement of the tourniquet at the thigh.[33] The technique is fundamentaly the same as that for intravenous regional anesthesia of the arm. A 7-cm pneumatic tourniquet should be used for adults with an occlusion pressure of 300 mm Hg. Use of the smaller 5-cm tourniquet may fail to provide complete arterial occlusion with pressures in excess of 450 mm Hg.[18] The greater saphenous vein just anterior to the medial malleolus can usually be cannulated with a 20- to 22-gauge needle and secured for vascular access of the local anesthetic agent.

With the tourniquet placed at the thigh, larger volumes of more dilute solutions are advocated. Lidocaine 0.25% to a total dose of 3.3 mg/kg is recommended.[33] This will provide the 75 to 100 ml of solution desired.

Use of the lower limb tourniquet just above the ankle has also been reported.[12] A double-cuff tourniquet was used and arterial occlusion pressures measured before the start of anesthesia. Cuffs were then inflated 100 mm Hg above occlusion pressure. A maximum volume of 40 to 50 ml of a dilute solution of local anesthetic agent was used (0.25–0.5% lidocaine or mepivacaine). No major complications were noted,[12,18,33] but occasional cases of tinnitus or signs of transient vascular absorption were noted. Because intravenous regional anesthesia is effective only during the period of tourniquet inflation, it, like general anesthesia, provides no postoperative analgesia.

INTRA-ARTICULAR BLOCKS

Intra-articular injections of local anesthetics, opioids, or combinations have become routine for perioperative pain management following arthroscopic knee surgery.[10,58] In an early comparison of femoral nerve block, intra-articular injection, or nothing, there was no difference in pain relief between intra-articular bupivacaine and the control, whereas only one of ten patients receiving a femoral nerve block had pain.[21] A number of recent reports enthusiastically recommend the use of this technique; however, the results are conflicting. Comparison of reports is difficult due to variability in underlying anesthetic techniques, different dosages and concentrations of local anesthetic, and frequent lack of control groups. Multivariate analysis in one study showed that gender, preoperative pain scores, and the type and length of surgical procedure were all significant in predicting postoperative pain, while the use of bupivacaine dropped out as a significant factor.[42] Two reports of intra-articular morphine or bupivacaine in patients undergoing arthroscopy under regional anesthesia indicated minimal efficacy. One found no decrease in postoperative pain medications in patients having spinal anesthesia and intra-articular morphine 1 mg, compared to a control group of patients having spinal anesthesia and intra-articular saline, although there was an effect in patients having intra-articular morphine combined with local anesthesia.[41] The other reported only two hours of improved pain relief with intra-articular bupivacaine compared to saline or 3 mg morphine in patients having epidural anesthesia.[47] In patients having general anesthesia, conflicting reports recommend intra-articular morphine alone[24,28] or conclude that intra-articular morphine and bupivacaine are equally efficacious, but both provide less analgesia than continuous lumbar plexus block for 24 hours postoperatively.[13] The safety of injecting large volumes of intra-articular bupivacaine has been ascertained,[25] and side effects are rare following intra-articular doses of morphine. Since these techniques are simple and low-risk and seem to afford pain relief under some conditions, they will likely be continued. Injection of other joints for postoperative pain relief is less commonly reported. In a prospective study of patients undergoing bilateral Keller's arthroplasty, however, the foot into which bupivacaine was placed into the pseudoarthrosis was significantly more pain-free than was the placebo side.[45] Carefully controlled studies will be necessary to determine which techniques are efficacious and under what clinical circumstances they should be applied.

LOCAL ANESTHETIC AGENTS

Although patient selection and regional block equipment have been discussed in Chapter 6, there are some considerations of local anesthetic agents that apply specifically to regional blockade of peripheral nerves. The extremes of the volume-concentration relationships that provide satisfactory anesthesia depend on the knowledge and technical expertise of the anesthesiologist.

Certain properties of the available local anesthetic agents must be exploited if the use of regional block of the lower extremity is to be maximally effective. Some of the more important of these properties are duration, concentration, toxicity, metabolism, and additives, such as epinephrine, carbon dioxide or bicarbonate, and hyaluronidase (see Chapter 4).

Consideration of the appropriate agent, concentration, and perhaps of an additive, should allow the anesthesiologist to provide an optimal nerve block of the lower extremity. In general, because many of the surgical procedures on the lower extremity require little or no muscle relaxation, weaker concentrations of solutions may be used to reduce total dose while providing sufficient volume. For example, with the combined 4-nerve block of the leg, it would be possible to use stronger concentrations on the sciatic and femoral blocks, and dilute to a weaker solution for primary sensory blockade of the lateral femoral cutaneous and obturator nerves.

It is equally important that the duration of analgesia be selected according to need. For example, a short surgical outpatient procedure may well be performed with 2-chloroprocaine, which would restore the patient to early ambulation, whereas bupivacaine or etidocaine might well be used for a patient who would benefit from prolonged analgesia and the sympathetic block of a sciatic nerve block. Residual neurologic involvement (hypoesthesia and dysesthesia) is not uncommon after nerve block with the very long-acting agents. This should be kept in mind in certain orthopedic procedures, especially those with plaster casts in which postsurgical neural involvement must be recognized.

Duration

The currently available local anesthetic agents may be separated into three general—albeit overlapping—categories: short-, intermediate-, and long-acting. The shortacting agents include procaine; 2-chloroprocaine, with or without epinephrine; lidocaine, without epinephrine; and prilocaine, without epinephrine. The intermediate group includes epinephrine-containing solutions of lidocaine and prilocaine; mepivacaine, with or without epinephrine; and perhaps tetracaine without epinephrine. The long-acting agents are effective over a longer period. They include dibucaine and tetracaine, with epinephrine, having a relatively long duration, and bupivacaine, etidocaine and ropivacaine, a very long duration. It should be recalled that very weak concentrations of a local anesthetic agent have a much shorter duration and that the very concentrated solutions have the longest duration of action.[14]

Perhaps the most complete data on peripheral nerve block, compiled by a single investigator, can be found in the work of Löfström, who used ulnar nerve blockade to evaluate the duration of local anesthetic agents.[35] In clinical studies from the other investigators, there were longer durations of cutaneous hypoesthesia to pinprick or pinch with both bupivacaine and etidocaine. Wencker and colleagues report analgesia of 770 minutes with bupivacaine and 764 minutes with etidocaine for axillary nerve block.[60] This study also showed that motor anesthesia exceeded analgesia with both agents. It must be noted that duration of surgical anesthesia—or postsurgical pain relief, for that matter—will be considerably shorter than the analgesia to pinprick quoted in most studies. In general, 45 to 90 minutes of surgical anesthesia can be achieved with the short-acting agents, 90 to 120 minutes with the intermediate agents, and 120 to 748 minutes with the long-acting group—although, of course, individual patient variables contribute to this parameter in many situations.

Concentration

Traditionally, it was thought that the very weak concentrations would block only the smallest nonmyelinated fibers, and provide mostly sympathetic nerve blockade or partial sensory analgesia, and that the strongest concentrations provided blockade of major motor fibers, with excessive concentrations producing neuritis or other nerve toxicity. It is now appreciated, primarily through controlled studies with the newest long-acting agents, that this traditional concept of concentration effect is invalid. Despite the difficulties inherent in arriving at clinically equipotent doses of local anesthetic agents, the work of Wencker, which noted differences in the motor-blocking properties of bupivacaine and etidocaine, has been confirmed by others.[60] Another observation by these investigators was that the sympathetic blockade by these agents varied, not only from agent to agent but also in degree of sensory and motor blockade—the sympathetic block with etidocaine apparently being of shorter duration than either its motor or its sensory blockade.

Toxicity

In practice, the maximum recommended dose of most local anesthetic agents has been the dose that was, presumably, safe to administer to a patient without fear of central nervous system (CNS) toxicity (i.e., seizures). This recommendation was based on animal studies. Although there is variability in the blood concentration at which seizures will occur, it is known that the site of administration does affect blood levels and therefore the hazard of toxicity (see Chapters 3 and 4). Many investigators have shown that levels are highest after intercostal nerve block, that levels after epidural block are 40% to 50% lower, and that extremity blocks (arm and leg) produce intermediate levels. The risk of toxicity is especially a concern after the combined nerve block of the lower extremity, chiefly through the relatively larger volumes of local anesthetic required to accomplish the block. Several recent studies reported plasma levels of local anesthetics following large doses used for combined lower extremity blocks. Mepivacaine, lidocaine, and bupivacaine administered in doses which exceeded the maximum recommended dosage by as much as 50% (bupivacaine) did not cause clinical toxicity or excessive plasma levels.[16,39,55] The use of epinephrine in the local anesthetic solutions has been shown to decrease plasma concentrations when high-dose bupivacaine is administered for combined blocks.[49] Nonetheless, it is extremely important that the anesthesiologist initially determine the total volume required for the block, in conjunction with the maximum total dose recommended for the agent, and then to dilute the concentration to comply with these requirements (see Chapters 3 and 4).

Metabolism

The metabolism of local anesthetic drugs has little specific application to nerve block of the lower extremity, other than the fact that certain conditions, such as hypercapnia and acidosis, have been shown to increase the likelihood of CNS toxicity for a particular dose of local anesthetic. Therefore, when maximum volume and total dose are determined, the systemic health of the patient should be noted carefully and dosage reduced accordingly. A more detailed discussion of toxicity and metabolism may be found in Chapters 3 and 4.

Additives

Epinephrine has been used with local anesthetic agents since the early 1900s, because it was assumed that duration of action would be extended and the blood concentration of the local anesthetic would be reduced, owing to delayed absorption. Recent work indicates that the beneficial effects of epinephrine for both duration and blood concentration depend on which local anesthetic is being used. Certainly, epinephrine is not necessary to extend the duration of etidocaine, bupivacaine, or ropivacaine. On the other hand, etidocaine and bupivacaine are used in high total doses for leg blocks, and, if epinephrine reduces blood levels at all, that is probably sufficient justification for its use.[6,49]

Hyaluronidase has been advocated to prevent large hematomas at the site of injection in arm and leg blocks.[40] Although no apparent problems have been reported from this use, there are also no reports of significant hematoma formation, so that its benefit, if any, is difficult to evaluate. Also undocumented is the effect that this additive may have on blood levels of the administered local anesthetic agents. Since it allows diffusion of blood (or drugs) through tissue planes, it is conceivable that this might increase vascular absorption of drug, and thus further increase marginally safe blood levels of local anesthetics.

Bromage has been especially enthusiastic about the addition of carbon dioxide to solutions of local anesthetic to hasten their clinical effectiveness.[7] Although carbon dioxide has been advocated primarily in epidural anesthesia, it is also effective for peripheral nerve block. More recently, the addition of bicarbonate to local anesthetic solutions has been recommended to achieve the same purpose.[63] Clinically, the speed of onset of nearly all of the local anesthetic agents, with the possible exception of 0.25% bupivacaine, is sufficiently rapid to provide surgical analgesia within the usual surgical preparation time—10 to 15 minutes.

REFERENCES

1. Bailey, S.L., Parkinson, S.K., Little, W.L., and Simmerman, S.R.: Sciatic nerve block: A comparison of single vs double injection technique. Reg. Anesth., *19:*9, 1994.
2. Berkowitz, A., and Rosenberg, H.: Femoral block with mepivacaine for muscle biopsy in malignant hyperthermia patients. Anesthesiology, *62:*651, 1985.
3. Berry, F.R.: Analgesia in patients with fractured shaft of femur. Anaesthesia, *32:*576, 1977.
4. Braun, H.: Anesthesia—Its Scientific Basis and Practical Use. 2nd ed. pp. 3. Philadelphia, Lea & Febiger, 1924.
5. Bridenbaugh, P.O., Moore, D.C., and Bridenbaugh, L.D.: Capillary PO_2 as a measure of sympathetic blockade. Anesth. Analg., *50:*26, 1971.
6. Bridenbaugh, P.O., *et al.*: Role of epinephrine in regional block anesthesia with etidocaine: A double-blind study. Anesth. Analg., *53:*430, 1974.
7. Bromage, P.R.: A comparison of the hydrochloride and carbon dioxide salts in lidocaine and prilocaine in epidural analgesia. Acta Anaesthesiol. Scand., *9:*55, 1965.
8. Brown, T.C.K., and Dickens, D.R.V.: A new approach to lateral cutaneous nerve of thigh block. Anaesth. Intensive Care, *14:*126, 1986.
9. Chang, P.C., Lang, S.A., and Yip, R.W.: Reevaluation of the sciatic nerve block. Reg. Anesth., *18:*18, 1993.
10. Chirwa, S.S., MacLeod, B.A., and Day, B.: Intra-articular bupivacaine (Marcaine) after arthroscopic meniscectomy: A randomized double-blind controlled study. Arthroscopy, *5:*33, 1989.
11. Dalens, B., Tanguy, A., and Vanneuville, G.: Sciatic nerve blocks in children: Comparison of the posterior, anterior, and lateral approaches in 180 pediatric patients. Anesth. Analg., *70:*131, 1990.
12. Davies, J.A.H., and Walford, A.J.: Intravenous regional anaesthesia for foot surgery. Acta Anaesthesiol. Scand., *30:*145, 1986.
13. De Andres, J., Bellver, J., Barrera, L., Febre, E., and Bolinches, R.: A comparative study of analgesia after knee surgery with intra-articular bupivacaine, intra-articular morphine and lumbar plexus block. Anesth. Analg., *77:*727, 1993.
14. De Jong, R.H.: Physiology and Pharmacology of Local Anesthesia. pp. 132–136. Springfield, IL, Charles C. Thomas, 1970.
15. Edwards, N.D., and Wright, E.M.: Continuous low-dose 3-in-1 nerve blockade for postoperative pain relief after total knee replacement. Anesth. Analg., *75:*265, 1992.
16. Elmas, C., and Atanassoff, P.G.: Combined inguinal paravascular (3-in-1) and sciatic nerve blocks for lower limb surgery. Reg. Anesth., *18:*88, 1993.
17. Guardini, R., Waldrom, B.A., and Wallace, W.A.: Sciatic nerve block: A new lateral approach. Acta Anaesthesiol. Scand., *29:*515, 1985.
18. Hagenouw, R.P.M., Bridenbaugh, P.O., van Egmond, J., and Stuebing, R.: Tourniquet pain: A volunteer study. Anesth. Analg., *65:*1175, 1986.
19. Hilgenhurst, G.: The bier block after 80 years: A historical review. Reg. Anesth., *15:*1, 1990.
20. Hood, G., Edbrooke, D.L., and Gerrish, S.P.: Postoperative analgesia after triple nerve block for fractured neck of femur. Anaesthesia, *46:*138, 1991.
21. Hughes, D.G.: Intra-articular bupivacaine for pain relief in arthroscopic surgery. Anaesthesia, *40:*84, 1985.
22. Hullander, M., Spillane, W., and Leivers, D.: The use of Doppler ultrasound to assist with sciatic nerve blocks. Reg. Anesth., *16:*282, 1991.
23. Ichiyanaghi, K.: Sciatic nerve block: Lateral approach with patient supine. Anesthesiology, *20:*601, 1959.
24. Joshi, G.P., McCarroll, S.M., O'Brien, T.M., and Lenane, P.: Intra-articular analgesia following knee arthroscopy. Anesth. Analg., *76:*333, 1993.
25. Katz, J.A., Kaeding, C.S., Hill, J.R., and Henthorn, T.K.: The pharmacokinetics of bupivacaine when injected intra-articularly after knee arthroscopy. Anesth. Analg., *67:*872, 1988.
26. Kempthorne, P.M., and Brown, T.C.K.: Nerve blocks around the knee in children. Anaesth. Intensive Care, *12:*14, 1984.
27. Khoo, S.T., and Brown, T.C.K.: Femoral nerve block: The anatomical basis for a single injection technique. Anaesth. Intensive Care, *11:*40, 1983.
28. Khoury, G.F., Chen, A.C., Garland, D.E., and Stein, C.: Intra-articular morphine, bupivacaine, and morphine/bupivacaine for pain control after knee videoarthroscopy. Anesthesiology, *77:*263, 1992.
29. Kilpatrick, A.W., Coventry, D.M., and Todd, J.G.: A comparison of two approaches to sciatic nerve block. Anaesthesia, *47:*155, 1992.
30. Kofoed, H.: Peripheral nerve blocks at the knee and ankle in operations for common foot disorders. Clin. Orthrop. *168:*97, 1982.
31. Labat, G.: Regional Anesthesia: Its Technic and Clinical Application. pp. 45. Philadelphia, W.B. Saunders, 1924.
32. Last, R.J.: Anatomy: Regional and Applied, Section 5. pp. 342. New York, Churchill Livingstone, 1978.
33. Lehman, W.L., and Jones, W.W.: Intravenous lidocaine for anesthesia in the lower extremity. J. Bone Joint Surg. Am., *66:*1056, 1984.
34. Löfström, B.: Nerve block at the knee-joint. *In* Illustrated Handbook in Local Anaesthesia. Chicago, Year Book Medical Publishers, 1969.
35. Löfström, B.: Ulnar nerve blockade for the evaluation of local anaesthetic agents. Br. J. Anaesth., *47:*297, 1975.
36. McCutcheon, R.: Regional anesthesia for the foot. Can. Anaesth. Soc. J., *12:*465, 1965.
37. McNichol, L.R.: Sciatic nerve block for children. Anaesthesia, *40:*410, 1985.
38. McNichol, L.R.: Lower limb blocks for children. Anaesthesia, *41:*27, 1986.
39. Misra, U., Pridie, A.K., McClymont, C., and Bower, S.: Plasma concentrations of bupivacaine following combined sciatic and femoral 3-in-1 nerve blocks in open knee surgery. Br. J. Anaesth., *66:*310, 1991.
40. Moore, D.C.: Regional Block. 4th ed. Springfield, IL, Charles C. Thomas, 1975.
41. Niemi, L., Pitkanen, M., Bjorkenheim, J.M., and Rosenberg, P.H.: In-

tra-articular morphine for pain relief after knee arthroscopy performed under regional anaesthesia. Acta Anaesthesiol. Scand., *38:*402, 1994.

42. Osborne, D., and Keene, G.: Pain relief after arthroscopic surgery of the knee: A prospective, randomized, and blinded assessment of bupivacaine and bupivacaine with adrenaline. Arthroscopy, *9:*177, 1993.
43. Parks, C.R., and Kennedy, W.F.: Obturator nerve block: A simplified approach. Anesthesiology, *28:*775, 1967.
44. Patel, N.J., Flashburg, M.H., Paskin, S., and Grossman, R.: A regional anesthetic technique compared to general anesthesia for outpatient knee arthroscopy. Anesth. Analg., *65:*185, 1986.
45. Porter, K.M., and Davies, J.: The control of pain after Keller's procedure—A controlled double blind prospective trial with local anesthetic and placebo. Ann. R. Coll. Surg. Engl., *67:*243, 1985.
46. Raj, P.P., Parks, R.I., Watson, T.D., and Jenkins, M.T.: New single position supine approach to sciatic-femoral nerve block. Anesth. Analg., *54:*489, 1975.
47. Raja, S.N., Dickstein, R.E., and Johnson, C.A.: Comparison of postoperative analgesic effects of intra-articular bupivacaine and morphine following arthroscopic knee surgery. Anesthesiology, *77:*1143, 1992.
48. Ringrase, N.H., and Cross, M.J.: Femoral nerve block in knee joint surgery. Am. J. Sports Med., *12:*398, 1984.
49. Robison, C., Ray, D.C., McKeown, D.W., and Buchan, A.S.: Effect of adrenaline on plasma concentrations of bupivacaine following lower limb nerve block. Br. J. Anaesth., *66:*228, 1991.
50. Rooks, M., and Fleming, L.L.: Evaluation of acute knee injuries with sciatic/femoral nerve blocks. Clin. Orthop., *179:*185, 1983.
51. Rorie, D.K., Byer, D.E., Nelson, D.O., and Sittipong, R., *et al.*: Assessment of block of the sciatic nerve in the popliteal fossa. Anesth. Analg., *59:*371, 1980.
52. Sarrafian, S.K., Ibrahim, I.N., and Breihan, J.H.: Ankle-foot peripheral nerve block for mid and forefoot surgery. Foot Ankle, *4:*86, 1983.
53. Selander, D., Dhuner, K.E., and Lundberg, E.: Peripheral nerve injury due to injection needles used for regional anesthesia. Acta Anaesthesiol. Scand., *21:*182, 1977.
54. Sharrock, N.E., Waller, J.F., and Fiero, L.E.: Midtarsal block for surgery of the forefeet. Br. J. Anaesth., *58:*37, 1986.
55. Simon, M.A., Gielen, M.J., and Lagerwerf, A.J.: Plasma concentrations after high doses of mepivacaine with epinephrine in the combined psoas compartment/sciatic nerve block. Anesthesia, *15:*256, 1990.
56. Singelyn, F.J., Gouverneur, J.A., and Gribomont, B.F.: Popliteal sciatic nerve block aided by a nerve stimulator: A reliable technique for foot and ankle surgery. Reg. Anesth., *16:*278, 1991.
57. Smith, B.E., Fischer, A.B.J., and Scott, P.U.: Continuous sciatic nerve block. Anaesthesia, *39:*155, 1984.
58. Stein, C., Comisel, K., Haimeri, E., *et al.*: Analgesic effect of intra-articular morphine after arthroscopic knee surgery. N. Engl. J. Med., *325:*1123, 1991.
59. Wassef, M.R.: Interadductor approach to obturator nerve blockade for spastic conditions of adductor thigh muscles. Reg. Anesth., *18:*13, 1993.
60. Wencker, K.H., Nolte, H., and Fruhstorfer, H.: Brachial plexus blockade for evaluation of local anaesthetic agents. Br. J. Anaesth., *47:*301, 1975.
61. Winnie, A.P.: Regional Anesthesia. Surg. Clin. North Am., *55:*861, 1975.
62. Winnie, A.P., Ramamurthy, S., and Durrani, Z.: The inguinal paravascular technic of lumbar plexus anesthesia. "The 3-in-1 block." Anesth. Analg., *52:*989, 1973.
63. Wong, K., Strichartz, G.R., Raymond, S.A.: On the mechanisms of potentiation of local anesthetics by bicarbonate buffer: Drug structure-activity studies on isolated peripheral nerve. Anesth. Analg., *76:*131, 1993.

Neural Blockade in Clinical Anesthesia and Management of Pain, Third Edition,
edited by M.J. Cousins and P.O. Bridenbaugh.
Lippincott–Raven Publishers, Philadelphia © 1998.

CHAPTER 12

Intravenous Regional Neural Blockade

Charles McK. Holmes

Intravenous regional anesthesia is a method of producing analgesia of the distal part of a limb by intravenous injection, while circulation to the limb is occluded.

HISTORY

The history of anesthesia of the arm has been reviewed in published reports.[63,64] Intravenous regional anesthesia was the first method whereby anesthesia of the arm could be achieved easily. The method was discovered by August Bier in 1908.[14] Bier was Professor of Surgery in Berlin, and he is best remembered as the first to make regular use of spinal anesthesia. To administer intravenous analgesia, he occluded the circulation in a segment of the arm with two tourniquets and then injected a solution of 0.5% procaine into a vein in the isolated segment. Many of the details mentioned by Bier in his paper are still relevant and are worth noting:

> It is important to empty the blood from the region to be anesthetized. This is done by winding an Esmarch[a] bandage proximally up the arm. The circulation is then occluded, above the level of the operation, by many turns of a soft rubber bandage. A similar bandage is applied below the site of the operation. A cannula is inserted in a suitable vein between the two tourniquets (Fig. 12-1). A 0.25% or 0.5% procaine solution in physiologic saline is used. Using the 0.5% strength, direct anesthesia (i.e., between the two bandages) comes on very rapidly. In the distal part of the limb, below the distal bandage, one gradually obtains conduction (indirect) anesthesia. After removal of the bandages, motor and sensory paralyses disappear within a few minutes. The onset of anesthesia in the deeper tissues is as rapid as in the skin, or sometimes more so. The procaine in physiologic saline passes rapidly through the vein walls and is absorbed (into the tissues); after re-establishment of the circulation it only slowly enters the general circulation. In only one case was a slight reaction to procaine observed on removing the bandages. To minimize the risk of reactions, one may loosen the proximal bandage to permit arterial inflow and thereby flush the procaine out by way of the wound (see also Chapter 1).

This method enjoyed wide popularity for a time, and somewhat similar intra-arterial and even intraosseous methods were described. Recently, the intra-arterial method has been revived,[74,75] and may still have a place, where no veins can be found. (It seems that the injection is somewhat more painful than the intravenous).

However, it was not long before simple and reliable techniques for brachial plexus block were developed, and the intravenous method declined in popularity. It was revived in 1963 by Holmes,[65] who used lidocaine because it appeared to give more reliable anesthesia than procaine. Currently, intravenous regional anesthesia (IVRA), sometimes referred to as *Bier block*, is regarded as one of the several alternative techniques for arm anesthesia.

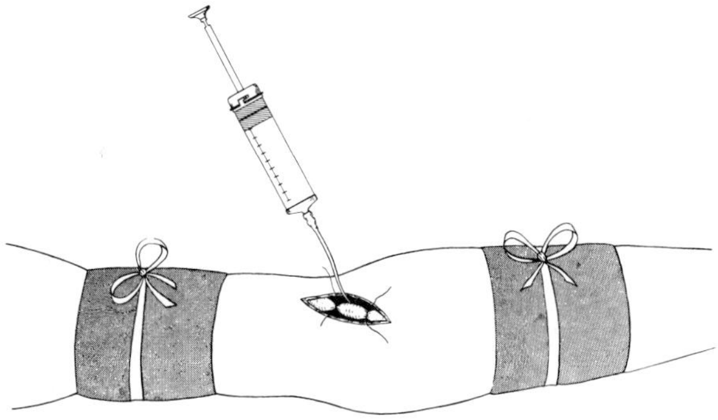

FIG. 12-1. Diagram of Bier's original method.

Advantages and Disadvantages

Advantages

Reliability. Correctly performed, the method is reliable and its success rate is high. Thorn-Alquist[109] has reported unsatisfactory analgesia in only 1% of 967 patients: Dunbar and Mazze[34] had a 96% success rate in 779 patients; and smaller series have reported 100% success rates (e.g., Tryba

C. McK. Holmes: Department of Anaesthesia, Mercy Hospital, Dunedin, New Zealand.

[a] von Esmarch was the Professor of Surgery in Berlin before Bier.

TABLE 12-1. *Success rates of four methods of obtaining arm analgesia in 368 patients (%)*

Method	Perfect result	Fair result	Failure	Complication	Phrenic nerve block
Axillary	76	19	5	9	–
Kulenkampff (supra-clavicular)	73	19	8	10	38
Perivascular (subclavian)	76	23	1	8	36
Interscalene	74	15	11	–	35

et al.[113] in 60 cases). In contrast, other methods of obtaining arm analgesia do not have such high success rates. In a retrospective study of 368 patients,[40] the success rates of four other methods were as shown in Table 12-1.

Ease of Performance. No specific anatomical knowledge is required; the intravenous regional technique requires only that the anesthesiologist insert a needle or cannula into a suitable vein. However, as with any other method involving the use of local anesthesia, the anesthesiologist must be thoroughly familiar with risks and complications and know how to manage them. They must also be skilled in the techniques of resuscitation and have all the necessary equipment readily available. The person performing the block should devote full attention to the patient and should not perform the surgery.

Safety. The reported incidence of adverse side effects is low. There is certainly no risk of such complications as total spinal anesthesia, phrenic nerve block (see Table 12-1); or pneumothorax as seen with other arm blocks. There is a risk of systemic toxicity, but this is no greater than with other arm block techniques.

Onset of analgesia is rapid, so that surgery or manipulation may begin within 5 to 10 minutes, and muscular relaxation is good, so fractures or dislocations can be reduced.

Controllable Duration of Action. The duration of action of the block is governed not by the duration of action of the local anesthetic agent being used, but rather by the time for which the tourniquet is kept inflated. Operations as long as 6 hours have been described,[68] and it would seem that there is no diminution of the block until the tourniquet is released.

Controllable Extent of Analgesia. The extent of the analgesia is limited proximally by the position of the tourniquet. The closer the tourniquet is to the periphery, the smaller the quantity of local anesthetic solution is required.

Rapidity of Recovery. Normal sensation and motor power return rapidly after cuff release, even if it is released well before the expiration of the agent's usual duration of nerve-blocking action. This rapid return to normal function is important because it helps to re-evaluate neurologic signs after fracture reduction. The patient who has had outpatient surgery will not be leaving the hospital with an anesthetized limb, and thus will not risk accidental injury, burns, and the like.

Infection Risk. There is no risk of infection, unlike the technique of direct injection of local anesthetics into the fracture site, which is generally not favored by orthopedic surgeons, despite some recent advocacy.[22]

Disadvantages

A Tourniquet Must be Used. This means that the method cannot produce analgesia of the entire limb but only of that portion of the limb distal to the tourniquet. The tourniquet must be kept inflated continuously; it is not possible to release it to enable bleeding vessels to be identified, unless more local anesthetic is injected after the tourniquet is reinflated.[8] The tourniquet may cause pain. Duration of surgery is limited by the time for which an arterial tourniquet is safe. The tourniquet itself may cause complications (*vide infra*), and at least one case of tourniquet paralysis is on record.[76]

Exsanguination. It is important to exsanguinate the limb prior to tourniquet inflation. This is generally done with an Esmarch bandage. If there is a fracture or laceration of the limb, pain may preclude the use of an Esmarch bandage. In such cases, elevation of the extremity for 2 to 3 minutes or use of an air-inflated splint will be satisfactory.[124]

Toxic Reactions. There is the possibility of a systemic reaction to the local anesthetic when it is released into the general circulation. There may even be a risk before the tourniquet is released (see following). The risk tends to be greater when larger quantities of local anesthetic agent are used, which, in turn, depends on the size of the limb and the position of the tourniquet. For this reason, analgesia of the whole leg with the use of a thigh tourniquet is not recommended, because the quantity of anesthetic solution required would be in excess of acceptable maximum dosage. An exception to this would be an amputation, because, provided the tourniquet was just above the amputation site, only a small amount of the anesthetic would remain to re-enter the circulation.

Inability to Provide a Bloodless Field. When analgesia of the hand or foot is produced with a tourniquet on the forearm or lower leg, there is likely to be gradual vascular engorgement, because of intraosseous blood flow not controlled by the tourniquet. If necessary, this may be controlled by a second tourniquet on the upper arm or thigh.

Rapidity of recovery with loss of analgesia may be considered a disadvantage in major surgical cases, and parenteral pain relief may be required early in the postoperative period.

Selection of Cases

Intravenous regional analgesia is most suited for surgery of the forearm and hand, including the manipulation of forearm fractures. Lesions at the elbow and above are usually better managed with some type of brachial plexus block. The intravenous regional method is also often unsatisfactory for anesthetizing the knee and calf region of the leg, because of the large quantity of solution required. Tourniquet pain is seldom a problem in short procedures, but may become so if the operation is prolonged. Methods of alleviating this discomfort will be discussed later in this chapter, but are not without some disadvantages.

In this author's opinion, intravenous regional anesthesia is therefore best suited for forearm, hand, ankle, and foot operations of relatively short duration.

Contraindications

Disease processes in which prolonged tourniquet times are contraindicated (e.g. sickle cell disease or trait), and tissue infection, such as extensive cellulitis, are contraindications to the use of the intravenous regional technique, as is known sensitivity to the agent. In addition, patients with a history of certain cardiac diseases may be considered unsuitable candidates for intravenous regional anesthesia. Untreated heart block is a particular contraindication, since sudden release of local anesthetic into the circulation may convert a partial heart block to a complete one, or may precipitate asystole. Bradycardia has been recorded following cuff release when lidocaine was used for intravenous regional block, even in normal patients.[34,71]

Technique

Standard Method for the Arm

Premedication. Premedication usually is not required, particularly if the proposed operation is likely to be of short duration. However, some form of sedation may be used for longer operations. Just prior to the performance of the block, an appropriate dose of a sedative, such as diazepam,[31] midazolam, or a neuroleptanalgesic may be given intravenously. This will help to reduce the patient's awareness of the operation and allow better tolerance of the inflated cuff, and it raises the threshold for toxic effects.[31]

Additional small intravenous increments of narcotics and/or sedatives may be given during long operations (see Chapter 6).

Preparation of the Patient. The patient should, normally, have fasted in the same manner as for those who have general anesthesia, since vomiting could represent a hazard if there are any complications, such as convulsions. Having ascertained that the patient accepts this form of analgesia and has no history of allergic reactions to local anesthetic drugs or has other contraindications, the anesthesiologist should explain the technique and should check the pulse occlusion pressure[123,124] on the operative side. The pulse occlusion pressure is best determined by a pulse oximeter on a finger. The oximeter should be transferred to the nonoperative side for monitoring during the surgery. The pneumatic tourniquet should be in good order, and must be fastened securely. The recommended cuff size is one that is 20% wider than the limb diameter; this means 12 to 14 cm wide for the average adult limb.[49] (Note that the cuffs on a double-cuff tourniquet are often only 5 to 6 cm wide.) The pressure gauge must be reliable: it is recommended that all such gauges be checked regularly against a mercury manometer. It is the author's preference, for reasons that will be elaborated later, not to use an automatic gas-powered tourniquet, nor to use one of the double-cuff tourniquets[67] originally designed for use with this method. Care should be taken to ensure that the cuff is applied smoothly and snugly around the arm. A further safeguard is to wrap a bandage around the tourniquet, to reduce the risk of it becoming loose or slipping. After the pulse occlusion pressure has been checked, the cuff may be left temporarily inflated above the diastolic pressure in order to distend the veins for insertion of the needle. As with any anesthetic administration, it should be routine to secure a route for intravenous fluids and supplemental drugs, usually in the other arm, and also to place a blood pressure cuff and pulse oximeter on that side so that the blood pressure, saturation, and pulse can be monitored during the procedure.

Choice of Vein. Usually a vein on the dorsum of the hand is selected. However, if no veins are visible there, a vein on the forearm or even at the antecubital fossa may be chosen. There is, however, some evidence that failure to obtain analgesia, or "patchy" analgesia, is more likely to occur when proximal veins are used.[106] A plastic cannula is preferred for the venipuncture, though a "butterfly" needle with a short extension tube may be used. A long intravenous catheter should not be used, because there is at least one recorded case in which the end of such a catheter was actually above the inflated cuff, resulting in the injection directly into the general circulation.[3] The cannula or needle is placed in the vein, flushed with saline, and taped securely. Care must be taken not to dislodge it during the exsanguination or subsequent injection. As with any venipuncture, there should be careful palpation for superficial arteries, to avoid intra-arterial injection.

Exsanguination. It has frequently been said that exsanguination of the limb assists in the production of complete analgesia. Not all workers agree.[30,111] The usual method is to wrap an Esmarch bandage snugly up the arm, starting, where possible, just proximal to the needle in the hand (Fig. 12-2). If this method is undesirable because of a fracture or wound, elevation of the arm or use of an air-inflated splint[125] is an acceptable alternative.

When the solution is injected, the veins become somewhat distended again for a time, and the surgical field is not as "bloodless" as it would be under a general anesthetic. To overcome this disadvantage, Rawal et al.[97] have proposed a novel method known as re-exsanguination, or "re-IVRA." This involves a reapplication of the Esmarch bandage after the limb is analgesic, with brief deflation and reinflation of the tourniquet. These authors showed that a better surgical field was obtained, without affecting the block. There was also better tolerance of the tourniquet. It is important to note, however, that those investigators[97] waited at least 15 minutes after injection of the local anesthetic and that the "brief" deflation period is actually deflation followed by *immediate* reinflation. Early deflation or delays in reinflation will likely lead to very high plasma levels of local anesthetic, if not an actual systemic toxic reaction.

The tourniquet is inflated to a pressure above the patient's pulse occlusion value. Although high pressures might be assumed to confer greater safely from leakage past the cuff, the discomfort is also likely to be related to the pressure. Therefore, the exact amount by which the tourniquet pressure should exceed the systolic pressure cannot clearly be stated because the patient's blood pressure may rise during the injection or during the operation. Some authors[26,56] advise a tourniquet pressure of 200 to 250 mm Hg, while a pressure of 150 mm Hg above systolic or 50 to 100 mm Hg above pulse occlusion pressure has also been recommended.[122,123] In all cases, disappearance of the radial pulse should be checked. The practice of cross-clamping the tubing of the cuff after inflation is not recommended; should the cuff have a small leak, it might not be detected. It is better to observe the cuff pressure at all times on the aneroid dial (Fig. 12-3).

Injection. Using a 50 ml syringe, 40 ml of 0.5% prilocaine, or lidocaine without preservative or vasoconstrictor, is injected slowly. The quantity may be varied according to the estimated mass of tissue below the tourniquet even though that mass may not correlate well with the patient's overall weight. For example, it may be necessary to use 50 ml for a muscular forearm of a 70 Kg patient, whereas a thin forearm of a 110 Kg patient may be satisfactorily anesthetized with a smaller amount. As the drug is injected, the skin usually becomes mottled, and analgesia develops rapidly. Muscular relaxation, usually quite profound, appears at the same time. If sufficient analgesia is not present 5 minutes after the injection of 40 ml, a further 10 ml should be given before removing the needle.

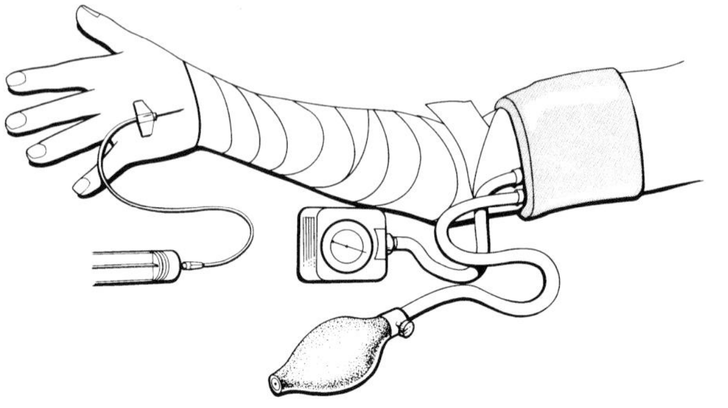

FIG. 12-2. Exsanguination with an Esmarch bandage before the injection.

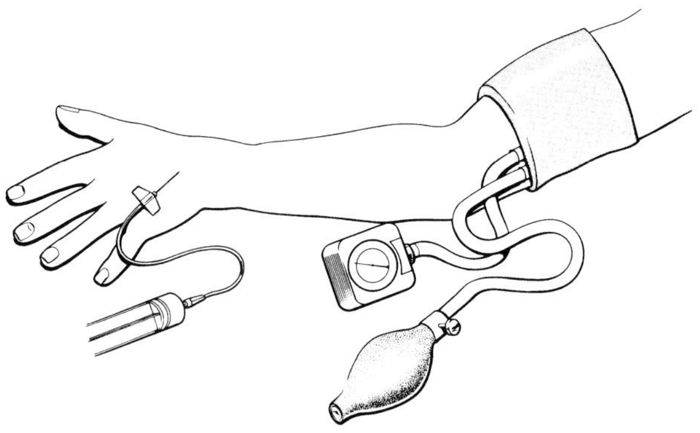

FIG. 12-3. The injection has been completed. The needle may be removed at this stage. Note the tourniquet tubing not clamped; the pressure is visible on the dial.

Tourniquet Discomfort. During the operation, the tourniquet must be kept inflated above the previously determined value. After a time, particularly in the unsedated patient, discomfort may develop at the site of the tourniquet. This may respond to a small intravenous dose of diazepam or an analgesic drug. An alternative or additional maneuver is to place another cuff below the first and to inflate it over the analgesic part of the arm, after which the upper cuff is deflated. Although this method is made easier if the double-compartment cuff[61,67] is used, for reasons that will be discussed later in this chapter, this device is not favored by the author. Another method that is said to relieve tourniquet discomfort is to apply a vibratory massager to the inflated cuff.[53]

Minimum tourniquet time is subject to debate, and will be discussed further. It is usually assumed that deflating the tourniquet soon after the injection would be equivalent to a rapid intravenous infusion of local anesthetic and could produce a toxic reaction. Without any direct evidence to the contrary, it is therefore recommended that the cuff remain inflated for a minimum of 15 minutes.

Tourniquet Release. The tourniquet is released at the end of the operation, and not before, since sensation returns rapidly. It is at this time that adverse reactions may occur, so the patient's pulse, oxygen saturation, blood pressure, and EKG should be monitored closely during the first few minutes after tourniquet release. Appropriate resuscitation equipment should be available, and the patient should be warned to expect transient generalized paresthesia and, sometimes, tinnitus. There appears to be no risk of delayed after effects.

MODIFIED METHOD FOR THE HAND

Many papers now attest to the value of this method for hand surgery, including one report of a series of outpatient

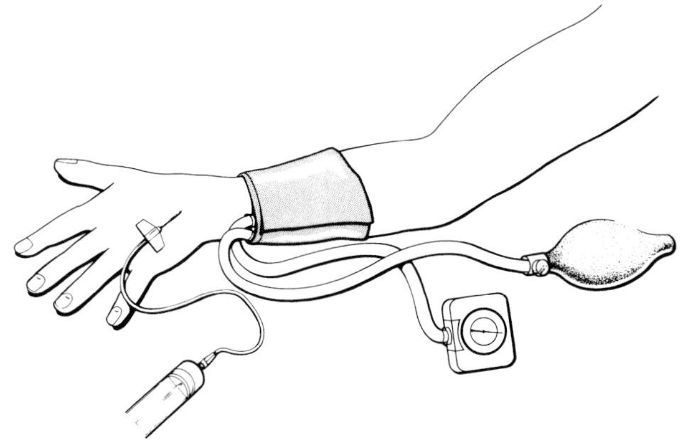

FIG. 12-4. The modified method for the hand. A second tourniquet might be placed on the upper arm, if necessary.

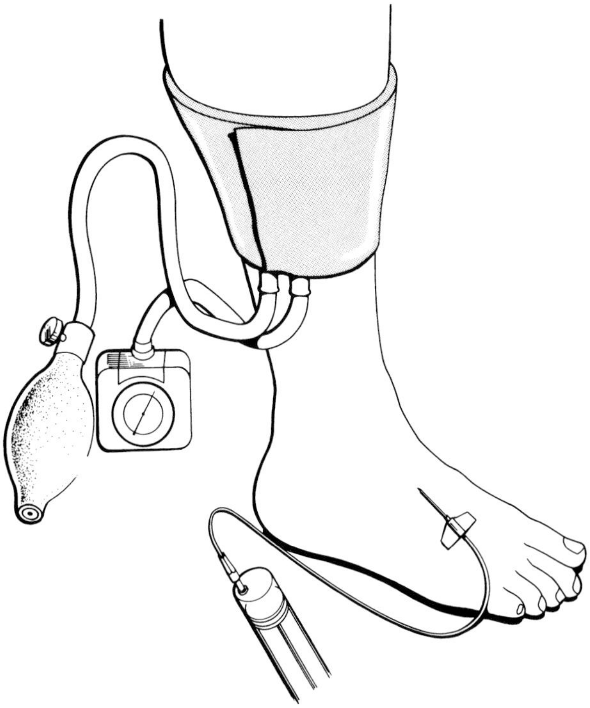

FIG. 12-5. The modified method for the foot.

operations for Dupuytren's disease.[73] The cuff is placed on the forearm, taking care to keep it below the head of the radius (Fig. 12-4). A difficulty sometimes encountered with this method is that blood flow through the radius and ulna causes gradual vascular congestion of the hand if the operation is other than quite short. Of course, since the quantity of solution is so small, the tourniquet could be released safely at any time, so a short procedure is quite feasible. For a longer operation, a second tourniquet on the upper arm may be needed to prevent this congestion. About 10 ml of solution will usually provide complete analgesia. Chan, Pun, Chan[21] and Rousso et al.[100] described the use of the forearm tourniquet, with another occluding cuff on the upper arm, while Plourde et al.[95] showed how the dose could be reduced to 1.5 mg/kg of 0.5% lidocaine, and still provide excellent anesthesia. A slight variation is described by both Roven[101] and Eastwood et al.[35] in which the injection is concentrated in the hand by the simple expedient of a rubber venipuncture tourniquet or a piece of Penrose tubing around the forearm.

An interesting variation of this is the method of digital regional anesthesia described by Ryding.[102] He showed that if a vein on the dorsum of a finger can be cannulated with a fine needle, that very good analgesia of the finger can be achieved with a small quantity of anesthetic, using a rubber tourniquet around the base of the finger. This method is quite appropriate for the treatment of conditions such as paronychia.

MODIFIED METHOD FOR THE FOOT AND ANKLE

There are now many papers describing foot and ankle surgery with the intravenous regional anesthesia method.[12,26,27,39,87,91,103,116] The same principles apply as for the hand (Fig. 12-5). The tourniquet should be placed well below the knee to avoid compressing the peroneal nerve on the neck of the fibula.

PROLONGED INTRAVENOUS REGIONAL ANESTHESIA

As mentioned earlier, intravenous regional anesthesia is better suited for short procedures. However, it may be used for prolonged operations if the patient is well sedated. The technique described by Brown and Weissman[18] consists of inserting an indwelling plastic catheter into a suitable vein away from the operation site and leaving it *in situ* during the operation. After about one hour, the tourniquet is deflated, and bleeding vessels may be secured during the short interval before sensation returns. The arm is then elevated, the tourniquet reinflated, and another dose of the local anesthetic injected. They found that to produce adequate analgesia, this dose may be only one-half the volume of the first. The procedure may be repeated if necessary. However, it is not proven that this short tourniquet release affects the incidence of tourniquet complications, and generally the governing factor in long operations is the time for which it is considered safe to leave a tourniquet inflated.

Pediatric Use (see Chapter 20)

The method is readily applicable for children who are old enough to comprehend a simple explanation of the procedure.[10,20,42,46,48,115] It is a very valuable procedure for the reduction of the common forearm fractures and similar lesions. The standard method is used, making sure the tourniquet is of an appropriate size for the circumference of the child's arm. Elevation is used for exsanguination in preference to an Esmarch bandage, to avoid any discomfort. The dose of prilocaine or lidocaine may be calculated on the basis of 3 mg/kg.

Use of Additive Substances

In an attempt to reduce the amount of local anesthetic required, or to improve the quality of the block, or both, various workers have tried the effects of adding analgesics and/or muscle relaxants. Armstrong, Power, and Wildsmith[7] found that fentanyl 0.1 mg added to 40 ml 0.5% prilocaine conferred no advantage, and caused nausea after tourniquet release. On the other hand, Pitkanen et al.[94] found that 0.2 mg did result in more patients having complete analgesia at 15 minutes, and a delayed onset of postoperative pain. Once again there was some nausea in the fentanyl groups however. Armstrong, Morton, and Nimmo[6] tried pethidine 100 mg in 40 ml 0.25% prilocaine. This did increase the speed of onset and the extent of sensory and motor block, reduced tourniquet pain, and subjectively improved the quality of the block. However, at tourniquet release, there was light-headedness and some nausea, precluding the clinical use of the modification. Abdulla and Fadhil[1] used both fentanyl 0.05 mg and pancuronium 0.5 mg combined with lidocaine 0.25%. This seemed to produce improved results. Similarly, de Mello[32] used fentanyl and atracurium with prilocaine. These modifications require further study before they can be recommended.

Choice of Local Anesthetic Agent

All the common local anesthetic agents including cocaine have been used for IVRA. Procaine was the standard drug used by the early researchers, but it is undoubtedly less effective than the modern agents. Lidocaine was used first by Holmes,[65] and many large series in which this agent was used have since been reported. Equally satisfactory analgesia (but not equal safety) is probably obtainable with all current local anesthetic drugs. However, it should be noted that the duration of action does not depend on the drug, but on the time for which the tourniquet is kept inflated. [Patchy analgesia is sometimes seen for a varying time after tourniquet release: this analgesia does appear to correlate with the known duration of action of the agent used.[38,81]]

It is also of interest to note that quite satisfactory analgesia can be obtained with 2-chloroprocaine, even though it is normally hydrolyzed rapidly in the blood. This agent is the least toxic and would, in theory, be the ideal choice. A higher incidence of thrombophlebitis occured in early studies with this agent and therefore it was not recommended.[57] A new preparation of 2-chloroprocaine has been tried recently for intravenous regional anesthesia, but still causes the thrombophlebitis problem.[93]

Prilocaine is the most rapidly metabolized of the amides, and is partially extracted by the pulmonary circulation. Given its efficacy by the intravenous route and the low incidence of thrombophlebitis associated with its use, it appears to have the most appeal of the drugs available (see Chapter 4). Prilocaine was first reported in 1964 by Hooper[66] in 64 cases. In a double-blind trial, Kerr[72] studied 22 patients who were given 0.5% prilocaine and 20 patients who were given 0.5% lidocaine. Nearly half the patients who received lidocaine had neurologic side effects (dizziness, tinnitus, muscular twitching), whereas there was only one minor episode of dizziness among the patients who received prilocaine. Eriksson[37] demonstrated that the effects seen on the electroencephalograms (EEGs) of patients given 200 mg of lidocaine IV (40 ml of 0.5%), although smaller in magnitude, were similar to those seen after direct intravenous injection of the same solution over a period of 2.3 minutes. Subjective symptoms could be correlated with the EEG changes and occurred in all subjects. With a similar amount of prilocaine, the EEG changes were considerably reduced, and there were no subjective symptoms. This could be explained partly by the lower plasma levels that occur after the administration of prilocaine, and partly by its lower inherent toxicity. Eriksson also showed that when intravenous regional anesthesia was produced with a mixture of 0.25% lidocaine and 0.25% of the prilocaine, the maximum plasma concentration of the prilocaine was less than that of the lidocaine. This effect has also been demonstrated by Thorn-Alquist.[110] Prilocaine must therefore be considered superior to lidocaine. The most impressive testimony for prilocaine is in a recent study by Bartholomew and Sloan,[11] who carried out a survey in Britain of over 45,000 cases. They found an incredible 99.989% absence of complications, and the 0.011% rate of complications related to minor side effects. They also detail two cases of accidental intravenous injection of prilocaine, with the patients both being totally unaware of the event, and suffering no symptoms.

Recent studies have considered the effect of alkalinizing prilocaine. The rationale is to increase the pKa, in order to facilitate membrane penetration. Such modification of local anesthetics is known to work in other situations. Armstrong and co-workers[4,5] and Solak et al.[106] have shown that the addition of sodium bicarbonate decreased the onset time, and improved the quality of anesthesia.

Bupivacaine was first used in intravenous regional anesthesia by Ware,[119,120] who recorded 14,000 cases without a single mishap.[121] Other authors have also used bupivacaine without problems.[47,70] A prospective double-blind trial[62] comparing prilocaine and bupivacaine showed no major side effects in all of the 200 patients included in the study, but 20% of the patients in the bupivacaine group had minor side effects, compared with 12% in the prilocaine group. Another double-blind trial of these two drugs was carried out by McKeown, Meiklejohn, and Scott,[85] in which six volunteers underwent intravenous regional anesthesia on four occasions each. Since bupivacaine has an *in vivo* potency four times that of prilocaine, 0.5% prilocaine was compared with 0.125% bupivacaine, and since Ware recommends 0.2% bupivacaine, this was compared with 0.8% prilocaine. On each occasion, 40 ml of one of these solutions was injected, and the results were compared. The authors found that although the higher doses gave more rapid onset and more profound blocks, they were associated with more marked toxicity (though no serious side effects were observed). These authors concluded that there was little to be gained by using the higher concentrations of either drug. Bupivacaine is now no longer recommended for this technique, nor is this use supported by its manufacturers.

Dose and Concentration. The dose of local anesthetic agent should be calculated according to the estimated mass of tissue below the tourniquet. A 40-ml dose is appropriate for an average-size arm with the tourniquet above the elbow, but this quantity may be altered proportionately for larger or smaller arms. However, since the incidence of toxic reactions is related to the blood level of the agent and since this in turn depends on, among other factors, the dose given in proportion to the total body weight, maximum doses according to body weight have been recommended (lidocaine, 1.5–3 mg/kg; prilocaine, 3–4 mg/kg; bupivacaine, 0.75–1.5 mg/kg).[34,57,84,120]

Pre-injection ischemia of 15 to 20 minutes' duration has been shown by Bell and co-workers[13] and Harris[57] to result in a significant reduction in the amount of solution required for satisfactory analgesia, but this modification does not appear to have achieved wide-spread popularity.

Varying concentrations from 0.15% up to 2% prilocaine have been used successfully. However, for a given total dose, a smaller volume would have to be used with the stronger solutions, which may result in rather patchy analgesia. Few dose-response studies have been performed, however. In a prospective double-blind study of 60 patients, Tryba, Zenz, and Hausmann[113] compared 4 mg/kg of prilocaine in concentrations of 0.8%, 1.5%, and 2.0%. They found that after the administration of the higher concentrations, analgesia persisting after tourniquet release was greater, the blood level of the agent was lower, and no side effects were observed. It should be noted that in this study the operations were around the wrist and that a tourniquet on the forearm was used in addition to the upper arm tourniquet. Hooper[66] recommended 20 ml of 1% prilocaine, but most workers have favored the 0.5% concentration.

Additives. It is important that all solutions of local anesthetic agents be free of epinephrine (adrenaline) and additives or preservatives. Thrombophlebitis has occurred from use of preservative-containing solutions. Those who provide their own dilute solutions of local anesthetics by adding normal saline to stronger concentrations of local anesthetics should be aware that vials of normal saline may contain preservatives or benzyl alcohol. It is a useful safety feature of prilocaine that the commercial preparation is not available with epinephrine and is preservative-free.

COMPLICATIONS (see Chapter 21)

> ". . . The most important requirement for avoiding untoward sequelae with any regional block is not the technique or the drug used but by whom and in what circumstances they are used."[b]

It should be stressed at the onset that many of the reports of complications relate to failure to adhere to the correct technique or to apply the appropriate resuscitative measures, or to some other factors not directly attributable to the method itself. Two interesting adverse reports that fall into this category deserve mention: A young woman lost her forearm and hand as a result of the injection of alcohol (almost certainly) instead of lidocaine, when intravenous regional anesthesia was being attempted[79], and a case of tourniquet paralysis with incomplete recovery is recorded.[76] However, all adverse reports must be set against the figure of "14,000 cases without mishap" mentioned by Ware,[121] the "10,000 cases without fatality" quoted by Colbern[23], the 20-year experience without mortality or major morbidity described by Brown, McGriff, and Malinkowski[19], and the 45,000 cases in the Bartholomew and Sloan survey.[11] The complications of intravenous regional anesthesia usually are caused by the systemic toxicity of the agent used (see Chapter 4). Local anesthetics principally affect the central nervous system (CNS), where they may be either stimulant or depressant, and the cardiovascular system, where they are depressant (see Chapters 2 and 4). It is noteworthy that the records of the Committee on Safety of Medicines show that prilocaine has caused no mortality (all uses, not just IVRA) over a 26-year period;[11] however, a problem unique to prilocaine is methemoglobinemia, though it is not a significant problem with intravenous regional anesthesia (*vide infra*).

A possible factor in some complications, and certainly documented in some cases of convulsions,[28,99] is leakage of the local anesthetic while the tourniquet is still apparently or actually inflated. Because of the adverse reactions that have been reported, two measures were taken in Britain. First, the use of automatic gas-operated tourniquets was advised against, and a "hazard notice"[33] was issued. Second, it was recommended that bupivacaine no longer be used for IVRA.

Deaths. Seven deaths attributed to intravenous regional analgesia were reported in Britain over the period 1979 to 1983.[58] Not all are well documented, but some common facts are known for some of the cases:[59] The patients were healthy, automatic tourniquets were used, bupivacaine was the drug, and the attending physician was not an anesthesiologist. Moreover, after having performed the block, the physician went on to perform the surgery himself. The mode of death is not clearly known in these cases, but some early cardiac depression was apparently a factor in some, raising the question of the relative cardiotoxicity of bupivacaine. This topic is discussed in Chapter 4.

[b] Moore, D.C.: Bipivacaine toxicity and Bier block: The drug, the technique, or the anesthetist. Anesthesiology *61*:782, 1984.

Central Nervous System Symptoms and Signs. These range from mild, transient giddiness, dizziness, or tinnitus to more serious phenomena such as muscular twitching, convulsions, and loss of consciousness. The latter signs are not common, however. In one series of 1,400 patients,[117] only 8 patients had CNS stimulation sufficient to require the administration of a barbiturate and only three of these had frank convulsions. All these patients had received a dose of lidocaine in excess of 5 mg/kg. Fleming[43,44] records "5 or 6" convulsions in another large series, again with lidocaine. Convulsions have been reported in many instances in which bupivacaine has been used:[28,29,54,60,99] but no convulsions have been reported with prilocaine.[122] Gürtner, Meyer, and Gürtner[50] monitored both the EEG and the EKG before, during, and after cuff release. They found no evidence of adverse effects on brain or cardiac function, after mepivacaine 0.5% 3mg/Kg. There was some drowsiness, however.

The highest frequency of minor CNS toxicity has been recorded by Harris,[57] who reported an incidence of 67.3% with 5 mg/Kg of prilocaine in a group of volunteers. A 50% incidence of CNS toxicity with lidocaine, 3 mg/kg, was recorded by Bell, Slater, and Harris[13] in a small group of volunteers. Most other workers have reported a lower incidence of 10% or less. Dunbar and Mazze[34] have recorded an incidence of 2.1% in 779 patients, with lidocaine or prilocaine.

Cardiovascular System Symptoms and Signs. These are usually also mild and transient. In 779 patients, Dunbar and Mazze[34] found no arrhythmias and only a slight drop in blood pressure or a slight bradycardia on release of the tourniquet. This is in keeping with the observations of most other workers. By contrast, however, Kennedy, Duthie, Parbrook, and Carr,[71] who monitored the ECG in all their 77 patients, found a 15% incidence of ECG changes, mostly of a minor nature, but recorded one cardiac arrest (successfully treated) that was preceded by bradycardia. They did not feel justified in continuing to use the technique (with lidocaine).

Methemoglobinemia is known to occur after the administration of prilocaine and may cause cyanosis (see Chapter 4). A significant rise in serum methemoglobin levels is not usually seen below a total dose of 600 mg of prilocaine, which is above the dose required for intravenous regional anesthesia.[80] Harris, Cole, Mital, and Laver[56] studied 58 volunteers given 5 mg/kg of prilocaine for intravenous regional anesthesia and found a small rise in methemoglobin from 0.33 ± 0.11 g per 100 ml (control) to 1.02 ± 0.33 g per 100 ml after tourniquet release. No cyanosis was observed. Bader et al.[9] state that about 10% of hemoglobin as methemoglobin is needed to produce detectable cyanosis, and in their study found peak levels of only 3%. Biscoping, Michaelis, and Hempelmann[15] found a mean level of 2.7% despite using 40 ml of 1.0% prilocaine. This level was sustained for some hours, which they attributed to delayed prilocaine release. McKeown and co-workers[84] report that they have "been using 0.5% prilocaine . . . in IVRA [intravenous regional anesthesia] for 15 years and have never seen methaemoglobinemia[sic] as a complication."

Factors That Influence the Incidence of Toxic Reactions

Leakage of Local Anesthetic Before Tourniquet Release. Many studies have now demonstrated that there may be leakage of anesthetic into the general circulation, even in the presence of an apparently well-inflated tourniquet cuff. There may be several reasons for this:

1. Leakage through intraosseous veins,
2. Leakage through ordinary veins,
3. Malfunctioning tourniquet.

Leakage Through Intra-osseous Veins. This was postulated by Shamay and Robin[104] to explain leakage of 14 C-labelled lidocaine, and also by Hanton and Punchihewa[54] in a clinical case in which convulsions developed. However, no direct evidence has been produced.

Leakage Through Ordinary Veins. For this to occur in the presence of a correctly inflated cuff, the venous pressure caused by the cuff presumably must exceed the pressure in the tissues. This was first shown by Raj and associates[96] in a study with radio-opaque solution, and has since been demonstrated by others.[99] Lawes and co-workers[77] measured pressures in a cephalic vein just below the cuff when injections were made in the dorsum of the hand. They found rapid injection could often cause venous pressures exceeding cuff pressure. However, Finegan and Bukht,[41] although demonstrating pressures as high as 190 mm Hg in a similar experiment, found none higher than the cuff pressure, when this was set at 150 mm Hg above systolic. Nevertheless, they felt it desirable to advise the use of wide cuffs that should fully encircle the arm (with a recommended width-to-length ratio of 1 to 3), that injections be made distally, that volumes of solution not exceed 60 ml, and that the injection be made slowly. Therefore, there is probably also an argument to avoid the saline "chasers" that some advocated in the past.[23] Additionally, Reynolds[98] recommends that exsanguination be as complete as possible. Finegan and Bukht[41] point out that as veins are filled, their cross-sectional shape changes from oval to circular, at which point they become relatively indistensible and pressure rises rapidly. Therefore, the more completely veins are emptied before the injection commences, the more volume they can accommodate without pressure rise. Grice et al.[49] distinguish between "gauge pressure" and "effective tourniquet pressure," this latter being the pressure that is transmitted to the veins and arteries of the limb. The main factor relating these two pressures is the width of the tourniquet in relation to the size of the limb; hence the desirability of having a cuff 20% wider than the limb diameter, as referred to earlier. These workers also define the "maximum venous pressure" (MVP), which is the maximum pressure that can be achieved during IV injection, no matter how forceful the injection. They show that MVP sometimes exceeded the systolic blood pressure, and that a wide cuff was better at preventing leakage than a narrow one. Their recommendations are for slow (90 seconds at least) injection, in a distal vein, using a wide cuff inflated to 300 mm Hg after Esmarch-bandage exsanguination.

In contrast to these studies, however, Lillie and co-workers[78], using 40 ml of technetium-labelled saline and a cuff pressure of 300 mm Hg, found no evidence of leakage in 5 volunteers. Injections were made at the antecubital fossa, but the injection speed and pressure were not stated.

Ogden[92] describes a case where, probably as a result of calcification of the vessels combined with the patient's obesity, the arm became congested despite a cuff pressure (double-cuff) of 320 mm Hg. The patient's blood pressure had been measured at 180/90 immediately beforehand, using an ordinary cuff. This problem is also discussed in more detail by Jeyaseelam and co-workers.[69] Davies and associates[28] studied the relation between the "occlusion pressure" (i.e., the cuff pressure at which the radial pulse disappears) and the systolic pressure. They found that in many cases the narrow-cuffed double tourniquets did not occlude the artery even at pressures 100 mm Hg greater that the systolic. Furthermore, "occlusion pressures" were usually different, depending on whether the proximal or distal duff was inflated. This difference was as great as 45 mm Hg. They therefore concluded that "occlusion pressure" should be measured

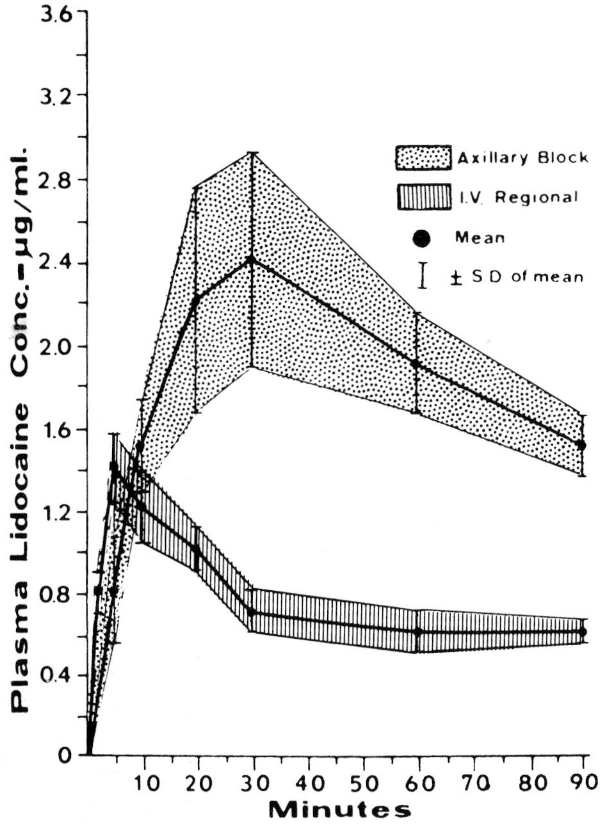

FIG. 12-6. A comparison of the blood levels of lidocaine after intravenous regional analgesia and axillary block. The horizontal axis refers to the time after tourniquet release for intravenous regional analgesia and time after injection of lidocaine for axillary block. (Mazze, R.I., and Dunbar, R.W.: Plasma lidocaine concentrations after caudal, lumbar epidural, axillary block and intravenous regional anesthesia. Anesthesiology, *27*:574, 1966.)

TABLE 12-2. *Plasma levels after tourniquet release*

Block	Dose of lidocaine (mg/kg)	Mean peak plasma level (µg/ml)
Intravenous regional anesthesia	3, 0.5%	1.5 ± 0.2
Axillary block	6–6.8, 1.5%[a]	2.5 ± 0.5
Lumbar epidural block	4.7–6.5, 1.5%[a]	3.1 ± 0.7
Caudal epidural block	5.8–7.5, 1.5%[a]	1.4 ± 0.6

[a] With 1:200,000 epinephrine

(Mazze, R. I., and Dunbar, R. W.: Plasma lidocaine concentrations after caudal, lumbar epidural, axillary block and intravenous regional anesthesia. Anesthesiology, *27*:574, 1966.)

with the same tourniquet and gauge that will be used for the procedure. A wide cuff is better than a double-cuff, but if the latter is used, "occlusion pressure" should be measured with both cuffs in turn, and the high reading should be chosen as the reference point. The pressure then used to inflate the cuff for the procedure must exceed the "occlusion pressure" by a margin that allows for rises in blood pressure during surgery.

Malfunctioning Tourniquet. This has certainly been a problem with automatic gas-operated tourniquets. Whether the problem has been mechanical or caused by operator error is not known in all the cases, but, as mentioned earlier, these devices have been advised against by a "hazard notice" in Britain.[33] Heath[59] states that they "are expensive and have if anything increased the incidence of tourniquet failure . . ." For this reason, they cannot be recommended unconditionally, but, if chosen, must be used with care and only after becoming fully conversant with the operating instructions.

Plasma levels of local anesthetic after tourniquet release have been studied by several authors. Using 0.5% lidocaine in a dose of 2.5 mg/kg and in most cases releasing the tourniquet after only 5 minutes, Hargrove, Hoyle, Parker, Beckett, and Boyes[55] found that maximum levels of anesthetic in venous blood from the other arm did not exceed 2 µg/ml. A similar figure of 1.5 0.2 µg/ml was found by Mazze and Dunbar[82] following 3 mg/kg of 0.5% lidocaine. They found considerably higher levels after axillary block and after lumbar epidural block (see Fig. 12-6, and Table 12-2).

Tucker and Boas,[114] who studied the plasma concentration of lidocaine in the contralateral artery, observed that the peak levels were 20% to 80% lower than those found after direct intravenous infusion of the same dose over 3 minutes. They also found the levels were lower (by about 40%) when the same dose was used for intravenous regional anesthesia in a 0.5% solution, rather than a 1% solution. If a cuff time of 10 minutes is assumed, pharmacokinetic calculations from this data indicate that after cuff release the drug reaches the systemic circulation in the following biphasic manner: There is an initial fast release of 30% of the dose, which is so rapid that reinflation of the cuff would only retard systemic uptake if it were performed within 30 seconds of cuff release, and then there is a slower washout of the remainder of the dose, so that up to 30 minutes after cuff release half the dose would still be retained in the limb.

These findings are supported by recent clinical data that indicate sustained high local anesthetic concentrations in the venous drainage from the blocked arm.[38] Thus, it is possible to reestablish anesthesia for approximately 10 to 30 minutes after cuff release by injecting half the original dose after reinflation of the cuff.

Eriksson[37] studied 5 volunteers who received IVRA on two occasions, once with prilocaine and once with lidocaine (40 ml of 0.5% in each case). The tourniquet was left inflated for 30 minutes after all injections. Sampling was from the contralateral brachial artery. The results are shown in Fig. 12-7, which demonstrates the consistently lower blood levels of prilocaine. These levels are lower than those usually considered toxic. A very similarly shaped curve, but for venous levels, is published by Bader et al.[9] Englesson, Eriksson, Wahlqvist, and Ortengren[36] found that symptoms were noted at a mean plasma level of 4.4 μg/ml in awake patients who received intravenous infusions of lidocaine, while Foldes, Molloy, McNall, and Koukal[45] found that toxic symptoms occurred at a plasma level of 5.3 μg/ml. In anesthetized patients, signs of toxicity were not seen below plasma levels of 10 μg/ml.[16]

Blood levels of bupivacaine were measured by Kalso and associates[70] following a mean dose of 1.8 mg/kg (range, 1.4–2.6 mg/kg) of 0.25% bupivacaine. They found mean level generally below 1.6 μg/ml (toxic level, 4–5 μg/ml), but even in some individuals with higher levels (maximum, 2.72 μg/ml) there were no CNS side effects. Ware and Caldwell,[118] in a study of 50 patients, gave 1.5 mg/kg of 0.2% bupivacaine, and found that the highest mean venous level was 840 ± 146 ng/ml, well below toxic levels. They saw no side effects other than transient drowsiness in one patient.

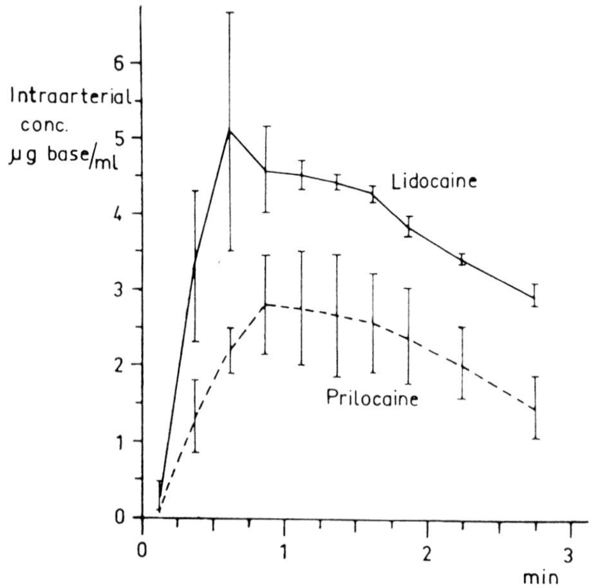

FIG. 12-7. The blood levels of lidocaine and prilocaine in the contralateral brachial artery after intravenous regional analgesia with a mixture of the two agents. (Eriksson, E.: The effects of intravenous local anesthetic agents on the central nervous system. Acta Anaesthesiol. Scand., *36* (Suppl.):79, 1969.)

By contrast, however, Tryba and co-workers,[112] in a prospective randomized study comparing 1 mg/kg bupivacaine with 4 mg/kg prilocaine, found that the plasma levels of bupivacaine were 3 times higher than those of prilocaine when expressed as a percentage of the toxic level. In one case, the bupivacaine level reached 85% of the toxic level. Tryba et al. suggest that their figures support their contention that bupivacaine not be used for intravenous regional anesthesia. Biscoping, Michaelis, and Hempelmann,[15] using 40 ml of 1.0% prilocaine, and sampling from the axillary vein by means of a long cannula passed up under the cuff, found a transient peak of 60 μg/ml, but this fell quickly to be below 20 μg/ml at 10 minutes.

The following factors may affect the peak blood level after tourniquet release: whether or not exsanguination is performed, time from injection to tourniquet release, mode of release, and arm movement after tourniquet release.

Exsanguination has been insufficiently studied. Adams, Dealy, and Kenmore[2] suggested that the more complete the exsanguination, the smaller the "reservoir" of lidocaine-containing blood to be flushed into the general circulation. Eriksson,[37] however, studied a few cases in which exsanguination had been performed with an Esmarch bandage, and he found no difference in plasma lidocaine level in these cases, compared with those in which the arm had only been elevated. Haasio, Hiippala, and Rosenberg[51] compared the effects of exsanguination using an Esmarch bandage with elevation for 2 minutes plus digital brachial artery occlusion. They found that the injection pressure rose significantly higher in the elevation group, but otherwise there were no significant differences between the groups in terms of toxicity.

Time to tourniquet release had been studied by several workers, but their findings have been variable. Mazze and Dunbar[82] found no correlation between peak venous levels and tourniquet time; indeed, the patient who had the longest tourniquet time had the third highest plasma lidocaine concentration (Fig. 12-8). However, this may have been related to errors inherent in venous sampling. Comparing tourniquet times of 15 to 30 minutes, Thorn-Alquist[110] found no difference in peak levels when sampling from the contralateral artery. Both of these studies used rather insensitive colorimetric assays for lidocaine. By contrast, Tucker and Boas,[114] again using arterial sampling, did find an inverse relationship between tourniquet time and peak plasma level (Fig. 12-9). This study used a sensitive gas chromatography assay for lidocaine.

Mode of Release of Tourniquet. Holmes[65] suggested that release and rapid reinflation of the tourniquet several times

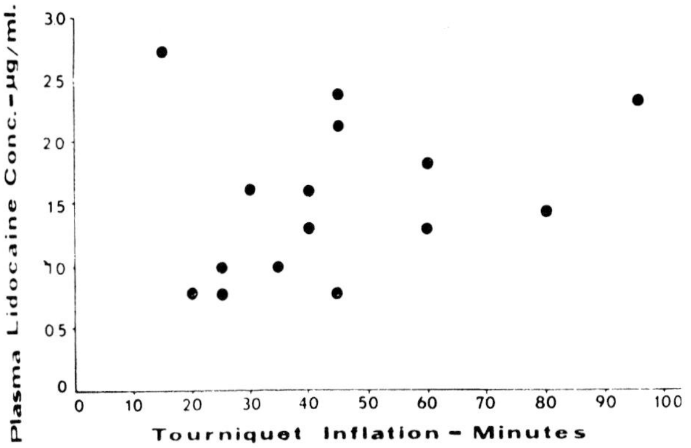

FIG. 12-8. Maximum plasma lidocaine concentration after tourniquet release, measured in venous blood, in relation to duration of tourniquet inflation. (Mazze, R.I., and Dunbar, R.W.: Plasma lidocaine concentrations after caudal, lumbar epidural, axillary block and intravenous regional anesthesia. Anesthesiology, *27*:574, 1966.)

would lessen the incidence of symptoms.[65] This maneuver has also been recommended by other workers. Merrifield and Carter[86] found a mean peak venous lidocaine level of 5.9±5.7 µg/ml when this procedure was performed, while with half the dose of lidocaine and without intermittent tourniquet release, the level was 4.7±0.2 µg/ml, which indicates a definite protective effect. Sukhani et al.[108] studied peak arterial concentrations (Cmax) in the contralateral radial artery, and the time to reach these peak levels (Tmax) following IV lidocaine. Various tourniquet "cycling" techniques did not influence Cmax, but did significantly prolong Tmax. The best technique appeared to be a sequence of release for 10 seconds, followed by a reinflation for one minute.

Arm movement immediately after tourniquet release should be discouraged because it has been shown to result in increased plasma levels of the drug.

Complications Related to the Use of a Tourniquet. When use of intravenous regional anesthesia is considered, the fact that a tourniquet must be used for the entire duration of the operation must be taken into account. There may be operations in which this is undesirable or even impossible, so that other methods of regional analgesia might be more appropriate. Also, there may be operations where the duration is considered too long for a tourniquet, although this is controversial because there does not appear to be any clear relationship between tourniquet time and complications. At least one case of tourniquet paralysis is recorded following intravenous regional anesthesia.[76]

Middleton and Varian[87] reviewed an estimated 630,000 tourniquet applications, and found an incidence of peripheral nerve damage of 1:8,000. The incidence was higher in procedures involving the upper limb (1:5,000) than in those involving the lower limb (1:13,000). In the upper limb, there were 27 patients with total palsy, 8 following the use of a pneumatic tourniquet and 19 following the use of an Esmarch bandage. All recovered. The tourniquet time varied from 20 minutes to 2½ hours. There were 19 patients with radial nerve palsy, in whom the tourniquet applications varied from 15 minutes to 1½ hours. All but one of these patients recovered. In the lower limb, there were 30 patients with palsy, all following the use of an Esmarch bandage. The tourniquet time varied from 30 minutes to 4½ hours, and all but one patient had an eventual full recovery. These authors studied the pressures that could be produced with an Esmarch bandage and found them variable and usually higher than supposed. However, they were not able to draw definite conclusions about the etiology of tourniquet paralyses. There did not seem to be any common factor in any of their cases. Moldaver[88] believed that direct mechanical pressure was more likely to be a factor than ischemia, and he cautioned against using a tourniquet in any area where a nerve could be compressed against bony structures.

The following general recommendations can therefore be made:

- A pneumatic tourniquet of a width 20% greater than the arm diameter should be chosen.
- The tourniquet should be applied where the nerves are best protected in the muscles.
- Excessive tourniquet pressure should be avoided by mea-

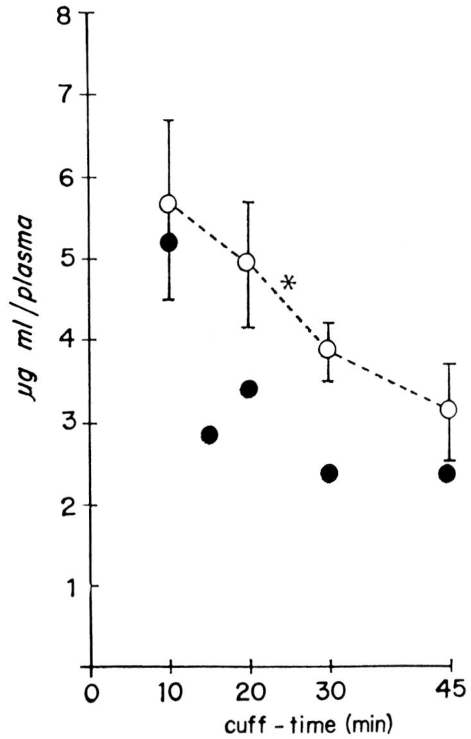

FIG. 12-9. Relation between cuff time and arterial plasma level of lidocaine, 1 minute after tourniquet release. *Open circles* represent mean data ± SD, solution; asterisk represents the difference significant at $p < 0.05$; *closed circles* indicate individual data with 0.5% solution. (Tucker, G.T., and Boas, R.A.: Pharmacokinetic aspects of intravenous regional anesthesia. Anesthesiology, *34*:538, 1971.)

suring the "occlusion pressure" before the operation and by maintaining a tourniquet pressure of no more than 50 to 100 mm Hg above this.

- The tubing should not be clamped between the cuff and the gauge because this would prevent a leaking cuff from being detected.
- The duration of application of the tourniquet should be as short as possible.

MODE OF ACTION

The mode of action of the local anesthetic agents in intravenous regional anesthesia has been the subject of much debate. There has been difficulty in separating the effects of the local anesthetic from those of ischemia alone. Direct pressure on nerves can cause anesthesia, and Miles, James, Clark, and Whitwam[88] and Shanks and McLeod[105] found quite marked effects from ischemia alone. In fact, Shanks and McLeod found that anesthesia, preceded by dysesthesia alone, usually developed in 5 to 30 minutes with ischemia alone, along with variable muscle weakness. However, all agree that the onset of anesthesia is much more rapid and complete when a local anesthetic is added.

Miles and colleagues[88] demonstrated that the latency of action potential in muscle was increased 55% by ischemia and 180% by ischemia plus lidocaine. They believed their results indicated that lidocaine acts on the peripheral part of the neuron. They showed that the muscle weakness was not reversible by neostigmine.

Shanks and McLeod,[105] however, using 1% lidocaine, concluded that the block was in the nerve trunks. They considered that the more pronounced effect of lidocaine on conduction in proximal segments of the nerve was the result of a greater concentration of the agent in the forearm, which would be in keeping with the radiographic studies of Fleming, Veiga-Pires, McCutcheon, and Emanuel[44] and Sorbie and Chacha,[107] who demonstrated that the local anesthetic proceeds rapidly in a proximal direction when it is injected in the dorsum of the hand.

Cotev and Robin,[25] in biopsy studies on dogs injected with 14C-labelled lidocaine, showed a selective accumulation of the agent in nerves and relatively little accumulation in muscle. They noted a biphasic washout of the drug, which they attributed to reactive hyperemia. In an elegant series of experiments, Raj, Garcia, Burleson, and Jenkins[96] demonstrated, by means of a lidocaine-Renografin-60 mixture, that the contrast concentrated principally around the elbow. No contrast was seen distal to the proximal phalanges. Anesthesia developed from the fingertips upward, reaching the elbow last. Contrast material confined to the hand, injected by way of the radial artery, did not produce anesthesia. When the block was established between two tourniquets, as in the original Bier method, nerve conduction above the block (median nerve in the axilla to thenar muscles) was decreased, whereas nerve conduction below the block (ulnar nerve at the wrist to hypothenar muscles) was unaltered. Anesthesia tended to develop earlier in the anteromedial aspect of the forearm and later in the posterolateral aspect.

Raj and colleagues[96] believe that these results show that the mode of action is on the larger nerve trunks. At the el-

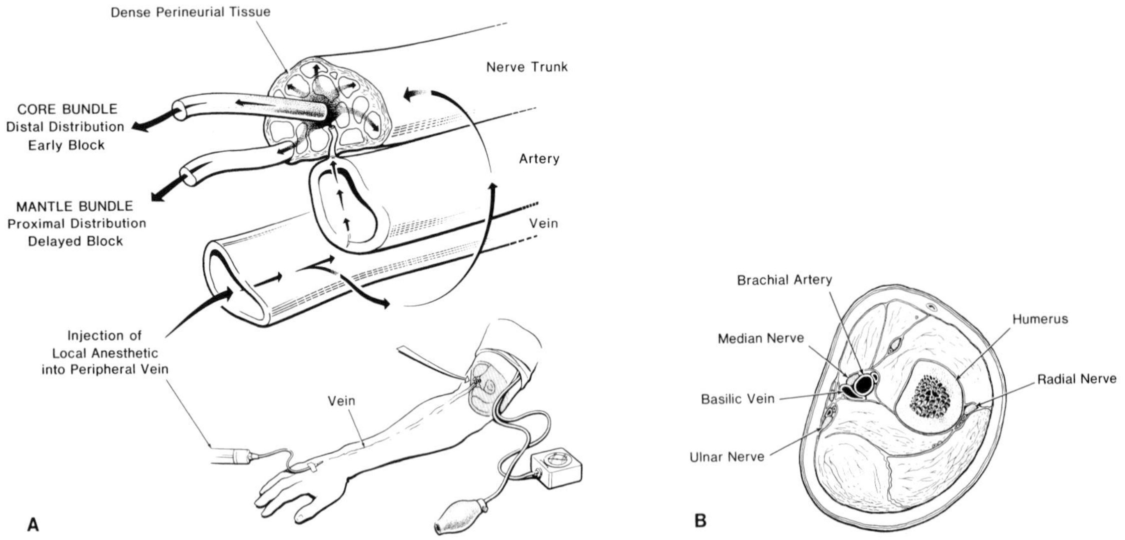

FIG. 12-10. Proposed mechanism of intravenous regional anesthesia. **A:** Local anesthetic injected into a dorsal hand vein travels to the large venous channels at the elbow. Here, it is transferred by arteries through the thick perineurium into the core of the major nerve trunks. From here, it diffuses outward so that the core bundles are blocked, initially resulting in "early distal block," and the mantle bundles (supplying proximal areas) are blocked last, resulting in "delayed proximal block." **B:** Note that, in a cross-section of the arm at the elbow, the median and ulnar nerves on the anteromedial aspect have rich vascular channels nearby. The radial nerve, on the posterolateral surface, has less vascularity in its vicinity. This may explain the later onset of analgesia in radial nerve distribution.

bow, the median and ulnar nerves are fairly close together and surrounded by large venous channels. The radial nerve is posterolateral and has fewer large vessels near it. Histologically, the peripheral nerve shows a thick perineurium, but with many vascular channels in the core of the nerve, in close proximity to the nerve fibrils. It would seem that these vascular channels carry the drug to the core of the nerve, from which it would diffuse toward the periphery. The greater number of venous channels close to the median and ulnar nerves, compared with the radial nerve, would explain the earlier onset of analgesia on the anteromedial aspect of the forearm (Fig. 12-10).

On the other hand, the speed of onset and, particularly, the rapidity of spread of analgesia are not like those seen with the block of a major nerve trunk.[17] Also, cases have been reported in which analgesia was complete everywhere except in a digit in which the local circulation was impaired: This does not support nerve trunk block.[8]

Furthermore, in a series of studies with technetium-labelled saline, Lillie and co-workers[78] showed that when the injection was made at the antecubital fossa, all the arm veins apparently filled, but hand-filling could be prevented with a forearm cuff. When prilocaine was injected, no analgesia of the hand was produced except in a small area corresponding to the distribution of the radial nerve. They argue that these results support the theory of block of small nerve endings, since no block of the major (medial and ulnar) trunks was seen during the 20-minute duration of the study.

Perhaps Bier should have the last word: ". . . [this] new method uses the vascular bed to bring the anesthetic agent to the nerve endings as well as the nerve trunks."[14]

INTRAVENOUS REGIONAL SYMPATHETIC BLOCK

Intravenous regional sympathetic block is similar to the intravenous regional anesthesia technique. The method was devised by Hannington-Kiff,[52,53] whose papers should be consulted for further details.

Premedication is usually unnecessary, but all the usual precautions should be taken. The blood pressure should be monitored, an intravenous infusion should be running, and the patient should be on a table capable of being tilted. If there is marked sympathetic dystrophy, there is often severe pain on injection, so much so that general anesthesia is preferred on the first occasion. However, general anesthesia is not usually required on subsequent occasions, provided the block is repeated before its effect has fully worn off. Nor is general anesthesia commonly necessary in cases where the block is being performed for Raynaud's disease.

The agent usually used is guanethidine, which is strongly bound to sympathetic nerve endings. An alternative method, which reduces the pain of injection, is to mix the guanethidine with 0.5% prilocaine. The cannula is placed in a hand vein, and the tourniquet is placed on the upper arm. Elevation is used for exsanguination, and the tourniquet is inflated to 50 to 100 mm Hg above the systolic pressure. The solution consists of 20 mg of guanethidine in 20 to 25 ml of physiologic saline. (For the leg, 40 mg of the drug is given in 40 ml of saline.) The tourniquet is kept inflated for 10 minutes and then released and reinflated several times while the blood pressure is monitored in the other arm. (A slight fall in blood pressure may occur.) Patients should be warned of the possibility of postural hypotension, which can occur up to 48 hours postblock. When guanethidine is not available, reserpine has been used effectively.

The effectiveness of the sympathetic block may be checked with a temperature probe. The advantages of this method are that it may be used after "postsympathectomy escape," that it may be used in patients who are taking anticoagulants, and that the potential complications of stellate ganglion block are avoided. Also avoided are the adhesions that can result from lumbar sympathetic block with phenol, which may render subsequent surgery difficult. The duration of effect is often as long as 4 to 6 weeks, and the block can be repeated (see also Chapter 13).

REFERENCES

1. Abdulla, W.Y. and Fadhil, N.M.: A new approach to intravenous regional anesthesia. Anesth. Analg. (Cleve.), *75:*597, 1992.
2. Adams, J.P., Dealy, E.J., and Kenmore, P.I.: Intravenous regional anesthesia in hand surgery. J. Bone Joint Surg., *46A:*881, 1964.
3. Anesthesia Conference (Clinical). N.Y. State J. Med., *66:*1344, 1966.
4. Armstrong, P., Brockway, M., and Wildsmith, J.A.W.: Alkalinisation of prilocaine for intravenous regional anaesthesia. Anaesthesia, *45:*11, 1990.
5. Armstrong, P., Watters, J., and Whitfield, A.: Alkalinisation of prilocaine for intravenous regional anaesthesia: Suitability for clinical use. Anaesthesia, *45:*935, 1990.
6. Armstrong, P.J., Morton, C.P., and Nimmo, A.F.: Pethidine has a local anaesthetic action on peripheral nerves *in vivo.* Anaesthesia, *48:*382, 1993.
7. Armstrong, P.J., Power, I., and Wildsmith, J.A.W.: Addition of fentanyl to prilocaine for intravenous regional anaesthesia. Anaesthesia, *46:*278, 1991.
8. Atkinson, D.I.: The mode of action of intravenous regional anaesthetics. Acta Anaesthesiol, Scand., *36* (Suppl.):131, 1969.
9. Bader, A.M., Concepcion, M., Hurley, R.J., and Arthur, G.R.: Comparison of lidocaine and prilocaine for intravenous regional anesthesia. Anesthesiology, *69:*409, 1988.
10. Barnes, C.L., Blasier, R.D., and Dodge, B.M.: Intravenous regional anesthesia: A safe and cost-effective outpatient anesthetic for upper extremity fracture treatment in children. J. Pediatr. Orthop., *11:*717, 1991.
11. Bartholomew, K., and Sloan, J.P.: Prilocaine for Bier's block: How safe is safe? Arch. Emerg. Med., *7:*189, 1990.
12. Bassinot, J.F., and Martinet, J.: Anésthésie locale intraveineuse pour chirurgie du pied et de la cheville. Ann. Fr. Anesth. Réanim. *6:*219, 1987.
13. Bell, H.M., Slater, E.M., and Harris, W.H.: Regional anesthesia with intravenous lidocaine. J.A.M.A., *186:*544, 1963.
14. Bier, A.: Ueber ein neuen Weg Lokalanasthesie an den gliedmassen zu Erzeugen. Verh. Dtsch. Ges. Chir., *37*(2):204, 1908.
15. Biscoping, J., Michaelis, G., and Hempelmann, G.: Das Verhalten der Plasmakonzentrationen von Prilocain nach intravenöser Regionalanaesthesie (IVRA) und ihre Beziehung zur Met-Hämoglobinämie. Reg. Anaesth. *11:*35, 1988.
16. Bromage, P.R., and Robson, J.G.: Concentrations of lignocaine in the blood after intravenous, intramuscular, epidural and endotracheal administration. Anaesthesia, *16:*461, 1961.

17. Brown, B.R.: Discussion on: The site of action of intravenous regional anesthesia. Anesth. Analg. (Cleve), *51:*776, 1972.
18. Brown, E.M., and Weissman, F.: A case report: Prolonged intravenous regional anesthesia. Anesth. Analg. (Cleve.), *45:*319, 1966.
19. Brown, E.M., McGriff, J.T., and Malinowski, R.W.: Intravenous regional anaesthesia (Bier block): Review of 20 years' experience. Can. J. Anaesth., *36:*307, 1989.
20. Carrell, E.D., and Eyring, E.J.: Intravenous regional anesthesia for childhood fractures. J. Trauma, *11:*301, 1971.
21. Chan, C.S., Pun, W.K., and Chan, Y.M.: Intravenous regional analgesia with a forearm tourniquet. Can. J. Anaesth., *34:*21, 1987.
22. Cobb, A.G., and Houghton, G.R.: Local anaesthetic infiltration versus Bier's block for Colles' fracture. Br. Med. J., *291:*1683, 1985.
23. Colbern, E.C.: The Bier block for intravenous regional anesthesia. Anesth. Analg. (Cleve.), *49:*935, 1970.
24. Committee on Safety of Medicines: Bupivacaine (Marcain plain) in intravenous regional anaesthesia (Bier's Block). Current Problems, *12:*, 1983.
25. Cotev, S., and Robin, C.: Experimental studies on intravenous regional analgesia using radioactive lidocaine. Acta Anaesthesiol. Scand., *36* (Suppl.):127, 1969.
26. Davies, J.A.H.: Intravenous regional analgesia with prilocaine for foot surgery: The effect of slow injections and high tourniquet inflation pressures. Anaesthesia, *44:*902, 1989.
27. Davies, J.A.H., and Walford, A.J.: Intravenous regional anaesthesia for foot surgery. Acta Anaesthesiol. Scand. *30:*145, 1986.
28. Davies, J.A.H., *et al.*: Intravenous regional analgesia. Anaesthesia, *39:*416, 1984.
29. Davies, J.A.H., Gill, S.S., and Weber, J.C.P.: Intravenous regional analgesia using bupivacaine. Anaesthesia, *36:*331, 1981.
30. Dawkins, O.S., *et al.*: Intravenous regional anaesthesia. Can. Anaesth. Soc. J., *11:*234, 1964.
31. De Jong, R.H., and Heavner, J.E.: Diazepam prevents local anesthetic seizures. Anesthesiology, *34:*523, 1971.
32. de Mello, W.F.: An alternative approach to intravenous regional anesthesia (IVRA). Anesth. Analg. (Cleve.), *76:*1173, 1993.
33. Departments of Health and Social Security: Automatic Tourniquets. HN (Hazard), *82:*7, 1982.
34. Dunbar, R.W., and Mazze, R.I.: Intravenous regional anesthesia. Anesth. Analg. (Cleve.), *46:*806, 1967.
35. Eastwood, D., Griffiths, S., Jack, J., Porter, K., and Watt, J.: Bier's block—an improved technique. Injury, *17:*187, 1986.
36. Englesson, S., Eriksson, E., Wahlqvist, S., and Ortengren, B.: Differences in tolerance to intravenous Xylocaine and Citanest (L67), a new local anaesthetic: A double-blind study in man. Proc. First Eur. Congr. Anaesth, *2:*206, 1, 1962.
37. Eriksson, E.: The effects of intravenous local anesthetic agents on the central nervous system. Acta. Anaesthesiol. Scand., *36* (Suppl.):79, 1969.
38. Evans, C.J., Dewar, J.A., Boyes, R.N., and Scott, D.B.: Residual nerve block following intravenous regional anaesthesia. Br. J. Anaesth., *46:*668, 1974.
39. Fagg, P.S.: Intravenous regional anaesthesia for lower limb orthopaedic surgery. Ann. R. Coll. Surg. Eng., *69:*274, 1987.
40. Farrar, M.D., Scheybani, M., and Nolte, H.: Upper extremity block: Clinical effectiveness and complications. Anaesthesia, *37:*368, 1982.
41. Finegan, B.A., and Bukht, M.D.: Venous pressures in the isolated upper limb during saline injection. Can. Anaesth. Soc. J., *31:*364, 1984.
42. Fitzgerald, B.: Intravenous regional anaesthesia in children. Br. J. Anaesth., *48:*485, 1976.
43. Fleming, S.A.: Safety and usefulness of intravenous regional anaesthesia. Acta Anaesth. Scand., *36*(Suppl.):21, 1969.
44. Fleming, S.A., Veiga-Pires, J.A., McCutcheon, R.M., and Emanuel, C.I.: A demonstration of the site of action of intravenous lignocaine. Can. Anaesth. Soc. J., *13:*21, 1966.
45. Foldes, F.F., Molloy, R., McNall, P.G., and Koukal, L.R.: Comparison of toxicity of intravenously given local anesthetic agents in man. J.A.M.A., *172:*1493, 1960.
46. Gingrich, T.F.: Intravenous regional anesthesia of the upper extremity in children. J.A.M.A., *200:*405, 1967.
47. Gooding, J.M., Tavakoli, M.M., Fitzpatrick, W.O., and Bagley, J.N.: Bupivacaine: Preferred agent for intravenous regional anaesthesia. South. Med. J., *74:*1282, 1981.
48. Granados, M., and Bernière, J.: L'anésthésie loco-régionale intraveineuse dans la chirurgie du membre supérieur chez l'enfant. Cah. Anesthesiol., *33:*211, 1985.
49. Grice, S.C., Morell, R.C., Balestrieri, F.J., Stump, D.A., and Howard, G.: Intravenous regional anesthesia: Evaluation and prevention of leakage under the tourniquet. Anesthesiology, *65:*316, 1986.
50. Gürtner, T.H., Meyer, C.H., and Gürtner, C.B.: Nebenwirkungen nach intravenöser Regionalanaesthesie (IVRA) auf ZNS und Herzrhythmus. Reg. Anaest., *9:*116, 1986.
51. Haasio, J., Hiippala, S., and Rosenberg, P.H.: Intravenous regional anaesthesia of the arm: Effect of the technique of exsanguination on the quality of anaesthesia and prilocaine plasma concentrations. Anaesthesia, *44:*19, 1989.
52. Hannington-Kiff, J.G.: Intravenous regional sympathetic block with guanethidine. Lancet, *1:*1019, 1974.
53. Hannington-Kiff, J.G.: Pain Relief. pp. 70. London, Heinemann Educational Books, 1974.
54. Hanton, R.J., and Punchihewa, V.G.: Intravenous regional analgesia using bupivacaine. Anaesthesia, *36:*350, 1981.
55. Hargrove, R.L., Hoyle, J.R., Parker, J.B., *et al.*: Blood lignocaine levels following intravenous regional analgesia. Anaesthesia, *21:*37, 1966.
56. Harris, W.H., Cole, D.W., Mital, M., and Laver, M.B.: Methemoglobin formation and oxygen transport following intravenous regional anesthesia using prilocaine. Anesthesiology, *29:*65, 1968.
57. Harris, W.H.: Choice of anesthetic agents for intravenous regional anesthesia. Acta Anaesthesiol. Scand., *36* (Suppl.):47, 1969.
58. Heath, M.L.: Bupivicaine [sic] toxicity and Bier blocks. Anesthesiology, *59:*481, 1983.
59. Heath, M.L.: Deaths after intravenous regional anaesthesia. Br. Med. J., *285:*931, 1982.
60. Henderson, A.M.: Adverse reaction of bupivacaine: Complication of intravenous regional analgesia. Br. Med. J., *281:*1043, 1980.
61. Hoffman, S., Simon, B.E., and Hartley, J.: A new tourniquet for intravenous regional anesthesia. Plast. Reconstr. Surg., *40:*243, 1967.
62. Hollingworth, A., Wallace, W.A., and Dabir, R.: Comparison of bupivacaine and prilocaine user in Bier's Block: A double-blind trial. Injury, *13:*331, 1982.
63. Holmes, C.McK.: The history and development of intravenous regional anaesthesia. Acta Anaesthesiol Scand., *36* (Suppl.):11, 1969.
64. Holmes, C.McK.: Anaesthetising the arm. N. Z. Med. J., *63:*24, 1964.
65. Holmes, C.McK.: Intravenous regional analgesia. Lancet, *1:*245, 1963.
66. Hooper, R.L.: Intravenous regional anaesthesia: A report of a new local anaesthetic agent. Can. Anaesth. Soc. J., *11:*247, 1964.
67. Hoyle, J.R.: Tourniquet for intravenous regional analgesia. Anaesthesia, *19:*294, 1964.
68. Ishibashi, T., Onchi, Y., and Okuda, T.: New method of local anesthesia for operations on the upper extremity. [in Japanese] Jpn. J. Anesthesiol. *15:*239, 1966.
69. Jeyaseelam, S., Stevenson, T.M., and Pfitzner, J.: Tourniquet failure and arterial calcification. Anaesthesia, *36:*48, 1981.
70. Kalso, E., Tuominen, M., Rosenberg, P.H., and Alila, A.: Bupivacaine blood levels after intravenous regional anesthesia of the arm. Reg. Anaesth., *5:*81, 1982.
71. Kennedy, B.R., Duthie, A.M., Parbrook, G.D., and Carr, T.L.: Intravenous regional analgesia: An appraisal. Br. Med. J., *1:*954, 1965.
72. Kerr, J.H.: Intravenous regional analgesia. Anaesthesia, *22:*562, 1967.
73. Kjeldal, I., and Nygaard, H.P.: Outpatient surgery for Dupuytren's disease under intravenous regional anaesthesia. J. Hand Surg. *13B:*257, 1988.
74. Koscielniak-Nielsen, Z.J., and Horn, A.: Intra-arterial regional analgesia for hand surgery. Anaesthesia, *48:*769, 1993.
75. Koscielniak-Nielsen, Z.J., and Stens-Pedersen, H.L.: Intra-arterial regional analgesia of the hand. Br. J. Anaesth., *66:*719, 1991.
76. Larsen, U.T., and Hommelgaard, P.: Pneumatic tourniquet paralysis following intravenous regional analgesia. Anaesthesia, *42:*526, 1987.
77. Lawes, E.G., Johnson, T., Pritchard, P., and Robbins, P.: Venous pressures during simulated Bier's block. Anaesthesia, *39:*147, 1984.
78. Lillie, P.E., Glynn, C.J., and Fenwick, D.G.: Site of action of intravenous regional analgesia. Anesthesiology, *61:*507, 1984.
79. Luce, E.A., and Mangubat, E.: Loss of hand and forearm following Bier block: A case report. J. Hand Surg., *8:*280, 1983.
80. Lund, P.C., and Cwik, J.C.: Propitocaine (Citanest) and methemoglobinemia. Anesthesiology, *26:*569, 1965.
81. Magora, F., Stern, L., Zylber-Katz, E., *et al.*: Prolonged effect of bupivacaine hydrochloride after cuff release in IV regional anaesthesia. Br. J. Anaesth., *53:*1131, 1980.

82. Mazze, R.L., and Dunbar, R.W.: Plasma lidocaine concentrations after caudal, lumbar epidural, axillary, and intravenous regional anesthesia. Anesthesiology, *27:*574, 1966.
83. Mazze, R.L., and Dunbar, R.W.: Intravenous regional anaesthesia: Report of 497 cases with a toxicity study. Acta Anaesthesiol. Scand., *36* (Suppl.):27, 1969.
84. McKeown, D.W., Duggan, J., Wildsmith, J.A., *et al.*: Which agent for intravenous regional anesthesia? Lancet, *2:*1503, 1983.
85. McKeown, D.W., Meiklejohn, B., and Scott, D.B.: Bupivacaine and prilocaine in intravenous regional anaesthesia. Anaesthesia, *39:*150, 1984.
86. Merrifield, A.J., and Carter, S.J.: Intravenous regional analgesia: Lignocaine blood levels. Anaesthesia, *20:*287, 1965.
87. Middleton, R.W.D., and Varian, J.P.: Tourniquet paralysis. Aust. N. Z. J. Surg., *44:*124, 1974.
88. Miles, D.W., James, J.L., Clark, D.E., and Whitwam, J.G.: Site of action of "intravenous regional anaesthesia." J. Neurol. Neurosurg. Psychiatry, *27:*574, 1964.
89. Moldaver, J.: Tourniquet paralysis syndrome. Arch. Surg., *68:*136, 1954.
90. Moore, D.C., Mather, L.E., and Bridenbaugh, L.D.: Bupivacaine (Marcaine): An evaluation of its tissue and systemic toxicity in humans. Acta Anaesthesiol. Scand., *21:*109, 1977.
91. Nusbaum, L.M., and Hamelberg, W.: Intravenous regional anesthesia for surgery on the foot and ankle. Anesthesiology, *64:*91, 1986.
92. Ogden, P.N.: Failure of intravenous regional analgesia using a double-cuff tourniquet. Anaesthesia, *39:*456, 1984.
93. Pitkanen, M.T., Suzuki, N., and Rosenberg, P.H.: Intravenous regional anaesthesia with 0.5% prilocaine or 0.5% chloroprocaine: A double-blind comparison in volunteers. Anaesthesia, *47:*618, 1992.
94. Pitkanen, M.T., Rosenberg, P.H., Pere, P.J., Tuominen, M.K., and Seppala, T.A.: Fentanyl-prilocaine mixture for intravenous regional anaesthesia in patient's undergoing surgery. Anaesthesia, *47:*395, 1992.
95. Plourde, G., *et al.*: Decreasing the toxic potential of intravenous regional anaesthesia. Can. J. Anaesth., *36:*498, 1987.
96. Raj, P.P., Garcia, C.E., Burleson, J.W., and Jenkins, M.T.: The site of action of intravenous regional anesthesia. Anesth. Analg. (Cleve.), *51:*776, 1972.
97. Rawal, N., Hallen, J., Amilon, A., and Hellstrand, P.: Improvement in IV regional anaesthesia by re-exsanguination before surgery. Br. J. Anaesth., *70:*280, 1993.
98. Reynolds, F.: Editorial. Anaesthesia, *39:*105, 1984.
99. Rosenberg, P.H., Kalso, E.A., Tuominen, M.K., and Linden, H.B.: Acute bupivacaine toxicity as a result of venous leakage under the tourniquet cuff during a Bier block. Anesthesiology, *58:*95, 1983.
100. Rousso, M., *et al.*: Low IV regional analgesia with bupivacaine for hand surgery. Br. J. Anaesth., *53:*841, 1981.
101. Roven, A.N.: The Bier block for hand surgery. Plast. Reconstr. Surg., *89:*769, 1992.
102. Ryding, F.N.: Digital regional analgesia. Anaesthesia, *36:*969, 1981.
103. Schürg, R., Biscoping, J., Bachmann, M.B., and Hempelmann, G.: Die intravenöse Regionalanaesthesie (IVRA) des Fuβes mit Prilocaine. Reg. Anaesth., *13:*118, 1990.
104. Shamay, C., and Robin, G.C.: Experimental studies on intravenous regional anaesthesia using radioactive lignocaine. Br. J. Anaesth., *38:*936, 1966.
105. Shanks, C.A., and McLeod, J.G.: Nerve conduction studies in regional intravenous analgesia using 1% lignocaine. Br. J. Anaesth., *42:*1060, 1970.
106. Solak, M., Akturk, G., Erciyes, N., *et al.*: The addition of sodium bicarbonate to prilocaine solution during IV regional anaesthesia. Acta Anaesthesiol. Scand., *35:*572, 1991.
107. Sorbie, C., and Chacha, P.: Regional anaesthesia by the intravenous route. Br. Med. J., *1:*957, 1965.
108. Sukhani, R., Garcia, C.J., Munhal, R.J., Winnie, A.P., and Rudvold, K.A.: Lidocaine disposition following intravenous regional anesthesia with different tourniquet deflation techniques. Anesth. Analg. (Cleve.), *68:*633, 1989.
109. Thorn-Alquist, A-M.: Intravenous regional anaesthesia. Acta Anaesthesiol. Scand., *15:*23, 1971.
110. Thorn-Alquist, A-M.: Blood concentration of local anaesthetics after intravenous regional anaesthesia. Acta Anaesthesiol. Scand., *13:*229, 1969.
111. Trias, A.: The use of intravenous regional anaesthesia in orthopaedic surgery. Acta Anaesthesiol. Scand., *36* (Suppl.):35, 1965.
112. Tryba, M., Hausmann, E., Zenz, M., and Wellhorner, H.H.: Toxizität von Prilocain und Bupivacain in der intravenösen Regionalanästhesie. Anasth. Intensivther. Notfallmed., *17:*207, 1982.
113. Tryba, M., Zenz, M., and Hausmann, E.: Prolonged analgesia after cuff release following IV regional analgesia with prilocaine. Br. J. Anaesth., *55:*631, 1983.
114. Tucker, G.T., and Boas, R.A.: Pharmacokinetic aspects of intravenous regional anesthesia. Anesthesiology, *34:*538, 1971.
115. Turner, P.L., *et al.*: Intravenous regional anaesthesia for the treatment of upper limb injuries in childhood. Aust. N. Z. J. Surg., *56:*153, 1986.
116. Valli, H., and Rosenberg, P.H.: Intravenous regional anaesthesia below the knee. Anaesthesia, *41:*1196, 1986.
117. Van Niekerk, J.P., and Tonkin, P.A.: Intravenous regional analgesia. S. Afr. Med. J., *40:*165, 1966.
118. Ware, R.J., and Caudwell, J.: Clinical and pharmacological studies of intravenous regional analgesia using bupivacaine. Br. J. Anaesth., *48:*1124, 1976.
119. Ware, R.J.: Intravenous regional analgesia using bupivacaine. Anaesthesia, *30:*817, 1975.
120. Ware, R.J.: Intravenous regional analgesia using bupivacaine: A double-blind comparison with ligocaine. Anaesthesia, *34:*231, 1979.
121. Ware, R.J.: Intravenous regional analgesia: The debate continues. Anaesthesia, *37:*958, 1982.
122. Wildsmith, J.A.W.: Intravenous regional analgesia: Essential safeguards. Anaesthesia, *37:*959, 1982.
123. Wilson, J.K., and Lyon, G.D.: Bier Block tourniquet pressure. Anesth. Analg. (Cleve.), *68:*823, 1989.
124. Winnie, A.P., and Ramamurthy, S.: Pneumatic exsanguination for intravenous regional anesthesia. Anesthesiology, *33:*664, 1970.
125. Wirth, E.R., and Kirk, W.O.: Cessation of blood flow in intravenous regional anesthesia. Anesth. Analg. (Cleve.), *67:*1015, 1988.

Neural Blockade in Clinical Anesthesia and Management of Pain, Third Edition,
edited by M.J. Cousins and P.O. Bridenbaugh.
Lippincott–Raven Publishers, Philadelphia © 1998.

CHAPTER 13

Sympathetic Neural Blockade of Upper and Lower Extremity

Harald Breivik, Michael J. Cousins, and J. Bertil Löfström

HISTORY AND GENERAL CONSIDERATIONS

The effects of sympathetic nerves in maintaining normal constrictor tone in the blood vessels of the skin have been known since the classic work of Claude Bernard in 1852. The well-known observation of increased skin temperature of the foot after surgical lumbar sympathectomy was first made by Hunter and Royle.[25] Surgical sympathectomy has been performed at some clinics, as reported by De Bakey in 1950, to promote healing of ischemic cutaneous ulcers and to relieve pain in the foot at rest (*rest pain*)[119]; however, at many vascular clinics today more emphasis is placed on vascular grafting procedures, and the refined surgical techniques undoubtedly have greatly improved the prognosis of the patient with occlusive vascular disease. Despite this movement away from sympathetic ablation, there is considerable potential benefit from sympathetic neural blockade as an adjunct to vascular surgery or as primary treatment for patients with rest pain who are not fit for, or not amenable to, vascular reconstruction. The large series of 1,666 patients with neurolytic lumbar sympathetic blocks reported in 1970 by Reid and colleagues bears testimony to this, and it is surprising that many clinics have largely neglected this important option in the treatment of vascular disease.[98]

Mandl first described the technique of lumbar sympathetic neural blockade in 1926, and his technique was clearly very similar to that for celiac plexus blockade described by Kappis in 1919.[59,83] A similar neglect of celiac plexus block for upper abdominal cancer has been apparent (see Chapter 31). The classic "anterior" approach to stellate ganglion blockade was initiated by Leriche[70] in 1934 and forms the basis of the technique described in this chapter.[7]

It is clear, then, that these techniques have all been available for more than 50 years. Surprisingly, precise documentation of their place in clinical medicine is only now becoming available, and much information remains to be obtained.

Sympathetic blockade is produced as an accompaniment to motor and sensory blockade during regional block for operative surgery (e.g., spinal and epidural anesthesia, brachial plexus block). It is maintained that "differential" sympathetic blockade without sensory and motor block can be produced with low concentrations of local anesthetic by means of epidural or spinal subarachnoid block (see below and Chapter 27). This has been used in the analysis of chronic pain. We believe that selective sympathetic ganglion block provides more reliable information (see Chapter 27). In the management of acute pain, epidural block at the appropriate segmental level relieves labor pain and the pain of renal colic by blocking visceral (sympathetic afferent) nociceptive and sympathetic efferent nerve fibers (see below and Fig. 13-1). However, the most specific application of sympathetic blockade appears to be in the use of selective blockade of the sympathetic ganglia (see following).

Because the sympathetic ganglia are, except in the thoracic region, relatively safely separated from somatic nerves, it is possible to achieve sympathetic blockade without loss of sensory or motor function. This offers the possibility of treating a variety of conditions in which reduced sympathetic activity might be beneficial. With careful technique, it is even possible to achieve permanent neurolytic blockade with essentially no loss of sensory and motor function. Thus, sympathetic blockade, at the three major levels indicated in Figure 13-2, is regarded as potentially one of the most rewarding series of techniques for diagnosis and management of acute and chronic pain syndromes and other conditions (see list on pp. 422). Our clinical experience has been that, of all neural blockade techniques, lumbar sympathetic

H. Breivik: Department of Anaesthesiology, The National Hospital (Rikshospitalet), N-0027 Oslo, Norway.

M. J. Cousins: Department of Anaesthesia and Pain Management, Royal North Shore Hospital, University of Sydney, St. Leonards, New South Wales 2065 Australia.

J. B. Löfström; Department of Anesthesiology, Linkoping University, S-581 85 Linkoping, Sweden.

block for rest pain and celiac plexus block for upper abdominal cancer, offer the most benefit at the lowest risk.

Celiac plexus blockade, superior hypogastric plexus block and ganglion impar block are described in Chapters 14 and 31, and lumbar sympathetic block and the remaining sympathetic ganglion blocks (stellate and thoracic) are described in this chapter, as is intravenous regional sympathetic block. Despite a duration of only up to 2 weeks, repeated intravenous regional sympathetic blocks are an attractive alternative to the higher-risk technique of thoracic sympathetic block or thoracic surgical or thoracoscopic sympathectomy.

It may be possible to use either unilateral or bilateral lumbar sympathetic block for some kinds of pelvic pain (particularly urogenital). This poses a much smaller risk than neurolytic subarachnoid block, with its possibility of loss of bladder function (see Chapter 31), and is less invasive than subarachnoid opioid plus bupivacaine catheter infusion. In order to take full advantage of sympathetic neural blockade, it is essential to bear in mind the general features of the anatomy and physiology of the peripheral sympathetic nervous system, as described in the next section, and the regional anatomy, as described with each of the techniques of sympathetic blockade. It is also important to use objective methods to evaluate the completeness of sympathetic blockade and its clinical effects, as shown on pages 423–426.

SYMPATHETIC NERVOUS SYSTEM

Anatomy and Physiology

The peripheral sympathetic nervous system begins as efferent preganglionic fibers in the intermediolateral column of the spinal cord, passing in the ventral roots from T1 to L2 (and perhaps some cervical roots) out of the spinal canal to run separately as white rami communicantes to the sympathetic chain, at the side of the vertebral bodies (Fig. 13-1). In the lower cervical region, the chain lies at the anterolateral aspect of the vertebral body and in the thorax is adjacent to the neck of the ribs, still relatively close to somatic roots (see Fig. 13-21). In the lumbar region, however, the chain angles forward to lie anterolateral to the body of the vertebra and is now separated from somatic roots by psoas muscle and psoas fascia (see Fig. 13-22). The preganglionic fibers pass a variable distance in the sympathetic chain to reach ganglia in the chain, or they may pass further to peripherally located ganglia (i.e., in the gut; Fig. 13-1). The inconstant level of relay in the chain itself may be responsible for a number of disappointing results from an apparently technically successful block. Sympathetic ganglia are segmentally located in the chest (T1–T11; T12). There are also three cervical ganglia, four to five lumbar ganglia, four sacral ganglia, and one coccygeal ganglion (the 'ganglion impar'). The postganglionic fibers are widely distributed, partly to join peripheral nerves (the gray communicantes) and partly to join vessels in different organs. The sympathetic chain not only receives efferent preganglionic but also afferent visceral fibers, which conduct pain from head, neck, and upper extremity (cervicothoracic ganglia); abdominal viscera (celiac plexus) (see Chapter 14); and urogenital system and lower extremity (lumbar ganglia; Fig. 13-2).

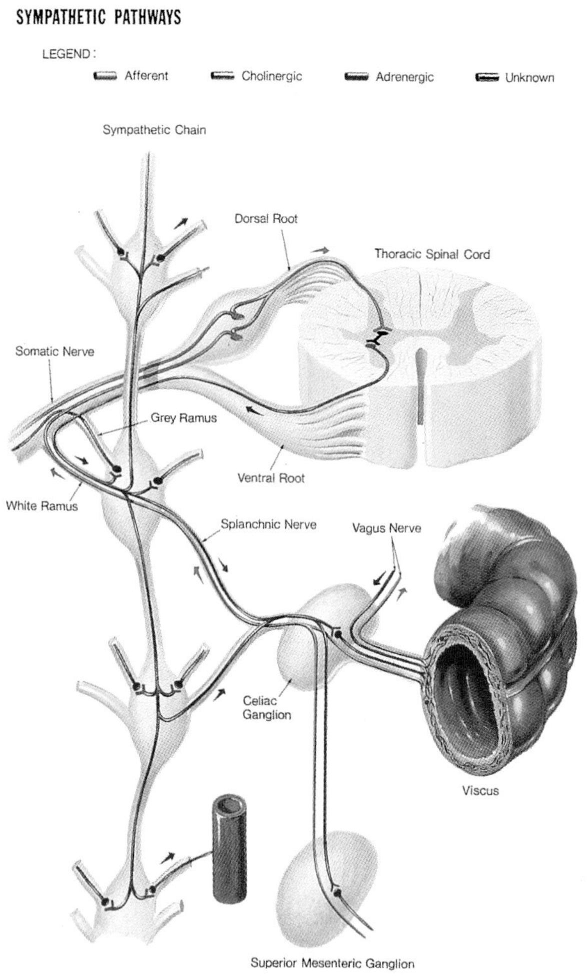

FIG. 13-1. Peripheral sympathetic nervous system. Cell bodies are located in the intermediolateral cell column of T1–L2 spinal segments. Efferent fibers (cholinergic) pass by way of the ventral root to a white ramus communicans and then to the paravertebral sympathetic ganglia or to more remotely located ganglia, such as the celiac ganglion. From each ganglion, they give rise to adrenergic fibers to supply viscera (celiac ganglion) or to join somatic nerves (from lumbar sympathetic ganglion) to supply efferent fibers to the limbs (sudomotor and vasomotor effects). In the case of lumbar sympathetic ganglia, the adrenergic fibers swing backward by a gray ramus communicans to join the somatic nerve. Afferent fibers travel by way of ganglia, such as celiac and lumbar sympathetic, without synapsing, and reach somatic nerves and then their cell bodies in the dorsal root ganglia. They then pass to the dorsal root and synapse with interneurons in the intermediolateral area of the spinal cord. These afferent fibers convey pain impulses from the viscera and are similar to nociceptive afferents except that they pass without synapsing through sympathetic ganglia.

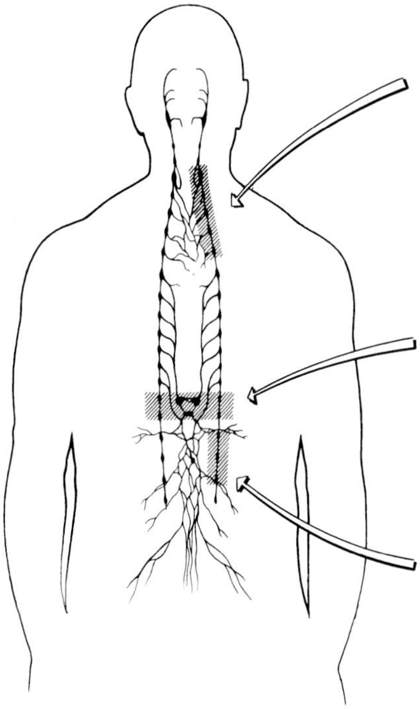

FIG. 13-2. An outline of the sympathetic nervous system. The three main levels of sympathetic blockade are shown along with major clinical uses. (Redrawn after Bonica, J.J.: The Management of Pain. Philadelphia, Lea & Febiger, 1953.)

Sympathetic Efferents to Blood Vessels

The great vessels (carotids, aorta, vena cava) receive direct postganglionic filaments from adjacent sympathetic ganglia (Fig. 13-3) and from plexuses (see Fig. 13-2). The main outflow of preganglionic fibers by means of the ventral roots may subsequently follow alternative courses: (i) synapse in the same level or adjacent ganglia and pass in somatic nerves to vessels; (ii) synapse in ganglia and pass directly to vessels via filaments; (iii) pass directly through sympathetic ganglia and synapse in prevertebral plexuses and then pass to vessels (Fig. 13-3); or (iv) pass through sympathetic ganglia and ascend or descend to synapse in ganglia above (e.g., cervical) or below (e.g., lower lumbar).

Vascular nerves and filaments from these diverse sources are united around individual vessels in extensive "perivascular adventitial plexuses," which in turn ramify into plexuses between adventitia and media and between media and intima. Plexuses are augmented by branches from nearby cranial or spinal nerves. Thus, there is great overlap from several spinal cord segments. Arteries and arterioles are more richly supplied than veins and venules. Although nerve fibers accompany venules, it is not known whether they serve a vasoconstrictor role.

Sympathetic fibers are generally found in a deep fascial plane and are less accessible than segmental nerves. Interruption of sympathetic nerve fibers by neural blockade can be achieved in the following ways: at the sympathetic chain by a sympathetic blockade, at peripheral nerves by a nerve block, at a vessel by perivascular infiltration, or to some extent by intradural or extradural injection of local anesthetic (see below). Sympathetic activity can also be blocked pharmacologically by an alpha-receptor blocker (phentolamine, dibenzyline); by a "depleter" of norepinephrine activity in sympathetic nerve ending (guanethidine or reserpine); or by a beta-receptor blocker, propranolol (β_1- and β_2-) or practolol (mainly β_1–receptor). Sympathetic nerve endings have both presynaptic and postsynaptic receptors (Fig. 13-4). Until recently, available alpha-receptor blockers acted upon both presynaptic and postsynaptic receptors. Blockade of presynaptic receptors interrupted the negative feedback that modifies norepinephrine (NE) release. More selective postsynaptic blockers (e.g., prazocin) are now available which have a much more sustained degree of alpha-blockade (Fig. 13-4).

Function

Vasoconstriction by Alpha Receptors. Arterioli (in the skin and in the splanchnic area), smaller arteries, and, in particular, peripheral veins, are normally under moderate vasoconstrictor influence. Pain, anxiety, and blood loss can provoke a very marked increase in arteriolar vasoconstrictor tone, mediated by the sympathetic nervous system; this change results in increased resistance, particularly in skin vessels, and thus influences the distribution of blood flow. In addition, there is an associated increase in vascular tone, which decreases the compliance of the venous system, reducing its blood content and increasing the venous pressure.

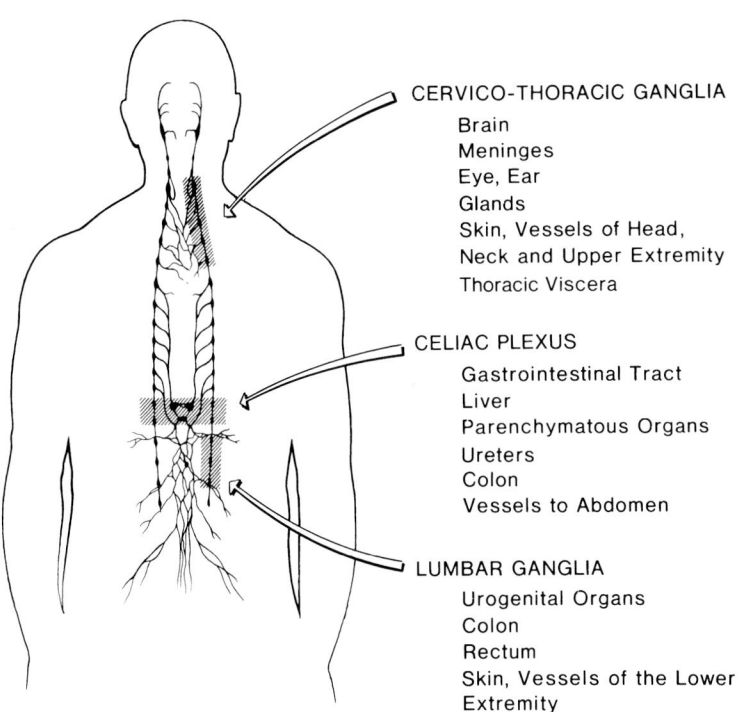

Heart Muscle Activity (Chronotropic and Inotropic Effect). β_1–stimulation causes increased heart rate and in-

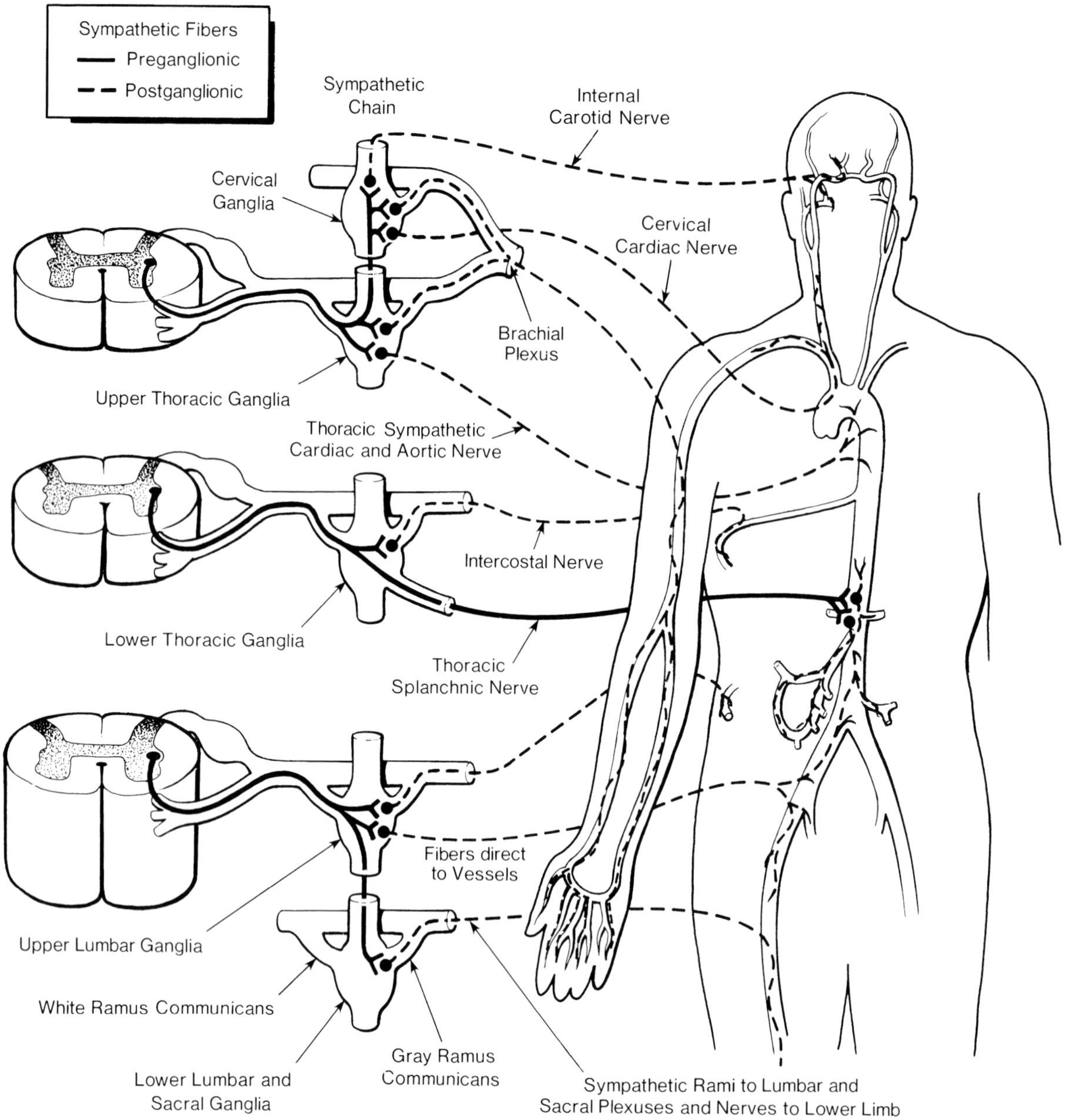

FIG. 13-3. Sympathetic nerve supply to blood vessels (see text).

creased cardiac contractility; thus high (T1–T4) thoracic sympathetic blockade may cause a marked reduction in cardiac output.

Bronchial Tone. β_2–stimulation causes bronchodilation so that it is theoretically possible for thoracic sympathetic blockade to cause bronchoconstriction, although this does not appear to be the case (see Chapter 8).

Vasodilatation. β_2–stimulation causes vasodilatation in some vascular beds (e.g., muscle); however, this is a minor effect and is overridden by local metabolic effects (see following).

Smooth Muscle Tone (e.g., in the Gut and in the Bladder). β_2–stimulation causes smooth muscle relaxation and sphincter contraction. Thus, sympathetic blockade results in smooth muscle contraction (a small, contracted gut) and sphincter relaxation. These effects provide excellent surgical access during procedures such as abdominoperineal resection. *Sudomotor* (sweat glands) and *hair follicles* have the same postganglion efferents as blood vessels; however, the neurotransmitter in sweat glands is *acetylcholine.*

Metabolic. The sympathetic nervous system has a metabolic effect that is said to explain the relaxation of smooth muscle in vessels (β_2) and in the gut, and its effect on the heart muscle. This metabolic effect is widespread and also affects carbohydrate and lipid distribution and utilization.[33]

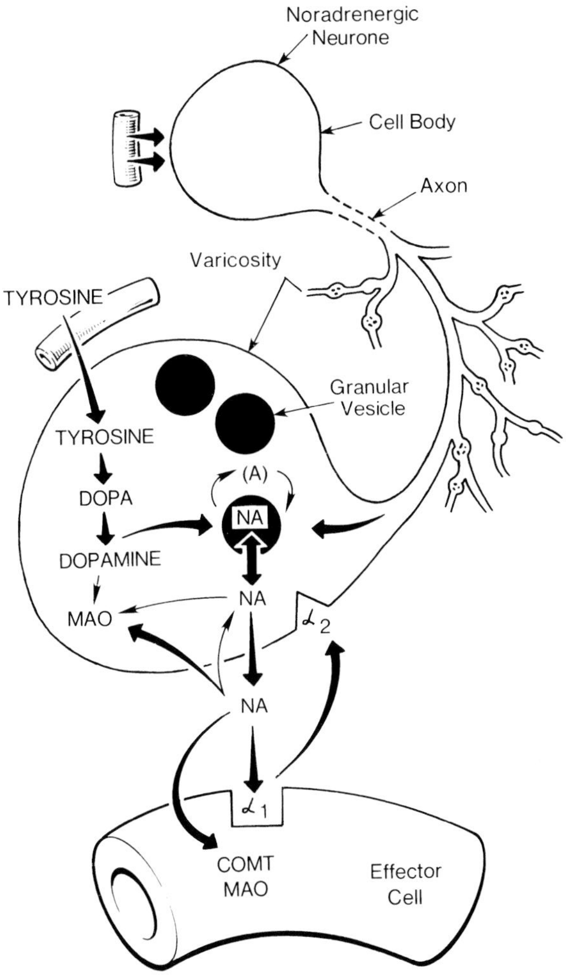

FIG. 13-4. Sympathetic nerve endings and receptors (see text). Diagram of synapse between a postganglionic sympathetic neuron and postsynaptic receptors on effector cells (e.g., smooth muscle of vessel wall). Stimulation of presynaptic (α_2) receptors by previously released norepinephrine (noradrenaline, NA) results in inhibition of further release of NA from the sympathetic neuron. Stimulation of α_1-receptors results in smooth muscle contraction. *MAO*, monoamine oxidase; *COMT*, catecholomethyltransferase.

Pain may be mediated through the sympathetic nervous system. Labor pain is transmitted by *afferent fibers* that traverse the lower thoracic sympathetic ganglia, whereas pain from upper abdominal viscera and the gut, as far as the descending colon, can be relieved adequately by celiac ganglion block. Pain from some pelvic viscera may be transmitted by the lumbar sympathetic ganglia (see Fig. 13-2). Sympathetic efferents may influence pain perception in the limbs.[39,57,95] After nerve or tissue trauma, release of neurotransmitters such as norepinephrine increases discharge from peripheral primary afferent nociceptors. Denervation hypersensitivity from augmented adrenoceptor activity may increase discharge from primary afferent nociceptors without increased sympathetic efferent nerve activity. (see Chapters 23, and 24). Also, microcirculatory changes caused by intense sympathetic activity may alter the biochemical environment and enhance nociceptor activity (Fig. 13-5). Sympathetic blockade may reverse such effects, provided it is done before abnormal nociceptive activity is permanently established rostral to the spinal cord (see following).

PHYSIOLOGIC EFFECTS ON PERIPHERAL BLOOD FLOW

A regional sympathetic block has its primary and most obvious effect on vasomotor activity. In a normal subject, this leads to dilatation of veins, promoting an accumulation of blood in the veins, and dilatation of the arterial vessels, which leads to a fall in the peripheral resistance and thus, if the perfusion pressure has not been altered, to an increased capillary blood flow.

In a normal subject, complete sympathetic block will be followed by visibly dilated veins or by increased blood flow, seen clinically in reduced capillary refill time or measured by plethysmography (Figs. 13-6 and 13-7), laser Doppler flowmetry,[4,5] or ^{133}Xe clearance, which measures capillary blood flow accurately (see below). Oscillometrically recorded, the peripheral pulse waves will be enlarged. Vasoconstrictor responses such as the "ice response" are abolished (Fig. 13-6). The blood flow increase will, to a large extent, be restricted to the skin, followed by an increase in skin temperature and a marked feeling of warmth in the extremity (Fig. 13-8).[119] Skin capillary oxygen tension and venous oxygen tension and saturation are also raised (see list on pp. 423). A widespread block will cause a peripheral pooling of blood, diminishing the venous return and producing a fall in cardiac output and blood pressure.

Muscle blood flow, being automatically regulated according to muscle metabolism, should not be affected by a sympathetic blockade at rest, at work, or after ischemia.[25] Thus reduced muscle flow (claudication) may not be helped by sympathetic block (Fig. 13-8). From what has been stated, it seems logical to use sympathetic blockade to improve the blood flow in a patient with insufficient peripheral skin blood flow because of vasospasm or arterial disease (i.e., rest pain) (Fig. 13-8).[24,25] It is not possible, however, to predict the effect of a sympathetic blockade in a patient with a diseased vascular system, as can be explained with the aid of the following illustrations. In Figure 13-9, an artery divides into two smaller branches. The total flow (Q_A) in the artery is proportionate to the perfusion pressure (P) and inversely proportionate to the peripheral resistance (PR). In each branch (B and C) the flows (Q_B and Q_C) are affected by the perfusion pressures, almost the same as in the artery (A) and inversely related to the regional resistance (RR_B and RR_C) in each branch. A blockade of the sympathetic fibers to branch B alone will have very little effect on the perfusion pressure (Fig. 13-10). As the regional resistance decreases in branch B, the flow through this vessel will increase. A unilateral

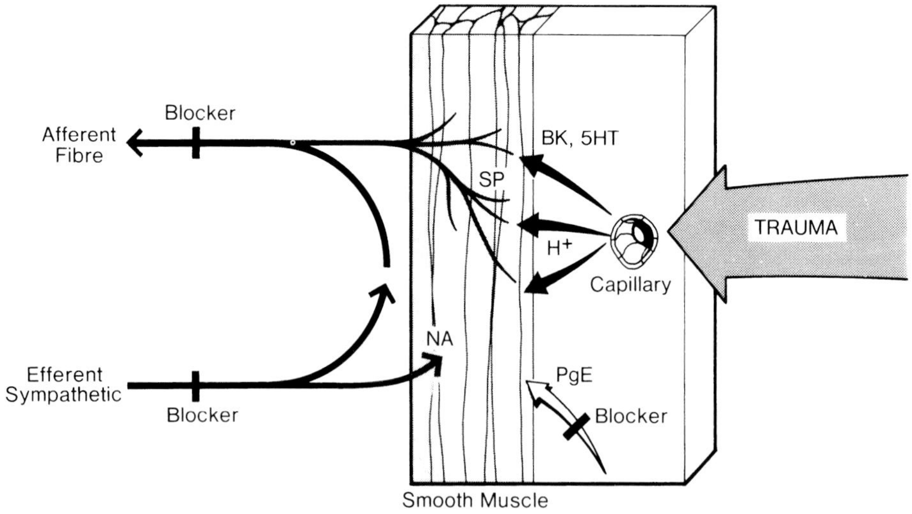

FIG. 13-5. Peripheral mechanisms of pain, sympathetic activity, and microcirculatory changes. Physical stimuli (e.g., trauma), the chemical environment (e.g., H^+ changes), algesic substance (e.g., serotonin [5HT] and bradykinin [BK], and microcirculatory changes (e.g., edema) may all modify peripheral nociceptor sensitivity. Increased nociceptor activity increases afferent fiber activity, with resultant increases in efferent sympathetic vasoconstriction, and also norepinephrine (noradrenaline [NA]) release with further increases in nociceptor sensitivity. Thus a repetitive cycle is set up. Substance P (SP) is probably the peripheral pain transmitter. Prostaglandins (PgE) also increase nociceptor sensitivity. Points of blockade of pain (shaded and marked "blocker") are as follows: 1. Afferent fibers (local anesthetics); 2. efferent sympathetic fibers (local anesthetics); and 3. prostaglandin synthesis (e.g., nonsteroidal anti-inflammatory drugs given orally). All three may relieve pain and produce an associated improvement in microcirculation by breaking the repetitive cycle. New approaches to pain relief include substance P depletion (e.g., by capsaicin). Additional points of blockade to produce vasodilation include the following: 1. Norepinephrine depletion at sympathetic nerve endings; 2. norepinephrine receptor blockade (see Fig. 13-32); 3. selective increase in levels of the prostaglandins PGE and PGE_1 (by intravascular infusion); and 4. calcium channel blockade (see Fig. 13-32).

FIG. 13-6. Skin plethysmography and ice response: Effect of sympathetic block. **A:** Before sympathetic block. Skin blood flow is similar (2 ml/100 ml/min) in both limbs, and the response to ice *(arrow)* is a similar reduction in the height of the pulse wave in both limbs. **B:** After sympathetic block. The blocked limb *(right)* shows a marked increase in the slope of the upward deflection of the pulse wave and an increase in height of the pulse wave; this reflects a tenfold increase of skin blood flow to 22 ml/100 ml/min. There is no change in blood flow in response to ice. In contrast, the unblocked limb *(left)* shows the same shape and height of the pulse wave, and there is a similar marked reduction in blood flow (40% decrease) in response to ice. (Cousins, M.J., Reeve, T.S., Glynn, C.J., Walsh, J.A., *et al.*: Neurolytic lumbar sympathetic blockade: Duration of denervation and relief of rest pain. Anaesth. Intensive Care, *7:*121, 1979). **C:** Apparatus for venous occlusion skin plethysmography *(VOP)*. The foot is enclosed in a constant temperature water bath, which surrounds a plethysmograph attached to a pressure transducer. A venous occlusion cuff is placed above the ankle. A typical trace is shown at right. Application of ice to the side of the neck results in a marked increase in sympathetic tone, with a decrease both in the upslope and in the area under the curve. (Reproduced with permission from Walsh, J.A., Glynn, C.J., Cousins, M.J., and Basedow, R.W.: Blood flow, sympathetic activity and pain relief following lumbar sympathetic blockade or surgical sympathectomy. Anaesth. Intensive Care, *13:*18, 1984.)

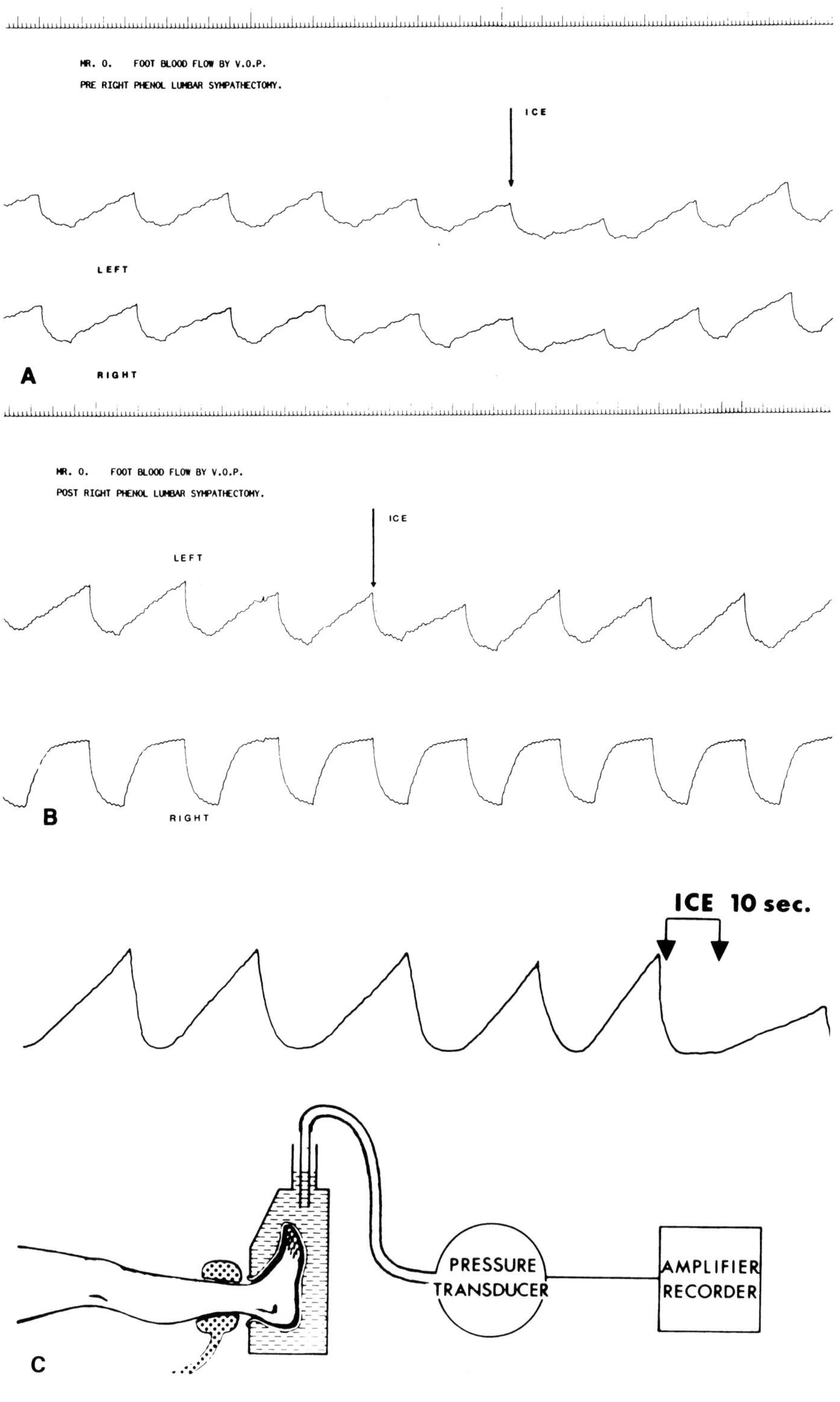
MR. O. FOOT BLOOD FLOW BY V.O.P.
PRE RIGHT PHENOL LUMBAR SYMPATHECTOMY.
ICE
LEFT
A
RIGHT
MR. O. FOOT BLOOD FLOW BY V.O.P.
POST RIGHT PHENOL LUMBAR SYMPATHECTOMY.
ICE
LEFT
B
RIGHT
ICE 10 sec.
PRESSURE TRANSDUCER
AMPLIFIER RECORDER
C

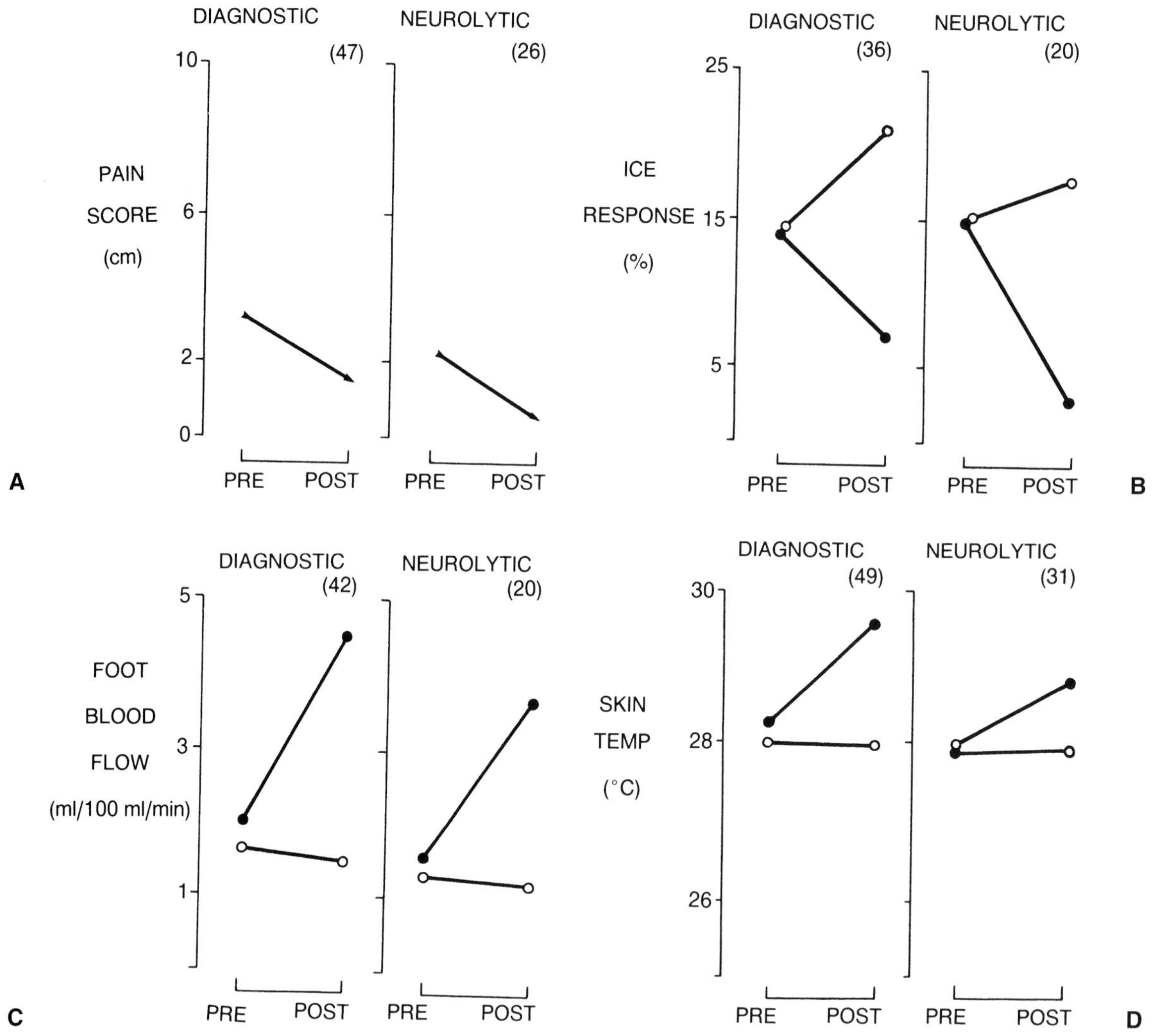

FIG. 13-7. A: Pain score. Pain score (mean on 10-cm analogue scale) prediagnostic and postdiagnostic local anesthetic (bupivacaine) and neurolytic (phenol) sympathetic blockade in 47 and 26 patients, respectively. Significant decreases in pain score resulted from diagnostic ($p < 0.001$) and neurolytic ($p < 0.001$) block. **B:** Vasoconstrictor ice response. Effect of diagnostic local anesthetic (bupivacaine, 36 patients) and neurolytic (phenol, 20 patients) sympathetic blockade on vasoconstrictor ice response (%) on treated (●) and control (○) limb (mean values). Significant decreases in ice response resulted from diagnostic ($p < 0.04$) and neurolytic ($p < 0.01$) block. **C:** Blood flow. Effect of diagnostic local anesthetic (bupivacaine, 42 patients) and neurolytic (phenol, 20 patients) sympathetic blockade on foot blood flow (m/100 ml/min) on treated (●) and control (○) limb (mean values). Significant increases in blood flow resulted from diagnostic ($p < 0.001$) and neurolytic ($p < 0.02$) block. **D:** Skin temperature. Effect of diagnostic local anesthetic (bupivacaine, 49 patients) and neurolytic block (phenol, 31 patients) on foot skin temperature (°C) on treated (●) and control (○) limbs (mean values). Significant increases in skin temperature resulted from diagnostic ($p < 0.001$) and neurolytic ($p < 0.01$) block. (Parts **A–D** are reproduced with permission from Walsh, J.A., Glynn, C.J., Cousins, M.J., and Basedow, R.W.: Blood flow, sympathetic activity and pain relief following lumbar sympathetic blockade or surgical sympathectomy. Anaesth. Intensive Care, *13:*18, 1984.)

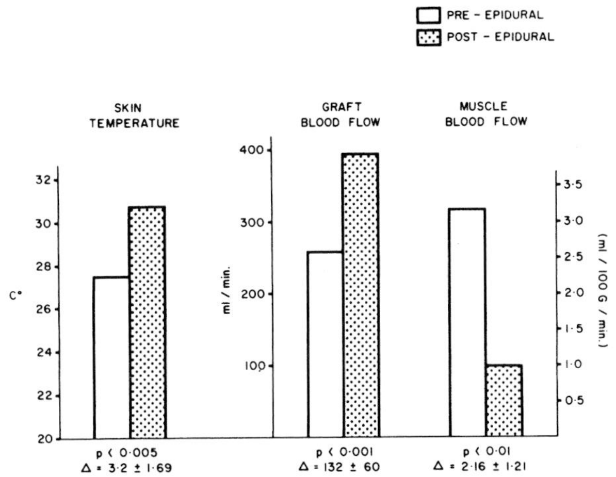

FIG. 13-8. Blood flow distribution after lumbar sympathetic blockade in arteriosclerotic patients at rest. Blood flow in the femoral artery (electromagnetic flow meter) is increased, as is skin blood flow (skin temperature); however, muscle blood flow (^{133}Xe clearance) is reduced. Note that this is a widespread sympathetic block (both lower limbs), which may sometimes even reduce the skin blood flow through diseased vessels (see Fig. 13-12). (Cousins, M.J., and Wright, C.J.: Graft muscle skin blood flow after epidural block in vascular surgical procedures. Surg. Gynecol. Obstet., *133*:59, 1971.)

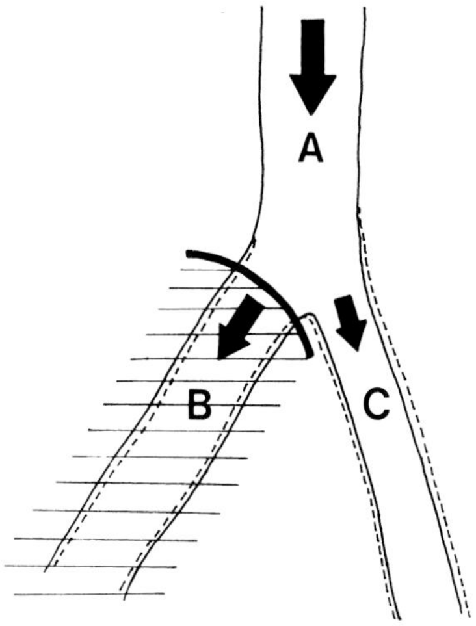

FIG. 13-10. A limited sympathetic blockade of fibers to branch *B* alone will little affect perfusion pressure. The flow in branch *B* will increase as the regional resistance is diminished. In branch *C* the flow will be slightly reduced as compensatory vasoconstriction occurs.

sympathetic blockade (in humans) is generally followed by a slight increase in vasomotor tone in the contralateral side, thus increasing the regional resistance and reducing the blood flow through this part of the vascular system.

In Figure 13-11, an arterial obstruction in branch B is shown. Such an obstruction will in itself diminish the blood flow by mechanically increasing the regional resistance; however, this might at least be compensated by an increase in the collateral blood flow. A widespread sympathetic blockade, as illustrated in Figure 13-12, will diminish the regional resistance, mainly in branch C with its undamaged vessels. The blood flow will be diverted into this part of the vascular tree, and thus blood will be stolen from the diseased part (branch B). Such stealing of blood is known to occur in patients with advanced arterial disease. In theory, stealing can occur at three different levels: A generalized vasodilatation in the body will steal blood from, for instance, one extremity; increased blood flow around the hip and in the pelvis will diminish the blood flow to the peripheral part of the lower extremity; or increased skin blood flow might steal blood from the muscles (see Fig. 13-8).[25,30,121]

In contrast, a localized vasodilatation that affects the collaterals to branch B and vessels beyond the arterial obstruction should increase blood flow to this region (Fig. 13-13).

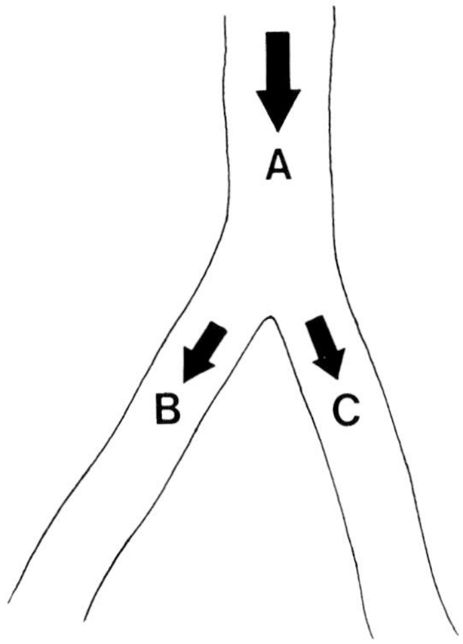

FIG. 13-9. The blood flows through an artery *(A)* or its branches *(B* and *C)* are proportionate to the perfusion pressures and inversely proportionate to total and regional resistances, respectively (see text).

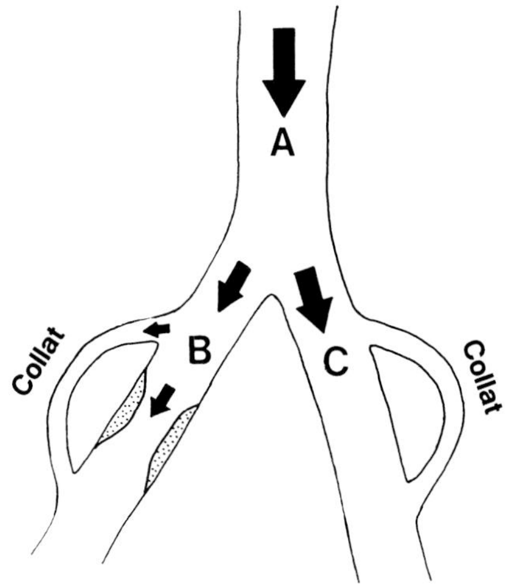

FIG. 13-11. An arterial obstruction in branch *B* will increase the resistance and thus hamper the blood flow. An increased flow through collaterals *(Collat)* may compensate for a fall in blood flow through the main channel (see text).

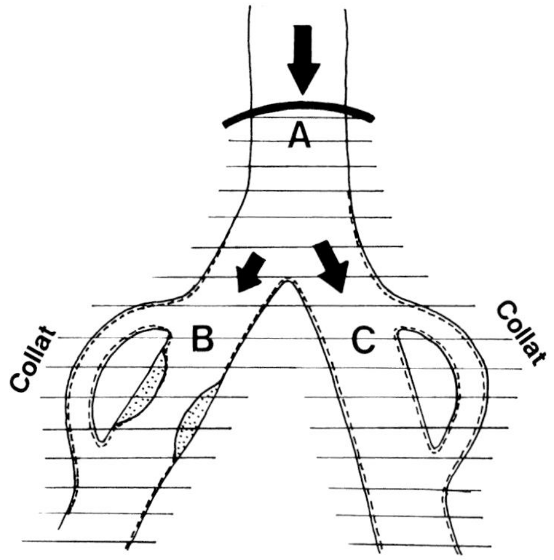

FIG. 13-12. A widespread sympathetic blockade of fibers to branches *B* and *C* will diminish resistance in undamaged vessels *(C)*, thereby potentially stealing blood from a diseased part *(B)* of the vascular tree.

If a decrease in vasomotor tone in the collaterals cannot be achieved, the maintenance of a good perfusion pressure is essential, as stressed by Lassen and Larsen.[68,69]

From this discussion, it is obvious that the clinical effect of a sympathetic block cannot easily be predicted. Only physiologic studies in patients and clinical experience will identify when a sympathetic block is indicated.

In patients with occlusive vascular disease, the prime indication for surgical or chemical sympathectomy is *rest pain* in a limb not amenable to direct arterial reconstruction.[119] Because of associated coronary artery disease, pulmonary disease, and other physical conditions, many of these patients are poor candidates for surgery and are thus better candidates for neurolytic sympathectomy.[24] However, the clinical results of both surgical and neurolytic sympathectomy, as reported in the literature, are contradictory. This might be explained by a poor selection of patients or by a lack of use of independent assessment of successful sympathetic ablation and its separate effects on blood flow and pain. This task may be simplified if one of the methods of evaluation in each category depicted in the list on page 423–426 is used.

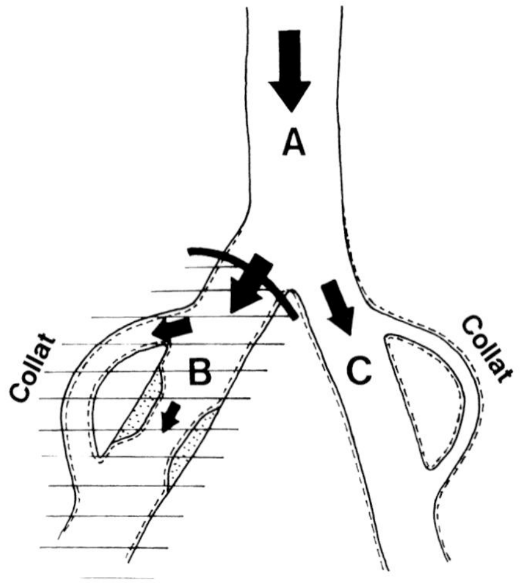

FIG. 13-13. A vasodilatation restricted to branch *B* and its collaterals *(Collat)* and vessels beyond the arterial obstruction should increase blood flow to this region.

The detrimental effects of generalized vasodilatation in patients with arteriosclerotic vascular disease that causes *rest pain* or intermittent claudication have been well described and are generally accepted today.[121]

It has been suggested that an increased skin blood flow should always occur in the presence of regional vasodilatation. This has also been reported in patients with obliterative arterial disease.[66,87,110]

Although skin blood flow is markedly under the control of sympathetic activity, a decreased blood flow has been demonstrated in patients with severe arteriosclerosis and, in particular, in patients with lower limb vascular disease who have a low ankle blood pressure before lumbar sympathetic blockade (below 60/20 mm Hg).[65,90,91,110,112,113] In these patients, the vascular lesions in the periphery are so extreme that, hypothetically, a "proximal stealing" always occurs, and thus a fall in the perfusion pressure peripherally is followed by a vasodilatation in vessels located proximally. Although rare, there are reports of worsening of pain and gangrene.[41] Remarkably enough, an increase in skin temperature is not always related to an increase in blood flow through the skin and may merely reflect venous pooling and local inflammatory changes.[113] During spinal anesthesia, changes in skin temperature are not closely correlated to changes in skin blood flow, as evaluated by laser Doppler flowmetry.[5,6]

The blood flow through muscle is automatically regulated according to metabolic needs. Thus, in intermittent claudication, the muscle tissue hypoxia and accumulation of metabolites at exercise should be followed by maximal dilatation of the muscle blood vessels, and therefore a sympathetic blockade should be of no value or may even worsen the symptoms because of "stealing" blood flow to the skin.[25,42,115] However, this is not necessarily so. Pain is a primary factor in provoking increased sympathetic activity. Hypothetically, this could result in vasoconstriction in the collateral vessels that supply the affected muscle (see Fig. 13-4). Sympathetic blockade under these circumstances may improve blood flow to muscle and thus explain why a beneficial effect of sympathectomy is observed in some patients with intermittent claudication.[66,89,98] This assumption and the clinical experience of several investigators are supported by a metabolic study in which deep venous blood was drawn before and at the maximum of a one-leg bicycle ergometer test in patients with intermittent claudication.[78] In one group of patients, with fairly high and segmentally located arterial lesions, who received sympathetic block (Group I), the rise in femoral venoarterial lactate difference during exercise was not as marked as before their sympathetic block, indicating an improvement in nutrient blood flow. By contrast, in a group of patients with multiple vascular lesions (Group II), no improvement in nutrient blood flow was achieved by sympathetic blockade. In Group I, 8 of 10 also experienced less ischemic pain on exercise during the sympathetic blockade. No patients in Group II experienced such pain relief. The most important effect of sympathetic blockade in Group I seemed to be pain relief during exercise, at least partly because of an improved blood flow and also enhancement of the development of collateral vessels, which is known to occur over time, providing opportunities for revascularization (see Table 13-3). It should be acknowledged that, with respect to pain evaluation, a placebo effect may occur, which has been reported with lumbar sympathetic blockade.[43]

Lumbar sympathetic blockade in connection with vascular surgery improves the flow through reconstructed vessels and should be of value in the immediate postoperative period.[26,64,66,99,117] Although less selective, this effect can also be achieved with epidural sympathetic block; however, the ganglion blockade is preferable, as discussed earlier in the chapter.[25]

The blockade of beta-fibers (sympathetic preganglionic fiber) during spinal and epidural blockade has recently been questioned.[5,23,77,80,81,82] Thus efferent sympathetic change has been studied with the help of skin conductance response (SCR) in which different stimuli (e.g., electrical stimulus, short, deep breath, verbal stimulation) have been used. In spinal analgesia, the sympathetic blockade starts at a level much lower than that of analgesia, in contrast to what has been previously stated in the literature.[48] Even at T1 blockade (which should have blocked all preganglionic fibers), an SCR response is often seen in the foot. This seems to indicate that the beta-fibers are not blocked as easily as previously thought. In most cases, when a T6 blockade has been achieved, a marked depression of the sympathetic responses is seen mainly in the foot (T12–L1). This partial sympathetic blockade, however, disappears much earlier than the analgesia, in most cases starting 20 to 40 minutes after the injection of the spinal anesthetic. Similar results have been seen when the skin blood flow has been studied with the help of laser Doppler flowmetry.[4,5] Also here, with a high blockade (T4–T6), an increased blood flow was seen only in the foot and in the thigh, at segment levels far below that of analgesia. A very high spinal analgesia is thus needed to make sure that marked depression of sympathetic activity in the lower extremity is produced. Changes in SCR response related to the height of an epidural blockade are very similar to those seen in spinal analgesia.[82]

The increase in limb blood flow resulting from epidural blocks has been clinically related to a lower incidence of postoperative thrombosis (see Chapter 8). This effect is most likely correlated with an increase in cardiac output, provoked by the local anesthetic itself (see Chapters 3, 4, and 8). The local anesthetics lidocaine and mepivacaine, when applied directly into the resistance vessels, produce a contraction, in contrast to what is seen during an intravenous (IV) infusion.[76]

The poor blocking of sympathetic fibers produced by an epidural blockade also explains the fact that a very high epidural blockade is required to ablate the stress responses during and after lower abdominal surgery. In upper abdominal surgery, epidural blockade is less effective in blocking the stress response. This can be markedly improved if a splanchnic blockade is added (see Chapter 5).

There is a variable degree of sympathetic blockade achieved by an intradural or extradural injection of a local anesthetic.[82] In contrast, in most instances, it is fairly easy to obtain a complete sympathetic blockade by an injection of the local anesthetic at sympathetic ganglia or postganglionic fibers.

It is obvious that a proper selection of patients for sympathetic blockade is of great importance. Because the number of patients with vascular disease is very large, complicated and time-consuming physiologic studies are not always feasible. The use of continuous catheter sympathetic blockade that lasts for 5 days is one method of obtaining a clinical evaluation of the effect of the blockade, which should at least detect patients whose symptoms are exacerbated after blockade.[63] A selective alternative is intravenous regional sympathetic block, which can eliminate technical failure and is a useful preliminary test for whether surgical sympathectomy or permanent blockade by chemical sympathectomy will be successful.[14,50] The prolonged duration (1–3 weeks) of intravenous sympathetic block allows adequate time for clinical assessment. A third alternative is to perform diagnostic block with long-acting local anesthetic mixed with contrast medium and to check adequacy of coverage of sympathetic chain under image intensifier; however, this has proved the least reliable of the three.[24,117]

In a clinical series, Kövamees and Löfström found that the most beneficial effect of sympathetic blockade was relief of *rest pain* (19/23, or 83%) with a somewhat lesser effect of improved healing of ulcers (23/55, or 42%) (see Table 13-2).[65] Increased walking tolerance (7/16, or 44%) was a significant benefit in a small group of patients with intermittent claudication. Sympathetic blockade was part of a general treatment program that included mobilization and wound treatment, and sometimes infusion of low molecular weight dextran. It was not possible to attribute an improvement to the sympathetic blockade alone. However, Cousins and colleagues[24] reported that duration of relief of rest pain was similar to duration of lumbar sympathetic blockade, strengthening the relation between pain relief and sympathetic denervation. In one study, pain relief was accompanied by increased skin temperature and skin blood flow (venous occlusion plethysmography), whereas sweating and vasoconstrictor ice response were decreased (see Fig. 13-7).[117] Another study indicated that nutritive blood flow was not increased but pain was relieved in a high percentage of patients.[28] Good results with relief of rest pain in the lower limbs have been reported by others.[9,28,56,98] Very little data are available on upper limb vascular disease, although case reports indicate beneficial results with sympathetic block in vasospastic disorders such as those in the list on page 422.

It would appear that the primary benefits that result from

sympathetic blockade are pain relief and improved healing of skin lesions; however, controlled studies of efficacy of sympathetic block are required to achieve a better definition of its role in the treatment of vascular disease of the lower and the upper limbs.

The pain-relieving effect of a sympathetic block in a patient with peripheral arterial disease is said to follow improved blood flow. Good pain relief often occurs, however, when no improvement in peripheral circulation can be noted;[28] possible mechanisms are discussed below (see also Fig. 13-6).

Clinical Conditions That Sympathetic Blockade May Benefit

To Produce Pain Relief

Renal colic (lumbar sympathetic block)
Obliterative arterial disease (lumbar sympathetic block)
Acute pancreatitis and pancreatic cancer (celiac plexus block)
Cancer pain from upper abdominal viscera (celiac plexus block)
Cardiac pain (thoracic sympathetic or stellate ganglion block)
Paget's disease of bone (stellate ganglion or lumbar sympathetic block)
Complex regional pain syndrome, CRPS type I[57] (formerly: reflex sympathetic dystrophy, minor post-traumatic syndrome, post-frostbite syndrome, shoulder/hand syndrome, Sudeck's atrophy)
Complex regional pain syndrome, CRPS type II[57] (formerly: causalgia)
Phantom limb pain
Central pain

To Improve Blood Flow in Vasospastic Disorders (Stellate or Lumbar Sympathetic Block)

Raynaud's disease
Accidental intra-arterial injections of thiopentone
Early frostbite
Obliterative arterial disease not suitable for vascular surgery[8,44]
Vascular surgery and reimplantation surgery (to improve postoperative blood flow)

To Improve Drainage of Local Edema (Stellate or Lumbar Sympathetic Block)

INDICATIONS FOR SYMPATHETIC BLOCKADE

The precise mechanism whereby the sympathetic nervous system is involved in peripheral pain has not yet been fully elucidated (see previous)[57]. It has been suggested that the cutaneous pain threshold, by means of a negative feedback loop, is influenced by sympathetic efferents (Fig. 13-5).[96] This may explain the often remarkable pain relief seen after sympathetic blocks in patients with threatening gangrene, despite a lack of improvement in skin blood flow. It is possible that increased efferent sympathetic activity increases activity in pain receptors by way of sympathetic fibers that are prevalent in proximity to sensory receptors. This provides an explanation of pain relief that may follow stellate ganglion block in patients with arteriopathy (e.g., associated with scleroderma) in the upper limb, despite the lack of change in blood flow.

There are also clinical observations that early herpes zoster pain and skin vesicles respond favorably to sympathetic blockade (see Chapter 27).[22,84] That they also respond well to a block of the appropriate somatic nerve is well established, and it is uncertain whether there is any specific sympathetic involvement in this condition. Results of sympathetic block in the treatment of postherpetic neuralgia are uniformly disappointing.

It is, of course, well documented that the pain of uterine contraction and cervical dilatation can be abolished by blockade of sympathetic afferents entering the spinal cord at T11–T12 (T10–L1). (These fibers are better classified as visceral nociceptive afferents, leaving sympathetic fibers only as efferents). This is usually achieved by extradural sympathetic blockade (see Chapter 18). Also, in a small series of patients with renal colic treated with extradural sympathetic block at L1, 9 of 14 patients passed their stones in 10 days and all were pain-free from the start of treatment; this series has now been increased to 32, all of whom obtained complete pain relief.[74] This compares favorably with other methods, and it has been suggested that relief of pain and reduction of ureteral spasm are brought about by sympathetic blockade of the first lumbar segmental outflow. Chronic pain from the urogenital tract has, in a few cases, been eliminated with chemical lumbar sympathectomy.[58] Cervicothoracic sympathetic blockade is also of value in the treatment of patients with severe angina pectoris, provided that the block extends down to the level of T4. The hazards, however, may often outweight the benefits.

In post-traumatic complex regional pain syndrome (CRPS), a sympathetic blockade is often followed by relief of the burning pain in the injured extremity and a feeling of softening of the tissues, primarily around the joints.[7,31,57,101] Symptoms of CRPS may be caused by hyperactivity in the sympathetic nervous system, or abnormal supersensitivity of adrenoceptors,[57,95] producing vasoconstriction, decrease in capillary surface area, redistribution of blood flow, fall in oxygen uptake (tissue hypoxia), increased vascular permeability, and lack of fluid mobilization.[57,72] A sympathetic blockade should then improve nutrient blood flow and decrease the accumulated fluid in the tissue, which explains the increased warmth and the rapid disappearance of tissue edema often seen during this form of treatment. Sympathetic block only produces significant residual clinical improvements if used early in this syndrome.

Sympathetic block is sometimes not helpful in post-traumatic pain syndromes for the following reasons:[39,57,95]

Although reflex hyperactivity of the sympathetic nervous system may be present in sympathetically maintained neuropathic pain, abnormal adrenoceptor hyperactivity may be more common: Increased or abnormal sensitivity to adrenergic agents in primary afferent nociceptors of damaged nerves may be a result of damaged sympathetic (motor) nerve fibers in mixed peripheral nerves. The resulting denervation hypersensitivity from augmented production of adrenergic receptors means that signs of sympathetic overactivity may be present locally with a normal (or low) sympathetic nervous system activity[57] (see also recent review[116]).

TESTING THE COMPLETENESS OF SYMPATHETIC BLOCKADE

In a patient with a healthy vascular system, a sympathetic blockade produces clear-cut subjective and objective effects on the peripheral circulation, as has been discussed in the previous section. In a patient with severe arterial disease, however, a complete sympathetic blockade can have been achieved with little or no demonstrable effect on the peripheral circulation.

Venous circulation is generally not involved in the disease process, and swelling of the veins can be a valuable indication of a successful block. Listed below are objective tests that can be used to provide an assessment of completeness of sympathetic block.

Results of all indirect methods that measure blood flow or temperature before and after sympathetic block depend on the initial condition: Low initial temperature (and blood flow) generally implies a large change after the block; a sympathetic block in a patient with high initial temperature (and blood flow) usually will result in only small changes after the block.[82]

Independent Tests of Sympathetic Function, Blood Flow, and Pain

Method of Evaluation

- *Sympathetic function*
  - Skin conductance response (SCR)[1,20,40,71,77]
  - Sweat test
    - Ninhydrin[32]
    - Cobalt blue[24]
    - Starch iodine
  - Skin plethysmography and "ice response"[24]
- *Blood flow*[45]
  - Plethysmography (muscle and skin)[87,88]
  - Xenon-133 clearance (muscle and skin)[46,55,115]
  - Sodium-24 clearance (muscle and skin)[54]
  - Antipyrine clearance[121]
  - Doppler technique (whole limb)[108,109]
  - Electromagnetic flow meter (whole limb)[25,26,66,99,118]
  - Laser Doppler flowmetry[4,5,62,63]
  - Pulse wave (skin)[3,45,60,61]
  - Temperature (skin)[78,79,90,91,110,113]
  - Size of ulcer (skin)[24]
  - Distal perfusion pressure[65,90,91,110–113]
  - Capillary oxygen tension (muscle or skin)[15]
  - Venous oxygen tension, saturation (muscle)[78]
  - Metabolism (muscle)[78]
- *Pain*
  - Pain score[24]
  - Analgesic requirements
  - Activity (e.g., claudication distance)

Skin Conductance Response

SCR was previously called the sympathogalvanic response (SGR). SCR tests not only efferent sympathetic activity but also afferent sensory activity and spinal and supraspinal inteneurons. Increased sympathetic activity, which in many people can be evoked by a short, deep breath or by pinching the skin, is followed by a change in skin conductance that can be recorded with a simple electrocardiograph. One ECG electrode is placed on the front and one on the back of the hand or foot (i.e., where sweat glands are abundant). A third grounding electrode is placed anywhere on the body. Before the electrodes are placed the skin must be scrubbed free of epithelial cells. In most patients, there will be a slow change in the baseline, which will come to rest after a few minutes. A short, deep breath or pinching will now, with a 1- to 2-second delay, be followed by a marked deflection that lasts for 4 to 5 seconds. This deflection does not occur if the sympathetic fibers of the extremity are blocked. A partial block of the response will be seen if the patient is atropinized (in clinically used doses). It is preferable to perform separate tests on two limbs simultaneously, thus making it possible to compare the blocked side with the unblocked side. This is essential if the SCR deflections are to be measured in the evaluation of indications for another sympathetic blockade (Fig. 13-14). It is well known that the baseline is far less stable and the deflections much more marked in young patients than in elderly patients. In elderly patients, it is also more difficult to provoke a sympathetic response, particularly in depressed people and in people who are freezing. Also, the SCR undergoes marked habituation, that is, each stimulus has a tendency to be followed by a smaller and smaller deflection. Each stimulus should therefore be 2 to 3 minutes apart. When habituation occurs, waiting for a few minutes, putting a warm blanket over the patient, and changing the stimulus from a deep, short breath to pinching or to verbal stimulation or, if available, to a more painful electrical stimulation, usually brings back a good response.

Ample experience with SCR has made it clear that it is not always possible to obtain a complete abolition with a sympathetic blockade, even though the vascular response seems to be maximal. It has been suggested that SCR can be used

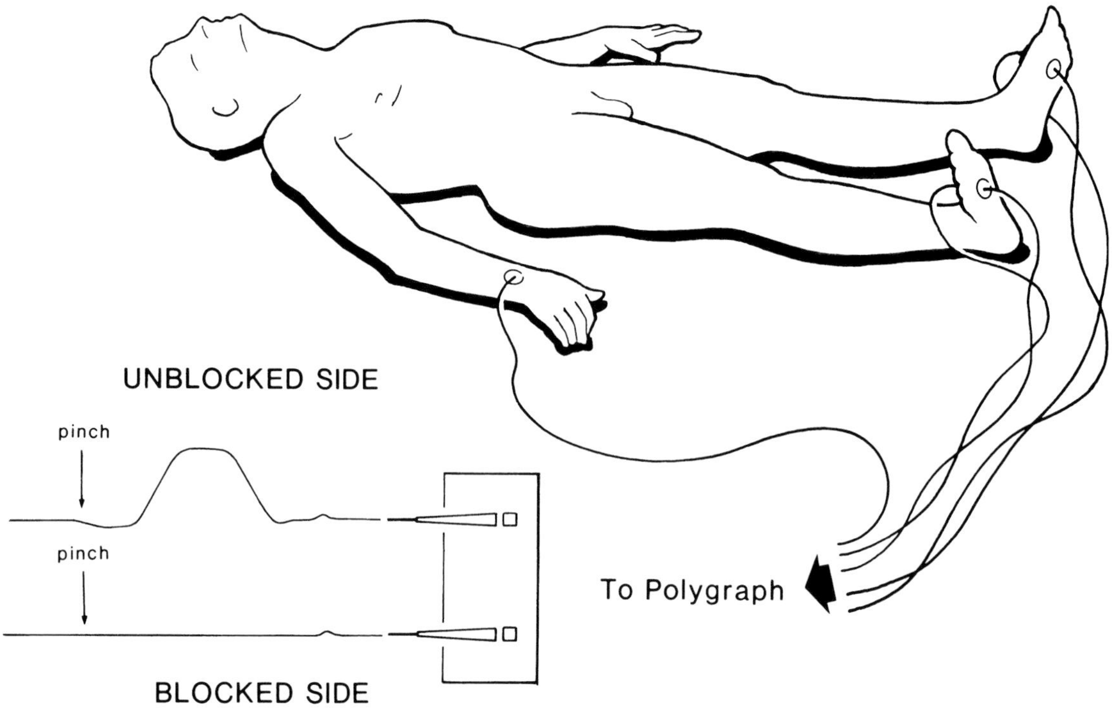

FIG. 13-14. Skin conductance response (SCR) or sympathogalvanic response. Electrodes are placed on the front and back of hands or feet, and a ground electrode is placed elsewhere on the body. Changes in baseline level on an ECG recorder indicate changes in sweat gland activity.

to predict the value of a sympathetic blockade in patients with arterial disease.[6,13] In this study, most patients with a good to moderate deflection on stimulation benefited from a sympathetic block. This was not seen in patients with little or no deflection. We have also used the SCR to check the completeness of sympathetic denervation following local anesthetic or chemical sympathectomy. When a permanent sympathetic blockade is under consideration and no, or only weak, skin resistance deflections are seen following SCR, a continuous sympathetic blockade is unlikely to be followed by any improvement in the peripheral circulation, although in some cases it may offer pain relief.

Skin Potential Response

The skin potential response (SPR) is an alternative to the SCR.[27] The SPR, like the SCR, has a rise time of 1 to 2 seconds and a fall time of 10 to 15 seconds. SPR has an amplitude of 5 mV. Like SCR, SPR is due to an increase in sympathetic activity and subsequent changes in sodium chloride flux in sweat gland ducts. The benefits claimed for SPR are that electrode size and placement are less critical than for SCR and no external signal source is required. However, a modified ECG recording equipment is needed because (i) most ECG machines have a frequency response of 0.1 to 100 Hz, whereas SPR requires 0.03 to 2 Hz. Also, 50 Hz interference may occur; (ii) SPR requires a wider range of input sensitivity than in standard ECG machines; (iii) ECG recorder paper speed of 25 mm/sec is too fast for SPR; and (iv) pre-gelled Ag–Agl electrodes are required ("Red Dot"—3M). A positive electrode is placed over palm or sole and a negative electrode over back of hand or foot. An indifferent electrode is attached at the wrist or ankle. Spontaneous changes in sympathetic tone result in negative, then positive, swings on the SPR recording. As with SCR, several factors influence the response: (i) degree of arousal—central nervous system (CNS) depression abolishes the response; (ii) drugs that alter sympathetic activity, for example, opiates and tranquilizers; (iii) anticholinergic drugs abolish the response since acetylcholine is the sudomotor transmitter; (iv) steroids interfere with sodium flux in sweat glands; and (v) ouabain affects sodium pumping in sweat glands.

Sweat Test

The sweat test is perhaps the most practicable test of sympathetic activity.

Ninhydrin Method. Fingerprints are taken (at intervals) before and after blockade.[32] After suitable preparation, which includes heating, the fingerprints are developed, and each functioning sweat gland can be seen and counted. This test is very accurate and its results reproducible; however, it is time-consuming and does not provide the clinician with an answer at the bedside.

Cobalt Blue Filter Paper Test. Filter papers are soaked in cobalt blue and then dried in an oven, after which they are kept in a desiccator until needed. Two filter papers are removed from the desiccator with forceps and placed on a

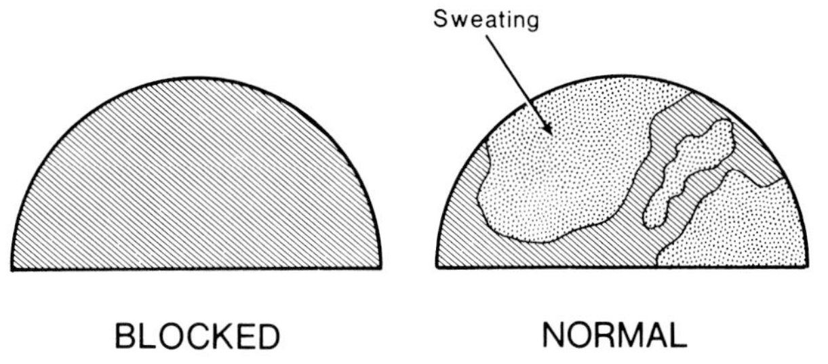

FIG. 13-15. Cobalt blue sweat test. The papers are blue *(shaded)* before the test. Sweating from the unblocked limb changes the color to pink *(stippled)*.

clean, dry surface, so that the patient can press both feet or hands onto the papers. Sweating is registered on the paper by a change in color from blue to pink. A limb with complete sympathetic block usually shows no color change (Fig. 13-15). Details for preparation of the filter papers are found in Appendix A of this chapter.

Starch-Iodine Test. The starch-iodine test works on a principle similar to that of the cobalt blue test. It has the advantage that the material can be spread over a complete limb. It is a messy technique, however, and not popular with patients.

Having ensured that sympathetic block is adequate, an independent assessment can then be made of the effect on blood flow. If this is combined with the ice test (see Fig. 13-6), a further evaluation of sympathetic function can be obtained and, if pain was present before blockade, pain relief can be independently assessed (see Fig. 13-7).

Assessment of Blood Flow Changes

Whole Limb Blood Flow

Indirect

Doppler Ankle/Brachial Index.[120] An ultrasound probe is used to facilitate blood pressure measurement with a standard cuff at brachial artery and also at the ankle. An ankle to brachial index is then calculated as follows:

$$\frac{\text{ankle}}{\text{brachial}} = \frac{80/50}{120/80} = 0.65$$

This reading is then repeated after sympathetic block.

Direct

Electromagnetic Flowmeter. This can be applied either directly to the blood vessel during surgery or percutaneously, using a "catheter tip" version.

Ultrasonic Flowmeter. Very small probes are now available that can be placed on the vessel wall at operation and left *in situ* postoperatively.

Muscle Blood Flow

Venous Occlusion Plethysmography. This has been used in the calf area under the assumption that the calf is mostly muscle with much less skin.

Clearance of Radioactive Substances after Direct Injection (e.g. ^{133}Xe). This provides one of the best measurements of nutritive blood flow (Fig. 13-16).[25]

Arterial Oxygen Concentration in Blood from Deep Calf Veins. This has also been used for an indirect estimate of oxygen delivery to calf muscle[78] Recently, a *mass spectrometer probe* has been developed to measure muscle tissue Po_2 directly.

Skin Blood Flow

Clearance of Radioactive Substances. This, injected directly into the skin, has been used (e.g., ^{133}Xe, ^{124}Na).

Laser Doppler Flowmeters. These provide a noninvasive assessment of changes in skin blood flow.[4,5]

Mass Spectrometer Microprobes and Skin "Cups." These are also being used in this situation to measure changes in skin Po_2 with different forms of treatment.

Occlusion Skin Plethysmography. This method has also been used in the area of the foot, hand, and digits, as described above (see Fig. 13-6).[24]

Skin Temperature Measurements. This technique, using a telethermometer and thermistor or thermocouple skin probes, provides an indirect but easily obtained estimate of changes in skin blood flow (Fig. 13-17). Liquid thermal crystals and heat-sensitive papers are also available.

Optical Density Skin Plethysmography (or Pulse Monitor). Several quite sensitive finger "pulse-meters" are now available and use several different wavelengths of light di-

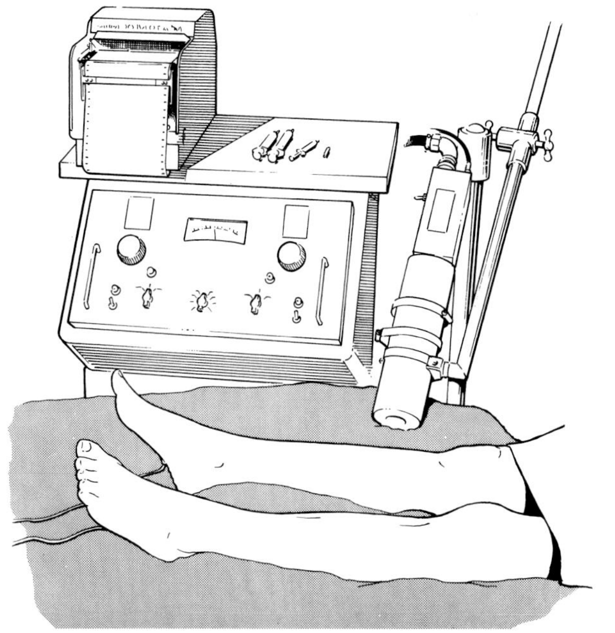

FIG. 13-16. Xenon-133 clearance technique for leg muscle blood flow. Xenon-133 is injected into the anterior tibial muscle and its clearance detected with a portable scintillation detector.

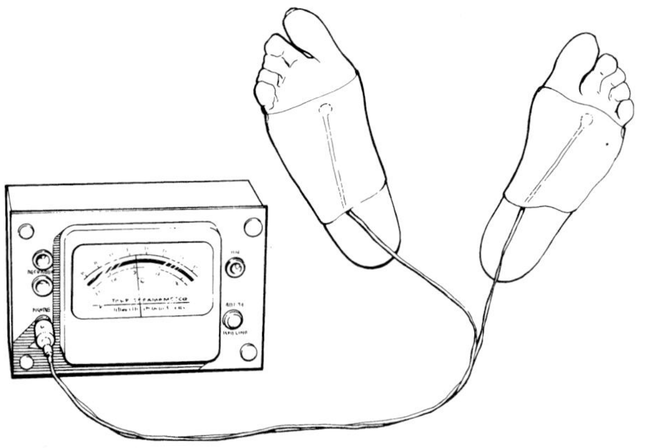

FIG. 13-17. Skin thermocouple probe and telethermometer. Simultaneous measurements are made on treated and untreated limb.

rected into the skin capillary bed. Capillary blood flow results in a cyclical change in optical density, yielding a wave form similar to that shown in Figure 13-6, and its amplitude is proportional to sympathetic activity.

Measurement of Size of Skin Ulcers. Progressive documentation of change in ulcer size is a very simple, practical method of checking progress after sympathetic block in patients with ischemic skin lesions.

Transcutaneous Oxygen Electrodes and Oximeters. These also provide an indirect assessment of skin blood flow by changes in oxygenation. Pulse oximeters can now easily be applied to fingers and toes.

Pain Assessment

As discussed in Chapters 24 and 25, there is still no objective method of pain assessment. Indirect methods such as the pain score (visual analogue scale), analgesic requirements, and improved level of activity are used; wherever possible these should be performed by an independent observer with a "double-blind" study design (see Chapter 25).

A baseline measurement/assessment before sympathetic block should be performed in each case for sympathetic activity, blood flow, and pain score by one of the methods described above. After sympathetic blockade, the completeness of sympathetic block, its effect on blood flow, and any effects on pain should be ascertained.

General Clinical Applications

The clinical situations in which sympathetic blockade may be considered are summarized in the list on page 422. The present lack of definitive data makes it highly desirable to carry out a diagnostic block before considering permanent blockade. In addition, one or more of the methods of independently assessing blockade, blood flow, and pain relief should be used.

General Contraindications

Patients on Heparin. Severe bleeding has been observed, particularly after lumbar sympathetic blockade in a heparinized patient. The bleeding occurs within the psoas fascia, producing minimal symptoms until frank shock occurs. Early symptoms are pain in the groin or pain when the leg is actively lifted and rotated outward. A hematoma may also pass through an intervertebral foramen into the spinal canal, after stellate or lumbar sympathetic block, causing pressure on nerves and vessels followed by neurologic symptoms (see also Chapter 8). Hematoma after stellate block has been reported to interfere with carotid blood flow (see Chapters 21 and 22).

Bilateral Injection During One Treatment Session. This probably should be avoided. Dosage tends to be high, and vascular responses may be a significant problem for this class of patient. Various side effects may pose an increased hazard if both sides are blocked. For example, bilateral recurrent laryngeal block after stellate block may cause stridor (see Chapter 21).

Bilateral Injection in the Lumbar Region for Permanent Blockade. This may cause loss of ejaculation[2] and should be avoided in young persons; however, impotence does not occur, and the patient does not become sterile.

Agents for Sympathetic Blockade

For short-term block, any of the conventional local anesthetics can be used. Addition of epinephrine to the local anesthetic solution will, to some extent, prolong the duration of action; however, the use of epinephrine in patients with severe vascular disease or vasospasm is questionable. Mepivacaine and bupivacaine, without epinephrine, have durations of 1½ to 3 and 3 to 10 hours, respectively. These durations are influenced only marginally by the addition of epinephrine, and therefore plain solutions are the solutions of choice.[15,92] It is useful to add contrast medium (2 ml of iohexol (Omnipaque®) or Conray-420®), as this allows confirmation of the adequacy of spread of solution (e.g., over L2–L4 ganglia; see Fig. 13-31).

The amount of local anesthetic agent needed in, for example, lumbar sympathetic blockade (1–5 ml, 0.5% mepivacaine or 0.25% bupivacaine at each level), even without epinephrine, poses a relatively small risk of a toxic reaction owing to local anesthetic absorption. There is, however, the ever present risk of acute intravascular injection and the other adverse effects of local anesthetic injection (see Chapter 4, Table 4-8).

For a permanent block (chemical sympathectomy), 6% to 7% phenol in water, 7% to 10% phenol in water-soluble (e.g., iohexol [Omnipaque®] Angiographin®) contrast medium, or 50% to 100% alcohol may be used. The last yields the highest incidence of neuralgia, and most authorities now prefer 7% to 10% phenol in Angiographin because it poses minimal resistance to injection, and its spread can be viewed under radiographic control.[9,24,36,117]

TECHNIQUES

Stellate Ganglion Block (Cervicothoracic Sympathetic Block)

Regional Anatomy

The cervical sympathetic chain lies in the fascial space, which is limited posteriorly by the fascia over the prevertebral muscles and anteriorly by the carotid sheath (Fig. 13-18).

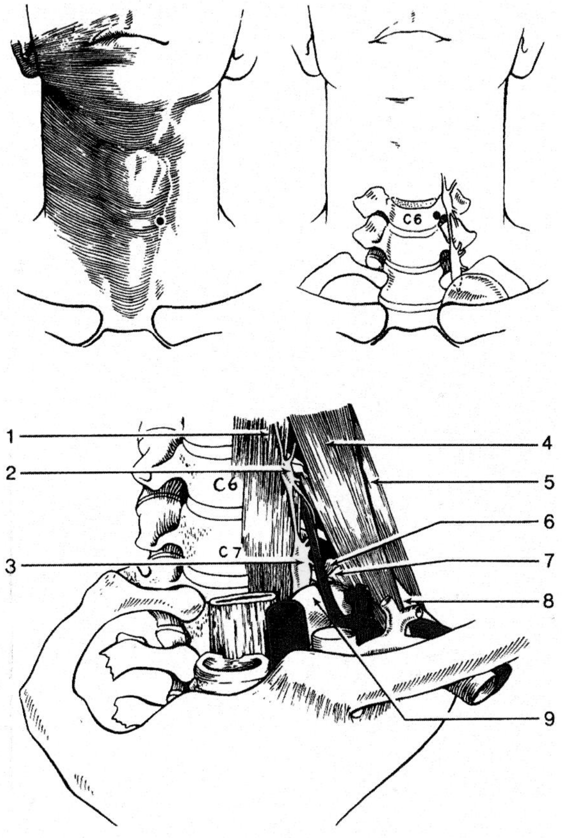

FIG. 13-18. Cervicothoracic sympathetic chain: Regional anatomy. **I:** Anterior view. Note stellate ganglion on neck of first rib and extending up to transverse process of C7. At this level, the cervicothoracic sympathetic chain has the vertebral artery on its anterolateral aspect with the pleura covering the lower third of the stellate ganglion. At the level of C6, the vertebral artery has dived posteriorly into the foramen intertransversarium and the pleura is well below. Note also that even at C6, a large volume of solution may diffuse posteriorly between the slips of origin of scalenus anterior to the roots of the brachial plexus **II:** Cross-section. Note the importance of lateral retraction of the carotid and extension of the neck to draw the esophagus medial to the needle path on the left side. It is necessary to withdraw the needle 2 to 5 mm after contacting the transverse process in order to clear the anterior aspect of the longus colli muscle. Correct needle direction onto the transverse process is very important, as is the avoidance of force with the risk of penetration of prevertebral fascia and intertransverse ligaments leading to entry into vertebral artery or dural cuff. (Modified from Bryce-Smith, R., and Macintosh, R. R.: Local Analgesia: Abdomen. Edinburgh, Livingstone Press, 1962.)

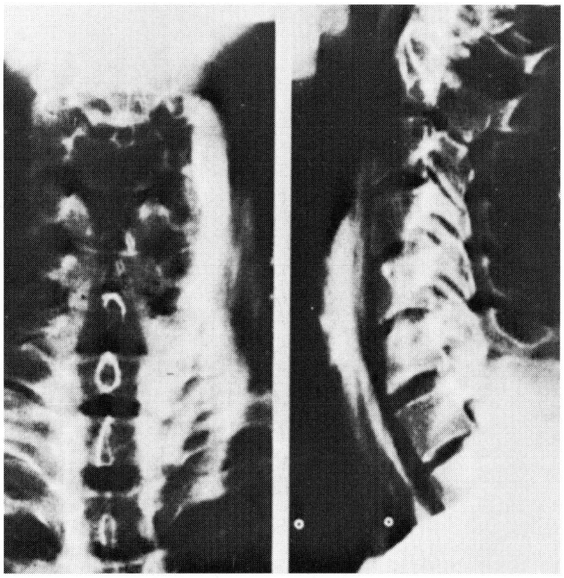

FIG. 13-19. The spread of 20 ml of local anesthetic solution injected in front of the prevertebral fascia at the 6th transverse process.

Although the sympathetic preganglionic fibers for the head, neck, and upper limb leave the spinal cord from segments as widely separated as T1 to T6, pathways converge and pass anteriorly to the neck of the first rib. Here, the first thoracic and inferior cervical ganglion may be separated or fused to form the stellate ganglion. In the latter case, the ganglion lies over the neck of the first rib. The ganglion is covered anteriorly in its lower part by the dome of the pleura, and in its upper part by the vertebral artery. Block of the stellate ganglion alone may provide disappointing results despite the correct anatomic placement of solution. This may be explained by the diverse origin of the sympathetic fibers in the thoracic cord and also by the fact that some thoracic preganglion fibers lie in other sympathetic ganglia and may bypass the stellate ganglion completely on their way into the head, neck, and upper extremity.[86] For best results, the local anesthetic solution has to fill the space in front of the prevertebral fascia down to at least T4. This can be achieved by an injection of 15 to 20 ml of weak local anesthetic solution in front of the transverse process of C6 (see Fig. 13-19). It is obvious that there is little advantage to be gained by needle placement at C7 and there is a greater risk of pneumothorax at this level. The term "cervicothoracic sympathetic block" thus seems more appropriate than "stellate ganglion block."

Procedure

A large number of techniques have been described. If the needle is aimed at C7 or the neck of the first rib, the risk of pneumothorax is considerable. On the other hand, the needle may be kept well above the pleura and reliance placed on the spread of a large volume of solution. This is the basis of the anterior approach first described by Leriche.[70]

"Paratracheal" (Anterior) Technique

The patient lies supine with the head slightly lifted forward on a thin pillow and tilted dorsally to stretch the esophagus away from the transverse processes on the left side; a rolled towel under the shoulders helps to increase access to the target area and also stretches the esophagus out of the way. The mouth should be slightly opened to relax the neck muscles.

The trachea and the carotid pulse are gently palpated by inserting two fingers between the sternocleidomastoid muscle and the trachea to find the most prominent cervical transverse process, C6—the Chassaignac tubercle, which lies at the level of the cricoid cartilage (Fig. 13-18). A skin wheal is raised with a fine needle over this transverse process. Two fingers are now gently pressed down to the C6 tubercle, pushing away the carotid artery laterally and the trachea toward the midline with the fingers slightly separated so that the tubercle lies just in between them (Fig. 13-18).

A 22-gauge, short-bevel, 4- to 5-cm-long needle, with a 20-ml syringe attached, is advanced through the skin and underlying tissues until it hits bone, that is, rests on the junction of C6 body and transverse process. The palpating fingers maintain their position; the hand holding the needle is kept braced against the patient, and the needle is withdrawn about 2 mm and fixed (Fig. 13-18).

Aspiration is performed before and after test doses of 0.5 ml × 4. Injection of even this small dose directly into the vertebral artery can result in a convulsion (see Chapter 4). A high resistance to injection may indicate periosteal injection, and a significant but lesser resistance indicates that the needle is still in prevertebral muscle, while radiating pain means the needle is too deep, that is, has penetrated a nerve root. While the needle is *in situ*, it is important that the patient not talk. If aspiration tests are negative and no sequelae follow, the full dose, 15 to 20 ml of local anesthetic, is injected (Fig. 13-20). In most instances, the patient will feel a lump in the throat and may often be temporarily hoarse; he or she should

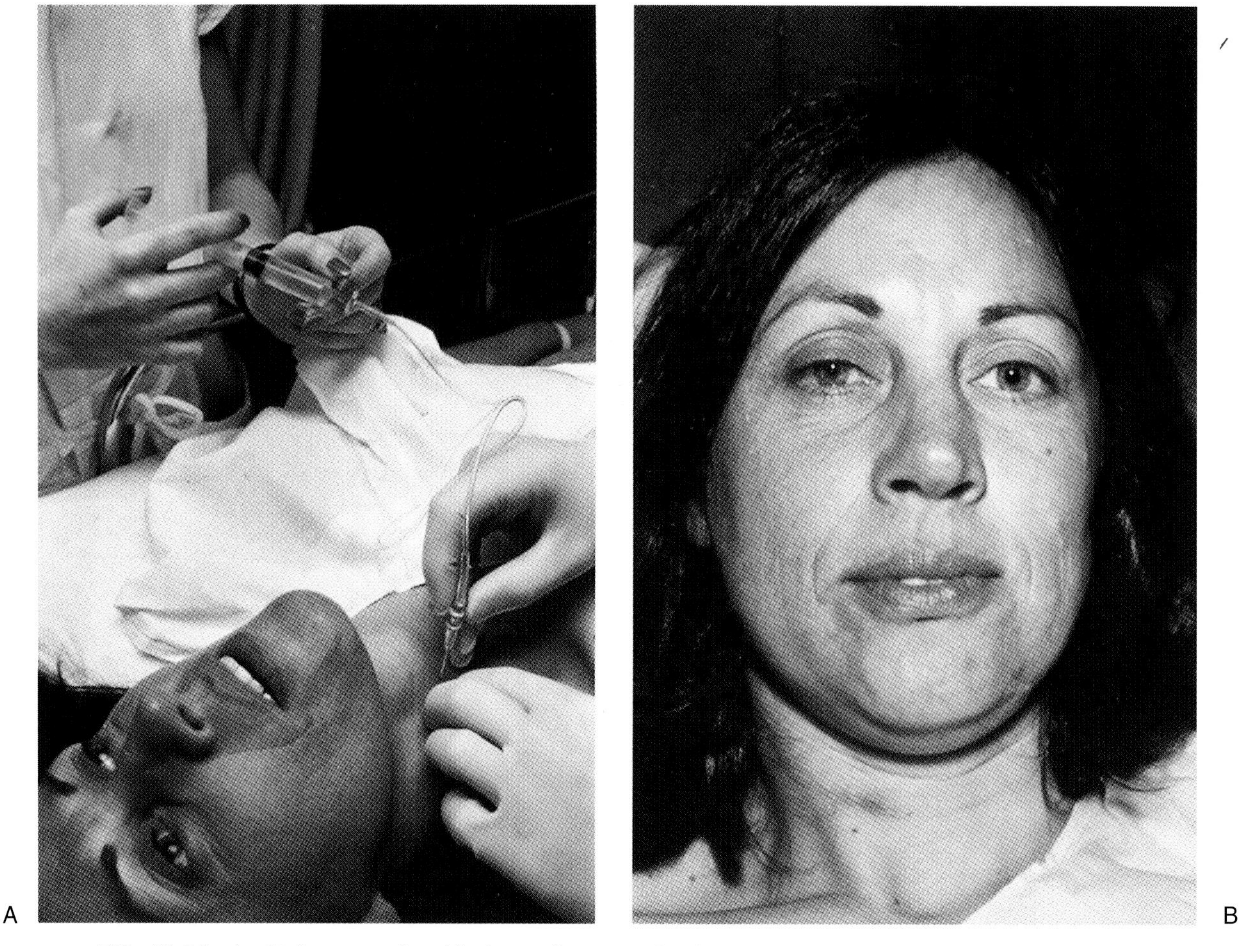

FIG. 13-20. A: Stellate ganglion block needle correctly placed. Note palpating hand *(left)* retracting carotid sheath laterally and hand-holding needle *(right)* braced against clavicle. An extension tubing is used so that an assistant may aspirate and inject. **B:** Horner's syndrome *(right)*. Note ptosis, miois, anhydrosis, and unilateral conjunctival engorgement.

be warned beforehand about these events. Because of these effects, patients are more comfortable sitting up. Fluids and food should be withheld while laryngeal reflexes are impaired.

Continuous Technique

A continuous technique has been described in which a thin radiopaque Teflon catheter is introduced under x-ray control with the paratracheal technique described above. The stylet is withdrawn and the catheter properly fixed.[73] It should be recognized, however, that movement of the catheter into proximity with vertebral artery, dural cuff, or other structures is possible.

Intravenous Sympathetic Block. This may be a more attractive technique when prolonged effect is required (see Chapter 12 and following).

Signs of a Successful Block

Horner's syndrome (Fig. 13-20) results if the cervical sympathetic fibers are blocked successfully: ptosis (drooping upper eyelid), miosis (small pupil), and enophthalmos (sinking of the eyeball). In addition, other features have been described, such as unilateral blockage of the nose (owing to engorgement of nasal mucosa), flushing of conjunctiva and skin, and anhydrosis (lack of sweating). The ptosis and conjunctival engorgement can be relieved by eyedrops of the alpha agonist neosynephrine. It should be noted that these signs may be present without complete sympathetic denervation of the upper limb, which may receive sympathetic supply from as far down as T9. The cobalt blue sweat test or SCR is the most useful in this situation (see list on pp. 423; see also Chapter 27).

Indications

The clinical indications for cervicothoracic sympathetic blocks are listed below.

Clinical Conditions That Cervicothoracic Sympathetic Blockade May Benefit Circulatory Insufficiency in the Arm, Due to:

Traumatic or embolic vascular occlusion or impaired circulation (e.g., intra-arterial thiopental)
Postembolectomy vasospasm
Raynaud's disease, scleroderma and other arteriopathies, frostbite[a]
Occlusive vascular disease: "acute on chronic" episodes

Pain

Complex Regional Pain Syndromes (CRPS) Type I and Type II[116] (see Chapter 23)
Causalgia following abdominal injury[104]
Herpes zoster
Phantom limb
Paget's disease
Neoplasm
Tropic changes in skin
Pain due to lesions in the CNS[75]

Other

Hyperhidrosis
Miscellaneous conditions in head region: stroke, Meniere's disease, tinnitus
Amblyopia due to quinine poisoning[107] (also causes retinal artery spasm and thrombosis)

These indications are based largely on anecdotal case reports, so that an initial diagnostic blockade should always be accompanied by a separate assessment, by one of the methods in the list on page 423 for sympathetic ablation, blood flow, and pain.

The most controversial indications are stroke and other conditions in the cranial distribution of the sympathetic chain, such as Meniere's disease. At present, no definitive data are available to demonstrate any benefit from sympathetic blockade.

Complications

Intra-arterial and intradural injections are dangerous complications (see following). It should be firmly stated that the negative aspiration test, as described above, does not exclude an intra-arterial or an intradural injection. To prevent the occurrence of these complications, one must realize that the needle should not meet any resistance, after it has passed through the skin, until it rests on what is obviously bone. If the needle is pushed through the prevertebral fascia and the ligaments connecting the transverse processes (this fascia and the ligament can usually be felt), the tip of the needle might be in or close to the vertebral artery or the dural sheath enclosing the cervical nerve roots. Spinal analgesia follows dural sheath injection.

Complications of Cervicothoracic (Stellate Ganglion) Sympathetic Blockade

Common

- Temporary hoarseness and feeling of a lump in the throat (recurrent laryngeal nerve block)
- Unpleasant effects of Horner's syndrome
- Hematoma may occur
- Neuralgia along chest wall and inner aspect of upper arm

[a] All three of these conditions should be treated at an early stage, for "acute or chronic" episodes.

Uncommon

Brachial plexus, rarely affected
Phrenic nerve block
Pneumothorax
Osteitis—transverse process

Severe

Injection into the vertebral artery—immediate CNS effects
Intradural injection—slow onset of symptoms

An injection of local anesthetic solution into the paravertebral fascia may also spread along the fascial plane to involve the brachial plexus.[19] Bilateral injection is inadvisable since inadvertent bilateral recurrent laryngeal nerve block may result in airway problems (loss of laryngeal reflex). Also, loss of cardioaccelerator activity may result in bradycardias and hypotension.

If a hematoma occurs, it might be necessary to inject below C6. This can usually be accomplished because it is possible to feel the prevertebral fascia and the ligaments over C7, after which the needle should be withdrawn several millimeters and the block completed as described above; the risk of pneumothorax increases.

Osteitis of the transverse process has been described after a stellate ganglion block, possibly because the needle traversed the esophagus before it reached the transverse process.[86]

Chemical Stellate Ganglion Block

An injection of 1 to 2 ml of 6% aqueous phenol or 10% phenol in iohexol (Omnipaque®) or Conray® dye (see following) at C6 will interrupt the cervical chain but will not produce a complete cervicothoracic sympathetic blockade. The arm may escape partially, and in these cases an injection of the sympathetic chain at T2 and T3 can be used as a supplement; however, this technique is not commonly practiced because of the proximity of pleura and somatic nerves (see also Chapter 31). A dural sheath may be entered, and injected solutions may migrate by means of the CSF to the nearby medulla, with its important control centers. A persistent Horner's syndrome may also be a problem.

Thoracic Sympathetic Block

Regional Anatomy

The sympathetic chain in the thoracic region lies close to the neck of the ribs, and thus is very close to the somatic roots (Fig. 13-21). In the cervical region, the sympathetic chain is separated from somatic roots by longus colli and anterior scalene muscles and, in the lumbar region, by psoas major. In contrast, no such muscle is present in the thoracic region, and the proximity of the pleura to the sympathetic chain adds a second hazard (Fig. 13-21).

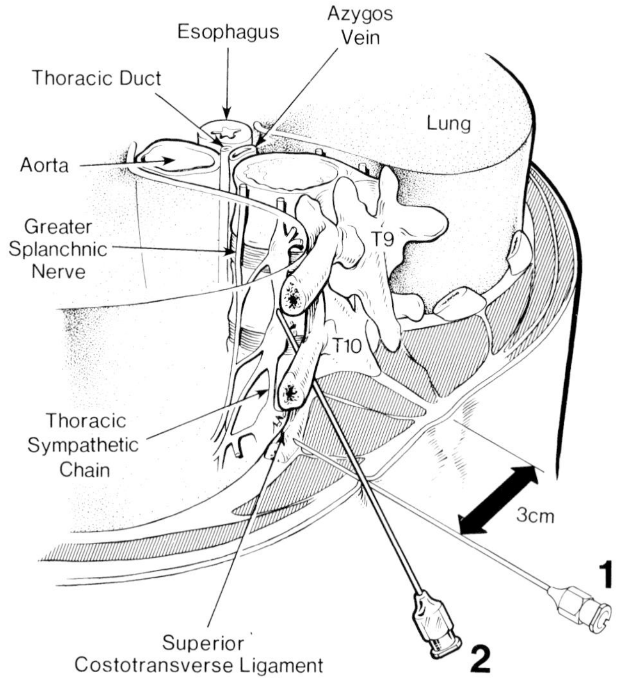

FIG. 13-21. Thoracic sympathetic (paravertebral) block. Needle insertion is 3 cm from the midline, opposite cephalad aspect of spinous process. Needle is initially inserted perpendicular to skin in all planes to reach rib or transverse process at a depth of about 2.5 to 3.5 cm. Sometimes the needle may need to be angled slightly superiorly or inferiorly to locate rib or transverse process. Needle is then directed cephalad above the rib, and a loss of resistance may be detected as the needle penetrates the costotransverse ligament. At this point the needle tip lies in the paravertebral space where both sympathetic and somatic thoracic nerves are located. Careful aspiration must be carried out for air (intrapleural), blood (intravascular), or CSF (intradural).

Technique

A 10-cm needle is introduced and angled toward the vertebral body two fingerbreadths (3 cm) from the midline opposite the T2 spinous process. As the needle is advanced, it either strikes rib or passes through the intercostal space and continues until it is held up by the body of the vertebra in the true paravertebral space (Fig. 13-21). It is generally easy to decide whether the bone encountered is rib or vertebral body, because the rib is more superficial and transmits through the needle a feeling of smoothness in contrast to the gritty roughness of the vertebral body; because of the anatomic problems outlined above, confirmation of position by image intensifier is highly desirable. When the needle reaches the vertebra, it is angled to pass less than 1 cm behind the crest of the vertebral body (Fig. 13-21). At this point, an injection of 2 ml of local anesthetic or, for permanent block, 6% phenol or absolute alcohol, is made, and a successful result is indicated if the patient has a warm dry hand and no evidence of Horner's syndrome. The use of image intensifier and injection, under

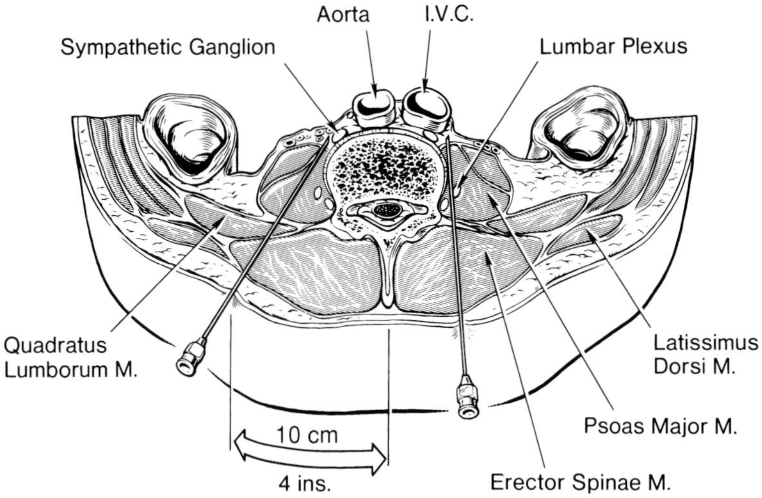

FIG. 13-22. Lumbar sympathetic block. Note that insertion of needle 10 cm from the midline enables the needle to reach the anterolateral angle of the vertebral body. Insertion of needle closer to the midline takes needle path close to somatic nerve roots and lateral to sympathetic chain. (Reproduced with permission from Cherry, D.A., Rao, D.M.: Lumbar sympathetic and coeliac plexus blocks—An anatomical study in cadavers. Br. J. Anaesth., *54*:1037, 1982.)

direct vision, of 10% phenol dissolved in iohexol (Omnipaque®) or Conray-420® (or Angiographin®) greatly increases the safety of this technique.

Indications

Some possible indications for permanent neurolytic sympathectomy for the upper limb syndromes are given in the list on page 429. Many clinics still prefer surgical sympathectomy, although a transaxillary (thoracic) approach is necessary to obtain complete sympathetic denervation of the upper limb; the use of thoracoscopic technique has been a significant advance. The results and complications of the neurolytic technique with an image intensifier remain to be assessed. Intrathoracic pain, such as status anginosus, has been treated by sympathetic block (by either stellate or thoracic approach); however, the availability of betablockers has diminished the appeal of sympathetic block, because the potential complications are very serious in a patient with severe myocardial disease. New options for status anginosus are cervical spinal cord stimulation (see Chapter 32) and epidural or intrathecal opioid and nonopioid drugs administration (see Chapter 29).

Complications

The two principal complications of this technique are pneumothorax and intrathecal injection[100] by way of the intervertebral foramen. Because of these two complications, this technique was used only minimally, until recent application of image-intensifier techniques allowed direct viewing of needle placement and appropriate spread of solution.

Lumbar Sympathetic Block

Regional Anatomy

The lumbar part of the sympathetic chain and its ganglia lie in the fascial plane close to the anterolateral side of the vertebral bodies, separated from somatic nerves by the psoas fascia and psoas muscle (Figs. 13-22 and 13-23). An injection of a large volume of fluid (e.g., 25 ml) anywhere in this space will, in most instances, fill the whole space. Theoretically, one injection at L2 or L3 should be enough to achieve adequate longitudinal spread. This single injection technique is now used by a number of experienced specialists in pain clinics (see below). However, in other clinics, injections are performed at two different levels, particularly with a neu-

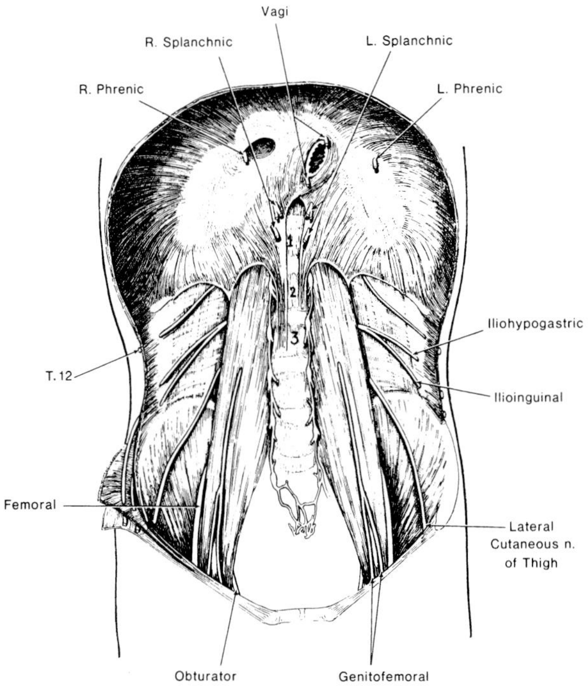

FIG. 13-23. Posterior abdominal wall, genitofemoral nerve. Note its course anterior to psoas major, thus being more vulnerable to neurolytic solution spreading laterally from the sympathetic chain. (Modified from Bryce-Smith, R., and Macintosh, R.R.: Local Analgesia: Abdomen. Edinburgh, Livingstone Press, 1962.)

rolytic agent such as phenol, to limit lateral spread at any one level, since this poses a risk of spread across psoas to the genitofemoral nerve, perhaps by a fibrous tunnel to a somatic nerve or, worse still, to a dural cuff region and thence to subarachnoid space (see Fig. 13-24).[17] When continuous blockade with catheters is used, it is also preferable to have two catheters because there is a tendency for a catheter to slide dorsally out of position.

In an anatomic study, lumbar sympathetic blocks were performed "blind" in cadavers to investigate the frequency of puncture of a major organ.[21] The technique of inserting the needles was based on that of Mandl (see following). With the cadaver in the lateral position, three 22-gauge, 15-cm needles were inserted about 10 cm (4 in) from the midline at the approximate levels of L1, L2, and L3. In thin cadavers, the distance of insertion of the needles from the midline was less, about 7.5 cm, whereas in obese subjects the distance was greater (up to 12.5 cm). Each needle was advanced onto the vertebral body, gradually positioned more anteriorly until it slipped beyond the anterolateral aspect of the vertebral body (see Fig. 13-22), and then advanced to the "hilt" to allow the cadaver to be positioned supine. The cadaver was then rolled over and the performance repeated on the other side.

Eighty needles were inserted in the direction of the lumbar sympathetic chain, and 95% passed either through the lumbar sympathetic chain or within 0.5 cm of it. In 90% of those occasions on which the chain was not traversed, the needles were lateral to the chain.

One needle passed through the hilum of the kidney, although in that cadaver there was a large osteophyte over an intervertebral disk that displaced the needle laterally. Two needles were found embedded in grossly osteoporotic vertebral bodies. All three of these placements would, doubtless, have been prevented by using a *c*-arm image intensifier like that used routinely in clinical practice. The position of the lumbar sympathetic chain was found to be remarkably constant on the anterolateral aspect of the vertebral bodies.

Almost all of the needles either passed through the sympathetic chain or lateral to it. As Figure 13-22 shows, the more lateral the insertion of the needle, the closer the tip should be to the lumbar sympathetic chain. There is also a

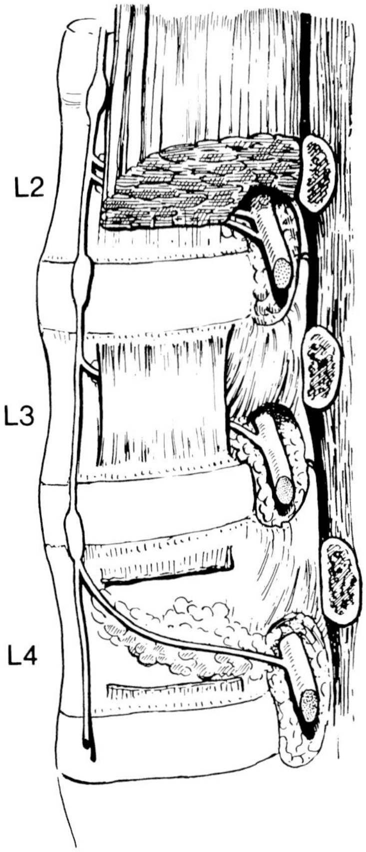

A

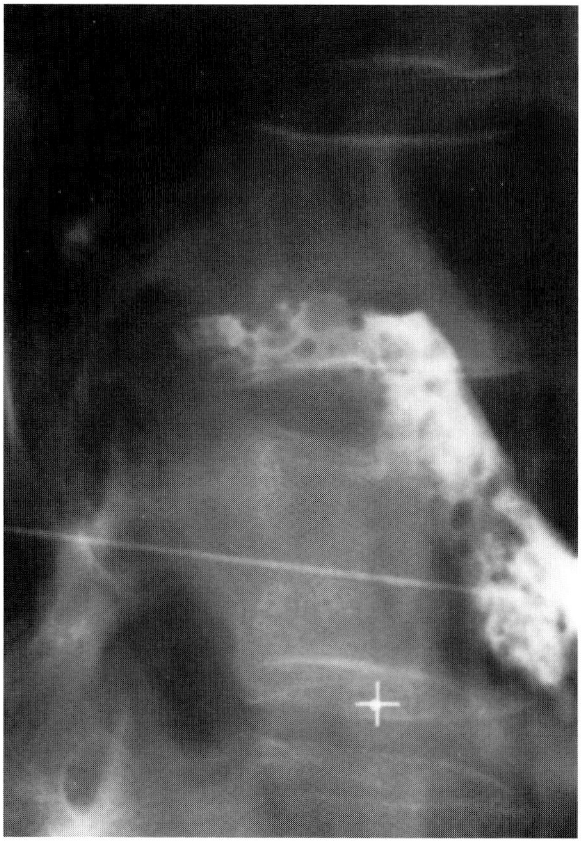

B

FIG. 13-24. A: Fibrous arch between paravertebral space and lumbar sympathetic chain. This pathway poses a potential for spread of neurolytic solution to somatic nerve roots, resulting in possible sensory loss or neuralgia. (Modified from Bryce-Smith, R., and Macintosh, R.R.: Local Analgesia Abdomen. Edinburgh, Livingstone Press, 1962.) **B:** Contrast medium injected too close to side of vertebral body spreading via fibrous arch.

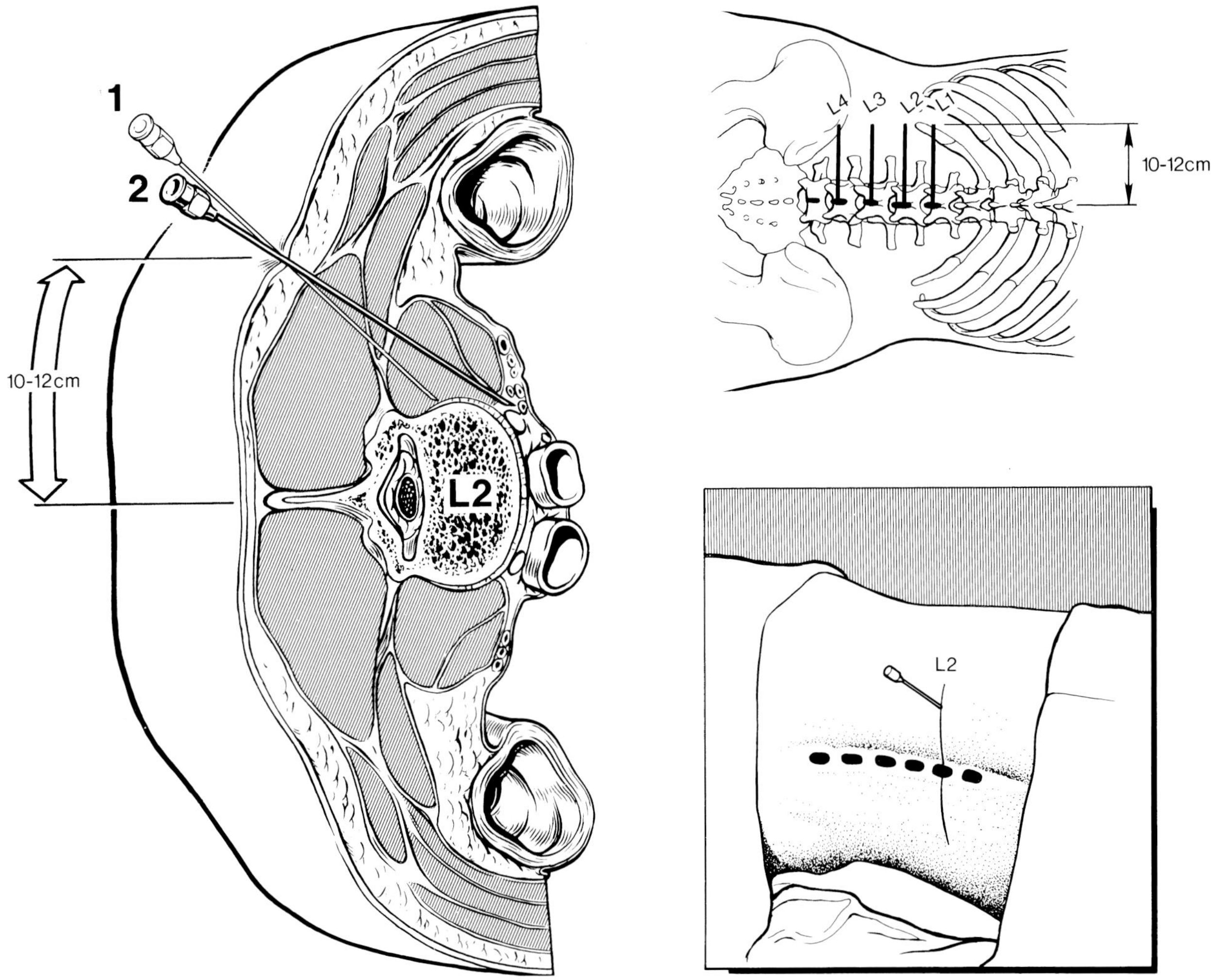

FIG. 13-25. Technique of lumbar sympathetic block. Note location of skin marks for L1 and L4 spinous processes, which then permit identification of L2 and L3. A line is drawn through the center of the spinous processes; this will lie below the transverse process of that vertebra. Needle insertion *(1)* is at the lateral margin of the erector spinae muscle (approximately 10 to 12 cm from midline). If it is desired to check the depth of the transverse process, the needle must be angled cephalad. Otherwise the needle is inserted approximately 45° toward the vertebral body until this structure is located. Then the needle is angled more steeply until it slips just past the vertebral body and through the psoas fascia *(2)* (see text). A single needle can be used instead of two or three needles; however, an increased volume must be injected.

lesser risk of piercing roots of the lumbar plexus or of contacting the transverse process.

Technique (Mandl) with Two Needles

The method of blocking the lumbar sympathetic chain was first introduced by Mandl in 1926 and was similar to that used by Kappis for injecting the celiac plexus.[59,83]

The spinous processes of L1 and L4 are marked as reference points. L1 is level with the line between the two points where the lateral side of the erector spinae muscles meets the 12th ribs; a line joining the posterior superior iliac crests passes through the lower part of the spine at L4 (see Fig. 13-25).

A subcutaneous wheal is raised about 8 to 10 cm laterally to the middle of the spinous processes of L2 and L4. Local anesthetic solution is injected subcutaneously (and with an intramuscular needle, against the transverse process above or below the site of injection by directing the needle 45° cranially or caudally and in between the transverse processes, if these are to be contacted).

A 20- to 22-gauge needle of approximately 12 cm in length (or an 18-gauge needle for continuous blockade) with a rubber marker is introduced through the skin until the tip of the needle has reached a transverse process. The marker is pushed down to the skin and the needle withdrawn. The distance from the skin to the transverse process is, in the normal adult, roughly half the distance from the skin to the lateral side of the vertebral body (10 cm). This may be a shorter distance if the patient has thin back muscles, and longer if the muscles are thick. The marker on the needle is moved toward the hub of the needle so that the distance from the tip to the marker is roughly twice the first marked distance.

The needle is reintroduced and directed slightly medially to pass between the transverse processes. When bone is reached, the marker should be almost flush with the skin, the bevel of the needle being directed toward the lateral side of the vertebral body. A slight change in angle of the needle will allow the tip of the needle to slide off the vertebra and to reach the sympathetic chain on the ventrolateral aspect of the vertebral body (see Fig. 13-22).[38] Correct position can be verified by using a loss-of-resistance test, with a syringe filled with air or saline. Penetration of the psoas fascia gives a resistance change not dissimilar to that of epidural block. Some specialists prefer to avoid the transverse process, so that the needle proceeds directly to the lateral aspect of the vertebral body (see following). A loss of resistance, at a shallower level, is often obtained between psoas and quadratus lumborum in the region of the transverse process (see Fig. 13-22). Placement of solution at this level would result in lumbar plexus block—highly undesirable if a neurolytic solution is used.

In clinical practice, the anesthesiologist often starts at L2 and, in a second step, introduces the needle at L4. When the needle is correctly placed at L2, the part of the needle outside the skin should be measured and the marker for L4 properly placed. In most patients, owing to the lumbar lordosis at L4, the distance from the skin to the vertebral body is usually a little greater than at L2. It is vitally important to aspirate to ensure that neither blood nor CSF is present, and to check that there is no resistance to injection; resistance could be due to the needle being in the wall of the aorta or vena cava, an abdominal viscus, or an intervertebral disk. Once again, radiographic confirmation (local anesthetic mixed with contrast medium) and injection under direct vision increase safety.[9,24,36,116]

In the most simple cases (e.g., renal colic), one injection of 20 to 30 ml, preferably of 0.25% bupivacaine with epinephrine, 1:200,000 (5 μg/ml), at L2 will completely eradicate pain. In patients with obliterative arterial disease, a diagnostic block with 1 to 5 ml of local anesthetic mixed with contrast medium, may be made at L2 and L4 under radiographic control. The continuous blockade technique is also very useful; needles are placed at L2 and L4, and, after the proper positioning of each needle, catheters are passed through the needles, which are then withdrawn over the catheters. The catheters are fixed along the erector spinae muscles. The cranial ends of the catheters, each with a needle and a Millipore filter, are placed in a sterile sponge in the supraclavicular fossa. The time interval between injections may be increased to 6 hours if bupivacaine is used. The continuous blockade is maintained for 5 days, during which the clinical effects of the blockade should be evaluated. In the case of the single-shot diagnostic block, the volume of local anesthetic in contrast medium should be the same as that proposed for neurolytic block. Also, a method of assessment from each category on the list on page 423 should be used immediately after the block. Often, diagnostic blocks are repeated if there is any doubt about results.[12]

In most instances, the procedure is short (<30 min) and fairly free of pain. Heavy premedication or general anesthesia is not necessary. Now and then, however, a needle may pass close to a segmental nerve, provoking "lightening" pain. The needle should always be advanced slowly and redirected slightly, if paresthesia should occur. The needle should not be directed too much toward the midline. We believe that it is better to be able to detect that the needle is close to a nerve in a lightly medicated patient than to accept the risk of undetected laceration of the nerve with a fairly large needle in a patient under general anesthesia. One case of severe segmental neuralgia, most likely the result of a nerve injury, supports this view.[24]

Single Injection Technique for Local Anesthetic or Neurolytic Block

Hatangdi and Boas describe the use of the tip of the 12th rib to act as a marker for needle insertion 2 to 3 cm below and medial to that point.[53] This allows easy access to the L3 vertebral body, and then placement next to sympathetic chain is verified, as above. Sufficient solution is injected (mixed with contrast medium) to cover L2, L3, and L4 levels. An alternative is to use the 12th rib to intersect a line drawn through

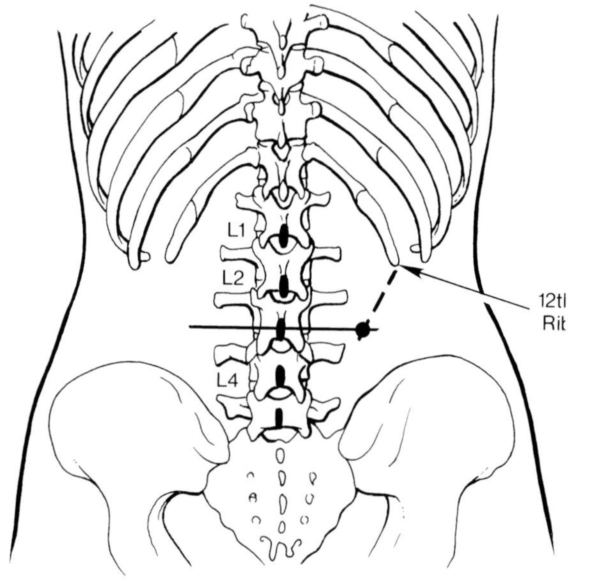

FIG. 13-26. Single needle technique of lumbar sympathetic block (see text). Note needle insertion 2 to 3 cm below and medial to the tip of the 12th rib. This should lie on a line through the center of L3 spinous process (see text). (Hatangdi, V.S., and Boas, R.V.: Lumbar sympathectomy: A single needle technique. Br. J. Anaesth., *57*:285, 1985.)

the middle of the L2 spinous process. Needle insertion at this point should be sufficiently lateral to obtain easy access to the L3 level. If desired, the transverse process can be avoided and the needle inserted directly onto the lateral aspect of the vertebral body. Sufficient solution is then injected to cover the sympathetic chain (Fig. 13-26).

Technique of Bryce-Smith

An alternative approach to local anesthetic lumbar sympathetic blockade has been described by Bryce Smith (1951).[16]

Because of the anterolateral position of the ganglia in the lumbar region, the course of the rami communicantes is long and winds around the vertebral body in a fibrous tunnel. This arch forms one of the origins of the psoas muscle and provides indirect access to the lumbar sympathetic chain (Fig. 13-27).

A wheal is raised three fingerbreadths lateral to the tip of the spinous process of L3, and a 12-cm needle is introduced at 70° and advanced toward the body of the vertebra; when the point of the needle reaches the body of the vertebra, it lies within the fibrous tunnel (Fig. 13-27). Fifteen to 20 ml of solution are deposited here, and this tracks forward to reach the sympathetic chain. This approach should not be used when neurolytic solutions are employed, because some of the fluid backtracks and causes a neuritis of the third lumbar nerve or enters a dural cuff and causes paraplegia.

Because this technique frequently leads to somatic block and does *not* provide a selective sympathetic block, it is also not indicated for diagnosis of pain syndromes.

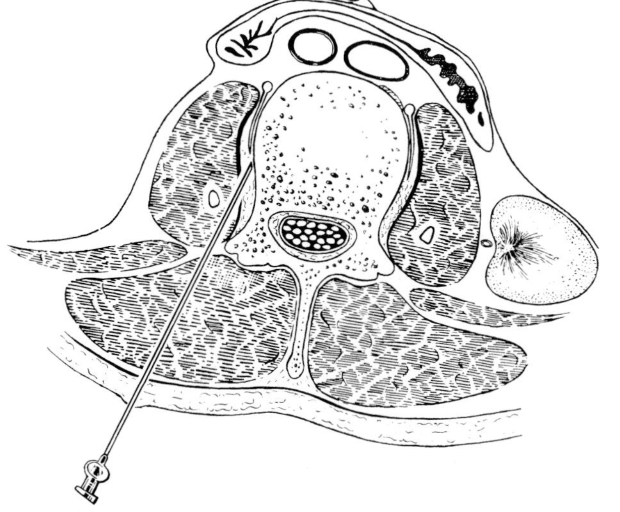

FIG. 13-27. Alternative technique for local anesthetic lumbar sympathetic block (see text). (Modified from Bryce-Smith, R., and Macintosh, R. R.: Local Analgesia: Abdomen. Edinburgh, Livingstone Press, 1962.)

Lumbar Sympathectomy with Neurolytic Agent

Neurolytic lumbar sympathectomy should be used for the treatment of vascular disease in consultation with a vascular surgeon. It is clear that even a successful sympathetic block in a patient with rest pain may result sometimes in demarcation of a nonviable area, such as a distal phalanx of a toe. This will require appropriate surgical treatment and should not be viewed as a disappointing side effect of the block, but rather as a necessary part of a rational treatment regimen.[18,93]

The use of lumbar sympathetic block with proper collaboration offers the following very considerable advantages:

Symptoms can be ameliorated without risk of surgery and anesthesia in a group of patients with a high incidence of severe ischemic heart disease, pulmonary disease, and other problems of old age. In the series reported by Reid and colleagues[98], there was a mortality of 1:1666 injections (less than 0.1%); this compares favorably with surgical sympathectomy, which has a mortality rate of at least 6% and as much as 20% in patients with severe vascular disease. In a recent series of 386 blocks, there was only 1 death within 1 week of blockade, and this patient had severe ischemic heart disease with congestive cardiac failure prior to blockade.[24]

Outpatient Treatment. Treatment may be performed on an outpatient basis, and elderly patients (usually 60–80 years of age) can be released after a short stay. This allows for considerable economy in hospital-bed use; surgical sympathectomy often requires 6 to 10 days in the hospital, when there are no complications.

Fewer Postoperative Thrombotic Phenomena. Such complications are reduced in the elderly because an operation and bed rest are avoided.

A large turnover of patients is possible (as many as 8 to 10 procedures in a single-day session).

If necessary, a bilateral procedure can be performed, with the second side blocked 1 week later, also on an outpatient basis.

Duration. Because the duration of sympathetic ablation is similar with surgical or neurolytic sympathectomy (mean, 6 months), the neurolytic technique offers an advantage. It can be repeated with very minimal morbidity. Nevertheless, the natural history of occlusive vascular disease is such that in one series only 5% required repeated blockade.[24]

Agents

Absolute alcohol has been used by several groups; however, it has a higher incidence of L1 neuralgia (see Chapter 31).[24] Seven percent phenol in water was used by Reid and colleagues in a very large series because of the low viscosity of the solution and ease of injection.[98] Seven percent to 10% phenol in iohexol (Omnipaque®), Conray-420® dye or Angiographin® has a similar low resistance to injection and the added advantage of being visible under image intensifier

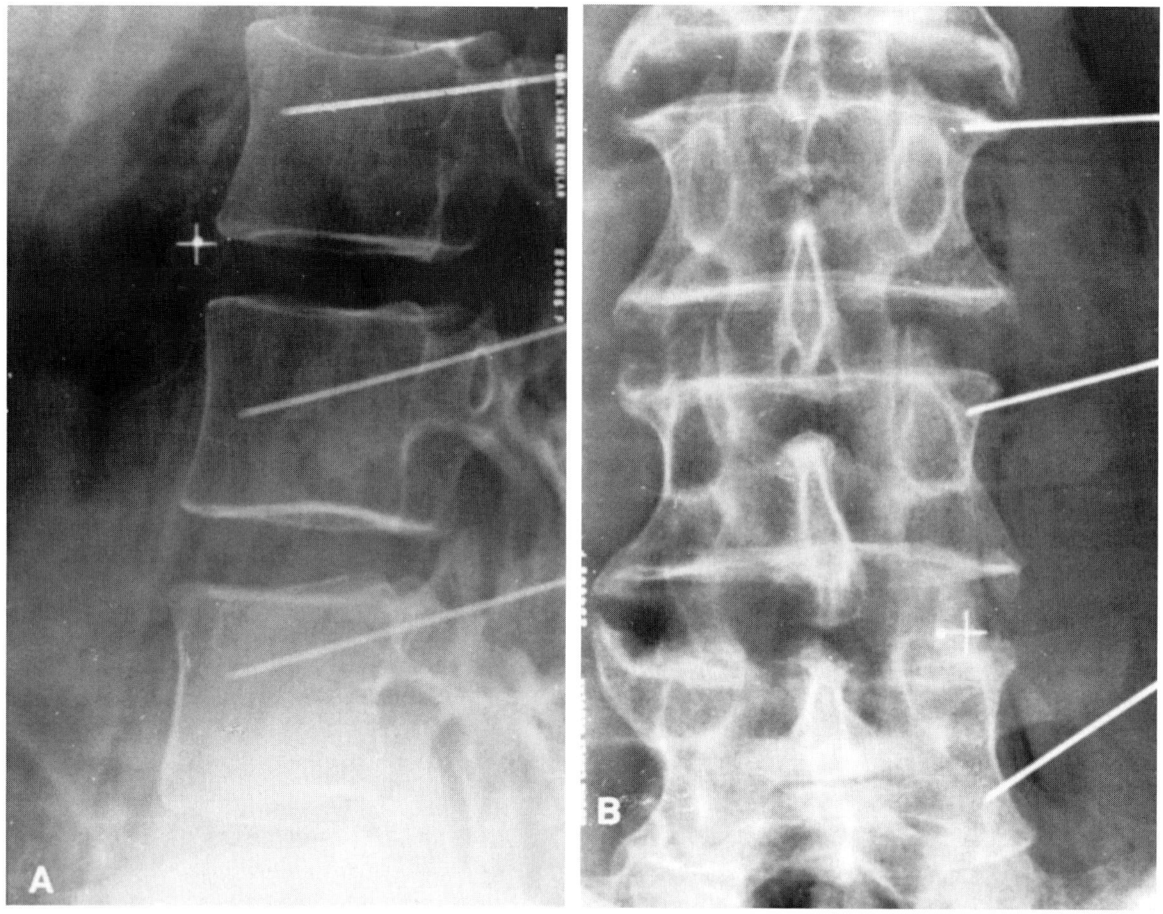

FIG. 13-28. A: X-ray: Needle placement, lateral view. **B:** X-ray: Needle placement, anteroposterior view.

(see Fig. 13-29).[9,24,36,117] When the patient is placed on his or her side under a vertical radiographic beam, it is also of value for the person to be tilted slightly, ventrally and dorsally, to check that the needle is fairly close to the vertebral column. One report advocates the semi-prone position with vertical x-ray screening to give a more precise view of needle position relative to vertebral body anterolateral aspect, with a single x-ray view.[62] If a biplanar image intensifier is available, then both lateral and anteroposterior views should be obtained (see Fig. 13-28). A convenient way to determine the spread is to dissolve phenol in an aqueous radiographic contrast medium (Omnipaque®, Conray-420®, or Angiographin®) and to inject it under direct radiographic control. This often allows confirmation of complete coverage of the lumbar sympathetic chain, with as little as 3 to 4 ml of solution (see Fig. 31-31).

Technique

The following modifications of local anesthetic blockade are advisable when neurolytic agents are used:

1. A radiopaque marker is placed on the skin,[50] and the level of needle insertion is checked under image intensifier. Needle position in the center of L2 and L4 vertebral bodies is checked with a lateral view (Fig. 13-28). Proximity of the needle to the disk space is avoided.
2. Needle position at the anterolateral angle of the L2 and L4 bodies is also checked in the lateral view (Fig. 13-28). Lack of movement of the needle during deep inspiration and expiration is checked carefully. With correct placement in psoas, needle tips should be immobile. Movement on respiration indicates placement lateral to psoas—possibly in the kidney.
3. An anteroposterior view is taken to check that each needle is close to the lateral aspects of the vertebral bodies (see Fig. 13-28).
4. Initially, 0.5 ml of contrast medium is injected and confirmation obtained that a sharp linear spread is occurring (Fig. 13-29). Resistance to injection and the appearance of a "blob" or fuzzy patch of contrast medium indicate injection into muscle or fascia, and injection is ceased (see Fig. 13–30).
5. As soon as linear spread is obtained, the injection is continued with neurolytic solution until each level has lin-

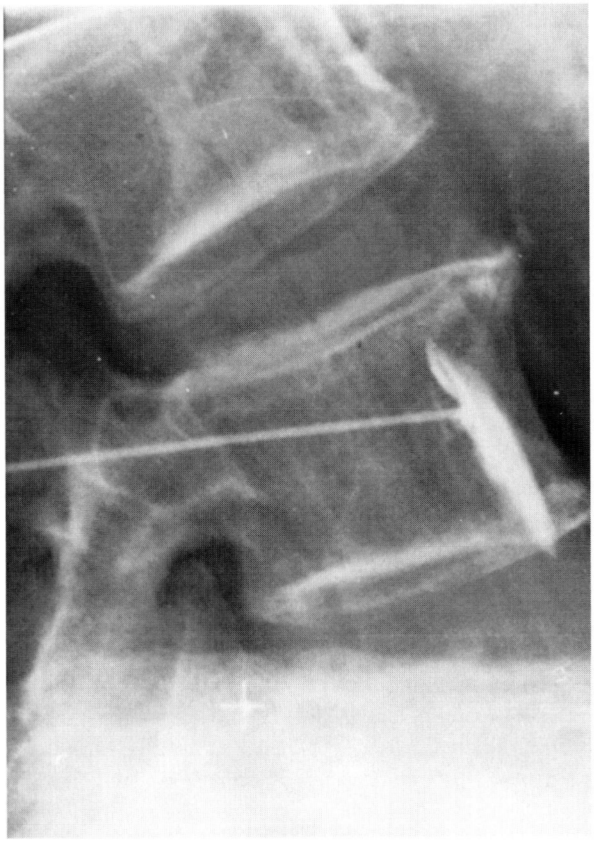

FIG. 13-29. Injection of 0.5 ml of contrast medium, showing correct linear spread along anterior aspect of psoas fascia.

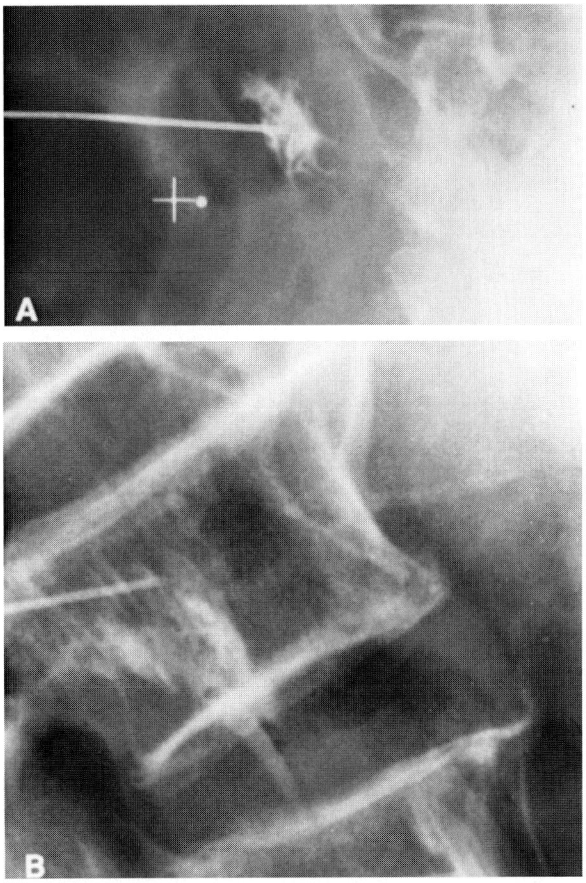

FIG. 13-30. A: X-ray showing injection of contrast medium into psoas major. **B:** X-ray showing injection too far posteriorly, probably between psoas and quadratus lumborum.

ear coverage. In most instances this requires no more than 2 ml and often as little as 1 ml of solution (see Fig. 13-31).

6. At the completion of the injection, an anteroposterior view is taken to confirm the spread of solution along the lateral aspect of the vertebral body (see Fig. 13-31).
7. Finally, 0.5 ml of air is injected immediately before removing each needle to prevent the needle's depositing neurolytic solution on somatic nerve roots during removal.

Patients are kept on their sides for 5 minutes to prevent the solution from spreading laterally toward the genitofemoral nerve or posteriorly between the slips of origin of the psoas major, and along the fibrous tunnel occupied by the rami communicates, toward somatic nerve roots.[16,17] Patients are then turned supine but instructed not to raise their heads for 30 minutes. Observations of skin temperature, blood pressure, and pulse are continued.

Recovery Procedure

Observations are continued for 1 hour in a recovery room, and, if stable, patients are permitted to sit to 45° and begin oral intake again. Blood pressure is checked sitting and then standing, and, if unchanged, patients are allowed to ambulate and the intravenous line is removed. Most outpatients are then able to go home, accompanied by a friend or relative. Patients with highly unstable cardiovascular disease are to be kept and maintained on an observation chart for at least 24 hours postblock.

Indications

The most common clinical indications for lumbar sympathetic blocks are listed as follows.

Clinical Conditions That Lumbar Sympathetic Blockade May Benefit

Circulatory insufficiency in the leg

Arteriosclerotic disease, severe pain +++, gangrene ++; intermittent claudication[a] ++ in selected cases; diabetic gangrene +, Buerger's disease +,

[a] Aortoiliac (small percentage responding) and femoropopliteal (higher percentage responding)

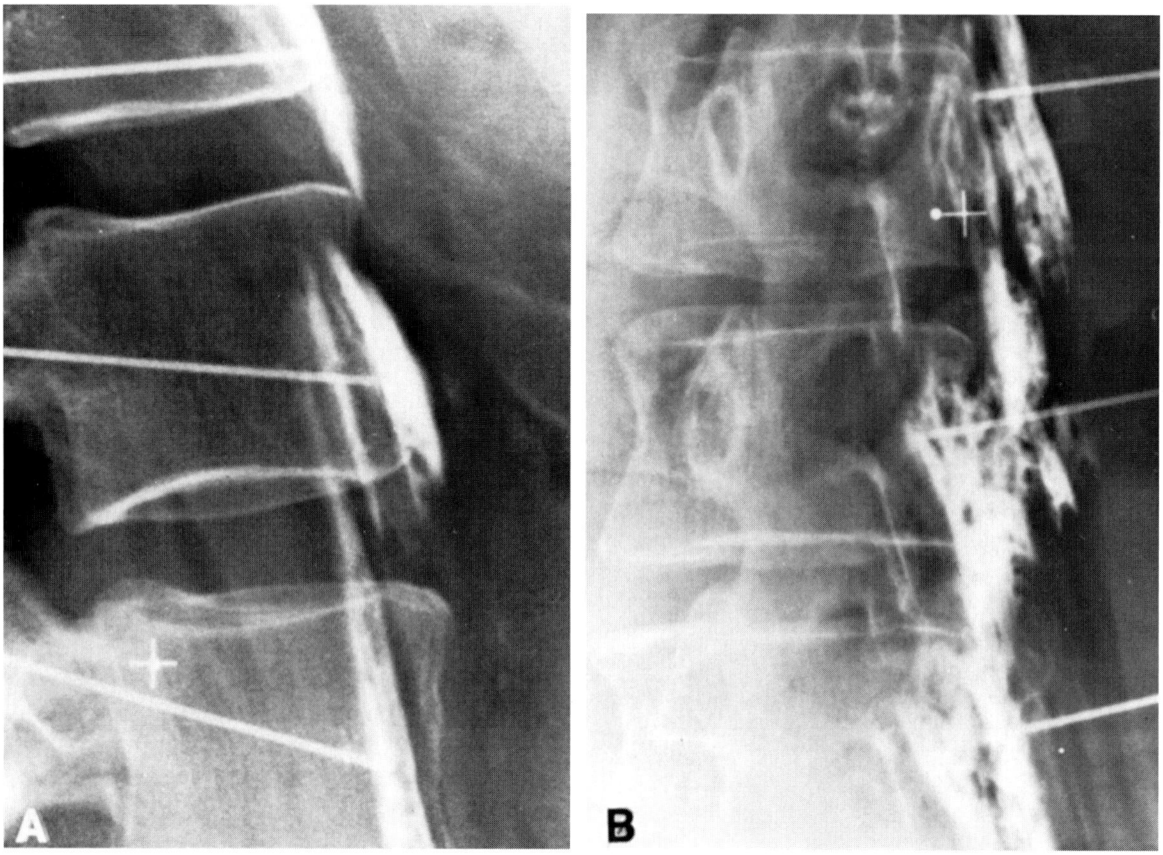

FIG. 13-31. **A:** Lateral view. Complete coverage of L2 and L4 vertebral body levels with injection of only 1 ml of 10% phenol on Conray 420 at each level. **B:** Anteroposterior view to show spread of solution following line of psoas muscle. Note limitation of lateral spread to reduce risk of genitofemoral nerve involvement.

After reconstructive vascular surgery, and
Arterial embolus

Pain

Renal colic,
Complex regional pain syndrome[b] Type I and Type II (see Chapter 23)
Herpes zoster,
Intractable urogenital pain in selected cases,
Phantom limb[b],
Amputation stump pain[b], and
Chilblains

General

Hyperhidrosis—reduced sympathetic activity to reduce sweating,
White leg phlegmasia alba dolens[c]
Trench foot[c]
Erythromelalgia[c], and
Acrocyanosis[c]

Some clinics have stopped using diagnostic blocks for patients with atherosclerotic vascular disease and rest pain, skin ulcers, or gangrene. Their rationale is that the incidence of adverse effects is extremely low and many of these patients tolerate multiple procedures poorly. In a recent series with measurement of pain, blood flow, and sympathetic activity, the results of diagnostic and neurolytic sympathetic blocks were essentially the same in every patient studied (see Fig. 13-7).[117] In younger patients with less well-defined chronic pain syndromes, however, diagnostic blocks should be performed before neurolytic sympathetic block. As discussed in the section on physiologic effects of sympathectomy, the best rationale for the use of lumbar sympathectomy in arterial disease is to obtain improved skin blood flow; however, pain relief may occur even without improved blood flow. Tables 13–1 to 13–3 summarize clinical data on the use of lumbar sympathectomy for pain and skin ulcers, as well as for other conditions in which its efficacy is more difficult to determine except by diagnostic block in each case.

TABLE 13-1. *Lumbar sympathetic block: examples of uses and results in three clinical series*

Study[a]	Number of cases
After vascular surgery ("continuous" local anesthetic lumbar sympathetic block)	70
Arterial embolism—no surgery	13 (7 improved)
Cytostatic perfusion (melanoma)	4
Frostbite	2
	89
Obliterative arterial disease (local anesthetic block followed by chemical sympathectomy in 72 cases)	122 (see Table 13-2)
Diagnostic local anesthetic followed by neurolytic agent[b]	
Rest pain and ischemic ulcers	386 (80% relieved)
Gangrene of lower extremity (pain relief and speeding up demarcation)	50 (55% relieved)
Reflex sympathetic dysfunction	12 (50%) relieved—those treated early)
Claudication	12 (50% relieved; only those with response to local anesthetic block received neurolytic block)
Neurolytic agent over 10-year period[c]	
Rest pain	194 (80% relieved)
Gangrene of lower extremity	40 (50% relieved)
Reflex sympathetic dysfunction (post-traumatic)	42 (45% relieved—those treated early)
Phantom limb	19 (60% relieved)

[a] Data from Löfström, B., and Zetterquist, S.: Lumbar sympathetic blocks in the treatment of patients with obliterative arterial disease of the lower limb. Int. Anesthesiol. Clin., *7*: 423, 1969.
[b] Data from Cousins, M. J., Reeve, T. S., Glynn, C. J., Walsh, J. A., *et al.*: Neurolytic lumbar sympathetic blockade: Duration of denervation and relief of rest pain. Anaesth. Intensive Care, *7*(2):121, 1979.
[c] Unpublished data from Lloyd, J. W., *et al.*

Complications

Complications of lumbar sympathetic blocks are extremely rare; however, a needle directed too far medially may pass into an intervertebral foramen, causing paraplegia. This may be recognized by the flow of cerebrospinal fluid (CSF), but it is not always the case. Thus, confirmation of correct placement by radiography is highly desirable (see also Chapter 22).

Complications of Lumbar Sympathetic Blockade[b]

Puncture of major vessel or renal pelvis, Subarachnoid injection,
Neuralgia—genitofemoral nerve (5% to 10% pain in the groin),
Somatic nerve, damage—neuralgia (1%),
Perforation of a disk,
Stricture of the ureter after phenol or alcohol injection,

[b] See Chapter 23; only useful *early* in these conditions
[c] Miscellaneous conditions in which reduced sympathetic activity may help to correct an abnormality in nutritive blood flow or venous or lymphatic drainage.

[b] Pain in the groin following injection is the most common untoward sequel. Subarachnoid tap is seen occasionally but is easily recognized and should not constitute a hazard. The remaining complications are very rare, when image intensifier control is used.

TABLE 13-2. *Results of lumbar sympathetic blockade in patients with obliterative arterial disease*

Primary symptoms	Number of patients		Results of initial continuous local anesthetic and neurolytic block: Pain relief 2+	1+	0	–
Gangrene arteriosclerotic	55	L.A.[a]	28		27	0
			∴28 phenol blocks			
			14	9	5	0
Diabetic neuropathic pain	28	L.A.	14		14	
			∴14 phenol blocks			
			8	4	2	0
Severe rest pain	23	L.A.	19	4	0	0
			23			
			∴ 18 phenol blocks (5 resolved with L.A.)			
			18	0	0	0
Intermittent claudication	16	L.A.	7	6	2	1
			12			
			∴ 12 phenol blocks (1 resolved with L.A.)			
			7		9	

[a] L.A., initial local anesthetic block. (Kövames, A., and Löfström, B.: Continuous lumbar sympathetic blocks in the treatment of patients with ischemic lower limbs. 10th Congress of Int. Cardiovascular Soc., 1971.)

Infection from catheter technique (extremely rare),
Ejaculatory failure (bilateral block in young males), and
Chronic back pain

After surgical and chemical sympathectomies, a pain or discomfort in the groin is often seen, hypothetically attributed to a genitofemoral nerve neuralgia. The discomfort may last 2 to 5 weeks.[9,24,29,97] This is so-called L1 neuralgia and is characterized by hyperesthesia in L1 distribution, and a burning pain. The patient often says that it is unbearable even to have clothes touch the thigh and may also describe the leg as "feeling as though it will explode." The condition responds well to transcutaneous electrical stimulation. The incidence is much higher with alcohol and appears to be least when the volume injected at any one level is the minimal amount necessary to achieve coverage of sympathetic ganglia, as checked by image-intensifier.[24]

TABLE 13-3. *Percentage of patients with occlusive vascular disease who responded to lumbar sympathetic block*

Rest pain (%)	Skin lesions (%)	Claudication (%)	References
	55	13	44, 45
	60	41	106
	64		8
57	45		61
71	55	20	49
62	100 (5/5)		87
63–51	35		105
48 (some)	33		42
57	43		102
	6		41
49 (complete relief)	50	–	24
80 (complete or partial relief)		–	24
–	–	0	43
–	–	0	88

INTRAVENOUS REGIONAL SYMPATHETIC BLOCK[51]

Site of Action and Efficacy

Intravenous regional sympathetic block[51] is based on the "Bier block," a local anesthetic intravenous regional block described in Chapter 12. The sympathetic blocking drug guanethidine (Ismelin®) has a high affinity for sympathetic nerve endings, where it displaces norepinephrine (NE) from presynaptic vesicles and prevents reuptake of NE. This causes a brief initial release of NE, followed by NE depletion (see Fig. 13-4), which results in long-lasting intravenous regional sympathetic blocks (IVRS) when the "Bier block" technique is used. Guanethidine has an advantage over reserpine, which has a similar action, except that reserpine crosses the blood-brain barrier and produces CNS effects, whereas guanethidine does not. Controlled studies now have documented the efficacy of IV regional guanethidine in increasing blood flow[10,47,85,114] and skin temperature[10,85] while decreasing the vasoconstrictor ice response[47] and reducing pain[10,14,85] in vascular disease[47] and reflex sympathetic dystrophies.[10,34,47] Sweating is not reduced[47,85] because it is mediated by cholinergic postganglionic sympathetic fibers.

A controlled study in volunteers compared guanethidine and reserpine, and found that only guanethidine significantly increased temperature after cold challenge and that this effect lasted 3 days.[85]

Duration of effect and efficacy of guanethidine was compared with stellate ganglion block in a randomized trial in patients with reflex sympathetic dystrophies.[10] In patients treated with stellate ganglion blocks, skin temperature and skin plethysmography measurements were significantly increased at 1 hour but not at later times. In patients treated with guanethidine, skin temperature was increased at 1 hour, 24 hours, and 48 hours postblock. Skin plethysmography measurements were significantly increased at 24 hours and remained so at 48 hours.[10]

Stellate blocks every other day (up to total of eight blocks) produced similar clinical effects to IV guanethidine block every 4 days (up to total of four blocks) in terms of pain score and clinical signs, when assessed at 1 month and 3 month follow-up.[10]

In a within-patient study of IV guanethidine blocks compared to placebo, skin temperature, and hand blood flow were significantly increased at 1 hour postblock.[47] At seven days postblock, hand blood flow, but not skin temperature, was increased. Vasoconstrictor response to ice was decreased at 1 hour and 7 days postblock.[47]

Thus there is good evidence that an intravenous regional sympathetic block offers the following: (i) It is less "invasive" and uncomfortable for patients; (ii) it results in significant modification of noradrenergic activity, that is, increased blood flow and decreased pain; and (iii) effects are longer-lasting than those of stellate blocks, 4 to 7 days, compared with less than 1 day. However, cholinergic activity is *not* modified.

A further application of IV sympathetic block is in (upper) limb angiography, where the vasodilatation greatly facilitates delineation of the vasculature.[114] It is also suggested as an aid to maintaining tissue perfusion in tissue-grafting operations.[114] In patients with severe vascular disease, in whom inflation of a tourniquet may be dangerous, guanethidine can be infused slowly into an artery by means of a narrow gauge needle, with effects similar to those of the IV technique.

Current and Future Options

In some countries, for example, the United States, an IV preparation of guanethidine is no longer available[c] since the drug has ceased to be of value, by this route, for hypertension. For this reason, we must examine other potential candidates for use in this valuable technique. Figure 13-32 gives a summary of sympathetic nerve transmission at the adrenergic nerve terminal, sites of action of neurotransmitters, and other factors influencing smooth muscle cells of the vasculature.

Interference with NF Synthesis. Methyldopa (Aldomet) was previously thought to have a predominantly peripheral action, leading to formation of a "false transmitter" α-methylnorepinephrine. It now seems, however, that this is metabolized to a powerful agonist methylepinephrine. Thus methyldopa is not an attractive choice for IV regional block.

Storage Vesicle Depletion and Block of NE Reuptake. Guanethidine and reserpine are the only drugs that have been evaluated and the only clinical options, where approved. Guanethidine and also bretylium block coupling of the action potential to NE release. Bretylium also blocks NE reuptake.

Reserpine is relatively ineffective and produces many side effects. Bretylium allows only 2 to 7 hours of pain relief after IVRS.[52] Many other drugs prevent NE reuptake, but none have been used for IVRS (e.g., tricyclic antidepressants, cocaine).

Block of Presynaptic (α_2) and Postsynaptic (α_1) Receptors. Phentolamine (Regitine) has been given in a dose of 10 mg IV for IVRS. Precise data on duration of effect are not available. Arnér[1] has shown that intravenous infusion of phentolamine can predict the therapeutic effect of IVRS with guanethidine ("the intravenous phentolamine test").

Block of Postsynaptic Receptors (α_1). Prazocin (Minipress®) is a relatively pure α_1-blocker. It does not interfere with the negative feedback on NE release that is mediated by means of α_2-receptors. There is no increase in NE release and no compensatory tachycardia seen with phentolamine. Duration of effect with IVRS is not known because an IV preparation has not been approved.

Other α_1-blockers are under development and include trimazosin and tarazosin. The latter may be of interest because of its reported long duration of effect. All of these drugs pose a potential for postural hypotension and water retention.

Block of NE Activity at Level of Vascular Smooth Muscle. This is a complex area, and precise sites of action are not delineated.

Prostaglandins (e.g., PGI_2). In most vascular beds there is a balance between dilatation effects produced by molecules such as PGE_1 and PGI_2 and vasoconstriction effects produced by thromboxanes. PGI_2 is five times more potent than PGE_1 in producing vasodilatation in coronary, renal, mesenteric, and skeletal muscle beds. Effects on arterioles are much greater than on veins. It is possible that the vascular effects are produced by inhibition of NE release from sympathetic nerve endings. There may also be a direct effect on smooth muscle. Both PGI_2 and PGE_1 inhibit platelet aggregation. It should be noted that PGE_1 causes uterine contraction, and is used to produce abortion. Both PGE_1 and PGI_2 have been used by IVRS in patients with severe peripheral vascular disease. Both were reported to give significant and long lasting improvement in blood flow and tissue oxygenation.[94,103] No preparations of these drugs are currently available for IVRS.

Hydralazine (Apresoline®) and Diazoxide (Hyperstat IV®). These two drugs have a direct effect on vascular smooth muscle that is as yet poorly defined. Effects on arterioles are greater than on veins. Experimental work has shown a

---

[c] In the United States and some other countries, guanethidine is available for "investigational" use by the IV route.

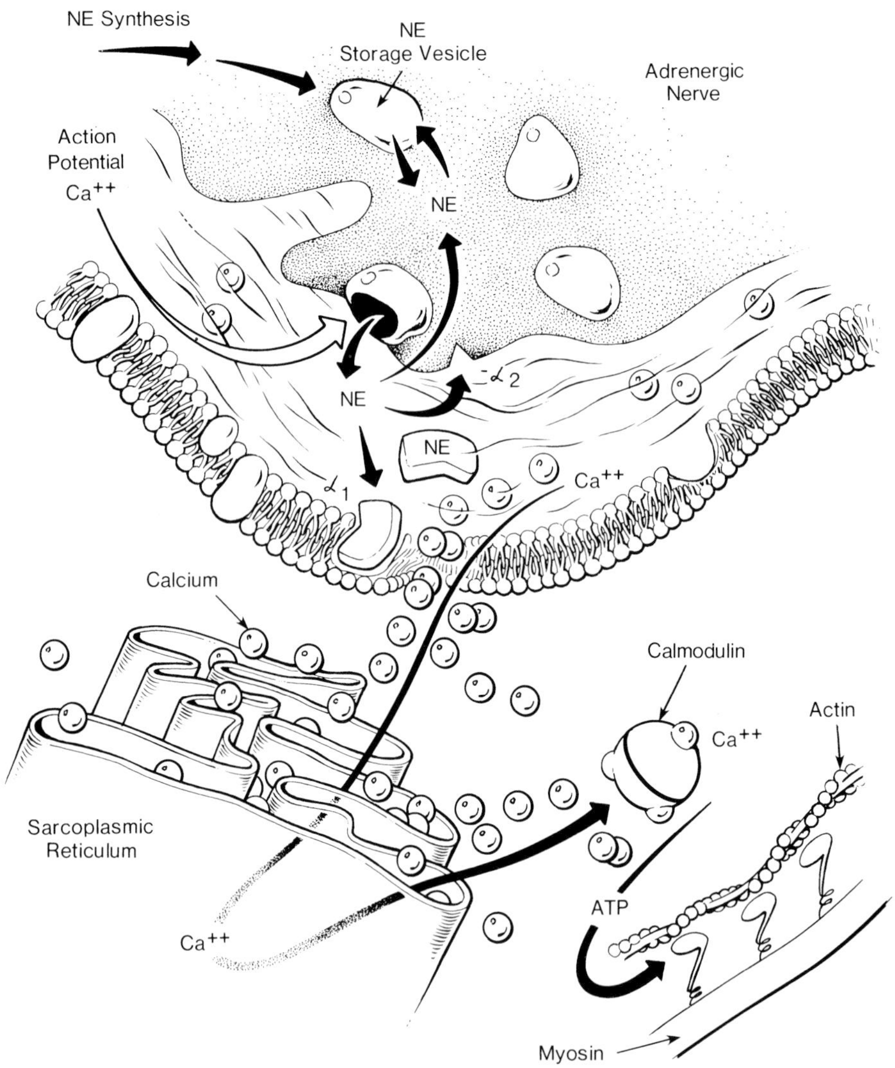

FIG. 13-32. Peripheral sympathetic neuroeffector synapse and potential sites of action of drugs for "intravenous regional sympathetic block" *(IVRS)*. A sympathetic nerve ending (adrenergic nerve terminal), synaptic cleft, cell membrane of smooth muscle of blood vessel wall, calcium channels, and contractile mechanism are shown. An action potential causes an influx of Ca^{++} into the nerve terminal, and the norepinephrine *(NE)* storage vesicle fuses with the plasma membrane to release NE. NE then activates α_1-excitatory receptors on smooth muscle (postsynaptic) and α_2-inhibitory receptors on plasma membrane (presynaptic). Alpha$_1$-receptor activation in the smooth muscle cell membrane results in an influx of Ca++, which binds to calmodulin. This regulatory protein molecule then binds to myosin, causing phosphorylation (via ATP) and initiation of the actin–myosin contractile process. *Potential sites of action for IVRS* are as follows: *1. Norepinephrine synthesis:* No drugs currently available for IVRS; *2. Blockade of NE release and reuptake:* guanethidine and bretylium block NE reuptake (also block coupling of action potential of NE release), resulting in storage granule depletion. Reserpine also blocks NE reuptake. *Note:* Tricyclics and cocaine block NE reuptake at plasma membrane of sympathetic nerve ending—NOT useful for IVRS. Also, other drugs may inhibit NE release into synaptic cleft: prostaglandin (PGE_1) and adenosine triphosphate (ATP); *3. Block of* α_2- and α_1-receptors (e.g., phentolamine); *4. Selective block of* α_1—receptors. Prazocin—not available yet as IV preparation. Trimazosin and tarazosin (long-acting) are still under development; *5. Effects on vascular smooth muscle* (e.g., diazoxide and hydralazine? action); *6. Calcium channel blocking drugs*; verapamil, nifedipine, diltiazem.

greater effect after intra-arterial than after intravenous infusion with respect to increased skin temperature and blood flow in limbs.

Neither drug has been evaluated by IVRS. Hydralazine can cause some serious side effects with highdose and long-term administration, for example, drug-induced lupus erythematosus, peripheral neuropathy, and pancytopenia. Both drugs produce a reflex increase in sympathetic activity as a result of hypotension. This has precipitated angina in susceptible patients.

Diazoxide is a relatively weak antagonist to NE and may have its action mediated by blocking calcium-dependent activation of action potentials in smooth muscle.

Calcium Entry ("Calcium Channel") Blocking Drugs. A very large number of drugs of this type are now available or are under development. In general, they interfere with the flux of calcium ion through smooth muscle cellular membranes, or with the uptake and release of calcium by intracellular membranes. Currently available drugs include verapamil, nifedipine, and diltiazem; however, many more drugs of very diverse structure are being investigated. Nifedipine appears to be more potent as a vasodilator than the other two, but has potent effects on myocardial muscle. It remains to be determined whether any of these drugs will bind firmly enough to vascular smooth muscle with IVRS technique to produce long-lasting vasodilatation, but with minimal cardiac effects. There are differences in site of action and physiochemical properties among these drugs that may influence their peripheral effects by IVRS technique. For example, nifedipine is a relatively pure slow channel (Ca^{++}) blocker acting at the "outer gate." Both verapamil and diltiazem appear to act on myosin kinase phosphorylation of myosin at the "inner gate." This prevents myosin-actin cross-bridging, and thus prevents muscle contraction.

Diltiazem may stimulate Ca^{++} extrusion from the cell, thus lowering sarcoplasmic Ca^{++}. Because of its deeper site of action and dual action, diltiazem may be more effective for IVRS. However, none of these drugs is approved for IVRS. Because of the role of Ca^{++} in secretory physiology, endocrine side effects may occur, in addition to cardiovascular side effects resulting from relative overdose.

Technique of Intravenous Regional Sympathetic Block (IVRS)

Guanethidine 10 to 30 mg is dissolved in 25 ml of normal saline for the upper limb and 30 ml for the lower limb. An IV cannula is placed in the nonaffected arm to be used in treatment of side effects. A second cannula is placed in the affected arm. A double cuff, or appropriate equipment, is used to exsanguinate the arm (see Chapter 12). The guanethidine is injected slowly and the cuff kept inflated for a minimum of 20 minutes. The cuff is then slowly deflated while monitoring the blood pressure. The patient remains supine until the blood pressure has been stabilized.

Some clinics dilute guanethidine in 20 ml of 0.5% prilocaine to make the injection more comfortable. An alternative technique is to infuse the guanethidine solution slowly into a peripheral artery over 10 to 15 minutes. The results are similar to IVRS, and the technique may be preferable if severe peripheral vascular disease is present.

REFERENCES

1. Arnér, S.: Intravenous phentolamine test: Diagnostic and prognostic use in reflex symmpathetic distrophy. Pain, *46:*17, 1991.
2. Baxter, A.D., and O'Kafo, B.A.: Ejaculatory failure after chemical sympathectomy. Anesth. Analg., *63:*770, 1984.
3. Beene, T.K., and Eggers, G.W.N., Jr.: Use of the pulse monitor for determining sympathetic block of the arm. Anesthesiology, *40:*412, 1974.
4. Bengtsson, M.: Changes in skin blood flow and temperature during spinal analgesia evaluated by laser Doppler flowmetry and infra-red thermography. Acta Anaesthesiol. Scand., *28:*625, 1984.
5. Bengtsson, M., Nilsson, G.E., and Löfström, J.B.: The effect of spinal analgesia on skin blood flow, evaluated by laser Doppler flowmetry. Acta Anaesthesiol. Scand., *17:*206, 1983.
6. Bengtsson, M., Löfström, J.B., and Malmqvist, L.-A.: Skin conductance responses during spinal analgesia. Acta Anaesthesiol. Scand., *29:*67, 1985.
7. Bergan, J.J., and Conn, J., Jr.: Sympathectomy for pain relief. Med. Clin. North Am., *52:*147, 1968.
8. Blain, A., Zadeh, A.T., Teves, M.L., and Bing, R.J.: Lumbar sympathectomy for arteriosclerosis obliterans. Surgery, *53:*164, 1963.
9. Boas, R.A., Hatangdi, V.S., and Richards, E.G.: Lumbar sympathectomy—A percutaneous chemical technique. In Bonica, J.J., *et al.* (eds.) Advances in Pain Research and Therapy. Vol. 1. pp. 685–689. New York, Raven Press, 1976.
10. Bonelli, S., Conoscente, F., Movilia, P.G., Restelli, L., *et al.*: Regional intravenous guanethidine vs. stellate ganglion block in reflex sympathetic dystrophies: A randomized trial. Pain, *16:*297, 1983.
11. Bonica, J.J.: The Management of Pain. Philadelphia, Lea & Febiger, 1953.
12. Bonica, J.J.: Clinical Application of Diagnostic and Therapeutic Nerve Blocks. Oxford, Blackwell Scientific Publications, 1958.
13. Boucher, J.R., Falardeau, M., Plante, R., Audet, J., *et al.*: Le reflexe sympatho-galvanique (RSG) et la sympathectomie. Can. Anaesth. Soc. J., *17:*504, 1970.
14. Breivik, H.: Intravenous regional sympathetic blockade with guanethidine. Tidsskr. Nor. Lægeforen., *99:*935, 1979.
15. Bridenbaugh, P.O., Moore, D.C., and Bridenbaugh, L.D.: Capillary Po_2 as a measure of sympathetic blockade. Anesth. Analg. (Cleve.), *50:*26, 1971.
16. Bryce-Smith, R.: Injection of the lumbar sympathetic chain. Anaesthesia, *6:*150, 1951.
17. Bryce-Smith, R., and Macintosh, R.R.: Local Analgesia: Abdomen. Edinburgh, Livingstone Press, 1962.
18. Campbell, J.N., Raja, S.N., Selig, D.K., *et al.*: Diagnosis and management of sympathetically maintained pain. *In* Fields, H.L., and Liebeskind, J., (eds): Progress in Pain Research and Management. pp. 85–100. Seattle, IASP Press, 1994.
19. Carron, H., and Litwiller, R.: Stellate ganglion block. Anesth. Analg. (Cleve.), *54:*567, 1975.
20. Christie, M.J.: Electrodermal activity in the 1980s: A review. J.R. Soc. Med. *74:*616, 1981.
21. Cherry, D.A., and Rao, D.M.: Lumbar sympathetic and coeliac plexus blocks–An anatomical study in cadavers. Br. J. Anaesth. *54:*1037, 1982.
22. Colding, A.: Treatment of pain. Organization of a pain clinic: Treatment of acute herpes zoster. Proc. R. Soc. Med., *66:*541, 1973.
23. Cook, P.R., Malmqvist, L.-Å., Bengtsson, M., *et al.*: Vagal and sympathetic activity during spinal analgesia. Acta Anaesthesiol. Scand., *34:*271, 1990.
24. Cousins, M.J., Reeve, T.S., Glynn, C.J., Walsh, J.A., *et al.*: Neurolytic lumbar sympathetic blockade: Duration of denervation and relief of rest pain. Anaesth. Intensive Care, *7*(2):121, 1979.
25. Cousins, M.J., and Wright, C.J.: Graft muscle skin blood flow after epidural block in vascular surgical procedures. Surg. Gynecol. Obstet., *133:*59, 1971.
26. Cronestrand, R., Juhlin-Dannfeldt, A., and Wahren, J.: Simultaneous measurements of external iliac artery and vein blood flow after reconstructive vascular surgery: Evidence of increased collateral circulation during exercise. Scand. J. Clin. Lab. Invest., *31* (Suppl. 128):167, 1973.
27. Cronin, K.O., and Kirsner, R.L.: Assessment of sympathectomy—The skin potential response. Anaesth. Intensive Care, *7:*353, 1979.
28. Cross, F.W., Cotton, L.T.: Chemical lumbar sympathectomy for ischemic rest pain. A randomized, prospective controlled clinical trial. Am. J. Surg., *150:*341, 1985.
29. Dam, W.H.: Therapeutic blockade. Acta Chir. Scand., *33* (Suppl.):89, 1965.

30. DeBakey, M.E., Burch, G., Ray, T., and Ochsner, A.: The "borrowing-lending" hemodynamic phenomenon (hemometakinesia) and its therapeutic application in peripheral vascular disturbances. Ann. Surg., *126:*850, 1947.
31. Detakats, G.: Sympathetic reflex dystrophy. Med. Clin. North Am., *49:*117, 1965.
32. Dhuner, K.G., Edshage, S., and Wilhelm, A.: Ninhydrin test—Objective method for testing local anaesthetic drugs. Acta Anaesthesiol. Scand., *4:*189, 1960.
33. Dollery, C.T., Paterson, J.W., and Conally, M.E.: Clinical pharmacology of beta-receptor-blocking drugs. Clin. Pharmacol. Ther., *10:*765, 1969.
34. Driessen, J.J., Van Der Werken, C., Nicolai, J.P.A., and Crul, J.F.: Clinical effects of regional intravenous guanethidine (Ismelin) in reflex sympathetic dystrophy. Acta Anaesthesiol. Scand., *27:*505, 1983.
35. Dunningham, T.H.: The treatment of Sudeck's atrophy in the upper limb by sympathetic blockade. Injury, *12:*139, 1980.
36. Eaton, A.C., Wright, M., and Callum, K.G.: The use of the image intensifier in phenol lumbar sympathetic block. Radiography, *46:*298, 1980.
37. Eriksen, S.: Duration of sympathetic blockade: Stellate ganglion versus intravenous regional guanethidine block. Anaesthesia, *36:*768, 1981.
38. Eriksson, E.: Illustrated Handbook in Local Anaesthesia. Copenhagen, Munksgaard, 1969.
39. Fields, H.L., and Robotham, M.C.: Multiple mechanisms of neuropathic pain: A clinical perspective. *In* Fields, H.L., and Liebeskind, J. (eds): Progress in Pain Research and Management. pp. 437–445. Seattle, IASP Press, 1994.
40. Fowles, D.C., Christie, M.J., and Edelberg, R., *et al.*: Publication recommendations for electrodermal measurements. Psychophysiology, *18:*232, 1981.
41. Froysaker, T.: Lumbar sympathectomy in impending gangrene and foot ulcer. Scand. J. Clin. Lab. Invest., *31* (Suppl. 128):71, 1973.
42. Fulton, R.L., and Blakeley, W.R.: Lumbar sympathectomy: A procedure of questionable value in the treatment of arteriosclerosis obliterans of the legs. Am. J. Surg., *116:*735, 1968.
43. Fyfe, T., and Quin, R.O.: Phenol sympathectomy in the treatment of intermittent claudication: A controlled clinical trial. Br. J. Surg., *62:*68, 1975.
44. Gillespie, J.A.: Future place of lumbar sympathectomy in obliterative vascular disease of lower limbs. Br. Med. J., *2:*1640, 1960.
45. Gillespie, J.A.: Late effects of lumbar sympathectomy on blood flow in the foot in obliterative vascular disease. Lancet, *1:*891, 1960.
46. Gillespie, J.A.: An evaluation of vasodilator drugs in occlusive vascular disease by measurement. Angiology, *17:*280, 1966.
47. Glynn, C.J., Basedow, R.W., and Walsh, J.A.: Pain relief following post-ganglionic sympathetic blockade with IV guanethidine. Br. J. Anaesth., *53:*1297, 1981.
48. Greene, N.M.: Preganglionic sympathetic blockade in man: A study of spinal anesthesia. Acta Anaesthesiol. Scand. *25:*463, 1981.
49. Haimovici, H., Steinman, C., and Karson, J.H.: Evaluation of lumbar sympathectomy in advanced occlusive arterial disease. Arch. Surg., *89:*1089, 1964.
50. Hannington-Kiff, J.G.: Pain Relief. pp. 68. London, Heinemann Press, 1974.
51. Hannington-Kiff, J.G.: Sympathetic nerve blocks in painful limb disorders. *In* Wall, P.D., and Melzack, R.: Textbook of Pain. 3rd ed. pp. 1032–1052. Edinburgh, Churchill Livingstone, 1994.
52. Hanowell, L.H., Kanefield, J.K., and Soriano, S.G.: A recommendation for reduced lidocaine dosage during intravenous regional bretylium treatment of reflex sympathetic distrophy. Anesthesiology *71:*811, 1989.
53. Hatangdi, V.S., and Boas, R.V.: Lumbar sympathectomy: A single needle technique. Br. J. Anaesth. *57:*285, 1985.
54. Herman, B.E., Dworecka, F., and Wisham, L.: Increase of dermal blood flow after sympathectomy as measured by radioactive sodium uptake. Vasc. Surg., *4:*161, 1970.
55. Hoffman, D.C., and Jepson, R.P.: Muscle blood flow and sympathectomy. Surg. Gynecol. Obstet., *127:*12, 1968.
56. Hughes-Davies, D.J., and Redman, L.R.: Chemical lumbar sympathectomy. Anaesthesia, *31:*1068, 1976.
57. Jänig, W. and Stanton-Hicks, M. (eds.): Reflex Sympathetic Dystrophy: A Reappraisal. Progress in Pain Research and Management. pp. 1–249. Seattle, IASP Press, 1996.
58. Johansson, H.: Chemical sympathectomy with phenol for chronic prostatic pain: A case report. Eu. Urol., *2:*98, 1976.
59. Kappis, M.: Sensibilitat und lokale Anasthesia im chirurginchen Gebiet der Bauchhohle mit besonderer Berucksichtigung der Splanchnicus-Anasthesie. Beitr. Z. Klin. Chir., *115:*161, 1919.
60. Kim, J.M., Arakawa, K., and von Linter, T.: Use of the pulse-wave monitor as a measurement of diagnostic sympathetic block and of surgical sympathectomy. Anesth. Analg. (Cleve.), *54:*289, 1975.
61. King, R.D., Kaiser, G.C., Lempke, R.E., and Shumacker, H.B.: Evaluation of lumbar sympathetic denervation. Arch. Surg., *88:*36, 1964.
62. Kirnö, K.: Regional analgesia and sympathetic nerve activity in man. Medical thesis, University of Göteborg, Sweden, Göteborg, 1992.
63. Klopfer, G.T.: Neurolytic lumbar sympathetic blockade: A modified technique. Anaesth. Intensive Care *11:*43, 1983.
64. Kovamees, A.: Skin blood flow in obliterative arterial disease of the leg: Effect of vascular reconstruction examined with xenon and iodine antipyrine clearance and skin temperature measurements. Acta Chir. Scand., (Suppl. 397): 1968.
65. Kovamees, A., Löfström, B., McCarthy, G., and Aschberg, S.: Continuous lumbar sympathetic blocks in the treatment of patients with ischemic lower limbs. 10th Congress of Int. Cardiovascular Soc., 1971.
66. Kovamees, A., Löfström, B., McCarthy, G., and Aschberg, S.: Continuous lumbar sympathetic blocks used to increase regional blood flow after peripheral vascular reconstruction. 18th Congress Eur. Soc. Cardiovascular Surg., 1974.
67. Langer, J., and Matthes, H.: Blockaden mit Lokalanasthetika im Bereich der Sympathikuskette. Z. Prakt. Anasth. Wiederbeleb Intensivther. *8:*93, 1973.
68. Larsen, O.A., and Lassen, N.A.: Medical treatment of occlusive arterial disease of the legs: Walking exercise and medically induced hypertension. Angiologia, *6:*288, 1969.
69. Lassen, N.A., *et al.*: Conservative treatment of gangrene using mineralocorticoid-induced moderate hypertension. Lancet, *1:*606, 1968.
70. Lériche, R., and Fontain, R.: L'anésthesie isolée du ganglion étoile: Sa technique ses indications ses resultats. Presse Med., *42:*849, 1934.
71. Lewis, L.W.: Evaluation of sympathetic activity following chemical or surgical sympathectomy. Anesth. Analg. (Cleve.), *34:*334, 1955.
72. Linde, B.: Studies on the vascular exchange function in canine subcutaneous adipose tissue with special reference to effects of sympathetic nerve stimulation. Acta Physiol. Scand., *433* (Suppl.): 1976.
73. Linson, M.A., Leffert, R., and Todd, D.P.: The treatment of upper extremity reflex sympathetic dystrophy with prolonged continuous stellate ganglion blockade. J. Hand Surg. *8:*153, 1983.
74. Lloyd, J.W., and Carrie, L.E.S.: A method for treating renal colic. Proc. R. Soc. Med., *58:*634, 1965.
75. Loh, L., Nathan, P.W., and Schott, G.D.: Pain due to lesions of central nervous system removed by sympathetic block. Br. Med. J., *282:*1026, 1981.
76. Löfström, J.B., Thorborg, P., and Lund, N.: Direct and indirect effect of some local anesthetics on muscle blood flow-tissue oxygen pressure. Reg. Anaesth., *10:*82, 1985.
77. Löfström, J.B., Malmqvist, L.-Å., and Bengtsson, M.: Can the "sympatho-galvanic reflex" (skin conductance response) be used to evaluate the extent of sympathetic block in spinal analgesia? Acta Anaesthesiol. Scand., *28:*578, 1984.
78. Löfström, B., and Zetterquist, S.: The effect of lumbar sympathetic block upon nutritive blood-flow capacity in intermittent claudication. A metabolic study. Acta Med. Scand., *182:*23, 1967.
79. Löfström, B., and Zetterquist, S.: Lumbar sympathetic blocks in the treatment of patients with obliterative arterial disease of the lower limb. Int. Anesthesiol. Clin., *7:*423, 1969.
80. Malmqvist, L.-Å., Bengtsson, M., Björnsson, G. *et al.*: Sympathetic activity and haemodynamic variables during spinal analgesia in man. Acta Anaesthesiol. Scand., *31:*467, 1987.
81. Malmqvist, L.-Å., Trygvasson, B., Bengtsson, M.: Sympathetic blockade during extradural analgesia with mepivacaine or bupivacaine. Acta Anaesthesiol. Scand., *33:*444, 1989.
82. Malmqvist, E.L.-Å.: Sympathetic neural blockade during regional analgesia: Clinical investigation in man. Linköping University medical dissertations. No. 366, Linköping, 1992.
83. Mandl, F.: Die Paravertebrate Injektion. Vienna, Springer-Verlag, 1926.
84. Masud, K.Z., and Forster, K.J.: Sympathetic block in herpes zoster. Am. Fam. Physician, *12:*142, 1975.

85. McKain, C.W., Bruno, J.U., and Goldner, J.L.: The effects of intravenous regional guanethidine and reserpine. J. Bone Joint Surg., *6:*808, 1983.
86. Moore, D.C.: Stellate Ganglion Block. Springfield, Charles C. Thomas, 1954.
87. Myers, K.A., and Irvine, W.T.: An objective study of lumbar sympathectomy: II. Skin ischaemia. Br. Med. J., *1:*943, 1966.
88. Myers, K.A., and Irvine, W.T.: An objective study of lumbar sympathectomy. I. Intermittent claudication. Br. Med. J., *1:*943, 1966.
89. Nielsen, J.: Thromboangitis obliterans (Buerger's disease). A study of the prognosis. Ugeskr. Laeger., *131:*1740, 1969.
90. Nielsen, P.E., Bell, G., Augustenborg, G., and Lassen, N.A.: Reduction in distal blood pressure by sympathetic nerve block in patients with occlusive arterial disease. Scand. J. Clin. Lab. Invest., *31* (Suppl. 128):59, 1973.
91. Nielsen, P.E., Bell, G., Augustenborg, G., Paaske-Hansen, O., *et al.*: Reduction in distal blood pressure by sympathetic block in patients with occlusive arterial disease. Cardiovasc. Res., *7:*577, 1973.
92. Nolte, H., Ahnefeld, F.W., and Halmagyi, M.: Die lumbale Grenzstrangblockad zur Beurteilung der Wirkungsdauer von Lokalanaesthetika. Acta Anaesthesiol. Scand., *23* (Suppl):618, 1966.
93. Ogawa, S.: Sympathectomy with neurolytics. *In* Hyodo, M., Oyama T., and Swerdlow, M. (eds.): The Pain Clinic IV. pp. 139–146. Utrecht, VSP Publishers, 1992.
94. Olsson, A.G., and Carlsson, A.L.: Clinical, hemodynamic and metabolic effects of intra-arterial infusions of prostaglandin E_1 in patients with peripheral vascular disease. Adv. Prostaglandin Thromboxane Res., *1:*429, 1976.
95. Perl, E.R.: A reevaluation of mechanisms leading to sympathetically related pain. *In* Fields, H.L., and Liebeskind, J. (eds.): Progress in Pain Research and Management, pp 129–150. Seattle, IASP Press, 1994.
96. Procacci, P., Francini, F., Zoppi, M., and Maresca, M.: Cutaneous pain threshold changes after sympathetic block in reflex dystrophies. Pain, *1:*167, 1975.
97. Raskin, N.H., Levinson, S.A., Hoffman, P.M., Pickett, J.B.E., III., *et al.*: Postsympathectomy neuralgia amelioration with diphenylhydantoin and carbamazepine. Am. J. Surg., *128:*75, 1974.
98. Reid, W., Watt, J.K., and Gray, T.G.: Phenol injection of the sympathetic chain. Br. J. Surg., *57:*45, 1970.
99. Scheinin, T.M., and Inberg, M.V.: Intraoperative effects of sympathectomy on ipsi- and contralateral blood flow in lower limb arterial reconstruction. Ann. Clin. Res., *1:*280, 1969.
100. Selander, D., and Sjostrand, J.: Longitudinal spread of intraneurally injected local anesthetics. Acta Anaesthesiol. Scand., *22:*622, 1978.
101. Sternschein, M.J., Myers, S.J., Frewin, D.B., and Downey, J.A.: Causalgia. Arch. Phys. Med. Rehabil., *56:*58, 1975.
102. Strand, L.: Lumbar sympathectomy in the treatment of peripheral obliterative disease. An analysis of 167 patients. Acta. Chir. Scand., *135:*597, 1969.
103. Szczeklik, A., Nizankowski, R., Splawinski, J., *et al.*: Successful therapy of advanced arteriosclerosis obliterans with prostacyclin. Lancet, *1:*1111, 1979.
104. Szeinfeld, M., Saucedo, R., and Pallares, V.S.: Causalgia of vascular etiology following an abdominal injury. Anesthesiology, *57:*46, 1982.
105. Szilagyi, D.E., Smith, R.F., Scerpella, J.R., and Hoffman, K.: Lumbar sympathectomy. Current role in the treatment of arteriosclerotic occlusive disease. Arch. Surg., *95:*953, 1967.
106. Taylor, G.W., and Calo, A.R.: Atherosclerosis of arteries of lower limbs. Br. Med. J., *1:*507, 1962.
107. Thomas, D.: Forced acid diuresis and stellate ganglion block in the treatment of quinine poisoning. Anaesthesia *39:*257, 1984.
108. Thulesius, O.: Beurteilung des schwergrades arterieller Durchblutungsstorungen mit dem Doppler-Ultraschallgerat. Angiologie, 13. Bern, Hans Huber, 1971.
109. Thulesius, O., and Gjores, J.E.: Use of Doppler shift detection for determining peripheral arterial blood pressure. Angiology, *22:*594, 1971.
110. Thulesius, O., Gjores, J.E., and Mandaus, L.: Distal blood flow and blood pressure in vascular occlusion: Influence of sympathetic nerves on collateral blood flow. Scand. J. Clin. Lab. Invest., *31* (Suppl. 128):53, 1973.
111. Tsuji, H., Shirasaka, C., Asoh, T., and Takeuchi, Y.: Influences of splanchnic nerve blockade on endocrine-metabolic responses to upper abdominal surgery. Br. J. Surg. *70:*437, 1983.
112. Uhrenholdt, A.: Relationship between distal blood flow and blood pressure after abolition of the sympathetic vasomotor tone. Scand. J. Clin. Lab. Invest., *31* (Suppl. 128):63, 1973.
113. Uhrendholdt, A., Dam, W.H., Larsen, O.A., and Lassen, N.A.: Paradoxical effect on peripheral blood flow after sympathetic blockades in patients with gangrene due to arteriosclerosis obliterans. Vasc. Surg., *5:*154, 1971.
114. Vaughan, R.S., Lawrie, B.W., and Sykes, P.J.: Use of intravenous regional sympathetic block in upper limb angiography. Ann. R. Coll. Surg. Engl., *67:*309, 1985.
115. Verstraete, M.: A critical appraisal of lumbar sympathectomy in the treatment of organic arteriopathy. Angiologia, *5:*333, 1968.
116. Walker, S.M., and Cousins, M.J.: Complex regional pain syndromes: Including "reflex sympathetic dystrophy" and "causalgia." Anaesth. Intens. Care, *25:*113, 1997.
117. Walsh, J.A., Glynn, C.J., Cousins, M.D., and Basedow, R.W.: Blood flow, sympathetic activity and pain relief following lumbar sympathetic blockade or surgical sympathectomy. Anaesth. Intensive Care, *13:*18, 1984.
118. Weale, F.E.: The hemodynamic assessment of the arterial tree during reconstructive surgery. Ann. Surg., *169:*484, 1969.
119. Wright, C.J., and Cousins, M.J.: Blood flow distribution in the human leg following epidural sympathetic blockade. Arch. Surg., *105:*334, 1972.
120. Yao, J.S.T., and Bergan, J.J.: Predicting response to sympathetic ablation (quoted in editorial). Lancet, *1:*441, 1974.
121. Zetterquist, S.: Muscle and skin clearance of antipyrine from exercising ischemic legs before and after vasodilating trials. Acta Med. Scand., *183:*487, 1968.

APPENDIX A

COBALT BLUE SWEAT TEST

General Requirements[a]

Whatman no. 41 filter papers 5.5 cm (halved) × 100
Cobalt chloride crystals (500 g)
Silica-gel crystals
Thermometer (and antiseptic)
Distilled water
Dressing forceps
Oven and tray
Blankets
Infrared lamps × 2 (or heat cradle)

Filter paper preparation

Dissolve 10 g of cobalt chloride in 100 ml of distilled water
Dip and drain halved filter papers, using forceps
Place on tray in oven at approximately 150° for 20 minutes (avoid excessive drying)
Remove with forceps from oven when pink color changes to bright blue
Seal in airtight jar with silica-gel crystals

Procedure

Record patient's oral temperature
Apply lamp for 30 minutes to trunk and arms (take care not to burn patient or heat face excessively)
Using forceps, place filter paper on firm dry surface, and apply both palms or plantar surfaces of feet, ensuring application as airtight as possible
Rerecord oral temperature, aiming to increase it by 0.3°F
Cease heat application if the above is recorded or if frank sweating is present

Comments. The procedure should be performed preblock and postblock because some patients have decreased sweating preblock (not including diabetic patients).

Ideally an area is also needed whereby the patient may bathe after treatment, because a profuse sweating reaction is desired to ensure that adequate heating of the patient has been achieved before adequate denervation exists.

Response	Filter Paper
Normal response (profuse sweating)	Blue → pink
Slight reduction (moderate sweating)	Blue → mottled pink/blue small area
Moderate reduction (slight sweating)	Blue → mottled pink/blue large area
Complete reduction (no sweating)	Remains blue

[a] Available from any large chemical supply house.

APPENDIX B

Name of preparation

10% phenol in iohexol (Omnipaque®), Conray-420® (or Angiographin®)

Ingredients

100 g of phenol A.R. (crystals)
IL Conray-420 (or Angiographin)

Equipment

1-liter glass measuring cylinder with stopper
1-liter vacuum flask
Scintered glass filter
Tufryn 0.45 μm 7-mm (Gelmann HT-450) membrane filter mounted in a Millipore swinnex 47-mm holder
Sterile disposable 50-ml syringe
Connector tube (about 9 in) for outlet of filter

Identity number

All washed with pyrogen-free water for injections filtered through a 0.2 μm filter, then dried in hot air oven, with all exposed outlets covered with aluminum foil.

Method of Manufacture

Weigh phenol into 1-liter measuring cylinder
Remove outer seals of Conray-420 bottles, leaving stoppers in place
Rinse exterior of these bottles with filtered water for injections
Place bottles in laminar flow cabinet after rinsing, and allow to dry in air stream
Remove stoppers with rinsed forceps
Pour Conray-420 into graduated cylinder containing phenol
Shake to dissolve phenol; make to volume and mix

Container/closure description

Container, 20-ml antibiotic vial
Stopper, red merco lacquered to suit
Crimp cap, gold aluminum long skirt to suit

Packing—equipment and method

Laminar flow cabinet
Filter through scintered glass into 1-liter vacuum flask
Pour into pyrex dish and load 50-ml syringe
Filter from syringe through 47-mm Tufryn filter with connector tube attached to outlet of filter holder and leading to vials.

C

Thorax and Abdomen

Neural Blockade in Clinical Anesthesia and Management of Pain, Third Edition,
edited by M.J. Cousins and P.O. Bridenbaugh.
Lippincott–Raven Publishers, Philadelphia © 1998.

CHAPTER 14

Celiac and Hypogastric Plexus, Intercostal, Interpleural, and Peripheral Neural Blockade of the Thorax and Abdomen

Dan J. Kopacz and Gale E. Thompson

In 1953, Sir Robert Macintosh introduced his book *Local Analgesia: Abdominal Surgery* with the following paragraph: "A local analgesic can provide ideal operating conditions when used alone; a fortiori[a] it will afford ideal conditions if a general anesthetic is given at the same time. Local analgesia, alone or combined with light general anesthesia, is therefore theoretically justified in every abdominal operation."[57] Now, more than 4 decades later, it is even more credible that Sir Robert's admonitions should provoke the common practice of routine, daily use of the nerve blocks described in this chapter. In one form or another, they are indeed applicable to *every* thoracic and abdominal surgical procedure.

There are several reasons for the tendency to pay lip service to regional anesthesia and then fail to use it. First, among many anesthesiologists, surgeons, and patients, there is an element of bias and emotion that has some of its origin in fact, but is perpetuated by fallacy. A single untoward event such as the famous Woolley and Roe case in England (1947)[15] for many years cast a pall over the practice of regional anesthesia. More recently, the cases of cauda equina syndrome after continuous spinal anesthesia have nearly eliminated this regional anesthetic technique from use.[89] This same kind of emotional overreaction to an untoward event has been played out in many countries in many slightly different ways. Ultimately it tends to lead to a halting, lame, conceptual approach to regional anesthesia. Second, there are really very few training environments in which one can develop expertise in performing nerve blocks. Regional anesthesia is not just a medical curiosity, and it is not to be practiced only infrequently on the high-risk patient. To be performed well, it must be used routinely! Thus, each time a surgical anesthetic is being selected, the anesthesiologist should consider first what kind of regional anesthetic technique might be adaptable to the case. Training programs must accentuate this kind of thinking and practice.[47] Finally, there is a tendency to evaluate the outcome of an anesthetic or surgical procedure in terms of survival. Survival is basic, of course, but there are various routes to any goal and the choice or type of anesthetic is of great importance. The patient may remember very little of the surgical scenario and be aware only that the "operation was a success." Data continues to be amassed from many sources to show that regional anesthesia can provide the basic foundation to allow a considerably less stressful operation, less deterioration in many physiologic functions, and improved postoperative analgesia (see Chapter 5).

In summary, certain basic precepts are essential to the successful use of the peripheral nerve blocks described in this chapter. These are:

- A personal conviction on the part of the anesthesiologist that regional anesthesia is indeed a safe, viable choice of anesthetic technique for any given surgical procedure.
- A thorough knowledge of anatomy.
- A thorough knowledge of the pharmacology of local anesthetic drugs.
- Adequate training in the use of regional anesthesia.
- A philosophy of using supplemental drugs at appropriate times and in adequate doses.
- A perceptive awareness of the possible side effects and complications of regional anesthesia. (*Note:* side effects are *not* complications.) (see Chapter 21).

D. J. Kopacz and G.E. Thompson: Department of Anesthesiology, Virginia Mason Medical Center, Seattle, Washington 98111.

[a] "All the more said of a conclusion that follows with even greater logical necessity than another already accepted in the argument"–*Webster's New World Dictionary*, College Edition.

An enlightened patient who has been counseled on the benefits and nature of regional anesthesia.

RATIONALE

Three fundamental arguments might be used to support the routine use of regional anesthesia:

It is the ideal form of balanced anesthesia.
It provides the best means of protection from the stress of surgery.
It is the optimum method of providing pain relief in the postanesthetic period.

BALANCED ANESTHESIA

The term "balanced anesthesia" has many connotations. Commonly, it implies that several different drugs are used to achieve hypnosis, amnesia, analgesia, muscle relaxation, or other conditions that we recognize as separate components of the phenomenon of anesthesia. Today the general tendency is to consider only inhaled or intravenous drugs when defining balanced anesthesia. The term was actually introduced by Lundy in 1926, and regional anesthesia played the key role in its description.[56] Elements of this concept were emphasized as early as 1915 by Crile.[17] Historically, therefore, it is most reasonable to consider regional anesthesia as the foundational component of balanced anesthesia. For instance, peripheral nerve block of the abdomen and chest can be considered the primary ingredient of a total anesthetic regimen because it provides most of the analgesia and muscle relaxation objectives of the total anesthetic. Addition of appropriate and complementary doses of either inhaled or intravenous drugs will then be dictated by such factors as the nature and duration of the surgical procedure, the patient's safety and desires, and operating room environmental considerations, including noise, temperature, teaching atmosphere, or conversation.

It is not uncommon for anesthesiologists to react negatively to the concept of combining regional nerve block with light general anesthesia. "Why give two anesthetics when one will do?" "You are doubling the risks of anesthesia." "It takes too much time." "It's not worth it," are frequently heard criticisms. Surprisingly, though, the same comments are not expressed about the potpourri of drugs used to accomplish general anesthesia. Often, these expressions merely reflect a lack of expertise or inclination to use regional anesthesia. In recent years, there have been numerous reports and findings that help restore balance to this controversy. There has been an increasing focus, for instance, on the potential dangers of general anesthetic drugs. Cardiovascular, renal, hepatic and thrombotic-fibrinolytic alterations, induced enzyme changes, ecologic hazards, and the possibility of increased malignancies have been acknowledged.[112] Until the fabled "ideal" or complete anesthetic agent is found, a variety of drugs will continue to be used to produce anesthesia. In practical terms, the local anesthetic drugs still should play the primary role in providing truly balanced anesthesia.

PROTECTION FROM SURGICAL STRESS

It is often said that a phenomenon that "cannot be quantitated, cannot be studied." Pain and stress are obvious examples of such phenomena. Surgical stress is not truly measurable, although we are slowly zeroing in on quantification of this elusive entity. Historically, George Crile's book *Anoci-association* contained many ideas about stress that were based on rudimentary knowledge. In simplified terms, he proposed that the use of local anesthetic drugs prevented noxious stimuli from invading the central nervous system; he believed they would prevent surgical shock, and that the opposite held for general anesthesia. He felt that general anesthesia allowed such impulses to penetrate the central nervous system (CNS) but obtunded the body's ability to respond. Intense central neuronal activity occurred, manifested by marked changes in vital signs and other stress indicators. He saw that such changes were greatly modified or even lacking in patients who had received regional anesthesia. As a result of this reduced stress, the patient appeared less fatigued and therefore was better suited to deal with other postoperative stresses. Recent demonstration in the laboratory setting of central sensitization and the intense interest in its blockade by 'preemptive analgesia' appears to justify Crile's early suspicions.[117] Clinically, we continue to form impressions about the degree of physiologic insult to patients during surgery. Many appear "washed out" or "beaten down" by the experience. This, of course, may be due to several factors, including the primary disease process, the surgical technique, or the conduct of the anesthetic. Whatever the stimulus and the response, it is important to consider possible ways to reduce the insult. Several surveys of anesthesiologists, surgeons, and primary care physicians have shown that these clinicians would favor regional anesthesia if they, themselves, or their patients required surgery.[44,86,87] It is likely that such opinions are shaped from clinical experiences that suggest that regional anesthesia is indeed the least stressful technique.

ANALGESIA IN THE POSTANESTHETIC RECOVERY PERIOD

It is just as important to achieve freedom from pain in the postoperative period as it is to control pain during surgery (see also Chapter 26). Anesthesiologists are increasingly concerned and involved in postoperative pain management beyond their more classic role of relieving pain only during surgery.[81] Patients have many fears about their surgical procedures, but they have an equal dread of pain following surgery. They can be reassured to an amazing degree if the anesthesiologist offers them one of the basic regional anesthetic techniques, which will allow them to regain consciousness but remain relatively pain-free in the immediate postoperative period. Currently available local anesthetic drugs will give analgesia for only 8 to 12 hours. New formulations that deposit these drugs in slow-release forms hold promise of substantially increasing this duration.[46,59] It is hoped that with further development, durations of action of 24 to 72 hours can be attained safely, while maintaining the characteristic of preferential blocking only of sensory nerves. The slight pain and the time involved in performing one or two blocks in the postoperative period would be more than offset by the benefits and duration of pain relief. This approach would tend to avoid the problems of apnea, hypotension, immobility, tachyphylaxis, fear of subarachnoid injection, and urinary retention encountered with continuous catheter epidural injections of local anesthetics or narcotics. Even with currently available drugs, intercostal nerve blocks have been repeated as many as 14 times in the postoperative period.[8] Despite the discomforts of turning and the multiple needle-sticks involved in this procedure, patients consistently preferred repeated blocks rather than sedation with narcotics. There is no doubt that analgesia is more profound and pain therapy more specific with intercostal blocks than with narcotics. Patients treated with repeated blocks have PaO_2 values that are slightly better, and their ability to cough and ambulate is especially impressive. The total hospital stay has been shortened in patients who received blocks, compared to those who were treated with narcotics for pain relief (see Chapter 26).

Other studies have examined the effects of intercostal blocks on lung volumes and gas flow rates following either abdominal or thoracic surgery. Unfortunately, it is often difficult to evaluate these studies and impossible to compare them because of differences in methodology. These differences include the site of incision, the number of nerves blocked, and the temporal relation of the blocks to the time of surgery. A few gross generalizations can be made. Most authors have used peak expiratory flow as a measure of the maximal expiratory effort that can be generated by a patient. When compared with opioid analgesia, intercostal block results in higher peak expiratory flows.[79] This is true whether measured immediately after surgery or on the following day. In healthy volunteers, Jakobson found that bilateral intercostal nerve blocks with 0.25% bupivacaine or 0.5% etidocaine caused no change in the normal pattern of breathing.[41] There were minor changes in several of the lung capacities and flows. Total lung capacity, forced vital capacity, and peak expiratory flow, all decreased by 4%. Functional residual capacity decreased by 8%, and peak expiratory airway pressure decreased by 7%. Interestingly, there was no difference in the effects of 0.25% bupivacaine and 0.5% etidocaine, even though one would expect a greater effect from etidocaine because of its more potent motor blocking effects when used for epidural anesthesia. In a similar study of healthy volunteers, Hecker et al. found similar minor changes when 1% lidocaine with epinephrine was used.[35] Ventilatory function was well maintained in these subjects even at extremes in demand imposed by graded increases in exercise on a cycle ergometer.

In general, intercostal nerve blocks are extremely effective in blocking motor function because of the small caliber of the nerves and because of the great length of the nerve in contact with the drug. When intercostal block does lead to respiratory failure, it is generally because pain relief from the block unmasks the ventilatory depression of previously administered narcotics.[16]

The approach of interpleural analgesia[85] for postoperative pain control has undergone a period of intense investigation. Anesthesia is attained primarily from blockade of multiple intercostal nerves by diffusion of local anesthetic through the parietal pleura, but several other mechanisms also may contribute. Details of the technique include placement of an epidural-type catheter via a Touhy needle anywhere between the 5th to 9th intercostal spaces. Twenty to 30 ml of 0.25% to 0.5% bupivacaine are then injected by means of the catheter at intervals of 4 to 18 hours. This technique has been used for multiple surgical procedures of the thorax and abdomen requiring either unilateral or bilateral incisions. The catheter may be left in place for several days or weeks as necessary for analgesia in both the acute and chronic pain settings. Although side effects and potential complications have tempered its use after the excitement of its original description, interpleural catheters remain as an option in the armamentarium of anesthesiologists treating pain.

PAIN PATHWAYS

Noxious stimuli from the thoracic and abdominal cavities are transmitted by nerve impulses carried along afferent fibers of the somatic, sympathetic, and parasympathetic divisions of the nervous system. The afferent somatic and sympathetic pain fibers converge on cells of secondary afferent neurons in the posterior horn of the spinal cord. After synapsing, they ascend in the spinothalamic tracts. Afferent impulses from the abdominal viscera pass through the celiac plexus by way of the vagus nerve to the medulla. Similarly, afferent parasympathetic innervation of the pelvic organs pass through the superior and inferior hypogastric plexi before reaching the spinal cord through the sacral parasympathetic fibers (S2–S4). Complete sensory anesthesia of thoracic and abdominal contents can be achieved only by blocking all afferent impulses from each of these three divisions of the nervous system. This is a formidable task to achieve with regional anesthesia alone. It is technically easier to block somatic nerve fibers, which are anatomically precise, as compared to autonomic pain fibers, which are diffuse, often ill-defined, and more difficult to isolate. Table 14-1 lists the many anatomic sites at which peripheral nerve block might be attempted for somatic and autonomic deafferentation of the thorax and abdomen. Pain from abdominal viscera can be perceived through sympathetic or parasympa-

TABLE 14-1. *Anatomic sites at which peripheral nerve block may be performed to produce sensory anesthesia of abdomen and thorax*

Component portion of nervous system	Specific nerves	Possible site of block
Parasympathetic	Vagus	Neck, esophageal hiatus, celiac plexus
	S2–S4	Pudendal, trans-sacral
Sympathetic	Thoracolumbar	Stellate ganglion, interpleural
	Sympathetic chain	Paravertebral sympathetic chain, celiac plexus, hypogastric plexus
Somatic	T1–T12 intercostal	Posterior angle of rib, thoracic paravertebral, interpleural
	Lumbar somatic	Lumbar paravertebral

thetic fibers. Physiologists and anatomists have difficulty in locating precisely or describing such fibers, but the clinical response of many patients demonstrates their existence. For instance, patients may respond to surgical manipulation of abdominal viscera even though they have spinal anesthesia to upper thoracic levels. Similarly, female patients may respond to uterine manipulation while under an epidural anesthetic that is perfectly adequate for skin incision and abdominal wall relaxation. Vagal afferent nerves must convey many of these impulses to brain stem levels and thence to the cerebral cortex. Although pain defies description, there appear to be differences in pain perceived via the autonomic nervous system as compared to pain perceived by means of the somatic nervous system.[34] The following list provides a way to characterize these differences.

Differences in Pain Experienced via the Somatic and Autonomic Divisions of the Nervous System

Somatic:

Precisely localized,
Sharp and definite,
Hurts where the stimulus is,
Associated with external factors,
Represented at cortical levels, and
Increases with increasing intensity of stimulus (e.g., to cut or burn skin will produce pain).

Autonomic:

Poorly localized,
Vague—may be colicky, cramping, aching, squeezing, and so forth,
May be referred to another part of the body,
Associated with internal factors,
Primarily reflex or represented at cord levels, and
Intensity of stimulus important but quality of stimulus also important (e.g., to cut or burn bowel will produce no pain, but distention of bowel will produce pain).

Regardless of the character of pain that a patient perceives or what neural pathway is involved, the anesthesiologist must respond to a patient's surgical pain on a moment-to-moment basis. It is often difficult to identify precisely which nerve or nerves are transmitting noxious impulses to the patient's level of perception. Regional anesthetic techniques may leave certain pain pathways open, either by design or by default. Only by close observation and anticipation of difficulties can the basic regional anesthetic be complemented properly, with some form of supplementary drug.

There may be significant side effects from blocking autonomic nerves. When the balance between sympathetic and parasympathetic tone is upset, the ensuing functional changes in heart, lung, and gut may be quite disturbing. Therefore, bilateral vagus nerve block or major sympathetic nerve blocks are better avoided, or at least undertaken with caution.[72] For abdominal surgery, intercostal nerve block may be combined with blockade of the visceral pain pathways at the level of the celiac plexus. Although celiac plexus blockade of sympathetic fibers may result in pooling of blood in the mesenteric vessels, it avoids interference with cardiac and pulmonary autonomic fibers.

PREMEDICATION AND SUPPLEMENTATION

The anesthesiologist who routinely advocates regional anesthesia will tend to use heavy premedication (see also Chapter 6). Administration of many types of nerve blocks can be eased if patients are relaxed, analgesic, and amnestic. Most patients want to sleep during the course of an operation. Sights, sounds, and conversations in the surgical suite that escape the attention of medical personnel may leave vivid impressions in the mind of a wide-eyed, alert patient. There is also a need to create an operating room environment in which teaching and other professional conversation can take place without unduly alarming patients.

All peripheral nerve block procedures for thoracic and abdominal analgesia use bony or vascular anatomic landmarks, and hence require no patient participation for proper execution of the block. Paresthesia, or nerve stimulation, does not need to be attained. Likewise, performance of these blocks may elicit significant skin and periosteal stimulation that can be obtunded easily by light sleep or sedation. This is not to say that these nerve blocks cannot be performed without sedation. In fact, that may be mandatory when their purpose is diagnostic or when these blocks are performed on seriously ill surgical patients. For routine surgery, however, the nerve blocks described in this chapter are best performed on patients who will not be able to recall the event. Achieving the proper degree of sedation for execution of the block, while maintaining the patient in a stable and amnesic state, is often as much of a challenge (and more underrated), than it is to actually perform the block itself. Premedication before arrival in the operating suite is no longer necessary, and generally no longer used in modern anesthesia practice. After the patient's arrival in the operating suite, an intravenous line should be established that supplies fluid and caloric requirements, but, in addition, serves as a means of titrating supplementary sedative drugs. Rapid, short duration, intravenous agents (fentanyl, midazolam, propofol, methohexital, etc.) are now available to produce a brief period of loss of awareness during completion of the nerve block, or to produce sleep during the operation. A wide variety of other drugs may be used, but it is important to titrate them in small intravenous doses, while observing closely for the desired action. The clinical situation dictates which one or ones should be used, depending on the need for amnesia, hypnosis, analgesia, or some combination of these effects.

The drugs and techniques used, if one wishes to produce loss of consciousness during intercostal and celiac plexus nerve block, deserve special comment. Ideally, these blocks should be performed in an induction room or other room that is separate from the noise and confusion of the operating room. It should be equipped with appropriate monitors and resuscitation materials. Upon completion of the nerve block, the patient should regain awareness quickly, which allows questioning and testing of the block while initiating additional monitoring procedures before the operation. Intravenous benzodiazepines may be doubly effective, first as sedative and amnesia producing agents, and second as a potential prophylactic against toxic effects of the local anesthetics. Large volumes and doses of local anesthetics are required for the blocks described in this chapter. Although benzodiazepines may protect from local anesthetic CNS toxicity in animals[20] one should not exceed maximum recommended doses of local anesthetics through a feeling of false security from use of these drugs. Early recognition is the key, and prompt use of resuscitation measures, especially oxygenation, must always remain the first priority in treatment of toxic reactions.

Inhalation agents must be used intraoperatively to supplement most regional nerve blocks used for thoracic and intra-abdominal surgery. For most patients, a combination of nitrous oxide and oxygen will ensure toleration of the endotracheal tube, adequate ventilation, oxygenation, and loss of consciousness. The anesthesiologist should not be chagrined at having to administer low, supplementary concentrations of more potent inhalation agents or neuromuscular blocking drugs, should it be necessary. This does not detract from the advantages to the patient of the nerve block, as one still avoids the need for large doses of relaxants or high concentrations of the inhalation agents. For superficial procedures which do not require muscle relaxation, a laryngeal mask airway is tolerated at lighter levels of anesthesia/sedation than is an endotracheal tube.[116] Again, regional nerve block should be considered a component of balanced anesthesia, with the required supplementation varying on a case-by-case basis. Music delivered by individual headphones is also an effective alternative to chemical or drug sedation for many patients.

LOCAL ANESTHETIC DRUGS (see Chapter 4)

There are many ways to classify anesthetic drugs. They may be viewed from a perspective of history, chemical structure, metabolism, dosage, or duration of action. The last is of utmost importance for the nerve blocks discussed in this chapter. Historically, the lack of effective long-acting local anesthetic drugs has been a major deterrent to the usefulness and application of many of the more important peripheral regional anesthetic techniques.[61] As noted earlier, among future pharmacological achievements, one can hope for development of a local anesthetic agent with a predictable duration of action of 48 to 72 hours. There are problems in developing such drugs, chief among them being concerns about cardiac depression and neurotoxicity. Currently available long-acting local anesthetic drugs display widespread variation in duration of block and the potential for tachyphylaxis.[21] Once such difficulties are overcome, however, anesthesia, which includes the postoperative as well as the intraoperative period, can be seriously considered. At present, there are short-acting (e.g., procaine, 2-chloroprocaine), intermediate-acting (e.g., lidocaine, mepivacaine), and long-acting (e.g., bupivacaine, ropivacaine) local anesthetic drugs. When ultra-long-acting drugs come into widespread use, the clinical role of the nerve blocks described here will be greatly enhanced.

CHOICE AND DOSAGE OF DRUG

Before starting any regional anesthetic, the purpose or goal of the block must be determined by asking questions such as the following: "Do I want profound motor block, or is sensory anesthesia adequate?" "How many nerves are to be blocked?" "Is the patient going to be further anesthetized following the block, or will no supplementary drugs be given?" "Does the patient have major cardiovascular, respiratory, hepatic, or renal disease?" "What is the patient's size, body build, and age?" "Are there any special demands of this surgeon or of the surgical procedure?" Only when such questions have been answered can the anesthesiologist determine the proper volume, concentration, and dosage of local anesthetic drug.[64] For instance, in preparing a solution of local anesthetic for bilateral intercostal and celiac plexus nerve block, the following calculations are made: (i) Total volume of solution required, (ii) Effective concentration of drug, (iii) Total (mg) dosage of drug, (iv) Volume of epinephrine to be added, and (v) Total dosage (μg) of epinephrine.

TABLE 14-2. *Some possible drug combinations for peripheral nerve blocks of abdomen and thorax*

Drug	Volume (ml)	Concentration (%)
Bupivacaine	60	0.5
Bupivacaine	60–100	0.25
Etidocaine	60–80	0.5
Tetracaine	60–100	0.15
Mepivacaine	60	1.0
Lidocaine	60	1.0

TABLE 14-3. *Final concentration of epinephrine derived from total dose and the volume with which it is mixed*

Epinephrine	Total volume of dilution	Final concentration
0.1 mg in	20 ml =	1:200,000
0.2 mg in	40 ml =	1:200,000
0.25 mg in	50 ml =	1:200,000
0.25 mg in	60 ml =	1:240,000
0.25 mg in	70 ml =	1:280,000
0.25 mg in	80 ml =	1:320,000
0.25 mg in	90 ml =	1:360,000
0.25 mg in	100 ml =	1:400,000

There are safe or ideal limits for each of these factors. It is obvious that all are interrelated. Volume multiplied by concentration determines total dose. Excesses of volume or concentration may possibly be tolerated by a particular patient, but toxic effects are more likely to occur. On the other hand, small volumes or low concentrations of drug will result in ineffective regional anesthesia. Any block might be inadequate in area, inadequate in duration, or inadequate in extent of motor or sensory fiber blockade. The local anesthetic must be tailored to the block and requires more than just a vague knowledge of local anesthetic drug dosages and effective concentrations. The total volume of drug necessary for bilateral intercostal nerve block varies from 40 to 80 ml of solution. This allows for deposition of 3 to 5 ml of solution under each of the ribs to be blocked. The effective concentration will depend primarily on the drug used and the desired degree of motor nerve blockade. Some commonly used combinations are provided in Table 14-2.

For each local anesthetic, there are approved recommendations for maximum total dose. These recommendations may vary from country to country, or region to region, according to the prevailing bias or custom. It is foolhardy to proceed to use any local anesthetic without an understanding of these limits. Many regional techniques (e.g., subarachnoid block) involve drug dosages that do not even begin to approach the maximum recommended dose. To perform the nerve blocks in this chapter, however, the anesthesiologist often will need to approach the maximum recommended dose to achieve a successful block (see also Chapter 4).

SYSTEMIC ABSORPTION

Blood levels of a local anesthetic are higher after intercostal and interpleural block than after any other of the commonly used regional anesthetic procedures. Tucker measured arterial plasma levels after epidural, caudal, intercostal, brachial plexus, and sciatic/femoral nerve block with a single injection of 500 mg of mepivacaine.[106] These blocks were performed with both 1% and 2% mepivacaine, with and without epinephrine. The highest plasma concentrations (5 to 10 μm/ml) were observed after intercostal nerve blocks without epinephrine. When a 1:200,000 concentration of epinephrine was added to the injected solution, plasma levels fell to the range of 2 to 5 μg/ml. These lower blood levels were similar to those found with all the other regional procedures he measured (see Chapter 3). Presumably due to the larger surface area of absorption, injection of 105 mg (21 ml, 0.5% with 1:200,000 epinephrine) of bupivacaine into the interpleural space results in significantly higher plasma local anesthetic levels than using the same solution for blockade of seven intercostal nerves.[109]

Systemic absorption of epinephrine may have a significant effect on both alpha- and beta-receptors and result in tachycardia, hypertension, and arrhythmias. Such changes usually are of little consequence in healthy patients if the total dose of epinephrine does not exceed 0.25 mg (Table 14-3). In patients with coronary artery disease and hypertension, the total dose should be limited to 0.25 mg or even avoided completely. On the other hand, it is arguable that epinephrine is an immediately available antidote to the cardiovascular depressant effects of local anesthetic drugs with which they are mixed.[67] Some practitioners include epinephrine in every nerve block for this reason. Likewise, one can use epinephrine as a probe or tracer drug to identify intravascular injections. This is perhaps most pertinent to epidural anesthesia, but the principle can be applied to any regional anesthetic technique. Ideally, epinephrine should be added fresh to the local anesthetic solution just before the time of injection. This ensures optimum pH of the final solution. Commercial preparations of local anesthetics that already contain epinephrine are strongly acidic, attributable to the addition of sodium bisulfite as an antioxidant for the epinephrine in the local anesthetic solution. Acidity promotes the ionized form of local anesthetic drugs and inhibits passage of drug molecules into the nerve cell membrane (see Chapter 2).

TECHNIQUES OF NERVE BLOCK

There are many specific details of the techniques used in performing peripheral nerve blocks to produce anesthesia of the thorax and abdomen. Proper technique begins with a thorough knowledge of anatomic relationships. To this foundation is applied the technical expertise required to do the block. The need to tailor the choice of local anesthetic to the contemplated nerve block has been emphasized previously. In a similar manner, the anesthesiologist can choose various combinations of peripheral nerve blocks to tailor the total anesthetic to the requirements of the surgical procedure. The most useful combination for upper abdominal surgery is that of intercostal nerve block and celiac plexus block. It is possible, however, to mix any of the following blocks in any manner suited to the anesthetic goal. By maintaining a broad perspective and an expanded armamentarium, the resourceful anesthesiologist will recognize many different situations in which the judicious application of one or more of these blocks might be of value.

INTERCOSTAL NERVE BLOCK

Anatomy

The intercostal nerves are the primary rami of T1 through T11. Many fibers from T1 unite with fibers from C8 to form the lowest trunk of the brachial plexus. These fibers leave the intercostal space by crossing the neck of the first rib, while a smaller bundle continues on a genuine intercostal course. The only other notable variation in intercostal nerves is the distribution of some fibers from T2 and T3 to the formation of the intercostobrachial nerve. Terminal distribution of this nerve is to the skin of the medial aspect of the upper arm. Somatic innervation of the area from the nipples to below the umbilicus is provided by segmental spinal nerves from T4–T11. The portion of chest wall above the nipples has overlapping innervation from the segmental spinal nerves of T2 and T3 and from peripheral branches from the cervical plexus (supraclavicular nerves, C3–C4). Because incisions for most thoracic and upper abdominal procedures generally do not extend above the T4 dermatome, anesthetizing of these nerves is not necessary. In the most accurate sense of the word, T12 is not an intercostal nerve because it does not run a course between two ribs; it might more appropriately be termed a subcostal nerve. Some of its fibers unite with fibers from the first lumbar nerve and are terminally represented as the iliohypogastric and ilioinguinal nerves.

A typical intercostal nerve has four significant branches (Fig. 14-1). The first are the paired gray and white rami communicantes, which pass anteriorly to and from the sympathetic ganglion and chain. The second branch arises as the posterior cutaneous branch and supplies the skin and muscles in the paravertebral region. The third branch is the lateral cutaneous division, which arises just anterior to the midaxillary line. This branch is of most concern to the anesthesiologist because it immediately sends subcutaneous fibers coursing both posteriorly and anteriorly to supply skin

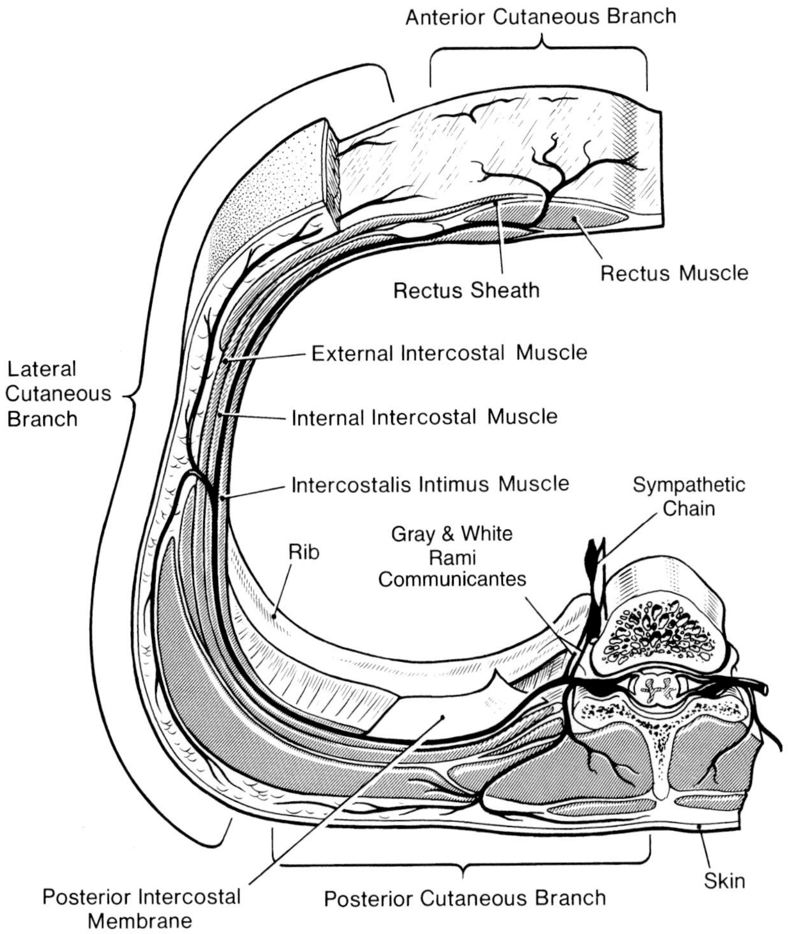

FIG. 14-1. An intercostal nerve and its branches. Approximate area of skin supplied by branches is also shown. There is evidence, however, that local anesthetic injected near the lateral cutaneous branch diffuses posteriorly to reach the posterior cutaneous branch (see also FIG. 14-4). Note also (i) the spinal nerves and dorsal root ganglia in the region of intervertebral foramen, with risk of perineurial spread into spinal fluid after intraneural injection in this region; (ii) direct injection into an intervertebral foramen may reach spinal fluid by means of a dural cuff; (iii) local anesthetic may gain access to epidural space by diffusing into an intervertebral foramen; and (iv) close to the midline the intercostal nerve lies directly on the posterior intercostal membrane and pleura. (v) Paravertebrally, solution may diffuse to rami communicantes and sympathetic chain.

of much of the chest and abdominal wall. The final branch of an intercostal nerve is the anterior cutaneous branch. In the upper five nerves, this branch terminates after penetrating the external intercostal and pectoralis major muscles to innervate the breast and front of the thorax. The lower six anterior cutaneous nerves terminate after piercing the sheath of the rectus abdominis muscle, to which they supply motor branches. Some final branches continue anteriorly and become superficial near the linea alba, to provide cutaneous innervation to the midline of the abdomen.

Medial to the posterior angles of the ribs, the intercostal nerves lie between the pleura and the fascia of the internal intercostal muscle. This fascial layer is also known as the posterior intercostal membrane. In the paravertebral region, there is only fatty connective tissue between nerve and pleura. At the angle of the rib (6 to 8 cm from the spinous processes), the nerve comes to lie between the internal intercostal muscle and the intercostalis intimus muscle. At this position, the costal groove is broadest and deepest. Cadaver studies have shown that the nerve itself remains subcostal only 17% of the time, has most frequently (73%) moved inferiorly into the midzone between ribs, and is often branching at this point.[32] The nerve is accompanied by intercostal veins and an artery, which lie superior to the nerve in the inferior groove of each rib (Fig. 14-2). The location of these vessels explains the tendency to high blood levels of local anesthetic agents following intercostal block. The costal groove becomes a sharp inferior edge of the rib, about 5 to 8 cm anterolateral to the angle of the rib. At this point, the intercostal groove ceases to exist, the lateral cutaneous branch is given off (see Fig. 14-1), and the intercostal nerve lies more inferiorly and moves toward the center of the intercostal space.

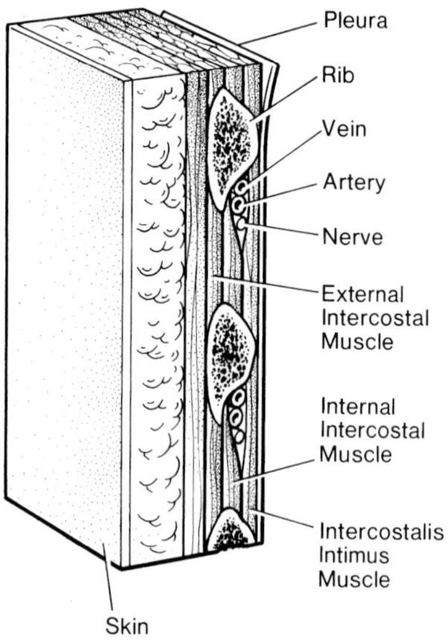

FIG. 14-2. Cross-section of rib and intercostal space. Section is shown in region of costal groove, which extends from near the head of the rib to 5 to 8 cm anterior to the angle of the rib. At the level of the angle of the rib, the intercostal nerve (one or more) lies inferior to vein and artery in the intercostal groove.

Technique

Intercostal nerve block may be performed at several possible sites along the course of the nerve. The most common, the posterior approach, offers several advantages, and is performed at a site in the region of the angle of the ribs just lateral to the sacrospinalis group of muscles, 7 to 8 cm lateral of the midline. At this location, the posterior intercostal membrane is impermeable. Lateral to this, the internal intercostal membrane becomes the internal intercostal muscle which may permit local anesthetic solution to diffuse out of the intercostal groove and into the external intercostal muscle. Furthermore, the ribs and intercostal spaces are thicker at the angle of the rib, allowing a larger margin of safety before pleura is contacted. For technical ease of performance and for an optimal teaching or learning experience, the patient is best placed in a prone position. This position also facilitates performace of celiac plexus block (or lumbar paravertebral block), which may be combined with bilateral intercostal nerve block for abdominal surgery. The premedicated patient is turned to a prone position after establishment of an intravenous infusion. A pillow is placed under the mid-abdomen to straighten the lumbar curve, and to increase the intercostal spaces posteriorly. The patient's arms are allowed to dangle off the sides of the gurney, which retracts the scapulae laterally and facilitates blockade of the intercostal nerves above T7.

The next step greatly facilitates nerve block and should be a routine part of nearly every regional anesthetic. This is the process of using skin markings to force a review of anatomic details and to define the site of needle insertion and direction for each block (Fig. 14-3). First, a vertical line should be drawn along the posterior vertebral spines. The next step is to palpate laterally to the edge of the sacrospinalis group of muscles, where the ribs are most superficial. This distance is somewhat variable, depending on body size, muscle mass, and physique, but is usually 6 to 8 cm from the midline. Lines are drawn somewhat parallel to the first line, but with a tendency to angle medially at the upper levels as the sacrospinalis muscles taper, so as to avoid the scapulae. The caudal end of the line should cross near the end of the shortened 12th rib, which is generally easy to palpate. Then, by successively palpating and marking the inferior edge of each rib (or interspaces between ribs) a diagram is completed along these two vertical lines (Fig. 14-3A). To avoid marking the same rib twice, markings on one side should correspond with the lines on the opposite side because the ribs are symmetrical. For abdominal surgery, six or seven (T5–T11 or T12) pairs of ribs are marked. For thoracic or other unilateral chest wall surgery, only the appropriate side and ribs are marked.

After positioning and marking of the patient, the local anesthetic solution is prepared. Epinephrine should be added

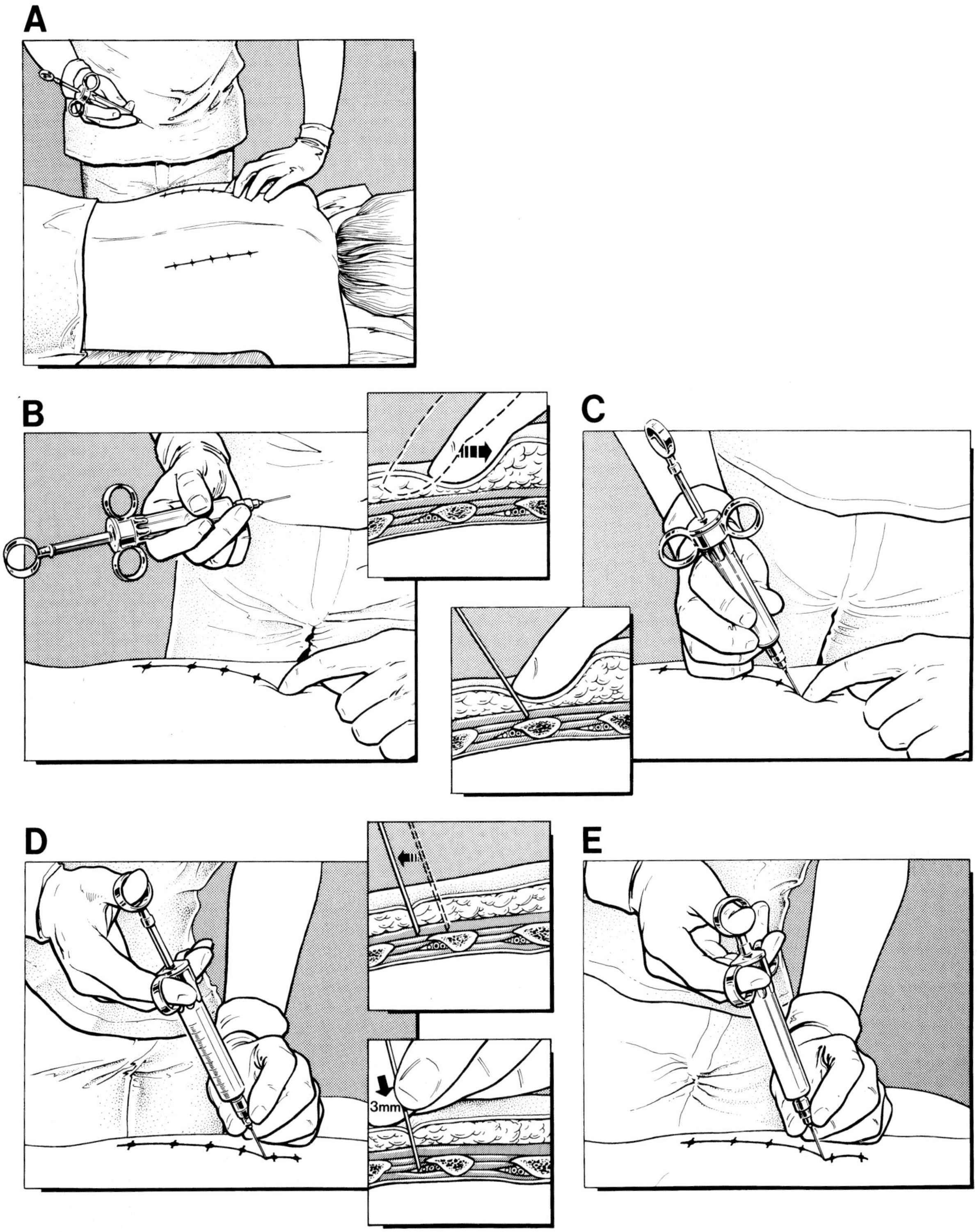

FIG. 14-3. Technique for intercostal block and corresponding deep anatomy (see text). **A:** Skin markings at lateral edge of sacrospinalis muscle (6 to 8 cm from midline). Note the medial curve of the line superiorly to avoid the scapulae. Ribs and interspaces are palpated. The lowest (most inferior) intercostal nerve is blocked first because the lower ribs are easy to palpate. (In **A–E** the diagrams show the second to last intercostal nerves to be blocked in this patient.) **B:** Skin at lower edge of rib retracted superiorly onto rib. **C:** Needle inserted onto rib (see also inset). Note finger palpating rib still in place and hand holding syringe firmly braced against back. **D:** The position of the hands now change. Note left hand now rests against the back and holds the needle as it is walked off the inferior edge of the rib and advanced 3 mm. Right hand is free to aspirate and inject. **E:** Injection completed with left hand still firmly against patient's back and controlling the needle.

to achieve a final concentration of 1:200,000, or less if the total dose of epinephrine required would exceed 0.25 mg (Table 14-3). The final solution is best prepared in a large mixing cup to afford ready access for refilling of the syringe during performance of the block.

Before starting the block, supplemental oxygen and intravenous sedation should be given to allow for patient comfort. Benzodiazepines, short-acting narcotics and barbiturates, propofol, and low doses of ketamine, are commonly used, either alone or in combination. Obviously, attention must be given to airway maintenance, oxygenation, and ventilatory adequacy in the prone patient. After an adequate level of sedation has been achieved, skin wheals are raised at each of the previously marked sites of injection. A disposable 30-gauge needle is ideal for raising these wheals. For maximal patient comfort, procaine or lidocaine might be chosen for the skin wheals because these drugs, injected subcutaneously, cause less pain than do the long-acting local anesthetics.[68]

Finally, the intercostal nerve blocks are performed successively at each of the skin wheal sites. To do this, a 2.5 to 4 cm, 22- or 23-gauge needle is attached to a full 10-ml Luer-Lok syringe. Disposable needles are of soft metal, and the tip may be bent with the repeated bony contact characteristic of this block, although they will penetrate the thick skin of the back more easily. A barbed needle will increase the risk of vascular or nerve damage and should be exchanged for a new needle if this occurs.

In the following sequence, hand and finger position is of utmost importance to assure safe control of the needle throughout the procedure (Fig. 14-3B–E). Standing at the patient's left side and beginning at the lowest rib, the index finger of the left hand is used to pull the skin perpendicular to the lower edge of the rib up and over the rib. While holding the syringe and needle in the right hand, which rests on the patient's back, the needle is introduced through the skin immediately off the tip of this retracting (left hand) finger, and advances the needle to contact the rib. Should there be difficulty in contacting the rib with the needle, the palpating left index finger should be used to redefine its depth and position. Care should be taken not to allow the needle to penetrate beyond this palpated depth. The right hand maintains firm contact between needle and rib, while the left hand is shifted to hold the needle's hub and shaft between the thumb, index, and middle fingers. Of utmost importance is the firm placement of the left hand's hypothenar eminence against the patient's back, so that unexpected patient movement does not cause further penetration with the needle. This also allows total control of needle depth as the left hand next walks the needle in the caudal direction off the lower edge of the rib. At that point, it is advanced 2 to 3 mm. A subtle 'give' or 'pop' of the fascia of the internal intercostal muscle may be felt. At this point 2 to 5 ml of the solution is slowly injected. A very slight jiggling motion may decrease the risk of significant intravascular injection and help ensure proper spread of solution into the fascial plane containing the nerve. After injection, the needle is removed to the subcutaneous tissue, the next higher rib is palpated with the left hand, and this process is repeated for each of the nerves to be blocked. In certain patients with severe barrel chest deformity or neurasthenic habitus, the intercostal injection may best be done with an even shorter 23- or 25-gauge needle.

The success rate of intercostal nerve block should approach 100%. Failure is usually due to too superficial an injection of solution. The average distance from posterior rib to pleura averages 8 mm,[74] so advancing a small distance (2 to 3 mm) after walking off the rib is safe. Another common error is to rotate the long axis of the syringe as it is being walked off the rib (Fig. 14-4). The needle should be kept at a slight 15° to 20° cephalad angle, which keeps the needle directed towards the intercostal groove, where the intercostal space is widest. If rotated into a caudad angle during the walk, the tendency is to inject the solution superficially in the intercostal space where it may not bathe the nerve.[66] When the technique described above is correctly followed, the firmly retracted skin over the rib will serve to ease the needle off the rib without need to resort to this rotary motion.

Intercostal nerve blocks can also be done at the midaxillary line while the patient is lying supine. This position is considerably more convenient in many situations (e.g., after induction of general anesthesia), but there is less margin of safety, the costal groove no longer exists, the nerve has often split into several main branches, and the lateral cutaneous branch of the nerve could be missed by the injected solution. Computed tomography studies show, however, that solutions spread readily along the subcostal groove for several centimeters and can come in contact with the origin or take-off of this large branch (see Figs. 14-1 and 14-4).

Another variation is to consider intercostal nerve block by jet injection.[94] Seddon used such a technique but found that present jet guns deliver only 1 ml at a time. Using that volume of a 1.5% bupivacaine solution gave considerable post-operative analgesia. It is perhaps worthy of further study.

Finally, placement of catheters in the intercostal space for intermittent injection or continuous infusion has been described. However, because of differing methods of investigation (patients vs. cadavers, distance of injection from midline, injection through needle or catheter), considerable controversy exists over the anatomic spread of solution injected into the intercostal space. This is confounded by the lack of a clear definition of where the paravertebral space ends, where the intercostal space begins, and whether a 'subpleural' or 'extrapleural' space exists between the two. Anatomically all of these entities are in continuity, and injection of sufficient volume at any of these points will lead to spread to the others.

Mowbray has shown that, because of autolysis, the length of spread of 3 ml of solution in cadavers is significantly greater (8.6 ± 1.8 cm in cadavers vs. 5.2 ± 1.4 cm in patients), and a spreading to more than one nerve can occur which is not noted in the living patient.[69] The significance of distance of injection from midline, or, more importantly, the

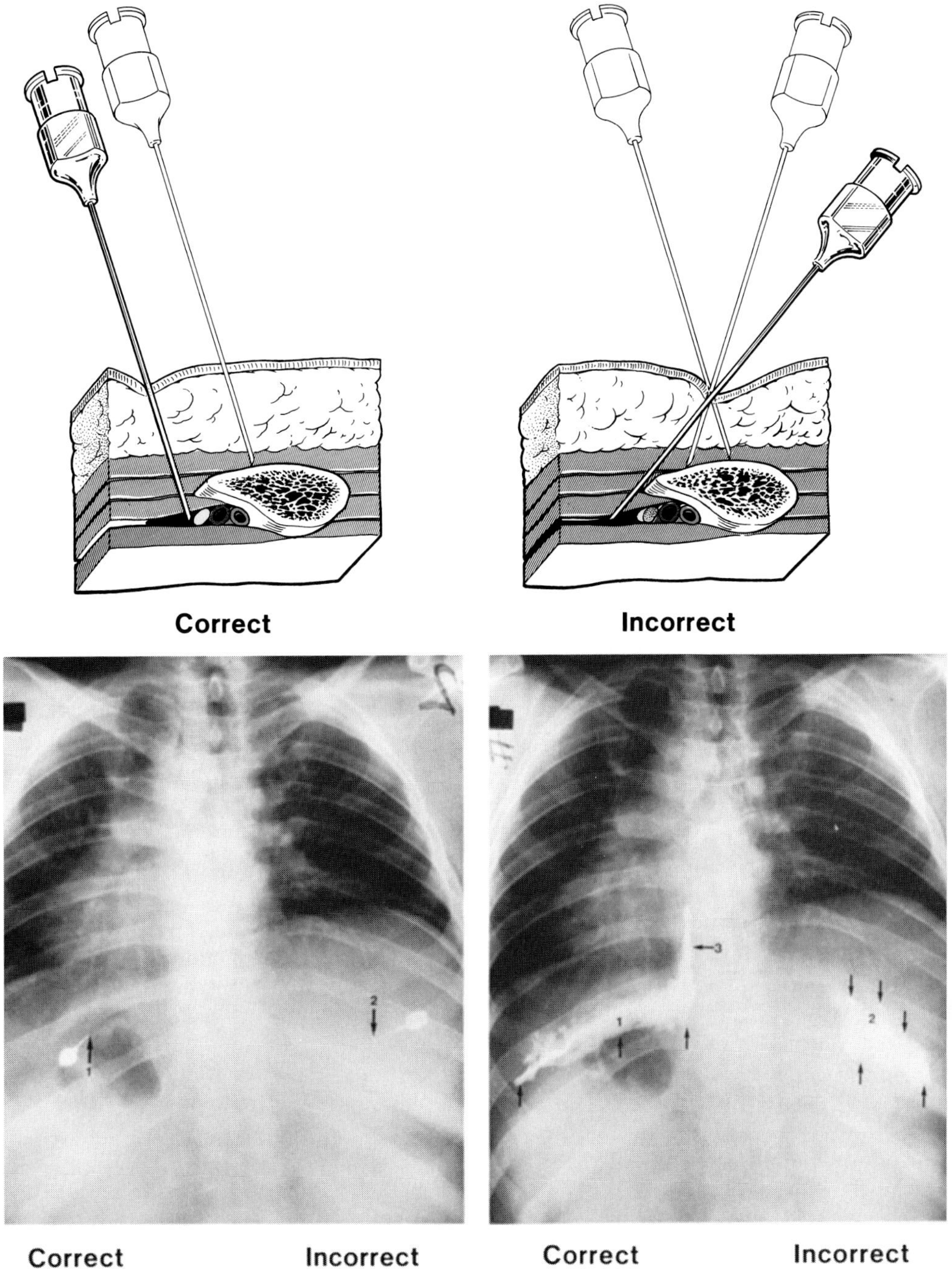

FIG. 14-4. Upper Panel: Comparison of correct *(left)* and incorrect *(right)* technique (see text). **Lower Panel:** X-ray showing correct needle insertion *(1)* compared to incorrect position *(2) (Left)*. X-ray showing injection of x-ray contrast medium *(Right)*. Injection from correctly placed needle results in spread along intercostal groove *(1)* and also into paravertebral space *(3)*. Injection from incorrectly placed needle results in a localized "blob" in intercostal muscles.[2] Arrows indicate extent of spread of solution.

point of injection relative to the angle of the rib and the attachment of the posterior intercostal membrane to the internal intercostal muscle, has been convincingly shown by Hord.[37] Injection of 5 ml through catheters placed at the angle of the rib and directed laterally,[1] are confined to a single intercostal space as their tips are well lateral of the medial border of the intercostalis intimis muscle. In contrast, injections through catheters directed medially[70] spread to contact 3 to 5 intercostal spaces because the tips of the catheters end up 2 to 3 cm medial of the medial border of the intercostalis intimus muscle, where solution can freely spread cephalad and caudad in the *extrapleural* space where the parietal pleura is less adherent to the ribs. Because of the eventual position of these catheter tips, they are probably more appropriately called 'continuous paravertebral catheters,' instead of 'continuous intercostal catheters.' Paravertebral catheters have been used successfully for management of unilateral postoperative pain, but are associated with an incidence of failure of 20% to 30%, and the possibility of temporary neuritis which has been noted.[14,18]

Surgical Applications

Relatively few surgical procedures can be performed under intercostal nerve block alone. Minor breast surgery,[3] extracorporeal lithotripsy,[58] and cardiac pacemaker insertion[80] have been described using intercostal blockade. Small umbilical and incisional hernias, and other minor procedures on the chest or abdominal wall, can be performed with intercostal blockade alone, but in general, some degree of supplemental anesthesia must complement the block for most other surgical procedures. For intra-abdominal procedures, celiac plexus block may be added to provide visceral anesthesia. Intercostal block may also be combined with brachial plexus block for more extensive operations on the breast, upper extremities, and axilla. For intrathoracic procedures, stellate ganglion block may be a nice addition to obtund visceral pain from lung parenchyma. Pain from pelvic structures is not relieved by intercostal block, and operations in that region are better done with spinal, caudal, or lumbar epidural techniques.

Nonsurgical Applications

Intercostal nerve block is extremely effective in providing pain relief for fractured ribs. Because vigorous palpation of broken ribs can be quite painful in the obese or in the patient with excessive local swelling, localization of the ribs and performance of the block can be aided by Doppler ultrasound.[108] Pleuritic pain and pain from flail chest also can be relieved in this manner. Blockade of two or three nerves is a simple way to prepare for insertion of thoracostomy or feeding gastrostomy tubes. Herpes zoster pain may be relieved and even treated in this way. Intercostal nerve block can be helpful in the differential diagnosis of visceral versus abdominal wall pain.

The most effective but least exploited use of this block is for postoperative control of pain (see Chapter 26). Perhaps the simplest demonstration of this technique is the amount of benefit derived from simply blocking the right 10th, 11th, and 12th intercostal nerves in patients having appendectomy.[12]

Complications (see Chapter 21)

The most feared complication of intercostal nerve block is pneumothorax. The actual incidence is extremely low, but many physicians avoid this block because of an imagined high frequency. Physicians in all stages of training performed more than 10,000 individual nerve blocks with a reported incidence of pneumothorax of only 0.073%.[62] Preoperative and postoperative chest films in 200 consecutive patients resulted in a pneumothorax incidence of 0.42% (1/2,610 intercostal nerve blocks). This pneumothorax was entirely asymptomatic (silent) and would most likely not have been detected had the chest X-rays not been taken as a routine part of the study.[63] Further retrospective analysis forces one to conclude that the true risks and mechanisms of pneumothorax have been greatly exaggerated. For instance, Moore reported the unexpected finding of contrast material within the pleural cavity in a roentgenographic study of block technique.[66] Further evidence of parietal pleural penetration is noted in two papers on continuous intercostal nerve blockade.[4,71] The authors were surprised to find catheters within the pleural space in cadaver studies and in cardiac surgical patients. Surgeons observed the catheter tip from within, after midline sternotomy. Nunn's observations of multiple dermatome block after a single injection might be explained by rationalizing that interpleural anesthesia was really being performed[74] (see next section). This internal pleural space approach to intercostal block forces us to reevaluate our more traditional perspectives. Treatment of pneumothorax, by needle aspiration or merely by careful observation, is usually all that is needed. Reabsorption of a small pneumothorax is also aided by administration of oxygen. Chest tube drainage should be performed only if there is failure to re-expand the lung with these preliminary maneuvers. Overzealous surgical treatment has often compounded an initial problem that might well have been resolved with simple measures.

A second complication relates to the toxic effects of absorbed local anesthetic and epinephrine following intercostal block. As previously mentioned, blood levels of the anesthetic drug after intercostal and interpleural blockade are higher than after any other regional anesthetic procedure. Systemic toxic reactions rarely occur in patients having diagnostic or therapeutic blocks, because smaller volumes of more dilute solution of drug are used. Greater amounts of more concentrated drug are injected to provide complete motor and sensory block in the surgical patient. These greater doses may result in delayed systemic toxicity, so that patients should be monitored closely for 15 to 20 minutes after completion of the block.

Peak plasma concentrations after intercostal blockade are dependent upon the local anesthetic agent used, the concentration and volume injected, and whether or not epinephrine is added (see also Chapter 3). Epinephrine seems to decrease plasma concentrations 30% to 50% for mepivacaine and bupivacaine, but does not influence the concentrations of ropivacaine and etidocaine when it is used for intercostal blockade.[43] As a general rule, a plasma concentration of 0.1 mcg/ml appears to result from the injection of every 10 mg of bupivacaine with epinephrine.

Performance of intraoperative intrathoracic intercostal injection appears to be associated with a higher incidence of complications. Multiple cases of total spinal anesthesia have been reported after intrathoracic intercostal blockade at the end of surgery with general anesthesia.[30,101] In most of these instances, the blocks were performed under direct vision, at a site more medial than would be chosen for the percutaneous approach. Injection of local anesthetic into a dural root cuff or directly into nerve tissue itself, with extensive intrafascicular spread, are proposed mechanisms for the resultant widespread blockade, which manifests as hypotension and bradycardia, dilated pupils, and prolonged anesthesia and paralysis.

Any regional anesthetic procedure, and especially intercostal nerve block, can lead to complications if the anesthesiologist becomes so involved in the mechanics of administering the nerve block that he neglects total patient care. The beginning practitioner of regional anesthesia tends to become so engrossed in technique and methods that he fails to see the patient as more than a portion of anatomic detail through which a needle is being inserted. Vital signs may not be heeded. This is especially dangerous when depressant drugs have been administered before the block. Complications from inattentiveness are not those of the nerve block *per se*, although respiratory embarrassment or cardiovascular problems are often wrongly ascribed as toxic effects of the local anesthetic.[6] The American Society of Anesthesiologists motto, "Constant vigilance," is extremely appropriate for proper use of any nerve block.

CELIAC PLEXUS NERVE BLOCK

Of the many regional block techniques available to the anesthetist, blockade of the celiac plexus is potentially one of the more valuable and probably underutilized. The reason for this lack of use is because it is exclusively an autonomic blockade and, in most surgical situations, must be combined with other somatic nerve blocks. Most anesthetists would prefer the more inclusive spinal or epidural block. Many anesthetists view celiac plexus block as valuable only in large pain clinics. Hamid et al. have demonstrated that, in combination with intermittent wound infiltration, bupivacaine attenuates the neuroendocrine response (measured by glucose and cortisol) when infused continuously through a catheter placed intraoperatively near the celiac plexus after major upper abdominal surgery.[31] Although the analgesia in this particular study was relatively ineffective, recent research focusing on the role of autonomic blockade in mediating stress and the endocrine response of surgery has rekindled interest in this block technique (see Chapter 5).

Anatomy

There seems to be significant confusion about the nomenclature of this portion of the autonomic nervous system. Textbooks have used terms such as solar plexus, the abdominal brain (of Bichat), celiac ganglia, and splanchnic plexus, to describe some or all of the same anatomy. Because the clinical and physiologic results of these nerve blocks must be evaluated, it is important to know whether the blocked structures are preganglionic or postganglionic, and which target organs will be affected by the block.

The celiac plexus is the largest of the great plexuses of the sympathetic nervous system. The cardiac plexus innervates structures which are primarily thoracic, the celiac plexus innervates abdominal organs, and the hypogastric plexus supplies pelvic organs. All three contain visceral afferent and efferent fibers. In addition, they hold parasympathetic fibers that pass through these ganglia after originating in cranial or sacral areas of the nervous system. Although the latter fibers may be found in these plexuses, all are primarily sympathetic nervous system structures. They contain no somatic fibers, but do innervate most of the abdominal viscera to include stomach, liver, biliary tract, pancreas, spleen, kidneys, adrenals, omentum, and small and large bowel. Although the terms plexus and ganglion often are used interchangeably, it is important to realize that plexus is a more inclusive term. A plexus is composed of a number of ganglia and nerve fibers that converge in a fairly well-defined anatomic location.

According to most standard anatomic textbooks, there are three splanchnic nerves—great, lesser, and least. The great splanchnic nerve arises from the roots of T5 or T6 to T9 or T10. It runs paravertebrally in the thorax, through the crus of the diaphragm to enter the abdominal cavity, and ends in the celiac (or semilunar) ganglion on that side. The lesser splanchnic nerve arises from T10 to T11 segments and passes lateral to, or with, the great nerve to the celiac ganglion. It sends postganglionic fibers to celiac and renal plexuses. The least splanchnic nerve arises from T11 and T12 segments and passes through the diaphragm to the celiac ganglion. It is worth remembering that all three splanchnic nerves are preganglionic and that the paired celiac (or semilunar) ganglia are where they synapse. The postganglionic fibers radiate to the abdominal viscera (Fig. 14-5).

Of more importance to performance of celiac plexus block is an understanding of the anatomy of the surrounding structures that will be subjected to the potential trauma of needles and drug. The celiac ganglia are situated in close relation to the first lumbar vertebrae. On the right side and anterior is the vena cava, and, on the left, anteriorly, is the aorta. The kidneys are lateral on either side. The paired ganglia are close to the midline on each side between the adrenal glands and are immediately above the pancreas. The postganglionic nerves are flat, and rest against the crus of the diaphragm. Covered partially by the vena cava on the right and the pancreas on the left, they become interconnected to form plexi. The plexus anterior to the aorta, around the base of the celiac artery and superior mesenteric artery, is referred to as the solar (or celiac) plexus.

In the past decade, some studies have added substantially to definition of the anatomy of this region. Ward and colleagues, in 1979, performed x-ray and careful autopsy examinations of 20 adult bodies.[113] The celiac ganglia were found to vary in number, size, and location. On either side, the number varied from one to five and the size from 0.5 to 4.5 cm in diameter. Ganglia on the left were uniformly lower

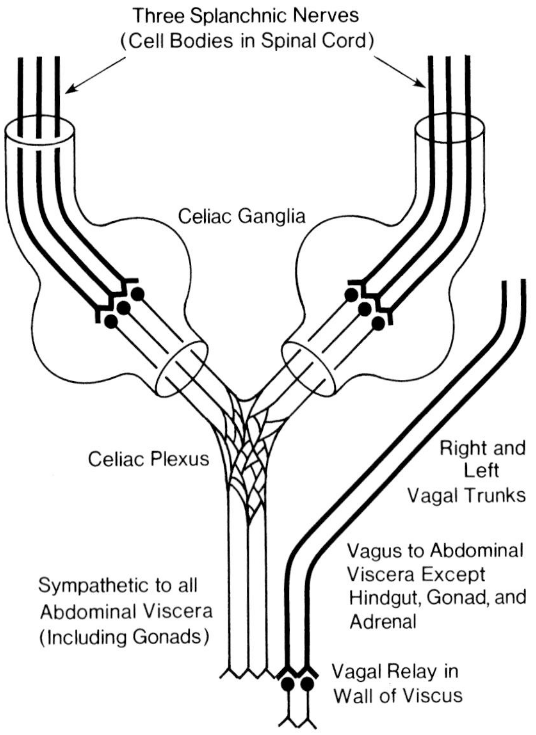

FIG. 14-5. Constituents of celiac plexus (see text). (Redrawn and reproduced with permission from Last, R.J.: Anatomy, Regional and Applied, 6th ed. pp. 315. Edinburgh, Churchill Livingstone, 1978.)

than on the right by an average of less than one vertebral level; the extreme was 1½ vertebral levels. On both sides, the ganglia were 0.6 to 0.9 cm below the celiac artery. The most consistent relationship of the ganglia was to the anterior vertebral margin, most frequently less than 1.5 cm anterior to this margin. In 1981, Moore et al.[65] verified needle placement and spread of injected solution by conventional x-ray and by computed tomography (CT) scan in 20 cancer patients. They noted that spread of the solution tended to be confined to the sides of the injection. They also noted that the anterior portion of the aortic plexus was 2 to 2.5 cm anterior to the anterior vertebral margin.

Technique

Celiac plexus nerve block is of special interest in that both bony and vascular landmarks can be used to good advantage in the performance of this block.[105] As with any nerve block, it is advisable to mark out a diagram on the skin that, projected mentally, can yield three-dimensional perspective for the ultimate placement of the needles. The easiest and most useful avenue of approach to the well-guarded celiac plexus is posterolateral. The patient is placed in a prone position with pillow under the abdomen, head turned flat to the table or cart, and arms dangling down at each side. The primary external topographic features are the 12th ribs and the inferior aspects of T12 and L1 spinous processes (Fig. 14-6). The figure formed by connecting the spine of T12 and L1 with points 7 to 8 cm lateral at the lower edges of the 12th ribs is that of a flattened isosceles triangle. The equal sides of this triangle serve as directional guides for the two needles. They are passed under the edge of each of the 12th ribs to approach the midline anterior to the body of L1. A 10- to 15-cm, 20-gauge needle is used, dictated by either the frailty or obesity of the patient. Skin wheals are raised 7 to 8 cm from the midline at the inferior edge of the 12th rib. Infiltration with a small amount of local anesthetic solution can be carried deeper for 1 to 3 cm. An awake patient should be warned about brief twinges of pain, which result from the advancing needle coming in contact with periosteum or lumbar nerves.

At first insertion, the needle is tilted about 45° from the horizontal, so that contact can be made with the lateral body of L1 at an average depth of 7 to 9 cm (Fig. 14-6). Bony contact at a more superficial level indicates that a vertebral transverse process has been encountered, requiring a slightly more caudal redirection of the needle. This must be recognized for what it is, because an incorrect judgment might lead to a superficial injection of anesthetic solution just 2 to 3 cm deep to the transverse process. An ensuing epidural, spinal, or psoas muscle injection could result in a widespread somatic nerve paralysis. This point is of special importance when neurolytic solutions are to be used. The depth of L1 will depend on the patient's size and on the location on the vertebral body at which contact is made (i.e., posterolateral or anterolateral). Once the vertebral body is identified at a usual depth of 8 to 10 cm, the needle is withdrawn to a subcutaneous level and its angle increased to allow the tip of the needle to pass 2 to 3 cm deeper than the previous point of bony contact. The needle's angle may have to be readjusted two or three times until it slides off the anterolateral side of the vertebral body. Determining the precise depth to which the needle should be advanced is of major importance. The simplest method is to advance the left-sided needle slowly, until sensitive fingertips feel aortic pulsations transmitted up the shaft (Fig. 14-6). Once this aortic depth is discovered, the right-sided needle can be inserted and readily advanced to a similar depth. Problems caused by bleeding from penetration of either aorta or inferior vena cava are extremely rare.

Once the needles have been positioned in the periaortic region, other confirmatory tests of needle placement should be performed to rule out improper position of the needle tip. For instance, leakage of blood, urine, ascites, or cerebrospinal fluid (CSF) will usually be spontaneous. If not, gentle aspiration should be performed in four quadrants and if all are negative, a 3 ml test dose of anesthetic solution is injected. This will provide additional confirmation of needle placement, since paralysis would rapidly follow unintended subarachnoid or epidural injection. The final confirmatory test depends on the anesthesiologist's sense of touch while injecting the final volume of anesthetic solution. In this regard,

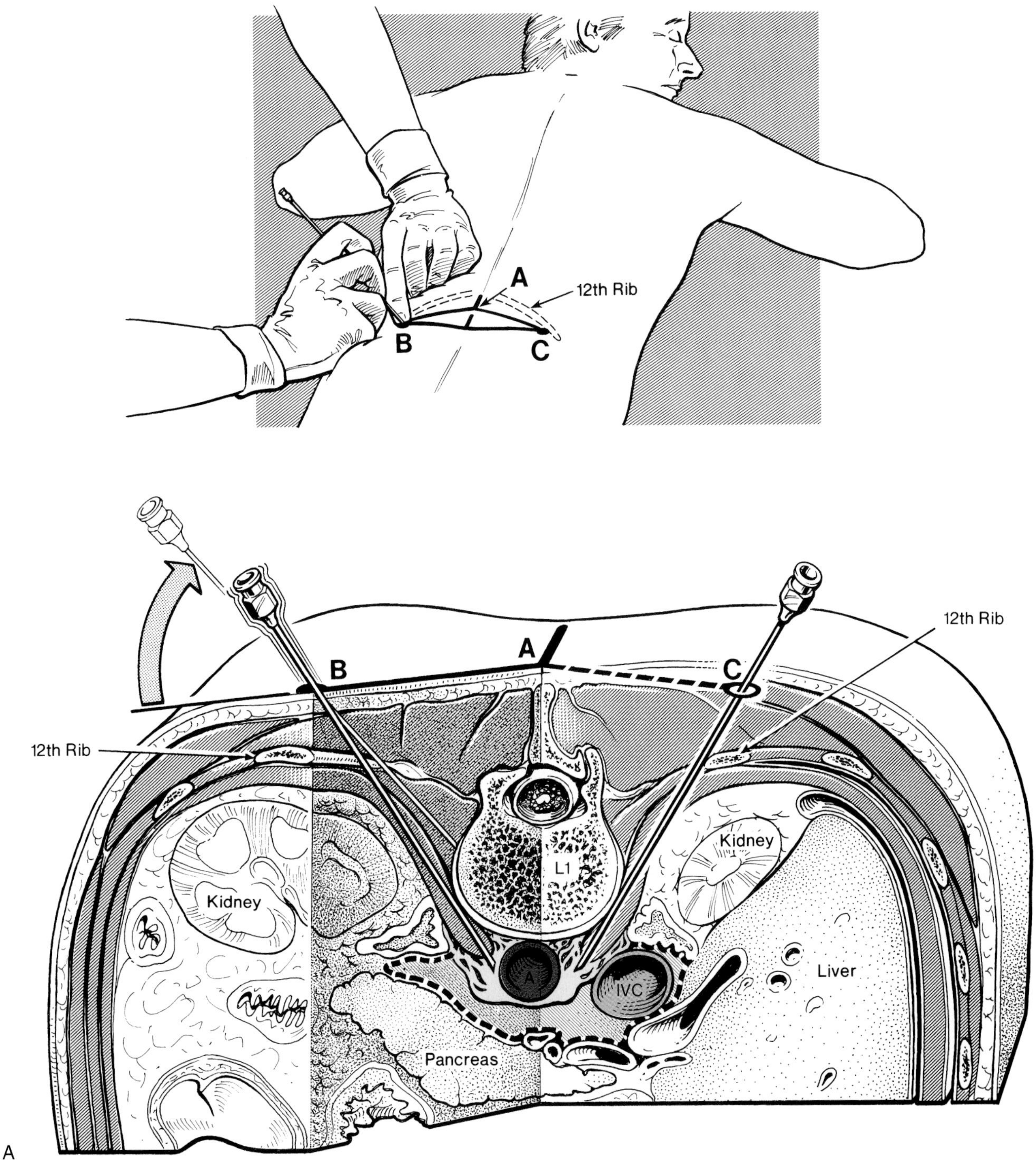

FIG. 14-6. A: Celiac plexus block. **Upper Panel:** Skin markings, position of patient, and initial insertion of needle. *Note:* Triangle formed by skin marks on lower border of 12th ribs (*B* and *C*) in line with inferior border of L1 spinous process and joined to inferior border of T12 (A). **Lower Panel:** Needle insertion and deep anatomy (see text). Skin markings and triangle (*A, B, C*) are still shown. Needle initially is directed in the plane of the line BA or CA, and at 45° to the horizontal axis of the body, to contact the lateral aspect of the L1 vertebral body. It passes inferior to the 12th rib and medial to the kidney. The angle of insertion to the *horizontal axis* of the body is then increased until the needle slips past the lateral aspect of the vertebral body, still in the line BA or CA, to reach the anterolateral aspect. On the left side, the aortic pulsations will be detected at the needle hub before puncturing the artery. Spread of a test dose of contrast medium (in the approximate area indicated by the light blue color) is a valuable guide to correct needle placement prior to diagnostic or therapeutic celiac block.

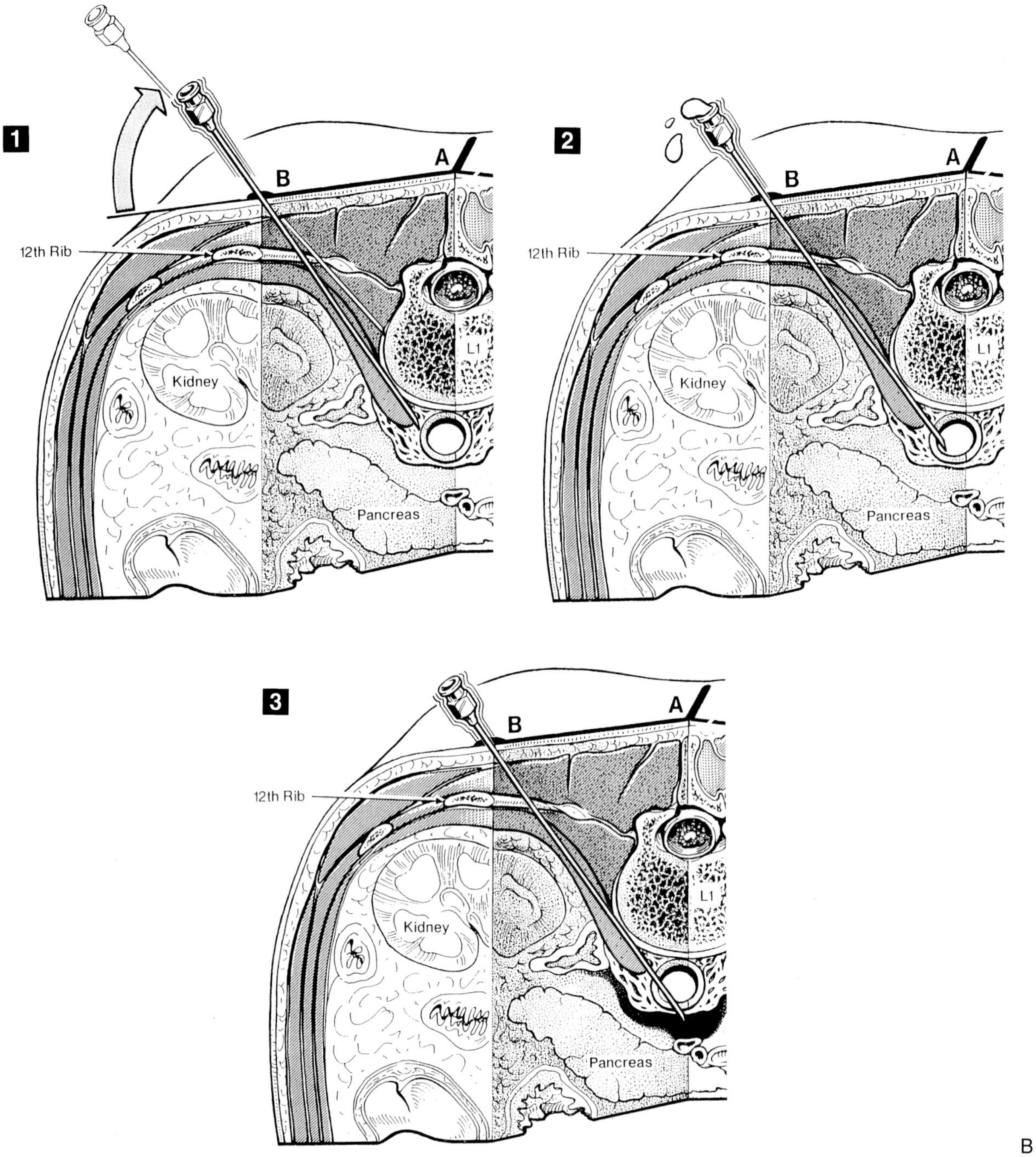

FIG. 14-6. *Continued.* **B:** Transaortic coeliac plexus block (see text).

the difference between a 20- and a 22-gauge needle is very pronounced. A 12-cm, 22-gauge needle requires such firm pressure during injection that it is difficult to appreciate whether resistance is due to the small needle bore or whether the site of injection is subperiosteal, within an intervertebral disc, or is otherwise abnormal. On the other hand, injection of 20 to 25 ml of solution through a 20-gauge needle affords little resistance[a]. This is to be expected if the injection is being properly performed in the loose retroperitoneal area where nerve fibers of the celiac plexus are located. Intraperitoneal injections could possibly occur, but this would require extremely lateral and deep placement of the needles. When neurolytic solutions are to be injected, use of a test dose should be meticulously performed, and the use of contrast media and an image intensifier (fluoroscopy or CT scan) is highly desirable (see also Chapter 31). Diagnostic (local anesthetic) and therapeutic (neurolytic agent) blockade can be performed at the same setting if the patient is kept lucid enough that it can be determined that relief is from the block and not the sedation. In this scenario, it is probably better to give a smaller volume initially (e.g., 6 to 10 ml local anesthetic through each needle), so that, once the block proves efficacious, the later injection of neurolytic agent does not spread excessively.

There have been reports of a number of other techniques for celiac plexus nerve block. Although the transaortic method of Ischia[39] would seem to have the theoretical advantage of spreading solution anterior to the aorta, this has yet to be demonstrated. Using a combination of fluoroscopy and fingertip feel, a 22-gauge needle is advanced to penetrate both walls of the aorta and to rest directly in the preaortic nerve network of the celiac plexus. A loss-of-resistance technique as the needle passes through the anterior aortic wall can also be employed.[27] Although this would seem to guarantee correct placement of local anesthetic or neurolytic solutions, these solutions may be diluted with extravasated blood and there is also the theoretical concern of dislodging atherosclerotic plaque in elderly patients. Postblock CT scans showed no retroperitoneal hematoma in six patients. Other authors have described variations of needle placement that emphasize the differences between transcrural celiac block and retrocrural splanchnic nerve block.[97] Perhaps the most bold is the ultrasound-guided (percutaneous) anterior approach, which does not seem to have any higher risk of complications, and may be of value in patients who cannot tolerate the prone position, or who are having radiologic biopsies performed simultaneously.[61] Anatomic variations make precise needle placement a difficult matter, even though fluoroscopy, standard x-rays, or CT guidance may be used (Fig. 14-7).[13] It is possible that the block may actually occur at nerve, ganglion, or plexus sites with any of the described techniques, and the reported results are quite similar for any of these various combinations (see also Chapter 31).

[a]Because aorta, gut, etc. "reseal" more readily after 22-gauge puncture, some clinicians prefer this needle.

Surgical Applications

The combination of intercostal and celiac plexus nerve block is ideal for surgery of the upper abdomen. Usually these two blocks are supplemented with light general anesthesia, since celiac block does not provide total anesthesia of all upper abdominal visceral sensation or reflexes. One special advantage to the surgeon is the diminution in bowel diameter, caused by block of sympathetic fibers and relative vagal overactivity, with increased peristalsis and gut constriction.

As with spinal or epidural anesthesia, there is a tendency for the sympathetic block of celiac plexus anesthesia to produce a fall in blood pressure. This is neither as frequent nor as severe as the hypotension following high spinal anesthesia; however, hypotension can persist into the postoperative period if long-acting local anesthetics are used. This potential problem can be treated by using a shorter-acting local anesthetic for the celiac block than for the intercostal block, by adequate replacement of blood and fluid losses during surgery, or by small doses of vasopressors. In general, the supine patient will be asymptomatic and physiologically stable even at pressures as low as 70 mm Hg systolic.

Nonsurgical Applications

Celiac plexus block can be used alone or in various combinations with intercostal nerve block to help in the differential diagnosis of visceral versus abdominal wall pain (see Chapter 27). The block can be of therapeutic value in acute pancreatitis by relieving spasm of ducts and sphincters in the pancreatic system.[49] When used in this regard, methylprednisolone may be mixed and injected along with the local anesthetic solution. The pains of hepatic artery embolization for metastatic malignancies, and of percutaneous interventional biliary manipulations, have been controlled with celiac plexus blockade.[53,55,115] Weinstabl et al. recently reported a provocative study of neurosurgical and head trauma patients receiving celiac plexus blockade in the treatment of posttraumatic disturbances in gastric emptying. All patients were at least 2 weeks past their original trauma, remained intubated and in the intensive care unit (ICU), and were considered at risk for aspiration because of large ($>$ 600 ml) daily gastric residual volumes, despite aggressive therapy. Relative to control patients, patients receiving a single bupivacaine (50 ml, 0.25%) celiac plexus block had a rapid and marked decrease in gastric volumes and were able to receive and tolerate enteral feedings immediately, with a duration of effect lasting 10 days.[114]

Although the efficacy of neurolytic celiac plexus block in pancreatic cancer pain management has been questioned, when compared to aggressive opiate regimens,[96] alcohol celiac plexus block appears to have fewer side effects.[60] It is the most effective of all therapeutic endeavors commonly used in the treatment of pancreatic cancer pain.[105] A comparison of the three posterior approaches (transaortic, classic retrocrural, and bilateral splanchnicectomy), appears to

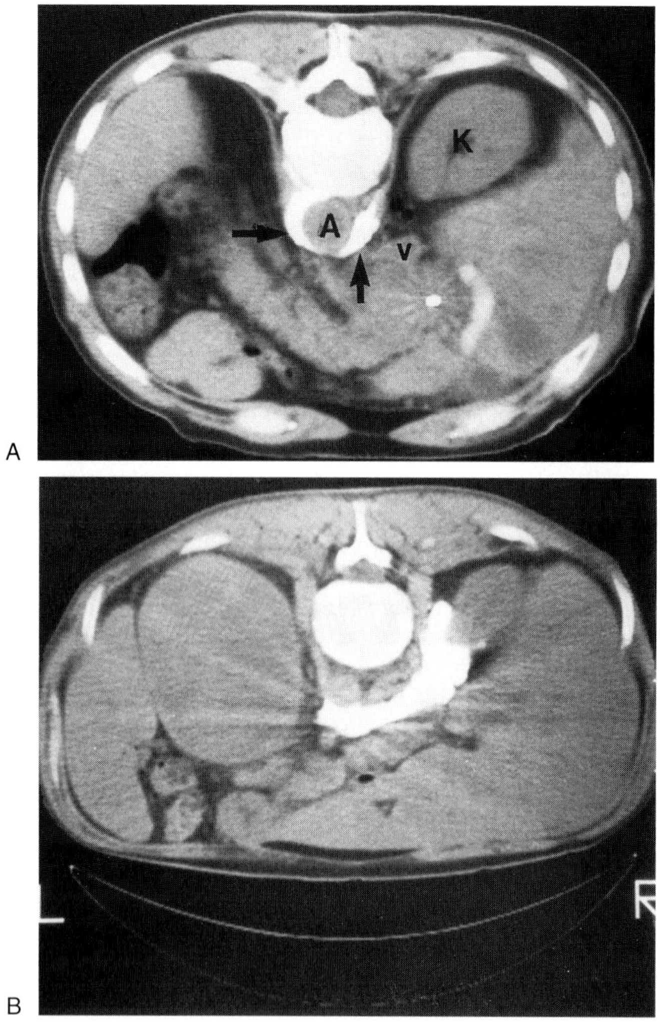

FIG. 14-7. Computed tomography (CT) scan of injection of contrast media during celiac plexus block. **A:** Needles have been inserted through the crus of the diaphragm (on right and left) and contrast medium injected. (In this case, 25 ml of a solution of 50% alcohol containing iothalamate was injected through each needle.) Note contrast almost surrounding aorta in a similar distribution to that shown in Figure 14-6. *A*, aorta; *V*, vena cava; *K*, kidney; *arrows*, spread of contrast media. **B:** Patient with large metastasis in left adrenal gland, seen as large mass to the left of vertebral body. The kidney and liver are seen on the right. *L*, left; *R*, right. In this situation, only one needle has been inserted through the crus of the diaphragm on the right side. Injection of 50 ml of the solution used in **A** results in an acceptable spread of solution. Insertion of a needle through the diaphragm on the left side would have a high chance of piercing the aorta. (Reproduced with permission from Moore, D.C.: Intercostal Nerve Block and Celiac Plexus Block for Pain Therapy. Advances in Pain Research and Therapy, Vol. 7. New York, Raven Press, 1984.)

show no significant differences in the results obtained; over 80% of patients report good and immediate relief, which lasts until death in approximately 75% of these patients.[10,38] Management of abdominal pain in non-pancreatic cancer patients, (73% good relief, 59% of these until death) though not quite as successful as in pancreatic cancer, warrants adoption of this technique for these patients as well.[9]

In contrast, alcohol celiac block does not lead to good, prolonged pain relief in patients with chronic pancreatitis or other chronic benign abdominal pain syndromes, although it may prove beneficial as a last resort in certain patients.[33]

Complications

Possible complications of celiac plexus block include hypotension, subarachnoid, epidural, intraosseous, or intrapsoas injection, intravascular injection, retroperitoneal hematoma secondary to bleeding from aorta or vena cava, and puncture of viscera (most often kidney), the lymphatic duct, abscesses, or cysts. Other complications reported after neurolytic blocks include paralysis, lower extremity dysesthesias, and sexual dysfunction. In such cases, the solution obviously had spread, to contaminate the lumbar plexus or central neuraxis. The rate of major neurologic complications after neurolytic blockade was 0.15% in a survey in England over a 5 year period.[19] Another, more remote, possibility is the impairment of blood supply from hematoma, radicular artery spasm, or perivascular pressure of injected solution. Some drop in blood pressure will occur in 30% to 60% of patients, depending on blood volume and physical status. It is usually not abrupt in onset. Misplaced injections are best prevented by experience, drawing the proper skin markings, and having the patient fully prone for the injection. Although celiac block can be performed on patients who are in a lateral or semiprone position, these positions make it more difficult to ensure proper orientation to anatomic details. Initial aspiration and the use of a test dose of local anesthetic solution are other precautionary measures against the complications of misplaced injections.

SPLANCHNIC NERVE BLOCK

Technique

The anatomy of the splanchnic nerves is described above. The splanchnic nerves can be blocked above the diaphragm, at the upper border of T12, with a technique similar to celiac plexus block. The needle is directed, however, to the anterolateral angle of the vertebral body of T12, to the same point on the vertebral body as in the lumbar sympathetic block (see Chapter 13). This block is not recommended for surgical application. For diagnosis and treatment of chronic abdominal pain, it is possible to obtain pain relief with a much smaller volume of solution than is the case with celiac block. Needle insertion is carried out under image intensifier control (Fig. 14-8A). Then a small volume (1 ml) of contrast media (e.g., angiographin) is injected to check that a linear spread is obtained, in anteroposterior and lateral views, along the anterolateral aspects of vertebral bodies immediately above the diaphragm (Fig. 14-8B). Either local anesthetic or neurolytic solution may be injected for diagnostic or therapeutic block, respectively. The neurolytic solution of choice is phenol in

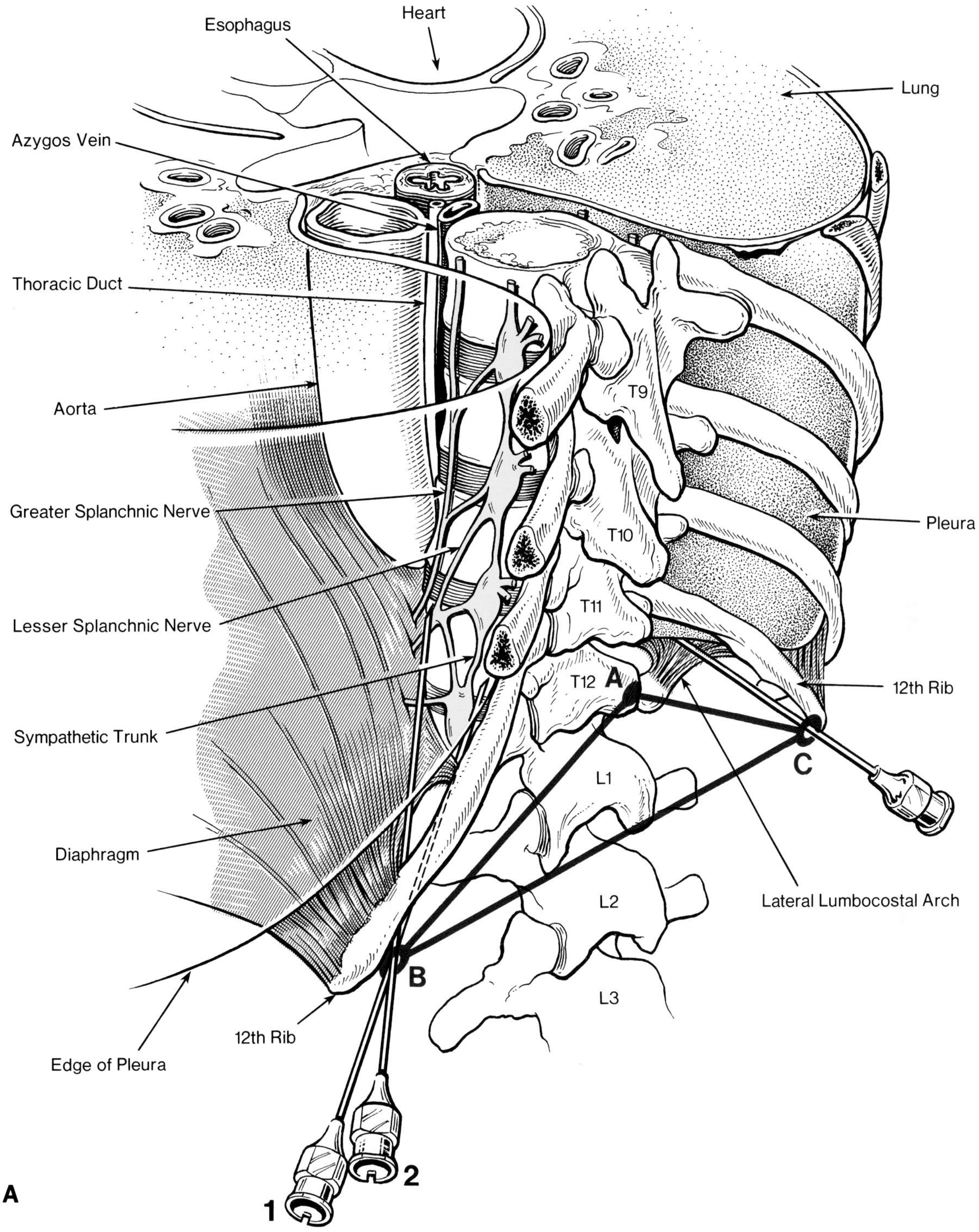

FIG. 14-8. A: Splanchnic nerve block, posterolateral view. Skin markings *B* and *C* are as in Figure 14-7. A is marked at the superior aspect of T12 spinous process. The technique of needle insertion is similar to that in Figure 14-7 but aimed along BA and CA to the superior aspect of T12. Note the proximity of pleura, and also the thoracic duct on left side.

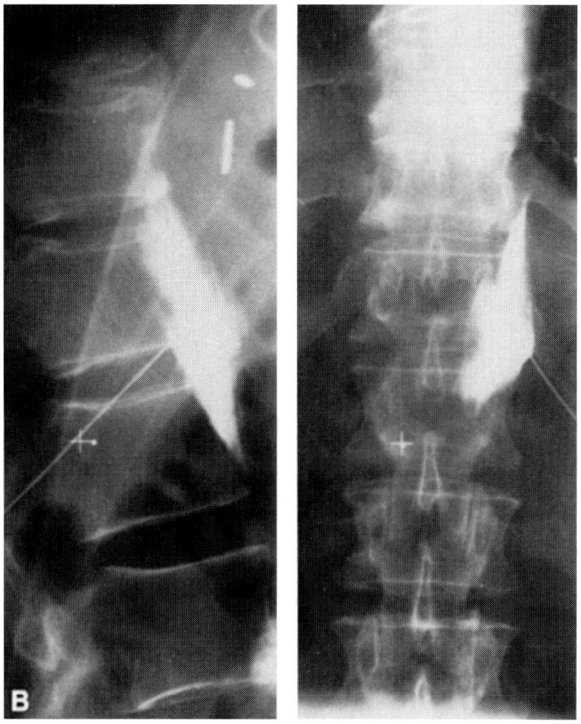

FIG. 14-8. *Continued.* **B:** Splanchnic nerve block: x-ray of spread of contrast medium, lateral view *(left)* and anteroposterior view *(right).* See text for details of block.

contrast media (e.g., 10% phenol in angiographin), which can be viewed directly as it spreads. Usually only 3 to 4 ml is required on each side.

Complications

Complications of this technique are similar to those of celiac block. Postural hypotension is less, however, because lumbar sympathetic ganglia are not blocked. The risk of pneumothorax is considerable, and it is important to keep the needle as close as possible to the vertebral body. The thoracic duct may be damaged, leading to chylothorax, or it may become obstructed, leading to lymphedema. Vascular puncture and hematoma formation may occur as in celiac block.

HYPOGASTRIC PLEXUS BLOCK

Although interruption of transmission through nerves in the hypogastric plexus in the treatment of a number of painful pelvic conditions has been accomplished surgically (presacral neurectomy), for many years, hypogastric plexus blockade by a percutaneous approach has only recently been described.[76] Because of the ease of applying epidural, caudal, or spinal anesthesia for surgery in the pelvic region, and because hypogastric plexus block is exclusively an autonomic blockade, it is likely that it will remain in the realm of pain management.

Anatomy

The (superior) hypogastric plexus constitutes the most caudal of the great plexi of the sympathetic nervous system. It is formed from pelvic visceral afferent and efferent sympathetic nerves from branches of the aortic plexus and fibers from the L2 and L3 splanchnic nerves. These pass through the plexus enroute to and from all pelvic viscerae (bladder, uterus, vagina, prostate, rectum) via the hypogastric nerves. The superior hypogastric plexus is retroperitoneal and distinctly situated at the sacral promontory, between the lower third of the fifth lumbar vertebrae and the upper third of the first sacral vertebral body, where it is accessible to blockade by a percutaneous needle. In this area, it is in close proximity to the bifurcation of the common iliac vessels. The inferior hypogastric plexi (right and left) are intertwined with the viscera of the pelvis, and for this reason, they cannot be isolated and separately blocked. However, as all of the sympathetic fibers must have passed first through the superior plexus, this is not a concern. They do receive parasympathetic fibers from S2–S4. Neither the superior nor the inferior hypogastric plexi contain somatic nerve fibers.

Technique

The patient is placed in the prone position, the same as for intercostal or celiac plexus blockade. In many respects, needle placement for hypogastric plexus block is identical to celiac plexus, but in the reverse direction (Fig. 14-9A). The target for a hypogastric plexus block is just anterior to the caudal end of the lumbar lordosis (L5–S1) instead of anterior to the cephalad end of the lordosis (L1) as in celiac plexus blockade. After the patient is adequately sedated, the skin is prepped with topical antiseptic, and the lumbosacral region is draped in a sterile manner. Bilateral skin wheals are raised 5 to 7 cm lateral to the L4–L5 interspace (intercristal line). A 10- to 15-cm, 20-gauge needle, with its bevel oriented in the medial direction, is introduced toward the midline at a 45° angle, and in the caudal direction at a 30° angle. Should the transverse body of L5 or iliac crest be encountered, first redirection slightly cephalad or caudad, then movement of insertion points 1 cm lateral or medial may be necessary. The needle is advanced until the body of L5 is contacted. The needle is then removed to the subcutaneous tissue, and maintaining the same caudal angle, redirected with slightly less medial angle and readvanced until it is felt to slide off the vertebral body. A slight loss of resistance from the psoas muscle fascia may be felt as the needle is advanced 1 cm more to reach its eventual position just anterior to the L5–S1 interspace (Fig. 14-9A). The second needle is placed in a similar manner on the opposite side. Fluoroscopic guidance is useful to facilitate passage of the needles and to demonstrate final positioning by injection of contrast. CT scan guidance may be beneficial in visualizing the common iliac vessels, or in determining whether exceptional anatomic alterations exist in the region, due to disease involvement. Contrast material (3

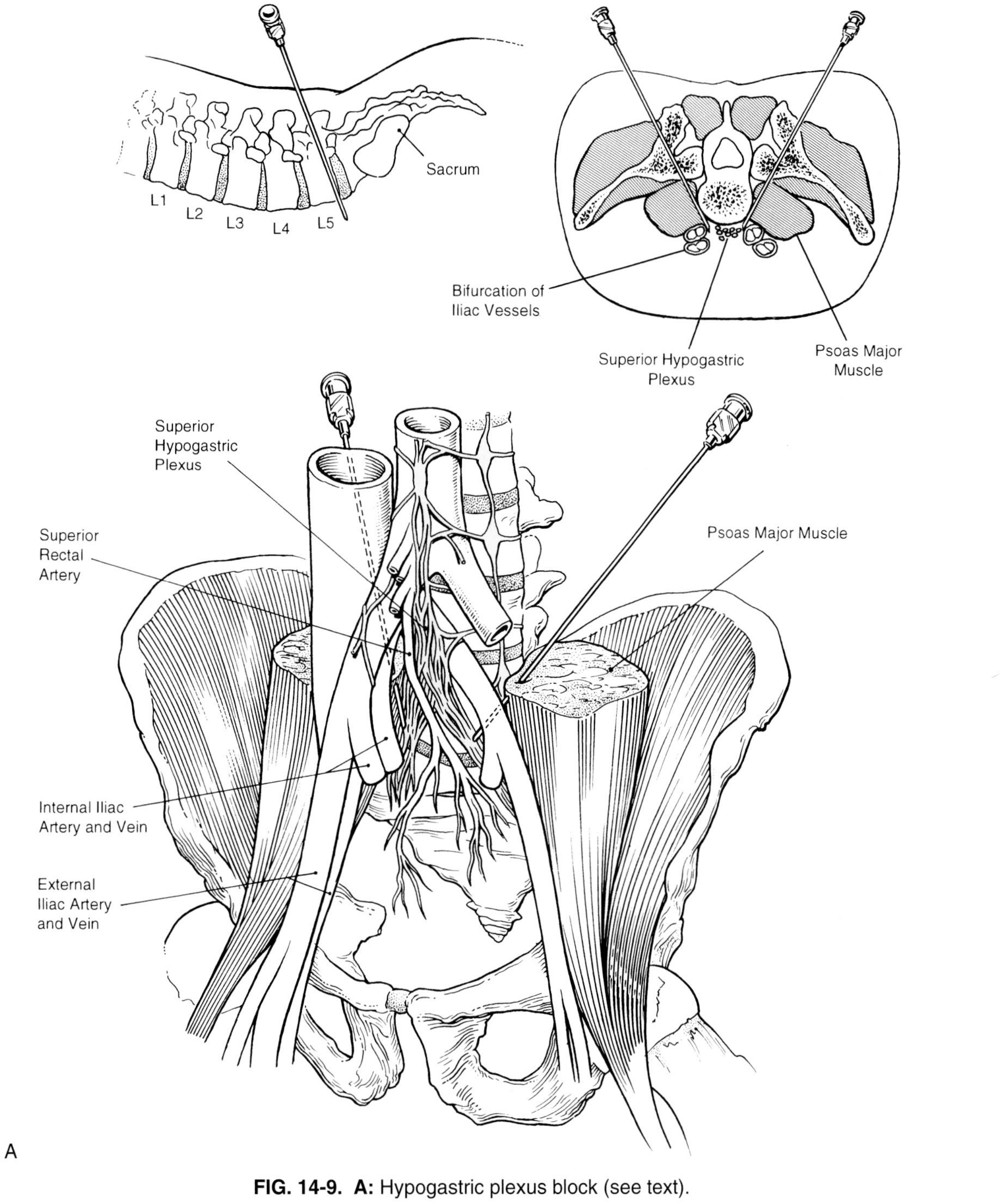

FIG. 14-9. A: Hypogastric plexus block (see text).

to 4 ml) should remain anterior to the vertebral bodies (Fig. 14–9B) with relatively smooth anterior (retroperitoneal space) and posterior (psoas muscle) borders on lateral images, and should meet but be confined to midline region on anteroposterior (AP) projections. A single-needle technique has been described, which may be useful for evaluation of nonmalignant conditions.[110] For malignant conditions where disease may prohibit adequate spread, the two-needle approach described above is recommended.[22]

Gentle aspiration should be performed in four quadrants, and if negative, a 3 ml test dose of epinephrine, containing local anesthetic, is injected to rule out intravascular or subarachnoid malpositioning. Substantial resistance to injection suggests improper positioning in the psoas muscle or the L5–S1 intervertebral disc. To confine solution to the plexus region, and to avoid spillage onto the nearby sacral somatic roots, injected volumes should be limited to 6 to 8 ml through each needle. For diagnostic/prognostic purposes,

B

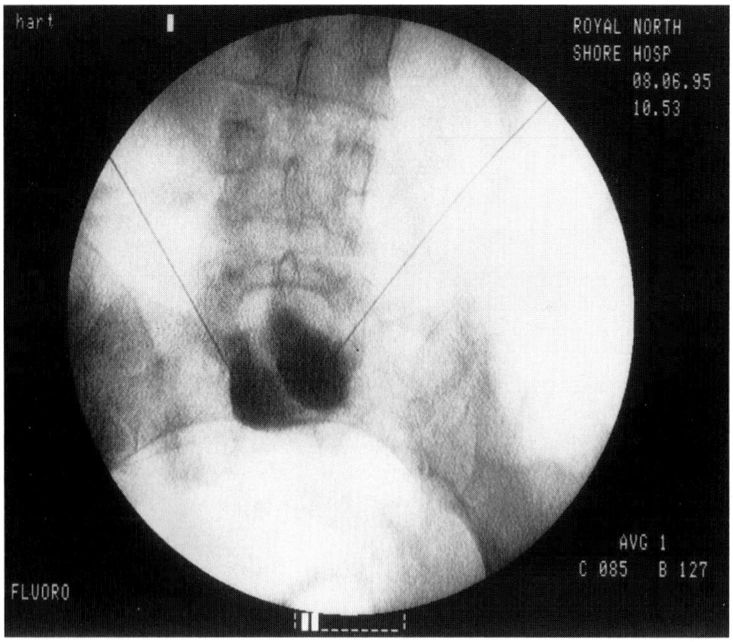

FIG. 14-9. *Continued.* **B:** Hypogastric plexus block. Anteroposterior radiograph (see text).

0.25% bupivacaine is recommended. When neurolytic agents are employed, use of a test dose should be performed meticulously, with repeated gentle aspiration through the remainder of injection. To date, neurolytic blockade has only been described using 10% phenol in water,[22] although 50% alcohol should be equally effective.

Surgical Applications

There are no reports of the efficacy of using hypogastric plexus blockade for surgical anesthesia. Because it is used exclusively as an autonomic block, it would have to be combined with other somatic blockade to provide adequate anesthesia. Theoretically, a combination anesthetic, including blockade of the hypogastric plexus, could block the autonomic 'stress' response of surgery in the pelvis, in ways analogous to celiac plexus blockade for abdominal surgery.

Non-surgical Applications

Hypogastric block may be useful in the differential diagnosis and treatment of chronic pelvic pain, particularly of neoplastic origin. Patients with pain due to cervical, endometrial, prostatic, testicular, and colorectal cancers have been treated with superior hypogastric blockade. Success (visual analogue guide for pain assessment [VAS] < 4 and significant reductions in opioid usage) appears to occur in 70%, with a duration until patient demise (3 to 12 months) in most reported patients. In three patients with pain felt to be secondary to complications of radiotherapy (enteritis, cystitis, proctitis), symptoms had not recurred after 2 years of follow-up.

Hypogastric plexus block can be considered in the evaluation and treatment of chronic benign pelvic pain conditions, but no data has yet been reported to support its efficacy.

Complications

Intramuscular, intravascular, subarachnoid, epidural, and intraperitoneal injection are all theoretically possible complications. Vascular puncture could lead to retroperitoneal hematoma formation, and neurologic damage could occur by direct needle trauma or with spillage of neurolytic solutions onto somatic nerves. Visceral puncture (ureter, bowel, uterus, and kidney) is possible. None of these possible complications have yet been reported. The incidence of these complications is therefore unknown, but should be minimized with strict adherence to technique.

INTERPLEURAL BLOCKADE

Anatomy

The visceral pleura invests the lung, following the fissures and indentations of the lobes. At the chest wall, diaphragm, and mediastinal margins of the lung, the pleura reflects back onto itself to form the parietal pleura, which follows the contours of the chest wall. Projected to the chest wall, anteriorly these lines of reflection emerge near the xiphoid, pass laterally to reach the midaxillary line at its intersection with the 10th rib, and cross the neck of the 12th rib to reach its posterior reflection about 4 cm from the midline. As these lines of reflection are fixed, interpleural anesthesia can, technically, be instituted anywhere within these boundaries.

Anesthesia is attained by diffusion of local anesthetic solution to nerves which run in proximity to the pleural surfaces. Anteriorly, laterally, and posteriorly, the parietal pleura is in close approximation to the intercostal nerves. Superiorly, the inferior roots of the brachial plexus pass a short distance over the cupola before reaching the first rib. Medially, the sympathetic chain, splanchnic, phrenic, and vagus nerves are also adjacent. The epidural and subarachnoid spaces are at a greater distance and are generally not felt to be a site of local anesthetic action during interpleural anesthesia. However, these structures are only separated from the parietal pleura by the fat and loose connective tissues of the epidural and paravertebral spaces, and should there be a significant breach of the parietal pleura, tracking of anesthetic solution to these structures is also possible.

Technique

Spread of local anesthetic solution within the interpleural space is dominated primarily by gravity, but to a lesser degree is influenced by volume and the location of the catheter itself.[40] These factors must be taken into account before placement of the catheter and injection of solution. Interpleural catheters most commonly are placed posteriorly with the patient in the lateral or semiprone position, but have also been placed near the midaxillary line or anteriorly with the patient supine. The hallmark of this technique is detection of the negative interpleural pressure, so placement should be performed either pre- or postoperatively in the awake patient, or during general anesthesia with the patient breathing spontaneously. Placement should be avoided during positive pressure ventilation, as the interpleural pressure is no longer negative, and the risk of pneumothorax, and its conversion to a tension pneumothorax, is greatly increased.[102]

When using the posterior approach, with the patient in either the lateral or prone position, the arm should be allowed to dangle in front of the body or off of the table to retract the scapula as far anteriorly as possible. After sterile prep and drape, the skin is first anesthetized at a point 8 to 10 cm lateral from the midline, overlying the top edge of a rib. Infiltration is carried deeper with a 4 cm, 22-gauge needle, until the rib is contacted (Fig. 14–10). The periosteum is quite sensitive, so additional injection of 1 ml of local anesthetic at this point will minimize discomfort. This 'finder' needle is removed and replaced with a 16- or 18-gauge Tuohy needle. After recontacting the rib, and with the hand which controls the needle maintaining firm contact with the patient's back, the needle is gently walked cephalad until it is felt to slide off the superior edge of the rib. The bevel should be aimed in the direction in which the catheter will be passed.

At this stage, one of two methods may be used safely. In the original technique, the stylet is removed and replaced with a "frictionless" (saline-lubricated or polished dry) glass 10 ml syringe containing 3 to 5 ml of air.[85] The needle-syringe unit is then advanced slowly, until entrance into the interpleural space is detected: the plunger will be pulled in as

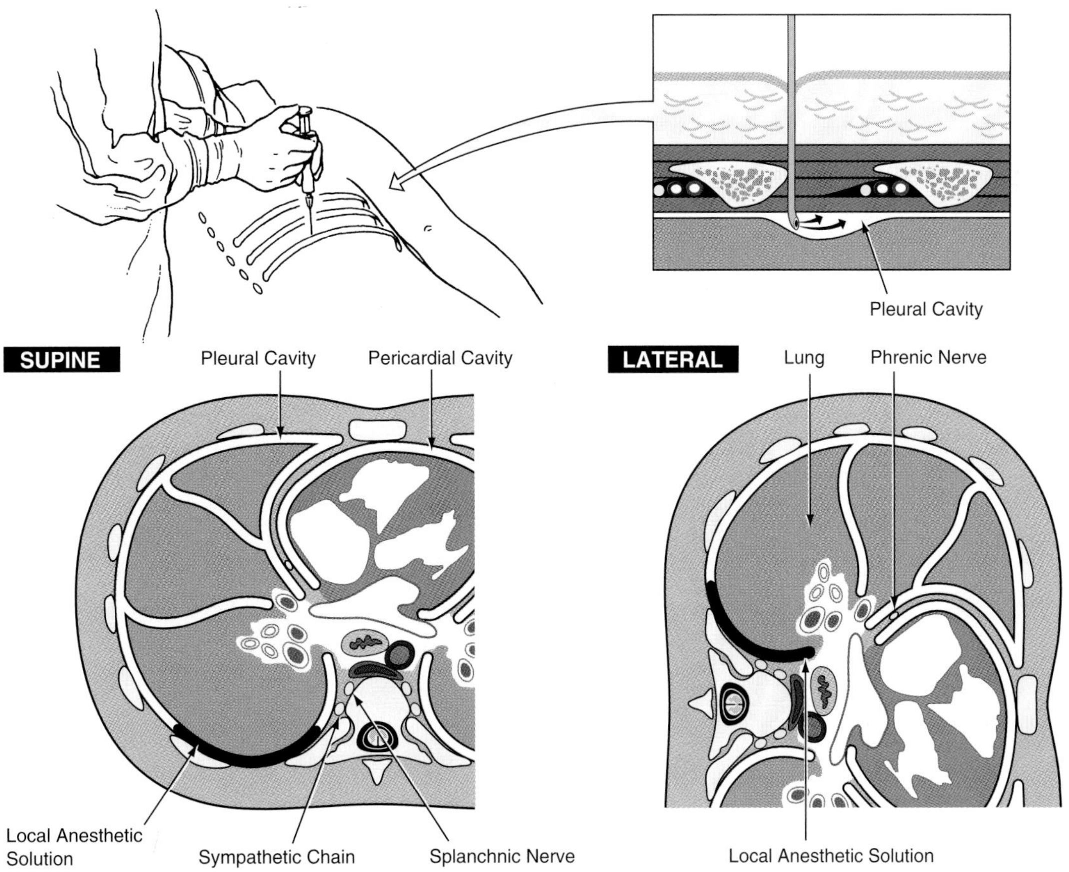

FIG. 14-10. Interpleural block (see text).

the negative interpleural pressure evacuates the air from the syringe (Figure 14-10). If awake, the patient should be warned that a brief twinge may be felt as the parietal pleura is penetrated. Gentle intermittent tapping of the plunger can assure that the needle is not being plugged, and that the plunger is not sticking in the barrel of the syringe. Both of these situations could result in the needle being advanced too far; no movement of the plunger would occur. If this technique is employed preoperatively, nitrous oxide should not be used during subsequent general anesthesia, because a significant expansion of the small pneumothorax which is created could occur.

Once in the interpleural space, the syringe is removed, and the interpleural catheter is gently passed 5 to 6 cm. The needle is removed then and an occlusive dressing is applied. Aspiration of the catheter may produce a small amount (<20 ml) of air or fluid. If blood or large amounts of air or fluid are obtained, the catheter should be removed and replaced, or the technique abandoned.

A second technique employs connecting a saline-containing syringe to the Tuohy needle after the stylet is removed.[5] Once connected, the plunger of the syringe is removed entirely, and close attention is directed to the meniscus at the saline-air interface. During slow advancement of the needle-syringe unit, entrance into the interpleural space is heralded by the 'falling column' of saline. A catheter is then passed into the open-ended syringe barrel, through the saline and needle, and into the interpleural space. The advantage of this technique is that no air is introduced or allowed to entrain into the interpleural space.

The use of loss-of-resistance to positive pressure should be strictly avoided; one cannot always be certain whether the loss is the interpleural space itself, or a 'false' loss-of-resistance which can occur between intercostal muscles or when the needle is advanced too far into lung parenchyma.

Prior to local anesthetic injection, the patient should be placed in a position to maximize the desired effect. As solution movement is governed by gravity, blockade will localize at the dependent point.[88] Positioning the patient with the operative side up causes solution to pool medially, which maximizes the amount of subsequent sympathetic blockade (Fig. 14-10, Lateral), while the supine and operative-side-down positions cause solution to accumulate near the intercostal nerves (Fig. 14-10, Supine), minimizing the amount of sympathetic blockade that is administered. A head-down positioning can increase the amount of cervical and upper thoracic sympathetic blockade and, in some instances, can produce anesthesia of the inferior roots of the brachial plexus.

As in epidural anesthesia, a small epinephrine-containing 'test dose' should be administered first to detect accidental intravascular placement. The total dose (20 to 30 ml) should be given in intermittent doses over 2 to 3 minutes, and the positioning maintained for 20 to 30 minutes to allow the anesthetic to "set." Bupivacaine 0.25% appears to have an onset and duration of action identical to the 0.5% concentration. In fact, the duration of action appears to be proportional to the mg amount of drug given (100 mg producing 8 hours of analgesia), not the concentration or volume.[100]

Surgical Applications

Although fear of pneumothorax and high serum local anesthetic levels have attenuated the initial enthusiasm, interpleural blockade remains a valuable anesthetic/analgesia option in selected clinical situations. Combination with light general anesthesia is often necessary. Interpleural analgesia is perhaps best utilized for open cholecystectomy, renal surgery, and unilateral breast procedures. After cholecystectomy, opioid requirements and VAS pain scales are reduced, and pulmonary parameters are improved when interpleural analgesia is used.[29,78]

Its usefulness during thoracotomy is controversial, because the duration of blockade appears to be significantly reduced when the parietal pleura is interrupted and a thoracostomy drainage tube is present.[28,103] However, instillation of local anesthetic through a chest tube (used as an interpleural catheter) may be a beneficial adjunct in the treatment of post-thoracotomy pain, if adequate analgesia is difficult to attain by other means and the tube can be clamped off for 20 minutes without patient hazard.

Bilateral interpleural catheters have been reported for upper abdominal surgery and bilateral pulmonary surgery through sternotomy.[51] The consequences of bilateral pneumothoraces, and the vigilance necessary to detect and treat rapidly, should they occur, are obvious.

Nonsurgical Applications

Interpleural catheterization has been used in many novel ways for nonsurgical means. Perhaps the best success is in treating the pain of multiple rib fractures, where dramatic improvement of pulmonary function results.[91] Case reports of treating upper limb ischemia and reflex sympathetic dystrophy, the pain of acute and chronic pancreatitis have been described.[2,75,83,84] Interpleural catheters have been used to treat spontaneous and iatrogenic pneumothoraces. Preliminary reports are optimistic in patients who have previously been very difficult to treat, including tumor invasion of the brachial plexus, vertebral metastases, and severe postherpetic neuralgia.[25,82] Catheters have been tunneled subcutaneously for the long-term management of thoracic pain in cancer patients.[108] Injection of phenol into the interpleural space was beneficial in managing a patient with esophageal cancer in whom other means of analgesia had been tried and found to be ineffective.[52] Although interpleural analgesia may not be a first choice in the treatment of many of these pathologic situations, its utilization may be beneficial in providing a drug or treatment "pause" which is frequently necessary in these circumstances.

Complications

The complications of interpleural injection of local anesthetic have been reviewed by Stromskag. Pneumothorax occurs in approximately 2.0%.[99] Many of the reported cases have occurred when patients were being mechanically ventilated, an active loss-of-resistance technique was used, the patient unexpectedly moved, or the Tuohy needle became accidentally occluded. The incidence of pneumothorax, with proper indications, and using sound technique, is most likely even less.

Serum local anesthetic levels reach a peak in 20 to 30 minutes, and tend to be higher than when equal amounts are injected for multiple intercostal nerve blocks. The analgesia also tends to be less intense and of shorter duration.[109] The addition of epinephrine does not decrease serum bupivacaine levels, nor does it increase the duration or intensity of blockade (see Chapter 3).

Phrenic nerve paresis does occur in some instances, but its incidence and clinical significance remain to be elucidated.[48,50] Ipsilateral bronchospasm has been reported in one patient.[95] Horner's syndrome occurs frequently, is reversible, and should not be unexpected, considering the sympathetic blockade which is possible. Cholestasis, documented by clinical and laboratory findings, has been described in three patients with right interpleural catheters used to treat upper extremity reflex sympathetic dystrophy (RSD[7]).

PARAVERTEBRAL LUMBAR SOMATIC NERVE BLOCK

Anatomy

When lumbar somatic nerve block is performed paravertebrally, it has many similarities to intercostal nerve block. Instead of using ribs as bony landmarks, however, the primary bony guide becomes the transverse process of the lumbar vertebral body—a "rudimentary" rib. The lumbar nerves exit their respective intervertebral foramina just inferior to the caudad edge of each transverse process. These nerves divide immediately into anterior and posterior branches. The small posterior branches supply the skin of the lower back and the paravertebral muscles. Of primary interest, however, are the anterior branches of the first four lumbar nerves. These nerves, together with a small branch from the 12th thoracic nerve, form the lumbar plexus. This plexus is conceived largely within the substance of the psoas major muscle, and most of the peripheral branches exit laterally in a plane between the psoas and quadratus lumborum muscles.

The major branches of the lumbar plexus (i.e., the iliohypogastric, ilioinguinal, and lateral femoral cutaneous nerves) continue laterally around the rim of the pelvis. Their terminal branches approach and pass near the anterior superior iliac spine. The femoral nerve passes almost directly caudad, after emerging from the lateral edge of psoas major. The obturator nerve emerges from the medial edge of psoas major, descends under the common iliac vessels, and finally emerges from the pelvis through the obturator foramen. The ultimate cutaneous distribution of each of these nerves is quite variable in the groin and anterolateral leg. There is also considerable overlap of cutaneous branches of individual nerves. The primary peripheral branches of the lumbar plexus are listed in Table 14-4 and illustrated in Figure 14-11. It is apparent that paravertebral nerve block of L1–L4 will result in sensory and motor block of the groin and much of the leg. For intra-abdominal, pelvic, or groin operations, only the upper two lumbar segments need to be blocked. In general, the lumbar nerves tend to slope sharply caudad as they emerge from the intervertebral foraminae. In doing so, they tend to course anterior to the tips of the transverse processes of the next lower lumbar vertebral bodies. A needle placed at the inferior edge of a transverse process will be close to nerves from two lumbar segments: Medially, it will

TABLE 14-4. *Origins and distribution of the lumbar plexus*

Peripheral nerve	Root segments
Iliohypogastric	T12, L1
Ilioinguinal	L1
Genitofemoral	L1, L2
Lateral femoral cutaneous	L2, L3
Femoral	L2, L3, L4
Obturator	L2, L3, L4

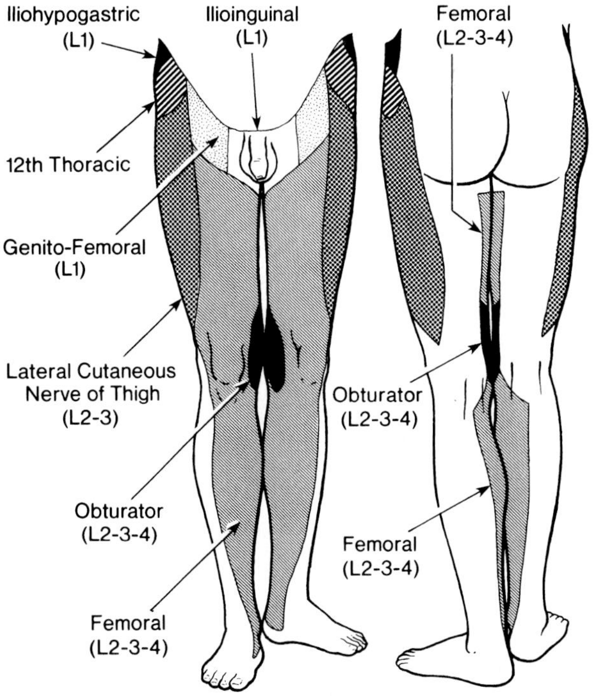

FIG. 14-11. Cutaneous branches of lumbar plexus and the areas of skin that they supply.

be close to the nerve exiting the vertebral foramen; laterally, it will be near the nerve from the next most cephalad vertebral level. Hence, local anesthetic solution injected at the proper depth inferior to one lumbar vertebral process actually can result in nerve block of two or more root segments.

Technique

The patient's prone position is identical to that described for intercostal and celiac plexus nerve block. The injection sites are marked while keeping in mind that the cephalad edge of a lumbar posterior spinous process lies opposite the caudad edge of its homologous transverse process. The distance between similar points on any two lumbar transverse processes is about 2 cm. Visualizing and then locating the transverse process is fundamental to a successful block. After palpating and marking each of the lumbar vertebral spinous processes, the anesthesiologist draws horizontal lines at the cephalad edge of each one, and projects them laterally. Two vertical lines should then be drawn parallel to, and 3 to 5 cm lateral from, the midline. The points of intersection of the vertical and horizontal lines mark the sites where skin wheals are raised (Fig. 14-12). In surgical patients, the block can be performed under the same sedation used for intercostal and celiac plexus block. An 8-cm, 22-gauge needle is inserted perpendicularly to the skin until it contacts the transverse process at a depth of 3 to 5 cm. The needle then should be withdrawn to a subcutaneous level, and redirected, to slide off the caudad edge of the transverse process. The needle is advanced another 2 to 3 cm beyond the point where it previously made contact with bone, and 6 to 10 ml of local anesthetic solution is injected as the needle is withdrawn 2 to 3 cm. Paresthesiae are not sought. This process is repeated at each of the lumbar levels at which anesthesia is desired. The useful concentrations of local anesthetic are the same as those used for intercostal block.

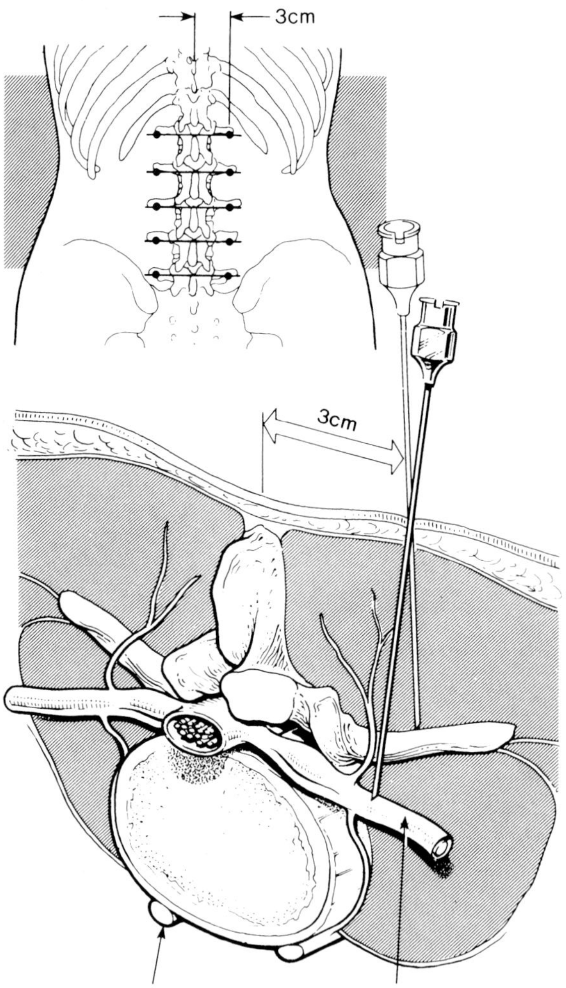

FIG. 14-12. Paravertebral lumbar somatic nerve block. **Upper Panel:** Skin markings are made by drawing lines across the cephalad aspect of spinous processes and then drawing vertical lines 3 cm from the midline. **Lower Panel:** A needle inserted perpendicular to the skin will contact the caudad edge of a transverse process. Angulation of the needle in a caudad direction to slide caudad to the transverse process will reach the spinal nerve 1 to 2 cm deeper than the transverse process.

Surgical Applications

Lumbar paravertebral nerve block can rarely be used as the sole anesthetic for surgery. It effectively complements intercostal and celiac plexus block for intra-abdominal surgery and pelvic procedures, particularly where the incision extends to the pubis. Groin operations, such as herniorrhaphy or femoral pseudoaneurysm repair or embolectomy, can be performed with lumbar block (particularly in anticoagulated patients where central neuraxial block is best avoided), but supplementation with local infiltration or intravenous drugs usually is necessary.

Nonsurgical Applications

When the block is used for diagnostic purposes, only small volumes of local anesthetic solution should be injected, so as to limit spread centrally or to adjacent lumbar nerves. Some physicians use fluoroscopy or a nerve stimulator to position the needle precisely and then inject only 0.5 to 1 ml of drug. This technique may be especially helpful in evaluating patients with back pain, in which the recurrent meningeal nerve may play a role. This branch is highly variable but tends to arise from the main nerve root just before separating into anterior and posterior parts. Another diagnostic use of paravertebral lumbar somatic block is in evaluating groin or genital pain, such as the nerve entrapment syndromes that sometimes follow/inguinal herniorrhaphy.

Complications

It is possible to inject into intravascular, epidural, or subarachnoid spaces, during performance of this block. Should the needle be inserted too far medially, it could enter a vertebral foramen or penetrate a dural sleeve to produce spinal anesthesia. There could also be perineural spread of solution into the epidural space, with a consequent variable degree of anesthesia over the lower extremities. Intravascular injection can be minimized by aspiration tests, and by avoiding large volume injections. The lumbar sympathetic chain may be anesthetized either from local block of gray and white rami communicantes, or by deeper penetration of local anesthetic drug to the sympathetic chain itself. Intraperitoneal injection, or puncture of retroperitoneal (kidney) or intra-abdominal organs, is possible, although only as a result of gross error.

PARAVERTEBRAL THORACIC SOMATIC NERVE BLOCK

Anatomy

In many ways, thoracic paravertebral nerve blockade is similar to lumbar paravertebral nerve block. A bony landmark is used to position the needle (or catheter) in proximity to the segmental spinal nerve; there are, however, some important differences. The risk of pneumothorax is a real possibility because of the proximity of the pleura and lung. One must remember also that the presence of ribs can make identification of bony landmarks confusing. Also, during performance of a lumbar paravertebral, the injection is into the body of the psoas muscle, where the nerve roots are forming the lumbar plexus. The psoas muscle also has been shown to form a caudal boundary to the thoracic paravertebral space and thus to confine thoracic paravertebral injections to the thoracic region.[54] However, paravertebral injections are not entirely restricted to the paravertebral space since solution has been shown to spread through the intervertebral foramina, where it then enters the epidural space and is free to course up and down or across the midline.[77] There is no muscle in the thorax analogous to the psoas muscle, and thoracic paravertebral injections are made into loose connective tissue which separates the parietal pleura from the bony architecture (rib, vertebral transverse process, and vertebral body). Finally, because of the smaller size of the thoracic vertebrae, the sympathetic chain and splanchnic nerves are in closer approximation to the final position of the needle. The psoas muscle in the lumbar region effectively contains the somatic nerves and a paravertebral injection within its fascia and isolates them from the sympathetic chain in the lumbar region. No such fascial layers separate the sympathetic chain from the somatic nerves in the thoracic region, so concomitant ipsilateral sympathetic blockade and somatic blockade can be anticipated.

Technique

Several modifications and techniques exist for thoracic paravertebral block. The first has been discussed previously in the section on intercostal blockade, and continuous intercostal catheterization. When an epidural catheter is passed 3 to 5 cm through a Tuohy needle, which has been placed into the intercostal space at the angle of the rib with its bevel directed medially, its lumen consistently will rest in or near the paravertebral space during subsequent dosing. It is sometimes beneficial to angle the needle slightly towards the midline to facilitate passage of the catheter, and to direct the needle itself somewhat tangential to the parietal pleura. A slight 'pop', or loss of resistance, may be felt as the posterior intercostal membrane is penetrated.

The second 'classic' approach requires localization of a thoracic vertebral transverse process as its prime landmark. The patient may be situated in the prone, lateral, or sitting positions. Because of the extreme angulation of the spinous processes of the thoracic vertebrae, a skin wheal is raised 3 cm lateral to the top of the spinous process of the vertebra above the chosen level. By inserting a 6 to 8 cm needle through the wheal and parallel to the midline, the transverse process is first located at a depth of 2 to 5 cm. To avoid accidental puncture of the pleura, it is imperative that the transverse process be found without the needle penetrating any deeper than necessary. If the transverse process is not contacted initially at a depth of 3 cm, it should be withdrawn, redirected slightly caudad, and then reinserted 3 cm. If the transverse process is still not contacted, the needle should be withdrawn again, and redirected slightly cephalad and advanced 3 cm. Only then should the needle be advanced deeper, in search of the transverse process.

Once the transverse process is located, the needle can be walked off either the cephalad or caudal edge of the process and advanced 1 to 2 cm further, where 6 to 10 ml of anesthetic solution is injected. An air-filled syringe can be connected to the needle after contact with the transverse process has been lost, and a 'loss-of-resistance' can be elicited as the needle penetrates the costotransverse ligament and enters the paravertebral space. The needle may be directed 20° to 30° medial to help avoid pleura, if the skin wheal had initially been placed too far lateral. This medial angulation also places the tip closer to the root as it emerges from the intervertebral foramen. Occasionally the vertebrae itself is contacted, at which point the needle is withdrawn 0.5 cm and the solution injected. Intentionally contacting the vertebrae has been employed by some, but is not recommended, as it is possible to enter an intervertebral foramen and the epidural or subarachnoid space, if the needle is advanced further without contacting bone. Walking off the top of the process will place the needle in proximity to the nerve root above, as it angles inferiorly before entering the intercostal groove.

A final modification involves intentionally locating the lamina first, by starting at a more medial point—1.5 cm lateral to the top of the spinous process, and walking caudad and lateral off the lamina into the costotransverse ligament. With this approach, a loss-of-resistance technique of passing through this ligament must be used, because the needle is directed lateral toward the pleura. Once loss-of-resistance occurs, solution is injected without any further advancement.

Surgical Applications

Except for superficial operations, thoracic paravertebral nerve block cannot be used as the sole anesthetic for surgery. When combined with light general anesthesia, it can be substituted for intercostal blockade and complements celiac plexus block for intra-abdominal surgery and thoracic procedures.

Nonsurgical Applications

Thoracic paravertebral block has been used effectively in the treatment of chronic post-thoracotomy pain, with relief from a single injection of local anesthetic lasting over 1 month in 60% of patients. Relief in treatment of chronic postmastectomy pain and postherpetic neuralgia are less successful.[45] Acute herpes zoster has been treated with thoracic paravertebral catheterization and continuous infusion of 0.25% bupivacaine at 5 ml/hr for 4 days.[42]

Like lumbar paravertebral somatic block, when used for diagnostic purposes, it is preferable to use only small volumes of local anesthetic solution, so as to limit spread centrally or to adjacent lumbar nerves. Some physicians seek specific paresthesia in the involved area and/or use fluoroscopy to position the needle precisely and then inject only 0.5 to 1 ml of drug.

Complications

Because of the proximity of the sympathetic chain and splanchnic nerves, ipsilateral sympathetic blockade can be expected. If bilateral blockade is performed, sympathetic blockade equivalent to spinal or epidural anesthesia to the thoracic region, and the possibility of hypotension, can be anticipated. Intravascular epidural and subarachnoid injections are possible. The incidence of solution tracking into the ipsilateral epidural space is as high as 70%, with bilateral epidural spread occurring in 7%.[77]

Pneumothorax has been reported, but its incidence is unknown. Furthermore, the safety of the different techniques of performing thoracic paravertebral blockade regarding their risk of pneumothorax is also unknown. Interpleural spread, without attendant puncture of visceral pleura, occurred in 7% of injections in one radiographic study.[77]

MISCELLANEOUS NERVE BLOCKS OF THE ABDOMEN AND CHEST

The somatic nerve blocks previously described in this chapter are performed at anatomic sites near the central neuraxis. There are many more peripheral sites along these nerve pathways for nerve block, but all are merely variations. The more distal the site on a peripheral nerve, the greater is the chance for incomplete block, because of factors such as spatial distribution, overlap of nerve territories, and the difficulty of reaching each of the multiple branches of an arborizing nerve with injected local anesthetic solution. These factors can be partially overcome by using large volumes of solution, by using multiple injections, and by selecting local anesthetic agents with high penetrability; however, it is easier to hit the trunk of a tree than to touch each of its branches, and the previously described blocks are therefore more useful and predictable. A small amount of anesthetic injected at a primary nerve trunk will provide the best quality anesthesia. The following blocks are described primarily for the sake of completeness of information, historical perspective, and to improve appreciation of anatomic detail of nerve distribution.

RECTUS BLOCK

Anatomy

As the lower five intercostal nerves course anteriorly, they surface eventually and terminate after penetrating the rectus abdominis muscle. These nerves enter the rectus sheath at the posterolateral border of the body of that muscle. The tendinous intersections of the rectus tend to create segmental distribution of individual intercostal nerves, but there is some overlap of adjacent fibers. Anteriorly, the rectus sheath is tough and fibrous from pubis to xiphoid. Posteriorly, it is strong and readily identifiable down to the level of the umbilicus, but then it fades into a thin sheath of transversalis fascia, which adheres closely to peritoneum below the semicircular line of Douglas. The posterior rectus sheath above the umbilicus is quite substantial and can serve as a "backboard" for injecting local anesthetic solution. This solution will be confined by the tendinous intersections, but within those limits will spread up and down to anesthetize the peripheral motor and sensory branches of the intercostal nerves.

Technique

The patient lies supine, and the anesthesiologist may stand at either side. From two to six sites are chosen for injections, the number depending on the location and size of surgical incision (Fig. 14-13). If performed while the patient is awake, skin wheals are raised at the middle of each segment of the rectus muscle body that can be palpated between tendinous intersections. A reusable or short bevel 5-cm, 22-gauge needle is passed through skin and subcutaneous tissue until it meets the firm resistance of the anterior rectus sheath. The block should be discontinued unless this sheath can be convincingly demonstrated by pushing on the needle. With controlled, steady pressure, the needle is pushed to penetrate this sheath with a definite snap. Advancing further passes the needle through the softer belly of the muscle, and as the needle approaches the posterior rectus sheath, the anesthesiologist will feel firm resistance again. Using this posterior

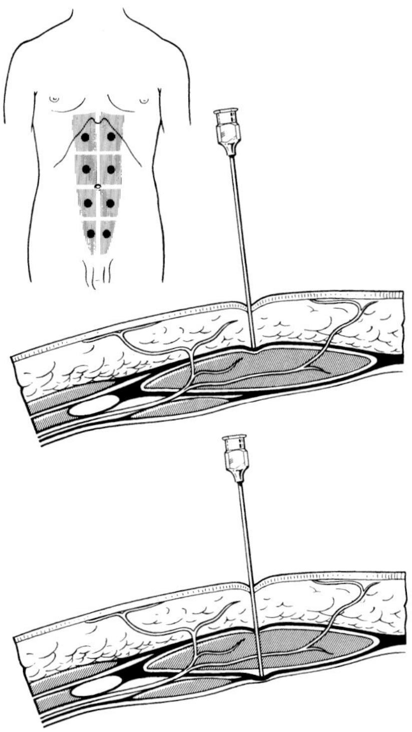

FIG. 14-13. Rectus block. **Upper:** Skin wheals are raised in the center of rectus segments. These are delineated by a vertical line through umbilicus and horizontal lines at umbilical level, and midway between umbilicus and xiphisternum, and umbilicus and pubis, respectively. **Middle:** Short bevel needle contacts resistance of anterior rectus sheath. **Lower:** Needle penetrates rectus muscle and is halted by resistance of posterior rectus sheath. Note the latter structure is absent below the line midway between umbilicus and pubis. Thus, these two rectus injections are made last.

sheath as a backboard, 10 ml of local anesthetic solution is injected. The process is repeated at each injection site. Blocks above the umbilicus should be performed first, and needle depth noted, before attempting any additional blocks below the umbilicus, where injection just after the loss-of-resistance of the anterior sheath may be safer and sufficient.

Surgical Applications

Rectus block alone will not provide enough anesthesia for most surgical procedures, and definitely will require supplementation if the abdominal cavity is to be explored. The block has proven useful in the management of surgical pain after incisional and umbilical hernias, postpartum and laparoscopic tubal ligation, Cesarean section when a midline incision is used,[104] and outpatient laparoscopy.[98]

Nonsurgical Applications

Rectus block may be useful in diagnosing abdominal nerve entrapment syndromes or localized myofascial problems.

Complications

It is difficult to identify the posterior rectus sheath where it lies near the xiphoid and pubis. Attempting this block at these levels may result in penetration of peritoneum and underlying organs such as liver, intestine, bladder, or uterus. In the patient with a distended abdomen, the thinly stretched rectus may prevent clear identification of anterior and posterior sheaths. A visible bulge in the abdominal wall upon injection indicates that the needle is too superficial, and a poor block will result. The block is difficult in the obese, cachectic, or elderly patient with poor abdominal muscle tone.

ILIAC CREST BLOCK

Anatomy

The peripheral extensions of the ilioinguinal, iliohypogastric, and 12th thoracic nerves follow a circular course that is somewhat determined by the bowl-like shape of the ilium. In sweeping around anteriorly, these branches pass near the anterior superior iliac spine—a prominent landmark even in the obese patient. At or near the level of the anterior superior iliac spine, the 12th thoracic and iliohypogastric nerves lie between the internal and external oblique muscles. The ilioinguinal nerve lies between transversus abdominis and internal oblique muscles initially and then penetrates internal oblique a variable distance medial to the anterior superior iliac spine (Fig. 14-14). They continue anteromedially and become superficial as they terminate in branches to skin and muscles of the inguinal region. Using the anterior superior iliac spine as a primary point of orientation, the anesthesiologist can perform an infiltration block known as iliac crest block. Success depends on spreading a large volume of anesthetic solution between abdominal wall muscle layers. The block is inadequate to provide total anesthesia for inguinal herniorraphy, because structures that enter the inguinal canal through the internal inguinal ring will not be anesthetized, but the surgeon can accomplish this adequately with direct local infiltration of the spermatic cord, during the procedure (see following).

Technique

The patient lies in the supine position. A point is marked on the skin roughly 3 cm medial and 3 cm inferior to the anterior superior iliac spine (Fig. 14-14). A skin wheal is raised and an 8-cm, 22-gauge needle inserted in a superolateral direction to contact the inner surface of the ilium (Fig. 14-14). Ten milliliters of local anesthetic solution is injected as the needle is slowly withdrawn. Then the needle should be reinserted at a somewhat steeper angle, to ensure penetration of all three lateral abdominal muscles. The injection is repeated as the needle is withdrawn. In the obese or heavily muscled patient, a third injection may be necessary at an even steeper angle. Subcutaneous infiltration superior to the skin wheal, from anterior superior iliac spine to umbilicus, will give a

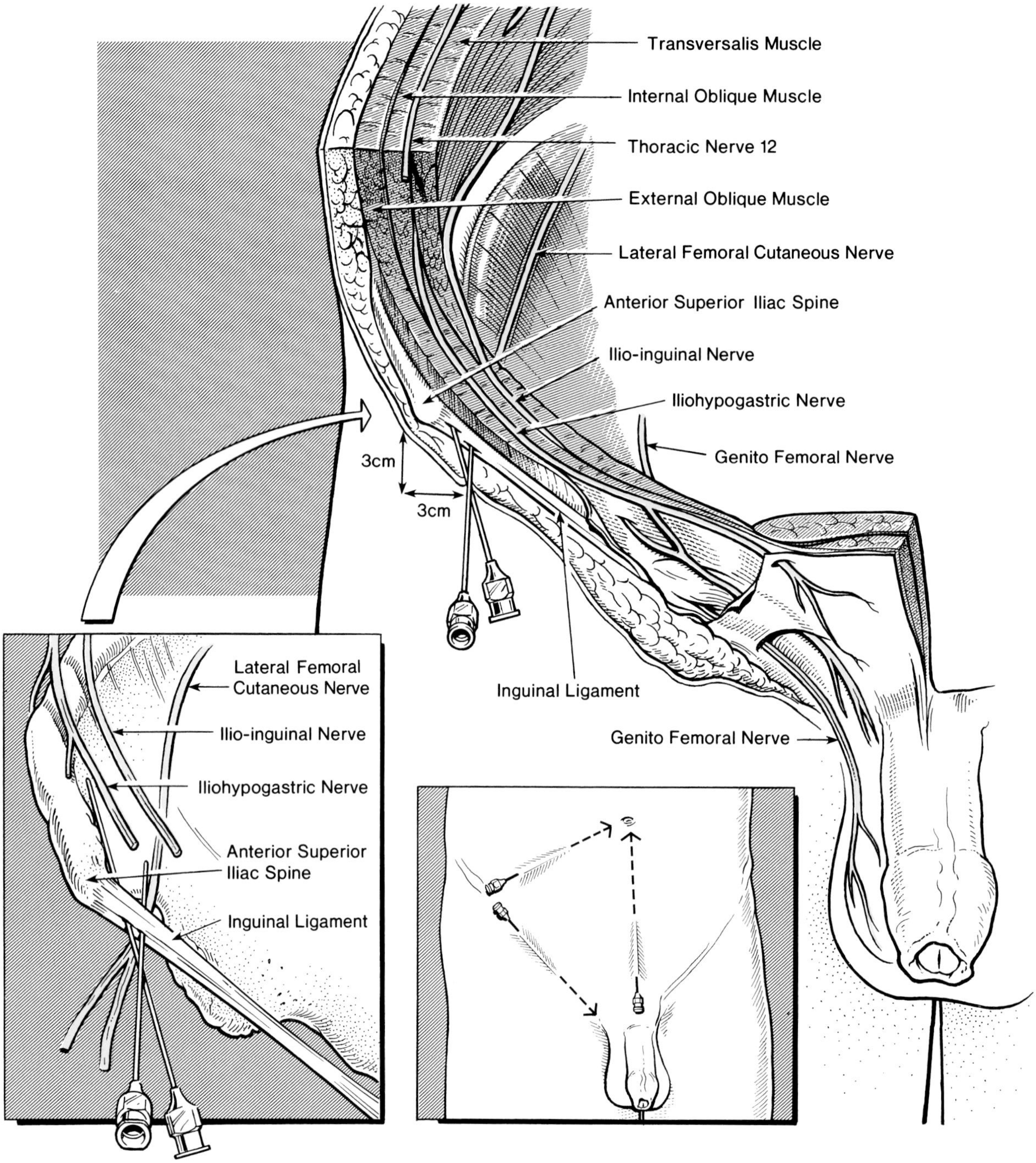

FIG. 14-14. Iliac crest block. **Upper Panel:** Note point of needle insertion 3 cm caudad to and 3 cm medial to anterior superior iliac spine (ASIS). Initial direction of needle is superolateral to reach the inner aspect of iliac bone. Then the needle is redirected approximately perpendicular to the long axis of the body (see also Fig. 14-13). Note the locations of nerves in relation to muscles of the abdominal wall (see text). An alternative technique is to insert the needle 3 cm along a line from ASIS to umbilicus (see Chapter 20, Fig. 20-5). **Lower Panel:** Bone and ligamentous landmarks in relation to nerves *(Left)*. Superficial infiltration for herniorrhaphy (see text) *(Right)*.

broader area of skin anesthesia as it catches some cutaneous branches of the last two or three intercostal nerves (Fig. 14-14). Infiltration is also extended along the line of the incision. Finally, midline infiltration, from umbilicus to pubis, may be used to block overlapping fibers from the opposite side (Fig. 14-14).

If herniorraphy is to be performed, a second skin wheal may be raised 2 to 3 cm above the midinguinal point. A 5-cm needle is inserted, perpendicular to the skin, to a depth of 3 to 5 cm. Ten to 15 ml of local anesthetic solution should be injected in fan-wise fashion. This produces anesthesia of the genitofemoral nerve, sympathetic fibers, and peritoneal sac. However, there is a risk of hematoma owing to trauma to the femoral artery. Thus it may be more appropriate and preferable for the surgeon to inject 2 to 3 ml of local anesthetic directly into the covering of the spermatic cord as soon as it is exposed.

Surgical Applications

Iliac crest block is an excellent first maneuver for the surgeon or anesthesiologist who performs infiltration anesthesia for inguinal herniorrhaphy.[92] Although the two injection sites described above may be adequate for herniorrhaphy, additional direct local infiltration may be needed to have a completely pain-free operation. It is especially difficult to anesthetize all the structures in the internal ring or the pubic ramus with a percutaneous injection.

The debate over the clinical existence of 'preemptive analgesia' (see Chapter 5) is particularly controversial in studies looking at inguinal hernia repair. Tverskoy first demonstrated, at one, two and ten days after surgery, marked decreases in analgesic requirements and in pain measurements at rest, during movement, and with pressure applied to the incision when spinal anesthesia or general anesthesia with presurgical wound infiltration were compared to general anesthesia alone.[107] The differences between spinal anesthesia and general anesthesia alone were less prominent than in those receiving general anesthesia and local infiltration, who had less pain with pressure applied to their incisions even at ten days after surgery. When specifically evaluating the timing of wound infiltration for the management of postoperative inguinal hernia pain, Ejlersen et al. have shown that the first demand for additional analgesics is significantly later (165 min vs. 225 min), and the percentage of patients not requiring analgesics at all (58% vs. 94%) are significantly less in patients receiving preincisional local anesthetic infiltration (1% lidocaine plain) compared to infiltration at the end of surgery.[26] However, Dierking was unable to demonstrate these differences in a study of nearly identical design.[24]

Bilateral ilioinguinal nerve block, using 10 ml plain 0.5% bupivacaine per side, during general anesthesia for Cesarean section has also been shown to significantly reduce pain scores and opiate requirements in the first 24 hours after surgery.[11]

Nonsurgical Applications

Iliac crest block may be useful in diagnosing nerve entrapment syndromes following herniorrhaphy.

Complications

Fairly large volumes of local anesthetic solutions can be injected with this block, and the anesthesiologist must use more dilute concentrations of drug (0.5% to 1.0% lidocaine or 0.125% to 0.25% bupivacaine with epinephrine) as well as watching for signs and symptoms of systemic toxic reaction. It is possible to penetrate peritoneum, intestine, or blood vessels. Aspiration should be performed before each injection. The solution can spread to produce anesthesia of the lateral buttocks, thigh, and front of the leg, in the distribution of the femoral or lateral femoral cutaneous nerves. This can interfere with ambulation and complicate an anticipated outpatient procedure.

CAVE OF RETZIUS BLOCK

Anatomy

The variable space located between urinary bladder and symphysis pubis is known as the cave of Retzius. This space contains a great venous plexus, as well as many terminating nerve fibers of the sacral plexus. An infiltration block of this area can be a useful adjunct to anesthesia for prostatectomy or bladder procedures. It will provide analgesia, decrease bleeding if vasoconstrictors are used, and facilitate the surgical dissection.

Technique

A skin wheal is raised 2.5 cm superior to the pubic symphysis. Subcutaneous infiltration can be performed laterally in the line of skin incision for retropubic prostatectomy. A 7- to 8-cm needle is then directed to the posterior aspect of the os pubis and anterior to the bladder. Ten ml of local anesthetic solution is injected as the needle reaches its maximum depth and is slowly withdrawn. This process is repeated with two lateral injections made through the same skin wheal (Fig. 14-15).

Surgical Applications

The block may be combined with rectus block and infiltration of the incision in the poor-risk patient for prostatectomy.

Nonsurgical Applications

The block occasionally is useful in patients who have severe pain due to bladder spasm after transurethral prostatectomy. There are few other useful nonsurgical applications for cave of Retzius block.

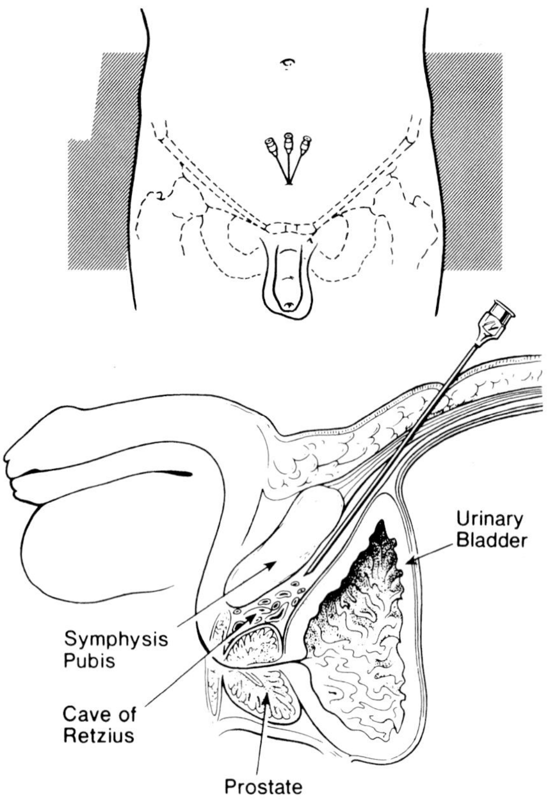

FIG. 14-15. Cave of Retzius block. **Upper Panel:** Needle insertion immediately superior to pubis, in midline and then with angulation to each side. **Lower Panel:** Lateral view, with patient supine. Note cave of Retzius, containing sympathetic nerves and pampiniform plexus of veins, at posteroinferior aspect of pubis. Note also angulation of needle at approximately 45° to long axis of body.

Complications

The chief concern is for excessive intravascular injection. Bladder puncture may occur, but it is unlikely unless the block is performed in a patient with distended bladder. Urinary retention is a theoretic concern, but this block usually is performed only in patients who already or will soon have indwelling catheters.

INTRA-ABDOMINAL NERVE BLOCK

Many anesthesiologists become frustrated with regional anesthesia for intra-abdominal operations because the patient experiences pain from manipulation of viscera or from the surgeon's exploring hands. This can occur even if the patient has evidenced no response to skin incision or dissection through the anterior abdominal wall. Once the peritoneal cavity has been entered, there are additional pathways over which pain is transmitted; these are the afferent pain fibers of the sympathetic and parasympathetic nervous systems. Light general anesthesia, heavy intravenous sedation, and rapid, delicate surgical technique are measures that can offset the problem. In addition, the surgeon might be persuaded to inject additional local anesthetic solution to provide the necessary anesthesia. A major drawback to this is that the surgeon must inject and wait, when he has an almost irresistible urge to proceed with the operation. Also, potentially toxic amounts of local anesthetic may be used and pain relief may still be incomplete. Despite these objections, the following three procedures might prove useful during the course of laparotomy.

Peritoneal Lavage

Lavage of the peritoneal cavity with large volumes of local anesthetic solution will result in analgesia; however, it is difficult to lavage all peritoneal surfaces and the solution must be left in the abdomen for 10 minutes. One hundred to 300 ml of solution (e.g., 0.15% lidocaine or 0.10% bupivacaine) are instilled into the peritoneal cavity after entrance into the cavity. Slight jostling of the abdomen may aid distribution. The Trendelenburg position aids the flow of the solution over the celiac area and the inferior surface of the diaphragm; this often improves analgesia. Some authors have observed marked shrinking of the intestine after this maneuver. Although local anesthetic solutions are absorbed readily from mucosal surfaces, serum local anesthetic levels are surprisingly low (highest level 2.2 mcg/ml after 500 mg of 0.5% lidocaine).[23] The laparoscope also provides an additional port of entry for the lavage solution. Instillation of either lidocaine or bupivacaine has been shown to reduce markedly the incidence and severity of referred shoulder pain after laparoscopy,[73] and is adequate as a sole anesthetic for laparoscopic tubal ligation,[23] if surgical manipulation is consciously gentle, and overdistention of the pneumoperitoneum is avoided. Combined with wound infiltration (or rectus sheath block), one can often provide an extensive pain-free period for patients after laparoscopic surgery.[36]

In contrast to laparoscopic procedures, the benefit of intraperitoneal local anesthetic after open laparotomy, is controversial. While some studies have demonstrated improvements in analgesia, a decreased hyperglycemic (stress) response, and improved colonic motility,[90] others have not shown these benefits,[111] even when local anesthetic is infused continuously through an intraperitoneal catheter.[93]

Vagus Nerve Block

The familiar abbreviation LARP (left anterior, right posterior) indicates that the left vagus is anterior and the right vagus is posterior at the esophageal hiatus. It is possible for the surgeon to infiltrate these nerves directly from the inferior side of the diaphragm. They are deep within the abdomen, and access is not simple; however, infiltration of 10 to 20 ml of dilute anesthetic solution at or near the level of the hiatus will provide marked diminution of sensation from the abdominal cavity.

Celiac Plexus Block

Numerous reports and observations have been made of the celiac plexus reflex during laparotomy. It is possible to infiltrate the celiac plexus directly with local anesthetic solution (20 to 40 ml). The surgeon may not always find this technically easy. Tumor masses, obesity, and the high posterior location of the celiac plexus in the abdomen, make direct visualization a challenge. In this situation, however, infiltration of a large volume of solution near the plexus may result in an adequate nerve block. A variation is to wash 40 to 60 ml of anesthetic solution into the upper posterior abdominal cavity. Dilute concentrations of local anesthetic are quite adequate and should be used as previously described.

REFERENCES

1. Ablondi, M., Ryan, J., O'Connell, C., and Haley, R.: Continuous intercostal nerve blocks for postoperative pain relief. Anesth. Analg., *45:*185, 1966.
2. Ahlburg, P., Noreng, M., Molgaard, J., and Egebo, K.: Treatment of pancreatic pain with interpleural bupivacaine: An open trial. Acta Anaesthesiol. Scand., *34:*156, 1990.
3. Atanassoff, P.G., Alon, E., Pasch, T., Ziegler, W.H., and Gautschi, K.: Intercostal nerve block for minor breast surgery. Reg. Anesth., *16:*23, 1991.
4. Baxter, A.D., Jennings, F.O., Harris, R.S., Flynn, J.F., and Way, J.: Continuous intercostal blockade after cardiac surgery. Br. J. Anaesth., *59:*162, 1987.
5. Ben-David, B., and Lee, E.: The falling column: A new technique for interpleural catheter placement. Anesth. Analg., *71:*1990.
6. Benumof, J., and Semenza, J.: Total spinal anesthesia following intrathoracic intercostal nerve blocks. Anesthesiology, *43:*124, 1975.
7. Billstrom, R., and Blomberg, H.M.: Cholestasis after interpleural bupivacaine for chronic upper limb pain. Anesth. Analg., *76:*1158, 1993.
8. Bridenbaugh, P., DuPen, S., Moore, D., Bridenbaugh, L., and Thompson G.: Postoperative intercostal nerve block analgesia versus narcotic analgesia. Anesth. Analg., *52:*81, 1973.
9. Brown, D.L.: A retrospective analysis of neurolytic celiac plexus block for nonpancreatic intra-abdominal cancer pain. Reg. Anesth., *14:*63, 1989.
10. Brown, D.L., Bulley, C.K., and Quiel, E.L.: Neurolytic celiac plexus block for pancreatic cancer pain. Anesth. Analg., *66:*869, 1987.
11. Bunting, P., and McConachie, I.: Ilioinguinal nerve blockade for analgesia after caesarean section. Br. J. Anaesth., *61:*773, 1988.
12. Bunting, P., and McGeachie, J.F.: Intercostal nerve blockade producing analgesia after appendicectomy. Br. J. Anaesth., *61:*169, 1988.
13. Cherry, D., and Rao, D.: Lumbar sympathetic and coeliac plexus blocks: An anatomic study in cadavers. Br. J. Anaesth. *54:*1037, 1982.
14. Conacher, I., and Kokri, M.: Postoperative paravertebral blocks for thoracic surgery. Br. J. Anaesth., *59:*155, 1987.
15. Cope, R.: The Woolley and Roe case: Woolley and Roe vs. Ministry of Health and Others. Anaesthesia, *9:*249, 1954.
16. Cory, P., and Mulroy, M.: Postoperative respiratory failure following intercostal block. Anesthesiology, *54:*418, 1981.
17. Crile, G., and Lower, W.: Anoci-association. Philadelphia, W.B. Saunders, 1915.
18. Crossley, A.W., and Hosie, H.E.: Radiographic study of intercostal nerve blockade in healthy volunteers. Br. J. Anaesth., *59:*149, 1987.
19. Davies, D.D.: Incidence of major complications of neurolytic coeliac plexus block. J.R. Soc. Med., *86:*264, 1993.
20. de Jong, R., and Bonin, J.: Benzodiazepines protect mice from local anesthetic convulsions and deaths. Anesth. Analg., *60:*385, 1981.
21. de Jong, R., and Cullen, S.: Buffer-demand and pH of local anesthetic solutions containing epinephrine. Anesthesiology, *24:*801, 1963.
22. de Leon-Casasola, O., Kent, E., and Lema, M.J.: Neurolytic superior hypogastric plexus block for chronic pelvic pain associated with cancer. Pain, *54:*145, 1993.
23. Deeb, R., and Viechnicki, M.: Laparoscopic tubal ligation under peritoneal lavage anesthesia. Reg. Anesth., *10:*24, 1985.
24. Dierking, G.W., Dahl, J.B., Kanstrup, J., Dahl, A., and Kehlet H.: Effect of pre- vs. postoperative inguinal field block on postoperative pain after herniorrhaphy. Br. J. Anaesth., *68:*344, 1992.
25. Dionne C.: Tumour invasion of the brachial plexus: Management of pain with intrapleural analgesia. Can. J. Anaesth., *39:*520, 1992.
26. Ejlersen, E., Andersen, H., Eliasen, K., and Mogensen, T.: A comparison between preincisional and postincisional lidocaine infiltration and postoperative pain. Anesth. Analg., *74:*495, 1992.
27. Feldstein, G.S., Waldman, S.D., and Allen, M.L.: Loss-of-resistance technique for transaortic celiac plexus block. Anesth. Analg., *65:*1092, 1986.
28. Ferrante, F.M., Chan, V.W., Arthur, G.R., and Rocco, A.G.: Interpleural analgesia after thoracotomy. Anesth. Analg., *72:*105, 1991.
29. Frenette, L., Boudreault, D., and Guay, J.: Interpleural analgesia improves pulmonary function after cholecystectomy. Can. J. Anaesth., *38:*71, 1991.
30. Gauntlett, I.S.: Total spinal anesthesia following intercostal nerve block. Anesthesiology, *65:*82, 1986.
31. Hamid, S.K., Scott, N.B., Sutcliffe, N.P., *et al.*: Continuous coeliac plexus blockade plus intermittent wound infiltration with bupivacaine following upper abdominal surgery: A double-blind randomised study. Acta Anaesthesiol. Scand., *36:*534, 1992.
32. Hardy, P.A.: Anatomical variation in the position of the proximal intercostal nerve. Br. J. Anaesth., *61:*338, 1988.
33. Hastings, R.H., and McKay, W.R.: Treatment of benign chronic abdominal pain with neurolytic celiac plexus block. Anesthesiology, *75:*156, 1991.
34. Haugen, F.: The autonomic nervous system and pain. Anesthesiology, *29:*785, 1968.
35. Hecker, B.R., Bjurstrom, R., and Schoene, R.B.: Effect of intercostal nerve blockade on respiratory mechanics and CO_2 chemosensitivity at rest and exercise. Anesthesiology, *70:*13, 1989.
36. Helvacioglu, A., and Weis, R.: Operative laparoscopy and postoperative pain relief. Fertil. and Steril., *57:*548, 1992.
37. Hord, A.H., Wang, J.M., Pai, U.T., and Raj P.P.: Anatomic spread of india ink in the human intercostal space with radiographic correlation. Reg. Anesth., *16:*13, 1991.
38. Ischia, S., Ischia, A., Polati, E., and Finco, G.: Three posterior percutaneous celiac plexus block techniques: A prospective, randomized study in 61 patients with pancreatic cancer pain. Anesthesiology, *76:*534, 1992.
39. Ischia, S., Luzzan, A., Ischia, A., and Faggion, S.: A new approach to the neurolytic block of the celiac plexus: The transaortic technique. Pain, *16:*333, 1983.
40. Iwama, H., Tase, C., Kawamae, K., Akama, Y., and Okuaki, A.: Catheter location and patient position affect spread of interpleural regional analgesia. Anesthesiology, *79:*1153, 1993.
41. Jakobson, S., Fridiksson, H., Hedenstrom, H., and Ivarsson, I. Effects of intercostal nerve blocks on pulmonary mechanics in healthy men. Acta Anaesthesiol. Scand. *24:*482, 1980.
42. Johnson, L.R., Rocco, A.G., and Ferrante, F.M.: Continuous subpleural-paravertebral block in acute thoracic herpes zoster. Anesth. Analg., *67:*1105, 1988.
43. Johnson, M.D., Mickler, T., Arthur, G.R., Rosenburg, S., and Wilson, R.: Bupivacaine with and without epinephrine for intercostal nerve block. J. Cardiothorac. Anesth., *4:*200, 1990.
44. Katz, J.: A survey of anesthetic choice among anesthesiologists. Anesth. Analg., *52:*373, 1973.
45. Kirvela, O., and Antila, H.: Thoracic paravertebral block in chronic postoperative pain. Reg. Anesth., *17:*348, 1992.
46. Kline, M., Boedeker, B., Burnham, K., Calkins, M., and Haynes, D.: Lecithin-coated bupivacaine microcrystals produce ultra-long duration local anesthesia. Reg. Anesth., *19:*2, 1994.
47. Kopacz, D.J., and Bridenbaugh, L.D.: Are anesthesia residency programs failing regional anesthesia? The past, present, and future. Reg. Anesth., *18:*84, 1993.
48. Kowalski, S.E., Bradley, B.D., Greengrass, R.A., Freedman, J., and Younes, M.K.: Effects of interpleural bupivacaine (0.5%) on canine diaphragmatic function. Anesth. Analg., *75:*400, 1992.

49. Kune, G., Cole, R., and Bell, S.: Observations on the relief of pancreatic pain. Med. J. Aust., *2:*789, 1975.
50. Lauder, G.R.: Interpleural analgesia and phrenic nerve paralysis. Anaesthesia, *48:*315, 1993.
51. Lee, E., and Ben, D.B.: Bilateral interpleural block for midline upper abdominal surgery. Can. J. Anaesth., *38:*683, 1991.
52. Lema, M.J., Myers, D.P., De Leon-Casasola, O., and Penetrante, R.: Pleural phenol therapy for the treatment of chronic esophageal cancer pain. Reg. Anesth., *17:*166, 1992.
53. Lieberman, R.P., Nance, P.N., and Cuka, D.J.: Anterior approach to celiac plexus block during interventional biliary procedures. Radiology, *167:*562, 1988.
54. Lonnqvist, P., and Hildingsson, U.: The caudal boundary of the thoracic paravertebral space: A study in human cadavers. Anaesthesia, *47:*1051, 1992.
55. Loper, K.A., Coldwell, D.M., Lecky, J., and Dowling, C.: Celiac plexus block for hepatic arterial embolization: A comparison with intravenous morphine. Anesth. Analg., *69:*398, 1989.
56. Lundy, J.: Balanced anesthesia. Minn. Med., *9:*399, 1926.
57. Macintosh, R., and Bryce-Smith, R.: Local Analgesia: Abdominal Surgery. Edinburgh, E. & S. Livingston, 1953.
58. Malhotra, V., Long, C.W., and Meister, M.J.: Intercostal blocks with local infiltration anesthesia for extracorporeal shock wave lithotripsy. Anesth. Analg., *66:*85, 1987.
59. Masters, D., Berde, C., Dutta, S., *et al.*: Prolonged regional nerve blockade by controlled release of local anesthetic from a biodegradable polymer matrix. Anesthesiology, *79:*340, 1993.
60. Mercadante, S.: Celiac plexus block versus analgesics in pancreatic cancer pain. Pain, *52:*187, 1993.
61. Montero, M.A., Vidal, L.F., Aguilar, S.J., and Donoso, B.L.: Percutaneous anterior approach to the coeliac plexus, using ultrasound. Br. J. Anaesth., *62:*637, 1989.
62. Moore, D., and Bridenbaugh, L.: Pneumothorax: Its incidence following intercostal nerve block. J.A.M.A., *174:*842, 1960.
63. Moore, D., and Bridenbaugh, L.: Pneumothorax: Its incidence following intercostal nerve block. J.A.M.A. *182:*1005, 1962.
64. Moore, D., Bridenbaugh, L., Thompson, G., Balfour, R., and Horton, W.: Factors determining dosages of amide-type local anesthetic drugs. Anesthesiology, *47:*263,1977.
65. Moore, D., Bush, W., and Burnett, L.: Celiac plexus block: A roentgenographic anatomic study of technique and spread of solution in patients and corpses. Anesth. Analg., *60:*369, 1981.
66. Moore, D., Bush, W., and Scurlock, J.: Intercostal nerve block: A roentgenographic anatomic study of technique and absorption in humans. Anesth. Analg., *59:*815, 1980.
67. Moore, D., and Scurlock, J.: Possible role of epinephrine in prevention or correction of myocardial depression associated with bupivacaine. Anesth. Analg., *62:*450, 1983.
68. Morris, R., McKay, W., and Mushlin, P.: Comparison of pain associated with intradermal and subcutaneous infiltration with various local anesthetic solutions. Anesth. Analg., *66:*1180, 1987.
69. Mowbray, A., and Wong, K.K.: Low volume intercostal injection: A comparative study in patients and cadavers. Anaesthesia, *43:*633, 1988.
70. Murphy, D.: Intercostal nerve block for fractured ribs and postoperative analgesia: Description of a new technique. Reg. Anesth., *8:*151, 1983.
71. Murphy, D.F.: Continuous intercostal nerve blockade: An anatomical study to elucidate its mode of action. Br. J. Anaesth., *56:*627, 1984.
72. Mushin, W.: Bilateral vagal block. Proc. R. Soc. Med., *38:*308, 1945.
73. Narchi, P., Benhamou, D., and Fernandez, H.: Intraperitoneal local anaesthetic for shoulder pain after day-case laparoscopy. Lancet, *338:*1569, 1991.
74. Nunn, J., and Slavin, C.: Posterior intercostal nerve for pain relief after cholecystectomy. Br. J. Anaesth., *52:*253, 1980.
75. Perkins, G.: Interpleural anaesthesia in the management of upper limb ischaemia: A report of three cases. Anaesth. Intensive Care, *19:*575, 1991.
76. Plancarte, R., Amescua, C., Patt, R.B., and Aldrete, J.A.: Superior hypogastric plexus block for pelvic cancer pain. Anesthesiology, *73:*236, 1990.
77. Purcell-Jones, G., Pither, C., and Justins, D.: Paravertebral somatic nerve block: A clinical, radiographic, and computed tomographic study in chronic pain patients. Anesth. Analg., *68:*32, 1989.
78. Rademaker, B.M., Sih, I.L., Kalkman, C.J., *et al.*: Effects of interpleurally administered bupivacaine 0.5% on opioid analgesic requirements and endocrine response during and after cholecystectomy: A randomized, double-blind, controlled study. Acta Anaesthesiol. Scand., *35:*108, 1991.
79. Rawal, N., Sjostrand, U., Dahlstrom, B., Nydahl, P., and Ostelius J.: Epidural morphine for postoperative pain relief: A comparative study with intramuscular narcotic and intercostal block. Anesth. Analg., *61:*93, 1982.
80. Raza, S.M., Vasireddy, A.R., Candido, K.D., Winnie, A.P., and Masters, R.W.: A complete regional anesthesia technique for cardiac pacemaker insertion. J. Cardiothorac. Vasc. Anesth., *5:*54, 1991.
81. Ready, L., Oden, R., Chadwick, H., *et al.*: Development of an anesthesiology-based postoperative pain management service. Anesthesiology, *68:*100, 1988.
82. Reiestad, F., McIlvaine, W.B., Barnes, M., *et al.*: Interpleural analgesia in the treatment of severe thoracic postherpetic neuralgia. Reg. Anesth., *15:*113, 1990.
83. Reiestad, F., McIlvaine, W.B., Kvalheim, L., Haraldstad, P., and Pettersen, B.: Successful treatment of chronic pancreatitis pain with interpleural analgesia. Can. J. Anaesth., *36:*713, 1989.
84. Reiestad, F., McIlvaine, W.B., Kvalheim, L., Stokke, T., and Pettersen, B.: Interpleural analgesia in treatment of upper extremity reflex sympathetic dystrophy. Anesth. Analg., *69:*671, 1989.
85. Reiestad, F., and Stromskag, K.: Interpleural catheter in the management of postoperative pain: A preliminary report. Reg. Anesth., *11:*89, 1986.
86. Rice, L., Trescot, A., Guzzetta, P., and Ruttimann, U.: Regional vs. general anesthesia: What would surgeons choose for themselves? Reg. Anesth., *11:*82, 1988.
87. Rice, L., Trescot, A., and Ruttimann, U.: Regional vs. general anesthesia: What do primary physicians select for their own surgery? Reg. Anesth., *13:*74, 1988.
88. Riegler, F.X., Vade, B.T., and Pelligrino, D.A.: Interpleural anesthetics in the dog: Differential somatic neural blockade. Anesthesiology, *71:*744, 1989.
89. Rigler, M.L., Drasner, K., Krejcie, T.C., *et al.*: Cauda equina syndrome after continuous spinal anesthesia. Anesth. Analg., *72:*275, 1991.
90. Rimback, G., Cassuto, J., Faxen, A., Hosgtrom, S., and Wallin, G.: Effect of intra-abdominal bupivacaine instillation on postoperative colonic motility. Gut, *27:*170, 1986.
91. Rocco, A., Reiestad, F., Gudman, J., and McKay, W.: Intrapleural administration of local anesthetics for pain relief in patients with multiple rib fractures. Reg. Anesth., *12:*10, 1987.
92. Ryan, J., Adye, B., Jolly, P., and Mulroy, M.: Outpatient inguinal herniorrhaphy with both regional and local anesthesia. Am. J. Surg., *148:*1984.
93. Scott, N., Mogensen, T., Greulich, A., Hjortso, N., and Kehlet, H.: No effect of continuous IP infusion of bupivacaine on postoperative analgesia, pulmonary function, and the stress response to surgery. Br. J. Anaesth., *61:*165, 1988.
94. Seddon, S.J., and Clayton, K.C.: Intercostal nerve block by jet injection. Anaesthesia, *39:*484, 1984.
95. Shantha, T.R.: Unilateral bronchospasm after interpleural analgesia. Anesth. Analg., *74:*291, 1992.
96. Sharfman, W.H., and Walsh, T.D.: Has the analgesic efficacy of neurolytic celiac plexus block been demonstrated in pancreatic cancer pain? Pain, *41:*267, 1990.
97. Singler, R.: An improved technique for alcohol celiac plexus nerve block. Anesthesiology, *56:*137, 1982.
98. Smith, B.E., Suchak, M., Siggins, D., and Challands, J.: Rectus sheath block for diagnostic laparoscopy. Anaesthesia, *43:*947, 1988.
99. Stromskag, K.E., Minor, B., Steen, P.A.: Side effects and complications related to interpleural analgesia: An update. Acta Anaesthesiol. Scand., *34:*473, 1990.
100. Stromskag, K.E., Reiestad, F., Holmqvist, E.L., and Ogenstad, S.: Intrapleural administration of 0.25%, 0.375%, and 0.5% bupivacaine with epinephrine after cholecystectomy. Anesth. Analg., *67:*430, 1988.
101. Sury, M., and Bingham, R.: Accidental spinal anaesthesia following intrathoracic intercostal nerve block. Anaesthesia, *41:*401, 1986.
102. Symreng, T., Gomez, M.N., Johnson, B., Rossi, N.P., and Chiang, C.K.: Intrapleural bupivacaine—technical considerations and intraoperative use. J. Cardiothorac. Anesth., *3:*139, 1989.
103. Symreng, T., Gomez, M.N., and Rossi, N.: Intrapleural bupivacaine

vs. saline after thoracotomy: Effects on pain and lung function—A double-blind study. J. Cardiothorac. Anesth., *3:*144, 1989.

104. Templeton, T.: Rectus block for postoperative pain relief. Reg. Anesth., *18:*258, 1993.
105. Thompson, G., Artin, R., Bridenbaugh, L., and Moore, D.: Abdominal pain and alcohol celiac plexus nerve block. Anesth. Analg., *56:*1, 1977.
106. Tucker, G.T., Moore, D.C., Bridenbaugh, P.O., Bridenbaugh, L.D., and Thompson, G.E.: Systemic absorption of mepivacaine in commonly used regional block procedures. Anesthesiology, *37:*277, 1972.
107. Tverskoy, M., Cozacov, C., Ayache, M., Bradley, E.J., and Kissin, I.: Postoperative pain after inguinal herniorrhaphy with different types of anesthesia. Anesth. Analg., *70:*29, 1990.
108. Vaghadia, H., and Jenkins, L.C.: Use of a Doppler ultrasound stethoscope for intercostal nerve block. Can. J. Anaesth., *35:*86, 1988.
109. van Kleef, J., Burm, A., and Vletter, A.A.: Single-dose interpleural vs. intercostal blockade: Nerve block characteristics and plasma concentration profiles after administration of 0.5% bupivacaine with epinephrine. Anesth. Analg., *70:*1990.
110. Waldman, S., Wilson, W., and Kreps, R.: Superior hypogastric plexus block using a single needle and computed tomography guidance: Description of a modified technique. Reg. Anesth., *16:*286, 1991.
111. Wallin, G., Cassuto, J., Hogstrom, S., and Hedner, T.: Influence of intraperitoneal anesthesia on pain and the sympathoadrenal response to abdominal surgery. Acta Anaesthesiol. Scand., *32:*553, 1988.
112. Walts, L., Forsythe, A., and Moore, J.: Critique: Occupational disease among operating personnel. Anesthesiology, *42:*1975.
113. Ward, E., Rorie, D., Nauss, L., and Bahn, R.: The celiac ganglion in man: Normal anatomic variations. Anesth. Analg., *58:*461, 1978.
114. Weinstabl, C., Porges, P., Plainer, B., *et al.*: Coeliac plexus block with bupivacaine reduces intestinal dysfunction in neurosurgical ICU patients. Anaesthesia, *48:*162, 1993.
115. Whiteman, M.S., Rosenberg, H., Haskin, P.H., and Teplick, S.K.: Celiac plexus block for interventional radiology. Radiology, *161:*836, 1986.
116. Wilkins, C., Cramp, P., Staples, J., and Stevens, W.: Comparison of the anesthetic requirement for tolerance of laryngeal mask airway and endotracheal tube. Anesth. Analg., *75:*794, 1992.
117. Woolf, C.J., and Chong, M.S.: Preemptive analgesia—treating postoperative pain by preventing the establishment of central sensitization. Anesth. Analg., *77:*362, 1993.

D

Head and Neck

Neural Blockade in Clinical Anesthesia and Management of Pain, Third Edition,
edited by M.J. Cousins and P.O. Bridenbaugh.
Lippincott–Raven Publishers, Philadelphia © 1998.

CHAPTER 15

Somatic Blockade of Head and Neck

Terence M. Murphy

Regional anesthesia for surgery of the head and neck has a long and successful history of use and application in dental surgery and otolaryngology, permitting surgical trespass around the airway in a safe manner. It was used more extensively for a variety of more invasive surgeries by Reclus and Pauchet[40] and Labat[1] in the days before routine endotracheal intubation. However, there are still many opportunities to utilize this technology, either as a replacement for general anesthesia, in selected patients (see examples below), or as an optimal analgesic supplement to general endotracheal anesthesia, both to reduce the amount of general anesthetic administered and to provide much improved postoperative pain relief. This latter priority, I'm glad to say, is receiving appropriate attention now for surgery elsewhere in the body, and I think utilization of the techniques described below would permit similar application in a variety of head and neck surgeries. The profound postoperative analgesia that can be delivered by a mandibular nerve block for a fractured mandible can provide a much more comfortable postoperative course for some unfortunate individual with his or her jaws wired together, affording better pain relief, and carrying less risk of airway compromise, as may occur with the alternative, often large, doses of respiratory depressant systemic analgesics.

One of the most frequently used and tested applications for regional anesthesia for head and neck surgery is, of course, in surgery of the eye and orbit (see Chapter 17). Traditionally, both the anesthesia and the surgery of this area were accomplished by the operating ophthalmologist. However, in recent times, anesthesiologists are being enlisted more and more to provide this anesthesia service, and although it is not taught in most residency programs, there is now a need for significant continuing medical education in this area for those anesthesiologists who work in such units.[49,19]

Because of the very compact anatomy, and the close relationship of cranial and cervical nerves to many vital structures, meticulous placement of the needle and small discrete doses of the anesthetic agent are required for accurate and safe regional anesthesia in this area. The landmarks for regional anesthesia in the head and neck are relatively constant, easily located, and predictable, for anesthesiologists prepared to acquire the skills necessary for these techniques, to ensure that satisfactory regional anesthesia can be consistently attained.

The trigeminal nerve and the cervical plexus provide cutaneous sensory innervation to the face, head, and neck. In addition, the glossopharyngeal and vagus nerves supply the pharynx and larynx. This chapter is concerned mainly with blocks of these cranial and cervical nerves to provide anesthesia for surgery, endoscopic procedures, and endotracheal anesthesia, as well as the use of such blocks in pain states.

The pharmacology of the agents used has considerable affect on regional anesthesia in any region of the body, but probably the greatest reason for failure is incorrect placement of the needle. Correct placement can be ensured only by a thorough understanding of the anatomy of the area in which the needle is inserted. Applied anatomical knowledge is of vital importance for success in regional anesthesia in general and particularly so in regional anesthesia of the head and neck. The anesthesiologist who wants to become skilled in these techniques would do well to consult the reading suggested at the end of the chapter[8,28,29] and to become completely familiar with the anatomy[24] by dissecting cadavers or reviewing prosected specimens whenever possible. Frequent recourse to a skull is advisable, both while learning how to perform these blocks and later, for review, just prior to such procedures.

APPLIED ANATOMY

Innervation of the Face

The anatomy and complexity of the nerve supply of the face in the adult is perhaps best understood in light of its development in the embryo, as the face forms around the prim-

T. Murphy: Formerly Department of Anesthesiology, University of Washington School of Medicine, Seattle, Washington 98195-6540.

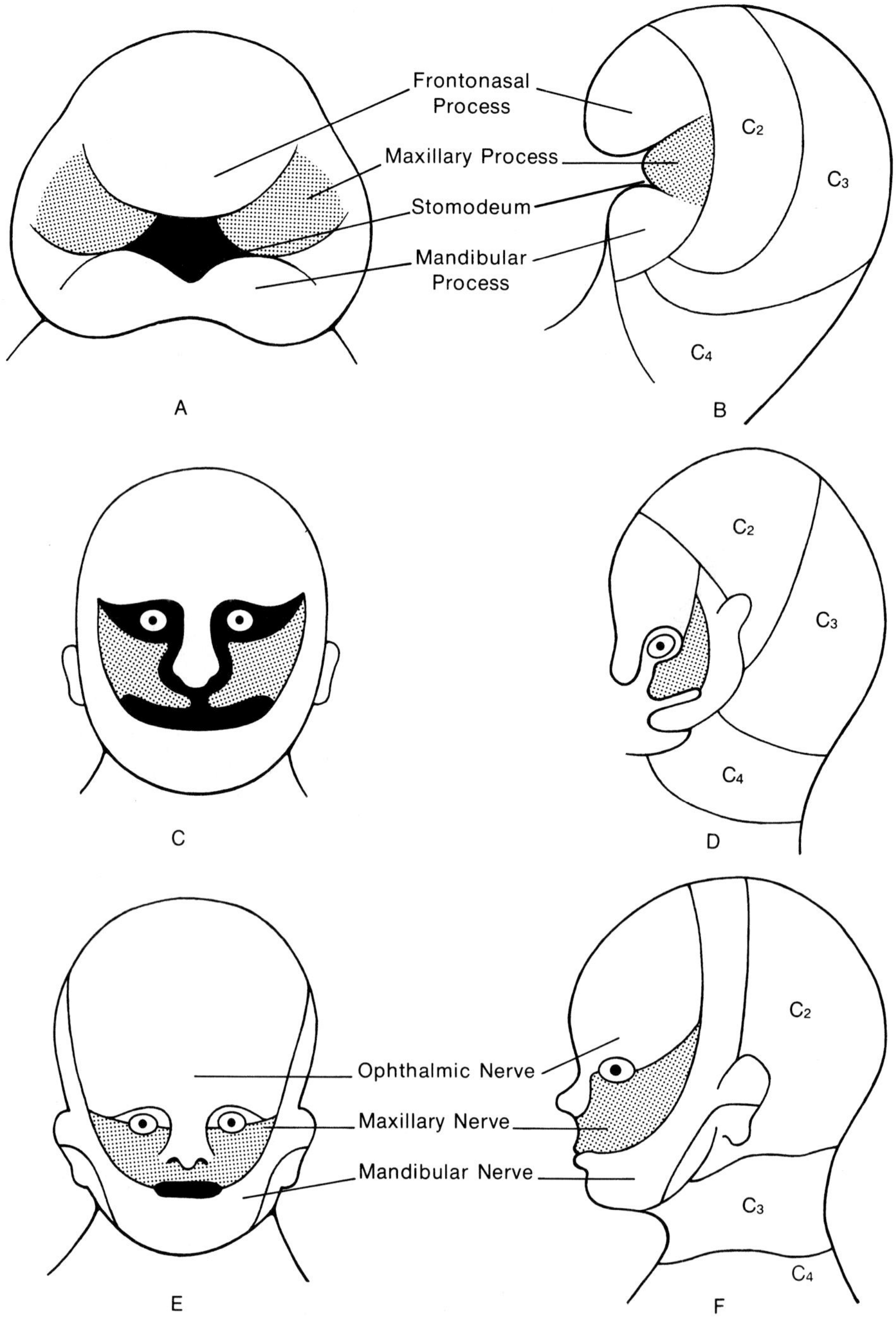

FIG. 15-1. Frontal and lateral views of development of dermatomes of the head and neck. **A, B:** The primitive stomodeum (mouth) is surrounded by the three parts of the developing face. **C, D:** The frontonasal process (supplied by the ophthalmic nerve) grows in from above, the maxillary processes (maxillary nerve) grow in from each side, and the mandibular process (mandibular nerve) forms the caudal margin. **E, F:** The frontonasal process forms the brow, eyebrows, upper eyelid, and nose in the fully developed face. The maxillary process forms both cheeks, lower eyelid, and upper lip. The mandibular process gives rise to the lower lip, the chin, and a strip of skin extending up the side of the face, often to the vertex, including the superior anterior two-thirds of the anterior surface of the ear. The cervical plexus derivatives of the second, third, and fourth cervical nerves supply the posterior part of the head and neck from the vertex down. Note in **F** that the skin over the angle of the jaw and the lower part of the auricle on the anterior surface and all of its posterior surface are supplied by cervical plexus dermatomes (C_2).

itive mouth (the stomodeum). Initially, the stomodeum is surrounded caudally by the mandibular arch (which is supplied by the mandibular nerve), laterally on each side by the maxillary processes (which are supplied by the maxillary division of the trigeminal nerve), and rostrally by the forebrain capsule, from which develops the frontonasal process (which is supplied by the first division of the trigeminal nerve, the ophthalmic nerve). The frontonasal process grows down into the primitive stomodeum from the forebrain capsule, and eventually this will form the nose of the mature embryo (Fig. 15-1). The two maxillary processes grow inward from either side and join together below the primitive nose, as shown, and they then form the rostral margin of the primitive mouth. Thus, in the mature face, the forehead, eyebrows, upper eyelids, and nose are supplied by the first ophthalmic division of the trigeminal nerve. The lower eyelid, cheek, and upper lip are supplied by the second division (i.e., the maxillary nerve), and the lower lip, chin, mandibular, and temporal regions are supplied by the third division, mandibular nerve. Because of the disproportionate growth of the cranial cavity in humans, these dermatomal distributions are distorted cranially, with the result that some skin innervated by the cervical plexus is drawn up over the angle of the mandible onto the face and posteriorly over the occipital area and the scalp as far forward as the vertex, as shown in Figure 15-2.

Trigeminal Nerve Distribution

The first division of the trigeminal nerve, the ophthalmic (V_1), is primarily distributed to the forehead and nose; the second division, the maxillary (V_2), supplies the upper jaw; and the third division, or mandibular nerve (V_3), supplies the lower jaw.

The gasserian ganglion lies posteromedially in the middle cranial fossa at the junction of its floor and the cavernous sinus just anterior to the ridge of the petrous temporal bone. The ganglion invaginates the dura and therefore lies in a dural pouch—Meckel's cave, which contains cerebrospinal fluid (CSF). An injection of local anesthetic or neurolytic agent into the ganglion area potentially can spread to, or accidentally be injected into, this pouch, and can therefore "spill" into the CSF. This could lead to the spread of analgesia to other adjacent cranial nerves (e.g., abducens, facial, etc.) and may even result in total spinal anesthesia. Therefore, meticulous aspiration and small (0.25 ml) test doses are mandatory. (The volume of Meckel's cave is about 0.5 ml.)

Ophthalmic Nerve

In its intracranial course, the trunk of the ophthalmic nerve does not lend itself to regional anesthesia. The intraorbital branches of the nasociliary nerve are blocked by retrobulbar block (see Chapter 17). The intraorbital branches, anterior ethmoidal and infratrochlear, can also be blocked in the orbit. The terminal divisions in the forehead and nose are suitable for peripheral nerve blocks of the face (see Fig. 15-3). The mandibular and maxillary divisions can be blocked as they leave the cranial cavity for their respective destinations (see clinical examples of same following).

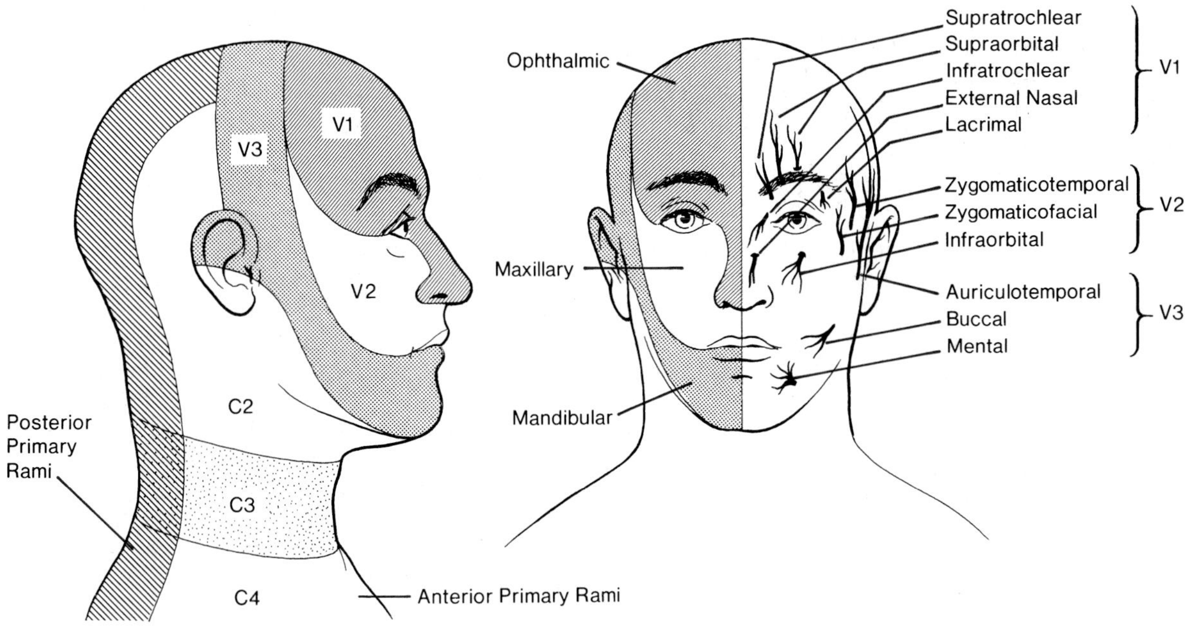

FIG. 15-2. Dermatomes and cutaneous nerves of head, neck, and face. Note that the supraorbital, infraorbital, and mental nerves all lie in the same vertical plane as the pupil, with the eye looking straight forward. The external nasal area is innervated by infratrochlear and external nasal (from anterior ethmoidal *n.*) branches of V_1 and the infraorbital branch of V_2. The internal nasal cavity is shown in Figure 15-4.

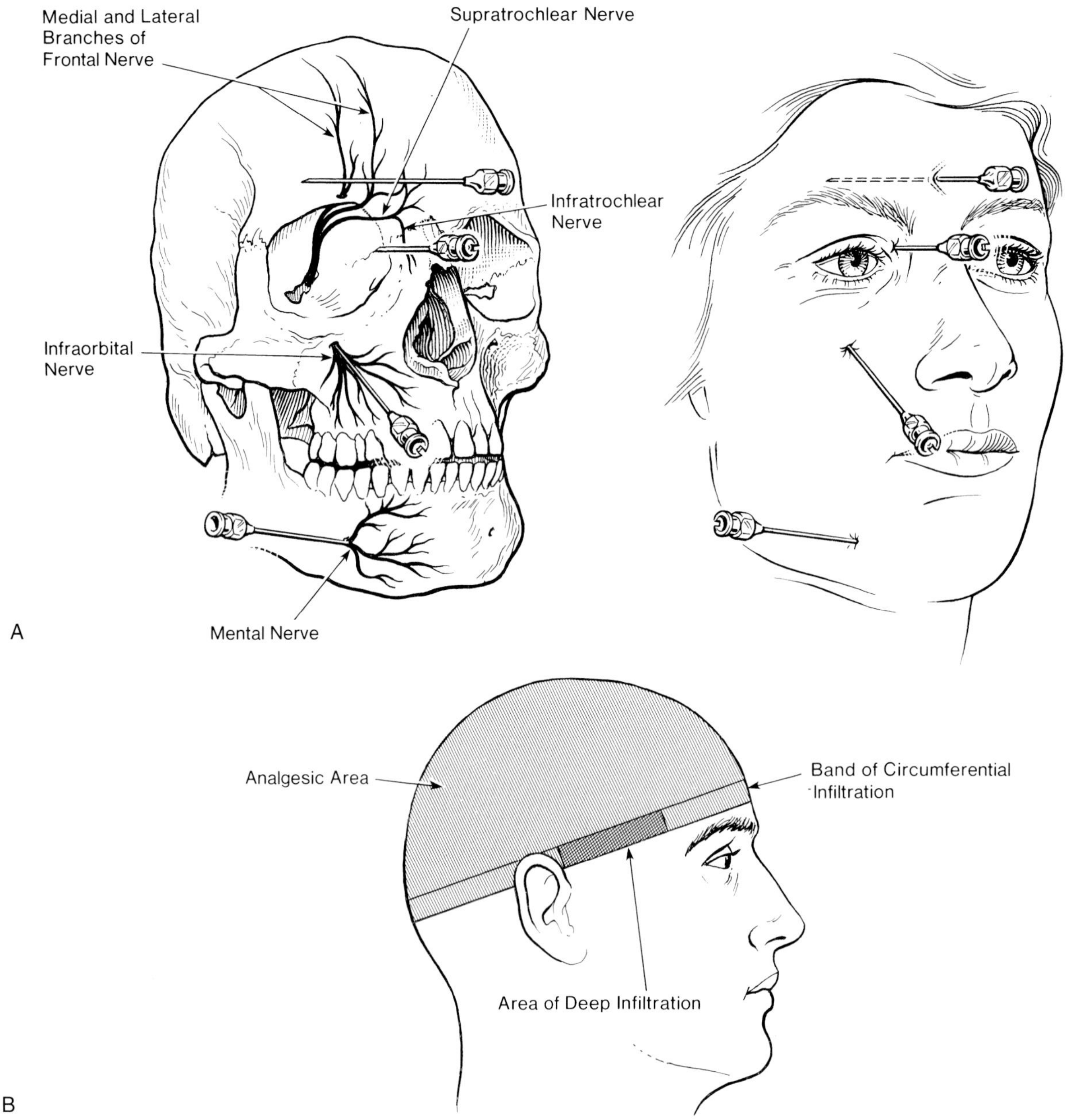

FIG. 15-3. A: Nerve block of the superficial branches of the trigeminal nerve. *The supraorbital and supratrochlear* branches of the first division (ophthalmic) can be blocked as they emerge above the orbit. A single needle insertion in the midbrow above the root of the nose can anesthetize the forehead bilaterally by infiltrations on either side through the same insertion. Note that this injection needs to be undertaken above the level of the eyebrow to prevent periorbital hematoma. The *infratrochlear nerve* (and also anterior ethmoidal nerve) is blocked by inserting a needle 1 cm above the inner canthus and just lateral to the medial wall of the orbit. The needle is directed posteriorly and slightly medially to a depth of about 2.5 cm. *The infraorbital nerve* is located one finger's breadth below the orbital rim in the same vertical position as the pupil with the eye looking forward. To enter the infraorbital foramen, advance the needle cephalad and laterally. It is not necessary, however, to enter the foramen, but just to infiltrate the nerve as it emerges at the foramen. *The mental nerve* is anesthetized again in the same vertical line as the pupil; to enter the mental foramen, direct the needle medially as shown in the diagram. The mental foramen lies at a different vertical level in the mandible at different ages (see text). **B:** *Circumferential infiltration of scalp* (see text). Note that infiltration is superficial except in the temporal region where infiltration deep to deep fascia is useful to help prevent movement of the temporalis muscle during surgery. If periosteum will be stimulated injection must be made deep to deep fascia.

Maxillary Nerve

To reach the upper jaw, this nerve leaves the cranial cavity through the anterior wall of the middle cranial fossa, via the foramen rotundum—and traverses the pterygomaxillary fossa (this compartment is also referred to as the pterygopalatine fossa, bounded anteriorly by the palatine bone medially, and the maxilla laterally; and posteriorly, by the pterygoid process of the sphenoid bone). The nerve crosses the fossa anterolaterally, to enter the floor of the orbit at the inferior orbital fissure. It can be blocked as it lies in the fossa, producing anesthesia of the upper jaw, the lateral nasal wall, and most of the nasal septum. The superior anterior part of both septum and lateral wall of nose receive contributions from the anterior ethmoidal branch of the ophthalmic nerve. The entire hard palate is supplied by the maxillary nerve via the sphenopalatine ganglion.

Mandibular Nerve

The mandibular nerve emerges from the cranial cavity through the floor of the middle cranial fossa, via the foramen ovale, to enter the infratemporal fossa. This fossa is a rectangular compartment bounded anteriorly by the posterior wall of the maxilla and posteriorly by the styloid apparatus and carotid sheath. The lateral wall is the ramus of the mandible, and the medial wall is composed anteriorly of the lateral pterygoid plate of the sphenoid bone and, posteriorly of the constrictor muscles of the pharynx. It has no floor, but its roof is the floor of the middle cranial fossa. In the infratemporal fossa, the mandibular nerve divides into its terminal branches. Block of the nerve at this site results in anesthesia of the ipsilateral lower jaw, the tongue, and lower teeth; the buccal surface of the cheek; and the skin overlaying the lower jaw, the temporal region, and the anterior superior two-thirds of the surface of the external ear. This nerve can be blocked relatively easily by introducing a needle into the infratemporal fossa through the coronoid notch of the mandible. It can also be blocked by an intraoral approach (see Chapter 16).

Innervation of Eyeball and Orbit

Innervation of the eye and neural blockade procedures for ocular branches of the trigeminal nerve and topical analgesia for eye surgery are discussed in Chapter 17.

Local and regional anesthesia lends itself very well to eye surgery, especially in those parts of the world where safe general anesthesia is not readily available. Regional anesthesia is much used also by many ophthalmologists in advanced medical communities for a variety of reasons, including satisfactory analgesia, surgical convenience and economy. This topic is dealt with in Chapter 17, and for the most part involves blockage of the sensory input to the globe. In addition to peribulbar or retrobulbar anesthesia, these patients also may require akinesia, i.e., paralysis of the facial and extraocular muscles, to prevent compression of the globe during open surgical procedures and to avoid risking extrusion of the globe contents. This is achieved by infiltrating the branches of the facial nerve as they cross the zygomatic bone, and involves infiltration of a weak local anesthetic solution, both laterally and inferiorly to the margin of the orbit. The facial nerve can also be anesthetized as it crosses the mandibular condyle, and can be identified anterior to the ear by asking the patient to open and close his or her mouth, a needle is inserted through the skin at the point overlying the junction of the superior and middle-third of the posterior edge of the ramus of the mandible; the nerve is infiltrated by the injection of 2 to 3 ml of local anesthetic solution at this point (see Chapter 17).

Although with more ambitious and lengthy ophthalmological surgical procedures, general anesthesia has been used more and more in this subspecialty field, local anesthesia still has much to commend it. A large review[4] of 10,000 ophthalmological operations identified a sub-group of 288 operations, on individuals with previous myocardial infarction, who had ophthalmologic surgery under regional anesthesia; there was no incidence of reinfarction. This suggests that regional anesthesia (which has been long used in ophthalmological surgery) may also offer a protective value to patients who have previously had myocardial infarction.

Innervation of the Nose

To anesthetize the external nose requires blockade at three sites: above the inner canthus of the eyelid, at the infraorbital foramen, and at the junction of nasal bone and cartilage. The nasal cavity can also be blocked conveniently at two primary sites: the sphenopalatine ganglion and the point of entry of the anterior ethmoidal nerve at the anterior end of the cribriform plate. Fortunately, both of these latter sites are high in the nasal cavity in the region known as the sphenoethmoidal recess. If the patient is positioned head down, local anesthetic solution, instilled by way of the nose, pools in this area. Thus, both sites of innervation can be blocked simultaneously. The small remaining area on the floor of the nasal cavity innervated by anterior superior alveolar nerve (V_2) requires local application, by holding the nares together after instilling local anesthetic, or by direct application (see following).

Innervation of Nasal Sinuses

Maxillary sinus
Maxillary nerve (V_2) and sphenopalatine ganglion
Ethmoidal sinus
Nasociliary nerve (from V_1) by way of anterior and posterior ethmoidal branches
Frontal sinus
Frontal nerve (from V_1).

Thus, drainage of the maxillary sinus by an oral approach (Caldwell-Luc) under neural blockade requires maxillary nerve block. Infiltration of the line of the incision over the canine fossa with epinephrine solution improves hemostasis. Sometimes, the operation of Caldwell-Luc extends to the ethmoidal sinus so that anterior ethmoidal block is also necessary.

Cutaneous Innervation of Head and Neck

The cutaneous supply of the head and neck derives from the three divisions of the trigeminal nerve (see following) and from the cervical plexus (see Fig. 15-2).

Cervical Plexus

The cervical plexus contributes to the supply of both the deep and the superficial structures of the neck. The first cervical nerve, C1, is a motor nerve to the muscles of the suboccipital triangle and has no sensory distribution to skin. The skin of the neck is supplied in sequential dermatomal pattern (like the trunk) by the cutaneous branches of C2–C4 by both anterior and posterior primary rami (see Fig. 15-2).

In the neck, all of the cutaneous supply derives from the cervical plexus and can be blocked by a single injection of the superficial cervical plexus, at the midpoint of the posterior border of the sternomastoid muscle, or by single injection blockade of the deep cervical plexus (see Fig. 15-10 and Chapter 10, Fig. 10-7). The latter also blocks the branches of the posterior primary rami, an advantage if analgesia is required toward the back of the neck; it is, however, associated with phrenic nerve palsy.

Blockade of the deep cervical plexus is essentially a paravertebral block in which the needle is inserted and positioned in relation to the transverse processes of the appropriate cervical vertebrae. Because of the obliquity of the transverse processes of the cervical vertebrae, it is important to direct the needle in a caudad fashion. To do otherwise risks entering the spinal canal at this site and thereby perhaps producing profound epidural or spinal anesthesia, or, even worse, damage to the spinal cord (see Fig. 15-11 and Chapter 10).

Because of the course of the vertebral artery—through the foramina transversaria in each transverse process—it is especially at risk and a potential site for inadvertent intravascular injections. Even a very small amount of local anesthetic agent (0.2 ml) injected into this vessel can produce profound toxic effects of convulsions, presumably because of high cerebral blood levels.[22]

In the region of the scalp, the nerves of supply have long superficial upward courses. Four sensory nerves pass in front of the ear to the scalp (supratrochlear and supraorbital from V_1; zygomaticotemporal from V_2; auriculotemporal from V_3), and four pass behind the ear (great auricular and greater, lesser, and least occipital nerves from cervical plexus). All eight nerves converge toward the vertex of the scalp and are effectively blocked if a band of local anesthetic is infiltrated from the glabella, above the ear to the occiput. Infiltration is made with 0.5 to 1% lidocaine immediately beneath the skin in the subcutaneous tissue. It is useful to inject some solution into the temporalis muscle, to prevent undue movement of the muscle during procedures on the scalp. Injection next to the periosteum is required only if bone is to be removed.

In the face, cutaneous branches are short, and they radiate. Thus, in this area, blockade of individual branches is more satisfactory than "barrage" block. For example, the skin below the eye as far as the upper lip can be anesthetized by infraorbital block (see following).

Styloid Apparatus—Glossopharyngeal Nerve

The styloid process is the landmark involved in blocking the glossopharyngeal nerve. It is the calcified rostral end of the stylohyoid ligament, and it varies considerably in length from patient to patient. Its tip lies approximately halfway between the angle of the mandible and the mastoid process and, provides a bony landmark when blocks of the glossopharyngeal nerve are planned (see Fig. 15-8). This nerve emerges from the jugular foramen posterior and medial to the styloid process. It exits from the foramen in very close relationship with the 10th and 11th cranial nerves and sweeps down parallel with the posterior border of the styloid process and at a slightly deeper plane. Therefore, by walking the needle until it just slips off the posterior aspect of the styloid process, the ninth cranial nerve can be blocked (usually along with the 10th and 11th as well). The large vascular conduits of the internal jugular vein and internal carotid artery are very closely related to this nerve at this point, and care must be taken to avoid injecting into these vessels.

The glossopharyngeal nerve supplies the posterior third of the tongue and the oropharynx from its junction with the nasopharynx at the level of the hard palate. It supplies the pharyngeal surfaces of the soft palate and the epiglottis, the fauces, and the pharyngeal wall, as far down as the pharyngoesophageal junction at the level of the cricoid cartilage (C6).

Innervation of the Larynx—Vagus Nerve

The vagus nerve supplies sensation to the larynx. The undersurface of the epiglottis and the laryngeal inlet down to the vocal folds are supplied by the internal laryngeal branch of the vagus. This nerve reaches the larynx by piercing the thyrohyoid membrane, which joins the thyroid to the hyoid cartilages. By blocking its parent nerve (the superior laryngeal branch of the vagus) below the tip of the greater cornu of the hyoid bone, the laryngeal inlet can be rendered insensitive down to the vocal cords. Below the cords, the larynx and trachea are supplied by the recurrent branch of the vagus that ascends in the neck, in the groove between the trachea and esophagus. Although the nerve can be blocked in this groove (and frequently is, as a "complication" of stellate ganglion block), anesthesia of the trachea is usually effected by spray techniques, either transorally or by percutaneous puncture at the cricothyroid membrane. The recurrent laryngeal nerve also supplies motor function to all the intrinsic muscles of the larynx (except the cricothyroid muscle), and bilateral motor block produces loss of phonation and loss of ability to close the glottis.

Innervation of Mouth and Pharynx

A detailed description of the innervation of teeth and mouth is given in Chapter 1, together with appropriate neural blockade techniques.

Innervation of Tonsil

The tonsil and its surroundings are innervated by the lesser palatine nerve (from V_2), the lingual nerve (from V_3), and by the glossopharyngeal nerve, by way of the pharyngeal plexus.

Thus, it is most practical to denervate the tonsillar fossa by infiltration around the tonsil, rather than by blocking individual nerves. This is usually preceded by asking the patient to suck viscous local anesthetic solutions. Alternatively, infiltration can be carried out in association with sedation or light general anesthesia.[7]

TRIGEMINAL NERVE BLOCK

Gasserian Ganglion Block

Gasserian ganglion block results in extensive anesthesia of the ipsilateral face, over the area shown in Figure 15-2. It was once used solely for surgery of the head and neck. With the advent of endotracheal intubation and more sophisticated techniques for general anesthesia, its appeal as a primary surgical anesthetic declined. However, it is still used diagnostically and therapeutically for neuralgias of the trigeminal system. It has merit as a diagnostic block, a permanent neurolytic block, and as a means of introducing heated probes for the newer techniques of thermogangliolysis.[26]

Anatomy

Lying at the apex of the petrous temporal bone at the junction of middle and posterior cranial fossa, the ganglion is situated in a fold of dura mater that forms an invagination around the posterior two-thirds of the ganglion. This invagination is a continuation of the CSF and bears the name of Meckel's cave or the Cavum trigeminale. It is reached with a needle by traversing the infra-temporal fossa and entering the middle cranial fossa, by way of the foramen ovale. Medially, the gasserian ganglion is bounded by the cavernous venous sinus, which contains the carotid artery, and the third, fourth, and sixth cranial nerves. Superiorly, it is the inferior surface of the temporal lobe of the brain, and posteriorly, the brain stem. Any of these structures might be damaged by the introduction of the needle through the foramen ovale. Also, because the ganglion is partially bathed in CSF, injections into the area might spread into the spinal fluid and, hence, produce a remote effect on other parts of the central nervous system (CNS). (See Fig. 15-4A).

Technique

An 8- to 10-cm, 22-gauge needle is required for gasserian ganglion block. The point of introduction of the needle is ap-

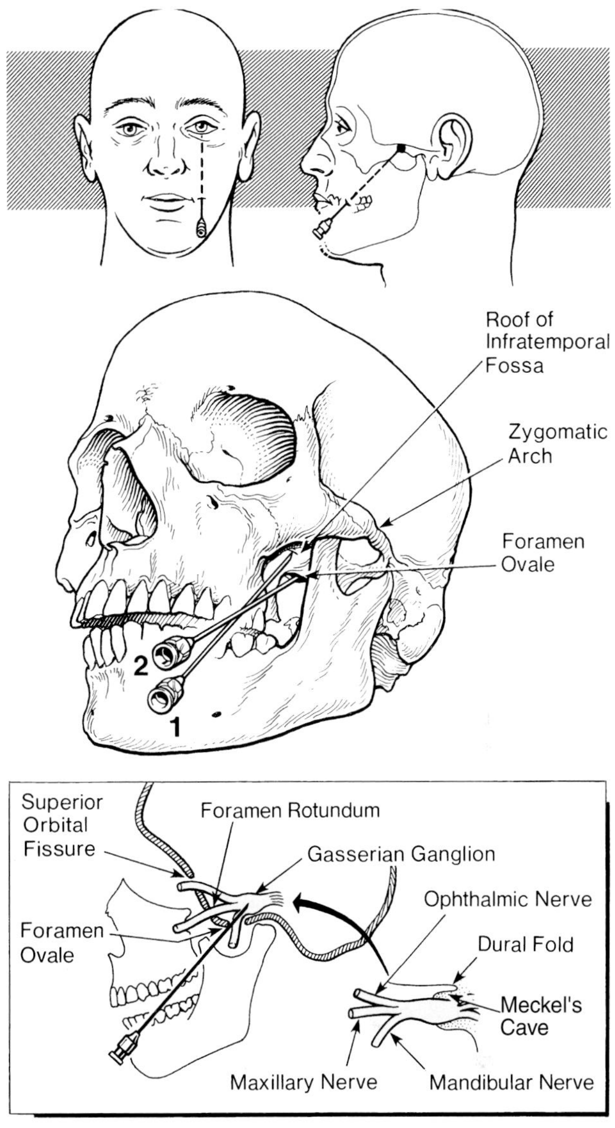

FIG. 15-4. A: Gasserian ganglion block. **Top Panel:**Note that the needle is inserted in the cheek about 1 cm posterior to the angle of the mouth as shown and directed toward the pupil in the anterior view and the midpoint of the zygoma in the lateral view. In patients with teeth, needle insertion in the cheek is superficial to the teeth of the upper jaw. In edentulous patients this may lie a variable distance between the angle of the mouth and a line midway between upper lip and nose. A palpating finger in the mouth helps to prevent needle penetration into the mouth. **Middle Panel:** As the needle is advanced into the infratemporal fossa, it will usually strike the roof of the infratemporal fossa initially *(1);* this is the correct depth to seek the foramen ovale. The needle is then directed slightly posteriorly *(2)* to obtain a mandibular nerve (V_3) paresthesia. **Lower, Panel:** The needle can then be advanced through the foramen ovale into the middle cranial fossa, where it will be adjacent to the gasserian ganglion, as shown. Note the relationships of the dural fold and Meckel's cave, containing cerebrospinal fluid. A needle advanced too far through the foramen ovale can enter the Meckel's cave, and subsequent injections could enter the cranial CSF and produce total spinal anesthesia (see text).

(figure continues on next page)

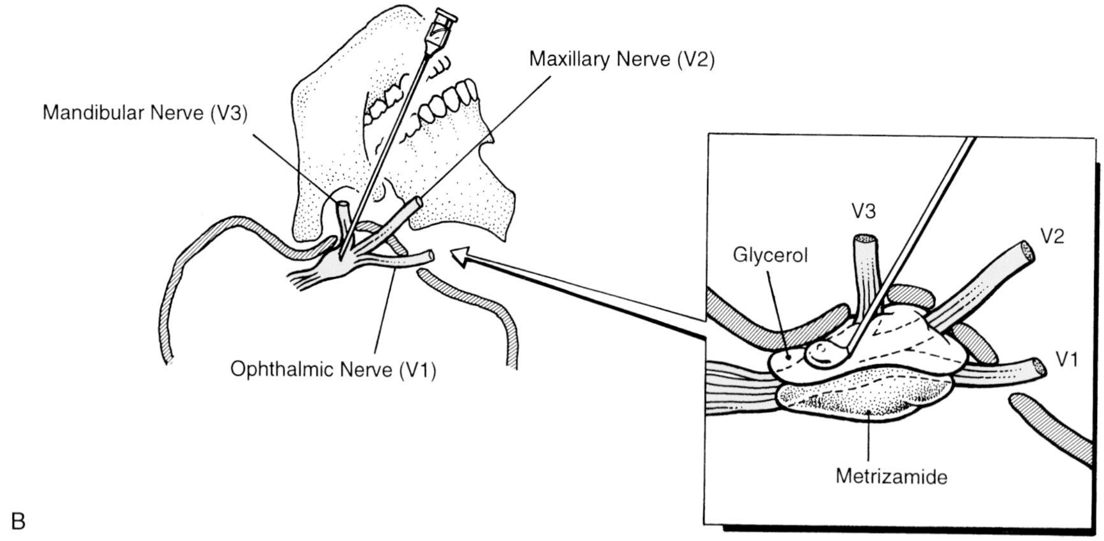

FIG. 15-4. *Continued.* **B:** *Gasserian ganglion neurolytic blockade with glycerol.* A needle is inserted via the foramen ovale as described in Fig 15-5A. However, in this technique the needle tip must penetrate the dural fold and then lie in the gasserian cistern of Meckel's cave (Fig 15-4A inset). CSF is aspirated to confirm placement in the gasserian cistern and then water-soluble contrast medium, such as Metrizamide, is injected to confirm correct placement, to outline Meckel's cave, and to indicate the volume required to bathe part or whole of the gasserian ganglion. In one approach to blocking V_3, or V_2 and V_3 the Metrizamide is removed and the injection made in the sitting position, or the patient sits up immediately after the injection. In an alternative approach, the Metrizamide is removed only to the extent that a residue covers V_1 in the supine position with the head extended; then the glycerol is injected while maintaining the same position; glycerol will sit on top of the Metrizamide (inset panel). In the unusual situation where V_1 and V_2 need to be blocked, while sparing V_3, Metrizamide is removed until only enough for one division remains and then glycerol is injected while the patient is in the sitting position, so that V_3 will be covered with the Metrizamide while the glycerol will sit on top of the Metrizamide, thus blocking V_1 and V_2.

proximately one finger's breadth posterior to the lateral margin of the mouth, next to the medial border of the masseter muscle. In edentulous patients, this landmark may not permit a sufficient angle of approach to enter the foramen ovale, and therefore a point of insertion more caudad is needed. The direction of the needle is both rostral and medial, to a point that coincides with the mid-point of the zygomatic arch when viewed from the lateral aspect, and the pupil from the anterior view (with the eyes looking straight forward), as in Figure 15-4A. It is important to keep a guiding finger in the oral cavity, palpating the cheek to ensure that the needle does not enter the mouth, which might, potentially, introduce contaminating bacteria into deeper structures. Such an approach usually causes the needle to impinge on the roof of the infratemporal fossa (i.e., the base of the skull, which is also the floor of the middle cranial fossa). The needle is then adjusted until it slips through the foramen ovale; usually just prior to this, a mandibular nerve paresthesia is obtained in the lower jaw or lip. This maneuver is optimally (but not necessarily) performed under radiographic control, so that the needle and its path through the foramen ovale can be visualized.

After the foramen ovale is entered, the needle should not be advanced more than 1 cm, and usually its advance is guided by the appropriate paresthesia. Initially, there will be a third-division mandibular paresthesia, but this can occur while the needle is still in the infratemporal fossa. A second division must be obtained, or a first-division paresthesia to the upper jaw or frontal area of the face, respectively, to confirm that the needle is in fact in the immediate vicinity of the gasserian ganglion. A stimulating device may be used to confirm the position of the needle in patients who are unable to locate the paresthesia accurately. This is, of course, a painful procedure, and it is appropriate to administer some intravenous analgesic—for example, .05 mg of fentanyl—as a preoperative medication. For diagnostic blocks, however, it is better not to cloud the sensorium with any analgesics whatsoever, in order to obtain a more accurate assessment of the block. Prior to injection, aspiration tests are mandatory to ensure that the needle has not entered a blood vessel or, in a more likely outcome, Meckel's cave with its CSF contents. If these aspiration tests are negative, then the anesthetizing agent, either a local anesthetic (1% lidocaine or the equivalent) or a neurolytic agent, is injected in small aliquots (e.g., 1/4 ml at a time) until the desired analgesic effect is obtained. If injection affords evidence of analgesia in only one of the divisions, then adjustment of the needle sometimes can affect spread to the other divisions—in patients in whom the needle is in the same vertical axis as the ganglion. However, there appear to be some patients in whom the ganglion lies at a more horizontal axis, and in these patients it is sometimes difficult, if not impossible, to obtain a first-division paresthesia.

Complications

Depending upon the manipulations needed to produce satisfactory block, the patient's face quite frequently will be painful for the following few days, and there is often bruising at the injection site. This usually responds well to treatment with systemic analgesics. Probably the most serious side-effect is injection of local anesthetic or neurolytic agent into the CSF contained within Meckel's cave and its resulting spillover into the circulating CSF of the cranial cavity. In our clinic, injections of as little as 1/4 of a ml of 1% lidocaine have resulted in unconsciousness and profound paralysis of the ipsilateral cranial nerve system, albeit temporary, but the patient needed cardiorespiratory support for a brief period (10 minutes). If a hyperbaric solution is used (e.g., lidocaine with epinephrine or phenol in glycerine), then the drug that emerges from Meckel's cavity will tend to flow over the free margin of the tentorium cerebelli to affect, immediately, the 6th, 8th, 9th, 10th, 11th, and 12th cranial nerves, and usually the patient loses consciousness. With neurolytic agents, there is a potential hazard of spread to these nerves, so that meticulous attention to aspiration tests, and perhaps even a test injection of a small dose of local anesthetic is appropriate before the injection of any neurolytic substances. If hypobaric solutions are used (e.g., lidocaine without epinephrine, or alcohol), then the flow will tend to be cephalad, probably involving the trochlear and oculomotor nerves initially, and almost certainly affecting consciousness to a variable extent.

Clinical Application of Gasserian Ganglion Blockade in Pain States

Local anesthetics injected into the ganglion can produce quite spectacular analgesia in certain pain states, e.g., tic douloureux (but only for short periods), and neurolytic blocks with alcohol were used in the past by some therapists for this condition. The pain relief is purchased at the significant price of hemifacial and corneal analgesia, with saliva often dribbling out of the ipsilateral numb side of the mouth. Such blocks, for long-term pain relief, are rarely done by therapists today.

Of more clinical usefulness has been the procedure of gangliolysis, or thermogangliolysis, because of its better 'track record.' For gangliolysis, an insulated needle is placed through the foramen ovale, using the techniques described above, usually under some form of light anesthesia (e.g., IV Propofol), and the patient is then permitted to awaken. At this point, electrical stimuli are delivered and the needle tip adjusted until paresthesias are elicited in the area of pain. A radio frequency lesion is made, using a thermistor, with the patient usually being reanesthetized with propofol before this otherwise painful procedure. As in many aspects of medicine, a conservative attitude toward tissue destruction is preferable, and initially, the anesthesiologist is only seeking a mild difference in sensory testing to pin-prick between the operative and the contralateral side of the face. If there is no evidence of the desired lesion, it can always be repeated immediately. Procedures can be accomplished on an outpatient basis.[26] This appears to be a successful maneuver in those 30% of tic douloureux patients who do not benefit from carbamazepine or other medication therapy, and approximately 80% will get at least one year's relief (see Chapter 32).[26]

An alternative to thermal coagulation for tic douloureux is provided by "bathing" the trigeminal ganglion in glycerol (0.1–0.3 ml). Proponents of this technique claim the relief is as satisfactory as thermal coagulation, with a greater degree of safety with regard to the production of excessive neural damage. Usual dose is 0.25 ml, but 0.3 ml may be needed for a large trigeminal cistern or in patients with multiple sclerosis and tic.

The technique for placing the needle into the area of the gasserian ganglion is as described above. However, in this method, the needle must be sited in the cul du sac of CSF that bathes the ganglion (Meckel's cave) and confirmed with metrizamide and fluoroscopy. The glycerol is injected into the cul de sac (after removal of metrizamide) by positioning the sitting patient appropriately, face down, to prevent, if possible, spillage of the glycerol into the posterior cranial fossa. Alternatively, the patient is positioned supine with the head extended. After entering the CSF in Meckel's cave, metrizamide is injected to bathe V_1 only, and then glycerol is injected to lie on top of the contrast medium, thus covering V_2 and V_3 (Fig. 15-4B).

Introduced by Häkanson[15] in 1981, with encouraging results, more recent reports have not been so successful.[9,48] However, it is claimed that glycerol gangliolysis is less likely to produce corneal anesthesia than are radio frequency lesions of the first division, and so it may have some advantages.[43]

Mullan[30] attempted therapy in this condition by passing a 14-gauge needle through the foramen ovale into Meckel's cave and inflating a number 4 Fogarty balloon catheter, for a window of time of up to 10 minutes, and reported similar successful results to those for other gangliolysis methods.

It seems that gangliolysis has improved success over neurolytic block, surgical neurectomy, and rhizotomy therapies, but which of the gangliolysis methods is superior is still debated amongst the proponents of the different techniques.[26]

Opthalmic Nerve Branches: Supraorbital and Supratrochlear Nerves

Supraorbital and supratrochlear nerve analgesia is a simple block that can produce excellent analgesia of the forehead and scalp back, from eyebrows to the vertex. (Retrobulbar block is described in Chapter 17.)

This is a simple and safe form of anesthesia for minor surgical procedures in this area (e.g., repair to lacerations, removal of cysts, etc.). The terminal divisions of the opthalmic branch of the trigeminal nerve involved are the supraorbital and supratrochlear branches, which emerge from within the orbit. The supraorbital branch, like the infraorbital and mental nerves, lies in the same vertical plane as that of the pupil when the patient is looking straight ahead (see Fig. 15-3). A block of this nerve is best effected above the eyebrow, after the nerve has emerged from the orbit through the supraorbital notch. A small dose of 2 to 4 ml of local anesthetic infiltrated between the skin and frontal bone will usually produce satisfactory anesthesia. The other terminal branch that supplies the forehead is the supratrochlear nerve, which emerges from the superomedial angle of the orbit and runs up on the forehead parallel to the supraorbital nerve, a finger's breadth or so, medial to it. This nerve is blocked as it emerges above the eyebrow, or can be involved by a medial extension of the anesthetic wheal used to block supraorbital nerve (or vice versa).

Clinical Example of Application of First-Division Trigeminal Block

CASE 15-1

A (very) senior medical personality was involved in an automobile accident. His head went through the windshield; he suffered a large gash over his forehead of approximately 7" in length, extending over both eyebrows, and a head injury that left the individual with significant confusion and perseveration. Because of the seniority of the individual, the presurgical repair consultation involved the whole spectrum of medical specialists. Obvious concern existed about the nature and extent of any brain injuries involved, and from an anesthetic point of view we wanted to provide a service which would not compromise brain function, or compromise adequate monitoring of brain function, if possible.

This circumstance lent itself very well to the simple provision of local anesthesia of the supraorbital and supratrochlear nerves bilaterally. A single skin wheal was produced in the mid-line craniad to eyebrow level, and using a 3", 22-gauge spinal needle, a `cuff' of 0.5% marcaine with 1:200,000 epinephrine was infiltrated in the loose areolar layer of the scalp to the midpoint of the eyebrow, encompassing infiltration of both the supraorbital and supratrochlear nerves bilaterally, through the same initial skin wheal in the midline. This resulted in a profound and satisfactory analgesia from the eyebrows up to the apex of the skull and a lengthy (2-hour) plastic surgical repair was accomplished, with the patient continuing to perseverate, but lying still and cooperating with the surgical procedure without need for administration of any additional centrally acting analgesics or sedatives. All in all, it was a very satisfactory delivery of anesthesia care which did not compromise the ongoing monitoring of this individual's cerebration.

I have also used this technique to repair a forehead laceration in my flyhalf at half time in a critically important rugby match, enabling him to rejoin the game immediately and continue to deliver splendid service to his inside center (modesty forbids me from identifying this latter individual, who given a 1/2 break by the sutured flyhalf in the final minutes, went on to score the winning touchdown! (Of course, had the injured player been a rugby forward no anesthetic would have been necessary for this minor surgery!)

Combined Infratrochlear and Anterior Ethmoidal Nerve Block

The nasociliary nerve divides into its terminal branches, anterior ethmoidal and infratrochlear, on the medial wall of the orbit 2.5 cm from the orbital margin. Both branches are blocked by inserting a 5-cm, 25-gauge needle 1 cm above the inner canthus. The needle is directed backward and slightly medially to pass just lateral to the inner wall of the orbit and medial to the eyeball and medial rectus muscle (Fig. 15-3). Depth of insertion is 2.5 cm, and at this point 1 ml of 2% lidocaine, or equivalent, is injected, while the needle is slowly withdrawn (see Chapter 17). Orbital veins are easily damaged, resulting in proptosis; thus, small-gauge needles should be used, and repeated insertion should be avoided. The infratrochlear nerve can be blocked by infiltrating at the superomedial border of the orbit and along its medial wall with 2 to 4 ml of local anesthetic. The external nasal branch of the anterior ethmoidal nerve can also be blocked, by infiltration at the junction of nasal bone with cartilage. Anterior ethmoidal and infratrochlear nerve blocks accompanied with an infraorbital nerve block can be very effective when they are performed bilaterally for plastic surgical procedures and reduction operations on the nose.

If the mucous membrane of the nose is likely to be stimulated, as it would be in reduction of a fractured nose, then branches of the anterior ethmoidal nerve and sphenopalatine ganglion that supply the septum and lateral wall of the nose should be blocked by topical application of local anesthetic (see Fig. 15-5).

Topical Analgesia of Nasal Cavities

As noted in the description of nerve supply, only two main sites require blockade: the sphenopalatine ganglion and the anterior ethmoidal nerve, both located in the region of the sphenoethmoidal recess (see Fig. 15-5).

Applicators. Macintosh[28] described a technique with 25% cocaine paste applied with nasal probes or applicators. Prior spraying of the nasal cavities with 0.5 ml of 5% cocaine

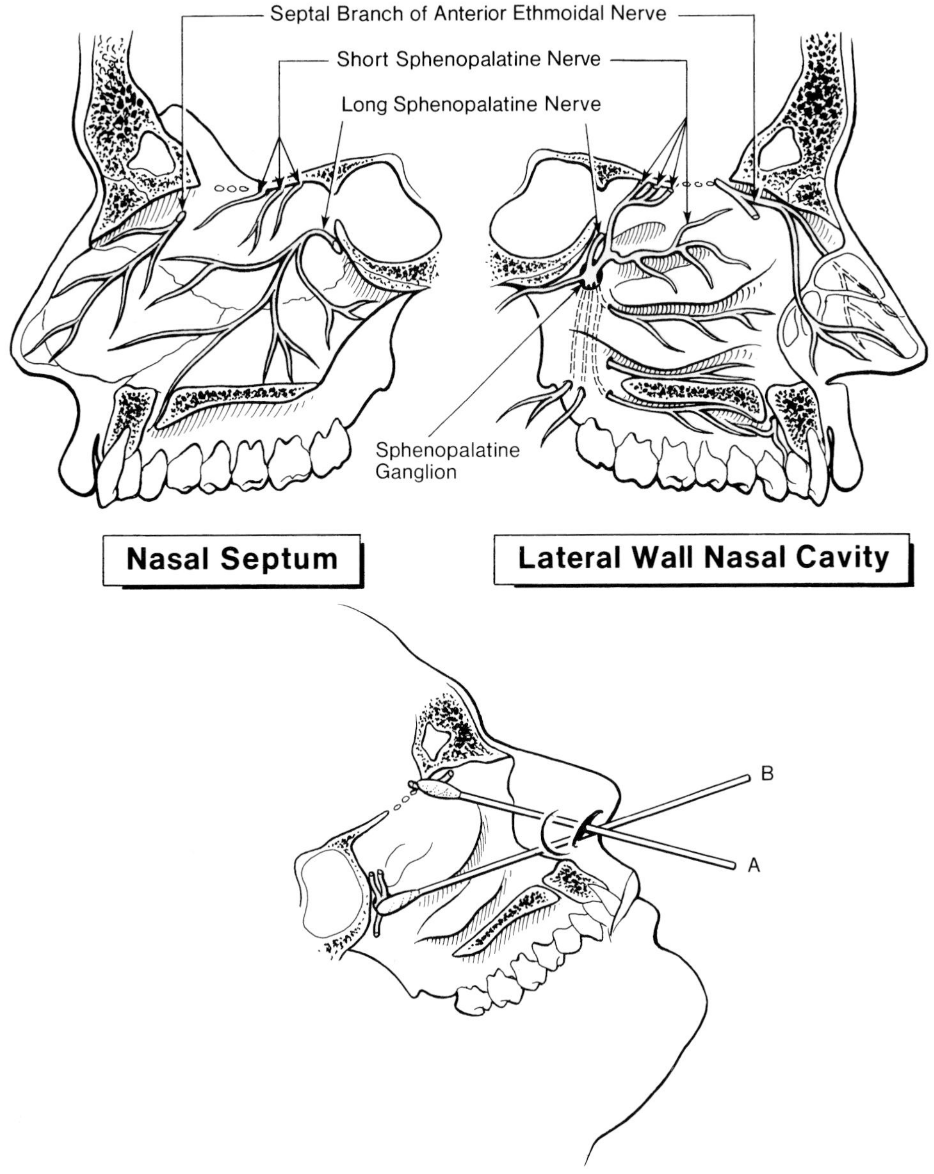

FIG. 15-5. Nerve supply of nasal septum and lateral wall of nasal cavity. Pledgets of cotton wool soaked in local anesthetic and inserted as shown to contact branches of the anterior ethmoidal nerve (*A*) and the sphenopalatine ganglion and nerves (*B*). Note pledget A is inserted parallel with the line of the external nose until it reaches the superior extent of the nasal cavity. Pledget *B* is inserted about 20° to 30° with the horizontal line through the floor of the nose, to reach the region sphenopalatine foramen.

solution on each side provides analgesia and some shrinking of the mucous membrane making the insertion of the applicators more comfortable for the patient. The anesthesiologist then employs a headlight and nasal speculum and gradually applies cocaine paste upward and backward in the nasal cavity. Initially insertion should be close to the septum to avoid injuring the lateral wall. Finally, one applicator is inserted parallel to the anterior border of the nasal cavity until it reaches the anterior end of the cribriform plate at a depth of approximately 5 cm. A second applicator is inserted at an angle of about 20° to the floor of the nose, until bone is felt at a depth of approximately 6 to 7 cm. The end of the applicator should now lie close to the sphenopalatine foramen.[11] The two applicators are left in place for 10 to 15 minutes, and the patient is asked to breathe through the mouth. Cocaine pastes of 10% are also available and are preferable if bilateral blocks are to be performed. It should be noted that the total administered dose of solution and paste should not exceed 200 mg (e.g., 1 ml 5% solution [50 mg] + 1.5 ml 10% paste [150 mg]). Because of the danger of cocaine overdose, some now prefer to use a 10% lidocaine spray for initial anesthesia (20 mg/puff) and then 5 to 10% lidocaine solution up to a maximum dose of 500 mg.

Instillation into sphenoethmoidal recess is unsatisfactory

if the mucous membrane is grossly thickened, or if other pathology exists. Also, it requires the patient to lie with the head upside down, which is distressing to many patients.

Technique. The mucous membrane is initially sprayed with local anesthetic solution, as described under Applications. The patient is then placed supine with a pillow under the shoulders and the neck extended so that the skull is upside down. The patient is told to breathe through the mouth. A blunt-nosed 10-cm cannula with a 120° angle at its midpoint is inserted through the nares until the angle lies at the external nares. The cannula is now swiveled, keeping close to the septum, until the end reaches the roof of the nose. Local anesthetic (e.g., 2 ml 5% cocaine or 2 ml 10% lidocaine) is injected. The procedure is repeated on the other side, and the position maintained for 10 minutes. Then the patient rolls supine, while holding the nares pinched, and lets the solution run out of the external nares. Injections into the nasal cavity do have significant potential for spread beyond same. Attempts to anesthetize the anterior ethmoidal nerve close to the cribriform plate have resulted in total spinal anesthesia[17] and it may be that this technique could be more safely performed with the application of anesthetic-soaked pledgets, inserted into the nose.

MAXILLARY NERVE

Block of Main Trunk in Pterygopalatine (Pterygomaxillary) Fossa

As it crosses the pterygopalatine fossa, the maxillary nerve is usually blocked by a lateral approach. The resulting block will produce profound anesthesia of the upper jaw and its teeth on the ipsilateral side of the face (Fig. 15-6).

Technique. The nerve is approached by way of the infratemporal fossa, and the needle is inserted in the skin at a point below the midpoint of the zygomatic arch overlying the coronoid notch of the mandible. Location of the point of needle insertion is aided by asking the patient to open the mouth wide and palpating the condyle of the mandible as it moves anteriorly to the midpoint of the zygoma. When the mouth is closed, the condyle leaves a clear entry path through the coronoid notch. An 8-cm, 22-gauge needle is inserted through the skin and subcutaneous tissues, which contain the parotid gland and possibly some of the rostral portions of the pes anserinus branches of the facial nerve destined for the orbicularis oculi muscles. An extensive subcutaneous infiltration of local anesthetic at this site may result in some temporary weakness of these muscles. Having traversed the coronoid notch of the mandible, the needle is directed medially until it reaches the medial wall of the infratemporal fossa, where it will strike the lateral surface of the lateral pterygoid plate, usually at a depth of about 5 cm. The needle is now walked anteriorly from the lateral pterygoid plate until it enters the pterygopalatine fossa, where it is advanced a further centimeter into the fossa. Usually, a paresthesia is not obtained or sought, and 5 ml of local anesthetic is injected into this fossa to produce anesthesia of the maxillary nerve. Authors have suggested that the sphenopalatine ganglion can be selectively blocked at this site[13] and used for treatment of refractory headaches. It is almost impossible to block selectively this ganglion without involving the second division of the trigeminal nerve. This more or less precludes the use of permanent blockade in this area, even if such headaches could be shown conclusively to be relieved by such blockade.

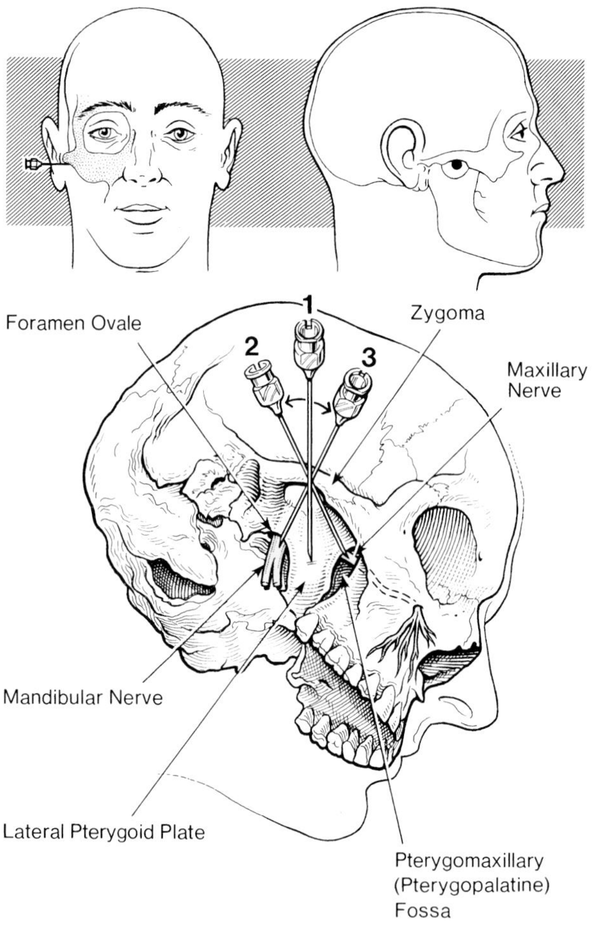

FIG. 15-6. Upper Panel: The coronoid notch is located below the midpoint of the zygoma. A finger is placed at this point and the patient asked to open his mouth. The condyle of the mandible should be palpable immediately, deep to the fingertip, as the mouth opens. The fingertip should then sink into the coronoid notch as the mouth is closed. **Lower Panel:** The maxillary and mandibular nerves are approached by way of the coronoid notch below the midpoint of zygoma. *(1)* The needle passes through the infratemporal fossa to reach the lateral pterygoid plate. Initial direction of the needle should be medial and slightly anterior. *(2)* The needle is then walked anteriorly until it passes into the pterygomaxillary (pterygopalatine) fossa, where the maxillary nerve is blocked. *(3)* The needle is then walked from position *(1)* posteriorly until it passes just posterior to the lateral pterygoid plate to block the mandibular nerve as it emerges from the foramen ovale. The needle point is kept at the same depth as the lateral pterygoid plate to prevent accidental introduction of the needle into the posterior pharynx.

Complications. Because of the highly vascular nature of the contents of the infratemporal fossa—containing as it does the five terminal branches of the maxillary artery with all their venae comitantes, plus the veins that drain the orbit by way of the inferior orbital fissure—a hematoma is frequently a sequel to this block. Such a hematoma can spread into the orbit and produce a profound black eye. The treatment of this is symptomatic, since it usually resolves in several days. Spread of local anesthetic to the optic nerve may occur, producing temporary blindness. The patient should, of course, be forewarned of these potential complications. This approach is not favored for neurolytic blockade because of proximity to the orbit. If maxillary division neurolytic blockade is required, it is common practice to employ the approach described under Gasserian Ganglion Block. Alternatively, some favor neurolytic blockade of its infraorbital branch if pain is confined to infraorbital nerve territory.

Clinical Example of Maxillary Nerve Block

CASE 15-2

A 15-year-old boy was scheduled for AM admit surgery to remove a foreign body from his left maxillary sinus area. It seems that as a child he had received a penetrating injury: a stick of wood had pierced his superior alveolar intraoral area during playtime activities and though the stick of wood was removed, it seems, in retrospect, that a portion of wood had been left inside his maxillary sinus. This had gone undetected for the best part of a decade, despite investigation as to why this young man's maxilla had failed to develop appropriately, creating a facial asymmetry. Following investigation using modern technology, evidence of a foreign body in the maxillary sinus area had been detected and surgical removal was planned.

The initial evaluation of this patient by one of our nurse anesthetists produced a report of a patient who was "utterly terrified, quivering, and shaking," at the forthcoming prospect of anesthesia and surgery. He had just entered the presurgical area from his home. The initial suggested plan for anesthesia care was to deliver general anesthesia (as expeditiously as possible).

However, on more detailed and appropriate history-taking, it appeared the young man was not terrified of the surgery, but was terrified of the anesthesia, having apparently had a close relative (a fond uncle) die from an anesthetic "complication," some years earlier. When it was explained to the patient that he could have the anesthesia performed locally and remain awake during the surgical procedure, a great sense of relief and tranquillity was restored to this otherwise terrified young man. A V_2 block in the pterygomandibular fossa produced good solid anesthesia of all the derivatives of the upper jaw, and a modified Caldwell-Luc approach to the anterior wall of his undeveloped maxilla permitted retrieval of the foreign body (and the fibrosed adnexa that had been lodged in his maxilla for almost a decade)! The patient and his family were effusive in their gratitude for the avoidance of general anesthesia.

Alternate Approach by Way of the Orbit. An alternative approach for blocking the maxillary nerve involves traversing the inferolateral borders of the orbit and depositing the local anesthetic in the pterygopalatine fossa superolaterally. A 6-cm, 22-gauge needle is inserted at the junction of the inferior and lateral borders of the orbit, and, keeping close to the bone, is advanced for a distance of 4 cm. It will then have entered the inferior orbital fissure, and its tip lies in the pterygopalatine fossa. No attempts are made to seek a paresthesia, and 5 ml of local anesthetic is injected at this site. This approach also may be complicated by hematoma production or spread of local anesthetic to the optic nerve, producing temporary blindness. The eye itself does not encroach directly upon the path of the needle in this block, being held off the floor of the orbit by the suspensory ligament of Lockwood.

Although this is not recommended as a first choice for second-division trigeminal block, it is an alternative when local conditions (e.g., trauma or infection) may preclude the conventional approach by the infratemporal fossa.

Alternate Approach by Way of the Infratemporal Fossa. Yet another alternative approach to the maxillary nerve is by way of the anterior aspect of the infratemporal fossa. Here, the needle is introduced anterior to the coronoid process of the mandible at a point below the anterior aspect of the zygomatic arch. This permits a medial approach toward the pupil of the eye, passing posterior to the posterior surface of the maxilla, directly into the pterygopalatine fossa. The needle should not be inserted to a depth greater than 5 cm, because this approach can lead unchecked into the optic nerve and by way of its foramen into the cranial cavity.[24] Although the bony landmarks for this block are usually constant, sometimes the zygomatic arch is relatively low in position, and if this is the case, then the second division of the trigeminal can actually be reached in the pterygo-mandibular fossa by advancing the needle superior to the zygoma.[35] In contrast, the approach by way of the coronoid notch involves an anterior direction, so that if the needle is advanced too deeply it will impinge on the posterior surface of the maxillary or palatine bones, and thereby, hopefully, be prevented from damaging deeper structures.

Block of Branches of Maxillary Nerves

Extraoral Block of Infraorbital Nerve. This technique is accomplished below the junction of the medial and middle thirds of the lower border of the orbit. This point lies in the same vertical plane as the pupil and the supraorbital and mental foramina (see Fig. 15-3). It is important to appreciate that the infraorbital foramen emerges in a caudad and medial direction, and to enter this foramen it is important to direct a 4-cm, 22- to 25-gauge needle laterally and cephalad. To block the nerve, however, infiltration of 1 to 2 ml of 1% lidocaine or the equivalent at its exit from the foramen is usually all that is needed, and it is not essential actually to enter the foramen. Block of this nerve will afford satisfactory anesthesia of the skin of the cheek medially to, and only partially including, the nose, which is also supplied by terminal branches of the first division of the trigeminal (i.e., infratrochlear and external nasal nerves). It will provide analgesia of the upper lip to the midline except in patients whose philtrum is derived from first-division dermatomes; in them, this middle portion of the upper lip will be supplied by the first division of the trigeminal nerve. This block is useful for superficial surgery in the dermal distribution of the nerve but will not, of course, produce any analgesia of deeper second-division structures, such as the teeth, unless the injection is made directly into the canal (see Chapter 16).

The two remaining branches of the maxillary division, zygomaticotemporal and zygomaticofacial, can be anesthetized by infiltration at the sites of emergence from the zygomatic bone, as shown in Figure 15-2. The indications for these are infrequently encountered, except for "ring blocks" of the scalp.

MANDIBULAR NERVE

Block of Main Trunk in the Infratemporal Fossa

The approach for blocking the main division in the infratemporal fossa is the same, initially, as that described for the maxillary nerve; that is, a 6-cm, 22-gauge needle is introduced below the midpoint of the zygomatic arch and passes through the coronoid notch of the mandible, directed medially across the infratemporal fossa until it impinges upon the bony medial wall (i.e., the lateral aspect of the lateral pterygoid plate) (Fig. 15-6). At this stage, the directions differ from those for a maxillary nerve block; for here the needle is walked posteriorly from the lateral pterygoid plate until a third-division paresthesia is obtained. If a paresthesia is not obtained, the needle, once it leaves the posterior aspect of the lateral pterygoid plate, can pierce the attached superior constrictor muscle and enter the pharynx. It should not, therefore, be inserted to a depth greater than the lateral pterygoid plate.

Third-division block here produces analgesia of the skin over the lower jaw (except at the angle) of the superior two-thirds of the anterior surface of the auricle, and of a strip of skin that often extends up to the temporal area (see Fig. 15-2). If sufficient concentration of local anesthetic is injected to result in motor blockade (1% lidocaine or equivalent), then the muscles of mastication will also be anesthetized, resulting in some incoordination of ipsilateral movements of the jaw. This is well tolerated after temporary blocks, but could be a long-term distressing complication of permanent blockade. The otic ganglion, lying in such intimate connection posterior to the mandibular division just below the foramen ovale, is inevitably blocked. This nerve supplies secretomotor fibers to the parotid gland, which pursue a peripatetic course from the inferior salivary nucleus; thus permanent impairment of secretion by this gland is a possible sequel of neurolytic blockade of the mandibular nerve.

Clinical Examples of Mandibular Nerve Block for the Fractured Mandible

The author working in an inner city hospital is frequently called upon to provide anesthesia for surgical repair of fractured mandibles produced in a variety of altercations that all too frequently occur in the local hostelries. When these surgical repairs are completed, the jaws usually are wired together, and in the recovery period, the patient obviously has a 'compromised' airway. The surgery will usually have been completed under nasotracheal intubation, and at the end of surgery, with the jaws wired together after extubation, there is a period of time when the airway may well be threatened, and if reintubation becomes necessary, it requires emergent release of the systems maintaining upper and lower jaw apposition. Also, there is often significant pain upon awakening, and, in providing analgesia, one always walks a tightrope between providing adequate analgesia, without compromising what is often a tenuous airway.

Since such individuals quite frequently have significant ethanol moieties circulating, their degree of cooperation with the recovery room staff can be less than complete, and along with the postoperative discomfort from the surgical site, they are often very difficult to manage. The delivery of a third-division mandibular nerve block, ideally preoperatively with a long-acting agent, or even postoperatively, in the recovery room area, can produce quite spectacular analgesia, and a very grateful and much more tranquil and cooperative patient, as the ethanol levels subside over the next several hours.

Block of Branches of Mandibular Nerve

Extraoral Block of Mental Nerve. The mental foramen, as mentioned above, lies in the same vertical line as the supraorbital and infraorbital foramen and the pupil, with the pupil in the midposition (Fig. 15-3). The position of the mental foramen varies with age and dentition, being more caudal on the mandibular ramus in youth and much nearer the alveolar margin of the mandible in the edentulous aged person. Although this nerve can be blocked by the intraoral route (see Chapter 16), it is possible to accomplish blockade extraorally. To enter the mental foramen, the needle must be directed anteriorally and caudad. However, it is not necessary actually to enter the foramen, and an infiltration, over the midpoint of the mandible in the vertical line of the pupil, is usually ample to produce analgesia of the lower lip and chin, and is effective anesthesia for operative procedures there.

Auriculotemporal Nerve. This nerve can be blocked as it ascends over the posterior root of the zygoma (see Fig. 15-2) behind the superficial temporal artery, and infiltration of 3 to 5 ml 1% lidocaine, or the equivalent, produces anesthesia of the upper two-thirds of the temporal fossa.

Alternative Approaches to Mandibular Nerve Block

In dental practice, where mandibular anesthesia is used for lower jaw procedures, it is frequently blocked by intraoral approaches which can be accomplished either with an open mouth[13] or with the jaws closed[14] (see Chapter 16). Juniper[20] has used cryotherapy to block inferior dental nerve at the mandibular lingula.

Glossopharyngeal Nerve Block

The ninth cranial nerve emerges via the jugular foramen in very close relationship to the vagus and accessory nerves, along with the internal jugular vein. It is blocked just below this point, and therefore both temporary and permanent blocks usually involve these other two cranial nerves, all three of which lie in the groove between the internal jugular vein and the internal carotid artery (Fig. 15-7). These two large vascular conduits may well be punctured during attempts to block these nerves at this site, resulting in either intravascular injection or hematoma. Even very small amounts (e.g., 1/4 ml of local anesthetic injected into the carotid artery at this point) can produce quite profound effects of convulsion and loss of consciousness. Therefore, as always, aspiration tests must be meticulous.

The landmarks for this block involve locating the styloid process of the temporal bone. This osseous process represents the calcification of the cephalic end of the stylohyoid ligament. This fibrous band, which passes from the base of the skull to the lesser cornu of the hyoid bone, ossifies to a different extent in different patients. Although it is relatively easy to identify in people with a large styloid process, if ossification has been limited, then the styloid process sometimes cannot be located with the exploring needle. Sometimes the process may be absent.

Technique

A 5-cm, 22-gauge needle is inserted at a point midway on a line joining the angle of the mandible to the tip of the mastoid process of the occipital bone (Fig. 15-7). The needle is advanced directly medially, until it locates the styloid process. In the event that the styloid process is not located, it is inserted to a depth of 3 cm. In patients who have had a radical neck dissection (and therefore are often candidates for this kind of block), the removal of the sternomastoid muscle places the styloid process, and its adjacent nerves and vessels, at a much more superficial location. In fact, in these patients, the styloid process can often be palpated in the interval between mastoid process and the posterior border of the mandible. The needle will then need to be inserted only 1 to 2 cm. Ideally, the styloid process is located as a bony endpoint and the needle adjusted posterior to this at the same depth as the process. An injection of 1 to 2 ml of 1% lidocaine or the equivalent will produce anesthesia of the glossopharyngeal, and the vagus and accessory nerves as well. At this site, it is not usually possible to block one of these three nerves selectively.

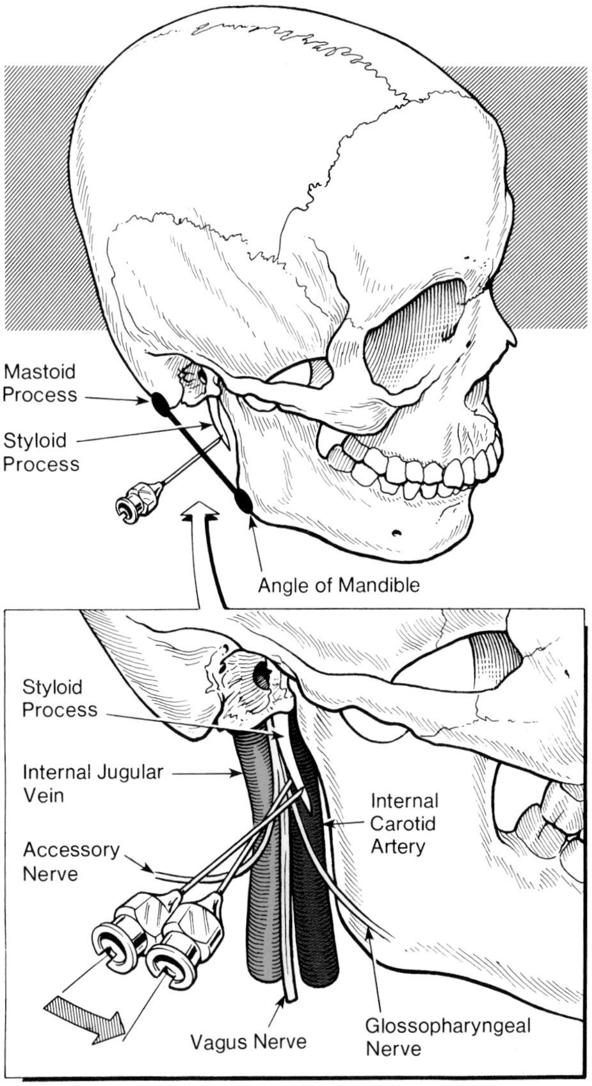

FIG. 15-7. Glossopharyngeal nerve block. **Upper Panel.** The needle is inserted at a point midway between the mastoid process and the angle of the mandible. **Lower Panel.** The needle is inserted at a right angle to the skin. At a depth of 2 to 3 cm the styloid process will be contacted (if present). The needle is then walked posteriorly off the styloid process. Local anesthetic deposited at this point will block glossopharyngeal, accessory, and vagus nerves. Note the proximity of the internal carotid artery and the internal jugular vein.

Glossopharyngeal nerve block is most frequently used for inoperable carcinomas that invade the distribution of the nerve in either the posterior third of the tongue or the pharyngeal trapezius muscles, and with numbness of the laryngeal inlet and trachea, and paralysis of the ipsilateral vocal cords (with resulting hoarseness).

The injection of neurolytic agents at this site, so close to the large vascular carotid and jugular conduits, is cause for concern because of the possibility of damage to the walls of these vessels, which might result in slough and necrosis, with potentially disastrous sequelae. However, such a complication has not yet been reported.

An alternative approach for intraorally blocking the glossopharyngeal nerve has been reported by Cooper et al.[10] This technique involves injecting local anesthetic into the midpoint of the posterior pillar of the fauces. This appears to offer considerable promise as a means of blocking the glossopharyngeal nerve distribution to the oropharynx, and, in combination with laryngeal nerve blocks (see below) and topical anesthesia, provides satisfactory analgesia for endoscopic procedures under regional anesthesia.

Vagus Nerve Block

The main trunk of the vagus nerve is rarely, if ever, blocked intentionally as a primary procedure. However, the branches of sensory distribution to the larynx can be blocked simply and efficiently, thereby rendering the laryngeal inlet and trachea insensitive to pain. This is very useful for intubations performed on conscious patients, and other endoscopic procedures. These branches can also be blocked permanently, for pain relief in terminal neoplastic disease in the area.

Superior Laryngeal Nerve Block

This branch of the vagus nerve is easily blocked as it sweeps around the inferior border of the greater cornu of the hyoid bone, which is readily palpable, even in the most obese patients. By pressing on the opposite greater cornu of the hyoid bone, the laryngeal structures can be displaced toward the side to be blocked (Fig. 15-8). A small 2.5-cm, 25-gauge needle is usually all that is required. It is walked from the inferior border of the greater cornu of the hyoid near its tip, and 3 ml of local anesthetic is infiltrated both superficially and deep to the thyrohyoid membrane. Penetration of this membrane is felt as a slight loss of resistance. The procedure is repeated on the other side. This will produce anesthesia over the inferior aspect of the epiglottis and the laryngeal inlet, as far down as the vocal cords. It will also produce motor blockade (if the concentration of lidocaine exceeds 1%, or the equivalent for other drugs) of the cricothyroid muscles.

Recurrent Laryngeal Nerve Block

To produce anesthesia below the cords, the simplest and most useful method is transtracheal puncture. Here, a relatively wide-bore needle (i.e., 20- or 22-gauge) is used so that air can be aspirated and rapid injection performed. The needle is introduced in the midline through the cricothyroid membrane. Entry of the needle into the trachea is identified by aspiration of air, and the patient will usually cough slightly at this stage. Rapid injection of 3 to 5 ml of local anesthetic will produce a dramatic cough in all but the most obtunded patients, and this spreads the local anesthetic up and down the trachea, yielding satisfactory topical anesthesia. It is usually necessary to use a higher concentration for this topical anesthesia than it is for nerve block, and 4% lidocaine is frequently chosen, although 2% lidocaine will produce adequate blockade but will take a little longer.

The nerve that supplies the wall of the trachea below that of the vocal cords is the recurrent laryngeal nerve. It is possible to block this nerve specifically (and, in fact, block of this nerve frequently occurs as a complication of stellate ganglion blocks).

In the event that blockade of the recurrent laryngeal nerve was ever required (e.g., for a possible neurolytic block for cancers of the vocal cords or below), then the nerve, which lies in the groove between esophagus and trachea, can be blocked at any cervical level below the cricoid cartilage. Attempts at this block would, of course, demand meticulous technique to avoid involvement of brachial plexus with an overly deep insertion of the needle.

Block of the auricular branch of the vagus has even been used for resolving bronchial asthma,[12] where the nerve exits from the base of the skull between the mastoid process and the external tympanic plate of the temporal bone.

Accessory Nerve (11th Cranial Nerve) Block

There are very few indications for blocking the accessory nerve. It is useful for trapezius muscle paralysis, as an adjunct to interscalene nerve blocks of the brachial plexus for surgery on the shoulder. With interscalene block alone, the patient has adequate analgesia of the operative site, but motor power is maintained in the trapezius muscle. He can, by shrugging his shoulders, inadvertently interfere with the surgical procedure; by blocking the accessory nerve in the posterior triangle of the neck, the trapezius muscle is paralyzed and the surgery often facilitated.

The posterior triangle of the neck is a compartment bounded anteriorly by the posterior border of sternomastoid muscle, laterally by the anterior border of the trapezius, and inferiorly by the middle third of the clavicle. The accessory nerve traverses this triangle in a very superficial location (Fig. 15-9). It emerges from the substance of the sternomastoid muscle at the junction of the superior and middle thirds of the posterior border of the muscle, and proceeds in a downward and lateral course across the triangle, to enter the trapezius muscle at the junction of the middle and inferior third of its anterior border. Anywhere along this course, it can successfully be blocked.[38] The accessory nerve lies superficial to the prevertebral fascia and therefore is lying deep

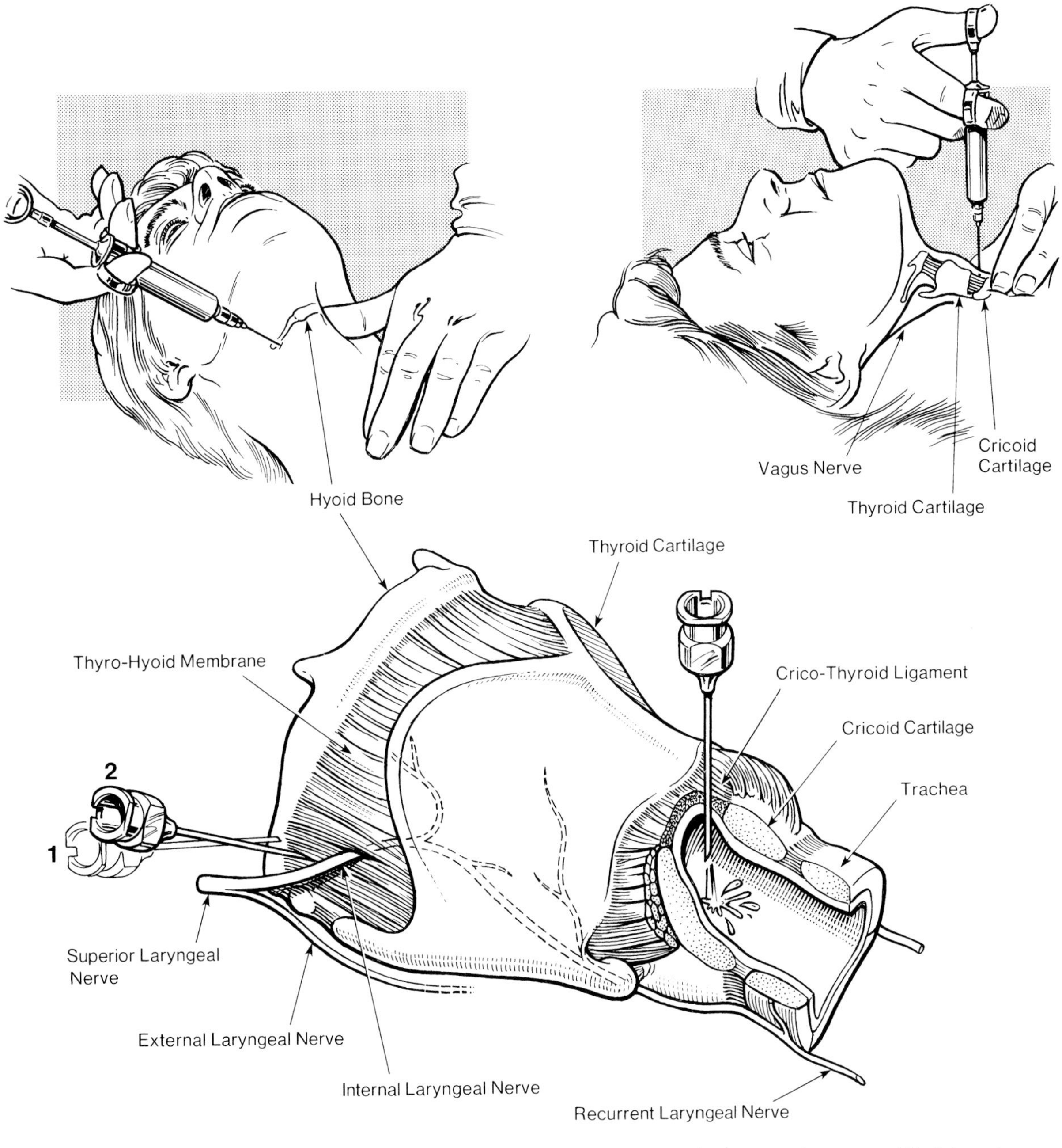

FIG. 15-8. Superior and recurrent laryngeal nerve block. The *superior laryngeal nerve* and its internal and external branches are blocked inferior to the lateral limits of the greater cornu of the hyoid bone. This landmark is brought into prominence by pressing medially on the contralateral cornu of the hyoid bone. *(1)* A needle is inserted onto the greater cornu of the hyoid bone and then walked off the inferior edge of the hyoid *(2)*. Needle depth is not increased beyond the depth of the hyoid to avoid the needle's piercing the larynx. Local anesthetic injected at *(2)* blocks the internal laryngeal nerve and produces anesthesia of the laryngeal inlet, down to the level of the vocal cords. The *recurrent laryngeal nerve* is blocked by introducing a needle through the cricothyroid membrane. Note one hand grasping the cricoid cartilage. The other hand is steadied against the patient's chin. Injection is made after aspirating for air. It is important that the local anesthetic be injected rapidly, and the needle immediately removed, since the patient will cough vigorously. Anesthesia is produced over the inferior surface of the vocal cords and the trachea.

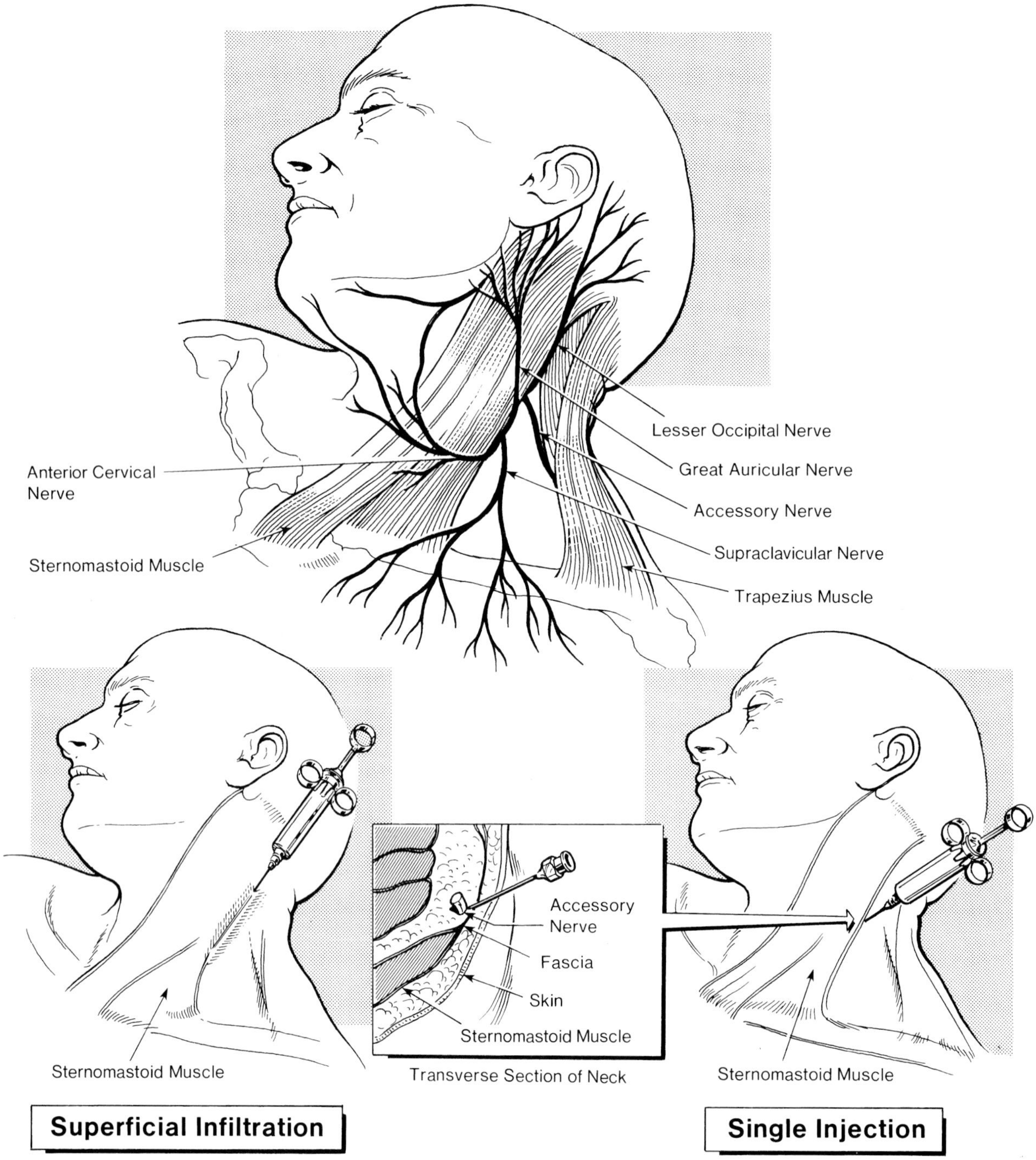

FIG. 15-9. The superficial cervical plexus, which is blocked in the posterior triangle of the neck as it emerges adjacent to the midpoint of the posterior border of the sternomastoid muscle. *Superficial infiltration* is extended along the middle third of the posterior border of the sternomastoid muscle. Note the close relationship of the accessory nerve as it emerges from the posterior border of the sternomastoid muscle at the junction of its middle and upper third, that is, just above the emerging superficial cervical plexus. *Single injection technique for accessory nerve block.* Note that the accessory nerve lies deep to the deep fascia of the neck and that this needs to be pierced as shown in the "*single injection,*" which is sometimes used as an adjunct to produce muscle paralysis of the trapezius muscle in shoulder operations. Successful block of the superficial cervical plexus results in analgesia corresponding to the C2, C3, and C4 dermatomes shown in Figure 15-2.

only to skin, platysma, and deep cervical fascia. Therefore, if a needle is introduced at the junction of the middle and superior thirds of the sternomastoid muscle at its lateral border, and an infiltration of 10 ml or so of local anesthetic is used, block can be accomplished. Accuracy can be increased if a stimulating device is used to locate the nerve. This nerve not infrequently is blocked inadvertently, when a superficial cervical plexus block is performed, and vice versa.

Ramamurthy et al.[38] has described a technique for blocking this nerve as it lies within the sternomastoid muscle. This is accomplished by infiltrating the substance of the muscle with 10 to 20 ml of local anesthetic below its attachment to the mastoid process. It is used for the therapy of spasms and painful conditions of the sternomastoid muscle itself.

Cervical Plexus Block

The cervical plexus is formed by loops between the anterior primary rami of the upper four cervical nerves. Its muscular branches are distributed to the prevertebral muscles, strap muscles of the neck, and, of course, the contributions to the phrenic nerve.

Superficial Cervical Plexus Block

The cutaneous distribution of the cervical plexus is to the skin of the anterolateral neck by way of the anterior primary rami of C2 to C4. These emerge as four distinct nerves from the posterior border of the sternomastoid muscle at approximately its midpoint, just below the emergence of the accessory nerve. The first branch radiates upward and backwards, as the lesser occipital nerve, to supply part of the posterior surface of the upper part of the ear and skin behind the ear; the second branch runs upward and forward, as the great auricular nerve, which supplies skin over the posterior surface of the ear and the anterior lower third of the ear, as well as over the angle of the mandible; the third branch, the anterior cutaneous nerve of the neck, supplies skin from the chin to the suprasternal notch; the fourth branches, the supraclavicular nerves, supply the skin over the inferior aspect of the neck and the clavicle and chest, down as far as the area overlying the second rib, while laterally, these supraclavicular nerves supply the skin over the deltoid muscle and posteriorly as far as the spine of the scapula. All four nerves can be blocked by infiltration at the midpoint of the posterior border

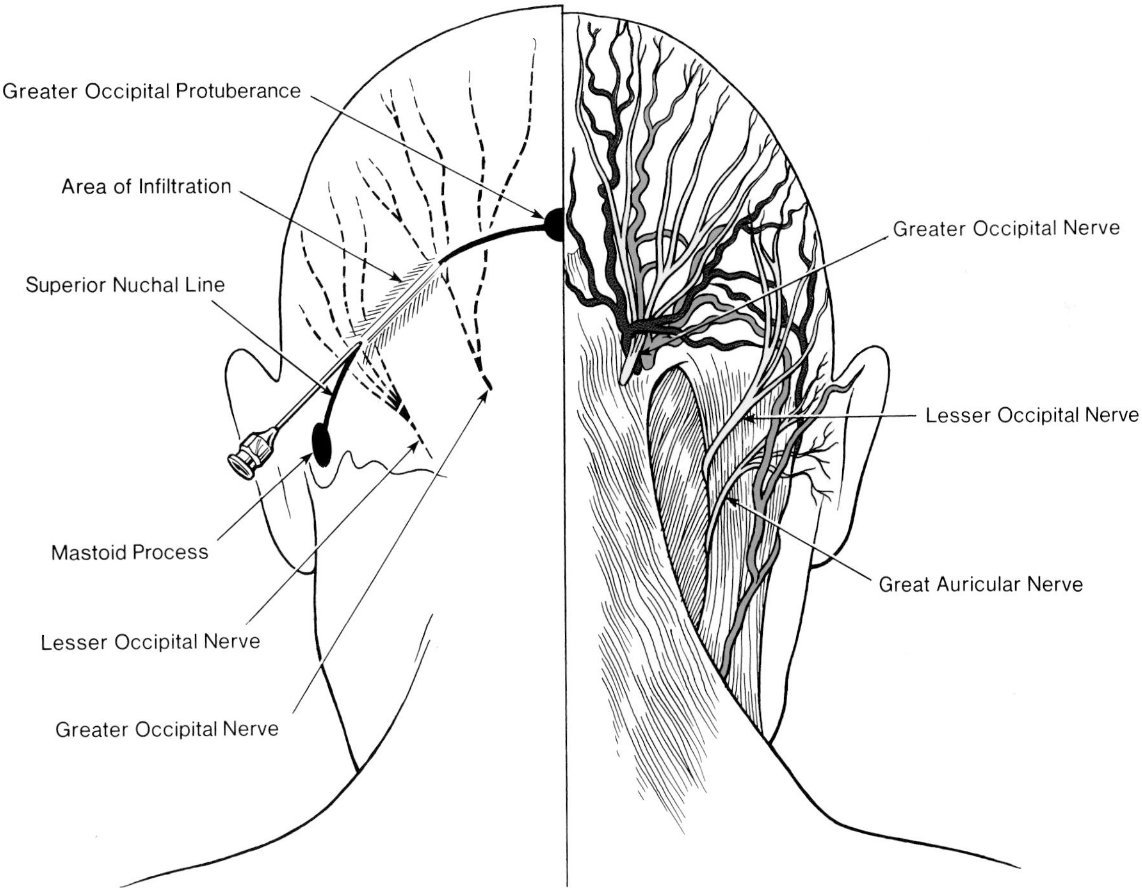

FIG. 15-10. Greater and lesser occipital nerve block. Note the greater and lesser occipital nerve branches crossing the superior nuchal line approximately halfway between the greater occipital protuberance and the mastoid process. Superficial infiltration along this line will produce analgesia of the posterior scalp. The greater occipital nerve can be located by identifying the pulsations of the posterior occipital artery, which crosses the nuchal line in company with the nerve.

of the sternomastoid (Fig. 15-9). Lidocaine, 1% (or the equivalent) (5 to 10 mls) infiltrated at this area, produces analgesia of the neck from the mandible to the clavicle, both anteriorly and laterally.

Block of Greater Occipital Nerve

The skin over the posterior extensor muscles of the neck and extending up over the occiput as high as the vertex, is supplied by the posterior rami of the cervical nerves. Of these, the greater occipital nerve is perhaps the most clinically significant. It is easily blocked as it crosses the superior nuchal line, approximately midway between the external occipital protuberance and the mastoid process (Fig. 15-10). It is located at this site by palpating the occipital artery that lies adjacent to it. Infiltration around the artery of 5 ml of 1% lidocaine or the equivalent will usually cause satisfactory block of this nerve and result in a band of anesthesia from the occiput to the vertex. This block is used along with blocks of the supraorbital, supratrochlear, auriculotemporal, and lesser

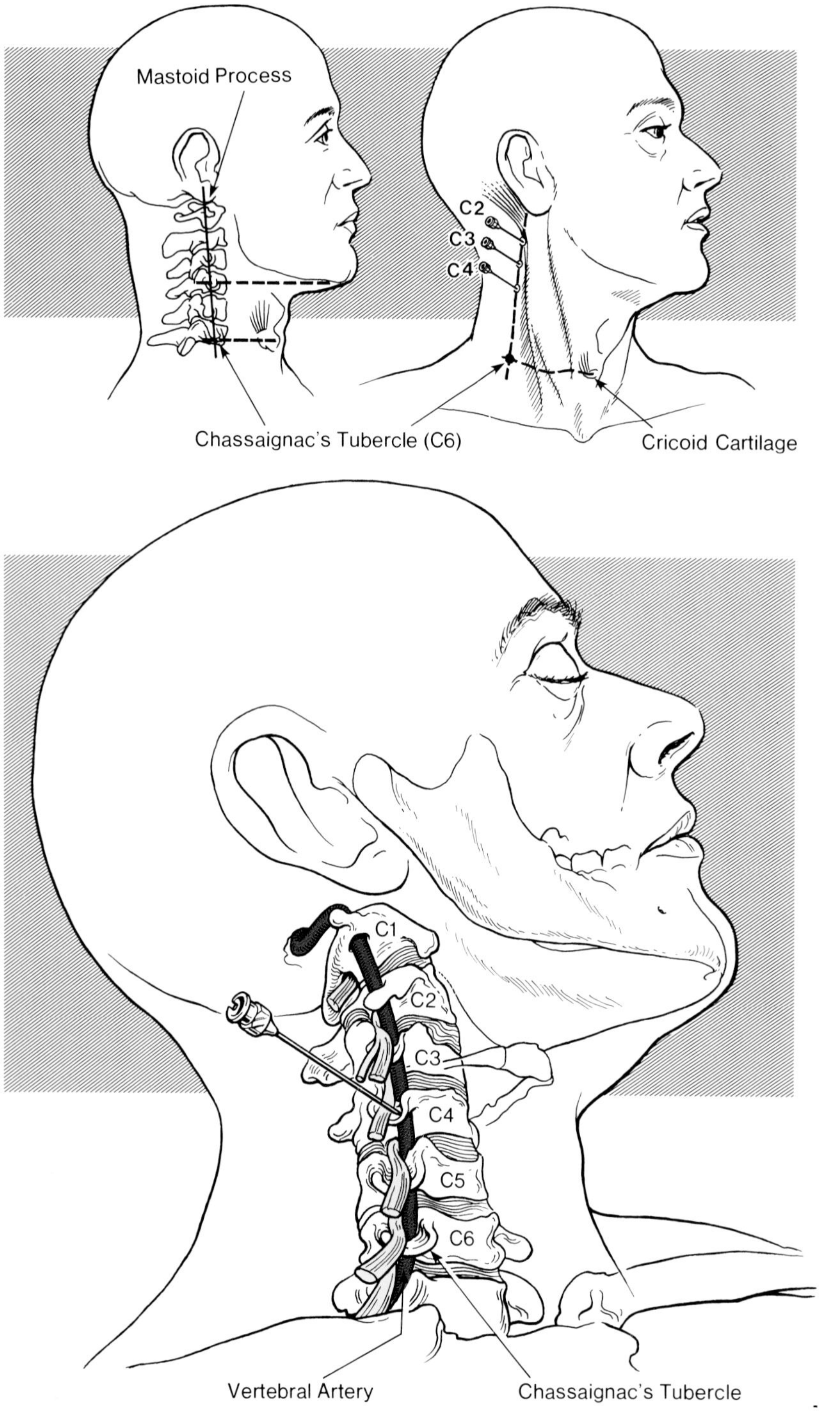

FIG. 15-11. Deep cervical plexus block. A line is drawn from mastoid process to Chassaignac's tubercle (C6). The latter lies on a line extended laterally from the cricoid cartilage. This line lies over the "gutters" in the superior surface of the transverse processes, upon which the cervical nerve roots pass laterally. The C4 nerve root is located at the junction of the vertical line and a line horizontally drawn to the lower border of the mandible, with the head in a neutral position. The C3 and C2 nerve roots can be located by dividing the distance between the mastoid and horizontal line into thirds (see *right upper panel*). The C5 nerve root lies midway between the "C6 line" and the line above. Individual cervical nerve roots may be blocked by injecting small volumes of local anesthetics, as shown in the upper right. Single injection block of cervical plexus can be obtained by a technique similar to interscalene brachial plexus block, since the cervical nerve roots are contained in a continuous space between the scalene muscles. A single needle is inserted on the vertical line at the C4 level, and directed medially and slightly caudad to contact the "gutter" of the transverse process (*lower panel*). Note that caudad direction is essential to avoid penetration of an intervertebral foramen, with possible injection into epidural space or dural sleeve (and thus direct entry to CSF). Note also the proximity of the vertebral artery passing through the foramina transversaria of the transverse processes.

occipital nerves to render the scalp anesthetized for surgery (see Fig. 15-3B). It is also a useful block in both diagnosis and treatment of occipital "tension" headaches. However, the mechanisms whereby such a block relieves these headaches is often more complex than the neural blockade *per se* (see Chapter 27).

Deep Cervical Plexus Block

Deep cervical plexus block is, in effect, a paravertebral nerve block of C2 to C4 spinal nerves as they emerge from the foramina in the cervical vertebrae. Each nerve lies in the sulcus in the transverse process of these vertebrae (Fig. 15-11). Three needles are traditionally used, being inserted at the levels of C2, C3, and C4. The sites of insertion are located by reference to a line that joins the tip of the mastoid process with Chassaignac's tubercle of C6, which is readily palpated at the level of the cricoid cartilage. The C2 transverse process is commonly located approximately one finger's breadth caudad to the mastoid process on this line, and C3 and C4 are at similar intervals caudally on the same line. A horizontal line through the lower border of the ramus of the mandible intersects this line at C4 (Fig. 15-11). Five-cm, 22-gauge needles are directed medially and caudad. The reason for the caudad direction is to avoid inadvertently entering the intervertebral foramen and producing a peridural or spinal block. The endpoint is the bony landmark of the transverse process, and paresthesias are obtained. Injection of 3 to 4 ml of 1% lidocaine or the equivalent on each nerve is generally adequate for anesthesia. Fortunately, the paravertebral space communicates freely in the cervical region, and the anesthetic solution spreads easily to adjacent levels. Deep cervical plexus block therefore can quite often be obtained with injections at just one level, with a larger volume of 6 to 8 ml. Deep cervical plexus block is a frequent sequel to the single needle interscalene approach for brachial plexus block; in fact, if digital pressure is maintained distally over the interscalene groove and the patient placed in a horizontal (or even head down posture), cervical plexus block can be predictably produced using the same needle insertion technique as for an interscalene brachial plexus block.

This block is sometimes useful for such procedures as thyroidectomy and tracheostomy under local anesthesia (although rarely, see below), and is also used effectively for unilateral carotid endarterectomy or for unilateral removal of cervical lymph nodes. A significant complication of the block is due to the proximity of the vertebral artery, because accidental direct intra-arterial injection may produce the profound and very rapid toxic side-effects of convulsions, unconsciousness and blindness;[44] therefore, aspiration tests are of great importance. Extension of the anesthetic into the epidural or subdural spaces is theoretically possible by either dural sleeves or leakage through intervertebral foramen; thus, patients who undergo such procedures must be observed very carefully. When the block is performed bilaterally, bilateral phrenic nerve block is a potentially serious hazard; therefore, the technique is not a practical proposition for thyroidectomy. Because the deep cervical plexus lies deep to the deep cervical fascia, spread to the cervical sympathetic chain should not occur. If, however, infiltration has spread anterior to the prevertebral fascia, then the cervical sympathetic chain will be involved, with resultant Horner's syndrome, and will spread also to the recurrent laryngeal nerve, resulting in hoarseness. Both of these complications in a failed block will indicate that, in fact, the anesthetic has been injected at a site superficial to the deep cervical fascia (Chapter 22).

Regional Anesthesia of the Ear

The pinnae of the ear are supplied by both cervical plexus and trigeminal nerves. The cervical plexus branch of the great auricular nerve (and maybe the lesser occipital), supplies the posterior surface of the ear and the lower third of the anterior surface. The superior two-thirds of the anterior surface is supplied by the auriculotemporal branch of the mandibular division of the trigeminal (Fig. 15-2).

The cervical plexus supply to the ear can be anesthetized by infiltration along the posterior aspect of the auricle over the mastoid process where 5 to 8 ml of local anesthetic is infiltrated (Fig. 15-12). The auriculotemporal contribution to the anterior surface of the ear can be anesthetized by infiltration over the posterior aspect of the zygoma (Fig. 15-12). A branch of the auriculotemporal nerve supplies the interior of the auditory canal over its superior aspect, and is injected at the junction between the bony and cartilaginous parts of the anterior wall of the auditory canal, where it can be reached with a 5- to 6-cm needle. Subcutaneous infiltration at this osseous cartilaginous junction is usually done with 2 ml of 1% lidocaine with 1/200,000 epinephrine.

The floor of the external auditory canal and the lower part of the tympanum are supplied by a branch of the vagus (the Alderman's Nerve).[a] This can be anesthetized by infiltrating the osseous cartilaginous junction of the external auditory canal over its lower aspect with 2 ml of 1% lidocaine with 1/200,000 epinephrine. The tympanum is best anesthetized by direct application of a 4 to 10% lidocaine spray, directing the spray at the roof of the auditory canal and permitting the solution to drain passively over the tympanum rather than directing the spray at the tympanum itself.

Cervical Epidural Anesthesia

In addition to the discrete regional blocks described for head and neck surgical procedures, it must be remembered that it is quite feasible to produce epidural blockade in the

[a] This is so called because in days past, when the city fathers had dined excessively at the community's expense, they would induce vomiting (and therefore make room for more free food and drink) by pouring hot water into the ear canal and, by reflexes precipitated by this branch of the vagus nerve, would have to regurgitate the food and drink consumed earlier and start again!

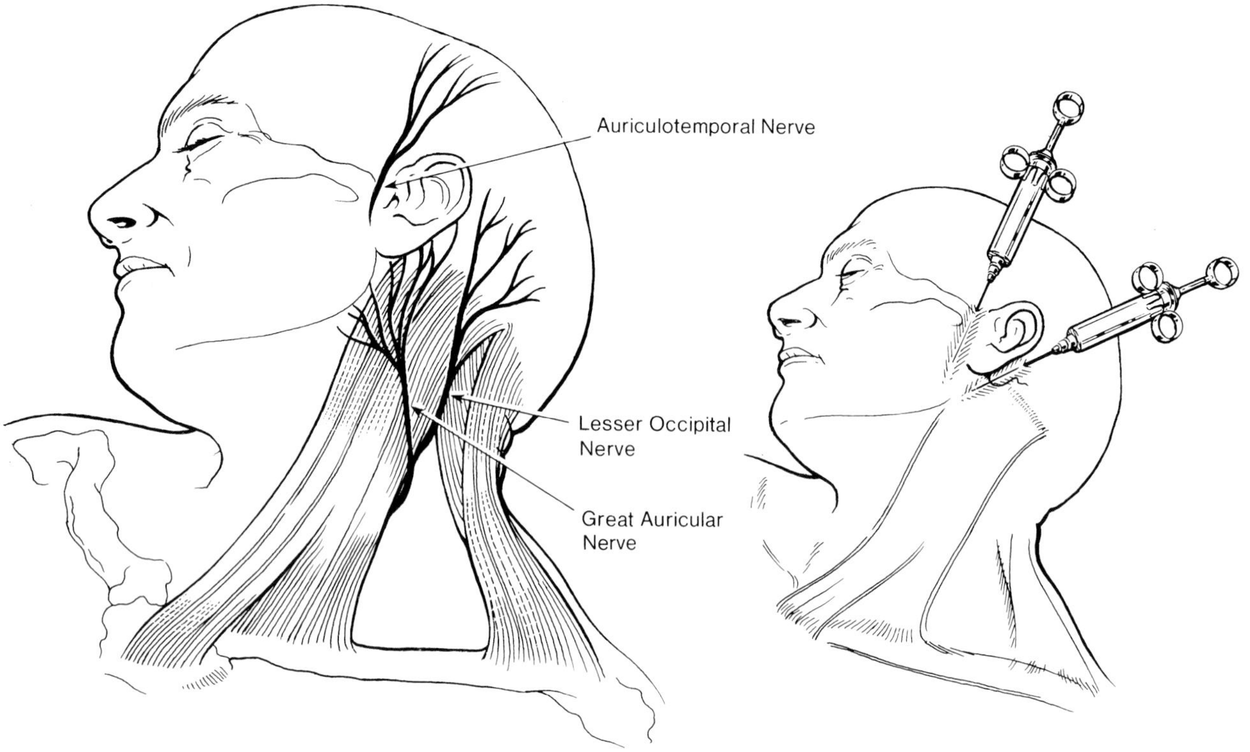

FIG. 15-12. Regional anesthesia of the ear. The *auriculotemporal nerve* (V_3) is blocked by infiltration over the posterior aspect of zygoma. The *great auricular nerve* and *lesser occipital nerve* (branches of the cervical plexus)are blocked by infiltration over the mastoid process posterior to the ear.

cervical regional which can facilitate extensive head and neck surgery.[47] This might be particularly appropriate, because many patients who are candidates for head and neck surgery belong to the older age group and have coexisting chronic obstructive pulmonary, and arteriosclerotic cardiovascular disease. Despite significant preoperative attempts to improve their cardiopulmonary conditions these patients frequently pose significant operative risks. Since the surgical procedures often are very lengthy, the opportunity for administering continuous local anesthetics is enhanced by an epidural catheter.

Because of the poor health of many elderly patients, invasive hemodynamic monitoring maybe required. Resting ventilation following cervical epidural block is similar to that following thoracic epidural block and, although there may be some statistically significant changes in both CO_2 accumulation and oxygenation, Takasaki et al.[45] deemed these not clinically significant in a group of surgical patients studied on whom this technique was used. Thus it may pose a useful form of analgesia for patients with compromised cardiorespiratory reserve who have a need for major prolonged head and neck reconstructive surgery.

Practical Applications

Regional anesthesia of the head and neck can be very useful for surgical anesthesia, for the diagnosis and therapy of various pain states,[11] and for postoperative pain relief. It has even been used to elucidate the mechanisms of voice production![42]

This anesthesia is, of course, eminently suited for minor plastic and other procedures on superficial structures in patients (e.g., patients with full stomachs or cardiorespiratory failure, etc.). It is well suited for outpatient surgery, and is also very useful as a supplement to light general anesthesia for many of the surgical procedures around the oral cavity, particularly so since regional block of the second or third division of the trigeminal nerve with a long-acting local anesthetic agent can afford excellent postoperative analgesia for patients who have had their jaws wired together, and, because of the threat to the airway, effective doses of narcotics are often withheld (see example above).

Some specific surgical procedures in the neck lend themselves well to regional anesthesia. *Thyroidectomy* does constitute a risk to the integrity of recurrent laryngeal nerve, and, using regional anesthesia, may be performed with an awake, cooperative patient, so that the patient's voice can act as an excellent monitor to the integrity of the nerve; however, as noted above, bilateral deep cervical plexus blocks are required for profound anesthesia of the thyroid region. These are, however, associated with the potential for some significant complications (vertebral arterial puncture, epidural or subarachnoid spread, and bilateral phrenic nerve block) all of which the experienced anesthesiologist can cope with, but since many of these procedures are performed by operators acting alone, who are not trained in anesthesiology, they may wish to conduct their surgeries with a `safer' form of anesthesia. It is feasible and sometimes necessary to modify these traditional blocks, and supplement them with local infiltration to accomplish a specific project. Therefore, by using, for example, superficial cervical plexus block, and infiltration of those elements of the thyroid capsule and its contents that probably have additional sensory somatic supply, and also by the autonomic nervous system, one can produce adequate analgesia of the area for surgical trespass.[48]

Carotid Endarterectomy

The patient's state of wakefulness is such a good indication of cerebral perfusion that some vascular surgeons prefer performing their carotid arterial surgeries with their patients awake. This can also be accomplished with deep cervical plexus block. Approximately 10% of carotid endarterectomies performed in the United States are done under some form of regional anesthesia. Some surgeons report a favorable experience, in more than 1,500 cases.[18] Allen et al.,[2] in a series of 679 operations concluded that it is also safer and more efficient, and uses less hospital resources.

Controversy has existed for some time concerning the relative merits of performing the operation of carotid endarterectomy under general or regional anesthesia. This operation poses significant risks to the patient for both cerebrovascular ischemia, as a result of interruption of blood flow during the procedure, and for the risks inherent in imposing major anesthetic and surgical stress on patients who commonly have significant and serious generalized cardiovascular disease. Although the operation traditionally has been done under general anesthesia, with indirect monitors of cerebral function (along with monitors of other bodily functions) there has been a renewed interest displayed in performing this procedure under regional anesthesia, with the patient awake and conscious, permitting direct monitoring of cerebral function by communicating with the patient throughout the procedure and particularly during the critical stages of clamping of the carotid arteries, with less need for carotid artery shunting, even in high-risk patients.[3,5]

Informed opinion is divided as to whether this form of anesthesia provides improved patient care, but there is significant information in the literature to suggest that it is very worthy of consideration.[6,34]

When the techniques of general, as opposed to regional, anesthesia have been compared for this operation, regional anesthesia appears to pose advantages with regard to the incidence of postoperative cerebral vascular stroke.[34] Because these patients have systemic cardiovascular disease, myocardial infarction is a risk to them, and in a series of 185 operations for this procedure done under local anesthetic, Prough et al.[36] reported no incidence of myocardial infarction. In another comparison between regional and general techniques for carotid endarterectomy, Jopling et al.[20] showed that the incidence of both postoperative hypertension and hypotension was lower in the group done under regional, as opposed to the group which had general anesthesia; this may indicate an improved postoperative cardiovascular status.

Controversy still exists in this regard, but with the reports currently available of some quite large series of patients managed quite successfully under regional anesthesia with awake monitoring, one of the significant objections to regional anesthesia in this technique (i.e., that patients or surgeons could not tolerate same), has been disproven. With appropriate patient (and surgeon) selection, this procedure can be quite satisfactorily performed under regional anesthesia, with a degree of mortality and morbidity that is no worse, and may even be better than, that performed under general anesthesia. It also appears that the monitoring required would be less complicated under regional anesthesia, and since the technique seems to involve less operative and surgical room time[20] it may also have economic advantages, because the treatment costs are less when performed in this manner. Significant reasons for this are less need for preoperative carotid arteriography and the postoperative course is a great deal smoother, such that these patients can usually be satisfactorily managed on routine postoperative surgical wards, and do not require a spell in the intensive (and expensive!) care unit.[23]

Endoscopy

It is perhaps in the field of endoscopy that regional anesthesia of the nasal, oral, pharyngeal, and laryngeal compartments has its most frequent application. There are a significant number of times in anesthesia use when intubation of the trachea most be ensured before obtaining the patient's normal protective reflexes. This "awake" intubation can be executed admirably either with local anesthetic spray or with nerve blocks. Such "awake" intubations are often necessary on patients with unstable necks (e.g., secondary to cervical fracture), and a combination of spray or laryngeal nerve blocks will permit orotracheal or nasotracheal intubation without having to risk undue flexion or extension movement in the neck, as occurs in routine laryngoscopy. Also, the integrity of an awake patient's CNS can be monitored during this maneuver (and confirmed after it is completed). In cases in which there may be difficulty with intubation, such as facial abnormalities or fractures, intubation under local analgesia does not preclude the use of any alternative (e.g. tracheostomy) if it fails. Such analgesia also lends itself well to diagnostic endoscopies of the pharynx, larynx, and even trachea for investigative and biopsy purposes (see also Chapter 16).

For patients with pain problems in the head and neck, regional analgesia permits elucidation of the pathway of the noxious stimulus (if any), and by an appropriate administration of different long- and short-acting local anesthetics, with placebo blocks, it is often possible to predict the therapeutic value of nerve section or neurolysis. In patients with cancers of the head and neck, blocks of the trigeminal, glossopharyngeal, laryngeal, or cervical plexus, either alone or in combination, can often afford excellent pain relief (see also Chapter 27).

Complications of Regional Anesthesia of Head and Neck

Applying regional anesthesia to the head and neck is an eminently safe procedure. However, like all other forms of therapy and intervention, a complication rate occurs, and as with the injection of local anesthetics into other parts of the body, it can be associated with an incidence of syncope, post-injection infection, local tissue trauma, hematoma and even allergic reactions.[31] There are also some specific complications which are peculiar to regional anesthetics in this area. These usually involve damage to adjacent structures, or spread to the central nervous system via direct or vascular spread, which can produce convulsions or extensive neuraxial anesthesia, requiring comprehensive resuscitation.

Accidental injection into one of the vascular conduits carrying blood directly to the brain (e.g. carotid or vertebral artery, or one of their branches) can produce significant transient losses of consciousness and/or convulsion, following accidental injection of small (0.5 ml or less) volumes of local anesthetic into the vertebral artery.[22] Total, reversible, blindness has also been described following similar inadvertant injections of small amounts (1 ml) of local anesthetic, accidentally, into a vertebral artery.[44] It is also possible for local anesthetic procedures to result in spread of local anesthetic into the neuraxis, either through direct penetration of the foramina of the skull or of intervertebral foramen in the cervical spine, producing total brain stem anesthesia.[32]

Infection is a rare complication of regional anesthesia in the head and neck, which is surprising, since many of the injections take place through the mucous membranes of the mouth and oropharnyx (which are notorious deposits of microorganisms). Lack of infection is, possibly, because local anesthetics are bacteriostatic and maybe even bacteriocidal.[32] There is scant reference in the literature to infectious complications, although two surprising cases of atlantoaxial subluxation were deemed to be caused by infection of the anterior transverse ligament following local anesthesia for tonsilectomy.[41]

Systemic toxic reactions to local anesthetic uptake can be produced by application of such agents to mucous membranes in the nose, oropharynx, and larynx, and attention to dose administered is critically important here, as in other forms of regional anesthesia. The use of benzocaine and prilocaine has been associated with episodes of methemoglobinemia induced following their application to mucous membranes in the throat and trachea.[33,39]

Introduction to Clinical Practice

Skill in regional anesthesia of this area of the body is a challenging and technically satisfying addition to the anesthesiologist's repertoire, it also provides optimal anesthesia for certain kinds of surgical procedures, and can provide long-lasting postoperative pain relief, and is important in pain-unit work.

In order to acquire the required level of expertise, it is useful to begin learning these techniques on anesthetized patients who have given prior consent. Successful blockade permits reduction, or deletion, of doses of supplemental anesthetics. If long-acting local anesthetics, such as bupivacaine or etidocaine, are employed, then the patient also receives the benefit of excellent postoperative analgesia in situations where analgesic doses of narcotics are contraindicated (e.g., surgery in close proximity to the airway).

Most operations in the head and neck area can be performed under the effects of some form of supplementary neural blockade. Only by routine supplementation of light general anesthesia by neural blockage in such cases can the success rate gradually improve. Unless this approach is used when needed, the anesthesiologist will find it difficult to provide an acceptable success rate for patients who have strong indications for head and neck procedures under neural blockade alone. It should be recognized that selection of the appropriate peripheral nerves for blockade can permit very effective and efficient analgesia for a wide range of plastic surgery procedures. Volumes of local anesthetic as small as 1 ml can be employed for individual nerves and then supplemented by minimal infiltration of the incision line, which is marked on the skin preoperatively. In one large plastic surgery unit, virtually all major plastic surgery of the face in elderly patients is carried out with peripheral neural blockade (Grey, personal communication).

The understanding of anatomy is of prime importance in executing any regional anesthetic, but especially so around the complex anatomical structures in the head and neck, in order to produce those blocks already described in the literature. It is important to realize too that if you understand anatomy well, you can create and deliver specific blocks that may not be in the normal anesthetic literature or repertoire, but may have an individual indication in a specific patient. We all from time to time meet unique patients with unique problems (and so we must sometimes produce unique blocks). For example, Haim and Urban recently described a specific block to denervate spasming rhomboid muscles.[17] This was achieved by applying basic anatomical knowledge, and using a stimulating needle to seek out the nerve to the rhomboids (dorsal scapular nerve), one of the three first branches of the brachial plexus (C5 and 6) as it lay within the substance of the middle scalene muscle.

Other innovative techniques have been devised by applying similar basic anatomical knowledge of this area for lateral chest wall pain by blocking the long thoracic nerve of Bell (nerve of supply to the serratus anterior muscle), another branch (C5, C6, and C7) of the brachial plexus roots, which can be located and blocked in the posterior triangle of the neck.[38]

In fact, with the use of stimulating needles, one can with a significant degree of accuracy and applied anatomy localize most nerves that carry a motor component.

Clinical Example of the Use of Combined Cranial and Cervical Nerve Blocks

CASE 15-3

A middle aged woman had been beset by her live-in `significant other' with a large carving knife. She suffered a single deep laceration that extended from the right infraorbital area across the angle of the mandible continuing dorsally across the root of the neck and sternomastoid muscle, finishing at a point caudad to the midpoint of the line joining her ipsilateral mastoid process to the greater occipital protuberance. There were also two lacerations on her forehead.

This woman needed an elaborate plastic surgical repair that would probably take significant time, and our surgeons were requesting that this be done under anesthesia in the operating room, because the extent of the laceration and plastic repair needed was more complex than could be coped with in the casualty department. The patient was refusing this treatment, and upon further inquiry at the preanesthetic visit she indicated that what she was most concerned about was the concept of general anesthesia. She appeared to have an inappropriate, but for her, very real, and morbid, fear of being 'put to sleep,' because she feared that she would not 'wake up.' She could not be convinced otherwise of the reversibility and safety of modern-day general anesthesia; a relative had died `under anesthesia' many years ago.

However, when reassured that this procedure could be done under regional anesthesia, keeping her awake, she was quite ready and willing to agree to it. This posed a regional anesthesia challenge; to perform this surgery under local infiltration would have required large volumes of local anesthetic, distorting the wound and probably interfering with the plastic repair. The wound extended from the right infraorbital nerve distribution (V_2), through the buccal nerve supply (V_3), involving both anterior cervical, great auricular, and lesser occipital, branches of the superficial cervical plexus and continuing in distribution to the occipital area, involving the posterior primary rami of the deep cervical plexus (C2).

Regional anesthesia was accomplished by a maxillary and mandibular nerve block, using the same needle stick through the coronoid notch of the mandible as was described above. The forehead was anesthetized with bilateral supraorbital and supratrachlear blocks, as described above, using 10 ml of local anesthetic. A deep cervical plexus block was then delivered at C4, using 7 ml of anesthetic agent. This resulted in dermal and deep tissue analgesia of all of the derivatives of the upper and lower jaw and the ipsilateral neck, both anterior and primary rami. Eminently satisfactory analgesia resulted, the patient, who was so grateful for being spared a general anesthetic, was exceedingly cooperative, lying still throughout a lengthy 2 and 1/2 hour surgical repair.

Regional anesthesia for head and neck surgery is not always necessary, and general anesthesia will often suffice, but there are from time to time `special circumstances' where regional anesthesia has a distinct advantage. Throughout this chapter, I have interspersed some examples taken from personal experiences over the years, where surgery could have been accomplished under general anesthesia, but for the specific patient, regional anesthesia was definitely indicated. If you have the skills needed in the descriptions of the blocks in this chapter, it will permit you to offer these services when needed; you will assure a more grateful patient.

REFERENCES

1. Adriani, J.: Labat's Regional Anesthesia: Techniques and Clinical Applications. 3d ed. Philadelphia, W.B. Saunders, pp. 138—179, 1969.
2. Allen, B.T., Anderson, C.B., Rubin, B.G., *et al.*: The influence of anesthetic technique on perioperative complications after carotid endarterectomy. J. Vasc. Surg. *19:*834, 1994.
3. Anthony T., Johansen K.: Optimal outcome for "high-risk" carotid endarterectomy. Am. J. Surg., *167:*469, 1994.
4. Backer, C.L., Tinker, J.H., Robertson, D.M., and Vlietstra, R.E.: Myocardial reinfarction following local anaesthesia for opthalmic surgery. Anesth. Analg., *59:*257, 1980.
5. Benjamin, M.E., Silva, M.B., Watt, C., *et al.*: Awake patient monitoring to determine the need for shunting during carotid endarterectomy. Surgery *114:*673, 1993.
6. Bolisjevac, J.E., and Farha, S.J.: Carotid endarterectomy: Results using regional anaesthesia. Am. Surg., *46:*403, 1980.
7. Boliston, T.A., and Upton, J.J.M.: Infiltration with lignocaine and adrenalin in adult tonsillectomy. J. Laryngol. Otol., *94:*1257, 1980.
8. Bonica, J.J.: The Management of Pain. Philadelphia, Lea and Febiger, 1990.
9. Burchiel, K.J.: Percutaneous retrogasserian glycerol rhizolysis in the management of trigeminal neuralgia. J. Neurosurg., *69:*361, 1988.
10. Cooper M., and Watson, R.L.: An improved regional anaesthetic technique for peroral endoscopy. Anesthesiology, *43:*372, 1975.
11. Devogel, J.C.: Cluster headache and sphenopalatine block. Acta Anaesthesiol. Belg., *32:*101, 1981.
12. Goel, A.C.: Auricular nerve block in bronchial asthma. J. Indian Med. Assoc., *76:*132, 1981.
13. Gow-Gates, G.A., and Watson, J.E.: The Gow-Gates mandibular block: Further understanding. Anesth. Prog., *24:*183, 1977.
14. Gustainis, J.F., and Peterson, L.J.: An alternative method of mandibular nerve block. J. Am. Dent. Assoc., *103:*33, 1981.
15. Häkanson, S.: Trigeminal neuralgia treated by injection of glycerol into the trigeminal cistern. Neurosurgery, *9:*638, 1981.
16. Haim, K., and Urban, B.: Dorsal scapula nerve block: Description of a technique and report of a case. Anesthesiology, *78:*361, 1993.
17. Hill, J.N., Gershon, N.I., and Garguiulo, P.O.: Total spinal blockade during local anesthesia of the nasal passages. Anesthesiology, *59:*144, 1983.
18. Imparato, A.M., Riles, T.S., Ramirez, A.A., Lamparello, P.J., and Mintzer, R.: Anaesthetic management in carotid artery surgery. Aust. N. Z. J. Surg., *55:*315, 1985.
19. Johnson, R.W., and Forrest, F.C.: Local and General Anesthesia for Ophthalmic Surgery. Butterworth-Heinemann, Oxford, 1994.
20. Jopling, M.W., deSanctis, C.A., and McDowell, D.E.: Anesthesia for carotid endarterectomy: A comparison of regional and general techniques. Anesthesiology, *59:*217, 1983.

21. Juniper, R.P.: Trigeminal neuralgia—Treatment of 3rd division by radiocontrolled cryoblockade of the inferior dental nerve at the mandibular lingular: A study of 31 cases. Br. J. Oral Maxillofac. Surg., *29:*154, 1991.
22. Kozody, R., Ready, L.B., and Barsa, J.E. *et al.*: Dose requirement of local anesthetic to produce grand mal seizure during stellate ganglion block. Can. Anaesth. Soc. J., *29:*489, 1982.
23. Kraiss, L.W., Kilberg, L., Critch, S., and Johansen K.H.: Short-stay carotid endarterectomy is safe and cost-effective. Am. J. Surg., *169:* 512, 1995.
24. Last, R.J. (ed.): Anatomy: Regional and Applied. Edinburgh, Churchill Livingstone, 1980.
25. Loeser, J.D.: What to do about tic douloureux. J.A.M.A., *239:*1153, 1978.
26. Loeser, J.D.: Tic douloureux and atypical face pain. *In:* Wall P.D., and Melzack R. (eds.) Textbook of Pain. pp 699–710, Churchill-Livingstone, New York, 1994.
27. Ludwig, B.O.: The role of local anaesthesia in the reduction of longstanding dislocation of the temperomandibular joint. Br. J. Oral Surg., *18:*81, 1980.
28. Macintosh, R., and Ostlere, M.: Local Analgesia for Head and Neck. E. and S. Livingstone, Edinburgh & London, 1967.
29. Moore, D.C.: Regional Block. 4th ed. Springfield, Charles Thomas, 1975.
30. Mullan, S., and Lichtor, T.: Percutaneous microcompression of the trigeminal ganglion for trigeminal neuralgia. J. Neurosurg., *59:*1007, 1983.
31. Murphy, T.M.: Complications of diagnostic and therapeutic nerve blocks. *In* Cooperman, L.H., and Orkin, F.K. (eds.): Complications in Anesthesiology. Philadelphia, Lippincott (in press).
32. Nique, T.A., and Bennett, C.R.: Inadvertent brainstem anesthesia following extraoral trigeminal V_2—V_3 blocks. Oral Surg., *51:*468, 1981.
33. Olsen, M.L., and McEvoy G.K.: Methemoglobinemia induced by local anesthesia. Am. J. Hosp. Pharm., *38:*89, 1981.
34. Peitzman, A.B., Webster, M.W., and Loubeau, J.M. *et al.*: Carotid endarterectomy under regional (conductive) anesthesia. Ann. Surg., *196:* 59, 1982.
35. Priman, J., and Etter, L.E.: Significance of variations of the skull in blocking the maxillary nerve—an anatomical and radiological study. Anesthesiology, *22:*42, 1961.
36. Prough, D.S., Schuderi, P.E., Stullken, E., and Davis, C.E.: Myocardial infarction following regional anaesthesia for carotid endarterectomy. Can. Anaesth. Soc. J., *31:*192, 1984.
37. Ramamurthy, S., Hickey, R., Maytorena, A., Hoffmann, J., and Kalantri, A.: Long thoracic nerve block. Anesth. Analg., *71:*197, 1990.
38. Ramamurthy, S., Akkinemi, B., and Winnie, A.P.: A simple method for spinal accessory nerve block. *In:* Abstracts of Scientific Papers–Annual Meeting, Chicago, American Society of Anesthesiologists, 1976.
39. Sandza, J.G., Roberts, R.W., Shaw, T.C., and Connors, J.P.: Symptomatic methemoglobinemia with a commonly used topical anesthetic cetacaine. Ann. Thorac. Surg., *30:*187, 1980.
40. Sherwood-Dunn, B.: Regional Anesthesia. pp. 37—109, Philadelphia, F.A. Davis, 1921.
41. Sipilia, P., Palva, A., Sorri, M., and Kauko, O.: Atlantoaxial subluxation: An unusual complication after local anesthesia for tonsillectomy. Arch. Otolaryngol., *107:*181, 1981.
42. Sorensen, D., Hori, Y., and Leonard, R.: Effects of laryngeal topical anesthesia on voice fundamental frequency perturbation. J. Speech Hear. Res., *23:*274, 1980.
43. Sweet, W.H.: Percutaneous methods of trigeminal neuralgia and other faciocephalic pain: Comparison with microvascular decompression. Semsin. Neurol., *8:*272, 1988.
44. Szeinfeld, M., Laurencio, M., and Pallares, V.S.: Total reversible blindness following stellate ganglion block. Anesth. Analg., *60:*689, 1981.
45. Takasaki, M., and Takahashi, T.: Respiratory function during cervical and thoracic extradural analgesia in patients with normal lungs. Br. J. Anaesth., *52:*1271, 1980.
46. Wittich, D.J., Berney, J.J., and Davis R.K.: Cervical epidural for head and neck surgery. Laryngoscope, *94:*615, 1984.
47. Yerzingatsian, K.L.: Thyroidectomy under local analagesia: The anatomical basis of cervical blocks. Ann. R. Coll. Surg. Engl., *71:*207, 1989.
48. Young, R.F.: Glycerol rhizolysis for treatment of trigeminal neuralgia. J. Neurosurg., *69:*39, 1988.
49. Zahl, K., and Meltzer, M.A. (eds.).: Regional anesthesia for intraoccular surgery: Opthalmological Clinics of North America, Philadelphia, W.B. Saunders, 1990.

Neural Blockade in Clinical Anesthesia and Management of Pain, Third Edition,
edited by M.J. Cousins and P.O. Bridenbaugh.
Lippincott–Raven Publishers, Philadelphia © 1998.

CHAPTER 16

Neural Blockade of Oral and Circumoral Structures

Intraoral Approach

C. Richard Bennett and Joseph A. Giovannitti Jr.

Local anesthesia of oral and circumoral structures has traditionally been provided by members of the medical profession using *extraoral* techniques. The dental profession, however, relies primarily on *intraoral* techniques to achieve its anesthetic goals. Either approach will usually provide satisfactory results, but there are those occasions in which one method is preferred over the other. The presence of anatomic anomalies, infection, or the nature of an injury, for example, may mitigate for or against a particular technique.

Generally, the extraoral approach is designed to provide anesthesia of a major nerve trunk (e.g., V_2, V_3). The effect of the blockade is to provide anesthesia of a rather wide area of the face, head, or neck. Not infrequently, however, anesthesia of a limited area of the oral cavity is indicated for therapeutic or diagnostic purposes. In these instances the intraoral approach will provide a safe, convenient, and easily mastered alternative to extraoral techniques.

In an attempt to expand the anesthesiologist's armamentarium, this chapter will discuss the most common intraoral techniques used by the dental profession to anesthetize the oral cavity. The techniques themselves are easily learned and, when administered properly, cause little if any physical discomfort to the patient. The anesthesiologist must be aware, however, of the existence of tremendous psychological factors associated with manipulations of the oral cavity. Anticipation of pain is the most common cause of anxiety associated with a dental visit and accounts for the avoidance behavior of 6 to 9 percent of the U.S. population who neglect needed dental care.[13] Perhaps after performing several intraoral nerve blocks, the physician will come to realize, the plight of the dentist in dealing with such an anatomically simple yet psychologically involved area as the oral cavity.

To discuss the psychological aspects of the oral cavity, dental phobias, "fear of the dentist," and the like, is beyond the scope of this chapter. Suffice it to say that on many occasions in which local anesthesia of the oral cavity (particularly via the intraoral approach) is to be provided, preoperative behavioral management strategies such as progressive relaxation, hypnosis, biofeedback, systematic desensitization, or chemically induced sedation must be provided. The effectiveness of any intraoral injection technique depends upon patient characteristics, operative requirements, and the clinician's skills. Each clinician should be aware of his skill limitations, as well as the effective limits of the technique selected. These limitations must be respected at all times, for if the clinical situation supersedes them, serious injury may result. Together, these factors make management of the apprehensive dental patient one of the most challenging problems in the health care delivery field.

PREPARATION

As with all anesthesia, certain requirements must be met before starting the procedure. It will be assumed that the findings of a recent history and physical examination have been reviewed and considered before selecting the anesthetizing technique and drugs that will be used. For the safety of the patient, it will also be assumed that the patient's physical condition and ability to tolerate the pending proce-

C.R. Bennett: Department of Anesthesiology, University of Pittsburgh, School of Dental Medicine, Pittsburgh, Pennsylvania 15261.

J.A. Giovanniti, Jr.: Departments of Oral and Maxillofacial Surgery and Pharmacological Sciences, Baylor College of Dentistry, Dallas, Texas 75246.

dure, and the presence of allergies or potentially interfering comedications, have been taken into account.

Special Injection Considerations

Patient Position

The intraoral injections to be described can best be carried out with the patient seated comfortably in the semireclining position (Fig. 16-1). (Most operating and many treatment tables can also be maneuvered into this position.) This position offers at least two advantages over the conventional upright or horizontal position. First, the convenience of the operator is facilitated. All areas of the oral cavity can be visualized easily and access is gained readily. Second, positional support to the patient's cardiovascular and respiratory systems is provided. Not infrequently, the person receiving an intraoral injection will suffer a bout of syncope during the course of anesthetic administration. Perhaps this relates to the psychological responses that take place when trespass of the oral cavity begins.

The semireclining position not only will aid venous return from both the lower extremities and upper torso, but will also facilitate respiration by relieving the diaphragm of pressure normally applied by the viscera when the patient is in the horizontal or Trendelenburg position. Using the semireclining position during injections can prevent syncopal episodes. The incidence of this annoying and often frightening (at least to the patient and surely to dental students) episode has been greatly reduced by the advent of lounge-type, contoured, dental chairs.

The description of all intraoral injection techniques to be covered will rely on anatomic landmarks for their points of reference. This may be in contrast to other textbooks in which an upright or horizontal patient position is assumed. Under those conditions, reference is often made to a syringe positioned perpendicular, parallel, or at an angle to the floor.

Tissue Preparation

Tissue preparation for regional anesthesia at extraoral sites usually involves disinfection of the area with a suitable preparatory solution, draping with sterile towels, and gloving by the operator. It would seem desirable to apply the same principles of "sterile technique" within the oral cavity. In practical terms, however, they are neither necessary nor attainable. Nevertheless, certain basic principles may be applied to minimize the risk of infection and mishap.

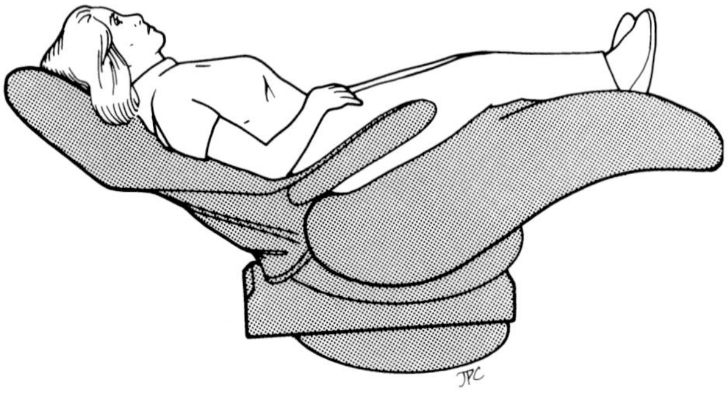

FIG. 16-1. Patient should be placed in semireclining position with legs and thorax slightly elevated.

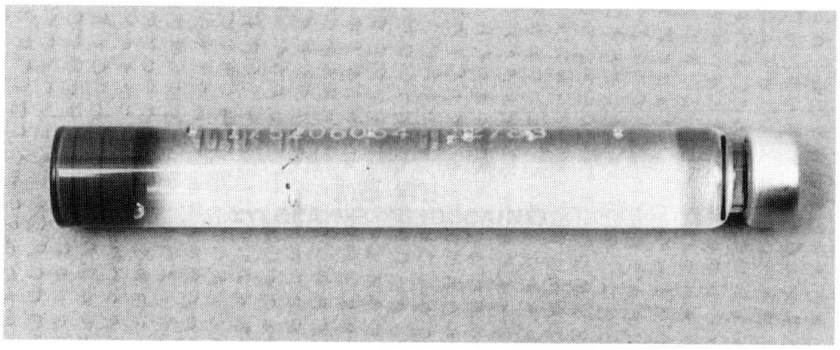

FIG. 16-2. Needle end (right) of the cartridge is sealed with a metal cap. A rubber plunger at the other end is used to expel the contents.

Before injection, the hands of the operator should be scrupulously cleansed and gloved. A surgical mask and eye protection should be worn to protect the operator from inadvertant exposure to blood, saliva, or mucus. Although sterile techniques cannot be strictly adhered to within the oral cavity, it is essential to exercise every precaution to ensure that infection is not introduced into deep structures.

Before inserting a needle into the tissues of the oral cavity, the operator should dry the area with a sterile cotton-tipped applicator or a 2-by-2 gauze sponge. The area should then be scrubbed with a suitable oral antiseptic agent and the antiseptic wiped from the tissue to prevent its introduction into the tissues during needle penetration.

Obviously, the administration of local anesthesia is one of the most frightening aspects of dental care. For this reason, it is recommended that tissue penetration be made as painlessly as possible. The application of a topical anesthetic (many flavored brands are available) before tissue penetration aids greatly in reducing discomfort.

ARMAMENTARIUM

Although basically similar to the armamentarium used for other types of neural blockade, the equipment used for intraoral anesthesia is sufficiently different and convenient enough to warrant comment. This is not to imply that "standard" equipment (plastic syringes and needles with Luer-Lok hubs) cannot or should not be used.

The materials used to obtain intraoral neural blockade may be subdivided as follows:[3]

1. Cartridges containing the anesthetic solution,
2. Syringes,
3. Needles, and
4. Auxiliary equipment and supplies.

Cartridge

The introduction of the local anesthetic cartridge for dental use was a major step forward because it ensured sterility

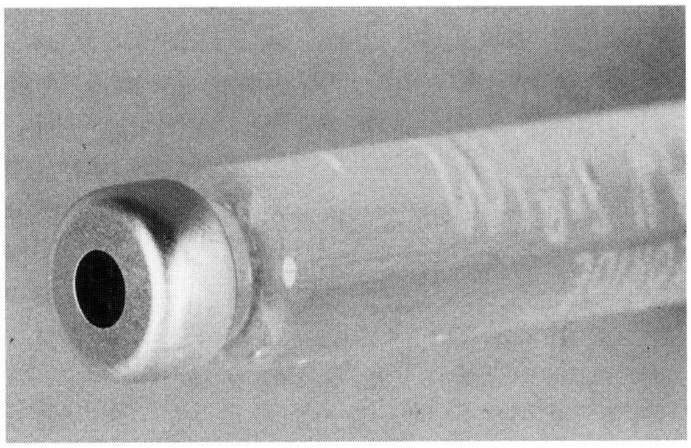

FIG. 16-3. Cartridge with aluminum cap over rubber diaphragm.

and uniformity of solution composition. The cartridge is a glass tube sealed at one end by a movable rubber stopper that can be forced into the tube by the plunger of the cartridge-type syringe (Fig. 16-2). The other end of the tube is sealed by an aluminum cap over a rubber diaphragm that is punctured by the cartridge end of the needle (Fig. 16-3). Cartridges are hermetically sealed and contain 1.8 ml of anesthetic solution.

Cartridges are supplied by the manufacturer in either vacuum-packed cans or sealed cartons. After the package containing the cartridges has been opened, it is recommended that cartridges be stored in their original container. Cartridges should not be placed or submerged in any germicide. Germicides will corrode the metal caps, and the potentially neurolytic germicide agent will eventually seep into the cartridge. The same may be said of the plunger end of the cartridge. In time, the germicide will penetrate the rubber stopper if the entire cartridge is submerged.

The contents of a dental cartridge include the local anesthetic drug, sodium chloride, and distilled water. Occasionally, a vasoconstrictor such as epinephrine or levonordefrin may be present, as well as sodium bisulfite, which acts as a preservative for the vasoconstrictor. Local anesthetic cartridges should never be heat-sterilized; this will cause breakdown of the vasoconstrictive agent. The contents of the local anesthetic cartridges are sterile from the manufacturer. If the cartridges are to be a part of a sterile system, they should be disinfected with an appropriate agent prior to handling. The shelf-life of a plain local anesthetic solution (no vasoconstrictor) in a dental cartridge is approximately 48 months. Local anesthetic solutions containing epinephrine and levonordefrin have shelf-lives of 18 months and 12 months, respectively.

Problems with Cartridges

Despite care taken in the manufacturing of local anesthetic cartridges, several minor problems may develop:

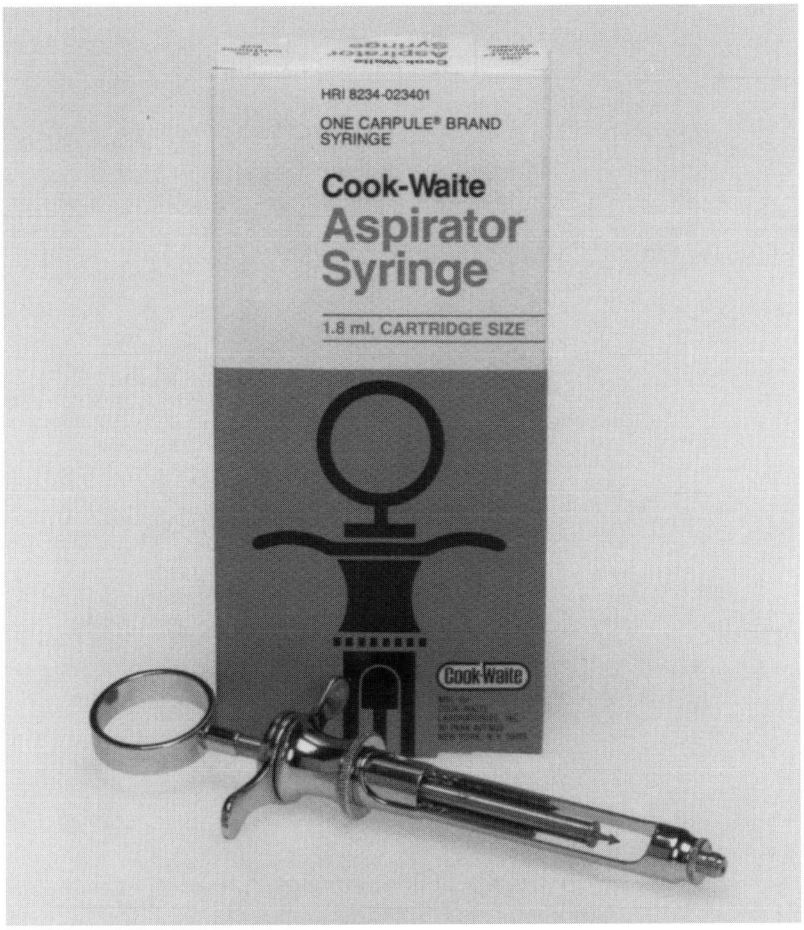

FIG. 16-4. Metal aspirating syringe that can be resterilized. (Courtesy of Cook-Waite Laboratories, Inc., New York).

1. Bubbles. Small bubbles (1 to 2 mm) may be noted within the cartridge. These bubbles are usually nitrogen gas, which has been bubbled into the anesthetic during the manufacturing process to prevent oxygen, which would cause deterioration of the vasoconstrictor, from entering the cartridge. The bubbles are harmless. However, large bubbles in cartridges with or without plungers extended beyond the end of the cartridge (extruded) are caused by freezing. Because the contents may no longer be considered sterile, they should be discarded or returned to the supplier.
2. Extruded plungers. Extruded plungers on cartridges that contain no bubbles usually indicate that the cartridge has been stored in disinfecting solution and that some of the solution has passed through the rubber stopper or diaphragm and contaminated the anesthetic solution. These, too, should be discarded.
3. Corrosion of aluminum cap. Corrosion of the cap is usually caused by immersing the cartridge in chemical disinfecting solutions that contain nitrate antirust materials. Cartridges with corroded caps should not be used.

Syringes

One of the most commonly used syringes for intraoral injections is the side-loading metal cartridge syringe (Fig. 16-4).

Before the needle is attached, the piston of the syringe is retracted and the cartridge inserted, plunger end first into the syringe (Fig. 16-5A). Next, the piston is pushed forward (not tapped; breakage of the glass cylinder might occur) with moderate pressure until the harpoon on the plunger (Fig. 16-5B) is firmly engaged in the rubber stopper. This will allow the stopper to be advanced and withdrawn when aspirating. The needle is then affixed to the threaded end of the syringe provided for this purpose (Fig. 16-5C). A few drops of solution are expressed to ensure that the unit is properly assembled and ready for use (Fig. 16-5D).

The syringe may be dismantled for cleaning. It may be reassembled and sterilized in the conventional manner.

There are several other types of cartridge syringes which may be used intraorally. The self-aspirating syringe is a variation of the conventional side-loading syringe just described. This syringe has no barbed plunger, but instead performs its aspirating function by depression of a thumb disk at its base. This action causes distortion of the cartridge diaphragm, which then rebounds as the thumb disk is released, producing aspiration. Subsequently, during the injection process, any release of plunger pressure will produce aspiration.

Needles

Needles for intraoral injection may range from 30 to 25 gauge and from 1.5 to 5 cm in length.

A needle that is used in conjunction with dental applica-

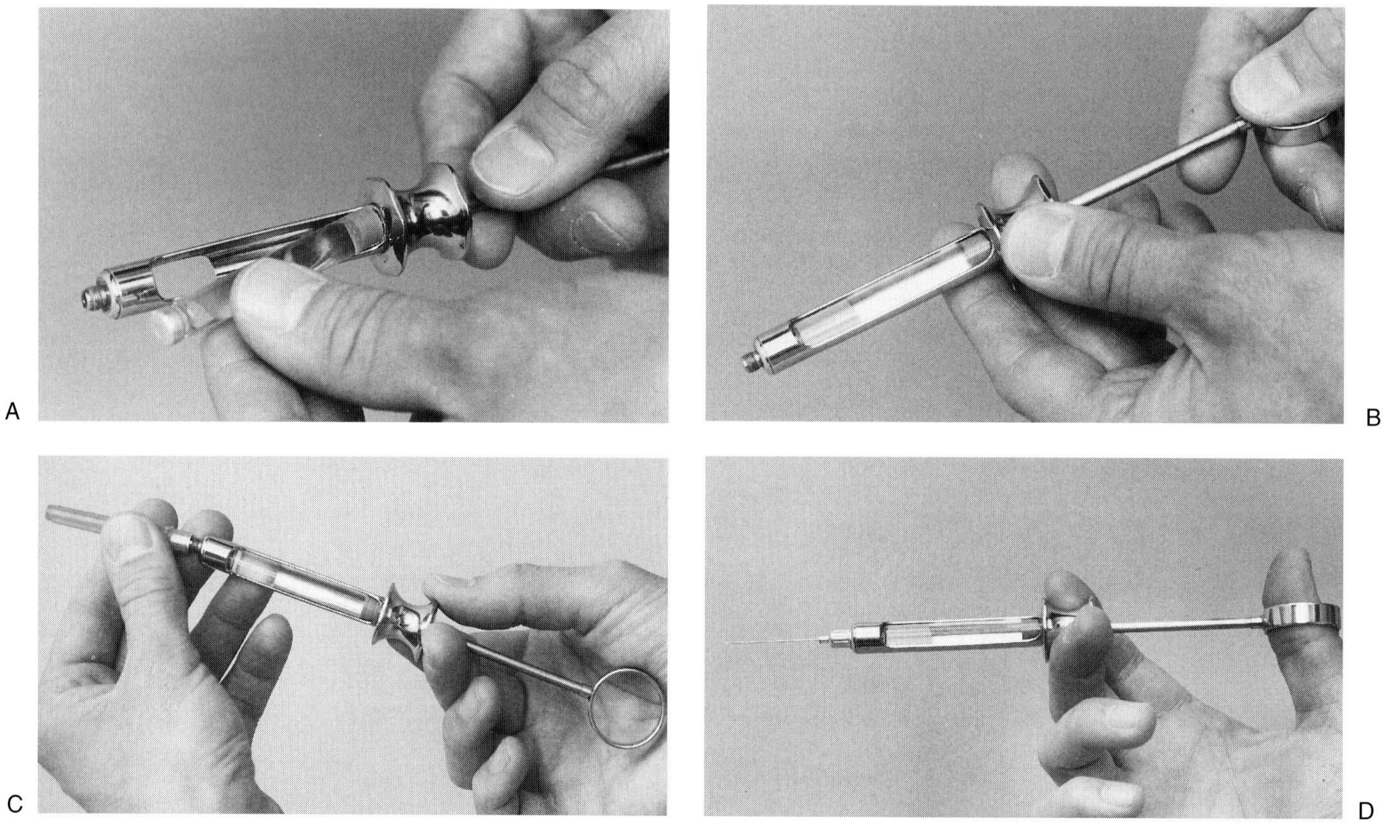

FIG. 16-5. A: Plunger is retracted and cartridge inserted into syringe. **B:** Piston is pushed forward until harpoon engages plunger. **C:** Needle is affixed to syringe top. **D:** Prepared syringe is ready for use.

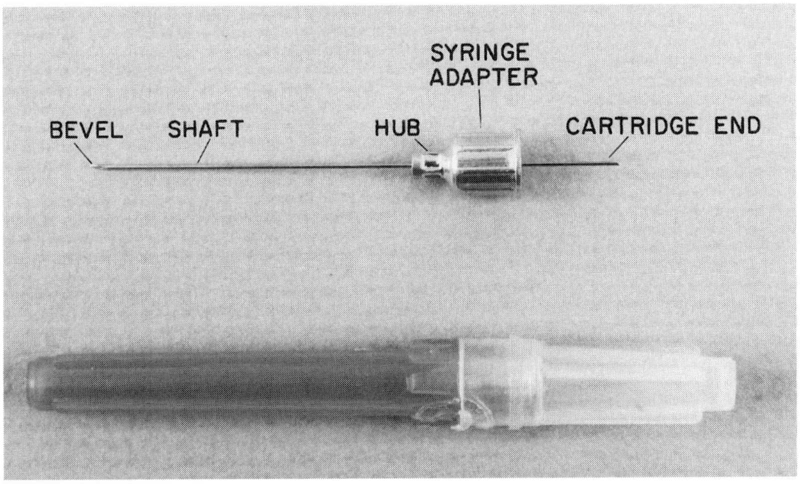

FIG. 16-6. Segments of dental needle.

tion is divided into 5 sections: the bevel, shank, hub, syringe adapter, and syringe end of the needle (Fig. 16-6). The gauge denotes the diameter of the lumen of the shank, while the length is measured from the hub to the point of the bevel.

For deep intraoral injections, the 25-gauge, 5 cm needle is preferred by most practitioners and advocated by most educators. This needle may be inserted painlessly and directed to the desired site with minimal deflection, yet is of sufficient gauge to allow reliable aspiration.

As noted above, the "dental needle" is equipped with a pointed extension that protrudes from the syringe adapter toward the barrel of the syringe. Once affixed to the syringe, this end of the needle protrudes through the rubber diaphragm of the cartridge, thus forming a sterile fluid path through which the anesthetic solution may be expressed from the cartridge.

Auxiliary Equipment and Supplies

Because complications and emergencies can occur during the use of regional anesthesia, it is imperative that all necessary equipment and supplies be on hand and readily available for emergency use. An emergency tray, containing necessary syringes, needles, and drugs, should be within easy reach. In addition, necessary adjuncts to airway maintenance and a manual ventilator should be on hand (see Chapter 6).

Although one may place anesthesia within the oral cavity, using relatively small doses and volumes of local anesthetic drugs, administration must not be approached carelessly. The head and neck, after all, constitute a very vascular area of the body. Unintentional intravascular injection or rapid absorption of even relatively small drug doses may precipitate sequelae of major proportion.

In addition, it is estimated that 90% of all medical emergencies occurring in dental offices are psychologically initiated (Monheim, L. M., personal communication). They frequently take place in conjunction with, but are not necessarily directly attributable to, the administration of local anesthesia.

Syncope, angina, hyperventilation syndrome, and precipitation of seizure activity in epileptic patients are a few of the reactions reported to have been precipitated by anticipation and fear associated with intraoral neural blockade (see also Chapter 4).[8]

LOCAL ANESTHETIC SOLUTIONS

Although any local anesthetic solution acceptable for neural blockade may be used within the oral cavity, only eight agents are currently marketed in cartridge form. Table 16-1

TABLE 16-1. *Local anesthetics in cartridge form*

Generic name	Trade name(s)	Vasoconstrictor
Bupivacaine 0.5%	Marcaine	1:200,000 epinephrine
Lidocaine 2%	Octocaine	Without vasoconstrictor
	Xylocaine	1:50,000 epinephrine
	Alphacaine	1:100,000 epinephrine
	Lignospan	
	Lignospan Forte	
Mepivacaine 2%	Carbocaine	1:20,000 Levonordefrin
Mepivacaine 3%	Carbocaine	Without vasoconstrictor
Mepivacaine	Isocaine	
Mepivacaine	Polocaine	
	Arestocaine	
	Scandanest	
Prilocaine 4%	Citanest Plain	Without vasoconstrictor
Prilocaine 4%	Citanest Forte	1:200,000 epinephrine
Etidocaine 1.5%	Duranest	1:200,000 epinephrine
Articaine 4%	Ultracaine D-S Forte	1:100,000 epinephrine
Articaine 4%	Ultracaine D-S	1:200,000 epinephrine
Propoxycaine 0.4%[a]	Ravocaine/ Novocaine	1:30,000 Levarterenol
Procaine 2%		

[a] Propoxycaine 0.4% and procaine 2% are combined in the same cartridge. Both compounds are ester-type anesthetic drugs. They are the only esters currently marketed in cartridge form. All other agents are amides.

TABLE 16-2. *Duration and maximum safe dosage of agents used in dentistry*

Drug	Duration pulpal/soft tissue	Maximum dose
Bupivacaine 0.4% 1:200,000 epinephrine	1–2h/>10h	1.3 mg/kg 90 mg max (10 cart)
Lidocaine 2% (without vasoconstrictor)	5–10 min/60–120 min	4.4 mg/kg 300 mg max (8.3 cart)
Lidocaine 2% 1:50,000 epinephrine	60–90 min/3–4 h	7.0 mg/kg 500 mg max (13.8 cart)[a]
Lidocaine 2% 1:100,000 epinephrine	60–90 min/3–4 h	7.0 mg/kg 500 mg max (13.8 cart)[a]
Mepivacaine 3%	20–40 min/2–3 h	6.6 mg/kg 400 mg max (7.4 cart)
Mepivacaine 2% 1:20,000 Levonordefrin	40–60 min/2–4 h	6.6 mg/kg 400 mg max (11.1 cart)[b]
Prilocaine 4%	10–15 min/2–4 h	7.9 mg/kg 600 mg max (8.3 cart)
Prilocaine 4% 1:200,000 epinephrine	60–90 min/2–4 h	7.9 mg/kg 600 mg max (8.3 cart)
Etidocaine 1.5% 1:200,000 epinephrine	1–2h/>10 h	8.0 mg/kg 400 mg max (14.8 cart)
Articaine 4% 1:100,000 epinephrine	75 min/2–4 h	7.0 mg/kg 500 mg max (7 cart)
Articaine 4% 1:200,000 epinephrine	45 min/2–4 h	7.0 mg/kg 500 mg max (7 cart)
Propoxycaine/procaine	10–20 min/2–3 h	6.6 mg/kg 400 mg max total ester (9.2 cart)

[a] Exceeds maximum recommended epinephrine dose
[b] Exceeds maximum recommended levonordefrin dose

lists these anesthetic agents (by generic and trade names) and the vasoconstrictors that they may contain.

As in other types of neural blockade, the choice of anesthetic agent and vasoconstrictor is based on factors such as physical status, age, and weight of the patient, duration required, and the need for hemostasis (see Table 16-2 for representative durations and recommended maximum safe dosages of agents used in dentistry).

In the past, local anesthetic cartridges also contained methylparaben as a germicide/preservative. Because of its documented allergenicity, however, many manufacturers have chosen to delete it from their preparations. To determine whether a particular brand of anesthetic contains methylparaben, one must consult the package insert or take note of the cartridge contents printed on the original container.

Bupivacaine (Marcaine Cook-Waite Laboratories, New York) marketed in dental cartridges contains monothioglycerol and ascorbic acid as antioxidants.[10]

VASOCONSTRICTORS

Vasoconstrictors are used primarily in the oral cavity to prolong the duration of anesthetic effect. Profound alpha-adrenergic agonism significantly reduces blood flow at the injection site, causing retention of the local anesthetic in the vicinity of the neuronal tissue. Its most pronounced effect is to increase the duration of lidocaine and mepivacaine in both the maxilla and mandible. By contrast, addition of a vasoconstrictor to bupivacaine or etidocaine does little to prolong their effects. These drugs produce a prolonged duration of anesthesia following mandibular block, primarily because of their high degree of lipid solubility. Their extreme lipid solubility works against these agents following maxillary infiltration injection, because rapid uptake by supraperiosteal tissues impedes diffusion of the drug to the superior alveolar nerves. Thus, even with the addition of a vasoconstrictor to bupivacaine or etidocaine, their usefulness for maxillary infiltration anesthesia is limited. Vasoconstrictors also play a role in reducing the potential for systemic toxicity of the injected local anesthetic, particularly lidocaine. They can also provide localized hemostasis for surgery.

The two most commonly used vasoconstrictors in dentistry are epinephrine and levonordefrin. In dental cartridges, epinephrine is contained in three concentrations, 5 micrograms per ml (1:200,000), 10 micrograms per ml (1:100,000), and 20 micrograms per ml (1:50,000). A standard dental cartridge with 1:100,000 epinephrine contains 18 micrograms of epinephrine. Levonordefrin is found only in dental cartridges containing mepivacaine, in a concentration of 50 micrograms per ml (1:20,000). A standard dental cartridge with 1:20,000 levonordefrin contains 90 micrograms of levonordefrin. Although levonordefrin is a relatively weaker adrenergic agonist than epinephrine, consideration should be given to the fact that the 1:20,000 concentration is 5 times greater than the standard concentration of epinephrine. Therefore, fewer cartridges con-

TABLE 16-3. *Maximum recommended dose of vasoconstrictors (70 kg)*

	Healthy	ASA II	ASA III
Epinephrine 1:100,000	3 mcg/kg 200 mcg max (11.1 cart)	1.5 mcg/kg 100 mcg/kg (5.5 cart)	0.75 mcg/kg 40 mcg/kg (2.22 cart)
Levonordefrin 1:20,000	7 mcg/kg (5.4 cart)	3.5 mcg/kg (2.7 cart)	1.5 mcg/kg (1.2 cart)

taining levonordefrin may be safely used in comparison with cartridges containing epinephrine. Table 16-3 gives generally accepted dosages for vasoconstrictors in healthy patients, as well as in those with cardiovascular system impairments.

The oral cavity is highly vascularized, and the systemic uptake of vasoconstrictors following intraoral injection is rapid. It has been demonstrated that a single dental cartridge of lidocaine 2% with 1:100,000 epinephrine will double the resting epinephrine titer within minutes.[4,6] Furthermore, the intraoral administration of eight dental cartridges of a 1 : 100,000 epinephrine solution (an easily attainable clinical situation) produces plasma epinephrine concentrations equivalent to those present during heavy exercise.[5] Thus, care should be taken when administering vasoconstrictor-containing local anesthetic solutions to patients with severe anxiety and/or cardiovascular disease. As a general rule, the minimum possible amount of vasoconstrictor should be used. One cartridge of a 1:100,000 epinephrine-containing solution should be well-tolerated even in patients with significant cardiovascular disease. Caution should also be exercised in patients taking nonspecific beta-adrenergic blockers, adrenergic neuron blockers, tricyclic antidepressants, and phenothiazine derivatives.

Vasoconstrictive agents should be used intraorally only when a plain local anesthetic solution fails to provide profound anesthesia, when the length of the planned procedure is longer than the expected duration of anesthesia with a plain solution, and when local hemostasis is required.

INTRAORAL INJECTION TECHNIQUES

Anatomy

Innervation of the head and neck is by way of the trigeminal and cervical nerves as depicted in Figure 16-7. More specifically, the trigeminal nerve supplies the face and anterior portions of the scalp by means of its ophthalmic (V_1), maxillary (V_2), and mandibular (V_3) divisions. All areas of the oral cavity are innervated by either V_2 or V_3 (see Chapter 15).

Techniques of Neural Blockade for the Maxillary Nerve and its Subdivisions

Anatomy of the Maxillary Division (V_2)

The maxillary nerve is entirely sensory (Fig. 16-8). It exits the skull through the foramen rotundum and enters the

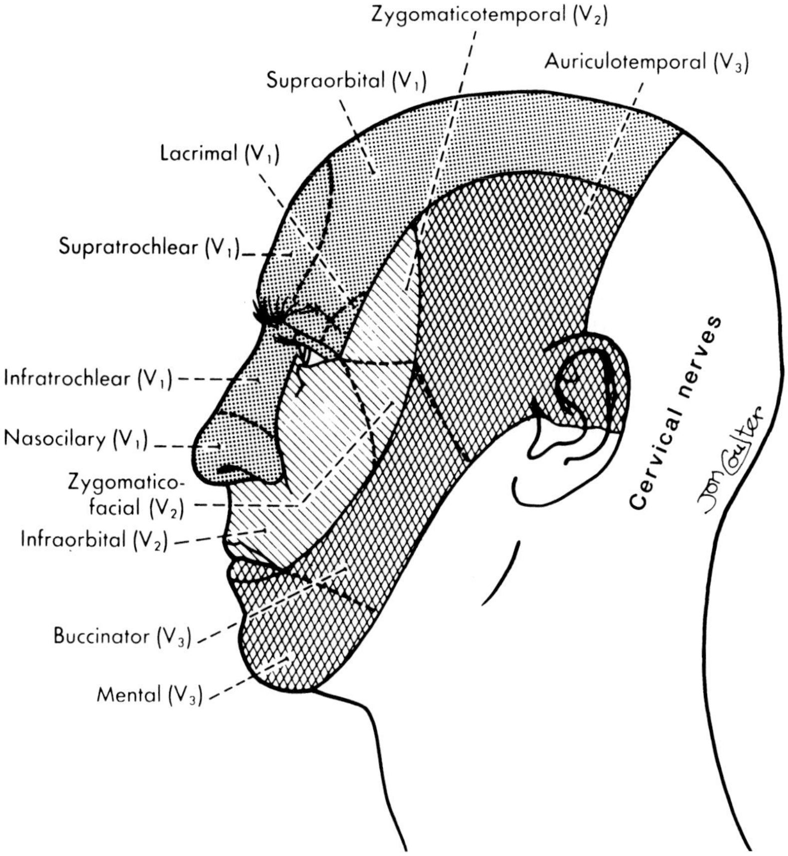

FIG. 16-7. Superficial sensory nerves of the head and neck.

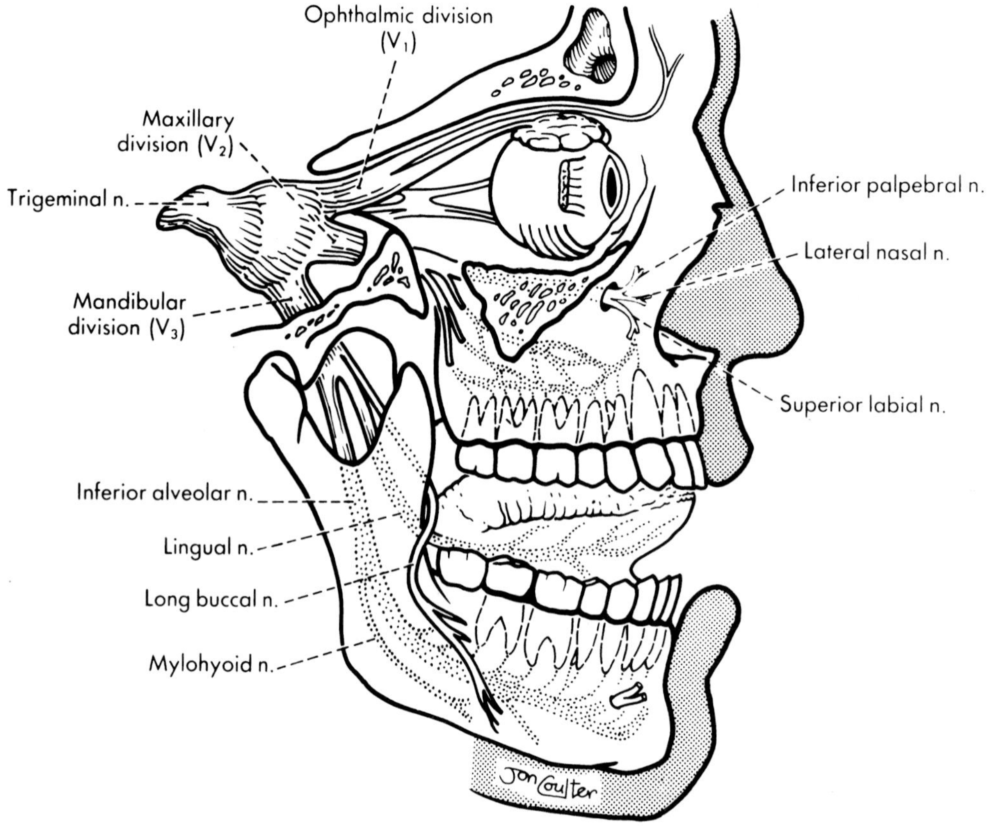

FIG. 16-8. Distribution of the trigeminal nerve.

pterygopalatine fossa, from where it progresses forward into the inferior orbital fissure and passes into the orbital cavity. Here it turns slightly laterally in the infraorbital groove on the orbital surface of the maxilla. As it continues forward, it passes through the infraorbital canal and exits onto the front of the maxilla through the infraorbital foramen.

The branches of the maxillary nerve are as follows:

Branches Within the Pterygopalatine Fossa

1. Pharyngeal branch—to mucosa of pharynx;
2. Middle and posterior palatine—to tonsil and soft palate;
3. Greater palatine—to mucosa of posterior palate;
4. Nasopalatine branch—to septal mucosa through incisive canal to the anterior hard palate;
5. Posterior and superior lateral nasal branch—to lateral walls of nasal cavity;
6. Posterior superior alveolar branch—to second and third maxillary molars as well as palatal and, distobuccal root of first molar, alveolus, and overlying buccal soft tissue. (The mesiobuccal root of the maxillary first molar is innervated by the middle superior alveolar nerve); and
7. Zygomatic branch—to skin of the temple and over the zygomatic bone.

At this point, the maxillary division becomes known as the infraorbital nerve.

Branches Within the Infraorbital Groove and Canal

1. Middle superior alveolar nerve—to anterior walls of the maxillary sinus, bicuspid teeth, buccal gingiva, and mucosa;
2. Anterior superior alveolar nerve—to incisor and cuspid teeth and labial soft tissue.

Terminal Branches on the Face

1. Inferior palpebral—to lower eyelid;
2. Lateral nasal—to skin of the side of the nose;
3. Superior labial—to cheek, skin, and mucosa of the upper lid.

It may be necessary to block one or more of the nerves or nerve branches listed in Table 16-4 for successful maxillary anesthesia.

Specific Intraoral Techniques

Local Infiltration

Soft tissues of the oral cavity may be satisfactorily anesthetized with local infiltration.

Technique. A 2.5-cm, 25-gauge needle is inserted beneath the mucous membrane into the connective tissue in the area to be anesthetized, and the solution is infiltrated slowly

TABLE 16-4. *Regional analgesia of the maxilla*

Nerves anesthetized	Areas anesthetized
Posterior superior alveolar nerve	Maxillary molars (except mesiobuccal root of first molar); buccal alveolar bone and soft tissues; lining of maxillary sinus corresponding to the molar teeth
Middle superior alveolar nerve	Mesiobuccal root of first molar; premolars; corresponding buccal alveolar bone and soft tissues; lining of maxillary sinus
Anterior superior alveolar nerve	Canines, lateral incisors, central incisors; corresponding buccal alveolar bone and soft tissues
Greater palatine nerve	Hard palate and overlying mucosa from molars to first bicuspids
Nasopalatine nerve	Hard and soft tissues of the entire anterior hard palate to the canines bilaterally
Infraorbital nerve	Lower eyelid, side of nose, upper lip; areas supplied by the middle and anterior superior alveolar nerves

throughout. Because in many areas of the oral cavity the mucosa is adherent to the underlying periosteum, care must be taken to avoid depositing large volumes of solution. Large volumes may strip the periosteum from the underlying bone or result in pressure-induced soft tissue ischemia. The result will be postinjection pain and, on occasion, tissue slough. Instrumentation is performed in the same tissue into which the anesthetic has been injected. An example of a local infiltration is an intrapapillary injection.

Block of Terminal Branches (Field Block or Infiltration)

Terminal branch block is indicated for anesthetizing anterior maxillary teeth or a limited area of the mandible. It is most commonly confined to the maxilla because the porosity of maxillary bone permits diffusion of the anesthetic solution through it. The technique is rarely successful in the mandible because of the density of the cortical plate of the bone. On occasion, successful anesthesia of the mandibular anterior teeth may be achieved with this technique, particularly if injections are made on children or adults who have a thin overlying cortical plate. The success of this technique depends on diffusion of the anesthetic solution through the periosteum and underlying bone, to come in contact with the nerves therein.

Technique. A 2.5-cm, 25-gauge needle is inserted through the mucous membrane and underlying connective tissue until it contacts the periosteum over the apex of the tooth (or teeth) in question (Fig. 16-9). One ml to 2 ml of solution should be injected slowly, allowing about 5 minutes for maximum effect. The maxillary incisors, cuspids, and bicuspids may be anesthetized in this manner. Maxillary molars will require other techniques, because their roots are divergent and the overlying bone is rather dense.

Infraorbital Nerve Block (Block of the Anterior and Middle Superior Alveolar Nerves)

Infraorbital nerve block is useful for providing anesthesia of the maxillary incisors, cuspids, and bicuspids, including their bony support and surrounding labial soft tissue. The lower eyelid, side of the nose, and upper lid will also be anesthetized.

Technique. The patient is instructed to look directly forward while the operator palpates the supraorbital and infraorbital notches. An imaginary straight line drawn vertically through these landmarks will pass through the pupil of the eye, infraorbital foramen, the bicuspid teeth, and the mental foramen (Fig. 16-10). When the infraorbital notch is located, the palpating finger (or thumb) should follow the vertical line inferiorly about 0.5 cm, at which point a shallow depression will be felt. The infraorbital foramen is located within the depression.

For a block on the right side, the thumb of the operator's left hand is placed over the previously located foramen and

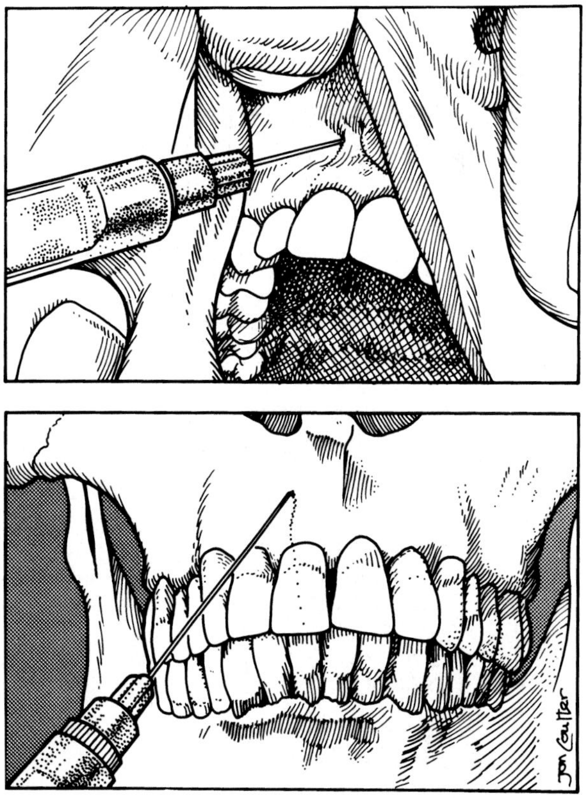

FIG. 16-9. Field block or infiltration. The needle is inserted through mucous membrane in the area of the tooth or teeth to be anesthetized.

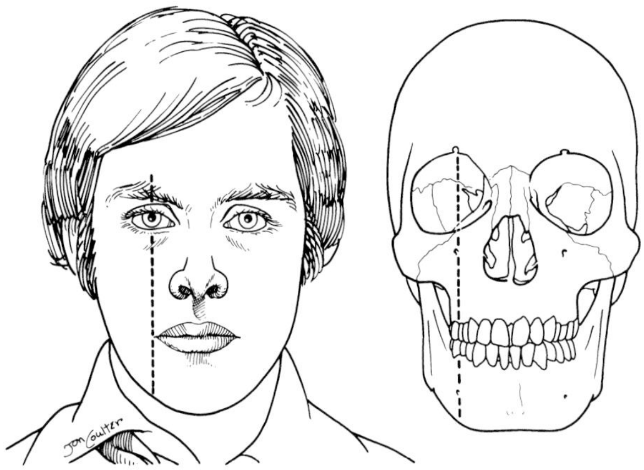

FIG. 16-10. Supraorbital notch, pupil of the eye, infraorbital notch, infraorbital frame, bicuspid teeth, and mental foramen lie on a straight vertical line.

the index finger is used to retract the lip (Fig. 16-11). A 4-cm, 25-gauge needle is then inserted along the imaginary vertical line until the foramen is reached. The needle should be inserted a sufficient distance (about 0.5 cm) from the labial plate, to bridge the canine fossa. The thumb in place over the foramen should be used to maneuver the needle into position so that it contacts the bone at the entrance to the foramen. The needle should not penetrate soft tissue for more than 2 cm. About 2 ml of solution is deposited. The skin over the infraorbital foramen should be massaged to promote the spread of the anesthetic solution into the foramen.

Tingling and numbness of the lower eyelid, side of the nose, and upper lip will always be produced, but is not necessarily an indication of a successful block. In order to anesthetize the anterior and middle superior alveolar nerves that supply the teeth, the solution must enter the infraorbital foramen and flow centrally through the infraorbital canal. Instrumentation of the teeth in question will demonstrate success or failure of the block.

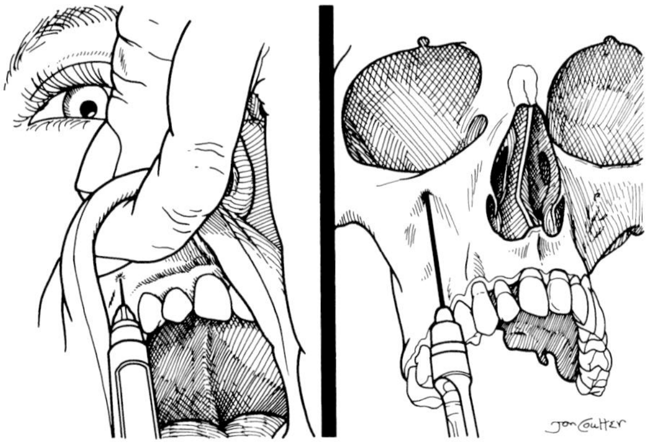

FIG. 16-11. The thumb is maintained in place over the infraorbital foramen.

Figure 16-12 depicts the anatomic relationships involved when performing the infraorbital nerve block.

Posterior Superior Alveolar Nerve Block

This nerve block provides anesthesia of the 3rd, 2nd, and 2/3 of the first maxillary molar as well as supporting hard and buccal soft tissue.

Since the first molar has dual innervation, the posterior superior alveolar nerve block must be coupled with infiltration over the mesiobuccal root to anesthetize it completely.

The posterior superior alveolar nerve arises from the maxillary nerve before it enters the body of the maxilla. It is located distal to the maxillary tuberosity.

Technique. For a block on the right side, the operator places the left forefinger on the buccal surface of the maxillary molars parallel to the occlusal plane. The finger is moved posteriorly until the zygomatic process of the maxilla is reached (Fig. 16-13). At this point, the finger is rotated so that the fingernail is adjacent to the alveolar mucosa and its bulbous portion is in contact with the posterior surface of the zygomatic process (Fig. 16-14). The index finger is now pointing in the exact direction the needle is to follow. The mouth should be opened only partially, because excessive opening may cause the coronoid process of the mandible to impinge upon the target area and/or impair visualization. A 4-cm, 25 gauge needle is inserted into the mucosa slightly posterior to the zygomatic arch, at a 45° angle to all three planes of orientation. The insertion is made for a distance of 1.5 to 2 cm, going upward, inward, and backward behind the tuberosity.

To avoid hematoma caused by unintentional trauma to the pterygoid venous plexus, the needle should be kept in contact with the posterior surface of the maxilla throughout the injection. Hematoma caused by a rent in an artery in this area will be rapidly manifest as swelling to the side of the face. Venous hematomas will develop more slowly. Either may produce swelling of surprising proportion. Cold compresses should be applied immediately if a hematoma is suspected.

The patient should not experience subjective signs of anesthesia, such as numbness or tingling, following this injection. Adequacy of the nerve block must be ascertained by instrumentation of the involved area without producing pain.

Maxillary Nerve Block (High Tuberosity Approach)

The entire second division of the trigeminal nerve may be anesthetized in a manner almost identical to that described for the posterior superior alveolar nerve block. The only difference is that to anesthetize the entire maxillary nerve a 4-cm needle should be inserted to a depth of about 4 cm. The entire contents of the cartridge (1.8 to 2 ml) should be deposited.

Anesthesia of the three terminal branches as they exit into the face confirms a successful neural blockade of the maxillary nerve.

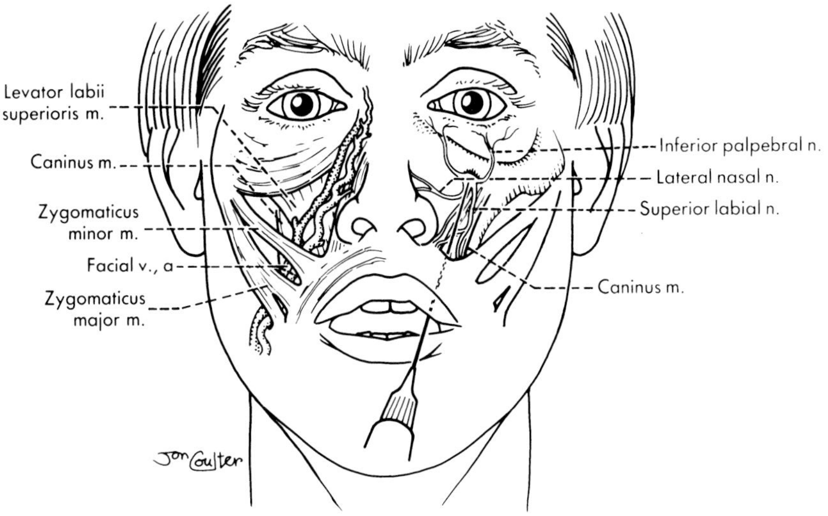

FIG. 16-12. Anatomic relationships relative to the infraorbital nerve block.

Nasopalatine Nerve Block

Anesthesia of the nasopalatine nerve will provide palatal hard and soft tissue anesthesia bilaterally from the bicuspids forward. The procedure for anesthetizing the nasopalatine nerve is relatively simple. Unfortunately, it is also relatively painful.

Technique. A 2.5-cm, 25-gauge needle is inserted into the incisive papilla just behind the maxillary central incisors (Fig. 16-15). The needle need not be introduced into the nasopalatine canal for successful anesthesia.

Because the soft tissue (particularly submucosal connective tissue) is sparse in this area, only a drop or two of solution can be injected. Care must be taken to avoid injecting too large a quantity of solution, lest postinjection pain and tissue slough ensue.

Greater (Anterior) Palatine Nerve Block

Anesthetizing the greater palatine nerve results in anesthesia of the posterior hard palate to the midline. This injection, too, is both relatively simple for the surgeon to master and painful for the patient.

Technique. The greater palatine nerve emerges into the palate through the greater palatine foramen and courses forward in a groove parallel to the molar teeth. The foramen is situated between the second and third maxillary molars about 1 cm from the teeth, toward the midline.

The foramen is approached from the opposite side with a 2.5-cm, 25-gauge needle that is kept as near to a right angle as possible, with the curvature of the palatal bone (Fig. 16-16). One-fourth to one-half ml is injected. For satisfactory palatal anesthesia, the greater palatine foramen and canal need not be entered.

Maxillary Nerve (Palatal Approach)

Using an approach similar to the one described for the anterior palatine nerve block, one may secure anesthesia of the entire distribution of the maxillary nerve. A 4-cm, 25-gauge needle is required.

Once the needle has penetrated the palatal mucosa, the

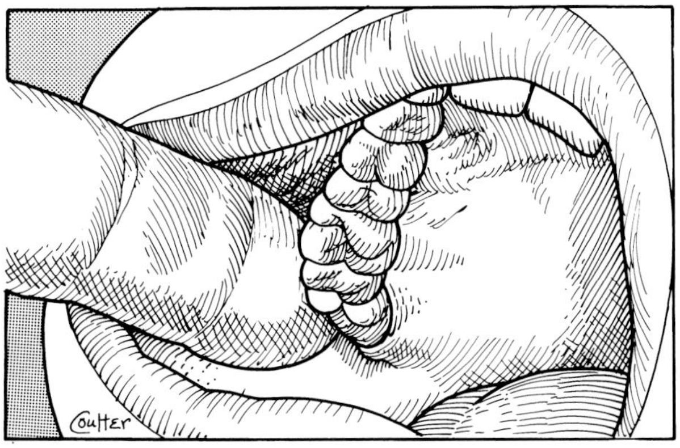

FIG. 16-13. The operator moves the left index finger posteriorly over the buccal surface of the maxillary molars until the zygomatic process of the maxilla is reached.

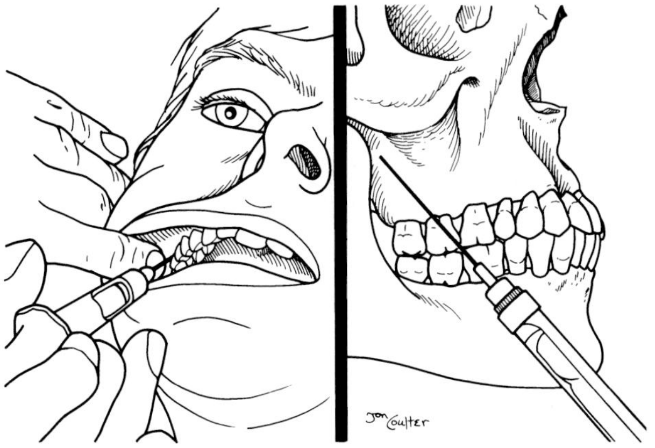

FIG. 16-14. Rotated finger points to path of needle insertion.

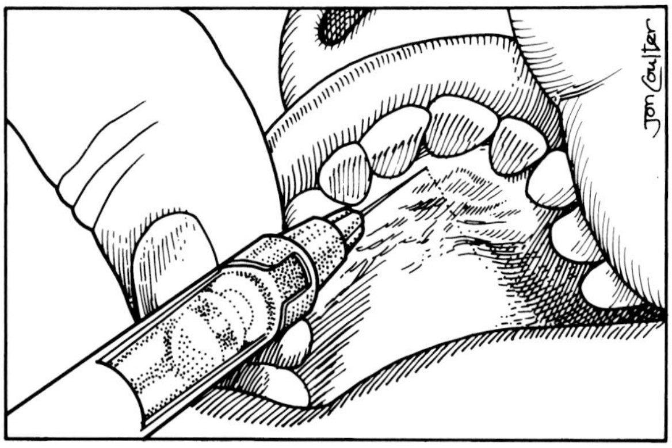

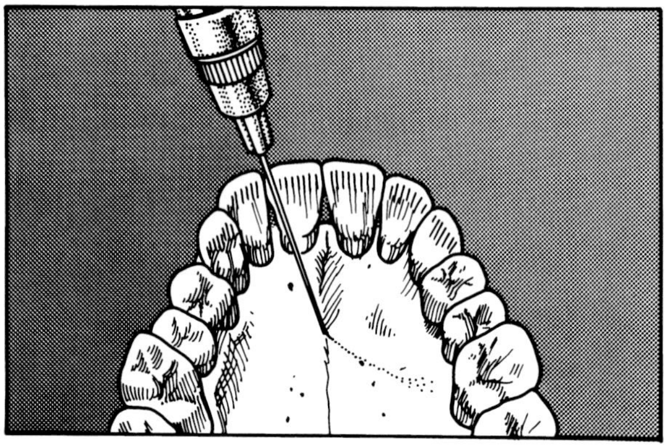

FIG. 16-15. Needle is inserted into the incisive papilla behind the maxillary central incisors.

greater palatine foramen is gently probed and the canal entered. The needle is advanced into the canal to a depth not to exceed 4 cm. Any resistance encountered should not be overcome with force, but the needle should be withdrawn and again advanced slowly. If continued resistance is met, regardless of how slight, the attempt should be discontinued.

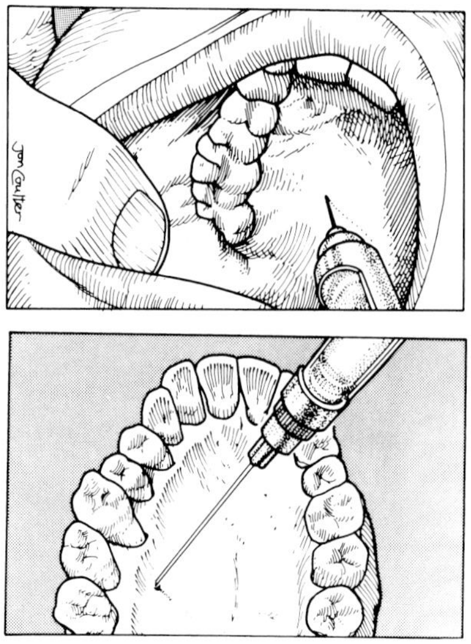

FIG. 16-16. Block of anterior palatine nerve. Needle is inserted from the opposite side, keeping it as near to a right angle as possible with the curvature of the palate.

Once resting within the canal at the desired depth, 2 ml of solution is deposited (see additional technique in ref. 14).

Techniques of Neural Blockade for the Mandibular Nerve and its Subdivisions

Anatomy of the Mandibular Division (V_3)

The mandibular division of the trigeminal nerve is both sensory and motor. The motor division does not emerge from the gasserian ganglion, but joins the sensory branch after it leaves the anteroinferior part of the gasserian ganglion. For a short distance they travel side by side, then form a single trunk to exit the skull through the foramen ovale. From this trunk, a motor branch passes to the internal pterygoid and two tensor muscles. The trunk then divides into anterior and posterior divisions.

The branches of the anterior division are as follows:

1. External pterygoid nerve—motor;
2. Masseter nerve—motor;
3. Temporal muscle nerve—motor; and
4. Long buccal nerve—sensory.

The long buccal nerve passes between the two heads of the pterygoid muscle, crosses the anterior border of the ramus at the level of the occlusal plane of the teeth, and supplies the skin and mucous membranes of the cheek and buccal gingiva, from the retromolar triangle to the bicuspid teeth.

The branches of the posterior division are as follows:

1. Auriculotemporal nerve—sensory to the parotid gland, temporomandibular joint, external auditory meatus, and scalp in the temporal region.
2. Lingual nerve—sensory to the lingual mucous membranes, anterior 2/3 of the tongue, and floor of the mouth. (The chorda tympani nerve from the seventh cranial nerve joins the lingual nerve shortly after its origin and supplies fibers of special sense to taste buds of the anterior 2/3 of the tongue.)
3. Inferior alveolar nerve—sensory to the mandibular teeth, body of the mandible, and labial gingiva anterior to the bicuspid teeth. This nerve passes downward on the medial side of the external pterygoid muscle and the medial side of the mandibular ramus. On the medial side of the ramus, in the pterygomandibular space, it enters the mandibular foramen. It then travels anteriorly within the body of the mandible. In the region of the mental foramen, the inferior alveolar nerve divides into 2 terminal branches:
   a. Mental nerve—leaves the body of the mandible through the mental foramen and is sensory to the skin of the chin and lower lip and mucous membrane lining the lower lip.
   b. Incisive nerve—continues anteriorly within the body of the mandible to supply anterior teeth and their supporting hard tissues.

It may be necessary to block one or more of the nerves or

TABLE 16-5. *Regional analgesia of the mandible*

Nerves anesthetized	Areas anesthetized
Inferior alveolar nerve	Mandibular teeth; surrounding hard and soft tissues unilaterally to the midline (does not innervate buccal soft tissue in the molar area)
Lingual nerve	Mucosa of floor of mouth, anterior 2/3 of tongue; lingual gingiva
Long buccal nerve	Mucosa of cheek; buccal mucosa and mucoperiosteum of molar region
Mental nerve	Buccal gingiva; mucoperiosteum from bicuspids to midline; skin of chin and lower lip (does not innervate teeth)
Incisive nerve	First bicuspid, canine, incisor unilaterally to the midline; areas innervated by the mental nerve

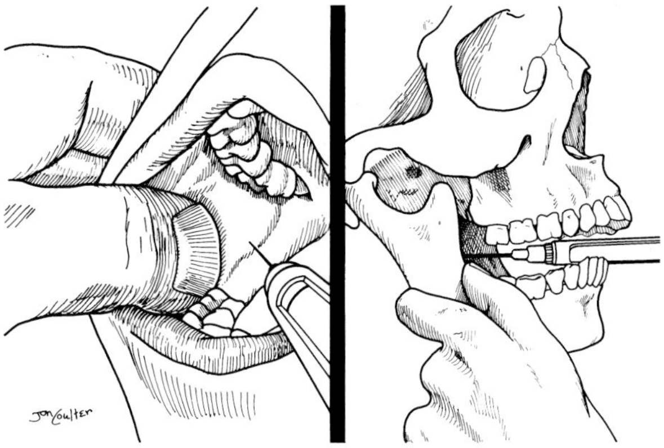

FIG. 16-18. The ramus is grasped between an intraorally placed thumb and an extraorally positioned index finger.

nerve branches listed in Table 16-5 for successful mandibular anesthesia.

Specific Intraoral Techniques

Classic Inferior Alveolar Nerve Block

This nerve block is used to provide hard tissue anesthesia in the mandible to the midline, and labial soft tissue anesthesia from the bicuspid teeth to the midline. For complete anesthesia of the mandible (e.g., for extraction of all teeth), this block must be supplemented with long buccal and lingual nerve blocks.

Technique. The patient is instructed to open the mouth as wide as possible. For a block on the right side, the operator palpates the mucobuccal fold in the area of the molar teeth with the left thumb. The thumb is then moved posteriorly until contact is made with the external oblique ridge on the anterior border of the ramus of the mandible. The deepest concavity on the anterior border of the ramus, the coronoid notch, is then identified. The coronoid notch is in a direct line with the lingula, the point at which the inferior alveolar nerve enters the ramus of the mandible (Fig. 16-17).

The palpating thumb is then moved medially onto the internal oblique ridge, the inner "edge" of the ramus. This manuever helps estimate the width of the ramus. The thumb is once again moved to the lateral side of the ramus, retracting soft tissues of the cheek while doing so. At this point, the left index finger grasps the posterior border of the mandible from the extraoral approach (Fig. 16-18). In this manner, the

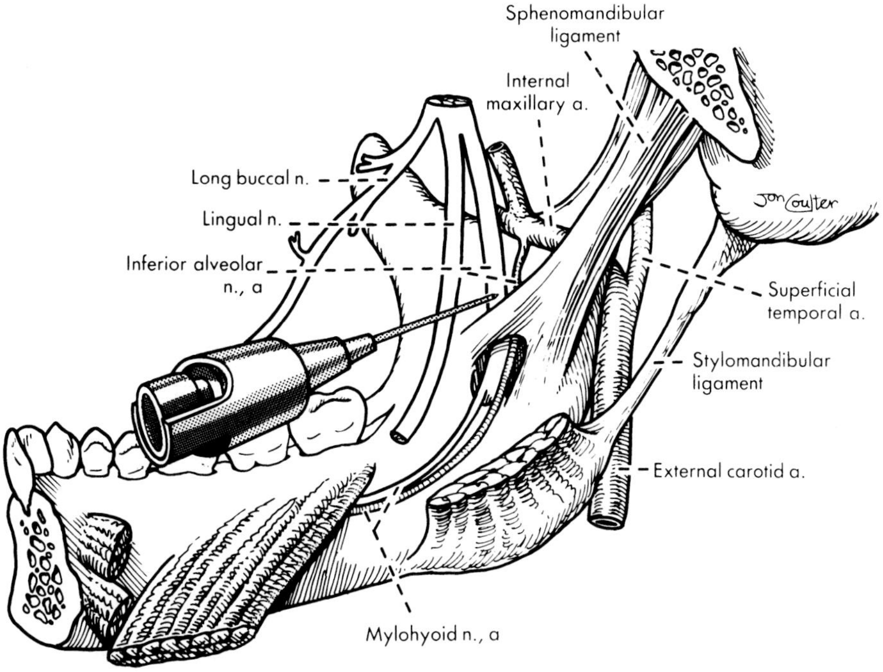

FIG. 16-17. Coronoid notch is in a direct line with the point at which the inferior alveolar nerve enters the ramus of the mandible.

operator is holding the ramus of the mandible between the thumb and index finger, thus allowing the operator to estimate the anteroposterior width of the ramus.

A syringe with a 4-cm, 25-gauge needle is then inserted parallel to the occlusal plane, at a height indicated by the coronoid notch just medial to the internal oblique ridge. The needle should approach the ramus at an angle that is parallel to the inner surface of the ramus (Fig. 16-19). Depth of insertion may be determined by estimating when the needle tip has been advanced half the distance between the thumb and index finger. When in proper position for deposition of solution, the needle tip will be close to the inferior alveolar nerve, artery, and vein.

After aspiration, about 2 ml of solution is deposited. Subjective symptoms of anesthesia include tingling and numbness of the lower lip.

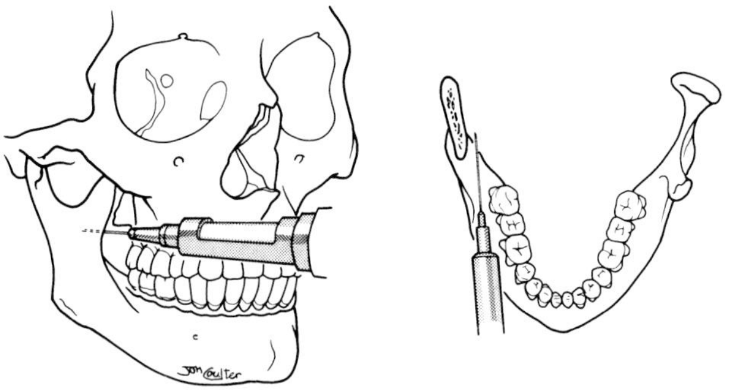

FIG. 16-20. With the teeth in occlusion, the needle is aligned parallel to the occlusal plane and positioned at the level just superior to the maxillary molars.

Closed-mouth (Akinosi) Approach to Mandibular Nerve Block

On occasion the need arises to anesthetize the mandibular nerve while the teeth are approximated in occlusion (e.g., jaws wired together following mandibular resection). This injection may be invaluable, for example, when removing intermaxillary fixation wires.

Since the height of needle insertion and deposition of anesthetic solution is considerably superior to the site for producing inferior alveolar nerve anesthesia, a true mandibular block will be secured,[1] that is to say, the long buccal, inferior alveolar, and lingual nerve distribution will be affected.

Technique. With the teeth in occlusion, the lips are retracted and the needle and syringe are aligned parallel to the occlusal plane at the level of the mucogingival junction of the maxillary molar teeth. The needle penetrates mucosa (Fig. 16-20) just medial to the ramus and is inserted to a depth of about 3 cm. Following negative aspiration, the entire contents of the cartridge are slowly deposited. Successful anesthesia will be confirmed by instrumentation of the mandibular distribution.

Two factors are apt to contribute to failure of this technique. First, the technique relies on a minimum number of bony landmarks for its execution. Depth of needle insertion, in particular, is a nebulous factor. In addition, improper angulation in a superior direction may result in partial or complete anesthesia of the maxilla, particularly if improper medial angulation occurs simultaneously.

Second, because of anatomic restrictions it is impossible to insert the needle parallel to the medial surface of the ramus. In effect, the deeper the needle penetration, the further from the "target" it gets.

Nevertheless, despite its drawbacks, this technique offers

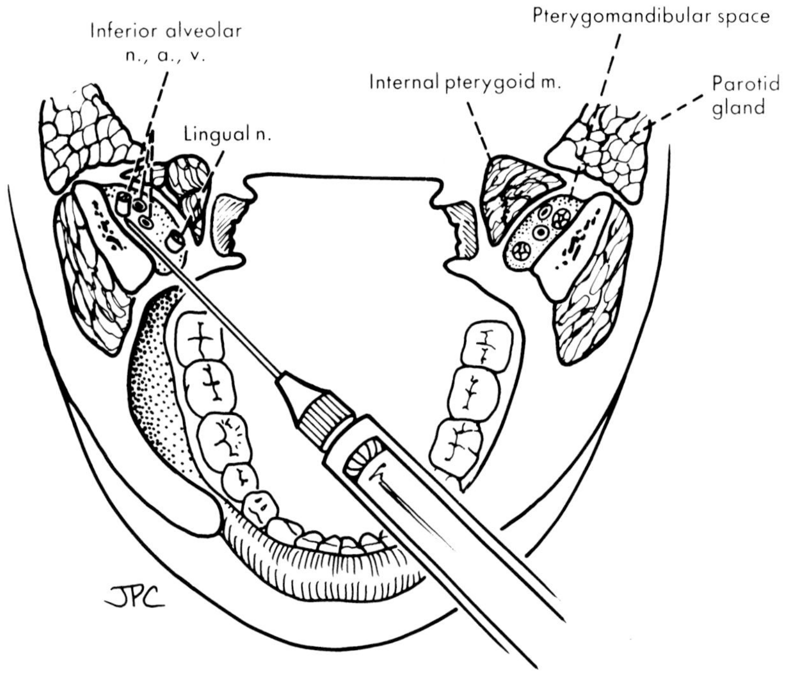

FIG. 16-19. Needle is inserted parallel to the medial surface of the ramus.

a suitable alternative to the classic approach to anesthesia of the mandible when circumstances dictate its need (see also Chapter 15, Fig. 15-6).

Lingual Nerve Block

The lingual nerve is close to the inferior alveolar nerve at its point of entry into the ramus of the mandible. For all intents and purposes, it is impossible to anesthetize the lingual nerve without simultaneously blocking the inferior alveolar nerve, and vice versa. For this reason, the injection technique for the lingual nerve block will not be discussed. (At any rate, it is identical to the inferior alveolar nerve block.)

Long Buccal Nerve Block

To provide complete mandibular anesthesia, the long buccal nerve block must supplement the inferior alveolar and lingual nerve blocks previously described. The long buccal nerve branches from the mandibular nerve at a point superior to the site for an inferior alveolar nerve block. A separate injection must be made to provide soft tissue anesthesia adjacent to the molar teeth (see Fig. 16-17).

Technique. The coronoid notch and external oblique ridge are identified in the manner described for the inferior alveolar nerve block. The cheek is retracted and the needle inserted through the soft tissue at the height of the occlusal plane. The needle is directed to the external oblique ridge and inserted until contact is made (Fig. 16-21).[2] One-fourth to 1/2 ml of solution is sufficient to anesthetize the long buccal nerve.

Mental Nerve Block

The mental nerve exits the body of the mandible through a foramen (mental foramen) located between the bicuspid teeth, near their apices. A block of this nerve provides soft tissue anesthesia of the chin, lower lip, and its underlying mucosa and gingiva.

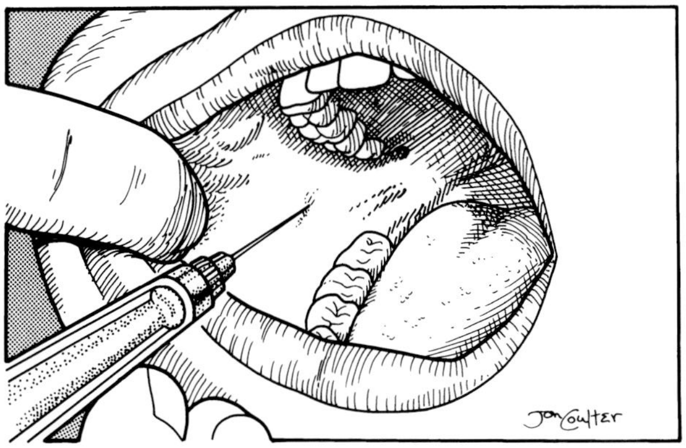

FIG. 16-21. Long buccal nerve block. The needle is inserted through the mucosa and directed toward the external oblique line at the level of the occlusal plane.

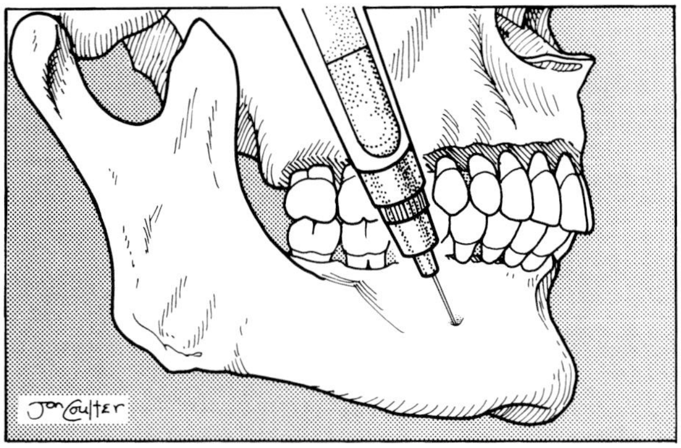

FIG. 16-22. To block the incisive nerve, direct the needle into the mental foramen and canal. The mental nerve will be blocked simultaneously.

Technique. A syringe with 2.5-cm needle attached is inserted through the mucosa and directed to a point approximating the apices of the bicuspid teeth (Fig. 16-22). One-half to 1 ml of solution is deposited.

Incisive Nerve Block

The incisive nerve is the continuation of the inferior alveolar nerve within the anterior body of the mandible. It supplies the anterior teeth and their supporting hard tissues.

Technique. Access to the incisive nerve is gained through the mental foramen and canal, a structure that opens in a down, forward, and inward direction. For satisfactory anesthesia of the incisive nerve, the mental foramen must be located, gently probed, and then entered by the needle tip. The needle must be directed into the canal at an angle parallel to its long axis.

After deposition of 1/4 to 1/2 ml of solution, anesthesia of the lower anterior teeth and their supporting structures will be produced. Because the mental nerve will be simultaneously anesthetized, anesthesia of the chin and lower lip will ensue.

ANCILLARY TECHNIOUES

Electronic Dental Anesthesia. Transcutaneous electrical nerve stimulation (TENS) has been used successfully since the early 1970s for the management of chronic pain syndromes and acute post-surgical pain. This same technology has been applied in dentistry to control the pain of intraoral instrumentation without use of local anesthetics. If effective, it would have obvious application in patients with needle phobias, and in those patients for whom local anesthetics or vasoconstrictors might be contraindicated, due to cardiac disease, intolerance, or allergy. Additional uses would be in the relief of muscle trismus or in the management of temporomandibular joint pain.

Two basic machines have been studied for electronic dental anesthesia: The classic high current (100 to 150 mA), low frequency (55 to 150 Hz) TENS unit with an H-wave generator, and a low current (4 mA), high frequency (15,000 Hz) device. Quarnstrom has determined that the high-current, low-frequency TENS unit provides the most reliable results.[11]

Technique. A TENS unit with either extraoral or intraoral electrodes may be used. Extraoral electrodes should be placed bilaterally on the affected jaw, over the infraorbital foramina in the maxilla, and over the mental foramina in the mandible. Intraoral electrodes consisting of conducting filaments embedded in cotton rolls are placed in the mucobuccal fold, directly adjacent to the affected teeth. The unit is turned on and the wave amplitude is set to a level predetermined by the manufacturer. The frequency is slowly increased until mild muscle contractions occur. Instrumentation or manipulation may begin at this point.

Electronic dental anesthesia results in clinically successful anesthesia in 80 to 90% of patients undergoing restorative dentistry.[9] However, the success rate decreases with the depth of restoration, for crown preparations, tooth extractions, or for molar teeth. It is not reliable for endodontic therapy. The efficacy of electronic dental anesthesia can be increased by the addition of nitrous oxide and aspirin-like drugs.[7,12] In order for electronic dental anesthesia to gain more widespread acceptance, further research is needed to determine the optimum frequency of stimulation and wave form. Attempts are underway to improve the quality and adherent properties of intraoral electrodes.

LOCAL COMPLICATIONS AND REASONS FOR FAILURE

Local Complications. Perhaps the most disconcerting localized complication following an intraoral injection is the production of *paresthesia* in the trigeminal system. It results from direct mechanical needle trauma to the nerve, or from injection of a contaminated anesthetic solution in close proximity to the nerve. Although relatively uncommon, paresthesia is most likely to occur following a conventional inferior alveolar nerve block injection. The altered sensation is usually transient and may resolve spontaneously within days, weeks, or months. In rare instances, the damage can be permanent. Maintaining good patient rapport and reassurance may prove to be effective therapeutic tools in the event of this complication.

Muscle Trismus. Another complication that may occur after an inferior alveolar nerve block is muscle trismus. The internal pterygoid muscle is most often affected. Limitation of muscular function after an intraoral injection may be caused by hematoma formation, direct muscle injury secondary to needle trauma, localized muscle necrosis secondary to the anesthetic drug or vasoconstrictor, infection in a fascial space, or the introduction of a foreign body. The treatment of intraoral trismus may include nonsteroidal anti-inflammatory agents, saline mouth rinses, antibiotics, and physical therapy.

Hematoma. Formation of hematomas is the result of direct needle trauma to a blood vessel, and is most likely to occur following a posterior superior alveolar nerve block injection. Signs and symptoms of hematoma include rapid swelling, a sensation of fullness in the area, facial asymmetry, and mild trismus. Management of a hematoma includes reassurance for the patient and application of ice to the affected area on the day of injury, followed in 24 hours by application of heat. When indicated, post-treatment antibiotics may also be necessary.

Mucosal Irritation. This may be produced by a number of different causes. Topical anesthetics, when applied to the mucosa for extended periods, may compromise the capillary integrity of the underlying tissue, and produce irritation. The injection of excessive volumes of local anesthetics with vasoconstrictors into tightly attached tissue may produce localized tissue ischemia and ulceration. The tissue overlying the hard palate is most frequently damaged in this manner. High pressure injection techniques, such as the periodontal ligament injection, have been reported to produce irritation and even necrosis of the interdental papilla, with exposure of the underlying bone. Self inflicted injuries, such as cheek-, lip-, and tongue-biting, are common causes of mucosal irritation, following local anesthesia, in children and occasionally in adults.

Infection. Though it is an extremely rare complication of local anesthesia, infection may result from injection into or through an infected area, the use of the same cartridge or needle in more than one patient, and multiple uses of the same needle in the same patient. Preparing the injection site with an antiseptic agent prior to injection may reduce the amount of bacteria at the site, but it is inconclusive as to whether this action helps prevent infection.

Needle Breakage. This is also very uncommon following local anesthetic administration. Single-use, disposable needles and high-quality manufacturing techniques have minimized this problem. However, unexpected patient movement, excessive lateral force by the operator, manufacturing defects, and intentional bending of the needle, all may result in needle breakage. The needle is most susceptible to breakage at the hub. It is, therefore, recommended that the needle never be inserted to this depth, because breakage at this point would result in loss of the needle into the tissue. The use of a 25-gauge needle will minimize the possibility of needle breakage.

Undesirable Nerve Block. Finally, inadvertent and undesirable nerve block may result from local anesthetic administration. This may result from gross misdirection of the needle, or an unusual pattern of anesthetic distribution. Undesirable nerves that may be temporarily affected include the facial nerve, with resultant transient hemifacial paralysis, and the recurrent laryngeal nerve with hoarseness and difficulty with speech. Both of these undesirable nerve blocks have been associated with the inferior alveolar nerve block.

Reasons for Failure. Although the success rate for obtaining profound regional anesthesia is extremely high, at times less than desirable results are achieved. There are many reasons for failure to achieve adequate anesthesia. Foremost among these is poor injection technique. The most common cause of a failed injection is improper identification of appropriate anatomic landmarks. This usually results in improper needle orientation or placement, which then leads to misdirection away from the target area.

Inappropriate needle selection may also contribute to failure. A needle that is too long or too short, coupled with uncertainty about the required depth of penetration, will lead to failure. In addition, the selection of a thin needle for certain injections may result in deflection away from the intended path of insertion. For this reason, a 25-gauge needle is preferable to a 27- or 30-gauge needle for intraoral injections.

The proper selection of the local anesthetic solution contributes to the success of intraoral local anesthesia. For example, plain local anesthetic solutions are taken up into the systemic circulation faster than local anesthetics containing vasoconstrictors. In the case of the highly vascular maxilla, it is advisable to use a local anesthetic with a vasoconstrictor, to ensure adequate working time, when infiltration injections are performed.

Occasionally, patients may experience some subjective signs of anesthesia but may not be able to withstand instrumentation without pain. This may be due in part to injection of an inadequate volume of anesthetic solution. Increasing the volume of injected solution will often remedy this problem. Increasing volume may also be of benefit in patients with anatomic variations.

Another cause of injection failure is intravascular injection of anesthetic solution. It is to be avoided, since it will rapidly remove the local anesthetic solution from the target area and prevent interaction with the nervous tissue. The intravascular injection of large quantities of local anesthetics and/or vasoconstrictors may lead to toxic reactions that could be life-threatening. Negative aspiration must always be performed prior to primary injection and each time the needle is repositioned.

Yet another possibility for failed local anesthesia is the presence of tissue inflammation. Since inflammation increases tissue blood flow, the systemic absorption of local anesthetic solutions is usually increased. Inflammation may also modify the activity of peripheral nerves by lowering the response threshold, changing the protein structure of the nerve, or enhancing conduction. Most significantly, inflammation lowers the tissue pH and creates an acidic environment in which the anesthetic solution must work. Lowered tissue pH significantly reduces the ability of local anesthetic drugs to block nervous tissue, and may render them ineffective.

Finally, when the above causes for failed anesthesia have been ruled out, the possibility of alternative innervation should be considered. Variant nerves may exist that supply structures not usually associated with them. This can occur in patients with an extremely high palate and long alveolar process. The nasopalatine nerve may exchange fibers with the anterior superior alveolar nerve, and contribute to the innervation of the incisor teeth. The long buccal nerve, although a branch of the third division of the trigeminal nerve, may innervate the buccal soft tissue in the maxillary molar area.

In the mandible, variant branches of the inferior alveolar nerve may leave the nerve before it enters the mandibular foramen. These branches are not blocked by the conventional inferior alveolar nerve block. A more superiorly oriented injection may be necessary for success in a case such as this. The mylohyoid nerve, which supplies sensory and motor function to the mylohyoid muscle and anterior belly of the digastric, may enter the mandible on the lingual side via a foramen in the bicuspid region. This occurs in about 10 percent of patients and may provide sensory innervation to the incisor teeth. Again, a conventional inferior alveolar block will not affect this nerve; however, a higher injection or lingual infiltration may result in success. The long buccal nerve, in most patients, assists in the supply of the mandibular molar and bicuspid teeth. The lingual nerve may assist in the supply of the mandibular bicuspids and first molar. Occasionally, the pharyngeal plexus of nerves, which normally supply the pharynx, may supply impacted mandibular third molars. Very rarely the cutaneous coli nerve, a branch of the cervical plexus, may enter the mandible on the inner surface of the lingual cortical plate and provide accessory innervation to the mandibular teeth.

SUMMARY

Discussed herein are the equipment, supplies, agents, and most common techniques used to provide local anesthesia of selective areas within the oral cavity. Although other techniques or modifications of those presented appear in a number of textbooks, it is hoped that the relatively simple, straightforward methods described will add significantly to the anesthesiologist's armamentarium.

REFERENCES

1. Akinosi, J.O.: A new approach to the mandibular nerve block. J. Oral Surg., *15:*83, 1977.
2. Bennett, C.R.: Conscious-sedation in Dental Practice. 2nd ed. St. Louis, C.V. Mosby, 1978.
3. Bennett, C.R.: Monheim's Local Anesthesia and Pain Control in Dental Practice. 7th ed. St. Louis, C.V. Mosby, 1984.
4. Cioffi, G.A., Chernow, B., Glahn, R.P., Terezhalmy, G.T., and Lake, C. R.: The hemodynamic and plasma catecholamine responses to routine restorative care. J. Am. Dent. Assoc., *111:*67, 1985.
5. Cryer, P.E.: Physiology and pathophysiology of the human sympathoadrenal neuroendocrine system. N. Engl. J. Med. *303:*436, 1980.
6. Dionne, R.A., Goldstein, D.S., and Wirdzek, P.R.: Effects of diazepam premedication and epinephrine-containing local anesthetic on cardiovascular and plasma catecholamine responses to oral surgery. Anesth. Analg., *63:*640, 1986.

7. Kajander, K.C.: Evaluation of low-intensity transcutaneous electrical nerve stimulation in combination with aspirin for reduction of controlled thermal sensation. Anesth. Prog., *35:*195, 1988.
8. Malamed, S.F.: Handbook of Medical Emergencies. 2nd ed. St. Louis, C.V. Mosby, 1982.
9. Malamed, S.F., Quinn, O.L., Torgersen, R.T., and Thompson, W.: Electronic dental anesthesia for restorative dentistry. Anesth. Prog. *36:* 192, 1989.
10. Marcaine Package Insert. New York, Cook-Waite Laboratories, 1985.
11. Quarnstrom, F.C.: Electrical dental anesthesia. Anesth. Prog., *39:*162, 1992.
12. Quarnstrom, F.C., Milgrom, P.: Clinical experience with TENS and TENS combined with nitrous oxide oxygen. Anesth. Prog. *36:*66, 1989.
13. Scott, D.S., and Hirschman, R.: Psychological aspects of dental anxiety in adults. J. Am. Dent. Assoc., *104:*27, 1982.
14. Wong, J.D., and Sved, A.M.: Maxillary nerve block anaesthesia via the greater palatine canal: A modified technique and case reports. Aust. Dent. J. *36:*15, 1991.

Neural Blockade in Clinical Anesthesia and Management of Pain, Third Edition,
edited by M.J. Cousins and P.O. Bridenbaugh.
Lippincott–Raven Publishers, Philadelphia © 1998.

CHAPTER 17

Neural Blockade for Ophthalmologic Surgery

Kathryn E. McGoldrick, Marianne E. Feitl, and Theodore Krupin

Orbital injection of local anesthetic was first performed in 1884, with cocaine, for enucleation of the globe.[44] However, it was not until the 1930s, when the less toxic procaine and, later, the amide anesthetics became available, that orbital block was commonly used for ophthalmic surgery. Atkinson's 1936 paper[6] popularized a technique that became firmly entrenched as the traditional retrobulbar block. Over the next five decades, anesthesiologists and ophthalmologists documented serious complications of retrobulbar blockade that can be either vision-threatening or life-threatening. Attempts to circumvent some of these complications led to the development in the mid-1980s of peribulbar block. However, peribulbar block can also be associated with serious adverse sequelae. Advances in cataract surgery that have enabled faster surgery with greater control and less trauma have allowed ophthalmologists to re-examine the use of topical anesthesia for this procedure, thereby obviating, in selected cases, the need for injection techniques.

Clearly, the requirements and complications of local anesthesia for intraocular and specialized extraocular surgical procedures are unique. A thorough understanding of the mechanism of neural blockade in ophthalmologic surgery is inextricably linked to detailed knowledge of the relevant anatomy. This chapter outlines the anatomy and techniques germane to the successful administration of local anesthesia for ophthalmic surgery. Moreover, in-depth discussion is presented of associated potential complications and their prevention.

K.E. McGoldrick: Department of Anesthesiology, Yale University School of Medicine, New Haven, Connecticut 06510; and Section of Ambulatory Surgery, Yale-New Haven Hospital, New Haven, Connecticut 06520.

M.E. Feitl: Department of Ophthalmology, University of Chicago, Chicago, Illinois 60614.

T. Krupin: Department of Ophthalmology, Northwestern University School of Medicine, Chicago, Illinois 60611.

ANESTHETIC REOUIREMENTS FOR OPHTHALMIC SURGERY

Intraocular Surgery

Anesthetic requirements for intraocular surgical procedures (eg, cataract extraction, penetrating keratoplasty, vitrectomy, etc.) include:

1. globe and conjunctival anesthesia;
2. globe lid and periorbital akinesia;
3. intraocular hypotonia.

Incomplete akinesia of the extraocular muscles and subsequent contraction of an extraocular muscle in an eye with a large, open, surgical wound can result in extrusion of intraocular contents. Incomplete akinesia of the eyelid can produce a similar complication secondary to orbicularis oculi muscular pressure on the globe.

Satisfactory local anesthesia should provide complete anesthesia of the globe and ocular adnexae. While the duration of the local anesthetic should be at least 11/2 to 2 hours, longer-acting agents also provide postoperative analgesia.

Normal intraocular pressure (IOP) generally is considered to be less than 21 mm Hg. Three main factors influence IOP:(i) external pressure on the eye by contraction of the orbicularis oculi muscle and the tone of the extraocular muscles, venous congestion of orbital veins (which may occur with vomiting and coughing), and conditions such as orbital tumor; (ii) scleral rigidity, which tends to increase with age; and (iii) changes in intraocular contents that are semisolid (lens, vitreous, or intraocular tumor) or fluid (blood and aqueous humor). Although these factors are all important in affecting IOP, the major control of intraocular tension is exerted by the fluid content, especially the aqueous humor.

Some surgeons administer preoperative hyperosmotic agents to dehydrate the eye and to lower IOP. Hyperosmotic agents used before injection of local anesthesia include intravenous (IV) mannitol (1 g/kg) administered through a filter to remove crystals 30 minutes prior to surgery or assorted oral drugs. Oral glycerine (1 g/kg) administered 1 hour preoperatively is said to have a less predictable ocular hypotensive effect than mannitol. Unfortunately, glycerine may trigger nausea or vomiting, and gastric fluid trapping increases the risk of aspiration. Oral isosorbide (1 g/kg) given 1 hour before surgery is not metabolized and results in less nausea and vomiting than does glycerine. Prophylactic antiemetic therapy is suggested prior to administering these oral agents.

Intraocular pressure should be measured after injection of local anesthetic agent and before the actual incision into the eye. Incomplete akinesia increases IOP by mechanical external pressure on the globe. Inhalation anesthetics purportedly cause dose-related decreases in IOP;[2] most central nervous system (CNS) depressants do also, including barbiturates,[39] neuroleptics,[37] opioids,[45] and propofol.[60] Although Everett and colleagues reported a reduction in IOP following retrobulbar injection, possibly owing to both relaxation of the extraocular muscles and decreased secretion of aqueous humor, retrobulbar anesthetic injection does not consistently lower IOP.[82] Indeed, excessive volume injected into the orbit may actually increase IOP, secondary to external pressure on the globe. A similar effect results if the injection is complicated by an orbital hemorrhage.

Extraocular Surgery

Requirements for pure sensory or combined sensory/motor blockade vary, according to the procedure being performed. Differential sensory blockade will permit surgical correction in the face of an unaltered motor component.

With extraocular procedures such as strabismus repair, for example, the importance of IOP recedes, and the specter of the oculocardiac reflex assumes significance.

OCULOCARDIAC REFLEX

Bernard Aschner and Guiseppe Dagnini first described the oculocardiac reflex in 1908. This reflex is triggered by pressure on the globe, and by traction on the extraocular muscles, as well as on the conjunctiva or on the orbital structures. (Indeed, a related reflex, the blepharocardiac reflex, may be elicited by stretching the eyelid muscle during placement of an eyelid retractor.[5]) Moreover, the reflex may be elicited by performance of a retrobulbar block,[8] by ocular trauma, and by direct pressure on tissue remaining in the orbital apex after enucleation.[42] The afferent limb is trigeminal, and the efferent limb is vagal. Although the most common manifestation of the oculocardiac reflex is sinus bradycardia, a vast array of cardiac dysrhythmias may appear, including junctional rhythm, ectopic atrial rhythm, atrioventricular blockade, ventricular bigeminy, multifocal premature ventricular contractions, wandering pacemaker, idioventricular rhythm, asystole, and ventricular tachycardia.[9,4,79] This reflex may occur during either local or general anesthesia; however, hypercarbia and hypoxemia are thought to augment the incidence and severity of the problem, as may inappropriate anesthetic depth.

Reports on the alleged incidence of the oculocardiac reflex are characterized by striking variability. Berler's study[8] reported an incidence of 50%, but other studies quote rates ranging from 16% to 82%.[9,87] Commonly, those articles disclosing a higher incidence included children in the study population, and children tend to have more vagal tone. Indeed, children and young adults undergoing eye muscle surgery under general anesthesia are most vulnerable to the oculocardiac reflex.

For pediatric strabismus surgery, current practice favors administration of IV atropine, 0.02 mg/kg, prior to manipulation of the extraocular muscles.[85] Alternatively, glycopyrrolate, 0.01 mg/kg administered IV, may produce less tachycardia than does atropine in this setting.[57] Although administration of retrobulbar anesthesia may provide some antidysrhythmic value by blocking the afferent limb of the reflex arc, such a regional technique is not devoid of potential complications, which include, but are not limited to, optic nerve damage, retrobulbar hemorrhage, and stimulation of the oculocardiac reflex arc by the retrobulbar block itself.

The incidence of the oculocardiac reflex is lower in geriatric patients. Prophylactic anticholinergic drugs offer no advantage in this group of patients and may, in fact, present major disadvantages. A variety of cardiac dysrhythmias[52,35] and several conduction abnormalities,[53] including ventricular fibrillation, ventricular tachycardia, and left bundle-branch block, have been attributed to IV atropine. Moreover, sinus tachycardia can trigger ischemia in a patient with coronary artery disease. Current recommended practice is to avoid prophylactic measures in this group of patients and to keep them well-ventilated and closely monitored. If a dysrhythmia appears, the surgeon should be asked to cease operative manipulation. Next, the patient's anesthetic depth and ventilatory status should be assessed. Frequently, heart rate and rhythm will return to baseline within 20 seconds. Moreover, Moonie and associates[61] noted that, with repeated manipulation, bradycardia is less likely to recur, probably secondary to fatigue of the reflex at the the cardioinhibitory center level. However, if the initial cardiac dysrhythmia is especially serious or if the reflex tenaciously recurs, atropine should be administered IV, but only after the surgeon stops ocular manipulation.

It is essential to appreciate that retrobulbar hemorrhage can produce a delayed oculocardiac reflex if the volume of blood deposited is sufficient to elevate IOP. Therefore, patients who have this complication should be placed on an electrocardiographic (ECG) monitor for several hours following the event.

PREOPERATIVE EVALUATION

Establishing Rapport and Assessing Medical Status

Preoperative preparation and evaluation of the patient begins with establishment of rapport and communication among the anesthesiologist, the surgeon, and the patient.

Most patients realize that surgery and anesthesia involve inherent risks, and they appreciate a candid discussion of complications, balanced with information concerning probability, or frequency, of serious sequelae. Such an approach, furthermore, fulfills the medicolegal responsibilities of the physician to obtain informed consent.

Obtaining a thorough medical history from the patient and performing a comprehensive physical examination are the foundations of safe patient care. A complete list of systemic and topical medications that the patient is currently or was recently taking must be elicited so that potential drug interactions can be anticipated and prevented. Additionally, if the patient will be admitted postoperatively, this list can ensure that essential medication will be administered during the hospitalization. Naturally, a history of any allergies to medicines, foods, latex, or adhesive tape should be documented. Knowledge of any personal or family history of adverse reactions to anesthesia is mandatory. Requisite laboratory studies will vary, depending on the age and physical status of the patient.

The anesthesiologist must be knowledgeable about the anesthetic implications of congenital and metabolic diseases with ocular manifestations. Diabetics, for example, frequently present with ocular complications, and the anesthesiologist must understand the systemic physiological disturbances that affect these patients. Indeed, the list of congenital and metabolic diseases with ocular pathology, that have important anesthetic implications, is impressive. A partial summary includes such syndromes as Crouzon, Apert, Goldenhar (oculoauriculovertebral dysplasia), Sturge-Weber, Marfan, Lowe (oculocerebrorenal syndrome), Down (trisomy 21), Wagner-Stickler, and Riley-Day (familial dysautonomia). Other diseases in this category are homocystinuria, myotonia dystrophica, and sickle cell disease. Comprehensive discussions of these syndromes can be found in these cited works.[54,55]

In addition, ophthalmic patients are often at the extremes of age, ranging from premature babies with retinopathy of prematurity and other ocular abnormalities to nonagenarians with cataracts, glaucoma, and retinal detachments. Hence, age-related considerations, such as altered pharmacokinetics and pharmacodynamics, apply. Moreover, elderly patients commonly suffer from thyroid dysfunction and cardiopulmonary, vascular, and renal diseases.

Selection of Anesthesia

The requirements of ophthalmic surgery include safety, profound analgesia, minimal bleeding, avoidance or obtundation of the oculocardiac reflex, awareness of drug interactions and of the relationship between ocular pathology and anesthetic effects, and a smooth emergence for the patient devoid of vomiting, coughing, or retching. For intraocular surgery, akinesia and prevention of intraocular hypertension are extremely important. In addition, the exigencies of ophthalmic surgery mandate that the anesthesiologist be positioned remote from the patient's airway, and this necessity can sometimes create logistic difficulties.

The few available studies suggest that the incidence of anesthetic morbidity[49] and mortality[10,19,68,69] is similar in patients undergoing ophthalmic surgery, under either local or general anesthesia. However, it must be acknowledged that patients were not well-matched in terms of age, pre-existing medical conditions, and types of ophthalmic surgery. Indeed, most ophthalmic procedures could be performed equally well in adults under either local or general anesthesia. (In children, general anesthesia is almost always selected.) When local anesthesia is elected, the ophthalmologist, or the anesthesiologist, administers the block; the anesthesiologist must also continuously monitor the patient's ECG and pulse oximeter, routinely check vital signs, and administer sedation appropriately. If a mature, cooperative patient and a gentle, communicative surgeon are involved, local anesthesia should provide satisfactory conditions for almost any ophthalmic operation of reasonable length. Local anesthesia is especially popular for anterior segment surgery of 2 hours' duration or less. Many posterior segment operations of similar length, however, may also be done under local anesthesia.

The choice of anesthesia should be individualized, according to the nature and duration of the procedure, the physical and psychological status of the patient, the ability of the patient to communicate and cooperate, and the personal preferences of the patient, the surgeon, and the anesthesiologist. Patients who are deaf or who speak a foreign language, and those with claustrophobia or excessive anxiety, are poor candidates for local anesthesia, as are those whose development is slowed. Other relative contraindications include tremors, chronic coughing, and inability to lie flat. In addition, a large penetrating eye injury, or perforated globe, is a contraindication to regional block of the orbit. Moreover, a previous operative complication that may have been related to administration of local anesthesia (e.g., blindness in one eye following a retrobulbar hemorrhage, an expulsive hemorrhage, or intraocular injection) suggests that general anesthesia should be strongly considered, if possible, for an operation on the sole remaining eye.

Although local anesthesia has many advantages, including minimal nausea and vomiting and superb postoperative analgesia, one must not be lulled into a false sense of security with this technique. Local anesthesia does not necessarily guarantee less physiologic trespass than does general anesthesia. Complications associated with retrobulbar block, for example, may result in blindness and even death; these will be discussed in detail later in this chapter.

Many advocate the administration of approximately 10 to 30 mg of methohexital IV or 0.3 to 0.5 mg/kg of propofol[25] IV immediately prior to performance of ocular regional anesthesia, provided no contraindications to either drug exist. These drugs should provide both analgesia and amnesia for needle insertion. Midazolam, 1 mg IV, is another useful agent to provide amnesia. What must be avoided, however, is the combination of local anesthesia with heavy sedation in the form of high doses of opioids, benzodiazepines, and hypnotics. Such polypharmacy is extremely undesirable because of the pharmacologic vagaries encountered in the geriatric population and the attendant risks of respiratory depression, airway obstruction, hypotension, behavioral aberrations, and prolonged recovery time. This unsatisfactory approach has all the disadvantage of an unintubated general anesthetic without the advantage of controllability that general anesthesia affords. Patients under conscious sedation, by definition, must be capable of cooperating, of responding rationally to instructions, and of maintaining airway patency. Nonetheless, excessive anxiety should be avoided because tachycardia and hypertension can have deleterious effects, especially in patients with coronary artery disease. The goal should be a calm, cooperative, aware patient. Moreover, patients with orthopedic deformities or arthritis must be meticulously positioned and given comfortable padding on the operating table. Supplemental oxygen should be delivered via a nasal cannula that also permits end tidal carbon dioxide ($ETCO_2$) sampling. A suction catheter can also be placed under the drapes to evacuate CO_2. The patient must be kept comfortably warm; the hazards of shivering are well known in patients with cardiac disease or, for that matter, in any patient having delicate eye surgery. Continuous ECG monitoring is crucial, lest performance of a retrobulbar block, pressure on the orbit, or tugging on the extraocular muscles, stimulates the oculocardiac reflex arc and produces dangerous cardiac dysrhythmias. Similarly, continuous oxygen saturation monitoring is essential.

TOPICAL ANESTHESIA

Agents and Complications

Topical anesthesia frequently is used to eliminate corneal and conjunctival reflexes, in order to obtain ocular measurements. In addition, these agents are used for removal of superficial foreign bodies, for suture removal, and for irrigation of the lacrimal system. Cocaine is frequently administered during dacryocystorhinostomy to provide analgesia, vasoconstriction, and shrinkage of the nasal mucous membranes.

Although many agents that cause surface analgesia are available for topical use (Table 17-1), the most widely used agents are proparacaine and tetracaine. All agents have a rapid onset of action, within 30 to 60 seconds, and a duration of action from 10 to 20 minutes.

TABLE 17-1. *Topical ophthalmologic anesthetic agents*

Agent	Concentration %
Proparacaine HCl (Opthaine, Ophthetic)	0.5
Tetracaine HCl (Pontocaine)	0.5
Benoxinate (Dorsacaine)	0.4
Dibucaine HCl (Nupercaine)	0.1
Phenacaine HCl (Holocaine, Tanicaine)	1.0
Piperocaine HCl (Metycaine)	2.0 solution 4.0 ointment
Cocaine	1.0–4.0

Ocular or serious systemic reactions to topical anesthetic agents are almost nonexistent, with the exception of cocaine. The only local anesthetic with vasoconstrictive properties, cocaine penetrates the eye, where it blocks the reuptake of catecholamines at the nerve terminal and has a sympathetic potentiating effect. Pupillary dilation occurs.

Although 1 gram of cocaine is considered to be the usual lethal dose for an adult, considerable variation occurs. The usual maximum dose of cocaine employed in clinical practice is 200 mg for a 70 kg adult, or 3 mg/kg. However, systemic reactions may appear with as little as 20 mg. It is clear that meticulous attention must be paid to the volume and concentration used because there is a narrow range from safety to toxicity to death. Meyers[58] described two cases of cocaine toxicity during dacryocystorhinostomy, emphasizing that cocaine is contraindicated in hypertensive patients or in patients receiving adrenergic-modifying drugs such as guanethidine, tricyclic antidepressants, or monoamine oxidase inhibitors. Additionally, sympathomimetics, such as epinephrine hydrochloride or phenylephrine hydrochloride, should not be given with cocaine.

Signs of cocaine toxicity can be evident in the respiratory, cardiovascular, and central nervous systems. Cocaine's effect on the CNS is biphasic: Initial stimulation is followed by depression as inhibitory synapses are stimulated.[78] The patient rapidly becomes excited, anxious, garrulous, and confused. Initially, reflexes are augmented. Headache is common. The pulse becomes rapid, and hypertension develops. Respiration becomes erratic. A chill may herald the sudden onset of hyperthermia. The pupils become dilated, and exophthalmos occurs. Nausea, vomiting, and abdominal pain are common. The patient may complain of something crawling on his or her skin. Delirium, Cheyne-Stokes breathing, convulsions, and, finally, unconsciousness occurs. Indeed, death may be very rapid following acute cocaine overdosage, and therapeutic maneuvers must be performed quickly.

Before administering cocaine, the physician should carefully search for possible contraindications, including the use of certain concurrent medications. To avoid toxic levels, dosages of dilute solutions should be calculated meticulously and administered carefully. If serious cardiovascular effects occur, IV labetalol may be given to counteract them.[28] Previously, propranolol had been used to control cocaine-induced hypertension.[75] However, a lethal hypertensive exacerbation has been ascribed to unopposed α stimulation.[71] Thus, labetalol offers the advantage of both α and β blockade. To combat the CNS symptoms of cocaine toxicity, IV barbiturates should be given. Cooling measures may be required to treat hyperthermia, including a cooling blanket and ice water or alcohol sponging. In the event of cardiopulmonary arrest, the usual resuscitative measures must be attempted.

All of the topical agents can be toxic to the corneal epithelium with frequent repeated administrations, and may delay the healing of corneal epithelial defects by inhibiting cell division and migration.[50] Therefore, topical anesthetics should be used for surgery or diagnostic tests and not for repeated symptomatic relief. Cocaine has the added disadvantage of causing loosening of the epithelium, which can result in large corneal erosions. Thus, cocaine has been replaced in many clinics by one of the alternatives shown in Table 17-1.

Usage for Cataract Surgery

Recent refinements in cataract surgery have been extremely impressive. During the last few decades, the transition from intracapsular surgery to planned extracapsular and then phacoemulsification has enabled surgeons to have greater control of the intraocular environment. Small incisions, scleral tunnel incisions, sutureless wounds, and now clear corneal incisions have minimized surgical trauma and accelerated healing and visual recovery. Moreover, the implantation of intraocular lenses through small incisions became possible with the development of continuous circular capsulorhexis and foldable implants.

Although Tomas Morena y Maiz of Peru first suggested the medical use of cocaine as a topical anesthetic in 1868, it was in 1884 that Koller and Freud in Vienna first instilled cocaine into the conjunctival sac for local ophthalmic analgesia. Then, in 1910, Julius Hirschberg reported on his extensive, favorable experience administering 2% cocaine chloride for topical anesthesia in cataract surgery.[34] The advances in cataract surgery mentioned earlier, which have enabled faster surgery, with greater control and less trauma, have allowed ophthalmologists to re-examine the use of topical anesthesia for this procedure. Phacoemulsification, with its small incisions, is obviously the procedure of choice in using topical anesthesia. Although planned extracapsular procedures can be performed under topical anesthesia, it is frequently advisable to use 1 to 2 ml of subconjunctival 1% lidocaine superiorly.

In 1990, R. Smith[80] of London performed extracapsular cataract extraction under topical anesthesia with 1% amethocaine drops and a supplemental subconjunctival injection of 2% lidocaine superiorly. In 1991, Richard Fichman[26] reported a series of cases of phacoemulsification under topical tetracaine. In 1991, Charles Williamson[92] developed a technique using phacoemulsification through a stepped clear corneal wound, under topical 4% lidocaine.

Topical anesthesia circumvents potential complications of peribulbar or retrobulbar block that can result in blindness or death. It also allows the patient to see well almost immediately after the surgery. Potential disadvantages of topical anesthesia include eye movement during surgery, patient anxiety and rarely allergic reactions. Immediate allergic reactions are manifested by hyperemia, stinging, itching and chemosis of the conjunctiva. Delayed hypersensitivity can occur as well. Proparacaine and especially cocaine have the greatest toxicity to the epithelium. Tetracaine, although less toxic, purportedly does not produce adequate deep anesthesia. Lidocaine has minimal epithelial toxicity and produces satisfactory deep analgesia of sufficient duration.[50]

Patient selection is critical and should be restricted to individuals who are alert, able to follow instructions, and can control their movements. Patients who are demented or photophobic, or who cannot communicate, are inappropriate candidates, as is one who has an inflamed eye. Similarly, patients with small pupils, which may require significant iris manipulation, or those who need large scleral incisions, may be contraindicated for topical anesthesia.

Williamson[93] describes his technique, beginning with the instillation of two drops of 0.5% tetracaine into the operative eye prior to the application of dilating drops. (Tetracaine prevents the stinging associated with mydriatics.) Then, before the patient is brought to the operating room, two sets of topical 4% lidocaine, four drops every 5 to 10 minutes, is begun. After the patient is positioned on the operating room table, four more drops of topical 4% lidocaine are instilled. A well-dilated pupil is necessary to prevent excessive iris manipulation. Orbital decompression devices are not used because they are uncomfortable and unnecessary; there is no solution in the orbit to cause external pressure. Minimal, if any, sedation is given because it is crucial that the patient be able to cooperate with the surgeon's instructions.

We look forward to statistical analyses of controlled studies with topical anesthesia. Nonetheless, as minimally invasive cataract and glaucoma surgery continue to evolve, it seems reasonable to expect that many more procedures can be done expertly with topical anesthesia.

ANESTHETIC AGENTS

Agents injected for local anesthesia in ophthalmic surgery Table 17-2 are basically the same as those used in other peripheral nerve blocks (see Chapter 4). Lidocaine has been the commonly used agent. In the last decade, however, there has been a tendency to use agents of longer duration, such as bupivacaine,[12] that reduce the need for postoperative analgesics and minimize eye movements immediately after surgery. These agents can be used alone or in combination with lidocaine, to take advantage of the rapid onset of lidocaine and the long duration of bupivacaine. In addition, the longer-duration agents can provide adequate anesthesia for the more lengthy and complex procedures such as combined vitrectomy and retinal reattachment surgery.

Epinephrine frequently is added to the injection solution for ophthalmologic neural blockade to counteract the vasodilator action of the anesthetic agent, and to reduce bleeding. Epinephrine can also serve as a marker of inadvertent intravenous injection and to facilitate augmentation and longer

TABLE 17-2. *Local anesthetic agents used in ophthalmology*

Agent	Concentration (%)	Maximum dose (mg)	Onset of action (min)	Duration of action
Procaine (Novocaine)	1–4	500	6–8	30–45 min
Mepivacaine (Carbocaine)	1–2	400	3–5	90–120 min
Lidocaine (Xylocaine)	1–2	400	4–6	30–60 min
Prilocaine (Citanest)	1–2	600	3–5	60–90 min
Bupivacaine (Marcaine)	0.25–0.75	175	3–5	4–12 h
Etidocaine (Duranest)	0.5–1	300	3–5	4–6 h

duration of action of lidocaine, mepivacaine, bupivacaine, or etidocaine. Dilute concentrations of 1:200,000 (1 mg:200 ml) should be used to avoid tissue injury secondary to ischemia. The authors discourage the use of premixed anesthetic solutions with epinephrine in the orbit, because of their high concentration of metabisulfite, an allergenic and neurotoxic substance. Rather, the authors recommend the addition of 0.1 ml of 1:1,000 epinephrine at time of use to 20 ml ampules or vials, or 0.15 ml of 1:1,000 to 30 ml vials, to produce 1:200,000 solutions. Retrobulbar epinephrine, however, may reduce blood flow to the optic nerve, and is best avoided in patients with glaucomatous optic nerve damage.

Ophthalmologists frequently inquire whether, in cardiac patients, epinephrine may be safely mixed with local anesthetic agents to cause vasoconstriction and prolongation of anesthesia. Donlon and Moss[17] emphasized that release of endogenous catecholamines secondary to suboptimal analgesia may vastly exceed the relatively minute amount of exogenous catecholamine injected. They state that 0.06 mg epinephrine (12 ml of 1:200,000) gives some systemic uptake but causes no untoward clinical effects.

The enzyme hyaluronidase is often added to the anesthetic solution to enhance solution diffusion through the tissues; this action is accomplished by hydrolysis of extracellular hyaluronic acid. For ophthalmic solutions, 7.5 to 15 turbidity-reducing units (TRU) per ml are used. The addition of hyaluronidase allows a more complete, consistent block with the use of less anesthetic solution, and thus less tissue distortion.

The myotoxic effects of local anesthetics on muscle fibers of humans and animals have been well-established.[46,83,27] Rainin and Carlson[70] reported three cases of permanent and one case of temporary vertical muscle paresis after injection of 0.75% bupivacaine directly into the extraocular muscles of four patients. Subsequently, Carlson and associates[11] showed that only 1 ml of 0.75% bupivacaine, 2% lidocaine, or 2% mepivacaine, injected retrobulbarly into rhesus monkeys, led to damage of the extraocular muscles closest to the site of injection, usually the inferior recti and oblique muscles. The same substances injected into human extraocular muscles caused massive lesions, which often occupied the bulk of the cross-section of the muscle. Within such lesions, all of the muscle fibers were uniformly destroyed.[11] Lidocaine appears preferentially to destroy white fibers, whereas bupivacaine is more toxic to red fibers. However, at higher concentrations of local anesthetics, this specificity is abolished, and all striated muscle is injured. Interestingly, other tissues such as smooth muscle, neurons, and connective tissue are unaffected by the same concentration of local anesthetic.

Clearly, intramuscular injection of local anesthetics above a threshold concentration[96] causes myonecrosis with loss of myotubules. Damaged fibers become hyalinized and are invaded by macrophages. However, cell nuclei appear to be spared. Regeneration[92,70,73] can begin after several days and is often complete in six weeks, if the microcirculation of the nerve and muscle are intact. In addition to being concentration dependent, myotoxicity is also dependent on the volume of muscle into which the local anesthetic is injected, and on limited epimysial or perimysial spread. Because damage is more likely to be irreversible if the blood supply to the muscle is damaged, injection into the extraocular muscles in the area of the hilum should be assiduously avoided. Early recognition of myotoxicity and selective patching of the eye during regeneration are important.

Ptosis following cataract surgery is not uncommon, and multiple factors have been implicated in its etiology.[51,23,40] These include the presence of a pre-existing ptosis, injection of anesthetic solution into the upper lid when performing facial nerve block, retrobulbar injection, injection of peribulbar anesthesia through the upper eyelid at the 12-o'clock position, ocular compression or massage, the eyelid speculum, placement of a superior rectus bridle suture with traction on the superior rectus-levator complex, creation of a large conjunctival flap, prolonged or tight patching in the postoperative period, and postoperative eyelid edema. As mentioned, direct intramuscular injection of local anesthetics may also account for many cases of transient and permanent ptosis.[70]

Feibel and colleagues[23] believe that the development of postcataract ptosis is multifaceted and that no single aspect of cataract surgery is the sole contributor. That the local anesthetic injection cannot be isolated as a primary factor is underscored by the observation that postsurgical ptosis is seen in patients undergoing surgery with general anesthesia.

ANATOMY OF THE ORBIT AND THE EYE

A thorough knowledge of the anatomy of the orbit and eye,[91,38] especially of the nerve supply to the orbital struc-

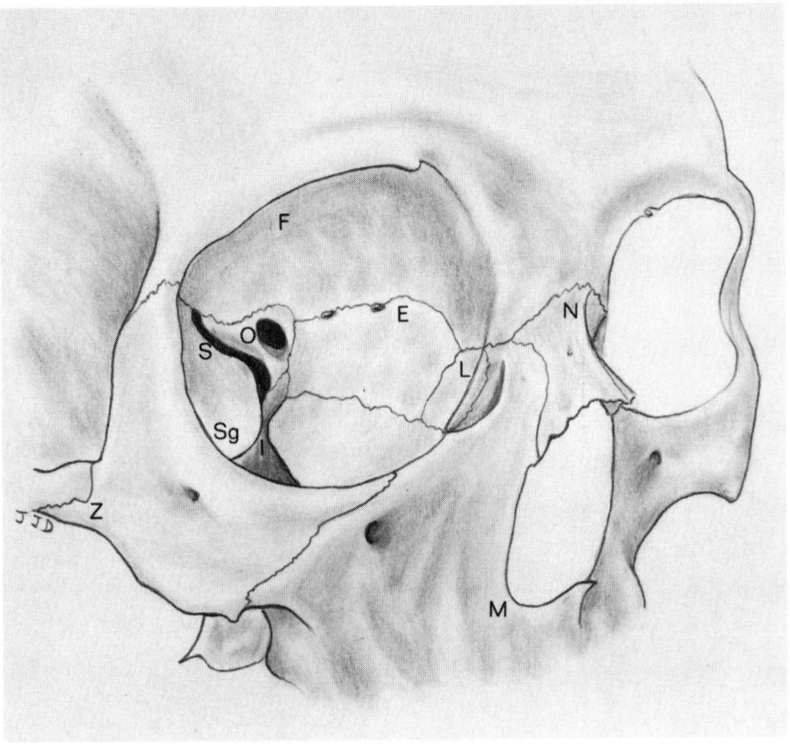

FIG. 17-1. *Bony orbit* showing the medial wall and floor. **N,** nasal bone; **M,** maxilla; **L,** lacrimal bone; **E,** ethmoid bone; **F,** frontal bone; **O,** optic foramen; **S,** superior orbital fissure; **Sg,** orbit plate of greater wing of sphenoid; **I,** inferior orbital fissure; **Z,** zygomatic bone. [Krupin, T., and Waltman, S.R., (eds): Complications in Ophthalmic Surgery. Philadelphia, J.B. Lippincott, 1984.]

tures, is essential to obtain effective neural blockade. Anatomy related to specific anesthetic blocks is detailed under the description of the regional block.

Orbit

The bony orbit has the shape of a pear with the stem directed toward the optic canal (Fig. 17-1). The orbit is covered by the outer periosteal layer of the dura mater (periorbita). Essentially, the orbit is intended as a socket for the eyeball. In addition, it contains the muscles, nerves, and vessels that enable the eye to function properly. A number of blood vessels and nerves supplying areas of the face around the orbital aperture pass through the orbit. Important surrounding anatomic entities include the anterior cranial fossa above, the maxillary sinus below, and the nasal cavity and ethmoidal air cells medially. There are nine canals and fissures in the orbit, the most important being the optic foramen, the superior

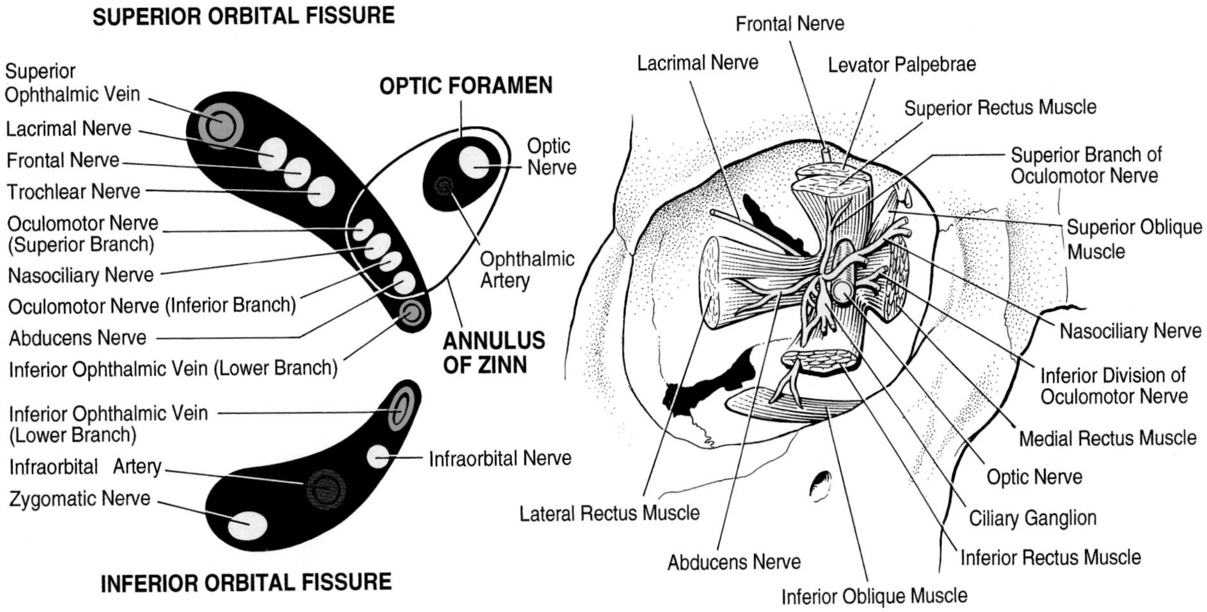

FIG. 17-2. *Bony orbit* with the superior and inferior orbital fissures and optic canal at the apex of the muscle cone.

TABLE 17-3. *Motor innervation to ocular adnexal muscles*

Nerve (Cranial Nerve)	Muscle innervation
Oculomotor (III)	Superior rectus
	Medial rectus
	Inferior rectus
	Inferior oblique
	Levator palpebrae superioris
Trochlear (IV)	Superior oblique
Abducens (VI)	Lateral rectus
Facial (VII)	
Upper zygomatic branch	Frontalis
	Orbicularis oculi upper lid
Lower zygomatic branch	Orbicularis oculi lower lid

and inferior orbital fissures, and the supraorbital and infraorbital foramina (Fig. 17-2).

Eye

The normal globe is about 24 mm in the anteroposterior diameter. This dimension is increased in myopic (nearsighted) eyes. The eyeball has three concentric layers: an outer fibrous layer (the cornea and sclera), a middle vascular layer (the iris, ciliary body, and choroid), and an inner neural layer (the retina). Intraocular contents are: aqueous humor in the anterior chamber (space lined by the cornea, iris, and pupil) and in the posterior chamber (space behind the iris and in front of the vitreous), the crystalline lens, and the vitreous humor (space behind the lens and in front of the retina).

The optic nerve (cranial nerve II) pierces the globe just above and 3 mm medial to the posterior pole. The nerve has a diameter of 1.5 mm and an intraorbital length of about 30 mm. The nerve exits the orbit by way of the optic foramen. The traditional upward and inward positiion of the globe during retrobulbar anesthesia (see following) results in stretching, as well as a downward and outward displacement of the optic nerve. This position may place the nerve in a vulnerable position for direct traumatization.[88,67]

Six extraocular striated muscles control the movements of the globe. The four rectus muscles (superior, medial, inferior, and lateral) originate from a common tendon ring that encircles the optic foramen (annulus of Zinn) with their tendinous insertion 5.5 to 7.5 mm from the limbus of the cornea. The superior oblique muscle originates above and medial to the optic foramen, runs medially to the trochlea, then bends backward to insert on the globe beneath the superior rectus muscle. The inferior oblique muscle originates medially from the periosteum of the lacrimal bone, runs beneath the inferior rectus muscle, and inserts on the posterolateral aspect of the globe. The 7th striated muscle in the orbit is the levator of the upper eyelid, which originates from the periosteum of the apex of the orbit above the superior

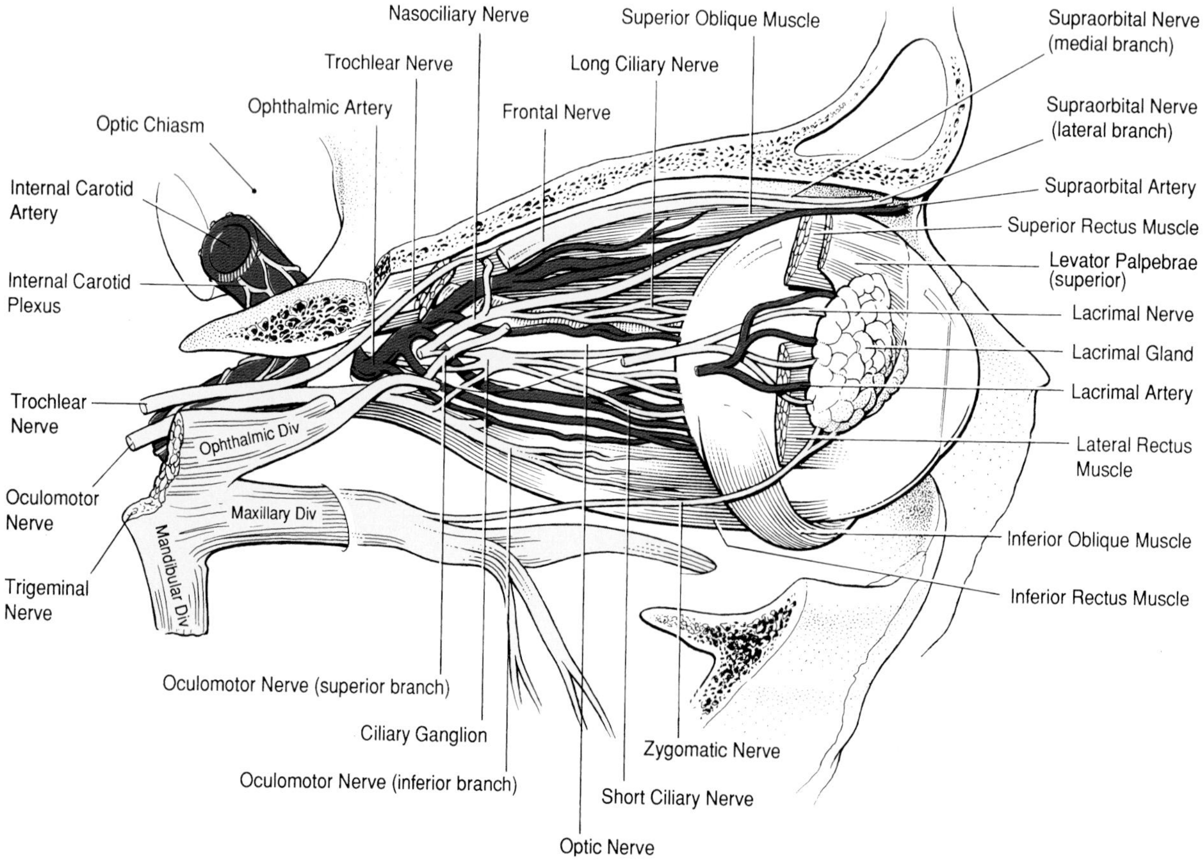

FIG. 17-3. A: *Orbital anatomy* as seen from the lateral approach.

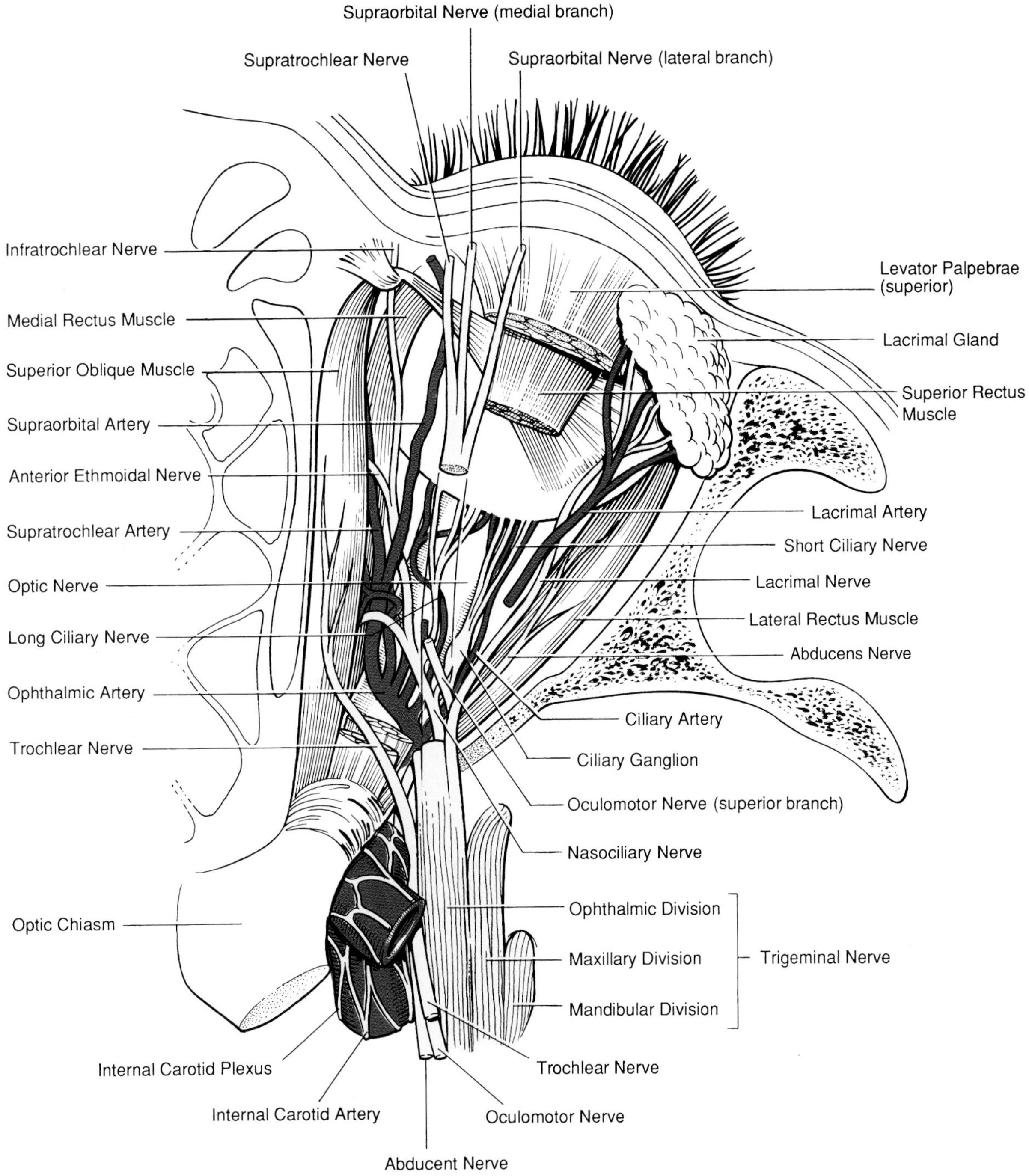

FIG. 17-3. *Continued.* **B:** *Orbital anatomy* as seen from above.

oblique muscle. The levator runs forward between the roof of the orbit and superior rectus muscle and spreads out into an aponeurosis that inserts into the skin and tarsal plate of the upper eyelid. Cranial nerves III, IV, and VI innervate these striated muscles (Table 17-3, and Fig. 17-3A, B).

Innervation of the Eye and Orbital Contents

The sensory supply to the eye and its adnexae is derived from the trigeminal nerve (cranial nerve V). This is a mixed nerve that comprises a large sensory part and a small motor part. The sensory portion of the nerve divides at the trigeminal ganglion into three branches: ophthalmic, maxillary, and mandibular (Table 17-4, Fig. 17-3 and 17-4).

The motor supply to the extraocular muscles and levator palpebrae muscle of the upper eyelid is provided by cranial nerves III, IV, and VI (see Table 17-3). The facial nerve (cranial nerve VII) supplies all the muscles of expression, including the orbicularis oculi in the eyelids. The nerve emerges through the stylomastoid foramen, just below the

TABLE 17-4. *Trigeminal (V cranial nerve) sensory innervation of the eye and adnexal structures*

Trigeminal Nerve Division	Branch	Sub-branch	Innervation
Ophthalmic	Frontal	Supratrochlear	Skin of lower forehead, skin root of nose, skin and conjunctiva of medial part of upper eyelid
		Supraorbital	Scalp and skin of forehead, skin and conjunctiva of upper eyelid
		Long ciliary	Cornea, iris, ciliary muscle
	Nasociliary	Infratrochlear	Medial upper and lower eyelid, skin and conjunctiva of inner canthus, caruncle, skin root of nose, lacrimal sac
		Long sensory root	Ciliary ganglion (cornea, iris, ciliary body via short ciliary nerves to the ganglion)
		Anterior ethmoid	Tip of nose
	Lacrimal		Outer upper and lower eyelid skin and conjunctiva, lateral canthus, and lacrimal gland
Maxillary	Infraorbital		Entire lower lid, medial and lateral parts of upper and lower lid, lacrimal sac, nasolacrimal duct, upper lip, skin over temple and lateral orbital wall
	Zygomatic		Skin of temporal area and lateral wall of the orbit

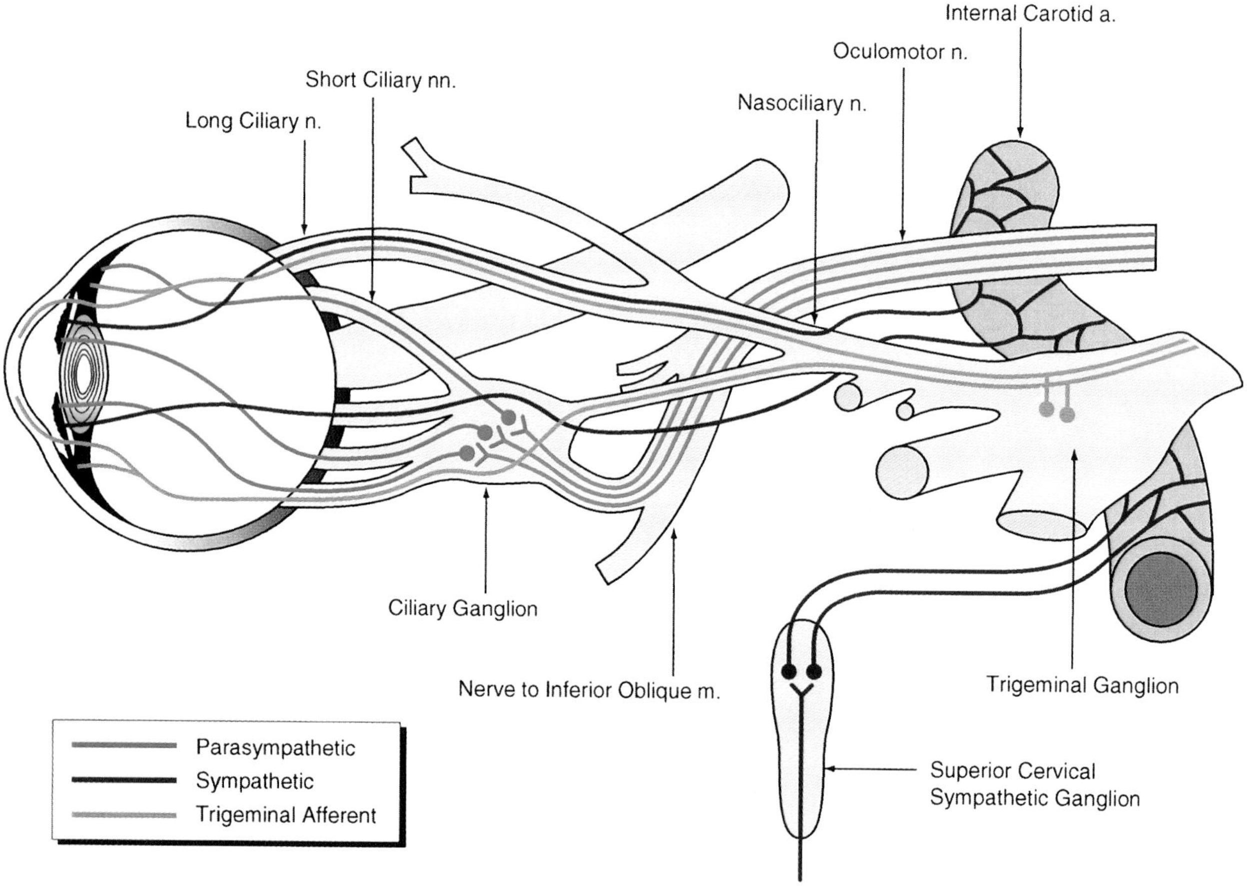

FIG. 17-4. *Innervation of the eye.*

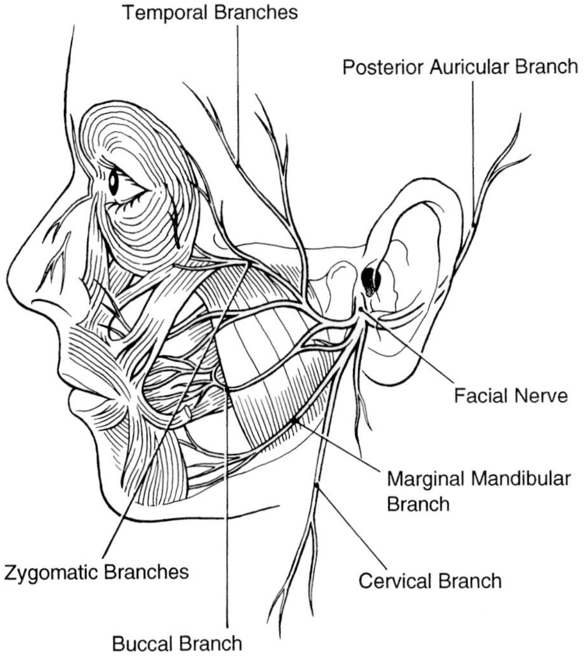

FIG. 17-5. *Facial nerve* and distribution of its branches.

osseous part of the outer ear. The facial nerve then turns forward and enters the parotid gland superficial to the neck of the mandible, where it divides into five branches: temporal, zygomatic, buccal, mandibular, and cervical. The temporal division supplies the upper part of the orbicularis oculi, the corrugator supercili, and the frontalis muscle. The zygomatic branch supplies the lower part of the orbicularis oculi muscle (Fig. 17-5).

The autonomic nervous system supplies the eye through the sympathetic and parasympathetic systems (Table 17-5, and Fig. 17-4).

AKINESIA OF THE ORBICULARIS OCULI MUSCLE

Akinesia of the eyelids is essential for all intraocular surgery to prevent squeezing of the lids and expulsion of intraocular contents. Paralysis of the orbicularis oculi muscle may be achieved either by local infiltration of the muscle or proximal infiltration of the branches of the facial nerve that supply it.

Van Lint Method

In 1914, van Lint was the first to describe akinesia of the orbicularis oculi for cataract extraction.[89] The classic van Lint technique involves inserting the needle at the lateral orbital rim and making a small intradermal wheal. The needle is then advanced into the deep tissues along the inferolateral orbital margin. As the needle is withdrawn, 2 to 4 ml of anesthetic are injected. The needle is then redirected along the superotemporal orbital margin. Again, anesthetic is injected as the needle is withdrawn. Pressure is then applied to the eye to promote diffusion of the anesthetic. This method has the side-effect of producing lid edema. Therefore, the technique has been modified by placing the injections more laterally to block the facial nerve as it crosses the periosteum of the orbital rim, and is followed by inferior and superior injections (Figure 17-6).

O'Brien Method

In 1927, O'Brien described a facial nerve block over the mandibular condyle, inferior to the posterior zygomatic process.[66] The condyle can be palpated as the patient moves his jaw. The needle is inserted about 1 cm to the level of the periosteum (Fig. 17-7). Anesthetic solution (2 to 3 ml) is injected as the needle is withdrawn. Because of the variable course of the facial nerve, the block may be incomplete. Hence, the following modifications have been recommended: After injecting over the condyle, partially withdraw the needle and redirect it inferiorly along the posterior edge of the ramus of the mandible. Then, inject the anesthetic solution while withdrawing the needle; reposition the needle anteriorly along the zygomatic arch, and inject the anesthetic while withdrawing the needle.

Atkinson Method

First described in 1953, the Atkinson method involves blocking the branches of the facial nerve to the orbicularis oculi as they cross the zygomatic arch (Fig. 17-8).[7] First, a skin wheal is made at the lower margin of the zygomatic arch below the lateral orbital rim. The needle is then directed superiorly and posteriorly along the zygoma (aimed just lateral to the midpoint between the tragus and lateral orbital rim). Anesthetic (5 to 10 ml) is injected as the needle is withdrawn.

TABLE 17-5. *Autonomic nervous system innervation to the eye*

System	Source	Nerves	Supply
Sympathetic	Superior cervical ganglion	Long ciliary nerve, (2) short ciliary nerves	Vascular system of choroid, ciliary body, iris (vasoconstrictors); motor impulses to iris dilator muscle
Parasympathetic	Oculomotor nerve (preganglionic fibers) to ciliary ganglion	Short ciliary nerves (postganglionic)	Ciliary body, motor impulse to the iris sphincter muscle and to the ciliary muscle

See also Fig. 17-4.

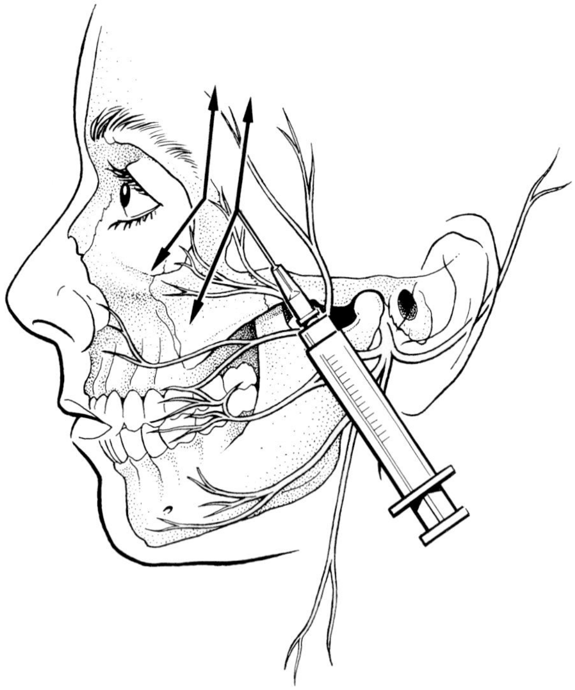

A

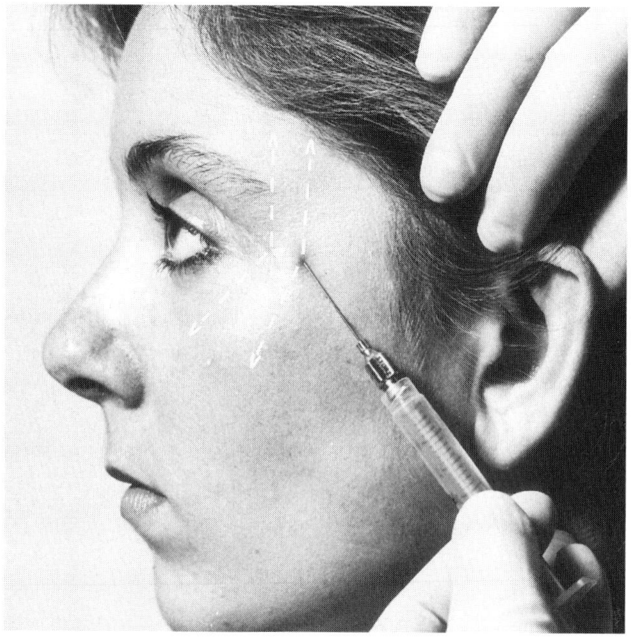

B

FIG. 17-6. **A:** *Anatomy of van Lint Technique* **B:** *Classic van Lint Technique* blocks the facial nerve at the lateral orbital rim. The modified technique (needle site) places the injection more lateral to avoid lid edema.

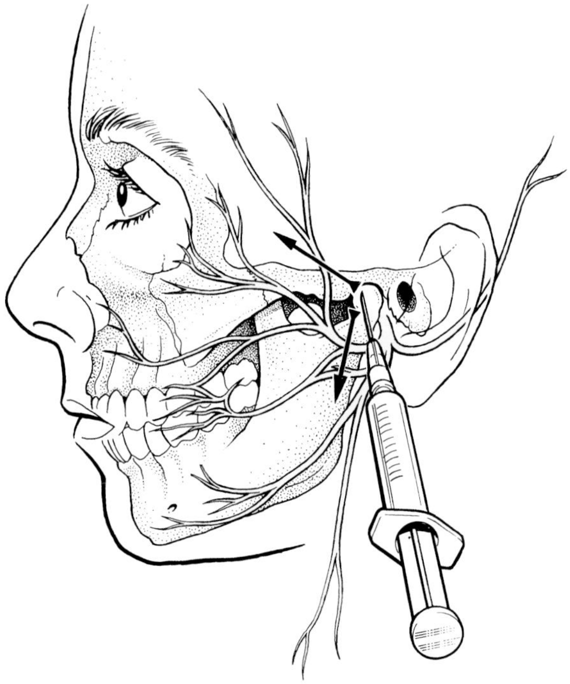

A

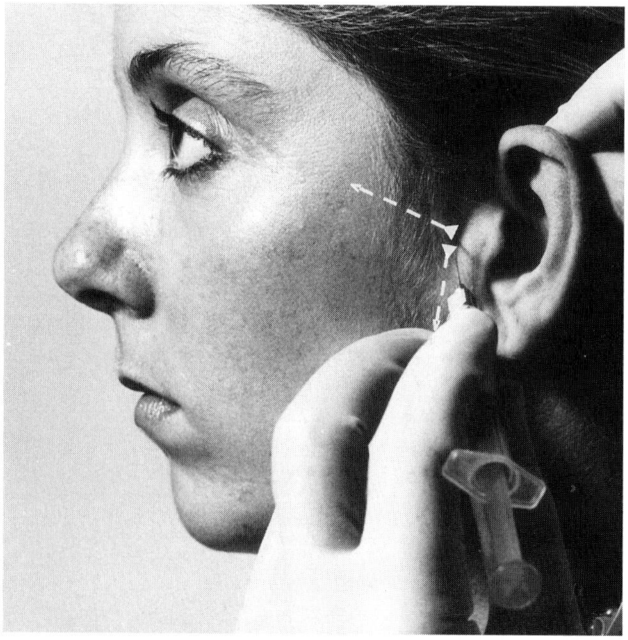

B

FIG. 17-7. **A:** *Anatomy of O'Brien technique* for facial nerve block. **B:** *O'Brien technique* for facial nerve block. Injection is performed over the mandibular condyle (tip of the needle). A modified technique (*dotted lines*) adds injections along the posterior edge of the mandible and anteriorly along the zygomatic arch.

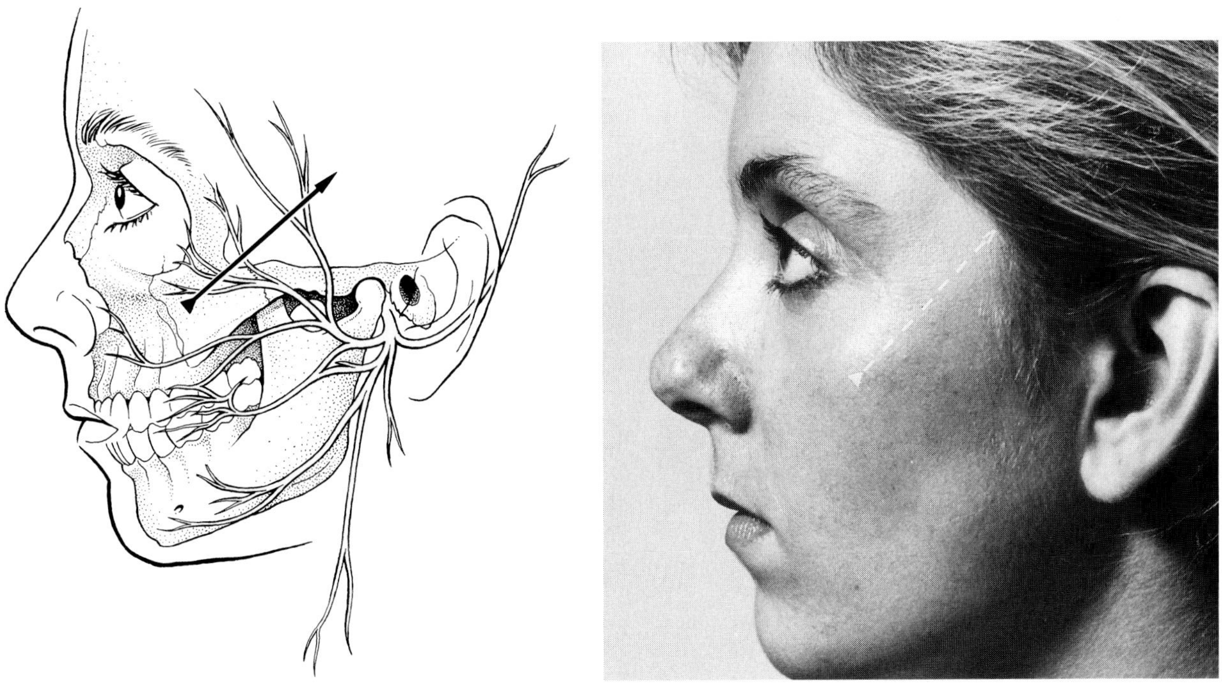

A B

FIG. 17-8. A: *Anatomy of Atkinson method* for facial nerve block. **B:** *Atkinson method* for facial nerve block.

Combined Methods

A number of injection techniques are described that combine the classic with the modified van Lint, O'Brien, and Atkinson methods. Inconsistencies of the different facial nerve blocks relate to individual variability in the course of the nerve, after it enters the parotid gland and subsequently divides into the five facial branches.

Nadbath-Rehman Method

Complete akinesia of the muscles innervated by the facial nerve may be achieved with the Nadbath-Rehman block,[63] initially described in 1963. The main trunk of the facial nerve is blocked at the concavity just below the external auditory meatus between the anterosuperior border of the mastoid process and the posterior border of the mandibular ra-

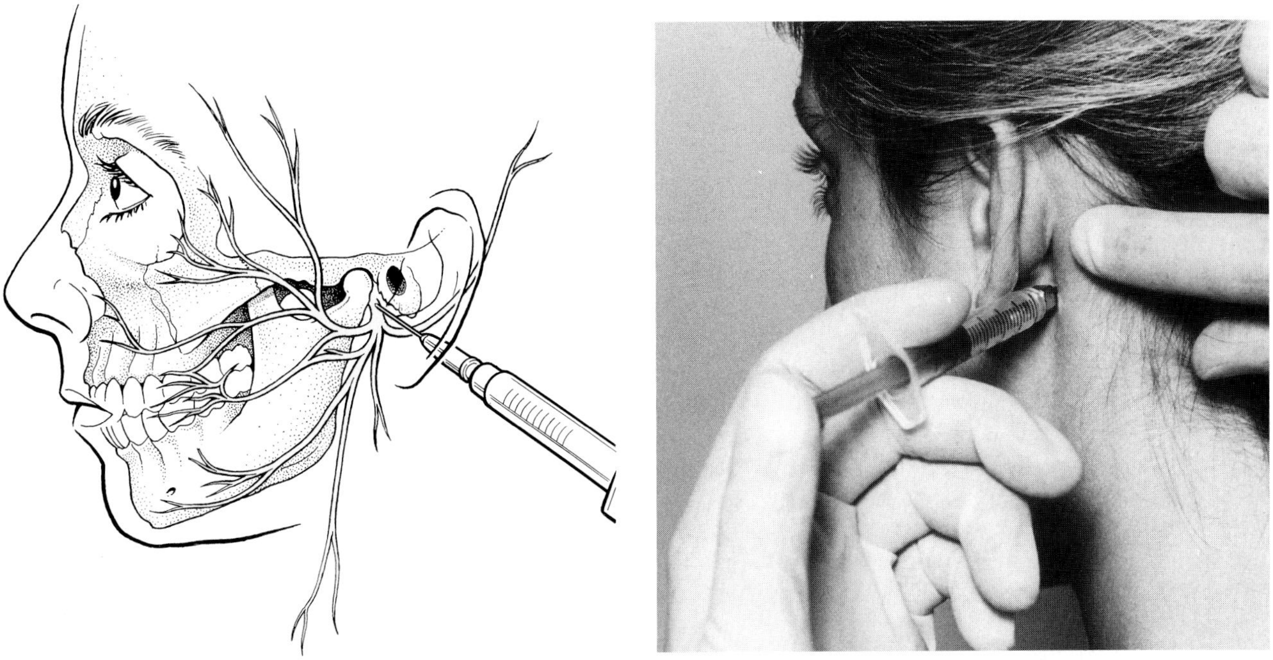

A B

FIG. 17-9. A: *Anatomy of Nadbath-Rehman facial nerve block.* **B:** *Nadbath-Rehman* facial nerve block.

mus (Fig. 17-9). The site can be identified by palpation, and confirmed by having the patient open and close his or her jaw. A 25 gauge, 12-mm needle is inserted into the skin, and an intradermal wheal is made. The needle is then advanced its full length, perpendicularly, into the tissue. The plunger is withdrawn to assure that the needle is not intravascular, and about 3 ml of anesthetic solution is injected as the needle is withdrawn. Gentle massage is applied to the injection site to diffuse the anesthetic. This technique produces complete facial nerve akinesia. The major advantage of this technique is the consistent course of the facial nerve from the stylomastoid foramen to the posteromedial surface of the parotid gland, before branching of the nerve. Akinesia of the lower facial musculature also occurs, and the patient must be informed of this associated occurrence during the preoperative interview and be reassured that the effect is transient. Patients may develop sudden dysphagia, hoarseness, respiratory distress, pooling of secretions, or laryngospasm.[94,14] Presumably these symptoms result from ipsilateral paralysis of the glossopharyngeal, vagus, and spinal accessory nerves, which exit the skull via the jugular foramen located a mere 10 mm medial to the stylomastoid foramen. Complete facial hemiparesis can be undesirable in the outpatient setting, because family members may misinterpret its effects as a stroke. Moreover, profound facial hemiparesis interferes with liquid and solid intake.

RETROBULBAR BLOCK

Technique

Retrobulbar injection of local anesthetic provides akinesia of the extraocular muscles by blocking cranial nerves III, IV, and VI, and anesthesia of the conjunctiva, cornea, and uvea, by blocking the ciliary nerves. These effects of retrobulbar anesthesia, combined with a separate block to provide akinesia of the orbicularis oculi muscle, permit intraocular surgery under local anesthesia.

Appropriate patient preparation, including monitoring, sedation, and positioning, has been discussed previously. Traditionally, patients had been instructed to look upward and inward during the retrobulbar injection, in order to place the inferior oblique muscle out of the trajectory of the retrobulbar needle. An additional advantage of superonasal gaze is that the patient looks away from the needle and the site of puncture. In 1981, however, Unsöld and colleagues,[88] using Computed tomography (CT) scanning of a cadaver orbit as the retrobulbar needle is inserted, exposed the hazards of the traditional Atkinson position of superonasal gaze during inferotemporal needle placement for retrobulbar block. They discovered that in this position, the optic nerve, ophthalmic artery and its branches, superior orbital vein, and the posterior pole of the globe rotated into the path of the retrobulbar needle. The chance of perforating the optic nerve or of piercing the meningeal sheath surrounding the optic nerve, thereby allowing local anesthesia to spread throughout the CNS, is also increased, because the nerve is put on stretch in this position. Hence, the current recommendation is to have the patient look in *primary gaze,* or *inferonasally.*[29,41]

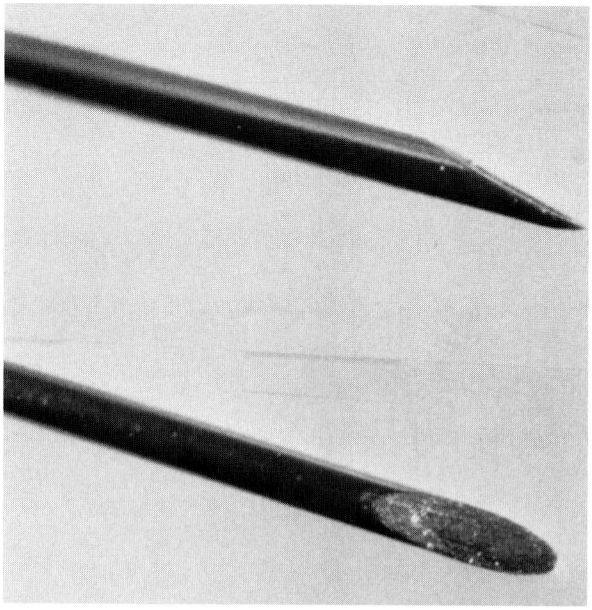

FIG. 17-10. Frontal and lateral views of the Atkinson needle for retrobulbar injection.

Conventional wisdom in ophthalmology had long maintained that the force required to perforate an eye during retrobulbar injection is noticeably greater with a specially designed blunt needle than with a standard hypodermic needle (Fig. 17-10). In 1993, Waller and colleagues[90] measured scleral perforation pressure with specific needle tips in preserved and unpreserved human cadaver eyes. These investigators confirmed that the noncutting edge, blunt-tipped needles do indeed have higher scleral perforation pressures than those with cutting edges (Table 17-6) (Nonetheless, there is

TABLE 17-6. *Scleral perforation pressures*

	Scleral Perforation Pressure (mmHg) Mean ± SD
Preserved Eyes	
30-gauge hypodermic	2 ± 0.5
27-gauge hypodermic	2 ± 0.5
18-gauge hypodermic	3 ± 1.3
23-gauge Atkinson	12 ± 2.6
Fresh Cadaver Eyes	
30-gauge hypodermic	1 ± 1
25-gauge hypodermic	2 ± 1
23-gauge Atkinson	10 ± 1
25-gauge Straus	12 ± 3.8
23-gauge Straus	12 ± 1
25-gauge Thornton	29 ± 4.5
23-gauge Thornton	35 ± 5
SD, standard deviation	

Reprinted with permission from Waller, S.G., Taboada, J. and O'Connor, P. Retrobulbar anesthesia risk: Do sharp needles really perforate the eyes more easily than blunt needles? Ophthalmology. *100*:506, 1993.

also a possibility that a perforating blunt needle tip does more serious retinal damage than its sharper counterpart.[29]) Moreover, large caliber (23-gauge) needles require more force to perforate the globe than do 25-gauge needles of the same tip design.[90] Thus, some clinics prefer to use fine disposable needles and small volume syringes to detect subtle changes in resistance.[31]

A "painless injection" may be achieved by first instilling local anesthetic eyedrops and then making an injection in the inferotemporal quadrant: The lower eyelid is retracted and a 30-gauge, 12-mm needle is inserted, tangentially to the globe, through the conjunctiva to a depth of 1 cm. The needle will have pierced the capsulopalpebral ligament, and 1 cc of local anesthetic inserted here will eliminate any pain from subsequent needle insertion for peribulbar or retrobulbar block, using the inferotemporal site of needle insertion. The retrobulbar needle is then inserted through the lower lid in the inferotemporal quadrant, at the junction of the lateral and middle thirds of the margin (Fig. 17-11). The needle (no longer than 31 mm[68]) is then directed perpendicular to the skin surface, with the bevel facing the globe to reduce the risk of perforation. After the needle passes the equator of the globe, it should be directed slightly lower than the orbital apex, toward the inferior part of the superior orbital fissure. The syringe should be aspirated before injection to be certain that the needle is not inside a vessel. Satisfactory retrobulbar block is achieved using injections of 1.5 to 2.0 ml of anesthetic solution into the muscle core. Many clinicians will inject larger volumes (4.0 to 5.0 ml) and use hyaluronidase to enhance diffusion through the orbit. These larger volumes

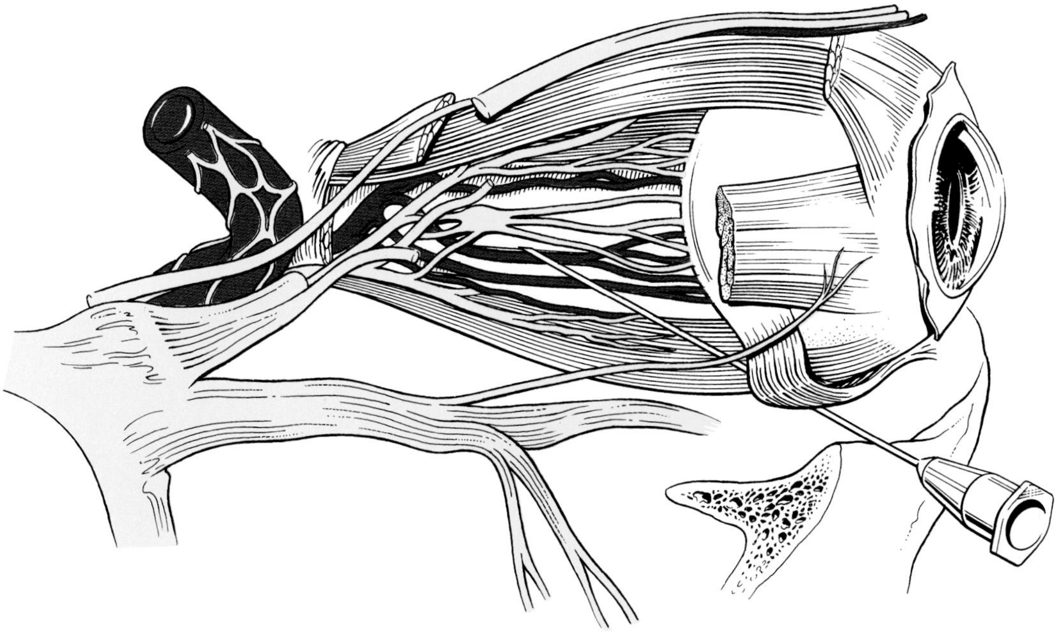

A

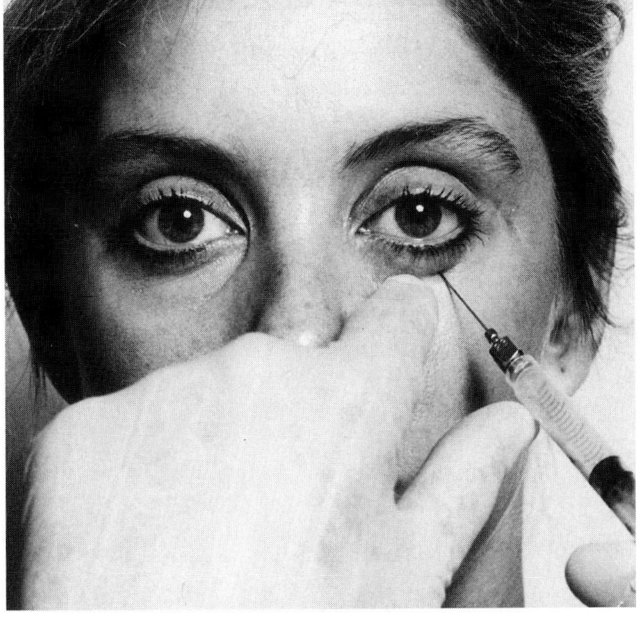

B

FIG. 17-11. A: *Anatomy of retrobulbar injection.* **B:** *Retrobulbar injection* with the eye in primary gaze. The index finger is palpating the orbital rim. The needle is directed slightly below the apex of the orbit (see text).

may produce additional pressure on the globe and chemosis of the conjunctiva. After the injection, firm intermittent digital pressure is applied for about 5 minutes to help distribute the anesthetic and lower IOP; some clinics prefer pressure devices that apply measurable pressure. If complete akinesia and adequate analgesia have not been achieved, it may be necessary to perform a supplemental retrobulbar injection, or a transconjunctival quadrant block, adjacent to the functioning extraocular muscle. The superior oblique muscle, located outside the annulus of Zinn, will not be paralyzed following retrobulbar blockade. Thus, the eye may intort when the patient is instructed to look down.

Although many clinicians perform the retrobulbar injection through the lower eyelid, a transconjunctival approach may be used also. The lower lid is pulled down and the needle inserted through the inferior cul-de-sac. Otherwise, the direction and technique are as described previously.

Complications

Retrobulbar injection is associated with both local and systemic complications[76] (Table 17-7). Perforation of the globe can occur during retrobulbar injection, despite the use of a blunted retrobulbar needle. Published studies from two retinal surgery practices show an approximate incidence of 1 in 1,000.[13,72] More recently, Waller et al.,[90] in a review of more than 4,000 charts, found no incidence of scleral perforation during retrobulbar or peribulbar injection. Risk factors for globe perforation include an anteroposterior (AP) length > 26 mm by ultrasound, commonly noted in high myopes, severe enophthalmos, previous scleral buckle, repeated surgeries, posterior staphyloma, repeated injections, and an uncooperative patient who moves. The patient typically has intense and immediate ocular pain with sudden loss of vision following perforation of the globe.[18] Approximately 50% of the time, the clinician will not recognize unintentional ocular perforation on administering the block, because the scleral perforation pressure may be so low as to be imperceptible, especially with sharp needles. In 30% of cases, the eye may feel hypotonic, possibly owing to loss of vitreous. In 10% of cases, the eye may feel very hard because of elevated IOP, following injection of local anesthetic into the globe. In this case, the scheduled surgical procedure must be postponed and appropriate retinal treatment undertaken.

Retrobulbar hemorrhage is the most common complication, occurring as often as 1 to 3% of the time after retrobulbar injection.[62] Vascular or hematologic disease may predispose a patient to develop a retrobulbar hemorrhage. In addition, systemic therapy with aspirin or anticoagulation therapy may be associated with this complication. Many ophthalmologists prefer that patients avoid aspirin for at least 10 days before intraocular surgery, with or without retrobulbar injection. If the patient is taking systemic anticoagulants, his or her internist should be consulted regarding cessation of, or lowering the dose of, anticoagulation treatment. Discontinuing anticoagulation can have serious medical consequences, and several studies suggest that cataract surgery can be safely performed under regional anesthesia without discontinuing anticoagulants,[56,30,74] especially if the prothrombin time is approximately 1.5 times control.[24] Signs and symptoms of retrobulbar hemorrhage include pain, increasing proptosis, and frequently subconjunctival or eyelid ecchymoses. The patient's IOP and central retinal artery pulsations should be monitored carefully by an ophthalmologist for signs of an impending retinal arterial occlusion. Because the oculocardiac reflex may be triggered several hours after the initial retrobulbar hemorrhage, ECG monitoring of the patient should be performed accordingly. If external pressure

TABLE 17-7. *Complications of retrobulbar anesthesia*

Complications	Signs and Symptoms	Mechanism
Ocular		
Perforation of the globe	Ocular pain, intraocular hemorrhage, restlessness	Direct trauma: myopic eye, posterior staphyloma, repeated injections
Retrobulbar hemorrhage	Subjunctival or eyelid ecchymosis, increasing proptosis, pain, ± increased IOP	Direct trauma (artery or vein)
Optic nerve damage	Visual loss, optic disc pallor	Direct injury to nerve or blood vessels, vascular occlusion
Systemic		
Intra-arterial injection	Cardiopulmonary arrest, convulsions	Retrograde flow to internal carotid and access to midbrain structures
Optic nerve sheath injection	Agitation, confusion, ptosis, mydriasis, dysphagia, dizziness, confusion, contralateral ophthalmoplegia, respiratory depression or arrest	Subdural or subarachnoid injection
Oculocardiac reflex	Bradycardia, other arrhythmias, asystole	Trigeminal nerve (afferent arc) to floor of fourth ventricle with efferent arc via vagus nerve

Reprinted with permission from Feitl, M.E., and Krupin, T.: Retrobulbar anesthesia. Ophthalmol. Clin North Am. *3*(1):83, 1990.

on the globe is sufficient to produce compression of the retinal arteries, then a deep lateral canthotomy should be performed to decompress the orbit rapidly. If this does not reestablish normal retinal blood flow, an anterior chamber paracentesis should be done to decompress the globe. Inadequate or delayed treatment of this complication may result in total loss of vision unilaterally. Some retrobulbar hemorrhages may be minimal, even subclincal, and on rare occasions the surgeon may consider continuing surgery. There is, however, significant risk of repeat hemorrhage intraoperatively, with devastating sequelae. Therefore, the recommended course following a recognized retrobulbar hemorrhage is to postpone surgery until all signs of the hemorrhage have resolved. Moreover, it may be prudent to plan general anesthesia for the rescheduled surgery.

Optic atrophy and permanent loss of vision may occur, even in the absence of retrobulbar hemorrhage.[20,43] Postulated mechanisms include direct injury to the nerve, injection into the nerve sheath with compressive ischemia, and intraneural sheath hemorrhage.[20,86] In addition, retinal vascular occlusion has been observed after retrobulbar injection, without evidence of a retrobulbar hemorrhage.[43,15] Each of these patients experiencing vascular occlusion without concomitant hemorrhage had a severe hematologic or vascular disorder. Another apparent risk factor is a previous episode. Therefore, it seems prudent to avoid future retrobulbar injection (and perhaps peribulbar injection) in a patient who has developed this rare complication.[15]

Systemic complications associated with retrobulbar blocks are rare, but potentially lethal. A partial list of these sequelae includes stimulation of the oculocardiac reflex arc, producing associated dysrhythmias, including asystole; intravascular injection of local anesthetic triggering initial CNS excitation[59] that can be followed by obtundation and cardiovascular collapse; and unintentional injection of local anesthetic into the CNS, that can result in respiratory arrest.

Although the amount of local anesthetic agent given with retrobulbar blockade is not usually sufficient to produce toxicity if unintentionally injected into a vein, this is not true for inadvertent intra-arterial injection. Indeed, only 1.8 ml of 2% lidocaine unintentionally injected into an artery of the head or neck region can produce profound toxicity.[3] These complications include virtually instantaneous seizures secondary to ophthalmic artery injection, with retrograde flow into the cerebral circulation.

From 1980 onward, several reports appeared in the literature documenting serious CNS depression following retrobulbar block. Although an incidence rate of 0.79% was reported in one paper,[95] other investigators suggest that the occurrence is more unusual, typically appearing once in 350 to 500 cases.[64,1,81,32] There is a continuum of sequelae, depending on the amount of drug that gains entrance to the CNS and the specific area to which the drug spreads.[37] Onset of symptoms is variable, ranging from 2 to 40 minutes.[33] The protean CNS signs may include violent shivering,[65] contralateral amaurosis, eventual loss of consciousness, apnea, and hemiplegia, paraplegia, quadriplegia, or hyperreflexia. Blockade of the 8th to 12th cranial nerves will result in deafness, vertigo, vagolysis, dysphagia, aphasia, and loss of neck muscle power. Although these signs may be present in various combinations, once it is apparent that the local anesthetic has spread to the CNS, the anesthesiologist must be prepared to provide immediate cardiopulmonary resuscitation, if necessary. When properly treated, these patients recover quickly and completely. However, delay in diagnosing and treating respiratory arrest, secondary to brain stem anesthesia, can result in death.

Much is now known about prevention of brain stem anesthesia. Attention has focused on ocular position when retrobulbar block is performed, and on the length of the needle selected. The traditional Atkinson position of superonasal gaze places the optic nerve in closer proximity to the advancing needle, where the needle tip can pierce the meningeal sheath surrounding the optic nerve, allowing local anesthesia to spread throughout the CNS. With the globe in primary gaze, or looking inferonasally,[47] the optic nerve is less vulnerable. Moreover, avoidance of deep penetration of the orbit is important to prevent this and other serious complications, including perforation of the globe. Even in the absence of penetration of the optic nerve sheath, central spread of local anesthetic from deep orbital injection *may* be a rare possibility.[77] Hence, the maximum needle length currently recommended for retrobulbar block is 31 mm (1.25 inches).[41]

PERIBULBAR BLOCK

Technique

Since the late 1980s, peribulbar block has gained increasing popularity. Peribulbar block is considered by many to be easier, safer, and less painful than retrobulbar block, because the muscle cone is not entered (Fig. 17-12), and the need for separate facial nerve block is eliminated because the relatively large volume (8 to 10 ml) of injected local anesthetic usually diffuses into the eyelids.[90]

Patient preparation, including monitoring and sedation, is as described for retrobulbar block. Davis and Mandel advocated a peribulbar or periconal technique in 1986,[16] and several modifications of their original protocol have since developed. In the most common technique, two injections are required; these are placed inferotemporally, and superonasally just below and medial to the supraorbital notch. There are differing views as to which injection should be made first; the lower lid puncture may be safer.[67] A 25-gauge, 1.25 inch needle is used and directed just beyond the equator of the globe. Following careful aspiration, 4 to 5 ml of anesthetic solution is injected in each site. Onset is usually slower than with retrobulbar blockade and may be delayed for as long as 15 to 20 minutes. Zahl and colleagues[97] reported that onset is accelerated by adding sodium bicarbonate to bupivacaine and hyaluronidase. However, others believe that pH adjustment of local anesthetic bottled at pH 6.0 or above to reach 7.4 has minimal effect.[36] In an area of rapid

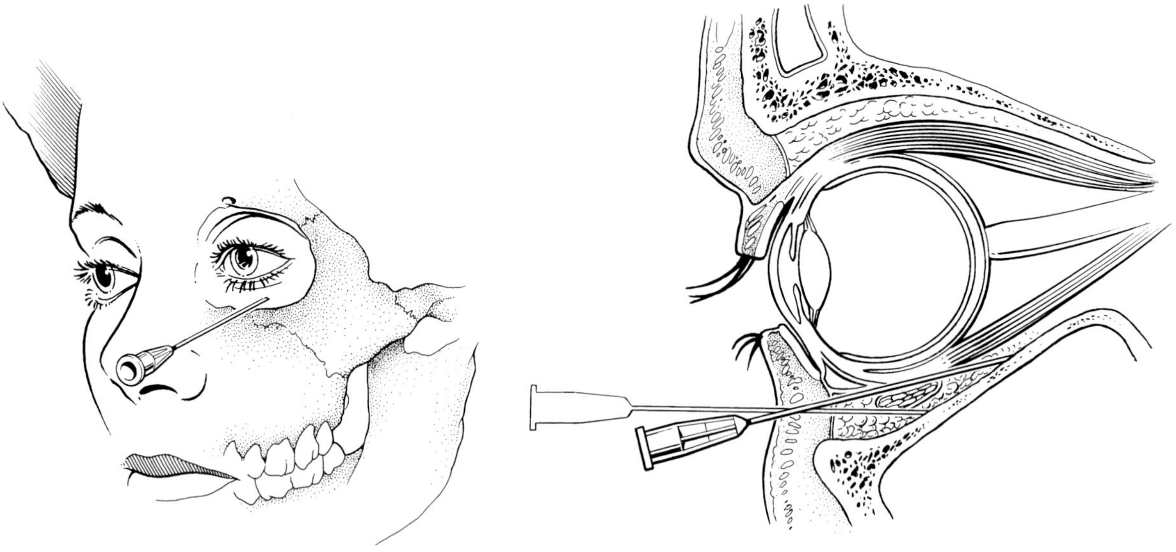

FIG. 17-12. ***Peribulbar block.*** With peribulbar block, the muscle cone is not entered. At both the superonasal injection site, and the inferotemporal site (shown here), anesthetic solution is deposited just past the equator.

blood flow[36] such as in orbital connective tissue, transcapillary extraction is also facilitated when concentration of base form predominates.

Ortiz et al.[67] confirmed, by a CT scan study, that superior midline and superotemporal puncture may cause perforation of the globe. Thus, these approaches are not used.

One approach is to use a single inferotemporal injection, and to supplement only if needed. Others use inferotemporal *or* superonasal injection first, and then, routinely, supplement with the other.

A further approach is to give a medial injection transconjunctivally, on the medial side of the caruncle, at the extreme medial side of the palpebral fissure. The bevel of the needle faces the medial orbital wall, and the needle passes posteriorly, in the transverse plane, directed at 5° angle away from the sagittal plane and towards the medial orbital wall. It is recommended that a 27-gauge, 20 to 25 mm disposable needle be used, and inserted until the hub reaches the plane of the iris.[41]

Some authors recommend the combination of inferotemporal retrobulbar (intracone) block and complimentary peribulbar (pericone) injection, with the medial caruncle technique favored.[31]

Complications

Peribulbar block typically has a higher failure rate (up to 50%[48]) than retrobulbar block. Additionally, the larger volume of anesthetic solution deposited in the orbit produces increased forward pressure on the eyeball, which some surgeons find objectionable. Eyelid ecchymoses occasionally appear. More serious complications have included peribulbar hemorrhage and perforation of the globe.

Recently, Feibel and colleagues[23] conducted a randomized, double-masked study of 317 patients and demonstrated that the incidence of postcataract ptosis is the same in both 2-injection peribulbar, or retrobulbar anesthesia. However, Esswein and von Noorden[21] retrospectively studied 9 patients with a permanent paresis of a vertical rectus muscle after cataract extraction. Peribulbar anesthesia was the most consistent feature in 7 of the 9 cases, and the authors postulated that permanent paresis of a vertical rectus muscle may be caused by a myotoxic effect of the local anesthetic. As typically performed, the peribulbar needle lies directly under the inferior rectus muscle and directly over the superior rectus muscle. To decrease the incidence of myotoxic complications when performing peribulbar injections, Esswein and von Noorden recommend avoiding the muscle belly, by injecting slightly medially and laterally to a vertical rectus muscle, using the lowest concentration and smallest quantity of local anesthetic needed to obtain analgesia and akinesia, injecting with a short, blunt-tipped needle, and waiting at least 30 minutes for effect before repeating injections.[21]

SENSORY NERVE BLOCKS

Frontal Nerve

The frontal nerve, while still in the orbit, divides into the supraorbital and supratrochlear nerves. A sensory frontal nerve block is very useful in adults undergoing frontalis suspensory surgery for ptosis repair. The block retains motility to the upper eyelid and globe, while providing sensory anesthesia to the upper eyelid and eyebrow. A local block can be performed on the frontal nerve within the orbit, or on its two branches near the orbit rim.

Frontal Nerve Block

A rigid 22-gauge, 4-cm needle is passed through the center of the eyelid just below the eyebrow and orbital margin. The needle is directed posteriorly, in a steplike fashion, along the roof of the orbit, until the entire 4-cm length of the needle has been passed (Fig. 17-13). This is the location where the frontal and lacrimal nerves enter the orbit. The needle is kept near the roof of the orbit to avoid penetration of the intermuscular septum, which would result in motor anesthesia of the levator and superior rectus muscles, as well as in sensory anesthesia. Not more than 0.5 ml of local anesthetic solution, with epinephrine but without hyaluronidase, is injected. Complications include penetration of the muscle cone and retrobulbar hemorrhage.

Supraorbital Nerve Block

The supraorbital nerve supplies the upper eyelid, the upper conjunctiva, the upper portion of the lacrimal fossa, the upper lacrimal duct, and the supraorbital portion of the forehead. The nerve runs from the superior orbital fissure immediately beneath the periorbita, along the orbital roof, to emerge from the orbit through the supraorbital foramen or notch. The notch is a separation in the superior orbital rim at the junction of its lateral 2/3 and medial 1/3, and is easily palpated. This landmark is on a line with the pupil when the eye is in the primary position. The nerve is blocked by inserting a needle through a skin wheal at the notch and injecting 2 to 3 ml of anesthesia solution (Fig. 17-14). Bleeding can occur from the accompanying supraorbital artery.

Supratrochlear Nerve Block

The supratrochlear nerve supplies the medial part of the upper eyelid, conjunctiva, and forehead. After branching from the frontal nerve, it runs medially to the supraorbital nerve just beneath the periorbita of the orbital roof. The nerve emerges from the orbit between the pulley (trochlea) of the superior oblique muscles and the supraorbital foramen or notch. The supratrochlear nerve can be blocked by inserting a needle 1 to 1.5 cm along the superomedial wall, just above the trochlea (Fig. 17-15). One to 1.5 ml of anesthetic is injected.

Nasociliary Nerve

The nasociliary branch of the ophthalmic nerve divides within the orbit into the anterior and posterior ethmoidal nerves and the infratrochlear nerve. The anterior ethmoidal nerve supplies the lateral wall of the nose in the area of the lacrimal fossa and the skin covering the ala nasi. The infratrochlear nerve runs just beneath the periorbita, along the medial orbital wall, and just above the medial rectus muscle. This nerve innervates the skin of the nose, the skin and the conjunctiva of the inner canthus, and the lacrimal sac. Infiltrative anesthesia of the infratrochlear and infraorbital (see following) nerves is used for surgery on the lacrimal sac (dacryocystorhinostomy).

Infratrochlear Nerve Block

The infratrochlear nerve is blocked by inserting a 25-gauge needle below the trochlea and just above the medial canthal ligament, along the medial orbital wall (Fig. 17-16). The needle is inserted to a depth of 2 to 2.5 cm, and 1.5 to 2.0 ml of anesthetic is injected. Introduction of the needle to a depth of 2.5 to 3.5 cm will also anesthetize the anterior ethmoidal nerve.

Terminal branches of the ophthalmic artery and small tributaries of the superior ophthalmic vein can be encountered

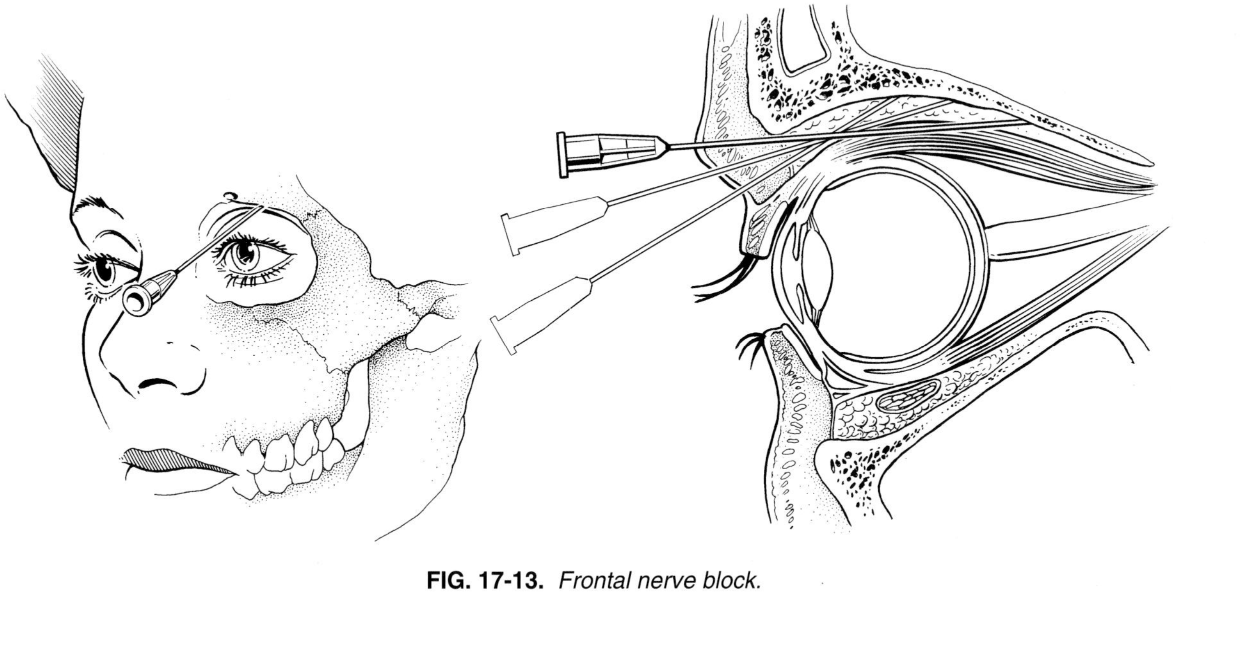

FIG. 17-13. *Frontal nerve block.*

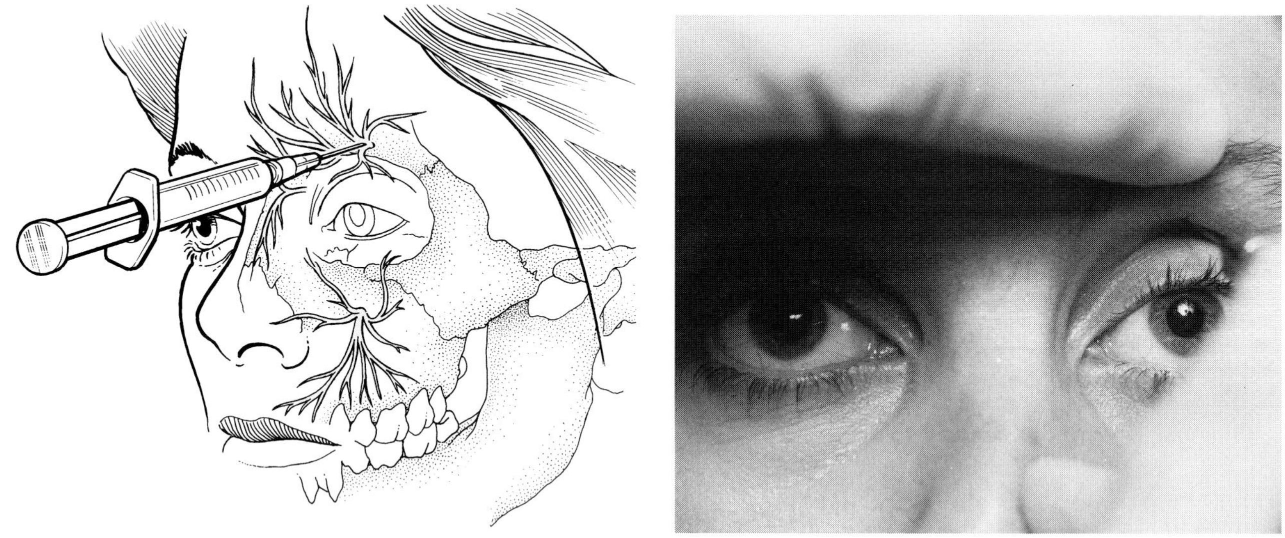

A B

FIG. 17-14. A: *Anatomy of Supraorbital nerve block.* **B:** *Supraorbital nerve block.* The needle is inserted at the supraorbital notch.

during an infratrochlear nerve block. Retrobulbar hemorrhage can occur in approximately 2% of blocks. If the hemorrhage is severe, the operation must be postponed.

Lacrimal Nerve

The lacrimal nerve is located at the superior part of the lateral orbital wall. The nerve supplies the lacrimal gland and the skin and conjunctiva of the lateral part of the upper eyelid. The nerve is anesthetized by introducing a 25-gauge needle through an intradermal wheal in the upper eyelid at the lateral wall of the orbit (Fig. 17-17). The needle is inserted along the lateral wall to a depth of 2.5 cm, and 2 ml of anesthetic solution is injected.

Maxillary Nerve

The maxillary nerve, the second division of the trigeminal nerve, runs through the orbit in the infraorbital groove. The nerve divides into the zygomatic and infraorbital nerves.

Zygomatic Nerve Block

The zygomatic nerve innervates the skin of the temporal area and the lateral wall of the orbit. Zygomaticotemporal and zygomaticofacial branches exit through small foramen in the zygomatic bone at the junction of the lateral and inferior orbital rims. Infiltrative anesthesia at these sites will block these nerves.

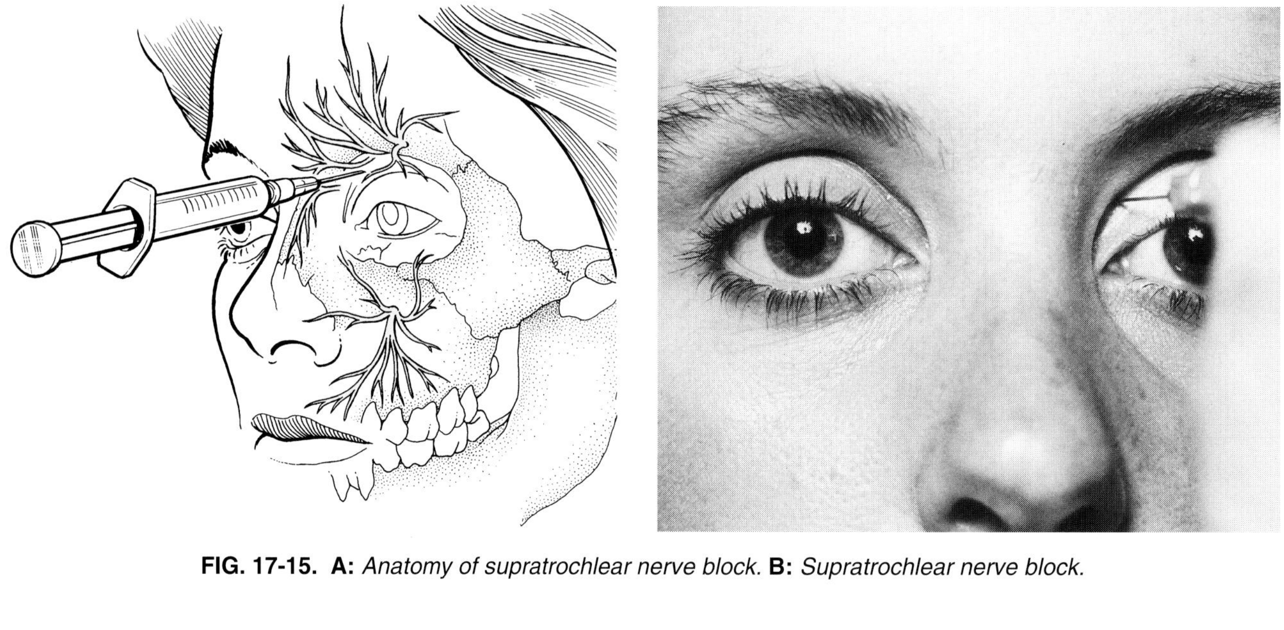

A B

FIG. 17-15. A: *Anatomy of supratrochlear nerve block.* **B:** *Supratrochlear nerve block.*

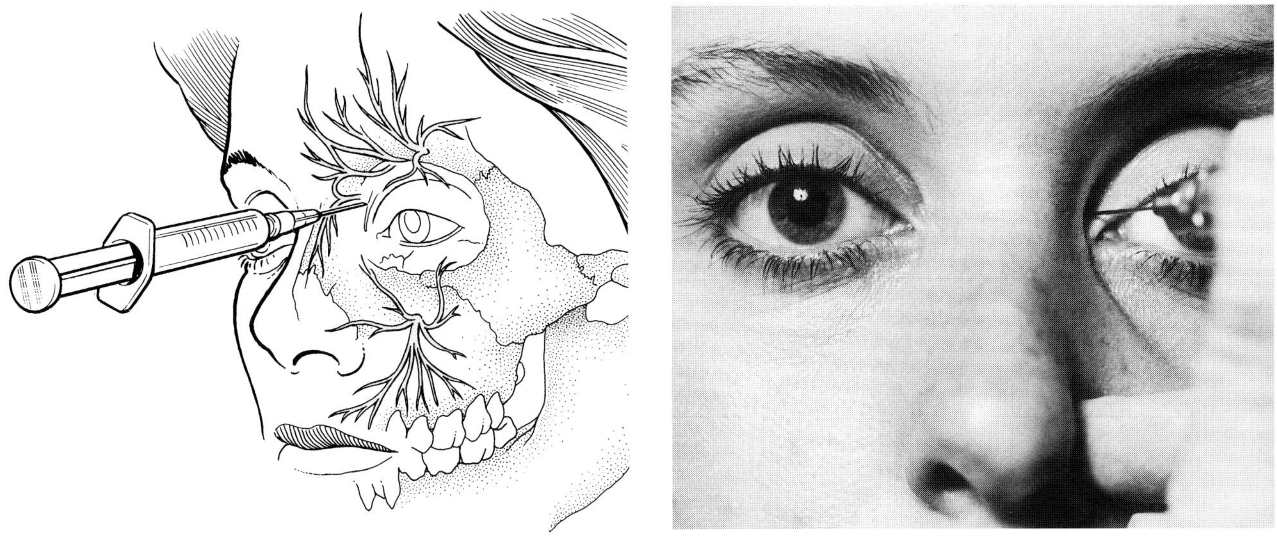

A B

FIG. 17-16. A: *Anatomy of infratrochlear nerve block.* B: *Infratrochlear nerve block.*

Infraorbital Nerve Block

The infraorbital nerve, within its canal, gives off alveolar nerves to the upper teeth, maxillary sinus, and nasal cavity. The infraorbital groove in the central orbital floor is bridged-over at its midportion to continue forward as the infraorbital canal. The nerve emerges on the face from the infraorbital foramen on the maxilla. The foramen is palpable as a small depression 1.5 cm below the inferior orbital rim. The foramen is on a line with the supraorbital notch and pupil. The nerve supplies the lower eyelid and cheek, inner canthus, and part of the lacrimal sac. Infraorbital combined with infratrochlear nerve block are used for dacryocystorhinostomy.

The infraorbital nerve can be blocked where it enters the canal on the orbital floor. A 2-ml injection of anesthetic is given along the floor, 1.0 to 1.5 cm behind the orbital rim. A block can also be done at the infraorbital foramen. The foramen is palpated on the maxilla, 1.5 cm below the orbital rim on a line with the supraorbital notch and pupil (Fig. 17-18). Anesthetic solution of 1.5 to 2.0 ml is injected at the external opening of the foramen or just within the canal.

Sub-Tenon's Space Block

Needle injection into sub-Tenon's space is made at the inferonasal aspect of the orbit. This produces better anesthesia

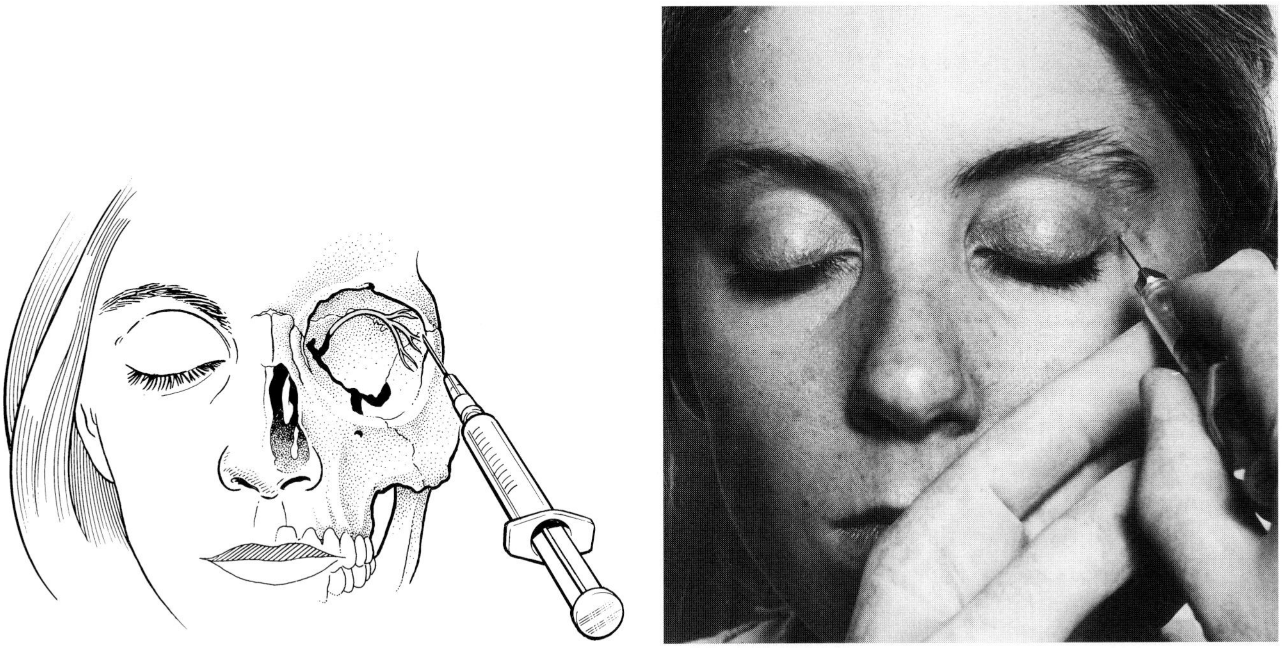

A B

FIG. 17-17. A: *Anatomy of lacrimal nerve block.* B: *Lacrimal nerve block.*

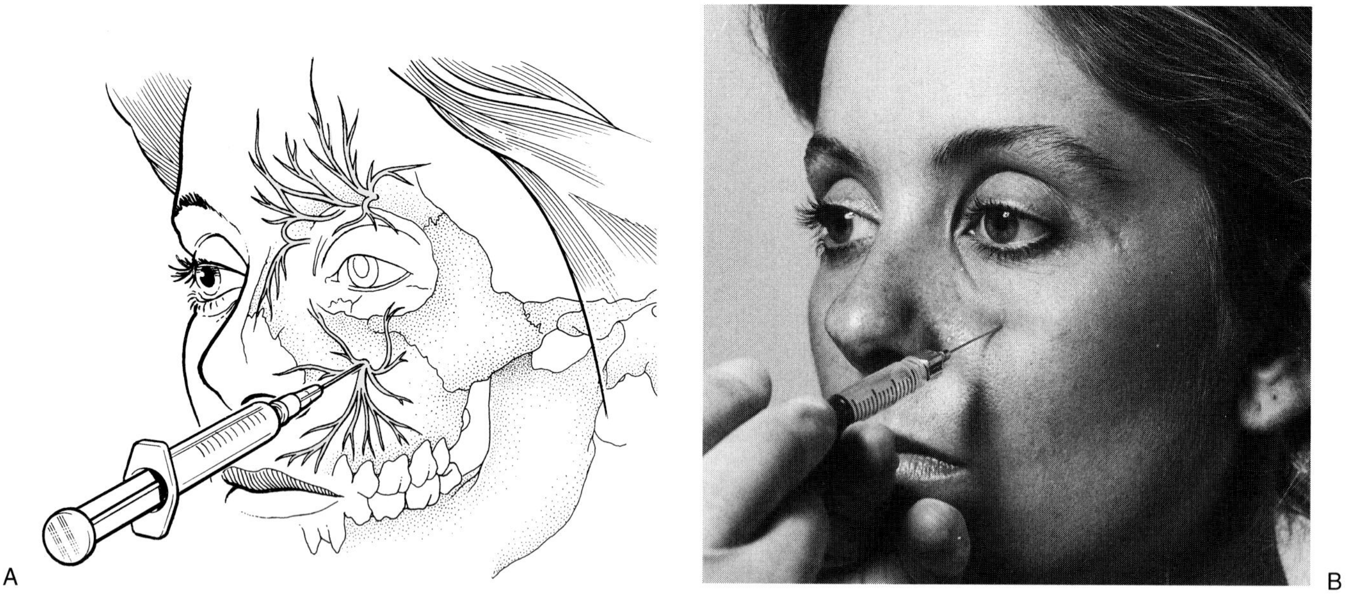

FIG. 17-18. A: *Anatomy of infra-orbital nerve block.* **B:** *Infra-orbital nerve block.*

of the iris and anterior segment than it does for subconjunctival injection. In the early 1990s, a new technique evolved[84] which employs infiltration of conjunctiva followed by opening up the sub-Tenon space with a pair of micro-scissors; then a blunt cannula is inserted and advanced about 1.7 cm, curving round the globe of the eye (Fig. 17-19). The degree of abolition of extraocular muscle movement is proportional to the volume and depth of injectate.

The anatomical basis of the sub-Tenon block is the fascial plane called Tenon's capsule. The extraocular muscles are connected by a sheet of condensed fascial tissue, and, external to this intermuscular septum, is a fascial plane, the Tenon's capsule. This capsule is a dense fascial layer which surrounds the globe of the eye and extraocular muscles all the way from the limbus to the optic nerve. A potential space exists between the sclera of the eye and Tenon's capsule. A small incision in conjunctiva 5 mm posterior to the limbus will pass through conjunctiva, Tenon's capsule and intermuscular septum. This gains access to the area known as sub-Tenon space.

Technique

Topical local anesthetic (Table 17-1) is applied to the cornea and conjunctiva, followed by one drop of epinephrine 0.1% (to reduce bleeding). The patient is asked to look out-

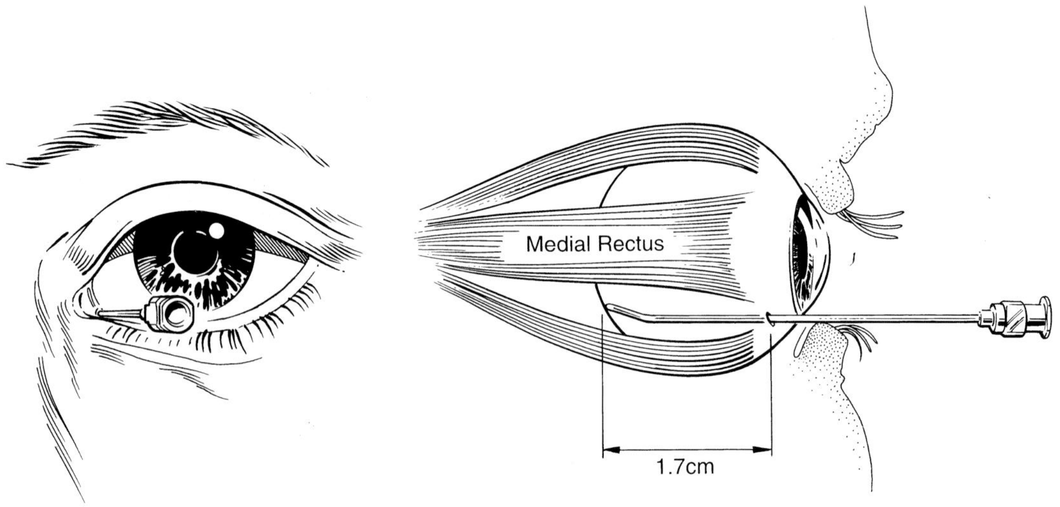

FIG. 17-19. *Sub-Tenon's space block.* Blunt Cannula (Southampton) is shown entering the conjunctiva at the inferonasal quadrant, approximately 5 mm from the limbus. An initial 'nick' in the conjunctiva is made to aid cannula insertion (see text). To aid access to the inferonasal conjunctiva, the patient is asked to look upwards and laterally with the eye to be blocked: This also aids passage of the blunt cannula. The final position of the cannula is shown in this figure with the eye in the anatomical position, to facilitate visualization of relationship of cannula to orbit.

wards and upwards with the eye to be blocked; this helps with access to the conjunctiva in the inferonasal quadrant, 5 mm from the limbus. At this point a blunt ophthalmological scissors (Wescott) is used to make a small 'nick' in the conjunctiva, and then a blunt Southampton curved cannula is used to deliver a small bleb of local anesthetic; this helps to elevate the Tenon's fascia. Moorfield's forceps are then used to grip the incised conjunctival edge, and the curved cannula is inserted onto bare sclera. The cannula is then glided along a path following the contour of the globe, until posterior to the equator, at a depth of about 1.7 cm from the limbus. Passage posterior to the equator may be aided by injecting 1 ml of local anesthetic at the level of the equator. A further 3 to 3.5 ml is injected posteriorly, depending on the size of the globe. Solution diffuses to cover the nerve supply of the cornea and conjunctiva, with variable cover of the nerve supply of extraocular muscles. Since there is no true separation of compartments in the orbit, solution may also diffuse into the intracone (retrobulbar) area.

ACKNOWLEDGMENT

The authors wish to thank Ms. Jacki Fitzpatrick for her expert assistance in typing the manuscript.

REFERENCES

1. Ahn, J.C., and Stanley, J.A.: Subarachnoid injection as a complication of retrobulbar anesthesia., Am. J. Ophthalmol., *103:*225, 1987.
2. Al-Abrak, M.H., and Samuel, J.R.: Effects of general anesthesia on intraocular pressure in man. Br. J. Ophthalmol., *58:*806, 1974.
3. Aldrete, J.A., Roma-Salas, F., Arora, S., *et al.*: Reverse arterial blood flow as a pathway for central nervous system toxic responses following injection of local anesthetics. Anesth. Analg., *57:*428, 1978.
4. Alexander, J.P.: Reflex disturbances of cardiac rhythm during ophthalmic surgery. Br. J. Ophthalmol., *59:*518, 1975.
5. Anderson, R.L.: The blepharocardiac reflex. Arch. Ophthalmol., *12:*56, 1978.
6. Atkinson, W.S.: Retrobulbar injection of anesthetic within the muscle cone. Arch Ophthalmol., *16:*494, 1936.
7. Atkinson, W.S.: Akinesia of the orbicularis. Am. J. Ophthalmol., *36:* 1255, 1953.
8. Berler, D.K.: Oculocardiac reflex. Am. J. Ophthalmol., *12*:56, 1963.
9. Bosomworth, P.P., Ziegler, C.H.: The oculocardiac reflex in eye muscle surgery. Anesthesiology, *19:*7, 1958.
10. Breslin, P.P.: Mortality in ophthalmic surgery. Int. Ophthalmol. Clin., *13*(2): Summer 1975.
11. Carlson, B.M., Emerich, S., Komorowski, T.E., Rainin, E.A., and Shepard, B.M.: Extraocular muscle regeneration in primates. Ophthalmology, *99:*582, 1992.
12. Chin, G.N., and Almquist, H.T.: Bupivacaine and lidocaine retrobulbar anesthesia: A double-blind clinical study. Ophthalmic Surg., *90:*369, 1983.
13. Cibis, P.A.: General discussion: Opening remarks. *In* Schepens, C.L., and Regan, C.D.J., (eds.): Controversial Aspects in the Management of Retinal Detachment. pp. 222. Boston: Little, Brown 1965.
14. Cofer, H.F.: Cord paralysis after Nadbath facial nerve block. Arch. Ophthalmol., *104:*337, 1986.
15. Cowley, M., Campochiaro, P.A., Newman, S.A., and Fogle, J.A.: Retinal vascular occlusion without retrobulbar or optic nerve sheath hemorrhage after retrobulbar injection of lidocaine. Ophthalmic Surg., *19:* 859, 1988.
16. Davis, D.B., and Mandel, M.R.: Posterior peribulbar anesthesia: An alternative to retrobulbar anesthesia. J. Cataract Refract Surg., *12:*182, 1986.
17. Donlon, J.V., Jr., and Moss, J.: Plasma catecholamine levels during local anesthesia for cataract operations. Anesthesiology., *51:*471, 1979.
18. Duker, J.S., Belmont, J.B., Benson, W.E., *et al.*: Inadvertent globe perforation during retrobulbar and peribulbar anesthesia: Patient characteristics, surgical management, and visual outcome. Ophthalmology, *98:*519, 1991.
19. Duncalf, D., Gartner, S., and Carol, B.: Mortality in association with ophthalmic surgery. Am. J. Ophthalmol., *69:*610, 1970.
20. Ellis, P.P.: Retrobulbar injections. Surv. Ophthamol., *18:*425, 1974.
21. Esswein, M.B., and von Noorden, G.K.: Paresis of a vertical rectus muscle after cataract extraction. Am. J. Ophthalmol., *116:*424, 1993.
22. Everett, W.G., Vey, E.K., and Veenis, C.Y.: Factors in reducing ocular tension prior to intraocular surgery. Trans. Am. Acad. Ophthalmol. Otolaryngols., *63:*286, 1959.
23. Feibel, R.M., Custer, P.L., and Gordon, M.O.: Postcataract ptosis: A randomized, double-masked comparison of peribulbar and retrobulbar anesthesia. Ophthalmology, *100:*660, 1993.
24. Feitl, M.E., and Krupin, T.: Retrobulbar anesthesia. Ophthalmol. Clin. North Am., *3*(1):83, 1990.
25. Ferrari, L.R., and Donlon, J.V.: A comparison of propofol, midazolam, and methohexital for sedation during retrobulbar and peribulbar block. J. Clin. Anesth., *4:*93, 1992.
26. Fichman, R.: American Society of Cataract and Refractive Surgery Meeting. April 1992.
27. Foster, A.H., and Carlson, B.M.: Myotoxicity of local anesthetics and regeneration of damaged muscle fibers. Anesth. Analg. *58:*727, 1980.
28. Gay, G.R., and Loper, K.A.: Control of cocaine-induced hypertension with labetalol. Anesth. Analg., *67:*92, 1988.
29. Grizzard, W.S., Kirk, N.M., Pavan, P.R., *et al.*: Perforating ocular injuries caused by anesthesia personnel. Ophthalmology, *98:*1011, 1991.
30. Hall, D.L., Steen, W.H., Drummond, J.W., and Byrd, W.A.: Anticoagulants and cataract surgery. Ophthalmic Surg., *19:*221, 1988.
31. Hamilton, R.C.: Techniques of orbital regional anaesthesia Br. J. Anaesth., *75:*88, 1995.
32. Hamilton, R.C., Gimbel, H.V., and Strunin, L.: Regional anaesthesia for 12,000 cataract extraction and intraocular lens implantation procedures. Can. J. Anaesth., *35:*615, 1988.
33. Hamilton, R.C.: Brain-stem anesthesia as a complication of regional anesthesia for ophthalmic surgery. Can. J. Ophthalmol., *27:*323, 1992.
34. Hirschberg, J.: History of Ophthalmology. 284, 1910.
35. Horgan, J.: Atropine and ventricular tachyarrhythmias. J.A.M.A., *223:* 693, 1973.
36. Hustead, R.F., and Hamilton, R.C.: Pharmacology. *In* Gills, J.P., Hustead, R.F., and Sanders, D.R., (eds.): Ophthalmic Anesthesia. pp. 69. Thorofare, New Jersey, Slack, Inc., 1993.
37. Ivankovich, A.D., and Lowe, H.J.: Influence of methoxyflurane and neuroleptanesthesia on intraocular pressure in man. Anesth. Analg., *48:* 933, 1969.
38. Johnson, R.W.: Anatomy for ophthalmic anesthesia. Br. J. Anaesth., *75:*80—87, 1995.
39. Joshi, C., and Bruce, D.L.: Thiopental and succinylcholine: Action on intraocular pressure. Anesth. Analg., *54:*471, 1975.
40. Kaplan, I.J., Jaffee, N.S., and Clayman, H.M.: Ptosis and cataract surgery. Ophthalmology, *92:*237, 1985.
41. Katsev, D.A., Drews, R.C., and Rose, B.T.: An anatomic study of retrobulbar needle path length. Ophthalmology, *96:*1221, 1989.
42. Kirsch, R.E., Samet, P., Kuzel, V., *et al.*: Electrocardiographic changes during ocular surgery and their prevention by retrobulbar injection. Arch. Ophthalmol., *58:*348, 1957.
43. Klein, M.I., Jampol, L.M., Condon, P.I., Rice, T.A., *et al.*: Central retinal artery occlusion without retrobulbar hemorrhage after retrobulbar anesthesia. Am. J. Ophthalmol., *93:*573, 1982.
44. Knapp, H.: On cocaine and its use in ophthalmic and general surgery. Arch. Ophthalmol., *13:*402, 1884.
45. Leopold, I.H., and Comroe, I.H.: Effect of intramuscular administration of morphine, atropine, scopolamine, and neostigmine on the human eye. Arch. Ophthalmol., *40:*285, 1948.
46. Libelius, R., Sonesson, B., Stamenovic, B.A., and Thesleff, S.: Denervation-like changes in skeletal muscle after treatment with a local anesthetic. J. Anat., *106:*297, 1970.
47. Liu, C., Youl, B., and Moseley, I.: Magnetic resonance imaging of the optic nerve in extremes of gaze: Implications for the positioning of the globe for retrobulbar anaesthesia. Br. J. Ophthalmol., *76:*728, 1992.
48. Loots, J.H., Koorts, A.S., and Venter, J.A.: Peribulbar anesthesia: A prospective statistical analysis of the efficacy and predictability of bupivacaine and lignocaine bupivacaine mixture. J. Cataract Refract. Surg., *19:*728, 1993.
49. Lynch, S., Wolf, G.L., and Berlin, I.: General anesthesia for cataract

surgery: A comparative review of 2,217 consecutive cases. Anesth. Analg., *53:*909, 1974.
50. Marr, W.G., Wood, R., Senterfit, L., and Sigelman, S.: Effect of topical anesthetics on regeneration of the corneal epithelium. Am. J. Ophthalmol., *43:*606, 1957.
51. Masket, S., (ed.). Consultation section. J. Cataract Refract. Surg., *17:* 854, 1991.
52. Massumi, R.A., Mason, D.T., Amsterdam, E.A., *et al.*: Ventricular fibrillation and tachycardia after intravenous atropine for treatment of bradycardias. N. Engl. J. Med., *287:*336, 1972.
53. McGoldrick, K.E.: Transient left bundle branch block during local anesthesia. Anesthesiol. Rev., *8* (6):36, 1981.
54. McGoldrick, K.E.: Pediatric ophthalmic surgery: Anesthetic considerations. *In*: McGoldrick, K.E. (ed.): Anesthesia for Ophthalmic and Otolaryngologic Surgery. pp. 190–209. Philadelphia, W.B. Saunders, 1992.
55. McGoldrick, K.E.: Ocular pathology and systemic diseases: Anesthetic implications. *In*: McGoldrick, K.E (ed.): Anesthesia for Ophthalmic and Otolaryngologic Surgery. pp. 210—234. Philadelphia, W.B. Saunders, 1992.
56. McMahan, I.B.: Anticoagulants and cataract surgery. J. Cataract Refract Surg., *14:*569, 1988.
57. Meyers, E.F., and Tomeldan, S.A.: Glycopyrrolate compared with atropine in prevention of the oculocardiac reflex during eye muscle surgery. Anesthesiology, *51:*350, 1979.
58. Meyers, E.F.: Cocaine toxicity during dacryocystorhinostomy. Arch. Ophthalmol., *98:*842, 1980.
59. Meyers, E.F., Ramirez, R.C., Boniu, K.I.: Grand mal seizures after retrobulbar block. Arch. Ophthalmol., *96:*847, 1978.
60. Mirakhur, R.K., Shepherd, W.F.I., and Darrah, W.C.: Propofol and thiopentone: Effects on intraocular pressure associated with induction of anaesthesia and tracheal intubation (facilitated with suxamethonium). Br. J. Anaesth., *59:*431, 1987.
61. Moonie, G.T., Rees, D.I., and Elton, D.: Oculocardiac reflex during strabismus surgery. Can. Anaesth. Soc. J., *11:*621, 1964.
62. Morgan, C.M., Schatz, H., Vine, A.K.M., *et al.*: Ocular complications associated with retrobulbar injections. Ophthalmology, *95:*660, 1988.
63. Nadbath, R.P., and Rehman, I.: Facial nerve block. Am. J. Ophthalmol., *55:*143, 1963.
64. Nicoll, J.M.V., Acharya, P.A., Ahlen, K., *et al.*: Central nervous system complications after 6,000 retrobulbar blocks. Anesth. Analg., *66:*1298, 1987.
65. Nicoll, J.M.V., Acharya, P.A., Edge, K.R., *et al.*: Shivering following retrobulbar block. Can. J. Anaesth., *35:*671, 1988.
66. O'Brien, C.S.: Akinesia during cataract extraction. Arch. Ophthalmol., *1:*447, 1929.
67. Ortiz, M., Vallis, R., Vallés, J., Blanco, D., and Vidal, F.: Topography of peribulbar anesthesia. Reg. Anesth., *20:*337, 1995.
68. Petruscak, J., Smith, R.B., and Breslin, P.P.: Mortality related to ophthalmological surgery. Arch. Ophthalmol., *89:*106, 1973.
69. Quigley, H.A.: Mortality associated with ophthalmic surgery. Am. J. Ophthalmol., *77:*518, 1974.
70. Rainin, E.A., and Carlson, B.M.: Postoperative diplopia and ptosis: A clinical hypothesis on the myotoxicity of local anesthetics. Arch. Ophthalmol., *102:*1337, 1985.
71. Ramoska, E., and Sacchetti, A.D.: Propranolol-induced hypertension in treatment of cocaine intoxication. Ann. Emerg. Med., *14:*1112, 1985.
72. Ramsay, R.C., and Knobloch, W.H.: Ocular perforatiion following retrobulbar anesthesia for retinal detachment surgery. Am. J. Ophthalmol., *86:*61, 1978.
73. Rao, V.A., and Kawatra, V.K.: Ocular myotoxic effects of local anesthetics. Can. J. Ophthalmol., *23:*171, 1988.
74. Robinson, G.A., and Nylander, A.: Warfarin and cataract extraction. Br. J. Ophthalmol., *73:*702, 1989.
75. Rappolt, R.T., Gay, G.R., and Inaba, D.S.: Propranolol in the treatment of cardiopressor effects of cocaine. N. Engl. J. Med., *295:*448, 1976.
76. Rubin, A.P.: Complications of local anesthesia for ophthalmic surgery. Br. J. Anaesth., *75:*93, 1995.
77. Shantha, T.R.: The relationship of retrobulbar local anesthetic spread to the neural membranes of the eyeball, optic nerve and arachnoid villi in the optic nerve (abstract). Anesthesiology, *73:*A850, 1990.
78. Schenck, N.L.: Cocaine: Its use and misuse in otolaryngology. Trans. Am. Acad. Ophthalmol. Otolaryngol., *80:*343, 1975.
79. Smith, R.B., Douglas, H., and Petruscak, J.: The oculocardiac reflex and sinoatrial arrest. Can. Anaesth. Soc. J., 19:138, 1972.
80. Smith, R.: Cataract extraction without retrobulbar injection. Br. J. Ophthalmol., *205:*107, 1990.
81. Stanley, J.A.: Subarachnoid injection of retrobulbar anesthetic as a complication of retrobulbar block. Saudi Bull. Ophthalmol., 2:13, 1987.
82. Starrels, M., Krupin, T., and Burde, R.M.: Bell's palsy and intraocular pressure. Ann. Ophthalmol., *7:*1067, 1975.
83. Steer, J.H., Mastaglia, F.L., Papadimitriou, J.M., and Bruggen, I.V.: Bupivacaine-induced muscle injury: The role of extracellular calcium. I. Neurol. Sci., *75:*205, 1986.
84. Stevens, J.D.: A new local anaesthesia technique for cataract extraction by one quadrant sub-Tenon's infiltration. Br. J. Ophthalmol., *76:*670, 1992.
85. Steward, D.J.: Anticholinergic premedication for infants and children. Can. Anaesth. Soc. J., *30:*325, 1983.
86. Sullivan, K.L., Brown, G.C., Forman, A.R., *et al.*: Retrobulbar anesthesia and retinal vascular obstruction. Ophthalmology, 90:373, 1983.
87. Taylor, C., Wilson, F.M., Roesch, R.: *et al.*: Prevention of the oculocardiac reflex in children: Comparison of retrobulbar block and intravenous atropine. Anesthesiology, *24:*646, 1963.
88. Unsöld, R., Stanley, J.A., and De Groot, J.: The CT-topography of retrobulbar anesthesia: Anatomic-clinical correlation of complications and suggestions of a modified technique. Albrecht von Graefes Arch. Klin. Exp. Ophthalmol, *217:*125, 1981.
89. van Lint, A.: Paralysie palpebrale temporaire provoquée par l'opération de la câtaracte. Ann. Ocul., (Paris), *151:*420, 1914.
90. Waller, S.G., Taboada, J., and O'Connor, P.: Retrobulbar anesthesia risk: Do sharp needles really perforate the eye more easily than blunt needles? Ophthalmology., *100:*506, 1993.
91. Warwick, R., (ed.). Wolff's Anatomy of the Eye and Orbit, 7th ed. Philadelphia, W.B. Saunders, 1977.
92. Williamson, C.H.: Cataract keratotomy with topical anesthesia. Ocular Surg News., *10*(15):44, 1992.
93. Williamson, C.H.: Clear corneal incision with topical anesthesia. *In* Gills, J.P., Hustead, R.F., and Sanders, D.R., (eds.): *Ophthalmic Anesthesia.* pp. 176. Thorofare, New Jersey, Slack, Inc., 1993.
94. Wilson, C.A., and Ruiz, R.S.: Respiratory obstruction following the Nadbath facial nerve block, Arch. Ophthalmol., *103:*1454, 1985.
95. Wittpenn, J.R., Rapoza, P., Sternberg, P., *et al.*: Respiratory arrest following retrobulbar anesthesia. Ophthalmology, *93:*867, 1986.
96. Yagiela, J.A., Benoit, P.W., Buoncristiani, R.D., *et al.*: Comparison of myotoxic effects of lidocaine with epinephrine in rats and humans. Anesth. Analg., *60:*471, 1981.
97. Zahl, K., Jordan, A., McGroarty, J., Gotta, A.W.: pH adjusted bupivacaine and hyaluronidase for peribulbar block. Anesthesiology, *72:*230, 1990.

Neural Blockade in Clinical Anesthesia and Management of Pain, Third Edition,
edited by M.J. Cousins and P.O. Bridenbaugh.
Lippincott–Raven Publishers, Philadelphia © 1998.

CHAPTER 18

Neural Blockade for Obstetrics and Gynecologic Surgery

Peter Brownridge, Sheila E. Cohen and M. Elizabeth Ward

NEURAL BLOCKADE FOR OBSTETRICS

An optimum obstetric anaesthesia and analgesia service is one which provides all forms of anaesthesia and analgesia for all women who wish or require such a service at all times.

Report of the National Medical Consultative Committee for Scotland, 1985.

Neural blockade plays an important role in modern obstetric practice. This reflects the needs of both consumers and obstetricians, since the main indications for neural blockade are to relieve pain and to provide conditions for an operative delivery. It is not surprising, therefore, that in many units a majority of women receive neural blockade at some stage during childbirth. While peripheral techniques are satisfactory for certain obstetric procedures, by far the best conditions, for practically all contingencies, can be met by using epidural and/or spinal blockade. Central neural blockade has become so well established because of its greater *safety,* compared with general anesthesia, when surgical delivery is required, and far better pain relief for labor compared with alternative analgesic techniques.

The proportion of babies born by cesarean section has risen during recent years to reach 20 to 25% in many centers. The need for anesthesia has increased accordingly. General anesthesia is relatively hazardous among the obstetric population, however, because pregnant patients sometimes are, unpredictably, more difficult to intubate, and they are also more prone to pulmonary aspiration. Despite considerable success in prevention of anesthesia-related maternal mortality in both the United Kingdom and the United States of America (anesthesia currently accounting for approximately 3 to 4% of maternal deaths in those countries), airway problems are still the most frequent cause of death directly due to anesthesia.[161,162,253] Risk appears greatest among women who require urgent anesthesia and who are already in labor. Neural blockade is safer than general anesthesia, because the patient's protective airway reflexes are maintained (provided consciousness is not lost) and intubation can be avoided. For these reasons, it has been recommended that regional anesthesia should be used whenever possible for emergency cesarean section.[161] The same recommendation applies equally to other obstetric procedures, like instrumental delivery and manual removal of the placenta.

Apart from safety considerations, there are other benefits associated with neural blockade for an operative delivery: both mother and partner can witness the birth; the baby is free from anesthetic drug depression; and the postoperative course is usually smoother and more pleasant for the mother.[426] Since the last edition of *Neural Blockade,* there have been several refinements in the management of cesarean section under regional anesthesia. These refinements, designed to improve both the quality and safety of anesthesia during an operative delivery, will be discussed later in the chapter. The relative merits of epidural versus spinal anesthesia also have become more clearly defined and there appears to be growing interest in deliberately combining both techniques.

Central neural blockade during labor not only provides unsurpassed analgesia, but allows the mother to be alert and co-operative.[514] This is a distinct advantage over systemic opioids and inhalation agents, which invariably are associated with clouding of consciousness and dysphoria. Central neural blockade also obtunds many of the adverse physiological responses to pain during labor and at cesarean section. Finally, central neural blockade can be adapted to meet changing obstetric needs once a catheter is introduced into the epidural or subarachnoid space.

P. Brownridge: Department of Anaesthesia and Intensive Care, Flinders Medical Center, The Flinders University of South Australia, Adelaide, South Australia 5042 Australia.

S.E. Cohen: Department of Anesthesia, Stanford University School of Medicine, Stanford, California 94305.

M.E. Ward: Department of Anaesthesia and Pain Management, Royal North Shore Hospital, University of Sydney, St. Leonards, New South Wales 2065 Australia.

Considering that continuous caudal analgesia for labor was introduced by Hingson and Edwards in 1942, it is surprising that the full potential of epidural analgesia has been exploited only in recent years. It is now universally accepted that perfectly satisfactory analgesia can be achieved during labor, using local anesthetic doses substantially less than those required for surgery. This avoids many of the unwanted side effects of traditional, dense, neural blockade. After all, the principal aim of neural blockade in labor is not to abolish sensation but to relieve suffering, preferably with as few side-effects as possible. Ideally, the degree of analgesia should be determined by the individual herself, with the most satisfactory results achieved when the patient can exercise some control over her analgesic requirements. This demand for flexibility in pain management has implications both in terms of drug choice (e.g., local anesthetic, opioid, alpha adrenergic agonist) and in drug delivery technique (e.g., intermittent injection, continuous infusion, or patient-controlled). Several regimens will be discussed in more detail later in the chapter.

The reason neural blockade is so commonly required, or requested, during childbirth and why it should be accessible to *all* parturients is apparent, and implies that an anesthesiologist must be readily available to all obstetric units (not just to provide anesthesia and analgesia, but also to provide resuscitation in obstetric emergencies). Unfortunately, financial and organizational constraints make such a proposition impractical in many units, particularly small ones. Despite recommendations from advisory bodies that there should be an epidural service in all specialist obstetric units,[568] a recent survey in the United Kingdom has shown that epidural analgesia is not available to all women who wish for it, or for whom it is recommended on medical grounds.[260] The survey revealed a five-fold difference in the use of epidural analgesia and indicated that unduly low rates were a reflection of inappropriate resource allocation, sociocultural variations, lack of trained staff, and lack of motivation for providing the services. If there are limitations in the range of services available, then at least these should be made known to the parturient before she arranges her place of delivery. She may prefer to go elsewhere!

While neural blockade is not entirely free of hazard among the obstetric population, most associated life-threatening complications (systemic toxicity, cardiac arrest, high spinal block, profound hypotension) are avoidable and/or treatable when proper procedures are followed. Non-fatal, yet still serious, complications (infection, neurological damage, persistent severe backache) appear to be extremely rare,[146,549] although there are no large, long-term, prospective studies available to provide an accurate assessment of the degree of risk. Less serious complications, such as dural puncture headache or mild backache, are more common, but usually resolve spontaneously or respond to simple treatment. The incidence of complications is often related to inexperience and/or a failure to meet proper standards of safety and supervision.

Experience has shown that the best results are achieved when the anesthesiologist is an integral member of the obstetric team.[428] The anesthesiologist should be experienced in obstetric anesthesia, have a firm grasp of physiologic and pharmacologic principles, and be aware of the myriad of medical complications which can arise during childbirth. Whenever possible, each unit should have an anesthesiologist appointed to formulate policies and guidelines, supervise teaching and training, organize a quality assurance program, arrange educational meetings, and form a liaison with other disciplines responsible for obstetric care. Deficiencies in communication (e.g., if the anesthesiologist was given insufficient notification about a potential clinical problem) often contribute to complications and should be audited.

Ideally, there should be broad agreement among attending medical and nursing staff regarding attitudes towards pain relief. It is confusing for patients when they receive conflicting information and advice about analgesia from different sources. In the absence of contraindications to a particular technique, the choice of pain relief should lie predominantly with the mother herself. Distribution of well-prepared, impartial information about pain relief should be an integral part of prenatal education. Such information can be conveyed in prenatal education classes and informal discussion

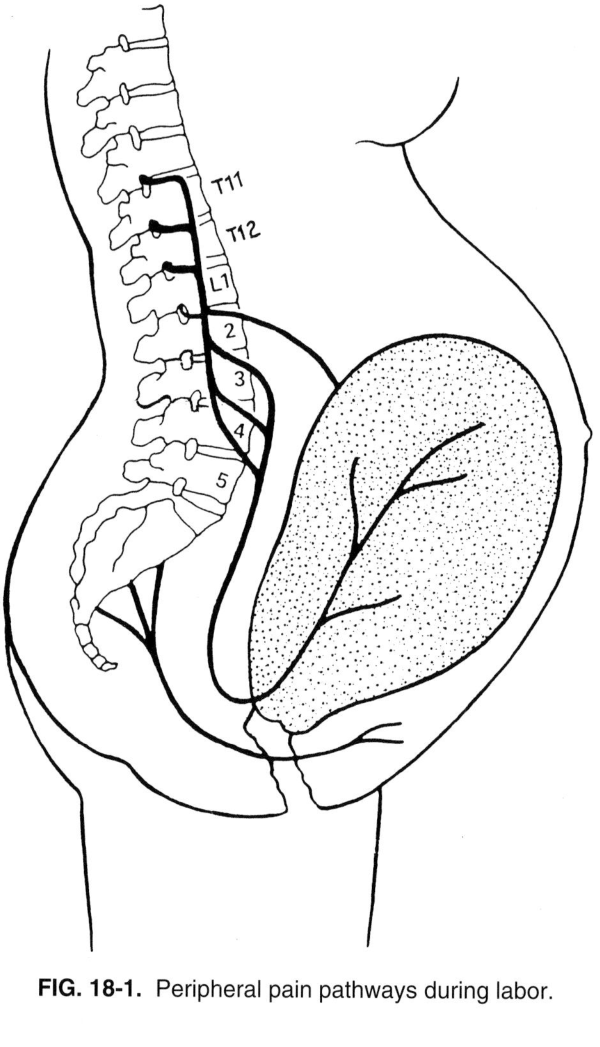

FIG. 18-1. Peripheral pain pathways during labor.

groups, booklets, and audiovisual productions. Prenatal education classes provide an ideal opportunity for the anesthesiologist to inform and reassure mothers about pharmacologic pain relief. These occasions are also educational for the anesthesiologist, who hears first-hand about the issues that concern child-bearing women.

PERIPHERAL PAIN PATHWAYS DURING LABOR

The peripheral pain pathways involved during labor were described first by Cleland in 1933.[120] It is convenient to discuss separately the pain associated with the first and second stages of labor, since these pathways are quite different (Fig. 18-1).

First Stage of Labor

Pain in the early parts of the first stage of labor is predominantly of visceral origin, secondary to uterine contractions and dilatation of the cervix. The intensity of pain is related to the strength of the contraction and the pressure thus generated. Noxious impulses from the cervix and uterus are transmitted by afferent nerves that accompany sympathetic pathways through, in turn, the pelvic, inferior, middle, and superior hypogastric plexuses; the lumbar sympathetic chain; the white rami of the spinal nerves of T10 to L1; and the posterior roots of these nerves to the cord. Pelvic parasympathetic innervation is not thought to be of any importance in the mediation of uterocervical pain.

In common with other forms of visceral pain, contraction pain is poorly localized and is referred to the abdomen, lower back and rectum. Low backache during the first stage of labor is almost certainly referred pain via the dorsal rami of T10 to L1, of which the lateral branches descend before becoming superficial and supplying the skin some 10 cm caudal to their spinal origin.[54,612] In addition to the pain of uterine contraction, descent of the fetal head into the pelvis in the latter part of the first stage causes pressure on pelvic structures and the roots of the lumbosacral plexus, producing pain via segments L2 and below. Thus, pain is often felt in the thighs, legs (L2–S1) and rectum, and is completely relieved only when neural blockade extends to the lower sacral nerve roots.

The fact that only three or four pairs of spinal nerve roots are involved in the mediation of uterine contraction pain makes the upper lumbar region of the spinal canal particularly suited for neural blockade in the first stage of labor.

Second Stage of Labor

Pain produced by stretching of the lower birth canal and perineum is transmitted by way of the pudendal nerve, de-

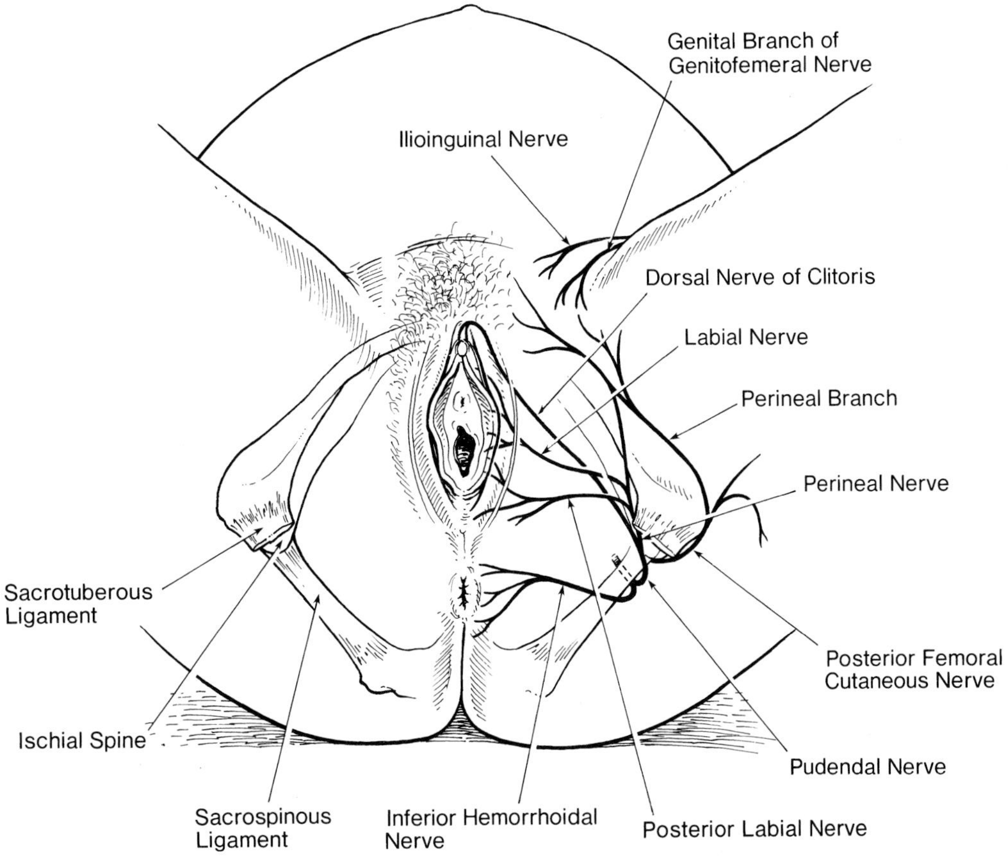

FIG. 18-2. Nerve supply to the perineum.

rived from the second, third, and fourth sacral nerves. Since this is a somatic nerve, pain experienced during delivery is intense and sharply localized. The pudendal nerve passes posteriorly to the junction of the ischial spine and sacrospinous ligament, and anteriorly to the sacrotuberous ligament. Successful pudendal block provides analgesia of the posterior 2/3 of the labia and of the perineum, including the anus (Fig. 18-2). The anterior third of the labia majora is supplied by the genitofemoral nerve.

APPLIED PHYSIOLOGY

Changes in respiratory, cardiovascular, and gastrointestinal function during pregnancy have particular implications for obstetric neural blockade. Only those relevant to the conduct of regional anesthesia are discussed here.

Respiratory Changes

Oxygen consumption increases during pregnancy by approximately 20% at term and is often doubled during labor.[493,538] This increase during pregnancy, however, is more than adequately compensated for by a 70% rise in alveolar ventilation.[151] Consequently, maternal $PaCO_2$ decreases to 30 to 32 mm Hg and a respiratory alkalosis develops with decreased plasma bicarbonate and buffering capacity. During labor, further hyperventilation occurs in response to pain[208] causing considerable hypocarbia and worsening of the respiratory alkalosis.[537] Minute volumes of 90 L per minute have been recorded during delivery.[125]

Despite upward displacement of the diaphragm by the gravid uterus, vital capacity, total lung capacity and inspiratory reserve volume remain unaltered.[584] This is because an increase in thoracic cage circumference adequately compensates for any diaphragmatic displacement. There is, however, a reduction in expiratory reserve volume (ERV) and functional residual capacity (FRC)[151] which is sufficient to cause some degree of airway closure in 50% of mothers at term in the supine position during normal tidal ventilation.[47,534] Obesity, recumbency and the lithotomy position aggravate this effect further.

There are several clinical implications of these respiratory changes for the anesthesiologist. As discussed later in this chapter, central neural blockade causes a progressive decrease in forced expiratory volume in 1 sec (FEV_1), forced vital capacity (FVC) and peak expiratory flow rate (PEFR) during cesarean section which may compromise the ability to cough effectively or clear inhaled vomit.[131,251]

1. In late gestation, the increase in pulmonary venous admixture, secondary to airway closure, may lead to a below normal PaO_2. This is particularly so in recumbent, obese patients. Stenger et al.,[573] for example, have shown lower maternal PaO_2 values and a wider scatter than in non-pregnant women of the same age. Oxygen supplementation must always be available for obstetric patients and should be used routinely during operative deliveries.
2. The increased oxygen requirements, combined with a diminished FRC, mean that hypoxemia occurs very rapidly in the presence of hypoventilation or apnea. It is important to recall that the degree of change in PaO_2 with ventilation follows a series of hyperbolic curves, depending on oxygen consumption (Fig. 18-3).[454] Thus, at an oxygen utilization of 400 ml per minute, PaO_2 shows a rapid decline once alveolar ventilation falls below approximately 7 L per minute. If controlled ventilation is required during pregnancy, a higher than usual minute volume is needed. Caution is also required whenever regional analgesia is performed following parenteral or inhalation analgesia, since the onset of effective pain relief may unmask their depressant effects on ventilation.
3. Hyperventilation and hypocarbia may reduce perfusion of certain organs. Cerebral blood flow, for example, is extremely sensitive to $PaCO_2$ changes, and hypocarbia is commonly associated with symptoms such as dizziness, disorientation, and light-headedness. Uterine and umbilical artery perfusion also may be reduced in the presence of extreme hypocarbia, thus contributing to the development of fetal acidemia.
4. Respiratory alkalosis can cause paresthesias and even frank tetany secondary to hypocalcemia. Prolonged acute hypocarbia also results in diminished plasma bicarbonate and buffer base concentrations, contributing to the development of metabolic acidosis during painful labors (see Figs. 18-5 and 18-6).[471,472]

Cardiovascular Changes

During pregnancy the heart is enlarged and rotated upwards and outwards. This produces radiographic and elec-

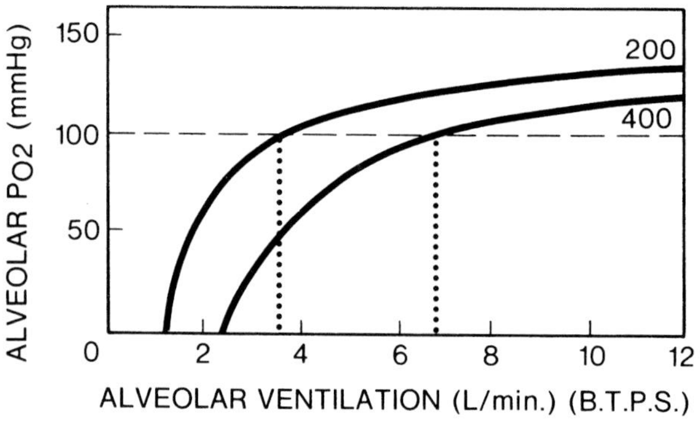

FIG. 18-3. The relationship between alveolar ventilation and alveolar PO_2 for values of oxygen consumption of 200 ml/min and 400 ml/min for a patient breathing air at normal barometric pressure. Note the alveolar ventilation required to maintain alveolar PO_2 above 100 mm Hg at the higher oxygen consumption in labor. (Modified from Nunn, J.F.: Applied Respiratory Physiology, pp. 386, London, Butterworths, 1977).

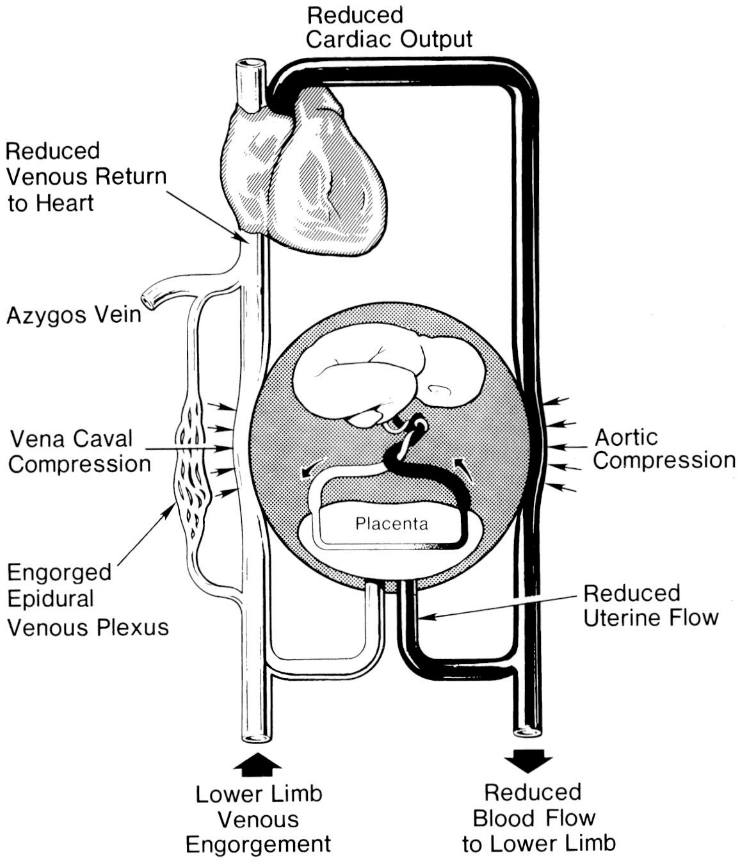

FIG. 18-4. Circulatory effects of aortocaval compression.

trocardiographic changes (right axis deviation, inverted T waves in V_2) which, although normal for pregnancy, may be interpreted as abnormal by the uneducated.

Pregnancy induces a "dynamic" circulation. A 30 to 50% increase in cardiac output and blood volume occurs in conjunction with a decrease in both systemic and pulmonary resistance.[118,341] These changes are such that blood pressure is normally unaltered, or slightly reduced. Adequate placental perfusion requires a uterine blood flow of 500 to 700 ml per minute at term.[33] Because uterine perfusion is largely pressure-dependent, hypotension from any cause, such as hypovolemia, reduced venous return or myocardial depression, must be treated promptly. Aortocaval compression by the gravid uterus is one of the most important (yet easily avoided) causes of decreased venous return, cardiac output and placental perfusion. This occurs whenever the mother assumes the supine position (Fig. 18-4). The potentially harmful sequelae of the supine position have been well documented.[48,179,184,326,550,614]

Most mothers tolerate the supine position without actually developing symptoms of hypotension, through compensatory mechanisms such as diversion of venous return from the lower limbs via the epidural and azygos veins, and an increase in peripheral resistance and heart rate. In only 10 to 15% of mothers are these compensatory mechanisms insufficient to maintain adequate cerebral perfusion. Classical symptoms of the "supine hypotensive syndrome" (pallor, sweating, nausea and faintness) develop in these women after several minutes in the supine position.[276,294]

Aortocaval compression is of particular importance to the anesthesiologist, because major regional and sympathetic blockade diminish the ability to compensate for a fall in cardiac output, rendering supine hypotension inevitable. The supine position must be avoided in late pregnancy at *all* times, whether symptoms suggesting hypotension are present or not. In labor, the mother should remain on her side, and at cesarean section either her position should be tilted, or her uterus mechanically displaced laterally (preferably to the left).

Aortocaval compression can jeopardize fetal well-being by reducing uterine blood flow, and possibly by interfering with placental venous drainage. Several studies have shown the deleterious effects of the supine posture on neonatal status both in labor[233,285,547] and at cesarean section.[29,148,176,234,595] Changes in fetal heart rate (FHR) are minimal when a lateral-tilt position is maintained during labor.[44,274,310,497,547] A further consequence of inferior vena caval compression is an increased venous return via other drainage pathways. In the spinal canal, this leads to engorgement of the epidural venous plexus of Bateson, which in turn diminishes the potential volume of the epidural space. This may explain, in part, why epidural local anesthetic dose requirements are reduced in late pregnancy and during labor (Fig. 18-4).[67] Epidural vascular engorgement also increases the risk of intravascular placement of the epidural needle or catheter, which raises the potential for toxicity with local anesthetics.

During labor, cardiac output and mean arterial pressure both increase as labor progresses. This is most marked during contractions, when cardiac outputs approaching 11 L/min have been recorded.[516] Hemodynamic changes of this order are of considerable relevance in the presence of certain cardiovascular disorders. Repeated Valsalva maneuvers during active bearing down at delivery also influence the circulation, especially when the normal sympathetic circulatory responses are obtunded by central neural blockade. A transiently greater fall in blood pressure occurs during phase 3 of the Valsalva maneuver, during voluntary pushing under epidural analgesia.[615] This can also affect placental perfusion and may explain why fetal acidemia develops more rapidly among mothers who bear down during a prolonged second stage compared with those who do not (see Fig. 18-6).[474]

Immediately after delivery, maternal blood volume is increased, secondary to an autotransfusion of up to 500 ml from the placenta. Hypertension, or pulmonary congestion and edema, can occur at this time, particularly in those most at risk, e.g., patients with heart disease and preeclampsia. Pulmonary congestion also can be precipitated after delivery, by vasopressor drugs (including ergometrine), and by drugs which cause fluid retention or circulatory overload, e.g., oxytocin and beta sympathomimetic agents.

Hematologic Changes

Several hematologic changes occur during pregnancy. Apart from reductions in hemoglobin concentration, hematocrit and blood viscosity[275,423] secondary to hemodilution, the most significant changes are those related to hemostasis. Thus, late pregnancy is associated with increased activation of the platelet, clotting and fibrinolytic systems.[225] The plasma fibrinogen concentration is almost doubled at term, and other clotting factors increase, though to a lesser degree.[475] This means that a state of hypercoagulability occurs during pregnancy and that the parturient is at increased risk of thromboembolism. Indeed, pulmonary embolism currently is a principal cause of maternal death in developed countries.

Thrombocytopenia at delivery in otherwise healthy women is apparently not uncommon; approximately 6% of women have platelet counts of less than 150,000/μl and 1% of less than 100,000/μl.[86] In the presence of preeclampsia, the incidence of thrombocytopenia is increased, with platelet counts of less than 150,000/μl occurring in 15 to 30% of patients.[40,548] Controversy exists about the advisability of performing central neural blockade in the presence of relative thrombocytopenia or a potential bleeding disorder. Several authorities have stipulated a cut-off platelet count below which regional anesthesia is contraindicated. Unfortunately, there is as yet no clinical evidence or rational basis on which to base such judgements. Others have insisted on the results of a bleeding time and full coagulation screen before considering epidural analgesia. While such tests can provide a useful indication of *disease severity,* none of them are able to identify which patients are at risk of developing an epidural hematoma. The bleeding time, in particular, is subject to wide observer variation, and when abnormal, may not reflect a significant bleeding tendency.[456]

The decision to withhold regional anesthesia on the grounds of mildly abnormal coagulation screening may be excessively conservative, since there is no published evidence to suggest that the risk of epidural hematoma is actually increased. However, as most anesthesiologists avoid regional anesthesia in the presence of a known bleeding disorder, such information is not available. When coagulation screening is abnormal, an evaluation should be made of the relative risks and benefits of regional anesthesia compared with alternative techniques.

Gastrointestinal Changes

The gravid patient is prone to pulmonary aspiration for several reasons: The intra-abdominal and intragastric pressures are raised; gastric emptying is delayed; esophageal reflux is more common; and stomach contents are highly acidic. In addition, during labor, nausea and vomiting are also exacerbated by pain, stress, and the administration of opioids, including epidural opioids.[195,223,447,628] Thus, the largest volumes of gastric contents occur in patients who have received opioid drugs, the smallest in those receiving epidural local anesthetics alone.[195,270,448]

While the risk of regurgitation and pulmonary aspiration is largely associated with general anesthesia, regional blockade is not entirely free from this danger. Aspiration can still occur if consciousness is depressed, secondary, for example, to the development of a high spinal block, systemic toxicity, hypovolemia, aortocaval compression, or concurrent medication. Vomiting may be precipitated by an episode of acute hypotension. Ergometrine also frequently causes vomiting, especially if given as an intravenous bolus.[410,414]

Various prophylactic measures have been recommended to reduce the risk of aspiration, including administration of oral antacids (e.g., 0.3 molar sodium citrate) immediately prior to surgery; oral or intravenous H_2 receptor antagonists;[532] substituted benzimidazoles (e.g., omeprazole);[196,421] and intravenous metoclopramide preoperatively to increase lower esophageal sphincter tone and increase gastric motility.[134,437] Preoperative gastric emptying, via an orogastric tube or by inducing emesis with apomorphine, is rarely performed now.

Uteroplacental Circulation and Oxygen Delivery

Uterine Blood Flow

The increase in maternal cardiac output that occurs during pregnancy is normally more than adequate to meet the requirements of the uteroplacental circulation (approximately 500 to 700 ml/min at term). Uterine blood flow varies directly with perfusion pressure (uterine arterial minus uterine venous pressure) and inversely with uterine vascular resistance. It is important to appreciate the factors which can influence these two parameters because fetal homeostasis and survival depend upon adequate placental perfusion.

Uterine perfusion pressure is reduced when systemic hypotension occurs from any cause, including hemorrhage, hypovolemia, decrease in cardiac output, sympathetic blockade and aortocaval compression. It should be noted that the uterine arteries originate *distal* to the portion of the aorta compressed by the gravid uterus when the patient lies in the supine position (i.e., at the level of the L4 vertebra; see Fig. 18-4).[48]

Uterine vascular resistance is influenced by both intrinsic and extrinsic factors. Thus, uterine arterial vasoconstriction can occur in response to sympathetic stimulation such as pain and anxiety.[235] The uterine vessels are particularly sensitive to direct-acting α-adrenergic drugs, and so these agents generally have been avoided.[498] When a vasopressor is indicated (for example, to treat hypotension secondary to regional anesthesia), ephedrine is the drug of choice, because its effect is predominantly that of a β-adrenergic agonist. Cardiac output and uterine blood flow improve consequently, as does arterial blood pressure.[499,559] More recent studies suggest that low doses of phenylephrine are acceptable alternatives in the treatment of hypotension, if ephedrine is ineffective or contraindicated (e.g., in the presence of cardiac disease and maternal tachycardia).[424,500,502]

The addition of epinephrine to local anesthetics in usual clinical concentrations (i.e., 1:200,000) has little influence upon placental perfusion.[26] Epidural analgesia in labor decreases circulating catecholamines, reduces sympathetic tone and abolishes hyperventilation; it may thereby improve placental perfusion (Fig. 18-5).

Although in the healthy parturient the placental vasculature is dilated maximally, in patients with pregnancy-induced hypertension uterine vascular resistance is increased and placental perfusion impaired. The pathophysiologic mechanisms are complex, but vasospasm is presumed to be an important factor, because epidural blockade improves placental blood flow even in the face of moderate falls in systolic blood pressure.[313]

Uterine vascular resistance is influenced *extrinsically* by uterine tone. Once the pressure generated by a contraction exceeds about 20 mm Hg, uterine blood flow decreases according to the magnitude of uterine pressure.[58,340] Uterine contractions must not be permitted to reach an amplitude or frequency sufficient to cause fetal asphyxia. Because excessive uterine contractility may become less obvious once pain relief is effective, the strength of contractions and fetal heart rate must be regularly monitored following neural blockade.

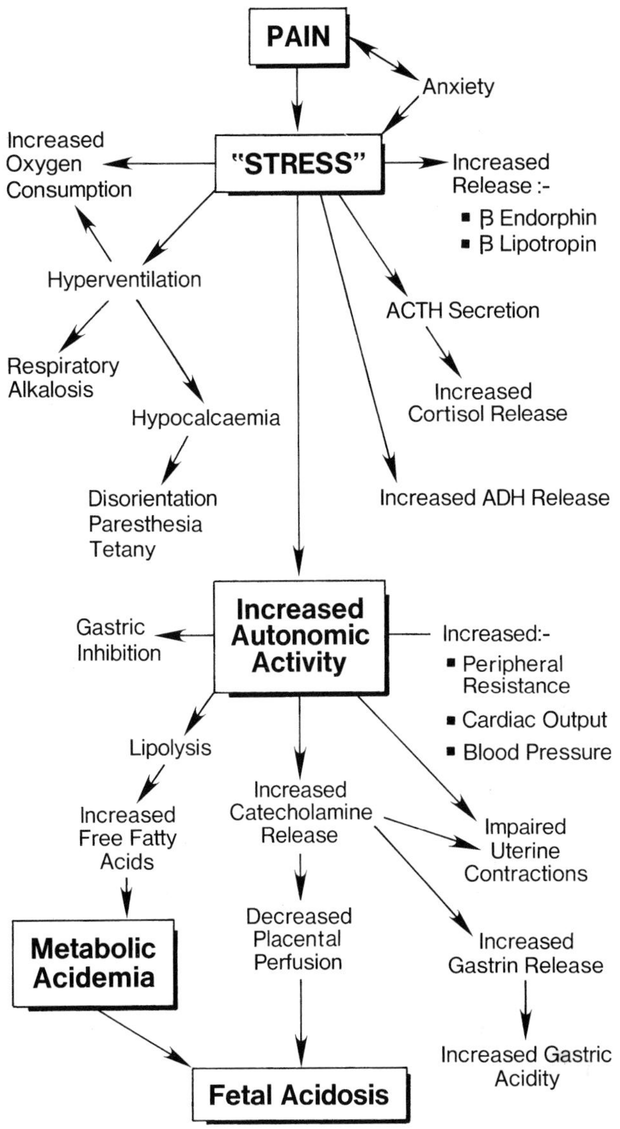

FIG. 18-5. Physiological changes secondary to pain in labor.

Oxygen Supply

Oxygen delivery to the fetus depends not only upon placental perfusion but also upon maternal arterial oxygen content. The latter relates to the product of hemoglobin concentration (×1.39—the oxygen capacity of hemoglobin in ml/g) and hemoglobin saturation. As noted earlier, hemoglobin concentration is lowered during normal pregnancy and PaO_2 is sometimes reduced due to an increase in pulmonary venous admixture. During pregnancy, there is a significant shift to the right of the oxyhemoglobin dissociation curve, compared with that of the non-pregnant state. This shift occurs as a result of an increase in the 2,3-diphosphoglycerate content of maternal red cells, which enhances oxygen release to all tissues, including the placenta.[523] In labor, however, excessive hyperventilation and hypocarbia may reverse this shift, and the result is impaired maternal-fetal oxygen transfer.

The fetus is adapted to survive at a much lower arterial oxygen tension (umbilical vein PaO_2 approximately 30 mm Hg) than is the adult. These adaptations include (i) a higher oxygen-carrying capacity (fetal hemoglobin [Hb-F] being approximately 17 g/100 ml); (ii) a greater affinity of Hb-F for oxygen, the Hb-F oxygen dissociation curve being shifted well to the left compared with adult Hb (i.e., P_{50} of 17 mm Hg as opposed to 27 mm Hg); and (iii) the Bohr effect, which favors Hb-F oxygen uptake within the placenta (accounting for 20 to 40% of maternal-fetal oxygen transfer). However, oxygen stores in the fetus are very limited and metabolic acidosis is readily incurred whenever oxygen transfer fails to meet oxygen requirements.

Although maternal arterial Hb is close to full saturation when breathing air, both maternal and fetal arterial PO_2 increase significantly when higher oxygen concentrations are inspired. Oxygen therapy should, therefore, be instituted without delay whenever fetal hypoxia is suspected. It should also be administered routinely during cesarean section performed under regional blockade.[501] Earlier fears that maternal PaO_2 in excess of 300 mm Hg might cause uterine vasoconstriction and fetal hypoxemia[522] have not been substantiated.[385,501]

Physiological Changes Secondary to Pain in Labor

The first stage of labor is associated with several physiological and biochemical perturbations which are largely pain-mediated, and are thus susceptible to effective analgesia, notably central neural blockade. Such perturbations have been observed in both the mother and the fetus and are summarized in Figure 18–5.

Maternal Changes. Plasma concentrations of beta-endorphin, beta-lipotrophin, gamma-lipotrophin and adrenocorticotrophic hormones, (all of which are derived from a common precursor), are increased during unmedicated labor.[9,74,203,232,332,583,640] It has been postulated that the release of beta-endorphin in rats may represent a mechanism for the modulation of pain in labor.[228] No change in pain threshold has been observed, however, among laboring women.[181,554]

Hormonal secretion from the adrenal cortex also increases during unmedicated labor,[83,85,311,377] whereas thyroid-stimulating hormone (TSH) concentrations remain unchanged.[311] Mothers who receive epidural analgesia have significantly lower plasma concentrations of all of the above hormones.[9,74,583] The actual *degree* of adrenocortical suppression depends on the extent of neural blockade and on the presence or absence of other stress-related factors, such as physical exertion and anxiety.[311,377]

A 3- to 5-fold increase in plasma catecholamines is also a concomitant of painful labor.[199,339] Consequently, the urinary excretion of catecholamines is increased.[312] These hormonal changes reflect an increase in adrenosympathetic activity, and explain why maternal blood pressure and peripheral resistance gradually rise as labor progresses. Again, they are obtunded by central neural blockade.[446]

Pain-mediated activation of the autonomic nervous system may contribute to the inhibition of gastric emptying and intestinal peristalsis which occurs in natural labor.[270] Release of the stomach hormone, gastrin, is stimulated during

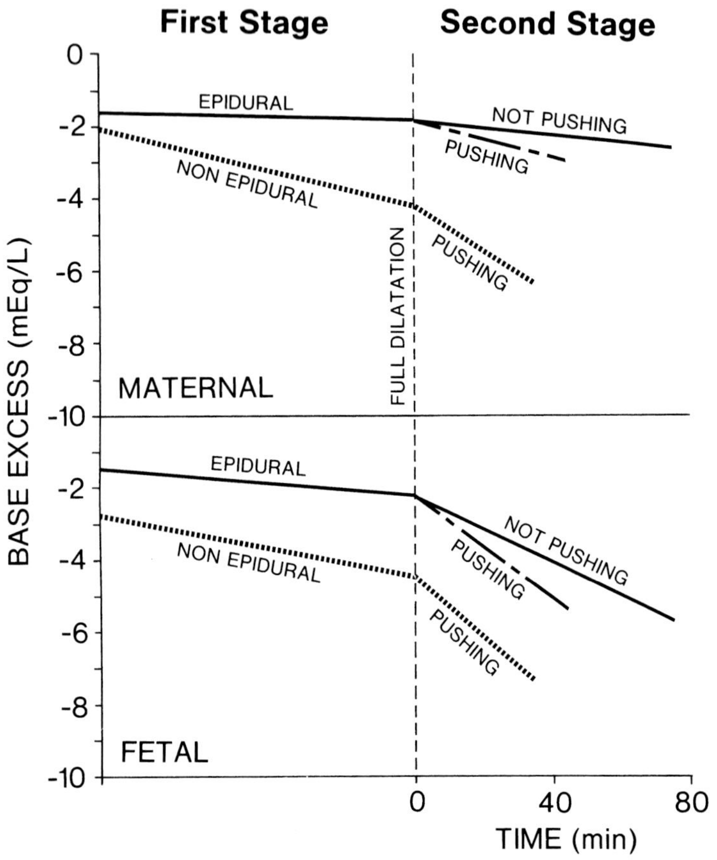

FIG. 18-6. Maternal and fetal acid-base changes during labor, comparing epidural and nonepidural analgesia. During the first stage of labor, both maternal and fetal changes are negligible with epidural analgesia. During the second stage, both maternal and fetal acidosis are accelerated due to active pushing. Although epidural block is associated with a longer duration of the second stage of labor, patients with epidural analgesia demonstrate minimal acidosis at full dilatation and a slower *rate* of development of acidosis, especially in the absence of pushing. (Adapted from Pearson and Davies: refs 471–474).

painful labor, causing increased gastric acid secretion.[254] In addition, excessive sympathetic activity is thought to aggravate incoordinate uterine contractility, which can develop during a prolonged labor.[373] In these circumstances, epidural analgesia may permit more normal uterine activity and hasten cervical dilatation.[417]

Pain during natural labor also influences acid-base balance. Maternal blood concentrations of free fatty acids and lactate gradually rise to reach a peak at delivery.[311,374,383,471,582] By contrast, when a woman in labor is given epidural blockade, only minor acid-base changes are observed during the first stage. The most likely explanation for the progressive maternal acidemia which occurs during painful labor is catecholamine-induced lipolytic metabolism, although starvation and a diminished buffering capacity, caused by metabolic compensation for a respiratory alkalosis, may also be contributing factors (Fig. 18-5).

Maternal metabolic acidosis in the second stage of labor is largely related to the degree of exertion during active pushing.[311,472] This occurs despite analgesia and is time-dependent. When labor is conducted under epidural analgesia, acidosis is less severe among mothers who do not actively push, compared with those who do (Fig. 18-6).[472]

Finally, once central neural blockade is established, hyperventilation in labor is virtually abolished.[471] Oxygen consumption is also consequently reduced.[244,538]

Quite apart from all of the above physiological perturbations, uterine contraction pain is often associated with nausea, fatigue, light-headedness, mental confusion, tingling sensation (secondary to hypocarbic hypocalcemia) and sweating. Epidural analgesia invariably abolishes these unpleasant symptoms and allows the mother to feel calm again.

Placentofetal Changes. Placental perfusion can be affected adversely by increased adrenosympathetic activity.[296] A norepinephrine infusion causes uterine vasoconstriction in the pregnant ewe,[527] and uterine blood flow decreases significantly during periods of stress in association with elevated plasma norepinephrine levels (Fig. 18-7).[562]

Whether the circulating catecholamine concentrations found during normal labor are enough to reduce placental perfusion awaits clarification. Epidural analgesia does, however, reduce maternal plasma catecholamine levels[557] and this may account for the improvement in placental perfusion that has been demonstrated following its use in labor.[272,309] The sympathetic blockade and decreased uterine vascular resistance associated with epidural analgesia presumably also contributes to improved perfusion. These effects of neural blockade can only be regarded as advantageous to the fetus.

At the onset of the second stage of labor, the fetus is less acidotic when epidural analgesia is used (Fig. 18-6),[473,474] although any suppression of the bearing-down reflex can lead to a prolonged period of pushing. This is not only unproductive and exhausting for the mother, but it exposes the fetus to increasing acidemia. In the second stage of labor, the mother should not be encouraged to push actively until the presenting part has descended as far as the perineum.

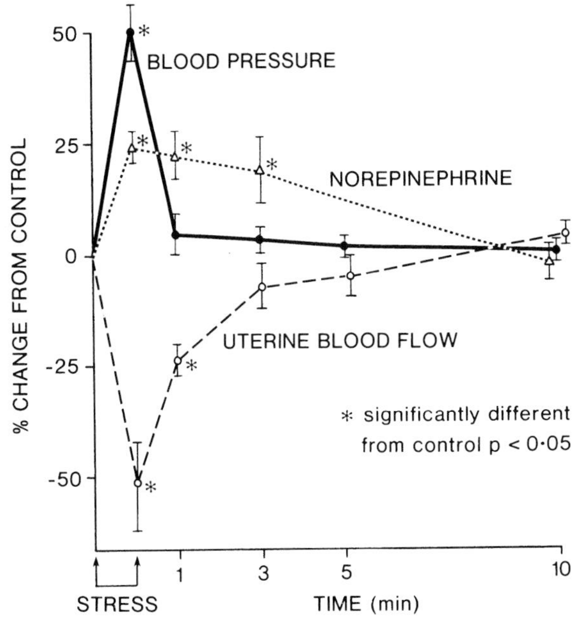

FIG. 18-7. Effects of stress on maternal arterial blood pressure, plasma norepinephrine concentration, and uterine blood flow in the pregnant ewe. (Shnider, S.M., Wright, R.G., Levinson, G., *et al.*: Uterine blood flow and plasma norepinephrine changes during maternal stress. Anesthesiology, *50*:524, 1979).

APPLIED PHARMACOLOGY

The physiological changes that occur during pregnancy alter the pharmacokinetic properties of most drugs. The volume of distribution and rate of renal clearance are both increased, while plasma protein binding is reduced. All drugs that are used in neural blockade cross the placenta by simple diffusion. Lipophilic drugs diffuse readily and so tend to undergo *flow-dependent* transfer, while polar drugs depend on their ability to penetrate the placental barrier and so are subject to *permeability-dependent* transfer.[506] Highly lipid soluble molecules, for example, approach equilibrium across the placenta within a single circulation,[247] whereas polar molecules and ions cross the placenta at a rate inversely proportional to their molecular size.[295]

While, strictly speaking, neural blockade is restricted to the use of local anesthetic agents, other drugs, such as opioids and adrenergic agonists, are also frequently used in the management of obstetric pain. For this reason, we must consider the role of these agents in this chapter as well.

Local Anesthetics

The placental transfer and disposition of local anesthetics administered to the mother have been the subject of several reviews.[167,348,358,411,476,488,498,543,591] It is clear that rapid equilibration occurs between local anesthetic concentrations in the two circulations, governed largely by the physicochemical properties of the agents used (see Chapter 3). Certain techniques and agents are more likely to achieve toxic blood levels than others. Direct fetal injection has been described following attempted paracervical, caudal and pudendal blocks, and even during perineal infiltration.[206] As local anesthetic toxicity is potentially lethal, its recognition and treatment (see Chapter 4) must be well understood by all staff who practice and supervise neural blockade in obstetrics.

It appears that pregnancy enhances the sensitivity of nerves to local anesthetics, an effect that is presumed to be due to elevated plasma progesterone concentrations.[87,159,319] Thus, the greater spread of central neural blockade in pregnancy may have a physiological as well as an anatomical basis. While it has been suggested that pregnancy may decrease the toxicity threshold to local anesthetics, this has not been substantiated with either lidocaine or mepivacaine in pregnant ewes.[432] The significant decrease in plasma protein binding of bupivacaine may explain the apparent increased sensitivity to this agent's toxicity in the parturient. In a study by Santos et al.[541] in sheep, convulsions occurred at lower *total* bupivacaine concentrations in pregnant than in nonpregnant animals. However, *free* drug concentrations were actually similar in both groups. Elevated plasma progesterone concentrations also may contribute to increased myocardial sensitivity to bupivacaine.

Ester-Linked Local Anesthetics

2-chloroprocaine. It has by far the shortest plasma half-life of all local anesthetics. In neonatal blood, the half-life is about 40 seconds, i.e., double the value for adult blood. Cumulative toxicity does not develop on account of its rapid hydrolysis. For these reasons, it has been recommended for epidural use during labor[267] and for paracervical block.[213] However, its shorter duration of action makes 2-chloroprocaine less attractive for continuous epidural analgesia (unless a continuous infusion is employed) since more frequent top-up doses are required. It also antagonizes the action of epidural bupivacaine,[132,238,265] epidural opioids[238,372] and epidural clonidine.[288]

In the past, 2-chloroprocaine has been associated with a number of neurologic complications following intrathecal injection.[160] Although it now appears that 2-chloroprocaine itself is no more neurotoxic than other local anesthetics, the antioxidant bisulfite present in older formulations can cause neurotoxic effects if given intrathecally. More recently, severe backache has been reported, among non-obstetric patients, following epidural analgesia using newer preparations of 2-chloroprocaine that contain ethylenediaminetetraacetic acid (EDTA).[293]

Tetracaine. Until recently, tetracaine was the most commonly used intrathecal agent in North America, but is not currently available in the United Kingdom or Australasia.

Amide-Linked Agents

Unlike ester-linked local anesthetics, the more commonly used amide-linked agents depend upon hepatic metabolism before they can be eliminated from the body. Accordingly, the elimination half-life is much longer than that of the esters. Maternal-fetal transfer of the unbound, undissociated form, following administration to the mother occurs readily and is dependent upon the maternal blood concentration of free drug. The fetal blood concentration reflects the dose that has been administered, the rate of maternal absorption, placental perfusion, fetal/neonatal and tissue disposition, metabolism and excretion. The basic principles of placental transfer and neonatal disposition are described in Chapter 3 and only the clinical implications are discussed here.

The fetal-to-maternal (F:M) ratio of local anesthetic plasma concentrations varies widely: Prilocaine has a ratio close to unity, whereas lidocaine and mepivacaine have values of 0.5 to 0.7. Bupivacaine and etidocaine have much lower F:M ratios of 0.2 to 0.3. Protein-binding in maternal blood limits the proportion of local anesthetic that is transferable to the fetus.[592] The F:M ratio is also influenced by the pH gradient between maternal and fetal blood. Fetal acidosis has been shown to cause an elevation in the F:M ratio of lidocaine,[72,73,429] mepivacaine[73] and bupivacaine[487] due to "ion-trapping." A decrease in fetal pH favors drug ionization and therefore retention within the fetal circulation. Local anesthetic toxicity is also enhanced in the presence of fetal acidosis.[429]

Although the elimination half-life of lidocaine is greater in the newborn than in the adult, due to the larger volume of distribution,[407] metabolic clearance is very similar on a weight-for-weight basis.[205] Plasma half-lives of mepivacaine[73] and bupivacaine[370] are also considerably longer in the neonate than the adult.

Toxic effects of local anesthetic agents in the fetus, as in the adult or neonate, are manifested by central nervous system and cardiovascular changes. Maternal toxicity has on occasion led to perinatal death following large doses,[498] and fetal cardiotoxicity may have been a contributory factor. More subtle central nervous system (CNS) changes have been revealed by neurobehavioral testing of the newborn (see following).

Lidocaine. It is used in obstetrics for all techniques of neural blockade, in many centers it is the preferred epidural agent for an operative delivery. When used to provide surgical anesthesia, it is preferable to add epinephrine (1:200,000 to 1:300,000) in order to limit placental transfer, prolong the duration of analgesia[4] and, in the case of epidural analgesia, improve local anesthetic spread to the sacral nerve roots.[440]

Mepivacaine. Placental transfer of mepivacaine is greater, and neonatal metabolism slower than that of lidocaine.[73] Neonatal neurobehavioral depression has been reported following the epidural administration of mepivacaine, and the potential for frank toxicity makes this agent relatively contraindicated for obstetric use.[431]

Prilocaine. It has the highest F:M ratio, which may exceed unity.[489] Although less toxic than lidocaine, methemoglobinemia has been reported in both mother and neonate.[30] In some cases, more than 10% of fetal hemoglobin has been converted to methemoglobin, an amount sufficient to produce neonatal cyanosis. These factors outweigh any advantages of prilocaine, except possibly for a single low dose pudendal block or perineal infiltration when delivery is imminent.

Bupivacaine. This is currently the amide agent of choice for epidural analgesia in labor. In concentrations of 0.25% or less, effective analgesia can be provided with minimal motor blockade.[82] The duration of action is convenient for use in labor and, unlike shorter-acting agents, tachyphylaxis is not clinically detectable.

For cesarean section, 0.5% bupivacaine is more popular than lidocaine in some centers. It has been suggested that bupivacaine is inherently more cardiotoxic than other local anesthetic agents, especially in higher concentrations.[25] However, a recent study of bupivacaine and ropivacaine in pregnant and non-pregnant sheep by Santos et al.[539] demonstrated that pregnancy did not increase the risk of local anesthetic systemic toxicity in either group. Nevertheless, as discussed in Chapter 4, extreme care must be taken to avoid accidental intravenous injection of large bolus doses of bupivacaine. Precautionary measures include the use of an epinephrine-containing test dose (3 ml of 1:200,000 solution) and incremental injections of the total dose.

Etidocaine. This agent provides motor blockade out of proportion to its sensory block and therefore is not suitable for epidural analgesia during labor. The rapid onset and good muscle relaxation, however, coupled with a very low F:M ratio, has made 1% etidocaine attractive for use in cesarean section.[363] It is not now available in most countries.

Ropivacaine. It is the first local anesthetic to be synthesized as a pure enantiomer, unlike bupivacaine and mepivacaine, which exist as racemic mixtures. Ropivacaine is chemically similar to bupivacaine, the butyl group being replaced by a propyl group. It has an identical pK_a to bupivacaine but is marginally less lipid soluble; both are more than 90% plasma protein bound.[525] The F:M ratio in sheep is approximately 0.2.[542] Further details of its clinical pharmacologic properties are presented in Chapter 4.

Most comparative studies of ropivacaine and bupivacaine for epidural anesthesia have shown no significant difference in onset, duration, or maximum sensory block height between the two agents, but ropivacaine appears to produce less intense, shorter duration motor block.[396] In addition, animal and human studies have confirmed that ropivacaine has lower CNS and cardiotoxic potential, when compared to bupivacaine.[396] These two features would seem to make ropivacaine an ideal agent for use in the obstetric patient.

At this time, only initial information is available concerning the use of ropivacaine in childbirth. Epidural ropivacaine 0.5% has been compared with bupivacaine 0.5% for cesarean section anesthesia.[158,239] Sensory block was similar for both agents, but motor blockade was reduced with ropivacaine. Neonatal outcome was similar between groups. An assessment by color Doppler ultrasound,[24] showed that uteroplacental and fetal circulation were not affected adversely by use of ropivacaine for cesarean delivery.

To date, there are three published studies,[185,397,574] and a preliminary report,[175] comparing ropivacaine with bupivacaine for labor analgesia. In all four studies, both local anesthetics were equally effective with respect to onset, intensity, and quality of pain relief. Moreover, no statistically significant difference in the incidence, intensity and duration of motor block between groups could be detected. Perhaps the method used to evaluate motor block in these studies was not sensitive enough. However, a recent study of bolus doses of epidural ropivacaine 0.25% and bupivacaine 0.25% for labor analgesia demonstrated significantly less motor block with ropivacaine.[220]

Stienstra et al.[574] suggested that ropivacaine may have an advantage over bupivacaine with respect to neonatal neurobehavioral performance. Similarly, Writer and colleagues,[631] in a prospective meta-analysis evaluating the influence of ropivacaine on neonatal outcome and labor progress, found that neonatal neurobehavioral performance at 24 hours was significantly better in the ropivacaine group. This study also found that there were significantly fewer instrumental deliveries in the ropivacaine group (27%) compared to the bupivacaine group (40%).[631]

More clinical experience with ropivacaine is needed to demonstrate conclusively its advantages over bupivacaine.

Effects of Local Anesthetics on the Uterus, Uterine and Umbilical Vessels and Fetal Heart Rate

Clinical studies on the effect of local anesthetics on uterine activity have produced conflicting results. It is unlikely that a direct effect on myometrial contraction will be observed in practice.[488] Isolated human uterine muscle begins to show a significant dose-related depression of contractility with lidocaine, for example, only at levels in excess of 25 μg/ml,[436] a level unlikely to be attained except in the event of gross toxicity or after paracervical block. Very high concentrations of local anesthetics *in vitro*, however, have been shown to cause *increased* uterine tone.[236]

Similarly, the actions of local anesthetics upon the uterine and umbilical vessels are of dubious clinical significance. *In vitro* studies have demonstrated a vasoconstricting effect of local anesthetics on uterine arteries. With lidocaine, this occurs only at concentrations in excess of 20 μg/ml.[226] In contrast, the umbilical arteries behave differently, depending upon the local anesthetic agent. Lidocaine and etidocaine dilate the umbilical vessels, whereas prilocaine and bupivacaine cause vasoconstriction.[593] All these effects have been recorded only at concentrations far exceeding blood concentrations associated with neural blockade (except possibly with paracervical block).

Local anesthetics theoretically can influence FHR by a variety of mechanisms including: direct depressant effects on fetal myocardium and central nervous system; maternal hypotension; constriction of uterine or umbilical vessels; and an increase in uterine tone. The reported frequency of FHR abnormalities following epidural analgesia in labor has varied widely. The relatively high incidence documented in early studies may have been related to inadequate intravenous fluids or to aortocaval compression. For example, Schifrin showed that late decelerations increased five-fold in the supine position, or when hypotension occurred.[547] When these factors were avoided, FHR changes related to epidural analgesia were minimal.[310,338,497,637] Abnormalities of FHR are more common during oxytocin infusion,[547] most likely reflecting decreased placental perfusion secondary to uterine contractions.

During cesarean section under epidural analgesia, little change in FHR variability has been reported with either lidocaine or bupivacaine.[360] Since larger local anesthetic doses are used for cesarean section than for labor, these results suggest that FHR changes following epidural analgesia are more likely to be a consequence of labor itself and not of the local anesthetic. This view is supported by the finding that FHR changes occur with a similar frequency after labor analgesia with intrathecal sufentanil, as after epidural techniques utilizing local anesthetics.[121]

Local Anesthetics and the Neurobehavioral Controversy

Frank neonatal local anesthetic toxicity is extremely rare, and Apgar scores and blood gas analyses are usually normal following uncomplicated neural blockade. However, these tests are useful only in detecting fairly severe depression of vital functions. Neurobehavioral assessments, which more closely scrutinize newborn behavior, have shown that subtle or delayed effects of obstetric anesthesia can be present even when more gross testing reveals no abnormalities. Neurobehavioral tests examine the neonate's muscle tone and reflex behavior, and also the more complex CNS functions, such as the ability to change the state of arousal, initiate complex motor acts and suppress meaningless environmental stimuli. The Early Neonatal Neurobehavioral Scale (ENNS)[544] and the Neurological and Adaptive Capacity Score (NACS)[27] have been used extensively to evaluate the effects of anesthesia on the newborn. Both are simplified versions of the more comprehensive and time-consuming Brazelton Neonatal Behavioral Assessment Scale,[61] differing from each other predominantly in the emphasis placed on the various aspects of neonatal behavior.

Concern about the effects of local anesthetics began when Scanlon and his associates compared the neonatal behavioral effects of maternal epidural analgesia with lidocaine and mepivacaine, and, in a second study, bupivacaine, with that of nonepidural controls.[544,545] Babies whose mothers had received lidocaine or mepivacaine were grouped together and scored less well on the first day of life on tests of muscle strength and tone than did infants whose mothers had received bupivacaine or no anesthesia. The authors described these infants as "floppy but alert," and correlated this finding with the persistence of lidocaine and, to a greater extent, mepivacaine, in the newborn.[73] Subsequently, the same group reported that chloroprocaine was similar to bupivacaine in its lack of neurobehavioral depression.[71]

In the United States, these findings resulted in the rejection of lidocaine for use in obstetric epidural anesthesia and the widespread adoption of bupivacaine and chloroprocaine. Subsequently, concerns regarding the potential toxicity of both these agents led to more critical evaluation of Scanlon's data.[152] One drawback of Scanlon's earliest study is that the epidural group consisted predominantly of patients who had received mepivacaine (n = 19) with a much smaller number (n = 9) having received lidocaine.[544] This is important, since umbilical cord concentrations of mepivacaine were significantly higher than those of lidocaine.[73] In spite of this, patients who received lidocaine and mepivacaine were grouped together for statistical analyses. Another criticism is that the second study was performed at a later date and lacked its own control group, comparisons being made with the nonepidural group of the earlier study. Interpretation of the data is also complicated by the fact that many patients in both the epidural and nonepidural groups received opioids or barbiturates. Thus, it was appropriate to question the validity of the conclusion that bupivacaine was superior to lidocaine; new investigations were clearly necessary.

Abboud and co-workers therefore compared neonatal condition following epidural anesthesia with lidocaine, chloroprocaine, and bupivacaine for both vaginal delivery and cesarean section.[5,6] No adverse effects were seen with any agent, and infants in all groups scored equally well on the ENNS. Similarly, Kileff and colleagues found no differences in the ENNS following epidural anesthesia for cesarean section with lidocaine compared with bupivacaine; in fact, infants whose mothers had received lidocaine suckled more vigorously at 24 hours of age.[329] Although one study found that babies performed marginally better on certain aspects of the Brazelton Assessment following chloroprocaine than following lidocaine, these findings were considered to be very subtle, and to be significantly less important in influencing neonatal outcome than other perinatal factors.[333]

Neurobehavioral testing also has been performed following systemic medication, and after other techniques of neural blockade. In general, global depression of the neurobehavioral examination occurs after the mother has been given general anesthesia and opioids, barbiturates or other sedative drugs. The degree and duration of depression is related to the dose to which the newborn has been exposed. Meperidine, for example, has been shown in several studies to produce significant neonatal neurobehavioral depression when administered to the laboring mother.[60,263] As might be expected, subarachnoid block with tetracaine resulted in higher scores on the ENNS than did general anesthesia with either ketamine or thiopental, presumably reflecting the minimal drug exposure involved with spinal anesthesia.[262]

Neurobehavioral testing, following paracervical block in which 0.25% bupivacaine was used, revealed no difference between the study group and control infants whose mothers had received, local infiltration, or spinal or pudendal block.[401] In contrast, Nesheim and colleagues reported poorer neurobehavioral scores following paracervical block (using bupivacaine) than following local infiltration only.[445] This study, however, is difficult to interpret, because paracervical block patients also received significant amounts of lidocaine for pudenal block and local infiltration, and both groups received intravenous sedatives or nitrous oxide. The effects of pudenal block by itself have been studied, comparing outcome following administration of either 0.5% bupivacaine, 1% mepivacaine, or 3% chloroprocaine. In surprising contrast to the findings when similar doses were used for epidural anesthesia, mepivacaine for pudendal block was associated with better performance on the ENNS than were the other agents.[403] Possible explanations for this are the lower neonatal blood concentrations, and shorter time from injection to delivery associated with pudendal block.

What are the long-term effects, if any, of abnormal neurobehavioral performance in the early neonatal period? Many studies in which an adverse effect has been attributed to anesthesia are complicated by the inclusion of mothers with abnormalities of pregnancy or delivery. Such problems are likely to affect adversely both newborn behavior and later development. In most of the studies of newborn neurobehavior following neural blockade discussed above, infants were totally normal by the second or third day of life. Ounsted et al. prospectively followed 570 children for four years after delivery, carefully evaluating neurologic and motor development.[460,461] No correlation was found between poor outcome and method of pain relief used for delivery, although emergency cesarean section and perinatal asphyxia were strongly associated with abnormal development. In another long-term study of the offspring of healthy mothers with uncomplicated pregnancies, cognitive ability at 5 years of age was not influenced by the method of anesthesia or analgesia used at delivery.[598]

In summary, therefore, the neonatal neurobehavioral effects of local anesthetics used for analgesia in childbirth appear to be of minimal significance. In this respect, it is more important to avoid maternal hypotension or hypoxia, which could cause the secondary problem of perinatal asphyxia and thereby affect the newborn.

Opioids

Several opioid drugs have been introduced into use for obstetric neural blockade. Epidural or intrathecal opioids provide excellent analgesia after cesarean section, using doses substantially less than those that are customarily required by other routes. In labor, epidural opioids are generally disappointing when used alone, but they can provide very effective pain relief when combined with a local anesthetic such as bupivacaine. Such local anesthetic-opioid drug combinations appear to be entirely compatible and, since they behave synergistically, both classes of drug can be used in relatively low doses. Intrathecal opioids alone appear to be more effective for labor analgesia and can be used in a combined spinal-epidural technique, or with a continuous spinal catheter.

Opioids are weak bases and are variably bound to plasma proteins, principally α_1-acid glycoprotein (AAG). Placental transfer occurs readily following all parenteral (including epidural) routes and the F:M ratio approaches unity rapidly in those opioids that have been studied. In some cases, the fetal plasma concentration falls less rapidly than the maternal plasma concentration, so that the F:M ratio rises with time and may exceed 1.0 for a while.[590] In the case of meperidine, neonatal elimination of the active metabolite, normeperidine, is slower than maternal.[434]

All opioids have the potential to depress neonatal neurobehavior, including respiration. Despite the large number of opioid drugs that have been introduced, however, there is no convincing evidence that any one is superior to another, in terms of fetal outcome, when they are given in *equipotent* doses. In any case, the dose requirements are relatively small when used in combination with epidural bupivacaine (and even less when given intrathecally) and most studies have found negligible neonatal effects, even with meperidine.[82] In the cases of fentanyl and sufentanil, fetal concentrations after epidural administration generally have not reached unity with maternal levels.[328,359,467] While further studies are needed to confirm, most centers consider that the benefits of spinal opioids in labor far outweigh any theoretically deleterious (yet readily reversible) depressant effects on the newborn.

α_2-Adrenergic Drugs

For a surgical delivery, epinephrine is often added to local anesthetics, to potentiate and prolong their effects.[68] Addition of epinephrine to lidocaine and mepivacaine reduces drug absorption, thereby enhancing the spread and quality of neural blockade, and lowering peak plasma concentrations.[394] With bupivacaine and etidocaine, epinephrine has only marginal effects on the duration of action,[137,509] and little effect on reducing the peak plasma concentration.[507]

The action of epinephrine on uterine tone, contractility and uterine blood flow remains controversial. Several studies have reported a reduction in uterine activity following epidural blockade and even pudendal block when epinephrine has been added to the local anesthetic.[138,310,386,497,594,636] Other factors, however, such as hypotension and aortocaval compression, inhibit contractions,[88] and it is not clear how much epinephrine *per se* contributes to uterine inhibition. Some authorities have recommended avoidance of epinephrine during labor,[12] whereas others consider the addition of 5 μg/ml to be harmless in the progress of labor.[53,413]

In normotensive patients, the uteroplacental and fetal circulations are not altered significantly by the addition of 5 μg of epinephrine to epidural local anesthetics.[23,26,178,394]

Among hypertensive patients with chronic fetal asphyxia, however, the addition of epinephrine increases vascular resistance in the uteroplacental circulation, indicating impaired blood flow.[21]

Recently, epinephrine (which possesses some α_2-adrenergic activity) has been shown to produce analgesia by a spinal mechanism. This may explain partly why some investigators have reported that the addition of epinephrine to epidural bupivacaine, with or without an opioid, seems to augment the quality and duration of analgesia during labor,[10,189,634] although this has not been confirmed by others.[366] The addition of epinephrine to epidural lidocaine significantly improves the quality of surgical anesthesia during cesarean section.[68]

The more specific α_2-adrenergic agonist, clonidine, can produce very effective postoperative analgesia after epidural or intrathecal administration alone, but the dose requirements are large (700 μg epidurally; 150 μg intrathecally) and side-effects, such as sedation, episodes of obstructive apnea, hypotension, bradycardia and mouth dryness, are common.[190,204,288,402,443] However, when combined with spinally-administered local anesthetics,[56,95] or opioids,[435,529] clonidine intensifies and prolongs the duration of analgesia using much smaller doses (100 to 200 μg). With these lower doses, the incidence of hypotension and other side effects seems to be much less. Eisenach and colleagues have demonstrated that epidural clonidine produces regional analgesia by a local, spinal action and a generalized inhibition of sympathetic nervous system activity.[188]

More recently, Capogna et al.[94] have shown that the addition of a small dose of clonidine, 75 or 150 μg, to epidural morphine 2 mg, significantly increases the duration of postoperative complete analgesia without increasing the incidence of side effects. Epidural clonidine has also been used in labor. Le Polain et al. found no improvement in either the quality, or the duration, of analgesia when clonidine, 30 μg, was added to bupivacaine, 12.5 mg, plus epinephrine, 25 μg, and sufentanil, 10 μg.[347] Using a larger dose of clonidine, 120 μg, with 0.125% bupivacaine, was associated with significant improvement in the duration of analgesia, but also with marked sedation.[457] In another study, epidural clonidine, 75 μg, was found to improve labor analgesia when combined with bupivacaine, 0.125%, but prolonged the duration of labor.[117] In none of these studies did the addition of clonidine increase the incidence of hypotension, FHR abnormalities, or a poorer neonatal outcome. However, the number of patients studied was small.

From the information currently available, it would seem that clonidine is unlikely to have a major place in epidural management during childbirth, except possibly as a low-dose adjunct to local anesthetics and/or opioids. In the future, more effective analgesia with use of higher doses of clonidine, but without hypotension, may be possible, since intrathecal neostigmine has been reported to antagonize hypotension and enhance analgesia associated with spinal clonidine.[279,623] In addition, cholinergic and α_2-adrenergic systems exhibit synergism with opioid mechanisms[16] (see also Chapter 29).

Systemic Drug Interactions

Certain nonanesthetic drugs are required frequently before and/or during the course of neural blockade; these have important effects on the body. They include vasopressors, oxytocics, prostaglandins, hypotensive agents, tocolytics and H_2 antagonists.

Vasopressor Agents

A vasopressor agent often is indicated to prevent or correct hypotension during central neural blockade, particularly during cesarean section performed under spinal anesthesia. Ephedrine, administered intravenously in small (5 mg) bolus doses,[157] or as an infusion (50 mg in 500 ml of crystalloid),[320] is regarded as the most appropriate vasopressor in obstetrics. Some authors have recommended a *prophylactic* ephedrine infusion during cesarean section.[320,619] Prophylactic *intramuscular* ephedrine is not recommended prior to epidural anesthesia because maternal hypertension and fetal asphyxia may occur,[520] especially if general anesthesia is required.[531] Many anesthesiologists still like to give a small dose of IV ephedrine (5 to 10 mg) immediately before spinal anesthesia, however, on the grounds that episodes of hypotension are more common and dramatic following a spinal, than following an epidural, anesthetic.

The net effect of ephedrine is to enhance uterine blood flow and to restore placental perfusion and maternal arterial blood pressure. Fetal acidosis secondary to hypotension is also arrested and often corrected.[559] Ephedrine has positive chronotropic activity and is transferred readily across the placenta. Both maternal and fetal tachycardia commonly occur, therefore, and increased fetal heart rate variability has been observed.[630] These effects are dose-related and, because they are not associated with fetal acidosis, they are regarded as being innocuous.[630] Recent findings suggest that ephedrine promotes fetal catecholamine release, stimulation of the neonatal central nervous system, and transitory, subclinical, changes in the electroencephalogram (EEG) pattern.[321]

While intravenous ephedrine usually is rapidly effective at correcting hypotension, it is not always so, and it can also cause palpitations. In these cases, a pure α_1-adrenergic agonist (e.g., phenylephrine, 20 to 100 μg;[424,578] methoxamine, 0.5 mg; or metaraminol, 0.25 mg), is recommended. These agents are very effective in treating ephedrine-resistant hypotension, and the maternal heart rate usually falls dramatically secondary to carotid baroreceptor stimulation. Despite theoretical concerns that these drugs might reduce uteroplacental perfusion, this does not appear to be of clinical importance during cesarean section *provided* small doses are used.[20,502,629]

Oxytocic Agents

Oxytocics are given commonly after delivery, to improve uterine contractility. Ergometrine, (0.25 to 0.5 mg), and oxytocin, (5 to 10 units), both reduce blood loss effectively,[423,419] although their cardiovascular effects when administered as an intravenous bolus are quite different (Table 18-1).

The vasoconstrictive action of ergometrine can seriously aggravate postpartum hypertension among patients with essential or pregnancy-induced hypertension or pheochromocytoma. Dangerous hypertension can occur following ergometrine administration to patients who have already received epinephrine or a vasopressor agent. This may be sufficiently severe to cause a cerebrovascular accident,[103] or pulmonary edema.[305]

Nausea, vomiting, and headache are much more common following ergometrine than oxytocin, and the latter is therefore preferred following delivery.[410] Despite theoretical concern about hypotension following oxytocin in the presence of regional anesthesia,[617] it seldom occurs in practice,[414] especially when the drug is administered as a dilute infusion,[305] or in bolus doses of less than 5 units. Ergometrine should be reserved for intramuscular use (which causes fewer side-effects) except when atonic uterine postpartum hemorrhage fails to respond to oxytocin.

Oxytocin infusions are used frequently in obstetrics for the induction or augmentation of labor, evacuation of the contents of the uterus in patients with hydatidiform mole, and termination of pregnancy in mid-trimester. However, even low doses of oxytocin are antidiuretic, and this effect has been demonstrated to occur within 15 minutes of the start of the infusion.[352] When prolonged infusions are given, water intoxication and hyponatremia may develop, resulting in convulsions and loss of consciousness.[18] Hyponatremia must be considered in the differential diagnosis, therefore, whenever convulsions occur during labor. The diagnosis should be suspected if the blood sodium concentration is less than 120 to 125 mmol/L. Water intoxication usually has been associated with oxytocin infusions in excess of 3.5 liters, with 5% dextrose as the vehicle.[201] Careful attention to fluid balance is required, therefore, and an isotonic solution is preferred as the vehicle for oxytocin infusions.

TABLE 18-1. *Side effects of intravenous oxytocin and ergometrine given as a bolus dose at delivery*

	Oxytocin 5–10 units	Ergometrine 0.25–0.5 mg
Cardiovascular[305,617]		
Peripheral resistance	↓ (transient)	↑ (prolonged)
Systemic blood pressure	↓ (transient)	↑ (prolonged)
Central venous pressure	↑ (transient)	↑ (prolonged)
Antidiuretic action[352]	Yes	No
Emetic action[410,414,419]	Rare	Common
Headache	Rare	Common

Prostaglandins

Prostaglandins occur naturally in numerous body tissues and both prostaglandin-$F_2\alpha$ ($PGF_2\alpha$) and prostaglandin-E_1 (PGE_1) and E_2 (PGE_2) increase during pregnancy. Both the E and F series of prostaglandins stimulate uterine contractions and have been used to ripen the cervix (PGE_2 gel), induce abortion (PGE_2), and arrest postpartum uterine hemorrhage ($PGF_2\alpha$), when other agents fail. Prostaglandins affect smooth muscle tone, causing side effects which can have serious implications for the parturient. PGE_2 is a bronchodilator, while $PGF_2\alpha$ causes significant bronchoconstriction, which can precipitate or exacerbate asthma in susceptible individuals.[207,567] The E and F series also have opposing effects on the cardiovascular system: $PGF_2\alpha$ causes vasoconstriction and significant increase in pulmonary vascular resistance, whereas PGE_2 can cause systemic and, occasionally, pulmonary, vascular hypotension.[283,553] Other side effects include gastrointestinal disturbances (nausea, vomiting, diarrhea) and transient pyrexia. Prostaglandins can be life-saving in the treatment of severe hemorrhage resulting from uterine atony. Prostaglandin-$F_2\alpha$ has been given intramyometrially, or intramuscularly (IM) and more recently has been replaced for this purpose by a synthetic 15-methyl derivative, 15-methyl-prostaglandin-$F_2\alpha$, which can be administered intravenously (IV), IM, or intramyometrially, in a 250 μg dose. The methyl analogue is more potent and exerts a more prolonged effect than the natural prostaglandin. In the recommended dosage, it is relatively free of cardiovascular effects and can even be given to hypertensive patients.[41]

Hypotensive Agents

Several drugs are used in the management of pregnancy-induced hypertension. These include hydralazine, diazoxide, methyldopa, magnesium sulfate, alpha and beta adrenergic antagonists, sodium nitroprusside, and in some centers, slow-calcium channel-blocking agents, such as nifedipine. The principles of pharmacologic management of hypertension during pregnancy have been reviewed by Lubbe.[362] Because the blood pressure can be very labile in such patients, regional anesthesia should be applied cautiously, and local anesthetics given in small incremental doses.

Tocolytic Agents

Beta sympathomimetic drugs have been used in the management of premature labor for more than 20 years. They act upon β_2-receptors on the surface of uterine muscle cells and cause relaxation by inhibiting myosin light-chain phosphorylation (i.e., tocolysis). In therapeutic intravenous infusion doses, unpleasant side effects are very common, and include apprehension, restlessness, skeletal muscle tremor, nausea, tachycardia and palpitations. Beta-mimetic agents increase heart rate and cardiac output, while lowering peripheral vascular resistance.[354] Normally, mean blood pressure changes little. These effects accentuate further the hyperdynamic circulatory state that exists in pregnancy, which explains why even with the relatively β_2-selective agents (ritodrine, terbutaline, salbutamol, hexoprenaline and fenoterol), cardiovascular complications such as myocardial ischemia and pulmonary edema have been reported.[635] Pulmonary edema, in association with β_2-sympathomimetic treatment of premature labor, has been described on at least 73 occasions, and has caused 7 deaths.[252] Additional factors that have been incriminated include multiple gestation, undiagnosed heart disease, fluid overload, corticosteroid therapy, myocardial depression secondary to general anesthesia, and intravenous ergometrine.

β_2-sympathomimetic agents also produce metabolic changes, including hyperglycemia, hypokalemia, hypocalcemia, and metabolic acidosis secondary to lactate accumulation.[135] These changes are secondary to β-receptor stimulation of gluconeogenesis and glycogenolysis.

In view of the potentially serious complications of tocolytic therapy, patients require close observation and monitoring in a unit where resuscitation facilities exist. Cardiac disease must be excluded and fluid balance, serum glucose, and potassium monitored frequently. The implications of tocolytic therapy to neural blockade are not entirely clear. Epidural blockade may be beneficial in the presence of fluid overload and also reduces endogenous catecholamine release in premature labor.[380] Caution must be exercised, however, to avoid fluid overload and further sudden changes in heart rate or peripheral resistance.

Sometimes, the obstetrician requests urgent uterine relaxation during cesarean section in order to extract the fetus more easily; for an inverted uterus after a vaginal delivery; during manipulations in breech or twin deliveries; or to aid in the extraction of a retained placenta. In these circumstances, a small intravenous bolus of nitroglycerine is most effective; uterine relaxation occurs within a minute and persists for a similar period of time.[163,391,479] The dose required to produce uterine relaxation has varied from 50 to 100 μg to 500 μg. Hypotension (if it occurs) is usually transient and does not require treatment. Occasionally, a further dose of nitroglycerine may be necessary if more prolonged relaxation is required, as, for example, in extraction of a retained placenta.

H_2-Antagonists

Both cimetidine and ranitidine interact with hepatic cytochrome P-450, but fears that this might seriously inhibit local anesthetic metabolism appear to be unfounded.[154]

TECHNIQUES OF NEURAL BLOCKADE

The blockade techniques commonly used are divided conveniently into two groups: central and peripheral (Fig. 18-8). Descriptions of the applied anatomy and methods for the central techniques are found elsewhere (see Chapters 7 to 9). The following peripheral techniques are used frequently in obstetric surgery: local infiltration, pudendal block, and paracervical block.

Local Infiltration

Local infiltration is used often during deliveries that require episiotomies. Subcutaneous infiltration is carried out along the episiotomy incision, followed by deposition of the local anesthetic solution in the ischiorectal fossa in a fan-shaped pattern. Dilute solutions, such as 0.5% to 1.0% lidocaine, usually are adequate for infiltration and should be used with epinephrine 1:200,000.

After pudenal block, the genitofemoral and ilioinguinal nerves, which supply the anterior 1/3 of the labia majora, are not blocked. Local bilateral subcutaneous infiltration in this area provides adequate analgesia (see Fig. 18-2). One of the disadvantages of extensive local infiltration is that large volumes of local anesthetic may be required. Even infiltration of the perineum with lidocaine prior to episiotomy results in significant transplacental transfer, despite modest doses and a short injection-to-delivery time.[482] The F:M ratio can be relatively high (i.e., >1.0) following perineal infiltration,

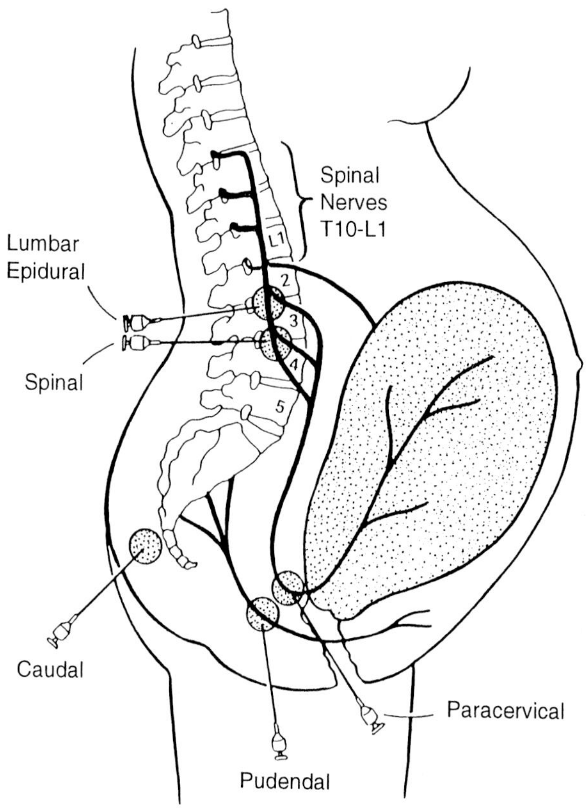

FIG. 18-8. Types of regional blocks that may be used to provide analgesia during obstetric and gynecological surgery.

and is correlated with the duration of the second stage of labor. This may represent a further example of enhanced local anesthetic transfer in the presence of fetal acidosis (see *amide-linked agents* earlier in this chapter).

Infiltration analgesia has also been used for cesarean section, but, because large volumes of local anesthetics are required, toxicity is a potential risk. Bonica has described a technique involving separate injections of subcutaneous, intrarectus, parietal peritoneal, visceral peritoneal and paracervical tissues.[53] However, spinal and epidural block have rendered infiltration methods obsolete, except in emergency situations when an anesthesiologist is not available immediately, or when the airway presents major difficulties, and regional anesthesia and awake intubation are impossible or contraindicated. Local infiltration may also be helpful in cases where regional anesthesia is inadequate and the block cannot be augmented or replaced.

Pudendal Block

Pudendal nerve block provides analgesia of the lower part of the vagina and perineum to allow an outlet forceps delivery and episiotomy (see Fig. 18-2). Two basic techniques are used in pudendal block: transvaginal and transperineal. The transvaginal technique has a higher success rate, probably owing to its simplicity.[331] In addition, it is less painful for the patient and produces a low incidence of complications. The transperineal pudendal block is now used infrequently, and only when the fetal head is fully descended onto the perineum.

Transvaginal Pudendal Block

With the patient in the lithotomy position, the ischial spine is palpated vaginally (see Fig. 18-9a). A 12- to 14-cm, 20-French gauge needle, attached to a 10 ml Luer-Lok syringe filled with local anesthetic solution is guided to the ischial spine through the vaginal wall by the index and middle fingers. Preferably, the needle is introduced through a needle guide (Iowa Trumpet or Kobak instrument), which limits its penetration. When the needle is in the sacrospinous ligament, compression of the syringe with local anesthetic solution meets with considerable resistance. As the needle tip passes through the ligament, loss of resistance is felt, and the area should then be infiltrated with local anesthetic solution. This procedure is then repeated on the other side.

Transperineal Pudendal Block

This approach requires a skin wheal about 2 to 3 cm posteromedial to the ischial tuberosity. The pudendal needle attached to the syringe, as described above, is guided to the ischial spine with the index finger usually placed in the vagina, or in the rectum, if the fetal head has fully descended to the perineum.

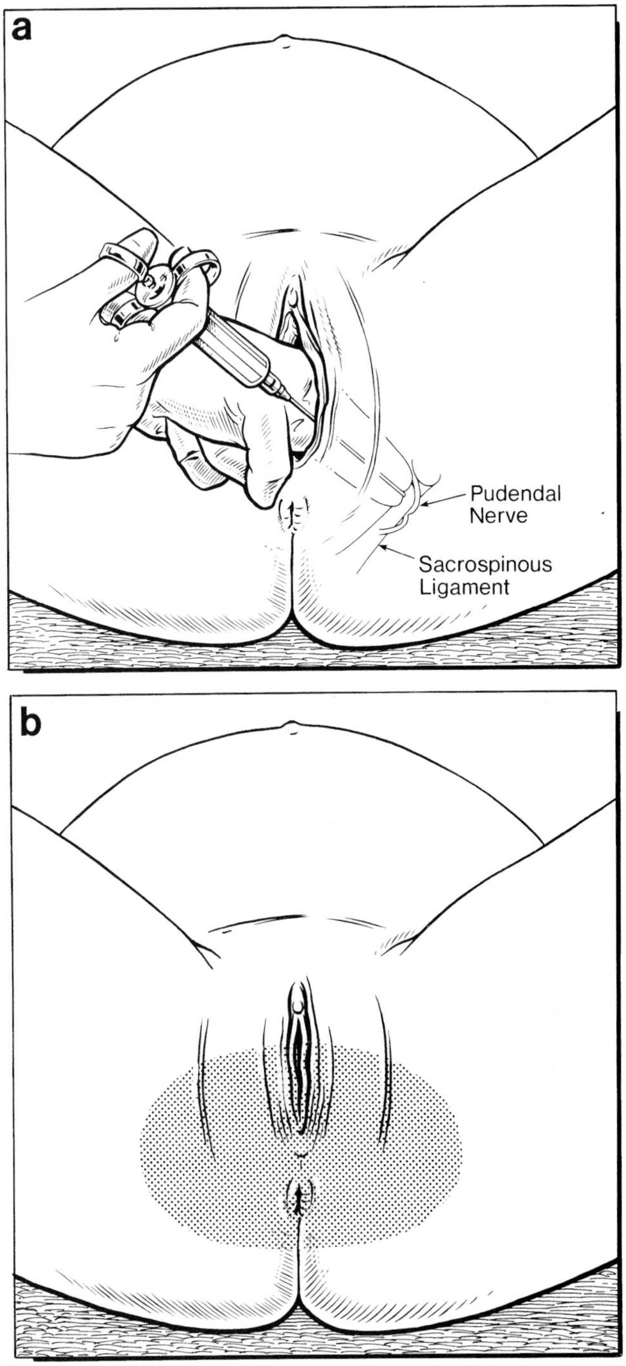

FIG. 18-9. a, b: Pudendal block by the transvaginal approach.

Lidocaine or mepivacaine (1%) with epinephrine (1:200,000) is the agent most commonly used for pudendal block. A total volume of 20 to 25 ml should be sufficient to produce the desired block, which usually lasts for 90 to 120 minutes. Chloroprocaine (1.5 to 2%) can also be used, but provides analgesia for only 60 to 90 minutes. Pudendal block produces analgesia in the posterior 2/3 of the labia and part of the buttock (see Fig. 18-9b). Analgesia of the anterior 1/3 of the labia requires local infiltration, as described above. As with all regional anesthetic techniques, it is important to make sure that intravascular injection is avoided by injecting slowly, attempting to aspirate the syringe and maintaining verbal contact with the patient.

The success rate of pudendal block undoubtedly is related to the experience of the clinician administering it. While success rates as high as 85% have been claimed,[546] one study reported a bilateral success rate of 50% with transvaginal blocks and only 25% with transperineal blocks, when they were performed by obstetric trainees.[552] Even when successful, the quality of analgesia is limited. In patients undergoing a mid-cavity or rotational forceps delivery, low subarachnoid or caudal analgesia is far more effective.[292] Pudendal block should only be performed by clinicians who are aware of the symptoms, signs, and treatment of local anesthetic toxicity (see Chapter 4).

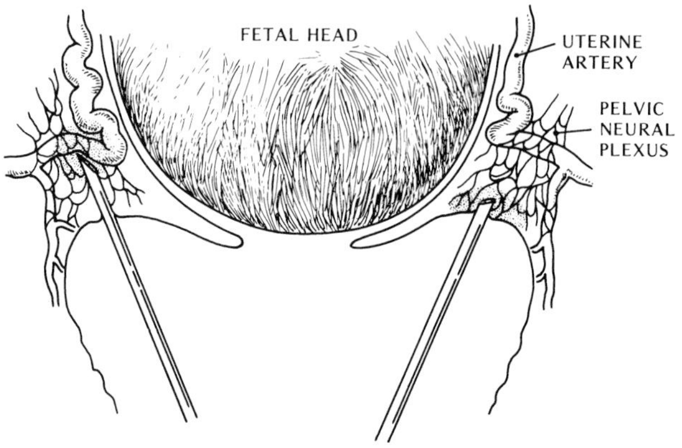

FIG. 18-10. Neurovascular anatomy associated with a paracervical block in obstetrics. The needle in the right fornix is short-bevelled and shows distribution of the local anesthetic. (Bloom, S.L., Horswill, C.W., and Curet, L.B.: Effects of paracervical blocks on the fetus during labor: A prospective study with the use of direct fetal monitoring. Am. J. Obstet. Gynecol., *114*:218, 1972).

Paracervical Block

First described by Gellert in Germany in 1926, paracervical block has been more popular in North America, Scandinavia, and continental Europe, than in the United Kingdom. Differing enthusiasm for the technique originally reflected differences in obstetric management. In those countries where paracervical block is popular, the obstetrician is involved directly with management during labor, whereas in the United Kingdom, uncomplicated labor (including analgesia) traditionally has been managed by a midwife.

The technique of paracervical block is relatively simple. To avoid intravascular injection, a 12- to 14-cm French gauge needle is used, with a guide (e.g., Iowa Trumpet), so that the needle point can only protrude 5 to 7 mm.[50] The guide, with needle tip protected, is directed into the lateral fornices between 3 and 4 o'clock, and between 8 and 9 o'-clock, by the index and middle fingers, so that the tip of the guide does not depress the vaginal mucosa excessively. An alternative technique employs a short bevelled needle with the guide omitted (Fig. 18-10).

Paracervical block provides effective analgesia for the first stage of labor, but this is of limited and variable duration (20 to 120 minutes),[231,237] and repeated blocks are needed during a long labor. The quality of pain relief is also less reliable than with epidural analgesia. The use of *continuous* paracervical block has not gained acceptance because it is difficult to maintain the tip of the catheter in the correct position. In addition, several cases of paracervical hematoma have developed into a neuropathy of the sacral plexus.[222]

The principal disadvantage of paracervical block is a high incidence of fetal arrythmias (particularly bradycardia), occurring within 10 minutes of injection in 5 to 70% of cases, sometimes accompanied by fetal acidosis and neonatal depression.[32,231,558] Unexplained fetal death has also been reported after paracervical block using mepivacaine and bupivacaine.[439,524] The etiology of the fetal depression is not entirely clear, but three different hypotheses have been proposed:

1. Direct depression of the fetal circulation by local anesthetics has been suggested.[12,32,579] Certainly, absorption from the paracervical area is rapid, with peak maternal and fetal blood levels occurring within 10 minutes,[476] the time at which FHR changes begin to appear. However, bradycardia has occurred even when fetal drug concentrations were low.[355] Freeman and co-workers[214] injected large doses of mepivacaine directly into anencephalic fetuses and found that although myocardial conduction depression invariably ensued, fetal bradycardia occurred only as a preterminal event. The poor correlation that exists between observed FHR changes and fetal local anesthetic concentration therefore makes a direct myocardial mechanism unlikely.
2. Paracervical block may cause uterine arterial vasoconstriction, which in turn leads to decreased placental perfusion, fetal hypoxia and bradycardia.[116,236] Bradycardia occurs most frequently with bupivacaine, and least often with chloroprocaine, thereby correlating with the effect of these drugs on uterine arteries. Local anesthetics appear to exert *in vitro* a dose-related *vasoconstrictive* effect upon the uterine artery at blood concentrations which occur clinically following paracervical block.[226,236]
3. Fetal hypoxia following paracervical block also may be secondary to an increase in uterine tone,[215,430,604] resulting from high concentrations of local anesthetics, although this concept has not been universally accepted.[116,408]
4. Other factors which may be contributory include mechanical distortion of uterine vessels, aortocaval compression, and the use of epinephrine. The incidence of FHR changes is not significantly altered, however, when epinephrine is added to local anesthetics.[558,579]

Whatever the mechanism of fetal bradycardia following

paracervical block, the incidence appears to be less following 2-chloroprocaine than with the amide-linked agents.[213,560,581,618] This may be related to the rapid hydrolysis of 2-chloroprocaine by plasma cholinesterase. Only trace concentrations of 2-chloroprocaine and its principal metabolite (2-chloroaminobenzoic acid) have been detected in the newborn following paracervical block.[483] However, 2-chloroprocaine has a short duration of action and several injections may be required during labor.[483] In many countries, it is not available. Lidocaine 1% is probably the most suitable agent for this block.

Paracervical block should be avoided in the presence of prematurity, uteroplacental insufficiency, or fetal distress, because the incidence of FHR changes is significantly higher in the presence of pre-existing FHR abnormalities.[342] It is difficult to avoid the conclusion that paracervical block has a limited role in modern obstetric practice, except in cases where central neural blockade is not feasible, or is unavailable. Continuous fetal heart rate monitoring should be used whenever paracervical block is performed.

CENTRAL NEURAL BLOCKADE DURING LABOR

> The most impressive effect (of epidural analgesia) is to bring tranquillity and humanity to the delivery suite, as well as happiness and dignity to a woman on one of the most important occasions in her life.
>
> Andrew Doughty, 1978.[174]

There can be no doubt that central neural blockade provides the most effective, consistently reliable, and versatile pain relief during childbirth. Compared with other forms of pain relief, epidural analgesia is associated with the highest levels of maternal satisfaction.[369] The lumbar (and to a much lesser extent, the caudal) epidural approach has proved to be the most practical and popular route of injection, although there has recently been some interest in the subarachnoid route, following the introduction of fine spinal catheters. Unlike the neural blockade techniques discussed so far, epidural analgesia can be extended to relieve both uterine pain (i.e., T10–L1) and pain related to distension of the lower birth canal (i.e., S2–S4) (see Fig. 18-8), as well as providing analgesia for episiotomy and forceps delivery.

Obstetric epidural pain management has become more sophisticated in recent years. Many centers, for example, now include an epidural opioid, in addition to local anesthetic during labor. While there seems to be general agreement that such opioid-local anesthetic combinations are clinically beneficial, it is difficult to compare results among centers because so many different opioids and dose regimens have been used. There are also differences in the manner in which epidural drugs are delivered (e.g., intermittent boluses, continuous infusions, patient-controlled doses). Each has its merits.[80] While such innovations pose some difficulties in the interpretation of study results, they do demonstrate the versatility and on-going evolution of epidural pain relief in obstetrics.

LUMBAR EPIDURAL ANALGESIA

Technical Considerations

Technical aspects of epidural analgesia are discussed fully in Chapter 8 and in standard obstetric anesthesia textbooks. Obstetric patients present additional challenges for the anesthesiologist: Spinal flexion is more difficult to achieve, especially if the patient is distressed and restless; some women find the sitting position uncomfortable during labor; the epidural space pressure becomes positive during uterine contractions; and epidural venous distension is present. Meticulous technique, therefore, is essential, if complications such as dural puncture and intravascular toxicity are to be avoided.

In laboring patients, the sensitivity and specificity of epinephrine as a marker for intravascular injection are limited because of the wide variability in maternal heart rate.[113,346] The sensitivity and positive predictive value of an epinephrine (10 to 15 μg) test dose can be improved by timing the injection to occur between contractions, limiting the observation period to 1 minute, noting the increase in heart rate relative to the peak heart rate in the 10 minutes or so before the test dose, and continuous heart rate monitoring. However, it has been estimated that between 27% to 45% of epidural catheters may be removed needlessly as a result of a positive test dose.[129] For these reasons, many centers consider routine test-dosing too cumbersome and not worthwhile in labor, when local anesthetic dosages are relatively low.

There is some evidence that the incidence of unilateral block, missed segments, and unsatisfactory analgesia is significantly less when closed-end (3 lateral holes) epidural catheters are used rather than open-end (single hole) catheters, especially among patients receiving *low-dose* epidural analgesia.[406]

Epidural dose requirements are generally accepted to be less during pregnancy,[67] although this has been disputed.[241] An exaggerated spread of local anesthetic may at term be caused by distension of the epidural venous plexus, either from vena caval occlusion, or secondary to uterine contractions (see Fig. 18-4). Fagraeus and associates observed facilitated spread of epidural analgesia even in early pregnancy, when mechanical factors related to the gravid uterus are unlikely to be significant.[198] These authors suggested that increased spread is more likely to be due to a reduction in buffer capacity, secondary to respiratory alkalosis, rather than to physical factors. As already mentioned, the nerve axon also appears to be rendered more sensitive to local anesthetics by progesterone during pregnancy.[87,159]

Pressure in the epidural space is increased during pregnancy, with higher values in the supine than the lateral position.[405] Epidural space pressure also rises during a uterine contraction,[66] although this effect is lessened following epidural analgesia.[405] Uterine contractions *per se,* however, have little influence on the physical spread of local anesthetic in the epidural space.[564]

Patient posture has minimal effect on the spread of epidural analgesia among patients who are not obese; a similar height of block is obtained whether she is placed in a lateral, or in a sitting, position.[404,451,521] In obese patients cephalad spread may[264] or may not[409] be limited to some degree in the sitting position.

Choice of Drug(s)

(a) Local Anesthetics

Bupivacaine has become widely established as the local anesthetic agent of choice during labor. Various regimens using concentrations ranging from 0.0625%[350] to 0.5%, with or without epinephrine, have been advocated. Weaker concentrations avoid undesirable dense motor blockade, but analgesia may be inadequate and its duration somewhat limited. The success rate for analgesia with bupivacaine 0.125%, for example, has ranged from as little as 30%[356,570] to more than 90%[49,586,599,637] of patients. The addition of epinephrine 1:200,000 improves the quality and duration of analgesia of the weaker concentrations of bupivacaine, but only at the expense of increased motor blockade.[356] Epidural chloroprocaine has also been used during labor, but the duration of action is brief (approximately 40 to 50 minutes following 3% chloroprocaine).[98,124] A mixture of chloroprocaine and bupivacaine does not provide any additional advantage over bupivacaine alone.[124] Lidocaine 1 to 2% with epinephrine is useful when more intense analgesia is required quickly for an instrumental delivery.

(b) Opioids

Used alone, epidural opioids generally have proven to be disappointing in childbirth, and supplementary analgesia invariably is needed during delivery. In the case of morphine, for example, doses in the range 2.5 to 5.0 mg were found ineffective in relieving uterine contraction pain in most cases,[145,291,371,633] although morphine 7.5 mg provides acceptable analgesia during the first stage of labor.[284] The long latency (up to 1 hour) and duration of action of epidural morphine also are problems. When controlled comparisons were made between epidural morphine and bupivacaine in the studies cited above, the local anesthetic proved to be far superior in providing pain relief.[284,291,633]

Side effects such as nausea, vomiting, sedation, and pruritus, frequently occur following epidural morphine. In one study comparing four different opioids, the incidence of pruritus was highest with morphine (60%).[17] In some patients, this symptom can be particularly severe.[371] The potential for respiratory depression occurring several hours after delivery is a further major reason for not using epidural morphine in labor.

Studies with the more lipid soluble opioids, meperidine, fentanyl and sufentanil, have yielded similar disappointing results, although the onset of analgesia is much more rapid (within 10 minutes). Both the efficacy and duration of analgesia are dose-dependent.[290,480,481,565] Meperidine, 25 mg, has an effective duration of less than an hour.[480,565] The addition of epinephrine 1:200,000 does not significantly improve the duration or quality of analgesia.[565] Compared with other opioids, however, meperidine very rarely causes pruritus[82] and is extremely effective in the treatment of shivering, during labor[78] and during cesarean section.[575]

In sufficiently large doses (150 to 200 μg), epidural fentanyl provides effective analgesia from uterine contraction pain within 10 minutes.[102,508] When used epidurally alone, fentanyl, 80 μg, is inferior to dilute concentrations of bupivacaine, and perineal analgesia is poor.[607] Like meperidine, it is also effective in reducing shivering.[390]

Epidural sufentanil provides dose-related analgesia for labor without any adverse neonatal effect;[572] the duration of analgesia with 5 to 15 μg doses is about an hour, with 40 to 50 μg doses lasting twice as long. However, analgesia in this study was probably enhanced by the epidural test dose of lidocaine with epinephrine that was given to all patients. In another study comparing labor analgesia with sufentanil, 10 μg, given intravenously, epidurally, or intrathecally, satisfactory analgesia only occurred with intrathecal administration.[90] Epidural alfentanil in bolus doses of 30 μg/kg, followed by a 30 μg/h infusion, results in poor analgesia.[224,259]

Local Anesthetic-Opioid Combinations

The use of local anesthetic-opioid drug combinations has become increasingly popular. There seems to be no limit to the number of opioid-bupivacaine mixtures and dosage regimens that have been introduced during the last decade. The actual choice of opioid drug seems to depend on local preferences and other indeterminable factors, rather than on firm clinical evidence.

The main attraction in using such drug combinations is the ability to reduce local anesthetic dosage and, consequently, the intensity of neural blockade. In this way, many of the dose-related side effects of epidural analgesia can be diminished considerably. These side-effects for the patient include: sensations of numbness and paresthesia; diminished awareness of the progress of labor and less urge to bear down at delivery; lower limb and pelvic floor muscle weakness; postural hypotension; shivering; and an increased likelihood for obstetric intervention (e.g., urinary catheterization and instrumental delivery). An instrumental delivery is a potent source of disappointment among women who hoped for a spontaneous birth.[427]

It is now generally considered that the benefits associated with the addition of an opioid drug outweigh potential opioid-related side-effects such as somnolence, nausea and vomiting, pruritus, and maternal and fetal respiratory depression. Although many of the reports cited below are based on very small study populations, worldwide experience using local anesthetic-opioid combinations is very extensive.

Bupivacaine-meperidine. The addition of meperidine, 25 mg, to bupivacaine, 12.5 mg, provides effective analgesia for approximately 90 minutes during the first stage of labor.[79,82,248] At these doses, lower limb motor blockade is barely detectable and opioid side-effects (particularly pruritus) are minimal.[82] Consequently, most patients who wish to bear weight, or ambulate, during labor are usually able to do so (see Fig. 18-11). The addition of meperidine also has been noted to produce an improved sense of patient well-being, independent of the analgesia achieved.[79]

Increasing the dose of meperidine to 50 or 100 mg provides analgesia that is equivalent to 0.25% bupivacaine for about 2 hours.[38,187] Larger doses, however, are associated with a higher incidence of side-effects such as nausea and sedation.[38]

Bupivacaine-fentanyl. The addition of fentanyl, 80 μg, to a test dose of bupivacaine provides a more rapid and complete onset of analgesia and significantly prolongs the duration of effect of the local anesthetic.[316,317] Such potentiation was noted only when fentanyl was administered by the epidural rather than the intramuscular route,[317] suggesting that the effect was due principally to a spinal action of the opioid drug. Cohen and associates found that the addition of 50 to 100 μg fentanyl to 0.25% bupivacaine produced the same degree of pain relief as 0.25% bupivacaine alone,[123] probably because the latter already provided excellent analgesia. A more interesting finding in this study was that 100 μg fentanyl added to 0.068% bupivacaine provided comparable analgesia to that obtained with 0.25% bupivacaine, with or without fentanyl.

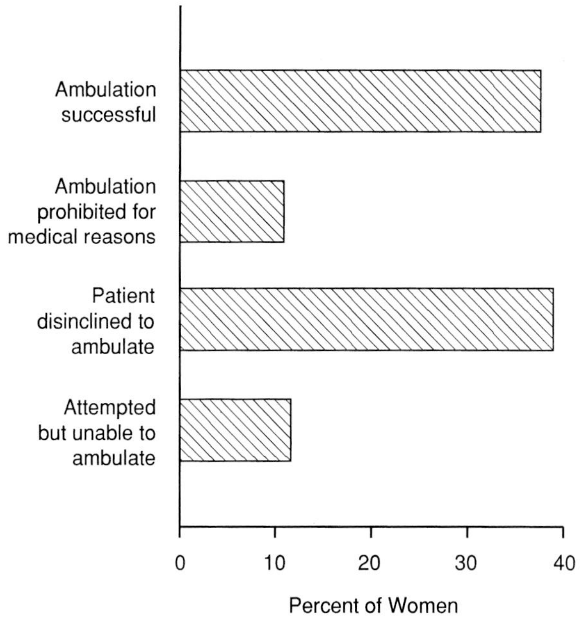

FIG. 18-11. Weight-bearing and ambulation during labor, using a low-dose epidural bupivacaine-meperidine mixture administered intermittently by midwives on a patient demand basis. (Unpublished data of 6,899 patients taken from the Obstetric Epidural Audit at Flinders Medical Centre, Adelaide, Australia).

Several other studies have shown that the addition of fentanyl (in a variety of different doses) to bupivacaine (also in a variety of different doses), whether administered by bolus, continuous infusion, or by a patient-controlled device, can significantly enhance both the duration and quality of analgesia when compared with bupivacaine alone.[106,110,112,306,366,450] The only significant side-effect reported in these studies appears to have been pruritus.

Bupivacaine-sufentanil. Epidural sufentanil, 20 to 30 μg, combined with 25.0 mg bupivacaine,[514] or sufentanil, 7.5 to 50 μg, with bupivacaine, 12.5 mg,[484,571,600,608] has been reported to provide better analgesia and less motor block during labor, than bupivacaine alone. Doses of 20 to 50 μg are relatively high, however, considering that systemically-administered sufentanil is 10 times as potent as fentanyl.[418] Satisfactory analgesia can be obtained using much smaller doses, for example 7.5 to 10 μg, added to a bolus of 0.125% bupivacaine, followed by a continuous infusion consisting of sufentanil, 0.25 μg/ml, combined with 0.0625% bupivacaine.[536] Again, pruritus appears to be a fairly common side effect (26% in one study).[608] Some deterioration in neonatal neurobehavior has been associated with sufentanil when used in very large doses, 30 to 80 μg, during cesarean section,[93] but neonatal depression has been absent with usual doses administered during the course of labor.[359,467]

Bupivacaine-alfentanil. One small study compared alfentanil, 5 μg/ml, and fentanyl, 2 μg/ml, combined with bupivacaine, 0.125%, as a continuous epidural infusion.[34] Analgesia was significantly better in the alfentanil group.

Bupivacaine-butorphanol. Unlike other opioid drugs discussed in this section, butorphanol is predominantly a kappa receptor agonist. The addition of epidural butorphanol, 1 to 3 mg, to bupivacaine, 25 mg, during labor, significantly increases the onset and duration of analgesia, compared to bupivacaine, 25 mg, alone.[2,8,287] It has been claimed that kappa agonists are associated with much less pruritus and nausea than opioids that depend on μ-agonism for their analgesic effect.[2,8,517] Unfortunately, these potential benefits of butorphanol are outweighed by an apparently higher incidence of somnolence and occasional dysphoria.[287] There has been recent concern that butorphanol is neurotoxic and may cause psychotomimetic side effects such as restlessness, agitation and muscle rigidity.[504]

Bupivacaine-methadone. In one study, methadone, 5 mg, improved the quality of analgesia provided by 0.25% bupivacaine and was associated with significantly less motor blockade, although it did not reduce the overall requirement for bupivacaine.[381]

Bupivacaine-diamorphine. Epidural diamorphine, 5 mg, when combined with bupivacaine, provided superior analgesia with fewer bupivacaine supplements, in one study among primigravidae in labor.[392] Another study found higher patient satisfaction among patients receiving an infusion of bupivacaine, 6.25 mg/h, mixed with diamorphine, 0.5 mg/h, than those receiving bupivacaine, 12.5 mg/h, alone, (although there was no difference in the amount of pain relief).[36] Diamorphine, 0.0025%, also compared favorably with fentanyl, 0.0002%, when added to bupivacaine, 0.125%, as a continuous infusion at a rate of 7.5 ml/hour in labor.[191] Pruritus was a common side-effect of diamorphine in these studies. Diamorphine is not available in many countries.

Maintenance of Epidural Analgesia after the Initial Dose

In practice, when epidural pain relief is available at the patient's request, and low doses are used, only a minority of women deliver within the duration of analgesia provided by the initial dose. Most women, therefore, require additional analgesia to be given by the epidural catheter. This can be provided in 3 different ways and each has its merits.[80]

Intermittent Bolus Injection. On-going analgesia is given by intermittent bolus (or, "top-up") injections, as required, by a nurse or medical practitioner. Provided further doses can be given *as requested* by the patient, intermittent injections present a very simple and convenient way of managing epidural analgesia during labor. In centers that permit nursing staff to administer epidural drugs, top-up doses can literally be given "on demand," but this is not usually the case in units where top-up doses can be given only by medical practitioners. When the latter restriction applies, there is likely to be some delay before analgesia can be re-established, and the patient may receive a stronger dose than is really required.

To some extent, delays in treatment can be overcome by giving top-up doses at regular (e.g., 90 minutes) intervals, rather than waiting for the patient to complain of pain.[495] However, regular dosing does not take into account the wide variation in analgesic requirements during labor. For some, pain relief may be inadequate, for others, too intense.

An alternative approach is to permit top-up doses to be given by the attending midwife (specially trained obstetric nurse) as, and when, required. By allowing the midwife to choose from a prescribed range of epidural drugs (e.g., a low-dose bupivacaine-opioid mixture; bupivacaine, 0.25%; bupivacaine, 0.5%), as well as to administer each top-up dose, according to individual need or circumstances, considerable flexibility in pain management can be achieved.[79] After all, the midwife develops a special rapport with the patient during childbirth and is well able to determine the patient's analgesic requirements as labor progresses.

The practice of permitting midwives or nurses to administer, let alone determine, epidural medication is controversial. The main concern has been one of safety. Nursing staff in some countries and/or individual hospitals are prohibited from giving epidural drugs of any description. It is beyond the scope of this chapter to discuss national differences in policies relating to midwife-managed epidural analgesia. When recommended practices are observed, however, the cumulative experience from at least two centers is reassuring (Table 18-2).[76,146] Bromage also refers to experience of over 30,000 epidurals safely managed by midwives in Montreal.[67]

Basic requirements for midwife-management of epidural analgesia in labor are summarized in Table 18-3. Additional recommendations have been suggested from time to time, such as aspirating and giving a test dose before each top-up dose and regular assessment of the upper sensory level of block.[307] The value of these additional tests has not been clearly established. Both false-positive and false-negative results can occur with a test dose, while it may be difficult to determine the upper level of sensory block when using local anesthetics in low dosage. Ultimately, safety depends on the degree of expertise, training, and familiarity of staff with epidural management and on the speed with which skilled assistance can be summoned in the event of an emergency.

Continuous Infusion Epidural Analgesia (CIEA). To ensure continuous analgesia and reduce the demands on medical personnel in centers in which nursing staff are not permitted to administer incremental doses, continuous epidural infusions via a mechanical infusion pump have been introduced. Infusates have included bupivacaine alone,[1,52,114,186,194,197,221,230,249,250,304,336,350,526,566,577] or bupivacaine combined with an opioid such as fentanyl,[110,112,156,306] sufentanil,[501,536] or alfentanil.[34] Recently, ropivacaine has been used for continuous epidural infusion for labor analgesia.[574,631] One comparative study of epidural infusions of 0.25% ropivacaine and bupivacaine found no differences between the two groups with respect to pain relief or motor blockade.[574] The second study[631] found a significantly lower incidence of instrumental deliveries in the ropivacaine group (see Local Anesthetics).

It has been claimed that CIEA is superior to intermittent bolus injections on several grounds, including: better and

TABLE 18-2. *Midwife-managed epidural analgesia in labor: incidence of potentially life-threatening complications*

Source	Crawford, J.S.[a]	Brownridge, P.[b]
Survey period	1968–1985	1975–1993
Number of epidurals administered	27,000	18,000
Number of top-up doses	>100,000	>65,000
Number of *potentially* life-threatening complications following a midwife administered dose	[c]3 (1:33,000)	nil

[a] From Crawford, J.S.: Some maternal complications of epidural analgesia for labour. Anaesthesia, *40*:1219, 1985.

[b] From Brownridge, P.: A three-year survey of an obstetric epidural service with top-up doses administered by midwives. Anaesth. Intensive Care, *10:* 298, 1982; and unpublished audited data.

[c] Includes two cases of systemic local anesthetic toxicity and one high spinal block. All cases resuscitated promptly and successfully.

TABLE 18-3. *Basic requirements for the management of epidural analgesia in labor*

Facilities and procedures
Adequate resuscitation, monitoring and anesthetic equipment immediately available and checked daily.
Protocols for management of complications (e.g., high spinal block, cardiovascular collapse, convulsions).
Staffing
A physician proficient in resuscitation readily available.
Attending midwives experienced in epidural management and in the recognition of complications.
Patient preparation
Exclude epidural contraindications (patient refusal, hypovolemia, bacteremia, coagulopathy).
Give explanation appropriate to the circumstances and obtain patient consent.
Ensure intravenous access.
Initial epidural injection
Sterile procedure.
Ensure the patient does not assume the supine posture.
Exclude subarachnoid or intravascular placement of needle/catheter (aspirate; give test dose).
Check blood pressure and fetal heart rate regularly. Treat hypotension if necessary (IV fluid load, IV ephedrine in 5 mg increments).
Evaluate patient response and check level of block.
Subsequent epidural management
Epidural medication may be administered and supervised by nursing staff (e.g., by intermittent injection, infusion device, PCEA) provided:
1. Facilities and staffing as outlined above are available.
2. Initial dose via the catheter has been administered by a physician.
3. Blood pressure and fetal heart rate are stable.
4. Epidural medication is clearly prescribed.
5. Epidural drugs are freshly prepared, double-checked and administered slowly.
6. Basic observations are recorded after each dose [e.g., blood pressure, fetal heart rate, assessment of degree of motor block and (?) height of block (using skin response to ice or pin-prick)].

more consistent analgesia; a lower incidence of hypotension; reduced dose requirements and less fetal drug exposure; greater safety; and reduced workload. Most of these reports, however, did not properly compare infusions with intermittent techniques, and it is doubtful in some cases whether bolus doses truly were given on demand. When they *were* properly compared, there was, in fact, very little to choose between the two regimens with regard to the quality of analgesia.[566] Moreover, a continuous infusion did not remove the need for additional bolus injections. The number of patients who required a bolus top-up in the reports cited above ranged from 24% to 83%. Not surprisingly, the need for additional analgesia when local anesthetics were used alone increased as the infusion dose was lowered.[350] At the time of writing, there are no published studies comparing the efficacy of intermittent epidural bolus doses of ropivacaine versus continuous infusion.

Infusion regimens do not necessarily decrease the epidural dose requirements either. On the contrary, most studies have shown the opposite to be the case when local anesthetics alone were used.[52,186,221,350,484,494,566] It follows, therefore, that the dose of drug received by the fetus is unlikely to be any less with CIEA than with intermittent injections. The incidence of hypotension also appears to be no different.[566]

It has been proposed that CIEA is intrinsically safer than intermittent bolus injections because accidental intravenous, subarachnoid or subdural injection is likely to be detected before serious patient harm occurs and because fewer bolus injections are needed.[526] While there may be some substance to these claims, it does not follow that CIEA demands less patient supervision or lower standards of care.

Patient-controlled Epidural Analgesia (PCEA). Advances in the design of patient-controlled infusion devices have recently been applied to epidural management during labor, with, or without, a background infusion.[202,211,218,219,366,462,463,494,609] PCEA permits the patient to balance her desired level of analgesia against any side-effects she may experience. The dose required to achieve this end is variable and often alters as labor progresses. It is not surprising, therefore, that one PCEA study found a 3-fold variation in bupivacaine use.[366] Gambling and associates compared PCEA with conventional top-up injections using 0.125% bupivacaine plus 1:400,000 epinephrine and found that the pain relief and hourly bupivacaine requirements were similar in both groups.[218] Previously, the same group compared PCEA with CIEA using 0.125% bupivacaine; in that study, the PCEA group received similar pain relief but significantly less local anesthetic than the CIEA group.[219] Ferrante and co-workers observed a similar dose-sparing effect with PCEA, when PCEA was compared with CIEA, using 0.125% bupivacaine plus fentanyl (2 μg/ml) infusion.[202]

An appropriate lockout interval is necessary when using PCEA, to allow for the delay in response after each dose demand. In the case of epidural bupivacaine plus a lipophilic opioid, a 10 to 15 minute lockout interval appears to be satisfactory.[366,462] Recent studies suggest that the addition of a background infusion confers no benefit over PCEA alone.[202,463] Patient monitoring must be just as vigilant using PCEA as with any other epidural technique.

The PCEA infusate is limited to a predetermined drug preparation. It is possible, therefore, to alter only the rate of delivery and not the nature of the drug(s) delivered. PCEA devices are costly and cumbersome to use, patient mobility is restricted and some mothers dislike being attached to too much technical equipment. Finally, PCEA is not entirely without risk; various errors and mechanical problems have been reported.[453,621]

Indications

By far the most common indication for epidural analgesia is the provision of pain relief. In addition, there are certain complications of pregnancy in which epidural analgesia is indicated on therapeutic grounds.

Preeclampsia and Hypertension

Preeclampsia (or pregnancy-induced hypertension) is a potentially serious complication specific to pregnancy which may arise *de novo,* or may be superimposed upon an underlying hypertensive disorder. Other causes of hypertension include: (i) essential hypertension; (ii) renal disease, e.g. glomerulonephritis; (iii) cardiovascular or autoimmune disease, for example, polyarteritis nodosa and lupus erythematosus; and (iv) adrenal disorders, for example, pheochromocytoma and primary aldosteronism. Preeclampsia is rarely manifest before 26 weeks of gestation. Classically, the diagnosis is suspected when at least 2 of the following 3 conditions arise: hypertension, proteinuria, and edema. Like other hypertensive states, symptoms may be absent until an advanced stage; these include headache, vomiting, epigastric pain, photophobia, and convulsions (eclampsia).

A detailed review of the etiology, pathogenesis, management, and treatment of preeclampsia is beyond the scope of this chapter. Failure of normal placental implantation results in reduced prostacyclin formation, and a rise in the vasoconstrictor, thromboxane A_2, which, further, leads to endothelial damage, reduced plasma volume, intravascular coagulation, and diminished organ perfusion.[70] Thus, there is widespread vascular dysfunction involving several organs, including the placenta.

The increase in systemic blood pressure that occurs in preeclampsia is largely secondary to a rise in systemic vascular resistance, although cardiac output usually is also increased. The underlying cause of this vasoconstrictive state is unknown. Although plasma catecholamine concentrations are significantly increased in preeclampsia,[3] other factors are likely to be more important. The failure of the circulation to dilate in the face of rising cardiac output is characteristic of preeclampsia. Despite an increase in total body water, the circulatory plasma volume can be contracted by as much as 25%.[367,492,569] The hematocrit and whole blood viscosity also are raised,[84,256,261] and these changes contribute further to the increase in peripheral resistance. Patients behave as if they are venoconstricted, becoming susceptible to circulatory congestion, and pulmonary edema, with excessive fluid administration.[367] Fluid management must balance input and output carefully, if necessary, with the guidance of central monitoring in severe cases. Both renal and uterine blood flow are decreased, usually in proportion to the severity of the disease.[169] These changes are associated with fibrin deposition, and lead to diminished glomerular filtration and intrauterine growth retardation. Liver function may be abnormal. Plasma colloid oncotic pressure is reduced[46] and this may contribute to the development of cerebral or pulmonary edema.[108] These circulatory changes are summarized in Figure 18-12.

Coagulation disorders often exist in preeclampsia, including a consumptive thrombocytopenia, hypofibrinogenemia and a prolonged plasma thrombin time.[491] In addition, the platelets may demonstrate abnormal function.[323] In severe cases, disseminated intravascular coagulation (DIC) may develop. The association of hemolysis, elevated liver enzymes and low platelets (commonly labeled the HELLP syndrome), is associated with a high incidence of morbidity, including hepatic rupture, acute renal failure, DIC, abruption and perinatal death.[563]

Preeclampsia is therefore a complicated disease and, despite a considerable improvement in prognosis over the years, it remains one of the major causes of maternal death in developed countries. Cerebral hemorrhage and pulmonary edema are the most common terminal events, although eclampsia, hepatic and renal failure, and DIC, are also contributory. The anesthesiologist should play an important role in the management of severe preeclampsia and therefore must understand the pathophysiology of the disease. The anesthesiologist must also be familiar with modern obstetric management of preeclampsia, because the patient may be receiving one or more of several potent drugs, which may interact with anesthesia and analgesia. These include sedatives and hypnotics, anticonvulsants, hypotensive agents, diuret-

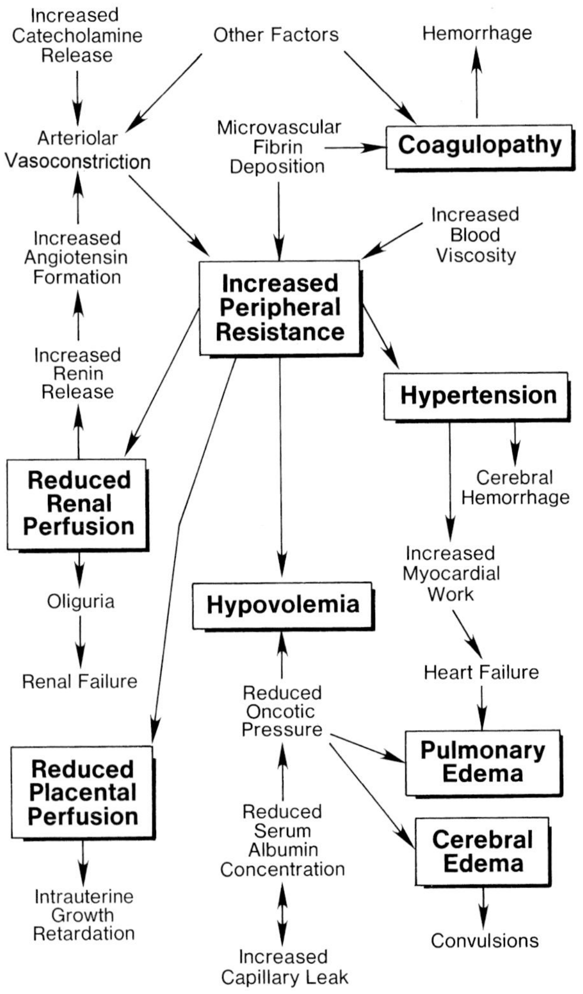

FIG. 18-12. Pathophysiological changes in preeclampsia (pregnancy-induced hypertension).

ics, low-dose aspirin, and, less commonly, heparin and corticosteroids.[362]

When vaginal delivery is planned in preeclampsia, epidural analgesia provides the best method of pain relief, while having several additional advantages. Diastolic blood pressure is reduced, on average, by over 20%[416] and placental perfusion is improved (provided that hypovolemia has been corrected and aortocaval compression is avoided).[309] This improvement in uterine blood flow presumably is due to sympathetic blockade and decreased endogenous catecholamine production. It is likely that renal perfusion is similarly improved, although this has not been confirmed.[300] Other physiological changes that occur during labor and that are largely secondary to pain or stress are also obtunded by epidural analgesia (see Fig. 18-6). Decreased maternal plasma catecholamine concentrations (which are known to be elevated in preeclampsia) prevent sudden fluctuations in blood pressure.[3,557] Moreover, an indwelling epidural catheter placed for labor analgesia allows a fast route for cesarean delivery anesthesia, if this becomes necessary.

Epidural analgesia allows an elective, controlled, instrumental delivery to be performed under ideal conditions, with perineal relaxation and minimal fetal trauma. There is also less need for maternal sedatives and opioids when epidural analgesia is employed. Nevertheless, epidural analgesia must not be used in the presence of hypovolemia. Cautious blood volume expansion, (with central venous or pulmonary artery wedge pressure monitoring in very severe cases), should precede or accompany the onset of autonomic blockade. The epidural block should be extended gradually, treating hypotension with additional fluids and small (2.5 to 5.0 mg) doses of IV ephedrine.

The choice of anesthesia for cesarean section in the presence of hypertension depends on several factors. Epidural anesthesia provides greater stability of systemic and pulmonary artery pressure compared with general anesthesia, in which sudden swings in arterial pressure occur at intubation and extubation.[266] In addition, use of epidural anesthesia avoids the need for airway instrumentation in a patient who has a higher than normal probability of being a difficult intubation, both with respect to her pregnancy and her preeclampsia. Postoperative epidural opioid or local anesthetic analgesia can also help the management of blood pressure following surgery.

The question of safety of central neural blockade in the presence of potentially altered coagulation, whether this results from treatment or from the disease itself, remains largely unresolved in the patient with preeclampsia. There are no hard and fast rules; however, some guidelines can be applied. If the platelet count is greater than 100,000/μl, it is likely that other indices of coagulation will be normal. In addition, if the recent platelet count is not dramatically lower than the previous value, and if there is no clinical evidence of coagulopathy, then regional anesthesia can be safely performed. It is important to bear in mind, however, that some patients with preeclampsia will have abnormal platelet function despite a normal platelet count. It has been shown that bleeding time is not predictive of the risk of hematoma formation,[456,518] and consequently, it is no longer performed by most obstetric anesthesiologists. To document downward trends, serial platelet counts and fibrinogen measurements are necessary. The decision to place an epidural catheter in a patient with rapidly developing severe preeclampsia should be made early on, while the patient's coagulation parameters are normal. If platelets fall to less than 100,000/μl, then a careful assessment of risk of spinal hematoma, versus benefits of regional anesthesia, must be carried out. Decisions about the use of regional anesthesia in this circumstance must be made on an individual basis, and often are matters of local practice and individual anesthesiologist's judgment. Just as critical as meticulous anesthetic technique and careful patient selection is the need for continued neurologic assessment. Early diagnosis and treatment of epidural or spinal hematoma is crucial (see also Chapters 8 and 21).

An increasing number of patients with preeclampsia are on low-dose aspirin therapy and, as mentioned above, many therefore have impaired platelet function, despite having a normal platelet count. Aspirin irreversibly inhibits the enzyme, cyclo-oxygenase, and consequently the production of thromboxane A_2, in platelets. With respect to the effects of aspirin, 60 mg daily, a large multicenter randomized placebo-controlled trial (CLASP) found no difference in the number of adverse reactions among women receiving aspirin, who also had epidural analgesia.[164] Low-dose aspirin therapy does not appear to influence the thromboelastography test and so it seems unlikely that aspirin increases the risk of developing an epidural hematoma.[459] A large prospective study recently performed by Horlocker et al.[280] showed that preoperative antiplatelet therapy does not increase the risk of spinal hematoma associated with central neural blockade.

Preterm Labor

Preterm labor occurs in 7 to 8% of pregnancies in the United States and is the leading cause of perinatal mortality. Parturients in preterm labor frequently are receiving tocolytic drugs (e.g., magnesium, beta-agonists, calcium channel blockers), which must be taken into account when planning anesthetic management.[109] The preterm fetus, particularly when gestational age is less than 30 weeks, is more susceptible to the stresses of labor and delivery. Asphyxia poses a greater hazard than to the term fetus, and intracranial hemorrhage is more common because of the soft cranium, fragile intracranial vessels, and a relative deficiency of clotting factors. When delivery becomes inevitable, the primary goal of obstetric management is to avoid trauma during delivery. Although the preferred route of delivery for very-low-birthweight infants remains controversial, a large percentage of preterm infants currently is delivered by cesarean section, often for complications such as fetal distress or breech presentation, which occur frequently in this population. Epidural anesthesia is considered the preferred method of analgesia for labor and vaginal delivery, because it avoids use of depressant drugs (to which the preterm fetus is particularly sensitive) and allows a controlled delivery. Animal studies suggest that preterm fetal lambs are similar with respect to the pharmacokinetic and pharmacodynamic effects of lidocaine[477] and may be more resistant to lidocaine toxicity than are animals of more advanced gestations.[580] However, in another study, lidocaine administration in the presence of asphyxia caused increased acidosis and deterioration of cardiovascular status in preterm fetal lambs, in contrast to term fetuses, in which it had no such effect.[433] Epidural anesthesia should be conducted using minimal doses of local anesthetics in early labor, extending the block in the second stage to produce perineal relaxation, if required, for episiotomy and forceps delivery. For cesarean section, regional anesthesia is preferred. A recent study assessing the influence of anesthetic technique on neonatal outcome in infants of less than 30 weeks' gestation demonstrated a 3-fold higher risk for low (0 to 3) one- and five-minute Apgar scores with general, as compared with, epidural anesthesia.[519] This relationship was present even when confounding factors that might have increased fetal risk were taken into account. Although spinal anesthesia has not been studied in this circumstance, similar neonatal outcome to that obtained with epidural anesthesia should be anticipated.

Breech Presentation

Formerly regarded as being contraindicated in breech presentations, several studies have now shown that epidural anesthesia is associated with superior conditions for delivery and improved neonatal outcome.[59,130,142,155,171] Initial fears that it would contribute to morbidity by increasing the breech extraction rate have not materialized. Retrospective studies of vaginal breech deliveries comparing epidural analgesia with "conventional" analgesia have found a small prolongation of labor, but no increase in the incidence of operative intervention; neonatal condition was actually better in deliveries in which epidural analgesia was employed.[59,130,142,155,171] A prospective study concluded that epidural analgesia did not prolong labor, that breech extraction was reduced, and that the acid-base status of the fetus was better than when labor was conducted with other methods of analgesia.[64] There are several possible explanations for these favorable results: since the mother is comfortable and cooperative, the progress of labor can be determined by thorough vaginal examinations; the otherwise common urge to push before full dilatation is obtunded; and good perineal relaxation provides optimal conditions for controlled delivery of the fetal head. As the need for emergency general anesthesia is also decreased, epidural analgesia should result in decreased maternal risk. For these reasons, epidural analgesia can be recommended whenever a vaginal breech delivery is proposed.[602]

Multiple Pregnancy

Multiple pregnancy used to be regarded as a contraindication to epidural analgesia on the grounds that a delay in the second stage of labor would lead to more frequent intervention and result in a contracted uterus that would jeopardize the second twin. Mortality and morbidity are greater among second twins and reflect contraction and even separation of the placental bed or cord prolapse, following delivery of the first infant. Multiple pregnancy also is commonly associated with premature labor and preeclampsia, which contribute further to a higher perinatal mortality. Obstetric intervention may be required urgently to expedite delivery of the second twin.

More recently, epidural analgesia for multiple births has been regarded favorably.[143,147,243,298,302,616] One large prospective study suggested that the provision of an epidural for either cesarean section or vaginal delivery was markedly beneficial to the second twin.[147] Although most of these studies reported a longer second stage of labor and increased operative intervention compared with other methods of analgesia, neonatal outcome was similar and the acid-base status of the second twin was usually as good as, or better than, that of its sibling.[147] Moreover, the facility with which obstetric intervention could be performed, without resource to the induction of urgent general anesthesia, was favorably noted in all these studies. Even locked twins have been successfully disimpacted under lumbar epidural blockade.[325]

Incoordinate Uterine Action

Failure to progress during labor in the absence of disproportion is commonly associated with incoordinate uterine activity. Labor is accordingly prolonged, painful, and exhausting for the mother, and the physiological changes associated with painful labor (Fig. 18-6) are accentuated with time. Uterine action invariably improves following epidural analgesia and frequently allows labor to progress normally.[373,417]

Maternal Medical Complications

Certain preexisting maternal medical conditions carry an increased risk of maternal and fetal complications, for example, cardiopulmonary diseases, diabetes, autoimmune disorders, and hepatic dysfunction. Severe illness in the obstetric patient may also occur coincidentally, or as a consequence of pregnancy. Examples of the former are trauma, burns, and malignancy; the latter category includes preeclampsia, peripartum hemorrhage, and pulmonary and amniotic fluid embolism. Cocaine and abuses of other substances, for example, amphetamines, opioids, and alcohol, may be iatrogenic causes of maternal and fetal compromise. Cocaine use may mimic other medical disorders, such as acute hypertensive disease of pregnancy. Severe, life-threatening illness may mandate the parturient's admission to an intensive care unit for treatment, where access to sophisticated monitoring equipment, ventilatory support and 1:1 nursing-to-patient care is available. An in-depth discussion of the treatment of severe medical disease in the parturient and its implications for the anesthetic management of labor and delivery is beyond the scope of this chapter, and the reader is referred elsewhere.[601]

In brief, epidural analgesia is generally recommended for labor in the presence of heart disease. Abolition of the physiological responses to pain (Fig. 18-6) is beneficial in patients with diminished cardiac reserve. Active bearing down at delivery also represents an additional workload on the heart. For these reasons, an elective instrumental delivery under epidural analgesia often is preferred. Epidural blockade is not theoretically indicated in patients with aortic stenosis or those with a right-to-left shunt, because of the adverse hemodynamic consequences of a decreased systemic vascular resistance; however, its successful use has been described for labor analgesia, with the emphasis that major hemodynamic changes must be avoided.[601] For cesarean delivery, general anesthesia provides a much more stable hemodynamic situation. Despite theoretical objections, epidural analgesia has been used safely in the presence of Eisenmenger's syndrome.[150] Regardless of anesthetic technique, appropriate use of invasive monitoring, and careful management of fluid balance are critical in these patients. Such monitoring must be continued post-delivery until hemodynamic stability has been maintained for a suitable length of time.

Epidural analgesia may be beneficial in patients with a history of chronic respiratory disease, intracranial surgery or cerebrovascular accident. Diabetes mellitus is also a relative indication.[413]

Fetal Abnormality and Intrauterine Death

It is only reasonable and humane to reduce pain as effectively as possible in grief-stricken patients. Accordingly, epidural analgesia should be available, although caution is required in patients with coagulopathy (see Preeclampsia).

Contraindications

With the passage of time, many earlier fears about the safety of epidural analgesia and its influence upon the progress of labor have been dispelled. Crawford has proposed that there remain only 3 absolute contraindications.[141] They include patient refusal, the presence of a severe coagulation defect, and local or generalized infection. Whether the latter should be an absolute contraindication is controversial. Other relative contraindications are discussed in Chapter 8.

In the past, it was feared that by abolishing pain, epidural analgesia might conceal the presence of intra-abdominal hemorrhage or other serious complications, thereby delaying treatment. It is now appreciated that these fears are not well-founded and that placental abruption[470] and uterine rupture[596] are still readily recognized under epidural blockade. A trial of labor in the presence of a uterine scar is not, therefore, a contraindication to epidural analgesia; indeed, it has been recommended.[399]

Failure of Analgesia

Many centers have shown that satisfactory epidural analgesia occurs in 85 to 90% of patients in labor.[49,76,140,141,173,269,274,413,422,496] Ideally, in order to provide pain relief from uterine contractions, local anesthetics should be injected as close as possible to the spinal nerve roots T10–L1 in the posterior midline position of the epidural space. The tip of an epidural catheter may sometimes be positioned away from the midline or even be passed through an intervertebral foramen into the paravertebral space.[597] Analgesia is then likely to be unilateral or incomplete. In this event, which can occur in almost 20% of patients,[76,105,173,269] some readjustment is usually all that is required to achieve satisfactory analgesia. These adjustments include turning the patient to the opposite side and giving a further dose, and partial withdrawal of the catheter or, in the case of persistent unilateral block, reinsertion (see also Chapter 8, Figs. 8-7 and 8-8).

Inadequate perineal analgesia for delivery is a more frequent nuisance, although it usually can be avoided by administering a larger dose of local anesthetic when delivery is imminent,[76,269,271] or by adding a lipid soluble opioid to the local anesthetic.[110,508] Some authorities have recommended giving a top-up dose in a sitting position before delivery,[67,173] although this practice has not been validated. Other centers do not aim to achieve perineal analgesia, preferring to supplement with local anesthetic infiltration, or a pudendal block, if required.[314]

Effect on the Course of Labor

It has become generally accepted that epidural analgesia does not prolong the duration of the first stage of labor.[141,417,486] A transitory decrease in uterine activity has been described,[496,622] but this is of little clinical importance. It is not clear whether or not the addition of epinephrine has any significant effect on uterine contractions.

The influence of epidural analgesia on the duration of the second stage of labor and on the necessity for an instrumental delivery remains controversial. Almost all of the case series cited in *Neural Blockade* have demonstrated an increased incidence of forceps delivery or vacuum extraction. This association is, however, complicated by several factors: (i) epidural analgesia is most commonly used among patients in whom spontaneous delivery is less likely to occur (e.g., fetal malposition, trial of labor); (ii) the decision to intervene is determined solely by the attending obstetrician, and there is considerable individual variation in this respect (e.g., in one unit, the forceps rate among obstetricians ranged between 10 and 70%);[174] and (iii) there is still controversy as to when the second stage should be considered to have begun and as to whether a time limit should be set before intervention is indicated. Obviously, all these factors have a considerable influence on the instrumental delivery rate. Despite these difficulties, a prospective trial has still shown a 5-fold increase in forceps delivery, and a 3-fold increase in malposition among mothers who received epidural analgesia using bupivacaine 0.5%.[281] Whether these results are applicable to modern epidural techniques, which use more dilute solutions of bupivacaine with opioids and cause less motor blockade, is questionable. Two recent studies have demonstrated a decreased incidence of instrumental delivery when dilute solutions of bupivacaine with opioids were compared with bupivacaine alone.[438,608] Although a low-cavity forceps delivery is generally regarded as being innocuous to the fetus, midforceps rotational deliveries have been associated with intracranial hemorrhage.[455]

Epidural analgesia may contribute directly to the higher incidence of intervention at delivery if perineal sensation has been abolished and if there has been sufficient loss of pelvic floor muscle tone to interfere with normal rotation of the fetal head. In an attempt to improve the rate of normal delivery, many centers use weaker concentrations of epidural local anesthetics,[112] or a limited "segmental block" for the first stage of labor only.[49,172,274,315,373,389] The latter practice may increase the likelihood of a spontaneous delivery, but delivery is more likely to be painful. Chestnut et al.[114] have shown that dense perineal analgesia associated with continuing an infusion of 0.125% bupivacaine throughout the second stage of labor increased the duration of the second stage and the incidence of forceps delivery without influencing malrotation or increasing the cesarean section rate. In contrast, continuing an infusion containing 0.0625% bupivacaine with fentanyl, 2 μg/ml, resulted in improved analgesia compared with patients who received saline placebo, but neither prolonged the second stage, nor increased the incidence of forceps delivery.[110] Despite the absence of surgical perineal anesthesia in 61% of patients in the study group (versus 85% in the placebo group), the majority of women were satisfied with their analgesia. Thus, it appears that many patients are prepared to trade off some degree of pain in the second stage in return for a spontaneous delivery.

Epidural analgesia should influence management at delivery, and readjustments in policy are often required when the technique is newly introduced. The mother should not be encouraged to push too early, and a longer second stage should be tolerated than in patients without regional blockade. Active intervention is indicated only if signs of fetal distress appear. Such policies have been shown to reduce the instrumental delivery rate considerably.[35,379]

It has recently been claimed by Thorp et al.[587,588,589] that epidural analgesia markedly increases the cesarean section rate for dystocia in nulliparous women. In their most recent study, 90 nulliparous women were randomized to receive either bupivacaine epidural analgesia or intravenous meperidine and promethazine.[588] Women who received epidural analgesia experienced prolongation of the first and second stages, a 2-fold increase in oxytocin augmentation and a cesarean section rate of 25%, compared with only 2.2% in women receiving systemic opioids; this effect was most marked in women receiving an epidural at a cervical dilatation of less than 5 cm. One criticism of this study is that decisions regarding obstetric management were not dictated by protocol, but were made by the individual obstetrician who was aware of the patient's analgesic technique.[165] Furthermore, little information is provided about anesthetic management, such as whether infusion rates were modified with the goal of minimizing motor blockade. Two studies by Chestnut et al.[111,115] investigating, respectively, patients receiving oxytocin, and those in spontaneous labor, tend to refute the claim that early epidural analgesia increases the risk of cesarean section. In both studies, patients requesting analgesia, with cervical dilatation of at least 3 cm but less than 5 cm, were randomized to receive either epidural bupivacaine, or epidural saline and intravenous nalbuphine. Epidural analgesia was managed with the goal of minimizing motor blockade and optimizing expulsive efforts. There were no differences in the incidence of cesarean section in either study between the early and late epidural groups, although the cesarean section rate was greater (18 to 19%) in women who required oxytocin for induction or augmentation of labor than in those in spontaneous labor (8 to 10%).

While Chestnut's studies did not compare epidural analgesia with no epidural analgesia, they do suggest that the effect of early epidural block is no different from that of a block performed in later labor. They also suggest that dysfunctional labor requiring oxytocin augmentation poses a greater risk for cesarean delivery. This conclusion is supported by a large (nonrandomized) study of 1,250 nulliparous women managed according to strict standardized criteria for the active management of labor.[97] Although epidural analgesia, oxytocin requirements, and the induction of labor conferred additive influences on the mode of delivery, the cesarean section rates were low: only 7.5% in primiparas with epidural analgesia, compared with 3.5% without regional block. Cesarean section rates were higher (12%) in women requiring oxytocin, and were similar, with or without epidural analgesia. Thus, any deleterious effect of epidural analgesia (if it exists) appears relatively small compared with that of dysfunctional labor.

Other Effects

Epidural analgesia prevents, or reverses, most of the pain-mediated physiological changes which are summarized in Figure 18-5. In addition, in some circumstances, uterine contractions can become more efficient and placental perfusion improved.[313] These aspects of epidural analgesia can be regarded only as beneficial to the fetus and the neonate. Epidural analgesia also appears to lower the incidence and severity of retinal hemorrhages in the newborn,[375,376] possibly by reducing pelvic floor muscle tone and pressure on the fetal head. It is not known whether intracranial hemorrhage is similarly reduced.

Side Effects and Complications

Epidural analgesia is associated inevitably with dose-related side-effects. Although minor, they can be a source of frustration and disappointment to the mother. For example, using traditional doses, weight-bearing and ambulation are not usually feasible and the lower limbs may become totally immobile. Ambulation has been found possible, however, under midwife supervision, using intermittent bupivacaine, 12.5 mg, with meperidine, 25 mg;[79] or an infusion of bupivacaine, 0.04%, with fentanyl[63] (see also section on combined spinal epidural [CSE] analgesia). Awareness of uterine contractions and of a full bladder may also be lost and the urge to bear down at delivery abolished altogether. The mother is therefore confined to bed and is more likely to require catheterization, episiotomy, and an instrumental delivery.

Symptoms of postural hypotension may develop when the patient is upright, and shivering occurs in up to 50% of mothers.[78,613] The latter can be reduced by warming epidural local anesthetics and intravenous fluids to body temperature,[400,556] or by giving a small dose of epidural opioid, such as meperidine[78] or fentanyl.[556] For reasons that are obscure, epidural analgesia seems to be associated with a small rise (less than 1°C) in maternal core body temperature as labor progresses.[91,216]

Nonobstetric complications of epidural analgesia (e.g., dural puncture, total spinal, unexpected "high epidural" blockade, bladder dysfunction, backache, neurological damage, and epidural hematoma or abscess) are discussed fully in Chapters 7, 8 and 21. For some reason, headache and back pain account for a relatively high proportion of obstetric, versus nonobstetric, anesthesia lawsuits in the United States.[107]

Prospective studies have shown that the incidence of backache and bladder dysfunction following epidural analgesia is no different from that which occurs after a pudendal block.[314,415] One postal survey, however, reported a higher incidence of long-term backache among women who received an epidural in labor than those who did not (18.9% versus 10.5%).[368] Interestingly, this relationship applied only to vaginal deliveries and not to elective cesarean section, suggesting that long-term backache may be related to muscular relaxation, and postural stresses incurred during labor, rather than to epidural analgesia per se. A more detailed recent survey from the United Kingdom reported a similar higher incidence of *new onset* backache among women who received epidural analgesia in labor (17.8% versus 11.7%), but in the majority of cases, backache was related to posture, and, in any case, was not severe.[535] In contrast, a large prospective study from the United States found no increase in backache following epidural blockade, either for vaginal or cesarean delivery.[62]

Neurologic complications following obstetric epidural analgesia are extremely rare and usually attributable to peripheral nerve lesions following an instrumental delivery, rather than to epidural analgesia per se.[269] A neurological consultation should nevertheless be sought if paresthesias or prolonged anesthesia occurs in the puerperium.

More serious complications, such as toxicity, total spinal, and unexpected "high epidural" blockade (see Chapters 8 and 21) have been reported, but are relatively rare in obstetrics. Some are avoidable and most are readily treatable with high standards of care and supervision. Nevertheless, their occurrence emphasizes the importance of having skilled staff in the labor ward and a physician experienced in resuscitation in close proximity.

CAUDAL EPIDURAL ANALGESIA

The caudal approach to the epidural space has become less popular in obstetrics during the past decade. Earlier, several large case series were published, reporting high success rates with few complications.[170,192,398,420] A cephalad spread sufficient to provide analgesia in the first stage of labor (i.e., to T10) is more difficult to achieve and requires larger doses than those needed with lumbar epidural analgesia. Also, dense blockade of the sacral nerves tends to occur early in labor, with the potential adverse effects discussed earlier. There seems to be a greater risk of systemic toxicity occurring with the caudal approach to the epidural space, possibly because of its greater vascularity and the relatively large dose of local anesthetic that is usually used (see also Chapter 9).

Caudal analgesia has been used as part of a 2-catheter technique in some centers, although it is doubtful whether this confers great advantage. By itself, caudal analgesia can be used for the provision of perineal analgesia when delivery is imminent, or when an instrumental delivery is planned. Under the latter conditions, many anesthesiologists would prefer to use a low subarachnoid block instead.

SUBARACHNOID ANALGESIA

Local Anesthetics

Subarachnoid blockade is the preferred technique when anesthesia of the lower birth canal is urgently required for an instrumental delivery, manual removal of a retained placenta, and/or repair of traumatic lacerations. Subarachnoid analgesia is more rapid and effective than either peripheral nerve blocks or caudal block on these occasions, and is much safer than general anesthesia.[77,100,144,413] All of the standard hyperbaric preparations are suitable (see Chapter 7). In patients undergoing perineal or vaginal surgery, or a low instrumental delivery, a sacral (saddle) block is adequate, but for a rotational forceps delivery or placental removal the patient should be positioned so as to ensure a block to T10. It is important to correct any hypovolemia with intravenous fluids before proceeding with subarachnoid block. Hyperbaric lidocaine, 25 to 30 mg, of a 1.5% or 2% solution in dextrose, provides ideal conditions for most obstetric procedures. If major blood loss has occurred, or if active hemorrhage is continuing, then general anesthesia may be a safer choice.

Continuous infusion of local anesthetic via a subarachnoid catheter ideally would allow prolonged, titratable, labor analgesia; however, routine spinal catheter use has been limited by post-dural puncture headache. The introduction of very fine gauge subarachnoid catheters rekindled interest in using intrathecal local anesthetics and/or opioids as a means of providing pain relief in labor.[45,289] One small preliminary study reported excellent analgesia using 1% lidocaine in 0.5 to 1.0 ml increments for maintenance, and hyperbaric lidocaine for delivery.[282] Another study reported equally good analgesia using an infusion of 0.125% bupivacaine, 1.5 ml/h, following an initial loading dose of bupivacaine, 2.5 mg.[393] In a few cases, perineal analgesia was achieved using 0.5% hyperbaric bupivacaine. However, following reports of cauda equina syndrome associated with hyperbaric local anesthetic injection, spinal microcatheters are no longer available for clinical use[200,510] (see also Chapter 21). It seems unlikely, therefore, that continuous spinal techniques will become acceptable in obstetric practice unless these problems can be overcome and anesthesiologists are assured that there is no increased risk of nerve damage, infection or dural puncture headache.

Opioids

There have been several studies concerning the use of intrathecal opioids during labor. Initial reports indicated that intrathecal morphine, 0.5 to 2.0 mg, relieved uterine contraction pain for several hours.[11,39] The onset of analgesia, however, was slow and supplementary pain relief was usually required for delivery.[11,39,551] Intrathecal morphine was also associated with a high incidence of side effects.[11,39,55,551] These include pruritus (72 to 100%), nausea (32 to 100%), somnolence (43 to 92%) and urinary retention (12 to 43%). Although serious respiratory depression did not occur in the studies cited above, the respiratory rate fell to 7 per minute in one patient, 14 hours after injection of morphine, 1 mg.[11]

While it was shown that some of the above opioid-related side effects could be reduced by an intravenous naloxone infusion (0.4 to 0.6 mg/h),[153] interest in intrathecal opioids waned until 1989, when Leighton et al.[345] described use of an intrathecal combination of fentanyl, 25 μg, and morphine, 0.25 mg. This was said to provide "rapid onset of profound, prolonged analgesia," although intense analgesia actually lasted only 2 to 4 hours, and patients who had not delivered within this time often required epidural analgesia in addition. However, this technique attracted much interest in the United States because of its apparent ease and a perception that supervision by an anesthesiologist was not necessary.

A subsequent prospective double-blind study by Honet et al.[278] of the lipid soluble agents fentanyl, sufentanil, and meperidine, given during labor via a microspinal catheter, demonstrated a more rapid onset and more profound degree of analgesia than occurred with morphine. Comparison of intrathecal fentanyl, 10 μg, sufentanil, 5 μg, and meperidine, 10 mg, revealed a similar onset and duration of analgesia with each treatment, although meperidine provided more reliable analgesia as labor progressed. These authors suggested that the local anesthetic effects of meperidine accounted for the greater degree of patient comfort using this drug, compared with fentanyl and sufentanil. All three drugs were said to be associated with minimal side effects.

Intrathecal opioids have also been used on a continuous basis. One small study reported that 55% of patients experienced good pain relief using intrathecal diamorphine, 0.2 to 0.4 mg, via a spinal catheter, but the incidence of side effects (pruritus, nausea, and somnolence) was high.[327] Two further studies, using intrathecal meperidine, 10 mg, reported pain relief within approximately 5 minutes and a mean duration of analgesia of 1 to 2 hours.[57,576] Side effects were similar to those reported with other opioids (although the incidence of pruritus was noted to be very low in both these studies). Possibly, the local anesthetic properties of meperidine account for the comparatively low incidence of pruritus with this agent.

To date, sufentanil and fentanyl have received most attention in the United States.[121,278,343,344,444] A comparison of IV, epidural and intrathecal sufentanil, 10 μg, found that adequate analgesia was obtained only with intrathecal injection, confirming that the opioid acts via a spinal rather than a systemic effect.[90] Another study comparing intrathecal sufentanil with epidural bupivacaine, 0.25%, found more profound labor analgesia with the former.[28] The same dose of intrathecal sufentanil has been shown to produce sensory changes, often extending up to the T4 level, without motor block, and was also associated with a minor degree of hypotension in 11 to 14% of patients.[121,246] Effective analgesia, however, is usually heralded by intense perineal pruritus. Other workers have also noted that mild hypotension is a common accompaniment to intrathecal sufentanil and fentanyl, with or without the addition of morphine.[180]

Some of the above findings (i.e., sensory block and hypotension) may seem surprising at first sight, in view of the presumed selective effects of opioids at the spinal μ-receptor. However, conduction block in isolated nerve preparations has been demonstrated not only with meperidine,[490] but also with high concentrations of fentanyl[229,490] and sufentanil.[229] It is possible, therefore, that these opioids may produce their effects, in part, through their local anesthetic activity. A recent study by Riley et al.,[512] however, found that the concentration of sufentanil among patients in labor did not influence analgesia or objective sensory changes, nor were sensory changes predictive of the duration of analgesia or hemodynamic changes. Intrathecal sufentanil does not block efferent sympathetic nerve fibers.[513] These data suggest that the effects of intrathecal sufentanil are *predominantly* mediated through spinal opioid receptors.

Other potentially serious adverse effects which have been described with the use of intrathecal opioids include respiratory depression and fetal bradycardia.[37,119,121,183,255] These side effects tend to occur within the first hour of intrathecal administration. Thus, as with any neural blockade technique, patients receiving intrathecal opioids during labor require careful monitoring.

COMBINED SPINAL EPIDURAL ANALGESIA

Use of intrathecal opioids as part of a combined spinal epidural technique (see Chapter 8, Fig. 8-31) has recently become popular for labor analgesia in some centers. Intrathecal opioid injection ensures rapid onset of intense analgesia, while placement of an epidural catheter permits analgesia to be maintained for extended periods, and provides flexibility to respond to the frequently changing circumstances of labor and delivery.

One study compared intrathecal morphine, 0.2 mg; epidural bupivacaine, 12.5 mg; and a combination of the two, using a needle-through-needle technique.[14] Patients who received the combined treatment had excellent pain relief within 20 minutes, while those who received either intrathecal morphine or epidural bupivacaine alone did not achieve adequate analgesia. Patients who received the combined treatment also required less local anesthetic during their labor, but those who received intrathecal morphine had a higher incidence of nausea, vomiting, and pruritus.

More recently, studies performed by Collis et al.[126,127] have shown that low-dose CSE analgesia can provide selective sensory block with preservation of motor power; maternal satisfaction was greater with the CSE technique, as compared to a standard epidural technique.[128] These investigators used an initial dose of intrathecal fentanyl 25 μg with bupivacaine 2.5 mg; this was followed by 10–15 ml of epidural bupivacaine 0.1% with fentanyl 2 μg/ml, half-hourly as required, to maintain analgesia. It has been shown that low dose combinations of bupivacaine and fentanyl for labor using CSE minimally impair dorsal column function.[469] Thus, provided the patient is appropriately assessed for diminished proprioception and motor function, ambulation during labor can be a safe option.

In the United States, a single dose of intrathecal sufentanil, 10 μg (or fentanyl, 25 μg) is most commonly used. This usually provides excellent analgesia within 3 to 6 minutes and a duration of approximately 2 hours, without any clinically detectable motor blockade.[121] If necessary, further analgesia can then be provided via the epidural catheter (following a suitable test-dose) using a low-dose bupivacaine-opioid drug combination. Campbell and associates[92] used a small dose of intrathecal bupivacaine, 2.5 mg, in addition to sufentanil, 10 μg, to prolong the duration of analgesia significantly, (148 ± 27 min.), as compared to intrathecal sufentanil alone (114 ± 27 min). The majority of parturients had no motor block.

In addition to the side-effects of intrathecal opioids which have been described above, there is a hypothetical risk of epidural catheter migration through the dural hole made by the spinal needle. However, provided that a fine-gauge spinal needle is used, this risk has been shown to be insignificant.[277,452] Post-dural puncture headache incidence is low (~3%) with uncomplicated CSE, and the need for epidural blood patch is similar to that after labor epidural.[452]

The combined spinal epidural technique is also described below, with reference to anesthesia for cesarean delivery.

ANESTHESIA FOR CESAREAN SECTION

> The delivery of the infant into the arms of a conscious and pain-free mother is one of the most exciting and rewarding moments in medicine.
> Donald D. Moir, 1976.[412]

For all intents and purposes, regional anesthesia for cesarean section is synonymous with central neural blockade. There is little indication today for local anesthetic infiltration or field block, and consequently these techniques will not be discussed any further.

Advantages of Central Neural Blockade for the Mother

Central neural blockade confers two major advantages over general anesthesia: (i) maternal consciousness is maintained, and (ii) the surgical site is temporarily denervated.

Maternal Awareness

Maintaining the patient's consciousness is by far the best safeguard against her developing airway obstruction and pulmonary aspiration, provided that (i) the upper airway reflexes are not depressed from any cause such as excessive sedation, syncope, or the development of a high block, and (ii) the patient is able to move into a position that allows vomitus to be removed quickly (for it is still possible for the supine conscious patient to aspirate material in the pharynx).[605]

Neural blockade permits the mother to see her baby immediately after birth and to share this event with her partner. This is of considerable psychological and emotional importance for many women and is the most common reason for patients to request regional, rather than general, anesthesia.[81] Infant suckling can often be established soon after delivery; this may explain a higher frequency of successful breast-feeding after central neural blockade than after general anesthesia.[351,426]

Sensory Denervation

As is the case with other abdominal surgery, the endocrine stress response is less when cesarean section is performed under regional anesthesia than under general anesthesia. Thus, when cesarean section is performed under regional anesthesia, maternal (but not fetal) catecholamine release is suppressed,[297] and plasma concentrations of glucose, adrenocorticotrophic hormone (ACTH), and cortisol, are substantially lower[353,361,442] (see also Chapter 5).

Other Benefits

Intraoperative blood loss is significantly less when cesarean section is performed under regional rather than general anesthesia.[227,337,412] Regional anesthesia is also associated with less postoperative morbidity, including gastrointestinal stasis, cough, pyrexia, fatigue, and depression.[426] In addition, epidural or spinal opioids can be administered to provide high-quality pain relief without sedation in the postoperative period. It is hardly surprising, therefore, that central neural blockade has become so popular among mothers for this operation.

Advantages of Central Neural Blockade for the Fetus/Neonate

The results of studies comparing the effects of anesthetic technique (regional versus general) on fetal heart rate, neonatal acid-base status, time to sustained respiration, ventilatory pattern, and Apgar score, are conflicting. Some studies have shown no significant differences,[7,43,177,209,212,273,299,465] whereas others have shown greater *initial* neonatal depression associated with general anesthesia.[193,268,458] In the event of a prolonged uterine incision-delivery interval (i.e., greater than 90 seconds), neonatal acid-base status deteriorates under general, but not under regional, anesthesia.[149] Infants presenting by the breech are also in better clinical condition when delivered under neural blockade.[149] Infants usually are more alert and responsive (as determined by neurobehavioral responses) when surgery is performed under regional, as opposed to general anesthesia[7] although one recent study found no difference in neonatal alertness between the two techniques.[322] In any case, such differences appear to be short-lived and of little importance to the overall well-being of the newborn.

Epidural versus Subarachnoid Anesthesia

The choice between subarachnoid and epidural block for cesarean section appears to be determined largely by local custom and preference. A recent prospective study comparing the two techniques found that they were equally acceptable.[606] Each technique has its merits (see Table 18-4).

The advantages of spinal anesthesia (when compared with epidural anesthesia) for cesarean section may be summarized as follows: (i) the onset of anesthesia is much quicker and more profound; (ii) there is no sparing of the sacral nerve roots (as sometimes occurs with epidural anesthesia); (iii) the local anesthetic dose requirements are considerably less and fetal uptake negligible;[334] and (iv) there is much less intraoperative shivering.[258] Spinal anesthesia produces a more profound motor block than epidural anesthesia, and there appears to be less need for intraoperative analgesic supplementation in the case of spinal anesthesia (20% versus 50% in one retrospective study).[511] A prospective study, however, found no difference between the two techniques regarding the level of sensory block and the incidence of visceral pain.[19] When urgent abdominal delivery is required, subarachnoid block is often a viable alternative to general anesthesia, including cases of fetal distress.[384]

Disadvantages of spinal anesthesia include: patient anxiety caused by the speed of onset of anesthesia; greater potential for the development of a high block; a higher incidence of hypotension[96,133,515,533] and vagal bradycardia[99] (and rarely, asystole); and the development of post-dural puncture headache (although the use of fine-gauge, pencil-point spinal needles has reduced the incidence of this complication).[528] Occasionally, the spread of neural blockade following a single dose spinal block is found to be inadequate. An epidural catheter, on the other hand, permits intraoperative dose adjustments to be made and provides access for on-going analgesia in the postoperative period.

Combined Spinal Epidural Anesthesia

It will be apparent from the above that there are certain advantages associated with both spinal and epidural anesthesia. For this reason, it has been suggested that further benefit might be obtained by deliberately combining the two techniques (see Fig. 18-13).[75,101]

Originally described, an epidural catheter is inserted in an upper lumbar interspace, immediately followed by a lower lumbar subarachnoid block. The epidural catheter is quickly taped over the skin and the patient is placed in a lateral tilt position, while the block takes effect. An alternative approach is to use a "needle-through-needle" technique, which can usually be performed more quickly and requires the patient to receive only one injection.[101,620] One study, however, has reported a higher failure rate using the needle-through-needle technique, as compared with separate injections.[365] Additional problems may arise if the anesthesiologist is distracted from giving full attention to the patient (e.g., while attempting to thread the epidural catheter) during the critical period of neural blockade onset. Finally, it appears possible for an epidural catheter to pass into the subarachnoid space via the spinal injection site, a potentially very serious complication if unrecognized.[610] However, a recent study has found this risk to be negligible.[277]

Several reports have confirmed the efficacy of combined spinal epidural blockade for cesarean section over epidural anesthesia alone.[505] In practice, the spinal component of the anesthetic alone is often perfectly adequate for surgery. If it *should* prove necessary to extend the upper level of sensory block, however, local anesthetic must be injected into the epidural catheter cautiously, since the dose requirement is sometimes surprisingly small (possibly due to cerebrospinal fluid [CSF] volume displacement).[51] It has been noted that the incidence of post-dural puncture headache appears to be much lower than expected when using a combined technique, possibly because postoperative epidural opioids pro-

TABLE 18-4. *Relative merits of subarachnoid vs. epidural anesthesia for cesarean section*

	Subarachnoid	Epidural
Speed of onset	Very rapid	Delayed
Upper limit of block	Variable, unpredictable	Usually satisfactory to T4
Lower limit of block	Usually satisfactory to S4	Variable, sacral sparing
Density of block	Profound	Variable, agent-dependent
Duration of motor block	Agent-dependent; may be prolonged	Agent-dependent; not usually prolonged
Systemic absorption	Negligible	Substantial; toxicity possible
Hypotension	Common; rapid onset	Variable; gradual onset
Shivering	Rare	Common
Dural puncture headache	Variable, unpredictable	Nil
Provision for postoperative analgesia	Nil	Ideal route for continuous analgesia

vide some prophylaxis against the headache.[77] In addition, the use of recently developed fine-gauge pencil-point spinal needles has been shown to result in a decreased incidence of post-dural puncture headache;[528] this will likely further enhance the appeal of combined spinal epidural techniques in the future.

Intraoperative Management

The patient must be nursed in a full lateral, or lateral tilt, position until delivery. On, or before, arrival to the operating area, a nonglucose-containing intravenous infusion should be set up and oxygen given by face mask to improve fetal oxygen reserve and acid-base status.[501] Routine monitoring should be established, including blood pressure manometry, electrocardiography and pulse oximetry, and fetal heart rate checked.

Neural blockade to T4 provides the best surgical conditions.[139] The most commonly used epidural local anesthetic agents for cesarean section are lidocaine (2%), bupivacaine (0.5 to 0.75%), etidocaine (1.0 to 1.5%) and chloroprocaine (3%). No clear advantage of one agent over another has been demonstrated and the choice seems to depend largely on individual preference. Chloroprocaine, lidocaine and etidocaine have a more rapid onset than bupivacaine.[182,301,632] It is generally agreed that epinephrine 1:200,000 should be added to epidural lidocaine and many add it to bupivacaine, mainly to decrease the risk of systemic toxicity.[68,335,394,624] In North America, many anesthesiologists add bicarbonate (1 mEq/ml per 10 ml) to lidocaine and sometimes to chloroprocaine to accelerate onset, particularly in an emergency.[168,217] It should be remembered, however, that this more rapid onset is associated with a higher incidence of hypotension.[468] For subarachnoid anesthesia, cinchocaine or tetracaine (8 to 12 mg hyperbaric), bupivacaine (12 to 15 mg hyperbaric or isobaric) and lidocaine (70 to 90 mg hyperbaric) have been used most commonly.

More recently, various opioid drugs have also been used in conjunction with both epidural (e.g., fentanyl, 100 μg[257,330,449,464]) and subarachnoid anesthesia (e.g., morphine, 0.2 mg,[13,15] sufentanil, 10 to 20 μg,[136] fentanyl, 10 to 25 mg[286,561]). Most studies reported significantly better analgesia when opioids were added to the local anesthetic, although pruritus was relatively common and some patients required naloxone for respiratory depression. There are even reports of cesarean section having been performed using intrathecal meperidine, 75 mg, as the sole agent.[89,318]

In addition to providing adequate surgical anesthesia and attending to other details, the patient requires encouragement, reassurance, and emotional support, during the operation. The anesthesiologist must be alert to any symptoms or side-effects that may cause alarm and anxiety, and attend to them promptly.

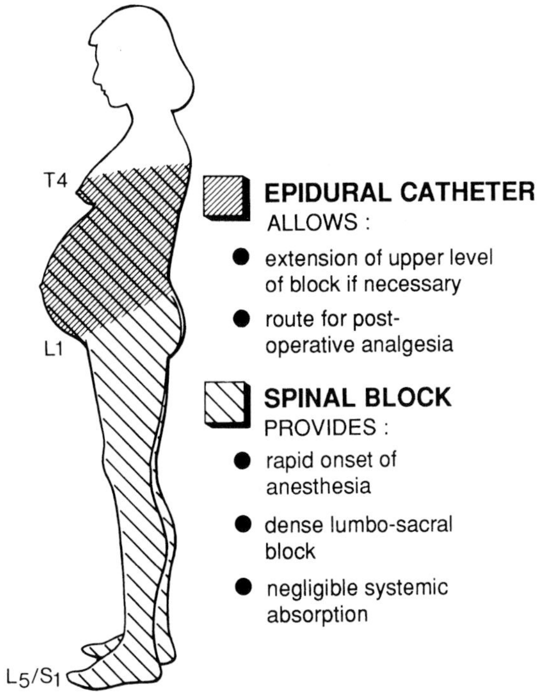

FIG. 18-13. Clinical advantages associated with the combined spinal epidural technique for cesarean section. [Brownridge, P.: Obstetric anaesthesia and caesarean section. *In* Brown, B.R. Jr., Prys-Roberts, C., (eds.): International Practice of Anaesthesia. Oxford, Butterworth-Heinemann, 1996.]

Prevention and Treatment of Hypotension

Hypotension is a potentially serious complication because it provokes alarming symptoms for the mother (syncope, nausea, and dyspnea) and may lead to a period of ischemia for the fetus. Fortunately, such episodes appear to be of little consequence provided they are short-lived and promptly treated.[157,382] The anesthesiologist must ensure that the circulating blood volume is adequate, that there is sufficient uterine displacement from the aorta and vena cava, and that there is no vagal inhibition of myocardial function due to cardiac sympathetic blockade. Uteroplacental and fetal hemodynamic status are not affected by well-controlled epidural analgesia for cesarean section in healthy patients using local anesthetics alone,[22] or with the addition of epinephrine.[23]

It is generally recommended that a fluid load of at least 1 liter of crystalloid or colloid solution is given intravenously before central neural blockade.[245,349,625] Dextrose infusions should be avoided, because they induce maternal and fetal hyperglycemia, and subsequently neonatal hypoglycemia after delivery.[242,324] Volumes in excess of 1 liter may help decrease the incidence of hypotension to some degree with epidural anesthesia,[349] but have little beneficial effect in the case of spinal anesthesia.[441,530] There is also a risk of developing pulmonary edema with excessive fluid-loading. Colloid solutions have no proven benefit over crystalloids for epidural anesthesia,[503] although 1 liter of albumin prevented hypotension with spinal anesthesia.[388] Some colloids (e.g., dextran, hemaccel) may precipitate anaphylaxis.

In any case, it is both futile and dangerous to try to treat hypotension by rapid intravenous infusion alone. As described earlier in this chapter, an intravenous pressor agent, such as ephedrine, is much more rational and effective treatment.[157,320,619] In fact, it has been shown that normal placental perfusion can be maintained with an ephedrine infusion, despite a moderate fall in blood pressure.[308]

Management of Pain

Supplementary analgesia may be required during periods of discomfort or pain, although the inclusion of opioids with the local anesthetic has decreased this need. Various measures have been described anecdotally including: nitrous oxide inhalation,[585] IV or epidural opioids, IV ketamine 0.1 to 0.2 mg/kg, and sedatives. Sedative drugs are best avoided, however, because they cause confusion and amnesia[425] and patient cooperation may be lost. If anesthesia is clearly inadequate before the operation begins, consideration should be given to repeating the block.

Central chest pain sometimes occurs after delivery, and this has usually been attributed to surgical peritoneal stimulation. More recently, however, it has been suggested that chest pain may be secondary to venous air embolism,[210,603] or myocardial ischemia.[466] While the incidence of such potentially alarming complications is apparently common when sophisticated monitoring is used (i.e., precordial doppler flowmetry and echocardiography), they are probably of little *clinical* importance. Episodes of electrocardiographic ST depression after delivery are common, but do not usually imply myocardial ischemia or impairment of myocardial function.[387,395,638] Nevertheless, a diagnosis of myocardial ischemia, or air or amniotic fluid embolism, must be considered if chest pain is accompanied by dyspnea, a decrease in arterial saturation, tachyarrythmia and persistent electrocardiogram (ECG) changes.

Other Symptoms

Nausea often occurs at some stage during cesarean section and usually reflects an episode of hypotension, bradycardia or peritoneal stimulation. Prompt treatment of hypotension with intravenous ephedrine significantly reduces the incidence of nausea from this cause.[157] Nausea and vomiting can also be reduced by giving intravenous metoclopramide, 10 mg,[364] or droperidol, 2.5 mg,[378] preoperatively, or droperidol, 0.5 mg, after delivery.[540] Metoclopramide may be preferable in patients receiving epidural or spinal opioids, as droperidol may lead to prolonged sedation and potentiate respiratory depression.[122]

Dyspnea may indicate patient anxiety, hypotension, the development of a high block, pulmonary congestion, or air or amniotic fluid embolism. A rapid evaluation will determine the most likely cause, and treatment should be initiated according to the diagnosis. The local anesthetic dose requirements for cesarean section are sometimes surprisingly small, especially among those who already have an established block or have a multiple pregnancy.[303] Spinal anesthesia performed *after* epidural blockade can also result in a very extensive block.[42] The anesthesiologist must always be prepared to induce general anesthesia to control ventilation if neural blockade extends sufficiently to cause respiratory embarrassment or patient distress.

Shivering can be reduced to some extent by warming intravenous fluids[627] and local anesthetic drugs[611] to body temperature. Opioid drugs (e.g., fentanyl, 25 μg,[357] sufentanil, 50 μg[555]) are also effective in decreasing the incidence and severity of shivering, when given epidurally. Intravenous meperidine, 50 mg, given after delivery has also been found effective in reducing intraoperative shivering.[104]

GYNECOLOGICAL PROCEDURES SUITABLE FOR NEURAL BLOCKADE

Dilatation and Curettage

Dilatation and curettage is frequently performed in the day-surgery setting when the indications are diagnostic or when a therapeutic abortion is to be performed. Although some feel that local anesthesia is suitable only for gestations of less than 12 weeks, others have reported use of a combined paracervical-intracervical block for mid-trimester dilatation and extraction.[626] The surgical procedure is preceded by the insertion of laminaria tents on the day before surgery, to permit gradual dilatation of the cervix.

Paracervical block is a useful technique for a number of reasons. It is relatively easy and contributes significantly to patient safety and early recovery. In addition, only one physician need be involved, and simplified medical facilities can be used. The dangers in this practice, however, should not be underestimated; toxic reactions have led to the death of 5 women receiving paracervical block for termination of pregnancy in the United States.[240] Full facilities and the necessary resuscitative skills are essential requirements for any physician contemplating its use (see Chapter 4). Because the procedure is short, lidocaine 1% with epinephrine can be used up to a maximum volume of 40 ml (400 mg). Chloroprocaine is a satisfactory alternative. Usually, a smaller dose is sufficient. Bupivacaine, 0.5%, also has been used,[626] but its longer duration is probably not necessary for such short procedures. Epinephrine contained in the local anesthetic does not appear to decrease uterine bleeding. In one study, supplementation of the block with intravenous fentanyl was associated with increased blood loss in gestations of greater than 17 weeks.[626]

Major Vaginal Surgery

Vaginal surgery can be conveniently separated into two categories, depending upon whether or not the ovarian pedicles are to be stretched or ligated (as in vaginal hysterectomy). These structures have a sensory nerve supply from the T10 level, and therefore regional anesthesia to above that level will be necessary. Any of the centrally acting blocks (caudal or lumbar epidural, or subarachnoid) is suitable, provided there are no contraindications to its use. The local anesthetic drugs commonly used for lumbar epidural anesthesia are lidocaine, 1.5% to 2%, 18 to 25 ml with epinephrine, 1:200,000, or bupivacaine, 0.5 to 0.75%. Most major vaginal surgery does not involve the ovarian structures, and therefore caudal epidural blockade is frequently suitable. Smaller doses of local anesthetic drugs can be used and will provide excellent anesthesia for the procedure. Once again, lidocaine, 1.5%, or bupivacaine, 0.5%, can be used, depending on the duration of the procedure. Despite adequate anesthesia, many patients also require light sedation, for example, with low dose intravenous infusion techniques, as described in Chapter 6.

Intra-abdominal Pelvic Surgery

Many of these operations are eminently suitable for regional block. The duration of the surgical procedure plays an important part in the choice of anesthesia, because some reconstructive surgery (tuboplasty, myomectomy) can be inordinately long procedures and the patient can become restless remaining in the same position. It is essential to ensure that the height of the block is sufficient; for these patients it should reach at least a level of T8. Of the three blocks previously mentioned, the lumbar epidural is used most frequently, either in a single-shot or continuous technique. Regional block is relatively contraindicated for extensive surgery to remove huge uterine or ovarian tumors, partly because the supine hypotensive syndrome can occur, but more importantly because the degree of difficulty in excising infiltrating tumors can result in significant blood loss or patient discomfort. Patients who undergo pelvic lymph node dissections, which are extensive procedures, frequently benefit from the use of a continuous lumbar epidural technique. The reduction in blood loss and improved surgical access owing to a small gut make surgery smoother; however, because the length of these procedures is often beyond the tolerance of most patients, it is necessary to supplement the regional block with light general anesthesia (see following).

The types and dosages of drugs used for intra-abdominal pelvic surgery are similar to those used in major vaginal surgery, in which traction on the ovarian structures is to be anticipated. The important feature in this situation is muscle relaxation; in order to achieve this, higher concentrations of lidocaine or bupivacaine are often used. Etidocaine, 1%, which produces intense motor blockade, is sometimes useful. Even with blockade to T8, however, some patients experience pain resulting from stimulation of vagal afferents. Thus, light general inhalational anesthesia, by means of a face mask, is often administered to supplement the epidural block (see Chapter 8). Equally attractive are newer techniques of low-dose intravenous infusion of opioid or sedative agents, or both (see Chapter 6). In more extensive procedures in which light general anesthesia is administered, endotracheal intubation is desirable to avoid airway difficulties, or hypoxia due to hypoventilation.

The major advantages of regional anesthesia for pelvic surgery are 2-fold: (i) there is a reduction in blood loss with an associated decrease in the surgical time; and (ii) the time to recovery from the anesthetic is considerably shortened, when compared with general anesthesia. Also, there appears to be an earlier return of appetite and improved gut motility when epidural analgesia is continued after operation. Epidural opioid analgesia can be used, and is particularly valuable after cancer surgery. It seems likely that the incidence of deep venous thrombosis also may be reduced after regional anesthesia (see Chapter 8).

Postpartum Tubal Ligation

If continuous lumbar or caudal epidural block has been used during labor, it is a simple procedure, postpartum, to administer additional local anesthetic to provide a suitable anesthetic level (T8) for tubal ligation. Lidocaine, 1.5% or 2%, with epinephrine, 1:200,000, or chloroprocaine, 3%, in volumes of 15 to 20 ml, are usually adequate. The incision for a postpartum tubal ligation is usually subumbilical and the procedure is short. It is important to ensure that cardiovascular stability is present and hydration adequate before administering the dose of local anesthetic, because a significant volume of blood frequently is lost during delivery. This is particularly important if a regional block is instituted for the first time postpartum, since the potential for hypotension is high when epidural block is induced in the presence of unrecognized blood loss. Spinal anesthesia using hyperbaric lidocaine, 50 to 75 mg, also provides excellent anesthesia for tubal ligation. Both epidural and spinal block may be safer than general anesthesia for surgery in the early postpartum period, because the mother is still at risk from aspiration at this time. Although the time at which normal gastrointestinal function returns to normal after pregnancy is not known, some anesthesiologists prefer to wait 6 to 8 hours after delivery before initiating a new anesthetic.

Laparoscopy

General anesthesia is most commonly employed for laparoscopy, because of fears of inadequate ventilation and aspiration during the period of pneumoperitoneum. Both local and epidural anesthesia have, however, been used with success and safety. Zellavos and colleagues[639] reported a series of 1,000 outpatient laparoscopic sterilizations, using a technique of subumbilical infiltration of the abdominal wall, with 2 ml of 1% lidocaine, following which pneumoperitoneum was achieved and each fallopian tube was sprayed by means of the operating laparoscope with 8 ml of the same solution. Penfield[478] used a somewhat more sophisticated technique on 1,200 patients, injecting lidocaine directly into the tubes with a 23-gauge needle-cannula inserted through the laparoscope. He also administered a paracervical block, to permit tolerance of the uterine sound. Both these studies report minimal patient discomfort and an extremely low incidence of complications, none of which was major. They also recommended use of nitrous oxide rather than carbon dioxide as the insufflating gas, since the latter was associated with more patient discomfort. It is important to note that in one study the average operating time was only 8 minutes,[639] emphasizing that surgical expertise is probably an essential component of success with this technique. Diamant and colleagues[166] and Brown and co-workers[69] demonstrated the lack of clinically significant changes in ventilation and blood gases during this procedure, although 2 (of 21) patients became agitated and 2 transiently apneic following sedation, in one study.[166] It is vital, therefore, that an anesthesiologist be available, along with adequate resuscitation equipment and surgical facilities, in the event that complications occur.

Epidural anesthesia using lidocaine, 1.5%, or chloroprocaine, 3%, also has been performed for laparoscopy with only mild shoulder pain and no serious anesthetic or surgical complications.[31,65] Again, blood gas values were not significantly changed during the procedure.[65] For both local and epidural anesthesia, the authors claim fewer anesthetic complications (such as cardiac arrhythmias, aspiration, sore throat, and vomiting), reduced costs, and more rapid discharge from hospital, compared with general anesthesia. With the vast number of outpatient laparoscopies currently being performed for tubal sterilization, and the diagnosis and treatment of infertility, local and regional anesthesia may become more generally accepted.

Summary

Neural blockade is ideal for gynecological surgical procedures. Regional anesthesia frequently reduces the amount of blood loss in the surgical field, and analgesia provided after surgery offers a smooth transition from the operative and postoperative period. Neurohumoral responses to surgery are reduced and recovery is more rapid (see Chapters 5 and 8).

REFERENCES

1. Abboud, T.K., Afrasiabi, A., Sarkis, *et al.*: Continuous infusion epidural analgesia in parturients receiving bupivacaine, chloroprocaine, or lidocaine—Maternal, fetal and neonatal effects. Anesth. Analg., *62:*421, 1983.
2. Abboud, T.K., Afrabiasi, A., Zhu, J., *et al.*: Epidural morphine or butorphanol augments bupivacaine analgesia during labor. Reg. Anesth., *14:*115, 1989.
3. Abboud, T.K., Artal, R., Sarkis, F., *et al.*: Sympathoadrenal activity: Maternal, fetal, and neonatal responses after epidural anesthesia in the pre-eclamptic patient. Am. J. Obstet. Gynecol., *144:*915, 1982.
4. Abboud, T.K., David, S., Nagappala, S., *et al.*: Maternal, fetal and neonatal effects of lidocaine with and without epinephrine for epidural anesthesia in obstetrics. Anesth. Analg., *63:*973, 1984.
5. Abboud, T.K., Khoo, S.S., Miller, F., *et al.*: Maternal, fetal and neonatal responses after epidural anesthesia with bupivacaine, 2-chloroprocaine, or lidocaine. Anesth. Analg., *61:*638, 1982.
6. Abboud, T.K., Kim, K.C., Noueihed, R., *et al.*: Epidural bupivacaine, chloroprocaine, or lidocaine for cesarean section—Maternal and neonatal effects. Anesth. Analg., *62:*914, 1983.
7. Abboud, T.K., Nagappala, S., Murakawa, K., David, S., *et al.*: Comparison of the effects of general and regional anesthesia for cesarean section on neonatal neurologic and adaptive capacity scores. Anesth. Analg., *64:*996, 1985.
8. Abboud, T.K., Reyes, A., Steffens, Z., *et al.*: Bupivacaine/butorphanol/epinephrine for epidural anesthesia in obstetrics: Maternal and neonatal effects. Reg. Anesth., *14:*219, 1989.
9. Abboud, T.K., Sarkis, F., Hung, T.T., *et al.*: Effects of epidural anesthesia during labor on maternal plasma beta-endorphin levels. Anesthesiology, *59:*1, 1983.
10. Abboud, T.K., Sheik-ol Eslam, A., Yanagi, T., *et al.*: Safety and efficacy of epinephrine added to bupivacaine for lumbar epidural analgesia in obstetrics. Anesth. Analg., *64:*585, 1985.
11. Abboud, T.K., Shnider, S.M., Dailey, P.A., *et al.*: Intrathecal administration of hyperbaric morphine for the relief of pain in labour. Br. J. Anaesth., *56:*1351, 1984.
12. Abouleish, E. (ed.): *In* Pain Control in Obstetrics, pp. 268, 286. Philadelphia, J.B. Lippincott, 1977.
13. Abouleish, E., Rawal, N., and Rashad, M.N.: The addition of 0.2 mg subarachnoid morphine to hyperbaric bupivacaine for cesarean delivery. Reg. Anesth., *16:*137, 1991.
14. Abouleish, E., Rawal, N., Shaw, J., *et al.*: Intrathecal morphine 0.2 mg versus epidural bupivacaine 0.125% or their combination: Effects on parturients. Anesthesiology, *74:*711, 1991.
15. Abouleish, E., Rawal, N., Tobon-Randall B., *et al.*: A clinical and laboratory study to compare the addition of 0.2 mg of morphine, 0.2 mg of epinephrine, or their combination to hyperbaric bupivacaine for spinal anesthesia in cesarean section. Anesth. Analg., *77:*457, 1993.
16. Abram, S.E., and Winne, R.P.: Intrathecal acetyl cholinesterase inhibitors produce analgesia that is synergistic with morphine and clonidine in rats. Anesth. Analg., *81:*501, 1995.
17. Ackerman, W.E., Juneja, M.M., Kaczorowski, D.M., and Colclough, G.W.: A comparison of the incidence of pruritus following epidural opioid administration in the parturient. Can. J. Anaesth., *36:*388, 1989.

18. Ahmad, A.J., Clark, E.H., and Jacobs, H.S.: Water intoxication associated with oxytocin infusion. Postgrad Med. J., *51:*249, 1975.
19. Alahuhta, S., Kangas-Saarela, T., Hollmén, A.I., and Edstrom, H.H.: Visceral pain during caesarean section under spinal and epidural anaesthesia with bupivacaine. Acta. Anaesthesiol. Scand., *34:*95, 1990.
20. Alahuhta, S., Räsänen, J., Jouppila, P., *et al.*: Ephedrine and phenylephrine for avoiding maternal hypotension due to spinal anaesthesia for caesarean section. Int. J. Obstet. Anesth., *1:*129, 1992.
21. Alahuhta, S., Räsänen, J., Jouppila, P., *et al.*: Uteroplacental and fetal circulation during extradural bupivacaine-adrenaline and bupivacaine for caesarean section in hypertensive pregnancies with chronic fetal asphyxia. Br. J. Anaesth., *71:*348, 1993.
22. Alahuhta, S., Räsänen, J., Jouppila, R., *et al.*: Uteroplacental and fetal haemodynamics during extradural anaesthesia for caesarean section. Br. J. Anaesth., *66:*319, 1991(a).
23. Alahuhta, S., Räsänen, J., Jouppila, R., *et al.*: Effects of extradural bupivacaine with adrenaline for caesarean section on uteroplacental and fetal circulation. Br. J. Anaesth., *67:*678, 1991(b).
24. Alahuhta, S., Räsänen, J., Jouppila, P., *et al.*: The effects of epidural ropivacaine and bupivacaine for cesarean section on uteroplacental and fetal circulation. Anesthesiology., *83:*23, 1995.
25. Albright, G.A.: Cardiac arrest following regional anesthesia with etidocaine or bupivacaine. Anesthesiology, *51:*285, 1979.
26. Albright, G.A., Jouppila, R., Hollmén, A.I., *et al.*: Epinephrine does not alter human intervillous blood flow during epidural anesthesia. Anesthesiology, *54:*131, 1981.
27. Amiel-Tison, C., Barrier, G., Shnider, S.M., *et al.*: A new neurological and adaptive capacity scoring system for evaluating obstetric medications in full-term newborns. Anesthesiology, *56:*340, 1982.
28. Anderson, M., D'Angelo, R., Phillip, J., *et al.*: Intrathecal sufentanil compared to epidural bupivacaine for labor analgesia. (Abstract) Anesthesiology, *79:*A970, 1993.
29. Ansari, I., Wallace, G., Clementson, C.A.B., *et al.*: Tilt caesarian section. J. Obstet. Gynaecol. Br. Commonw., *77:*713, 1970.
30. Arens, J.F., and Carrera, A.E.: Methemoglobin levels following peridural anesthesia with prilocaine for vaginal deliveries. Anesth. Analg., *49:*219, 1970.
31. Aribarg, A.: Epidural analgesia for laparoscopy. J. Obstet. Gynaecol. Br. Commonw., *80:*567, 1973.
32. Asling, J.H., Shnider, S.M., Margolis, A.J., *et al.*: Paracervical block anesthesia in obstetrics. II: Etiology of fetal bradycardia following paracervical block anesthesia. Am. J. Obstet. Gynecol., *107:*626, 1971.
33. Assali, N.S., Brinkman, C.R., and Nuwayhid, B.: Uteroplacental circulation and respiratory gas exchange. *In* Gluck L., (ed.): Modern Perinatal Medicine. pp. 67. Chicago, Year Book Medical Publishers, 1974.
34. Bader, A.M., Ray, N., and Datta, S.: Continuous epidural infusion of alfentanil and bupivacaine for labor and delivery. Int. J. Obstet. Anesth., *1:*187, 1992.
35. Bailey, P.W., and Howard, F.A.: Epidural analgesia and forceps delivery: Laying a bogey. Anaesthesia, *38:*282, 1983.
36. Bailey, R., Ruggier, R., and Findley, I.L.: Diamorphine-bupivacaine mixture compared with plain bupivacaine for analgesia. Br. J. Anaesth., *72:*58, 1994.
37. Baker, M.N., and Sarna, M.C.: Respiratory arrest after second dose of intrathecal sufentanil. Anesthesiology, *83:*231, 1995.
38. Baraka, A., Maktabi, M., and Noueihid, R.: Epidural meperidine-bupivacaine for obstetric analgesia. Anesth. Analg., *61:*652, 1982.
39. Baraka, A., Noueihid, R., and Hajj, S.: Intrathecal injection of morphine for obstetric analgesia. Anesthesiology, *54:*136, 1981.
40. Barker, P., Callander, C.C.: Coagulation screening before epidural analgesia in pre-eclampsia. Anaesthesia, *46:*64, 1991.
41. Baskett, T.F., and Writer, W.D.: Postpartum Hemorrhage. *In* Datta, S., (ed.). Anesthetic and Obstetric Management of High-Risk Pregnancy. 2nd ed. pp. 110. St Louis, Mosby–Year Book, 1996.
42. Beck, G.N., and Griffiths, A.G.: Failed extradural anaesthesia for caesarean section: Complication of subsequent spinal block. Anaesthesia, *47:*690, 1992.
43. Belfrage, P., Irestedt, L., Raabe, N., and Arner, S.: General anaesthesia or lumbar epidural block for caesarean section? Effects on the foetal heart rate. Acta Anaesthesiol. Scand., *21:*67, 1977.
44. Belfrage, P., Raabe, N., Thalme, B., and Berlin, A.: Lumbar epidural analgesia with bupivacaine in labor: Determination of drug concentration and pH in fetal scalp blood, and continuous fetal heart rate monitoring. Am. J. Obstet. Gynecol., *121:*360, 1975.
45. Benedetti, C., and Tiengo, M.: Continuous subarachnoid analgesia in labour. Lancet, *335:*225, 1990.
46. Benedetti, T.J., and Carlson, R.W.: Studies of colloid osmotic pressure in pregnancy-induced hypertension. Am. J. Obstet. Gynecol., *135:*308, 1979.
47. Bevan, D.K., Holdcroft, A., Loh, L., *et al.*: Closing volume and pregnancy. Br. Med. J., *1:*13, 1974.
48. Bieniarz, J., Crottogini, J.J., Curuchet, E., *et al.*: Aortocaval compression by the uterus in late human pregnancy. Am. J. Obstet. Gynecol., *100:*203, 1968.
49. Bleyaert, A., Soetens, M., Vaes, L., *et al.*: Bupivacaine 0.125 percent, in obstetric analgesia: Experience in three thousand cases. Anesthesiology, *51:*435, 1979.
50. Bloom, S.L., Horswill, C.W., and Curet, L.B.: Effects of paracervical blocks on the fetus during labor, a prospective study with the use of direct fetal monitoring. Am. J. Obstet. Gynecol., *114:*218, 1972.
51. Blumgart, C.H., Ryall, D., Dennison, B., and Thompson-Hill, L.M.: Mechanism of extension of spinal anaesthesia by extradural injection of local anaesthetic. Br. J. Anaesth., *69:*457, 1992.
52. Bogod, D.G., Rosen, M., and Rees, G.A.D.: Extradural infusion of 0.125% bupivacaine at 10 ml/h to women during labour. Br. J. Anaesth., *59:*325, 1987.
53. Bonica, J.J.: *In* Principles and Practice of Obstetric Analgesia and Anesthesia, pp. 531. Philadelphia, F.A. Davis, 1967.
54. Bonica, J.J.: Peripheral mechanisms and pathways of parturition pain. Br. J. Anaesth., *51:*3S, 1979.
55. Bonnardot, J.P., Maillet, M., Colau, J.C., *et al.*: Maternal and fetal concentration of morphine after intrathecal administration during labour. Br. J. Anaesth., *54:*487, 1982.
56. Bonnet, F., Catoire, P., Brun Buison, V., *et al.*: Effects of oral and subarachnoid clonidine on spinal anesthesia with bupivacaine. Reg. Anesth., *15:*211, 1990.
57. Boreen, S., Leighton, B.L., Kent, H., and Norris, M.C.: Intrathecal meperidine for labor analgesia: Preliminary communication. Int. J. Obstet. Anesth., *1:*149, 1992.
58. Borell, V., Fernstrom, I., Ohlson, L., and Wiquist, N.: Influence of uterine contractions on the uteroplacental flow at term. Am. J. Obstet. Gynecol., *93:*44, 1965.
59. Bowen-Simpkins, P., and Fergusson, I.L.: Lumbar epidural block and the breech presentation. Br. J. Anaesth., *46:*420, 1974.
60. Brackbill, Y., Kane, J., Manniello, R.L., and Abramson, D.: Obstetric meperidine usage and assessment of neonatal status. Anesthesiology., *40:*116, 1974.
61. Brazelton, T.B.: *In* Neonatal Behavioural Assessment Scale. London, Spastics International Medical Publications, William Heinemann, 1973.
62. Breen, T.W., Ransil B.J., Groves P.A., and Oriel, N.E.: Factors associated with back pain after childbirth. Anesthesiology, *81:*29, 1994.
63. Breen, T.W., Shapiro, T., Glass, B., *et al.*: Epidural anesthesia for labor in an ambulatory patient. Anesth. Analg., *77:*919, 1993.
64. Breeson, A.J., Kovacs, G.T., Pickles, B.G., and Hill, J.G.: Extradural analgesia: The preferred method of analgesia for vaginal breech delivery. Br. J. Anaesth., *50:*1227, 1978.
65. Bridenbaugh, L.D., and Soderstrom, R.M.: Lumbar epidural block anesthesia for outpatient laparoscopy. J. Reprod. Med., *23:*85, 1979.
66. Bromage, P.R.: Continuous lumbar epidural analgesia for obstetrics. Can. Med. Assoc. J., *85:*1136, 1961.
67. Bromage, P.R.: Epidural Analgesia. pp. 141, 548. Philadelphia, W.B. Saunders, 1978.
68. Brose, W.G., and Cohen, S.E.: Epidural lidocaine for cesarean section: Effect of varying epinephrine concentration. Anesthesiology, *69:* 936, 1988.
69. Brown, D.R., Fishburne, J.I., Robertson, V.O., and Hulka, J.V.: Ventilatory and blood gas changes during laparoscopy with local anesthesia. Am. J. Obstet. Gynecol., *124:*741, 1976.
70. Brown, M.A.: Pregnancy-induced hypertension: Current concepts. Anaesth. Intensive Care, *17:*185, 1989.
71. Brown, W.U.: Guest discussion. *In* Hodgkinson, R., Marx, G.F., Kim, S.S., *et al.*: Neonatal neurobehavioral tests following vaginal delivery under ketamine, thiopental, and extradural anesthesia. Anesth. Analg., *56:*548, 1977.
72. Brown, W.U. Jr., Bell, G.C., and Alper, M.H.: Acidosis, local anesthetics and the newborn. Obstet. Gynecol., *48:*27, 1976.
73. Brown, W.U., Bell, G.C., Lurie, A.O., *et al.*: Newborn blood levels of lidocaine and mepivacaine in the first postnatal day following maternal epidural anesthesia. Anesthesiology, *42:*698, 1975.

74. Browning, A.J., Butt, W.R., Lynch, S.S., *et al.*: Maternal and cord plasma concentrations of beta-lipotrophin, beta-endorphin and gamma-lipotrophin at delivery: Effect of analgesia. Br. J. Obstet. Gynaecol., *90:*1152, 1983.
75. Brownridge, P.: Central neural blockade and caesarian section. Part I: Review and case series. Anaesth. Intensive Care, *7:*33, 1979.
76. Brownridge, P.: A three-year survey of an obstetric epidural service with top-up doses administered by midwives. Anaesth. Intensive Care, *10:*298, 1982.
77. Brownridge, P.: Spinal anaesthesia revisited: An evaluation of subarachnoid block in obstetrics. Anaesth. Intensive Care., *12:*334, 1984.
78. Brownridge, P.: Shivering related to epidural blockade with bupivacaine in labour, and the influence of epidural pethidine. Anaesth. Intensive Care, *14:*412, 1986.
79. Brownridge, P.: Epidural bupivacaine-pethidine mixture: Clinical experience using a low-dose combination in labour. Aust. N. Z. J. Obstet. Gynaecol., *28:*17, 1988.
80. Brownridge, P.: Epidural medication after the initial dose: Reflections on current methods of administration during labour. Anaesth. Intensive Care, *18:*300, 1990.
81. Brownridge, P., and Jefferson, J.: Central neural blockade and caesarian section. II: Patient assessment of the procedure. Anaesth. Intensive Care, *7:*163, 1979.
82. Brownridge, P., Plummer, J., Mitchell, J., and Marshall, P.: An evaluation of epidural bupivacaine with and without meperidine in labour. Reg. Anesth., *17:*15, 1992.
83. Buchan, P.C.: Emotional stress in childbirth and its modification by variations in obstetric management. Acta Obstet. Gynecol. Scand., *59:* 319, 1980.
84. Buchan, P.C.: Pre-eclampsia—A hyperviscosity syndrome. Am. J. Obstet. Gynecol., *142:*111, 1982.
85. Buchan, P.C., Milne, M.K., and Browning, M.C.K.: The effect of continuous epidural blockade on plasma 11-hydroxycorticosteroid concentrations in labour. J. Obstet. Gynaecol. Br. Commonw., *80:*974, 1973.
86. Burrows, R.F., and Kelton, J.G.: Thrombocytopenia at delivery: A prospective survey of 6,715 deliveries. Am. J. Obstet. Gynecol., *162:* 731, 1990.
87. Butterworth, J.F., Walker, F.O., and Lysak, S.Z.: Pregnancy increases median nerve susceptibility to lidocaine. Anesthesiology, *72:*962, 1990.
88. Caldeyro-Barcia, R.: Effect of position changes on the intensity and frequency of uterine contractions during labor. Am. J. Obstet. Gynecol., *80:*284, 1960.
89. Camann, W.R., and Bader, A.M.: Spinal anesthesia for cesarean delivery with meperidine as the sole agent. Int. J. Obstet. Anesth., *1:*156, 1992.
90. Camann, W.R., Denney, R.A., Holby, E.D., and Datta, S.: A comparison of intrathecal, epidural, and intravenous sufentanil for labor analgesia. Anesthesiology, *77:*884, 1992.
91. Camann, W.R., Hortvet, L.A., Hughes, N., *et al.*: Maternal temperature regulation during extradural analgesia for labour. Br. J. Anaesth., *67:*556, 1991.
92. Campbell, D.C., Camann, W.R., and Datta, S.: The addition of bupivacaine to intrathecal sufentanil for labor analgesia. Anesth. Analg., *81:*305, 1995.
93. Capogna, G., Celleno, D., and Tomassetti, M.: Maternal analgesia and neonatal effects of epidural sufentanil for cesarean section. Reg. Anesth., *14:*282, 1989.
94. Capogna, G., Cellano, D., Zangrillo, A., *et al.*: Addition of clonidine to epidural morphine enhances postoperative analgesia after cesarean delivery. Reg. Anesth., *20:*57, 1995.
95. Carabine, U.A., Milligan, K.R., and Moore, J.: Extradural clonidine and bupivacaine for postoperative analgesia. Br. J. Anaesth., *68:*132, 1992.
96. Caritis, S.N., Abouleish, E., Edelstone, U.I., and Mueller-Heubach, E.: Fetal acid-base state following spinal or epidural anesthesia for cesarean section. Obstet. Gynecol., *56:*610, 1980.
97. Carli, F., Creagh-Barry, P., Gordon, H., *et al.*: Does epidural analgesia influence the mode of delivery in primiparae managed actively? A preliminary study of 1,250 women. Int. J. Obstet. Anaesth., *2:*15, 1993.
98. Carlsson, C., Dahlgren, N., Magnusson, J., and Hanson, A.: Epidural block with chloroprocaine during labour. Acta Anaesthesiol. Scand., *24:*469, 1980.
99. Carpenter, R.L., Caplan, R,A., Brown, D.L., *et al.*: Incidence and risk factors for side effects of spinal anesthesia. Anesthesiology., *76:*906, 1992.
100. Carrie, L.E.S.: Spinal anaesthesia—an alternative route. *In* Doughty, A., (ed.). Epidural Analgesia in Obstetrics, pp. 179. London, Lloyd-Luke, 1980.
101. Carrie, L.E.S.: Extradural, spinal or combined block for obstetric surgical anaesthesia. Br. J. Anaesth., *65:*225, 1990.
102. Carrie, L.E.S., O'Sullivan, G.M., and Seegobin, R.: Epidural fentanyl in labour. Anaesthesia, *36:*965, 1981.
103. Casady, G.N., Moore, D.C., and Bridenbaugh, L.D.: Post-partum hypertension after use of vasoconstrictor and oxytocic drugs. J.A.M.A., *172:*1011, 1960.
104. Casey, W.F., Smith, C.E., Katz, J.M., *et al.*: Intravenous meperidine for control of shivering during caesarean section under epidural anaesthesia. Can. J. Anaesth., *35:*128, 1988.
105. Caseby, N.G.: Epidural analgesia for the surgical induction of labour. Br. J. Anaesth., *46:*747, 1974.
106. Celleno, D., and Capogna, G.: Epidural fentanyl plus bupivacaine 0.125% for labour: Analgesic effects. Can. J. Anaesth., *35:*375, 1988.
107. Chadwick, H.S., Posner, K., Caplan, R.A., *et al.*: A comparison of obstetric and nonobstetric anesthesia malpractice claims. Anesthesiology, *74:*242, 1991.
108. Chesley, L.: *In* Hypertensive Disorders of Pregnancy. pp. 363. New York, Appleton-Century-Crofts, 1978.
109. Chestnut, D.H., and Dailey, P.A.: Anesthesia for preterm labor and delivery. *In* Shnider, S.M., Levinson, G., (eds.): Anesthesia for Obstetrics. 3rd ed. pp. 337. Baltimore, Williams and Wilkins, 1993.
110. Chestnut, D.H., Laszewski, L.J., Pollack, K.L., *et al.*: Continuous epidural infusion of 0.0625% bupivacaine–0.0002% fentanyl during the second stage of labor. Anesthesiology, *72:*613, 1990.
111. Chestnut, D.H., McGrath, J.M., Vincent, R.D., *et al.*: Does early administration of epidural analgesia affect obstetric outcome in nulliparous women who are in spontaneous labor? Anesthesiology, *80:* 1201, 1994(a).
112. Chestnut, D.H., Owen, C.L., Bates, J.N., *et al.*: Continuous infusion epidural analgesia during labor: A randomized, double-blind comparison of 0.0625% bupivacaine/0.0002% fentanyl versus 0.125% bupivacaine. Anesthesiology, *68:*754, 1988.
113. Chestnut, D.H., Owen, C.L., Brown, C.K., *et al.*: Does labor affect the variability of maternal heart rate during induction of epidural anesthesia? Anesthesiology, *68:*622, 1988.
114. Chestnut, D.H., Vandewalker, G.E., Owen, C.L., *et al.*: The influence of continuous epidural bupivacaine analgesia on the second stage of labor and method of delivery in nulliparous women. Anesthesiology, *66:*774, 1987.
115. Chestnut, D.H., Vincent, R.D., McGrath, J.M., *et al.*: Does early administration of epidural analgesia affect obstetric outcome in nulliparous women who are receiving intravenous oxytocin? Anesthesiology, *80:*1193, 1994(b).
116. Cibils, L.A., and Santonja-Lucas, J.J.: Clinical significance of fetal heart rate patterns during labor: III: Effect of paracervical block anesthesia. Am. J. Obstet. Gynecol., *130:*73, 1978.
117. Cigarini, I., Kaba, A., Bonnet, F., *et al.*: Epidural clonidine combined with bupivacaine for analgesia in labor: Effects on mother and neonate. Reg. Anesth., *20:*113, 1995.
118. Clark, S.L., Cotton, D.B., Pivarnik, J.M., *et al.*: Position change and central hemodynamic profile during normal third-trimester pregnancy and postpartum. Am. J. Obstet. Gynecol., *164:*883, 1991.
119. Clarke, V.T., Smiley, R.M., and Finster, M.: Uterine hyperactivity after intrathecal injection of fentanyl for analgesia during labor: A cause of fetal bradycardia? Anesthesiology, *81:*1083, 1994.
120. Cleland, J.G.P.: Paravertebral anesthesia in obstetrics. Surg. Gynecol. Obstet., *57:*51, 1933.
121. Cohen, S.E., Cherry, C.M., Holbrook, R.H., *et al.*: Intrathecal sufentanil for labor analgesia—sensory changes, side effects, and fetal heart rate changes. Anesth. Analg., *77:*1155, 1993.
122. Cohen, S.E., Rothblatt, A.J., and Albright, G.A.: Early respiratory depression with epidural narcotic and intravenous droperidol. Anesthesiology, *59:*559, 1983.
123. Cohen, S.E., Tan, S., Albright, G.A., and Halpern, J.: Epidural fentanyl/bupivacaine mixtures for obstetric analgesia. Anesthesiology, *67:*403, 1987.
124. Cohen, S.E., and Thurlow, A.: Comparison of a chloroprocaine-bupivacaine mixture with chloroprocaine and bupivacaine used individually for obstetric epidural analgesia. Anesthesiology, *51:*288, 1979.

125. Cole, P.V., and Nainby-Luxmoore, P.C.: Respiratory volumes in labour. Br. Med. J., *1:*1118, 1962.
126. Collis, R.E., Baxandall, M.L., Srikantharajah, I.D., *et al.*: Combined spinal epidural analgesia with ability to walk throughout labour. Lancet, *341:*767, 1993.
127. Collis, R.E., Baxandall, M.L., Srikantharajah, I.D., *et al.*: Combined spinal epidural analgesia: Technique, management and outcome of 300 mothers. Int. J. Obstet. Anesth., *3:*75, 1994.
128. Collis, R.E., Davies, D.W.L., and Aveling, W.: Randomised comparison of combined spinal-epidural and standard epidural analgesia in labour. Lancet., *345:*1413, 1995.
129. Colonna-Romano, P., Lingaraju, N., Godfrey, S.D., and Braitman, L.E.: Epidural test dose and intravascular injection in obstetrics: Sensitivity, specificity, and lowest effective dose. Anesth. Analg., *75:*372, 1992.
130. Confino, E., Ismajovich, B., Rudick, V., and David, M.P.: Extradural analgesia in the management of singleton breech delivery. Br. J. Anaesth., *57:*892, 1985.
131. Conn, D.A., Moffatt, A.C., McCallum, G.D.R., and Thorburn, J.: Changes in pulmonary function tests during spinal anaesthesia for caesarean section. Int. J. Obstet. Anesth., *2:*12, 1993.
132. Corke, B.C., Carlson, C.G., and Dettbarn, W.D.: The influence of 2-chloroprocaine on the subsequent analgesic potency of bupivacaine. Anesthesiology, *60:*25, 1984.
133. Corke, B.C., Datta, S., Ostheimer, G.W., *et al.*: Spinal anaesthesia for caesarean section: The influence on neonatal outcome. Anaesthesia, *37:*658, 1982.
134. Cotton, B.R., and Smith, G.: Single and combined effects of atropine and metoclopramide on the lower oesophageal sphinter pressure. Br. J. Anaesth., *53:*869, 1981.
135. Cotton, D.B., Strassner, H.T., Lipson, L.G., and Goldstein, D.A.: The effects of terbutaline on acid base, serum electrolytes, and glucose homeostasis during the management of preterm labor. Am. J. Obstet. Gynecol., *141:*617, 1981.
136. Courtney, M.A., Bader, A.M., Hartwell, B., *et al.*: Perioperative analgesia with subarachnoid sufentanil administration. Reg. Anesth., *17:* 274, 1992.
137. Covino, B.G., and Vassallo, H.G.: Pharmacokinetic aspects of local anesthetic agents. *In* Local Anesthetics: Mechanism of Action and Clinical Use. pp. 103. New York, Grune and Stratton, 1976.
138. Craft, J.B., Jr., Epstein, B.S., and Coakley, C.S.: Effect of lidocaine with epinephrine versus lidocaine (plain) on induced labor. Anesth. Analg., *51:*243, 1972.
139. Craft, J.B., Roizen, M.F., Dao, S.D., *et al.*: A comparison of T4 and T7 dermatomal levels of analgesia for caesarean section, using the lumbar epidural technique. Can. Anaesth. Soc. J., *29:*264, 1982.
140. Crawford, J.S.: Lumbar epidural block in labour: A clinical analysis. Br. J. Anaesth., *44:*66, 1972(a).
141. Crawford, J.S.: The second thousand epidural blocks in an obstetric hospital practice. Br. J. Anaesth., *44:*1277, 1972(b).
142. Crawford, J.S.: An appraisal of lumbar epidural blockade in patients with a singleton fetus presenting by the breech. J. Obstet. Gynaecol. Br. Commonw., *81:*867, 1974.
143. Crawford, J.S.: An appraisal of lumbar epidural blockade in labour in patients with multiple pregnancy. Br. J. Obstet. Gynaecol., *82:*929, 1975.
144. Crawford, J.S.: Experience with spinal analgesia in a British obstetric unit. Br. J. Anaesth., *51:*531, 1979.
145. Crawford, J.S.: Experiences with epidural morphine in obstetrics. Anaesthesia, *36:*207, 1981.
146. Crawford, J.S.: Some maternal complications of epidural analgesia for labour. Anaesthesia, *40:*1219, 1985.
147. Crawford, J.S.: A prospective survey of 200 consecutive twin deliveries. Anaesthesia, *42:*33, 1987.
148. Crawford, J.S., Burton, M., and Davies, P.: Anaesthesia for section: Further refinements of a technique. Br. J. Anaesth., *45:*726, 1973.
149. Crawford, J.S., and Davies, P.: Status of neonates delivered by elective caesarean section. Br. J. Anaesth., *54:*1015, 1982.
150. Crawford, J.S., Mills, W.G., and Pentecost, B.L.: Pregnant patient with Eisenmenger's syndrome. Case report. Br. J. Anaesth., *43:*1091, 1971.
151. Cugell, D.W., Frank, N.R., Gaensler, E.A., and Badger, T.L.: Pulmonary function in pregnancy: Serial observations in normal women. Am. Rev. Tuberc. Pulm. Dis., *67:*568, 1953.
152. Dailey, P.A., Baysinger, C.L., Levinson, G., and Shnider, S.M.: Neurobehavioral testing of the newborn infant. Clin. Perinatol., *9:*191, 1982.
153. Dailey, P.A., Brookshire, G.L., Shnider, S.M., *et al.*: Naloxone decreases side effects after intrathecal morphine for labor. Anesth. Analg., *64:*658, 1985.
154. Dailey, P.A., Hughes, S.C., Rosen, M.A., *et al.*: Effect of cimetidine and ranitidine on lidocaine concentrations during epidural anesthesia for cesarean section. Anesthesiology, *69:*1013, 1988.
155. Darby, S., Thornton, C.A., and Hunter, D.J.: Extradural analgesia in labour when the breech presents. Br. J. Obstet. Gynaecol., *83:*35, 1976.
156. D'Athis, F., Mâcheboeuf, M., Thomas, H., *et al.*: Epidural analgesia with a bupivacaine-fentanyl mixture in obstetrics: Comparison of repeated injections and continuous infusion. Can. J. Anaesth., *35:*116, 1988.
157. Datta, S., Alper, M.H., Ostheimer, G.W., and Weiss, J.B.: Method of ephedrine administration and nausea and hypotension during spinal anesthesia for cesarean section. Anesthesiology, *56:*68, 1982.
158. Datta, S., Camann, W., Bader, A., and VanderBurgh, L.: Clinical effects and maternal and fetal plasma concentrations of epidural ropivacaine versus bupivacaine for cesarean section. Anesthesiology, *82:* 1346, 1995.
159. Datta, S., Lambert, D.H., Gregus, J., and Gissen, A.J.: Differential sensitivities of mammalian nerve fibres during pregnancy. Anesth. Analg., *62:*1070, 1983.
160. De Jong, R.: The chloroprocaine controversy. Am. J. Obstet. Gynecol., *140:*237, 1981.
161. Department of Health. Report on Confidential Enquiries into Maternal Deaths in England and Wales, 1982–1984. London: Her Majesty's Stationery Office, 1989.
162. Department of Health. Report on Confidential Enquiries into Maternal Deaths in the United Kingdom, 1988–1990. London: Her Majesty's Stationery Office, 1992.
163. De Simone, C.A., Norris, M.C., and Leighton, B.L.: Intravenous nitroglycerine aids extraction of a retained placenta. Anesthesiology, *73:*787, 1990.
164. De Swiet, M., and Redman, C.W.G.: Aspirin, extradural anaesthesia and the MRC collaborative low-dose aspirin study in pregnancy (CLASP). Br. J. Anaesth., *69:*109, 1992.
165. Dewan, D.M., and Cohen, S.E.: Epidural analgesia and the incidence of cesarean section—Time for a closer look. Anesthesiology, *80:* 1189, 1994.
166. Diamant, M., Benumof, J.L., Saidman, L.J., *et al.*: Laparoscopic sterilization with local anesthesia: complications and blood-gas changes. Anesth. Analg., *56:*335, 1977.
167. DiFazio, C.A.: Metabolism of local anaesthetics in the fetus, newborn and adult. Br. J. Anaesth., *51:*29S, 1979.
168. DiFazio, C.A., Carron, H., Grosslight, K.R., *et al.*: Comparison of pH-adjusted lidocaine solutions for epidural anesthesia. Anesth. Analg., *65:*760, 1986.
169. Dixon, H.G., Browne, J.C.M., and Davey, D.A.: Choriodecidual and myometrial blood flow. Lancet, *2:*369, 1963.
170. Dogu, T.S.: Continuous caudal analgesia and anesthesia for labor and vaginal delivery: A review of 4,071 confinements. Obstet. Gynecol., *33:*92, 1969.
171. Donnai, P., and Nicholas, A.D.: Epidural analgesia: Fetal monitoring and the condition of the baby at birth with breech presentation. Br. J. Obstet. Gynaecol., *82:*360, 1975.
172. Doughty, A.: Selective epidural analgesia and the forceps rate. Br. J. Anaesth., *41:*1058, 1969.
173. Doughty, A.: Lumbar epidural analgesia—the pursuit of perfection: With special reference to midwife participation. Anaesthesia, *30:*741, 1975.
174. Doughty, A.: Epidural analgesia in labour: The past, the present and future. Proc. R. Soc. Med., *71:*879, 1978.
175. Douglas, M.J., Weeks, S.B., Writer, W.D., *et al.*: A double-blind comparison between epidural ropivacaine 0.25% and bupivacaine 0.25% for the relief of childbirth pain: Report of a multicenter study. (Abstract) Reg. Anesth., *19:*2S (Suppl.) 12, 1994.
176. Downing, J.W., Coleman, A.J., Mahomedy, M.C., *et al.*: Lateral table tilt for caesarean section. Anaesthesia, *29:*696, 1974.
177. Downing, J.W., Houlton, P.C., and Barclay, A.: Extradural analgesia for caesarean section: A comparison with general anaesthesia. Br. J. Anaesth., *51:*367, 1979.
178. Dror, A.: Maternal hemodynamic responses to epinephrine-containing

local anesthetics in mild pre-eclampsia. Reg. Anesth., *13:*107, 1988.
179. Drummond, G.B., Scott, S.E.M., Lees, M.M., and Scott, D.B.: Effects of posture on limb blood flow in late pregnancy. Br. Med. J., *4:*587, 1974.
180. Ducey, J.P., Knape, K.G., Talbot, J., *et al.*: Intrathecal narcotics for labor cause hypotension. (Abstract) Anesthesiology, *77:*A997, 1992.
181. Dunbar, A.H., Price, D.D., and Newton, R.A.: An assessment of pain responses to thermal stimuli during stages of pregnancy. Pain, *35:*265, 1988.
182. Dutton, D.A., Moir, D.D., Howie, H.B., *et al.*: Choice of local anaesthetic for extradural caesarean section—Comparison of 0.5% and 0.75% bupivacaine and 1.5% etidocaine. Br. J. Anaesth., *56:*1361, 1984.
183. Eberle, R.L., Norris, M.C., Mallozi Eberle, A., *et al.*: The effect of maternal position on fetal heart rate during epidural or intrathecal analgesia for labor. [Abstract], Anesthesiology, *83:*A944, 1995.
184. Eckstein, K.L., and Marx, G.F.: Aortocaval compression and uterine displacement. Anesthesiology, *40:*92, 1974.
185. Eddleston, J.M., Holland, J.J., Griffin, R.P., *et al.*: A double-blind comparison of 0.25% ropivacaine and 0.25% bupivacaine for extradural analgesia in labour. Br. J. Anaesth., *76:*66, 1996.
186. Eddleston, J.M., Maresh, M., Horsman, E.L., and Young, H.: Comparison of the maternal and fetal effects associated with intermittent or continuous infusion of extradural analgesia. Br. J. Anaesth., *69:*154, 1992.
187. Edwards, N.D., Hartley, M., Clyburn, P., and Harmer, M.: Epidural pethidine and bupivacaine in labour. Anaesthesia, *47:*435, 1992.
188. Eisenach, J., Detweiler, D., and Hood, D.: Hemodynamic and analgesic actions of epidurally administered clonidine. Anesthesiology, *78:*277, 1993.
189. Eisenach, J.C., Grice, S.C., and Dewan, D.M.: Epinephrine enhances analgesia produced by epidural bupivacaine during labor. Anesth. Analg., *66:*447, 1987.
190. Eisenach, J.C., Lysak, S.Z., and Viscomi, C.M.: Epidural clonidine analgesia following surgery. Anesthesiology, *71:*640, 1989.
191. Enever, G.R., Noble, H.A., Kolditz, D., *et al.*: Epidural infusion of diamorphine with bupivacaine in labour: A comparison with fentanyl and bupivacaine. Anaesthesia, *46:*169, 1991.
192. Epstein, H.M., and Sherline, D.M.: Single-injection caudal anesthesia in obstetrics. Obstet. Gynecol., *33:*496, 1969.
193. Evans, C.M., Murphy, J.F., Gray, O.P., and Rosen, M.: Epidural versus general anaesthesia for elective caesarean section: Effect on Apgar score and acid-base status of the newborn. Anaesthesia, *44:*778, 1989.
194. Evans, K.R., and Carrie, L.E.S.: Continuous epidural infusion of bupivacaine in labour. Anaesthesia, *34:*310, 1979.
195. Ewah, B., Yau, K., King, M., and Reynolds, F.: Effect of epidural opioids on gastric emptying in labour. Int. J. Obstet. Anesth., *2:*125, 1993.
196. Ewart, M.C., Yau, G., Gin, T., *et al.*: A comparison of the effects of omeprazole and ranitidine on gastric secretion in women undergoing elective caesarean section. Anaesthesia, *45:*527, 1990.
197. Ewen, A., Mcleod, D.D., Mcleod, D.M., *et al.*: Continuous infusion epidural analgesia in obstetrics: A comparison of 0.08% and 0.25% bupivacaine. Anaesthesia, *41:*143, 1986.
198. Fagraeus, L., Urban, B.J., and Bromage, P.R.: Spread of epidural analgesia in early pregnancy. Anesthesiology, *58:*184, 1983.
199. Falconer, A.D., and Powles, A.B.: Plasma noradrenaline levels during labour. Anaesthesia, *37:*416, 1982.
200. FDA Safety Alert. Cauda equina syndrome associated with use of small-bore catheters in continuous spinal anesthesia. May 29, 1992.
201. Feeney, J.G.: Water intoxication and oxytocin. Br. Med. J. *285:*243, 1982.
202. Ferrante, F.M., Lu, L., Jamison, S.B., and Datta, S.: Patient-controlled epidural analgesia: Demand dosing. Anesth. Analg., *73:*547, 1991.
203. Fettes, I., Fox, J., Kuzniak, S., *et al.*: Plasma levels of immunoreactive betaendorphin and adrenocorticotrophic hormone during labor and delivery. Obstet. Gynecol., *64:*359, 1984.
204. Filos, K.S., Goudas, L.C., Patroni, O., and Polyzou, V.: Intrathecal clonidine as a sole analgesia agent for pain relief after cesarean section. Anesthesiology, *77:*276, 1992.
205. Finster, M., and Pedersen, H.: Placental transfer and fetal uptake of drugs. Br. J. Anaesth. *51:*25S, 1979.
206. Finster, M., Poppers, P.J., Sinclair, J.C., *et al.*: Accidental intoxication of the fetus with local anesthetic drug during caudal anesthesia. Am. J. Obstet. Gynecol., *92:*922, 1965.
207. Fishburne, J.I., Jr., Brenner, W.E., Braaksma, J.T., and Hendricks, C.H.: Bronchospasm complicating intravenous prostaglandin-$F_2\alpha$ for therapeutic abortion. Obstet. Gynecol., *39:*892, 1972.
208. Fisher, A., and Prys-Roberts, C.: Maternal pulmonary gas exchange. Anaesthesia., *23:*350, 1968.
209. Fisher, J.T., Mortola, J.P., Smith, B., *et al.*: Neonatal pattern of breathing following cesarean section: Epidural versus general anesthesia. Anesthesiology., *59:*385, 1983.
210. Fong, J., Gadalla, F., Pierri, M.K., and Druzin, M.: Are doppler-detected venous emboli during cesarean section air emboli? Anesth. Analg., *71:*254, 1990.
211. Fontenot, R.J., Price, R.L., Henry, A., *et al.*: Double-blind evaluation of patient controlled epidural analgesia during labour. Int. J. Obstet. Anesth., *2:*73, 1993.
212. Fox, G.S., Smith, J.B., Namba, U., and Johnson, R.C.: Anesthesia for cesarean section: Further studies. Am. J. Obstet. Gynecol., *133:*15, 1979.
213. Freeman, D.V., and Arnold, N.I.: Paracervical block with low doses of chloroprocaine—fetal and maternal effects. J.A.M.A., *231:*56, 1975.
214. Freeman, R.K., Gutierrez, N.A., Ray, M.L., *et al.*: Fetal cardiac response to paracervical block anesthesia. Am. J. Obstet. Gynecol., *113:* 583, 1972.
215. Freeman, R.K., and Schifrin, B.S.: Whither paracervical block? Int. Anesthesiol. Clin., *11:*69, 1973.
216. Fusi, L., Maresh, M.J.A., Steer, P.J., and Beard, R.W.: Maternal pyrexia associated with the use of epidural analgesia in labour. Lancet, *1:*1250, 1989.
217. Galindo, A.: pH adjusted local anesthetics: Clinical experience. Reg. Anesth. *8:*35, 1986.
218. Gambling, D.R., McMorland, G.H., Yu, P., and Laszlo, C.: Comparison of patient-controlled epidural analgesia and conventional intermittent "top-up" injections during labor., Anesth. Analg., *70:*256, 1990.
219. Gambling, D.R., Yu, P., Cole, C., *et al.*: A comparative study of patient controlled epidural analgesia (PCEA) and continuous infusion epidural analgesia (CIEA) during labour. Can. J. Anaesth., *35:*249, 1988.
220. Gatt, S.P., Crooke, D.K., Anderson, A., and Lockley S.M.: Pain relief and sensory and motor block in mothers receiving epidural ropivacaine 0.25% and bupivacaine 0.25% for analgesia in labour—A double-blind, parallel, randomised comparison of efficacy. (Abstract). 17th Annual Meeting of the European Academy of Anaesthesiology, Helsinki, 1995.
221. Gaylard, D.G., Wilson, I.H., and Palmer, H.G.R.: An epidural infusion technique for labour. Anaesthesia, *42:*1098, 1987.
222. Gaylord, T.G., and Pearson, W.J.: Neuropathy following paracervical block in the obstetric patient. Obstet. Gynecol., *60:*521, 1982.
223. Geddes, S.M., Thorburn, J., and Logan, R.W.: Gastric emptying following caesarean section and the effect of epidural fentanyl. Anaesthesia, *46:*1016, 1991.
224. Gepts, E., Heytens, L., and Camu, F.: Pharmacokinetics and placental transfer of intravenous and epidural alfentanil in parturient women. Anesth. Analg., *65:*1155, 1986.
225. Gerbasi, F.R., Bottoms, S., Farag, A., and Mammen, E.: Increased intravascular coagulation associated with pregnancy. Obstet. Gynecol., *75:*385, 1990.
226. Gibbs, C.P., and Noel, S.C.: Response of arterial segments from gravid human uterus to multiple concentrations of lignocaine. Br. J. Anaesth., *49:*409, 1977.
227. Gilstrap, L.C., Hauth, J.C., Hankins, G.D.V., and Patterson, A.R.: Effect of type of anesthesia on blood loss at cesarean section. Obstet. Gynecol., *69:*328, 1987.
228. Gintzler, A.R.: Endorphin-mediated increases in pain threshold during pregnancy. Science, *210:*193, 1980.
229. Gissen, A.G., Guigino, L.D., Datta, S. *et al.*: Effects of fentanyl and sufentanil on peripheral mammalian nerves. Anesth. Analg., *66:*1272, 1987.
230. Glover, D.J.: Continuous epidural analgesia in the obstetric patient: A feasibility study using a mechanical infusion pump. Anaesthesia, *32:* 499, 1977.
231. Goins, J.R.: Experience with mepivacaine paracervical block in an obstetric private practice. Am. J. Obstet. Gynecol., *167:*342, 1992.
232. Goland, R.S., Wardlaw, S.L., Stark, R.I., and Frantz, A.G.: Human plasma β-endorphin during pregnancy, labor, and delivery. J. Clin. Endocrinol. Metab., *52:*74, 1981.
233. Goodlin, R.C.: Importance of the lateral position during labor. Obstet. Gynecol., *37:*698, 1971(a).

234. Goodlin, R.C.: Aortocaval compression during cesarean section. Obstet. Gynecol., *37:*702, 1971(b).
235. Greiss, F.C., and Gabble, F.L.: Effect of sympathetic nerve stimulation on the uterine vascular bed. Am. J. Obstet. Gynecol., *97:*962, 1967.
236. Greiss, F.C., Still, J.G., and Anderson, S.G.: Effects of local anesthetic agent on the uterine vasculature and myometrium. Am. J. Obstet. Gynecol., *124:*889, 1976.
237. Grenman, S., Erkkola, R., Scheinin, M., *et al.*: Epidural and paracervical blockades in obstetrics: Catecholamines, arginine vasopressin and analgesic effect. Acta Obstet. Gynecol. Scand., *65:*699, 1986.
238. Grice, S.C., Eisenach, J.C., and Dewan, D.M.: Labor analgesia with epidural bupivacaine plus fentanyl: enhancement with epinephrine and inhibition with 2-chloroprocaine. Anesthesiology, *72:*623, 1990.
239. Griffin, R.P., and Reynolds, F.: Extradural anaesthesia for caesarean section: A double-blind comparison of 0.5% ropivacaine with 0.5% bupivacaine. Br. J. Anaesth., *74:*512, 1995.
240. Grimes, D.A., and Cates, J.: Deaths from paracervical anesthesia used for first-trimester abortion. N. Engl. J. Med., *295:*1397, 1976.
241. Grundy, E.M., Zamora, A.M., and Winnie, A.P.: Comparison of spread of epidural anesthesia in pregnant and nonpregnant women. Anesth. Analg., *57:*544, 1978.
242. Grylack, L.J., Chu, S.S., and Scanlon, J.W.: Use of intravenous fluids before cesarean section: Effects on perinatal glucose, insulin and sodium homeostasis. Obstet. Gynecol., *63:*654, 1984.
243. Gullestad, S., and Sagen, N.: Epidural block in twin labour and delivery. Acta Anaesthesiol. Scand., *21:*504, 1977.
244. Hägerdal, M., Morgan, C.W., Sumner, A.E., and Gutsche, B.B.: Minute ventilation and oxygen consumption during labor with epidural analgesia. Anesthesiology, *59:*425, 1983.
245. Hallworth, D., Jellicoe, J.A., and Wilkes, R.G.: Hypotension during epidural anaesthesia for caesarean section: A comparison of intravenous loading with crystalloid and colloid solutions. Anaesthesia, *37:*53, 1982.
246. Hamilton, C.L., and Cohen, S.E.: High sensory block after intrathecal sufentanil for labor analgesia. Anesthesiology, *83:*1118, 1995.
247. Hamshaw-Thomas, A., and Reynolds, F.: Placental transfer of bupivacaine, pethidine and lignocaine in the rabbit: Effect of umbilical flow rate and protein content. Br. J. Obstet. Gynaecol., *92:*706, 1985.
248. Handley, G., and Perkins, G.: The addition of pethidine to epidural bupivacaine in labour—Effect of changing bupivacaine strength. Anaesth. Intensive Care, *20:*151, 1992.
249. Hanson, A.L., and Hanson, B.: Continuous mini-infusion of bupivacaine into the epidural space during labor. Reg. Anesth., *10:*139, 1985.
250. Hanson, B., and Matouskova-Hanson, A.: Continuous epidural analgesia for vaginal delivery in Sweden. Acta. Anaesthesiol. Scand., *29:* 712, 1985.
251. Harrop-Griffiths, A.W., Ravalia, A., Browne, D.A., and Robinson, P.N.: Regional anaesthesia and cough effectiveness: A study in patients undergoing caesarean section. Anaesthesia, *46:*11, 1991.
252. Hawker, F.: Pulmonary oedema associated with beta$_2$-sympathomimetic treatment of premature labour. Anaesth Intensive Care., *12:* 143, 1984.
253. Hawkins, J., Koonin, L., Palmer, S., *et al.*: Anesthesia-related maternal deaths in the United States: A twelve-year review 1979–1990. (Abstract) Anesthesiology, *79:*A982, 1993.
254. Hayes, J.R., Ardill, J., Kennedy, T.L., *et al.*: Stimulation of gastric release by catecholamines. Lancet, *1,* 1972.
255. Hays, R.L., and Palmer, C.M.: Respiratory depression after intrathecal sufentanil during labor. Anesthesiology, *81:*511, 1994.
256. Hehre, F.W., Hook, R., and Hon, E.H.: Continuous lumbar peridural anesthesia in obstetrics: the fetal effects of transplacental passage of local anesthetic agents. Anesth. Analg., *48:*909, 1969.
257. Helbo-Hansen, H.S., Bang, U., Lindholm, P., and Klitgaard, N.A.: Maternal effects of adding epidural fentanyl to 0.5% bupivacaine for caesarean section. Int. J. Obstet. Anesth., *2:*21, 1993.
258. Helbo-Hansen, S., Bang, U., Garcia, R.S., *et al.*: Subarachnoid versus epidural bupivacaine 0.5% for caesarean section. Acta Anaesthesiol. Scand., *32:*473, 1988.
259. Heytens, L., Cammu, H., and Camu, F.: Extradural analgesia during labour using alfentanil. Br. J. Anaesth., *59:*331, 1987.
260. Hibbard, B.M., and Scott, D.B.: The availability of epidural anaesthesia and analgesia in obstetrics. Br. J. Obstet. Gynaecol., *97:*402, 1990.
261. Hobbs, J.B., Oats, J.N., Palmer, A.A., *et al.*: Whole blood viscosity in preeclampsia. Am. J. Obstet. Gynecol., *142:*288, 1982.
262. Hodgkinson, R., Bhatt, M., Kim, S.S., *et al.*: Neonatal neurobehavior tests following cesarean section under general and spinal anesthesia. Am. J. Obstet. Gynecol., *132:*670, 1978.
263. Hodgkinson, R., Bhatt, M., and Wang, C.N.: Double-blind comparison of the neuro-behaviour of neonates following the administration of different doses of meperidine to the mother. Can. Anaesth. Soc. J., *25:*405, 1978.
264. Hodgkinson, R., and Husain, F.J.: Obesity, gravity, and spread of epidural anesthesia., Anesth. Analg., *60:*421, 1981.
265. Hodgkinson, R., Husain, F.J., and Bluhm, C.: Reduced effectiveness of bupivacaine 0.5% to relieve labor pain after prior injection of chloroprocaine 2%. (Abstract) Anesthesiology, *57:*A201, 1982.
266. Hodgkinson, R., Husain, F.J., and Hayashi, R.H.: Systemic and pulmonary blood pressure during caesarean section in parturients with gestational hypertension. Can. Anaesth. Soc. J., *27:*839, 1980.
267. Hodgkinson, R., Marx, G.F., Kim, S.S., and Miclat, N.M.: Neonatal neurobehavioural tests following vaginal delivery under ketamine, thiopental and extradural anesthesia. Anesth. Analg., *56:*548, 1977.
268. Hodgson, C.A., and Wauchob, T.D.: A comparison of spinal and general anaesthesia for elective caesarean section: effect on neonatal condition at birth. Int. J. Obstet. Anesth., *3:*25, 1994.
269. Holdcroft, A., and Morgan, M.: Maternal complications of obstetric epidural analgesia. Anaesth. Intensive Care, *4:*108, 1976.
270. Holdsworth, J.D.: Relationship between stomach contents and analgesia in labour. Br. J. Anaesth., *50:*1145, 1978.
271. Hollmén, A.: Regional techniques of analgesia in labour. Br. J. Anaesth., *51:*17S, 1979.
272. Hollmén, A.I., Jouppila, R., Jouppila, P., *et al.*: Effect of extradural analgesia using bupivacaine and 2-chloroprocaine on intervillous blood flow during normal labour. Br. J. Anaesth., *54:*837, 1982.
273. Hollmén, A.I., Jouppila, R., Koivisto, M., *et al.*: Neurologic activity of infants following anesthesia for cesarean section. Anesthesiology, *48:* 350, 1978.
274. Hollmén, A., Jouppila, R., Pihlajaniemi, R., *et al.*: Selective lumbar epidural block in labour: A clinical analysis. Acta Anaesthesiol. Scand., *21:*174, 1977.
275. Holly, R.G.: Anaemia in pregnancy. Obstet. Gynecol., *5:*562, 1955.
276. Holmes, F.: Incidence of the supine hypotensive syndrome in late pregnancy. J. Obstet. Gynaecol. Br. Commonw., *67:*254, 1960.
277. Holmström, B., Rawal, N., Axelsson, K., and Nydahl, P.A.: Risk of catheter migration during combined spinal epidural block: Percutaneous epiduroscopy study. Anesth. Analg., *80:*747, 1995.
278. Honet, J.E., Arkoosh, V.A., Norris, M.C., *et al.*: Comparison among intrathecal fentanyl, meperidine, and sufentanil for labor analgesia. Anesth. Analg., *75:*734, 1992.
279. Hood, D.D., Eisenach, J.C., Mallak, K., and Tuttle, R.: The analgesic interaction between intrathecal neostigmine and epidural clonidine in humans. (Abstract) Anesthesiology, *83:*A883, 1995.
280. Horlocker, T.T., Wedel, D.J., Schroeder, D.R., *et al.*: Preoperative antiplatelet therapy does not increase the risk of spinal hematoma associated with regional anesthesia. Anesth. Analg., *80:*303, 1995.
281. Hoult, I.J., MacLennan, A.H., and Carrie, L.E.S.: Lumbar epidural analgesia in labour: Relation to fetal malposition and instrumental delivery. Br. Med. J., *1:*14, 1977.
282. Huckaby, T., Skerman, J.H., Hurley, R.J., and Lambert, D.H.: Sensory analgesia for vaginal deliveries: A preliminary report of continuous spinal anesthesia with a 32-gauge catheter. Reg. Anesth., *16:*150, 1991.
283. Hughes, W.A., and Hughes, S.C.: Hemodynamic effects of prostaglandin E_2. Anesthesiology, *70:*713, 1989.
284. Hughes, S.C., Rosen, M.A., Shnider, S.M., *et al.*: Maternal and neonatal effects of epidural morphine for labor and delivery. Anesth. Analg., *63:*319, 1984.
285. Humphrey, M., Houslow, D., Morgan, S., and Wood, C.: The influence of maternal posture at birth on the foetus. J. Obstet. Gynaecol. Br. Commonw., *80:*1074, 1973.
286. Hunt, C.O., Naulty, J.S., Bader, A.M., *et al.*: Perioperative analgesia with subarachnoid fentanyl-bupivacaine for cesarean delivery. Anesthesiology, *71:*535, 1989.
287. Hunt, C.O., Naulty, J.S., Malinow, A.M., *et al.*: Epidural butorphanol-bupivacaine for analgesia during labor and delivery. Anesth. Analg., *68:*323, 1989.
288. Huntoon, M., Eisenach, J.C., and Boese, P.: Epidural clonidine after cesarean section. Appropriate dose and effect of prior local anesthetic. Anesthesiology, *76:*187, 1992.

289. Hurley, R.J., and Lambert, D.H.: Continuous spinal anesthesia with a microcatheter technique: preliminary experience. Anesth. Analg., *70:* 97, 1990.
290. Husemeyer, R.P., Cummings, A.J., Rosonkiewicz, J.R., and Davenport, H.T.: A study of pethidine kinetics and analgesia in women in labour following intravenous, intramuscular, and epidural administration. Br. J. Clin. Pharmacol., *13:*171, 1982.
291. Husemeyer, R.P., O'Connor, M.C., and Davenport, H.T.: Failure of epidural morphine to relieve pain in labour. Anaesthesia, *35:*161, 1980.
292. Hutchins, C.J.: Spinal analgesia for instrumental delivery: A comparison with pudendal nerve block. Anaesthesia, *35:*376, 1980.
293. Hynson, J.M., Sessler, D.I., and Glosten B.: Back pain in volunteers after epidural anesthesia with chloroprocaine. Anesth. Analg., *72:*253, 1991.
294. Ikeda, T., Ohbuchi, H., Ikenoue, T., and Mori, N.: Maternal cerebral hemodynamics in the supine hypotensive syndrome. Obstet. Gynecol., *79:*27, 1992.
295. Illsley, N.P., Hall, S., Penfold, P., and Stacey, T.E.: Diffusional permeability of the human placenta. Contrib. Gynecol. Obstet., *13:*92, 1985.
296. Irestedt, L., Lagercrantz, H., and Belfrage, P.: Causes and consequences of maternal and fetal sympathoadrenal activation during parturition. Acta Obstet. Gynecol. Scand., (Suppl.), *118:*111, 1984.
297. Irestedt, L., Lagercrantz, H., Hjemdahl, P., *et al.*: Fetal and maternal plasma catecholamine levels at elective cesarean section under general or epidural anesthesia versus vaginal delivery. Am. J. Obstet. Gynecol., *142:*1004, 1982.
298. James, F.M., Crawford, J.S., Davies, P., and Naiem, H.: Lumbar epidural analgesia for labor and delivery of twins. Am. J. Obstet. Gynecol., *127:*176, 1976.
299. James, F.M. III, Crawford, J.S., Hopkinson, R., *et al.*: A comparison of general anesthesia and lumbar epidural analgesia for elective cesarean section. Anesth. Analg., *56:*228, 1977.
300. James, F.M. III, and Davies, P.: Maternal and fetal effects of lumbar epidural analgesia for labor and delivery in patients with gestational hypertension. Am. J. Obstet. Gynecol., *126:*195, 1976.
301. James, F.M. III, Dewan, D.M., Floyd, H.M., *et al.*: Chloroprocaine vs. bupivacaine for lumbar epidural analgesia for elective cesarean section. Anesthesiology, *52:*488, 1980.
302. Jaschevatzky, O.E., Shalit, A., Levy, Y., and Grunstein, S.: Epidural analgesia during labour in twin pregnancy. Br. J. Obstet. Gynaecol., *84:*327, 1977.
303. Jawan, B., Lee, J.H., and Chong, Z.K.: Spread of spinal anaesthesia for caesarean section in singleton and twin pregnancies. Br. J. Anaesth., *70:*639, 1993.
304. Johnsrud, M., Dale, P.O., and Lovland, B.: Benefits of continuous infusion epidural analgesia throughout vaginal delivery. Acta Obstet. Gynecol. Scand., *67:*355, 1988.
305. Johnstone, M.: The cardiovascular effects of oxytocic drugs. Br. J. Anaesth., *44:*826, 1972.
306. Jones, C., Paul, D.L., Elton, R.A., and McLure, J.H.: Comparisons of bupivacaine and bupivacaine with fentanyl in continuous extradural analgesia during labour. Br. J. Anaesth., *63:*245, 1989.
307. Jones, M.J.T., Bogod, D.G., Rees, G.A.D., and Rosen, M.: Midwive's assessment of the upper sensory level after epidural blockade. Anaesthesia, *43:*557, 1988.
308. Jouppila, P., Jouppila, R., Barinoff, T., and Koivula, A.: Placental blood flow during caesarean section performed under subarachnoid blockade. Br. J. Anaesth., *56:*1379, 1984.
309. Jouppila, P., Jouppila, R., Hollmén, A., and Koivula, A.: Lumbar epidural analgesia to improve intervillous blood flow during labor in severe pre-eclampsia. Obstet. Gynecol., *59:*158, 1982.
310. Jouppila, P., Jouppila, R., Kaar, K., and Merila, M.: Fetal heart rate patterns and uterine activity after segmental epidural analgesia. Br. J. Obstet. Gynaecol., *84:*481, 1977.
311. Jouppila, R., and Hollmén, A.: The effect of segmental epidural analgesia on maternal and foetal acid-base balance, lactate, serum potassium and creatine phosphokinase during labour. Acta Anaesthesiol. Scand., *20:*259, 1976.
312. Jouppila, R., Hollmén, A., Jouppila, P., and Karki, N.: Segmental epidural analgesia and urinary excretion of catecholamines during labour. Acta Anaesthesiol. Scand., *21:*50, 1977.
313. Jouppila, R., Jouppila, P., Hollmén, A., and Kuikka, J.: Effect of segmental extradural analgesia on placental blood flow during normal labour. Br. J. Anaesth., *50:*563, 1978.
314. Jouppila, R., Pihlajaniemi, R., Hollmén, A., and Jouppila, P.: Segmental epidural analgesia and postpartum sequelae. Ann. Chir. Gynaecol. Fenn. *67:*85, 1978.
315. Jouppila, R., Jouppila, P., Karimen, J.M., and Hollmén, A.: Segmental epidural analgesia in labour: Related to the progress of labour, fetal malposition and instrumental delivery. Acta Obstet. Gynaecol. Scand., *58:*135, 1979.
316. Justins, D.M., Francis, D., Houlton, P.G., and Reynolds, F.: A controlled trial of extradural fentanyl in labour. Br. J. Anaesth., *54:*409, 1982.
317. Justins, D.M., Knott, C., Luthman, J., and Reynolds, F.: Epidural versus intramuscular fentanyl: Analgesia and pharmacokinetics in labour. Anaesthesia, *38:*937, 1983.
318. Kafle, S.K.: Intrathecal meperidine for elective caesarean section: A comparison with lidocaine. Can. J. Anaesth., *40:*718, 1993.
319. Kaneko, M., Saito, Y., Kirihara, Y., and Kosaka, Y.: Pregnancy enhances the antinociceptive effects of extradural lignocaine in the rat. Br. J. Anaesth., *72:*657, 1994.
320. Kang, Y.G., Abouleish, E., and Caritas, S.: Prophylactic intravenous ephedrine infusion during spinal anesthesia for cesarean section. Anesth. Analg., *61:*839, 1982.
321. Kangas-Saarela, T., Hollmén, A.I., Tolonen, U., and Eskelinen, P.: Does ephedrine influence newborn neurobehavioral responses and spectral EEG when used to prevent maternal hypotension during caesarean section? Acta Anaesthesiol. Scand., *34:*8, 1990.
322. Kangas-Saarela, T., Koivisto, M., Jouppila, R., *et al.*: Comparison of the effects of general and epidural anaesthesia for caesarean section on the neurobehavioral responses of newborn infants. Acta Anaesthesiol. Scand., *33:*313, 1989.
323. Kelton, J.G., Hunter, D.J.S., and Neame, P.B.: A platelet function defect in preeclampsia. Obstet. Gynecol., *65:*107, 1985.
324. Kenepp, N.B., Kumar, S., Shelley, W.C., *et al.*: Fetal and neonatal hazards of maternal hydration with 5% dextrose before caesarean section. Lancet, *1:*1150, 1982.
325. Kenney, A., Koh, L.S., and Pole, Y.L.: A case of locked twins managed under lumbar epidural analgesia. Anaesthesia, *33:*32, 1978.
326. Kerr, M.G., Scott, D.B., and Samuel, E.: Studies of the inferior vena cava in late pregnancy. Br. Med. J., *1:*532, 1964.
327. Kestin, I.G., Madden, A.P., Mulvein, J.T., and Goodman, N.W.: Analgesia for labour and delivery using diamorphine and bupivacaine via a 32-gauge intrathecal catheter. Br. J. Anaesth., *68:*244, 1992.
328. Kick, O., Vertommen, J.D., Van Aken, H., and Gryseels, J.: Sufentanil: Maternal and neonatal plasma levels after epidural administration during labor and delivery. (Abstract). Anesthesiology, *75:*A837, 1991.
329. Kileff, M.E., James, F.M. III, Dewan, D.M., and Floyd, H.M.: Neonatal neurobehavioral responses after epidural anesthesia for cesarean section using lidocaine and bupivacaine. Anesth. Analg., *63:*413, 1984.
330. King, M.J., Bowden, M.I., and Cooper, G.M.: Epidural fentanyl and 0.5% bupivacaine for elective caesarean section. Anaesthesia, *49:*285, 1990.
331. Kobak, A.S., Evans, E.F., and Johnson, G.R.: Transvaginal pudendal block. Am. J. Obstet. Gynecol., *71:*981, 1956.
332. Kofinas, G.D., Kofinas, A.D., and Tavakoli, F.M.: Maternal and fetal β-endorphin release in response to the stress of labor and delivery. Am. J. Obstet. Gynecol., *152:*56, 1985.
333. Kuhnert, B.R., Harrison, M.J., Linn, P.L., and Kuhnert, P.M.: Effects of maternal epidural anesthesia on neonatal behavior. Anesth. Analg., *63:*301, 1984.
334. Kuhnert, B.R., Zuspan, K.J., Kuhnert, P.M., *et al.*: Bupivacaine disposition in mother, fetus and neonate after spinal anesthesia for caesarean section. Anesth. Analg., *66:*407, 1987.
335. Laishley, R.S., Morgan, B.M., and Reynolds, F.: Effect of adrenaline on extradural anaesthesia and plasma bupivacaine concentrations during caesarean section. Br. J. Anaesth., *60:*180, 1988.
336. Lamont, R.F., Pinney, D., Rodgers, P., and Bryant, T.N.: Continuous versus intermittent epidural analgesia: A randomised trial to observe obstetric outcome. Anaesthesia, *44:*893, 1989.
337. Lao, T.T., Halpern, S.H., and Crosby, E.T.: Anesthesia and blood loss in preterm cesarean section: comparison between general and regional anesthesia. Int. J. Obstet. Anesth., *2:*85, 1993.
338. Lavin, J.P., Samuels, S.V., Miodovnik, M., *et al.*: The effects of bupivacaine and chloroprocaine as local anesthetics for epidural anesthesia on fetal heart rate monitoring parameters. Am. J. Obstet. Gynecol., *141:*717, 1981.

339. Lederman, R.P., McCann, D.S., Work, B., and Huber, M.J.: Endogenous plasma epinephrine and norepinephrine in last-trimester pregnancy and labor. Am. J. Obstet. Gynecol., *129:*5, 1977.
340. Lees, M.H., Hill, J.D., Ochsner, A.J., *et al.*: Maternal placental and myometrial blood flow of the rhesus monkey during uterine contractions. Am. J. Obstet. Gynecol., *110:*68, 1971.
341. Lees, M.M., Scott, D.B., and Kerr, M.G.: Haemodynamic changes associated with labour. J. Obstet. Gynaecol. Br. Commonw., *77:*29, 1970.
342. LeFevre, M.L.: Fetal heart rate pattern and post-paracervical fetal bradycardia. Obstet. Gynecol., *64:*343, 1984.
343. Leicht, C.H., Evans, D.E., and Durkan, W.J.: Intrathecal sufentanil for labor analgesia: Results of a pilot study. (Abstract). Anesthesiology, *73:*A981, 1990.
344. Leicht, C.H., Evans, D.E., Durkan, W.J., and Noltner, S.: Sufentanil vs. fentanyl intrathecally for labor analgesia. (Abstract). Anesth. Analg., *72:*S159, 1991.
345. Leighton, B.L., De Simone, C.A., Norris, M.C., and Ben-David, B.: Intrathecal narcotics for labor revisited: The combination of fentanyl and morphine intrathecally provides rapid onset of profound analgesia. Anesth. Analg., *69:*122, 1989.
346. Leighton, B.L., Norris, M.C., Sosis, M., *et al.*: Limitations of epinephrine as a marker of intravascular injection in laboring women. Anesthesiology, *66:*688, 1987.
347. Le Polain, B., De Kock, M., Scholtes, J.L., and Van Lierde, M.: Clonidine combined with sufentanil and bupivacaine with adrenaline for obstetric analgesia. Br. J. Anaesth., *71:*657, 1993.
348. Levinson, G., and Shnider, S.M.: Placental transfer of local anesthetics: Clinical implications. *In* Marx, G.F. (ed.): Parturition and Perinatology, pp. 173. Philadelphia, Williams and Wilkins, 1973.
349. Lewis, M., Thomas, P., and Wilkes, R.G.: Hypotension during epidural analgesia for caesarean section. Anaesthesia, *38:*250, 1983.
350. Li, D.F., Rees, G.A.D., and Rosen, M.: Continuous extradural infusion of 0.0625% or 0.125% bupivacaine for pain relief in primigravid labour. Br. J. Anaesth., *57:*264, 1985.
351. Lie, B., and Juul, J.: Effect of epidural vs. general anesthesia on breastfeeding. Acta Obstet. Gynecol. Scand., *67:*207, 1988.
352. Liggins, G.C.: Antidiuretic effects of oxytocin, morphine and pethidine in pregnancy and labour. Aust. N. Z. J. Obstet. Gynaecol.,*3:*81, 1963.
353. Lindahl, S., Norden, N., Nybell-Lindahl, G., and Westgren, M.: Endocrine stress response during general and epidural anaesthesia for elective caesarean sections. Acta Anaesthesiol. Scand., *27:*50, 1983.
354. Lipshitz, J.: Beta adrenergic agonists. Seminars in Perinatology, *5:* 252, 1981.
355. Liston, W.A., Adjepon-Yamoah, K.K., and Scott, D.B.: Foetal and maternal lignocaine levels after paracervical block. Br. J. Anaesth., *45:*750, 1973.
356. Littlewood, D.G., Buckley, P., Covino, B.G., *et al.*: Comparative study of various local anaesthetic solutions in extradural block in labour. Br. J. Anaesth., *51:*47S, 1979.
357. Liu, W.H.D., and Luxton, M.C.: The effect of prophylactic fentanyl on shivering in elective caesarean section under epidural anaesthesia. Anaesthesia, *46:*344, 1991.
358. Lofstrom B.: Aspects of the pharmacology of local anaesthetic agents. Br. J. Anaesth., *43:*194, 1970.
359. Loftus, J.R., Hill, H., and Cohen, S.E.: Epidural fentanyl and sufentanil with bupivacaine for labor: Maternal and neonatal effects. (Abstract) Anesthesiology, *75:*A856, 1991.
360. Loftus, J.R., Holbrook, R.H., and Cohen, S.E.: Fetal heart rate after epidural lidocaine and bupivacaine for cesarean section. Anesthesiology, *75:*406, 1991.
361. Loughran, P.G., Moore, J., and Dundee, J.W.: Maternal stress response associated with caesarean delivery under general and epidural anaesthesia. Br. J. Obstet. Gynaecol., *93:*943, 1986.
362. Lubbe, W.F.: Hypertension in pregnancy: Pathophysiology and management. Drugs, *28:*170, 1984.
363. Lund, P.C., Cwik, J.C., Gannon, R.T., and Vassallo, H.G.: Etidocaine for caesarean section-effects on mother and baby. Br. J. Anaesth., *49:* 457, 1977.
364. Lussos, S.A., Bader, A.M., Thornhill, M.L., and Datta, S.: The antiemetic efficacy and safety of prophylactic metoclopramide for elective cesarean delivery during spinal anesthesia. Reg. Anesth., *17:* 126, 1992.
365. Lyons, G., Macdonald, R., and Mikl, B.: Combined epidural/spinal anaesthesia for caesarean section: Through the needle or in separate spaces? Anaesthesia, *47:*199, 1992.
366. Lysak, S.Z., Eisenach, J.C., and Dobson, C.E.: Patient-controlled epidural analgesia during labor: A comparison of three solutions with a continuous infusion control. Anesthesiology, *72:*44, 1990.
367. Mabie, W.C., Ratts, T.E., and Sibai, B.M.: The central hemodynamics of severe pre-eclampsia. Am. J. Obstet. Gynecol., *161:*1443, 1989.
368. MacArthur, C., Lewis, M., Knox, E.G., and Crawford, J.S.: Epidural anaesthesia and long-term backache after childbirth. Br. Med. J., *301:* 9, 1990.
369. MacArthur, C., Lewis, M., and Knox, E.G.: Evaluation of obstetric analgesia and anaesthesia: Long-term maternal recollections. Int. J. Obstet. Anesth., *2:*3, 1993.
370. Magno, R., Berlin, A., Karlsson, K., and Kjellmer, I.: Anesthesia for cesarean section IV: Placental transfer and neonatal elimination of bupivacaine following epidural analgesia for elective cesarean section. Acta Anaesthesiol. Scand., *20:*141, 1976.
371. Magora, F., Olshwang, D., Eimerl, J., *et al.*: Observations on extradural morphine analgesia in various pain conditions. Br. J. Anaesth., *52:* 247, 1980.
372. Malinow, A.M., Mokriski, B.L.K., Wakefield, M.L., *et al.*: Anesthetic choice affects postcesarean epidural fentanyl analgesia. (Abstract). Anesth. Analg.,*67:*S138, 1988.
373. Maltau, J.M., and Andersen, H.T.: Epidural anaesthesia as an alternative to caesarean section in the treatment of prolonged, exhaustive labour. Acta Anaesthesiol. Scand., *19:*349, 1975.
374. Maltau, J.M., Andersen, H.T., and Skrede, S.: Obstetrical analgesia assessed by free fatty acid mobilisation. Acta Anaesthesiol. Scand., *19:*245, 1975.
375. Maltau, J.M., and Egge, K.: Epidural analgesia and perinatal retinal haemorrhages. Acta Anaesthesiol. Scand., *24:*99, 1980.
376. Maltau, J.M., Egge, K., and Moe, N.: Retinal hemorrhages in the preterm neonate: A prospective randomised study comparing the occurrence of hemorrhages after spontaneous versus forceps delivery. Acta Obstet. Gynecol. Scand., *63:*219, 1984.
377. Maltau, J.M., Eielson, O.V., and Stokke, K.T.: Effects of stress during labor on the concentration of cortisol and estriol in maternal plasma. Am. J. Obstet. Gynecol., *134:*681, 1979.
378. Mandell, G.L., Dewan, D.M., Howard, G., and Floyd, H.M.: The effectiveness of low-dose droperidol in controlling nausea and vomiting during epidural anesthesia for cesarean section. Int. J. Obstet. Anesth., *1:*65, 1992.
379. Maresh, M., Choong, K.-H., and Beard, R.W.: Delayed pushing with lumbar epidural analgesia in labour. Br. J. Obstet. Gynaecol., *90:*623, 1983.
380. Marks, R.J., and DeChazol, R.C.S.: Ritodrine-induced pulmonary oedema in labour. Anaesthesia, *39:*1012, 1984.
381. Martin, C.S., McGrady, E.M., Colquhoun, A., and Thornburn, J.: Extradural methadone and bupivacaine in labour. Br. J. Anaesth., *65:* 330, 1990.
382. Marx, G.F., Cosmi, E.V., and Wollman, S.B.: Biochemical status and clinical condition of mother and infant at cesarean section. Anesth. Analg., *48:*986, 1969.
383. Marx, G.F., and Greene, N.M.: Maternal lactate, pyruvate and excess lactate production during labour and delivery. Am. J. Obstet. Gynecol., *90:*786, 1964.
384. Marx, G.F., Luykx, W.M., and Cohen, S.: Fetal-neonatal status following caesarean section for fetal distress. Br. J. Anaesth.,*56:*1009, 1984.
385. Marx, G.F., and Mateo, C.V.: Effects of different oxygen concentrations during general anaesthesia for elective caesarian section. Can. Anaesth. Soc. J., *18:*587, 1971.
386. Matadial, L., and Cibils, L.A.: The effect of epidural anesthesia on uterine activity and blood pressure. Am. J. Obstet. Gynecol., *125:*846, 1976.
387. Mathew, J.P., Fleisher, L.A., Rinehouse, J.A., *et al.*: ST segment depression during labor and delivery. Anesthesiology, *77:*635, 1992.
388. Mathru, M., Rao, T.L.K., Kartha, R.K., *et al.*: Intravenous albumin for prevention of spinal hypotension during cesarean section. Anesth. Analg., *59:*655, 1980.
389. Matouskova, A., Dottori, O., Forssman, L., and Victorin, L.: An improved method of epidural analgesia with reduced instrumental delivery rate. Acta Obstet. Gynecol. Scand., *54:*231, 1975.
390. Matthews, N.C., and Corser, G.: Epidural fentanyl for shaking in obstetrics. Anaesthesia, *43:*783, 1988.

391. Mayer, D.C., and Weeks, S.K.: Antepartum uterine relaxation with nitroglycerine at caesarean delivery. Can. J. Anaesth., *39:*166, 1992.
392. McGrady, E.M., Brownhill, D.K., and Davis, A.G.: Epidural diamorphine and bupivacaine in labour. Anaesthesia, *44:*400, 1989.
393. McHale, S., Mitchell, V., Howsam, S., and Carli, F.: Continuous subarachnoid infusion of 0.125% bupivacaine for analgesia during labour. Br. J. Anaesth., *69:*634, 1992.
394. McLintic, A.J., Danskin, F.H., Reid, J.A., and Thorburn, J.: Effect of adrenaline on extradural anaesthesia, plasma lignocaine concentrations and the feto-placental unit during elective caesarean section. Br. J. Anaesth., *67:*683, 1991.
395. McLintic, A.J., Pringle, S.D., Lilley, S., *et al.*: Electrocardiographic changes during cesarean section under regional anesthesia. Anesth. Analg., *74:*51, 1992.
396. McClure, J.H.: Ropivacaine. Br. J. Anaesth., *76:*300, 1996.
397. McCrae, A.F., Jozwiak, H., and McClure, J.H.: Comparison of ropivacaine and bupivacaine in extradural analgesia for the relief of pain in labour. Br. J. Anaesth., *74:*261, 1995.
398. Meehan, F.P.: Continuous caudal analgesia in obstetrics. Proc. R. Soc. Med., *62:*185, 1969.
399. Meehan, F.P., Moolgaoker, A.S., and Stallworthy, J.: Vaginal delivery under caudal analgesia after caesarean section and other major uterine surgery. Br. Med. J., *2:*740, 1972.
400. Mehta, P., Theriot, E., Mehrotra, D., *et al.*: Shivering following epidural anesthesia in obstetrics. Reg. Anesth., *9:*83, 1984.
401. Meis, P.J., Reisner, L.S., Payne, T.F., and Hobel, C.J.: Bupivacaine paracervical block: Effects on the fetus and neonate. Obstet. Gynecol., *52:*545, 1978.
402. Mendez, R., Eisenach, J.C., and Kashtan, K.: Epidural clonidine analgesia after cesarean section. Anesthesiology, *73:*848, 1990.
403. Merkow, A.J., McGuiness, G.A., Erenberg, A., and Kennedy, R.L.: The neonatal neuro-behavioral effects of bupivacaine, mepivacaine, and 2-chloroprocaine used for pudendal block. Anesthesiology, *52:* 309, 1980.
404. Merry, A.F., Cross, J.A., Mayadeo, S.V., and Wild, C.J.: Posture and spread of extradural analgesia in labour. Br. J. Anaesth., *55:*303, 1983.
405. Messih, M.N.A.: Epidural space pressures during pregnancy. Anaesthesia, *36:*775, 1981.
406. Michael, S., Richmond, M.N., and Birks, R.J.S.: A comparison between open-end (single-hole) and closed-end (three lateral holes) epidural catheters. Anaesthesia, *44:*578, 1989.
407. Mihaly, G.W., Moore, R.G., Thomas, J., *et al.*: The pharmacokinetics of anilide local anaesthetics in neonates. I: Lignocaine. Eur. J. Clin. Pharmacol., *13:*143, 1978.
408. Miller, F.C., Quesnel, G., Petrie, R.H., *et al.*: The effects of paracervical block on uterine activity and beat-to-beat variability of the fetal heart rate. Am. J. Obstet. Gynecol., *130:*284, 1978.
409. Milligan, K.R., Cramp, P., Schatz, L., *et al.*: The effect of patient position and obesity on the spread of epidural analgesia. Int. J. Obstet. Anesth., *2:*134, 1993.
410. Milne, M.K., and Murray Lawson, J.I.: Epidural analgesia for caesarian section. A review of 182 cases. Br. J. Anaesth., *45:*1206, 1973.
411. Mirkin, B.L.: Perinatal pharmacology, placental transfer, fetal localization, and neonatal disposition of drugs. Anesthesiology, *43:*156, 1975.
412. Moir, D.D.: Anaesthesia for caesarian section: An evaluation of a method using low concentrations of halothane and 50 percent oxygen. Br. J. Anaesth., *42:*136, 1970.
413. Moir, D.D.: *In* Obstetric Anaesthesia and Analgesia. pp. 51. London, Bailliere Tindall, 1976.
414. Moir, D.D., and Amoa, A.B.: Ergometrine or oxytocin: Blood loss and side effects at spontaneous vertex delivery. Br. J. Anaesth., *51:*113, 1979.
415. Moir, D.D., and Davidson, S.: Postpartum complications of forceps delivery performed under epidural and pudendal nerve block. Br. J. Anaesth. *44:*1197, 1972.
416. Moir, D.D., Victor-Rodrigues, L., and Willocks, J.: Epidural analgesia during labour in patients with pre-eclampsia. J. Obstet. Gynaecol. Br. Commonw., *79:*465, 1972.
417. Moir, D.D., and Willocks, J.: Management of inco-ordinate intrauterine action under continuous epidural analgesia. Br. Med. J., *3:*396, 1967.
418. Monk, J.P., Beresford, R., and Ward, A.: Sufentanil: A review of its pharmacological properties and therapeutic use. Drugs, *36:*286, 1988.
419. Moodie, J.E., and Moir, D.D.: Ergometrine, oxytocin and extradural analgesia. Br. J. Anaesth., *48:*571, 1976.
420. Moore, D.C., Bridenbaugh, L.D., Bridenbaugh, P.O., and Tucker, G.T.: Caudal and epidural blocks with bupivacaine for childbirth: Report of 657 parturients. Obstet. Gynecol., *37:*667, 1971.
421. Moore, J., Flynn, R.J., Sampaio, M., *et al.*: Effect of single-dose omeprazole on intragastric acidity and volume during obstetric anaesthesia. Anaesthesia, *44:*559, 1989.
422. Moore, J., Murnaghan, G.A., and Lewis, M.A.: A clinical evaluation of the maternal effects of lumbar extradural analgesia for labour. Anaesthesia, *29:*537, 1974.
423. Mor, A., Yang, W., Schwarz, A., and Jones, W.C.: Platelet counts in pregnancy and labor: A comparative study. Obstet. Gynecol., *16:*338, 1960.
424. Moran, D.H., Perillo, M., LaPorta, R.F., *et al.*: Phenylephrine in the prevention of hypotension following spinal anesthesia for cesarean delivery. J. Clin. Anesth., *3:*301, 1991.
425. Morgan, B.M., Aulakh, J.M., Barker, J.P., *et al.*: Anaesthesia for caesarean section—A medical audit of junior anaesthetic staff practice. Br. J. Anaesth., *55:*885, 1983.
426. Morgan, B.M., Aulakh, J.M., Barker, J.P., *et al.*: Anaesthetic morbidity following caesarean section under epidural or general anaesthesia. Lancet, *1:*328, 1984.
427. Morgan, B.M., Bulpitt, C.J., Clifton, P., and Lewis, P.J.: Analgesia and satisfaction in childbirth (The Queen Charlotte's 1,000-mother survey). Lancet, *2:*808, 1982.
428. Morgan, B.M., Magni, V., and Goroszenuik, T.: Anaesthesia for emergency caesarean section. Br. J. Obstet. Gynaecol., *97:*420, 1990.
429. Morishima, H.O., and Covino, B.G.: Toxicity and distribution of lidocaine in nonasphyxiated and asphyxiated baboon fetuses. Anesthesiology, *54:*182, 1981.
430. Morishima, H.O., Covino, B.G., Yeh, M-N., *et al.*: Bradycardia in the fetal baboon following paracervical block anesthesia. Am. J. Obstet. Gynecol., *140:*775, 1981.
431. Morishima, H.O., Daniel, S.S., Finster, M., *et al.*: Transmission of mepivacaine hydrochloride across the human placenta. Anesthesiology, *27:*147, 1966.
432. Morishima, H.O., Finster, M., Arthur, R., and Covino, B.G.: Pregnancy does not alter lidocaine toxicity. Am. J. Obstet. Gynecol., *162:* 1320, 1990.
433. Morishima, H.O., Pedersen, H., Santos, A.C., *et al.*: Adverse effects of maternally administered lidocaine on the asphyxiated preterm fetal lamb. Anesthesiology, *71:*110, 1989.
434. Morselli, P.K., and Rovei, V.: Placental transfer of pethidine and norpethidine and their pharmacokinetics on the newborn. Eur. J. Clin. Pharmacol., *18:*25, 1980.
435. Motsch, J., Graber, E., and Ludwig, K.: Addition of clonidine enhances postoperative analgesia from epidural morphine: A double-blind study. Anesthesiology, *73:*1067, 1990.
436. Munson, E.S., and Embro, W.J.: Lidocaine, monoethylglycinexylidide, and isolated human uterine muscle. Anesthesiology, *48:*183, 1978.
437. Murphy, D.F., Nally, B., Gardiner, J., and Unwin, A.: Effect of metoclopramide on gastric emptying before elective and emergency caesarean section. Br. J. Anaesth., *56:*1113, 1984.
438. Murphy, J.D., Hendersen, K., Bowden, M.I., *et al.*: Bupivacaine versus bupivacaine plus fentanyl for epidural analgesia: Effect on maternal satisfaction. Br. Med. J., *302:*564, 1991.
439. Murphy, P.J., Wright, J.D., and Fitzgerald, T.B.: Assessment of paracervical nerve block anaesthesia during labour. Br. Med. J., *1:*526, 1970.
440. Murphy, T.M., Mather, L.E., Stanton-Hicks, M.D'A., *et al.*: Effects of adding adrenaline to etidocaine and lignocaine in extradural anaesthesia. 1: Block characteristics and cardiovascular effects. Br. J. Anaesth., *48:*893, 1976.
441. Murray, A.M., Morgan, M., and Whitwam, J.G.: Crystalloid versus colloid for circulatory preload for epidural caesarean section. Anaesthesia., *44:*463, 1989.
442. Namba, Y., Smith, J.B., Fox, G.S., and Challis, J.R.G.: Plasma cortisol concentrations during caesarean section. Br. J. Anaesth., *52:*1027, 1980.
443. Narchi, P., Benhamou, D., Hamza, J., and Bouaziz, H.: Ventilatory effects of epidural clonidine during the first 3 hours after caesarean section. Acta Anaesthesiol. Scand., *36:*791, 1992.
444. Naulty, J.S., Barnes, D., and Becker, R.: Continuous subarachnoid sufentanil for labor analgesia. (Abstract). Anesthesiology, *73:*A964, 1990.

445. Nesheim, B.I., Lindbaek, E., Storm-Mathisen, I., and Jenssen, H.: Neurobehavioural response of infants after paracervical block during labour. Acta Obstet. Gynecol. Scand., *58:*41, 1979.
446. Neumark, J., Hammerle, A.F., and Biegelmayer, C.: Effects of epidural analgesia on plasma catecholamines and cortisol in parturition. Acta Anaesthesiol. Scand., *29:*255, 1985.
447. Nimmo, W.S., Wilson, J., and Prescott, L.F.: Narcotic analgesics and delayed gastric emptying during labour. Lancet, *1:*890, 1975.
448. Nimmo, W.S., Wilson, J., and Prescott, L.F.: Further studies of gastric emptying during labour. Anaesthesia, *32:*100, 1977.
449. Noble, D.W., Morrison, L.M., Brockway, M.S., and McClure, J.H.: Adrenaline, fentanyl, or adrenaline and fentanyl as adjuncts to bupivacaine for extradural anaesthesia in elective caesarean section. Br. J. Anaesth., *66:*645, 1991.
450. Noble, H.A., Enever, G.R., and Thomas, T.: Epidural bupivacaine dilution for labour: A comparison of three concentrations infused with a fixed dose of fentanyl. Anaesthesia, *46:*549, 1991.
451. Norris, M.C., and Dewan, D.M.: Effect of gravity on the spread of extradural anaesthesia for caesarean section. Br. J. Anaesth., *59:*338, 1987.
452. Norris, M.C., Grieco, W.M., Borkowski, M., *et al.*: Complications of labor analgesia: Epidural versus combined spinal epidural techniques. Anesth. Analg., *79:*529, 1994.
453. Nottcut, W.: Overdose of opioid from PCA pumps. Br. J. Anaesth., *69:*450, 1992.
454. Nunn, J.F.: *In* Applied Respiratory Physiology. 2nd ed. pp. 386. London, Butterworths, 1977.
455. O'Driscoll, K., Meagher, D., MacDonald, D., and Geoghegan, F.: Traumatic intracranial haemorrhage in first born infants and delivery with obstetric forceps. Br. J. Obstet. Gynaecol., *88:*577, 1981.
456. O'Kelly, S.W., Lawes, E.G., and Luntley, J.B.: Bleeding time: Is it a useful clinical tool? Br. J. Anaesth., *68:*313, 1992.
457. O'Meara, M.E., and Gin, T.: Comparison of 0.125% bupivacaine with 0.125% bupivacaine and clonidine as extradural analgesia in the first stage of labour. Br. J. Anaesth., *71:*651, 1993.
458. Ong, B.Y., Cohen, M.M., and Palahniuk, R.J.: Anesthesia for cesarean section—Effects on neonates. Anesth. Analg., *68:*270, 1989.
459. Orlikowski, C.E.P., Payne, A.J., Moodley, J., and Rocke, D.A.: Thromboelastography after aspirin ingestion in pregnant and nonpregnant subjects. Br. J. Anaesth., *69:*159, 1992.
460. Ounsted, M.: Pain relief during childbirth and development at 4 years. J. R. Soc. Med., *74:*629, 1981.
461. Ounsted, M., Scott, A., and Moar, V.: Delivery and development: To what extent can one associate cause and effect? J. R. Soc. Med., *73:* 786, 1980.
462. Paech, M.J.: Patient-controlled epidural analgesia during labour: Choice of solution. Int. J. Obstet. Anesth., *2:*65, 1993.
463. Paech, M.J.: Patient-controlled epidural analgesia in labour—Is a continuous infusion of benefit? Anaesth. Intensive Care, *20:*15, 1992.
464. Paech, M.J., Westmore, M.D., and Speirs, H.M.: A double-blind comparison of epidural bupivacaine and bupivacaine-fentanyl for caesarean section. Anaesth. Intensive Care, *18:*22, 1990.
465. Palahniuk, R.J., Scatliff, J., Biehl, D., *et al.*: Maternal and neonatal effects of methoxyflurane, nitrous oxide and lumbar epidural anaesthesia for caesarean section. Can. Anaesth. Soc. J., *24:*586, 1977.
466. Palmer, C.M., Norris, M.C., Giudici, M.C., *et al.*: Incidence of electrocardiographic changes during cesarean delivery under regional anesthesia. Anesth. Analg., *70:*36, 1990.
467. Palot, M., Visseaux, H., Botmans, C., *et al.*: Placental transfer and neonatal distribution of fentanyl, alfentanil and sufentanil after continuous epidural administration for labor. (Abstract). Anesthesiology, *77:*A991, 1992.
468. Parnass, S.M., Curran, M.J.A., and Becker, G.L.: Incidence of hypotension associated with epidural lidocaine using alkalinized and nonalkalinized lidocaine for cesarean section. Anesth. Analg.,*66:* 1148, 1987.
469. Parry, M.G., Bawa, G.P.S., Poulton, B., and Fernando, R.: Comparison of dorsal column function in parturients receiving epidural and combined spinal epidural (CSE) for labour and elective caesarean section. (Abstract) Int. J. Obstet. Anesth., *5:*213, 1996.
470. Paterson, M.E.L.: The aetiology and outcome of abruptio placentae. Acta Obstet. Gynecol. Scand., *58:*31, 1979.
471. Pearson, J.F., and Davies, P.: The effect of continuous lumbar epidural analgesia on the acid-base status of maternal arterial blood during the first stage of labour. J. Obstet. Gynaecol. Br. Commonw., *80:*218, 1973(a).
472. Pearson, J.F., and Davies, P.: The effect of continuous lumbar epidural analgesia on maternal acidbase balance and arterial lactate concentration during the second stage of labour. J. Obstet. Gynaecol. Br. Commonw., *80:*225, 1973(b).
473. Pearson, J.F., and Davies, P.: The effect of continuous lumbar epidural analgesia upon fetal acidbase status during the first stage of labour. J. Obstet. Gynaecol. Br. Commonw., *81:*971, 1974(a).
474. Pearson, J.F., and Davies, P.: The effect of continuous lumbar epidural analgesia upon fetal acid-base status during the second stage of labour. J. Obstet. Gynaecol. Br. Commonw., *81:*975, 1974(b).
475. Pechet, L., and Alexander, B.: Increased clotting factors in pregnancy. N. Engl. J. Med., *265:*1093, 1961.
476. Pedersen, H., Morishima, H.O., and Finster, M.: Uptake and effect of local anesthetics in mother and fetus. Int. Anesthesiol. Clin.,*16:*4, 73, 1978.
477. Pedersen, H., Santos, A.C., Morishima, H.O., *et al.*: Does gestational age affect the pharmacokinetics and pharmacodynamics of lidocaine in mother and fetus? Anesthesiology, *68:*367, 1988.
478. Penfield, A.J.: Laparoscopic sterilization under local anesthesia—1,200 cases. Obstet. Gynecol., *49:*725, 1976.
479. Peng, A.T.C., Gorman, R.S., Shulman, S.M., *et al.*: Intravenous nitroglycerin for uterine relaxation in the postpartum patient with retained placenta. Anesthesiology, *71:*172, 1989.
480. Perris, B.W.: Epidural pethidine in labour: A study of dose requirements. Anaesthesia, *35:*380, 1980.
481. Perris, B.W., and Malins, A.F.: Pain relief in labour using epidural pethidine with adrenaline. Anaesthesia, *36:*631, 1981.
482. Philipson, E.H., Kuhnert, B.R., and Syracuse, C.B.: Maternal, fetal, and neonatal lidocaine levels following local perineal infiltration. Am. J. Obstet. Gynecol., *149:*403, 1984.
483. Philipson, E.H., Kuhnert, B.R., Syracuse, C.B., *et al.*: Intrapartum paracervical block anesthesia with 2-chloroprocaine. Am. J. Obstet. Gynecol., *146:*16, 1983.
484. Phillips, G.: Continuous infusion epidural analgesia in labor: The effect of adding sufentanil to 0.125% bupivacaine. Anesth. Analg., *67:* 462, 1988.
485. Phillips, G.H.: Epidural sufentanil/bupivacaine combinations for analgesia during labor: Effect of varying sufentanil doses. Anesthesiology, *67:*835, 1987.
486. Phillips, J.C., Hochberg, C.J., Petrakis, J.K., and Van Winkle, J.D.: Epidural analgesia and its effects on the "normal" progress of labor. Am. J. Obstet. Gynecol., *129:*316, 1977.
487. Pickering, B., Biehl, D., and Meatherall, R.: The effect of foetal acidosis on bupivacaine levels in utero. Can. Anaesth. Soc. J., *28:*544, 1981.
488. Poppers, P.J.: Evaluation of local anaesthetic agents for regional anaesthesia in obstetrics. Br. J. Anaesth., *47:*322, 1975.
489. Poppers, P.J., and Finster, M.: Use of prilocaine hydrochloride for epidural analgesia in obstetrics. Anesthesiology, *29:*1134, 1968.
490. Power, I., Brown, D.T., and Wildsmith, J.A.W.: The effect of fentanyl, meperidine and diamorphine on nerve conduction *in vitro.* Reg. Anesth., *16:*204, 1991.
491. Pritchard, J.A., Cunningham, F.G., and Mason, R.A.: Coagulation changes in eclampsia: Their frequency and pathogenesis. Am. J. Obstet. Gynecol., *124:*855, 1976.
492. Pritchard, J.A., and Stone, S.R.: Clinical and laboratory observations in eclampsia. Am. J. Obstet. Gynecol., *99:*754, 1967.
493. Prowse, C.M., and Gaensler, E.A.: Respiratory and acid-base changes during pregnancy. Anesthesiology, *26:*381, 1965.
494. Purdie, J., Reid, J., Thorburn, J., and Asbury, A.J.: Continuous extradural analgesia: Comparison of midwife top-ups, continuous infusions and patient-controlled administration. Br. J. Anaesth., *68:*580, 1992.
495. Purdy, G., Currie, J., and Owen, H.: Continuous extradural analgesia in labour. Comparison between "on demand" and regular "top-up" injections. Br. J. Anaesth., *59:*319, 1987.
496. Raabe, N., and Belfrage, P.: Lumbar epidural analgesia in labour: A clinical analysis. Acta. Obstet. Gynecol. Scand., *55:*125, 1976.
497. Raabe, N., and Belfrage, P.: Epidural analgesia in labour. IV: Influence on uterine activity and fetal heart rate. Acta Obstet. Gynecol. Scand., *55:*305, 1976.
498. Ralston, D.H., and Shnider, S.M.: The fetal and neonatal effects of regional anesthesia in obstetrics. Anesthesiology., *48:*34, 1978.
499. Ralston, D.H., Shnider, S.M., and De Lorimer, A.A.: Effects of equipotent ephedrine, metaraminol, mephentermine and methoxamine on uterine blood flow in the pregnant ewe. Anesthesiology., *40:* 354, 1974.

500. Ramanathan, S., Friedman, S., Moss, P., *et al.*: Phenylephrine for the treatment of maternal hypotension due to epidural anesthesia. Anesth. Analg., *63:*262, 1984.
501. Ramanathan, S., Gandhi, S., Arismendy, J., *et al.*: Oxygen transfer from mother to fetus during cesarean section under epidural anesthesia. Anesth. Analg., *61:*576, 1982.
502. Ramanathan, S., and Grant, G.J.: Vasopressor therapy for hypotension due to epidural anesthesia for cesarean section. Acta. Anaesthesiol. Scand., *32:*559, 1988.
503. Ramanathan, S., Masih, A., Rock, I., *et al.*: Maternal and fetal effects of prophylactic hydration with crystalloids or colloids before epidural anesthesia. Anesth. Analg., *62:*673, 1983.
504. Rawal, N., Nuutinen, L., Raj, P.P., *et al.*: Behavioral and histopathological effects following intrathecal administration of butorphanol, sufentanil, and nalbuphine in sheep. Anesthesiology, *75:*1025, 1991.
505. Rawal, N., Schollin, J., and Wesstrom, G.: Epidural versus combined spinal epidural block for caesarean section. Acta. Anaesthesiol. Scand., *32:*61, 1988.
506. Reynolds, F.: Placental transfer of drugs. Int. J. Obstet. Anesth., *2:* 108, 1991.
507. Reynolds, F., Hargrove, R.I., and Wyman, J.B.: Maternal and foetal plasma concentrations of bupivacaine after epidural block. Br. J. Anaesth., *45:*1049, 1973.
508. Reynolds, F., and O'Sullivan, G.: Epidural fentanyl and perineal pain in labour. Anaesthesia, *44:*341, 1989.
509. Reynolds, F., and Taylor, G.: Plasma concentrations of bupivacaine during continuous epidural analgesia in labour: The effect of adrenaline. Br. J. Anaesth., *43:*436, 1971.
510. Rigler, M.L., Drasner, K., Krejcie, T.C., *et al.* Cauda equina syndrome after continuous spinal anesthesia. Anesth. Analg., *72:*275, 1991.
511. Riley, E.T., Cohen, S.E., Macario, A., *et al.*: Spinal versus epidural anesthesia for cesarean section: A comparison of time efficiency, costs, charges and complications. Anesth. Analg., *80:*709, 1995.
512. Riley, E.T., Cohen, S.E., Ratner, E.F., *et al.*: Intrathecal sufentanil: Relationships between diluent volume, sensory and blood pressure changes, and duration of analgesia. (Abstract). Society for Obstetric Anesthesia and Perinatology, 26th Annual Meeting, 1994.
513. Riley, E.T., Walker, D., Hamilton, C.L., and Cohen, S.E.: A comparison of intrathecal sufentanil and bupivacaine with regard to changes in temperature and blood pressure. (Abstract). Anesthesiology, *83:* A939, 1995.
514. Robinson, J.O., Rosen, M., Evans, J.M., *et al.*: Maternal opinion about analgesia for labour: A controlled trial between epidural block and intramuscular pethidine combined with inhalation. Anaesthesia, *35:* 1173, 1980.
515. Robson, S.C., Boys, R.J., Rodeck, C., and Morgan, B.: Maternal and fetal haemodynamic effects of spinal and extradural anaesthesia for elective caesarean section. Br. J. Anaesth., *68:*54, 1992.
516. Robson, S.C., Dunlop, W., Boys, R.J., and Hunter, S.: Cardiac output during labour. Br. Med. J., *295:*1169, 1987.
517. Rodriguez, J., Payne, M., Afrabiasi, A., *et al.*: Continuous infusion epidural anesthesia during labor: A randomized double-blind comparison of 0.0625% bupivacaine/0.002% butorphanol and 0.125% bupivacaine. Reg. Anesth., *15:*300, 1990.
518. Rogers, R.P.C., and Levin, J.: A critical reappraisal of the bleeding time. Semin. Thromb. Hemost., *16:*1, 1990.
519. Rolbin, S.H., Cohen, M.M., Levinton, C.M., *et al.*: The premature infant: Anesthesia for cesarean delivery. Anesth. Analg., *78:*912, 1994.
520. Rolbin, S.H., Cole, A.F.D., Hew, E.M., *et al.*: Prophylactic IM ephedrine before epidural anaesthesia for caesarean section: Efficacy and actions on fetus and newborn. Can. Anaesth. Soc. J., *29:*148, 1982.
521. Rolbin, S.H., Cole, A.F.D., Hew, E.M., and Virgint, S.: Effect of lateral position and volume on the spread of epidural anaesthesia in the parturient. Can. Anaesth. Soc. J., *28:*431, 1981.
522. Rorke, M.J., Davey, D.A., and Du Toit, H.F.: Foetal oxygenation during caesarean section. Anaesthesia, *23:*585, 1968.
523. Rorth, M., and Bille-Brahe, N.E.: 2,3 Diphosphoglycerate and creatinine in the red cell membrane during pregnancy. Scand. J. Clin. Lab. Invest., *28:*271, 1971.
524. Rosefsky, J.B., and Petersiel, M.E.: Perinatal deaths associated with mepivacaine paracervical block anesthesia in labor. N. Engl. J. Med., *278:*530, 1968.
525. Rosenberg, P.H., Kyttä, J., and Alila, A.: Absorption of bupivacaine, etidocaine, lignocaine and ropivacaine into n-heptane, rat sciatic nerve, and human extradural and subcutaneous fat. Br. J. Anaesth., *58:* 310, 1986.
526. Rosenblatt, R., Wright, R., Denson, D., and Raj, P.: Continuous epidural infusions for obstetric analgesia. Reg. Anesth., *8:*10, 1983.
527. Rosenfeld, C.R., and West, J.: Circulating response to systemic infusion of norephinephrine in the pregnant ewe. Am. J. Obstet. Gynecol., *127:*376, 1977.
528. Ross, A., and Popham, P.: Post-dural puncture headache and spinal anesthesia. Int. Anesthesiol. Clin., *32:*137, 1994.
529. Rostaing, S., Bonnet, F., Levron, J.C., *et al.*: Effect of epidural clonidine on analgesia and pharmacokinetics of epidural fentanyl in postoperative patients. Anesthesiology, *75:*420, 1991.
530. Rout, C.C., Akoojee, S.S., Rocke, D.A., and Gouws, E.: Rapid administration of crystalloid preload does not decrease the incidence of hypotension after spinal anaesthesia for elective caesarean section. Br. J. Anaesth., *68:*394, 1992.
531. Rout, C.C., Rocke, D.A., Brijball, R., and Koovarjee, R.V.: Prophylactic intramuscular ephedrine prior to caesarean section. Anaesth. Intensive Care, *20:*448, 1992.
532. Rout, C.C., Rocke, D.A., and Gouws, E.: Intravenous ranitidine reduces the risk of acid aspiration of gastric contents at emergency cesarean section. Anesth. Analg., *76:*156, 1993.
533. Russell, I.F.: Spinal anaesthesia for caesarean section: The use of 0.5% bupivacaine. Br. J. Anaesth., *55:*309, 1983.
534. Russell, I.F., and Chambers, W.A.: Closing volume in normal pregnancy. Br. J. Anaesth., *53:*1043, 1981.
535. Russell, R., Groves, P., Taub, N., *et al.*: Assessing long-term backache after childbirth. Br. Med. J., *306:*1299, 1993.
536. Russell, R., and Reynolds, F.: Epidural infusions for nulliparous women in labour: A randomised double-blind comparison of fentanyl/bupivacaine and sufentanil/bupivacaine. Anaesthesia, *48:*856, 1993.
537. Saling, E., and Ligdas, P.: The effect on the foetus of maternal hyperventilation during labour. J. Obstet. Gynaecol. Br. Commonw., *76:* 877, 1969.
538. Sangoul, F., Fox, G.S., and Houle, G.L.: Effect of regional analgesia on maternal oxygen consumption during the first stage of labor. Am. J. Obstet. Gynecol., *121:*1080, 1975.
539. Santos, A.C., Arthur, G.R., Wlody, D., *et al.*: Comparative systemic toxicity of ropivacaine and bupivacaine in nonpregnant and pregnant ewes. Anesthesiology, *82:*734, 1995.
540. Santos, A.C., and Datta, S.: Prophylactic use of droperidol for control of nausea and vomiting during spinal anesthesia for cesarean section. Anesth. Analg., *63:*85, 1984.
541. Santos, A.C., Pedersen, H., Harman, T.W., *et al.*: Does pregnancy alter the systemic toxicity of local anesthetics? Anesthesiology, *70:*991, 1989.
542. Santos, A.C., Pedersen, H., Sallusto, J.A., *et al.*: Pharmacokinetics of ropivacaine in nonpregnant and pregnant ewes. Anesth. Analg., *70:* 262, 1990.
543. Scanlon, J.W., and Alper, M.H.: Perinatal pharmacology and evaluation of the newborn. Int. Anesthesiol. Clin., *11:*163, 1973.
544. Scanlon, J.W., Brown, W.U., Weiss, J.B., and Alper, M.H.: Neurobehavioral responses of newborn infants after maternal epidural anesthesia. Anesthesiology, *40:*121, 1974.
545. Scanlon, J.W., Ostheimer, G.W., Lurie, A.O., *et al.*: Neurobehavioral responses and drug concentrations in newborns after maternal epidural anesthesia with bupivacaine. Anesthesiology, *45:*400, 1976.
546. Schierup, L., Schmidt, J.F., Jensen, A.T., and Rye, B.A.O.: Pudendal block in vaginal deliveries: Mepivacaine with and without epinephrine. Acta Obstet. Gynecol. Scand., *67:*195, 1988.
547. Schifrin, B.S.: Fetal heart rate patterns following epidural anaesthesia and oxytocin infusion during labour. J. Obstet. Gynaecol. Br. Commonw., *79:*332, 1972.
548. Schindler, M., Gatt, S., Isert, P., *et al.*: Thrombocytopenia and platelet functional defects in pre-eclampsia: Implications for regional anaesthesia. Anaesth. Intensive Care, *18:*169, 1990.
549. Scott, D.B., and Hibbard, B.M.: Serious non-fatal complications associated with extradural block in obstetric practice. Br. J. Anaesth., *64:* 537, 1990.
550. Scott, D.B., and Kerr, M.G.: Inferior vena caval pressure in late pregnancy. J. Obstet. Gynaecol. Br. Commonw., *70:*1044, 1963.
551. Scott, P.V., Bowen, F.E., Cartwright, P., *et al.*: Intrathecal morphine as sole analgesic during labour. Br. Med. J., *2:*351, 1980.
552. Scudamore, J.H., and Yates, M.J.: Pudendal block—A misnomer? Lancet, *1:*23, 1966.
553. Secher, N.J., Thayssen, P., Arnsbo, P., and Olsen, J.: Effect of

prostaglandin E_2 and F_2 alpha on the systemic and pulmonary circulation in pregnant anesthetized women. Acta Obstet. Gynecol. Scand., *61:*213, 1982.
554. Sengupta, P., and Nielsen, M.: The effect of labour and epidural analgesia on pain threshold. Anaesthesia, *39:*982, 1984.
555. Sevarino, F.B., Johnson, M.D., Lema, M.J., *et al.*: The effect of epidural sufentanil on shivering and body temperature in the parturient. Anesth. Analg., *68:*530, 1989.
556. Shehabi, Y., Gatt, S., Buckman, T., and Isert, P.: Effect of adrenaline, fentanyl and warming of injectate on shivering following extradural analgesia in labour. Anaesth. Intensive Care., *18:*31, 1990.
557. Shnider, S.M., Abboud, T.K., Artal, R., *et al.*: Maternal catecholamines decrease during labor after lumbar epidural anesthesia. Am. J. Obstet. Gynecol., *147:*13, 1983.
558. Shnider, S.M., Asling, J.H., Hall, J.W., and Margolis, A.J.: Paracervical block anesthesia in obstetrics. I: Fetal complications and neonatal morbidity. Am. J. Obstet. Gynecol., *107:*619, 1970.
559. Shnider, S.M., DeLorimer, A.A., Hall, J.W., *et al.*: Vasopressors in obstetrics. I: Correction of fetal acidosis with ephedrine during spinal hypotension. Am. J. Obstet. Gynecol., *102:*911, 1968.
560. Shnider, S.M., and Gildea, J.: Paracervical block anesthesia in obstetrics. Am. J. Obstet. Gynecol., *116:*320, 1973.
561. Shnider, S.M., and Levinson, G.: Anesthesia for cesarean section. *In* Shnider, S.M., and Levinson, G., (eds.): Anesthesia for Obstetrics. 3rd ed. pp. 216. Baltimore, Williams and Wilkins, 1993.
562. Shnider, S.M., Wright, R.G., Levinson, G., *et al.*: Uterine blood flow and plasma norepinephrine changes during maternal stress. Anesthesiology, *50:*524, 1979.
563. Sibai, B.M., Taslimi, M.M., El-Nazer, A., *et al.*: Maternal-perinatal outcome associated with the syndrome of hemolysis, elevated liver enzymes, and low platelets in severe pre-eclampsia-eclampsia. Am. J. Obstet. Gynecol., *155:*501, 1986.
564. Sivakumeran, C., Ramanathan, S., Chalon, J., and Turndorf, H.: Uterine contractions and the spread of local anesthetics in the epidural space. Anesth. Analg., *61:*127, 1982.
565. Skjoldebrand, A., Garle, M., Gustafsson, L.L., *et al.*: Extradural pethidine with and without adrenaline during labour: Wide variation in effect. Br. J. Anaesth., *54:*415, 1982.
566. Smedstad, K.G., and Morison, D.H.: A comparative study of continuous and intermittent epidural analgesia for labour and delivery. Can. J. Anaesth., *35:*234, 1988.
567. Smith, A.P.: The effects of intravenous infusions of graded doses of prostaglandin-$F_2\alpha$ and E_2 on lung resistance in patients undergoing termination of pregnancy. Clin. Sci., *44:*17, 1973.
568. Social Services Committee. Second Report, 1979–1980 Perinatal and Neonatal Mortality, London: Her Majesty's Stationery Office, 1980.
569. Soffronoff, E.C., Kauffman, B.M., and Connaughton, J.F.: Intravascular volume determinations and fetal outcome in hypertensive disease of pregnancy. Am. J. Obstet. Gynecol., *127:*4, 1977.
570. Stainthorp, S.F., Bradshaw, E.G., Challen, P.D., and Tobias, M.A.: 0.125% bupivacaine for obstetric analgesia? Anaesthesia, *33:*3, 1978.
571. Steinberg, R.B., Dunn, S.M., Dixon, D.E., *et al.*: Comparison of sufentanil, bupivacaine and their combination for epidural analgesia in obstetrics. Reg. Anesth., *17:*131, 1992.
572. Steinberg, R.B., Powell, G.M., Hu, X., and Dunn, S.M.: Epidural sufentanil for analgesia for labor and delivery. Reg. Anesth., *14:*225, 1989.
573. Stenger, V., Eitsman, D., Anderson, T., *et al.*: Observations on placental exchange of the respiratory gases in pregnant women at cesarean section. Am. J. Obstet. Gynecol., *88:*45, 1964.
574. Stienstra, R., Jonker, T.A., Bourdrez, P., *et al.*: Ropivacaine 0.25% versus bupivacaine 0.25% for continuous epidural analgesia in labour: A double-blind comparison. Anesth. Analg., *80:*285, 1995.
575. Sutherland, J., Seaton, H., and Lowry, C.: The influence of epidural pethidine on shivering during lower-segment caesarean section under epidural anaesthesia. Anaesth. Intensive Care, *19:*228, 1991.
576. Swayze, C.R., Skerman, J.H., Walker, E.B., and Sholte, F.G.: Efficacy of subarachnoid meperidine for labor analgesia. Reg. Anesth., *16:*309, 1991.
577. Taylor, H.J.C.: Clinical experience with continuous epidural infusion of bupivacaine at 6 ml per hour in obstetrics. Can. Anaesth. Soc. J., *30:* 277, 1983.
578. Taylor, J.C., and Tunstall, M.E.: Dosage of phenylephrine in spinal anesthesia for caesarean section. Anaesthesia, *46:*314, 1991.
579. Teramo, K.: Effects of obstetrical paracervical blockade on the fetus. Acta. Obstet. Gynecol. Scand.,*50:* (Suppl.):16, 1971.
580. Teramo, K., Benowitz, M., Heymann, M.A., and Rudolph, A.M.: Gestational differences in lidocaine toxicity in the fetal lamb. Anesthesiology., *44:*133, 1976.
581. Teramo, K., and Widholm, O.: Studies of the effect of anesthetics on the fetus. Part I: The effect of paracervical block with mepivacaine upon foetal acid-base values. Acta. Obstet. Gynecol. Scand. (Suppl.), *46:*1, 1967.
582. Thalme, B., Belfrage, P., and Raabe, N.: Lumbar epidural analgesia in labour. I: Acid-base balance and clinical condition of mother, fetus and newborn child. Acta. Obstet. Gynecol. Scand., *53:*27, 1974.
583. Thomas, T.H., Fletcher, J.E., and Hill, R.G.: Influence of medication, pain and progress in labour on plasma beta-endorphin-like immunoreactivity. Br. J. Anaesth., *54:*401, 1982.
584. Thomson, K.J., and Cohen, N.E.: Vital capacity observations in normal pregnant women. Surg. Gynecol. Obstet., *66:*591, 1938.
585. Thorburn, J., and Moir, D.D.: Epidural analgesia for elective caesarean section-technique and its assessment. Anaesthesia, *35:*3, 1980.
586. Thorburn, J., and Moir, D.D.: Extradural analgesia: The influence of volume and concentration of bupivacaine on the mode of delivery, analgesic efficacy, and motor block. Br. J. Anaesth., *53:*933, 1981.
587. Thorp, J.A., Eckert, L.O., Ang, M.S., *et al.*: Epidural analgesia and cesarean section for dystocia: risk factors in nulliparas. Am. J. Perinatol., *8:*402, 1991.
588. Thorp, J.A., Hu, D.H., Albin, R.M., *et al.*: The effect of intrapartum epidural analgesia on nulliparous labor: A randomized, controlled, prospective trial. Am. J. Obstet. Gynecol., *169:*851, 1993.
589. Thorp, J.A., Parisi, V.M., Boylan, P.C., and Johnston, D.A.: The effect of epidural analgesia on cesarean section for dystocia in nulliparous women. Am. J. Obstet. Gynecol., *161:*670, 1989.
590. Tomson, G., Garle, R.I.M., Thalme, B., *et al.*: Maternal kinetics and transplacental passage of pethidine during labour. Br. J. Clin. Pharmacol., *13:*653, 1982.
591. Tucker, G.T.: Plasma-binding and disposition of local anesthetics. Int. Anesthesiol. Clin., *13:*33, 1975.
592. Tucker, G.T., Boyes, R.N., Bridenbaugh, P.O., and Moore, D.C.: Binding of anilide-type local anesthetics in human plasma II: Implications in vivo with special reference to transplacental distribution. Anesthesiology, *33:*304, 1970.
593. Tuvemo, T., and Willdeck-Lund, G.: Smooth muscle effects of lidocaine, prilocaine, bupivacaine and etidocaine on the human umbilical artery. Acta Anaesthesiol. Scand., *26:*104, 1982.
594. Tyack, A.J., Parsons, R.J., Millar, D.R., and Nicholas, A.D.: Uterine activity and plasma bupivacaine levels after caudal epidural analgesia. J. Obstet. Gynaecol. Br. Commonw., *80:*896, 1973.
595. Ueland, K., Gills, R., and Hansen, J.M.: Maternal cardiovascular dynamics. I: Cesarean section under subarachnoid block anesthesia. Am. J. Obstet. Gynecol., *100:*42, 1968.
596. Uppington, J.: Epidural analgesia and previous caesarean section. Anaesthesia, *38:*336, 1983.
597. Usubiaga, J.E., Reis, A., and Usubiaga, L.E.: Epidural misplacement of catheters and mechanisms of unilateral blockade. Anesthesiology, *32:*158, 1970.
598. Van den Berg, B.J., Levinson, G., Shnider, S.M., *et al.*: Evaluation of long-term effects of obstetric medication on clinical development. (Abstract). Society for Obstetric Anesthesia and Perinatology Annual Meeting, 1980.
599. Vanderick, G., Geerinckx, K., Van Steenberge, A.L., and De Muylder, E.: Bupivacaine 0.125% in epidural block analgesia during childbirth: Clinical evaluation. Br. J. Anaesth., *46:*338, 1974.
600. Van Steenberge, A., Debroux, H.C., and Noorduin, H.: Extradural bupivacaine with sufentanil for vaginal delivery: A double-blind trial. Br. J. Anaesth., *59:*1518, 1987.
601. Van Zundert, A., and Ostheimer, G.W., (eds.): *In* Pain Relief and Anesthesia in Obstetrics. New York, Churchill Livingstone, 1996.
602. Van Zundert, A., Vaes, L., Soetens, M., *et al.*: Are breech deliveries an indication for lumbar epidural analgesia? Anesth. Analg., *72:*399, 1991.
603. Vartikar, J.V., Johnson, M.D., and Datta, S.: Precordial doppler monitoring and pulse oximetry during cesarean delivery: Detection of venous air embolism. Reg. Anesth., *14:*145, 1989.
604. Vasicka, A., Robertazzi, R., Raji, M., *et al.*: Fetal bradycardia after paracervical block. Obstet. Gynecol., *38:*500, 1971.
605. Vaughan, R.S., Rees, G.A.D., and Williams, G.L.: An unusual case of Mendelson's syndrome. Br. J. Anaesth., *52:*459, 1980.

606. Vegfors, M., Cederholm, I., Gupta, A., *et al.*: Spinal or epidural anaesthesia for elective caesarean section? Int. J. Obstet. Anesth., *1:*141, 1992.
607. Vella, L.M., Willatts, D.G., Knott, C., *et al.*: Epidural fentanyl in labour: An evaluation of the systemic contribution to analgesia. Anaesthesia, *40:*741, 1985.
608. Vertommen, J.D., Vandermeulen, E., Van Aken, H., *et al.*: The effects of the addition of sufentanil to 0.125% bupivacaine on the quality of analgesia during labor and on the incidence of instrumental deliveries. Anesthesiology, *74:*809, 1991.
609. Viscomi, C., and Eisenach, J.C.: Patient-controlled epidural analgesia during labour. Obstet. Gynecol., *77:*348, 1991.
610. Vucevic, M., and Russell, I.F.: Spinal anaesthesia for caesarean section: 0.125% plain bupivacaine 12 ml compared with 0.5% plain bupivacaine 3 ml. Br. J. Anaesth., *68:*590, 1992.
611. Walmsley, A.J., Giesecke, A.H., and Lipton, J.M.: Contribution of extradural temperature to shivering during epidural anaesthesia. Br. J. Anaesth., *58:*1130, 1988.
612. Warwick, R., and Williams, P.L. (eds.): Dorsal rami of the spinal nerves. *In* Gray's Anatomy. 35th ed. pp. 1032 Norwich, Longman, 1973.
613. Waters, H.R., Rosen, N., and Perkins, D.H.: Extradural blockade with bupivacaine. Anaesthesia, *25:*184, 1970.
614. Weaver, J.B., Pearson, J.F., and Rosen, M.: The effect of posture and epidural block upon limb blood flow and radial artery pressure in term pregnant women. Br. J. Obstet. Gynaecol., *82:*844, 1975.
615. Weaver, J.B., Pearson, J.F., and Rosen, M.: Response to a Valsalva manoeuvre before and after epidural block. Anaesthesia, *32:*148, 1977.
616. Weeks, A.R., Cheridjian, V.E., and Mwanje, D.K.: Lumbar epidural analgesia in labour in twin pregnancy. Br. Med. J., *2:*730, 1977.
617. Weis, F.R., Markello, R., Mo, B., and Bochiechio, P.: Cardiovascular effects of oxytocin. Obstet. Gynecol., *46:*211, 1975.
618. Weiss, R.R., Halevy, S., Almonte, K.O., *et al.*: Comparison of lidocaine and 2 chloroprocaine in paracervical block: Clinical effects and drug concentration in mother and child. Anesth. Analg., *62:*168, 1983.
619. Wennberg, E., Frid, I., Haljamäe, H., and Norén, H.: Colloid (3% dextran 70) with or without ephedrine infusion for cardiovascular stability during extradural caesarean section. Br. J. Anaesth., *69:*13, 1992.
620. Westbrook, J.L., Donald, F., and Carrie, L.E.S.: An evaluation of a combined spinal/epidural needle set utilising a 26-gauge, pencil-point spinal needle for caesarean section. Anaesthesia, *47:*990, 1992.
621. White, P.F.: Mishaps with patient-controlled analgesia. Anesthesiology, *66:*81, 1987.
622. Willdeck-Lund, G., Lindmark, G., and Nilsson, B.A.: Effect of segmental epidural analgesia upon the uterine activity with special reference to the use of different local anaesthetic agents. Acta. Anaesthesiol. Scand., *23:*519, 1979.
623. Williams, J.S., Tong, C., and Eisenach, J.C.: Neostigmine counteracts spinal clonidine-induced hypotension in sheep. Anesthesiology, *78:* 301, 1993.
624. Wilson, C.M., Moore, J., Ghaly, R.G., *et al.*: Plasma concentrations of bupivacaine during extradural anaesthesia for caesarean section. Anaesthesia, *43:*12, 1988.
625. Wollman, S.B., and Marx, G.F.: Acute hydration for prevention of hypotension of spinal anesthesia in parturients. Anesthesiology, *29:*374, 1968.
626. Woodward, G.: Intraoperative blood loss in midtrimester dilatation and extraction. Obstet. Gynecol., *62:*69, 1983.
627. Workhoven, M.N.: Intravenous fluid temperature, shivering, and the parturient. Anesth. Analg., *65:*496, 1986.
628. Wright, P.M.C., Allen, R.W., Moore, J., and Donnelly, J.P.: Gastric emptying during lumbar extradural analgesia in labour: Effect of fentanyl supplementation. Br. J. Anaesth., *68:*248, 1992.
629. Wright, P.M.C., Iftikhar, M., Fitzpatrick, K.T., *et al.*: Vasopressor therapy for hypotension during epidural anesthesia for cesarean section: Effects on maternal and fetal flow velocity ratios. Anesth. Analg., *75:*56, 1992.
630. Wright, R.G., Shnider, S.M., Levinson, G., *et al.*: The effect of maternal administration of ephedrine on fetal heart rate and variability. Obstet. Gynecol., *57:*734, 1981.
631. Writer, W.D., Ahlen, K., Hedlund, C., and Heeroma, K.: Ropivacaine compared to bupivacaine for epidural labour analgesia: A prospective meta-analysis. (Abstract) ISRA Congress, Auckland, 1996.
632. Writer, W.D.R., Dewan, D.M., and James, F.M. III.: Three percent 2-chloroprocaine for cesarean section: Appraisal of a standardised dose technique. Can. Anaesth. Soc. J., *31:*559, 1984.
633. Writer, W.D.R., James, F.M. III, and Scott-Wheeler, A.: Double-blind comparison of morphine and bupivacaine for continuous epidural analgesia in labor. Anesthesiology., *45:*215, 1981.
634. Yau, G., Gregory, M.A., Gin, T., and Oh, T.E.: Obstetric epidural analgesia with mixtures of bupivacaine, adrenaline, and fentanyl. Anaesthesia, *45:*1020, 1990.
635. Ying, Y.-K., and Tejani, N.A.: Angina pectoris as a complication of ritodrine hydrochloride therapy in premature labor. Obstet. Gynecol., *60:*385, 1982.
636. Zador, G., Lindmark, G., and Nilsson, B.A.: Pudendal block in normal vaginal deliveries: Clinical efficacy, lidocaine concentrations in maternal and fetal blood, fetal and maternal acid-base values and influence of uterine activity. Acta. Obstet. Gynecol. Scand. (Suppl.), *34:* 51, 1974.
637. Zador, G., and Nilsson, B.A.: Low-dose intermittent epidural anaesthesia in labour: Influence on labour and fetal acid-base status. Acta. Obstet. Gynecol. Scand. (Suppl.), *34:*17, 1974.
638. Zakowski, M.I., Ramanathan, S., Baratta, J.B., *et al.*: Electrocardiographic changes during cesarean section: A cause for concern? Anesth. Analg., *76:*162, 1993.
639. Zellavos, H., Shah, Y., and Moody, L.: Outpatient laparoscopy with local anesthesia. Int. J. Gynaecol. Obstet., *17:*379, 1980.
640. Zivny, J., Kobilkova, J., Vorlicek, F., *et al.*: Plasma β-endorphin-like immunoreactivity during pregnancy, parturition, puerperium and in newborn. Acta. Obstet. Gynecol. Scand., *65:*129, 1986.

Neural Blockade in Clinical Anesthesia and Management of Pain, Third Edition,
edited by M.J. Cousins and P.O. Bridenbaugh.
Lippincott–Raven Publishers, Philadelphia © 1998.

CHAPTER 19

Neural Blockade for Outpatients

Michael F. Mulroy and L. Donald Bridenbaugh

Regional anesthesia techniques for surgical patients have grown in popularity because they provide dramatic improvements in postoperative pain relief and hospital discharge times. These advantages help reduce costs and maximize use of hospital resources. As a major component of hospital cost reduction, outpatient surgery has grown to the point where it now accounts for approximately 55% of all surgical procedures performed in the United States. Use of regional anesthesia in the outpatient setting can also increase efficiency and cost effectiveness, improve recovery, provide post-operative analgesia, and shorten time to discharge.[15]

The advantages of avoiding general anesthesia have been recognized since the advent of outpatient surgery. The first reports of ambulatory surgery involved hernia repairs done under local infiltration in a surgeon's office.[56] Local infiltration has been used extensively in physicians' offices, especially by plastic surgeons and dentists. The more complex techniques of spinal, epidural, and peripheral nerve block anesthesia, are also advantageous in outpatient surgery units.

ADVANTAGES OF REGIONAL ANESTHESIA

1. *Avoiding Emesis.* Reviews of ambulatory surgery experience consistently identify nausea and vomiting as "the big little problem,"[27] the most frequent anesthesia-related cause of delay in discharge,[21,35,57] and in unplanned admission, which ranges from 0.5 to 2% in published series.[20] It is also a primary source of patient dissatisfaction in ambulatory surgery recovery.[39] Nausea is most frequently associated with use of general anesthesia and is generally conceded to occur in 20 to 30% of patients.[55] Narcotic use may be associated with an incidence of vomiting as high as 40%.[9,19] Although this can be reduced by the use of antiemetics, these drugs can prolong recovery by producing somnolence, and can also lead to other delayed side effects, such as dysphoria, after discharge.[34] Although the intravenous agent propofol results in significantly less nausea and vomiting than inhalation agents, the incidence is still as high as 15% to 24%.[16,52] Desflurane offers no improvement over previous inhalation anesthetics, with an incidence of 40 to 50% emesis.[19,31] The incidence of emesis is clearly lower after regional anesthesia techniques, especially if excessive narcotic premedication is avoided. If nausea does occur with the hypotension associated with a central neuraxial block, it is usually short-lived, easily remedied, and does not prolong discharge times.
2. *Relieving Pain.* Postoperative pain is usually the second major cause of unplanned admission after outpatient surgery. General anesthetic agents, especially those chosen for rapid emergence, do not provide residual analgesia unless narcotics are added. Long-acting local anesthetics (such as bupivacaine), used for upper or lower extremity blocks, can produce 4 to 24 hours of analgesia, which will allow the patient to travel home in comfort.[14] This period of analgesia provides a more positive experience and reduces the use of oral narcotic analgesics, which are also associated with nausea that delays discharge. Infiltration of the wound after hernia repair,[45] or other major abdominal surgery, can also reduce postoperative pain and reliance on narcotics. This technique is underutilized, and deserves more encouragement by the anesthesiologist and surgeon in the outpatient setting.
3. *Reduced Nursing Care.* With fewer side effects of general anesthesia (especially emesis and pain), and with a higher degree of mental alertness on admission, the regional anesthesia patient easily represents a reduced nursing burden in the postanesthesia care unit (PACU). In fact, patients with minor peripheral nerve blocks in many institutions bypass the first-stage recovery areas and are transferred directly to step-down units.
4. *Shortening Discharge Time.* With side effects mini-

M.F. Mulroy and L.D. Bridenbaugh: Department of Anesthesiology, Virginia Mason Medical Center, Seattle, Washington 98111.

mized, recovery time can be reduced. The time to discharge and the total cost of recovery have been shown to be shorter with regional techniques, compared to general anesthesia, especially when nausea is associated with the general anesthetic.[15] Patel reported that peripheral nerve block of the leg, with either of 2 techniques, was superior to general anesthesia in providing rapid discharge after arthroscopy.[40] Randel reported that epidural anesthesia also provided more rapid discharge than did either general or spinal anesthesia for arthroscopy.[43] Patients with epidural blockade could eat and ambulate faster, and thus were ready to leave the unit sooner.

The ideal demonstration of alertness, post-operative analgesia, and rapid discharge, occurs with the use of axillary block for hand surgery. Allen showed that patients receiving axillary blocks were discharged an hour sooner than similar patients undergoing the same operation with propofol-nitrous oxide general anesthesia, given by mask.[1] The arm block patients required no supplemental analgesics and less nursing care. Retrospective reviews of large series of patients have shown the advantages of rapid discharge with interscalene block for shoulder surgery,[8,13] as well as axillary block for hand surgery.[14]

The more rapid return of alertness after regional anesthesia is intuitively comprehensible, if heavy sedation is avoided. Peripheral nerve blocks allow for almost immediate discharge from the ambulatory unit, but spinal or epidural blockade may delay discharge until motor function has returned in the lower extremity. Several studies have shown discharge times in the area of 2 hours following chloroprocaine, or 3 hours following lidocaine block,[38] which compare favorably to the 120 to 200 minute delays seen with isoflurane or desflurane,[19] or even the 120 minutes required for "street fitness" after propofol.[17] Although these newer general anesthetic agents have been shown to produce significantly more rapid early recovery than the previous outpatient general anesthetics, return of full mental alertness is still delayed, often because of the need to use analgesic or antiemetic drugs in the recovery period.[58]

The appropriate application of regional techniques requires changes in the selection of techniques and shorter-duration local anesthetic drugs. These modifications will be discussed in this chapter. The actual block techniques and pharmacological characteristics of the drugs have been described in detail elsewhere.

PATIENT SELECTION

Although patients considered eligible for outpatient surgery are usually suitable candidates for almost any type of anesthesia, the use of a neural blockade technique requires more informed patient acceptance, cooperation, and understanding than is needed for a general anesthetic. An extremely apprehensive patient is likely to need larger doses of sedation, which can negate the relative advantage of a block technique. Cooperation and understanding are necessary especially if an operation is to be performed solely under local anesthesia. Patients must be willing to undergo surgery while awake, and submit to the relative discomfort of infiltration of the local anesthetic, with a pure local anesthetic technique, but with this, patients can obtain the advantages described above, and avoid the greater risks of general anesthesia.

Most outpatients will be of physical status ASA I or II (American Society of Anesthesiology patients classifications), but may also be the poor-risk patient (ASA physical status III or IV). More poor-risk patients are being treated in the outpatient setting in recent years, to avoid complications of hospitalization. The rapid return to normal status in this situation is ideal for many patients with lung disease, diabetes, etc. If the medical condition is stable and the surgical procedure does not change the medical problems that the patient was managing at home before surgery, then certainly he or she can continue to be managed at home after the surgery and recovery from anesthesia.

Small children cannot be expected to cooperate as adults do, and should not be treated under local or regional anesthesia without appropriate supplemental sedation. The age at which children can tolerate local anesthesia will vary individually, and with the ability of the physician to gain the child's confidence. Regional techniques can provide excellent pain relief for infants and children, and their use should be encouraged whenever possible.

Some patients with anatomic abnormalities, or who are very obese, may present technical difficulties in performing the blocks. Discretion is the better part of valor. The additional time required may negate the advantages of regional techniques. For the grossly obese, a controlled general anesthetic with mechanical ventilation may be preferable to an extensive central neuraxial block with heavy sedation, which may further impair ventilation.

Many physicians using local anesthesia in their offices or emergency centers frequently ignore the need for patients to remain NPO after midnight or the necessity for an appropriate and current history, physical examination, and laboratory studies. This, again, is not to be condoned. Surgical or anesthetic complications can and do occur in simple procedures under local or regional anesthesia. Individuals practicing on an outpatient basis must be prepared to treat and legally to defend any complication (see Chapter 21).

SURGEON AND ANESTHESIOLOGIST

Skill and patience are the primary requirements for physicians involved in procedures to be performed on outpatients receiving regional anesthesia. The surgeon must be supportive of regional techniques, both in preoperative discussion with the patient and during intraoperative management of the procedure. The surgeon must occasionally be willing to wait a few minutes for the block to become effective; he or she must conduct the surgery gently, realizing that the patient may perceive pressure as pain. Surgeons who are convinced of the advantages of regional anesthesia techniques in providing greater alertness, less nausea, and earlier recovery for their patients are willing to tolerate occasional inconveniences and may even suggest regional anesthesia to their patients.

The anesthesiologist must also demonstrate skill and patience. Skill can be acquired and maintained only if the anesthesiologist is sufficiently interested in regional blocks to undergo a period of training that involves considerable practice. Even for an expert, a successful block will not be obtained in all cases, and the beginner must certainly expect a number of failures. It is helpful to acquire the needed experience by performing regional blocks as supplementary analgesia in patients for whom general anesthesia is part of the anesthetic routine. The anatomy of landmarks can be learned from a textbook, but experience can be gained only by repeated administration. It is well accepted that multiple attempts, and some failures, must be endured with the attempt to master any technical skill. It has been shown that the learning curves for central neuraxial blocks in residency training are similar to the process of gaining proficiency in endotracheal intubation in residency.[30] As subspecialists, we should devote the same patience and persistence to these beneficial techniques as we do to the necessary ones of airway management. Patience is mandatory, because a block may take as long as 30 minutes to perform and become completely effective. No surgery should be performed until the effect of the block has been tested.

SELECTION OF TECHNIQUE

The technique chosen must depend on the site of surgery and the anticipated duration of the procedure. For operations on the extremities, peripheral nerve blocks with intermediate- or long-duration local anesthetics will usually provide adequate duration of anesthesia, as well as residual analgesia for discharge home. Prolonged duration of neural blockade in this situation is usually an advantage, especially if opioid analgesics (and the possible nausea or vomiting) can be avoided in the PACU. Nevertheless, some patients are disturbed by prolonged numbness of an extremity, and the intermediate duration drugs may be preferable. For lower-extremity block, prolonged anesthesia may interfere with ambulation, and the relatively shorter duration and greater ease of performance of spinal or epidural anesthesia must be considered when considering a peripheral nerve block of the leg.

For central neuraxial blockade, the considerations are changed, since prolonged spinal or epidural anesthesia may delay discharge, due to failure to ambulate or urinate. For that reason, shorter-duration local anesthetics are preferable, with the use of local infiltration, when possible, as a supplement to provide prolonged analgesia. Another consideration is the potential for specific side-effects, such as pneumothorax with supraclavicular block, which may be undiagnosed in an outpatient. (see Chapters 10, 11, and 21).

PREMEDICATION AND SEDATION (SEE CHAPTER 6)

Most patients are more nervous than they will admit, and the attitude of medical personnel is of enormous psychological importance in relieving this anxiety. Some patients will benefit from a pharmacological sedative; however, this may lead to lack of cooperation, and the result is a patient who requires prolonged supervision and may be unfit to go home. Although rapport, gentleness, and skill in performing the block usually make premedication unnecessary, preoperative sedation for regional anesthesia may be appropriate.

Midazolam, 1 to 2 mg, may be given orally, intramuscularly, or (most frequently) intravenously. The amnestic effect of the benzodiazepines is an excellent asset to regional anesthesia, often ablating the recall of unpleasant needle insertions or paresthesias. The sedative-amnestic effect can limit its usefulness if the patient becomes confused and can no longer cooperate with the anesthesiologist who is performing a block technique. Heavy sedation can also prolong time to discharge, and, thus, moderate doses are recommended, usually not to exceed 5 mg in a healthy adult.[48] The duration of midazolam sedation generally is 30 minutes, but higher doses (as for conscious sedation) will prolong recovery. The availability of flumazenil is not a justification for excessive doses!

For uncomfortable procedures (which probably include all multiple needle insertions!), sedation and amnesia are not enough. Analgesia should be provided. The short-acting narcotic fentanyl, in 50 to 100 mcg doses, is ideal for outpatient use because it attenuates patient discomfort associated with the performance of the blocks or eliciting of a paresthesia, but does not limit patient cooperation. Again, excessive doses are to be avoided because of the risk of respiratory depression and the potential for increased nausea and vomiting.[48] Respiratory depression is increased when fentanyl is combined with midazolam in these circumstances.[4] Oxygen desaturation occurs frequently, and the use of supplemental oxygen during the performance of blocks and during surgery is advisable.[49] The short-acting analgesics alfentanil and remifentanil might be appealing, but their duration is too brief to be useful for performance of most blocks.

If further intraoperative sedation is needed, small quantities of intravenous midazolam or fentanyl may be titrated. A further alternative is the use of an intravenous propofol infusion in doses of 25 to 50 mcg/kg/min. At this infusion rate, sedation is provided with minimal hangover and recovery delay. Methohexital is another alternative which involves lower cost, but may require longer recovery and produce an unwanted excitement or "anti-analgesic" phase.[18]

As for monitoring, the ASA guidelines apply.[2] Pulse oximetry is an ideal monitor for patients receiving narcotic sedation, as it provides warning of respiratory depression and arterial oxygen desaturation. It also is an excellent pulse counter for detection of unintentional intravascular injection of local anesthetic, if epinephrine is added to the solution. Electrocardiogram (ECG) and blood pressure monitoring must be available, even for local infiltration cases. Ideally, all patients should have vital signs measured and recorded from the moment the block is started. For major regional techniques, the special risk is systemic toxic reaction to the local anesthetics, and close observation of the patient's mental status is the primary monitoring required, especially during the 30-minute interval following peripheral injection when the blood levels are continuing to rise. Because of the risk of toxicity, as well as the more common risk of respiratory depression from sedative medications, a dedicated observer trained in advanced life support must be available to monitor mental status, especially with local anesthesia and sedation provided by the surgeon. Mechanical monitors (such as ECG or oximetry) are not sufficient to detect rising blood levels of local anesthetic and impending toxicity. (see Chapter 6).

Since local infiltration of small doses of local anesthetics normally will not interfere with the physical or mental condition of a patient, under certain circumstances it may be permissible to observe only the following basic requirements:

1. A patient must never be left alone.
2. Regular verbal contact with the patient must be maintained to ensure consciousness and comfort.
3. Whether every patient receiving a nerve block should have an intravenous needle in place as well as oscilloscopic monitoring of the heart is a matter of physician judgement, and would depend on the amount of local anesthetic drugs, the site injected, technique, and the patient's physical status.
4. Pulse and blood pressure should be measured and recorded before starting the block, and then as clinically indicated.
5. Resuscitation equipment and knowledgeable, helpful, personnel must be available to treat a complication in the event that it does occur.

LOCAL ANESTHETIC DRUGS

In choosing the appropriate local anesthetic drug for outpatient nerve block anesthesia, duration of action is the primary consideration. Procaine and 2-chloroprocaine are the briefest in action, but chloroprocaine may be too short in duration. Procaine is adequate for local infiltration but diffuses through tissue poorly and is unreliable for major nerve block and peridural anesthesia. For subarachnoid anesthesia, procaine provides a duration of anesthesia even shorter than lidocaine. The dose required is usually 50% greater than the lidocaine requirement for a similar block level (Table 19-1). It is commercially available in a 10% solution, but should be diluted to a maximum concentration of 5%, to avoid potential neurotoxicity. It can be used as an isobaric solution when diluted with an equal volume of cerebrospinal fluid (CSF), or a hypobaric solution when diluted with sterile water. Mixing with 10% glucose will produce a hyperbaric solution.

TABLE 19-1. *Doses for spinal anesthesia*

	Lower extremity	Abdominal
Procaine	50–75 mg	75–100
Lidocaine	40–50	60–75
Bupivacaine	4–6	6–8

Lidocaine is the most commonly used drug for subarachnoid anesthesia of slightly longer duration. For hypobaric applications, the 2% commercial preparation can be diluted with an equal volume of sterile water. Forty mg is usually sufficient to produce perianal anesthesia, when the patient is in the jackknife position at injection. The 2% solution can be used alone as an isobaric preparation. Lidocaine is available in a premixed hyperbaric solution of 5% local anesthetic with 7.5% dextrose. This higher concentration has been associated with reports of transient radicular irritation, presenting as pain in the anterior thighs for 24 hours following subarachnoid injection at the L2 level.[46] Although this concentration of lidocaine has been used extensively in patients for many years, experimental study has suggested that it is toxic to amphibian nerves if applied directly under laboratory conditions.[5] Further study is needed to resolve this discrepancy between clinical experience and these data, but the current recommendation is that the 5% solution should be diluted with an equal volume of saline, or CSF, before injection.

The duration of lidocaine spinal anesthesia is dose dependent, and is prolonged by the addition of epinephrine. It produces an average duration of 90 minutes at the knee when used plain, or 120 minutes when epinephrine is added.[36] (Fig. 19-1) Epinephrine does prolong the time required for urination, and thus may delay discharge.[11] The use of 10 to 20 mcg of fentanyl as an adjuvant to lidocaine spinal anesthesia will produce prolonged pain relief similar to epinephrine, but without a delay in voiding.[32] (Table 19-2)

2-Chloroprocaine is not used for intravenous regional block because it may result in phlebitis.[25] Chloroprocaine is an excellent choice for both epidural analgesia and anesthesia because of its rapid onset and short duration in the outpatient setting. Previous problems of neurotoxicity after unintentional subarachnoid injection have been remedied by the removal of 0.2% sodium bisulfite as a preservative. The current formulation of 2-chloroprocaine, with ethylenediamintetra-acetic acid (EDTA) as a preservative, has been associated with a few reports of severe back pain, after the use of large volumes in healthy young outpatients. This complaint appears to be most frequently associated with volumes of greater than 30 cc. The use of smaller volumes is associated with no greater incidence of back pain than with lidocaine.[51] It appears prudent to limit 2-chloroprocaine to procedures of 60 minutes duration or less, or for use as a "top up" medication after a lidocaine epidural, when only a slightly longer period of analgesia is required.

The intermediate-acting amino-amide anesthetics lido-

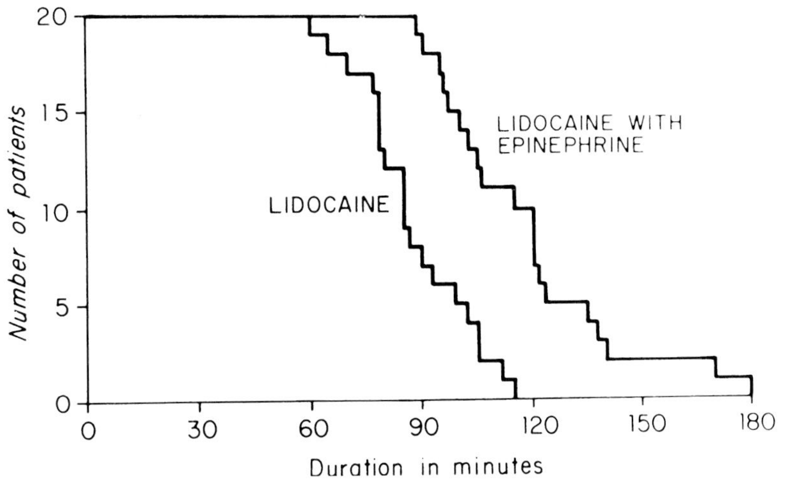

FIG. 19-1. Duration of lidocaine spinal anesthesia in the leg, with and without epinephrine. (Moore, D.C., Chadwick, H.S., and Ready, L.B.: Epinephrine Prolongs lidocaine spinal: Pain in the operative site most accurate method of determining local anesthetic duration. Anesthesiol. Clin., *20*:71, 1982, with permission.)

caine and mepivacaine appear to be safe and reliable for epidural anesthesia in the usual clinical doses and do not unduly prolong recovery, if epinephrine is not administered concomitantly. The risk of undesirable rapid systemic absorption must be considered when deleting the customary 1:200,000 concentration of epinephrine from local anesthetic solutions. For initiating epidural anesthesia, 2% lidocaine or 1.5% mepivacaine is useful, whereas lower concentrations are more appropriate for reinjection of epidural catheters or for peripheral nerve blockade. The duration of action of equivalent doses is somewhat longer with mepivacaine than with lidocaine. (Fig. 19-2)

The new local anesthetic cream, eutectic mixture of local anesthetics (EMLA), has been shown to be useful in providing subcutaneous analgesia in children, for the placement of intravenous catheters. It does not appear to be effective for other procedures such as lithotripsy, but may have some application in plastic surgery. (see Chapter 4).

Bupivacaine, tetracaine, ropivacaine and etidocaine generally have little use in outpatient surgery because of their long duration of action. They can be useful in providing prolonged postoperative analgesia, when used for wound infiltration or arm blocks. Their use without epinephrine for spinal anesthesia may be appropriate for an early morning case of anticipated long duration. Local anesthetic drugs are discussed in detail in Chapter 4. No matter which drug is chosen, one basic principle is imperative and is generally accepted: only the smallest volume of the local anesthetic drug in a solution of the lowest possible concentration that will give the desired effect should be used.

NEURAL BLOCKADE TECHNIQUES

The specific details and diagrams for performing the various nerve blocks are found in other chapters in this text and

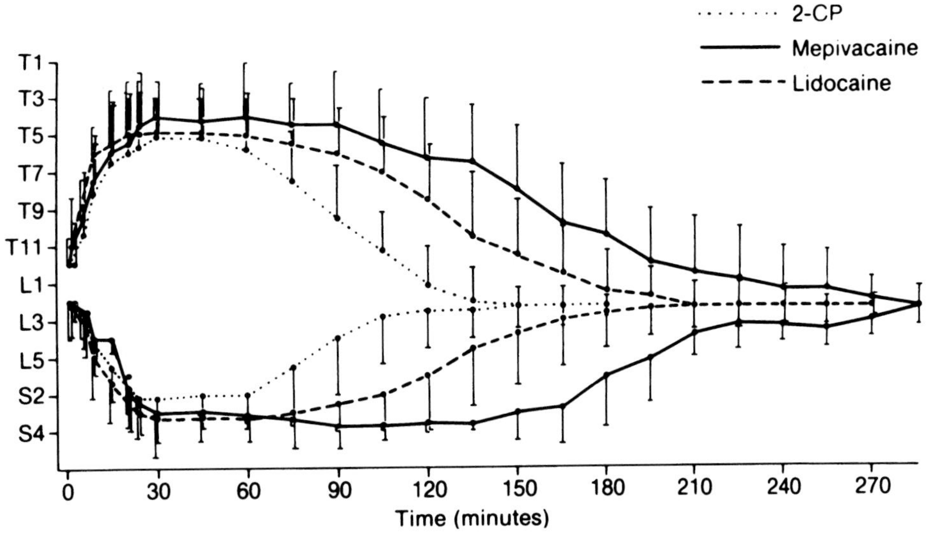

FIG. 19-2. Duration of epidural anesthesia with chloroprocaine, lidocaine, and mepivacaine, 20 cc volumes with epinephrine added. (From Kopacz, D. J., and Mulroy, M.F.: Chloroprocaine and lidocaine decrease hospital stay and admission rate after outpatient epidural anesthesia. Reg. Anesth., *15*:30, 1990, with permission.)

should be referred to by individuals unfamiliar with a certain technique.

Of the techniques suitable for outpatient application, *local infiltration* of the operative site is the safest and simplest. Intracutaneous and subcutaneous infiltration with a suitable dilute concentration of an intermediate-acting local anesthetic drug is sufficient for removal of superficial scars or lesions. An expansion of this technique is the "field block" by subcutaneous infiltration blocking of minor nerves that supply a particular area. This is most commonly used for hernia blocks, penile blocks for circumcisions, or breast blocks for excision of breast lumps. These procedures are usually performed by the surgeon and provide significant postoperative analgesia as well as satisfactory operative anesthesia, if careful infiltration of both deep and superficial layers is performed.[60] The addition of epinephrine to the local anesthetic solution can be helpful in obtaining hemostasis, as well as in reducing plasma levels of drug if a large volume or dose is required. Addition of epinephrine is contraindicated in procedures on the digits or penis.

Retrobulbar or peribulbar block for cataract surgery[59] is the ideal example of a peripheral nerve block that provides excellent surgical anesthesia, good post-operative pain relief, and, thus, rapid discharge from the hospital (see Chapter 17). In most institutions, these blocks are performed by surgeons, but anesthesiologists can perform them in an adjacent room and reduce turnover time in busy outpatient units. Although sedation often is needed for placement of the block, it is usually not needed intraoperatively, and these patients can leave the operating room in a wheelchair for the second-stage recovery unit and early discharge.

For the anesthesiologist, the simplest and most reliable anesthesia is the *intravenous regional technique* usually ascribed to August Bier (see Chapter 12). It is suitable for most superficial surgical procedures on extremities that take less than 90 minutes to perform (the limiting factor being tourniquet time). The major hazard of this technique is the accidental or premature release of the tourniquet, or inadequate tourniquet pressure, with resulting excessive blood levels of the local anesthetic drug. Close monitoring is essential, and 2-stage release of the tourniquet is required if tourniquet time is less than 40 minutes. It is recommended that the tourniquet pressure be at least 100 mm Hg above the patient's normal systolic pressure, if leakage of the local anesthetic drug under the tourniquet into the systemic circulation is to be prevented. The use of a wide blood pressure cuff as well as slow injection of the local anesthetic in a peripheral vein, following full exsanguination of the arm, has been shown to reduce the potential for leakage of local anesthetic under the cuff.[22] This technique is unsuitable when a tourniquet is contraindicated, for example, in amputations or vascular access procedures. It is useful for excision of neuromas, release of carpal tunnel compression, and other orthopedic and general procedures (see Chapter 12). This technique does not provide any residual analgesia, but does give full return of arm function before discharge.

If more intense local anesthesia of the upper extremity is required, regional block of the *brachial plexus* is favored. The plexus can be approached in the interscalene groove, as it crosses the first rib, or in the axilla (see Chapter 10). Each technique has its advantages and proponents. The supraclavicular approach is avoided by some in outpatients because of the small but disabling incidence of pneumothorax. Interscalene blockade is less likely to suffer this complication, and is useful for shoulder procedures.[8,13] The axillary approach provides good anesthesia to the forearm, as long as care is taken to block the musculocutaneous nerve by infiltration. The major hazard of these techniques is unintentional intravascular injection. A major advantage, however, is the provision of prolonged analgesia through the use of long-acting local anesthetics for the discharge home. The corollary of this is that the extremity must be padded carefully and the patient cautioned to protect it as long as the numbness persists. The details for performing these techniques are all described in Chapter 10.

Unilateral or bilateral *intercostal nerve blocks* are ideally suited for surgical procedures of the abdomen and chest wall (see Chapter 14). This procedure does involve a small risk of pneumothorax but does not limit ambulation or function and does not create the sympathetic blockade seen with central (peridural or spinal) blocks. Early ambulation and discharge make this a particularly effective choice for outpatients.

In the leg, any combination of *sciatic, femoral, lateral femoral cutaneous, and obturator* nerve blocks is possible for lengthy and involved procedures (see Chapter 11). These blocks are particularly appropriate anesthesia for fractures and dislocations of the ankle or distal leg, and especially for arthroscopy. Femoral nerve block interferes with ambulation by disrupting quadriceps muscle function, and may not be useful for routine arthroscopy. It is effective in providing analgesia for more painful procedures such as anterior cruciate ligament repair, and may allow earlier discharge as long as ambulation is assisted with crutches. A lateral femoral cutaneous nerve block frequently is the technique of choice for obtaining analgesia when a procedure is planned to take skin for minor skin grafts.

An excellent alternative is blockade of the sciatic nerve at the knee in the *popliteal fossa.*[44] By including blockade of the femoral nerve over the tibial head, total anesthesia of the lower leg below the knee can be obtained without loss of control of the extremity, although the patient will require crutches and generous padding of the foot to allow safe discharge.

Use of *ankle block* for surgery on the foot[33,47] is especially valuable for procedures on the sole of the foot, such as cuts, foreign bodies, and plantar warts, because this is a very sensitive area but tough and difficult to infiltrate locally. It also provides anesthesia for extensive foot surgery, such as bunionectomies. A midcalf tourniquet, if properly applied, is well tolerated by most patients for at least 30 minutes; this is helpful for most procedures on the foot.

TABLE 19-2. *Duration of 50 mg lidocaine spinal anesthesia*

Solution	Height of block	Duration (minutes ± SD)				
		2 Segment regression	T12 Surg anesth	Motor block	L1 regression	S2 regression
1.5% plain (isobaric)	T6 (T3–L2)	56 ± 5	20 ± 13	71 ± 8	104 ± 5	130 ± 18
1.5% dextrose (hyperbaric)	T3 (T7–L1)	39 ± 5	29 ± 10	30 ± 8	73 ± 10	99 ± 11
5% hyperbaric + epinephrine	T4	56 ± 11	45 ± 30	108 ± 30	96 ± 42	156 ± 43
5% with dextrose only	T3 (C8–T5)	50 ± 16	49 ± 30	88 ± 20	109 ± 6	150 ± 8
5% hyperbaric fentanyl 20 μg	T3	70	75 ± 32	89 ± 31	100 ± 31	157 ± 11

Adapted from data of Chiu, A., Liu, S., Carpenter, R.L., *et al.:* The effects of epinepherine on lidocaine spinal anesthesia: A crossover study. Anesth. Analg., *80:*735, 1995; and Halpern, S. and Preston, R.: Postdural puncture headache and spinal needle design: Meta-analyses. Anesthesiology, *81:*1376, 1994.

Spinal and epidural anesthesias are the simplest and most reliable of the regional techniques. They can delay ambulation and produce more physiologic side-effects. Nevertheless, they are useful in outpatients. Spinal (subarachnoid block), using 50 to 75 mg of lidocaine or 6 to 10 mg tetracaine without epinephrine, can provide from 30 to 90 minutes of rapid and dense anesthesia, with longer duration in the perineal area or leg Table 19-2. A major limitation of spinal anesthesia has been the incidence of post-lumbar puncture headache, which approaches 10% overall in inpatients but can be reduced to less than 1% by the use of a 25- or 27-gauge spinal needle and by restricting the technique to older patients. The use of even smaller needles increases the technical difficulty of the procedure, and does not appear to offer further advantages. The use of the rounded tip needles (Whitacre, Sprotte) has been shown to reduce the incidence of headache even further,[23] even in the younger patients, and has facilitated the use of spinal anesthesia in the outpatient setting. If a headache does occur, treatment with epidural blood patch on an outpatient basis is effective in remedying this complication without the need for a hospital admission.

In younger patients whose potential for headache is higher, or the patient who is reluctant to accept spinal blockade, *epidural* anesthesia is a suitable alternative. Both caudal and lumbar epidural anesthesia are more difficult technically and slightly less reliable than subarachnoid block, but have worked very successfully for perineal, lower-extremity orthopedic, and gynecologic procedures.[7] Epidural anesthesia is also very effective for lithotripsy operations, providing alertness and rapid discharge.[29] Another application of epidural anesthesia is in the repair of inguinal or femoral hernias.[45] The surgeon may delay the onset of postoperative pain by supplementing short-acting epidural anesthetic by wound infiltration with a long-acting local anesthetics drug, such as 0.25% bupivacaine. This technique is preferable to reliance on a hernia block, since the latter often includes femoral nerve anesthesia, which may be prolonged and limit ambulation. Patients who have adequate surgical anesthesia with a combination of epidural and local infiltration may be discharged comfortably to their homes, with a supply of oral NSAID± opioid to use when analgesia abates.

PEDIATRIC REGIONAL TECHNIQUES (SEE CHAPTER 20)

Regional techniques can also be applied to pediatric patients in the outpatient setting to provide the advantages of postoperative analgesia and rapid discharge, as in the adult. The major difference is that in a pediatric patient the block is usually performed during a general anesthetic because younger children generally do not tolerate local anesthetic injection while awake, or as the sole anesthetic for a procedure. The primary applications in this age group for outpatient surgery are aimed at providing pain relief in the healthy child being discharged home the same day. Several techniques have been described. The simplest application is local infiltration, as it is with adults. An alternative for a child is simply to irrigate the wound with local anesthetic; this appears to have efficacy equal to injection techniques for hernia surgery.[10]

Ilioinguinal nerve block is extremely simple, and useful after hernia repair or scrotal procedures. A 25-gauge needle is introduced into the abdominal wall 1 cm above and medial to the anterior superior iliac spine, and a volume of local anesthetic injected in a fan-wise direction to block the ilioinguinal nerve fibers traveling between the transverse and internal oblique abdominal muscles, and the iliohypogastric fibers running superficially to the muscles. A dose of 2 mg/kg of 0.25 to 0.5% bupivacaine is effective.[24]

Caudal block is also useful. The sacral hiatus is much more easily appreciated in children than in adults, and the cornua on either side can be seen and easily palpated. A small (23- to 25-gauge) needle can be easily introduced, with aseptic technique, through the skin and through the sacrococcygeal membrane, to enter the caudal canal. The needle is introduced first at about a 60° angle, and then lowered to a 20° angle, once it has gone through the membrane. The bevel should be introduced only a few millimeters, since the dural sac in children extends low in the caudal canal. Once absence of blood or CSF aspiration is confirmed, local anesthetic is injected. This block is usually performed with the infant asleep, and requires very little time in experienced hands. (see Chapters 9 and 20).

The dose of local anesthetic for children has been the subject of controversy, with several recommendations based on age or weight. A useful formula is that 0.5 ml/kg will usually produce adequate sacral and perineal analgesia. Twice that amount will block lower thoracic segments.[3] Bupivacaine in a 0.25% concentration (with epinephrine) provides reliable analgesia for 2 to 5 hours.[54] Lower concentrations will provide less motor block, but most pediatric anesthesiologists are comfortable with sending a child home with some lower extremity weakness, as long as the parents understand the need to support and protect the numb extremities. The total dose of local anesthetic should not exceed 3 mg/kg of bupivacaine or 5 mg/kg of lidocaine. The technique is useful for analgesia for hernia repair, curcumcision, hypospadius repair, and lower extremity surgery. (see Chapter 20).

Another alternative for penile operations is a *penile block.* There are 2 techniques advocated. The simplest is the subcutaneous ring block, injecting local anesthetic superficial to the fascia of the penile shaft at its base. Alternatively, 1 to 2 cc of local anesthetic can be injected deep to the fascia (Buck's fascia) on either side of the dorsal midline.[53] This will provide analgesia for procedures on the distal shaft, although the proximal shaft and the base of the penis are innervated by the genitofemoral and ilioinguinal nerves, which must be blocked by superficial infiltration. In either case, 0.25% bupivacaine provides excellent analgesia; epinephrine is never added to solutions in this area. (see Chapter 20).

This discussion has covered only some of the commonly used techniques of regional anesthesia in outpatient surgery. In addition, there are multitudes of specialized blocks, such as the supraorbital or infraorbital nerve blocks, scalp blocks for procedures on the face, ear, and tongue, which are difficult to anesthetize locally, and superficial cervical plexus blocks for head and neck procedures. (see Chapter 15). Many diagnostic and therapeutic nerve blocks for pain can be adapted for use in outpatients. The specific techniques for performing any of the individual nerve blocks are detailed in other sections of *Neural Blockade.* The use of regional anesthesia in outpatients is limited only by the imagination and ability of the anesthesiologists and the surgeons involved.

POSTOPERATIVE RECOVERY

Before discharge, the patient should recover sufficiently from anesthesia to approach his or her preoperative physical and mental status. This does not imply full recovery, particularly if a peripheral blockade technique has been used, because the block will in all likelihood still be effective. If the patient is properly instructed, however, he or she can usually be sent home during this period. The risk of a delayed toxic reaction decreases rapidly after 30 minutes and is not a consideration after 1 hour. Careful instruction must be given in order to avoid injury. In addition, patients must be provided with an appropriate sling or other protection for the numb extremity or anesthetized area. If a sympathetic block is included, elevation of the vasodilated extremity is especially useful.

Those who have received epidural or spinal block must have full recovery of motor function before discharge. If all sensory anesthesia has regressed, particularly with a full return of perineal sensation, then sympathetic blockade and orthostatic hypotension should not be a problem on ambulation.[42] Urinary retention is not a frequent problem, but can occur after axial blockade, especially in older males and in patients who have had operations with groin or perineal incisions. The frequency of retention is related to the duration of the local anesthetic agent,[6,45] and, thus, short-duration drugs should be chosen for axial blocks. With drugs such as lidocaine, the incidence of retention has even been reported as lower than with general anesthesia.[41] Although many outpatient units require voiding before discharge, this is often awkward and stressful for the young outpatient. The bladder can be assessed by physical examination or ultrasound, and simple catheter drainage performed if distention is present. Following this (or if no distention is present), most patients can be discharged home with instructions to return to the emergency room should problems develop later.[12]

Because most of the patients who have had regional block anesthesia have had minimal premedication or sedation, they spend a shorter time in the postoperative recovery unit than those who have had general anesthesia. Studies conducted in an ambulatory surgery unit comparing the recovery time and complications of general anesthesia and epidural anesthesia, when used for outpatient laparoscopies, demonstrated a significant advantage for this type of anesthesia.[37]

When the effects of the neural blockade wear off, the patient may need an analgesic, which should be prescribed as part of the postoperative care. It is well worth stressing that a very effective analgesic for operations on extremities is provided by elevation and immobilization. Routine oral narcotic analgesics are often associated with the onset of nausea in the PACU, and should be avoided if possible. If narcotics are demanded urgently by a patient in the immediate postoperative period, the possibility of a complication should be considered because minor surgical procedures normally will not be followed by severe pain. The use of alternative analgesics, such as nonsteroidal anti-inflammatory drugs like ketorolac, has been shown to reduce narcotic requirements without producing nausea or respiratory depression. Ketorolac has been effective in reducing narcotic requirements in the outpatient setting, and may be sufficient by itself to provide analgesia for minor surgical procedures. It is particularly effective in orthopedic and urologic procedures, although contraindicated in the presence of significant coagulopathy or renal disease. Doses of 30 mg intravenously (15 mg in elderly patients) will provide 6 hours of analgesia. Recent practice suggests that doses of 15 mg intramuscularly, with 10 mg in the elderly patient, are equally effective.

The use of local infiltration with local anesthetics is another excellent alternative. A field block or local infiltration of the wound at the termination of surgery can be accomplished with a long-acting local anesthetic drug, which will allow a fairly long postoperative period of analgesia while the patient is recovering. This is especially effective in pediatric patients. Instillation of bupivacaine into knee joints following arthroscopy will also reduce narcotic requirements.[50] The use of morphine in joints may be helpful in situations where inflammation is present,[28] but the reports of its effectiveness are inconclusive.[26]

In most institutions in which procedures are being performed on outpatients, patients are provided with a form that warns of possible sequelae, a brief instruction sheet on postoperative care, appointments with the responsible physician, and advice about food or drink. The form emphasizes the need for patients to be accompanied by a responsible adult, not only to and from the surgical center, but at home for the first 24 hours. Any other relevant information can also be given at that time, including warnings about possible complications and the availability of a 24-hour telephone contact. A similar instruction sheet is given to the patient on discharge from the outpatient facility.

SUMMARY

At present, about 55 to 60% of the surgical procedures in the United States either are being performed or could be performed on an outpatient basis. The principles of anesthetic management for outpatients are the same as those for inpatients, bearing in mind that most of the procedures will be short, the surgical procedure itself should not necessitate postoperative hospitalization, and the operating facilities may be limited—all making neural blockade an excellent anesthetic choice. The customary modifications that have been made for anesthetic management of the outpatient under neural blockade include (i) the selection of patients, surgeons, and anesthetists qualified and motivated toward nerve block anesthesia; (ii) written preoperative instructions and information to all patients because of the short period available for evaluation and rapport; (iii) little or no preanesthetic medication; (iv) use of regional block anesthetic techniques wherever possible, including infiltration of the wound with a long-acting local anesthetic drug to decrease the need for postoperative narcotics; (v) written postoperative instructions and a method for telephone or return follow-up on discharge; and (vi) no limitation as to the ASA physical status of the patients or the techniques of anesthesia. If the above considerations are followed, the use of neural blockade in outpatients will be a most satisfying experience.

REFERENCES

1. Allen, H.W., Mulroy, M.F., Fundis, K., and Carpenter, F.L.: Regional versus propofol general anesthesia for outpatient hand surgery. Anesthesiology, *79:*A1, 1993.
2. American Society of Anesthesiologists, House of Delegates: Standards for Basic Intra-operative Monitoring. Park Ridge (IL), ASA, October 21, 1986. amended October 13, 1993.
3. Armitage, E.N.: Regional anaesthesia in pediatrics. Clin. Anaesth., *3:* 553, 1985.
4. Bailey, P.L., Pace, N.L., Ashburn, M.A., *et al.*: Frequent hypoxemia and apnea after sedation with midazolam and fentanyl. Anesthesiology, *73:*826, 1990.
5. Bainton, C.R., and Strichartz, G.R.: Concentration dependence of lidocaine-induced irreversible conduction loss in frog nerve. Anesthesiology, *81:*657, 1994.
6. Bridenbaugh, L.D.: Catheterization after long- and short-acting local anesthetics for continuous caudal block for vaginal delivery. Anesthesiology, *46:*357, 1977.
7. Bridenbaugh, L.D., and Soderstrom, R.M.: Lumbar epidural block anesthesia for outpatient laparoscopy. J. Reprod. Med., *23:*85, 1979.
8. Brown, A.R., Weiss, R., Greenberg, C., Flatow, E.L., and Bigliani, L.U.: Interscalene block for shoulder arthroscopy: Comparison with general anesthesia. Arthroscopy, *9:*295, 1993.
9. Campbell, W.I.: Analgesic side effects and minor surgery: Which analgesic for minor day-case surgery? Br. J. Anaesth., *64:*617, 1990.
10. Casey, W., Rice, L.J., Hannallah, R.S., *et al.*: comparison between bupivacaine instillation versus ilioinguinal/iliohypogastric nerve block for postoperative analgesia following inguinal herniorrhaphy in children. Anesthesiology, *72:*637, 1990.
11. Chiu, A., Liu, S., Carpenter, R.L., *et al.*: The effects of epinephrine on lidocaine spinal anesthesia: A crossover study. Anesth. Analg., *80:*735, 1995.
12. Chung, F.: Are discharge criteria changing? J. Clin. Anesth., *5:*64S, 1993.
13. D'Alessio, J.G., Rosenblum, M., Shea, K.P., and Freitas, D.G.: A retrospective comparison of interscalene block and general anesthesia for ambulatory surgery shoulder arthroscopy. Reg. Anesth., *20:*62, 1995.
14. Davis, W.J., Lennon, R.L., and Wedel, D.J.: Brachial plexus anesthesia for outpatient surgical procedures on an upper extremity. Mayo Clin. Proc., *66*(5):470, 1991.
15. Dexter, F., and Tinker, J.H.: Analysis of strategies to decrease postanesthesia care unit costs. Anesthesiology, *82:*94, 1995.
16. Ding, Y., Fredman, B., and White, P.F.: Recovery following outpatient anesthesia: Use of enflurane versus propofol. J. Clin. Anesth., *5:*447, 1993.
17. Doze, V.A., Westphal, L.M., and White, P.F.: Comparison of propofol with methohexital for outpatient anesthesia. Anesth. Anag., *65:*1189, 1986.
18. Dundee, J.W.: Alterations in response to somatic pain associated with anaesthesia. II. The effect of thiopentone and pentobarbitone. Br. J. Anaesth., *32:*407, 1960.
19. Ghouri, A.F., Bodner, M., and White, P.F.: Recovery profile after desflurane-nitrous oxide versus isoflurane-nitrous oxide in outpatients. Anesthesiology, *74:*419–424, 1991.
20. Gold, B.S., Kitz, D.S., Lecky, J.H., and Neuhaus, J.M.: Unanticipated admission to the hospital following ambulatory surgery. J.A.M.A., *262:* 3008, 1989.
21. Green, G., and Jonsson, L.: Nausea: The most important factor determining length of stay after ambulatory anesthesia. A comparative study of isoflurane and/or propofol techniques. Acta Anaesthesiol. Scand., *37:*742, 1993.
22. Grice, S.C., Morell, R.C., Balestrieri, F.J., Stump, D.A., and Howard, G.: Intravenous regional anesthesia: Evaluation and prevention of leakage under the tourniquet. Anesthesiology, *65:*316, 1986.
23. Halpern, S., and Preston, R.: Postdural puncture headache and spinal needle design: Meta analyses. Anesthesiology, *81:*1376, 1994.
24. Hannallah, R.S., Broadman, L., Belman, A.B., Abramowitz, M.D., and Epstein, B.S.: Comparison of caudal and ilioinguinal/iliohypogastric nerve blocks for control of post-orchiopexy pain in pediatric ambulatory surgery. Anesthesiology, *66:*832, 1987.
25. Harris, W.H.: Choice of anesthetic agents for intravenous regional anesthesia. Acta Anaesthesiol. Scand., *36*(Suppl.): 47, 1969.
26. Heard, S.O., Edwards, W.T., Ferrari, D., *et al.*: Analgesic effect of intra-articular bupivacaine or morphine after arthroscopic knee surgery: A randomized, prospective, double-blind study. Anesth. Analg., *74:* 822, 1992.
27. Kapur, P.A.: Editorial: The big "little problem." Anesth. Analg., *73:* 243, 1991.
28. Khoury, G.F., Chen, A.C., Garland, D.E., and Stein C.: Intra-articular morphine, bupivacaine, and morphine/bupivacaine for pain control after knee videoarthroscopy. Anesthesiology, *77:*263, 1992.

29. Kopacz, D., and Mulroy, M.F.: Chloroprocaine and lidocaine decrease hospital stay and admission rate after outpatient epidural anesthesia. Reg. Anesth., *15:*30, 1990.
30. Kopacz, D.J., and Neal, J.M.: Learning regional anesthesia techniques: How many is enough? Reg. Anesth., *19:*37, 1994.
31. Lebenom, M.M.H., Pandit, S.K., Kothary, S.P., *et al.*: Desflurane vs. propofol anesthesia: A comparative analysis in outpatients. Anesth. Analg., *76:*936, 1993.
32. Liu, S.S., Chiu, A.A., Carpenter, R.L., *et al.*: Fentanyl prolongs lidocaine spinal anesthesia without prolonging recovery. Anesth. Analg., *80:*730, 1995.
33. McCutcheon, R.: Regional anesthesia of the foot. Can. Anaesth. Soc. J., *12:*465, 1965.
34. Melnick, B., Sawyer, R., and Krarmbelkar, D., *et al.*: Delayed side-effects of droperidol after ambulatory general anesthesia. Anesth. Analg., *69:*748, 1989.
35. Meridy, H.W.: Criteria for selection of ambulatory surgical patients and guidelines for anaesthetic management: A retrospective study of 1553 cases. Anesth. Analg., *61:*921, 1982.
36. Moore, D.C, Chadwick, H.S., and Ready, L.B.: Epinephrine prolongs lidocaine spinal: Pain in the operative site most accurate method of determining local anesthetic duration. Anesthesiology, *67:*416, 1987.
37. Mulroy, M.F., and Bridenbaugh, L.D.: Regional anesthetic techniques for outpatient surgery. Int. Anesthesiol. Clin., *20:*71, 1982.
38. Neal, J.M., Deck, J.J., Lewis, M.A., and Kopacz, D.J.: A double-blind comparison of epidural 2-chloroprocaine vs. lidocaine for outpatient knee arthroscopy. Anesthesiology, *79:*A12, 1993.
39. Orkin, F.: What do patients want? Preferences for immediate postoperative recovery. Anesth. Analg., *74:*S225, 1992.
40. Patel, N.J., Flashburg, M.H., Paskin, S., and Grossman, R.: Regional anesthetic technique compared to general anesthesia for outpatient knee arthroscopy. Anesth. Analg., *65:*185, 1986.
41. Petros, J.G., Rimm, E.B., Robillard, R.J., and Argy, O.: Factors influencing postoperative urinary retention in patients undergoing elective inguinal herniorrhaphy. Am. J. Surg., *161:*431, 1991.
42. Pflug, A.E., Aasheim, G.M., and Foster, O.: Sequence of return of neurological function and criteria for safe ambulation following subarachnoid block (spinal anaesthetic). Can. Anaesth. Soc. J., *25:*133, 1978.
43. Randel, G.I., Levy, L., Kothary, S.P., *et al.*: Epidural anesthesia is superior to spinal or general for outpatient knee arthroscopy. Anesthesiology, *71:*A769, 1989.
44. Rorie, D.K., Nelson, D.O., Sittipong, R., and Johnson, K.A.: Assessment of block of the sciatic nerve in the popliteal fossa. Anesth. Analg., *59:*37, 1980.
45. Ryan, J.A., Adye, B.A., Jolly, P.C., and Mulroy, M.F.: Outpatient inguinal herniorraphy with both regional and local anesthesia. Am. J. Surg., *148:*313, 1984.
46. Schneider, M., Ettlin, T., Kaufmann, M., *et al.*: Transient neurologic toxicity after hyperbaric subarachnoid anesthesia with 5% lidocaine. Anesth. Analg., *76:*1154, 1993.
47. Schurman, D.J.: Ankle block anesthesia for foot surgery. Anesthesiology, *44:*348, 1976.
48. Shafer, A., White, P.F., Urquhart, M.L., and Doze, V.A.: Outpatient premedication: Use of midazolam and opioid analgesics. Anesthesiology, *71:*495, 1989.
49. Smith, D.C., and Crul, J.F.: Oxygen desaturation following sedation for regional analgesia. Br. J. Anaesth., *62:*206, 1989.
50. Smith, I., Hemelrijck, J.V., White, P.F., and Shively, R.: Effects of local anesthesia on recovery after outpatient arthroscopy. Anesth. Analg., *73:*536–539, 1991.
51. Stevens, R.A., Urmey, W.F., Urquhart, B.L., and Kao, T.C.: Back pain after epidural anesthesia with chlorprocaine. Anesthesiology, *78:*492, 1993.
52. Van Hemelrijck, J., Smith, I., and White, P.F.: Use of desflurane for outpatient anesthesia—A comparison with propofol and nitrous oxide. Anesthesiology, *75:*197, 1991.
53. Vater, M., and Wandless, J.: Caudal or dorsal nerve block? A comparison of two local anesthetic techniques for post-operative analgesia following day-case circumcision. Acta Anaesthesiol. Scand., *29:*175, 1985.
54. Warner, M.A., Kunkel, S.E., Offord, K.O. Atchison, S.R., and Dawson, B.: The effects of age, epinephrine, and operative site on duration of caudal analgesia in pediatric patients. Anesth. Analg. *66:*995, 1987.
55. Watcha, M.F., and White, P.F.: Postoperative nausea and vomiting. Anesthesiology, *77:*162, 1992.
56. Waters, R.M.: The down-town anaesthesia clinic. Am. J. Surg., *33:*71, 1919.
57. White, P.F., and Shafer, A.: Nausea and vomiting: Causes and prophylaxis. Semin. Anesth., *6:*300, 1988.
58. White, P.F.: Studies of desflurane in outpatient anesthesia. Anesth. Analg., *75:*S47, 1992.
59. Wong, D.H.W.: Regional anaesthesia for intraocular surgery. Can. J. Anaesth. *40:*635, 1993.
60. Yndgaard, S., Holst, P., Bjerre-Jepsen, K., *et al.*: Subcutaneously versus subfascially administered lidocaine in pain treatment after inguinal herniotomy. Anesth. Analg., *79:*324, 1994.

Neural Blockade in Clinical Anesthesia and Management of Pain, Third Edition,
edited by M.J. Cousins and P.O. Bridenbaugh.
Lippincott–Raven Publishers, Philadelphia © 1998.

CHAPTER 20

Neural Blockade for Pediatric Surgery

Lynn M. Broadman and Linda Jo Rice

Neural blockade has been employed in pediatric patients since Bier's 1899 report of a spinal anesthetic in an 11-year-old.[19] At a time when open-drop chloroform was the technique of choice for general anesthesia, the introduction of spinal anesthesia effected a considerable reduction in morbidity and mortality in infants and children undergoing surgical procedures.[61] Eather noted in 1975 that regional anesthetic techniques were underutilized in pediatric patients for 3 major reasons: lack of experience, fear of adverse effects, and lack of patient co-operation.[50]

In the 1980s, many anesthesiologists rediscovered benefits of regional anesthesia in adult patients. Anesthesiologists who gained their skills in applying regional anesthesia to adult patients began to stretch that skill into the pediatric population. By the 1990s, increasing regional anesthesia expertise in adult patients, coupled with the appreciation that infants and children *do* suffer pain led to increased utilization of pediatric regional techniques.[7,42,69,127]

Most regional techniques employed in infants and children are placed following the induction of general anesthesia, with the goal of providing postoperative analgesia.[130] Lack of co-operation by pediatric patients will never be eliminated; however, improved sedation agents and the recognition that regional anesthesia, combined with a light general anesthetic is both safe and efficacious, allow more children to receive the benefit of this approach to balanced anesthesia.[142] Regional analgesia techniques are particularly useful for ambulatory surgery patients, in whom pain is a major reason for unanticipated hospital admission.[55]

L.M. Broadman: Departments of Anesthesiology and Pediatrics, West Virginia University School of Medicine, Morgantown, West Virginia 26506.

L.J. Rice: Department of Anesthesiology, All Children's Hospital, St. Petersburg, Florida 33704-4641.

GENERAL CONSIDERATIONS

Children vary in size, and aspects of their anatomy change as they grow. The dura and spinal cord reach lower levels in infants than in older patients (Table 20-1). In addition, the epidural space is shallower, and the epidural fat is looser and more areolar, so that spread of local anesthetics is more even and passage of catheters for continuous analgesia is easier. Ligaments and fasciae are thinner; it may be more difficult to feel fascial planes and aponeuroses with the needle tip, because of less resistance. In small children, the nerves are thinner, allowing easier diffusion of the local anesthetic solution and a more rapid onset of action. Myelination of nerves may also be incomplete. These factors allow adequate blockade to be achieved with lower concentrations of local anesthetic.

The adjunct intraoperative analgesia that regional blocks provide is of secondary benefit to most anesthesiologists and to most parents.[128] Benefits of combining regional techniques with a light general anesthetic include:

1. Faster awakening at the end of the case, as the adjunct intraoperative analgesia allows less of the volatile agent to be employed intraoperatively.
2. Suppression of undesirable autonomic reflexes, such as laryngospasm during circumcision and perianal procedures.
3. Limb immobilization in the immediate perioperative period following nerve or tendon graft.
4. Decreased "stress response" to surgery (see Chapter 5).

There are relatively few indications for use of a regional technique as a sole anesthetic in a pediatric patient. The situations where regional techniques with light or no sedation are useful include:

1. Premature infants who are at increased risk for postoperative apnea, and who require surgery below the umbilicus.

TABLE 20-1. *Anatomic differences of importance in spinal and epidural anesthesia in children and adults*

Anatomic variable	Neonate	Infant	Small child	Older child	Adult
Position of lower end of spinal cord	L3		L1 at 12 months		L1
Position of lower end of dural sac	S4		S2		S2
CSF/kg	4 ml	4 ml	3 ml	2 ml	2 ml
Condition of epidural fat	Loose	Loose	Loose	± Loose	Firmly packed

CSF, cerebrospinal fluid.

2. Children with neuromuscular disease who have reduced respiratory reserve. It is important for the family to understand that a regional anesthetic will not worsen the patient's underlying condition.
3. Children with chronic airway or pulmonary disease, such as tracheomalacia, asthma or cystic fibrosis.
4. Children at risk of malignant hyperthermia.
5. Older children who wish to remain awake. Many older children undergoing arthroscopic surgery are interested in their surgeries and want to watch the procedures.

The excellent postoperative pain relief afforded by regional techniques is of particular advantage in the ambulatory surgery patient, for whom narcosis, with its resulting drowsiness and possible nausea, may delay discharge. In the inpatient, continuous catheter techniques such as caudal, epidural or peripheral nerve infusions have been shown to provide effective, prolonged analgesia.[74,106] Blocks have been used for analgesia following cleft lip or palate repair or tonsillectomy.[24,86] Regional blocks are also useful for nonsurgical pain, such as cancer pain, sickle cell pain, pain of fractured femur, and reflex sympathetic dystrophies.[88,142,164,172] Finally, regional blockade may be useful in relieving vascular spasm or providing prolonged sympathectomy.[9,53,76]

Parental acceptance of regional anesthetic techniques in children is very high. Broadman reviewed 687 children who received blocks following sedation or induction of general anesthesia.[28] More than 10% were less than 1 year of age, while 60% were under the age of 6 years. Two hundred families were selected at random for phone interview from 3 to 9 months after the anesthetic; 90% of the parents would allow their child to have another regional anesthetic.

Dalens and Hasnaoui noted in a study of 750 children undergoing caudal block that conscious children tolerated surgery poorly from a psychological point of view, though they were free of pain.[41] Fourteen of the 46 patients who did not receive general anesthesia became restless and irritable within 30 minutes, while 6 additional children became restless by the end of the surgical procedure. At a time when we recognize that children benefit from sedation during minor procedures, we should not be surprised that children do not like to lie still and awake in a boring, uncomfortable, scary, place like an operating room.[136]

Regional blocks do, however, have limitations. These techniques require skill and practice in their performance, particularly on smaller infants. This skill may not be present in all practitioners. In addition, since these blocks are most often employed as an intraoperative adjunct to a light general anesthetic, performance of the block may benefit from an assistant who monitors the child while the anesthesiologist places the block. With increasing experience, and use of the laryngeal mask airway, this need for an assistant may decrease, although it is always easier to perform a block with skilled assistance available.

Contraindications for the use of regional techniques in children are similar to those in adults: lack of parental or (older) patient consent, presence of infection at the proposed site of injection, hypovolemia, coagulopathy, and inappropriate anatomy.

DOSAGE OF LOCAL ANESTHETICS IN CHILDREN

The recommendations for safe maximal dosage in children are scaled-down doses for weight based on maximum doses for the 70-kg male adult. The purpose of maximum recommended doses is to prevent the administration of excessive amounts of drug which could result in toxicity (see Chapter 4).[141] This definition is difficult in pediatric patients, for a number of reasons. Early signs of toxicity, such as confusion or dizziness, as well as late signs such as seizures, may be masked by general anesthesia. The blood levels at which toxic signs occur are not clearly defined in humans, and are defined for awake, adult, humans, when they are available (see Chapter 3).

Table 20-2 outlines the generally accepted doses per kilogram. It is important to realize that when the volume and concentration of local anesthetic needed for a block has been determined, the total mgs of drug should also be calculated. If the total mass of drug is too high, either the concentration or volume may be reduced. Further information regarding doses for continuous infusion of local anesthetic will be provided under each individual block described in this chapter.

In general, it is important to avoid motor blockade of the lower extremities in ambulatory patients. Motor blockade not only delays discharge, but also distresses young children, who may not like the "numb" feeling and may harm themselves trying to ambulate when they have poor control over their lower extremities.

TABLE 20-2. *Local anesthetic agents and doses in children*

Agent	Topical use: Concentration (%)	Topical use: Dose (mg/kg)[a]	Injection: Plain solution dose (mg/kg)	Injection: Dose with epinephrine (mg/kg)[a]
Bupivacaine			2.5–3	2.5–3
Lidocaine	2–10	3[b]	5	7–10
Mepivacaine		5	5	7
Prilocaine			5–7	7–9
			(Dose not to exceed 600 mg, single dose only)	
Etidocaine			3	3–4
Chloroprocaine and Procaine			7	10
Tetracaine (Amethocaine)	0.5–2	2	1.5	1.5
Cocaine	3–10	2		

[a] These doses are the same on a milligram per kilogram basis as in adults and are based on measurements of plasma levels after safe clinical use, compared to adult toxic plasma levels.

[b] This low dose is preferable below the age of 3 years, because plasma levels following topical use at this age are relatively higher than those for older children.

PLASMA CONCENTRATIONS AND TOXICITY (see Chapter 4)

Local anesthetic pharmacology has not been well evaluated in pediatric patients.[16] Because infants and children vary in their response to drugs, it would seem advisable to stay well within traditional maximum limits (Table 20-2). Reports of seizures following continuous infusions of local anesthetics in the caudal space point out that these drugs cannot be used with impunity.[3,15,113] In addition, local anesthetic/epinephrine toxicity is an increasing concern, especially in infants.[66,89,110,157]

Concomitant administration of volatile agents affects toxicity of local anesthetics.[56,62,79] Badgwell and co-workers, in a study of bupivacaine toxicity and the influence of volatile agents on plasma levels of bupivacaine in young pigs, found that younger animals had higher seizure and dysrhythmia thresholds than older animals, but that plasma levels of bupivacaine were also higher.[10] Heavner and colleagues also noted that hypercarbia and hypoxia enhance bupivacaine toxicity in young pigs, cautioning that vigilant attention to airway management is of paramount importance when placing a block in an infant.[81] Kyttä and colleagues employed a combination of lidocaine and bupivacaine in piglets, finding that the toxicity of the two local anesthetics is additive when used in combination.[98] The "test dose for intravascular injection" is unreliable in children undergoing volatile agent anesthesia (see following).

Children Are Not More Resistant to Local Anesthetic Toxicity Than Are Adults!

Plasma protein concentrations are quite low in the neonate, and plasma protein binding does not approach adult levels until after the first year of life, enabling more of the drug to remain active.[31] Neonates may manifest symptoms of neurologic toxicity at blood concentrations of lidocaine as low as 2.5 μg/ml, whereas toxicity in the adult is unlikely at a concentration less than 5 μg/ml. The younger the child is, the higher are the blood levels of other local anesthetics.[59,60] Using bupivacaine 3 mg/kg for single-dose caudal analgesia, Eyres et al. found peak blood concentrations of 1.5 μg/ml in the 1-year-old.[57] Ecoffey and colleagues, using lidocaine 5 mg/kg, observed maximum blood concentrations between 1.6 and 2.5 μg/ml, well below the adult toxic concentration of 5 μg/ml.[51]

The metabolism of local anesthetics is greatly reduced in the neonate, both because of decreased plasma pseudocholinesterase and decreased hepatic microsomal activity. Children eliminate drugs faster than newborns and infants, but more slowly than adults do. This slower rate of elimination requires particular attention to continuous infusions of local anesthetic.

The relatively larger cardiac output of pediatric patients is a factor in the rapid increase of local anesthetic blood levels, especially in the vessel-rich groups, such as the brain and heart. Physiologic differences between adult and pediatric patients balance such that local anesthetic uptake provides for peak blood levels about 20 minutes following injection (similar to adults), but there may be a shorter duration of anesthesia in children than in adults. Early central nervous system manifestations of toxicity may not be apparent or may be misinterpreted in awake infants and toddlers. The first signs of local anesthetic toxicity in a pediatric patient may be dysrhythmias or cardiovascular collapse.[66,110,157]

PROBLEMS WITH THE TEST DOSE

There is no effective test dose for intravascular injection in children undergoing general anesthesia with volatile agents. Desparmet and colleagues studied 65 children ranging in age from 1 month to 11 years.[48] Following induction of mask halothane/nitrous oxide anesthesia, with stable end-tidal halothane concentration of 1%, 20 children received *intravenous* injection of 10 μg/kg of atropine, followed 5 minutes later with lidocaine 0.1 mg/kg with 1:200,000 epinephrine (0.5 μg/kg), while 20 children received the same regimen without the atropine. Twelve children received atropine premedication followed by lidocaine 1% without epinephrine, while 12 received the intravenous lidocaine alone.

The children who received the intravenous epinephrine-containing solution without atropine premedication did not have consistent increases in heart rate. Although these workers noted that 94% of children receiving atropine premedication, followed by intravenous epinephrine, demonstrated a brief heart rate increase of greater than 10 beats per minute (peaking at 45 seconds and lasting to 60 seconds post-injection), it must be emphasized that this injection was performed with a stable end-tidal halothane concentration of 1%. Increases in heart rate of 10 beats per minute or greater may be noted following needle placement in children who are not so deeply anesthetized. Perillo and colleagues performed a similar study, comparing intravenous isoproterenol in doses of 0.05 μg/kg and 0.075 μg/kg.[124] As in the epinephrine study, increases in blood pressure were not consistent.

Brendel and others compared the doses of epinephrine and isoproterenol employed in the above studies, with intravenous lidocaine alone.[26] A blinded observer who watched the electrocardiogram (ECG) as the intravenous solution was injected failed to identify a significant percentage of the "mock test-doses." As in adults, it is important to administer the local anesthetic in incremental doses rather than to rely completely on a test dose.

There have been recent reports of cardiac events in infants weighing less than 10 kg who received caudal blocks. Two infants (4 and 8 kg) had episodes of ventricular tachycardia and brief cardiovascular collapse following attempted caudal blockade with bupivacaine-epinephrine solutions.[157] There were negative aspirations in both circumstances. The authors believed that the malignant cardiac rhythms were due to epinephrine toxicity, and that slow fractional administration of local anesthetic is important.

Freid and others also noted changes following unintentional intravascular injection of bupivacaine with epinephrine in infants, reporting 5 cases in which ST-T wave changes and relative *bradycardia,* during administration of a test dose, alerted the authors to possible intravascular injection.[66] In each instance, the caudal block was stopped, and the needle was removed and replaced, with successful blockade in 4 cases. Caudal blockade was abandoned after repeated ECG changes in the 5th case. The authors have observed these changes only in infants, but advocate electrocardiographic monitoring as superior to simple counting of the heart rate. Maxwell and colleagues employed phenytoin in successful treatment of a neonate with bupivacaine-induced cardiac toxicity.[110]

SPECIFIC BLOCKS AND THEIR USE IN CHILDREN

Any regional block technique described elsewhere in *Neural Blockade* can be employed in pediatric patients, provided the anesthesiologist bears in mind the anatomical, physiologic, pharmacologic, and psychologic differences related to the child's size and stage of development. Detailed descriptions of the techniques should be studied before proceeding with the block. The blocks described below will be discussed with particular reference to their use in children.

CAUDAL ANALGESIA (see Chapter 9)

Extensive clinical experience attests to the ease of performance, reliability, and safety of this popular pediatric block, especially in patients weighing over 10 kg.[41,159] However, this block is deceptively simple to perform, and one must have respect for the rare, but potentially serious, complications that can occur with any regional technique.[66,71,110]

"Single-dose" caudals are simple to perform and easily adaptable to modern anesthesia practice.[55] Although many pediatric surgical procedures are in the T10–S5 dermatomal distribution, caudal approach to the epidural space makes analgesia for higher dermatomes achievable at the expense of a larger dose of local anesthetic.[114]

Anatomy

As in adults, the infant's sacrum is a triangular bone formed by the fusion of five sacral vertebrae. The vertebral arches become completely ossified and unite with one another and with the vertebral bodies by the age of 8 years. The sacral hiatus, situated at the lower end of the sacrum, is the nonfusion of the 5th sacral vertebral arch. The large bony processes on either side are the sacral cornua, while the coccyx lies immediately caudad. The sacral hiatus is covered by the sacrococcygeal membrane (see Chapter 9, Fig. 9-1).

In most infants and prepubertal children, these landmarks are easily palpable. There is considerable variation in the anatomy of the sacral hiatus because of developmental defects of the sacral canal roof; this may account for the small percentage of caudal block failures in children less than 7 years of age and the larger percentage in older patients.[41]

As the sacral hiatus is relatively more cephalad in infants, the distance between the sacral hiatus and the end of the dural sac is relatively short (Table 20-1). As previously mentioned, the infant's epidural space offers less resistance to the cephalad spread of injected local anesthetics or to advancement of a caudal catheter, than does that of the adult.[23,73,125]

Single-Dose Caudal Block Placement

Following placement of the child in the lateral position, identify the hiatus by placing a finger in the depression between the sacral cornua, and rocking back and forth to identify the cephalad bony edge of the fused arch of S4.

Following careful skin preparation, asepsis must be maintained by wearing sterile gloves or by palpating the skin through a sterile alcohol swab. Once the caudal space is entered using a short (2.5 cm), 23-gauge needle attached to a syringe containing the appropriate volume of local anesthetic solution, the technique is the same as in adults (see Chapter 9, Fig. 9-6). The needle must be placed exactly in the midline at a 60° angle to the coronal plane, perpendicular to all other planes. The bevel of the needle should be directed ventrally to minimize the chance of piercing the anterior sacral structures. The needle is advanced, and a distinct "pop" is felt as the sacrococcygeal membrane is pierced. The needle may then be lowered to an angle of 20° and advanced an additional 2 to 3 mm, to make sure that the entire bevel surface is in the caudal space. Further advancement of the needle will increase the chances of dural puncture. Use of a short intravenous extension tube or butterfly needle to decrease the chance of needle advancement, with pressure on the syringe plunger, may be useful.

After attempted aspiration demonstrates the absence of blood or CSF, the appropriate amount of local anesthetic is injected in small increments. If the surgical procedure is to be performed in the prone position, the caudal block may be placed after the child has been positioned for surgery. A roll under the hips is useful for block placement in this position.

If blood is noted on aspiration, the needle should be removed completely and the anatomy reidentified. Because the distance between the sacrococcygeal ligament and the anterior table of the sacrum is very small in infants, attempted redirection of the needle, or simple withdrawal until there is no more blood aspirated, may leave the tip of the needle subcutaneous or intraosseous. Even after needle replacement, the local anesthetic should be injected in small aliquots with careful monitoring for signs of systemic toxicity. If a dural puncture is noted (a rare event), it would be prudent to abandon attempts at caudal blockade, because of the risk of total spinal block; an alternate regional technique[47] should be selected.

Meticulous attention to the child is vital, during performance of this block, particularly if endotracheal intubation is not planned, and a small child is placed in the lateral position with general anesthesia maintained via mask or laryngeal mask airway. Having an assistant is useful for monitoring of the patient and for assistance in technical aspects of block placement.

Agents and Dosage

Busoni and Andreuccetti evaluated correlation of spread of the local anesthetic to age and weight, and noted that weight was a better predictor in newborns and infants, while age was a better guide in older children.[32] Clinically, the most workable formula is that suggested by Armitage (Table 20-3).[6] He notes that because there is not an opportunity to repeat a single-dose block, the initial dose must be large enough to produce the required level of analgesia. It is of note that most studies for groin incision surgery, such as hernia repair, employ volumes of 0.75 ml/kg of 0.25% bupivacaine.

TABLE 20-3. *Volumes for single dose caudal block*

Volumes (ml/kg)[a]	Dermatomal level
0.5	Sacral
0.75	Inguinal
1.0	Lower thoracic
1.25	Mid-thoracic

(Modified from Armitage, E.N.: Local anaesthetic techniques for prevention of postoperative pain, Br. J. Anaesth. *58*:790, 1986.)

[a] Volumes of 0.25% bupivacaine.

Wolf and colleagues employed bupivacaine 0.75 ml/kg in 105 pediatric ambulatory surgical patients undergoing herniorrhaphy, orchidopexy, or hypospadias repair and found no difference in duration of postoperative analgesia between 0.25% and 0.125% bupivacaine.[167] These workers also found that 50% of these inpatient children needed no supplemental analgesics 12 hours after caudal block. If a dilute concentration of local anesthetic is desired, it is important to employ preservative-free normal saline as the diluent.

Fisher and others indicate no prolongation of analgesia with the addition of epinephrine, while an earlier study noted both the addition of epinephrine and infiltration of sacral surgical site produced prolonged analgesia.[63,160] However, both studies relied on parental questioning on the first postoperative day, to establish duration of analgesia. This is in contrast to the study by Wolf and colleagues, where children were not discharged from the hospital until the day after their inguinal surgery, thus allowing for more objective observation.[167] These studies, plus the larger study by Dalens and Hasnaoui, noted no impact of caudal blockade with local anesthetic on the time to micturition.[41]

Jamali and others found that addition of clonidine to the caudal analgesic mixture more than doubled the analgesic time.[85] There were no differences in respiratory rate, SpO_2 values, hemodynamic parameters, sedation, or sleep time.

Mazoit and others studied pharmacokinetics in infants receiving 2.5 mg/kg of bupivacaine for caudal analgesia, and found that serum and plasma levels were both in the range of 0.5 to 1.9 μg/ml, while Stow and colleagues noted time to peak plasma concentration of around 20 minutes.[111,150] Eyres and coworkers measured plasma bupivacaine concentrations after caudal injection of 3 mg/kg of bupivacaine 0.25% solution in 45 children and found mean blood levels ranging from 1.2 to 1.4 μg/ml.[57] Yaster and associates showed that peak plasma levels of lidocaine of 1.1 to 3.2

μg/ml were detected 30 to 40 minutes after the caudal administration of 5 mg/kg.[171] In all 4 studies, the peak plasma levels of both bupivacaine and lidocaine were less than those that are considered to be toxic in adults.

There appears to be an increased risk of unrecognized intravascular injection in infants weighing less than 10 kg. Veyckemans and others reported a series of 1,100 caudal blocks in children younger than 7 years, 463 of which were in infants less than 10 kg in weight.[159] These workers had 76 bloody taps, with 8 systemic reactions recognized (defined as an increased heart rate greater than 20 beats per minute, usually with electrocardiogram changes, cutaneous vasoconstriction, and severe arterial hypertension). All 8 were in infants less than 10 kg in weight; 6 had negative aspirations for blood and were considered as "concealed bloody taps." Epinephrine 1:200,000 was always added freshly to the local anesthetic. All episodes responded to hyperventilation with oxygen; there were no convulsions or episodes of cardiovascular collapse. In addition to the above report, there have been other reports of cardiac events in infants weighing less than 10 kg who received caudal blocks (see Introduction).

Clinical Use

Caudal blockade has been shown to result in minimal intraoperative changes in cardiorespiratory function in children.[80,123] Dalens and Hasnaoui reported that successful blockade was much more likely in children less than 7 years of age (7/626 failures versus 19/124 patients over 7 years of age).[41] They also noted that awake children did not psychologically tolerate the operating room environment, even in the presence of excellent anesthesia; restlessness was more pronounced in those patients who had a motor as well as a sensory block.

Spear noted the efficacy of single-dose caudal blockade as the sole anesthetic for high-risk infants undergoing inguinal herniorrhaphy, as did Gunter and others.[72,148] Splinter and colleagues, and Hannallah and co-workers, found that caudal and ilioinguinal-iliohypogastric blocks produced similar analgesia following inguinal surgery.[75,149] Moores and colleagues point out that rectal nonsteroidal anti-inflammatory drugs (NSAIDs) may be equally effective to caudal blockade for postoperative analgesia, while Ryhänen and others indicate that NSAIDs may even be superior to caudal blocks in terms of duration of analgesia.[119,135] Further research in this area is important in comparing alternative analgesic regimens.

Safety and Possible Complications

Although clinical experience with pediatric caudal block is quite extensive, reports of large series have been published only very recently. Gunter, in 1991, surveying 119 children's hospitals and anesthesiology residency programs, included over 150,000 caudal blocks, with an estimated incidence of catastrophic complications of 1:40,000.[71] Experience at Children's National Medical Center (CNMC) from 1983 to 1993 in over 7,800 infants and children included 2 recognized dural punctures and 1 high spinal in a premature graduate who received a caudal block following a failed spinal anesthetic. Such complications as hypotension and urinary retention have not been reported in any study. All authors stress that the key to the safety of the procedure is knowledge of the anatomy in children, meticulous attention to detail in selection and preparation of the site, and careful aspiration before drug injection.

Willis believes that the two problems most commonly associated with caudal blocks are lack of success and pain on injection (see Chapter 9). In children, lack of success is due primarily to injecting an inadequate volume of drug. Although infection is frequently listed among the complications of caudal block, it is rarely noted in clinical practice.[137,151] This may be particularly due to modern, single-use needles or other changes in technique.

Intravenous injection can be prevented by repeated gentle aspiration after each needle movement. Use of excessive force to attempt aspiration may fail to show blood, if the suction force collapses the vein. Most bloody aspirates are due to intraosseous, rather than intravenous, placement of the needle. The cancellous mass of sacral bone is covered by a wafer-thin, brittle, layer of cortex that can be damaged easily. This complication is best avoided by inserting the needle in the line of the sacral canal, avoiding excessive force, and keeping the bevel of the needle directed ventrally, so that it slides over the anterior plate of the sacrum. Referral to the section on test-dosing underscores the danger of assuming that a negative test-dose or lack of visual evidence of bloody tap guarantees that the needle is not intravascular.

Because of the lower extension of the dural sac, the risk of dural puncture theoretically is higher in infants than in adults or older children. That complication, however, is technique-dependent and easily recognized if gentle aspiration is performed following placement of the needle and prior to the first injection of drug.

Continuous Caudal Technique

Continuous caudal techniques are often employed in infants and toddlers, rather than continuous epidural techniques, because:

1. The caudal space is easier to access in this age group than the lumbar epidural space.
2. Caudal catheters are passed more easily cephalad, to either the lumbar or thoracic epidural space, in young children.
3. There may be a reduced chance of causing direct spinal cord trauma with the caudal approach than there would be with lumbar or thoracic epidural placement.

Continuous caudal techniques may be used to provide surgical anesthesia in high-risk infants undergoing inguinal herniorrhaphy; a combined general/regional technique may be used in older infants and children.[38,82] Analgesia may be provided with intermittent or continuous administration of local anesthetic solution or a dilute local anesthetic/opioid combination.[46,92] Alternatively, opioids alone can be employed to provide profound postoperative analgesia in older children.[94]

Placement of Caudal Catheters

As for most other blocks, caudal catheters usually are placed in pediatric patients after the induction of general anesthesia. In situations where a continuous caudal technique is to be employed as the sole anesthetic technique, such as for inguinal herniorrhaphy in the high-risk neonate, general anesthesia and sedation are avoided.[82] Topical local anesthesia with eutectic mixture of local anesthetics (EMLA) cream applied over the infant's sacral hiatus, and over a prospective intravenous access site, can facilitate regional block placement in this case.

There are commercially available kits with 20-gauge Tuohy or Crawford needles and 24-gauge catheters, as well as kits with 18- and 19-gauge 3.75 to 5 cm Tuohy needles, through which a 20-gauge(adult) catheter can be passed. Alternatively, a 22-gauge intravenous catheter-over-needle can be employed; a "pop" is felt as the needle/catheter combination pierces the sacrococcygeal membrane, and the catheter is threaded over the needle into the caudal space. An intravenous administration set or microtubing is then attached to the catheter hub, allowing serial injections through the caudal catheter for initial block, as well as administration of additional doses of local anesthetic during the surgical procedure. These intravenous catheters are not a satisfactory substitute for conventional caudal/epidural catheters in the postoperative setting, as they will kink at the hub in an active, pain-free, child.

Air loss-of-resistance techniques for caudal or epidural blockade are to be avoided in pediatric patients, because of the risk of venous air embolism.[70] McGown, in a series of 500 pediatric caudal blocks, reported an incidence of inadvertent entry into a caudal epidural vessel of 7%, while Dalens and Hasnaoui experienced an incidence of blood return of 10.6% in their series of 750 caudal blocks, when long needles were employed.[41,114]

Negative aspiration does not rule out the potential for a catheter tip to lie within a blood vessel, and children can develop a life-threatening venous air embolism from small quantities of air. In fact, children may be at more risk than adults, because of their high incidence of probe-patent foramen ovale (up to 50% in children less than 5 years of age).

Placement of Lumbar and Thoracic Catheters via the Caudal Space

Lumbar and thoracic epidural catheters allow the achievement of narrower bands of segmental anesthesia with reduced volumes of local anesthetic solutions. However, these techniques are more challenging, technically, in young children. One solution to this problem is to place a catheter via the caudal space and thread this catheter cephalad until it comes to rest in a region proximal to the surgical field. It should be pointed out that such long advancement of a catheter may lead to dural puncture or nerve damage, in addition to malposition.

Bösenberg and others took advantage of the difference in epidural fat between young children and adults, to thread caudal catheters into the thoracic region.[23] These workers placed 16-gauge intravenous catheters into the caudal spaces of 20 neonates and infants and advanced 18-gauge epidural catheters as far as the level of T-8, confirming placement by abdominal radiographs. In 19 of 20 infants, the epidural catheter was placed within one vertebra of the desired level. On 14 of 20 occasions, slight resistance was felt during attempted passage of the catheter and it became necessary to flex the spines of these infants, to facilitate catheter advancement. Placement of the catheter with the infant in the lateral, rather than in the prone, position is therefore recommended. The same authors demonstrated in infant cadavers that catheters which were forcibly advanced against resistance either coiled up or doubled back in the epidural space. It is unknown when the epidural fat consistency alters to that of an adult.

Securing the caudal catheter is very important, both because of the possibility of soilage in infants as well as the need to provide security in an active toddler. The authors employ 2 clear, occlusive, dressings to protect the catheter. One is placed caudad to the catheter over the gluteal crease and serves to prevent the rostral spread of urine, feces, and other contaminants. The second occlusive dressing covers the catheter about 2.0 cm in all directions and is adherent to the cephalad portion of the first dressing. An alternative method is to cover the site with an occlusive dressing, and erect a barrier, using a larger, waterproof, transparent drape with adhesive on a single edge.[112] The barrier flap is secured to the infant's back just below the distal end of the catheter dressing, and turned upward against the back. The infant is then diapered and the free end of the flap is folded onto the outside of the diaper.

Removal of a catheter that has been advanced far into the epidural space must be done with care.[125] One should be careful to apply gentle traction; if resistance is encountered, flexion or extension of the child's back at the lumbar curve usually will facilitate catheter removal.

EPIDURAL BLOCK (see Chapter 8)

Dalens and colleagues showed that a single-dose epidural could be employed, in conjunction with a light general anesthetic, to provide both adjunct anesthesia and postoperative analgesia for infants and young children.[38] These workers, employing a short-beveled Potts-Cournand needle, experienced inadvertent dural puncture in 4 of the 52 children, 2 days to 7 years of age, in whom this technique was used.

One of the most frequently mentioned reasons for placement of epidural catheters in infants and children is the fear of fecal contamination and subsequent infection if caudal catheters are employed.[152] As mentioned in the continuous caudal section, this concern seems to be more theoretical than real if appropriate dressing and monitoring of the caudal site takes place.[151]

Anatomy

The depth of the epidural space from the skin increases as the child grows; Eyres and colleagues estimate that this distance is about 1.0 mm/kg, while Ecoffey, reports that the skin-epidural distance ranges between 10 to 18 mm at the lumbar level and 7 to 14 mm at the thoracic level in infants 3 to 36 months of age.[52,59]

Technique

As has been mentioned, use of air for loss-of-resistance in pediatric patients has been associated with venous air embolism.[140] Schwartz and others reported circulatory collapse in a 9-month-old infant who received 3.0 ml of air into the lumbar space.[143] Studies in dogs found that 0.5 ml/kg/min of air injected into the epidural space was associated with cardiovascular collapse; this is approximately the same volume of air injected into the infant in the Schwartz case report.[2]

An alternate technique using an intravenous micro-drip infusion set has been employed for identification of the epidural space.[96,170] The infusion set was prepared with saline and connected to the hub of an epidural needle placed into the interspinous ligament. The microdrip chamber was kept at about 1 meter above the skin puncture site, and a small bubble of air remained in the tubing at its junction with the epidural needle hub. As the needle was advanced, the bubble suddenly moved from the tubing into the needle and normal saline began to drip from the chamber. Although there were 4 inadvertent dural punctures in this series of 350 patients, 3 occurred within the first 30 cases.

Specialized equipment is available for the performance of epidural anesthesia in pediatric patients. Short (2.5 to 4.0 cm) Tuohy needles with proportionately shorter bevels are available in both 20-gauge (with 24-gauge catheters)and 18-gauge (for use with adult catheters). A smaller glass syringe is also available. Although standard adult equipment can be employed in very small children, the length and large bevel of the needle and the larger, heavy, glass syringe are awkward.

TABLE 20-4. *Doses for continuous caudal and epidural blockade*

Route	Agent concentration %	Dose (bupivacaine) mg/kg
Continuous Caudal/	bupivacaine 0.1% fentanyl 1–2 mcg/ml	0.2–0.25 mg/kg/hr (infants) 0.4–0.5 mg/kg/hr (older)
Epidural	bupivacaine 0.1%/ morphine	0.2–0.25 mg/kg/hr 0.005 mg/kg/hr
	lidocaine 0.5%/ fentanyl	1.5 mg/kg/hr 0.5–2.5 mcg/kg/hr

TABLE 20-5. *Six safety tips for local anesthetic infusions*

1. Children are probably not "more resistant" to local anesthetic toxicity than adults.
2. Do not rely on premonitory symptoms or signs for detection of toxicity.
3. Do not exceed recommended doses or infusion rate.
4. Do not expect low-placed lumbar or caudal epidural local anesthetic infusions to provide the sole analgesia after surgery in upper abdominal or thoracic dermatomes.
5. For epidural bupivacaine infusions, after a loading dose of 2 to 2.5 mg/kg, infusion rates should probably not exceed 0.4 to 0.5 mg/kg/hr for older infants, toddlers and children, or 0.2 to 0.25 mg/kg/hr for neonates.
6. Reduce infusion rates further for patients with risk factors for seizures.

(Modified from: Berde, C.B.: Convulsions associated with pediatric regional anesthesia. Anesth. Analg. *75:*164, 1992.)

Agents and Doses

The limitations of the test dose with epinephrine are identical to limitations elsewhere in the central neuraxis. Various dosages, volumes, and concentrations of both local anesthetics and opioid solutions have been employed (Table 20-4). Reports of seizures following continuous infusion of local anesthetics into the epidural or caudal space led Berde to make recommendations regarding total dose/hour of bupivacaine (Table 20-5).[15] Yaster and colleagues employ lidocaine, with daily monitoring of blood levels, rather than bupivacaine.[171]

SPINAL ANESTHESIA (see Chapter 7)

The largest series of spinal anesthetics in children is that of Berkowitz and Greene, who reported a series of 350 spinal anesthetics in children and adolescents.[18] More recently, spinal anesthesia has been recommended for infants at high risk for postoperative apnea following general anesthesia.[11,77,95,121,161,163]

Anatomy

The neonatal spinal cord reportedly ends at anywhere from T12 to L3, lower than the adult L1 level, which makes it preferable to perform the lumbar puncture at the L4 or L5 interspace; the approximate depth of the subarachnoid space is 1 to 1.5 cm from the skin.[22]

Technique

Most neonatal and pediatric spinal anesthesia needles have a Quincke point; fortunately, children rarely suffer post-dural puncture headaches (PDPH).[21] The authors employ a 22-gauge, 3.75 cm Quincke needle, for infants and children up to 15 kg, and switch to an adult, 26-gauge needle, for older children and adolescents.

Commercially available disposable trays, including clear-hubbed needles of both sizes and a clear, fenestrated drape, are available. Performance of this block (or a caudal or epidural) in an awake infant will require 2 assistants; one securely restrains the infant while the second tends to the airway and comforts the infant. Positioning the infant in a sitting position will increase the cerebrospinal fluid (CSF) hydrostatic pressure. The assistant holding the patient in position must provide firm restraint and assure that the infant's neck remains extended; flexion of the neck of a preterm infant may decrease the transcutaneous oxygen tension ($TcPO_2$) by as much as 28 mm Hg.[68]

The spinal needle is inserted using a midline approach. A bloody tap may occur if the needle is not advanced exactly in the midline. The characteristic "pops" as the needle pierces posterior spinal ligaments and the dura are less distinct in the preterm infant than in older patients. Use of a 22-gauge needle allows brisk, free, flow of CSF, with concomitant recognition of proper needle placement. Once CSF has appeared, the syringe containing local anesthetic is carefully attached and the drug is injected. It is imperative that the assistant continues to restrain the patient firmly, because it is easy to dislodge the needle and to inject the local anesthetic solution subcutaneously.

After the needle is removed, the patient is placed in the supine position. Care is taken not to place the feet higher than the head; for example, one should not immediately lift the infant's legs to place an electrocautery grounding pad on the back. Motor blockade should be evident within 1 to 2 minutes.

Dohi and colleagues noted that patients less than 5 years of age show little or no change in blood pressure with spinal anesthesia, even without fluid loading.[49] However, children older than 6 years demonstrated widely variable decreases in blood pressure, similar to observations in adults. Harnik and colleagues and Rice and others have observed similar cardiovascular stability in patients younger than 1 year.[77,129] Abajian and others recommend placing the intravenous catheter in a lower extremity after the spinal anesthetic has been administered, rather than struggling with venipuncture to administer fluids before spinal anesthesia is established.[1] Oberlander and colleagues postulated that there is a compensatory reduction in vagal efferent activity in response to partial blockade of sympathetic outflow to the heart, based on their study that monitored heart rate variability in 8 neonates undergoing spinal anesthesia.[121] These workers also confirmed that neonates do not have hemodynamically significant venodilation during spinal anesthesia.

Agents and Doses

The duration of spinal anesthesia in young children is shorter than in older children or adults. The sensory level of anesthesia produced by all doses of hyperbaric drugs is almost uniformly T4, unless the patient is placed in the Trendelenberg position after performance of the block, in which case the level of anesthesia may rise above T4.[169] Larger doses, however, do produce longer neural blockade (Table 20-6).

TABLE 20-6. *Choice of local anesthetic doses for subarachnoid block based on anticipated duration of surgery*

Duration of surgery (min)	Drug solution	Dose (mg/kg)
30	Lidocaine 5%/dextrose 7.5%/epinephrine	3.0
60	Tetracaine 1%	0.4–1
90	Tetracaine 1%/epinephrine	0.4–1

Sedation should be avoided in high-risk infants, as the use of respiratory depressants may negate the value of the regional technique.[95,163] Usually, a soothing touch and a pacifier are all the infant needs to remain quiet during surgery if the NPO period prior to surgery has been minimal. Analgesia from the spinal anesthetic may not be enough to provide adequate surgical conditions; therefore, upper extremity restraint is an important part of this anesthetic technique in an infant.[126] Appropriate sedation may be employed in older children and adolescents prior to placement of the spinal anesthetic.

Doses have not been well established for children over 3 years of age. It is important to note that doses for spinal anesthesia in this age group are not based on a mg/kg formula as in infants. It is suggested that the anesthesiologist employ conservative doses extrapolated from experience in adults.

Clinical Use

Spinal anesthesia has been employed most often for hernia repair in postpremature infants who are at risk for apnea and periodic breathing in the postoperative period following general anesthesia.[146] During the procedures in one series of spinal anesthetics in 34 older children,[20] the children, depending on their ages, were either sedated or entertained with cartoons played on a video cassette recorder. The patients were prehydrated with 6 ml/kg of lactated Ringer's solution before placement of the spinal anesthetic, and no incident of hypotension occurred. One 2-1/2-year-old patient, however, did experience post dural puncture headache (PDPH).

Safety and Efficacy

A report of spinal anesthesia in 20 infants recovering from respiratory distress syndrome included monitoring of sensory-evoked potentials in 8 infants.[77] This information suggested that the onset and the resolution of spinal anesthesia of the immature spinal cord can be recorded by an electric marker.

Welborn and colleagues, in their comparison of high-risk

infants undergoing inguinal hernia repair under spinal anesthesia, caution that the advantage of this technique is removed when sedation is added.[163] Krane and others compared spinal and general anesthesia without sedation, and found fewer episodes of respiratory abnormalities in the premature graduates who received regional anesthesia without sedation.[95]

Even without sedation, postoperative apnea can still occur in high-risk infants following regional anesthesia. These episodes probably were not due to the anesthetic technique, since they occurred 12 to 32 hours after surgery.[37] However, in light of these reports, it would be prudent to observe high-risk patients in a high-dependency nursing area, for at least 12 hours following surgery, even with a regional anesthetic and no sedation. Interestingly, reports are beginning to appear in the surgical literature about the safety of this technique, in spite of the fact that no monitoring beyond observation was utilized by these authors.[156,158]

The incidence of PDPH in pediatric patients is vanishingly small, with only a few PDPH reported in children under 12 years of age. Lumbar puncture with a 20- or 22-gauge needle is a frequently performed diagnostic procedure in pediatric patients, and is often used to provide chemotherapy in children. Even under these circumstances, PDPH is infrequent, and rarely requires treatment.[21] Epidural blood patch provides effective treatment for PDPH in pediatric patients.[97] The use of sedation as well as EMLA cream may be beneficial; practitioners should consider each child's age and level of maturation when determining whether conscious or deep sedation will be required. The volume of autologous blood recommended varies from 0.5 to 0.75 ml/kg, and should be injected slowly.

CENTRAL NEURAXIS OPIOIDS (see also Chapter 29)

Probably no other aspect of pediatric postoperative pain management has shown more growth and development in the past decade than the use of central neuraxis opioid and local anesthetic infusions. Delayed respiratory depression is always possible, whether the opioid is administered via the caudal, epidural, or spinal route, especially in young infants. This is particularly true with concomitant administration of systemic opioids.

Many practitioners believe that intravenous morphine provides postoperative analgesia equivalent to caudal bupivacaine. Wolf and Hughs investigated 32 patients younger than 4 years of age who were undergoing abdominal surgery.[168] Half of the children received a caudal infusion of 0.25% bupivacaine, while the other half received a loading dose of intravenous morphine (0.15 mg/kg)followed by a morphine infusion of 5 to 10 μg/kg/hr. The authors note that while differences in ventilatory frequency and oxygenation were statistically significant, they did not appear to have any clinical consequences.

Studies such as these emphasize that each child's postoperative analgesia plan must be individualized. Risk-benefit ratios, patient acuity, the expected intensity of the postoperative pain, and the institutional level of expertise with various analgesia modalities, must all be considered. Rosen and others have shown that children undergoing cardiac surgery benefit from caudal morphine because of decreased need for inotropic support, and the benefit of intense analgesia.[132] One group in this study received conventional opioid therapy; although this group was judged to be pain-free both during surgery and in the intensive care unit postoperatively, they had higher levels of stress hormones and required more inotropic support than did those children who received caudal morphine prior to the onset of surgery. This is the first controlled study in which central neuraxis opioid management was compared to more conventional analgesic techniques in non-healthy children. As in adults, sick children may benefit more from aggressive pain management than do healthy children (see also Chapter 5).[131]

Epidural/Caudal Opioids

All opioids have been employed in the extradural space, with the same lipophilic/hydrophilic considerations as in older patients. Attia and colleagues studied the pharmacokinetics and CO_2 sensitivity to epidural morphine in children following abdominal or urologic surgery.[8] The pharmacokinetic parameters observed after epidural morphine in older children were similar to those previously measured in adults, including a significant decrease in the minute ventilatory response to $P_{ET}CO_{2\text{-}55}$ for more than 22 hours following epidural morphine administration.

As in adults, fentanyl and sufentanil require continuous administration rather than bolus administration, because of the short duration of postoperative analgesia obtained.[102] In addition, because these lipophilic opioids provide intense analgesia in the areas of administration without extensive spread, placement of the catheter tip near the dermatomal level of the surgical site is imperative. Infusions of dilute bupivacaine (0.0625 to 0.1%), with the addition of 1 to 2 mcg/ml of fentanyl, at rates of 0.15 to 0.3 ml/kg/hr have been employed.[14] Total volume required depends upon the location of the epidural catheter tip in relation to the surgical site and the extent of the surgical field.

Rostral spread of caudally administered morphine allows this drug to provide postoperative analgesia for upper abdominal and thoracic surgeries. Krane and others demonstrated that caudal morphine in a dose of 0.033 mg/kg provides excellent analgesia, with less incidence of respiratory depression than larger doses.[93,94] Valley and Bailey reported the use of caudal morphine 0.07 mg/kg diluted with normal saline in 138 children undergoing major cavity surgery.[155] Children weighing less than 5 kg received 3 ml of solution, while those weighing 5 to 15 kg received 5 ml and those weighing over 15 kg received 10 ml of solution. Of note is the high incidence of respiratory depression; 11/138 children, 10 of whom were under 1 year of age. Most had received concomitant systemic opioids along with the extradural opioids. The mean time from the administration of caudal morphine until the onset of respiratory depression in this group was 3.8 hours; no respiratory depression occurred in any child later than 12 hours after the last dose. All respiratory depression was managed successfully with naloxone 5 to 20 μg/kg, followed by infusions of 2 to 10 μg/kg/hr.

Rosen suggests a regimen of morphine 0.04 mg/kg in the same volumes as used by Valley, followed by a continuous infusion of 0.15 to 0.2 ml/kg/hr with a dose of 6 to 8 μg/kg/hr.[132] He suggests administration of intravenous morphine 25 μg/kg as needed for rescue analgesia. Nausea, vomiting, and pruritus have been treated with intravenous nalbuphine in doses of 25 μg/kg, while respiratory depression should be reversed with intravenous naloxone 10 μg/kg.

Bailey and colleagues compared the efficacy of caudal, epidural, and intravenous butorphanol in reducing the incidence of adverse side-effects associated with the administration of epidural morphine, and found that there was no difference in the incidence of adverse side-effects among the children who had received butorphanol and those who had not.[12] Lawhorn and Brown found a decreased incidence of opioid-related complications when butorphanol 40 μg/kg was added to epidural morphine 80 μg/kg.[100]

As noted in the section on caudal analgesia, the addition of clonidine to epidural morphine appears to provide prolonged analgesia without increasing side effects.[85]

Spinal Opioids (see Chapter 29)

Intrathecal opioids are employed much less frequently in pediatric patients than are epidural opioids, probably because caudal/epidural blockade is a more common regional anesthetic technique in this population than is subarachnoid blockade. However, there are some instances in which intrathecal opioids have been employed to advantage in specific pediatric populations. Harris and colleagues studied 50 children 2 to 9 years of age undergoing selective dorsal root rhizotomy surgery for treatment of severe spasticity resulting from cerebral palsy.[78] While this surgery can reduce spasticity dramatically, the postoperative course often is complicated by refractory pain and muscle spasm. Subarachnoid morphine was administered at the completion of the surgery, under direct visualization at the S2 level. Nearly 50% of the children experienced nausea, vomiting, and mild facial pruritus. The authors concluded that low dose intrathecal morphine (7 to 15 μg/kg) provided equivalent analgesia to higher doses.

Nichols and colleagues studied the disposition and respiratory effects of intrathecal morphine in 10 infants and children undergoing craniofacial surgery.[120] All of these children required cerebrospinal fluid (CSF) drainage as part of the surgical procedure, accomplished by placing a subarachnoid catheter at the L4–L5 interspace. The same catheter was used to administer subarachnoid morphine (2 μg/kg)prior to the conclusion of surgery, and then to sample and measure the CSF concentration of morphine at 6, 12, and 18 hours. Corresponding plasma concentrations of morphine were determined by radioimmunoassay. Intrathecal morphine produced a reduction in both the slope and the intercept of the ventilatory response curve, greatest 6 hours after morphine administration, and only partially recovered 12 and 18 hours later. This study documents that infants and children may experience respiratory depression for at least 18 hours following subarachnoid morphine administration, and that appropriate monitoring and safeguards are essential.

PEDIATRIC EXTREMITY BLOCKS

The basic techniques used to perform extremity blocks in infants and children are similar to those used in adults, with two major differences:

1. Awake children are less likely to cooperate with block needle placement than are adults, and it is highly unlikely that children will be able to understand the concept of reporting a paresthesia. Infants cannot cooperate at all, of course. Consequently, use of a peripheral nerve stimulator is an important alternative for identification of the peripheral nerve.
2. Children fear needles. Therefore, either general anesthesia or appropriate levels of sedation should be employed before placement of the block.

As always, doses of local anesthetics should be calculated in terms of both volume and total mg/kg of drug, to avoid exceeding recommended doses (Table 20-7).

Sedation (see Chapter 6)

For most elective procedures, general anesthesia is induced by mask and then the blocks are placed. Following block placement, the inspired concentration of volatile anesthetic agent can be reduced to minimal levels if the block is expected to provide the surgical anesthetic. An alternate approach in older children requires establishment of intravenous access and deep sedation with intravenous propofol 1 to 1.5 mg/kg, followed by a continuous infusion of propofol (100 to 150 μg/kg/min). The propofol infusion may be continued (75 to 125 μg/kg/min), or curtailed, depending upon the child's age and the clinical situation. Administration of deep sedation or mask general anesthesia is contraindicated in traumatized children, or in other settings where airway protection and full stomach precautions must take precedence over the fear of needles. In these circum-

TABLE 20-7. *Volume of local anesthetic for peripheral nerve blocks in pediatric patients*

Block	Volume (ml/kg)
Interscalene/Parascalene brachial plexus	0.25
Axillary brachial plexus	0.33
Sciatic nerve	0.15–0.2
Inguinal paravascular ("3-in-1" block)	0.5

(From Broadman, L.M.: Regional anesthesia for the pediatric outpatient. Anesth. Clin. North Am., *5*:53, 1987).

stances, the block should be performed on an unsedated or very lightly sedated child. Parental presence may be quite helpful in calming and allaying the anxiety of the child in such circumstances. Again, the use of the peripheral nerve stimulator may be very helpful (see Chapter 6).

Upper Extremity (see Chapter 10)

These blocks may be used for all surgical procedures of the upper extremity. As in adults, there are several approaches to brachial plexus blockade.

Anatomy

Surface anatomy in children differs from that in adults, with less soft tissue overlaying the bony landmarks, and they are therefore more readily palpated. Otherwise, the anatomy of the plexus sheaths and major blood vessels is the same as in the adult.

Axillary Block

Many practitioners prefer the axillary approach to the brachial plexus because of its safety and ease of performance. Although the technique is the same for children as adults, it is often surprising to note how superficial the nerves are in young children, when one performs this block for the first time.[33] Inappropriately deep injection of local anesthetic is the most common reason for a failed block. As opposed to adults, the musculocutaneous nerve usually is blocked with this approach in pediatric patients. The approach also has been employed for placement of catheters for continuous infusion of local anesthetic.[162]

Interscalene/Parascalene Block

The interscalene approach to the brachial plexus is the best technique for procedures in children involving the shoulder and upper arm, and is suitable, too, for cases where the child is unable to abduct the arm because of pain or injuries. Again, the technique is similar to that used in adults. A peripheral nerve stimulator is used in lieu of paresthesiae. In cooperative children, it is helpful to palpate and mark the interscalene groove before administering heavy sedation or general anesthesia.

Dalens and others have demonstrated in infants and children that the parascalene approach to the brachial plexus provides more satisfactory anesthesia with fewer complications than does the supraclavicular approach.[39] One-half of the children received a supraclavicular block, while the other half received a parascalene block. All were performed by the same anesthesiologist, using insulated needles and a peripheral nerve stimulator. Analgesia was complete in 88% of the children in the supraclavicular block group, while 97% of the parascalene group had adequate analgesia. Forty-two children in the supraclavicular block group developed a Horner's syndrome (70%), while only 2 children in the parascalene group developed one.

Intravenous Regional Anesthesia (see Chapter 12)

Intravenous regional anesthesia can be used easily in cooperative and older children, although there are reports of this block being used in children as young as 3 years of age. This technique is used most frequently to reduce and set simple upper extremity fractures and dislocations, often by nonanesthesiologists in the emergency department.[36,122]

A butterfly needle or cannula is inserted into the hand, and the extremity is exsanguinated by gravity (use of an Esmarch is usually too painful for the awake child to endure). Tourniquet pressures should be 180 to 240 mm Hg for the upper limb, and 350 for the lower limb. The dose is 3 mg/kg of preservative-free 0.5% lidocaine or prilocaine; as in adults, the tourniquet should not be released for at least 20 minutes following injection of local anesthetic. Toxicity issues from defective tourniquet or premature tourniquet release are similar to those in adults.

Peripheral Blocks

The radial, median, and ulnar nerves can be blocked easily either at the level of the antecubital fossa or at the wrist, using techniques similar to those used in adults. Small volumes of local anesthetics (0.5 to 1 ml), and fine-bore needles, are employed in young children.

Lower Extremity Blocks (see Chapter 11)

The multiple injections required to produce lumbar and sacral plexus anesthesia in infants and children make individual nerve blocks of the lower extremity less popular than the more reliable and technically easier caudal, epidural and spinal techniques. However, there are circumstances where it is advantageous to block individual nerves.[25,83,117] Ankle blocks may be very useful in older children for procedures such as debridement of ingrown toenail.

Sciatic Nerve Block

Although the sciatic nerve can be blocked successfully in anesthetized children, using the anterior approach and a loss-of-resistance technique, most anesthesiologists recommend the use of a peripheral nerve stimulator.[116] This block may also be employed in combination with a femoral or lumbar plexus block to provide effective anesthesia of the entire lower extremity.

Use of the peripheral nerve stimulator is suggested in pediatric patients. If motor activity is noted above the level of the knee as the stimulating needle is advanced, it is very likely due to direct stimulation of the gluteal muscles. Such motor activity cannot be accepted as sciatic nerve stimulation. Injection in the face of motor activity above the level of the knee probably will result in failure of the block. The nerve stimulator is connected and the needle is advanced at right angles to the skin in all planes until dorsiflexion of the foot (tibial nerve), or plantar flexion (common peroneal nerve), is noted. Once the strongest contraction has been obtained, local anesthetic solution is administered in a similar manner as that already described. The size of the needle will depend on the size of the patient; a 22-gauge spinal needle may be used in the adolescent, whose gluteal muscle may be quite thick. The entire length of the needle, however, need not be used.

Techniques for blockade of the sciatic nerve are similar in children and adults, although the variable sizes of pediatric patients do require some adjustment in needle placement. For the posterior approach to the sciatic nerve, the patient is placed in the lateral position, with the leg to be blocked uppermost and flexed, so that the foot is at the level of the popliteal fossa of the opposite leg (see Chapter 11, Fig. 11-5). This position stretches the nerve so that it will roll less. Labat's line is formed by dropping a perpendicular line inferiorly from the midpoint of a line drawn between the superior border of the greater trochanter and the posterior superior iliac spine. The Winnie modification adjusts for the patient's height by drawing a line between the greater trochanter and the sacral hiatus. The intersection of the Winnie line and Labat's line approximates the location of the sciatic nerve as it exits the pelvis through the greater sciatic notch. As the sciatic nerve exits the greater sciatic notch and begins its course down the leg, it passes a point approximately equidistant from the ischial tuberosity and the greater trochanter. Both of these landmarks are readily palpable in children; in addition, a deep notch can be felt between them. The sciatic nerve lies in this notch.

The anterior approach to the sciatic nerve in pediatric patients is described by McNicol and by Dalens and others.[45,116] With the patient lying supine, a line is drawn from the anterior superior iliac spine to the pubic tubercle (Fig. 20-1). A second line is drawn parallel to the first, medially from the greater trochanter of the femur. A perpendicular line is dropped from the medial and middle parts of the proximal line to the distal line. The needle is then walked off the medial edge of the femur, until it enters the thigh muscles. Gentle pressure is applied to the barrel of a syringe attached to the needle as it passes through the thigh muscles, until there is a loss of resistance when the needle enters the sciatic neurovascular compartment. If a nerve stimulator is used, the end point is identical to that in the posterior approach. Dalens and others have compared several approaches to this block in pediatric patients, and have found a higher success rate with the posterior approach than with the anterior.[45]

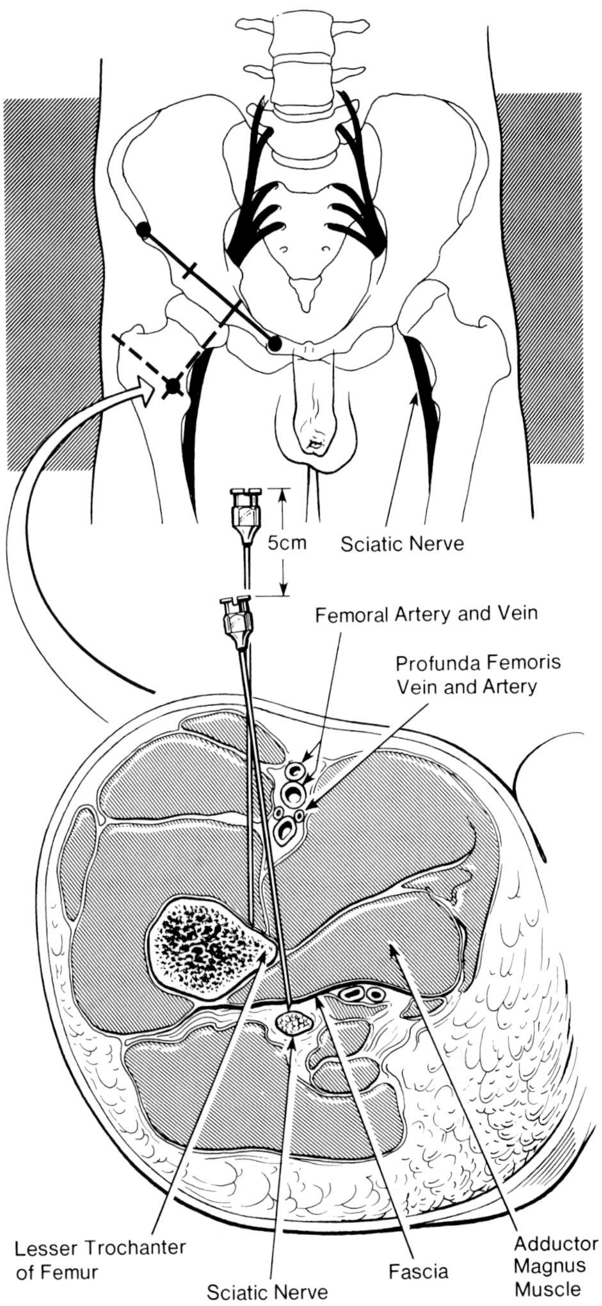

FIG. 20-1. Anterior approach to sciatic nerve block (see text). Cross-section of the leg at the level of the lesser trochanter to show the relationship between the sciatic nerve and the femur, and the fascia separating it from adductor magnus.

Femoral Nerve Block

Although Winnie popularized the inguinal perivascular technique (the "3-in-1" block) for lumbar plexus anesthesia, Dalens and colleagues have pointed out recently that one can obtain a complete block of all the components of the plexus only if large volumes of local anesthetic solution are injected deep to the fascia iliaca.[40,43,166] Therefore, these workers suggest that the fascia iliaca block is an effective one for the lumbar plexus in children.

The femoral nerve is located lateral to the femoral artery, deep to both fascia lata and fascia iliaca. Femoral nerve blocks alone can be used to provide instantaneous pain relief and muscle relaxation in children with femoral shaft frac-

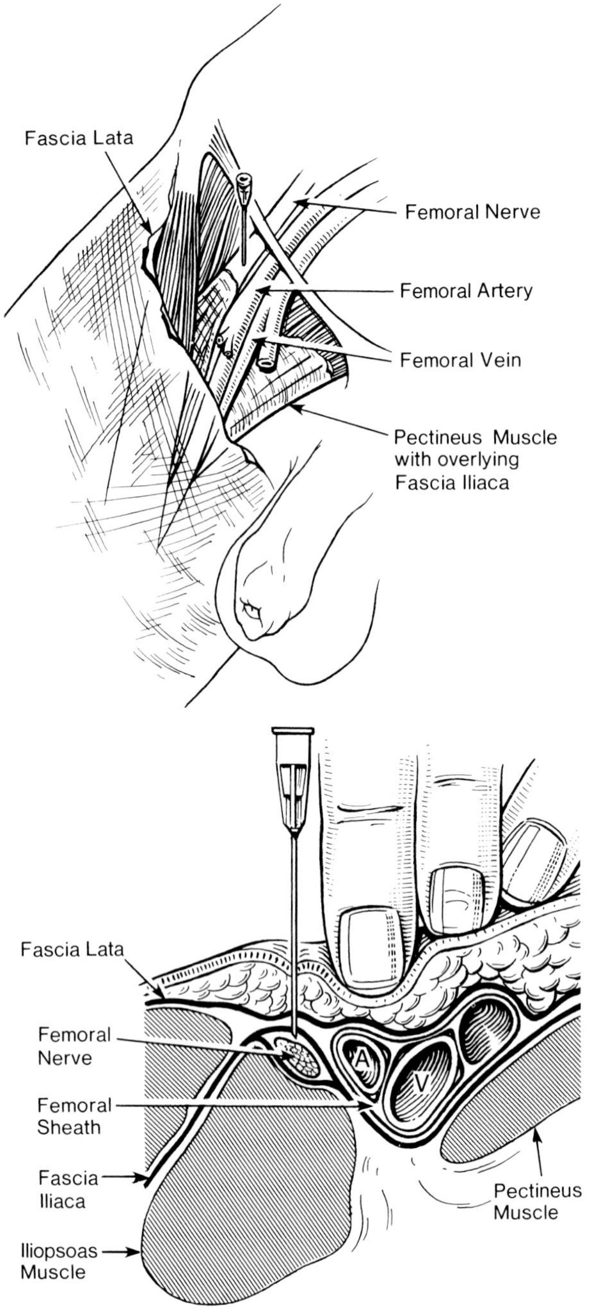

FIG. 20-2. Femoral nerve block (see text). The femoral nerve lies in a canal immediately lateral to the femoral artery just below the inguinal ligament. It lies deep to fascia lata and fascia iliaca. Loss of resistance can be felt twice when a short beveled needle is inserted through these two layers. The femoral artery and vein lie deep to fascia lata but superficial to fascia iliaca. (Khoo, S.T., and Brown, T.C.K.: Anaesth. Intensire Care, *11*:40, 1983.)

tures (Fig. 20-2).[91] Such blocks are performed often in emergency departments. The femoral artery is located with the left hand, and the skin is prepared. The needle, with a nerve stimulator electrode attached, is advanced perpendicularly to the skin, just lateral to the arterial pulsation, until the two "pops" are felt, or until the quadriceps muscle begins to contract at the patella. One must not be distracted by a sartorius contraction, because the tip of the needle is not at the optimal location at the time this occurs. Once the quadriceps muscle contracts, the needle is withdrawn slowly until the contraction ceases, then advanced slowly until the strongest contraction is noted. At this point, after negative aspiration for blood, 0.5 to 1.0 ml of local anesthetic solution should abolish the twitch. Once this occurs, the remainder of the solution is injected. Aspiration should be performed frequently during injection. Continuous blockade of the femoral nerve

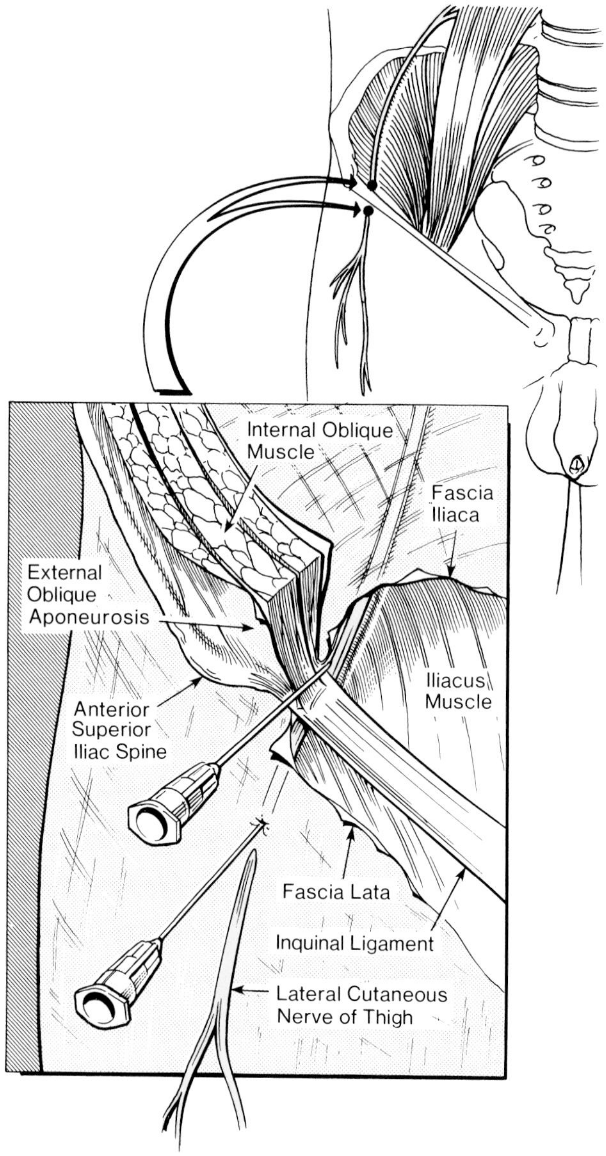

FIG. 20-3. Lateral cutaneous nerve of thigh block (see text). The lateral cutaneous nerve of the thigh passes inferiorly on iliacus muscle covered by iliacus fascia. Just medial to the anterior superior iliac spine it turns anteriorly to pass just below the inguinal ligament and runs deep to the fascia lata until it emerges subcutaneously. The lateral cutaneous nerve can be blocked (**1**) just medial to the anterior superior iliac spine, when loss of resistance is felt on passing through the external oblique aponeurosis and on emerging through the internal oblique muscle or (**2**) 1 to 2 cm below the anterior superior iliac spine by injecting deep to fascia lata.

can also be used to provide protracted postoperative analgesia.[106]

Lateral Cutaneous Nerve of the Thigh Block

Lateral cutaneous nerve of the thigh block can be used to perform muscle biopsies and skin graft donations from the anterior aspect of the thigh.[105] The technique for this individual nerve block is similar to that used in adults, with injection just medial to the anterior superior iliac spine (Fig. 20-3). The first loss of resistance will be felt as the needle passes through the external oblique aponeurosis, and the second as the needle emerges through the external oblique muscle and enters the fascial canal containing the nerve. If a lumbar plexus block is performed in conjunction with a sciatic nerve block, one can provide surgical anesthesia and postoperative analgesia for all lower extremity procedures.[40]

Nerve Blocks at the Knee

Nerve blocks at the level of the knee have been employed for postoperative analgesia as well as to provide excellent motor blockade for physical therapy in children with severe muscle spasms.[25,90] Tibial nerve block can be performed with the patient prone, by placing a needle just lateral to the midpoint of a line drawn from the apex of the popliteal fossa and the midpoint of a line drawn between the femoral condyles (Fig. 20-4). The nerve lies about 0.5 cm deep to the fascia covering the popliteal fossa; use of a peripheral nerve stimulator may be helpful.

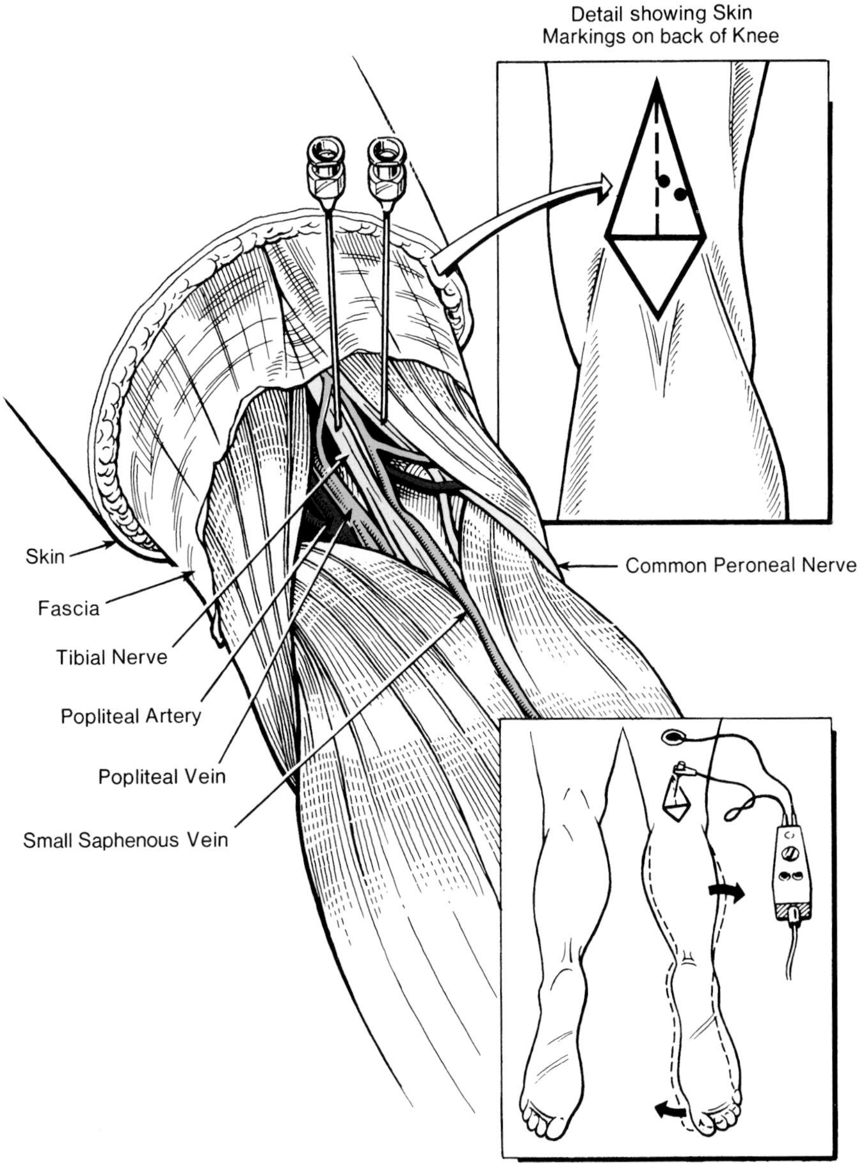

FIG. 20-4. Tibial and common peroneal nerve block (see text). The tibial and common peroneal (lateral popliteal) nerves diverge in the popliteal fossa, which is bounded by biceps femoris muscle laterally and semimembranosus muscle medially. They can be blocked as they pass through the triangle formed by these muscles and a line drawn between the femoral condyles. As the needle is inserted, a loss of resistance should be felt as the needle penetrates the fascia overlying the popliteal fossa.

The common peroneal nerve leaves the tibial nerve at the apex of the popliteal fossa, and runs laterally just medial to the biceps femoris muscle and deep to the popliteal fossa. The block should not be performed at the neck of the fibula, because neuralgia is more likely to occur. The saphenous nerve can be blocked by infiltration just posterior to the medial border of the tibia in the vicinity of the long saphenous vein just below the knee (see also Chapter 11, Fig. 11-11).

ILIOINGUINAL/ILIOHYPOGASTRIC NERVE BLOCK (see Chapter 14)

This simple block produces profound postoperative analgesia following outpatient hernia repair in children.[99,145] Children who received this block following the induction of anesthesia but prior to inguinal hernia repair required significantly less systemic analgesic, even after 48 hours. This technique can be used for other procedures requiring an inguinal incision (e.g., hydrocelectomy and orchiopexy).[75] However, wound infiltration at the end of surgery, or simple instillation of bupivacaine at the completion of surgical dissection, also provides postoperative analgesia.[34,118] Addition of oral or rectal nonsteroidal anti-inflammatory agents can augment the analgesia supplied by the ilioinguinal nerve block (see also Chapter 14, Fig. 14-14).[107]

Technique

Both ilioinguinal and iliohypogastric nerves can be blocked easily by a simple infiltration of the abdominal wall in the area medial to the anterior superior iliac spine (Fig. 20-5). A 25-gauge needle is used to puncture the skin 1/2 inch medial and 1/2 inch inferior to the anterior superior iliac spine, just above the inguinal ligament. Three "pops" will be felt as the skin, external, and internal oblique fascias are pierced; several fan-shaped injections of 3 to 5 ml of bupivacaine, 0.25 to 0.5%, are made as the needle is withdrawn, plus a subcutaneous wheal. Alternatively, if the block is performed at the completion of surgery, the area to be infiltrated may be approached through the lateral edge of the groin incision. Transient femoral paresis has been reported following this block, however. If femoral blockade should occur, observation is all that is required until the femoral block dissipates.[134]

Casey and others demonstrated that analgesia may be obtained by instilling 5 ml of bupivacaine, 0.25%, into the

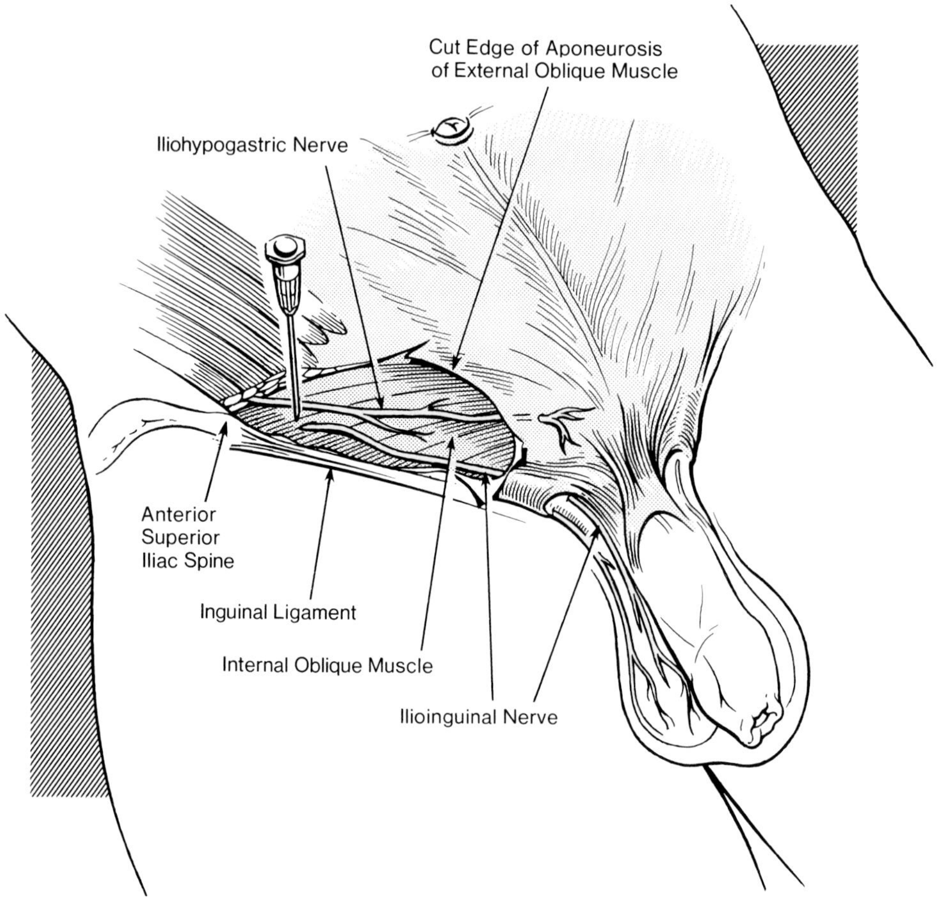

FIG. 20-5. Ilioinguinal and iliohypogastric nerve block (see text). The ilioinguinal nerve emerges though the internal oblique muscle about 1 to 2 cm medial to the anterior superior iliac spine. It lies deep to the external oblique aponeurosis, which can be felt when a short beveled needle is passed through it.

wound following completion of surgical dissection, but prior to hernia repair.[34] This simple instillation of local anesthetic to exposed ilioinguinal nerve as well as muscle fibers provided analgesia identical to that provided by wound edge infiltration performed at the end of the surgical procedure.

Stow and colleagues evaluated plasma bupivacaine concentrations following caudal analgesia (bupivacaine 2mg/kg)or ilioinguinal nerve block (1.5 mg/kg).[150] Peak concentrations occurred between 20 and 30 minutes, and plasma concentrations were low (0.25 to 0.72 μg/ml). Others have evaluated serum bupivacaine concentrations following ilioinguinal-iliohypogastric block and wound edge infiltration, and have found similarly low concentrations.[118]

PENILE BLOCK

Blockade of the dorsal nerves of the penis provides effective analgesia for penile surgery, such as hypospadias repair or circumcision. Skin flushing, mild cyanosis, and vomiting, are common in newborns who have undergone circumcision without anesthesia; penile block reduced these physiologic stresses.[165] Peak serum lidocaine levels, noted at 60 minutes, were less than those seen in infants whose mothers had received epidural analgesia.[144] Others have demonstrated the efficacy of penile block in older boys undergoing circumcision.[29,44]

Anatomy

The distal 2/3 of the penis is innervated by the dorsal nerves, which are bilateral and adjacent to the midline (Fig. 20-6). The dorsal nerves are distal twigs of the pudendal nerves, which arise from the sacral plexus (S2, 3, 4). At the base of the penis, these nerves divide into multiple filaments that encircle the shaft before reaching the glans. The dorsal penile nerves are covered by Buck's fascia and lie alongside

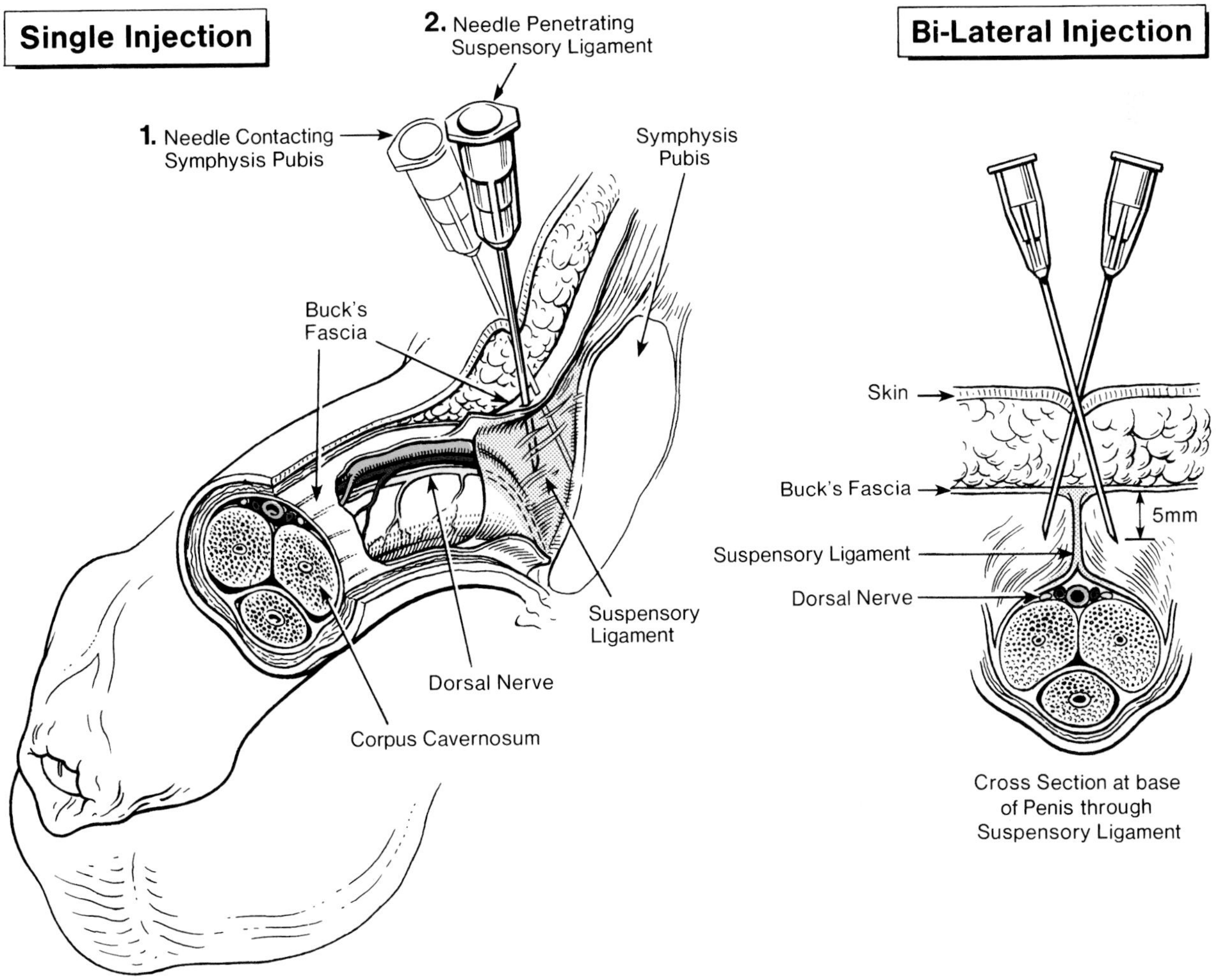

FIG. 20-6. Dorsal nerve of penis block (see text). The dorsal nerves of the penis, derived from the pudendal nerve, run anteriorly below the pubis on the corpora cavernosa. They are most commonly blocked as they traverse the triangular space bounded by the pubic symphysis, the corpora cavernosa, and Buck's facia. In the transverse section the nerves lie deep to the suspensory ligament of the penis, at which point it splits to surround the penis. **Left:** Lateral view. **Right:** Cross-section. The needle must penetrate Buck's fascia. The injection is then made on either side of the suspensory ligament: through a single midline insertion or through bilateral insertions. *Note:* Size has been expanded to aid visualization.

the dorsal artery and veins of the penis, and the midline structures. The base and proximal part of the penis are innervated by the genitofemoral and ilioinguinal nerves.

Technique

The most popular penile block technique is injection of the dorsal nerves of the penis. Dorsal penile nerve block involves one or two injections of 1 to 2 ml of local anesthetic deep to Buck's fascia. Fontaine and coworkers employed a block in the newborn involving 0.4 ml of local anesthetic injected at the 10 o'clock and 2 o'clock positions at the base of the penis.[64] Brown and colleagues, investigating the anatomic basis of this block, by using injected radiologic contrast medium and dissection techniques, noted that the double-injection technique provided a more satisfactory diffusion of local anesthetic than did a single injection.[30]

Dalens and co-workers described penile blockade via the subpubic space in children, thereby blocking the nerves before their entry into the base of the penis.[44] There is less chance of injuring neurovascular or other penile structures with this technique. The Dalens method involves insertion of a 25-gauge needle 0.5 to 1 cm on either side of the midline, directed approximately 70° to the skin. The needle is then advanced medial and caudal at approximately 20°. Two injections of 0.1 mg/kg of bupivacaine or lidocaine are necessary, because the 2 subpubic compartments do not communicate.

An easier technique for penile blockade was described by Broadman and coworkers.[29] The subcutaneous ring block involves circumferential subcutaneous infiltration of the base of the penis with 0.25% bupivacaine. It is critical to avoid epinephrine-containing solutions for any penile block technique. The penis is an end organ; vasoconstriction with epinephrine may seriously compromise its circulation.

No complications have been reported with the ring block. However, Sara and Lowry noted two occurrences of gangrene of the tip of the penis after blocks using the dorsal penile nerve block technique.[138] The authors postulate that perfusion was probably impaired by hematoma formation resulting from the puncture of blood vessels. Berens reported a 2-day-old who was given a dorsal penile nerve block with an epinephrine-containing solution resulting in profound vasoconstriction and ischemia of the genitalia.[17] A caudal block was employed to provide a sympathectomy for treatment of this complication.

Topical lidocaine has been used to produce penile analgesia after circumcision, although the dorsal nerve block may provide more effective analgesia.[5,35] In two studies by Tree-Trakarn and colleagues, lidocaine spray, ointment, and jelly were found to be equally effective in reducing pain and avoiding the need for postoperative analgesics, and lidocaine jelly proved an effective after-hospital treatment for such pain.[153,154] Lidocaine spray was the preparation preferred by the children, because it could be applied repeatedly without contact with the wound. As was previously mentioned, EMLA cream has also been found effective for topical anesthesia of the glans penis.[101]

INTERCOSTAL NERVE BLOCKS (see Chapter 14)

These blocks are useful in pediatric patients not only for the relief of postoperative pain, but also for relief of pain from rib fractures following chest trauma. Blocking the upper thoracic nerves provides analgesia to the chest wall and blocking the lower provides analgesia to the abdominal wall.

Anatomy and technique of performance of intercostal blockade are similar in infants, children, and adults. The distance from the rib margin to the pleura may be no greater than 2 mm in the young child; consequently very short needles are most appropriate.

Rothstein and colleagues demonstrated that intercostal nerve blocks could be used to provide safe and effective pain relief in children following unilateral thoracic surgeries.[133] These investigators administered 2, 3, and 4 mg/kg of bupivacaine 0.5% with 1 : 200,000 epinephrine by performing percutaneous intercostal nerve blocks at 5 levels. Plasma bupivacaine concentrations were measured at 5-minute intervals for 15 minutes, then at 30, 60, 120, and 180 minutes following block placement. Mean plasma levels were dose-dependent and ranged from 0.77 μg/kg when 2 mg/kg was administered, to 1.87 μg/kg when 4 mg/kg was employed. The authors noted that the volume of distribution of bupivacaine was greater and clearance was more rapid in children than in adults, and recommended that no more than 3 mg/kg of bupivacaine be employed for intercostal blockade.

Bricker at al. repeated the Rothstein study in neonates and infants less than 6 months of age; however, all blocks were placed by the surgeon under direct visualization prior to chest closure, and 1.5 mg/kg of bupivacaine was employed.[27] These workers found no difference between neonatal (0.82 μg/kg) and infant (0.91 μg/kg) blood levels following intercostal blockade.

INTERPLEURAL BLOCK (see Chapter 14)

The interpleural block may be used to provide analgesia following thoracotomy or upper abdominal surgery, or for patients with thoracic trauma or rib fractures. McIlvaine and colleagues reported the successful use of bupivacaine via interpleural infusion to provide postoperative analgesia in 14 pediatric patients, ranging in age from 5 months to 18 years, undergoing anterior spinal fusion or aortic coarctation surgery.[115] No patient required supplemental analgesia during the 24-hour infusion of bupivacaine 0.25% with 1:200,000 epinephrine at a rate of 0.5 ml/kg/hr. Although plasma bupivacaine levels exceeded 4 μg/ml in 5 of the children, and 7 μg/ml in one child, no systemic toxic effects of the local anesthetic were noted in any child.

This block has limitations in the pediatric population for three reasons:

1. Plasma bupivacaine levels frequently exceed the accepted adult toxic limit of 4 μg/ml after a 24-hour infusion of what is considered to be an accepted infusion rate and total dose of bupivacaine.
2. The analgesia is posture-dependent and children must remain in bed in the supine position to obtain effective analgesia.
3. There is a substantial risk of developing a pneumothorax if a percutaneous technique is employed in a child who does not have a tube thoracostomy on the side where the interpleural catheter is placed. The technique for placement is similar to that in adults.

PARAVERTEBRAL BLOCK

Lönnqvist recently has demonstrated that a catheter can be placed in order to provide continuous paravertebral block.[103] Eng and Sabanathan have utilized percutaneous placement of catheters to infuse bupivacaine at a rate of 0.5 mg/kg/hr to provide profound postoperative analgesia to children following thoracotomy.[54]

Technique (see Chapter 11, Fig. 11-2)

The anesthetized child is turned into the lateral position, with the side to be blocked placed uppermost, and the skin of the back is punctured 1 to 2 cm lateral to the spinous processes of T7–T9. The epidural needle should be inserted at a right angle to the skin and advanced until contact is made with the transverse process. The needle is then walked off the superior border of the transverse process, and the paravertebral space is identified by using a saline loss-of-resistance technique. Loss of resistance is noted as the needle tip pierces the costotransverse ligament, and 2 to 3 cm of catheter is threaded. A test dose of 1.5 ml of 0.25% bupivacaine with epinephrine, 1 : 200,000, is administered, followed by a bolus dose of 0.5 ml/kg and an infusion of 0.25 ml/kg/hr.

Because of the risks of pneumothorax and laceration of blood vessels and the potential for sudden high plasma levels of local anesthetic, paravertebral blocks have very few indications in pediatric patients; even in experienced hands, this technique is much less popular than other regional procedures such as epidural block.[104]

TOPICAL ANESTHESIA

Skin

The solid, pure, bases of lidocaine and prilocaine constitute a eutectic mixture (EMLA) that forms an emulsion when mixed together.[67] A concentration of 80% lidocaine-prilocaine is achieved by a cream that has only a 5% concentration of local anesthetic. The high concentration of lidocaine and prilocaine in an unionized form in this high-water-content medium stimulates transdermal spread (see Chapter 4).

EMLA is applied to dry, intact, skin, covered with an occlusive dressing, and left for an hour. Under those circumstances, EMLA penetrates intact skin and provides anesthesia to a depth of 5 mm. It is therefore very useful for painful superficial procedures in the unsedated child.[108] EMLA has also been used for neonatal circumcision, and to facilitate the lysis of prepucial adhesions in older boys.[13]

Children who are using EMLA for the first time will still be afraid of the needle. Maunuksela and Korpela noted a significant difference in 4- to 10-year-old children who reported no pain following EMLA, and those who reported severe pain after receiving a placebo.[108] Soliman and colleagues, on the other hand, found no difference in children's self-report pain scores following venipuncture, in a study comparing EMLA with intradermal lidocaine.[147] Lack of cooperation by both groups of children during venipuncture indicated that the emotional component of anticipating pain was strong even when the child stated that his "skin was sleepy." Even in infants and toddlers, the use of EMLA greatly decreases pain behaviors during invasive procedures.

EMLA should be used with caution in infants less than 3 months of age, or in patients who are taking sulfonamides or other methemoglobin-inducing medications, because of the potential of methemoglobinemia.[84] However, venous plasma levels of methemoglobin after application of 2 ml of EMLA for 4 hours were only 2% of the total hemoglobin. Other local anesthetic preparations are currently being evaluated as alternatives to EMLA.[65]

TAC (tetracaine 0.5%, adrenaline 1:2000, cocaine 11.8%) is used in emergency departments to provide analgesia for children with superficial lacerations.[87] A cotton ball is saturated with TAC solution and taped over the wound surface for 15 to 20 minutes before suturing. Systemic cocaine toxicity has been reported in children after misuse of TAC (excessive doses, mucosal application, and application to burned skin). Both cocaine and adrenaline are vasoconstrictors; consequently this compound should not be employed on end-organs such as digits, nose and penis.

Mucous Membrane

Topical anesthesia may be employed in the nose and nasopharynx before passage of a nasotracheal tube, as well as in the mouth to reduce the response to an oral airway, or in the larynx and trachea before passage of a bronchoscope. The considerations in choosing agents for these purposes in adults apply also in children.[4,58] An appropriate dose of lidocaine for topical spray would be 2 mg/kg. Prolonged seizures have been reported with viscous lidocaine; again, it is important to be aware of the dose of local anesthetic administered into this highly vascular area.[4]

Topical anesthesia is a great help during bronchoscopy. The local anesthetic may be applied by hand spray, jet spray, syringe and perforated cannula, or pledget. When possible, the container should hold only the maximum safe amount of anesthetic to be used. The delivery of most atomizers varies greatly with the position in which it is held.

Topical anesthesia also may be useful in cystoscopic procedures. An aqueous jelly applied to the urethra often enables the anesthesiologist to use very light supplemental general anesthesia.

Local Infiltration

Local anesthesia may be the best technique for intravenous catheter placement, vascular cutdown, and other superficial procedures on premature or sick newborns. In such cases, the infant is held in position by well-padded restraints, and 0.5% lidocaine or 0.5% bupivacaine is infiltrated along the line of incision.

Wound edge infiltration can also provide postoperative analgesia, such as with hernia repair or pyloromyotomy. Surgeons frequently employ subcutaneous injection of local anesthetics and epinephrine, to decrease blood loss. A total of 2.5 mg/kg of bupivacaine 0.25% or 0.5%, or a total of 5 mg/kg of 0.25% or 0.5% lidocaine may be utilized.[16,89] Addition of epinephrine increases the permissible amount of lidocaine because of its vasoconstrictive effect and consequent decrease in blood levels of local anesthetic.

REFERENCES

1. Abajian, J.C., Mellish, R.W.P., Brown A.F., *et al.*: Spinal anesthesia for surgery in the high-risk infant. Anesth. Analg., *63:*359, 1984.
2. Adornato, D.C., Goldenberg, P.L., Ferrario, C.M., *et al.*: Pathophysiology of intravenous air embolism in dogs. Anesthesiology, *49:*120, 1978.
3. Agarwal, R., Gutlove, D.P., and Lockhart, C.H.: Seizures occurring in pediatric patients receiving continuous infusion of bupivacaine. Anesth. Analg., *75:*284, 1992.
4. Amitai, Y., Zylber-Katz, E., Avital, A., Zangen, D., and Noviski, N.: Serum lidocaine concentrations in children during bronchoscopy with topical anesthesia. Chest, *98:*1370, 1990.
5. Andersen, K.H.: A new method of analgesia for relief of circumcision pain. Anaesthesia, *44:*118, 1989.
6. Armitage, E.N.: Local anaesthetic techniques for prevention of postoperative pain., Br. J. Anaesth., *58:*790, 1986.
7. Arthur, D.S., and McNicol, L.P.: Local anaesthetic techniques in paediatric surgery. Br. J. Anaesth., *58:*760, 1986.
8. Attia, J., Ecoffey, C., Sandouik, P., *et al.*: Epidural morphine in children: Pharmacokinetics and CO_2 sensitivity. Anesthesiology, *65:*590, 1986.
9. Audenaert S.M., Vickers, H., and Burgess, R.C.: Axillary block for vascular insufficiency after repair of radial club hands in an infant. Anesthesiology, *74:*368, 1991.
10. Badgwell, J.M., Heavner, J.E., and Kytta, J.: Bupivacaine toxicity in young pigs is age dependent and is affected by volatile agents, Anesthesiology, *73:*297, 1990.
11. Bailey, A., Valley, R., and Peacock, J.: Regional anaesthesia in high risk infants. Can. J. Anaesth., *39:*203, 1992.
12. Bailey, A.B., Valley, F.D., Fried, R.F., *et al.*: Epidural morphine combined with epidural butorphanol for postoperative analgesia. Anesthesiology, *79:*A1136, 1993.
13. Benini, F., Johnston, C., Faucher, D., and Aranda, J.V.: Topical anesthesia during circumcision in newborn infants. J.A.M.A., *270:*850, 1993.
14. Berde, C.B., Sethna, N.F., Yemen, T.A., *et al.*: Continuous epidural bupivacaine-fentanyl infusions in children following ureteral reimplantation. Anesthesiology, *73:*A1128, 1990.
15. Berde, C.B.: Convulsions associated with pediatric regional anesthesia. Anesth. Analg., *75:*164, 1992.
16. Berde, C.B.: Toxicity of local anesthetics in infants and children. J. Pediatr., *122:*S14, 1993.
17. Berens, R., and Pontus, S.P.: A complication associated with dorsal penile nerve block. Reg. Anesth., *15:*309, 1990.
18. Berkowitz, S., and Greene, B.A.: Spinal anesthesia in children: Report based on 350 patients under 13 years of age. Anesthesiology, *12:*376, 1950.
19. Bier, A.: Experiments regarding the cocainization of the spinal cord. Z. Chir., *51:*361, 1899.
20. Blaise, G., and Roy, W.L.: Spinal anaesthesia for minor paediatric surgery. Can. Anaesth. Soc. J., *33:*227, 1986.
21. Bolder, P.M.: Postlumbar puncture headache in pediatric oncology patients. Anesthesiology, *65:*696, 1986.
22. Bonadio, W.A., Smith, D.S., Metrou, M., *et al.*: Estimating lumbar puncture depth in children. N. Engl. J. Med., *319:*952, 1988.
23. Bösenberg, A.T., Bland, B.A.R., Schülte-Steinberg, O., and Downing, J.W.: Thoracic epidural anesthesia via the caudal route in infants. Anesthesiology, *69:*265, 1988.
24. Bösenberg, A.T., and Kimble, F.W.: Infraorbital nerve block in neonates for cleft lip repair: Anatomical study and clinical application. Br. J. Anaesth., *74:*506, 1995.
25. Bösenberg, A.T.: Lower limb nerve blocks in children using unsheathed needles and a nerve stimulator. Anaesthesia, *50:*206, 1995.
26. Brendel, J.K., Yemen, T.A., and Berry, F.A.: Intravenous injection of local anesthetic: Identification with isoproterenol and epinephrine in children during halothane anesthesia. Reg. Anesth., *18:*49, 1993.
27. Bricker, S.R.W., Telford, R.J., and Booker, P.D.: Pharmacokinetics of bupivacaine following intraoperative intercostal nerve block in neonates and infants aged less than 6 months. Anesthesiology, *70:*942, 1989.
28. Broadman, L.M., and Hannallah, R.S.: Regional anesthesia in children—An analysis of risk and parental acceptance. Reg. Anesth., *10:* 33, 1985.
29. Broadman, L.M., Hannallah, R.S., Belman, A.B., *et al.*: Post-circumcision analgesia—A prospective evaluation of subcutaneous ring block of the penis. Anesthesiology, *67:*399, 1987.
30. Brown, T.C.K., Weidner, N.J., and Bouwmeester, J.: Dorsal nerve of penis block—anatomical and radiological studies. Anaesth. Intensive Care, *17:*34, 1989.
31. Burrows, F.A., Lerman, J., and LeDez, K.M.: Alpha$_1$-acid glycoprotein and the binding of lidocaine in children with congenital heart disease. Can. J. Anaesth., *37:*883, 1990.
32. Busoni, P., and Andreuccetti, T.: The spread of caudal analgesia in children: A mathematical model. Anaesth. Intensive Care, *14:*140, 1986.
33. Campbell, R.J., Ilett, K.F., and Dusci, L.: Plasma bupivacaine concentrations after axillary block in children. Anaesth. Intensive Care, *14:*343, 1986.
34. Casey, W.F., Rice, L.J., Hannallah, R.S., *et al.:* A comparison between bupivacaine instillation versus ilioinguinal/iliohypogastric nerve block for postoperative analgesia following inguinal herniorrhaphy in children. Anesthesiology, *72:*637, 1990.
35. Chambers, F.A., Lee, J., Smith, J., and Casey, W.: Post-circumcision analgesia: Comparison of topical analgesia with dorsal nerve block using the midline and lateral approaches. Br. J. Anaesth., *73:*437, 1994.
36. Colizza, W.A., and Said, E.: Intravenous regional anaesthesia in the treatment of forearm and wrist fractures and dislocations in children. Can. J. Surg., *36:*225, 1993.
37. Cox, R.G., and Goresky, G.V.: Life-threatening apnea following spinal anesthesia in former pre-term infants. Anesthesiology, *73:*345, 1990.
38. Dalens, B., Tanguy, A., and Haberer, J.P.: Lumbar epidural anesthesia for operative and postoperative pain relief in infants and young children. Anesth. Analg., *65:*1069, 1986.
39. Dalens, B., Vanneuville, G., and Tanguy, A.: A new approach to the brachial plexus in children: Comparison with the supraclavicular approach. Anesth. Analg., *66:*1264, 1987.
40. Dalens, B., Tanguy, A., and Vanneuville G.: Lumbar plexus blocks in children: A comparison of two procedures in 50 patients. Anesth. Analg., *67:*750, 1988.
41. Dalens, B., and Hasnouai, A.: Caudal anesthesia in pediatric surgery: Success rates and adverse effects in 750 consecutive patients. Anesth. Analg., *68:*83, 1989.
42. Dalens, B.: Regional anesthesia in children. Anesth. Analg., *68:*654, 1989.
43. Dalens, B., Vanneuville, G., and Tanguy, A.: Comparison of the fascia iliaca compartment block with the 3-in-1 block in children. Anesth. Analg., *69:*705, 1989.

44. Dalens, B., Vanneuville, G., and Dechelotte, P.: Penile block via the subpubic space in 100 children, Anesth. Analg., *69:*41, 1989.
45. Dalens, B., Vanneuville, G., and Tanguy, A.: Sciatic nerve blocks in children: Comparison of the posterior, anterior and lateral approaches in 180 pediatric patients. Anesth. Analg., *70:*131, 1990.
46. Desparmet, J., Meistelman, C., Barre, J., and Saint-Maurice, C.: Continuous epidural infusion of bupivacaine for postoperative pain relief in children. Anesthesiology, *67:*108, 1987.
47. Desparmet, J.F.: Total spinal after caudal anesthesia in an infant. Anesth. Analg., *70:*665, 1990.
48. Desparmet, J., Mateo, J., Ecoffey, C., *et al.*: Efficacy of an epidural test dose in children anesthetized with halothane. Anesthesiology, *72:* 249, 1990.
49. Dohi, S., Naito, H., and Takahashi, T.: Age-related changes in blood pressure and duration of motor block in spinal anesthesia. Anesthesiology, *50:*319, 1979.
50. Eather, K.F.: Regional anesthesia for infants and children. Int. Anesthesiol. Clin., *13:*19, 1975.
51. Ecoffey, C., Desparmet, J., Berdeaux, A., *et al.*: Pharmacokinetics of lignocaine in children following caudal anaesthesia. Br. J. Anaesth., *56:*1399, 1984.
52. Ecoffey, C., Doubousset, A.M., and Samii, K.: Lumbar and thoracic anesthesia for urologic and upper abdominal surgery in infants and children. Anesthesiology, *65:*87, 1986.
53. Edwards, W.T., and Burney, R.G.: Use of repeated nerve blocks in management of an infant with Kawasaki's disease. Anesth. Analg., *67:*1008, 1988.
54. Eng, J., and Sabanathan, S.: Continuous paravertebral block for postthoracotomy analgesia in children. J. Pediatr. Surg., *27:*556, 1992.
55. Epstein, B.S., and Hannallah, R.S.: The pediatric patient. *In* Wechsler, B, ed: Anesthesia for ambulatory surgery. pp. 131. Philadelphia, J.B. Lippincott Company, 1991.
56. Eyres, R.L., Kidd, J., Oppenheim, R., and Brown, T.C.K.: Local anaesthetic plasma levels in children. Anaesth. Intensive Care, *6:*243, 1978.
57. Eyres, R.L., Bishop, W., Oppenheim, R., *et al.*: Plasma bupivacaine concentrations in children during caudal epidural analgesia. Anaesth. Intensive Care, *11:*20, 1983.
58. Eyres, R.L., Bishop, W., and Brown, T.C.K.: Plasma lignocaine levels following topical laryngeal application. Anaesth. Intensive Care, *11:*20, 1983.
59. Eyres, R.L., Hastings, C., Brown, T.C.K., *et al.*: Plasma bupivacaine concentrations following lumbar epidural anaesthetic in children. Anaesth. Intensive Care., *14:*131, 1986.
60. Eyres, R.L.: Local anaesthetic agents in infancy. Paediatr. Anaesth., *5:*213, 1995.
61. Farr, R.E.: Local anesthesia in infancy and childhood. Arch. Pediatr., *37:*381, 1920.
62. Finholt, D.A., Stirt, J.A., DiFazio, C.A., *et al.*: Lidocaine pharmacokinetics in children during general anesthesia. Anesth. Analg., *65:* 279, 1986.
63. Fisher, Q.A., McComiskey, C.M., and Hill, J.L., *et al.*: Postoperative voiding interval and duration of analgesia following peripheral or caudal nerve blocks in children. Anesth. Analg., *76:*173, 1993.
64. Fontaine, P., and Toffler, W.L.: Dorsal penile nerve block for newborn circumcision. Am. Fam. Physician, *43:*1327, 1991.
65. Freeman, J.A., Doyle, E., Im, N.T., and Morton, N.S.: Topical anaesthesia of the skin: A review. Paediatr. Anaesth., *3:*129, 1993.
66. Freid, E.B., Bailey, A.G., and Valley, R.D.: Electrocardiographic and hemodynamic changes associated with unintentional intravascular injection of bupivacaine with epinephrine in infants. Anesthesiology, *79:*394, 1993.
67. Gajraj, N.M., Pennant, J.H., and Watcha, M.F.: Eutectic mixture of local anesthetics (EMLA) cream. Anesth. Analg., *78:*574, 1994.
68. Gleason, C.A., Martin, R., Anderson, J.V., *et al.*: Optimal position for a spinal tap in preterm infants. Pediatrics, *71:*31, 1983.
69. Goresky, G.V., Klassen, K., and Waters, J.H.: Postoperative pain management for children. Anesthesiol. Clin. North Am., *9:*801, 1991.
70. Guinard, J-P., and Borboen, M.: Probable venous air embolism during caudal anesthesia in a child. Anesth. Analg., *76:*1134, 1993.
71. Gunter, J.: Caudal anesthesia in children: A survey. Anesthesiology, *75:*A936, 1991.
72. Gunter, J.B., Watcha, M.F., Forestner, J.E., *et al.*: Caudal epidural anesthesia in conscious premature and high-risk infants. J. Pediatr. Surg., *26:*9, 1991.
73. Gunter, J.B., and Eng, C.: Thoracic epidural anesthesia via the caudal approach in children. Anesthesiology, *76:*935, 1992.
74. Haber, B.W., and Berde, C.B.: Spinal opioids for pediatric pain management. *In* Sinatra, R.S., Hord, A.B., Ginsberg, S., *et al.*, eds.: Acute pain, mechanisms and management. pp. 470. St. Louis, Mosby–Year Book, 1992.
75. Hannallah, R.S., Broadman, L.M., Belman, A.B., *et al.*: Comparison of caudal and ilioinguinal/iliohypogastric nerve blocks for control of post-orchiopexy pain in pediatric ambulatory surgery. Anesthesiology, *66:*832, 1987.
76. Hargreaves, D.M., Spargo, P.M., and Wheeler, R.A.: Caudal blockade in the management of aortic thrombosis following umbilical artery catheterisation. Anaesthesia, *47:*493, 1992.
77. Harnik, E.V., Goy, G.R., Potolicchio, S., *et al.*: Spinal anesthesia in premature infants recovering from respiratory distress syndrome. Anesthesiology, *64:*95, 1986.
78. Harris, M.M., Kahana, M.D., and Park, T.S.: Intrathecal morphine for postoperative analgesia in children after selective dorsal root rhizotomy. Neurosurgery, *28:*519, 1991.
79. Hastings, C.L., Brown, T.C.K., Eyres, R.L., *et al.*: The influence of age on lignocaine pharmacokinetics in young puppies. Anaesth. Intensive Care, *14:*135, 1986.
80. Hatch, D.J., Hulse, M.G., and Lindahl, S.G.E.: Caudal analgesia in children: Influence on ventilatory efficiency during halothane anaesthesia. Anaesthesia, *39:*873, 1984.
81. Heavner, J.E., Dryden, C.F., Sanghani, V., *et al.*: Severe hypoxia enhances central nervous system and cardiovascular toxicity of bupivacaine in lightly anesthetized pigs. Anesthesiology, *77:*142, 1992.
82. Henderson, K., Sethna, N.F., and Berde, C.B.: Continuous caudal anesthesia for inguinal hernia repair in former preterm infants. J. Clin. Anesth., *5:*129, 1993.
83. Hughes, P.J., and Brown, T.C.K.: An approach to posterior femoral cutaneous nerve block. Anaesth. Intensive Care., *14:*350, 1986.
84. Jakobson, B., and Nilsson, A.: Methemoglobinemia associated with prilocaine-lidocaine cream and trimethoprim sulfomethoxazole: A case report. Acta Anaesthesiol., Scand., *29:*453, 1985.
85. Jamali, S., Monin, S., Begon, C., *et al.*: Clonidine in pediatric caudal anesthesia. Anesth. Analg., *78:*663, 1994.
86. Jebelees, J.A., Reilly, J.S., Gutierrez, J.F., *et al.*: The effect of preincisional infiltration of tonsils with bupivacaine on the pain following tonsillectomy under general anesthesia. Pain, *47:*305, 1991.
87. Jeter, J.H., and Mueller, D.: TAC gel—a sterile formulation. Ann. Emerg. Med., *23:*600, 1994.
88. Johnson, C.M.: Continuous femoral nerve blockade for analgesia in children with femoral fractures. Anaesth. Intensive Care, *22:*281, 1994.
89. Karl, H.W., Swedlow, D.B., Lee, K.W., *et al.*: Epinephrine-halothane interactions in children. Anesthesiology, *58:*142, 1983.
90. Kempthorne, P.M., and Brown, T.C.K.: Nerve blocks around the knee in children. Anaesth. Intensive Care, *12:*14, 1984.
91. Khoo, S.T., and Brown, T.C.K.: Femoral nerve block—The anatomic basis for a single injection technique. Anaesth. Intensive Care, *11:*40, 1983.
92. Krane, E.J., Jacobson, L.E., Lynn, A.M., *et al.*: Caudal morphine for postoperative analgesia in children: A comparison with caudal bupivacaine and intravenous morphine. Anesth. Analg. *66:*647, 1987.
93. Krane, E.J.: Delayed respiratory depression in a child after caudal epidural morphine. Anesth. Analg., *67:*79, 1988.
94. Krane, E.J., Tyler, D.C., and Jacobson, L.E.: The dose response of caudal morphine in children. Anesthesiology, *71:*48, 1989.
95. Krane, E.J., Haberkern, C.M., and Jacobson, L.E.: Postoperative apnea, bradycardia, and oxygen desaturation in formerly premature infants: Prospective comparison of spinal and general anesthesia. Anesth. Analg., *80:*7, 1995.
96. Kumagai, M., and Yamashita, M.: Sacral intervertebral approach for epidural anaesthesia in infants and children: Application of "drip and tube" method. Anaesth. Intensive Care, *23:*469, 1995.
97. Kumar, V, Maves, T., and Barcellos, W.: Epidural blood patch for treatment of subarachnoid fistula in children. Anaesthesia, *46:*117, 1991.
98. Kyttä, J., Heavner, J.E., Badgwell, J.M., and Rosenberg, P.H.: Cardiovascular and central nervous system effects of coadministered lidocaine and bupivacaine in piglets. Reg. Anesth., *16:*89, 1991.
99. Langer, J.C., Shandling, B., and Rosenberg, M.: Intraoperative bupivacaine during outpatient hernia repair in children: A randomized double blind trial. J. Pediatr. Surg., *22:*267, 1987.

100. Lawhorn, C.D., and Brown, R.E.: Epidural morphine with butorphanol in pediatric patients. J. Clin. Anesth., *6:*91, 1994.
101. Lee, J.J., and Forrester. P.: EMLA for postoperative analgesia for day case circumcision in children: A comparison with dorsal nerve of penis block. Anaesthesia, *47:*1081, 1992.
102. Lejus, C., Roussière, G., Testa, S., *et al.*: Postoperative extradural analgesia in children: Comparison of morphine with fentanyl. Br. J. Anaesth., *72:*156, 1994.
103. Lönnqvist, P.A., and Hesser, U.L.: Location of the paravertebral space in children and adolescents in relation to surface anatomy assessed by computed tomography. Paediatr Anaesth., *2:*285, 1992.
104. Lönnqvist, P.A.: Plasma concentrations of lignocaine after thoracic paravertebral blockade in infants and children. Anaesthesia, *48:*958, 1993.
105. Maccani, R.M., Wedel, D.J., Melton, A., *et al.*: Femoral and lateral femoral cutaneous nerve block for muscle biopsy in children. Paediatr. Anaesth., *5:*223, 1995.
106. Malawar, M.M., Buch, R., Khurana JS, *et al.*: Postoperative infusional continuous regional analgesia. Clin. Orthop., *266:*227, 1991.
107. Mannion, D., Armstrong, C., O'Leary, G., and Casey, W.: Paediatric post-orchidopexy analgesia—Effect of diclofenac combined with ilioinguinal-iliohypogastric nerve block. Paediatr. Anaesth., *4:*327, 1994.
108. Maunuksela, E-L., and Korpela, R.: Double-blind evaluation of a lignocaine-prilocaine cream (EMLA)in children. Br. J. Anaesth., *58:* 1242, 1986.
109. Maxwell, L.G., Yaster, M., Wetzel, R.C., and Niebyl, J.R.: Penile nerve block for newborn circumcision. Obst. Gynecol., *70:*415, 1987.
110. Maxwell, L.G., Martin, L.D., and Yaster, M.: Bupivacaine-induced cardiac toxicity in neonates: Successful treatment with intravenous phenytoin. Anesthesiology, *80:*682, 1994.
111. Mazoit, J.X., Denson, D.D., and Samii K.: Pharmacokinetics of bupivacaine following caudal anesthesia in infants. Anesthesiology, *68:* 397, 1988.
112. McClain, B.C., and Reed, S.A.: Barrier flaps for caudal anesthesia in pediatric patients. Anesthesiology, *1:*48, 1989.
113. McCloskey, J.J., Haun, S.E., and Deshpande, J.K.: Bupivacaine toxicity secondary to continuous caudal epidural infusion in children. Anesth. Analg., *75:*287, 1992.
114. McGown, R.G.: Caudal analgesia in children: Five hundred cases for procedures below the diaphragm. Anaesthesia, *37:*806, 1982.
115. McIlvaine, W.B., Chang, J.H.T., and Jones, M.: The effective use of intrapleural bupivacaine for analgesia after thoracic and subcostal incisions in children. J. Pediatr. Surg., *23:*1184, 1988.
116. McNicol, L.R.: Sciatic nerve block for children—Sciatic nerve block by the anterior approach for postoperative pain relief. Anaesthesia, *40:* 410, 1985.
117. McNicol, L.R.: Lower limb blocks for children. Anaesthesia, *41:*27, 1986.
118. Mobley, K.A., Wandless, J.G., and Fell, D.: Serum bupivacaine concentrations following wound infiltration in children undergoing inguinal herniotomy. Anaesthesia, *46:*500, 1991.
119. Moores, M.A., Wandless, J.G., and Fell, D.: Paediatric postoperative analgesia: A comparison of rectal diclofenac with caudal bupivacaine after inguinal herniotomy. Anaesthesia, *45:*156, 1990.
120. Nichols, D., Yaster, M., Lynn, A., *et al.*: Disposition and respiratory effects of intrathecal morphine in children. Anesthesiology, *79:*733, 1993.
121. Oberlander, T.F., Berde, C.B., Lam, K.H., *et al.*: Infants tolerate spinal anesthesia with minimal overall autonomic changes: Analysis of heart rate variability in former premature infants undergoing hernia repair. Anesth. Analg., *80:*20, 1995.
122. Olney, B.W., Lugg, P.C., Turner, P.L., *et. al.*: Outpatient treatment of upper extremity injuries in childhood using intravenous regional anaesthesia. J. Pediatr. Orthop., *8:*576, 1988.
123. Payen, D., Ecoffey, C., Carli, P., *et al.*: Pulsed Doppler ascending aortic, carotid, brachial, and femoral artery blood flows during caudal anesthesia in infants. Anesthesiology, *67:*681, 1987.
124. Perillo, M., Sethna, N.F., and Berde, C.B.: Intravenous isoproterenol as a marker for epidural test-dosing in children. Anesth. Analg., *76:* 178, 1993.
125. Rasch, D.K., Webster, D.E., Pollard, T.G., and Gurkowski, M.A.: Lumbar and thoracic epidural analgesia via the caudal approach for postoperative pain relief in infants and children. Can. J. Anaesth., *37:* 359, 1990.
126. Rice, L.J., and Britton, J.T.: Neonatal spinal anesthesia. Anesth. Clin. North Am., *10:*129, 1992.
127. Rice, L.J., and Britton, J.T.: Neural blockade for pediatric pain management. *In* Sinatra, R.S., Hord, A.H., Ginsberg, B., *et al.*, (eds): Acute pain, mechanisms and management. pp. 483. St. Louis, Mosby–Year Book., 1992.
128. Rice, L.J., and Britton, J.T.: Pediatric postoperative analgesia. Semin. Anesth., *XII:*27,1993.
129. Rice, L.J., DeMars, P.D., Crooms, J., *et al.*: Duration of spinal anesthesia in infants under one year of age: Comparison of three drugs. Reg. Anesth., *19:*325, 1994.
130. Rice, L.J.: Regional anesthesia. *In* Motoyama, E., and Davis, P., (eds.): Smith's anesthesia for infants and children. Ed 6. pp. 403. St. Louis, C.V. Mosby Co., 1996.
131. Rosen, K.R., and Rosen, D.A.: Caudal epidural morphine for control of pain after open heart surgery in children. Anesthesiology, *70:*418, 1989.
132. Rosen, D.A., Broadman, L.M., Pyles, L., *et al.*: The use of pre-emptive caudal morphine to improve outcome in children undergoing cardiac surgery. Reg. Anesth., (press).
133. Rothstein, P., Arthur, G.R., Feldman, H.S., *et al.*: Bupivacaine for intercostal nerve blocks in children: Blood concentrations and pharmacokinetics, Anesthesiology, *65:*625, 1986.
134. Roy-Shapira, A., Amoury, R.A., Ashcraft, K.W., *et al.*: Transient quadriceps paresis following local inguinal block for postoperative pain control. J. Pediatr. Surg., *20:*554, 1985.
135. Ryhänen, P., Adamski, J., Puhakka, K., *et al.*: Postoperative pain relief in children: A comparison between caudal bupivacaine and intramuscular diclofenac sodium. Anaesthesia, *49:*57, 1994.
136. Sandler, B.S., Weyman, C., and Conner, K.: Midazolam versus fentanyl as premedication for painful procedures in children with cancer. Pediatrics, *89:*631, 1992.
137. Sang, C.N., Berde, C.B., *et al.*: A multicenter study of safety and risk factors in pediatric regional anesthesia. Anesthesiology, *81:*A1386, 1994.
138. Sara, C.A., and Lowry, C.J.: A complication of circumcision and dorsal nerve block of the penis. Anaesth. Intensive Care, *13:*79, 1984.
139. Scott, D.B.: "Maximum recommended doses" of local anaesthetic drugs. Br. J. Anaesth., *63:*373, 1989.
140. Sethna, N.F., and Berde, C.B.: Venous air embolism during identification of the epidural space in children. Anesth. Analg., *76:*925, 1993.
141. Sethna, N.F., and Wilder, R.T.: Regional anesthetic techniques for chronic pain. *In* Schechter, N.G., Berde, C.B., and Yaster, M. (eds.): Pain in infants, children, and adolescents. pp. 281. Baltimore, Williams and Wilkins, 1993.
142. Sethna, N.F., and Berde, C.B.: Pediatric regional anesthesia. *In* Gregory, G.A., (ed.): Pediatric Anesthesia. pp. 281. New York, Churchill-Livingstone, 1994.
143. Schwartz, N., and Eisenkraft, J.B.: Probable venous air embolism during epidural placement in an infant. Anesth. Analg., *76:*1136, 1993.
144. Sfez, M., Le Mapihan, Y., Mazoit, X., and Dreux-Boucard, H.: Local anesthetic serum concentrations after penile nerve block in children. Anesth. Analg., *71:*423, 1990.
145. Shandling, B., and Steward, D.J.: Regional analgesia for postoperative pain in pediatric outpatient surgery. J. Pediatr. Surg., *15:*477, 1980.
146. Sims, C., and Johnson, C.M.: Postoperative apnea in infants. Anaesth. Intensive Care, *22:*40, 1994.
147. Soliman, I.E., Broadman, L.M., Hannallah, R.S., *et al.*: Comparison of the analgesic effects of EMLA (Eutectic Mixture of Local Anesthetics) to intradermal lidocaine infiltration prior to venous cannulation in unpremedicated children. Anesthesiology, *68:*804, 1988.
148. Spear, R.M.: Dose-response in infants receiving caudal anesthesia with bupivacaine. Paediatr. Anaesth., *1:*47, 1991.
149. Splinter, W.M., Bass, J., and Komocar, L.: Regional anaesthesia for hernia repair in children: Local vs caudal anaesthesia. Can. J. Anaesth., *42:*197, 1995.
150. Stow, P.J., Scott, A., Phillips, A., *et al.*: Plasma bupivacaine concentrations during caudal analgesia and ilioinguinal-iliohypogastric nerve block in children. Anaesthesia, *43:*650, 1988.
151. Strafford, M.A., Wilder, R.T., and Berde, C.B.: The risk of infection from epidural analgesia in children: A review of 1620 cases. Anesth. Analg., *80:*234, 1995.
152. Tobias, J.D., Lowe, S., O'Dell, N., and Holcomb, G.W.: Thoracic epidural anaesthesia in infants and children. Can. J. Anaesth., *40:*879, 1993.

153. Tree-Trakarn T., and Pirayavaraporn, S.: Postoperative pain relief for circumcision in children: Comparison among morphine, nerve block, and topical analgesia. Anesthesiology, *62:*519, 1985.
154. Tree-Trakarn, T., Pirayavaraporn, S., and Lertakyamanee, J.: Topical analgesia for relief of post-circumcision pain. Anesthesiology, *67:* 395, 1987.
155. Valley, R.D., and Bailey, A.G.: Caudal morphine for postoperative analgesia in infants and children: A report of 138 cases. Anesth. Analg., *72:*120, 1991.
156. Vane, D.W., Abajian, J.C., and Hong, A.R.: Spinal anesthesia for primary repair of gastroschisis: A new and safe technique for selected patients. J. Pediatr. Surg., *29:*1234, 1994.
157. Ved, S.A., Pinosky, M., and Nicodemus, H.: Ventricular tachycardia and brief cardiovascular collapse in two infants after caudal anesthesia using a bupivacaine-epinephrine solution. Anesthesiology, *79:* 1121, 1993.
158. Veverka, T.J., Henry, D.N., and Milroy, M.J.: Spinal anesthesia reduces the hazard of apnea in high-risk infants. Am. Surg., *57:*531, 1991.
159. Veyckemans, F., Van Obbergh, L.J., and Gouverneur, J.M.: Lessons from 1,100 pediatric caudal blocks in a teaching hospital. Reg. Anesth., *17:*119, 1992.
160. Warner, M.A., Kunkel, S.E., Offord, K.O., *et al.*: The effects of age, epinephrine, and operative site on duration of caudal analgesia in pediatric patients. Anesth. Analg., *66:*995, 1987.
161. Webster, A.C., McKishnie, J.D., Kenyon, C.F., *et al.*: Spinal anaesthesia for inguinal hernia repair in high-risk neonates. Can. J. Anaesth., *38:*281, 1991.
162. Wedel, D.J., Krohn, J.S., and Hall, J.A.: Brachial plexus anesthesia in pediatric patients. Mayo Clin. Proc., *66:*583, 1991.
163. Welborn, L.G., Rice, L.J., Hannallah, R.S., *et al.*: Postoperative apnea in former preterm infants: Prospective comparison of spinal and general anesthesia. Anesthesiology, *72:*838, 1990.
164. Wilder, R.T., Berde, C.B., Wolohan, M., *et al.*: Reflex sympathetic dystrophy in children: Follow-up of 70 patients. Anesthesiology, *75:* 693, 1991.
165. Williamson, P.S., and Williamson, M.L.: Physiological stress reduction by a local anesthetic during newborn circumcision. Pediatrics, *71:* 36, 1983.
166. Winnie, A.P., Ramamurthy, S., and Durrani, Z.: The inguinal paravascular technique of lumbar plexus anesthesia: The "3-in-1" block. Anesth. Analg., *52:*984, 1973.
167. Wolf, A.R., Valley, R.D., Fear, D.W., *et al.*: Bupivacaine for caudal analgesia in infants and children: The optimal effective concentration. Anesthesiology, *69:*102, 1988.
168. Wolf, A.R., and Hughs, D.: Pain relief for infants undergoing abdominal surgery: Comparison of infusions of I.V. morphine and extradural bupivacaine. Br. J. Anaesth., *70:*10, 1993.
169. Wright, T.E., Orr, R.J., Haberkern, C.M., *et al.*: Complications during spinal anesthesia in infants: High spinal blockade. Anesthesiology, *73:*1290, 1990.
170. Yamashita, M., and Tsuji, M.: Identification of the epidural space in children. Anaesthesia, *46:*872, 1991.
171. Yaster, M., Aronoff, D., Kornhauser, D.M., *et al.*: The pharmacokinetics of lidocaine during caudal anesthesia in children. Anesthesiology, *63:*A465, 1985.
172. Yaster, M., Tobin, J.R., Billett, C., *et al.*: Epidural analgesia in the management of severe vaso-occlusive sickle cell crisis. Pediatrics, *93:* 310, 1994.

Neural Blockade in Clinical Anesthesia and Management of Pain, Third Edition,
edited by M.J. Cousins and P.O. Bridenbaugh.
Lippincott–Raven Publishers, Philadelphia © 1998.

CHAPTER 21

Complications of Local Anesthetic Neural Blockade

Phillip O. Bridenbaugh and Denise J. Wedel

It is often difficult for the anesthesiologist to be objective when discussing complications of any kind. The word itself has a negative connotation and is used frequently to imply fault, failure, or even negligence. Although elements of these may be present in many complications, there is virtually nothing in life, medicine, anesthesia, or neural blockade that is totally without risk of complication—cause not withstanding. The safest approach to a discussion of complications of local anesthetic neural blockade, therefore, is to have a clear understanding of what the complications of a given procedure might be, and be prepared to prevent or diagnose and treat them appropriately.

Unfortunately, many unsuccessful procedures or poor results are automatically attributed to "complications." This may preserve the anesthesiologist's reputation, but, unfortunately, tends to reflect poorly on the procedure. One might state it another way: Is there really a high complication rate with neural blockade, or is it just a low success rate in the hands of many?

Often, normal responses to neural blockade are called complications, for example, hypotension with high spinal anesthesia. One must differentiate, therefore, between normal side effects and true complications. *Webster's Dictionary* defines a complication as "a difficult factor or issue, often appearing unexpectedly and changing existing plans, methods or attitudes." Clearly, hypotension with a high spinal block may be sudden, but it should not *usually* be unexpected. Conversely, *Webster's* defines a side effect as "a secondary and usually adverse effect." Certainly much of what occurs with neural blockade is physiologic side effect as opposed to unexpected complication.

P.O. Bridenbaugh: Department of Anesthesia, University of Cincinnati College of Medicine, Cincinnati, Ohio 45267-0531.

D.J. Wedel: Department of Anesthesiology, Mayo Clinic, Rochester, Minnesota 55905.

CAUSES OF COMPLICATIONS

One classic way of discussing the complications of a given entity is by cause. For neural blockade, therefore, one might discuss complications owing to equipment, drugs, and, perhaps, human error. Such an approach makes it more difficult to anticipate the complications and side effects of new or different techniques. A more systematic approach is to discuss causes as something common to all neural blockade techniques and then proceed to their logical classification.

If, as defined, side effects were anticipated and therefore prevented, the resultant complications would also be avoided. The causes of these unanticipated side effects can be separated into three general categories: All may be referred to as errors in judgment as they relate to (i) technique, (ii) drugs, and (iii) management of the patient.

TECHNIQUE

Errors in judgment related to technique are concerned with selecting the nerve block technique (if in fact one is appropriate) that best fits the needs of the patient and the surgeon, and the abilities of the anesthesiologist. This is often the precursor, but quite different from actual technical errors in performing the block. Clearly, abstinence is the best way to avoid complications, but, if one is carefully selective in the application of nerve block procedures, the inverse ratio of high success with few complications will prevail. Anesthesiologists are taught, however, that regional anesthesia is the anesthesia of choice for poor-risk and trauma patients. The morbidity and the mortality associated with regional anesthesia often occur through flawed selection of the poor-risk or emergency patient, for example, the morbidly obese, the belligerent patient, or the full-stomach hypovolemic patient, who may require the sort of nerve block that the anesthesiologist has seldom done. Even if the technique is suited to the patient, it may not be suited to the abilities of the anesthesiologist.

DRUGS

A successfully accomplished technique puts the needle next to the nerves to be blocked. The successful nerve block relies on the selection of the correct local anesthetic agent or, more frequently, the right concentration or volume. Poor judgment leads to a partial block (inadequate concentration or volume) or one that wears off before the surgery finishes (wrong drug). All too frequently, patients are selected for a nerve block because of a relative contraindication to general anesthesia, that is, a full stomach or difficult intubation. The risk of complications secondary to an inadequate block is clearly greater in this circumstance. The opposite error in drug selection is that of excess volume or concentration, or both, leading to toxicity or prolonged neural blockade. The use of 0.75% bupivacaine, for example, for an arm block in an outpatient will subject the patient to many hours of a vasodilated, useless extremity or the risk of a grand mal seizure from drug overdose 30 minutes after completing the block.

PATIENT MANAGEMENT

The end result of any nerve block, no matter how successfully administered, is dependent upon how well the patient's total anesthetic experience is managed. The successful management of the patient can become extremely difficult and complex if there have been preceding errors in judgment relating to just the neural blockade portion of the patient's anesthetic care.

Most patients require some measure of supplemental sedation, amnesia, or analgesia, or all three, in order to be psychologically satisfied with their anesthetic experience. Inappropriate selection of drugs, such as the dissociative agents, can convert a responsible and cooperative patient into a restless, belligerent, or even unmanageable and disoriented one, who must then be given a full general anesthetic.

Conversely, overdose of sedative or hypnotic agents may result in loss of consciousness, airway obstruction, and hypoxia, and the patient will need resuscitative intubation and ventilation. Technicians may be skilled at doing perfect nerve blocks, but trained anesthesiologists must learn how to select and manage patients in whom a regional anesthetic technique will be an important adjunct to their total successful anesthetic management.

CLASSIFICATION OF COMPLICATIONS AND SIDE-EFFECTS

Discussions of the complications of a major area of medical practice, such as neural blockade, too often include an outline or structure that will cover all the complications of all the procedures. The most thorough, repetitive, and tedious approach is to make a list of all reported or theoretical complications for each of the nerve block techniques. Other authors have approached the discussion by etiology, that is, complications owing to equipment, to drugs, and to human error. There are, however, many complications for which we do not know the cause. Furthermore, such an approach does not allow one to predict what complications might occur with new techniques.

The approach here is to suggest that there is an anatomic and therefore physiologic commonality for the nerve block techniques that allows one to predict which complications might occur, and the magnitude and frequency of such complications. Because most of the nerves to be blocked are surrounded by major blood vessels and lie in proximity to major body organs (i.e., lung, liver, kidney), it seems reasonable to classify complications into three major systemic groups: (i) vascular complications, (ii) respiratory complications, and (iii) neurologic complications. A fourth miscellaneous group will collect those complications or side-effects not having a relationship to the other three systems.

VASCULAR COMPLICATIONS AND SIDE EFFECTS

At nearly every site of the body where neural blockade is accomplished, the nerves to be blocked are surrounded by arteries and veins forming the neurovascular bundle. Naturally, the larger or more proximal the nerve, the greater is the likelihood that the surrounding vessels are also large. There has been a tendency in the past to classify all vascular complications as unintentional intravenous injection of local anesthetics in sufficient volume or dose to precipitate a grand mal seizure. Less frequent, but just as important, are complications from intra-arterial injections and hematoma formation.

Arterial Injection

The deceptive difference between intravenous and intra-arterial injection comes as a result of our failure to realize that although all venous blood empties into the heart and goes through the lungs before going to the target organ (i.e., the brain), drugs injected into the internal carotid or vertebral arteries go directly to the brain. Therefore, a very small dose of local anesthetic will result in central nervous system (CNS) toxicity. All other arterial injections feed into the venous circulation and will behave similarly to intravenous injections. The potential for this complication was noted by Moore in his textbook *Stellate Ganglion Block* in 1954.[78] Since that time, isolated case reports have appeared in the literature, usually after stellate ganglion block. If one reflects on the anatomy of the vertebral and internal carotid arterial system (Fig. 21-1), however, it is apparent that a similar complication may result from insertion of needles into any part of the head and neck of a patient. Certainly retrobulbar block, interscalene block, cervical plexus block, vagal nerve block, and, perhaps, even, local infiltration for insertion of

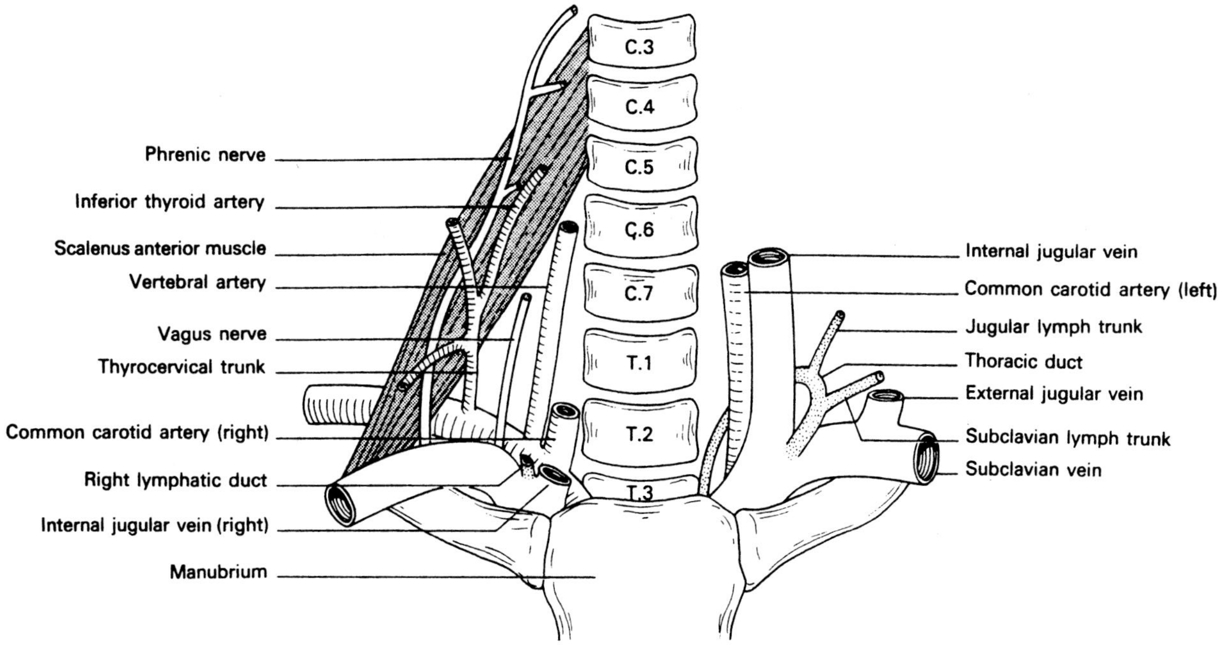

FIG. 21-1. Relationship of carotid and vertebral arteries to neural structures of the neck. (Thompson, J.S.: Core Textbook of Anatomy. pp. 228. Philadelphia, J. B. Lippincott, 1977.)

central lines, are but a few of the techniques that could result in an intra-arterial-induced local anesthetic seizure.

Korevaar and co-workers[61] stressed the small doses required to precipitate toxicity by comparing the actual doses of 7 previous case reports with their estimated toxic dose. The minimum toxic dose injected into a vertebral or internal carotid artery as a bolus can be estimated by accepting that 15% of the cardiac output that goes to the brain is equally divided among the four arteries supplying the brain. Therefore, 15% of the minimum intravenous toxic dose divided by four will be the estimated bolus toxic dose intra-arterially (Table 21-1).

Convulsions are not the only complication of bolus injection into the internal carotid or vertebral artery: total blindness, aphasia, hemiparesis, and unconsciousness of a transient and completely recoverable nature have also been reported.[101,109] It is equally probable that local anesthetic injections around the head and neck may enter small arteries, and, by retrograde flow, pass into the cerebral circulation. Tomlin, in a review of death during outpatient dental anesthetics, commented on the case of a 22-year-old woman who, after receiving an inferior alveolar dental nerve block with 1.5 ml of 2% lignocaine with 1:80,000 norepinephrine, lost consciousness, paled, convulsed, had a cardiac arrest, and died.[114] In an effort to demonstrate retrograde flow by bolus injection into small arteries, Aldrete[2] performed lingual artery lidocaine injections in baboons and measured lidocaine levels in the internal carotid artery. Six seconds after lingual artery injection, the lidocaine levels in the internal carotid artery were 28 μg/ml. Injection of microspheres further illustrated retrograde flow.

Injections made into brachial and femoral arteries also demonstrated retrograde flow into the internal carotid system. This study, along with clinical reports, suggests that ophthalmologists, dentists, otorhinolaryngologists, and other surgeons who inject local anesthetics around the head and neck should aspirate gently and repeatedly, and inject slowly, to avoid such complications.

TABLE 21-1. *Anesthetic agents and toxic doses*[a]

Local anesthetic agent	Minimum toxic intravenous dose (mg/kg)	Estimated intra-arterial toxic dose[a] (mg)	Reported toxic doses (mg)
Procaine	19.2	43.2	100
Tetracaine	2.5	5.6	2.5
Lidocaine	6.4	14.4	10 16 90
Bupivacaine	1.6	3.6	32.5 7.5

[a] Estimated for injection into a vertebral or internal carotid artery for a 60-kg subject.

(Korevaar, W.C., Burney, R.G., and Moore, P.A.: Convulsions during stellate ganglion block: A case report. Anesth. Analg., *58*:330, 1979.)

Intravenous Injection

As previously noted, most clinicians, from the time they were taught how to do a venipuncture, were taught that inviolate dictum, "Aspirate before you inject." The humorous but irrational extreme of this dictum can be observed in practitioners who insert a needle subcutaneously causing pain to the patient, and faithfully aspirate before making a skin wheal with a local anesthetic agent. The scientific world anxiously awaits the first report of a toxic reaction secondary to intravascular injection of a skin wheal.

Although direct intravenous injections are much more likely than intra-arterial, the larger volumes or doses required for CNS toxicity afford some protection from this complication. A cautious anesthesiologist and a conscious patient *usually* can detect the prodrome of CNS toxicity before frank seizures occur (see Chapter 4). Certainly, unintentional intravenous injection is possible with all of the regional block techniques, with the remote exception of subarachnoid block. In point of fact, as one listens to anesthesia colleagues or reads the literature on CNS and cardiovascular toxicity of local anesthetics, it becomes apparent that most of these unintentional intravenous injections result from injection through an indwelling epidural catheter. Many novices to the use of indwelling epidural or caudal catheters are unaware of the gentleness with which aspiration must be accomplished if blood (or cerebrospinal fluid [CSF]) is to be aspirated at all—let alone the full length of the catheter to the aspirating syringe. It is common that the strong negative pressures exerted at the tip of the catheter by an enthusiastic anesthesiologist on the proximal end of a 20-ml syringe will collapse vein or dura instantly and nothing will be returned, only to result in complications when too much local anesthetic is injected too quickly. A moderate practice suggests use of a small test dose of local anesthetic containing 1 : 200,000 epinephrine with appropriate cardiovascular monitors followed by slow injection of 5-ml increments of local anesthetic, to reach the final preselected total dose (see Chapter 4).

Another, more subtle, form of intravenous toxicity was reported by the practitioners of intravenous regional anesthesia (see Chapter 12). Heath,[48] in a letter to the editors of *Anesthesiology,* drew attention to the fact that from 1979 to early 1983, "seven patients have died in the United Kingdom as a result of Bier blocks in which bupivacaine was used." The role of bupivacaine in those fatalities is not the issue here (see Chapters 4 and 12). Other factors that contribute to such complications relate to the fact, first, that many practitioners other than trained anesthesiologists are performing Bier blocks, even in offices, emergency rooms, and outpatient facilities, where neither equipment nor trained personnel are available to treat seizures or perform resuscitation.[43] Death and, much more commonly, CNS toxicity from intravenous regional anesthesia, may result from errors of technique or drug dosage, along with failure of resuscitation. Disasters have certainly resulted from tourniquet failure, illustrating the point that tourniquet equipment should be well maintained and checked frequently for maintenance of accurately displayed pressures.[93] However, the injected solution can "leak" beneath even a correctly inflated cuff. After a patient had seizures and cardiovascular collapse with intravenous regional anesthesia, despite an accurate tourniquet pressure of 120 mm Hg over systolic (180/300 mm Hg), Rosenberg and colleagues[97] performed phlebographic studies in three patients and three volunteers. In 4 of the 6 subjects, contrast medium leakage was seen proximal to the tourniquet. To continue the study of the problem of leakage under the tourniquet, Lawes and colleagues[64] measured the pressures generated in the venous system of the arm during injection of a simulated intravenous regional anesthetic. Had the practitioners adhered to the recommended tourniquet pressure of 50 mm Hg over systolic 3 of 4 subjects would have sustained periods of venous pressure in excess of tourniquet pressure, thus allowing leakage of injected solution under the cuff and into the systemic circulation. Even with the tourniquet inflated to 250 mm Hg, 1 of 4 subjects would still have had leakage under the cuff. These situations of high venous pressure are more likely to occur if the injection is made rapidly or into a proximal vein, if the volume injected is large, or if the extremity is inadequately exsanguinated.[46] The effect of speed of injection and method of exsanguination was studied by Duggan and associates.[29] They noted that venous pressures were dependent upon the methods of exsanguination, with highest pressures occurring when no exsanguination was done and lowest with exsanguination by Esmarch bandage, regardless of the rate of injection. The slow rate of injection always produced significantly lower peak pressures than did the faster rate at all degrees of exsanguination (Table 21-2). The severity of the clinical response depends on the dose and concentration of

TABLE 21-2. *Effect of rate of injection and preinjection exsanguination on mean peak venous pressures*

Rate of injection	Preinjection exsanguination	Mean peak venous pressures (mm Hg ± SD)	Range
0.833 ml^{-1}	Nil	213.33 ± 48.34	280–150
	Elevation	161.67 ± 44.80	230–105
	Elevation and Esmarch	105.83 ± 25.38	130–70
0.42 ml^{-1}	Nil	151.67 ± 47.40	210–90
	Elevation	95.00 ± 26.83	140–60
	Elevation and Esmarch	70.83 ± 21.31	100–50

(Duggan, J., McKeown, D.W., and Scott, D.B.: Venous pressures generated during IV regional anaesthesia [IVRA]. Br. J. Anaesth., *55:*1158P, 1983.)

local anesthetic being injected which is able to gain access to the systemic circulation. One should not, however, overlook the obvious: that sudden or early tourniquet release, or both, are still the most common cause(s) of CNS or cardiovascular complications associated with intravenous regional anesthesia.

Hematoma

Only in the past decade or so has the practitioner of regional anesthesia become concerned about the risks of hematoma formation coincident with or subsequent to neural blockade. The major concern with hematoma formation is not whether it will occur, but where. Hematoma after most peripheral nerve blocks is uncommon and usually of little consequence. The major awareness of this potential complication focuses on the subarachnoid and epidural spaces (see Chapters 7 and 8) and in retrobulbar block[34] (see Chapter 17), where diagnosis is more difficult, treatment complicated, and complications serious. With the nearly ubiquitous use of nonsteroidal anti-inflammatory drugs (NSAIDs) in the general population and the perioperative use of a variety of anticoagulants for prevention of deep vein thrombosis, the major question has become, "When, if ever, is it safe to use spinal or epidural anesthesia in patients who are receiving anticoagulant therapy?" In a report of over 100 spontaneous epidural hematomas, 25% were associated with anticoagulation therapy.[108] Owens[84] reviewed 34 cases of spinal hematoma after lumbar puncture that had been reported in the world literature. Six involved the administration of an anesthetic. Fourteen patients had received anticoagulants, though only 2 were given anticoagulants prior to needle placement. Another 2 patients were treated with NSAIDs immediately before or after lumbar puncture. In addition, 11 patients had evidence of coagulopathy or significant thrombocytopenia. In summary, 27 of the 34 patients (79%) with spinal hematomas associated with lumbar puncture had evidence of hemostatic abnormality. A recent review of the literature discusses the use of spinal and epidural anesthesia in the anticoagulated patient.[121] Table 21-3 summarizes the pharmacologic activities of commonly used anticoagulants and NSAIDs.

Intravenous Heparin

Individual patient sensitivity to heparin varies. Highly sensitive patients exhibit both greater increases in coagulation time and prolongation of effect after heparin administration; they may also be at higher risk for hemorrhagic complications, compared to patients with normal or low sensitivity. Factors affecting heparin sensitivity include general medical condition, diet, cardiac status, renal function, and liver disease. Cooke and co-workers[20] measured blood heparin levels in 10 consecutive patients, who received 5,000 units of heparin before elective hip operations; they found a wide variation in dose response (Fig. 21-2).

Heparin has a half-life in circulating blood of 1 1/2 to 2 hours and is cleared within 4 to 6 hours of administration of a therapeutic dose. Protamine in the dose of 1 mg for every 100 units of heparin will reverse the anticoagulant effects, although careful titration is advised. Laboratory testing to determine the degree of anticoagulation should be performed on heparinized patients prior to neural blockade. The activated partial thromboplastin time (APTT) is reproducible, has a rapid endpoint, is sensitive to low doses of heparin, and can be performed at a convenient time in a central laboratory. The activated clotting time (ACT) is also a sensitive test with reproducible results, has a short endpoint, and can be automated.

Rao and El-Etr[87] reported on 3165 patients receiving continuous epidural, and on 847 receiving continuous subarachnoid anesthesia, for lower-extremity vascular surgery over a

TABLE 21-3. *Pharmacologic activities of anticoagulants and NSAIDs[a]*

Agent	Effect on coagulation variables: BT	PT	APTT	Time to peak effect	Time to normal hemostasis post therapy	Comments
Intravenous heparin	↑	↑	↑↑↑	minutes	4–6 hours	Monitor ACT, APTT; delay heparinization for 1 hour after needle placement
Subcutaneous heparin	↑	↑	↑↑	40–50 minutes	4–6 hours	APTT may remain normal, monitor anti-Xa activity
Warfarin	–	↑↑↑	↑	4–6 days (3 days with loading dose)	4–6 days	Monitor PT
Aspirin	↑↑↑	—	—	hours	7 days	Bleeding time not reliable predictor of platelet function
Other NSAID	↑↑↑	—	—	hours	3–5 days	
Thrombolytic agent	↑↑↑	↑	↑	minutes	1–2 days	Usually heparinized in addition. Monitor closely.

BT, bleeding time; PT, prothrombin time; APTT, activated thromboplastin time; ACT, activated clotting time; ↑, clinically insignificant increase; ↑↑, possibly clinically significant increase; ↑↑↑, clinically significant increase

[a] From Hindman, B.J.: Usefulness of the post-aspirin bleeding time. Anesthesiology, *64*:368, 1986.

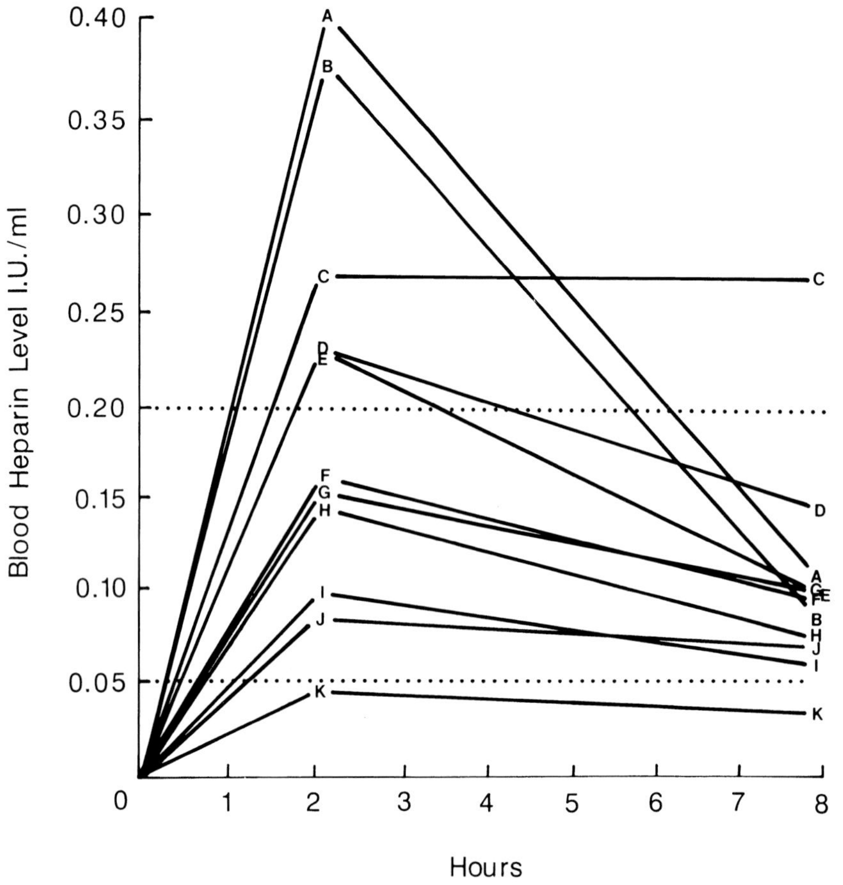

FIG. 21-2. Blood heparin levels following subcutaneous injection of 5,000 units of heparin in 10 consecutive patients. (Cooke, E.D.: Monitoring during low dose heparin prophylaxis. N. Engl. J. Med., *294:*1066, 1976.)

6-year-period (1973 to 1978). Patients with a history of preexisting coagulation abnormalities, thrombocytopenia or preoperative anticoagulation therapy were excluded. Preoperative anticoagulation studies were also performed. All of their patients received heparin anticoagulation, to twice baseline ACT levels, approximately 1 hour after insertion of the anesthetic catheter. The heparin dose was repeated every 6 hours following measurement of the ACT throughout the period of anticoagulation therapy. The catheters were removed the following day 1 hour prior to administration of the maintenance dose of heparin. There was no incidence of peridural or subarachnoid hematoma. In summary, while the patients in this study safely underwent placement of indwelling epidural or spinal catheters, followed by systemic heparinization, the heparin activity was closely monitored and the indwelling catheters were removed at a time when circulating heparin levels were relatively low.

A report on the use of intrathecal morphine[73] in 40 cardiac surgical patients 50 minutes before heparinization also showed no evidence of neurologic sequelae (see also Chapter 8).

Although the 2 previous studies suggest that central neural blockade followed by heparinization can be conducted safely, Ruff and Dougherty[98] reported documented spinal hematomas in 7 of 342 stroke patients who underwent a diagnostic lumbar puncture with a 20-gauge needle, followed by anticoagulation with heparin. There were also 18 patients with severe or radicular back pain lasting more than 48 hours. The authors identified traumatic needle placement, initiation of anticoagulation within 1 hour of lumbar puncture or concomitant aspirin therapy as risk factors.

Subcutaneous Heparin

The risk of spinal hematoma in patients on low-dose heparin (heparin 5,000 units subcutaneously every 8 to 12 hours) remains controversial and largely unstudied. Following subcutaneous injection of 5,000 units of heparin, maximum anticoagulation effect is observed in 40 to 50 minutes and usually returns to baseline within 4 to 6 hours. The APTT may remain in the normal range and often is not monitored.

Lowson and Goodchild[68] reviewed 99 epidural and 37 spinal anesthetics performed on patients who received heparin 5,000 units 2 hours prior to elective abdominal procedures. Heparin prophylaxis was continued into the postoperative period. When epidural blood vessel puncture occurred (5%), the needle or catheter was replaced at a different interspace. There were no neurologic complications. Similarly, Allemann et al.[3] studied 82 spinal and 105 epidural anesthetics (66 of which involved an epidural catheter) performed on patients undergoing orthopedic procedures who had received subcutaneous heparin 2 hours preoperatively. Again there were no reported cases of spinal hematoma.

However, there are at least two reported cases of epidural

hematoma occurring in patients on low-dose heparin who underwent lumbar puncture or epidural blockade.[23,25] In both cases, blood was encountered during catheter placement, and an epidural hematoma with complete paraplegia developed within 24 hours.

Low Molecular Weight Heparin

Low molecular weight heparin (LMWH) is a heterogenous mixture of polysaccharide chains that can be separated into fragments of various molecular weights. Since each fractionation contains heparins of different molecular weights, each must be evaluated as a specific pharmacological substance. LMWH exhibits a dose-dependent antithrombotic effect that is assessed by measuring the anti-Xa activity level. The advantages of LMWH over unfractionated heparin include a higher and more predictable bioavailability after subcutaneous administration, a longer biological half-life, and a smaller impact on platelet function.

Berqvist et al.[11] reviewed 44 articles on LMWH used for thromboprophylaxis. LMWH was administered in conjunction with spinal or epidural anesthesia in 9,013 patients; there were no spinal hematomas in this series. One case of spinal hematoma associated with LMWH has been reported. The patient had minimal bleeding during insertion of an epidural catheter, and 3 hours later, after the third LMWH injection, developed irreversible paraplegia. An epidural hematoma extending from T_9-L_4 was evacuated without neurologic improvement.[116]

Oral Anticoagulants

Oral anticoagulants are often administered prior to major joint surgery, in anticipation of continuing these agents during the postoperative period for venous thrombosis prophylaxis. As with heparin, patients show varying sensitivities to oral anticoagulants. The effects of these drugs are not apparent until a significant depression of the synthesis of biologically active factors has occurred, usually 2 to 3 days. The anticoagulant effects persist for 4 to 6 days after termination of therapy, while new, biologically active, vitamin K factors are synthesized. In an emergent situation, the anticoagulant effects can be reversed by transfusing fresh frozen plasma and injecting vitamin K.

Odoom and Sih reported on 1,000 lumbar epidural blocks in 950 patients undergoing vascular surgery during a 3-year period between 1977 and 1980.[82] A significant difference in this series from that of Rao was that all of these patients were receiving preoperative oral anticoagulation therapy. No side-effects were observed in any patient that could be related to hemorrhage or hematoma formation in the epidural space.

In a recent report by Horlocker et al.[53] 192 epidural catheters were placed in patients undergoing total knee arthroplasty. All patients received warfarin perioperatively, and catheters were left in place for up to 96 hours, to provide pain relief. The authors noted that the mean prothrombin time was not prolonged until the third postoperative day. No spinal hematomas occurred.

Antiplatelet Agents

NSAIDs are often self-administered for pain relief or prescribed for the treatment of rheumatoid arthritis or other bone and joint conditions in the orthopedic and aged populations. Low-dose aspirin therapy is recommended as prophylaxis for a variety of common medical conditions, resulting in almost universal use of this agent. While the effects of NSAIDs are relatively short-lived and measured in days, the antiplatelet effects of aspirin may last for a week or longer after ingestion. Locke and colleagues[67] reported a case of spontaneous acute spinal epidural hematoma unassociated with trauma, conventional anticoagulant therapy, coagulopathy, or vascular abnormalities. They attributed the etiology to two doses of aspirin, two tablets each.

Conversely, however, Benzon[10] prospectively studied 100 consecutive patients on low, intermediate, and high doses of aspirin for less than 1 week, less than 1 month, and greater than 1 month. The average bleeding time and the incidence of prolonged bleeding time were not significantly different in any of the groups. Benzon performed 246 epidural and spinal blocks on 87 patients (8 who had bleeding times prolonged to 10.5 minutes) without any signs or symptoms of epidural hematoma. A large retrospective study, suggesting that central neural blockade is safe in patients taking these medications, has been confirmed prospectively.[51,52,54] Appropriate preoperative evaluation of such patients includes determination of whether they have histories of abnormal bleeding or bruising, which might indicate that further evaluation is needed. The bleeding time is not a good predictor of the risk of bleeding.[37,50]

Thrombolytic Agents

Thrombolytic therapy is used frequently in the treatment of myocardial infarction, pulmonary embolism, deep venous thrombosis, and peripheral artery occlusion. These patients often receive concomitant intravenous heparin to maintain an APTT of 1.5 to 2 times normal. Thrombolytic agents actively dissolve fibrin clots that have already been formed. Exogenous plasminogen activators such as streptokinase and urokinase not only dissolve thrombus, but also affect circulating plasminogen, leading to decreased levels of both plasminogen and fibrin. In a study involving 290 patients with acute myocardial infarction who were treated with thrombolytic therapy (streptokinase or rt-PA), and subsequently heparinized, fibrinogen and plasminogen were maximally depressed at 5 hours after thrombolytic therapy and remained significantly depressed at 27 hours.[88] Hemorrhagic events occurred in 1/3 of the patients, and major hemorrhagic events, defined as a decrease in hemoglobin of 5 g/dl, occurred in approximately 1/2 of the patients. The primary bleeding site was the catheterization or other puncture site in

70% of the hemorrhages. The authors recommended avoiding invasive procedures in patients receiving thrombolytic therapy.

Two cases of spinal hematoma in patients with indwelling epidural catheters who received thrombolytic agents have been reported in the literature.[26,83]

Hematomas may occur for a variety of reasons, not all related to low-dose heparin. Scott and associates[100] reported two cases of acute, *spontaneous* spinal hematoma, and noted that about 100 additional cases had been reported since the original report by Hughling Jackson in 1869. The hematoma is not considered spontaneous if it is associated with a bleeding disorder, trauma, or other causes. Hematoma may also occur secondary to full anticoagulation therapy. Harik and colleagues[45] reported the 2nd case of complete spontaneous recovery from subarachnoid hemorrhage of more than 100 cases found in the literature at that time. Similarly, lumbar puncture or needle trauma into the subarachnoid or epidural space may result in hematoma. Rengarchy[92] and Greensite[44] reported such cases and noted very few similar cases in the literature.

Still unresolved is the question of when it is safe to use spinal and epidural anesthesia in the face of altered coagulation. Hard and fast rules are impossible and inappropriate; however, there seems to be some common ground for caution that has been expressed in the aforementioned reports. First, of course, is an awareness by the anesthesiologist of what medications the patient is taking and effect of the medications on coagulation. If there is any evidence that the patient has received such drugs in the past *or will receive such drugs* intraoperatively, then appropriate coagulation studies should be accomplished. Acceptable deviations from the norm become very individualized and matters of local practice. Patients considered not suitable for continuous epidural or spinal by some authors[82,87] include those with pre-existing neurologic disease, blood dyscrasias, infection at the puncture site, and preoperative full anticoagulant therapy.

Equally as important as proper patient selection and careful anesthetic technique is the requirement for constant intraoperative and postoperative monitoring of neurologic stability. Many authors stress that failure to make an early diagnosis of hematoma, or diagnosis not followed by immediate decompression, is likely to result in little or incomplete neurologic improvement. The real risk in using these techniques is less in the occurrence than in the failure to diagnose and treat accurately and quickly. It has been suggested that patients should be monitored daily in the hospital after removal of the epidural or spinal catheter.[82] Whenever the patients return to outpatient clinics, they should undergo appropriate neurologic examination. Finally, it is most important to note that the presence of a severe or prolonged backache, with or without neurologic signs, local tenderness, fever, or leukocytosis, is an indication for early spinal computerized tomography or magnetic resonance scan. Any clinical or radiologic evidence of cord compression should be followed by an immediate laminectomy and decompression, since complete recovery becomes less likely as surgery time is delayed (see Table 21-4 for other signs and symptoms of epidural and spinal hematoma).

TABLE 21-4. *Signs and symptoms of spinal and epidural hematoma*

Local and radiating pain at site of hematoma
Headache or stiff neck, or both, with subarachnoid hematoma
Bilateral numbness and weakness (paraparesis/quadriparesis)
Loss of bowel and bladder sphincter function
Decreased or lost reflexes distal to lesion
Blood-stained CSF after lumbar puncture
Defect on myelography

CSF, cerebrospinal fluid

More devastating, and fortunately very rare, are intracranial hematomas after subarachnoid puncture for either diagnostic or anesthetic purposes, especially in patients without pre-existing intracranial disease. Newrick and Read[80] noted 12 such patients in 5 previous reports in the literature and discussed 2 cases of theirs. Two recent reports document intracranial hemorrhagic events following repeated spinal anesthetics in elderly males.[14,120] The case report of Erola and associates[36] noted herniation of the uncus rather than hemorrhage. Although rare, the presumed pathophysiology is similar and carries a clear clinical implication.

The brain is suspended in cerebrospinal fluid with the additional support of vessels and venous sinuses (see Fig. 21-5). When the amount of cerebrospinal fluid is decreased by spinal tap or leakage through the needle hole in the dura, the brain tends to sag, especially when the patient is upright. The downward traction on pain-sensitive cerebral vessels is assumed to produce the clinical situation of "post-dural puncture headache (PDPH)." If allowed to persist untreated, the most serious consequences of cerebrospinal fluid leak, with further sagging of the brain, is rupture of small cerebral vessels resulting in subdural hematoma. The time-interval from the dural puncture to serious neurologic symptoms may be from a few days to 4 months. If not evacuated, these hematomas have been fatal. Similar to the spinal and epidural hematomas, even when evacuated, recovery has been nil to incomplete in most cases.

The clinical implication in this rare but devastating complication is the presenting feature of typical PDPH (discussed later in this chapter). It would seem that early and aggressive treatment of this early but minor complication would prevent these hemorrhages and should become part of our practice. The presence of a low-pressure headache may be a relative contraindication to repeated spinal anesthesia. There seems to be no benefit in delayed symptomatic, prolonged, and ineffective treatment of these headaches. Early neurologic examination and follow-up are essential.

RESPIRATORY COMPLICATIONS AND SIDE EFFECTS

Clinical impressions about the respiratory complications of neural blockade are, unfortunately, too simplistic and misinformed. Most practitioners believe that as long as they avoid doing supraclavicular brachial plexus blocks or intercostal nerve blocks, which "everyone knows have a high incidence of pneumothorax," they will have no respiratory complications to worry about. In point of fact, the incidence of pneumothorax is much less than they expect, and there are other problems which need to be considered.

Excluding *central* respiratory depression, there are 2 primary mechanisms whereby neural blockade may produce respiratory complications: (i) interference with the neuromuscular mechanics of ventilation; and (ii) interference with the thoracic volume of the lungs. Practically speaking, the first complication arises from blockade of the cervical nerve roots or phrenic nerves that are the motor nerves to the diaphragm or, in isolated cases, abolition of the motorpower to the abdominal and intercostal muscles of respiration. The second complication of thoracic volume comes through pneumothorax, hemothorax, or hydrothorax, all of which serve to reduce functional lung volume. The true incidence of these complications is difficult to determine, although recent studies using ultrasonography have clarified the frequency and effect of phrenic nerve block.[118] The patient with normal pulmonary function can tolerate easily loss of his respiratory muscles if his diaphragm is intact or, conversely, loss of unilateral diaphragmatic function if the other muscles are intact. It is the respiratory cripple subjected to these side effects of neural blockade who has a problem. This illustrates the difference between a side effect and a complication. High spinal, epidural, interscalene, supraclavicular and intercostal nerve blocks will block those muscles of respiration functionally, a physiologic side effect that is not a complication until applied to the wrong patient or not diagnosed and treated properly.

Interference with Mechanics of Respiration

Many thousands of nerve blocks (interscalene, intercostal, thoracic epidural, for example) have been done for relief of postoperative and traumatic pain. There is also significant evidence in the literature that this form of analgesia is less depressing to ventilation than either narcotics or no treatment at all; however, there are reports that blockade of the nerves to the muscles of respiration in elderly patients, and in patients who have chronic obstructive pulmonary disease, may be harmful. Engberg[35] compared narcotics with unilateral and bilateral intercostal nerve blocks for pain relief after subcostal and midline incisions. Whereas the use of unilateral intercostal blocks had a positive effect on pulmonary function, the bilateral intercostal blockade in elderly patients was suspected of contributing to postoperative pulmonary complications. There have been two similar case reports[19,21] of elderly patients who received intercostal nerve blocks immediately after operation and who were pain-free with apparently adequate ventilation, but in less than 50 minutes both required reintubation and ventilation, owing to inadequate ability to sustain themselves with spontaneous ventilation. Neither patient had pneumothorax or any other new radiographic evidence of pulmonary complications. Thus, it appears that intercostal block should be used with caution in this very select group of patients. Clearly, a select number of unilateral nerves blocked with weaker (nonmotor blocking) concentrations of local anesthetic solutions would still be preferred therapy over no pain relief or high-dose narcotics.

Since the earliest days of neural blockade, there has been an awareness of the importance of the diaphragm to good ventilation, and therefore to the potential respiratory complications that might arise from blockade of its motor nerve supply—the phrenic nerves. The difficulty for the clinician is in trying to predict either the incidence or the magnitude of this risk. Labat[1] states in his early book *Regional Anesthesia* that "*bilateral* blocking of the cervical plexus is not attended by any appreciable or dangerous functional disturbances due to block of the phrenic nerves. The paresis (of the diaphragms)—caused by a bilateral cervical plexus block—is apparently insufficient to interfere with ventilation. Perhaps the intercostal muscles compensate for the decreased diaphragmatic activity." Similar statements have been made by other authors about the seriousness of this complication, especially unilateral diaphragmatic paralysis; however, most do caution against doing nerve blocks that might result in bilateral involvement. It is even more difficult to arrive at an incidence of this complication, since the incidence clearly varies with technique, method of diagnosis, concentration of local anesthetic solution, and skill of the anesthesiologist. More important is an awareness of the anatomy of the cervical nerve roots and phrenic nerves above the clavicle, so that appropriate precautions may be taken whenever any practitioner injects local anesthetic solutions into the neck, for whatever reason.

The phrenic nerve (C3,4,5) is the most important branch of the cervical plexus. In addition to providing motor innervation to the diaphragm, it transmits proprioceptive sensory fibers from the central part of the diaphragm. In addition, it supplies filaments to pleura and pericardium. The principal component of the nerve is derived from the anterior primary ramus of C4, but contributions are provided by C3 and C5. The 3 roots join at the lateral border of the scalenus anterior muscle when the full constituted nerve passes downward and medially across the face of the muscle covered by a very thin prevertebral fascia, and then over the subclavian artery and behind the vein to enter the thorax (Fig. 21-3). After encountering a case of respiratory failure caused by phrenic nerve block secondary to brachial plexus block, Knoblanche[60] studied 15 select patients having supraclavicular brachial plexus block with x-ray examination of the diaphragm 3 hours after successful block. Ten of the 15 patients (67%) demonstrated diaphragmatic paralysis, and 5 had Horner's syndrome following injection of 30 milliliters of 0.5% bupivacaine.

The interscalene approach to the brachial plexus has a reported incidence of complete ipsilateral phrenic nerve block, ranging from 36% to 100%, with the higher incidence documented by ultrasonography.[118] Urmey and McDonald reported a 25% reduction in pulmonary function in patients un-

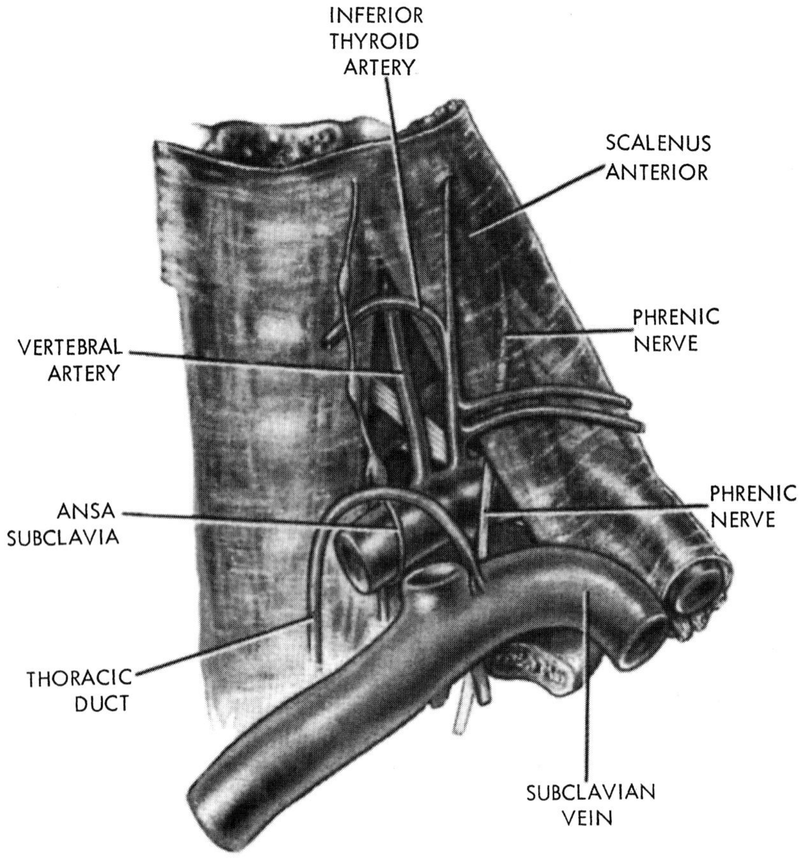

FIG. 21-3. Relationship between the phrenic nerve and the scalene muscles and subclavian vessels. (Last, R.J.: Anatomy: Regional and Applied. pp. 376. New York, Churchill Livingstone, 1978.)

dergoing interscalene block anesthesia.[117] While this is usually a benign, self-limited, condition, persistence of phrenic nerve paresis for several years following interscalene block has been reported.[8] Careful attention to technique, decreased volumes and concentrations of local anesthetic, and anticipation of potential problems should diminish the impact of this complication.

If not carefully done, virtually any nerve block or local anesthetic infiltration with significant volumes in the area of the cervical nerve roots or scalenus muscles could result in blockade of the phrenic nerve, including deep cervical plexus block, interscalene brachial plexus block, supraclavicular brachial plexus block, stellate ganglion block, and probably even superficial cervical plexus block. Just as in the case of intercostal nerve block, if respiratory compromise from a paralyzed diaphragm could be a risk to a given patient, then bilateral blocks should not be done; if unilateral paralysis is deemed risky, then abstinence or dilute (nonmotor blocking) concentrations and small volumes of local anesthetic solutions should be used.

Interference with Thoracic Volume

The majority of these complications are, obviously, pneumothoraces caused by needle puncture of the pleural surface. Although this has been identified most often with supraclavicular brachial plexus block and intercostal nerve block, it may also occur with stellate ganglion block, interscalene plexus block, deep cervical plexus block, subclavian plexus block, and paravertebral thoracic nerve blocks (somatic and sympathetic). Just as was true with phrenic nerve block, true incidence of pneumothorax with any technique is unknown. Most of the reports in the literature varied widely from author to author and are now decades old (Table 21-5). More recent reports account for the unusual complications that also interfere with lung and thoracic volume. As an added complication of regional blocks in the face of anticoagulation, a case of hemopneumothorax following subclavian perivascular brachial plexus block has been reported by Mani and colleagues[72] in a patient who received heparin therapy intraoperatively and postoperatively. The patient became dyspneic and complained of chest pain on the third postoperative day; radiography showed massive hemopneumothorax. About 1,700 ml of blood-stained fluid was aspirated. Although spontaneous hemothorax has been reported with anticoagulant therapy, the presence of an associated 10% pneumothorax on the same side as the brachial block suggests needle trauma to the lung. A reminder of the additional risks of performing neural blockade on the left side of the neck came from the report of Thompson and co-workers.[111] One day after unsuccessful attempts at left stellate ganglion block, the patient returned to the hospital complaining of dyspnea and chest pain. Radiography revealed a left pneumothorax with a fluid level. Two aspirations over 1 hour's time produced 1,375 ml of milky fluid reported to be chyle. Although all physicians are cautioned about injury to

TABLE 21-5. *Reported incidence of pneumothorax after various nerve blocks*

Nerve block	Incidence (%)
Supraclavicular brachial plexus block	0.6–2
Stellate ganglion block	
Anterior approach	0.25
Anterolateral approach	0.5–8
Posterior approach	3–13
Thoracic paravertebral (somatic) block	0–6
Thoracic paravertebral (sympathetic) block	1.4–7.9

the thoracic duct in the left neck, it is a rare clinical complication. It is important for anesthesiologists to realize that iatrogenic trauma to the thoracic duct is not unique to neural blockade but has been reported as a complication of subclavian vein catheterization in the placement of hyperalimentation lines.[113] Further illustrating the fact that other than nerve-blocking needles may result in air or fluid in the chest is the report of Ghani and Berry[42] of right hydrothorax after left external jugular vein catheterization for fluid infusion.

Two important clinical considerations must be kept in mind regarding needle puncture of the lung, without regard to fault. If any of the patient's care after such trauma involves positive intrapleural pressure (e.g., endotracheal anesthesia or ventilation), then one must be alert to the possibility of a tension pneumothorax, which can be further complicated by the use of nitrous oxide. Such an occurrence could result in an intraoperative crisis if not recognized early and treated properly. Less serious, but of no small consequence, is the fact that even intermittent positive pressure breathing from respiratory therapy may convert a small asymptomatic pneumothorax into a large and clinically significant one, requiring chest tube drainage.

The role of chest radiography in the diagnosis of pneumothorax, empirically, or when clinically indicated, is variable according to personal or specialty practice standards. Apropos of the previous reports on central venous line placement is the recommendation by those authors that the position of all central lines be verified radiographically. Pneumothorax, depending upon the magnitude of the pleural trauma, may not appear radiographically for 6 to 12 hours. Therefore, routine chest x-rays in the recovery room may not be helpful. If one accepts the philosophy that most clinically significant pneumothoraces are symptomatic and that there is an incidence of less than 5%, then there is little justification for empiric chest x-rays, as opposed to individual clinical indications.

Treatment or management of pneumothorax is also variable and often determined by a consultant surgeon rather than an anesthesiologist. Moore[79] recommends that pneumothoraces of approximately 20% or less are likely to resolve spontaneously and therefore require no treatment. Anything over 20% should be aspirated. Those only slightly larger and asymptomatic may be aspirated with a needle; the larger and symptomatic ones probably will require chest tube and suction drainage. Periodic follow-up radiographs should be taken to ensure that there has been no recurrence of pneumothorax post-therapy.

NEUROLOGIC COMPLICATIONS AND SIDE-EFFECTS

Neurologic complications are clearly associated with the most notoriety and misinformation of all the complications of neural blockade. They include the rare but often disastrous complications to the spinal cord and surrounding structures, and the more frequent complications of headache and peripheral nerve disturbances. Despite the fact that these serious and often permanent complications happen at a rate that is severalfold less than mortality with general anesthesia, they remain as a daily reminder to all and therefore have a more negative impact on respective nerve block techniques than mortality has on general anesthesia techniques. Maintaining a global perspective on all the complications of anesthesia and surgery is equally important; it is critically necessary to demonstrate that all neurologic sequelae are not necessarily due to the neural blockade technique. Nicholson and McAlpine[81] quote two large surgical series of 50,000 and 30,000 patients, respectively. Seventy-two patients in the former series and 31 patients in the latter developed postoperative neural complications, usually peripheral nerve and usually related to positioning of the patient. A report on nerve injury associated with anesthesia from the data base of the American Society of Anesthesiologists's Closed Claims Study (1990) stated that 227 of 1,541 (15%) of the claims reviewed were for nerve injury.[62] Postoperative ulnar neuropathy, usually following general anesthesia, was the most common nerve injury, representing 1/3 of all nerve injuries. Brachial plexus injuries (23%) and lumbosacral nerve root injuries (16%) were less common. The authors reported that the exact cause of injury was often unclear. Only lumbosacral nerve injuries were associated with predominantly regional anesthetic techniques.

Delayed Systemic Toxicity

At first glance, it may seem unusual to separate *acute* (intravascular) systemic toxicity (previously discussed in this chapter) from delayed (absorption) systemic toxicity. The acute problem, however, is a complication of unintentional vascular injection, whereas delayed systemic toxicity is really a neurologic consequence of relative overdose of local anesthetic agent. Most anesthesiologists memorize a single maximum allowable dose of each local anesthetic agent on a milligram-per-body-weight basis and are quite unaware of all the technical, physiologic, pharmacologic, and pathologic variables that might predispose a patient to toxicity at "normal" doses (see Chapter 4). Less appreciated than toxicity from single-injection overdose is the very delayed CNS toxicity that may result from toxic blood levels achieved through cumulative overdose (see Chapter 3). The potential for more serious or even fatal complications from this type of CNS toxicity is a result of the very late and insidious onset of the convulsions and the very long time they may persist. Whereas the direct intravascular injection of a local anesthetic agent will precipitate an immediate but very transient convulsion, the CNS toxicity secondary to relative overdose (single or cumulative) may not occur for 20 minutes or for several hours. This also means that the patient having the immediate seizure probably will be attended by the practitioner administering the block, who, presumably, has the equipment and the ability to provide appropriate resuscitation. With delayed onset of toxicity, patients may have been moved to nontreatment areas, and the administering practitioner in all likelihood has left to attend to other anesthetic duties, and the unattended patient is left vulnerable to a prolonged seizure. All patients who have received a single large dose, or who are receiving intermittent or continuous doses of local anesthetics, must be attended by trained personnel in areas where complications may be treated quickly and appropriately. Such occurrences after cumulative dose local anesthetics are most likely to happen in obstetric or postoperative pain patients. Thorburn and Moir[112] reported two patients who had bupivacaine epidural analgesia for labor followed by cesarean section, and who manifested seizure activity after 10 hours (357.5 mg) and 9 hours (356.25 mg), respectively. Similar situations may result in surgical anesthesia in which a major nerve block is missed and repeated by another anesthesiologist, using full doses of local anesthetic; if still unsatisfactory, the surgeon infiltrates even more of the "local," and the patient convulses. Although *neural* absorption of local anesthetic cannot be guaranteed, the *vascular* bed is ubiquitous and virtually assures that every milligram of administered local anesthetic will contribute to a higher blood level.

An obvious preventive measure to this "total dose—high blood level" problem would be the monitoring of plasma levels of the local anesthetics. The seizure level of these agents has been studied extensively (see Chapters 3 and 4), and the ability to measure blood levels is clinically possible. Unfortunately, the precise seizure level for a given patient is neither predictable nor constant; in addition to body weight, it depends on site of injection, presence of vasoconstrictors, lipid solubility, pKa and protein binding of the injected drug, pH of the patient's blood, and the patient's cardiac, renal, and hepatic function. Hasselstrom and Mogensen[47] reported a toxic reaction to bupivacaine in a patient whose plasma bupivacaine level was 1.1 μg/ml. The accepted toxic threshold for bupivacaine is in the range of 4 μg/ml or greater. It seems, therefore, that plasma level monitoring by itself will not prevent all toxic reactions. On the other hand, monitored levels approaching 4 μg/ml or greater should alert the clinician to take corrective action.

COMPLICATIONS IN SUBARACHNOID AND EPIDURAL SPACES

Before discussing the major permanent complications, a comment on the clinical syndrome known as "total spinal" anesthesia is in order. Most anesthesiologists realize that if large volumes or doses of local anesthetic are injected unintentionally into the subarachnoid space, the patient will become apneic, unresponsive, and usually hypotensive, requiring immediate supportive therapy. Usually after a period of time commensurate with duration of action of the injected drug, the spinal anesthetic regresses and the patient recovers. The element of concern to the clinician, however, is the fact that uneventful recovery does not always occur. Reasons for this are not all known, but failure to recognize and treat this condition properly certainly provides a setting for serious, irreversible complications. The anesthesiologist usually recognizes the unintentional subarachnoid injection during placement of an epidural or caudal anesthetic. Unfortunately, however, there are many other situations in neural blockade in which local anesthetics may be placed into the subarachnoid or epidural space and not be recognized.

These unexpected complications usually result from paravertebral nerve block techniques such as deep cervical plexus block, retrobulbar block, interscalene block, stellate ganglion block, intercostal nerve block, infraclavicular nerve block, thoracic and lumbar somatic and sympathetic nerve blocks, and celiac ganglion block. Hill and co-workers[49] reported a case of total spinal blockade during local anesthesia of the nose by the surgeon. Had not the patient failed to answer a question, the surgical drapes covering her comatose apneic state would not have been removed and a fatality may have resulted. Similar unexpected spinal or segmental epidural anesthetics have resulted from intrathoracic intercostal nerve block by surgeons before closing.[41] Not surprising, then, is the occurrence of epidural[63] and total spinal[6,32] anesthesia after interscalene arm block. Spinal anesthesia associated with interscalene block can result from inappropriately deep needle placement into the intervertebral foramen or injection into the dural cuff along a nerve root. Usually the apnea and loss of consciousness are short-lived, and the patient recovers without sequelae. Caudad needle orientation and intermittent dosing with frequent aspiration are preventive measures. Finally, in discussing the unsuspected onset of neurologic (or vascular) complications, one needs to keep in mind that epidural catheters may migrate into blood vessels or the subarachnoid space, resulting in toxic reaction or total spinal from what previously had been a functional epidural anesthetic.[85]

An unfortunate and severe complication with serious neurologic sequelae associated with unintentional subarachnoid injection of 2-chloroprocaine for epidural anesthesia was reported in the United States (see Chapter 4).[89,91] Of interest is that the resulting neuropathology varied from prolonged motor and sensory effect, to cauda equina syndrome, to adhesive arachnoiditis. In an effort to gain a true perspective on the serious neurologic complications after spinal and epidural, Kane[58] did an extensive search of the literature on this topic. His review serves to illustrate an important fact that all physicians must keep in mind. The multiple case reports of various complications that abound in the literature draw our

TABLE 21-6. *Survey reports of epidural anesthesia*

Reference[a]	Number of patients	Anesthetics	Procedures	Neurologic sequelae
Bleyaert (3)	3,000	Bupivacaine, 0.125%, 1:800,000 epinephrine	Obstetric	None
Moore (4)	11,080	Bupivacaine, 0.25%, 0.5%, or 0.75%, with or without epinephrine	Surgical, obstetric, diagnostic	None
Holdcroft (5)	1,000	Bupivacaine, 0.5%, or lidocaine, 1.5% (32 patients)	Obstetric	1 foot drop; 1 paresthesia of thigh
Moore (6)	7,286	Lidocaine + tetracaine with epinephrine in 6,270 patients; various agents in remaining cases	Surgical, obstetric	1 bilateral paralysis of quadriceps muscles
Lund (7)	10,000	Lidocaine, 2% (8,000 patients); chloroprocaine, 3% (700 patients); hexylcaine, 2% (200 patients)	Surgical, obstetric, diagnostic	1 paresis of 1 leg (subarachnoid hexylcaine); 4 paresthesias of thigh; 1 persistent numbness; 3 bladder or rectal incontinence
Eisen (8)	9,532	Lidocaine	Obstetric	16 paresthesias; 9 numbness of thigh; 1 paraplegia (1 of 5,091 surgical cases)
Bonica (9)	3,885	Various; mostly lidocaine	Surgical, obstetric, diagnostic	1 hypalgesia of trunk, weakness of leg (subarachnoid lidocaine); 1 paresthesias, numbness weakness of leg

[a] Refers to references listed within Kane's original article (see citation below).
(Kane, R.E.: Neurologic deficits following epidural or spinal anesthesia. Anesth. Analg., *60*:151, 1981.)

attention to the *kinds* of complications that may occur. Reviews such as this or those of Usubiaga[119] and Dawkins,[24] to name only a few, indicate the frequency and varied circumstances under which these might occur. Kane's review found three patients with permanent paralysis or paresis in a series of 50,000 epidural anesthetics (Table 21-6); in 65,000 spinal anesthetics, one permanent paralysis occurred (Table 21-7). Usubiaga studied more than 750,000 epidural anesthetics and concluded an incidence of 1 neurologic complication per 11,000 anesthetics. Of 32,718 cases reviewed, Dawkins reported an incidence of transient neurologic lesions of 0.1% and permanent lesions of 0.02%.

The kinds of neurologic sequelae causing permanent disturbances and their etiology are not always precise because only surgical or autopsy examination will provide tissue diagnosis. Paralysis or paresis may be due to cord ischemia or infarct secondary to hematoma, abscess, or anterior spinal artery occlusion. This may be caused by severe hypotension of any etiology and not just of spinal or epidural anesthesia. Direct injury to the spinal cord, roots, and their coverings may be traumatic or chemical. Chemical contaminants such as detergents, preservatives, and neurolytics act as irritants and may induce meningeal or arachnoid inflammatory responses. Excessive doses or concentrations of local anes-

TABLE 21-7. *Survey reports of spinal anesthesia*

Reference[a]	Number of patients	Anesthetics	Procedure	Neurologic sequelae
Kortum (23)	2,592	Bupivacaine, 0.5%	Surgical	1 lumbar plexus injury
Bergman (24)	10,000	Lidocaine, mepivacaine, bupivacaine	Various	None
Phillips (25)	10,440	Lidocaine	Obstetric, surgical	8 persistent peripheral neuropathy
Moore (26)	11,574	Tetracaine, dibucaine: with epinephrine or phenylephrine in 8,852	Surgical, obstetric	1 persistent muscular weakness of legs, impotence
Sadov (27)	20,000	Tetracaine, procaine, dibucaine	Various	1 paraplegia due to spinal tumor; 3 meningitis
Dripps (28); Vandam (29–31)	10,098	Tetracaine, procaine, dibucaine: with epinephrine in 2,000		No major neurologic sequelae; 2 foot drop; 1 leg weakness (trauma); 12 exacerbation of previous neurologic disease
Brown (32)	600	Tetracaine	Surgical	2 peroneal paresis, unilateral

[a] Refers to references listed within Kane's original article (see citation below).
(Kane, R.E.: Neurologic deficits following epidural or spinal anesthesia. Anesth. Analg., *60*:152, 1981.)

thetics and vasoconstrictors have also been incriminated in this process. Previously undiagnosed spinal tumors, or other spinal abnormalities, may be "revealed" at the time of spinal or epidural anesthesia (see Chapter 8).

Adhesive arachnoiditis and cauda equina syndrome are rare complications which have been linked to the use of spinal microcatheters when greater than normal doses of local anesthetic (primarily hyperbaric lidocaine) were administered because of initial inadequate blockade.[95,96] The authors concluded that though the etiology was unclear, the neural damage might have been caused by maldistribution of relatively high doses of local anesthetic to the sacral nerve roots. These catheters have been removed from the market for re-evaluation. Clinical signs of chronic adhesive arachnoiditis include bowel and bladder dysfunction, sensory loss in the perineum, and variable lower-extremity paresis, and can present slowly over days to weeks. The variable nature of the complaints and onset can result in a delay in diagnosis. CSF examination and radiographic studies may not be helpful in determining the etiology of this problem, but should be performed to rule out other anatomical or infectious causes. A cystometrogram will often show increased bladder volume and reduced sensation of urgency. Electromyography may also be helpful in determining the extent of involvement and confirming the clinical findings.

Recently, high concentrations of lidocaine have also been implicated in transient neurologic deficits when injected intrathecally as a single dose.[5,105] Repeated applications of local anesthetics via an indwelling intrathecal catheter, or by multiple single-shot spinal injections, to improve on a patchy or failed block, may be a potentially unsafe practice. Suggested precautions include: (i) aspiration of CSF before and after drug injection; (ii) evaluation of the extent of sacral blockade to ascertain preferential distribution to that site; (iii) limitation of the drug dosage to a maximum precalculated "safe" dosage; (iv) avoiding reinforcement of the same drug distribution if an injection must be repeated, by changing the (drug, patient's position, or changing drug baricity, etc.); and (v) if CSF cannot be aspirated after injection, by avoiding full dose repetition unless no sign of neural blockade (including in the sacral area) is present.[27]

Another potentially serious complication of spinal or epidural anesthesia that occurs somewhere between 0.1% to 0.82% is the subdural injection of local anesthetic solutions.[66] Clinically, the injection of substances into the "extra arachnoid" (or subdural)space was reported as a complication of myelography in the early 1960s with an incidence of 10% to 13%.[55,56,95,99]

The subdural (extra arachnoid) space is a potential space between dura and arachnoid. Unlike the epidural space, the

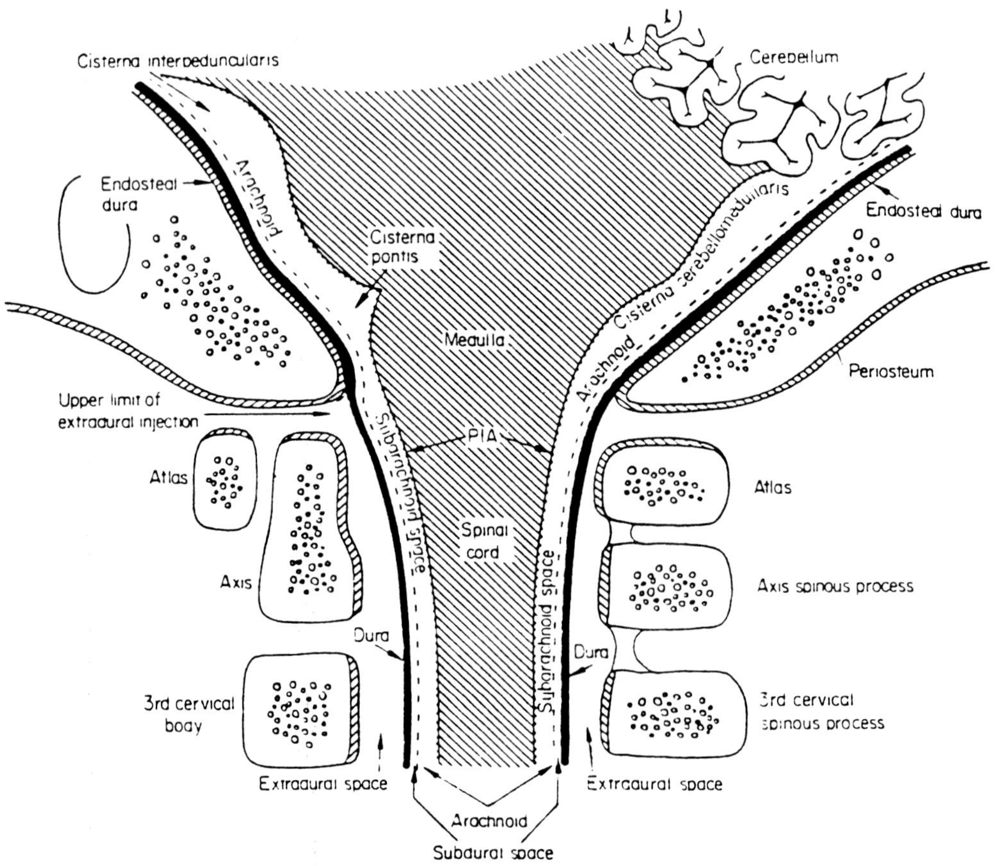

FIG. 21-4. Diagrammatic representation of the layers covering the spinal cord to show the site of the cervical subdural space and its extension into the cranial cavity. (Mehta, M., and Maher, R.: Injection into the extra arachnoid subdural space. Anaesthesia, *32*:762, 1977.)

subdural space extends intracranially Fig. 21-4. It contains a minute quantity of serous fluid to moisten the opposing membranes; but no CSF. It does not communicate directly with the subarachnoid space but extends laterally over the nerve roots and ganglion. The space is wider in the cervical region than elsewhere and closely adjacent to the nerve roots, where unintentional entry by an epidural needle or catheter is more likely to occur.[76] Further elaboration of the anatomy of the subdural space was reported using spinaloscopy at the L-2-3 level in autopsy cases.[12] Of 15 autopsy subjects, the subdural space in 10 subjects was opened easily. In another interspace, an epidural catheter was introduced through a Tuohy needle into the subdural space in 8 of the 15 subjects. An important observation is the thin nature of the arachnoid which was perforated by epidural catheters and through which catheters could be visualized. Clinical conclusions of this study are limited because of the differences in physiologic parameters between the antemortem and postmortem states. It does confirm, however, that the subdural space is capable of accepting the bevel of a Tuohy needle as well as an epidural catheter.

The clinical manifestations of subdural drug placement are variable and depend on such things as preceding dural puncture, rotation of needle, and dose of drug injected into the subdural space. A retrospective study of 2,182 lumbar epidural steroid injections attempted to determine the incidence of inadvertent subdural block where major criteria included failure to aspirate CSF and an unexpected widespread sensory block. Minor criteria were a delayed onset of 10 or more minutes, variable motor block and sympatholysis out of proportion to anesthetic dose. Eighteen patients were identified.[68] General conclusions included sensory levels higher than expected from doses injected, only 60% incidence of motor block, no aspiration of CSF, onset times from 5 to 30 minutes, and 60% incidence of hypotension (>30% drop from baseline). Contrary to the expressed rationalizations of some clinicians, the subdural space is not a silent repository to which all missed spinals and epidurals may be attributed (see Chapter 7).

Infection

Bacterial infection is a possible risk in all neural blockade, but, like hematoma, it is of greatest concern if it occurs around the spinal cord and its coverings or spaces. Micro-organisms may be transmitted by syringes, catheters, needles, and injected agents. They may come from the anesthesiologist or from the patient, with a septic process of the skin, tissue, or blood. The most common infections are localized to skin and subcutaneous tissue in patients with chronic pain who have had indwelling catheters left in place for days to weeks. The serious neural infections of abscess, meningitis, and arachnoiditis are quite rare.

The most common organisms seen in bacterial meningitis are staphylococcus aureus, coliform species and pseudomonas. Bacterial meningitis presents 24 to 48 hours after needle placement with fever, stiff neck, and signs of meningeal irritability. Analysis of spinal fluid should be performed early so that appropriate antibiotic treatment can be instituted. Partial treatment with antibiotics prior to CSF examination may confuse the diagnosis. Kilpatrick and Girgis[59] reported 17 cases of meningitis after spinal anesthesia over a 5-year period in a ward in Cairo, Egypt, treating 1,429 meningitis patients. Only 10 of the 17 had positive CSF cultures: Eight were *Pseudomonas aeruginosa,* 1 was *Staphylococcus aureus,* and 1 was *Streptococcus mitis.* These organisms were *not* cultured from the other patients who had not had spinal anesthesia. They concluded that meningitis in patients after recent spinal anesthesia commonly is due to unusual or nosocomial organisms and recommended aggressive, meticulous, bacteriologic evaluation and early treatment.

Abscess formation following epidural or spinal anesthesia can be superficial, requiring limited surgical drainage and intravenous antibiotics, or can occur deep in the epidural space with associated cord compression. The latter is fortunately a rare complication, but requires aggressive, early surgical management in order to achieve a satisfactory outcome. Usubiaga[119] reported seven cases of infection associated with epidural anesthesia, noting that most reports came in earlier years. Beaudoin and Klein[9] reported a patient who developed back pain following five spinal anesthetics, and who was found, 4 weeks after the last spinal, to have a large epidural abscess. CSF examination was sterile and normal except for elevated protein content (0.9 g/liter). They presumed infection of a hematoma but could not determine whether the source of contamination was blood-borne or external. Superficial infections present with local tissue swelling, erythema and drainage, often associated with fever, but rarely causing neurologic problems unless untreated. Epidural abscess formation usually presents several days after neural blockade, with clinical signs of severe back pain, local tenderness, and fever associated with leukocytosis. Radiologic evidence of an epidural mass in the presence of variable neurologic deficit is diagnostic. Magnetic resonance imaging is advocated as the most sensitive modality for evaluation of the spine when infection is suspected.[70] Surgical intervention within 12 hours is associated with the best chance of neurologic recovery. Injection of epidural steroids and underlying disease processes associated with immunocompromise theoretically increase the risk of infection.[108] Patients should be observed carefully for signs of infection when a continuous epidural catheter is left in place for prolonged periods. Injection of local anesthetic or insertion of a catheter in an area at high risk for bacterial contamination, such as the sacral hiatus, may also increase the risk for abscess formation, emphasizing the importance of meticulous aseptic technique.

Recent animal data suggest that appropriate antibiotic therapy prior to dural puncture in the presence of bacteremia may decrease the risk of CSF contamination.[18] Human data are scarce, although Bader reported the use of epidural anesthesia in 279 pregnant patients with chorioamnionitis, three with documented bacteremia, without adverse infectious complications.[4] The importance of a localized infection at a site distant from the site of needle insertion in the etiology of epidural or intrathecal infectious complications is unknown, but at best such an association is highly theoretical. However, the rare reports of adverse events serve as a warning to the practitioner who initiates epidural or spinal anesthesia in the face of a local or systemic infection. Although fever, by itself, may have many causes other than bacteremia, and therefore may not mitigate against such anesthetics, extreme caution and thought should be used when doing these blocks in septic patients.

Headache

The most minor, but also the most common, complication of spinal anesthesia, and perhaps of epidural anesthesia, is post-dural puncture headache (PDPH). It is important to the image of spinal anesthesia that the age-old term "spinal headache" be discarded in favor of "PDPH," because this specific syndrome more frequently occurs subsequent to dural puncture for myelogram, diagnostic neurologic or radiologic studies, and even to unintentional puncture with epidural anesthesia. Despite significant progress in preventing or treating some complications of neural blockade, little has changed in the prevention and treatment of postdural puncture headaches over the past 2 decades. The most frequently cited preventive factors are the use of small and/or pencil-point needles and selection of older patients. Most authors writing on the topic still quote authors and series dating back 3 to 4 decades. Driessen and colleagues[28] prospectively studied 613 patients in whom a total of 783 spinal anesthetics had been performed. Twenty-three patients (2.9%) developed a typical postdural puncture headache. A later study by Eckstein and associates[33] of 1,009 patients compared the 22-gauge and 25-gauge Quincke tip spinal needle with a 22-gauge Whitacre tip needle. The smaller needle caused only 1/2 as many headaches as the larger needle. There was no difference between the 22-gauge Quincke tip and the 22-gauge Whitacre tip. The overall incidence of headaches was about 5%. Interestingly, and contrary to common belief, the highest frequency of headaches was reported in female patients in the 5th decade. An increase with younger age patients was *not* noted. Definite bloody taps were associated with significantly higher rates. Several more recent studies also show an acceptable rate of PDPH in young patients when small needles are used for dural puncture.[40,69,74] Recent studies comparing small (25- to 29-g) diamond-point to pencil-point (22- to 24-g) needles failed to show significant differences in the overall incidence of PDPH in widely varying patient populations.[65,69,71,110] One study reported a significantly higher incidence when the diamond-point needle was inserted perpendicular to the dural fibers[110] and another showed a higher incidence of "moderate to severe" headache with the standard needle point.[65] A comparison of midline and paramedian techniques, using a pencil-point needle, showed a higher incidence of headache with the paramedian approach in older patients.[56] Interestingly, intrathecal catheters placed through large gauge epidural needles (18-g) did not have a higher incidence of headache compared to either a continuous catheter through a 20-gauge needle or a single-shot 22-gauge diamond point needle.[75] Although nearly all series report a higher incidence of postlumbar puncture headaches in obstetric patients receiving spinal anesthesia, the reasons are not clear. Ravindran and co-workers[90] studied the effect of "bearing down" at the time of delivery. They found no difference in the incidence of headache in the two groups (9% versus 10%).

Little new has been added to the therapeutic regime, with conservative treatment and autologous epidural blood patch still being the favored technique, (see Chapter 7). Early diag-

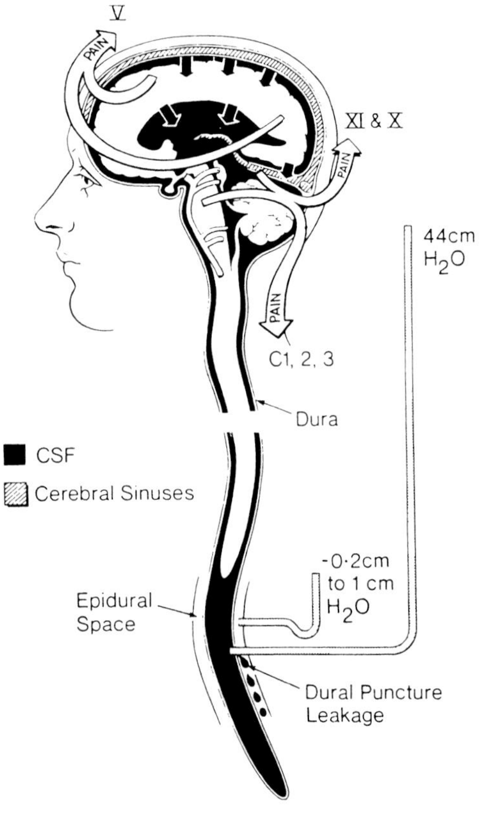

FIG. 21-5. Pathophysiology of dural puncture headache. Barometric figures are those to be expected in the subarachnoid and epidural spaces in the upright position at the site of lumbar puncture. The pressure differential favors CSF leakage. Note that CSF pressure is approximately atmospheric at the base of the brain. CSF leakage leads to descent of the brain in the upright position (*dark arrows*) on pain-sensitive intracranial vessels and the tentorium. Pain is referred (*open arrows*) above the tentorium via the trigeminal nerve (*V*) to the frontal region, and below the tentorium via the glossopharyngeal and vagal nerves (*IX, X*) to the occiput and via the upper cervical nerves (*C1, 2, 3*) to the neck and shoulders. (Brownridge, P.: The management of headache following accidental dural puncture in obstetric patients. Anaesth. Intensive Care., *11*:9, 1983.)

nosis and treatment are essential because, as noted earlier in this chapter, there are case reports of intracerebral hematomas in patients with prolonged, untreated, postpuncture headaches, presumably from significant losses of CSF. A summary of proposed factors in postdural puncture headache is shown in Figure 21-5.

COMPLICATIONS OF PERIPHERAL NERVE BLOCKS

Less dramatic than, but equally important as, the complications of the spinal cord, its coverings, and spaces, are the complications related to the peripheral nerves. Many advocates of regional anesthesia stress the need for paresthesias as an integral part of the nerve block technique to ensure successful anesthesia. Conversely, critics of the paresthesia approach to neural blockade have been equally vocal about the damage that could, theoretically, result from repeated needle trauma to the nerves. Clinical reports by many authors of thousands of peripheral nerve blocks of all types render this criticism more theoretical than real. Reports by Selander and colleagues,[104] however, provided sufficient evidence to cause anesthesiologists to reexamine the risks of eliciting paresthesias during nerve blocks. They studied the frequency of nerve lesions after axillary plexus block performed with nerve location, either by paresthesias or by axillary artery pulsation. Their study included 290 patients in the paresthesia group and 243 in the arterial group. It should be noted, however, that paresthesias were elicited in 40% of patients in the arterial group. All patients received 1% mepivacaine containing 1 : 200,000 epinephrine. Symptoms varied from light dysesthesias lasting a few weeks to severe dysesthesias with aching and paresis lasting more than 1 year (Table 21-8). The presumed etiology of these nerve complications was either direct nerve trauma from the needle or drug-induced injury following direct intraneural injection. To elucidate these differences, the same group[103] studied the effects of intrafascicular or topical application of bupivacaine on isolated rabbit sciatic nerve. Whereas the topical application to the nerve of saline, bupivacaine, and bupivacaine plus epinephrine caused no detectable nerve injury, the intrafascicular injections resulted in axonal degeneration and damaged blood nerve barrier.

Axonal degeneration was the same after physiologic saline as after plain bupivacaine in low concentrations. It did increase, however, with increasing concentrations of bupivacaine and with the epinephrine-containing solutions (Table 21-9). They concluded that intraneural injections should be avoided and, whenever possible, solutions should be used which do not contain epinephrine. Earlier work by Selander,[102] using the same sciatic nerve preparation, studied the effect of the angle of the needle bevel on nerve injury. One needle was the conventional sharp-pointed needle (14°-bevel) and the other, a very blunt-tipped (45°-bevel) needle. Their results showed that whereas the sharp needle tended to cut the nerve fiber in both the parallel and horizontal approaches, the 45° short-bevel needle tended to push the nerve fiber away and, therefore, produced less axonal damage (see Chapter 6, Table 6-2). A more recent study of needle impalement in rat sciatic nerves associated more severe, frequent, and longer duration nerve injuries with short bevel needles. The least traumatic injuries occurred when a long bevel needle was inserted parallel to the nerve fibers.[94] The results of this study suggest that recommendations that paresthesia techniques should be avoided in all patients may not be justified.

The clinical importance of these studies is to stress not only that each variable—drug, needle, and epinephrine—may by itself cause axonal damage, but, combined in the form of an intraneural injection of a significant volume of solution, will be likely to cause serious problems. Meticulous technique, combined with a clear understanding of pertinent underlying medical conditions (e.g. diabetes mellitus), and application of local anesthetic pharmacology with an emphasis on tissue toxicity, will aid in prevention of nerve trauma. Barutell and colleagues[7] reported the case of a 49-year-old woman who received 8 ml of 1% prilocaine for interscalene brachial plexus block. "The patient suffered a sharp paresthesia—when the needle was inserted, and, at the same time, a brisk jerk of the hand occurred. Neither spinal fluid nor blood escaped. The paresthesia became worse

TABLE 21-8. *Number of patients with symptoms of postanesthetic nerve lesion*

	Number of patients	Nerve lesion Patients	Nerve lesion %
Paresthesia group	290	8	2.8
Artery group	243	2	0.8
Total	533	10	1.9

(Selander, D., Edshage, and S., Wolff, T.: Paresthesiae or no paresthesiae? Acta Anesthesiol. Scand., *23*:29, 1979.)

TABLE 21-9. *Axonal degeneration after intrafascicular injection of 0.05 ml*

Agent	Concentration (mg/ml)	Axonal degeneration[a] 0 → +	+ +	+ + +
Physiologic saline		11	4	1
Bupivacaine	5	10	6	—
Bupivacaine	10	4	7	5
Bupivacaine with epinephrine, 5 μg/ml	5	—	11	5

[a] Degrees of axonal degeneration: 0 → +: none or insignificant; + +: significant but <50% of axons; + + +: ≥50% of axons.

(Selander, D., Brattsand, R., Lundborg, G., *et al.*: Local anesthetics: Importance of mode of application, concentration and adrenaline for the appearance of nerve lesions. Acta Anesthesiol. Scand., *23*:129, 1979.)

when the injection of the local anaesthetic began, but in spite of this injection was continued . . . When 8 ml had been injected, the patient suddenly became hoarse—loss of consciousness and respiratory failure followed." The day after operation, the patient had a paralysis of the extensor muscles of her fingers and of the flexor and intrinsic muscles of the hand. These deficits never resolved. This case is extremely important in illustrating the dictum that one should never continue injecting local anesthesia if a patient complains of severe pain. Retraction or movement of the needle 1 to 2 mm will ensure that it is not intraneural, and such complications should be avoided.

Because most of the complications to peripheral nerves manifest in the postoperative period, it is essential that patients be followed by the anesthesiologist in the prolonged postoperative period, through close communication with the primary surgeon. Winchell[122] reported on 854 consecutive patients receiving upper arm block for upper extremity surgery who were evaluated on their first and second postoperative visits to the surgeon for evidence of neuropathy. They found 3 patients with unequivocal evidence of nerve damage, for an incidence of 0.36%. It is equally important that possible causes other than a given nerve block technique be included in the etiologic diagnoses. All patients, but especially trauma patients, should have neurologic examination results noted on their chart. In addition to anesthetic causes, faulty positioning of the patient, tight casts and dressings, intraoperative tourniquet use and surgical trauma may result in damage to peripheral nerves. Nicholson and McAlpine,[81] in writing about neural injuries associated with surgical positions and operations, quote series of 50,000 and 30,000 patients, respectively. Seventy-two patients in the first series developed postoperative nerve complications believed to be related to the period during which the patient was anesthetized. Brachial plexus palsy was the most common injury occurring in 23 of 28 patients who had undergone open heart surgery. Other nerves involved included peroneal, radial, ulnar, median, and sciatic. In the study of 30,000 patients (1940 to 1945), 31 patients had paresis of one or more nerves during the postoperative period—26 in the upper extremity and 5 in the lower (all common peroneal nerve). A review of nerve injury associated with anesthesia from the American Society of Anesthesiologists[7] Closed Claims Study database reported that 227 of 1,541 (15%) of the claims were for nerve injury.[62] The most common lesion was ulnar neuropathy, usually following general anesthesia. Brachial plexus injuries (23%) and lumbosacral nerve root injuries (16%) were seen less frequently, and only lumbosacral nerve injuries were associated with predominantly regional anesthetic techniques.

Three cases of femoral neuropathy as a complication of lithotomy position under spinal anesthesia reported by Tondare and co-workers[115] illustrate one of the most troublesome areas for the diagnosis of postsurgical complications. These authors reported on three patients who sustained unilateral peripheral femoral neuropathy of 4 to 8 weeks' duration, after vaginal hysterectomy operations in the lithotomy position, lasting 2 to 21/2 hours. They attributed the complication to the extreme abduction of the thighs with external rotation at the hip, causing ischemia of the femoral nerve as it is kinked beneath the tough inguinal ligament. All too often, if a patient has had spinal or epidural anesthesia, the surgical and nursing staff will suggest to the patient that the complications are a result of anesthesia. The anesthesiologist who makes careful postoperative rounds can become aware of these latent complications and solicit appropriate neurologic consultations. Most unilateral peripheral nerve problems will not be a result of spinal, caudal, or epidural anesthesia, but from some more peripheral cause.

One of the proposed explanations for peripheral nerve injury has been that smaller nerves, especially when they lie over bone or in restricted fascial compartments, are more vulnerable to ischemia or traumatic injury (e.g., pressure), or both. Some practitioners have discouraged block of nerves at the knee (see Chapter 11) and digits for that very reason. Nerves in tight places also will not slide away as easily from the advancing block needle and are therefore more vulnerable to intraneural injection. Born[13] reported a series of 49 patients receiving 0.5% bupivacaine for wrist and metacarpal nerve blocks. Seven patients developed hyperesthesia in the blocked nerve distribution, lasting from 1 week to 4 months. Relatively large total volumes of solution were used, and three of the patients had 1 : 200,000 epinephrine added to their solutions. This then reinforces the admonition of teachers of regional block: that is, when blocking small nerves, use small volumes of weak concentrations of local anesthetic solutions *without* epinephrine. In addition, extreme caution should be used to avoid nerve trauma or intraneural injections.

MISCELLANEOUS COMPLICATIONS OF NEURAL BLOCKADE

Although the manifestations of the complications to be noted herein will likely be neurologic or vascular, they arise from a variety of causes in the performance of neural blockade and tend to be discrete entities; they thus are grouped together in a miscellaneous category to include such diverse topics as allergy, methemoglobinemia, backache, and equipment failure.

Allergy to Local Anesthetics

Many patients, and all too often their physicians and dentists, believe themselves allergic to local anesthetic (see Chapter 4) and subject themselves to a life of inconvenience or therapeutic confusion every time they require a procedure done under "local." In point of fact, although allergic reactions to the ester family of local anesthetics are known to occur, they are not common. Even more relevant in today's practice of infiltration and regional neural blockade, using amide types of local anesthetics, is the fact that clinically manifest allergic reactions in this group of drugs are extremely rare. Brown and colleagues[15] reported a patient who presented with a history "years ago" of a reaction to lignocaine. They skin-tested, uneventfully, with 0.2 ml of 0.5% prilocaine, but when they skin-tested with 0.2 ml of 0.5% bupivacaine the patient immediately developed a tight chest, rash, and visual disturbances. Immunologic studies showed a decrease in plasma complement C4 concentration, which they thought indicated the reaction was immunologically mediated. Soon thereafter, Fisher and Pennington[39] reported on a patient who had a very positive history of lidocaine and prilocaine allergy in whom they performed a variety of dilutional intradermal tests. The tests confirmed her clinical sensitivity and suggested no allergy to bupivacaine, which she subsequently received without untoward effect (Table 21-10) . They emphasize that skin tests for one group of local anesthetics give no information about any other and that all should be tested.

Methemoglobinemia

An increased level of methemoglobin has been a recognized complication of receiving the local anesthetic agent prilocaine since its introduction in the early 1960s (See Chapters 3 and 4) . Although as little as 1.52% may cause visible cyanosis, it is of little consequence. The formation of methemoglobin is dose-related, with doses of >8 mg/kg for peripheral nerve blocks required to produce symptoms. This phenomenon is of minimal importance to clinicians, because the drug has become less commonly used for intravenous regional anesthesia and infiltration. Duncan and Kobrinsky[30] reported extremely high levels of methemoglobin in a neonate who received 7.5 mg of 4% prilocaine for surgical infiltration during a palate repair.

Different patients may metabolize the drug differently. Therefore, should cyanosis occur in any patient who has received prilocaine, a methemoglobin determination should be obtained. The cyanosis of methemoglobinemia has a late onset—a few hours after injection—and therefore may be missed as the causative factor when diagnosed by recovery room nurses and surgical staff.

TABLE 21-10. *Intradermal testing in a patient after severe anaphylactoid reactions to local anesthetic*

	Dilution			
Drug	1:10,000	1:1,000	1:100	1:10
1% procaine	NT[a]	NT	—	0.8[b]
1% xylocaine	14/40	14/40	NT	NT
1% mepivacaine	0/0	0/0	0/0	0/0
1% bupivacaine	0/0	0/0	0/0	0/0
0.5% amethocaine	5/15	12/28	NT	NT
1% prilocaine	10/45	15/45	NT	NT

[a] NT = not tested.
[b] Expressed as wheal size over flare size (mm).
(Fisher, M., and Pennington, J.C.: Allergy to local anaesthesia. Br. J Anaesth., *54*:893, 1982.)

Backache

Pain of any kind is a subjective complaint, the cause of which may be as obscure as its symptoms. Headache and backache are two such relatively frequent pain problems, usually associated with spinal, epidural, and paravertebral neural blockade. Since headache of neural blockade origin is a more specific syndrome attributed to postdural puncture, it is discussed in detail in Chapter 7. Backache, however, may also follow surgery under general anesthesia. An early study evaluated patients who received either spinal or general anesthesia and found no significant difference in incidence of backache between the two techniques. It is generally accepted that backache most commonly occurs after procedures in which there is flattening of the normal lumbar curve owing to relaxation of the paraspinous muscles (with either muscle relaxants or local anesthetics), allowing stretch of the joint capsules and spinous ligaments. Such an effect is exaggerated if the patient is further manipulated, as might occur during the lithotomy position. Regional anesthesia probably has been unfairly incriminated as the cause of this problem for two reasons: First, there is a high use of regional anesthesia for surgical procedures employing the lithotomy position (e.g., urology, obstetrics, and gynecology); and second, there is the natural cause-and-effect reaction of many patients who reason that "I received a needle puncture in my back (especially if traumatically done) and developed pain in my back after surgery; therefore, the needle must have caused the back pain." Moir and Davidson[77] compared 50 patients receiving pudendal nerve block for vaginal delivery with 50 patients who received epidural analgesia and noted 32% incidence of backache in the pudendal group and 22% in the epidural group. Crawford,[22] in analyzing 923 lumbar epidural blocks for labor, noted that 45% of his patients complained of backache on one or more of the first 6 postnatal days. In 32% of the total series, backache began on the day after delivery. He believed that in most patients, there was no evidence that it was related to the epidural block.

Reports of severe, spasmodic, back pain associated with epidural chloroprocaine followed the introduction of the ethylenediaminetetraacetic acid (EDTA) containing Nesacaine-MPF formulation.[38] Hynson and co-workers described the same symptoms in volunteers having epidural anesthesia with 3% chloroprocaine but not with lidocaine or saline injections.[55] Possible contributory factors cited were the presence of EDTA, large injected volumes, low pH and local infiltration with chloroprocaine. In a prospective study of 100 patients, Stevens et al.[107] injected chloroprocaine solutions of various pH volumes with and without EDTA, using lidocaine as a control. They reported no difference in superficial back pain; however, the group receiving the large volume of EDTA containing chloroprocaine had worse pain. They recommended limiting total volumes to less than 25 ml to decrease the incidence of this problem. The exact mechanism has not been elucidated.

The importance of discussing this relatively benign complication is not to encourage practitioners to deny further that nerve block techniques may cause such a problem; rather, it is extremely important that the patients undergoing these procedures by informed preanesthetically that backache may occur as a result of the procedure (surgery, anesthesia, *and* position) but that it is usually transient and can be treated successfully with analgesics.

Faulty Equipment and Technique

These are not complications, but rather the cause of some relatively minor complications. Perhaps the most notable is that of the "sheared catheter." The majority of reports indicate the cause of this complication is the withdrawal of the epidural catheter back into a needle, with the sharp edge of the needle shearing the catheter (Fig. 21-6). Occasionally, catheters that have been in the patient for some time will break off at the skin surface. Despite the universal dictum "Never pull a catheter back through a needle," these complications still occur. There is, however, increasing agreement among practitioners of epidural anesthesia that if a catheter is sheared or broken off in the epidural space, it does not necessarily have to be removed surgically. Most of the current catheters are made of inert materials and are not likely to cause tissue reaction or injury to vessels and organs. The patient should be informed of the occurrence and be given the recommendation that it be left in place unless it subsequently becomes a problem. However, if the catheter breaks off in the subcutaneous tissues, it may serve as a wick for infection into the deep structures. In these cases, surgical removal may be necessary.

Inserting the catheter beyond the recommended 2 to 4 cm may result in coiling and subsequent knotting of the catheter in the epidural space. This problem usually will present as difficulty in removing the catheter, which will gradually attentuate as traction is applied. Epidural cathethers are made of materials with high tensile strength, so that it is sometimes possible to apply gentle, continuous, traction on the catheter, until the knot becomes attenuated enough to allow it to be pulled intact through the structures overlying the epidural space. While the risk of this maneuver is that the catheter will break, other options are limited.

Earlier authors cautioned about broken needles and the damage that might occur. Recommendations for removal of broken needles still prevail, since they might migrate from the site of entry and lead to more serious complications. Modern needles are resistant to breakage, but buckling and breaking of epidural needles due to excessive axial force has been reported.[31] A minor, but often unappreciated, complication of the current long-beveled disposable needles used for neural blockade is their predisposition to "spur" upon striking a bony surface. The result, when examined closely (Fig. 21-7), is a needle tip resembling a small fish hook. Clearly, such a needle tip passing in and out of nerves, arteries, and veins could cause significant damage. It is impor-

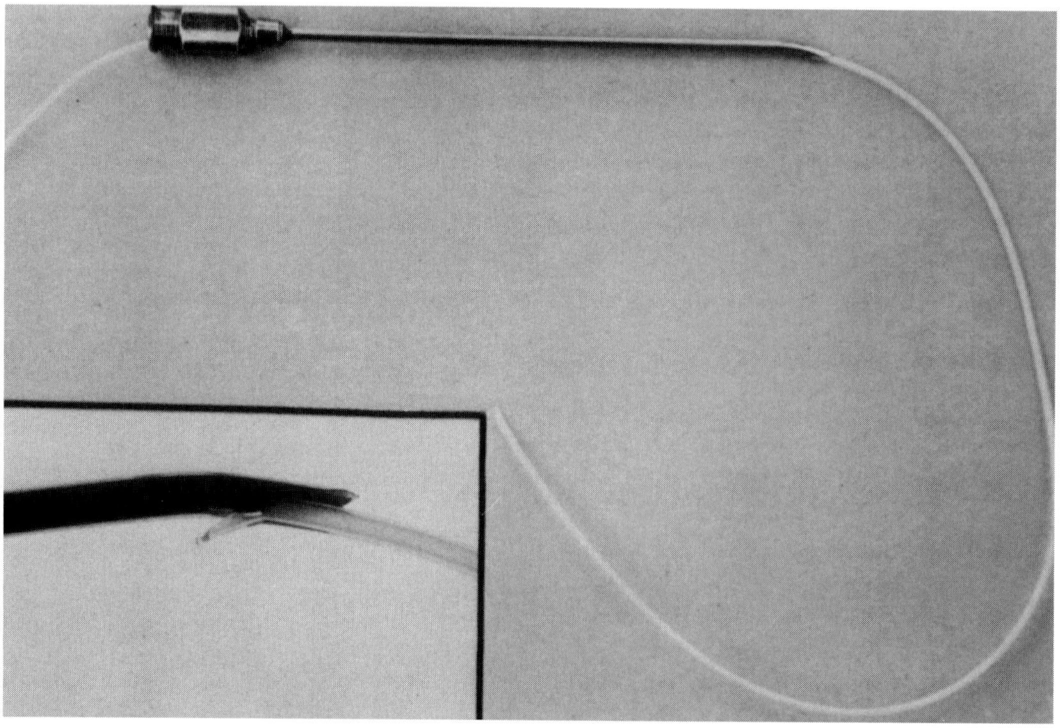

FIG. 21-6. A needle "shearing off" a catheter.

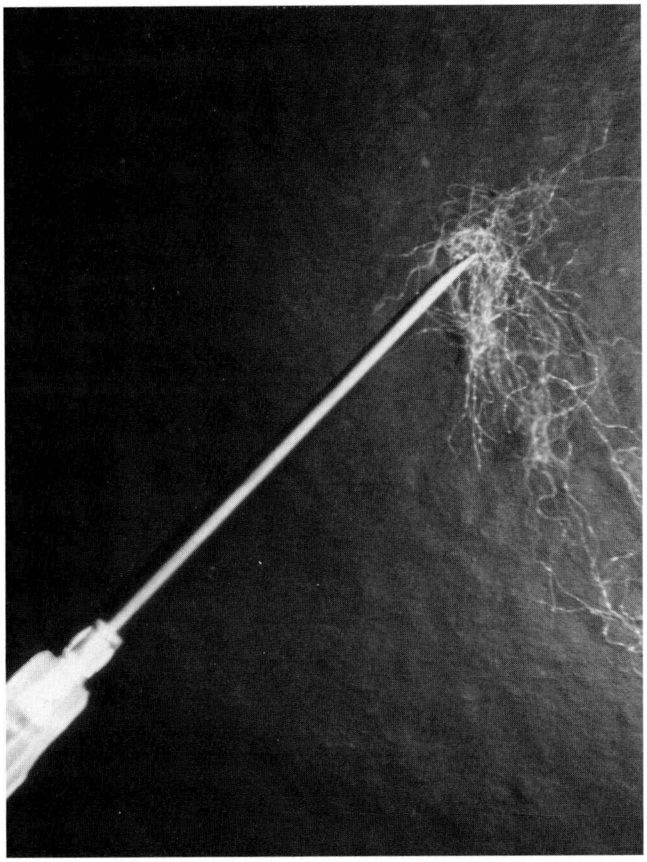

FIG. 21-7. Needle with barb or "fish hook."

tant, therefore, that such needles be tested frequently by passing the tip over gauze or cotton, and that they be discarded for a new one at the first indication of spur formation.

PROPHYLAXIS OR TREATMENT OF COMPLICATIONS

It was suggested at the beginning of this chapter that many of the complications of neural blockade were a result of errors in judgment, related to choice of patient, technique, drug, concentration, volume, supplementation with sedation, and so forth. The most effective prophylaxis is to avoid, whenever possible, situations that could lead to an increased risk of complications. Of prime importance, therefore, is a careful and thorough preanesthetic evaluation of the patient to be anesthetized, to determine whether he or she has, for example, altered anatomy, coagulopathies, altered blood volume, and any restrictions to supplementation or resuscitation, and special attention should, in these cases, be given to features of the preselected regional block technique.

Equally important in the preanesthetic evaluation is a discussion with the patient of the proposed technique, its benefits, and its significant risks, necessary to provide a legitimate informed consent. This discussion should be in sufficient detail that patients understand, in advance, their role in co-operating with the administration of the anesthetic and how it will be managed intraoperatively (see Chapter 6). Many complications incur the potential for medicolegal problems through patient-physician misunderstanding or lack of rapport.

Perhaps most important in preventing complications is insurance of adequate and functional equipment not only for performance of the anesthetic but also for resuscitation, the latter being extremely important for nerve blocks performed in offices and outpatient settings. Unfortunately, centers or practitioners who perform regional blocks infrequently will attempt to assemble a disarray of obsolete needles and syringes on an "as needed" basis and then will wonder at their high incidence of failures and complications. Everyone who undertakes the practice of neural blockade, no matter how minor, should be trained in cardiopulmonary resuscitation and should have immediate access to the essential equipment and supplies. Incurring complications can be avoidable; failure to diagnose and treat those complications appropriately may be negligence.

Although many of the complications discussed herein will occur almost immediately or within the anesthetic period, others, such as neuropathies, headache, and pneumothorax, occur some days later in the postsurgical period. It is important, therefore, that all patients undergoing neural blockade be visited a sufficient number of times postanesthetically so that the documented record will show evidence of the anesthesiologist's awareness of any complications that may occur. Most postanesthesia complications are erroneously attributed to an anesthetic cause by other physicians and nurses in the absence of adequate anesthesia follow-up during the postsurgical period. Early diagnosis, consultation with appropriate specialists, and early initiation of corrective therapy are medicolegal and professional responsibilities of all anesthesiologists. This, coupled with good patient rapport and recordkeeping, will ensure the maximum beneficial outcome from any complication following regional anesthesia.

REFERENCES

1. Adriani, J.: Labat's Regional Anesthesia. 3rd ed. pp. 192. Philadelphia, W.B. Saunders, 1967.
2. Aldrete, J.A., Romo-Salas, P., Arora, S., *et al.*: Reverse arterial blood flow as a pathway for central nervous system toxic responses following injection of local anesthetics. Anesth. Analg., *57:*428, 1978.
3. Allemann, B.H., Gerber, H., and Gruber, U.F.: Spinal conduction anesthesia in the face of subcutaneously administered heparin-dihydro ergot for thromboembolism prophylaxis. Anaesthetist, *32:*80, 1983.
4. Bader, A.M., Gilbertson, L., Kirz, L., and Datta, S.: Regional anesthesia in women with chorioamnionitis. Reg. Anesth., *17:*84, 1992.
5. Bainton, C.R., and Strichartz, G.R.: Concentration dependence on lidocaine-induced irreversible conduction loss in frog nerve. Anesthesiology, *81:*657, 1994.
6. Baraka, A., Hanna, M., and Hammoud, R.: Unconsciousness and apnea complicating parascalene brachial plexus block: Possible subarachnoid block. Anesthesiology, *77:*1046, 1992.
7. Barutell, C., Vidal, F., Raich, M., and Montero, A.: A neurological complication following interscalene brachial plexus block. Anaesthesia, *35:*365, 1980.
8. Bashein, G. Robertson, H.T., and Kennedy, W.F. Jr.: Persistent

phrenic nerve paresis following interscalene brachial plexus block. Anesthesiology, *63:*102, 1985.
9. Beaudoin, M.G., and Klein, L.: Epidural abscess following multiple spinal anaesthetics. Anaesth. Intensive care, *12:*163, 1984.
10. Benzon, H.T., Brunner, E.A., and Vaisrub, N.: Bleeding time and nerve blocks after aspirin. Reg. Anesth., *9:*86, 1984.
11. Berqvist, D., Lindblad, B., and Matzsch, T.: Low molecular weight heparin for thromboprophylaxis and epidural/spinal anaesthesia—Is there a risk? Acta Anaesthesiol. Scand., *36:*605, 1992.
12. Blomberg, R.G.: The lumbar subdural extra-arachnoid space of humans: An anatomical study using spinaloscopy in autopsy cases. Anesth. Analg., *66:*177, 1987.
13. Born, G.: Neuropathy after bupivacaine wrist and metacarpal nerve blocks. J. Hand Surg., *9A:*109, 1984.
14. Böttiger, B.W., and Diezel, G.: Acute intracranial subarachnoid haemorrhage following repeated spinal anaesthesia. Anaesthesist, *41:*152, 1992.
15. Brown, D.T., Beamish, D., and Wildsmith, J.A.W.: Allergic reaction to an amide local anaesthetic. Br. J. Anaesth., *53:*435, 1981.
16. Brown, E.M., and Elman, D.S.: Postoperative backache. Anesth. Analg., *40:*683, 1961.
17. Brownridge, P.: The management of headache following accidental dural puncture in obstetric patients. Anaesth. Intensive Care, *11:*4, 1983.
18. Carp, H., and Bailey, S.: The association between meningitis and dural puncture in bacteremic rats. Anesthesiology, *76:*739, 1992.
19. Casey, W.F.: Respiratory failure following intercostal nerve blockade. Anaesthesia, *39:*351, 1984.
20. Cooke, E.D.: Monitoring during low-dose heparin prophylaxis. N. Engl. J. Med., *294:*1066, 1976.
21. Cory, P.C., and Mulroy, M.F.: Postoperative respiratory failure following intercostal block. Anesthesiology, *54:*418, 1981.
22. Crawford, J.S.: Lumbar epidural block in labor: A clinical analysis. Br. J. Anaesth., *44:*66, 1972.
23. Darnat, S., Guggiari, M., Grob, R., Guillaume, A., and Viars, P.: Lumbar epidural haematoma following the setting-up of an epidural catheter. Ann. Fr. Anesth. Reanim., *5:*550, 1986.
24. Dawkins, C.J.M.: An analysis of the complications of extradural and caudal block. Anesthesia, *24:*554, 1969.
25. Dean, W.M., and Woodside, J.R.: Spinal hematoma compressing cauda equina. Urology, *13:*575, 1979.
26. Dickman, C.A., Shedd, S.A., Spetzler, R.F., Shetter, A.G., and Sonntag, V.K.H.: Spinal epidural hematoma associated with epidural anesthesia: Complications of systemic heparinization in patients receiving peripheral vascular thrombolytic therapy. Anesthesiology, *72:* 947, 1990.
27. Drasner, K., and Rigler, M.I.: Repeat injection after a "failed spinal": At times, a potentially unsafe practice. Anesthesiology, *75:*713, 1991.
28. Driessen, A., Mauer, W., Fricke, M., Kossmann, B., and Schleinzer, W.: Prospective studies on the pathologic mechanism of postspinal headache in a select group of patients. Anaesthetist, *29:*38, 1980.
29. Duggan, J., McKeown, D.W., and Scott, D.B.: Venous pressures generated during IV regional anaesthesia (IVRA). Br. J. Anaesth., *55:* 1158P, 1983.
30. Duncan, P., and Kobrmsky, N.: Prilocaine-induced methemoglobinemia in a newborn infant. Anesthesiology, *59:*75, 1983.
31. Dunn, S.M., Steinberg, R.B., O'Sullivan, P.S., Goolishian, W.T., and Villa, E.A.: A fractured epidural needle: Case report and study. Anesth. Analg., *75:*1050, 1992.
32. Dutton, R.P., Eckhardt, W.F. 3rd., and Sunder, N.: Total spinal anesthesia after interscalene blockade of the brachial plexus. Anesthesiology, *80:*939, 1994.
33. Eckstein, K.L., Rogacev, Z., Vincente-Eckstein, A., and Grahovac, A.: Prospective comparative study of postspinal headache in young patients (less than 51 years) . Reg. Anesth., *5:*57, 1982.
34. Edge, K.R., and Nicoll, J.M.: Retrobulbar hemorrhage after 12,500 retrobulbar blocks. Anesth. Analg., *76:*1019, 1993.
35. Engberg, G.: Relief of postoperative pain with intercostal blockade compared with the use of narcotic drugs. Acta Anaesthesiol. Scand., *70 (Suppl.)* 1136, 1978.
36. Erola, M., Kaukinen, L., and Kaukinen, S.: Fatal brain lesion following spinal anaesthesia. Acta Anaesthesiol. Scand., *25:*115, 1981.
37. Ferraris, V.A., and Swanson, E.: Aspirin usage and perioperative blood loss in patients undergoing unexpected operations. Surg. Gynecol. Obstet., *156:*439, 1983.
38. Fibuch, E.E., and Opper, S.E.: Back pain following epidurally administered nesacaine-MPF. Anesth. Analg., *69:*113, 1989.
39. Fisher, M., and Pennington, J.C.: Allergy to local anaesthesia. Br. J. Anaesth., *54:*893, 1982.
40. Frenkel, C., Altscher, T., Groben, V., and Hörnchen, U.: Incidence of post-dural puncture headache in a young patient population. Anaesthesist, *41:*142, 1992.
41. Gallo, J.A., Lebowitz, P.W., Battit, G.E., and Bruner, J.M.R.: Complications of intercostal nerve blocks performed under direct vision during thoracotomy. J. Thorac. Cardiovasc. Surg., *86:*628, 1983.
42. Ghani, G.A., and Berry, A.J.: Right hydrothorax after left external jugular vein catheterization. Anesthesiology, *58:*93, 1983.
43. Gould, J.E., Casey, W.F., and Reynolds, F.: Bupivacaine intravenous anaesthesia and resuscitation (Letters). Anaesthesia, *39:*612, 1984.
44. Greensite, F.S., and Katz, J.: Spinal subdural hematoma associated with attempted epidural anesthesia and subsequent continuous spinal anesthesia. Anesth. Analg., *59:*72, 1980.
45. Harik, S.I., Raichle, M.E., and Reis, D.J.: Spontaneously remitting spinal epidural hematoma in a patient on anticoagulants. N. Eng. J. Med., *284:*1355, 1971.
46. Hassan, E.K., Hutton, P., and Black, A.M.S.: Dangers of cubital fossa injections for Bier's blockade. Br. J. Anaesth., *55:*1158P, 1983.
47. Hasselstrom, I.J., and Morgensen, T.: Toxic reaction of bupivacaine at low plasma concentration. Anesthesiology, *61:*99, 1984.
48. Heath, M.L.: Bupivacaine toxicity and Bier blocks (Letter) . Anesthesiology, *59:*480, 1983.
49. Hill, I.N., Gershon, N.I., and Gargiulo, P.O.: Total spinal blockade during local anesthesia of the nasal passages. Anesthesiology, *59:*144, 1983.
50. Hindman, B.J.: Usefulness of the post-aspirin bleeding time. Anesthesiology, *64:*368, 1986.
51. Horlocker, T.T.: Central neural blockade for patients receiving anticoagulants. *In* Clinical Anesthesia Updates. Vol. 5. No. 2. Philadelphia, J. B. Lippincott Company, 1994.
52. Horlocker, T.T., Wedel, D.J., Offord, K.P., *et al.*: Do preoperative antiplatelet drugs increase the risk of hemorrhagic complication associated with regional anesthesia. Anesth. Analg., *70:*631, 1995.
53. Horlocker, T.T., Wedel, D.J., and Schlichting, J.L.: Postoperative epidural analgesia and oral anticoagulant therapy. Anesth. Analg., *79:* 89, 1994.
54. Horlocker, T.T., Wedel, D.J., and Offord, K.P.: Does preoperative antiplatelet therapy increase the risk of hemorrhagic complications associated with regional anesthesia? Anesth. Analg., *70:*631, 1990.
55. Hynson, J.M., Sessler, D.I., and Glosten, B.: Back pain in volunteers after epidural anesthesia with chloroprocaine. Anesth. Analg., *72:*253, 1991.
56. Janik, R., and Dick, W.: Influence of different puncture techniques on incidence of postspinal headache: Median or paramedian approach. Anaesthesist, *41:*137, 1992.
57. Jones, M.D., and Newton, T.H.: Inadvertent extra-arachnoid injections in myelography. Radiology., *80:*818, 1963.
58. Kane, R.B.: Neurologic deficits following epidural or spinal anesthesia. Anesth. Analg., *60:*150, 1981.
59. Kilpatrick, M.E., and Girgis, N.I.: Meningitis: A complication of spinal anesthesia. Anesth. Analg., *62:*513, 1983.
60. Knoblanche, G.E.: The incidence and aetiology of phrenic nerve blockade association with supraclavicular brachial plexus block. Anaesth. Intensive Care, *7:*346, 1979.
61. Korevaar, W., Burney, R.G., and Moore, P.A.: Convulsions during stellate ganglion block: A case report. Anesth. Analg., *58:*329, 1979.
62. Kroll, D.A., Caplan, R.A., Posner, K., Ward, R.J., and Cheney, F.W.: Nerve injury associated with anesthesia. Anesthesiology, *73:*202, 1990.
63. Kumar, A., Battit, G.F., Fraese, A.B., and Long, M.C.: Bilateral cervical and thoracic epidural blockade complicating interscalene brachial plexus block. Anesthesiology, *35:*650, 1971.
64. Lawes, E.G., Johnson, T., Prichard, P., and Robbins, P.: Venous pressures during simulated Bier's block. Anaesthesia, *39:*147, 1984.
65. Lim, M., Cross, G.D., and Sold, M.: Postdural puncture headache: A comparison between the 29 G Vygon and 24 G Sprotte needles. Anaesthesist, *41:*539, 1992.
66. Lubenow, T., Keh-Wong, E., Kristof, K., Ivankovich, O., and Ivankovich, A.D.: Inadvertent subdural injection: A complication of an epidural block. Anesth. Analg., *67:*175, 1988.

67. Locke, G.E., Giorgio, A.J., and Biggers, S.L.: Acute spinal epidural hematoma secondary to aspirin-induced prolonged bleeding. Surg. Neurol., *5:*292, 1976.
68. Lowson, S.M., and Goodchild, C.S.: Low-dose heparin therapy and spinal anesthesia. Anaesthesia, *44:*67, 1989.
69. Lynch, J., Arhelger, S., Krings-Ernst, I., Ground, S., and Zech, D.: Whitacre 22-gauge pencil-point needle for spinal anaesthesia: A controlled trial in 300 young orthopaedic patients. Anaesth. Intensive Care, *20:*322, 1992.
70. Mamourian, A.C., Dickman, C.A., Drayer, B.P., and Sonntag, V.K.H.: Spinal epidural abscess: Three cases following spinal epidural injection demonstrated with magnetic resonance imaging. Anesthesiology, *78:*204, 1993.
71. Manchanda, V.N., Murad, S.H.N., Shilyansky, G., and Mehringer, M.: Unusual clinical course of accidental subdural local anesthetic injection. Anesth. Analg., *62:*1124, 1983.
72. Mani, M., Ramamurthy, N., Rao, T.L.K., *et al.*: An unusual complication of brachial plexus block and heparin therapy. Anesthesiology, *48:*213, 1978.
73. Mathews, E.T., and Abrams, L.D.: Intrathecal morphine in open heart surgery. Lancet., *2:*543, 1980.
74. Mayer, D.C., Quance, D., and Weeks, S.K.: Headache after spinal anesthesia for cesarean section: A comparison of the 27-gauge Quincke and 24-gauge Sprotte needles. Anesth. Analg., *75:*377, 1992.
75. Mazze, R.I., and Fujinaga, M.: Postdural puncture headache after continuous spinal anesthesia with 18-gauge and 20-gauge needles. Reg. Anesth., *18:*47, 1993.
76. Mehta, M., and Maher, R.: Injection into the extra-arachnoid subdural space. Anaesthesia *32:*760, 1977.
77. Moir, D.D., and Davidson, S.: Postpartum complications of forceps delivery performed under epidural and pudendal nerve block. Br. J. Anaesth., *44:*1197, 1972.
78. Moore, D.C.: Stellate Ganglion Block. pp. 110. Springfield, IL, Charles C. Thomas, 1954.
79. Moore, D.C.: Regional Block. 4th ed. pp. 240. Springfield, IL, Charles C. Thomas, 1965.
80. Newrick, P., and Read, P.: Subdural haematoma as a complication of spinal anesthetic. Br. Med. J., *285:*341, 1982.
81. Nicholson, M.J., and McAlpine, F.S.: Neural injuries: Association with surgical positions and operations. *In* Martin, J. T., ed., Positioning in Anesthesia and Surgery. pp. 193. Philadelphia. W.B. Saunders, 1978.
82. Odoom, J.A., and Sih, I.L.: Epidural analgesia and anticoagulant therapy: Experience with 1,000 cases of continuous epidurals. Anaesthesia, *38:*254, 1983.
83. Onishchuk, J.L., and Carlsson, C.: Epidural hematoma associated with epidural anesthesia: Complications of anticoagulant therapy. Anesthesiology, *77:*1221, 1992.
84. Owens, E.L., Kasten, G.W., and Hessel, E.A.: Spinal hematoma after lumbar puncture and heparinization. Anesth. Analg., *65:*1201, 1986.
85. Park, R.: A migrating epidural cannula (Letter). Anaesthesia, *39:*289, 1984.
86. Pearson, R.M.G.: A rare complication of extradural analgesia. Anaesthesia, *39:*460, 1984.
87. Rao, T.K.I., and El-Etr, A.A.: Anticoagulation following placement of epidural and subarachnoid catheters. Anesthesiology, *55:*618, 1981.
88. Rao, A.K., Pratt C., Berke, A., *et al.*: Thrombolysis in myocardial infarction trial—Phase I. J. Am. Coll. Cardiol., *11:*1, 1988.
89. Ravindran, R.S., Bond, V.K., Tasch, M.D., *et al.*: Prolonged neural blockade following regional analgesia with 2-chloroprocaine. Anesth. Analg., *59:*447, 1980.
90. Ravindran, R.S., Viegas, O.J., Tasch, M.D., *et al.*: Bearing down at the time of delivery and the incidence of spinal headache in parturients. Anesth. Analg., *60:*524, 1981.
91. Reisner, L.S., Hochman, B.N., and Plumer, M.H.: Persistent neurologic deficit and adhesive arachnoiditis following intrathecal 2-chloroprocaine injection. Anesth. Analg., *59:*452, 1980.
92. Rengarchy, S.S., and Murphy, D.: Subarachnoid hematoma following lumbar puncture causing compression of the caudal equina. J. Neurosurg., *41:*252, 1974.
93. Reynolds, F.: Bupivacaine and intravenous regional anaesthesia (Editorial). Anaesthesia, *39:*105, 1984.
94. Rice, A.S.C., and McMahon, S.B.: Peripheral nerve injury caused by injection needles used in regional anaesthesia: Influence of bevel configuration, studied in a rat model. Br. J. Anaesth., *69:*433, 1992.
95. Rigler, M.L., Drasner, K., Krejcie, T.C., *et al.*: Cauda equina syndrome after continuous spinal anesthesia. Anesth. Analg., *72:*275, 1991.
96. Robinson, R.A., Stewart, S.F.C., Myers, M.R., *et al.*: In vitro modeling of spinal anesthesia. Anesthesiology, *81:*1053, 1994.
97. Rosenberg, P.H., Kalso, E.A., Tuominen, M.K., and Linden, H.B.: Acute bupivacaine toxicity as a result of venous leakage under the tourniquet cuff during Bier block. Anesthesiology, *58:*95, 1984.
98. Ruff, R.L., and Dougherty, J.H.: Complications of lumbar puncture followed by anticoagulation. Stroke, *12:*879, 1981.
99. Schultz, E.H., and Brogdon, B.G.: The problem of subdural placement in myelography. Radiology, *79:*91, 1962.
100. Scott, D.B., Quisling, R.G., and Miller, C.A.: Spinal epidural hematoma. J.A.M.A., *235:*513, 1976.
101. Scott, D.L., Ghia, J.N., and Teeple, E.: Aphasia and hemiparesis following stellate ganglion block. Anesth. Analg., *62:*1038, 1983.
102. Selander, D., Dhuner, K.S., and Lundberg, G.: Peripheral nerve injury due to injection needles used for regional anesthesia. Acta Anaesthesiol. Scand., *21:*182, 1977.
103. Selander, D., Brattsand, R., Lundborg, G., *et al.*: Local anesthetics: Importance of mode of application, concentration, and adrenaline for the appearance of nerve lesions. Acta Anaesthesiol. Scand., *23:*127, 1979.
104. Selander, D., Edshage, S., and Wolff, T.: Paresthesiae or no paresthesiae? Acta Anaesthesiol. Scand., *23:*27, 1979.
105. Snyder, R., Hue, G., Flugstad, P., and Viarengo, C.: More cases of possible neurologic toxicity associated with single subarachnoid injections of 5% hyperbaric lidocaine (Letter). Anesth. Analg., *78:*411, 1994.
106. Spurny, O.M., Rubin, S., Wolff, J.W., *et al.*: Spinal epidural hematoma during anticoagulant therapy. Arch. Intern. Med., *114:*103, 1964.
107. Stevens, R.A., Urmey, W.F., Urquhart, B.L., and Kao, T.C.: Back pain after epidural anesthesia with chloroprocaine. Anesthesiology, *78:* 492, 1993.
108. Strong, W.E.: Epidural abscess associated with epidural catheterization: A rare event? Report of two cases with markedly delayed presentation. Anesthesiology, *74:*943, 1991.
109. Szienfeld, M., Laurencio, M., and Pallares, V.S.: Total reversible blindness following stellate ganglion block. Anesth. Analg. *60:*689, 1989.
110. Tarkkila, P.J., Heine, H., Tervo, R-R.: Comparison of Sprotte and Quincke needles with respect to postdural puncture headache and backache. Reg. Anesth., *17:*283, 1992.
111. Thompson, K.J., Melding, P., and Hatangdi, V.S.: Pneumochylothorax: A rare complication of stellate ganglion block. Anesthesiology, *55:*589, 1981.
112. Thorburn, J., and Moir, D.D.: Bupivacaine toxicity in association with extradural analgesia for caesarean section. Br. J. Anaesth., *56:*551, 1984.
113. Thurer, R.J.: Chylothorax: A complication of subclavian vein catheterization and parenteral hyperalimentation. J. Thorac. Cardiovasc. Surg., *71:*465, 1976.
114. Tomlin, P.J.: Death in outpatient dental anesthetic practice. Anaesthesia, *29:*551, 1974.
115. Tondare, A.S., Nadkarn, A.V., Sathe, C.H., and Dave, V.B.: Femoral neuropathy: A complication of lithotomy position under spinal anesthesia. Can. Anaesth. Soc. J., *30:*84, 1983.
116. Tryba, M.: Und die teilnehmer des workshops uber hamostaseologische probleme bie regionalanaesthesien: Haemostaseologische voraussetzungen zur durch-fuhrung von regionalanaesthesien. Reg. Anaesth., *12:*127, 1989.
117. Urmey, W.F., and McDonald, M.: Hemidiaphragmatic paresis during interscalene brachial plexus block: Effects on pulmonary function and chest wall mechanics. Anesth. Analg., *74:*352, 1992.
118. Urmey, W.F., Talts, K.H., and Sharrock, N.F.: One hundred percent incidence of hemidiaphragmatic paresis associated with interscalene brachial plexus anesthesia as diagnosed by ultrasonography. Anesth. Analg., *72:*498, 1991.
119. Usbiaga, J.E.: Neurological complications following epidural anesthesia. Int. Anesthesiol. Clin., *13:*1, 1975.
120. van de Kelft, E., de la Porte, C., Meese, G., and Adriaensen, H.: Intracranial subdural hematoma after spinal anesthesia. Acta Anaesthesiol. Belg., *42:*177, 1991.
121. Vandermeulen, E.P., Van Aken, H., and Vermylen, J.: Anticoagulants and spinal-epidural anesthesia. Anesth. Analg., *79:*1165, 1994.
122. Winchell, S.W., and Wolfe, R.: The incidence of neuropathy following upper extremity nerve blocks. Reg. Anesth., *10:*12, 1985.

Neural Blockade in Clinical Anesthesia and Management of Pain, Third Edition,
edited by M.J. Cousins and P.O. Bridenbaugh.
Lippincott–Raven Publishers, Philadelphia © 1998.

CHAPTER 22

Complications of Neurolytic Neural Blockade

J. Edmond Charlton and William A. Macrae

The use of any agent which relies upon nonspecific destruction of tissue for its clinical effect is bound to be hazardous. Where the clinical intent is to destroy nervous tissue, the potential for harm becomes even greater and adverse effects may be long-lasting and serious. It might be asked why any sensible clinician would want to use techniques that have such potential for harm?

The answer is simply that when pain is uncontrolled by conventional methods, alternative methods of pain control need to be sought. Not everyone has instantly available neurosurgery or immediate access to radiofrequency lesion generators and advanced imaging techniques. Neurolytic blocks are simple, low-technology procedures with a high success rate and may be of enormous benefit. Ventafridda and colleagues[82] used neurolytic blockade in 29% of patients entered into a two-year validating study for the World Health Organization (WHO) analgesic ladder for cancer pain relief. Patients in whom the analgesic ladder failed to provide adequate analgesia were those who received neurolytic blockade.

The clinician must know the pros and cons of each procedure if a sensible choice is to be made, and this includes a detailed knowledge of the potential complications. No choice can be made about neurolytic blocks without weighing up the incidence of complications against other factors, which must include the quality of pain relief obtained and the speed and ease with which the result is obtained. Some procedures mentioned in this chapter are of historical interest in the developed world but may still be in use where resources are limited.

Practical Considerations

In order to minimize the potential for complications, the first requirement is a sound understanding of the anatomy and physiology. Clinicians have sought to reduce the potential for harm by using smaller volumes of neurolytic agent than those used in the corresponding local anesthetic block. This should reduce the likelihood of overflow and spillover onto surrounding structures. In addition, the mandatory use of radiological control with biplane screening or advanced imaging, and the use of neurolytic agents dissolved in contrast media to permit visualization of spread whilst the injection is being made, have increased the safety of these procedures. Many experts would argue that a record of these images should be kept for medicolegal purposes. A further reduction in the dangers of neurolytic blockade is likely as a result of the employment of alternative methods of managing severe pain. Clinicians are happier to use large doses of opioids and other drugs for longer periods than previously. The use of selective radiofrequency lesioning or neurosurgery may offer more suitable alternatives to neurolytic nerve block for certain high risk procedures, such as the trigeminal ganglion or thoracic sympathetic chain ablation. It is likely that the overall use of neurolytic block techniques is falling, but it is unlikely that use will cease altogether. Less frequent use should make the clinician even more vigilant and careful in the performance of the procedures. It should be remembered that other agents may be injected accidentally which may subsequently prove to be neurolytic and there is a need to know what the likely sequelae of such an event may be.

The Agents

The most commonly used neurolytic agents are phenol and alcohol and these are covered in detail elsewhere in this text (see Chapters 30, 31). Other neurolytic agents such as ammonium chloride and chlorocresol are of historical interest only. As far as can be determined, the effect of both phenol and alcohol upon neural tissue is a nonspecific and identical destruction of the neural architecture and any other tissues which may be involved. The extent and severity of the damage will be related to the internal structure of the nerve at the point of injection, the amount of material injected and the effects of the agent itself (see also Chapter 30).

J.E. Charlton: Department of Pain Management and Anaesthesia, Royal Victoria Infirmary, Newcastle upon Tyne NEI 4LP United Kingdom.

W.A. Macrae: The Pain Clinic, Ninewells Hospital, Dundee DDI 9SY United Kingdom.

Sunderland has stated that the neural damage sustained by injection of sclerosing substances varies in severity from rapidly reversible changes that cause only transient loss of function to permanent constrictive scarring in and about the nerve, sufficient to prevent recovery of the nerve.[74]

Another important consideration is the possibility of vascular damage caused by the neurolytic agent (see Chapter 30). If the blood supply to the nerve is compromised, even greater damage may be the result. There is a widely quoted but unconvincing piece of evidence that phenol may have a greater affinity for vascular tissues than neural tissue.[55] Whether or not this is true, the fact remains that neurolytic agents such as phenol and alcohol will destroy all types of tissue, and thus infinite care is required in their use. More recent work has shown that both alcohol and phenol cause a contractile response in blood vessels which may account for loss of function in tissues exposed to these agents.[10] Overflow onto other nerves may lead to prolonged motor deficit and loss of protective sensation in a group of people in whom any loss of function may represent a tragedy.

In most circumstances, it is prudent to use a diagnostic or prognostic block before performing neurolytic block (see Chapter 27). Unexpected spread of local anesthetic may cause temporary and reversible difficulties, but the same spread by a neurolytic agent may be serious. Subclinical weakness may become paralysis, and if spread to phrenic nerve occurs in a patient with compromised respiratory function, the overall result could be life-threatening.

Block Performance

Diagnostic blockade has several advantages. It will permit the patient and the clinician to assess the effect of the block; it will offer the opportunity to assess possible side-effects; and it may reveal unsuspected variations from the normal anatomy (see Chapter 27), if the block fails to work. Carrying out diagnostic blockade will not guarantee success with succeeding neurolytic blocks because the needle may be placed differently; equally, complications encountered during diagnostic blockade may be avoided during subsequent neurolytic blocks. Another method of reducing the number and magnitude of complications of neurolytic block is to inject a test-dose of local anesthetic once the needle is judged to be in satisfactory position. The amount of local anesthetic injected will be dependent upon the proposed block and should be sufficient to give a recognizable response. Adequate assessment can only be carried out if the patient is awake or lightly sedated, so that he or she can respond appropriately.

As a general rule, it is advisable to carry out diagnostic blockade before most neurolytic blocks. This is especially so if there is doubt about which nerve is involved, or whether blocking it will give adequate pain relief. In addition, it is wise to carry out diagnostic block, where blocking other nerves unintentionally may cause problems, for example, where blockade of phrenic nerve may lead to respiratory embarrassment in patients with pre-existing pulmonary disease, or where the patient may have a pre-existing motor weakness which may progress to paralysis if damage to motor nerves occurs inadvertently. Thus it may be argued that the least possible volume should be chosen that will produce an observable clinical effect. The use of large amounts of local anesthetic prior to a neurolytic block may have the effect of diluting the neurolytic agents used and it may also cause the agent to spread over a larger area and make complications more likely (see also Chapter 31).

It is axiomatic that proper consent should be obtained before any diagnostic or therapeutic blockade. This is especially important where neurolytic block is concerned, and the consent form and patient's records should indicate that the patient is aware of, and has been informed about, common side effects. It is the authors' belief that mention should be made of major side effects and problems, too, as this will ensure that consent for neurolytic blockade is both informed and given freely with adequate knowledge about the intended procedure.

After a neurolytic block has been carried out, the result should be assessed over a day or two. Most neurolytic blocks regress over this period and an apparently satisfactory result may be less so with the passage of time. In addition, unwanted side effects or spread to other neural structures may decrease quite rapidly. It has been suggested that this diminution in the amount of tissue destruction is due to a biphasic effect of the agents employed.[54] If there are unwanted side effects, it is most important to keep the patient fully informed about the problems. Management should be directed at relieving pain, preventing disuse atrophy, and reassuring the patient. By and large, nerves damaged by neurolytic solutions tend to regenerate in time, except for the optic nerve, and all steps should be taken to make recovery as comfortable and complete as possible.

The possibility of legal action is an ever-present accompaniment to the performance of neurolytic blockade. This is so especially if the block is carried out for the relief of nonmalignant pain. The grounds on which an action may be brought include:

1. Complications caused by the injection.
2. The patient did not consent to the procedure.
3. The procedure was carried out inexpertly.
4. The wrong procedure was performed.
5. Treatment of the complication(s)was inadequate.

In general, the most common complication of neurolytic block is persistent pain. This may be due to a modification of the underlying disease process and it may be due also to a chemical neuritis caused by the neurolytic agent. This seems to occur more frequently with alcohol. Pain at the injection site is probably due to local tissue irritation and may be reduced by ensuring that no neurolytic agent tracks through to the skin by flushing the needle through with saline or local anesthetic as it is removed after the block. Swelling, cellulitis, and sloughing of tissues have all been reported after neurolytic block, and persistence of the pain suggests a possible complication such as a slough or sterile abscess formation; there are particular risks involved when a block is being performed at a superficial site such as the intercostal nerve or over the coccyx.[77]

Intravascular injection of phenol is very unpleasant for the patient and should be avoided if at all possible by careful repeated aspiration during the procedure. Phenol is reported to stimulate the central nervous system (CNS), causing muscle tremors and eventually convulsions (Benzon, 1979, Felsenthal; 1974). Reid and colleagues reported that intravascular 10% phenol caused "severe tinnitus and flushing within a few seconds but recovery is rapid and complete."[68] Personal experience suggests that even small amounts (1 ml) of 10% phenol in a contrast medium injected intravascularly can cause prolonged and unpleasant feelings of nausea, sickness, and weakness. Intravascular injection of alcohol is reported as being "entirely pleasurable and will require no specific therapy."[13]

Neurolytic nerve block is used on patients who may have had major vascular surgery (see Chapter 13). Both phenol and alcohol may disrupt the integrity of certain vascular prosthetic grafts. Gale and co-workers[27] have shown that Dacron (Meadox Medicals, Oakland, NJ) woven grafts are degraded by concentrations of alcohol of at least 50%, and, to a lesser extent, by phenol of at least 6%. Gore-Tex (W. L. Gore Associates, Flagstaff, AZ) grafts show only minimal change. They suggest that it may be prudent to try other therapeutic modalities, before embarking upon neurolytic blockade, where a prosthetic graft is near to the site of the block.

SPECIFIC BLOCKS

Subarachnoid Neurolytic Blocks

The accessibility of the spinal nerve roots has led to widespread use of this technique in the past. However, it is not possible to perform selective blockade—even with infinite care and skill—sensory, motor, and autonomic blockade will occur in varying proportions. This will, of course, lead to unwanted complications, which are usually only temporary, but in some instances they may be both prolonged and very unpleasant. An additional drawback is the limited length of action frequently seen with subarachnoid neurolytic blocks.

As with virtually all neurolytic procedures, there are no prospective, randomized controlled trials to support their use. However, there exists a substantial body of clinical opinion that supports the use of subarachnoid neurolytic blocks to relieve the pain of advanced malignancy that is not responding to other forms of treatment (see Chapter 31). It is not possible to give accurate figures about the incidence of complications, because the patients who have received subarachnoid neurolytic blocks have many variables which may affect the number and sort of complications seen. Variables include the underlying diagnosis: whether the pain is arising from primary or secondary tumor, the type of treatment the patient is receiving, and the presence or absence of pre-existing neurological damage arising from the disease process. It is easy to blame an intervention like a neurolytic block for a dramatic change in physical findings or symptomatology, but in many cases this may represent an extension of the disease process or a side effect of accompanying treatment.[37] Scrupulous examination and assessment before the procedure will enable an evaluation to be made about the likelihood of such problems.

The plain truth is that comparative studies will not be carried out, because neurolytic block will continue to be used as part of a management plan in patients who are unresponsive to conventional treatment. This will always be a small number and humanitarian demands dictate that the treatment should not be withheld so that the patient can be part of a "properly constructed" trial. To form some idea of the likelihood of complications, we are left to rely upon clinical anecdote, and most clinical anecdote relates only to unusual problems encountered in small series; or to a low level of unpleasant sequelae in large series. The overall morbidity of a given technique remains unclear.

Problems with subarachnoid neurolytic blockade are most likely to be related to the site and extent of blockade. Most conventional texts suggest that neurolytic blocks should be aimed at a small number of segments and repeated on a number of occasions if extensive denervation is required. The practical importance of this advice is that it will reduce the changes of excessive damage to other structures. About 1/2 of patients receiving subarachnoid phenol or alcohol have some kind of upset after the procedure. This is usually a systemic upset such as feeling unwell, or suffering from nausea or headache; less commonly they may experience burning pains or paresthesias. These latter problems may last between a day and 2 or 3 weeks. Virtually all these problems are self-limiting and Swerdlow analyzed the length of time complications were present in 300 patients who received over 450 neurolytic blocks[76,77] (Table 1).

The problems that are likely to give rise to the most anxiety are paralysis of motor function or bladder and bowel dys-

TABLE 22-1. *Subarachnoid neurolytic blockade: complications lasting more than three days in 300 patients*

48 had one or more complications that persisted more than 3 days; 21 had received more than one intrathecal injection.
28 had one or more complications that persisted more than 1 week.
19 had one or more complications that persisted more than 2 weeks.
10 had one or more complications that persisted more than 1 month.
(All patients were followed for 3 months, or to death, if this occurred earlier).

From Swerdlow, M.: Complications of Neurolytic Blockade. *In* Cousins, M.J., and Bridenbaugh, P.O. (eds.): Neural Blockade in Clinical Anesthesia and Management of Pain. 2nd Ed. J.B. Lippincott, Philadelphia, 1988.

function. There seems to be little to choose between phenol and alcohol as the agent employed, and the agent chosen may be dependent upon the preference of the anesthetist. It is the authors' impression that complications had to be fairly extensive before they were reported, and that many minor degrees of weakness and numbness have gone unreported and without remark by clinician or patient. Nathan[53,54] reported a 12% incidence of sphincter dysfunction after subarachnoid phenol. Bonica stated that 25% of patients had bladder, bowel, or lower limb dysfunction after subarachnoid neurolytic injection. These figures seem high and may reflect the less conservative approach to neurolytic blockade that existed before radiological control became mandatory.

Paresis is most likely with higher cervicothoracic blocks and bladder or sphincter problems usually are limited to lumbar blocks. However, Swerdlow[78] reports a patient who developed bladder paralysis after a phenol block at T11, following three uncomplicated neurolytic blocks at lower levels, and a second patient who developed bladder paresis after a phenol block at T7.

Problems with bladder control can be relatively common following neurolytic block. Tank and co-workers reported that half of 37 patients had a transient loss of bladder control after receiving intrathecal alcohol blocks for severe sacral plexus pain.[78] Three of their patients had permanent loss. Papo and Visca[57] noted five permanent and 10 temporary interruptions of bladder function after phenol saddle block in 39 patients. Injection of neurolytic agents into the cervical part of the subarachnoid space has been reported to cause respiratory arrest although the doses used seem high and must have been contributory.[32,75]

The potential vagaries that accompany neurolytic blockade have been highlighted in a case report by Capuzzo and colleagues.[12] The injection of 1.5 ml of contrast at L1–L2 was followed by caudal spread. Injection of 0.7 ml of 10% phenol with some head-down tilt resulted in cranial nerve involvement from which the patient gradually recovered over 48 hours. However, bladder and anal sphincter control were absent until death two months later. Porges and Zdrahal[59] reported blocking the lowest sacral roots for pain relief in inoperable rectal cancer with both alcohol and phenol in glycerine. When using alcohol, they found that higher components of the sacral roots could become involved when cerebrospinal fluid (CSF) pressure was low, presumably by alteration in flow of neurolytic agents within the spinal canal. They suggest increasing pressure by instilling synthetic CSF prior to the block.

Published results of the use of intrathecal phenol are rare and none are recent. The reported incidence of side effects in these papers is shown in Table 2.

Reports of complications with intrathecal alcohol are even more rare. Although Derrick[23] and Hay[30] have both reported large personal series, the overall incidence of side-effects and permanent complications is extremely low (Table 3). It would be unwise to speculate on why this might be so, but great experience is one obvious factor which will reduce the likelihood of problems. Use of other neurolytic agents such as ammonium sulphate or chlorocresol is associated with a far higher incidence of side-effects, but all reports are more than 50 years old.

As might be expected, a neuritis can follow subarachnoid alcohol, injection. Katz[39] has suggested that the mechanism is due to spilling of the alcohol into the epidural space during subarachnoid injection; however, it is difficult to believe that placement of alcohol near unprotected nerves will not cause a neuritis; what is surprising is that it happens infrequently. Meningeal irritation can follow subarachnoid alcohol and may last several days. Swerdlow[77] reports that headache, neck rigidity, and pain over the vertebral column may be accompanied by increased CSF pressure. Treatment is bed rest, analgesia and removal of CSF. Surgery, radiotherapy and tumor growth are all factors which may have already compromised the blood supply to the cord, and neurolytic block may be the final step in a tragic reduction in

TABLE 22-2. *Reported complications of intrathecal phenol[a]*

Bladder dysfunction	9.0%
Rectal sphincter dysfunction	2.0%
Headache	3.0%
Paresis	12.9%
Dysesthesia	8.0%

[a] Combined results of 704 patients.

From Papo, I. and Visca, A.: Phenol subarachnoid rhizotomy for the treatment of cancer pain. A personal account of 290 cases. Advances in Pain Research and Therapy, *2:*339, 1979; Stovner, J. and Endresen, R.: Intrathecal phenol for cancer pain. Acta Anaesthesiol. Scand., *16:*17, 1972; Mark, V.H., White, J.C., Zervas, N.T., *et al.:* Intracathel use of phenol for the relief of chronic severe pain. N. Eng. J. Med., *267:* 589, 1962; White, J.C., and Sweet, W.H.: Pain and the Neurosurgeon. Springfield, IL., Charles C. Thomas, 1969; Mehta, M.: Intractable Pain. London, W.B. Saunders, 1973; Nathan, P.W.: Pain in cancer: Comparison of results of cordotomy and chemical rhizotomy. *In* Pusek, I., Kune, Z. (eds.): Present Limits of Neurosurgery. Amsterdam, Excerpta Medica, 1972; and Lifshitz, S., Debacker, L.J., and Buchsbaum, A.J.: Subarachnoid phenol block for pain relief in gynecologic malignancy. Obstet. Gynecol. *48:*316, 1976.

TABLE 22-3. *Reported complications of subarachnoid alcohol[a]*

Bladder dysfunction	3.5%
Rectal sphincter dysfunction	0.0%
Headache	0.0%
Paresis	3.9%
Dysesthesia	3.8%

[a] Combined results of 574 patients.

From Derrick, W.S.: Subarachnoid alcohol block for the relief of intractable pain. Acta Anaesthesiol. Scand. *24:*(Suppl.), 167, 1966; and Hay, R.C.: Subarachnoid alcohol block in the control of intractable pain. Anesth. Analg., *41:*12, 1962.

blood flow as thrombosis of the anterior and posterior spinal arteries has been reported.[80,34]

Not before time, the use of subarachnoid hypertonic saline has fallen into disuse. This technique was as terrifying to the administrator as it was unpleasant for the patient. Huge increases in pulse rate and blood pressure would occur in virtually every case and deaths from myocardial infarction and other causes were reported.

Extradural Neurolytic Blockade

Strangely, few reports of the use of neurolytic blockade by this route have been published. Swerdlow[77] reports Grunwald[29] as describing over 200 patients treated with extradural 6% to 10% aqueous phenol. Urinary incontinence occurred in 26% and lasted longer than 2 weeks in 8%. There was bowel incontinence in 10% and muscular weakness in 6.3%; these complications lasted longer than 2 weeks in 3.6% and 1.4%, respectively. Bromage[7] reported 55 epidural neurolytic injections. Complications were few in number and all were temporary; they were temporary muscle weakness, mild paraparesis, and transient urinary retention in 2 cases.

Personal experience suggests that extradural aqueous phenol can be injected, after positioning of the catheter at the dermatomal segment appropriate to the pain, in small aliquots, 1 to 2 ml, depending upon the site of the catheter tip. Smaller quantities will yield an adequate spread in the cervical and thoracic regions, whereas larger volumes may be required in the lumbar region when treating pelvic and lower limb pain. Recently, Racz and his colleagues have described an epidural catheter specifically for the administration of epidural neurolytic injections.[1] This catheter can be guided under radiological control into the desired position. Unpleasant surprises can be avoided by checking the spread of solution with local anesthetic and/or contrast medium before performing the neurolytic block. The theory is that it is possible to reduce the incidence of side effects by carrying out small, repeated, denervations, using small amounts. Practice seems to indicate that this may be true and side effects regress after a day or so, and if the catheter is left in situ, further denervation can be carried out after readjusting the position of the catheter. Complications have included transient loss of bladder and bowel function, unilateral motor weakness and sensory loss in the dermatomes blocked.

N-butyl-p-aminobenzoate (BAB), a highly lipid-soluble congener of benzocaine, has been given epidurally to relieve pain in cancer patients. This agent appears to relieve pain, but insufficient data have been collected to determine whether BAB is neurolytic or not (see also Chapters 4 and 31).[41]

PERIPHERAL NERVE NEUROLYTIC BLOCKADE

Head and Neck

Classic *Gasserian ganglion block* with neurolytic agents (see Chapter 15) is becoming much rarer as treatment of pain arising in the distribution of the Vth cranial nerve is more commonly carried out by use of surgical techniques (see Chapter 32). The high incidence of devastating side effects is another reason that alternative management techniques have been sought. Posterior fossa decompression, radiofrequency lesioning and glycerol injections[68] all have better safety records than neurolytic ablation. It should be borne in mind before contemplating any neurolytic technique around the head and neck that there is a mortality associated with these procedures.[72]

Techniques of blockade should be immaculate; injections should be slow and controlled, and a precise dosage should be given. An isolated needle should always be used, because the majority of problems are associated with spread of injected material. A diagnostic block always should be carried out before injection of a neurolytic agent for the treatment of pain in a trigeminal distribution. This is because the resultant anesthesia of the face can be very upsetting to the patient, who should always have the opportunity to experience this beforehand. The patient can be reassured that some sensation will return and the same is true for many of the other common side effects, such as Horner's syndrome, weakness of the muscles of mastication,[18] and spillover onto adjacent cranial nerves and their branches.

Problems have been reported with oculomotor, abducens,[67] auditory, cochlear-vestibular, facial, and other nerves, accompanied by either temporary or permanent loss of function. Table 4 shows complications of alcohol Gasserian ganglion block reported in two series.[31,47]

When blockade of the facial nerve occurs, the muscle paralysis may be temporary or permanent.[52,67] In addition, the eye will not close properly and this may lead to corneal ulcers or keratitis. Because there is a high incidence of corneal anesthesia, there is a need to provide long-term pro-

TABLE 22-4. *Complications of alcohol Gasserian ganglion block*

Complication	Henderson (196 injections)	Miles (130 injections)
Oculomotor palsy (temporary)	6	4
Abducens palsy (temporary)	2	—
Glossopharyngeal palsy (temporary)	1	—
Corneal anaesthesia	69	20
Permanent anaesthesia (cheek/nose)	66	?
Nasal ulceration	12	2
Blindness	1	—
Corneal ulceration	?	2
Trigeminal motor weakness	—	1

From Henderson, W.R.: Trigeminal neuralgia: The pain and its treatment. Br. Med. J. *1*:7, 1967; and Miles, J.: Trigeminal neuralgia. *In* Lipton, S. (ed.): Persistent Pain. Vol. 2. London, Academic Press, 1980.

tection of the eye, and earlier series had a high incidence of keratitis following trigeminal ablation. One of the most unpleasant side effects quoted by Swerdlow[77] is anesthesia dolorosa and persistent paresthesias in the anesthetic area, although this too, is more of a feature of earlier series.[64,71] Neurolytic techniques should not be used around the orbit, since they carry the risk of permanent blindness if they reach the optic nerve. However, where the eye is painful and already blind, neurolytic block with phenol has been advocated as a method of management.[3] The authors suggest that the 1.5 ml of aqueous phenol used was less painful than the equivalent volume of alcohol, and less likely to give long-term painful sequelae.

Blockade of the *supraorbital nerve* carries with it the risk of diffusion into the orbit and the possibility of permanent blindness. The volume injected around a superficial nerve like this should never be more than 0.5 ml, to minimize the risk of spread and to lower the incidence of skin sloughing and necrosis.

Neurolytic blockade of *branches of the trigeminal nerve* can lead to other changes in addition to those already mentioned. Ulceration and sloughing of skin, the ala of the nose, and the soft and hard palate have all been reported. Whether these problems are as a result of the effect upon the target nerve, or of the neurolytic agent upon the blood supply, remains in doubt. At least 1 fatality due to intravascular injection has been reported.[33] Spread near branches of the facial nerve will lead to permanent paralysis of facial muscles.

In those rare instances where neurolytic blockade of the *glossopharyngeal nerve* has been attempted, it is almost impossible not to involve vagus, accessory, and hypoglossal nerves, as they are in very close contact in the area of the jugular foramen where this block is normally carried out. Paresis of this nerve will paralyze the pharyngeal muscles and will lead to severe problems with swallowing; thus, bilateral blockade should not be carried out. There are many major vascular structures (carotid artery and internal jugular vein) which can be compromised.

Phenol injection into the cisterna magna has been described for the relief of pain in the face and head.[6] The majority of patients had some form of complication, usually a reversible nerve paresis, but in 18% there was permanent trigeminal nerve damage.

Plexus and Major Nerve Neurolytic Blockade

Neurolytic blockade of neural structures of this nature is not recommended unless there are simply no other procedures likely to bring pain relief. Paresis or paralysis of the motor component of plexus or nerve will follow and for the patient, even the prospect of pain relief may not offset the dismay of having a paralyzed limb without feeling. In anesthetic practice, the presence of sheaths around nerve plexuses and major nerves is used to ensure spread of local anesthetic and an effective block. Small volumes of neurolytic agent are likely to be ineffective; large volumes are likely to spread along the sheaths to other structures, such as root cuffs or the major blood vessels that accompany virtually every major plexus and nerve. These structures may be endangered and thrombosis, erosion, sloughing, ulceration, and hemorrhage may occur. Unless the function of the nerves is already compromised, and unless other methods of pain relief have been seen to fail, this sort of treatment should not be considered.

Minor Peripheral Nerve

Intercostal block and blockade of specific peripheral nerves have all been suggested as methods of producing pain relief. Intercostal nerve block frequently is followed by a distressing neuritis, especially if alcohol has been used. Some older practitioners have suggested that this is because the denervation is partial and that the solution is to carry out more extensive denervation. There is no evidence to support this view, and the advent of better techniques of pain control, such as cervical cordotomy, has led to these techniques falling into disuse. Because of the superficial nature of this group of nerves, tissue-sloughing and ulceration was common. Where intercostal blockade is carried out by the paravertebral route, there is the danger of injecting neurolytic fluid into a root cuff or CSF and causing damage to the spinal cord.[62] Neurolytic peripheral nerve blocks have the additional disadvantage of not being very effective.[63]

SYMPATHETIC NEUROLYTIC BLOCKADE

Cervical Blocks

Neurolytic stellate ganglion block has been suggested to improve local blood flow where ulceration and sloughing has occurred following neurolytic head and neck blockade. The procedure should always be carried out under radiological control and with tiny volumes of neurolytic solution in contrast medium. The high incidence of nerve irritation seen with this technique can be minimized by adding a small quantity of methylprednisolone to the injectate. It is not undertaken often probably because of the potential for complications. Therapeutic stellate ganglion block has been reported to cause blockade of the recurrent laryngeal, vagus, and phrenic nerves, brachial plexus; it has also spread both spinally and epidurally and has led to pneumothorax, damage to the thoracic duct, discitis and abscesses. Complications reported following neurolytic block are less extensive, but the potential for any of those mentioned clearly exists. Probably the worst problem reported is extensive infarction of the spinal cord.[75]

Lumbar Blocks

Complications can arise from the effect of the sympathectomy itself or from the procedure. Although the careful use of good technique can avoid most of the problems associated with the procedure, it is important to realize that certain phenomena which are relatively common, such as postsympathectomy neuralgia or hypotension, are the result of a successful sympathectomy and will occur inevitably in a proportion of patients. Backache is common, though short-lived, and is an almost inevitable result of the passage of the needle (see also Chapter 13).

The anatomy of the lumbar sympathetic trunk in man is extremely variable and as this has a great bearing upon the cause of many complications it is worth a brief review. In theory there should be 5 ganglia on each side, lying anterolateral to the vertebral bodies and separated from the somatic roots by the psoas muscles and fascia. In practice, this is seldom the case. Cowley and Yeager[17] found that the number of ganglia varied from 1 to 8 with the 2nd and 3rd ganglia most likely to be present. The outflow and connections of the pre- and postganglionic fibers also vary considerably. Experimentally the preganglionic sympathetic fibers regenerate more quickly and easily than somatic nerves. The postganglionic neurons are unable to regenerate following resection, but it is possible that renervation may follow unilateral sympathectomy because of crossover from the other side.[69] Umeda et al.[81] studied the position of the lumbar sympathetic ganglia and the lumbar arteries in order to determine the best needle position for chemical sympathectomy. The most likely position for the lumbar sympathetic ganglion was found to be between the lower 1/3 of L2 and the upper 1/3 of L3. The lumbar arteries usually crossed the sympathetic chain at the midpoint of the vertebral body. It is clear that in order to have the best chance of achieving a sympathetic block with the smallest amount of neurolytic solution, and to avoid a potentially hazardous intravascular injection, the needle tips should be placed at the lower third of L2 and the upper third of L3. Imaging and recording of needle placement is mandatory.

In an interesting study, Cherry and Rao[15] performed blind percutaneous lumbar sympathectomy (i.e., without x-ray control) on cadavers and analyzed the position of the needles. Using the standard technique, 95% of needles passed through the lumbar chain, or within 0.5 cm of it. Of those needles that missed, 90% were lateral to the chain. One needle passed through a kidney; however, in that case, a large osteophyte was present. Two needles were imbedded in osteoporotic vertebral bodies. In a study investigating celiac plexus block Moore et al.[51] showed that if the needle is introduced through the skin more than 7.5 cm lateral to the midline, there is a risk of hitting a kidney. In sympathectomy, the risk of renal puncture is less, because the path of the needle may pass below the kidneys. Weyland and colleagues[83] confirmed that likelihood of renal puncture decreased with more medial insertion of the needle. They concluded that to reduce the risk of accidental trauma to major organs the paravertebral distance of insertion of the needles should not exceed 6, 7, and 10 cm for lumbar sympathetic blocks at the levels of L2, L3, and L4, respectively.

The lumbar sympathetic nerves supply efferents to the lower extremities, controlling vasoconstriction, sudomotor activity, piloerection, and some sexual function. Following a successful lumbar sympathectomy, there is an increase in blood flow to the lower limb. The majority of this flow is through shunts and does not contribute to muscle flow significantly (see Chapter 13). Skin temperature will rise, partly because of increased skin blood flow, but mainly because of a reduction in counter current cooling caused by the shunting. The result of these changes is a decrease in venous return, which in turn causes a fall in cardiac output and blood pressure. Most patients can compensate within a few days by increasing their circulating volume, but in some cases, hypotension can be a problem. All patients should be warned about it, and immediately following the procedure blood pressure should be checked while the patients are lying and while standing. Patients should be assessed for suitability for day case sympathectomy with this in mind, and those who cannot be accompanied home and looked after adequately at home should be admitted for overnight observation. Occasionally, acute hypotension can be a problem after the procedure, and ephedrine and intravenous fluids must be available for treatment of this potentially serious complication.

Post-sympathectomy Neuralgia

The most common complication is post-sympathetic neuralgia. Proposed mechanisms have been the subject of a recent review.[42] The reported incidence has varied widely between studies, from around 30% to 50%.[45,49] Whether the sympathectomy is achieved by open surgical resection or percutaneous techniques does not seem to influence the incidence.[60,65,66] Cousins et al.,[16] using a percutaneous technique, found an incidence of 40% using alcohol, but only 20% using phenol. In the first large series on chemical sympathectomy, Reid et al.[66] reported an incidence of 9% of injections and 14.6% of patients. A prospective study on postsympathectomy neuralgia following open surgical sympathectomy, reported an incidence of 35% overall. There was no relation to demographic features or diagnosis, nor indication for sympathectomy. The pain usually started 10 to 14 days following sympathectomy and was of abrupt onset at full intensity. The mean duration was 23 days and it lasted 1 to 5 weeks in all but one of their patients, in whom the pain lasted for 3 months. The pain tended to be worse at night, and most described it as a deep, dull, boring, pain.[65]

Patients can also experience paresthesias, a burning pain, and allodynia. The location of the pain may be in the anterior, anterolateral, or medial aspect of the thigh and knee. Raskin et al.[65] reported good pain relief with carbamazepine and phenytoin. Cousins et al.[16] reported good results with transcutaneous nerve stimulation and more recently Buche et al.[11] reported good results in 10 patients using epidural fentanyl and methylprednisolone. Unfortunately, none of these studies are randomized control trials, and in a condition which tends to remit spontaneously, results must therefore be interpreted with caution.

Other Problems

Sexual function is normally subserved through the first lumbar ganglion, the destruction of which causes a failure of ejaculation with no effect on orgasm, libido, or potency.[69,2] Sexual dysfunction in females and bladder function disturbance has been reported following open sympathectomy and there is no reason to believe that these problems could not occur also after neurolytic block.[25]

Fatalities have occurred following sympathectomy. Following open sympathectomy, Erichsen[25] reported a mortality of 2.1% in a series of 241 patients, although most of these were bilateral. Postlethwaite[60] had a mortality of 1% following open sympathectomy. Chemical sympathectomy seems to be associated with a lower mortality rate, and in the series of 1,028 patients described by Reid and colleagues[66] there was only 1 death. They state in their paper, "It is surprising that deaths have not been more frequent, as many of these patients are poor surgical risks and some have died from coronary thrombosis or cerebral vascular incidents prior to admission, or in some cases after admission but before phenol injection." In the study of 386 patients carried out by Cousins and co-workers,[16] 1 died within a week of chemical sympathectomy. There are few data on long-term survival after lumbar sympathectomy. It must be borne in mind that most patients coming for sympathectomy have peripheral vascular disease, which is a widespread systemic problem. In studies at the Vascular Clinic at Ninewells Hospital, Dundee, (Spence V., personal communication), patients with peripheral vascular disease were investigated for other problems. Seventy-five percent of patients were found to have coronary artery disease and 1/3 had hemodynamically significant disease in their carotid arteries. Gillespie[28] found an overall mortality of 25% within 1 to 7 years. Most of these were due to strokes or myocardial infarction.

Many other complications have been reported, including paraplegia, presumably due to thecal spread through a root cuff,[70] renal or ureteric damage which has led to nephrectomy or formation of a urinary fistula,[26,77] intrapleural injection, Horner's syndrome[85] and bilateral block from unilateral injection.[61]

Celiac Plexus Blocks

Like the lumbar sympathetic chain, the celiac axis has variable anatomy and some form of imaging must be undertaken with every block to ensure correct placement. Moore and co-workers[51] carried out an extensive anatomical study to determine the optimal approach to the celiac axis. Taking the classic approach of Kappis as their starting point, they showed that by limiting the point of needle entry to no more than 7.5 cm lateral to the midline, the risk of hitting the kidney could be markedly reduced. Since then, other authors have described approaches to the celiac axis using the transaortic[36] or anterior approaches[50,86] or with a catheter technique.[35] For any new technique to become popular, it should be easy to perform, be as effective as existing techniques, and have a low incidence of side effects. This is, of course, true of all the recently described techniques. It remains to be seen whether greater experience will lead to an increase in the number of problems encountered with new techniques of celiac plexus block.

No matter what route is employed, the fact remains that celiac plexus block is retroperitoneal, and there is no fixed route of spread, with the solution tending to follow the line of least resistance. It has been claimed that the use of computed tomography or magnetic resonance imaging will reduce further the incidence of side effects.[51] Ultrasound has its advocates and it has been stated that phenol and glycerol mixtures provide the advantage of excellent contrast.[40] Some form of radiological or ultrasound control is necessary to warn of spread of solution towards nerve roots or other vital structures, as it is recognized that dangers with celiac plexus block are accentuated by the relatively large volumes of solution used. It is claimed that the supradiaphragmatic, greater splanchnic nerve block will bypass problems caused by anatomical distortion of the target area resulting from tumor spread, infection or previous surgery.[5] This approach would permit the use of smaller volumes of neurolytic solution. However, a disadvantage may be an increased incidence of pneumothorax and pleuritic pain (see Chapter 14).

Eisenberg et al.[24] have carried out a meta-analysis of the use of neurolytic celiac plexus block for the treatment of cancer pain. They noted that the frequency of adverse effects was very variable due to inconsistency in published reports; however, backache and local pain will occur in 96% of patients. Intravascular injection and hemorrhage are ever-present complications because of the proximity of the great vessels; pneumothorax is, also, for similar anatomical reasons.[9]

Hypotension and diarrhea are common accompaniments to a successful block and usually are self-limiting. However, severe hypotension may occur in up to 38% of patients, who may have become relatively dehydrated due to advanced illness, and resuscitative measures such as intravenous infusions, compression stockings, and abdominal binders may need to be used until homeostasis is reestablished.[24] Care is needed after the block and pulse and blood pressure should be monitored on a routine basis to ensure circulatory stability before allowing patients to sit, and again before allowing them to stand, and before starting to walk.

Increased bowel motility is common in up to 60% of patients for the first few days after the block, but gradually reverts to normal in most cases.[86] Occasionally, diarrhea may be intractable following celiac plexus block and can be treated with octreotide.[20]

Problems encountered with celiac plexus block include unilateral[79,43] and bilateral paralysis[14,21] with and without loss of sphincter control,[19] foot drop[8] irritation of the first lumbar nerve,[38] hematuria[51] and failure to ejaculate.[4] Suggested mechanisms for the paraplegia have been advanced by De Conno et al.[21] and Brown and Rorie.[10]

Hypogastric Plexus Blocks

This block targets the sympathetic nerves as they overlie the sacral promontory and can be blocked to reduce pain arising from the pelvic contents. No serious complications have been reported as yet but experience is limited.[22,58] It may be assumed that urinary and bowel problems are likely and that neural damage and hemorrhage are other potential problems.

REFERENCES

1. Arter, O.E., and Racz, G.B.: Pain management of the oncologic patient. Semin. Surg. Oncol. *6:*162, 1990.
2. Baxter, A.D., and O'Kafo, B.A.: Ejaculatory failure after chemical sympathectomy. Anesth. Analg., *63:*770, 1984.
3. Birch, M., Strong, N., Brittain, P., and Sandford-Smith, J.: Retrobulbar phenol in blind painful eyes. Ann. Ophthalmol. *25:*267, 1993.
4. Black, A.C., and Dwyer, B.: Coeliac plexus block. Anaesth Intensive Care., *1:*315, 1979.
5. Boas, R.A.: Sympathetic blocks in clinical practice. International Anesthesiology Clinics, *149:*16, 1978.
6. Bortoluzzi, M., and Marini, G.: Phenol injection into cisterna magna for relief of advanced intractable cancer pain in the faciocephalic area. J. Neurosurg. Sci., *30:*167, 1986.
7. Bromage, P.R.: Epidural Analgesia. Philadelphia, W. B. Saunders, 1978.
8. Brown, D.L.: Neurolytic celiac plexus block for nonpancreatic intra-abdominal cancer pain. Reg. Anesth., *14:*63, 1989.
9. Brown, D.L., Bulley, C.K., and Quiel, E.L.: Neurolytic celiac plexus block for pancreatic cancer pain. Anesth. Analg. *66:*869, 1987.
10. Brown, D.L., and Rorie, D.K.: Altered activity of isolated segmental lumbar arteries of dogs following exposure to ethanol and phenol. Pain, *65:*139, 1994.
11. Buche, M., Randour, P., Mayne, A., Jouken, K., and Schoevaerdts, J.C.: Neuralgia following sympathectomy. Ann. Vasc. Surg., *2:*279, 1988.
12. Cappuzzo, M., Gritti, G., and Vassalli, A.: Anomala diffusione di fenolo in un caso di neurolisi subarachnoidea. Algos., *1:*58, 1984.
13. Challenger, J. Sympathetic nervous system blocking. *In* Swerdlow, M. (ed.)., Relief of Intractable Pain. Excerpta Medica, Amsterdam. 1974.
14. Cherry, D.A., and Lamberty, J.: Paraplegia following coeliac plexus block. Anaesth. Intensive Care. *12:*61, 1984.
15. Cherry, D.A., and Rao, D.M.: Lumbar sympathetic and coeliac plexus blocks: An anatomical study in cadavers. Br. J. Anaesth., *54:*1037, 1982.
16. Cousins, M.I., Reeve, T.S., Glynn, C.J., Walsh, J.A., and Cherry, D.A.: Neurolytic lumbar sympathetic blockade: Duration of denervation and relief of rest pain. Anaesth. Intensive Care. *7:*121, 1979.
17. Cowley, R.A., and Yeager, G.H.: Anatomic observations on the lumbar sympathetic nervous system. Surgery, *25:*880, 1949.
18. Crimeni, R.: Clinical experience with mepivacaine and alcohol in neuralgia of the trigeminal nerve. Acta Anaesthesiol. Scand., *24*(Suppl.), 173, 1966.
19. Davies, D.D.: Incidence of major complications of neurolytic coeliac plexus block. J. R. Soc. Med., *86:*264, 1993.
20. Dean, A.P., and Reed, W.D.: Diarrhoea—An unrecognised hazard of coeliac plexus block. Aust. N. Z. J. Med., *21:*47, 1991.
21. De Conno, F., Caraceni, A., Aldrighetti, L., *et al.*: Paraplegia following coeliac plexus block. Pain, *55:*383, 1993.
22. de Leon-Casasola, O.A., Kent, E., and Lema, M.J.: Neurolytic superior hypogastric plexus block for chronic pelvic pain associated with cancer. Pain, *54:*145, 1993.
23. Derrick, W.S.: Subarachnoid alcohol block for the relief of intractable pain. Acta Anaesthesiol. Scand., *24:*(Suppl.)167, 1966.
24. Eisenberg, E., Carr, D.B., and Chalmers, T.C.: Neurolytic celiac plexus block for treatment of cancer pain: A meta-analysis. Anesth. Analg., *80:*290, 1995.
25. Erichsen, H.G.: Lumbar sympathectomy in obliterative arteriosclerosis. Scand. J. Thorac. Cardiovasc. Surg. *13:*333, 1979.
26. Fraser, I., Windle, R., Smart, J.G., and Barrie, W.W.: Ureteric injury following chemical sympathectomy. B. J. Surg., *71:*349, 1984.
27. Gale, D.W., Valley, M.A., Rogers, J.N., and Poterack, K.A.: Effects of neurolytic concentrations of alcohol and phenol on Dacron and Gore-Tex vascular prosthetic grafts. Reg. Anesth., *19:*395, 1994.
28. Gillespie, J.A.: Future place of lumbar sympathectomy in obliterative vascular disease of lower limbs. Br. Med. J., *2:*1640, 1960.
29. Grunwald, I.: Neurolise com fenol: Uso da via peridural no tratamento da dolor de cancer. Rev. Bras. Anestesiol. *26:*628, 1976.
30. Hay, R.C.: Subarachnoid alcohol block in the control of intractable pain. Anesth. Analg., *41;*12, 1962.
31. Henderson, W.R.: Trigeminal neuralgia: The pain and its treatment. Br. Med. J. *1:*7, 1967.
32. Holland, A.J.C., and Youseff, M.A.: A complication of subarachnoid phenol blockade. Anaesthesia, *34:*260, 1979.
33. Horowitz, N.H., and Rizzoli, H.V.: Postoperative Complications in Neurosurgical Practice. pp. 666. Baltimore, Williams and Wilkins, 1967.
34. Hughes, J.T.: Thrombosis of the posterior spinal arteries. Neurology (Minneapolis), *20:*659, 1970.
35. Humbles, F.F., and Mahaffey, J.E.: Teflon epidural catheter placement for intermittent celiac plexus blockade and celiac plexus neurolytic blockade. Reg. Anesth. *15:*103, 1990.
36. Ischia, S., Luzzani, A., Ischia, A., Magon, F., and Toscano, D.: Subarachnoid neurolytic block (L5–S1)and unilateral percutaneous cervical cordotomy in the treatment of pain secondary to pelvic malignant disease. Pain, *20:*139, 1984.
37. Ischia, S, Ischia, A., Polati, E., and Finco, G.: Three posterior percutaneous celiac plexus block techniques. A prospective, randomized study in 61 patients with pancreatic cancer pain. Anesthesiology., *76:*534, 1992.
38. Jones, R.R.: Technique for injection of splanchnic nerves with alcohol. Anesth. Analg., *36:*75, 1957.
39. Katz, J.: Pain, theory and management. *In* Scurr, C.B., and Feldman, S. (eds.).: Scientific Foundations of Anaesthesia. pp. 226. London, Heinmann, 1970.
40. Kirvela, O., Svedstrom, E., and Lundbom, N.: Ultrasonic guidance of lumbar sympathetic and celiac plexus block: A new technique. Reg. Anesth. *17:*43, 1992.
41. Korsten, H.H., Ackerman, E.W., Grouls, R.J.: *et al.* Long-lasting epidural sensory blockade by n-methyl-p-aminobenzoate in the terminally ill intractable cancer pain patient. Anesthesiology, *75:*950, 1991.
42. Kramis, R.C., Roberts, W.J., and Gillette, R.G.: Post-sympathectomy neuralgia: Hypotheses on peripheral and central neuronal mechanisms. Pain, *64:*1, 1996.
43. Leung, J.W.C., Bowen-Wright, M., Aveling, W., *et al.*: Coeliac plexus block for pancreatitis. Br. J. Surg., *70:*730, 1983.
44. Lifshitz, S., Debacker, L.J., and Buchsbaum, A.J.: Subarachnoid phenol block for pain relief in gynecologic malignancy. Obstet. Gynecol. *48;*316, 1976.
45. Litwin, M.S.: Post-sympathectomy neuralgia. Arch. Surg., *84:*591, 1962.
46. Mark, V.H., White, J.C., Zervas, N.T., *et al.*: Intrathecal use of phenol for the relief of chronic severe pain. N. Engl. J. Med. *267:*589, 1962.
47. Mehta, M.: Intractable Pain. London, W. B. Saunders, 1973.
48. Miles, J.: Trigeminal neuralgia. *In* Lipton, S. (ed.): Persistent Pain. Vol. 2. London, Academic Press, 1980.
49. Mockus, M.B., Rutherford, R.B., Rosales, C., and Pearce, W.H.: Sympathectomy for causalgia. Arch. Surg.: *122:*668, 1987.
50. Montero, M.A., Vidal, L.F., and Inaraja, M.L.: The percutaneous anterior approach to the coeliac plexus using CT guidance. Pain., *34:*285, 1988.
51. Moore, D.C., Bush, W.H., and Burnett, L.L.: Celiac plexus block: A roentgenographic, anatomic study of technique and spread of solution in patients and corpses. Anesth. Analg. *60:*369, 1981.
52. Mousel, L.H.: Treatment of intractable pain of the head and neck. Anesth Analg., *46:*705, 1967.
53. Nathan, P.W.: Pain in cancer: Comparison of results of cordotomy and chemical rhizotomy. *In* Pusek, I., Kune, Z. (eds).: Present Limits of Neurosurgery. Amsterdam, Excerpta Medica, 1972.
54. Nathan, P.W., and Sears, T.A.: Effects of phenol on nervous conduction. J. Physiol. *150:*565, 1960.
55. Nour-Eldin, F.: Preliminary report: Uptake of Phenol by vascular or brain tissue. Microvas. Res. *2:*224, 1970.

56. Papo, I., and Visca, A.: Phenol rhizotomy in the treatment of cancer pain. Anesth. Analg. *53:*99, 1974.
57. Papo, I., and Visca, A.: Phenol subarachnoid rhizotomy for the treatment of cancer pain. A personal account of 290 cases. Advances in Pain Research and Therapy, *2:*339, 1979.
58. Plancarte, R., Amescua, C., Patt, R.B., and Aldrete, J.A.: Superior hypogastric plexus block for pelvic cancer pain. Anesthesiology, *73:*236, 1990.
59. Porges, P., and Zdrahal, F.: Intrathecal alcohol neurolysis of the lower sacral roots in inoperable rectal cancer. Anaesthesist, *34;*627, 1985.
60. Postlethwaite, J.C.: Lumbar sympathectomy. Br. J. Surg. *60:*878, 1973.
61. Purcell-Jones, G., and Justins, D.M.: Delayed contralateral sympathetic blockade following chemical sympathectomy—a case history. Pain, *34:*61, 1988.
62. Purcell-Jones, G., Pither, C.E., Justins, D.M.: Paravertebral somatic nerve block: A clinical, radiographic and computed tomographic study in chronic pain patients. Anesth. Anal., *68:*32, 1989.
63. Ramamurthy, S., Walsh, N.E., Schoenfeld, L.S., and Hoffman, J.: Evaluation of neurolytic blocks using phenol and cryogenic block in the management of chronic pain. J. Pain Symptom. Manage. *4:*72, 1989.
64. Ramb, H.: Die alkoholinjektion ins Ganglion Gasseri bei der trigeminusneuralgie. Dtsch Med. Wochenschr. *74:*826, 1949.
65. Raskin, N.H., Levinson, S.A., Hoffman, P.M., Pickett, J.B.E., and Fields, H.L.: Postsympathectomy neuralgia. Am. J. Surg., *128:*75, 1974.
66. Reid, W., Kennedy, Watt, J., and Gray, T.G.: Phenol injection of the sympathetic chain. Br. J. Surg., *57:*45, 1970.
67. Ruge, D., Brochner, R., and Davis, L.: A study of the treatment of 637 patients with trigeminal neuralgia. J. Neurosurg. *15:*528, 1958.
68. Saini, S.S.: Retrogasserian anhydrous glycerol injection therapy in trigeminal neuralgia: Observations in 552 patients. J. Neurol. Neurosurg. Psychiatry, *50:*1536, 1987.
69. Simeone, F.A.: The anatomy of the lumbar sympathetic trunks in man. J. Cardiovasc. Surg., *20:*283, 1979.
70. Smith, R.C., Davidson, N.M., and Ruckley, C.V.: Hazard of chemical sympathectomy. Br. Med. J., *1:*552, 1978.
71. Sperling, E., Stender, A.: Tic Douloureux und Gessichtsschmerz (Therapeutische und Pathogenetische Betrachtungen) Dtsch. Zahn. Mund. Keiferheilkd. Zentralbl., *173:*161, 1955.
72. Stender, A.: Excerpta Medica Congress Series. Washington, D.C., *36,* 1961.
73. Stovner, J., and Endresen, R.: Intrathecal phenol for cancer pain. Acta Anaesthesiol. Scand., *16:*17, 1972.
74. Sunderland, S.: Nerves and nerve injuries. Edinburgh, E. & S. Livingstone, 1978.
75. Superville-Sovak, B., Rasminsky, M., and Finlayson, M.H.: Complications of phenol neurolysis. Arch. Neurol., *32:*226, 1975.
76. Swerdlow, M.: Intrathecal and Extradural Block. *In* Swerdlow M. (ed.): Relief of Intractable Pain. 2nd Ed. Amsterdam, Excerpta Medica, 1978.
77. Swerdlow, M.: Complications of Neurolytic Neural Blockade. *In* Cousins, M.J., and Bridenbaugh, P.O., eds.: Neural Blockade in Clinical Anesthesia and Management of Pain. 2nd ed. pp. 719–735. J.B. Lippincott, Philadelphia, 1988.
78. Tank, T.M., Dohn, D.F., and Gardner, W.J.: Intrathecal injections of alcohol and phenol fo relief of intractable pain. Cleve. Clin. Q., *30:*111, 1963.
79. Thompson, G.E., Moore, D.C., Bridenbaugh, L.D., and Artin, L.Y.: Abdominal pain and alcohol celiac plexus nerve block. Anesth. Analg. *56:*1, 1977.
80. Totoki, T., Kato, T., Nomoto, Y., *et al.*: Anterior spinal artery syndrome—A complication of cervical intrathecal phenol injection. Pain, *6:*99, 1979.
81. Umeda, S., Arai, T., Hatano, Y., Mori, K., and Hoshino, K.: Cadaver anatomic analysis of the best site for chemical lumbar sympathectomy. Anesth. Analg., *66:*643, 1987.
82. Ventafridda, V., Tamburini, M., Caraceni, A., De Conno, F., and Naldi, F.: A validation study of the WHO method for cancer pain relief. Cancer., *15;*850, 1987.
83. Weyland, A., Weyland, W., Carduck, H.P., Hildebrandt, J., and Kettler, D.: Optimization of the image intensifier-assisted technique of lumbar sympathetic block: Computer tomographic simulation of a paravertebral puncture access. Anaesthesist., *42:*710, 1993.
84. White, J.C., and Sweet, W.H.: Pain and the Neurosurgeon. Springfield, IL, Charles C. Thomas, 1969.
85. Wills, M.H., Korbon, G.A., and Arasi, R. Horner's syndrome resulting from a lumbar sympathetic block. Anesthesiology, *68:*613, 1988.
86. Zenz, M., Kurz-Muller, K., Strumpf, M., and May, B.: The anterior sonographic-guided celiac plexus blockade: Review and personal observations. Anaesthesist, *42:*246, 1993.

PART III

Neural Blockade in the Management of Pain

Neural Blockade in Clinical Anesthesia and Management of Pain, Third Edition,
edited by M.J. Cousins and P.O. Bridenbaugh.
Lippincott–Raven Publishers, Philadelphia © 1998.

CHAPTER 23.1

Introduction to Pain Mechanisms

Implications for Neural Blockade

Philip J. Siddall and Michael J. Cousins

This chapter provides an overview of current concepts of pain and some of the implications that these concepts have for pain management. It should be stated at the outset that the biological response to a noxious stimulus is not pain.[64] The International Association for the Study of Pain has defined pain in this way: "Pain is an unpleasant sensory and emotional experience associated with actual or potential tissue damage, or described in terms of such damage."[79] It must always be remembered that the perception of pain is a complex interaction that involves sensory, emotional, and behavioral factors.[76] A detailed review of neurobiological mechanisms involved in pain perception is found in Chapter 24. However, the role of psychological factors, which include a person's emotional and behavioral responses, must always be considered as an important component in the perception and expression of pain. The psychological aspects of pain perception are described in Chapter 25. The person in pain must always be seen in the context of interactions between biological and psychosocial processes. Any pain management attempts that do not reckon with these interactions will lead inevitably to frustration and failure.

The biological processes involved in pain perception are no longer viewed as a simple "hard-wired" system with a pure "stimulus-response" relationship. The more recent conceptualization of pain considers the changes which occur within the nervous system following any prolonged, noxious stimulus. For example, trauma to any part of the body, and nerve damage in particular, can lead to changes within other regions of the nervous system which influence subsequent responses to sensory input. There is increasing recognition that long-term changes occur within the peripheral and central nervous system following noxious input. This plasticity of the nervous system then alters the body's response to further peripheral sensory input.

Recognition of these changes has fostered the concept that pain is divided into two entities: physiological and pathophysiological or clinical.[113] Physiological pain describes the situation in which a noxious stimulus activates peripheral nociceptors, which then transmit sensory information through several relays until it reaches the brain and is recognized as a potentially harmful stimulus (Fig. 23.1-1, Table 23.1-1). More commonly, the insult to the body which produces pain also causes inflammation, and tissue or nerve injury. The pathophysiological processes which occur following injury result in a stimulus-response pattern that is quite different from that seen following physiological pain and has therefore been termed pathophysiological or clinical pain (Fig. 23.1-2, Table 23.1-2). It is the elucidation of these pathophysiological processes that has the most relevance for our understanding and management of pain in the clinical setting.

P.J. Siddall and M.J. Cousins: Department of Anaesthesia and Pain Management, University of Sydney, Royal North Shore Hospital, St. Leonards, New South Wales 2065 Australia.

PAIN MECHANISMS

Peripheral Mechanisms

Primary Afferent Nociceptors

The primary afferent nociceptor is generally the initial structure involved in nociceptive processes. Most body structures contain nerve endings which are responsive to mechanical, thermal, and chemical stimuli (see Chapter 24). Depending on the response characteristics of the nociceptor, stimulation results in propagation of impulses along the afferent fiber toward the spinal cord. The receptors associated with transmission of noxious information can be grouped into two main categories: Aδ fiber mechanothermal and C fiber polymodal nociceptors (see Chapter 24, Figure 24-8).

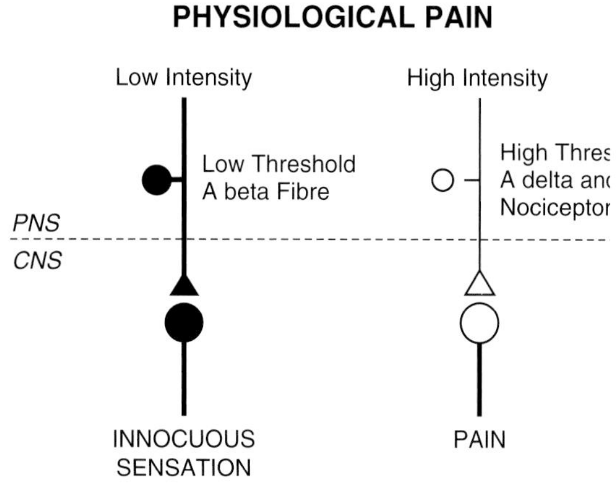

FIG. 23.1-1. Under "physiological" conditions, low intensity, non-noxious stimuli activate low-threshold receptors to generate innocuous sensations, and high intensity, noxious stimuli activate high-threshold nociceptors which may lead to the sensation of pain. PNS, peripheral nervous system; CNS, central nervous system [From Woolf, C.J., and Chong, M.S.: Pre-emptive analgesia-treating postoperative pain by preventing the establishment of central sensitization. Anesth. Analg., *77*:362, 1993.]

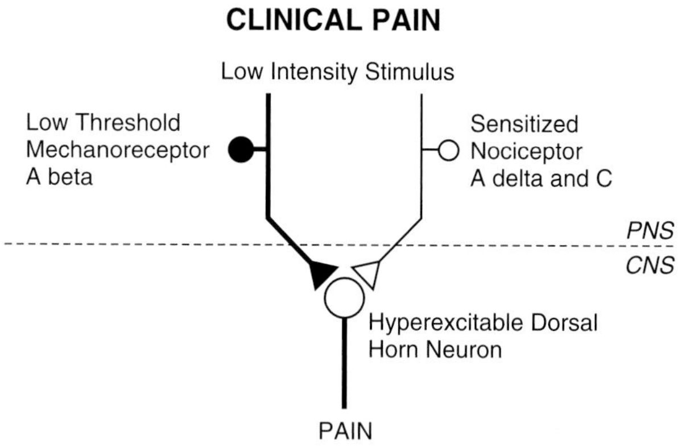

FIG. 23.1-2. In the clinical situation, central and peripheral changes lead to abnormal excitability in the nervous system. This means that low-intensity stimuli can produce pain. *PNS*, peripheral nervous system; *CNS*, central nervous system [From Woolf C.J., and Chong, M.S.: Pre-emptive analgesia-treating postoperative pain by preventing the establishment of central sensitization. Anesth. Analg. *77*:362, 1993.]

Many forms of pain arise from direct activation or sensitization of primary afferent neurons, especially C fiber polymodal nociceptors.[14] However, the process of nociceptor activation sets in train other processes which contribute to and modify responses to further stimuli. For example, a relatively benign noxious stimulus such as a scratch to the skin initiates an inflammatory process in the periphery, which then changes the response properties to subsequent sensory stimuli (Fig. 23.1-3). Under normal conditions, thermal, mechanical, and chemical stimuli activate high threshold nociceptors which signal this information to the first relay in the spinal cord. However, under clinical conditions, application of a noxious stimulus is usually prolonged, traumatic, and associated with tissue damage. Tissue damage results in inflammation, which directly affects the response of the nociceptor to further stimulation.

Peripheral Sensitization

Part of the inflammatory response is the release of intracellular contents from damaged cells and inflammatory cells such as macrophages, lymphocytes, and mast cells. Nociceptive stimulation also causes a neurogenic inflammatory response with the release of substance P, neurokinin A, and calcitonin gene-related peptide (CGRP) from the peripheral terminals of nociceptive afferent fibers.[59] Release of these peptides results in a changed excitability of sensory and sympathetic nerve fibers, vasodilatation, and extravasation of plasma proteins, as well as acting on inflammatory cells to release chemical mediators. These interactions induce release of a "soup" of inflammatory mediators such as potassium, serotonin, bradykinin, substance P, histamine, cytokines, nitric oxide, and products from the cyclo-oxygenase and lipoxygenase pathways of arachidonic acid metabolism (Fig. 23.1-4).[38,44,85] These chemicals then sensitize high-threshold nociceptors which results in the phenomenon of peripheral sensitization (see Chapter 24 and Fig. 24–4).

After sensitization, low-intensity mechanical stimuli which would not normally cause pain are now perceived as painful. There is also an increased responsiveness to thermal stimuli at the site of injury. This zone of primary hyperalgesia surrounding the site of injury is due to peripheral changes and is a feature which is commonly observed following surgery and other forms of trauma.

TABLE 23.1-1. *Features of physiological pain*

Pain (Aδ and C fibers) can be differentiated from touch (Aβ fibers)
Pain serves a protective function
Pain acts as a warning of *potential* damage
Pain is transient
Pain is well localized
Stimulus-response pattern is the same as with other sensory modalities, e.g., touch

TABLE 23.1-2. *Features of clinical pain*

Pain can be elicited by Aδ and C as well as Aβ fibers
Pain is "pathological," i.e., it is associated with inflammation, neuropathy, etc.
Occurs in the context of peripheral sensitization
Occurs in the context of central sensitization
Pain outlasts the stimulus
Pain spreads to nondamaged areas

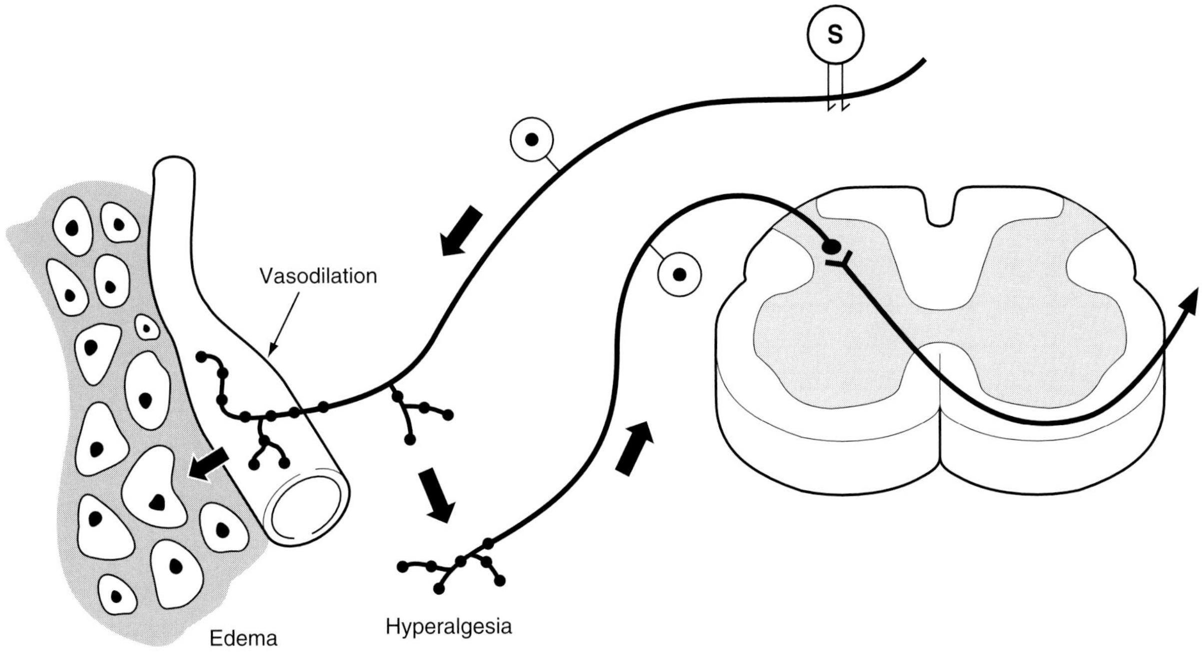

FIG. 23.1-3. Effect of antidromic impulses in primary afferents. Stimulation *(S)* of the cut end of primary afferent fibers results in the release of chemical mediators from the peripheral terminals which produce vasodilation (flare), edema (wheal), and hyperalgesia: (triple response of Lewis). (From Fields, H.L.: Pain. New York, McGraw-Hill, 1987.)

NSAIDs

Nonsteroidal anti-inflammatory drugs (NSAIDs) are commonly used for peripheral analgesia to reduce the inflammatory response.[103] Agents such as aspirin, paracetamol, and other NSAIDs provide their anti-inflammatory action by blocking the cyclo-oxygenase pathway. It is now apparent that cyclo-oxygenase exists in two forms, COX_1 and COX_2. While COX_1 is always present in tissues, including the gastric mucosa, COX_2 is induced by inflammation.[91] This presents an opportunity for development of agents which have a selective anti-inflammatory effect without gastric side-effects. Besides the peripheral action of NSAIDs, there is increasing evidence that they exert their analgesic effect through central mechanisms.[102,103]

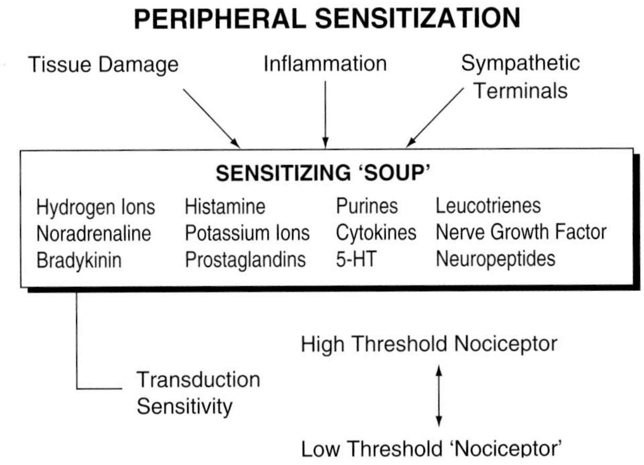

FIG. 23.1-4. The sensitivity of high-threshold nociceptors can be modified in the periphery by a combination of chemicals that act as a "sensitizing soup." These chemicals are produced by damaged tissue as part of the inflammatory reaction and by sympathetic terminals. 5-HT, 5-hydroxytryptamine. (From Woolf, C.J., and Chong, M.S.: Preemptive analgesia-treating postoperative pain by preventing the establishment of central sensitization. Anesth. Analg., *77*:362, 1993.)

NSAIDs are used extensively in treatment of acute postoperative pain.[78] While there has been some concern about the risks of NSAIDs, they continue to have a useful role as analgesics in the perioperative period. Naproxen,[23] diclofenac,[57] and ketorolac[83] have all been used either pre- or postoperatively with a demonstrated reduction in postoperative pain and reduced opioid requirements (see Chapter 26). The different sites of action found with NSAIDs and opioids would also suggest additive, or possibly even synergistic, effects; in clinical practice they are often used in combination.

Peripheral Action of Opioids

Opioids traditionally have been viewed as centrally acting drugs. However, there is now evidence that endogenous opioids act on peripheral sites following tissue damage.[95,97] Opioid receptors are manufactured in the cell body (dorsal root ganglion) and transported toward the central terminal in the dorsal horn and toward the periphery (Fig. 23.1-5). The peripheral receptors become active following local tissue

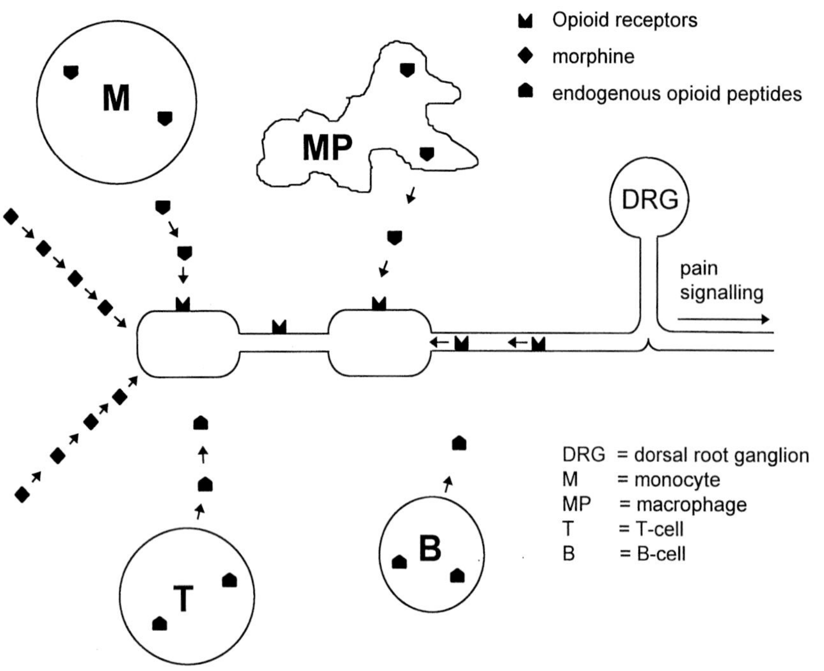

FIG. 23.1-5. Peripheral inflammation results in production of opioid receptors by the dorsal root ganglion *(DRG)* and transport of opioid receptors toward the peripheral terminal. Peripheral opioid receptors are activated by exogenous application of morphine and endogenous opioid peptides released by monocytes *(M)*, T-cells *(T)*, B-cells *(B)*, and macrophages *(MP)*. (From Stein, C.: Morphine-A local "analgesic." Pain: Clinical Updates., *3*:1, 1995.)

damage. This occurs with unmasking of opioid receptors and arrival of immunocompetent cells that possess opioid receptors; these can synthesize opioid peptides. It is this ability that stimulated interest in peripheral administration of opioids, such as intra-articular administration following knee surgery or arthroscopy,[48,96] or topical administration of morphine.[100] Despite initial enthusiasm for this technique, some have expressed doubt about the usefulness and cost-benefit of intra-articular morphine, particularly following arthroscopy or minor knee surgery.[1] However, opioids with physicochemical properties favoring peripheral action are under development and, if successful, such drugs may be useful for regional application.

Peripheral Nerve Injury

Nociceptors are not simply inert conductors of sensory information. Recent studies have demonstrated that section of, or damage to, a peripheral nerve results in a number of biochemical, physiological, and morphological changes that act as a focus of pain in themselves.[33,84] Nerve damage results in an increased production of peptides, such as nerve growth factor (NGF), which regulate neuronal growth. However, following nerve damage, NGF may play a part in development of altered responsiveness to sensory input.[60]

Neuroplasticity changes aimed at maintaining sensory input may occur at peripheral and/or spinal level (Fig. 23.1-6). These biochemical changes cause nerve fibers to undergo morphological and physiological changes. The damaged end of the nerve fiber sprouts and may produce a spontaneously firing neuroma (see Chapter 24). It may also demonstrate changed properties in response to various stimuli (Fig. 23.1-7). These properties include sensitivity to mechanical stimuli, spontaneous firing, and sensitivity to noradrenaline (norepinephrine).[33] Similar changes occur within the cell body of the afferent nociceptor, the dorsal root ganglion.[34] Reduction in the blood supply to myelinated fibers ends in demyelination and production of ectopic impulses. These impulses may give rise in the perception of sharp, shooting, or burning pain to patients with conditions such as diabetic neuropathy. Other clinical conditions that may have a peripheral neuropathic component include post-herpetic neuralgia and post-amputation pain; however there is almost invariably a central component (see following).

A number of agents are used with varying degrees of success in the management of peripheral neuropathic pain.[46,86] These include tricyclic antidepressants,[66,68] anticonvulsants such as carbamazepine and sodium valproate,[72] clonidine,[119] opioids,[87] local anesthetics such as lignocaine (lidocaine),[6] and antiarrhythmic agents, such as mexiletine.[17] In addition to these agents, now used extensively in the management of peripheral neuropathic pain, several new agents may be promising, but have not as yet been systematically evaluated. These include new antidepressants such as venlafaxine and nefazodone, and new anticonvulsants such as gabapentin, vigabatrin, and lamotrigine.

Systemic administration of local anesthetic agents can culminate in a marked reduction of neuropathic pain,[6] because relatively low concentrations of local anesthetic can reduce ectopic activity in damaged nerves at levels below the concentration required to produce conduction block.[34] A puzzling feature of the response of peripheral neuropathic

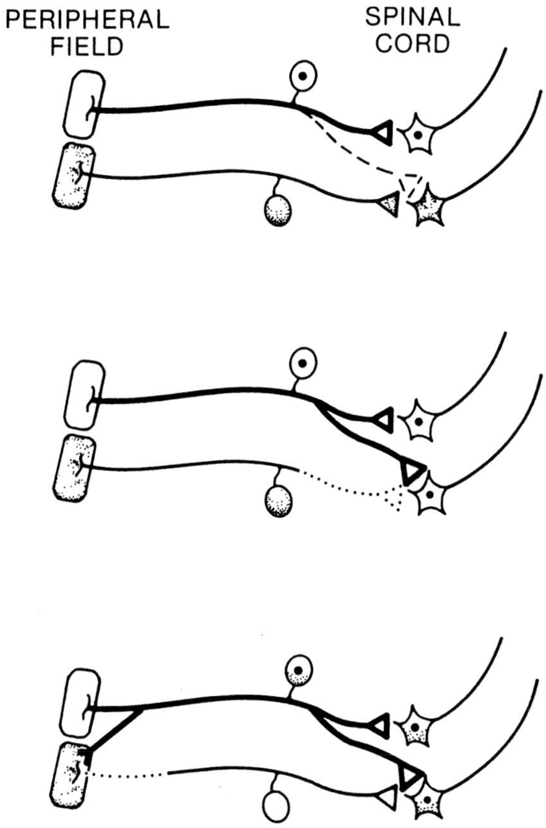

FIG. 23.1-6. Neuroplasticity following damage to primary afferent fibers. **Top:** Normal connectivity of primary afferent. Primary afferents innervate a defined peripheral region and activate a specific population of spinal cord neurons. In addition, the primary afferent has central connections that are normally ineffective *(dashed line).* In the normal situation, each spinal cord cell responds only to stimulation of its own peripheral field. **Middle:** When the central process of a primary afferent that innervates an adjacent peripheral field *(stipple)* is interrupted *(dotted line),* the formerly ineffective central connection of the intact primary afferent *(heavy line)* becomes effective. Both spinal cord cells now respond only to stimulation of the innervated peripheral field (not stippled). **Lower:** When the peripheral process of the adjacent primary afferent is cut *(dotted line)*, changes occur in the spinal cord that are similar to those produced by cutting the central process. In addition, the peripheral process of the intact primary afferent *(heavy line)* sprouts and grows into the denervated peripheral region *(stipple).* In this case, both spinal cord cells respond to stimulation of both peripheral fields. (From Fields, H.L.: Pain. New York, McGraw-Hill, 1987.)

pain to systemic administration of local anesthetics is the time course of pain relief. While intrathecal or peripheral nerve blockade results in temporary reduction in pain behavior in an animal model of neuropathic pain, systemic administration of lidocaine results in a reduction in mechanical hyperalgesia that persists for one week.[18] This finding challenges previously accepted explanations for the mechanisms of local anesthetics in reducing neuropathic pain, and also suggests possible clinical application.[98]

Sympathetic Nervous System

The sympathetic nervous system also has an important role in generation and maintenance of chronic pain states.[51,52,71] Nerve damage and even minor trauma can lead to a disturbance in sympathetic activity (Fig. 23.1-8), which then leads to a sustained condition (now termed a "complex regional pain syndrome," replacing the previously used term, "reflex sympathetic dystrophy"[80]). Complex regional pain syndromes are associated with features of sympathetic dysfunction, including vasomotor and sudomotor changes, abnormalities of hair and nail growth, osteoporosis, sensory symptoms of spontaneous burning pain, hyperalgesia and allodynia, and, often, disturbance of motor function (see Appendix A).

Basic studies have demonstrated that several changes involving the sympathetic nervous system may be responsible for development of these features.[52] Inflammation can result in the sensitization of primary nociceptive afferent fibers by prostanoids that are released from sympathetic fibers[59] (Fig. 23.1-9). Following nerve injury, sympathetic nerve stimulation or administration of noradrenaline can excite primary afferent fibers via an action at α-adrenoceptors; there is also innervation of the dorsal root ganglion by sympathetic terminals[69] (see Chapter 24, Fig. 24-14). This means that activity in sympathetic efferent fibers can lead to abnormal activity or responsiveness of the primary afferent fiber.

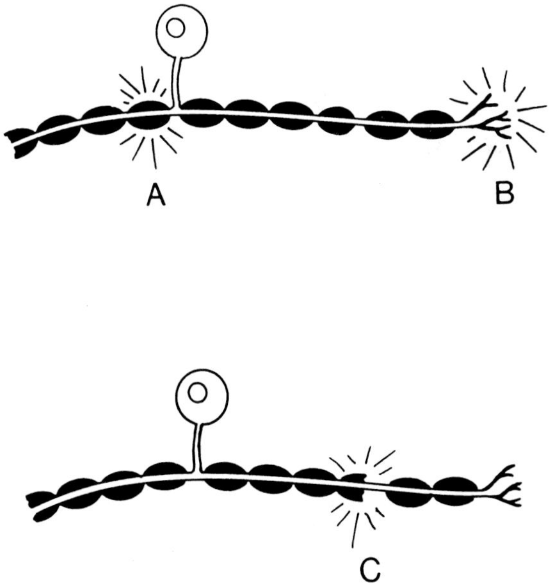

FIG. 23.1-7. Sites of ectopic discharge in damaged primary afferent nociceptors. **Top:** A transected nerve begins to regenerate, sending out sprouts *(B)* that are mechanically sensitive, sensitive to α-adrenergic agonists, and spontaneously active. In addition, a secondary site of hyperactivity *(A)* develops near the cell body in the dorsal root ganglion. **Bottom:** Ectopic impulses may arise from a short patch of demyelination on a primary afferent *(C).* (From Fields, H.L.: Pain. New York, McGraw-Hill, 1987.)

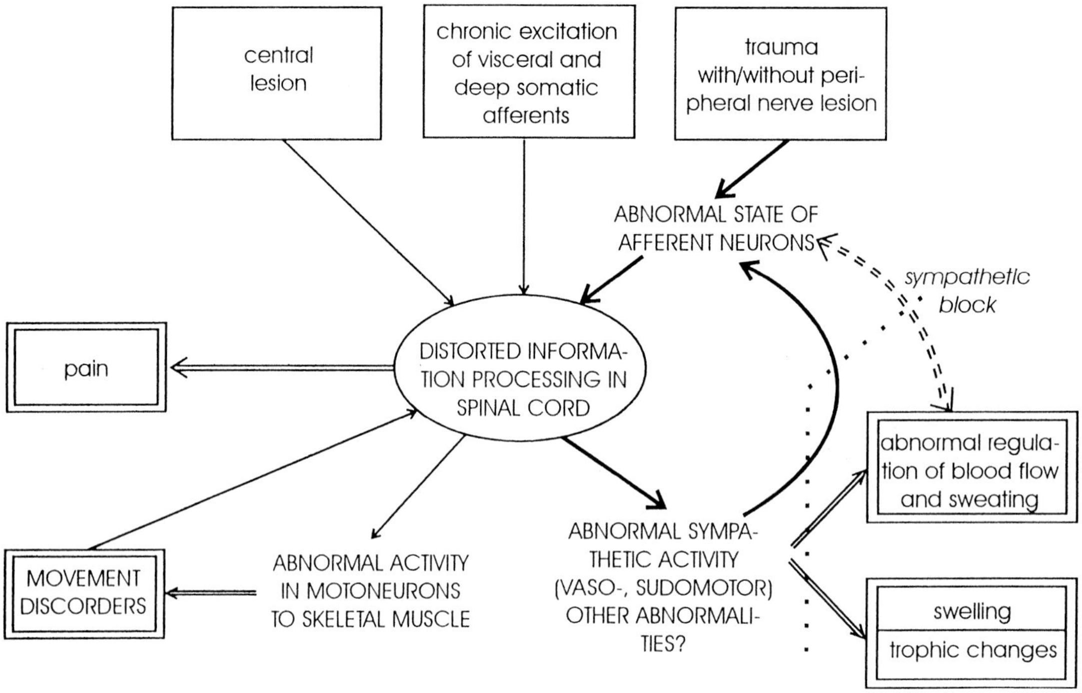

FIG. 23.1-8. General hypothesis about the neural mechanisms of the generation of CRPS I and II following peripheral trauma, with and without nerve lesions, chronic stimulation of visceral afferents (e.g., myocardial infarction) and deep somatic afferents and, rarely, central trauma. The clinical observations are double-framed. Note the vicious circle *(arrows in bold black).* An important component of this circle is the excitatory influence of postganglionic sympathetic axons on primary afferent fibers in the periphery. [From: Jänig, W.: The puzzle of "reflex sympathetic dystrophy": Mechanisms, hypotheses, open questions. *In* Jänig, W., and Stanton-Hicks, M. (eds.): Reflex Sympathetic Dystrophy: A Reappraisal. Seattle, IASP Press, 1996.]

Complex regional pain syndromes may be sympathetically maintained or sympathetically independent (see also Chapter 27). Pain problems that are sympathetically maintained may respond to sympathetic blockade by agents administered systemically, epidurally, regionally, or around the sympathetic ganglion[15] (see Chapter 13).

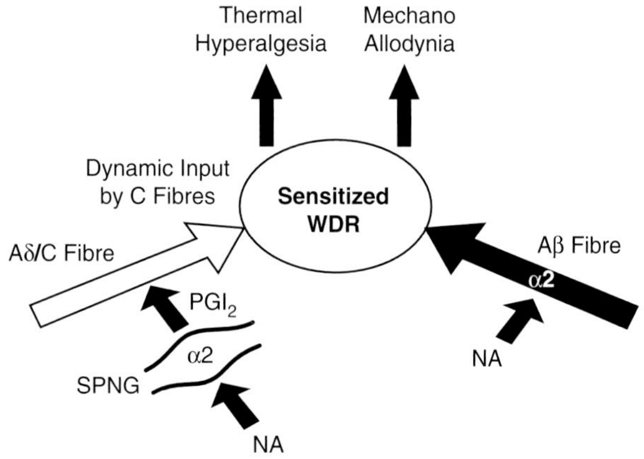

FIG. 23.1-9. Inflammation and nerve injury leads to sensitization of wide dynamic range (WDR) neurons in the dorsal horn. This process involves sensitization of nociceptive primary afferents by release of prostanoids *(PGI2)* from sympathetic fibres and activation of Aβ fiber α_2 adrenoceptors by noradrenaline *(NA).* The effect of these interactions is a resultant thermal hyperalgesia and mechanical allodynia.

Silent Nociceptors

Silent nociceptors have been identified in a number of different tissues and species and once again bear testimony to the dynamic nature of sensory function: They are a class of unmyelinated primary afferent neurons that do not respond to excessive mechanical or thermal stimuli under normal circumstances.[70] However, in the presence of inflammation and chemical sensitization, they become responsive, discharge vigorously even during ordinary movement, and display changes in receptive fields.[90] This class of nociceptors may be an additional factor important in the development of sensitization following inflammation (see also Chapter 24).

Dorsal Horn Mechanisms

Termination Sites of Primary Afferents

The dorsal horn is the site of termination of primary afferents and there is a complex interaction among afferent fibers, local intrinsic spinal neurons, and the endings of descending fibers from the brain[16] (see following, Fig. 23.1-18, Chapter 24, and Fig. 24-8). Primary afferent nociceptors terminate primarily in laminae I, II, and V,[61] where they connect with several classes of second-order neurons in the dorsal horn of the spinal cord (see following and Fig. 23.1-17). Some fibers ascend and descend several segments in Lissauer's tract before terminating on neurons that project to higher centers (see Chapter 24 and Fig. 24-9).

There are two main classes of second-order dorsal horn neurons associated with sensory processing. The first class of neurons is termed "nociceptive specific" or "high-threshold"; the second class is termed "wide dynamic range" or "convergent." The two classes have different response properties to afferent input and are located in different regions of the dorsal horn. Nociceptive specific neurons are located within the superficial laminae of the dorsal horn and respond selectively to noxious stimuli.[20] Wide dynamic range neurons generally are located in deeper laminae and respond to both noxious and non-noxious input[109] (see following and Fig. 23.1-17).

Wide dynamic range neurons normally do not signal pain in response to a tactile stimulus at a non-noxious level. However, if they become sensitized and hyperresponsive, they may discharge at a high rate following a tactile stimulus (see Chapter 24 and Fig. 24-12). If the activity of the wide dynamic range neuron exceeds a threshold level following this stimulus, then the non-noxious tactile stimulus will be perceived as painful and give rise to the phenomenon of allodynia.[65]

Neurotransmitters

Pharmacological studies have helped to identify the many neurotransmitters and neuromodulators involved in pain processes in the dorsal horn[107] (see Chapter 24 and Fig. 24-13). The excitatory amino acids glutamate and aspartate have a major role in nociceptive transmission in the dorsal horn.[21] The excitatory amino acids act at N-methyl D-aspartate (NMDA), non-NMDA receptors such as AMPA (α-amino-3-hydroxy-5-methyl-4-isoxazolepropionic acid), kainate, and metabotropic glutamate receptors[88,107] (Fig. 23.1-10).

Several of the peptides released by primary afferents have a role in nociception. These include substance P, neurokinin A, and calcitonin gene-related peptide (CGRP). Substance P and neurokinin A act on neurokinin receptors. There are a number of other receptors that are involved in nociceptive transmission or modulation; they include opioid (μ, κ, and

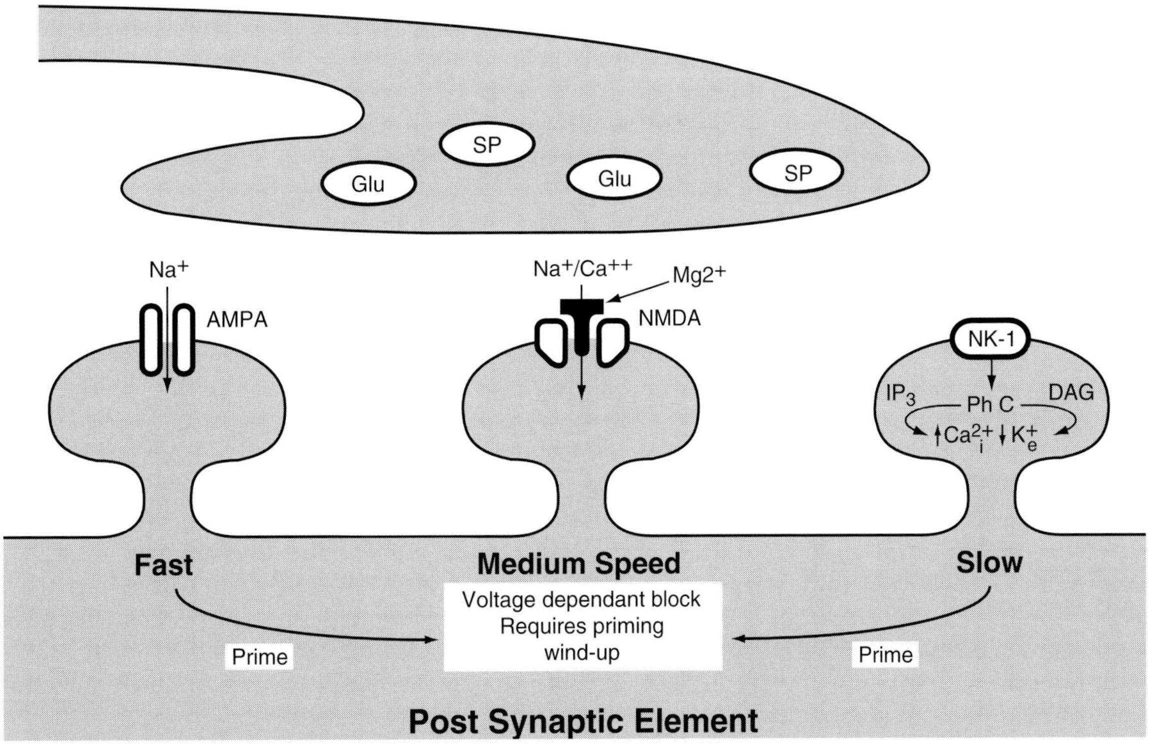

FIG. 23.1-10. Release of glutamate (Glu) and substance P (SP) from the terminals of nociceptive primary afferents activates AMPA and neurokinin 1 (NK-1) receptors respectively on the post synaptic membrane. Activation of these receptors results in sodium (Na^+) influx at the AMPA receptor and activation of second messengers (IP3, Ph C, DAG). These processes then act to prime the NMDA receptor with removal of the magnesium plug and sodium and calcium (Ca^{++}) influx. *AMPA*, α-amino-3-hydroxy-5-methyl-4-isoxazolepropionic acid; *IP3*, inositol triphosphate; *DAG*, diacylglycerol; *NMDA*, N-methyl D-aspartate; *Ph C*, phospholipase C.

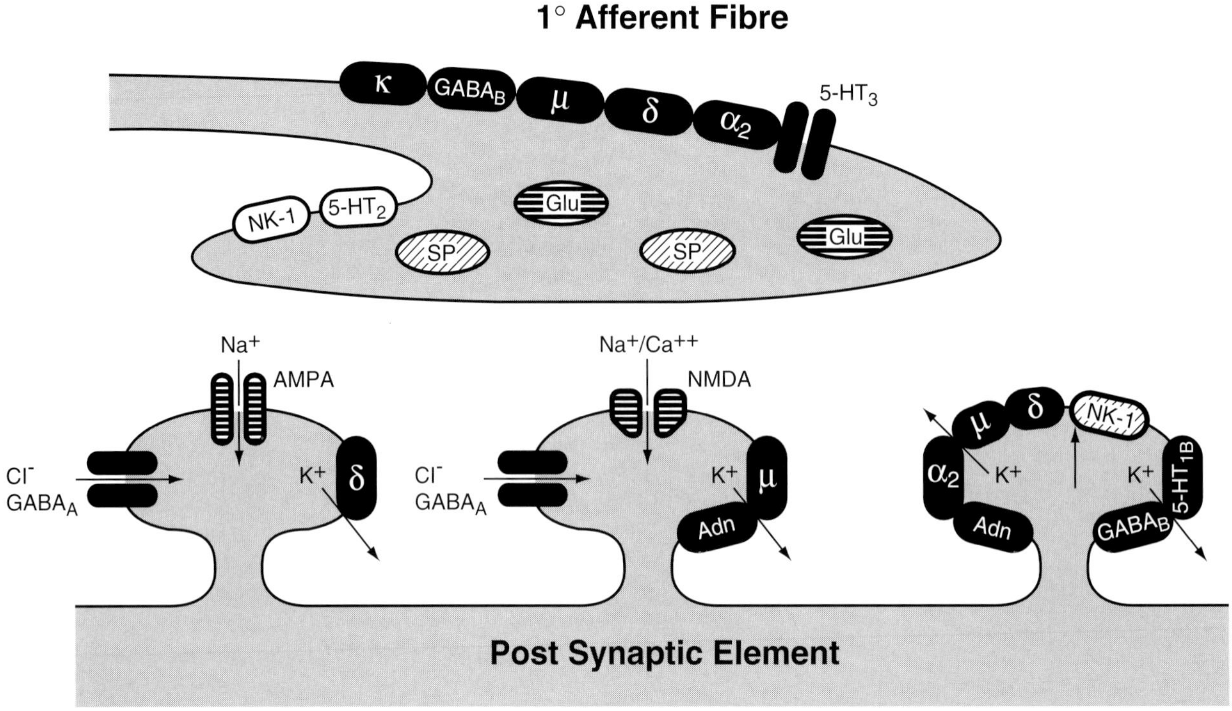

FIG. 23.1-11. Possible arrangement of receptors on pre- and postsynaptic structures in the dorsal horn of the spinal cord. *5-HT*, serotonin; α_2, alpha 2 adrenoceptor; *Adn*, adenosine; *AMPA*, α-amino-3-hydroxy-5-methyl-4-isoxazolepropionic acid; *GABA*, gamma aminobutyric acid; *Glu*, glutamate; *NMDA*, N-methyl D-aspartate; *NK-1*, neurokinin 1; κ, δ, μ, opioid receptors; *SP*, substance P. [From Wilcox, G.L.: Excitatory neurotransmitters and pain. *In* Bond, M.R., Charlton, J.E., and Woolf, C.J. (eds.): Proceedings of the 6th World Congress on Pain, Pain Research and Clinical Management Series. Vol. 4. pp. 97–117, Amsterdam, Elsevier, 1991.]

δ), alpha adrenergic, gamma-amino-butyric acid (GABA), serotonin (5HT), and adenosine receptors (Fig. 23.1-11).

Traditional approaches in pain management have focused on classical ligand-receptor blockade as a means to reduce nociceptive or neuropathic input. The rapid progress in our understanding of the molecular and genetic mechanisms involved in nociception provides a new and potentially useful approach to pain management. Using this approach, it may be possible to develop drugs that regulate gene expression and selectively modify the expression of specific receptors that are involved in the transmission of nociceptive and neuropathic messages.[4]

NMDA receptor

It appears that non-NMDA receptors such as the AMPA receptors may mediate responses in the "physiological" processing of sensory information. However, with prolonged release of glutamate or activation of neurokinin receptors, a secondary process occurs which appears to be crucial in the development of abnormal responses to further sensory stimuli. This sustained activation of non-NMDA or neurokinin receptors "primes" the NMDA receptor so that it is in a state ready for activation (Fig. 23.1-10).

There is evidence that NMDA receptors are involved in a number of phenomena that may contribute to the medium or long-term changes observed in chronic pain states. These phenomena include the development of "wind-up,"[29] facilitation, central sensitization,[115] changes in peripheral receptive fields, induction of oncogenes, and long-term potentiation.[22] Long-term potentiation, in particular, refers to the changes in synaptic efficacy that occur as part of the process of memory, and may play a role in the development of a cellular "memory" for pain or enhanced responsiveness to noxious inputs. Furthermore, it appears that NMDA antagonists can attenuate these responses,[115] indicating a role for NMDA antagonists in the prevention of chronic pain states.

While there are drugs available such as ketamine and the experimental drug, MK-801, which appear to block NMDA receptor-mediated changes,[37,101,115] the side effects associated with their use have meant that they have limited use in the clinical situation. Nevertheless, there still remains a potential for the development of clinically suitable NMDA receptor antagonists; and several agents are being investigated either for analgesia or for use in other medical conditions.[63]

Intracellular Events

Activation of NMDA receptors appears to set in train a cascade of secondary events in the cell which has been acti-

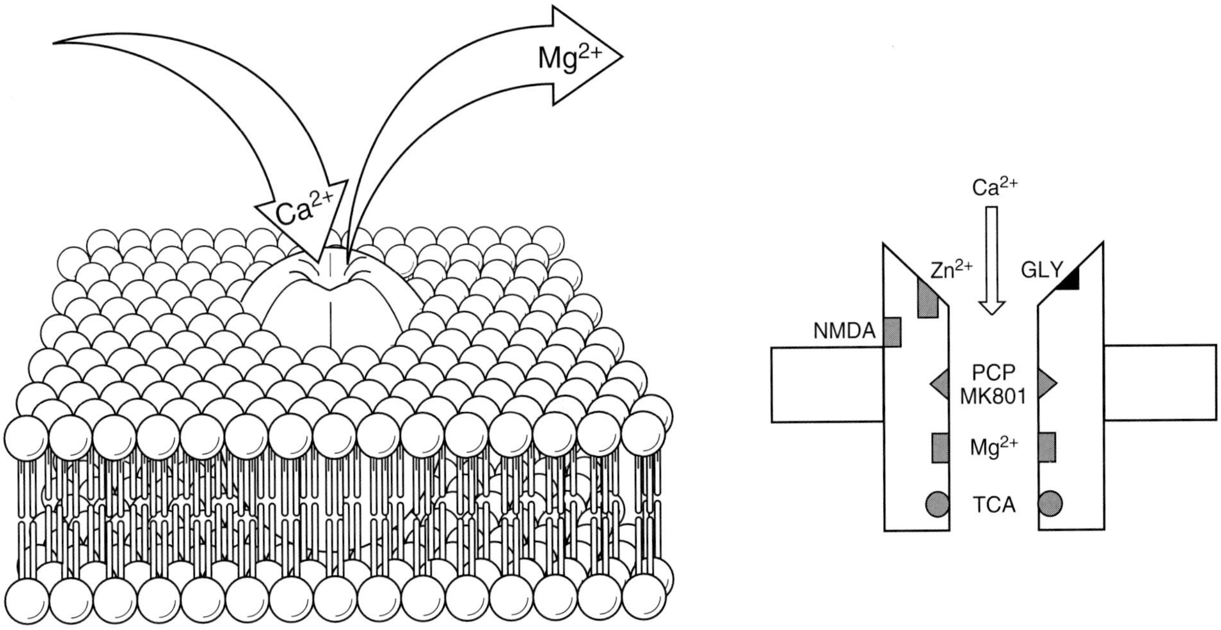

FIG. 23.1-12. Representation of the NMDA (N-methyl D-aspartate) receptor complex. Removal of the magnesium plug leads to calcium influx. The NMDA receptor complex contains a number of sites, activation of which results in modulation of receptor activity. These sites include: glycine *(GLY)*, dizocilpine *(MK-801)*, phencyclidine *(PCP)*, magnesium *(Mg^{2+})*, tricyclic antidepressant *(TCA)*, and zinc *(Zn^{2+})*.

vated. These events lead to changes within the cell which increase the responsiveness of the nociceptive system and lead to some of the phenomena described above.[36] The NMDA receptor channel in its resting state is blocked by a magnesium plug. Priming of the NMDA receptor, by corelease of glutamate and the peptides acting on the neurokinin receptors, leads to removal of the magnesium plug and subsequent calcium influx into the cell, precipitating secondary events such as oncogene induction,[81] production of nitric oxide (NO),[47] and activation or production of a number of second messengers including phospholipases, polyphosphoinosites (IP_3, DAG), cGMP, ecosanoids, and protein kinase C[21] (Figs. 23.1-12, 23.1-13, 23.1-14).[21] These second messengers then act directly to change the excitability of the cell or

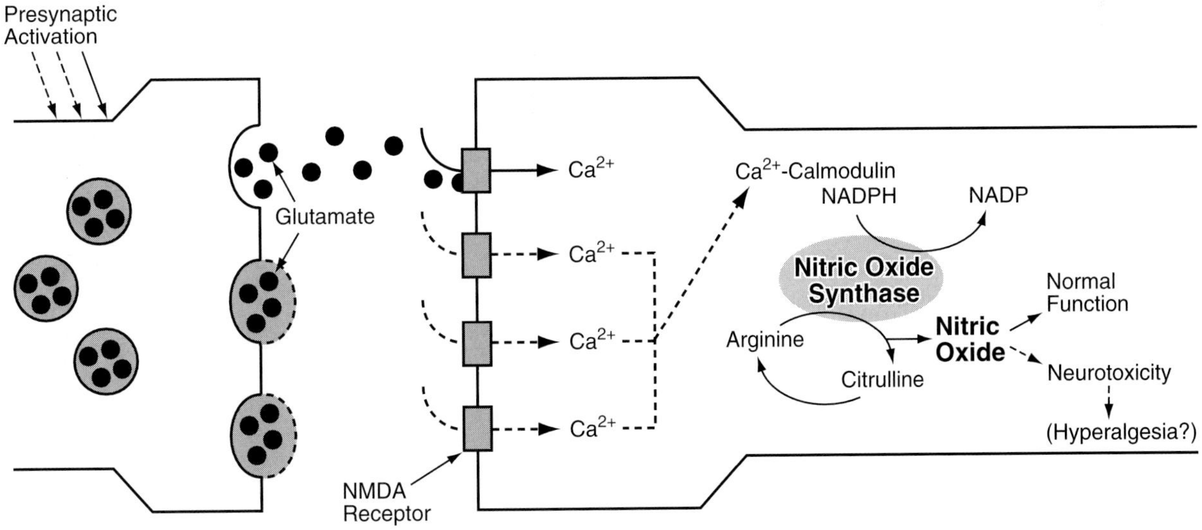

FIG. 23.1-13. Diagram illustrating postsynaptic events following release of glutamate from central terminals of primary afferents in the spinal cord. Following priming of the NMDA receptor complex, subsequent glutamate release results in NMDA receptor activation with subsequent calcium influx. Intracellular calcium then acts on a calmodulin-sensitive site to activate the enzyme nitric oxide synthase (NOS). In the presence of a cofactor NADPH, NOS uses arginine as a substrate to produce nitric oxide and citrulline. Nitric oxide has a role in normal cellular function but increased production may be involved in hyperalgesia and may lead to neurotoxicity.

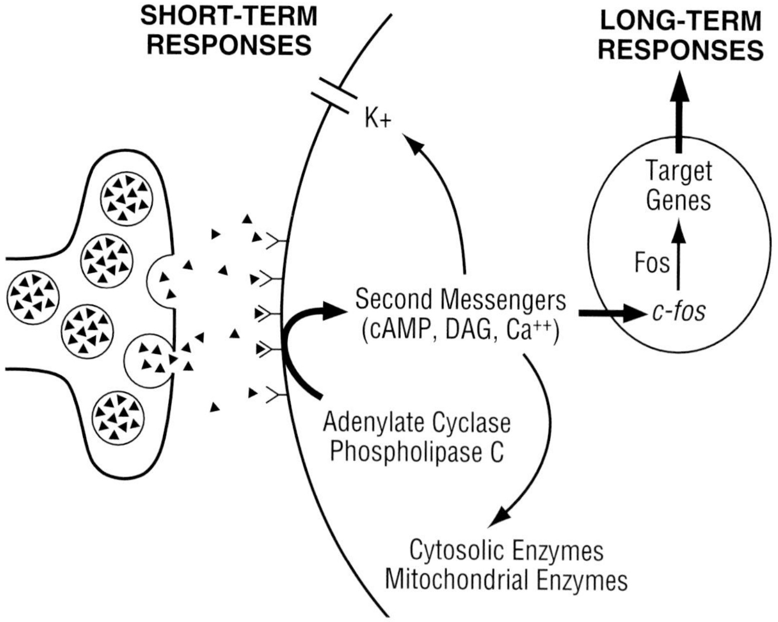

FIG. 23.1-14. Neurotransmitter release from the central terminal of peripheral afferents results in activation of receptor sites on the postsynaptic membrane. Activation of phospholipase C and adenylate cyclase leads to the production of the second messengers cyclic AMP and diacylglycerol (DAG). Mobilization of these second messengers may result in a decrease in K^+ efflux and elevation of intracellular calcium. The increase in intracellular calcium results in the induction of the proto-oncogene c-fos, production of Fos protein, and a presumed action on target genes to alter long-term responses of the cell to further stimuli.

induce the production of oncogenes which may result in long term alterations in the responsivity of the cell. Prolonged stimulation, presumably through sustained and therefore excitotoxic release of glutamate, may result in cell death.

The exact role of NO in nociceptive processing is still unclear and it does not appear to be important in acute nociception.[67] However, production of NO is implicated in the induction and maintenance of chronic pain states,[74] and may be one of the factors responsible for the cell death which has been demonstrated to occur under these conditions (Fig. 23.1-13). It has been suggested that NO acts as a positive feedback mechanism in the maintenance of pain[74] (see Chapter 24 and Fig. 24-13). Blockade of NO in neuropathic animal pain models results in a decrease in the behavioral correlates of pain.[75,106]

The production of arachidonic acid metabolites as part of the cascade that occurs following NMDA receptor activation also raises an interesting potential avenue of intervention that is already being explored.[40] Although the peripheral effects of NSAIDs have been emphasized in the past, it appears that there may be a role for the spinal administration of NSAIDs. Spinal NSAIDs either act directly on receptors, such as the strychnine-insensitive glycine site of the NMDA receptor complex, or influence the production of metabolites within the cell (Fig. 23.1-12).

Central Sensitization

As described above, it is now known that changes occur in the periphery following trauma which lead to the phenomenon of peripheral sensitization and primary hyperalgesia. The sensitization that occurs can only partly be explained by the changes in the periphery. Following injury, there is an increased responsiveness to normally innocuous mechanical stimuli (allodynia) in a zone of secondary hyperalgesia in uninjured tissue surrounding the site of injury. In contrast to the zone of primary hyperalgesia, there is no change in the threshold to thermal stimuli. These changes are believed to be a result of processes that occur in the dorsal horn of the spinal cord following injury;[9] this is the phenomenon of central sensitization (Fig. 23.1-15).

These changes indicate that, in the presence of pain, the central nervous system is not hard wired, but plastic, and that attempts to modify pain must take these changes into account. A barrage of nociceptive input, such as occurs with surgery, results in changes to the response properties of dorsal horn neurons.[19] It has been demonstrated that a painful stimulus at a level sufficient to activate C fibers, not only activates dorsal horn neurons but neuronal activity also progressively increases throughout the duration of the stimulus.[77] Therefore, with clinical pain associated with nociceptive input, there is not a simple stimulus-response relationship, but a wind-up of spinal cord neuronal activity (see Chapter 24, Fig. 24-12). Wind-up is dependent on activation of the NMDA receptor,[37,115] and therefore has the potential to be modified by agents acting at this site. This wind-up may make these neurons more sensitive to other input and is a component of central sensitization (Figs. 23.1-10 and 23.1-11).

Several other changes have been noted to occur in the dorsal horn with central sensitization.[39] First, there is an expansion in receptive field size, so that a spinal neuron will respond to stimuli that would normally be outside the region which responds to nociceptive stimuli. Secondly, there is an increase in the magnitude and duration of the response to stimuli which are above threshold in strength. Lastly, there is a reduction in threshold, so that stimuli which are not normally noxious activate neurons which normally transmit no-

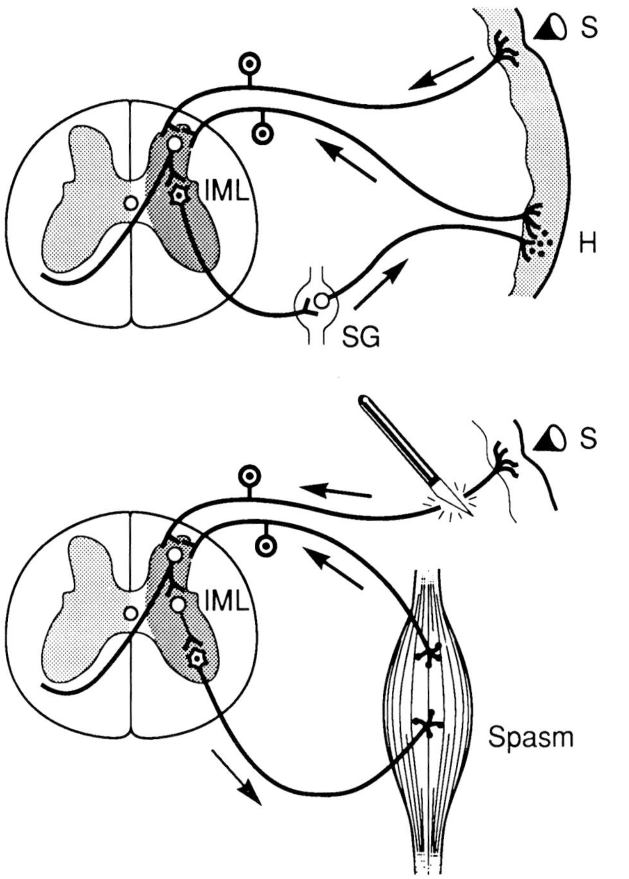

FIG. 23.1-15. Depiction of increased spinal neuron activity (hyperactivity) in response to various stimuli. **Top:** Nociceptive stimulus delivered at the skin surface *(S)* activates a primary afferent nociceptor that, in turn, activates the sympathetic preganglionic neuron in the intermediolateral column *(IML).* The preganglionic neuron activates the noradrenergic postganglionic neuron in the sympathetic ganglion *(SG),* which sensitizes, and can activate primary afferent nociceptors *(H)* that feed back to the spinal cord, maintaining the pain. Peripheral injury is associated with an increase in spinal neuron activity, so that there is an enhanced responsiveness to subsequent input. **Bottom:** Section of a peripheral nerve (e.g., following trauma) results in pronounced and long-lasting increases in spinal cord activity. Tissue injury also produces increased activity of spinal neurons causing activation of ventral horn neurons and muscle spasm. Prolonged muscle spasm activates muscle nociceptors that feed back to the spinal cord to sustain the spasm. (Modified from Fields, H.L.: Pain. New York, McGraw-Hill, 1987.)

ciceptive information. These changes may be important both in acute pain states such as post-operative pain and in the development of chronic pain.[107]

The demonstration of the phenomenon of wind-up,[77] has had a major impact on the current conceptualization of pain and has led to a surge of interest in approaches such as pre-emptive analgesia. Much of the philosophy and rationale behind pre-emptive analgesia lies in an attempt to reduce the development of sub-acute or chronic pain by abolishing or reducing acute pain and thus preventing the changes associated with wind-up. However, the development of chronic pain may have more to do with the phenomenon of long-term potentiation (LTP) than it does with wind-up. Long-term potentiation is the strengthening of the efficacy of synaptic transmission that occurs following activity across that synapse; it shares many of the physiological and biochemical features that are associated with development of chronic pain. It is dependent on activation of NMDA receptors,[22] and LTP3 in particular, which has a longer time constant (20 to 30 days), and is associated with the induction of immediate early genes, including fos-related genes,[2] which are often used as markers in basic pain studies.

Nerve damage results in enhancement of calcium flux, nitric oxide production, and protein kinase C (PKC) generation. PKC has a particularly potent effect in increasing activity at the NMDA receptor, thus causing a vicious circle. Intrathecal, or systemic, administration of morphine for neuropathic pain may also increase NMDA activity, while at the same time decreasing the efficacy of morphine at the mu opioid receptor.[101,111] Thus, unwittingly, morphine administration in neuropathic pain may contribute progressively to increasing the pain (Fig. 23.1-16) (see Chapter 24, pp. 761–762).

It has also been demonstrated that morphological changes occur within the dorsal horn following peripheral nerve injury. Peripheral nerve injury results in a redistribution of central terminals of myelinated afferents with sprouting of these terminals from lamina III to lamina II.[58,112] If func-

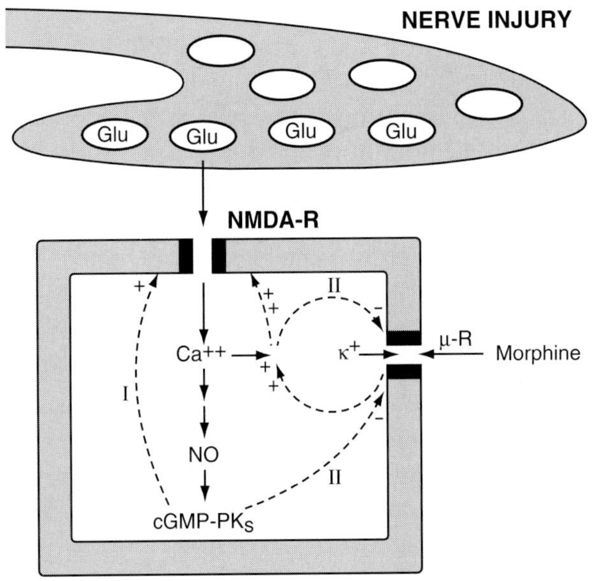

FIG. 23.1-16. Nerve injury leads to release of glutamate *(Glu)* from the central terminals of primary nociceptive afferents. Glutamate activates the N-methyl D-aspartate *(NMDA)* receptor which leads to calcium influx and increased production of nitric oxide *(NO).* An increase in nitric oxide leads to activation of cyclic GMP and various protein kinases *(PK_s).* These substances then act as a feedback mechanism at the NMDA receptor (positive feedback) and μ opioid receptor (negative feedback). This means that subsequent administration of morphine results in a "vicious circle," with further positive feedback at the NMDA receptor (see text).

tional contact is made between these terminals which normally transmit non-noxious information and neurons that normally receive nociceptive input, this may provide a framework for the pain and hypersensitivity to light touch (allodynia) that is seen following nerve injury (Fig. 23.1-17).

Modulation at a Spinal Level

Transmission of nociceptive information is subject to modulation at several levels of the neuraxis, including the dorsal horn (see Chapter 24). Afferent impulses arriving in the dorsal horn initiate inhibitory mechanisms which limit the effect of subsequent impulses. Inhibition occurs through the effect of local inhibitory interneurons and descending pathways from the brain (Fig. 23.1-18). In the dorsal horn, incoming nociceptive messages are modulated by endogenous and exogenous agents which act on opioid, α-adreno, GABA, and glycine receptors located at pre- and postsynaptic sites (Figs. 23.1-11 and 23.1-18).

Opioid Receptors

Opioids are widely used and are generally efficacious in the management of pain. Although found both pre- and post-

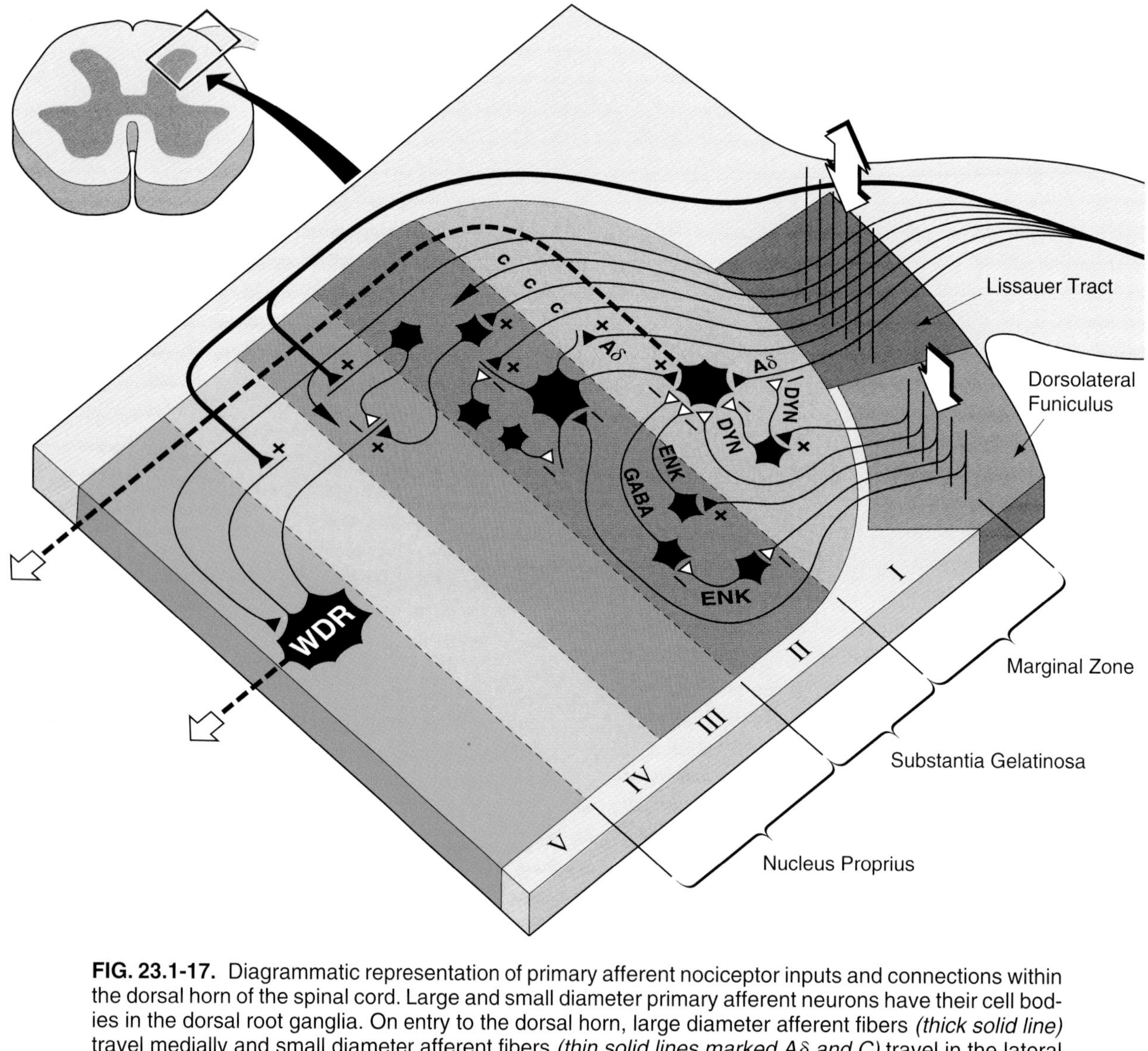

FIG. 23.1-17. Diagrammatic representation of primary afferent nociceptor inputs and connections within the dorsal horn of the spinal cord. Large and small diameter primary afferent neurons have their cell bodies in the dorsal root ganglia. On entry to the dorsal horn, large diameter afferent fibers *(thick solid line)* travel medially and small diameter afferent fibers *(thin solid lines marked Aδ and C)* travel in the lateral portion of the entry zone. The spinal terminals of the small fibers enter the cord and have collateral branches, which may ascend and descend the spinal cord for several segments, in Lissauer's tract, before synapsing in the dorsal horn. Aδ fiber afferents terminate in lamina I (marginal zone) and C fiber afferents terminate in lamina II (substantia gelatinosa). Local interneurons may produce synaptic inhibition of small diameter afferents and post-synaptic inhibition of projection neurons. Interneurons may have an excitatory action. Modulation also occurs as a result of descending influences arising from fibers in the dorsolateral funiculus. These descending fibers make contact with either projection neurons or interneurons. Neurotransmitters released from interneurons include gamma aminobutyric acid *(GABA)*, enkephalin *(ENK)*, and dynorphin *(DYN)*.

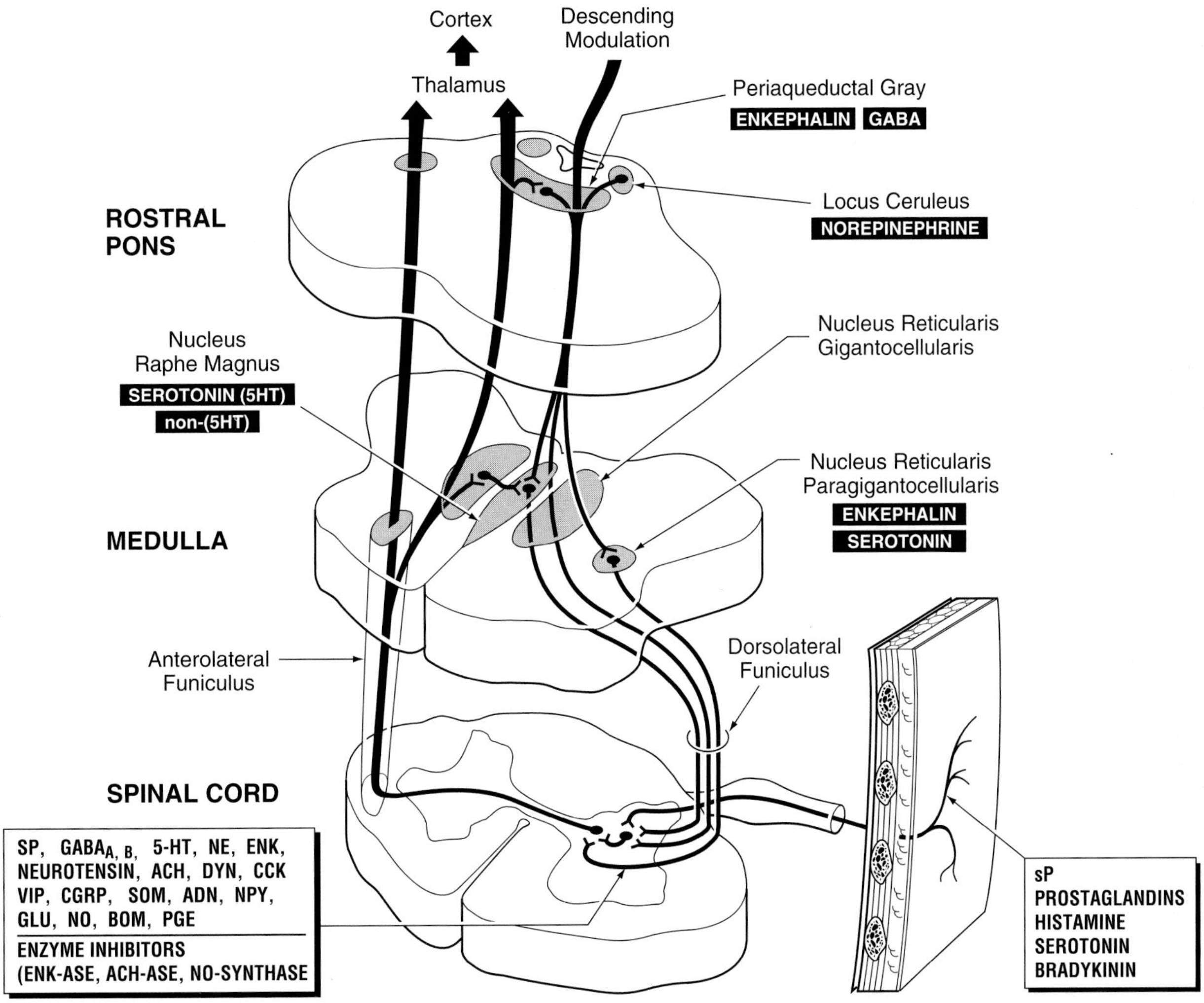

FIG. 23.1-18. Simplified schema of afferent sensory pathways *(left)* and descending modulatory pathways *(right).* Stimulation of nociceptors in the skin surface leads to impulse generation in the primary afferent. Concomitant with this impulse generation, increased levels of various endogenous algesic agents (substance P, prostaglandins, histamine, serotonin, bradykinin) are detected near the area of stimulation in the periphery. Primary afferent nociceptors relay to projection neurons in the dorsal horn, which ascend in the anterolateral funiculus to terminate in the thalamus. En route, collaterals of the projection neurons activate multiple higher centers, including the nucleus reticularis gigantocellularis *(NRG).* Neurons from the NRG project to the thalamus and also activate the nucleus raphe magnus *(NRM)* and periaqueductal gray *(PAG)* of the midbrain. Descending fibers from the PAG project to the NRM and reticular formation adjacent to the NRM. These neurons activate descending inhibitory neurons which are located in these regions and travel via the dorsolateral funiculus to terminate in the dorsal horn of the spinal cord. Descending projections also arise from a number of brain stem sites including the locus ceruleus *(LC).* A number of neurotransmitters are released by afferent fibers, descending terminations, or local interneurons in the dorsal horn and modulate peripheral nociceptive input. These include substance P *(SP),* gamma aminobutyric acid *(GABA),* serotonin *(5-HT),* norepinephrine *(NE),* enkephalin *(ENK),* neurotensin, acetylcholine *(ACH),* dynorphin *(DYN),* cholecystokinin *(CCK),* vasoactive intestinal peptide *(VIP),* calcitonin-gene-related peptide *(CGRP),* somatostatin *(SOM),* adenosine *(ADN),* neuropeptide Y *(NPY),* glutamate *(GLU),* nitric oxide *(NO),* bombesin *(BOM)* and prostaglandins *(PGE).* Inhibitors of enzymes such as enkephalinase *(ENK-ASE),* acetylcholinesterase *(ACH-ASE)* and nitric oxide synthase *(NO-SYNTHASE)* may act to modify the action of these neurotransmitters.

synaptically in the dorsal horn, the majority (about 75%) are located presynaptically.[10] Activation of presynaptic opioid receptors results in a reduction in the release of neurotransmitters from the nociceptive primary afferent.[49] However, the changes that occur with inflammation and neuropathy can produce significant changes in opioid sensitivity that involve a number of mechanisms. These include: the mechanisms shown in Figure 23-16; an interference with opioid analgesia by cholecystokinin (CCK);[116] loss of presynaptic opioid receptors;[10] and the formation of the morphine metabolite, morphine-3-glucuronide,[94] which may antagonize the analgesic action normally produced by opioid receptor activation.

It has also been demonstrated that the NMDA receptor is involved in the development of tolerance to opioids[8] (see Fig. 23.1-16). Animal studies indicate that administration of an NMDA antagonist reduces the development of tolerance to morphine[111] and prevents the withdrawal syndrome in morphine-tolerant rats.[101] Therefore, agents which act as NMDA antagonists, such as dextromethorphan, have the potential to interfere with the development of pain states, potentiate the action of opioids,[3] and prevent the development of opioid tolerance (see also Chapter 29).

Alpha Adrenoceptors

Activation of α-adrenoceptors in the spinal cord has an analgesic effect either by endogenous release of noradrenaline by descending pathways from the brain stem; or by exogenous spinal administration of agents such as clonidine.[117] Furthermore, α-adrenoceptor agonists appear to have a synergistic effect with opioid agonists.[73] There are a number of α-adrenoceptor subtypes and the development of selective α-adrenoceptor subtypes agonists has the potential to provide effective new analgesic agents with reduced side effects.

GABA and Glycine

Both GABA and glycine are involved in tonic inhibition of nociceptive input and loss of their inhibitory action can result in features of neuropathic pain such as allodynia.[93] Although both $GABA_A$ and $GABA_B$ receptors have been implicated at both pre- and postsynaptic sites, it has been demonstrated that $GABA_A$-receptor-mediated inhibition occurs through largely postsynaptic mechanisms.[62] In contrast, $GABA_B$ mechanisms may be preferentially involved in presynaptic inhibition through suppression of excitatory amino acid release from primary afferent terminals. This finding may help to understand the disparity between laboratory findings which demonstrate that $GABA_B$ receptor agonists such as baclofen have an antinociceptive action[110] and clinical experience, which has found that intrathecal baclofen is of limited use in the management of chronic pain.[45] Particularly in neuropathic pain, where there is increased excitability of second-order neurons, with no direct relationship to the amount of excitatory amino acids (EAAs) released by primary afferents, intrathecal administration of $GABA_A$ agonists may be more effective.

Ascending Tracts

Spinal Structures

Second-order projection neurons in the dorsal horn, as well as some in the ventral horn and central canal region, project to supraspinal structures through several tracts (see Chapter 24). These include the spinothalamic, spinoreticular, and spinomesencephalic tracts, which ascend the spinal cord in the contralateral anterolateral quadrant. Although this would suggest that section of these tracts using an anterolateral cordotomy should be a useful procedure in abolishing or relieving pain, results are variable and often transient. There is a latent ipsilateral pathway which progressively takes over from the contralateral spinothalamic pathway following cordotomy, and this may account for eventual failure, and sometimes lack of, analgesia.

Several other procedures are employed to disrupt specific tracts within the spinal cord. These include cordotomy, extralemniscal myelotomy and commissural myelotomy.[118] Once again, excellent relief can be obtained in the short term, but long-term results are often disappointing, and complications include return of pain, motor weakness, and loss of bladder and bowel function. Therefore, these procedures are usually limited to treatment of cancer pain. Lesioning of the dorsal root entry zone (DREZ) has proven to be effective for neuropathic pain associated with brachial and lumbar plexus avulsion.[89] The duration of pain relief of many years seems to be an exception to the rule that neuroplasticity limits the duration after lesions in the nervous system; for example, radiofrequency lesions of the trigeminal ganglion relieve the pain of trigeminal neuralgia for 6 to 12 months, but, inevitably, pain returns.

Supraspinal Structures

Second-order neurons ascend the spinal cord to terminate in many supraspinal structures throughout the brain stem, thalamus, and cortex (Fig. 23.1-19 and see also Chapter 24). In the thalamus, these relays have been divided into 2 main groups: i. Those involved in the sensory discriminative component of pain (ventrocaudal or ventroposterior nuclei of the thalamus); and ii. Those regions involved in the affective-motivational aspects of pain (medial nuclei of the thalamus).[108] Animal studies indicate that there is a large spinothalamic projection, with terminations within the ventral posterior thalamic nucleus, and that neurons within this region respond preferentially to noxious stimuli.[56] These findings suggest that nuclei in this area act as a relay for the transmission of nociceptive information. A recent report by Craig et al.[27] claims to identify a nucleus within the thalamus that is specific for pain and temperature sensation.[105] However, it is interesting that stimulation of the ventrocaudal nucleus (analogous to the ventral posterior nucleus in animals and supposedly part of the "pain" pathway) in awake humans rarely results in pain, except in those who have central deafferentation pain.[30]

Positron emission studies have identified a number of subcortical structures that are presumed to be involved in nociceptive transmission and pain perception. These include thalamus, putamen, caudate nucleus, hypothalamus, amygdala, periaqueductal gray, hippocampus, and cerebellum. While previous physiological and anatomical experiments have

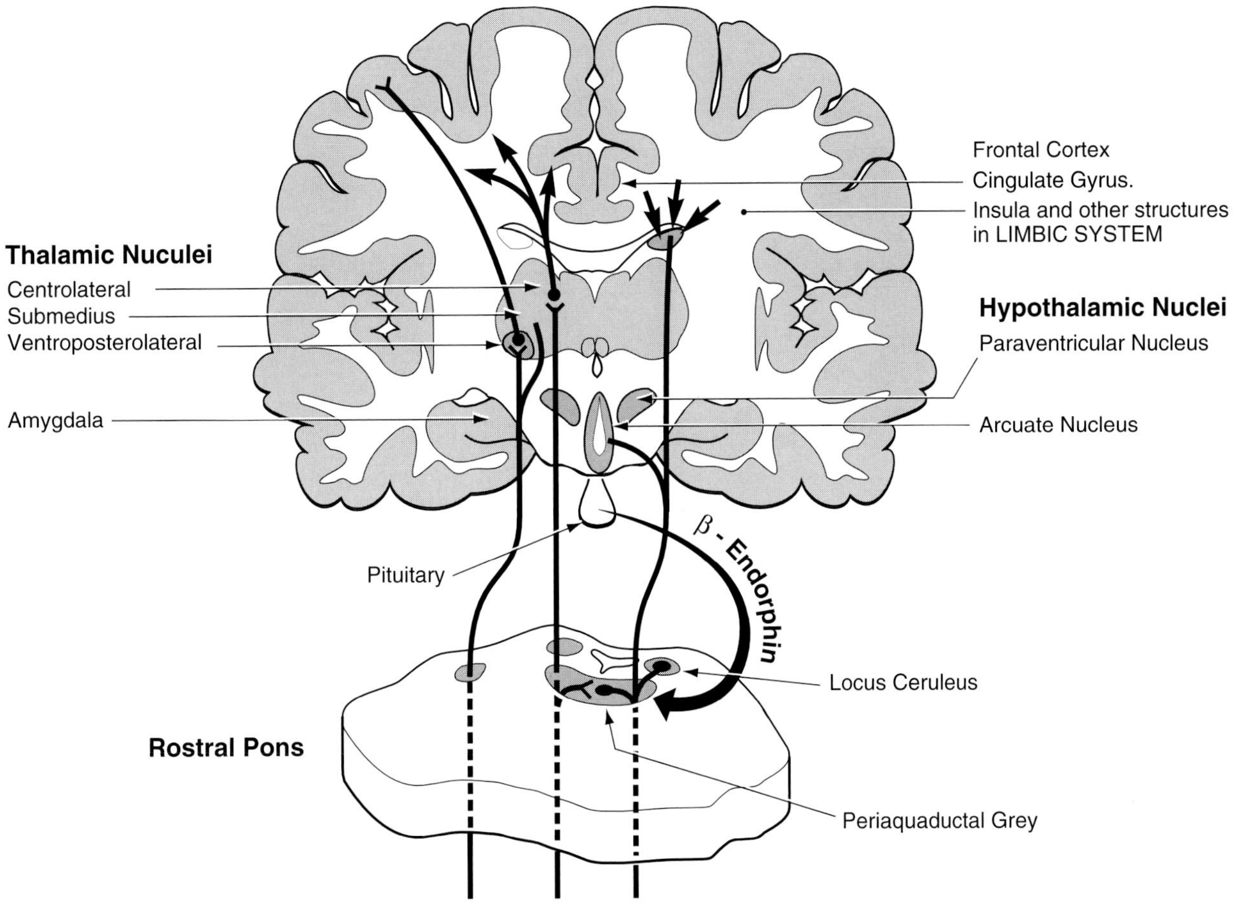

FIG. 23.1-19. Rostral projections of nociceptive processing. Ascending projections *(left)* travelling in the anterolateral funiculus, as well as projections from the medulla, pons, and midbrain terminate in the thalamic nuclear complex. The ventroposterolateral *(VPL),* centrolateral, and submedian nuclei receive nociceptive information. The VPL projects to the somatosensory cortex. The centromedian nucleus projects more diffusely, including projections to regions of the limbic system. The descending fibers *(right)* inhibit the transmission of nociceptive information between primary afferents and projection neurons in the dorsal horn. The periaqueductal gray *(PAG)* receives projections from a number of brain regions including the amygdala, frontal and insular cortex, and the hypothalamus. In addition to direct neural connections, endorphins synthesized in the pituitary are released into the cerebrospinal fluid and blood, where they can exert an inhibitory effect at multiple centers including the PAG.

suggested that some of these structures are responsible for pain transmission, the role of others is unclear. Also of interest is the finding from positron emission tomography (PET) studies that an acute, experimental, painful stimulus results in an increase of activity in the thalamus,[54] while patients with chronic pain due to cancer[35] and chronic neuropathic pain[50] demonstrate a decrease in activity in the thalamus.

Cortical Structures

It has been tempting to divide higher neural centers involved in pain-processing into those which are involved in the sensory-discriminative component of pain perception (somatosensory cortex), and those associated with the affective component of pain perception (cingulate cortex). However, this may be an oversimplification, and the role of the cortex in pain perception remains unclear.

The effect of cortical stimulation and lesions on pain perception is confusing and intriguing. It has been known for many years that patients who have had a complete hemispherectomy can have almost normal pain sensation.[7] In the awake human, stimulation of primary somatosensory cortex typically evokes nonpainful sensations.[108] Neurosurgical lesions of cortical regions produce varying effects, depending on the region ablated.[53] Lesions of the frontal lobe and cingulate cortex result in a condition in which pain perception remains. However, the suffering component of pain appears to be reduced; the person reports pain only when queried and spontaneous requests for analgesia are reduced. These effects contrast with those seen following lesions of the medial thalamus and hypothalamus; following lesions of these regions there is pain relief, but without demonstrable analgesia.

Both PET and functional magnetic resonance imaging (fMRI) have been helpful in elucidating supraspinal mechanisms of pain processing, although there is some inconsistency in results, which may be due to the stimuli used in different studies. Using both techniques, painful stimuli result in activation of sensory, motor, premotor, parietal, frontal, occipital, insular, and anterior cingulate regions of the cortex.[31,54,99] While it is by no means clear, it has been suggested, on the basis of PET findings, that the parietal regions of the cortex are responsible for evaluation of the temporal and spatial features of pain, and that the frontal cortex, including anterior cingulate, is responsible for the emotional response to pain.[99]

Descending Inhibition

Since the turn of the century, considerable interest has focused on the presence of descending inhibitory influences which modulate sensory input. This concept was developed further by Melzack and Wall with the proposal of the gate theory. It is now known that there are powerful inhibitory influences on nociceptive transmission acting at many levels of the neuraxis (see Chapter 24). These descending influences arise from a number of supraspinal structures, including hypothalamus, periaqueductal gray matter (PAG), locus coeruleus, nucleus raphe magnus, and nucleus paragigantocellularis lateralis (Figs. 23.1-18, 23.1-19). Descending inhibition involves the action of endogenous opioid peptides as well as other neurotransmitters, including serotonin and noradrenaline, and GABA.[42] Many of the traditional strategies available in pain management, such as the use of opioids, act via these inhibitory mechanisms. Elucidation of inhibitory mechanisms has prompted the use of new techniques which aim to stimulate these inhibitory pathways. It has also provided a clearer rationale for techniques already in use and used empirically. These include the use of techniques such as deep brain stimulation, transcutaneous electrical nerve stimulation, acupuncture, and epidural spinal cord stimulation.

ETIOLOGY AND FEATURES OF ACUTE AND CHRONIC PAIN

Acute and chronic pain may arise from cutaneous, deep somatic, or visceral structures. Careful mapping of the principal superficial dermatomes is important for effective use of neural blockade techniques. Dermatomes are shown in Chapter 8, Figure 8-35. Visceral pain is much more vaguely localized than somatic pain and has other unique features (Table 23.1-3). Convergence of visceral and somatic afferents has been proven, and this helps to explain referred pain. Also, important viscerosomatic reflexes have been identified (Fig. 23.1-20).

The relief of visceral pain requires blockade of visceral nociceptive fibers that travel to the spinal cord by way of the sympathetic chain. The viscera and the spinal cord segments associated with their visceral nociceptor afferents are shown in Table 23.1-4. Visceral pain is referred to the body surface areas, as shown in Figure 23.1-21. It should be noted that there is considerable overlap for the various organs. Thus it is not surprising that there is a substantial error rate in the diagnosis of visceral pain. Also, there are important viscerosomatic and somaticovisceral reflexes that may make diagnosis and treatment difficult (Fig. 23.1-20). Pain pathways for gynecologic pain have been poorly understood; they are shown in Figure 23.1-22.

Temporary relief of visceral pain by blockade of the somatic referred area poses potential problems of interpretation of diagnostic local anesthetic nerve blocks (see Chapter 27). The processes of peripheral and central sensitization, which have been described previously in this chapter, may be shared by somatic as well as visceral structures. This may account for the heightened response of visceral structures to a relatively benign stimulus following inflammation or tissue damage: visceral hyperalgesia.

Features of Acute Pain

There are important differences between most types of acute pain and chronic pain. In acute pain, the nervous system usually is intact; the pain is caused by trauma, surgery,

TABLE 23.1-3. *Visceral pain compared with somatic pain*

	Somatic	Visceral
Site	Well localized	Poorly localized
Radiation	May follow distribution of somatic nerve	Diffuse
Character	Sharp and definite	Dull and vague (may be colicky, cramping, squeezing, etc.)
Relation to stimulus	Hurts where the stimulus is; associated with external factors	May be "referred" to another area; associated with internal factors
Time relations	Often constant (sometimes periodic)	Often periodic and builds to peaks (sometimes constant)
Associated symptoms	Nausea usually only with deep somatic pain owing to bone involvement	Often nausea, vomiting, sickening feeling

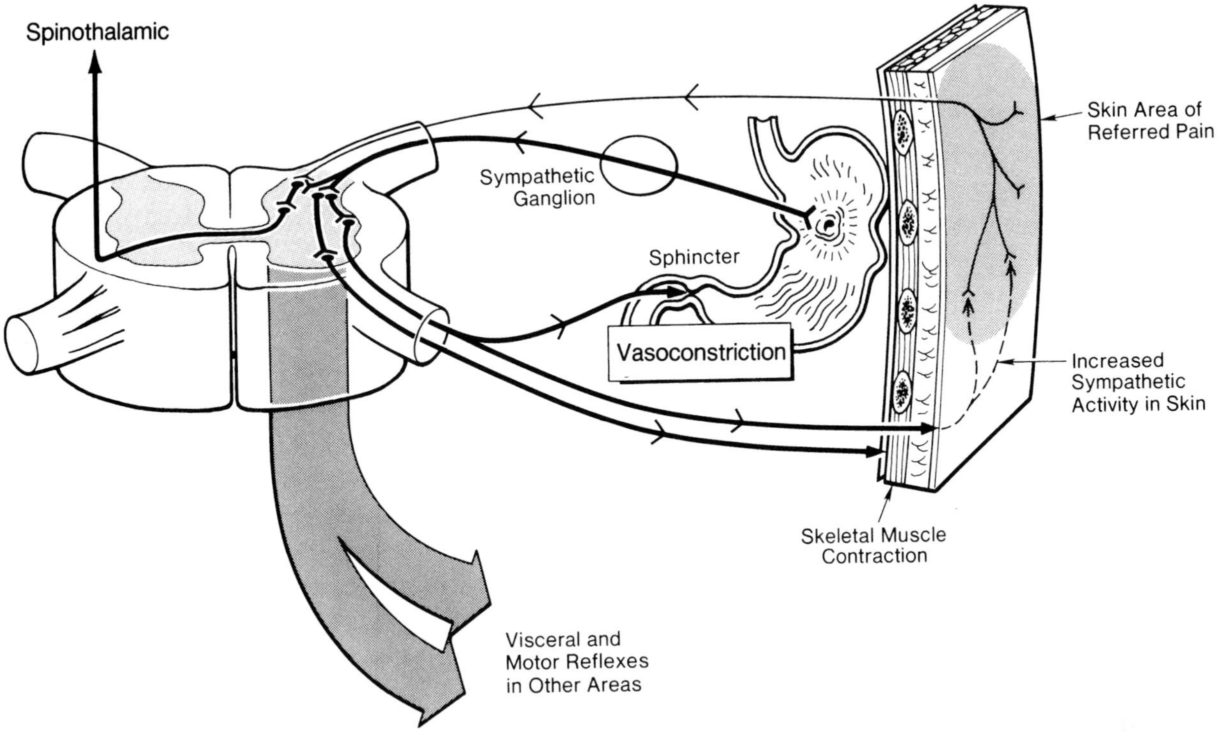

FIG. 23.1-20. Visceral pain: Convergence of visceral and somatic nociceptive afferents. Visceral nociceptive afferents converge on the same dorsal horn neuron as do somatic nociceptive afferents. Visceral noxious stimuli are then conveyed, together with somatic noxious stimuli, by means of the spinothalamic pathways to the brain. Note the following: *1.* Referred pain is felt in the cutaneous area corresponding to the dorsal horn neurons upon which visceral afferents converge. This is accompanied by allodynia and hyperalgesia in this skin area. *2.* Reflex somatic motor activity results in muscle spasm, which may stimulate parietal peritoneum and initiate somatic noxious input to dorsal horn. *3.* Reflex sympathetic efferent activity may result in spasm of sphincters of viscera over a wide area, causing pain remote from the original stimulus. *4.* Reflex sympathetic efferent activity may result in visceral ischemia and further noxious stimulation. Also, visceral nociceptors may be sensitized by norepinephrine release and microcirculatory changes. *5.* Increased sympathetic activity may influence cutaneous nociceptors, which may be at least partly responsible for referred pain. *6.* Peripheral visceral afferents branch considerably, causing much overlap in the territory of individual dorsal roots. Only a small number of visceral afferent fibers converge on dorsal horn neurons compared with somatic nociceptor fibers. Also, visceral afferents converge on the dorsal horn over a wide number of segments. Thus, dull, vague, visceral pain is very poorly localized. This is often called deep visceral pain.

acute medical conditions, or a physiological process (e.g., labor). Facial grimaces and signs of increased autonomic activity and other potentially harmful effects may be evident: for example, hypertension, tachycardia, vasoconstriction, sweating, increased rate and decreased depth of respiration, skeletal muscle spasm, increased gastrointestinal secretions, decreased intestinal motility, increased sphincter tone, urinary retention, venous stasis, and potential for thrombosis, and possible pulmonary embolism; anxiety, confusion and delirium (see Chapters 5 and 26). Also, the pain usually ceases when the wound heals or the medical condition improves. Patients are usually aware that the pain will improve as they recover, and that an end to pain is in sight. This may not be so if patients are ill-prepared and poorly informed (see Chapter 25).

Some severe and prolonged acute pain may become progressively more like chronic pain (see below). Some patients with chronic pain may have superimposed acute pain (e.g., when they require further surgery or develop a bone fracture owing to metastatic cancer).[43] Such patients may not have an intact nervous system and may have marked pre-existing psychological problems, opioid tolerance, and other conditions.

Extensive somatic and sympathetic blockade may be required to relieve acute pain associated with some types of major surgery. For example, the following may be required for pain after thoracoabdominal esophagogastrectomy with cervical anastomosis: C3-C4 *and* T2-T12 *sensory* nerves (somatic structures in neck, thorax, and abdomen); *cervicothoracic sympathetic chain and celiac plexus* (intrathoracic and abdominal viscera); C3, C4 *phrenic nerve sensory afferents* (pain from incision in central diaphragm referred to shoulder tip).

Segmental and suprasegmental reflex responses to acute

TABLE 23.1-4. *Viscera and their segmental nociceptive nerve supply*

Viscus	Spinal segments of visceral nociceptive afferents[a]
Heart	T1–T5
Lungs	T2–T4
Esophagus	T5–T6
Stomach	T6–T10
Liver and gall bladder	T6–T10
Pancreas and spleen	T6–T10
Small intestine	T9–T10
Large intestine	T11–T12
Kidney and ureter	T10–L2
Adrenal glands	T8–L1
Testis, ovary	T10–T11
Urinary bladder	T11–L2
Prostate gland	T11–L1
Uterus	T10–L1

[a] These travel with sympathetic fibers and pass by way of sympathetic ganglia to the spinal cord. However, they are not sympathetic (efferent) fibers. They are best referred to as visceral nociceptive afferents. *Note:* Parasympathetic afferent fibers may be important in upper abdominal pain (vagal fibers, celiac plexus).

pain result in muscle spasm, immobility, vasospasm, and other adverse effects, as described above (see Chapters 5 and 26). This may intensify the pain by way of various vicious cycles (see Fig. 23.1-20), which include increased sensitivity of peripheral nociceptors (see Chapter 24). Acute pain that is unrelieved causes anxiety and sleeplessness, which in turn increase pain (see Chapter 26); anxiety and feelings of helplessness, both before and after surgery, elevate pain levels. Prevention and relief are valuable adjuncts to other treatments. Psychological journals contain much of relevance to acute pain (see Chapter 25). After major surgery, severe trauma, or painful medical conditions (e.g., pancreatitis), acute pain can persist for more than 10 days.[11] In such situations, the pain and its sequelae become similar to chronic pain. It is not uncommon for such patients to show anger, depression, and other characteristics of chronic pain[11,25] (see Chapter 25). Thus, one should be wary of drawing too sharp a distinction between acute and chronic pain: as acute pain persists, more emphasis may need to be placed on psychological approaches, as well as the traditional physical and pharmacological approaches to treatment.

Features of Chronic Pain

It has been agreed arbitrarily that chronic pain is that pain which persists past the time of healing or for more than roughly 3 months.[80] However, severe acute pain can become essentially chronic after only about 10 to 14 days (see previously). Chronic pain progressively leads to limitation of physical, mental, and social activities, with accompanying anger, depression, and family and socioeconomic disruption. It seems that sympathoadrenal responses habituate, or become exhausted, in chronic pain and then vegetative responses emerge: sleep disturbance, irritability, loss of appetite for food and sex, decreased motor activity, mental depression (see Chapter 25). The facial expression of patients with chronic pain may be subdued, sad, or even sleepy, owing to excessive medication. This may give the impression that pain cannot be present. Patients with chronic pain often are exhausted from lack of sleep and from extreme demands on their mental and physical resources. Severe psychoneurosis and other psychological disturbances may result

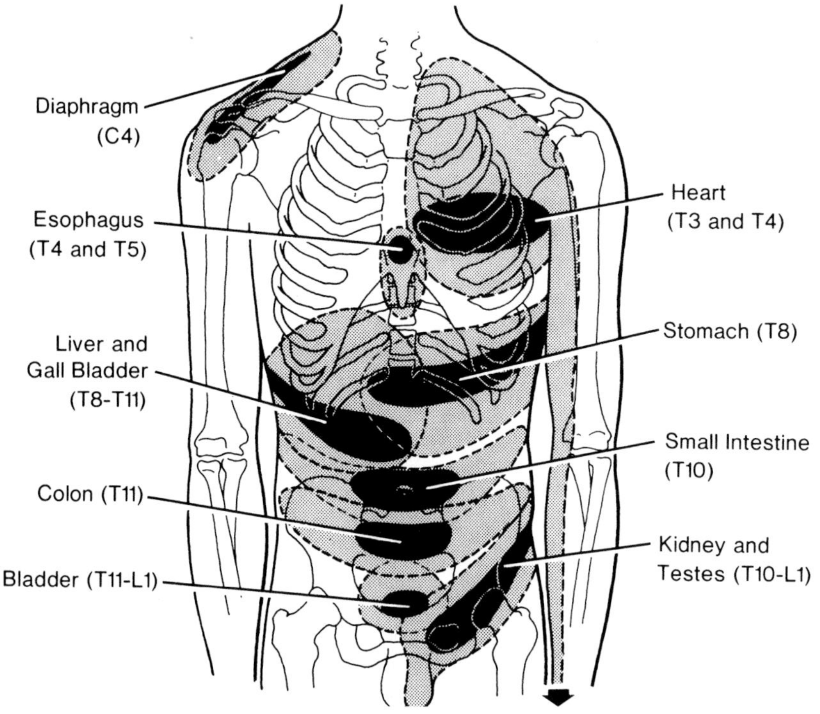

FIG. 23.1-21. Viscerotomes. Approximate superficial areas to which visceral pain is referred, with related dermatomes in brackets. The dark areas are those most commonly associated with pain in each viscus. The *gray areas* indicate approximately the larger area that may be associated with pain in the viscus. [From Cousins, M.J.: Visceral pain. *In* Andersson, S., Bond, M., Mehta, M., and Swerdlow, M. (eds.): Chronic Non-Cancer Pain: Assessment and Practical Management. Lancaster, MTP Press, 1987.]

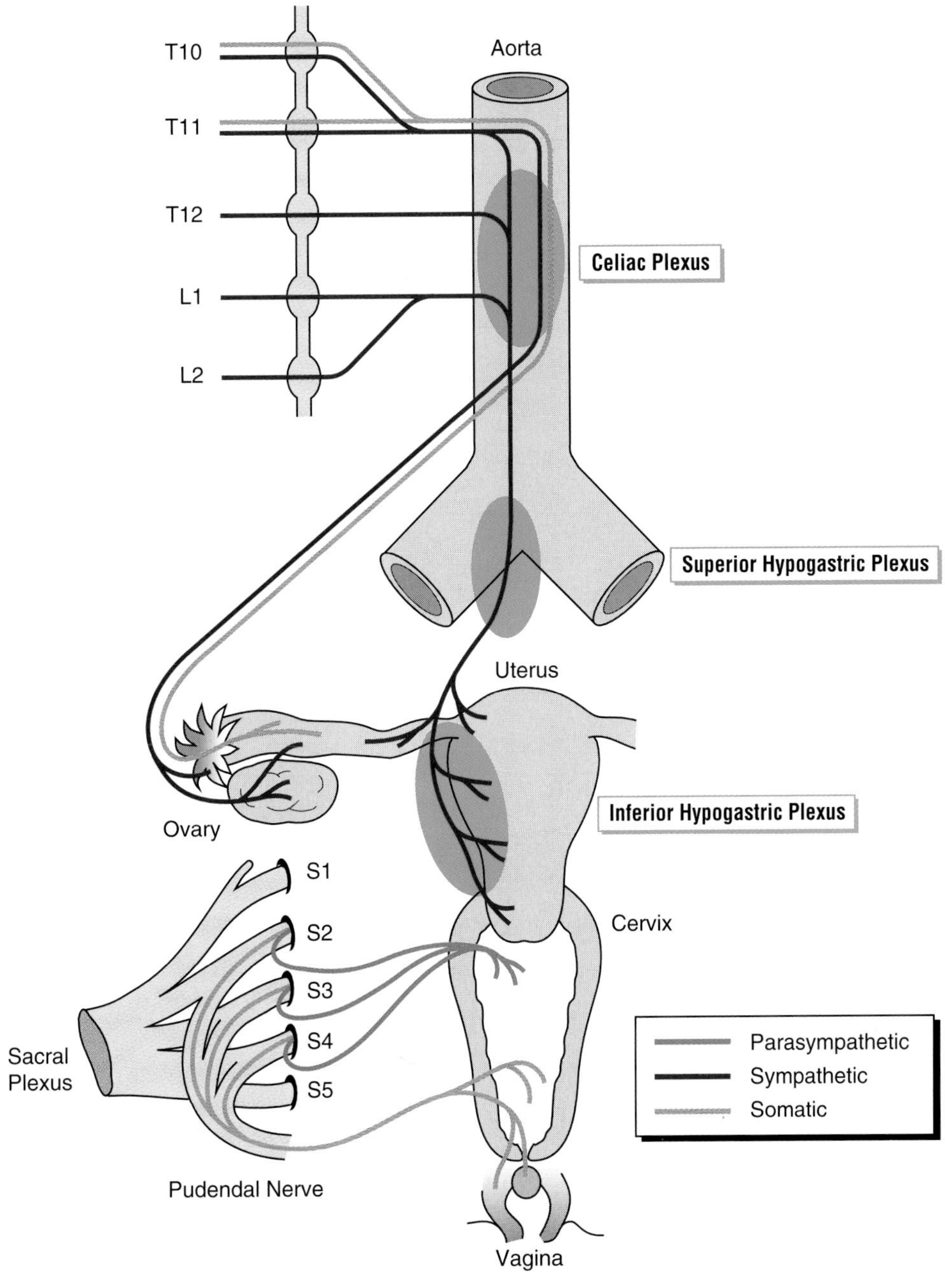

FIG. 23.1-22. Pain pathways in gynecologic pain. Somatic afferents from lower vagina are also shown. [From Cousins, M.J., and Wilson, P.R.: Gynecologic pain. *In* Coppleson, M. (ed.): Gynecologic Oncology. Edinburgh, Churchill-Livingstone, 1981.]

from severe unrelieved chronic pain. These may be rapidly and completely reversed on relief of the pain. Treatment must address these components of chronic pain syndromes (see Chapter 25). Outstanding progress in understanding neurological mechanisms of pain has helped greatly in treatment of chronic pain (see Chapter 24, 26, 27, and 28–34).

CLASSIFICATION OF CHRONIC PAIN

Diagnosis and treatment of chronic pain has been helped greatly by the development of a "Classification of Chronic Pain: Description of Chronic Pain Syndromes and Definitions of Pain Terms."[80] It will aid treatment by improving immensely recognition of various chronic pain syndromes. It will also encourage the use of a universal language of pain, and thus will permit precise reporting and gathering of vital statistical and epidemiological information about chronic pain. The Definitions of Pain Terms are reproduced in their entirety in Appendix A (see end of this chapter). It should be stressed that the definition of pain is equally applicable to acute and chronic pain. "The Classification of Chronic Pain Syndromes" is reproduced in part, with the kind permission of Professor Harold Merskey and Professor Nikolai Bogduk, and the publishers, IASP Press, Seattle. The scheme for cod-

TABLE 23.1-5. *Types of pain in patients with cancer*

I. Patients with acute cancer-related pain
   a. Associated with the diagnosis of cancer
   b. Associated with cancer therapy (surgery, chemotherapy, or radiation)
II. Patients with chronic cancer-related pain
   a. Associated with cancer progression
   b. Associated with cancer therapy (surgery, chemotherapy, or radiation)
III. Patients with pre-existing chronic pain and cancer-related pain
IV. Patients with a history of drug addiction and cancer-related pain
   a. Actively involved in illicit drug use
   b. In methadone maintenance programs
   c. With a history of drug abuse
V. Dying patients with cancer-related pain

Incidence of different types of pain is approximately as follows: Directly caused by cancer (78%); caused by treatment (19%); indirectly related or unrelated to cancer (3%). However, many patients have multiple pains (e.g., a high percentage, (30% to 40%) of patients have myofascial syndromes) *in addition* to cancer-related pain. (Data from Foley, K.M.: The treatment of cancer pain. N. Engl. J. Med *313*:84, 1985.)

ing is given in detail and then some complete examples of classifications and descriptions of pain syndromes are given. The reader is strongly encouraged to consult the full classification for the full range of descriptions.[80]

Several points pertinent to neural blockade can be made.

1. The scheme for coding encourages precise description of region of body, system involved, temporal characteristics of pain, intensity, time since onset, and etiology. This helps to identify pain syndromes that may be responsive to neural blockade, and pinpoints anatomic regions involved.
2. The classification refers first to *generalized* syndromes (e.g., peripheral neuropathy) that may have important underlying medical diseases (e.g., amyloid, diabetes). Some of these may be amenable to treatment of the disease as a means of pain treatment, and are frequently, but not invariably, unresponsive to neural blockade. Some may require a good knowledge of the disease process in order to treat the pain effectively *and safely*. *Regionalized* pain syndromes are described, and some of these are amenable to neural blockade.

TABLE 23.1-6. *Pain syndromes in patients with cancer: pain directly caused by cancer[a] (primary or metastatic)*

Mechanism	Common sites and characteristics of pain
Infiltration of bone by tumor	Dull, constant aching; ± muscle spasm
Base of skull (jugular foramen, clivus, sphenoid sinus)	Early onset pain in occiput, vertex, frontal areas, respectively
Vertebral body (subluxation atlas, metastases C7–T1, L1 sacral)	Early onset pain in neck and skull, neck and shoulders, midback, lower back, and coccyx, respectively ± neurologic deficit
Metastatic fracture close to nerves	Acute onset pain + muscle spasm
Hypercalcemia (associated with multiple bone metastases)	Sudden increase in pain ± confusion ± drowsiness
Infiltration or compression of nerve tissue by tumor	
Peripheral nerve (± peripheral and perivascular lymphangitis)	Burning constant pain in area of peripheral sensory loss ± dysesthesia and hyperalgesia ± signs of sympathetic over-activity. See neuropathy definition
Plexus, e.g., lumbar	Radicular pain to anterior thigh and groin (L1–L3) or to leg and foot (L4–S2)
e.g., sacral	Dull aching midline perianal pain + sacral sensory loss and fecal and urinary incontinence
e.g., brachial	Radicular pain in shoulder and arm ± Horner's syndrome (superior pulmonary sulcus or Pancoast syndrome)
Meningeal carcinomatosis	Constant headache ± neck stiffness or low back and buttock pain
Epidural spinal cord compression (± vertebral body infiltration)	Severe neck and back pain locally over involved vertebra, or radicular pain
Obstruction of hollow viscus e.g., gut, genitourinary tract	Poorly localized, dull, sickening pain, typical visceral pain
Occlusion of arteries and veins by tumour	Ischemic pain like rest pain (skin) or claudication (muscle) or pain ± venous engorgement
Stretching of periosteum or fascia, in tissues with tight investment, by tumefaction	Severe localized pain (e.g., periosteum) or typical visceral pain (e.g., ovary)
Inflammation owing to necrosis and infection of tumors (± superficial ulceration)	Severe localized pain (e.g., perineum), visceral pain (e.g., cervix)
Soft tissue infiltration	Localized pain; unsightly and foul-smelling if ulcerated
Raised intracranial pressure	Severe constant headache, behavioral changes, confusion, etc.

[a] A subcategory can be defined as *Pain related to the cancer*, e.g., muscle spasm, constipation, bedsores, lymphedema, candidiasis, herpetic and postherpetic neuralgia, deep venous thrombosis, pulmonary embolism.

TABLE 23.1-7. *Pain syndromes in patients with cancer: pain associated with cancer therapy*

Mechanism	Common sites and characteristics of pain
Following surgery	
Acute postoperative pain	Wound or referred pain; back or other sites (owing to posture during surgery)
Nerve trauma	Neuralgic pain in area of peripheral nerve or spinal nerve
Entrapment of nerves in scar tissue	Superficial wound scar hypersensitivity of area supplied by scarred nerves (e.g., perineum)
Amputation of limb or other area (e.g., breast)	Localized stump pain (neuroma) or phantom pain referred to absent region
Following radiotherapy	
Acute lesions or inflammation of nerves or plexuses	Pain associated with motor and sensory loss (e.g., brachial plexus, lumbar plexus distribution); diffuse limb pain, 6 months to many years after radiation ± lymphedema and local skin changes ± sensory loss ± motor loss (difficult to distinguish from tumor recurrence)
Radiation fibrosis of nerves or plexuses	
Myelopathy of spinal cord	Brown-Sequard syndrome (ipsilateral sensory and contralateral motor loss) with pain at level of spinal cord damage, or referred pain
Peripheral nerve tumors owing to radiation	Painful enlarging mass in area of radiation along line of peripheral nerve or plexus
Following chemotherapy	
Vinca alkaloid (vincristine > vinblastine, taxol)-induced peripheral neuropathy	Burning pain in hands and feet associated with symmetrical polyneuropathy
Steroid pseudorheumatism owing to slow as well as rapid withdrawal of steroid treatment	Diffuse joint and muscle pain with associated tenderness to palpation but no inflammatory signs Pain resolves when steroid reinstituted
Aseptic necrosis of bone (femoral or humoral head) with chronic steroid therapy	Pain in knee, leg, or shoulder with limitation of movement; bone scan changes delayed after pain onset
Postherpetic neuralgia, following herpes zoster infection in area of tumor or area of radiotherapy with onset during chemotherapy	Continuous burning pain in area of sensory loss or painful dysesthesias or intermittent, shock-like pain

3. The use of neural blockade is appropriate and effective only in some of these many syndromes (see Chapters 27, 28, 29, 31, and 32). Those using neural blockade should be familiar with all of the syndromes in the classification and with the treatments other than neural blockade that are effective for some syndromes. In particular, it should be recognized that there are many well-described pain syndromes where psychological factors play a major role. However, in some of these, neural blockade may be useful as an *adjunct* to psychological measures (see Chapters 27, 28, and 33).
4. The classification and coding system can be used to obtain precise information about the efficacy of neural blockade in many pain syndromes in which it has as yet not been *objectively* evaluated.

Pain Syndromes in Cancer Patients

Treatment of cancer pain has been helped by clear descriptions of major categories of pain problems that occur commonly in cancer patients, and etiologic factors in cancer pain[12,13,43] (Tables 23.1-5 through 23.1-9). It will be clear that neural blockade offers an effective means of treatment of only some of these syndromes. Failure to assess *and reassess* cancer pain in the light of these potential etiologies will end in poor results from use of neural blockade. It should be remembered that central pain, including deafferentation pain, can occur in patients with cancer.[104] This is not responsive, on a continued basis, to neural blockade, except sometimes to stimulation techniques (see Chapter 32). Precise description of the origin *and pattern* of cancer pain is important. For example, it has been reported that intermit-

TABLE 23.1-8. *Pain syndromes in patients with cancer: pain unrelated to cancer or cancer therapy*

Mechanism	Common sites and characteristics of pain
Neuropathy (e.g., diabetic)	Burning pain in hands, feet
Degenerative disc disease	Back pain ± radicular pain
Rheumatoid arthritis	Joint pain, on movement
Diffuse osteoporosis	Back pain, limb pain (may be like causalgia)
Posture abnormalities after surgery	Back pain and muscle spasm ± radicular pain
Myofascial syndromes owing to anxiety	Local pain in muscle with muscle spasm ± referred pain; trigger areas in muscle
Headache	Typical migraine or tension type

TABLE 23.1-9. *Pain syndromes in patients with cancer: pain exacerbated or entirely caused by psychological factors*

Psychological factor	Possible causes
Anxiety	Sleeplessness Fear of death; loss of dignity (loss of self-control) Fear of surgical mutilation; uncontrollable pain Fear of the future; loss of social position and work Confused understanding of disease owing to poor communication Family and financial problems
Depression	Sleeplessness Loss of physical abilities Sense of helplessness Disfigurement Loss of valued social position, financial problems
Anger	Frustration with therapeutic failures Resentment of sickness Irritability caused by pain and general discomfort
A vicious circle usually develops:	

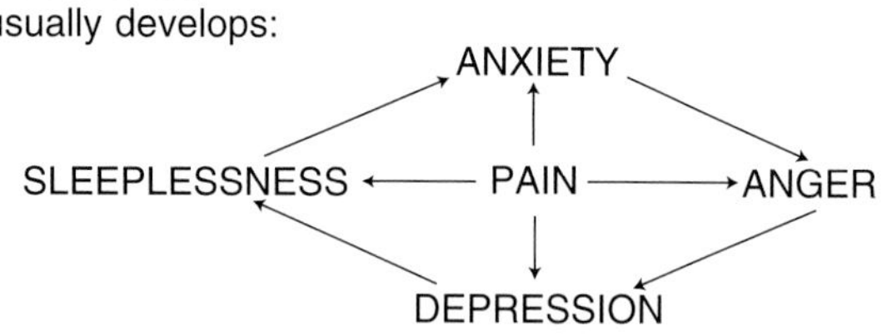

tent visceral pain responds poorly to spinal opioids (see Chapter 29).

PAIN MANAGEMENT: CLINICAL ISSUES

Peripheral Nerve Blockade

Peripheral nerve blockade is used often as a diagnostic procedure to predict outcome for nerve section or neuroablative procedures. However, it has been demonstrated that isolated, uncontrolled, nerve blocks have little diagnostic or predictive value in the assessment of sciatic pain due to lumbosacral disease.[82] The recent evidence for physiological and morphological changes within the spinal cord following sustained peripheral input suggests that there are pitfalls in diagnostic neural blockade. First, chronic pain due to peripheral nerve damage may no longer be dependent on peripheral input. Unfortunately, there is no evidence that treatments aimed at the periphery modify established central sensitization. Thus, for example, a long standing intercostal neuralgia will not be expected to respond to intercostal neurectomy; indeed the pain may increase as the processes of central sensitization may be enhanced. Secondly, diagnostic nerve blocks seek to identify a pain source and can thereby isolate the person from the disease process thought to be responsible for the pain. Using diagnostic nerve blocks in this way can mean that little recognition is made of the complex psychological issues that can underlie the chronic pain presentation. It may even mean that a psychological diagnosis is made on the basis of the person's response to a diagnostic procedure. For these reasons, diagnostic procedures must be done in the context of a multidisciplinary assessment, with an understanding of the complex biological and psychological components of chronic pain and placebo response to interventions (see Chapters 27, 28, and 33).

Spinal Administration of Agents

Elucidation of the types of receptors present pre- and postsynaptically around nociceptive transmission neurons in the dorsal horn has led to the use of spinal drug administration as a pain management technique. The application of relatively low doses of agents acting at specific receptor types within the spinal cord with the relative avoidance of side effects has been a major advance in the management of some pain problems. Some people who have been unresponsive to administration of oral agents have had greatly improved relief with the use of infusion devices which administer agents such as morphine or clonidine, either alone or in combination, directly into the intrathecal space. In selected cases, intrathecal administration of a combination of morphine and clonidine has been effective in treatment of some types of neuropathic pain, including pain following spinal cord injury[92] (see Chapter 29).

Although their use is largely experimental at this stage, the availability of spinal drug administration has led to interest in the use of agents not traditionally considered for use by the spinal route. NSAIDs have an action at the glycine receptor of the NMDA receptor complex and tricyclic antidepressants also have an action at a receptor within the NMDA complex. Both types of agents have been administered by the spinal route with some success (see Chapter 29).

However, the success that has been achieved by targeting spinal receptors directly has not been without some problems. Many agents, while promising in the laboratory, have severe side effects or are toxic when administered by the spinal route, and are therefore unsuitable for this method of administration. Although it was believed early in the use of the technique that dose escalation was not a problem, it has been found that some people using opioids require increasing doses to maintain adequate analgesia. Chronic administration of intrathecal opioids can also result in hormonal changes and there are reports of paradoxical pain in some people, especially at higher dose levels[32] (see Chapter 29).

Pre-emptive Analgesia

Discovery of the changes associated with the phenomenon of central sensitization has led to attempts to prevent these changes. It has been demonstrated that early postoperative pain is a significant predictor of long-term pain.[55] It was hoped that steps which would reduce or abolish noxious input to the spinal cord during a painful event such as surgery would reduce or minimize spinal cord changes and thereby lead to reduced pain postoperatively and long-term. However, it is still not known what duration or degree of noxious input is required before these long-term changes occur.

It is also not known how much long-term changes are dependent on the afferent barrage during surgery, and how much they are dependent on continuing inputs from the wound after surgery. At both stages, there will be sustained noxious input, and therefore both stages have the capacity to produce central sensitization. However, it would be expected that intervention which pre-empts central sensitization and seeks to prevent it, rather than attempts to treat it after it has occurred, would be more successful (see Chapter 26).

This concept has led to an increasing interest in the use of pre-emptive analgesia. Local anaesthetics, opioids, and NSAIDs have been used alone or in combination and have been administered locally, epidurally, intrathecally, or systemically. They have also been administered pre-, intra-, and postoperatively. Many trials have purported to show that pre-emptive analgesia results in reduced pain, decreased analgesic requirements, improved morbidity, and decreased hospital stay.[28,114] However the variability in agent, and timing and method of administration, as well as differences in the type of surgery and anesthetic procedures, has made it difficult to compare trials which examine the effectiveness of pre-emptive analgesia. There have also been several problems with the design of these studies, that has made it difficult to draw definite conclusions concerning outcomes. Therefore, despite studies which appear to indicate the advantages of pre-emptive analgesia, the logical appeal of this approach and its ready application to the clinical arena, two recent reviews[28,114] both conclude that further trials are necessary before a definitive statement can be made about its benefits and advantages.

Most studies have focused on the effect of pre-emptive analgesia in reducing pain in the early postoperative period. However pre-emptive analgesia may also be important in reducing the incidence of chronic pain. One study which has generated interest was the finding by Bach and colleagues,[5] that preoperative epidural blockade of patients undergoing lower-limb amputation resulted in a lower incidence of phantom limb pain at 6 and 12 months following surgery, when compared to the control group which had intraoperative block alone. Although it has been pointed out that there are several inadequacies in the design of this study,[28] it does demonstrate that pre-emptive analgesia may have the potential to prevent the development of chronic pain states, and further studies should be carried out to address this important question. A second study reports that the degree of pain after thoracic surgery predicts long-term post-thoracotomy pain.[55]

Conclusion

There has been substantial progress in our understanding of pain mechanisms in recent years. Our understanding of the pharmacology and physiology of nociceptive processes and the identification of neurotransmitters and pathways involved in nociceptive transmission has led to the development of new agents and more effective use of agents that were previously available. The recognition and characterization of nervous sytem changes that occur with pain has also had a profound influence on our conceptualization of pain, and indicates the potential that exists to modify or prevent the development of chronic pain states, by managing acute pain more effectively and in different ways.

REFERENCES

1. Aasbo, V., Raeder, J.C., Grogaard, B., and Roise, O.: No additional analgesic effect of intra-articular morphine or bupivacaine compared with placebo after elective knee arthroscopy. Acta Anaesthesiol. Scand., *40:*585, 1996.
2. Abraham, W.C., Mason, S.E., and Demmer, J., *et al.*: Correlations between immediate early gene induction and the persistence of long-term potentiation. Neuroscience, *56:*717, 1993.
3. Advokat, C., and Rhein, F.Q.: Potentiation of morphine-induced antinociception in acute spinal rats by the NMDA antagonist dextrorphan. Brain Res., *699:*157, 1995.
4. Akopian, A.N., Abson, N.C., and Wood, J.N.: Molecular genetic approaches to nociceptor development and function. Trends Neurosci., *19:*240, 1996.
5. Bach, S., Noreng, M.F., and Tjellden, N.U.: Phantom limb pain in amputees during the first 12 months following limb amputation. Pain, *33:*297, 1988.
6. Backonja, M.M.: Local anesthetics as adjuvant analgesics. J. Pain Symptom Manage., *9:*491, 1994.
7. Barber, T.X.: Toward a new theory of pain: Relief of chronic pain by prefontal leucotomy, opiates, placebos, and hypnosis. Psychol. Bull., *56:*430, 1959.
8. Basbaum, A.I.: Mechanisms of substance P-mediated nociception and opioid-mediated antinociception. *In* Stanley, T.H., and Ashburn, M.A. (eds.): Anesthesiology and Pain Management. pp. 1–17. Dordrecht, Kluwer Academic, 1994.
9. Bennett, G.J., Kajander, K.C., Sahara, Y., Iadarola, M.J., and Sugimoto, T.: Neurochemical and anatomical changes in the dorsal horn of rats with an experimental painful peripheral neuropathy. *In* Cervero, F., Bennett, G.J., and Headley, P.M. (eds.): Processing of Sensory Information in the Superficial Dorsal Horn of the Spinal Cord. pp. 463–471, Amsterdam, Plenum Press, 1989.
10. Besse, D., Lombard, M.C., Zakac, J.M., Roques, B.P., and Besson, J.-M.: Pre- and postsynaptic distribution of mu, delta, and kappa opioid receptors in the superficial layers of the cervical dorsal horn of the rat spinal cord. Brain Res., *521:*15, 1990.
11. Bonica, J.J.: Biology, pathophysiology, and treatment of acute pain. *In* Lipton, S., and Miles, J. (eds.): Persistent Pain, Vol. 5. pp. 1–32, Orlando, Grune & Stratton, 1985.
12. Bonica, J.J.: Treatment of cancer pain: Current status and future needs. *In* Fields, H.L. (ed.): Advances in Pain Research and Therapy, Vol. 9. pp. 589–616, New York, Raven Press, 1985.
13. Bonica, J.J., and Ventafridda, V.: Pain of advanced cancer. *In* Fields, H.L. (ed.): Advances in Pain Research and Therapy, Vol. 2. New York, Raven Press, 1979.
14. Meyer, R.A., Campbell, J.N., and Raja, S.N.: Peripheral neural mechanisms of nociception. *In* Wall, P.D., and Melzack, R. (eds.): Textbook of Pain, 3rd. Ed. pp. 13–44, Edinburgh, Churchill Livingstone, 1994.
15. Campbell, J.N., Raja, S.N., Selig, D.K., Belzberg, A.J., and Meyer, R.A.: Diagnosis and management of sympathetically maintained pain. *In* Fields, H.L., and Liebeskind, J.C. (eds.): Progress in Pain Research and Management, Vol. 1. pp. 85–100, Seattle, IASP Press, 1994.
16. Cervero, F., and Iggo, A.: The substantia gelatinosa of the spinal cord: A critical review. Brain, *103:*717, 1980.
17. Chabal, C., Jacobson, L., Mariano, A., Chaney, E., and Britell, C.W.: The use of oral mexiletine for the treatment of pain after peripheral nerve injury. Anesthesiology, *76:*513, 1992.

18. Chaplan, S.R., Bach, F.W., Shafer, S.L., and Yaksh, T.L.: Prolonged alleviation of tactile allodynia by intravenous lidocaine in neuropathic rats. Anesthesiology, *83:*775, 1995.
19. Chi, S.-I., Levine, J.D., and Basbaum, A.I.: Effects of injury discharge on the persistent expression of spinal cord fos-like immunoreactivity produced by sciatic nerve transection in the rat. Brain Res., *617:*220, 1993.
20. Christensen, B.N., and Perl, E.R.: Spinal neurons specifically excited by noxious or thermal stimuli: Marginal zone of the dorsal horn. J. Neurophysiol., *33:*293, 1970.
21. Coderre, T.J.: The role of excitatory amino acid receptors and intracellular messengers in persistent nociception after tissue injury in rats. Mol. Neurobiol., *7:*229, 1993.
22. Collingridge, G., and Singer, W.: Excitatory amino acid receptors and synaptic plasticity. Trends Pharmacol. Sci., *11:*290, 1990.
23. Comfort, V.K., Code, W.E., Rooney, M.E., and Yip, R.W.: Naproxen premedication reduces postoperative tubal ligation pain. Can. J. Anaesth., *39:*349, 1992.
24. Cousins, M.J.: Visceral pain. *In* Andersson, S., Bond, M., Mehta, M., and Swerdlow, M. (eds.): Chronic Non-Cancer Pain: Assessment and Practical Management. pp. 119. Lancaster, MTP Press, 1987.
25. Cousins, M.J., and Phillips, G.D. (Eds.): Acute Pain Management. Clinics in Critical Care Medicine, Edinburgh, Churchill Livingstone, 1986.
26. Cousins, M.J., and Wilson, P.R.: Gynecologic pain. *In* Coppleson, M. (ed.): Gynecologic Oncology. pp. 1013. Edinburgh, Churchill Livingstone, 1981.
27. Craig, A.D., Bushnell, M.C., Zhang, E.T., and Blomqvist, A.: A thalamic nucleus specific for pain and temperature sensation. Nature, *372:*770, 1994.
28. Dahl, J.B., and Kehlet, H.: The value of pre-emptive analgesia in the treatment of postoperative pain. Br. J. Anaesth., *70:*434, 1993.
29. Davies, S.N., and Lodge, D.: Evidence for involvement of N-methylaspartate receptors in 'wind-up' of class 2 neurons in the dorsal horn of the rat. Brain Res., *424:*402, 1987.
30. Davis, K.D., Kiss, Z.H.T., Tasker, R.R., and Dostrovsky, J.O.: Thalamic stimulation-evoked sensations in chronic pain patients and in nonpain (movement disorder) patients. J. Neurophysiol., *75:*1026, 1996.
31. Davis, K.D., Wood, M.L., Crawley, A.P., and Mikulis, D.J.: fMRI of human somatosensory and cingulate cortex during painful electrical nerve stimulation. Neuroreport, *7:*321, 1995.
32. De Conno, F., Caraceni, A., Martini, C., *et al.*: Hyperalgesia and myoclonus with intrathecal infusion of high-dose morphine. Pain, *47:*337, 1991.
33. Devor, M.: The pathophysiology of damaged peripheral nerves. *In* Wall, P.D., and Melzack, R. (eds.): Textbook of Pain. 3rd Ed. pp. 79–100. London, Churchill Livingstone, 1994.
34. Devor, M., Wall, P.D., and Catalan, N.: Systemic lidocaine silences ectopic neuroma and DRG discharge without blocking nerve conduction. Pain, *48:*261, 1992.
35. Di Piero, V., Jones, A.K.P., and Ianotti, F., *et al.*: Chronic pain: A PET study of the central effects of percutaneous high cervical cordotomy. Pain, *46:*9, 1991.
36. Dickenson, A.H.: NMDA receptor antagonists as analgesics. *In* Fields, H.L., and Liebeskind, J.C. (eds.): Pharmacological Approaches to the Treatment of Chronic Pain: New Concepts and Critical Issues. Progress in Pain Research and Management. Vol. 1. pp. 173–187, Seattle, IASP Press, 1996.
37. Dickenson, A.H., and Sullivan, A.F.: Evidence for a role of the NMDA receptor in the frequency dependent potentiation of deep rat dorsal horn nociceptive neurons following C fiber stimulation. Neuropharmacology, *26:*1235, 1987.
38. Dray, A., Urban, L., and Dickenson, A.: Pharmacology of chronic pain. Trends Pharmacol. Sci., *15:*190, 1994.
39. Dubner, R., and Ren, K.: Central mechanisms of thermal and mechanical hyperalgesia following tissue inflammation. *In* Boivie, J., Hansson, P., and Lindblom, U. (eds.): Touch, Temperature, and Pain in Health and Disease: Mechanisms and Assessments, Vol. 3. pp. 267–277. Seattle, IASP Press, 1994.
40. Eisenach, J.C.: Aspirin, the miracle drug—spinally, too? Anesthesiology, *79:*211, 1993.
41. Fields, H.L.: Pain. New York, McGraw-Hill, 1987.
42. Fields, H.L., and Basbaum, A.I.: Central nervous system mechanisms of pain modulation. *In* Wall, P.D., and Melzack, R. (eds.): Textbook of Pain, 3rd Ed. pp. 243–257. Edinburgh, Churchill Livingstone, 1994.
43. Foley, K.M.: The treatment of cancer pain. N. Engl. J. Med., *313:*84, 1985.
44. Forster, R.W., and Ramage, A.G.: The action of some chamical irritants on somatosensory receptors of the cat. Neuropharmacology, *20:*191, 1981.
45. Fromm, G.H.: Baclofen as an adjuvant analgesic. J. Pain Symptom. Manage., *9:*500, 1994.
46. Galer, B.S.: Neuropathic pain of peripheral origin—Advances in pharmacologic treatment. Neurology, *45:*S 17, 1995.
47. Garthwaite, J., Charles, S.L., and Chess-Williams, R.: Endothelium-derived relaxing factor release on activation of NMDA receptors suggests role as intercellular messenger in the brain. Nature, *336:*385, 1988.
48. Haynes, T.K., Appadurai, I.R., Power, I., Rosen, M., and Grant, A.: Intra-articular morphine and bupivacaine analgesia after arthroscopic knee surgery. Anaesthesia, *49:*54, 1994.
49. Hori, Y., Endo, K., and Takahashi, T.: Presynaptic inhibitory action of enkephalin on excitatory transmission in superficial dorsal horn of rat spinal cord. J. Physiol., *450:*673, 1992.
50. Iadarola, M.J., Max, M.B., and Berman, K.F., *et al.*: Unilateral decrease in thalamic activity observed with positron emission tomography in patients with chronic neuropathic pain. Pain., *63:*55, 1995.
51. Jänig, W.: The puzzle of "reflex sympathetic dystrophy": Mechanisms, hypotheses, open questions. *In* Jänig, W., and Stanton-Hicks, M. (eds.): Reflex Sympathetic Dystrophy: A Reappraisal. pp. 1–24, Seattle, IASP Press, 1996.
52. Jänig, W., and McLachlan, E.M.: The role of modifications in noradrenergic peripheral pathways after nerve lesions in the generation of pain. *In* Fields, H.L., and Liebeskind, J.C. (eds.): Progress in Pain Research and Management. Vol. 1. pp. 101–128. Seattle, IASP Press, 1994.
53. Jannetta, P.J., Gildenberg, P.L., Loeser, J.D., Sweet, W.H., and Ojemann, G.A.: Operations on the brain and brain stem for chronic pain. *In* Bonica, J.J. (ed.): The Management of Pain. Vol. 2. pp. 2082–2103. Philadelphia, Lea & Febiger, 1990.
54. Jones, A.K.P., Brown, W.D., Friston, K.J., Qi, L.Y., and Frackowiak, R.S.J.: Cortical and subcortical localization of response to pain in man using positron emission tomography. Proc. R. Soc. Lond. B. Biol. Sci., *244:*39, 1991.
55. Katz, J., Jackson, M., Kavanagh, B.P., and Sandler, A.N.: Acute pain after thoracic surgery predicts long-term post-thoracotomy pain. Clin. J. Pain., *12:*50, 1996.
56. Kenshalo, D.R., Jr., Giesler, G.J., Jr., Leaonard, R.B., and Willis, W.D.: Responses of neurons in primate ventral posterior lateral nucleus to noxious stimuli. J. Neurophysiol., *43:*1594, 1980.
57. Laitinen, J., and Nuutinen, L.: Intravenous diclofenac coupled with PCA fentanyl for pain relief after total hip replacement. Anesthesiology, *76:*194, 1992.
58. Lekan, H.A., Carlton, S.M., and Coggeshall, R.E.: Sprouting of A-beta fibers into lamina II of the rat dorsal horn in peripheral neuropathy. Neurosci. Lett., *208:*147, 1996.
59. Levine, J.D., Fields, H.L., and Basbaum, A.I.: Peptides and the primary afferent nociceptor. J. Neurosci., *13:*2273, 1993.
60. Lewin, G.R., and Mendell, L.M.: Nerve growth factor and nociception. Trends Neurosci., *16:*353, 1993.
61. Light, A.R., and Perl, E.R.: Spinal termination of functionally identified primary afferent neurons with slowly conducting myelinated fibers. J. Comp. Neurol., *186:*133, 1979.
62. Lin, Q., Peng, Y.B., and Willis, W.D.: Role of GABA receptor subtypes in inhibition of primate spinothalamic tract neurons-difference between spinal and periaqueductal gray inhibition. J. Neurophysiol., *75:*109, 1996.
63. Lipton, S.A.: Prospects for clinically tolerated NMDA antagonists: Open-channel blockers and alternative redox states of nitric oxide. Trends Neurosci., *16:*527, 1993.
64. Loeser, J.D., and Cousins, M.J.: Contemporary pain management. Med. J. Aust., *153:*208, 1990.
65. Loh, L., Nathan, P.W.: Painful peripheral states and sympathetic blocks. J. Neurol. Neurosurg. Psychiatry, *41:*664, 1978.
66. Magni, G.: The use of antidepressants in the treatment of chronic pain: A review of the current evidence. Drugs, *42:*730, 1991.
67. Malmberg, A.B., and Yaksh, T.L.: Spinal nitric oxide synthesis inhibition blocks NMDA-induced thermal hyperalgesia and produces antinociception in the formalin test in rats. Pain, *54:*291, 1993.
68. Max, M.B., Lynch, S.A., Muir, J., Shoaf, S.E., Smoller, B., and Dub-

ner, R.: Effects of desipramine, amitriptyline, and fluoxetine on pain in diabetic neuropathy. N. Engl. J. Med., *326:*1250, 1992.

69. McLachlan, E.M., Janig, W., Devor, M., and Michaelis, M.: Peripheral nerve injury triggers noradrenergic sprouting within dorsal root ganglia. Nature, *363:*543, 1993.
70. McMahon, S., and Koltzenburg, M.: The changing role of primary afferent neurones in pain. Pain, *43:*269, 1990.
71. McMahon, S.B.: Mechanisms of sympathetic pain. Br. Med. Bull., *47:*584, 1991.
72. McQuay, H.J., Carroll, D., Jadad, A.R., Wiffen, P.J., and Moore, A.: Anticonvulsants drugs for management of pain: A systematic review. Br. Med. J., *311:*1047, 1995.
73. Meert, T.F., and De Kock, M.: Potentiation of the analgesic properties of fentanyl-like opioids with α_2-adrenoceptor agonists in rats. Anesthesiology, *81:*677, 1994.
74. Meller, S.T., and Gebhart, G.F.: Nitric oxide (NO) and nociceptive processing in the spinal cord. Pain, *52:*127, 1993.
75. Meller, S.T., Pechman, P.S., Gebhardt, G.F., and Maves, T.J.: Nitric oxide mediates the thermal hyperalgesia produced in a model of neuropathic pain in the rat. Neuroscience *50:*7, 1992.
76. Melzack, R.: Psychological aspects of pain: Implications for neural blockade. *In* Cousins, M.J., and Bridenbaugh, P.O. (eds.): Neural Blockade in Clinical Anesthesia and Management of Pain. 2nd Ed. pp. 845–860. Philadelphia, J.B. Lippincott Company, 1988.
77. Mendell, L.M.: Physiological properties of unmyelinated fiber projection to the spinal cord. Exp. Neurol., *16:*316, 1966.
78. Merry, A., and Power, I.: Perioperative NSAIDs: Towards greater safety. Pain Reviews, *2:*268, 1995.
79. Merskey, H.: Pain terms: A list with definitions and notes on usage. Recommended by the IASP Subcommittee on Taxonomy. Pain, *6:*249, 1979.
80. Merskey, H., and Bogduk, N.: Classification of chronic pain: Descriptions of chronic pain syndromes and definitions of pain terms. 2nd Ed. Seattle, IASP Press, 1994.
81. Morgan, J.I., and Curran, T.: Role of ion flux in the control of c-fos expression. Nature, *322:*552, 1986.
82. North, R.B., Kidd, D.H., Zahurak, M., and Piantadosi, S.: Specificity of diagnostic nerve blocks: A prospective, randomized study of sciatica due to lumbosacral disease. Pain, *65:*77, 1996.
83. O'Hara, D.A., Fragen, R.J., Kinzer, M., and Pemberton, D.: Ketorolac tromethamine as compared with morphine sulfate for the treatment of postoperative pain. Clin. Pharmacol. Ther., *41:*556, 1987.
84. Ollat, H., Cesaro, P.: Pharmacology of neuropathic pain. Clin. Neuropharmacol., *18:*391, 1995.
85. Perl, E.R.: Sensitization of nociceptors and its relation to sensation. *In* Bonica, J.J., and AlbeFessard, D. (eds.): Advances in Pain Research and Therapy. pp. 17–28. New York, Raven Press, 1976.
86. Portenoy, R.K.: Management of neuropathic pain. Current and Emerging Issues in Cancer Pain: Research., 369, 1993.
87. Portenoy, R.K., Foley, K.M., and Inturrisi, C.E.: The nature of opioid responsiveness and its implications for neuropathic pain: New hypotheses derived from studies of opioid infusions. Pain, *43:*273, 1990.
88. Price, D.D., Mao, J.R., and Mayer, D.J.: Central neural mechanisms of normal and abnormal pain states. *In* Fields, H.L., and Liebeskind, J.C. (eds.): Pharmacological Approaches to the Treatment of Chronic Pain: New Concepts and Critical Issues. Progress in Pain Research and Management. Vol. 1. pp. 61–84, Seattle, IASP Press, 1994.
89. Rath, S.A., Braun, V., Soliman, N., Antoniadis, G., and Richter, H.P.: Results of DREZ coagulations for pain related to plexus lesions, spinal cord injuries, and postherpetic neuralgia. Acta Neurochir., *138:*364, 1996.
90. Schaible, H.-G., and Schmidt, R.F.: Direct observation of the sensitization of articular afferents during an experimental arthritis. *In* Dubner, R., Gebhardt, G., and Bond, M.R. (eds.): Proceedings of the 5th World Congress on Pain. Vol. 3. pp. 44–50. Amsterdam, Elsevier, 1988.
91. Seibert, K., Zhang, Y., and Leahy, K., *et al.*: Pharmacological and biochemical demonstration of the role of cyclooxygenase 2 in inflammation and pain. Proc. Natl. Acad. Sci. U.S.A., *91:*12013, 1994.
92. Siddall, P.J., Gray, M., Rutkowski, S., and Cousins, M.J.: Intrathecal morphine and clonidine in the management of spinal cord injury pain: A case report. Pain, *59:*147, 1994.
93. Sivilotti, L., and Woolf, C.J.: The contribution of $GABA_A$ and glycine receptors to central sensitization: Disinhibition and touch-evoked allodynia in the spinal cord. J. Neurophysiol., *72:*169, 1994.
94. Smith, M.T., Watt, J.A., and Cramond, T.: Morphine-3-glucuronide: A potent antagonist of morphine analgesia. Life Sci., *47:*579, 1990.
95. Stein, C.: Peripheral mechanisms of opioid analgesia. Anesth. Analg., *76:*182, 1993.
96. Stein, C.: Morphine: A local "analgesic." Pain: Clinical Updates, *3:*1, 1995.
97. Stein, C., Millan, M.J., and Shippenberg, T.S.: Peripheral opioid receptors mediating antinociception in inflammation: Evidence for involvement of mu, delta, and kappa receptors. J. Pharmacol. Exp. Ther., *248:*1269, 1989.
98. Strichartz, G.: Protracted relief of experimental neuropathic pain by systemic local anesthetics—how, where, and when. Anesthesiology, *83:*654, 1995.
99. Talbot, J.D., Marrett, S., Evans, A.C., *et al.*: Multiple representations of pain in human cerebral cortex. Science, *251:*1355, 1991.
100. Tennant, F., Moll, D., and Depaulo, V.: Topical morphine for peripheral pain. Lancet, *342:*1047, 1993.
101. Trujillo, K.A., and Akil, H.: Inhibition of morphine tolerance and dependence by the NMDA receptor antagonist MK-801. Science, *251:*85, 1991.
102. Urquhart, E.: Central analgesic activity of nonsteroidal antiinflammatory drugs in animal and human pain models. Semin. Arthritis Rheum., *23:*198, 1993.
103. Walker, J.S.: NSAID: An update on their analgesic effects. Clin. Exp. Pharmacol. Physiol., *22:*855, 1995.
104. Wall, P.D.: Cancer pain: Neurogenic mechanisms. *In* Fields, H.L. (ed.): Advances in Pain Research and Therapy. Vol. 9. pp. 575–587. New York, Raven Press, 1985.
105. Wall, P.D.: Pain in the brain and lower parts of the anatomy (letter). Pain, *62:*389, 1995.
106. Wiesenfeld-Hallin, Z., Hao, J.X., Xu, X.J., and Hokfelt, T.: Nitric oxide mediates ongoing discharge in dorsal root ganglion cells after peripheral nerve injury. J. Neurophysiol., *70:*2350, 1993.
107. Wilcox, G.L.: Excitatory neurotransmitters and pain. *In* Bond, M.R., Charlton, J.E., and Woolf, C.J. (eds.): Proceedings of the 6th World Congress on Pain. Pain Research and Clinical Management Series. Vol. 4. pp. 97–117. Amsterdam, Elsevier, 1991.
108. Willis, W.D.: The Pain System. The Neural Basis of Nociceptive Transmission in the Mammalian Nervous System. Basel, Karger, 1985.
109. Willis, W.D., and Coggeshall, R.E.: Sensory Mechanisms of the Spinal Cord. New York, Plenum Press, 1991.
110. Wilson, P.R., and Yaksh, T.L.: Baclofen is antinociceptive in the spinal intrathecal space of animals. Eur. J. Pharmacol., *51:*323, 1995.
111. Wong, C.S., Cheng, C.H., Luk, H.N., Ho, S.T., and Tung, C.S.: Effects of NMDA receptor antagonists on inhibition of morphine tolerance in rats—binding at mu-opioid receptors. Eur. J. Pharmacol., *297:*27, 1996.
112. Woolf, C., Shortland, P., and Coggeshall, R.E.: Peripheral nerve injury triggers central sprouting of myelinated afferents. Nature, *355:*75, 1992.
113. Woolf, C.J.: Recent advances in the pathophysiology of acute pain. Br. J. Anaesth., *63:*139, 1989.
114. Woolf, C.J., and Chong, M.S.: Preemptive analgesia-treating postoperative pain by preventing the establishment of central sensitization. Anesth. Analg., *77:*362, 1993.
115. Woolf, C.J., and Thompson, S.W.N.: The induction and maintenance of central sensitization is dependent on N-methyl-D-aspartic acid receptor activation; Implications for the treatment of post-injury pain hypersensitivity states. Pain, *44:*293, 1991.
116. Xu, X.-J., Puke, M.J.C., Verge, V.M.K., Wiesenfeld-Hallin, Z., Hughes, J., and Hokfelt, T.: Up-regulation of cholecystokinin in primary sensory neurons is associated with morphine insensitivity in experimental neuropathic pain in the rat. Neurosci. Lett., *152:*129, 1993.
117. Yaksh, T.L., and Reddy, S.V.R.: Studies in the primate on the analgetic effects associated with intrathecal actions of opiates, alpha-adrenergic agonists and baclofen. Anesthesiology, *54:*451, 1981.
118. Zeidman, S.M., and North, R.B.: General neurosurgical procedures for management of chronic pain. *In* Raj, P.P. (ed.): Current Review of Pain. pp. 103–115. Philadelphia, Current Medicine, 1994.
119. Zeigler, D., Lynch, S.A., Muir, J., Benjamin, J., and Max, M.B.: Transdermal clonidine versus placebo in painful diabetic neuropathy. Pain, *48:*403, 1992.

APPENDIX A: CLASSIFICATION OF CHRONIC PAIN

Reproduced with permission of the International Association for the Study of Pain (IASP) and IASP Press, and the Editors Harold Merskey and Nikolai Bogduk. The material reproduced is a small portion of the publication "Classification of Chronic Pain: Descriptions of Chronic Pain Syndromes and Definitions of Pain Terms. 2nd Edition, IASP Press" (1994).[80] The reader is strongly encouraged to consult the full document.

PAIN TERMS

Pain

An unpleasant sensory and emotional experience associated with actual or potential tissue damage, or described in terms of such damage.

Note: Pain is always subjective. Each individual learns the application of the word through experiences related to injury in early life. Biologists recognize that those stimuli which cause pain are liable to damage tissue. Accordingly, pain is that experience we associate with actual or potential tissue damage. It is unquestionably a sensation in a part or parts of the body, but it is also always unpleasant and therefore also an emotional experience. Experiences which resemble pain but are not unpleasant, e.g., pricking, should not be called pain. Unpleasant abnormal experiences (dysesthesias) may also be pain but are not necessarily so because, subjectively, they may not have the usual sensory qualities of pain.

Many people report pain in the absence of tissue damage or any likely pathophysiological cause; usually this happens for psychological reasons. There is usually no way to distinguish their experience from that due to tissue damage, if we take the subjective report. If they regard their experience as pain and if they report it in the same ways as pain caused by tissue damage, it should be accepted as pain. This definition avoids tying pain to the stimulus. Activity induced in the nociceptor and nociceptive pathways by a noxious stimulus is not pain, which is always a psychological state, even though we may well appreciate that pain most often has a proximate physical cause.

Allodynia

Pain due to a stimulus which does not normally provoke pain.

Note: The term *allodynia* was originally introduced to separate from hyperalgesia and hyperesthesia, the conditions seen in patients with lesions of the nervous system where touch, light pressure, or moderate cold or warmth evoke pain when applied to apparently normal skin. *Allo* means "other" in Greek and is a common prefix for medical conditions that diverge from the expected. *Odynia* is derived from the Greek word "odune" or "odyne," which is used in "pleurodynia" and "coccydynia" and is similar in meaning to the root from which we derive words with -algia or -algesia in them. Allodynia was suggested following discussions with Professor Paul Potter of the Department of the History of Medicine and Science at The University of Western Ontario.

The words "to normal skin" were used in the original definition but later were omitted in order to remove any suggestion that allodynia applied only to referred pain. Originally, also, the pain provoking stimulus was described as "non-noxious." However, a stimulus may be noxious at some times and not at others, for example, with intact skin and sunburned skin, and also, the boundaries of noxious stimulation may be hard to delimit. Since the Committee aimed at providing terms for clinical use, it did not wish to define them by reference to the specific physical characteristics of the stimulation, e.g., pressure in kilopascals per square centimeter. Moreover, even in intact skin there is little evidence one way or the other that a strong painful pinch to a normal person does or does not damage tissue. Accordingly, it was considered to be preferable to define allodynia in terms of the response to clinical stimuli and to point out that the normal response to the stimulus could almost always be tested elsewhere in the body, usually in a corresponding part. Further, allodynia is taken to apply to conditions which may give rise to sensitization of the skin, e.g., sunburn, inflammation, trauma.

It is important to recognize that allodynia involves a change in the quality of a sensation, whether tactile, thermal, or of any other sort. The original modality is normally non-painful, but the response is painful. There is thus a loss of specificity of a sensory modality. By contrast, hyperalgesia (q.v.) represents an augmented response in a specific mode, viz., pain. With other cutaneous modalities, hyperesthesia is the term which corresponds to hyperalgesia, and as with hyperalgesia, the quality is not altered. In allodynia the stimulus mode and the response mode differ, unlike the situation with hyperalgesia. This distinction should not be confused by the fact that allodynia and hyperalgesia can be plotted with overlap along the same continuum of physical intensity in certain circumstances, for example, with pressure or temperature.

See also the notes on hyperalgesia and hyperpathia.

Analgesia

Absence of pain in response to stimulation which would normally be painful.

Note: As with allodynia (q.v), the stimulus is defined by its usual subjective effects.

Anesthesia dolorosa

Pain in an area or region which is anesthetic.

Causalgia

A syndrome of sustained burning pain, allodynia, and hyperpathia, after a traumatic nerve lesion, often combined with vasomotor and sudomotor dysfunction and later trophic changes.

Central pain

Pain initiated or caused by a primary lesion or dysfunction in the central nervous system.

Dysesthesia

An unpleasant abnormal sensation, whether spontaneous or evoked.

Note: Compare with pain and with paresthesia. Special cases of dysesthesia include hyperalgesia and allodynia. A dysesthesia should always be unpleasant and a paresthesia should not be unpleasant, although it is recognized that the borderline may present some difficulties when it comes to deciding as to whether a sensation is pleasant or unpleasant. It should always be specified whether the sensations are spontaneous or evoked.

Hyperalgesia

An increased response to a stimulus which is normally painful.

Note: Hyperalgesia reflects increased pain on suprathreshold stimulation. For pain evoked by stimuli that usually are not painful, the term allodynia is preferred, while hyperalgesia is more appropriately used for cases with an increased response at a normal threshold, or at an increased threshold, e.g., in patients with neuropathy. It should also be recognized that with allodynia the stimulus and the response are in different modes, whereas with hyperalgesia they are in the same mode. Current evidence suggests that hyperalgesia is a consequence of perturbation of the nociceptive system with peripheral or central sensitization, or both, but it is important to distinguish between the clinical phenomena, which this definition emphasizes, and the interpretation, which may well change as knowledge advances.

Hyperesthesia

Increased sensitivity to stimulation, excluding the special senses.

Note: The stimulus and locus should be specified. Hyperesthesia may refer to various modes of cutaneous sensibility, including touch and thermal sensation without pain, as well as to pain. The word is used to indicate both diminished threshold to any stimulus and an increased response to stimuli that are normally recognized.

Allodynia is suggested for pain after stimulation which is not normally painful. Hyperesthesia includes both allodynia and hyperalgesia, but the more specific terms should be used wherever they are applicable.

Hyperpathia

A painful syndrome characterized by an abnormally painful reaction to a stimulus, especially a repetitive stimulus, as well as an increased threshold.

Note: It may occur with allodynia, hyperesthesia, hyperalgesia, or dysesthesia. Faulty identification and localization of the stimulus, delay, radiating sensation, and after-sensation may be present, and the pain is often explosive in character. The changes in this note are the specification of allodynia and the inclusion of hyperalgesia explicitly. Previously, hyperalgesia was implied, since hyperalgesia was mentioned in the previous note and hyperalgesia is a special case of hyperesthesia.

Hypoalgesia

Diminished pain in response to a normally painful stimulus.

Note: Hypoalgesia was formerly defined as diminished sensitivity to noxious stimulation, making it a particular case of hypoesthesia (q.v.). However, it now refers only to the occurrence of relatively less pain in response to stimulation that produces pain. Hypoesthesia covers the case of diminished sensitivity to stimulation that is normally painful.

The implications of some of the above definitions may be summarized for convenience as follows:

Allodynia:	lowered threshold:	stimulus and response mode differ
Hyperalgesia:	increased response:	stimulus and response mode are the same

Hyperpathia:	raised threshold: increased response:	stimulus and response mode may be the same or different
Hypoalgesia:	raised threshold: lowered response:	stimulus and response mode are the same

The above essentials of the definitions do not have to be symmetrical and are not symmetrical at present. Lowered threshold may occur with allodynia but is not required. Also, there is no category for lowered threshold and lowered response—if it ever occurs.

Hypoesthesia

Decreased sensitivity to stimulation, excluding the special senses.

Note: Stimulation and locus to be specified.

Neuralgia

Pain in the distribution of a nerve or nerves.

Note: Common usage, especially in Europe, often implies a paroxysmal quality, but neuralgia should not be reserved for paroxysmal pains.

Neuritis

Inflammation of a nerve or nerves.

Note: Not to be used unless inflammation is thought to be present.

Neurogenic pain

Pain initiated or caused by a primary lesion, dysfunction, or transitory perturbation in the peripheral or central nervous system.

Neuropathic pain

Pain initiated or caused by a primary lesion or dysfunction in the nervous system.

Note: See also Neurogenic Pain and Central Pain. Peripheral neuropathic pain occurs when the lesion or dysfunction affects the peripheral nervous system. Central pain may be retained as the term when the lesion or dysfunction affects the central nervous system.

Neuropathy

A disturbance of function or pathological change in a nerve: in one nerve, mononeuropathy; in several nerves, mononeuropathy multiplex; if diffuse and bilateral, polyneuropathy.

Note: Neuritis (q.v.) is a special case of neuropathy and is now reserved for inflammatory processes affecting nerves. Neuropathy is not intended to cover cases like neurapraxia, neurotmesis, section of a nerve, or transitory impact like a blow, stretching, or an epileptic discharge. The term *neurogenic* applies to pain due to such temporary perturbations.

Nociceptor

A receptor preferentially sensitive to a noxious stimulus or to a stimulus which would become noxious if prolonged.

Note: Avoid use of terms like pain receptor, pain pathway, etc.

Noxious stimulus

A noxious stimulus is one which is damaging to normal tissues.

Note: Although the definition of a noxious stimulus has been retained, the term is not used in this list to define other terms.

Pain Threshold

The least experience of pain which a subject can recognize.

Note: Traditionally the threshold has often been defined, as we defined it formerly, as the least stimulus intensity at which a subject perceives pain. Properly defined, the threshold is really the experience of the patient, whereas the intensity measured is an external event. It has been common usage for most pain research workers to define the threshold in terms of the stimulus, and that should be avoided. However, the threshold stimulus can be recognized as such and measured. In psychophysics, thresholds are defined as the level at which 50% of stimuli are recognized. In that case, the pain threshold would be the level at which 50% of stimuli would be recognized as painful. The stimulus is not pain (q.v.) and cannot be a measure of pain.

Pain Tolerance Level

The greatest level of pain which a subject is prepared to tolerate.

Note: As with pain threshold, the pain tolerance level is the subjective experience of the individual. The stimuli which are normally measured in relation to its production are the pain tolerance level stimuli and not the level itself. Thus, the same argument applies to pain tolerance level as to pain threshold, and it is not defined in terms of the external stimulation as such.

Paresthesia An abnormal sensation, whether spontaneous or evoked.

Note: Compare with dysesthesia. After much discussion, it has been agreed to recommend that paresthesia be used to describe an abnormal sensation that is not unpleasant, while dysesthesia be used preferentially for an abnormal sensation that is considered to be unpleasant. The use of one term (paresthesia) to indicate spontaneous sensations and the other to refer to evoked sensations is not favored. There is a sense in which, since paresthesia refers to abnormal sensations in general, it might include dysesthesia, but the reverse is not true. Dysesthesia does not include all abnormal sensations, but only those which are unpleasant.

Peripheral Neurogenic Pain Pain initiated or caused by a primary lesion or dysfunction or transitory perturbation in the peripheral nervous system.

Peripheral Neuropathic Pain Pain initiated or caused by a primary lesion or dysfunction in the peripheral nervous system.

SCHEME FOR CODING CHRONIC PAIN DIAGNOSES

The digital portion of the codes is explained first, followed by the letters used as suffixes.

The first digit (Axis I), concerned with the regions, has generally not been difficult to complete. If a patient has pain in more than one region, two codes should be completed for that patient.

The second digit (Axis II) also has generally not been difficult to complete, but the details in this area are open to debate. For example, migraine has been coded, in accordance with the belief of some specialists, as a disorder of the central nervous system, but others might think that it should be coded as a disorder of the vascular system. Again, we should emphasize the practical aspect of the matter: provided that the code is available and useful to those who accept criteria for migraine in accordance with the descriptions provided, the theoretical position adopted in regard to the second digit is not necessarily important.

The third digit (Axis III) deals with the characteristics of the pain episode. It is not controversial, but some judgment is required in deciding whether a condition is continuous with exacerbations or merely continuous.

The fourth digit (Axis IV) has to be filled in for each patient according to his or her particular report as to the severity or chronicity of his or her illness. Accordingly, it is shown as an X throughout the tabulation of codes in association with descriptions here.

The fifth digit (Axis V) is open to most argument because there is a great uncertainty about many of the mechanisms involved in the production of pain in different conditions. Again, it should be said that provided that the coding arrangements give each syndrome a specific and individual number or code, it is not important whether the ultimate truth of the cause of the syndrome be expressed in that code or not. In any case, since some syndromes have the same final code for the five digits, it has become necessary to distinguish them by adding a letter-a, b, c, etc.—in the sixth place. In certain instances the letter "a" has been used to indicate acute conditions compared with chronic conditions that share the same five digits. The leading example of this is acute tension headache. For the most part, however, the letter "a" in the sixth place merely indicates the first of several conditions to be described with the same five digits.

The letters S and R are used after the digits for the codes that identify spinal and radicular pain, respectively. Where both occur *in the same location*, the letter C, for combined spinal and root pain, is preferred.

A full list of those codes allocated so far is provided below. Before examining the value of the coding system, the reader may find it helpful to look at descriptions of conditions with which he or she is familiar and to consider if the codes do justice, or in his or her view any sort of injustice, to them. After that it may be worthwhile to compare the codes for the general syndromes with each other, and then compare with each other those where the same condition affects different parts of the body.

Give priority to the main site of the pain.

Axis I: Regions: Record main site first; record two important regions separately. If there is more than one site of pain, separate coding will be necessary. More than three major sites can be coded, optionally, as shown.

Head, face, and mouth	000
Cervical region	100
Upper shoulder and upper limbs	200
Thoracic region	300
Abdominal region	400
Lower back, lumbar spine, sacrum, and coccyx	500
Lower limbs	600
Pelvic region	700
Anal, perineal, and genital region	800
More than three major sites	900

Axis II: Systems

Nervous system (central, peripheral, and autonomic) and special senses; physical disturbance or dysfunction	00
Nervous system (psychological and social)*	10
Respiratory and cardiovascular systems	20
Musculoskeletal system and connective tissue	30
Cutaneous and subcutaneous and associated glands (breast, apocrine, etc.)	40
Gastrointestinal system	50
Genito-urinary system	60
Other organs or viscera (e.g., thyroid, lymphatic, hemopoietic)	70
More than one system	80
Unknown	90

Note: The system is coded whose abnormal functioning produces the pain, e.g., claudication = vascular. Similarly, the nervous system is to be coded only when a pathological disturbance in it produces pain. Thus pain from a pancreatic carcinoma = gastrointestinal; pain from a metastatic deposit affecting bones = musculoskeletal.

* To be coded for psychiatric illness without any relevant lesion.

Axis III: Temporal Characteristics of Pain: Pattern of Occurrence

Not recorded, not applicable, or not known	0
Single episode, limited duration (e.g., ruptured aneurysm, sprained ankle)	1
Continuous or nearly continuous, nonfluctuating (e.g., low back pain, some cases)	2
Continuous or nearly continuous, fluctuating severity (e.g., ruptured intervertebral disc)	3
Recurring irregularly (e.g., headache, mixed type)	4
Recurring regularly (e.g., premenstrual pain)	5
Paroxysmal (e.g., tic douloureux)	6
Sustained with superimposed paroxysms	7
Other combinations	8
None of the above	9

Axis IV: Patient's Statement of Intensity: Time Since Onset of Pain*

Not recorded, not applicable, or not known		.0
Mild	—1 month or less	.1
	—1 month to 6 months	.2
	—more than 6 months	.3
Medium	—1 month or less	.4
	—1 month to 6 months	.5
	—more than 6 months	.6
Severe	—1 month or less	.7
	—1 month to 6 months	.8
	—more than 6 months	.9

* Decide the time at which pain is recognized retrospectively as having started, even though the pain may occur intermittently. Grade for intensity in relation to the level of current pain problem.

Axis V: Etiology

Genetic or congenital disorders (e.g., congenital dislocation)	.00
Trauma, operation, burns	.01
Infective, parasitic	.02
Inflammatory (no known infective agent), immune reactions	.03
Neoplasm	.04
Toxic, metabolic (e.g., alcoholic neuropathy, anoxia, vascular, nutritional, endocrine), radiation	.05
Degenerative, mechanical*	.06
Dysfunctional (including psychophysiological)†	.07
Unknown or other	.08
Psychological origin (e.g., conversion hysteria, depressive hallucination).	.09

Note: No physical cause should be held to be present, nor any pathophysiological mechanism

*For example, biliary colic or lumbar puncture headache would be mechanical.

† For example, migraine, irritable bowel syndrome, tension headache. *Note:* Include syndromes where a pathophysiological alteration is recognized. Emotional causes may or may not be present.

Examples:

Mild postherapetic neuralgia of T5 of T6 6 months' duration	303.22e
Severe tension headache More than 6 months' duration	033.97c
Severe primary dysmenorrhea Duration not recorded	765.07b

CHRONIC PAIN SYNDROMES: DIAGNOSIS AND CODING

A. Relatively Generalized Syndromes

I. Relatively Generalized Syndromes	
1. Peripheral Neuropathy	203.X2a (arms, infective)
	203.X3a (arms, inflammatory or immune reactions)
	203.X5a (arms, toxic, metabolic, etc.)
	203.X8a (arms, unknown or other)
	603.X2a (legs, infective)
	603.X3a (legs, inflammatory or immune reactions)
	603.X5a (legs, toxic, metabolic, etc.)
	603.X8a (legs, unknown or other)
	X03.X4d (Von Recklinghausen's disease)
2. Stump Pain	203.X1a (arms)
	603.X1a (legs)
3. Phantom Pain	203.X7a (arms)
	603.X7a (legs)
4. Complex Regional Pain Syndrome, Type I (Reflex Sympathetic Dystrophy)	203.X1h (arms)
	603.X1h (legs)
5. Complex Regional Pain Syndrome, Type II (Causalgia)	207.X1h (arms)
	607.X1h (legs)
6. Central Pain	
If three or more major sites are involved, code first digit as 9:	903.X5c (vascular)
	903.X1c (trauma)
If only one or two sites are involved, code according to specific site or sites (e.g., for head or face, code 003.X5c, etc.)	903.X2c (infection)
	903.X3c (inflammatory)
	903.X4c (neoplasm)
	903.X8c (unknown)

7. Syndrome of Syringomyelia (when affecting head or limb; code additional entries for other areas)	007.X0 (face) 207.X0 (arm) 607.X0 (leg)
8. Polymyalgia Rheumatica	X32.X3a
9. Fibromyalgia (Fibrositis)	X33.X8a
10. Rheumatoid Arthritis	X34.X3a
11. Osteoarthritis	X38.X6a
12. Calcium Pyrophosphate Dihydrate Deposition Disease (CPPD)	X38.X0 or X38.X5a
13. Gout	X38.X5b
14. Hemophilic Arthropathy	X34.X0a
15. Burns	X42.X1 or X82.X1
16. Pain of Psychological Origin	
16.1. Muscle Tension	X33.X7b
16.2. Delusional or Hallucinatory	X1X.X9a
16.3. Hysterical, Conversion, or Hypochondriacal	X1X.X9b
16.4. Associated with Depression	X1X.X9d
17. Factitious Illness and Malingering	No code: see note in text
18. Regional Sprains or Strains (code only)	X33.X1d
19. Sickle Cell Arthropathy (code only)	X34.X0c
20. Purpuric Arthropathy (code only)	X34.X0d
21. Stiff Man Syndrome (code only)	934.X8
22. Paralysis Agitans (code only)	902.X7
23. Epilepsy (code only)	X04.X7
24. Polyarteritis Nodosa (code only)	X5X.X3
25. Psoriatic Arthropathy and Other Secondary Arthropathies (code only)	X34.X8c
26. Painful Scar (code only)	X4X.X1b
27. Systemic Lupus Erythematosis Systemic Sclerosis and Fibrosclerosis, Polymyositis and Dermatomyositis (code only)	X33.X3b
28. Infective Arthropathies (code only)	X33.X3c
29. Traumatic Arthropathy (code only)	X33.X1a
30. Osteomyelitis (code only)	X32.X2f
31. Osteitis Deformans (code only)	X32.X5b
32. Osteochondritis (code only)	X32.X5c
33. Osteoporosis (code only)	X32.X5d
34. Muscle Spasm (code only)	X37.X7
35. Local Pain, No Cause Specified (code only)	X7X.XXa or X3X.X8e
36. Guillain-Barré Syndrome	901.X3

B. Relatively Localized Syndromes[a] of the Head and Neck (Examples)

II. Neuralgias of the Head and Face	
1. Trigeminal Neuralgia (Tic Douloureux)	006.X8a
2. Secondary Neuralgia (Trigeminal) from Central Nervous System Lesions Arnold-Chiari Syndrome(code only)	006.X4 (tumor) 006.X0 (aneurysm) 002.X2b (congenital)
3. Secondary Trigeminal Neuralgia from Facial Trauma	006.X1
4. Acute Herpes Zoster (Trigeminal)	002.X2a
5. Postherpetic Neuralgia (Trigeminal)	003.X2b
6. Geniculate Neuralgia (VIIth Cranial Nerve): Ramsay Hunt Syndrome	006.X2
7. Neuralgia of the Nervus Intermedius	006.X8c
8. Glossopharyngeal Neuralgia (IXth Cranial Nerve)	006.X8b
9. Neuralgia of the Superior Laryngeal Nerve (Vagus Nerve Neuralgia)	006.X8e
10. Occipital Neuralgia	004.X8 or 00.4X1 (if subsequent to trauma)
11. Hypoglossal Neuralgia (code only)	006.X8
12. Glossopharyngeal Pain from Trauma (code only)	003.X1a
13. Hypoglossal Pain from Trauma (code only)	003.X1b
14. Tolosa-Hunt Syndrome (Painful Ophthalmoplegia)	002.X3a
15. SUNCT Syndrome (Shortlasting, Unilateral, Neuralgiform Pain with Conjunctival Injection and Tearing)	006.X8j

16. Raeder's Syndrome (Raeder's Paratrigeminal Syndrome)	002.X4 (tumor)
	002.X1a (trauma)
Type I	002.X3b (inflammatory, etc.)
Type II	002.X8 (unknown)
III. Craniofacial Pain of Musculoskeletal Origin	
1. Acute Tension Headache	034.X7a
2. Tension Headache: Chronic Form (Scalp Muscle Contraction Headache)	033.X7c
3. Temporomandibular Pain and Dysfunction Syndrome (also called Temporomandibular Joint Disorder)	034.X8a
4. Osteoarthritis of the Temporomandibular Joint (code only)	033.X6
5. Rheumatoid Arthritis of the Temporomandibular Joint	032.X3b
6. Dystonic Disorders, Facial Dyskinesia (code only)	003.X8
7. Crushing Injury of Head or Face (code only)	032.X1
IV. Lesions of the Ear, Nose, and Oral Cavity	
1. Maxillary Sinusitis	031.X2a
2. Odontalgia: Toothache 1. Due to Dentino-Enamel Defects	034.X2b
3. Odontalgia: Toothache 2. Pulpitis	031.X2c
4. Odontalgia: Toothache 3. Periapical Periodontitis and Abscess	031.X2d

[a]*Note:* This list is abbreviated and provides only a sample of "localized" pain syndromes and their codes.

DETAILED DESCRIPTIONS OF PAIN SYNDROMES: EXAMPLES

Relatively Generalized Syndromes

GROUP I: RELATIVELY GENERALIZED SYNDROMES

Peripheral Neuropathy (I-1)

Definition

Constant or intermittent burning, aching, or lancinating limb pains due to generalized or focal diseases of peripheral nerves.

Site

Usually distal (especially the feet) with burning pain, but often more proximal and deep with aching. Focal with mononeuropathies, in the territory of the affected nerve (e.g., meralgia paresthetica).

System

Peripheral nervous system.

Main Features

Prevalence: common in neuropathies of diabetes, amyloid, alcoholism, polyarteritis, Guillain-Barré Syndrome (for which see I–36), neuralgic amyotrophy, Fabry's disease. Age of Onset: variable, usually after second decade. Pain Quality: (a) burning, superficial, distal pain often with dysesthesia, constant. May be in the territory of a single affected nerve; (b) deep aching, especially nocturnal, constant; and (c) sharp lancinating "tabetic" pains, especially in legs, intermittent.

Associated Symptoms

Sensory loss, especially to pinprick and temperature; sometimes weakness and muscle atrophy (especially in neuralgic amyotrophy); sometimes reflex loss; sometimes signs of loss of sympathetic function; smooth, fine skin; hair loss.

Laboratory Findings

(a) Features of the primary disease, e.g., diabetes; and (b) features of neuropathy: reduced or absent sensory potentials, slowing of motor and sensory conduction velocities, EMG evidence of muscle denervation.

Usual Course

Distal burning and deep aching pains are often long-lasting, and the disease processes are relatively unresponsive to therapy. Pain resolves spontaneously in weeks or months in self-limited conditions such as Guillain-Barré syndrome or neuralgic amyotrophy.

Complications

Drug abuse, depression.

Social and Physical Disabilities

Decreased mobility.

Pathology

Nerve fiber damage, usually axonal degeneration. Pain especially occurs with small fiber damage (sensory fibers). Nerve biopsy may reveal the above, plus features of the specific disease process, e.g., amyloid.

Summary of Essential Features and Diagnostic Criteria

Chronic distal burning or deep aching pain with signs of sensory loss with or without muscle weakness, atrophy, and reflex loss.

Differential Diagnosis

Spinal cord disease, muscle disease.

Code

203.X2a	Arms: infective
203.X3a	Arms: inflammatory or immune reactions
203.X5a	Arms: toxic, metabolic, etc.
203.X8a	Arms: unknown or other
603.X2a	Legs: infective
603.X3a	Legs: inflammatory or immune reactions
603.X5a	Legs: toxic, metabolic, etc
603.X8a	Legs: unknown or other
X03.X4d	Von Recklinghausen's disease

REFERENCES

Thomas, P.K., Pain in peripheral neuropathy: clinical and morphological aspects. *In* Ochoa, J. and Culp, W. (eds.): Abnormal Nerves and Muscles as Impulse Generators. Oxford University Press, New York, 1982.

Asburn, A.K., and Fields, H.L.: Pain due to peripheral nerve damage: an hypothesis. Neurology, *34:* 1587, 1984.

Stump Pain (I-2)

Definition

Pain at the site of an extremity amputation.

Site

Upper or lower extremity at the region of amputation. Pain is not referred to the absent body part but is perceived in the stump itself, usually in region of transected nerve(s).

System

Peripheral nervous system; perhaps central nervous system.

Main Features

Sharp, often jabbing pain in stump, usually aggravated by pressure on, or infection in, the stump. Pain often elicited by tapping over neuroma in transected nerve or nerves.

Associated Symptoms

Refusal to utilize prosthesis.

Signs

Pain elicited by percussion over stump neuromata.

Laboratory Findings

None.

Usual Course

Develops several weeks to months after amputation; persists indefinitely if untreated.

Relief

(a) Alter prosthesis to avoid pressure on neuromata; (b) resect neuromata so that they no longer lie in pressure areas; and (c) utilize neurosurgical procedures such as rhizotomy and ganglionectomy or spinal cord or peripheral nerve stimulation in properly selected patients.

Complications

Refusal to use prosthesis.

Social and Physical Disabilities

Severe pain can preclude normal daily activities; failure to utilize prosthesis can add to functional limitations.

Pathology

Neuroma at site of nerve transection.

Essential Features

Pain in stump.

Differential Diagnosis

Phantom limb pain, radiculopathy.

Code

203.Xla	Arms
603.Xla	Legs

Phantom Pain (I-3)

Definition

Pain referred to a surgically removed limb or portion thereof.

Site

In the absent body part.

System

Central nervous system.

Main Features

Follows amputation, may commence at time of amputation or months to years later. Varies greatly in severity from person to person. Reports of prevalence vary from $< 1\%$ to $> 50\%$ of amputees. Believed to be more common if loss of limb occurs later in life, in limbs than in breast amputation, in the breast before the menopause rather than after it, and particularly if pain was present before the part was lost. Pain may be continuous, often with intermittent exacerbations. Usually cramping, aching, burning; may have superimposed shocklike components. Seems to be less likely if the initial amputation is treated actively and a prosthesis is promptly utilized. Phantom limb pain is almost always associated with distorted image of lost part.

Associated Symptoms

Aggravated by stress, systemic disease, poor stump health.

Signs

Loss of body part.

Usual Course

Complaints persist indefinitely; frequently with gradual amelioration over years.

Relief

No therapeutic regimen has more than a 30% long-term efficacy. TENS, anticonvulsants, antidepressants, or phenothiazines may be helpful. Sympathectomy or surgical procedures upon spinal cord and brain, including stimulation, are sometimes helpful.

Social and Physical Disabilities

May preclude gainful employment or normal daily activities.

Pathology

Related to deafferentation of neurons and their spontaneous and evoked hyperexcitability.

Essential Features

Pain in an absent body part.

Differential Diagnosis

Stump pain.

Code

203.X7a	Arms
603.X7a	Legs

Complex Regional Pain Syndromes (CRPS)

This title is being introduced to cover the painful syndromes which formerly were described under the headings of "Reflex Sympathetic Dystrophy" and "Causalgia." There has been dissatisfaction with the term "reflex sympathetic dystrophy" because not all the cases seem to have sympathetically maintained pain, and not all were dystrophic. The conditions usually follow injury which appears regionally and have a distal predominance of abnormal findings, exceeding the expected clinical course of the inciting event in both magnitude and duration and often resulting in significant impairment of motor function. The syndrome broadly corresponding to what was formerly described as reflex sympathetic dystrophy is now termed CRPS Type I (Reflex Sympathetic Dystrophy), and causalgia is described as CRPS Type II (Causalgia).

In the previous edition of this classification, causalgia was presented before reflex sympathetic dystrophy. However, because the present descriptions recognize that causalgia begins with a nerve injury but develops the signs of CRPS Type I as well, it has been felt better to give the description of CRPS Type I before that of causalgia. This means that the initial identifying numbers in the classification have been changed, CRPS Type I becoming syndrome I-4; CRPS Type II becoming syndrome I-5.

Sympathetically maintained pain (SMP) may be found in association with these syndromes. It is taken to be pain that is maintained by sympathetic efferent innervation or by circulating catecholamines. This is a feature of several types of painful conditions and is not an essential requirement of any one condition. It is understood that pain relieved by a specific sympatholytic procedure may be considered SMP. This does not imply a mechanism for the pain but simply follows the common clinical observation that in certain cases sympatholytic interventions will lead to a reduction of pain. It is also notable that a patient may have SMP and *sympathetically independent pain* (SIP) at the same time. SMP may occur in some patients with CRPS, but certainly does not occur in all.

Complex Regional Pain Syndrome, Type I (Reflex Sympathetic Dystrophy) (I-4)

Definition

CRPS Type I is a syndrome that usually develops after an initiating noxious event, is not limited to the distribution of a single peripheral nerve, and is apparently disproportionate to the inciting event. It is associated at some point with evidence of edema, changes in skin blood flow, abnormal sudomotor activity in the region of the pain, or allodynia or hyperalgesia.

Site

Usually the distal aspect of an affected extremity or with a distal to proximal gradient.

System

Peripheral nervous system; possibly the central nervous system.

Main Features

Pain often follows trauma, which is usually mild and is not associated with significant nerve injury. It may follow a fracture, a soft tissue lesion, or immobilization related to visceral disease, e.g., angina or stroke. The onset of symptoms usually occurs within one month of the inciting event. The pain is frequently described as burning and continuous and exacerbated by movement, continuous stimulation, or stress. The intensity of pain fluctuates over time, and allodynia or hyperalgesia may be found which are not limited to the territory of a single peripheral nerve. Abnormalities of blood flow occur, including changes in skin temperature and color. Edema is usually present and may be soft or firm. Increased or decreased sweating may appear. The symptoms and signs may spread proximally or involve other extremities. Impairment of motor function is frequently seen.

Associated Symptoms and Signs

Atrophy of the skin, nails, and other soft tissues, alterations in hair growth, and loss of joint mobility may develop. Impairment of motor function can include weakness, tremor, and, in rare instances, dystonia. Symptoms and signs fluctuate at times. Sympathetically maintained pain may be present and may be demonstrated with pharmacological blocking or provocation techniques. Affective symptoms or disorders occur secondary to the pain and disability. Guarding of the affected part is usually observed.

Laboratory Findings

Noncontact skin temperature measurement indicates a side-to-side asymmetry of greater than 1°C. Due to the unstable nature of the temperature changes in this disorder, measurements at different times are recommended. Measurements of skin blood flow may show an increase or a reduction. Testing of sudomotor function, both at rest and evoked, indicates side-to-side asymmetry. The bone uptake phase of a three-phase bone scan may reveal a characteristic pattern of subcutaneous blood pool changes. Radiographic examination may demonstrate patchy bone demineralization.

Usual Course

Variable.

Relief

In cases with sympathetically maintained pain, sympatholytic interventions may provide temporary or permanent pain relief.

Complications

Phlebitis, inappropriate drug use, and suicide.

Social and Physical Impairment

Inability to perform activities of daily living and occupational and recreational activities.

Pathology

Unknown.

Diagnostic Criteria

1. The presence of an initiating noxious event, or a cause of immobilization.
2. Continuing pain, allodynia, or hyperalgesia with which the pain is disproportionate to any inciting event.
3. Evidence at some time of edema, changes in skin blood flow, or abnormal sudomotor activity in the region of the pain.
4. This diagnosis is excluded by the existence of conditions that would otherwise account for the degree of pain and dysfunction.

Note: Criteria 2–4 must be satisfied.

Differential Diagnosis

CRPS Type II (causalgia) unrecognized local pathology (e.g., fracture, strain, sprain), traumatic vasospasm, cellulitis, Raynaud's disease, thromboangiitis obliterans, thrombosis.

Code

203.Xlh	Arms
603.Xlh	Legs

Complex Regional Pain Syndrome, Type II (Causalgia) (I-5)

Definition

Burning pain, allodynia, and hyperpathia usually in the hand or foot after partial injury of a nerve or one of its major branches.

Site

In the region of the limb innervated by the damaged nerve.

Main Features

The onset usually occurs immediately after partial nerve injury but may be delayed for months. The nerves most commonly involved are the median, the sciatic, the tibial, and the ulnar. Causalgia of the radial nerve is very rare. Spontaneous pain occurs which is described as constant and burning, and is exacerbated by light touch, stress, temperature change or movement of the involved limb, visual and auditory stimuli (e.g., sudden sound or bright light), and emotional disturbances. The intensity of the pain may fluctuate over time, and allodynia-hyperalgesia occur but are not limited to the territory of a single peripheral nerve. Abnormalities in skin blood flow may develop, including changes in skin temperature and skin color. Edema is usually present and may be soft or hard, and either hyperhidrosis or hypohidrosis may be present. The symptoms and signs may spread proximally, and infrequently may involve other extremities. Impairment of motor function is frequently seen.

Associated Symptoms and Signs

Atrophy of the skin, nails, and other soft tissues, alterations in hair growth, and loss of joint mobility may occur. Impairment of motor function may include weakness, tremor, and in rare instances, dystonia. The symptoms and signs may fluctuate. Sympathetically maintained pain may be present. Affective disorders appear. Guarding of the affected part is usually found.

Laboratory Findings

Noncontact measurement of skin temperature indicates a side-to-side asymmetry of greater than 1.1°C. Because of the unstable nature of the temperature changes in this disorder, measurements at different times are recommended. Testing of sudomotor function both at rest and evoked indicates side-to-side asymmetry. The bone uptake phase with three-phase bone scan reveals a characteristic pattern of periarticular uptake. Radiographic examination may demonstrate patchy bone demineralization.

Usual Course

Variable.

Relief

In cases with sympathetically maintained pain, sympatholytic interventions may provide temporary or permanent pain relief.

Complications

Phlebitis, inappropriate drug use, and suicide.

Social and Physical Impairment

Inability to perform activities of daily living and occupational and recreational activities.

Pathology

Unknown.

Diagnostic Criteria

1. The presence of continuing pain, allodynia, or hyperalgesia after a nerve injury, not necessarily limited to the distribution of the injured nerve.
2. Evidence at some time of edema, changes in skin blood flow, or abnormal sudomotor activity in the region of the pain.
3. This diagnosis is excluded by the existence of conditions that would otherwise account for the degree of pain and dysfunction.

Note: All three criteria must be satisfied.

Differential Diagnosis

CRPS Type I (Reflex Sympathetic Dystrophy), unrecognized local pathology (e.g., fracture, strain, sprain), traumatic vasospasm, cellulitis, Raynaud's disease, thromboangiitis obliterans, thrombosis.

Code

207.X1h	Arms
607.X1h	Legs

Central Pain (I-6)

Definition

Regional pain caused by a primary lesion or dysfunction in the central nervous system, usually associated with abnormal sensibility to temperature and to noxious stimulation.

Site

The regional distribution of the pain correlates neuro-anatomically with the location of the lesion in the brain and spinal cord. It may include all or most of one side, all parts of the body caudal to a level (like the lower half of the body), or both extremities on one side. It may also be restricted simply to the face or part of one extremity.

System

Central nervous system.

Main Features

Age of Onset: all ages may be affected. The onset may be instantaneous, but usually occurs after a delay of weeks or months, rarely a few years, and the pain increases gradually. *Pain Quality*: many different qualities of pain occur, the most common being burning, aching, pricking, and lancinating. Often the patient experiences more than one kind of pain. Dysesthesias are common. The pain is usually spontaneous and continuous, and exacerbated or evoked by somatic stimuli such as light touch, heat, cold, or movement. Some patients have no pain at rest, but suffer from evoked pain, paresthesias, and dysesthesias. The pain can be augmented by startle stimuli (e.g., sudden sound or light), by visceral activity (e.g., micturition), or by anxiety and emotional arousal. The pain may be superficial or deep. *Intensity*: varies from mild but irritating to intolerable.

Associated Symptoms and Signs

There may be various neurological symptoms and signs such as monoparesis, hemiparesis, or paraparesis, together with somatosensory abnormalities in the affected areas. Impaired sensibility for temperature and noxious stimulation are leading signs. Increased threshold for at least one modality is most common, and this is frequently accompanied by dysesthetic or painful reactions to somatic stimuli, particularly touch and cold. Such reactions commonly meet the criteria for allodynia, hyperalgesia, and hyperpathia. In some patients it is difficult to show the altered sensibility with standard clinical tests. The threshold for tactile, vibration, and kinesthetic sensibility may be increased or normal.

Laboratory Findings

MRI or CT may show a relevant lesion.

Usual Course

In some cases, improvement occurs with time, but in most patients the pain persists.

Relief

TENS may give relief in a few patients but can also transiently exacerbate the pain. Anticonvulsant drugs help in some instances, especially carbamazepine and particularly for paroxysmal elements of the pain. Certain antidepressants (e.g., amitriptyline) seem to give the best relief, and some think that phenothiazines (e.g., chlorpromazine, fluphenazine) may be helpful.

Social and Physical Disabilities

This pain is a great physical and psychological burden to most patients. In consequence, their social life and work are often much impaired. Allodynia in response to external stimuli and movements may hamper rehabilitation and prevent activities, thus making the patient physically handicapped.

Pathology

Cerebrovascular lesions (infarcts, hemorrhages), multiple sclerosis, and spinal cord injuries are the most common causes. Central pain is also common in syringomyelia, syringobulbia, and spinal vascular malformation, and may occur after operations like cordotomy. Increasing evidence indicates that central pain only occurs in patients who have lesions affecting the spino-thalamocortical pathways, which are important for temperature and pain sensibility. The lesion can be located at any level along the neuraxis, from the dorsal horn of the spinal cord to the cerebral cortex. The lesion sometimes may involve the medial lemniscal pathways.

Diagnostic Criteria

Regional pain attributable to a lesion or disease in the central nervous system and accompanied by abnormal sensibility for temperature and pain, most often hyperpathia.

Differential Diagnosis

Nociceptive, peripheral neurogenic, and psychiatric causes of pain should be excluded as far as possible. Sensory abnormalities will in most cases allow a diagnosis for positive reasons.

Code

If three or more major sites are involved, code first digit as 9:

903.X5c	Vascular
903.X1c	Trauma
903.X2c	Infection
903.X3c	Inflammatory
903.X4c	Neoplasm
903.X8c	Unknown

If only one or two sites are involved, code first digit according to specific site or sites; for example, for head or face, code 003.X5c.

Syndrome of Syringomyelia (I-7)

Definition

Aching or burning pain usually in a limb, commonly with muscle wasting due to tubular cavitation gradually developing in the spinal cord.

Site

Pain in shoulder, arm, chest, or leg, rarely in the face, occasionally bilateral.

System

Central nervous system.

Main Features

Pain is usually unilateral and continuous in an area that corresponds to the site of cavitation of spinal cord or brainstem, most frequently in the shoulder-girdle and arm. It may be a periodic diffuse dull ache but sometimes, and particularly when the pain is situated in forearm and hand, may have an intense burning quality. The pain may be severe and referred to deep structures in the limb, not responding to rest or minor sedation.

Associated Symptoms

Muscular weakness in affected region.

Signs

There is commonly muscle-wasting beginning in small muscles of the hand and ascending to the forearm and shoulder-girdle with fasciculation and an early loss of tendon reflexes. Scoliosis kyphosis may occur. Characteristically, pain and temperature sensations are impaired but other sensations are intact. The area of sensory impairment typically has a shawl distribution over the front and back of the upper thorax. A Horner's syndrome may appear.

Usual Course

The disease usually begins in the second or third decade and slowly progresses.

Social and Physical Disability

The disease may be present for 15 to 20 years, progressing slowly, but still compatible with an active, self-supporting life. After 15 or 20 years the problems of pain, weakness, and general infirmity usually result in increasing invalidism, eventually leading to total dependency.

Pathology

A tubular cavitation develops slowly in the spinal cord, extending over many segments. The most common location is in the lower cervical cord near the central canal. There is loss of anterior horn cells and interruption of spinothalamic fibers. The cavity may be lined by a thick layer of glial tissue. Cavities may be bilateral and asymmetric and may communicate with an enlarged central canal. Ascent of the cavity into the brain stem produces syringobulbia. The canal may extend the entire length of the cord. Associated findings may be ectopic cerebellar tonsils, hydrocephalus, cerebellar hypoplasia, and astrocytoma or ependymoma of the spinal cord.

Essential Features

Pain in the relevant distribution of slowly progressing muscle weakness and wasting and impairment of sensation to pinprick and temperature, while other sensory modalities remain intact.

Differential Diagnosis

Other conditions which have to be considered are: (1) amyotrophic lateral sclerosis, (2) multiple sclerosis, (3) tumor of the spinal cord, (4) skeletal anomalies of the cervical spine, (5) platybasia, and (6) cervical spondylosis.

Code

007.X0	Face
207.X0	Arm
607.X0	Leg

Polymyalgia Rheumatica (I-8)

Definition

Diffuse aching, and usually stiffness, in neck, hip-girdle, or shoulder-girdle, usually associated with a markedly raised sedimentation rate, sometimes associated with giant cell vasculitis, and promptly responsive to steroids.

System

Musculoskeletal system.

Main Features

Incidence about 54 per 100,000 in those over 30 years of age. Deep muscular aching pain usually begins in the neck, shoulder-girdle, and upper arms, but may only involve the pelvis and proximal parts of the thighs. Morning stiffness and stiffness after inactivity are prominent features.

Associated Symptoms

Malaise, fatigue, depression, low-grade fever, weight loss, and giant cell arteritis.

Aggravating Factors

Movement.

Signs

No muscle tenderness or weakness.

Laboratory Findings

Anemia of chronic disease, raised sedimentation rate (usually greater than 50 mm/hour Westergren).

Relief

Dramatic response to oral corticosteroids, usually in low doses, e.g., 5–20 mg prednisone daily.

Complications

Blindness from giant cell arteritis.

Pathology

Giant cell vasculitis.

Essential Features

Diffuse pain with malaise, elevated sedimentation rate, response to steroids.

Diagnostic Criteria

1. Symmetrical proximal limb myalgia and severe stiffness.
2. Symptoms lasting longer than two weeks.
3. Age of onset: 50 years or older.
4. Erythrocyte sedimentation rate (Westergren) 40 mm or higher.
5. Morning stiffness exceeding one hour.

The diagnosis is to be made if three or more of the above criteria are present, or if one of the above criteria and pathologic evidence of giant cell arteritis is present.

Differential Diagnosis

Polymyositis, fibrositis, hyperthyroidism.

Code

X32.X3a

REFERENCES

Bird H.A., Esselinkcz, W., Dixon, A.St.J., Mowat, A.G., and Wood, P.H.N.: An evaluation of criteria for polymyalgia rheumatica. Ann. Rheum. Dis., *38:* 434, 1979.

Ayoub, W.T., Franklin, C.M., and Torretti, D.: Polymyalgia rheumatica: duration of therapy and long-term outcome. Am. J. Med., *37*: 309, 1985.

Fibromyalgia (or Fibrositis) (I–9)

N.B.: We consider Myofascial Pain Syndrome (diffuse or not) to have a somewhat different meaning and think it adds confusion to use the term when discussing fibromyalgia.

Definition

Diffuse musculoskeletal aching and pain with multiple predictable tender points.

Site

Multiple anatomic areas.

System

Musculoskeletal system (muscles, ligaments, tendons, joints).

Main Features

Primary fibromyalgia, without important associated disease, is uncommon compared to concomitant fibromyalgia. It may occur in childhood but is most common in the fourth and fifth decades. The sex ratio is 6:1 female to male. Concomitant fibromyalgia occurs with any other musculoskeletal condition, where it may act to intensify the pain of the associated condition. The syndrome is chronic, and remissions are uncommon. *Pain*: Widespread aching of more than three months' duration, often poorly circumscribed and perceived as deep, usually referred to muscle or bony prominences. Most common areas are cervical, thoracic, and lumbar. Although pain in the trunk and proximal girdle is aching, distal limb pain is often perceived as associated with swelling, numbness, or stiff feeling. Day-to-day fluctuation in pain intensity and shifting from one area to another are characteristic, although the pain is usually continuous. Stiffness is present in 80% and is perceived as an increased resistance to joint movement, particularly toward the end of the range of movement. Both pain and stiffness are maximal within the broad sclerotomic and myotomic areas of reference of the lower segments of the cervical and lumbar spine. *Fatigue* is present in 80%, and is often severe enough to interfere with daily activities. Sleep disturbance is present in 75%, and waking is unrefreshed or tired. *Multiple tender points*: Discrete local areas of deep tenderness widely dispersed throughout the body and involving a variety of otherwise normal tissues are a pathognomonic feature provided about 60% of examined sites are tender. Tender points are found within muscle and over tendons, muscle insertions, and bony prominences. Tender point sites are "tender" in many normal individuals but are reported as "painful," often with grimace or withdrawal when palpated, in those with fibromyalgia. The predictable location of these tender points and their multiplicity are essential features of the syndrome.

Associated Symptoms and Signs

Paresthesias: Most often involving the upper extremities, are found in 60%.

Headaches: Noted in 53%.

Irritable Bowel Syndrome: Noted in 30%.

Anxiety: Noted in 48%.

Skinfold Tenderness: The rolling of the skin and subcutaneous tissues of the upper scapula region between the examiner's thumb and index finger elicits tenderness in 60%.

Reactive Hyperemia: Redness of the skin developing after palpation of tender points over the trapezius and contiguous regions is found in half the patients.

Autonomic Phenomena: Reactive hyperemia is the most commonly recognized feature, but temperature changes and mild soft tissue swelling involving the distal upper extremities are also frequently reported.

Aggravating and Relieving Features

Cold, poor sleep, anxiety, humidity, weather change, fatigue, and mental stress intensify symptoms in 60% to 70%. Symptoms are typically made worse or brought on by prolonged or vigorous work activity. Warmth (78%) temporarily improves symptoms.

Signs

Tender points, widely and symmetrically distributed, are the characteristic sign of the syndrome. They are not found in other musculoskeletal syndromes.

Relief

Relief may be provided by reassurance and explanation about the nature of the syndrome and possible mechanisms of pain: anxiety may thus be reduced, expensive and hazardous investigations and treatments limited, and use of medication reduced. Low-dose amitriptyline, cyclobenzaprine, and aerobic exercise have been shown, in placebo controlled, double-blind studies, to improve symptoms.

Pathology

Nonspecific muscle changes have been found in some biopsy studies. Blood flow during exercise is reduced, and decreased oxygen uptake in muscles has been noted. Two studies have found increased levels of substance P in the cerebrospinal fluid of patients. In general, these findings, some of which may be secondary phenomena, have been insufficient to explain the major signs and symptoms of the syndrome.

Etiology

Unknown. The syndrome may begin in childhood or early life without obvious association. It also is noted frequently following trauma, and has been known to develop after apparent viral illness. Finally, it may appear insidiously in later life. Thus the syndrome may be the final common pathway, perhaps as hyperalgesia, for a number of causative factors. Trauma or degenerative changes in the cervical or lumbar regions might precipitate the syndrome. Intrinsic changes in levels of neurotransmitters might play a factor. A syndrome similar to fibromyalgia can be induced temporarily with experimental reduction in non-REM sleep. Low-grade symptoms may be increased by mental stress or fatigue. An association with *previous* major depression in patients and families has suggested a genetic factor.

Classification Criteria for Primary and Concomitant Fibromyalgia (from Wolfe et al. 1990)

1. History of Widespread Pain

Definition

Pain is considered widespread when all of the following are present: pain in the left side of the body, pain in the right side of the body, pain above the waist and below the waist. In addition, axial skeletal pain (cervical spine or anterior chest or thoracic spine or low back) must be present. In this definition, shoulder and buttock pain is considered as pain for each involved side. "Low-back" pain is considered lower segment pain.

2. Pain in 11 of 18 Tender Point Sites on Digital Palpation

Definition

Pain, on digital palpation, must be present in at least 11 of the following 18 tender point sites:

Occiput: bilateral, at the suboccipital muscle insertions.
Low Cervical: bilateral, at the anterior aspects of the intertransverse spaces at C5-C7.
Trapezius: bilateral, at origins above the scapula spine near the medial border.
Supraspinatus: bilateral at origins above the scapula spine near the medial border.
Second Rib: bilateral, at the second costochondral junctions, just lateral to the junctions on upper surfaces.
Lateral Epicondyle: bilateral, 2 cm distal to the epicondyles.
Gluteal: bilateral, in upper outer quadrants of buttocks in anterior fold of muscle.
Greater Trochanter: bilateral, posterior to the trochanteric prominence.
Knees: bilateral, at the medial fat pad proximal to the joint line.

Digital palpation should be performed with an approximate force of 4 kg.

For a tender point to be considered "positive," the subject must state that the palpation was painful. "Tender" is not to be considered painful.

For classification purposes, patients will be said to have fibromyalgia if both criteria are satisfied. Widespread pain must have been present for at least three months. The presence of a second clinical disorder does not exclude the diagnosis of fibromyalgia.

Code

X33.X8a

REFERENCES

Wolfe, F., Smythe, H.A., Yunus, M.B., *et al.:* The American College of Rheumatology 1990 criteria for the classification of fibromyalgia: report of the Multicenter Criteria Committee. Arthritis Rheum., *33:* 160, 1990.

Bennett, R.M. and Goldenberg, D.L. (eds.): The fibromyalgia syndrome, Rheumatic Disease Clinics of North America. Vol. 15. No. 1. Philadelphia, W.B. Saunders, 1989.

Note: Specific Myofascial Pain Syndromes

Synonyms: fibrositis (syndrome), myalgia, muscular rheumatism, nonarticular rheumatism.

Specific myofascial syndromes may occur in any voluntary muscle with referred pain, local and referred tenderness, and a tense shortened muscle. The pain has the same qualities as that of the diffuse syndromes. Passive stretch or strong voluntary contraction in the shortened position of the muscle is painful. Satellite tender points may develop within the area of pain reference of the initial trigger point. Other phenomena resemble those of the diffuse syndromes. Diagnosis depends upon the demonstration of a trigger point (tender point) and reproduction of the pain by maneuvers which place stress upon proximal structures or nerve roots. This suggests that the syndrome is an epiphenomenon secondary to proximal pathology such as nerve root irritation. Relief may be obtained by stretch and spray techniques, tender point compression, or tender point injection including the use of "dry" needling.

Some individual syndromes are described here, e.g., sternocleidomastoid and trapezius. Others may be coded as required according to individual muscles that are identified as being a site of trouble.

Rheumatoid Arthritis (I-10)

Definition

Aching, burning joint pain due to systemic inflammatory disease affecting all synovial joints, muscle, ligaments, and tendons in accordance with diagnostic criteria below.

Site

Symmetrical involvement of small and large joints.

System

Musculoskeletal system and connective tissue.

Main Features

Diffuse aching, burning pain in joints, usually moderately severe; usually intermittent with exacerbations and remissions. The condition affects about 1% of the population and is more common in women. Diagnostic criteria of the American Rheumatism Association describe and further define the illness. They are as follows: (1) morning stiffness, (2) pain on motion or tenderness at one joint or more, (3) swelling of one joint, (4) swelling of at least one other joint, and (5) symmetrical joint swelling.

All of the above have to be of at least six weeks' duration. Further criteria include: (6) subcutaneous nodules, (7) typical radiographic changes, (8) positive test for rheumatoid factor in the serum, (9) a poor response in the mucin clot test in the synovial fluid, (10) synovial histopathology consistent with rheumatoid arthritis, and (11) characteristic nodule pathology.

Classical rheumatoid arthritis requires seven criteria to be diagnosed. Definite rheumatoid arthritis may be diagnosed on five criteria, and probable rheumatoid arthritis on three criteria.

Associated Symptoms

Morning stiffness usually greater than half an hour's duration; chronic fatigue. Inflammation may affect eyes, heart, lungs.

Signs

Tenderness, swelling, loss of range of motion of joints, ligaments, tendons. Chronic destruction and joint deformity are common.

Laboratory Findings

Anemia, raised ESR (erythrocyte sedimentation rate), rheumatoid factor in the serum in the majority of cases.

Relief

Usually good relief of pain and stiffness can be obtained with nonsteroidal anti-inflammatory drugs, but some patients require therapy with gold or other agents.

Pathology

Chronic inflammatory process of synovium, ligaments, or tendons. There may be systemic vasculitis.

Essential Features

Aching, burning joint pain with characteristic pathology.

Diagnostic Criteria

1. Morning stiffness in and around joints lasting at least one hour before maximal improvement.

Editors' Note: The foregoing represents only a selection of the many Chronic Pain Syndromes in the *Classification of Chronic Pain, 2nd Edition* (IASP Press, 1994). The reader is encouraged to consult the source document.

Neural Blockade in Clinical Anesthesia and Management of Pain, Third Edition,
edited by M.J. Cousins and P.O. Bridenbaugh.
Lippincott–Raven Publishers, Philadelphia © 1998.

CHAPTER 23.2

Introduction to Pain in Pediatric and Neonatal Patients

Suellen M. Walker

The management of pain in pediatric practice has expanded, and has undergone marked changes in recent years. It is now well accepted that neonates and infants not only are developmentally capable of responding to painful stimuli, but that untreated pain may have detrimental short- and long-term effects. Tools are available for assessment of pain in children at differing developmental stages, and the measurement of pain is becoming part of routine 'vital observations.' Increased knowledge of the pharmacokinetics and pharmacodynamics of local anesthetics in infants and children, the development of acute pain services, increased training of medical and nursing staff in pain management, and improved monitoring, have all contributed to the safe adoption of neural blockade techniques such as epidural infusions for pediatric patients.

DEFINITION

The definition of pain by the International Association for the Study of Pain (IASP) refers to the sensory and emotional experience of pain, which is described by the patient in terms relating to actual or potential tissue damage. The applicability of this definition in neonates and preverbal or developmentally delayed children who are not capable of self-report has been questioned recently.[3] Even in older children, the relationship between experiencing and reporting pain will be influenced by the developmental stage of the child, the person eliciting the self-report and the method used, and the individual's perception of the consequences of reporting pain.[3]

In the absence of self-report of pain, evidence for the perception and subsequent response to painful stimuli has been based on physiological[1,29,32] and behavioral studies.[49,79] Both areas of study show responses early in life, even in very premature infants, suggesting that the sensation of pain requires no previous experience and appears early, as it is an important signaling system for tissue damage.[3] Both functional and behavioral responses undergo ongoing modification as experience increases.

DEVELOPMENT OF NOCICEPTION

Study of development of pain mechanisms and responses to noxious stimuli in animal and human models has important implications in the management of pain. It is now well established that nociception occurs in neonates, and untreated pain has harmful effects. Our understanding of pain patterns seen in the adult can also be enhanced by an appreciation of the development of nociception, particularly the importance of inhibitory mechanisms, and the impact of interconnections between A fibers and C fibers in the dorsal horn.

Nociceptive Processing

The anatomical, functional, and neurochemical mechanisms for nociceptive processing are present in neonates. The time frame of the structural development of pain pathways has been summarized by Fitzgerald[29,31] and Anand,[1] and is depicted schematically in Figure 23.2-1. Cutaneous sensory receptors appear in the perioral area at 7 weeks' gestation, spread to the hands and feet by 11 weeks, and to all cutaneous and mucous surfaces by 20 weeks' gestation. At 13 weeks, dorsal horn development commences, with the laminar arrangement, synaptic interconnections, and neurotransmitter vesicles being present by 30 weeks. As connections between the thalamus and neocortex develop, between 20 to 24 weeks, cortical perception of pain may be present even in the smallest premature infant.[47] Functional maturity of the cerebral cortex is suggested by fetal and neonatal elec-

S.M. Walker: Department of Anaesthesia and Pain Management, Royal North Shore Hospital; and Pain Management and Research Centre, University of Sydney, St. Leonards, New South Wales 2065 Australia.

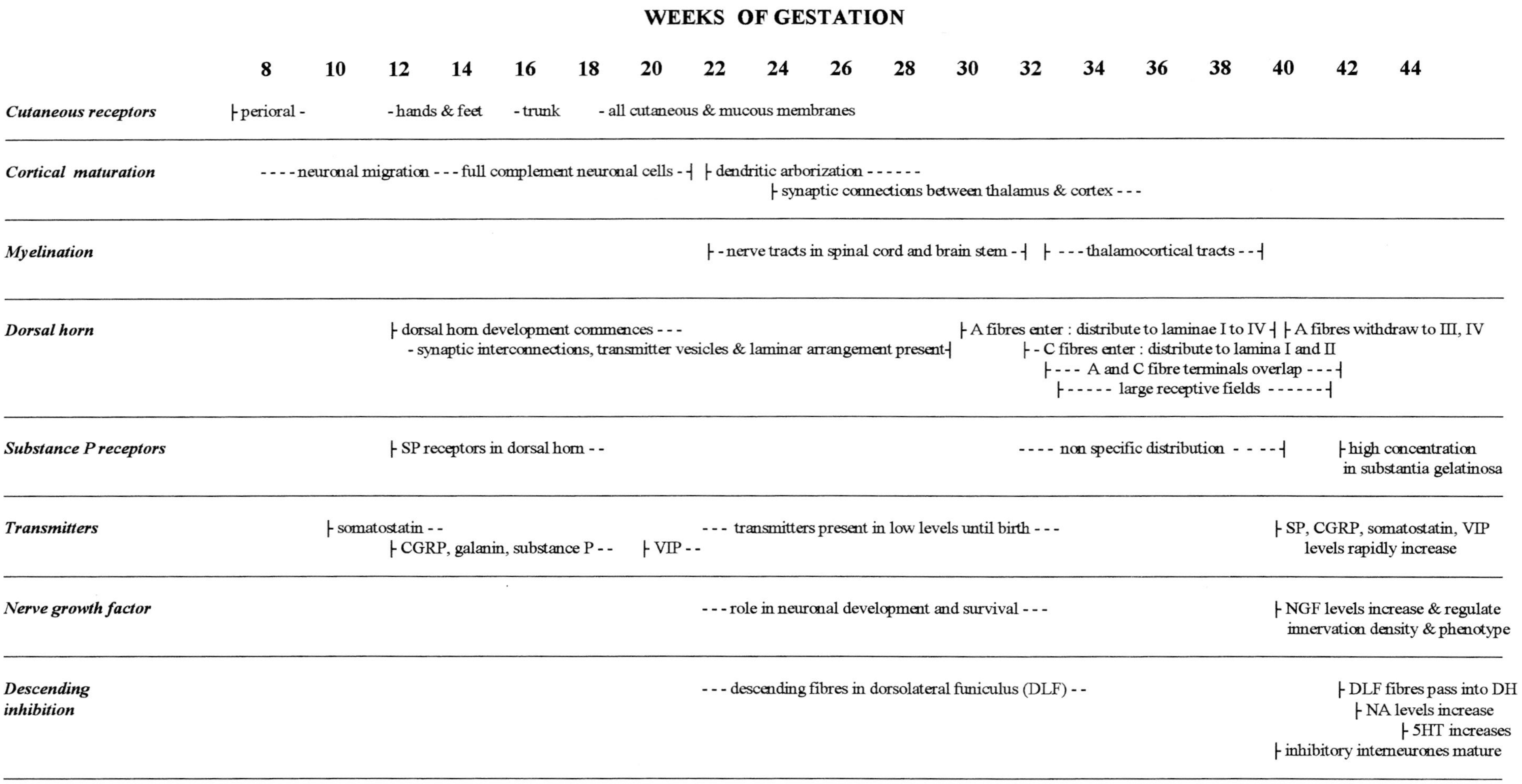

FIG. 23.2-1. Schematic diagram of the development of nociceptive mechanisms in the fetus and neonate.[2,29,30,31,33,34] Nociceptive pathways begin to develop early in fetal life; all anatomical and neurochemical components are present well before full term at 40 weeks; and further differentiation and modulation occurs in the early postnatal period. *SP,* substance P; *CGRP,* calcitonin gene-related peptide; *VIP,* vasoactive intestinal peptide; *NGF,* nerve growth factor; *DLF,* dorsolateral funiculus; *NA,* noradrenaline/norepinephrine; *5HT,* serotonin; *DH,* dorsal horn.

troencephalographic patterns (bilateral synchronous activity from 26 weeks), high levels of cerebral glucose utilization in sensory areas, and behavioral activity (periods of sleep and wakefulness occur from 28 weeks).[1]

Immature myelination previously was equated with reduced pain perception; however, the slower conduction is offset by the shorter axonal length to be travelled by nerve impulses in the small body of the infant. During the second trimester, nerve tracts in the spinal cord become myelinated, by 30 weeks pain pathways to brain stem and thalamus are completely myelinated, and thalamocortical pain fibers are myelinated by 37 weeks' gestation.[29]

Considerable growth and reorganization of pain pathways occurs in the neonatal period.[30]

Peripheral Mechanisms

Polymodal nociceptors responding to intense mechanical, thermal, and chemical stimuli are present at birth, as are high- and low-threshold mechanoreceptors, although the latter are initially less mature.[36] Despite having established sensory receptor properties at birth, C fibers initially are unable to produce neurogenic edema, which may reflect the low levels of substance P and calcitonin gene-related peptide (CGRP) released by C fibers in the early postnatal period.[29] There is poor recruitment of blood-borne inflammatory cells and the local inflammatory response is immature. Local resident macrophages play a more important role in neonatal inflammation, and as these cells are capable of releasing cytokines and growth factors (including nerve growth factor [NGF]) the normal development of sensory innervation may be affected in areas of inflammation.[29]

Dorsal Horn Mechanisms

The laminar arrangement of the dorsal horn undergoes significant changes in early postnatal life. Large-diameter cutaneous A-fibers enter the dorsal horn, and initially their terminals extend dorsally from lamina V through to laminae I and II.[33] Afferent C fibers then enter the dorsal horn and terminate in the substantia gelatinosa, and for several weeks occupy laminae I and II with A fibers. This overlap is increased after neonatal sciatic nerve section in rats, as both axotomized A fibers and invading intact A fibers sprout dorsally into denervated substantia gelatinosa.[76] C fibers initially are electrophysiologically and neurochemically immature and produce only sub-threshold depolarizations in the spinal cord. However, noxious mechanical stimulation or non-specific chemical irritants which activate afferent A fibers produce reflex activity at this stage.[30] As C fibers mature postnatally, the A fibers withdraw to a more restricted distribution in laminae III and IV.[33]

The neurotransmitters glutamate and substance P are colocalized in C-fiber terminals in the dorsal horn, and although they are present early in fetal life, the levels are low at first.[31] The synaptic activity of C fibers matures during the first two postnatal weeks, as levels of transmitters (SP, CGRP, somatostatin, and vasoactive intestinal peptide [VIP] increase in the dorsal horn, and substance P receptors move from an initial nonspecific distribution to reach a high concentration in the substantia gelatinosa.[1] Initially, N-methyl-D-aspartate (NMDA) receptors are also widely distributed through the dorsal horn. Early in postnatal life, the affinity of NMDA receptors for glutamate and the increase in intracellular calcium which follows NMDA activation are increased. Thus, NMDA-mediated wind-up and central sensitization may be even more apparent in the neonate.[30] The lowering of cutaneous thresholds in infants undergoing repeated procedures in intensive care[5,35] may, in part, reflect changes in central excitability.[5]

Inhibitory Nociceptive Mechanisms

Dorsal horn inhibitory mechanisms (both descending and interneuronal) are poorly developed at birth. Local inhibitory mechanisms in the dorsal horn are immature at birth as inhibitory interneurons are the last fibers to develop, enkephalin levels are low, and opioid receptor sensitivity is initially low (but increases 3-fold in the first two weeks after birth[1]). Receptive fields are large as A-β afferents are not restricted to laminae III and IV of the dorsal horn, but extend dorsally up to laminae 1 and II.[5,33] The descending inhibitory pathways pass in the dorsolateral funiculus which is present early in fetal life, but connections into the dorsal horn do not develop until 10 to 19 days after birth.[34] In addition, levels of the inhibitory pathway transmitters, noradrenaline and serotonin, are initially low.[5] GABA and glycine are inhibitory transmitters in adults (see Chapter 23.1), but can depolarize immature spinal neurones causing increases in intracellular calcium[73] and therefore may have an excitatory action in neonates. Lack of inhibition results in exaggerated and generalized responses to both low- and high-threshold sensory inputs, which gradually become more specific as the nervous system matures.[5,31]

Inhibition suppresses excitatory mechanisms that may reemerge later in life under pathological conditions.[30] In adults, following central sensitization, nociception can be evoked by innocuous or A-β afferent inputs resulting in allodynia (see Chapter 23.1). This is the *usual* situation in the neonate, because the flexion reflex can be activated by noxious and non-noxious stimuli initially, and only later becomes more specific. The sprouting of A fibers into more superficial laminae of the dorsal horn following nerve injury in adults[92] may reflect the early developmental interaction at this site.

Immediate Responses to Noxious Stimuli

Physiological and Biological Responses

Nociception results in immediate physiological, humoral, and immune responses in the neonate, which may be associated with harmful effects. Increase in heart rate, blood pressure and intracranial pressure, and decreases in transcutaneous PO_2 occur during painful procedures in neonates, but can be reduced with adequate analgesia.[2,8] A marked stress response to surgery, with increases in cortisol, catecholamines, aldosterone, glucagon and other steroid hormones, has been shown in neonates undergoing surgery with inadequate anesthesia. Neonates receiving deep anesthesia had decreased morbidity (related to sepsis, metabolic acidosis, disseminated intravascular coagulation) and also decreased mortality.[2]

Behavioral Responses

Clinicians often rely on interpretation of overt behaviors to indicate the presence and severity of a patient's pain; particularly in neonates, infants, and young children. Behavioral responses (facial actions, cry characteristics, body movements, and posture) incorporate many inputs,[7,79] and only indirectly reflect pain experience; it may be difficult to differentiate pain from generalized distress. However, clear differences in behavioral and physiological responses to tissue damage and handling have been shown (e.g., real versus sham heel stick[50,51]). In preterm infants, responses become more recognizable with increasing gestational age; specific facial expressions and increases in heart rate are seen in infants from as young as 26 to 28 weeks.[22,50,51] The cutaneous thresholds for flexor withdrawal reflexes are very low in preterm infants, and receptive fields are large. With increasing gestational age, the cutaneous threshold increases and receptive fields reduce in size.[5] In term neonates, responses are still generalized, but within the first two to three postnatal weeks, specific nociceptive responses that are only elicited by high intensity stimuli become apparent. Thus, behavioral responses vary depending on the developmental stage of the child, and can be correlated with our knowledge of the developing pain transmission system. Generalized responses to both low-and high-threshold stimuli in preterm and term neonates may reflect the lack of local and descending inhibitory mechanisms and the widespread distribution of receptors. Behavioral responses are gradually modified, become more specific, occur in response to higher threshold stimuli, and have more rapid recovery as local and descending inhibitory mechanisms increase. In addition, receptive fields decrease as the distribution of nerve terminals and receptors come to approximate those seen in the adult.

Behavioral responses to neonatal circumcision can be reduced with the use of local anaesthesia.[8,27] Crying and facial actions are reduced during the procedure,[8] but behavioral differences are evident on the following day. Infants receiving a dorsal penile nerve block with lignocaine prior to circumcision remained more attentive and demonstrated a greater ability to quiet themselves, compared to a control group given saline.[27]

Long-Term Effects

Pathophysiological Changes

Inadequately treated pain may lead to long-term pathophysiological effects. Primary afferent activity leads to N-methyl-D-aspartate (NMDA) excitatory postsynaptic potentials which, in neonates, are greater in magnitude and may result in increased development of central sensitization. Induction of the c-fos proto-oncogene, a marker of persistent neuronal changes, can be seen from birth. Increasingly noxious stimuli resulted in increased fos protein, suggesting that expression is proportional to stimulus intensity and duration.[94] Clinically, hyperalgesia has been observed following repeated heel pricks[29] in neonates, and ongoing hypersensitivity and lowered mechanical thresholds have been found in previously injured regions.[30]

Long-term structural and functional reorganization may result from noxious stimuli in neonates. Skin wounds in neonatal rats have been shown to result in hyperinnervation (innervation density increases up to 300%) which persists long after the wound has healed and is associated with reductions in mechanical threshold on behavioral sensory testing.[70] Increases in NGF levels, which are greater than the degree of upregulation seen in adults, occur following skin wounding and may underlie the hyperinnervation.[20] These effects are most marked when the wound is performed in immediate postnatal life, then decline to the weaker and transient effect seen in the adult. Collateral sprouting in the periphery after nerve section is more marked in the neonate[71] and involves not only C fibers as seen in the adult, but also A fiber sprouting.[70] Thus, the plasticity of cutaneous nervous distribution, particularly at critical stages of development, is demonstrated.[70]

Damage to cutaneous sensory axons results in death of dorsal root ganglion cells due to loss of trophic support (NGF), leading to deafferentation in the spinal cord, arrest of second-order neuron growth, and sprouting of neurones from nearby intact fibers. Centrally, collateral sprouting in the dorsal horn after nerve injury is also more marked in the neonate and occurs in both A fibers and C fibers.[30,76] Connections in the thalamus and cortex may be altered, with potential distortion of body map representation.

Behavioral Changes

Early pain experience is one of the many factors affecting the development of pain behaviors. Premature infants who require intensive care undergo a variety of painful procedures including venipuncture, insertion of monitoring lines, intubation, and surgery, which may be performed with inadequate analgesia. These insults occur at varying stages of development of the nociceptive pathways, and premature infants may display long-term behavioral changes in response to subsequent painful stimuli. Extremely low birthweight (ELBW, <1000g) children who required prolonged neonatal intensive care have been shown to have higher somatization (i.e., somatic complaints of unknown origin) compared to matched full-term healthy neonates, when tested at three to four years of age.[42] At 18 months corrected conceptual age, extremely low birth weight toddlers who had required prolonged neonatal intensive care were subjectively rated by parents as less sensitive to pain than a matched group of full birth weight infants.[44] In low and full birth weight infants, pain sensitivity was mainly a function of temperament, but this relationship was not found for ELBW toddlers, suggesting that pain behavior development had been altered.[44]

Prolonged behavioral changes have also been observed following neonatal circumcision performed without analgesia. Circumcised boys had significantly higher observer and behavioral pain scores, and longer crying bouts following routine vaccination at four to six months of age.[82]

Therefore, premature and term neonates and infants are capable of responding to noxious stimuli. This response may initially be generalized, nonspecific, and of high intensity due to the widespread distribution of receptors and slower maturation of inhibitory mechanisms. Pain warrants treatment from a humanitarian view point, but also because short- and long-term morbidity can result if analgesic treatment is inadequate.

ASSESSMENT OF PAIN IN CHILDREN

Pain perception includes not only the sensory responses associated with a noxious stimulus (i.e., nociception), but also an emotional or affective component which contributes to the overall 'pain experience.' Despite an apparent equivalent noxious stimulus, individuals vary in the level of pain experienced depending on their age, gender, cognitive level, previous pain experience, and family and cultural background. Pain perception also is influenced by cognitive factors which include: the child's expectations and understanding of the source of pain and his or her degree of self control; behavioral factors such as the responses of parents or staff and the use of physical restraints; and emotional factors including the level of anxiety, fear, and frustration felt by the child.[58]

All measures of pain or distress are affected by the age and developmental stage of the child. In infants, toddlers, and cognitively impaired children, clinicians must rely on the interpretation of behavioral (verbal, facial, and motor) or physiological responses to presumed painful stimuli. Such measures are affected by the developmental age of the child and by learned responses[7] and provide only indirect or inferential evidence regarding pain experience. Crying may relate to generalized distress, parental separation, or hunger; and an increase in heart rate may be due to other physiological factors, such as sepsis or hypovolemia. As a child develops, changes in cognitive strategies increase their ability to modulate their behavioral response to noxious stimuli.[7] However, children vary in the coping strategies they adopt, which may be passive or avoidant on one hand or active and information seeking on the other, with active coping becoming more likely with increasing age. Children develop a pain 'language' as their vocabulary and experience increases, and can increasingly report the quality and intensity of their pain.[91]

An ideal pain assessment scale should be sensitive to changes in pain intensity, reliable, simple to use for patients and staff, be recorded regularly, and used to direct and assess the efficacy of analgesic interventions. Different scales vary in their ability to fulfill these criteria, and an appropriate tool should be chosen, based on the developmental stage of the child and the required application (e.g., clinical or research purposes).

Pain assessment may be based on recording physiological changes, observing behavior, or on the child's self report of pain.

1. *Physiological methods.* Changes in heart rate, respiratory rate, blood pressure, palmar sweating, transcutaneous oxygen pressure, and adrenocortical hormones have been recorded in association with invasive procedures in infants,[1,2] and the degree of change can be reduced with appropriate use of analgesics. However, physiological changes are nonspecific. A generalized and complex response to "pain stress,"[7] rather than a specific response to pain intensity is inferred, but other factors such as hypovolemia and sepsis will also affect these parameters. Changes in heart rate and blood pressure are useful for detecting acute responses to noxious stimuli in situations where the child is monitored constantly (e.g. neonatal intensive care and intraoperatively), but provide little information about ongoing pain. Measurement of hormone levels does not provide immediate information, and is applicable only in research settings.
2. *Behavioral/Observational methods.* A large number of pain assessment tools have been developed, based on the observed behavioral responses of children to pain. A distinct set of facial changes and characteristics of cry can be recognized in neonates undergoing heel lance.[43] More complex scales involve scoring observed verbal and motor behaviors, and measured parameters, such as heart rate.[53,55,58,59,68] The Observer Pain Scale grades severity from 1 to 5; and in the Objective Pain Scale, five parameters (blood pressure, crying, movement, agitation, and verbal response) are scored as 0, 1, or 2. The Children's Hospital of Eastern Ontario Pain Scale (CHEOPS)[59] scores cry, facial expression, verbal response, torso and leg position, and CRIES[53] (Crying, Requirement for oxygen, Increased vital signs, Expression and Sleeplessness). These scales result in some standardization and provide a guide for parameters to be included in assessment. Clinically, the child's family or guardian provide additional information about the usual behavioral responses of the child, and can often grade pain as absent, mild, moderate, or severe. Some children become withdrawn and quiet in response to pain, particularly in a hospital environment, and may be assessed

incorrectly. Children may not exhibit distress in direct proportion to the intensity of their pain,[58] and consolability is an important factor to include, in an effort to discriminate pain behaviors from hunger or separation anxieties.[55]

3. *Direct report methods.* Children as young as three years can report the level of their pain if tools are geared to their developmental stage and language skills.[68] Examples include selecting the number of poker chips, or choosing the face from a series of photographs,[6] or line drawings,[13] which correlate with their perceived pain intensity. It should not be assumed that faces scales represent a linear relationship, and there may be confusion between the sensory and affective components of pain.[55] Toddlers can verbalize 'hurt,' and as the child becomes older he or she can increasingly describe not only the unpleasant aspect of pain, but also its sensory attributes (quality, duration, intensity, location). Visual analog scales with a line from no-pain to worst-pain experienced can be used in older children. More recently, colored analog scales with blue at the no-pain end, ranging to red at the severe-pain end of the scale, have been validated.[58]

Because so many assessment tools are available, it is important that each institution has a protocol for the measure it chooses to use; and determines that staff are adequately trained to ensure reliable measurement and interpretation of pain scores. In a study following tonsillectomy, behavioral assessment (CHEOPS) was found to be more reliable than self-report (Oucher) in the postanesthesia recovery room, due to residual effects of general anesthesia. However, when patients returned to the day surgery unit, self-report was more accurate.[81] Thus a tool must be chosen which is appropriate for the developmental stage of the child, and for the setting in which it is used.

NEURAL BLOCKADE IN CHILDREN: CLINICAL ISSUES

Postoperative Pain

Peripheral nerve blocks are used frequently in pediatric practice to provide perioperative analgesia and reduce general anesthetic requirements (see Chapter 20). Polymer matrices incorporated with bupivacaine are being developed which provide sustained release of local anesthetic. This preparation has the potential to provide prolonged reversible blockade of peripheral nerves following a single injection or application.[56]

Epidural Analgesia

The caudal epidural space is easy to reach in children, by injection through the sacrococcygeal ligament, and single-dose perioperative injections of local anesthetic have a long history of use in pediatric practice (see Chapter 20). Recognition of the benefits of regional anesthesia in providing postoperative pain relief, increased knowledge of the pharmacology of local anesthetics in children, and the availability of smaller epidural needles and catheters has led to an increase in the use of epidural infusion techniques in children. Safe adoption of perioperative epidural analgesia for children requires experienced anesthetists, excellently trained recovery room and ward staff, adequate follow-up and monitoring in the ward, and the availability of specialized staff, both for consultation and to manage complications.

Local Anesthetics

Long-acting local anesthetics such as bupivacaine are most often used to provide perioperative regional anesthesia. An appropriate volume and concentration of local anesthetic must be selected for each patient, based on the weight of the child, type of surgery (site and duration), desired density of block, and postoperative requirements for analgesia. Local anesthetic toxicity in children may result from inadvertent intravascular or intraosseous injection, or the use of greater than recommended doses.[93] After a loading dose of 2 to 2.5 mg/kg of bupivacaine, infusion rates of 0.4 to 0.5 mg/kg/hr for older infants and children, and 0.2 to 0.25 mg/kg/hr for neonates have been recommended.[9,23,25,26] Retropleural[84] or interpleural[39,78,88] local anesthetic has been used in children and neonates to provide analgesia following thoracotomy. As with epidural blockade, local anesthetic toxicity is a potential complication, particularly in low birthweight neonates,[39] and care must be taken with bolus and infusion dosages.

Adrenaline (Epinephrine)

The addition of adrenaline to local anesthetic solutions reduces the peak plasma concentration of bupivacaine following single caudal injections, and prolongs the duration of analgesia (particularly in younger children).[87] However, the risk of arrhythmias may be increased following intravascular injection, if the local anesthetic solution contains adrenaline.[38,85,87] Adrenaline-containing solutions often are used for epidural test-doses in adults, because intravascular injection of small volumes is detected by an increase in heart rate. This indicator has been found to be unreliable in children anesthetized with halothane. Intravenous atropine 10 μg/kg five minutes before injection of a test dose of lignocaine with adrenaline 1:200,000 (5 μg/ml) resulted in an earlier and greater increase in heart rate (18 versus 10 beats/minute), and thus may improve the ability to detect intravascular injection with adrenaline-containing solutions.[24] Isoproterenol has also been suggested as an additive to epidural local anesthetic to provide an indicator of intravascular injection. A mean maximum increase of 21.5 +/− 9.5 beats per minute following intravenous 0.075 μg/kg isoproterenol was seen in 22 of 23 children during halothane anesthesia.[67] However, further studies of neural toxicity of isoproterenol and dose-response evaluation are required before these results can be extrapolated to epidural injection.

Non-opioid Spinal Analgesics

Increased knowledge of the physiology and pharmacology of pain transmission in the spinal cord (see Chapter 23.1) has increased the range of analgesic agents being administered intrathecally or epidurally. Combining such agents with local anesthetic solutions may reduce the concentration of local anesthetic required (thus reducing the potential for urinary retention and motor block) and/or increase the duration of analgesia. It must be remembered that the toxicology of many agents by epidural administration is not fully elucidated. Also, many trials are conducted in patients undergoing procedures such as inguinal hernia repair, in whom analgesia could be provided by a less invasive ilioinguinal/iliohypogastric nerve block, or by surgical infiltration of the wound with local anesthetic. The ratio of risk-to-benefit of new therapies requires careful study before general application in pediatric practice.[41]

Administration of *morphine* by a single caudal epidural injection provides prolonged analgesia (10 to 14 hours), but has the potential to cause delayed respiratory depression, vomiting, and pruritus.[52] The high lipid solubility of *fentanyl* results in a short duration of action and segmentalized analgesia following epidural administration. Therefore, this agent is well suited to epidural infusion techniques. Addition of fentanyl (0.4 to 0.6 μg/kg/hr) to local anesthetic infusions reduces the concentration of local anesthetic required and improves the efficacy of analgesia.

Addition of *clonidine* 2 μg/kg to epidural bupivacaine or mepivacaine has been shown to increase the duration of analgesia.[21,48,54] Cardiovascular parameters were not significantly altered by the addition of clonidine, but there was an increased duration of sedation.[48,54]

Caudal administration of *ketamine* 0.5 mg/kg has been shown to provide analgesia when administered alone, and to prolong the duration of analgesia when combined with local anesthetic.[21,65] Caudal midazolam has been compared with bupivacaine 0.25% and a combination of both agents.[64] Although analgesia appeared satisfactory in all groups, there was no clear evidence of an advantage with midazolam.

Epidural Catheters

In young children, catheters introduced via the caudal space can be advanced to the thoracic epidural space. Initially, passage of 18-gauge catheters was described in infants,[16] and more recently 24-gauge catheters *with a stylet* were successfully advanced to the thoracic level (T12 to T6) in children up to 10 years of age.[46] Radiographic examination confirmed passage to the measured spinal level in the majority of cases. Due to the proximity of the anus and risk of infection, care must be taken with the dressing of caudal catheters and their use must be limited to two or three days.[26]

Attempts to advance unstiffened 19-gauge catheters in children aged 0 to 8 years (weight 5 to 38 kg) from *lumbar* (L4–L5) insertion have been shown to be unreliable,[14] as only 22% of catheters reached the desired level (T10–T12). If threading was difficult, catheters did not pass beyond L4–L5; but ease of advancement did not correlate with success in reaching T10–T12. The majority of catheters were found to circle near the point of entry or even to form a figure eight. Catheters must not be threaded against resistance; this may represent impingement against a nerve root, or increase the chance of the catheter kinking or doubling back.[14,16,46]

Choice of Technique

Recent controversies about epidural techniques in children relate to difficulties in detecting intravascular injection in anesthetized children, the use of thoracic epidurals, the risk of neurological problems, and gas embolism using loss of resistance to air.[40]

As epidural needles and catheters are inserted in anesthetized children, lancinating pain or paresthesia as a marker of nerve root irritation is absent. The risk of nerve root damage may be reduced by use of appropriate needles, slow careful insertion, and not injecting against resistance. The procedure should be abandoned if neural injury is suspected, or if undue technical difficulties are encountered.[40] The best method of attaining epidural analgesia of thoracic dermatomes in children remains controversial. The anesthetist must balance the risks of segmental insertion at levels above the termination of the spinal cord in an anesthetised patient against the risks of advancing a catheter which may not reach the desired level, or which may potentially cause nerve root or vascular damage by kinking and circling in the epidural space.

Five cases of serious neurological sequelae were reported in a retrospective questionnaire review of 24,005 pediatric regional anesthetics performed between 1982 and 1991 in 10 French and Belgian institutions.[37] Two patients became tetraplegic and two paraplegic with magnetic resonance image (MRI) evidence of spinal cord abnormalities; and one patient developed neurological impairment following a circulatory arrest secondary to local anesthetic toxicity. All five patients were infants less than three months of age. Blocks were performed by experienced anesthetists, but technical difficulties with identification of the epidural space were noted in two cases, and blood was aspirated during insertion in a patient who subsequently developed an epidural hematoma.

Acute cardiorespiratory deterioration related to venous air embolism has been reported following the use of air to identify the epidural space.[45,74] Children may be at greater risk of vascular perforation (large needle relative to epidural space, epidural venous plexus distended in children with positive pressure ventilation, catheters threaded for greater distance); intravascular placement is more difficult to identify (high flow resistance in smaller-gauge needles and catheters, collapsible, thin-walled veins); and the effects are more severe (large volume per kg in smaller children, probe patent foramen ovale present in 50% of children up to five years of age so there is greater potential for arterial embolization). If air is used, only a small volume should be present in the syringe, to minimize injection into the epidural space. Saline rather than air has been recommended for loss-of-resistance identification of the epidural space,[75] but debate continues, because many anesthetists are experienced with the use of air,[17,18] and injection of saline can make a cerebrospinal fluid leak, due to dural puncture, more difficult to identify or can dilute the injected local anesthetic, if large volumes are used.

There is now widespread experience with the safe and effective use of epidural infusions for postoperative analgesia in children. Issues relating to the dose and type of analgesic used, and the technique of insertion, require evaluation by individual anesthetists according to their own skills, the level of postoperative supervision available in the hospital, and the perceived risks and benefits for individual patients.

Complex Regional Pain Syndrome Type 1 (RSD)

Complex Regional Pain Syndrome Type (CRPS)1 (previously known as 'reflex sympathetic dystrophy [RSD]') is a syndrome that usually follows an initiating noxious event: spontaneous pain or allodynia/hyperalgesia occur in a regional distribution not limited to the territory of a single peripheral nerve, and the degree of pain is apparently disproportionate in severity to the inciting event (see Chapter 23.1). It is associated at some point with evidence of edema, changes in skin blood flow, or abnormal sudomotor activity in the region of the pain.[15,77,86] CRPS Type 1 occurs in children but is under-recognized, and often diagnosed late.

In adults, upper limb involvement is most common, but in children the lower extremity is more frequently involved[12,28,66] (84% of 395 cases[90]). There is also a marked predominance of affected females to males (4:1[90]) in pediatric cases. The peak incidence is between 9 and 13 years of age, but CRPS has been reported in a three-year-old.[72] The prognosis for CRPS in children is more favorable, because few progress to atrophic changes or to osteoporosis.[28,66] Active physiotherapy and resumption of weight-bearing is imperative; disuse will increase symptoms.

Sympatholytic procedures have a role in children with CRPS, to provide pain relief and allow physiotherapy and mobilization. In adult practice early sympathetic blockade is advocated, but the timing of invasive procedures in children is debated. Olsson[66] reported complete recovery in 60% of patients and improvement in a further 25% of 55 children who underwent intravenous regional block with guanethidine, early in the course of CRPS. However, the duration of follow-up is not stated, and some patients were excluded from the treatment group. By contrast, the treatment algorithm of Wilder et al.[90] reserves sympathetic blocks for patients unresponsive to noninvasive therapies (physiotherapy, transcutaneous electrical nerve stimulation [TENS], cognitive behavioral pain management techniques, and tricyclic antidepressants). Sympathetic blocks were associated with the highest rate of resolution of symptoms but were required in only 37 of the 70 patients. No correlation was found between the duration of symptoms and the likelihood of relief of symptoms following a sympathetic block, but these children had long-standing disease (average 12 months) prior to diagnosis. As lower limb symptoms predominate, a lumbar paravertebral sympathetic block (see Chapter 13) is the most common procedure, and often requires general anesthesia to be performed in children. In patients with severe recurrent symptoms, a continuous epidural or sympathetic block (via a paravertebral catheter) may be required. Epidural clonidine (0.2 μg/kg/hr) has been used successfully, in combination with dilute local anesthetic, for refractory CRPS.[69]

Cancer Pain

The nature of pain related to cancer differs markedly in pediatric and adult populations (Table 23.2-1). Pain may be directly tumor-related (e.g. infiltration of bone or raised intracranial pressure) but usually remits with primary treatments such as chemotherapy and radiotherapy. In a series of 92 children and adolescents, the median time to resolution of pain, following commencement of definitive anticancer therapy, was 10 days.[63] The majority of childhood tumors are hematological and have a better prognosis with aggressive therapy, when compared to infiltrative carcinomas in adults.

Children often find diagnostic and therapeutic procedures to be the most difficult part of having cancer (Table 23.2-2).[61] Blood-sampling, intravenous access for chemotherapy, lumbar punctures, and bone marrow aspirates are ongoing, and are often repeated sources of pain. Interventions for managing procedure-related pain and distress require consideration of the type of procedure, the anticipated level and duration of pain, and individual factors such as the age, and emotional and physical condition of the patient. Adequate analgesia must be provided, ranging from local anesthesia and oral agents, to intravenous sedation or general anesthesia. As children often have a degree of anxiety associated with repeated procedures, an anxiolytic such as midazolam and the use of nonpharmacological techniques (distraction, imagery, relaxation techniques, parental presence) are useful supplements to analgesia agents.[4]

The cancer treatment may also be associated with painful complications. Severe oral mucositis may occur following chemotherapy and radiotherapy, and requires topical anesthetic agents combined with opioids by continuous infusion or patient-controlled analgesia. Because patients often have a long disease-free survival, neuropathic pain resulting from radiation, chemotherapeutic agents, or surgery may require ongoing management. In one series, treatment-related toxicity accounted for two-thirds of the pain reported by inpa-

TABLE 23.2-1. *Differences between pediatric and adult cancer*

	Children	Adult
Incidence	uncommon (1% of total)	common (99% of total)
Tumor type	mostly hematological leukemia: 30% lymphoma: 13% cerebral: 18% neuroblastoma: 11%	mostly solid tumors
Outcome	mostly curable	mostly incurable
Treatment	aggressive	variable
Palliative care	usually short (weeks)	often months to years
Bony metastases	uncommon	common
Disease-related pain	often remits with treatment 10–50% of patients	may be progressive 70–80% of patients
Procedure-related pain	frequent and recurrent	less problematic

tients and 80% of the pain reported by outpatients; whereas fewer patients reported pain unrelated to recent diagnostic procedures (50% of inpatients and 25% of outpatients).[62]

Tumor recurrence which is unresponsive to therapy tends to progress rapidly,[57,61] and may be associated with further pain. Provision of analgesia is a crucial aspect of palliative care, and the adequacy of treatment must be regularly reassessed; there is great individual variation in response to analgesics and in the incidence of side effects. World Health Organization guidelines have been developed for the management of cancer pain in children.[60] As in adult practice, the analgesic ladder should be followed with stepwise prescription of analgesics according to pain severity. The oral route should be used if possible, and regular rather than PRN administration of analgesics for continuous pain should be planned. Adjuvant therapy should be considered at all stages, and includes the use of tricyclic antidepressants and anticonvulsant drugs for the management of neuropathic pain, and corticosteroids for tumor-related raised intracranial pressure.

Massive doses of opioids or invasive procedures are most frequently required in children with solid tumors and associated spread to peripheral nerves or spinal cord compression.[19,57] Although only a small number of children with terminal malignancy require invasive pain management techniques, epidural or intrathecal infusions of opioids and/or local anaesthetics should be considered if side effects of oral opioids are excessive, or if pain is inadequately controlled with less invasive measures.[10,19,57,83] With careful monitoring, the risk of infection related to long-term epidural catheters for patients with terminal disease is low.[80] Neurolytic blockade (e.g. celiac plexus block[11]) is rarely required in children, but may have a role in selected cases with terminal disease and pain uncontrolled by other measures.[10,11,19]

TABLE 23.2-2. *Cancer pain syndromes in children*

Pain directly due to cancer
- Common childhood malignancies respond rapidly to treatment and disease related pain often remits
- Bone pain is most common: Generalized marrow infiltration by leukemia, neuroblastoma metastases; or direct bone invasion by osteosarcoma, Ewings sarcoma
- Tumor recurrence which is unresponsive to therapy tends to progress rapidly, resulting in early death

Pain due to diagnostic or therapeutic procedures
- Intravenous cannulation
- Blood sampling
- Bone marrow aspirates
- Lumbar punctures
- Postoperative pain

Pain related to treatment
- Mucositis secondary to chemotherapy or radiotherapy
- Neuropathy
  - Drug-induced peripheral neuropathy (vincristine)
  - Radiation-induced nerve injury following surgery, eg. amputation
- Postoperative pain
- Infection
- Bone changes secondary to corticosteroids

CONCLUSION

Increased understanding of the development of nociceptive pathways has emphasized the importance of adequately treating pain in neonates and infants, and has also increased our understanding of the pathophysiology of pain at all ages. Adequate assessment of pain in neonates and infants requires appreciation of the developmental stage of the child and incorporation of information from physiological and behavioral responses. Neural blockade techniques have an expanding role in the management of acute pain in children, in addition to a more limited but important role in chronic and cancer pain states.

REFERENCES

1. Anand, K.J.S., and Hickey, P.R.: Halothane-morphine compared with high-dose sufentanil for anesthesia and postoperative analgesia in neonatal cardiac surgery. N. Engl. J. Med., *326:*1, 1992.
2. Anand, K.J.S., and Hickey, P.R.: Pain and its effects in the human neonate and fetus. N. Engl. J. Med., *317:*1321, 1987.

3. Anand, K.J.S., and Craig, K.D.: New perspectives on the definition of pain (editorial). Pain, *67:*3, 1996.
4. Anderson, C.T.M., Zeltzer, L.K., and Fanurik, D.: Procedural pain. *In* Schechter, N.L., Berde, C.B., and Yaster, M. (eds.): Pain in Infants, Children, and Adolescents, pp. 435–458, Baltimore, Williams & Wilkins, 1993.
5. Andrews, K., and Fitzgerald, M.: The cutaneous withdrawal reflex in human neonates: Sensitization, receptive fields, and the effects of contralateral stimulation. Pain, *56:*95, 1994.
6. Aradine, C.R., Beyer, J.E., and Tomkins, J.M.: Children's pain perception before and after analgesia: A study of instrument construct validity and related issues. J. Pediatr. Nurs, *3:*11, 1988.
7. Barr, R.G.: Pain experience in children: Developmental and clinical characteristics. *In* Wall, P.D., and Melzack, R. (eds.): Textbook of Pain, 3rd Ed. pp. 739–765, Edinburgh, Churchill Livingstone, 1994.
8. Benini, F., Johnston, C., Faucher, D., and Aranda, J.V.: Topical anesthesia during circumcision in newborn infants. J.A.M.A., *270:*850, 1993.
9. Berde, C.B.: Convulsions associated with pediatric regional anesthesia. Anesth. Analg. *75:*164, 1992.
10. Berde, C., Ablin, A., Glazer, J., Miser, A., Shapiro, B., Weisman, S., and Zeltzer, P.: Report on the subcommittee on disease-related pain in childhood cancer. Pediatrics, *86:*818, 1990.
11. Berde, C.B., Sethna, N.F., Fisher, D.E., Kahn, C.H., Chandler, P., and Grier, H.E.: Celiac plexus blockade for a 3-year-old boy with hepatoblastoma and refractory pain. Pediatrics, *86:*779, 1990.
12. Bernstein, B.H., Singsen, B.H., Kent, J.T., Kornreich, H., King, K., Hicks, R., and Hanson, V.: Reflex neurovascular dystrophy in children. J. Pediatr., *93:*211, 1978.
13. Bieri, D., Reeve, R.A., Champion, G.D., Addicoat, L., and Ziegler, J.B.: The faces pain scale for the self-assessment of the severity of pain experienced by children: Development, initial validation, and preliminary investigation for ratio scale properties. Pain, *41:*139, 1990.
14. Blanco, D., Llamazares, J., Rincon, R., Ortiz, M., and Vidal F.: Thoracic epidural anesthesia via the lumbar approach in infants and children. Anesthesiology, *84:*1312, 1996.
15. Boas, R.A.: Complex regional pain syndromes: Symptoms, signs, and differential diagnosis. *In* Janig, W., and Stanton-Hicks, M. (eds.): Reflex Sympathetic Dystrophy: A Reappraisal. Progress in Pain Research and Management. Vol. 6. pp. 79–92, Seattle, IASP Press, 1996.
16. Bosenberg, A.T., Bland, B.A.R., Schulte-Steinberg, O., and Downing, J.W.: Thoracic epidural anesthesia via caudal route in infants. Anesthesiology, *69:*265, 1988.
17. Bosenberg, A.T.: Recent developments in paediatric regional anaesthesia. Curr. Opin. Anaesthesiol., *9:*233, 1996.
18. Busoni, P., and Messeri, A.: Loss-of-resistance technique to air for identifying the epidural space in infants and children. Use an appropriate technique! (Letter). Paediatr. Anaesth., *5:*397, 1995.
19. Collins, J.J., Grier, H.E., Kinney, H.C., and Berde, C.B.: Control of severe pain in children with terminal malignancy. J. Pediatr., *126:*653, 1995.
20. Constaninou, J., Reynolds, M.L., Woolf, C.J., Safieh-Garabedian, B., and Fitzgerald, M.: Nerve growth factor levels in developing rat skin: Upregulation following skin wounding. Neuroreport, *5:*2281, 1994.
21. Cook, B., Grubb, D.J., Aldridge, L.A., and Doyle, E.: Comparison of the effects of adrenaline, clonidine, and ketamine on the duration of caudal analgesia produced by bupivacaine in children. Br. J. Anaesth., *75:*698, 1995.
22. Craig, K.D., Whitfield, M.F., Grunau, R.V., Linton, J., and Hadjistavropoulos, H.D.: Pain in the preterm neonate: Behavioral and physiological indices. Pain, *52:*287, 1993.
23. Dalens, B. (ed.): Regional Anesthesia in Infants, Children, and Adolescents. London, Williams & Wilkins 1995.
24. Desparmet, J., Mateo, J., Ecoffey, C., and Mazoit, X.: Efficacy of an epidural test dose in children anesthesized with halothane. Anesthesiology, *72:*249, 1990.
25. Desparmet, J., Meistelman, C., Barre, J., and Saint-Maurice, C.: Continuous epidural infusion of bupivacaine for postoperative pain relief in children. Anesthesiology, *67:*108, 1987.
26. Desparmet, J.F.: Central blocks in children and adolescents. *In* Schechter, N.L., Berde, C.B., and Yaster, M. (eds.): Pain in Infants, Children, and Adolescents, pp. 245–260, Baltimore, Williams & Wilkins, 1993.
27. Dixon, S., Snyder, J., Holve, R., and Bromberger, P.: Behavioral effects of circumcision with and without anesthesia. J. Dev. Behav. Pediatr., *5:*246, 1984.
28. Fermaglich, D.R.: Reflex sympathetic dystrophy in children. Pediatrics, *60:*881, 1977.
29. Fitgerald, M., and Anand, K.J.S.: Developmental neuroanatomy and neurophysiology of pain. *In* Schechter, N.L., Berde, C.B., and Yaster, M. (eds.): Pain in Infants, Children, and Adolescents, pp. 11–31, Baltimore, Williams & Wilkins, 1993.
30. Fitzgerald, M.: Developmental biology of inflammatory pain. Br. J. Anaesth., *75:*177, 1995.
31. Fitzgerald, M.: Neurobiology of fetal and neonatal pain. *In* Wall, P.D., and Melzack, R. (eds.): Textbook of Pain, 3rd ed. pp. 153–163, Edinburgh, Churchill Livingstone, 1994.
32. Fitzgerald, M.: The developmental neurobiology of pain. *In* Bond, M.R., Charlton, J.E., and Woolf, C.J. (eds.): Proceedings of the 6th World Congress on Pain, Pain Research and Clinical Management. Vol. 4. pp. 253–261, Amsterdam, Elsevier, 1991.
33. Fitzgerald, M., Butcher, T., and Shortland, P.: Developmental changes in the laminar termination of A fiber cutaneous sensory afferents in the rat spinal cord dorsal horn. J. Comp. Neurol., *348:*225, 1994.
34. Fitzgerald, M., and Koltzenburg, M.: The functional development of descending inhibitory pathways in the dorsolateral funiculus of the newborn rat spinal cord. Dev. Brain Res., *24:*261, 1986.
35. Fitzgerald, M., Millard, C., and MacIntosh, N.: Cutaneous hypersensitivity following peripheral tissue damage in newborn infants and its reversal with topical anesthesia. Pain, *39:*31, 1989.
36. Fitzgerald, M.: Cutaneous primary afferent properties in the hind limb of the neonatal rat. J. Physiol., *383:*79, 1987.
37. Flandin-Blety, C., and Barrier, G.: Accidents following extradural analgesia in children: The results of a retrospective study. Paediatr. Anaesth., *5:*41, 1995.
38. Freid, E.B., Bailey, A.G., and Valley, R.D.: Electrocardiographic and hemodynamic changes associated with unintentional intravascular injection of bupivacaine with epinephrine in infants. Anesthesiology, *79:*394, 1993.
39. Giaufre, E., Bruguerolle, B., Rastello, C., Coquet, M., and Lorec, A.M.: New regimen for interpleural block in children. Paediatr. Anaesth., *5:*125, 1995.
40. Goldman, L.J.: Complications in regional anaesthesia (editorial). Paediatr. Anaesth., *5:*3, 1995.
41. Goresky, G.V.: The clinical utility of epidural midazolam for inguinal hernia repair in children. Can. J. Anaesth., *42:*755, 1995.
42. Grunau, R.V., Whitfield, M.F., Petrie, J.H., and Fryer, E.L.: Early pain experience, child and family factors, as precursors of somatization: A prospective study of extremely premature and fullterm children. Pain, *56:*353, 1994.
43. Grunau, R.V.E., Johnston, C.C., and Craig, K.D.: Neonatal facial and cry responses to invasive and non-invasive procedures. Pain, *42:*295, 1990.
44. Grunau, R.V.E., Whitfield, M.F., and Petrie, J.H.: Pain sensitivity and temperament in extremely low-birth-weight premature toddlers and preterm and full-term controls. Pain, *58:*341, 1994.
45. Guinard, J.P., and Borboen, M.: Probable venous air embolism during caudal anesthesia in a child. Anesth. Analg., *76:*1134, 1993.
46. Gunter, J.B., and Eng, C.: Thoracic epidural anesthesia via the caudal approach in children. Anesthesiology, *76:*935, 1992.
47. Houck, C.S., Troshynski, T., and Berde, C.B.: Treatment of pain in children. *In* Wall, P.D., and Melzack, R. (eds.): Textbook of Pain, 3rd ed. pp. 1419–1434, Edinburgh, Churchill Livingstone, 1994.
48. Ivani, G., Mattioli, G., Rega, M., Conio, A., Jasonni, V., and De Negri, P.: Clonidine-mepivacaine mixture vs plain mepivacaine in paediatric surgery. Paediatr. Anaesth., *6:*111, 1996.
49. Johnston, C.C., Stevens, B., Craig, K.D., and Grunau, R.V.E.: Developmental changes in pain expression in premature, full-term, two- and four-month-old infants. Pain, *52:*201, 1993.
50. Johnston, C.C., Stevens, B., Yang, F., and Horton, L.: Developmental changes in response to heelstick in preterm infants: A prospective cohort study. Dev. Med. Child Neurol., *38:*438, 1996.
51. Johnston, C.C., Stevens, B.J., Yang, F., and Horton, L.: Differential response to pain by very premature neonates. Pain, *61:*471, 1995.
52. Krane, E.J., Tyler, D.C., and Jacobsen, L.E.: The dose response of caudal morphine in children. Anesthesiology, *71:*48, 1989.
53. Krechel, S.W., and Bildner, J.: CRIES: a new neonatal postoperative pain measurement score. Initial testing of validity and reliability. Paediatr. Anaesth., *5:*53, 1995.
54. Lee, J.J., and Rubin, A.P.: Comparison of a bupivacaine-clonidine mixture with plain bupivacaine for caudal analgesia in children. Br. J. Anaesth., *72:*258, 1994.

55. Marvin, J.A.: Pain assessment versus measurement. J. Burn Care Rehabil., *16:*348, 1995.
56. Masters, D.B., Berde, C.B., Dutta, S.K., Griggs, C.T., Hu, D., Kupsky, W., and Langer, R.: Prolonged regional nerve blockade by controlled release of local anesthetic from a biodegradable polymer matrix. Anesthesiology, *79:*340, 1993.
57. Maunuksela, E., Saarinen, U.M., and Lahteenoja, K.M.: Prevalence and management of terminal pain in children with cancer: Five-year experience in Helsinki, Finland. *In* Tyler, D.C., and Krane, E.J. (eds.): Advances in Pain Research Therapy. Vol. 15. pp. 383–390. New York, Raven Press, 1990.
58. McGrath, P.A.: Pain in the pediatric patient: Practical aspects of assessment. Pediatr. Ann., *24:*126, 1995.
59. McGrath, P.J., Johnson, G., Goodman, J.T., Schillinger, J., Dunn, J., and Chapman, J.: CHEOPS: A behavioral scale for rating postoperative pain in children. *In* Fields, H.L., Dubner, R., and Cervero, F. (eds.): Advances in Pain Research and Therapy. Vol. 9. pp. 395–402, New York, Raven Press, 1985.
60. McGrath, P.A.: Development of the World Health Care Organization guidelines on cancer pain relief and palliative care in children. J. Pain Symptom Manage., *12:*87, 1996.
61. Miser, A.: Management of pain associated with childhood cancer. *In*: Schechter, N.L., Berde, C.B., and Yaster, M. (eds.): Pain in Infants, Children, and Adolescents. pp. 411–423. Baltimore, Williams & Wilkins, 1993.
62. Miser, A.W., Dothage, A., Wesley, R.A., and Miser, J.S.: The prevalence of pain in a pediatric and young adult cancer population. Pain, *29:*73, 1987.
63. Miser, A.W., McCalla, J., Dothage, J.A., Wesley, M., and Miser, J.S.: Pain as a presenting symptom in children and young adults with newly diagnosed malignancy. Pain, *29:*85, 1987.
64. Naguib, M., El Gammal, M., Elhattab, Y.S., and Seraj, M.: Midazolam for caudal analgesia in children: Comparison with caudal bupivacaine. Can. J. Anaesth., *42:*758, 1995.
65. Naguib, M., Sharif, M.Y., Seraj, M., El Gammal, M., and Dawlatly, A.A.: Ketamine for caudal analgesia in children: Comparison with caudal bupivacaine. Br. J. Anaesth., *67:*559, 1991.
66. Olsson, G.I., Arner, S., and Hirsch, G.: Reflex sympathetic dystrophy in children. *In* Tyler, D.C., and Krane, E.J. (eds.): Advances in Pain Research and Therapy. Vol. 15. pp. 323–331, New York, Raven Press, 1990.
67. Perillo, M., Sethna, N.F., and Berde, C.B.: Intravenous isoproterenol as a marker for epidural testdosing in children. Anesth. Analg., *76:*178, 1993.
68. Porter, F.: Pain assessment in children: Infants. *In* Schechter, N.L., Berde, C.B., and Yaster, M. (eds.): Pain in Infants, Children, and Adolescents. pp. 87–96, Baltimore, Williams & Wilkins, 1993.
69. Rauck, R.L., Eisenach, J.C., Jackson, K., Young, L.D., and Southern, J.: Epidural clonidine treatment for refractory reflex sympathetic dystrophy. Anesthesiology, *79:*1163, 1993.
70. Reynolds, M.L., and Fitzgerald, M.: Long-term sensory hyperinnervation following neonatal skin wounds. J. Comp. Neurol., *358:*487, 1995.
71. Reynolds, M.L., Fitzgerald, M.: Neonatal sciatic nerve section results in thiamine monophosphate but not substance P or calcitonin gene-related peptide depletion from the terminal field in the dorsal horn of the rat: the role of collateral sprouting. Neuroscience, *51:*191, 1992.
72. Richlin, D.M., Carron, H., Rowlingson, J.C., Sussman, M.D., Baugher, W.H., Goldner, R.D.: Reflex sympathetic dystrophy: Successful treatment by transcutaneous nerve stimulation. J. Pediatr., *93:*84, 1978.
73. Riechling, D.B., Kyrozis, A., Wang, J., and MacDermott, A.B.: Mechanisms of GABA and glycine depolarization-induced calcium transients in rat dorsal horn neurons. J. Physiology, (London), *476:*411, 1994.
74. Schwartz, N., and Eisenkraft, J.B.: Probable venous air embolism during epidural placement in an infant. Anesth. Analg., *76:*1136, 1993.
75. Sethna, N.F., and Berde, C.B.: Venous air embolism during identification of the epidural space in children (editorial). Anesth. Analg., *76:*925, 1993.
76. Shortland, P., and Fitzgerald, M.: Neonatal nerve section results in rearrangement of the central terminals of saphenous and axotomized sciatic nerve afferents in the dorsal horn of the spinal cord of the adult rat. Eur. J. Neurosci., *6:*75, 1994.
77. Stanton-Hicks, M., Janig, W., Hassenbusch, S., *et al.*: Reflex sympathetic dystrophy: Changing concepts and taxonomy. Pain, *63:*127, 1995.
78. Stayer, S.A., Pasquariello, C.A., Schwartz, R.E., Balsara, R.K., and Lear, B.R.: The safety of continuous pleural lignocaine after thoracotomy in children and adolescents. Paediatr. Anaesth., *5:*307, 1995.
79. Stevens, B.J., Johnston, C.C., and Horton, L.: Factors that influence the behavioral pain responses of premature infants. Pain, *59:*101, 1994.
80. Stratford, M.A., Wilder, R.T., and Berde, C.B.: The risk of infection from epidural analgesia in children: A review of 1,620 cases. Anesth. Analg., *80:*234, 1995.
81. Sutters, K.A., Levine, J.D., Dibble, S., Savedra, M., and Miaskowski, C.: Analgesic efficacy and safety of single-dose intramuscular ketorolac for postoperative pain management in children following tonsillectomy. Pain, *61:*145, 1995.
82. Taddio, A., Goldbach, M., Ipp, M., Stevens, B., and Koren, G.: Effect of neonatal circumcision on pain responses during vaccination in boys. Lancet, *344:*291, 1994.
83. Tobias, J.D.: Indications and application of epidural anesthesia in a pediatric population outside the perioperative period. Clin. Pediatr., *32:*81, 1993.
84. Vane, D.W., Pietropaoli, J.A., Smail, F.D., Hong, A.R., and Abaijan, J.C.: Continuous retropleural infusion for analgesia after thoracotomy in newborn infants. Pediatr. Surg. Int., *10:*311, 1995.
85. Ved, S.A., Pinosky, M., and Nicodemus, H.: Ventricular tachycardia and brief cardiovascular collapse in two infants after caudal anesthesia using a bupivacaine-epinephrine solution. Anesthesiology, *79:*1121, 1993.
86. Walker, S.M., and Cousins, M.J.: Complex regional pain syndromes: Including 'reflex sympathetic dystrophy' and 'causalgia.' Anaesth. Intensive Care, *25:*113, 1997.
87. Warner, M.A., Kunkal, S.E., Offord, K.O., Atchison, S.R., and Dawson, B.: The effects of age, epinephrine and operation site on duration of caudal anaesthesia in pediatric patients. Anesth. Analg., *66:*995, 1987.
88. Weston, P.J., and Bourchier, D.: The pharmacokinetics of bupivacaine following interpleural nerve block in infants of very low birth-weight. Paediatr. Anaesth., *5:*219, 1995.
89. Wilder, R.T., Berde, C.B., Wolohan, M., *et al.*: Reflex sympathetic dystrophy in children. J. Bone Joint Surg., *6:*910, 1992.
90. Wilder, R.T.: Reflex sympathetic dystrophy in children and adolescents: Differences from adults. *In* Janig, W., and Stanton-Hicks, M. (eds.): Reflex Sympathetic Dystrophy: A Reappraisal. Progress in Pain Research and Management. Vol. 6., pp. 67–78. Seattle, IASP Press, 1996.
91. Wilkie, D.J., Holzemer, W.L., Tesler, M.D., Ward, J.A., Paul, S.M., and Savedra, M.C.: Measuring pain quality: Validity and reliability of children's and adolescents' pain language. Pain, *41:*151, 1990.
92. Wolf, C., Shortland, P., and Coggeshall, R.E.: Peripheral nerve injury triggers central sprouting of myelinated afferents. Nature, *355:*75, 1992.
93. Yaster, M., Tobin, J.R., and Maxwell, L.G.: Local anesthetics. *In* Schechter, N.L., Berde, C.B., and Yaster, M. (eds.): Pain in Infants, Children, and Adolescents. pp. 179–194., Baltimore, Williams & Wilkins, 1993.
94. Yi, D.K., and Barr, G.A.: The induction of Fos-like immunoreactivity by noxious thermal, mechanical and chemical stimuli in the lumbar spinal cord of infant rats. Pain, *60:*257, 1995.

Neural Blockade in Clinical Anesthesia and Management of Pain, Third Edition,
edited by M.J. Cousins and P.O. Bridenbaugh.
Lippincott–Raven Publishers, Philadelphia © 1998.

CHAPTER 24

Physiologic and Pharmacologic Substrates of Nociception and Nerve Injury

Tony L. Yaksh

From a teleologic standpoint, certain classes of unconditioned stimuli that interact with visceral, somatic, or muscular receptor systems give rise to a complex syndrome of behavior in the unanesthetized organism that we refer to as pain. This syndrome is frequently characterized by vocalization or efforts to escape. An important, though not unique, characteristic is that "stimuli become adequate as excitants of pain when they are of such intensity as to threaten damage to the skin." Such stimuli were referred to by Sherrington as being nociceptive.[713] To generalize on this phenomenon, we note that other unconditioned stimuli, such as electrical stimuli, that do not produce evident damage will produce the same behavioral syndrome. We would thus conclude that these stimuli have activated portions of the circuitry that mimic the input produced by the stimulus that physically damages the organism. Similarly, displacement of a joint beyond its normal range of motion, reversible ischemia of cardiac muscle or gallbladder sphincter contraction, although not necessarily leading to acute and immediate damage, produces similar response syndromes (e.g., vocalization, guarding), which suggest that the organism's response to the input provided by that stimulus is similar to its response to the tissue-damaging stimulus. The substrate by which these classes of information gain access to the central nervous system will be one of the principal subjects of this chapter. The behavior of the organism in context thus provides corollaries which define the "painful" nature of the stimulus. In some instances, the behavioral response reflects a defined pain state (e.g., a pain report, vocalization, guarding), but the stimulus appears inappropriate. Thus, a modestly intense stimulus may evoke a response normally associated with a more intense input or a light touch may result in behavior that is normally only associated with a tissue injury. In the first case, we might define this behavioral state as reflecting a hyperalgesia, whereas in the second case, the syndrome may be referred to as a hyperpathia or allodynia. The apparent alteration of the linkage between stimulus intensity and response is now commonly appreciated and constitutes an important example of the dynamic characteristics of systems that process sensory information. As will be seen, the presence of dynamic control systems and long-term changes in connectivity induced by repetitive afferent input or by nerve injury can induce a powerful alteration in the stimulus-response relationship. The appreciation of the complex relation between stimulus and response indeed represents one of the major advances in conceptualization of the pain response that has occurred in the past 15 to 20 years. It is now apparent that one cannot consider the afferent limb through which "pain" information travels (e.g., the pain pathway) without considering the systems that modulate at every level that very transmission.

T. L. Yaksh: Department of Anesthesiology, University of California San Diego, La Jolla, California 92093-0818.

NOCICEPTION: THE BEHAVIORAL CORRELATES

Acute Stimulus

It is commonly appreciated that acute mechanical distortion (pressure), increases in temperature applied to the body surface, or acute distention of a hollow viscus will evoke (i) unlearned but organized escape response with decreasing latency/increasing reliability,[340,386] and (ii) the appearance of physiologic reflexes that are evoked by small afferent input (e.g., autonomic responses—blood pressure/heart rate)[596,685] or spinal somatic reflexes (e.g. tail flick, skin twitch).[245,684] In humans, experimental stimuli, such as acute thermal or electrical stimuli, will similarly evoke responses reporting pain with greater rated intensity and with greater certainty as the electrical,[144,145,147,817] thermal,[87,287] or mechanical[404,405] stimulus intensity is increased. These acute, focal stimulus exposures, both in humans and in animals, have several properties:

1. The focus of the behavior and the pain referral is typically limited to the site of stimulus exposure (e.g., it is somatotopically limited).
2. With an intense focal stimulus it is possible that the observer will frequently report an acute sharp sensation (first pain) followed by a dull throbbing (second pain).[494,652]
3. If the stimulus is limited to a brief exposure and if the stimulus does not itself produce a local injury, the response measure (latency, pain report) can be shown to be relatively stable over an extended sequence of exposures.
4. If the stimulus is extended, results in a persistent state of activity (as with a chemical stimulus that activates small afferents), or results in a local injury (e.g., tissue damage or a local burn), the pain report/behavior will show a time-dependent change, suggesting an increase in the response generated by the stimulus.[652] This will be discussed below.

In general, then, it can be seen that with an acute high-intensity stimulus there can be a relatively faithful representation of the magnitude of the stimulus and its interaction with the body surface. However, as will be discussed further in subsequent sections, the acute stimulus event with no tissue injury is in fact an anomaly that probably does not exist outside of well-controlled environmental situations (e.g., a psychophysical laboratory). Under normal circumstances, there is a prolonged and ongoing input that is driven by the nature of the stimulus that has led to tissue injury.

Protracted Stimulus

If there is a local tissue injury as a result of the stimulus, it can be shown that the magnitude of the subsequent response generated by a subsequent test stimulus is markedly enhanced and a previously innocuous stimulus is reported as aversive. This post-injury state is referred to as primary hyperalgesia. In this state, there is (i) a reduction in the threshold to produce a pain response, (ii) an augmented response to a suprathreshold stimulus, and (iii) an ongoing pain report. Importantly, this sensitization is observed for essentially all modalities (e.g., thermal and mechanical) and tends to be localized to the immediate locality of the injury.[480,560]

In contrast to the above, shortly after the induction of a local injury, it can be shown that a region surrounding the local injury appears, and is substantially larger than the injury, in which low-threshold tactile (but not thermal) stimuli will evoke a significant pain report.[495] Human psychophysical studies have pursued the characteristics of this event systematically by the use of intradermally injected capsaicin. This agent is known to selectively activate C primary afferents.[57] In these studies, it has been shown that intradermal capsaicin will evoke a local primary hyperalgesia that dissipates within the hour and also a large, persistent, secondary hyperalgesia in which low-threshold tactile stimulation (but not thermal) will evoke a pain report.[480,717,756] The mechanism of this sensitization will be considered later; however, it should be noted that: (i) the secondary hyperalgesia lies considerably beyond the edge of the injury flare (e.g., the axon reflex),[469] (ii) the allodynia is mediated by large afferents (e.g., mechanically evoked pain diminished by a tourniquet blocking large afferents;[480] and (iii) the evolution of the secondary hyperalgesic state is prevented by a local anesthetic block of the region injected with capsaicin prior to the injection of capsaicin, but not after.[479] These latter observations suggest that in the face of a local injury, there is a locally mediated enhancement of the organism's response to a given stimulus. This primary hyperalgesia is accompanied by the appearance of an extended area of sensitization in which low-intensity mechanical stimuli evoke a pain response. Animal models have similarly been employed in which a local injury, such as that induced by the injection of formalin or carrageenan into the skin,[340,806] the generation of an acute arthritic state[584,698] or a local burn (as with ultraviolet [UV]),[778] can evoke a prominent facilitation of pain behavior.

These observations in humans and animals have striking significance in the treatment of pain states, as they suggest that the prior interventions may reduce the magnitude of the postinjury stimulus. Accordingly, as will be noted later, the systems that are activated by such protracted afferent input themselves have unique properties.

NOCICEPTIVE PROCESSING: ROSTRALLY PROJECTING SUBSTRATES

The following sections discuss the substrates through which information generated by high-intensity stimuli gains access to higher centers. Anatomically, the substrates may be broadly considered in terms of the primary afferents—the spinal cord, the brain stem (medulla, mesencephalon, diencephalon), and the cortex. In each case, one must consider the presumptive evidence associating activity in elements of that substrate with the afferent and efferent connections of that substrate and the behavioral sequelae that might be predicted secondary to the physiologic manipulations (lesion, stimulation) of that substrate.

Primary Afferent Systems

Addressed below are the anatomic, physiologic, and pharmacologic characteristics of afferents as they appear to relate to nociceptive transmission.

Myelinated and Unmyelinated Afferents

Afferent fibers can be broadly classified according to whether they are myelinated or unmyelinated. Large-diameter peripheral afferents enveloped in Schwann cell sheets range in diameter from about 6 to 14 μm in the human cutaneous nerve. Nonmyelinated fibers range in diameter from 0.2 to 2.0 μm and, although not possessing the Schwann cell investment, are commonly co-located in proximity with other small fibers within a common Schwann cell sheath (bundles of Remak). Myelinated to unmyelinated fiber ratios in cutaneous nerves are about 1:3 to 1:5 in humans.[226,608] Thus, while the largest of myelinated fibers represent the largest area in a cross-section of nerve, numerically they are likely to constitute a relatively small proportion of the afferent pathways. The peripheral terminals of these axons ramify extensively in the subcutaneous layer, sending collaterals into the dermis. In this process some fibers lose their Schwann cell investment and become nonmyelinated. Conduction velocities of myelinated fibers thus decrease and approach that of unmyelinated fibers when measured near their site of termination.[389,390,541]

Afferent axons in the skin ramify profusely,[128] losing their perineural sheath. Large-diameter fibers, commonly excited by low-intensity mechanical stimuli, may develop specialized terminals with distinctly organized encapsulations constructed of non-neuronal elements.[66,101,827] However, the vast majority of nerve terminals, and certainly those deriving from unmyelinated fibers, show little evidence of specialization.[827] Unmyelinated terminals show extensive branching in a horizontal layer in the superficial dermis, and several axon branches may be invested by a single Schwann cell. Axon collaterals enter the epidermal layer with the basement membrane of the nerve terminal becoming contiguous with that of the epidermis. Unmyelinated fiber terminals are directed toward the stratum corneum, and there they lie between the juxtaposed epidermal cells.[127,149] A similar organization is observed in different target tissues such as the cornea (Fig. 24-1). In tooth pulp and knee joint, both myelinated and unmyelinated fibers appear to lose their Schwann cell sheath and show prominent local branching.[18,359] These nonspecialized or so-called free nerve endings commonly display agranular vesicles and numerous mitochondria (Fig. 24-1).[127,359,382,750–752] As will be discussed in the comments on the peripheral pharmacology of afferents, these vesicle populations provide the substrate for the release of locally active agents at the *distal* terminals of the sensory axon. It appears likely that certain "free" nerve endings are characteristically sensitive to physical stimuli that evoke pain behavior: (i) activation of small-diameter myelinated and unmyelinated fibers is associated with tissue damage (see following), and most small-diameter fibers apparently end in unencapsulated terminals; and (ii) electrical, mechanical, thermal, or chemical stimuli, when applied to certain structures such as the cornea or the tooth pulp which possess no encapsulated endings, will evoke a pain report.[17,18,147,487]

Primary Afferent Neuron Morphology

Primary sensory neurons are pseudo-unipolar, with the soma located in the dorsal root ganglion (DRG) or, as in the fifth nerve, in the trigeminal ganglion. The DRG may be divided into two categories[23]: (i) large, lightly staining cells (type A), which give rise to large-diameter myelinated fibers, and (ii) small darkly staining cells (type B) from which derive the small-diameter myelinated or unmyelinated primary afferent axons.[647,871] Morphologically, type A and type B neurons have been differentiated on the basis of structural components such as relative content of granular and smooth endoplasmic reticulum and of ribosomes, neural filaments and microtubules, Golgi apparatus, and lysosomal bodies.[499a] Histochemical differences also exist. Fluoride-resistant acid phosphatase,[164,178,464–466] cholinesterase,[419,420] and a number of peptides appear to be preferentially located in type B cells (see below). Because axon terminals do not possess ribosomes with which to manufacture peptides and proteins, such materials are synthesized in the soma[220] and transported to the distal terminals of the neuron by means of an energy-dependent axon transport system.[609,611] Differences have not been observed between myelinated and unmyelinated fibers in the velocity or character of axon transport,[107,610] and the ability to conduct an action potential does not depend on the viability of axon transport systems. However, changes in the transport of materials to the distal terminals appear to play several important roles in the maintenance of the axon. Blockade of axon transport (as with certain neuropathy-inducing agents such as colchicine or vinblastine), results in trophic changes in axon structure.[467] Moreover, the likely role of certain peptides in primary afferent neurotransmission and the inability of nerve terminals to synthesize peptides argue for the importance of such a transport system.

Correlation of Behavior and Sensory Afferent Activity

Direct Activation of Axons. Zotterman,[881] using multiple unit recording, observed that high-intensity electrical stimulation in the periphery activated rapidly and slowly conducting fibers. Based on conduction velocity of cutaneous sensory nerves, fibers were subsequently designated as A-beta (approximately 30–100 m/sec) and A-delta (approximately 4–30 m/sec). The C component consisted of those fibers conducting at less than 2.5 m/sec.[280] This classic definition is shown in the recording presented in Figure 24-2. Based on dissection, muscle afferents have been divided into the following groups on the basis of axon diameter: group 1, greater than 12 μm; group II, 6 to 12 μm; group III, 1 to 6 μm; and group IV, less than 1 μm.[510] Given the close relationship between axon diameter in myelinated/unmyelinated axons and conduction velocities, the following relationships are normally accepted: group I, no sensory homolog; group II, A-beta; group III, A-delta; and group IV, C (see Table 24-1).

Electrical stimulation that produced synchronous volleys in high-threshold cutaneous afferents (and therefore slowly conducting and of small diameter) evoked massive sympathetic discharges and pseudo-affective responses even in lightly anesthetized animals,[881] suggesting that the activation was associated with a noxious stimulus. In humans, stimulation that evoked only fast-conducting volleys in cutaneous nerves gave rise to sensations of tickling or light pressure, whereas stimulation that evoked fast and slow components resulted in pain.[167,759] High-intensity stimulation

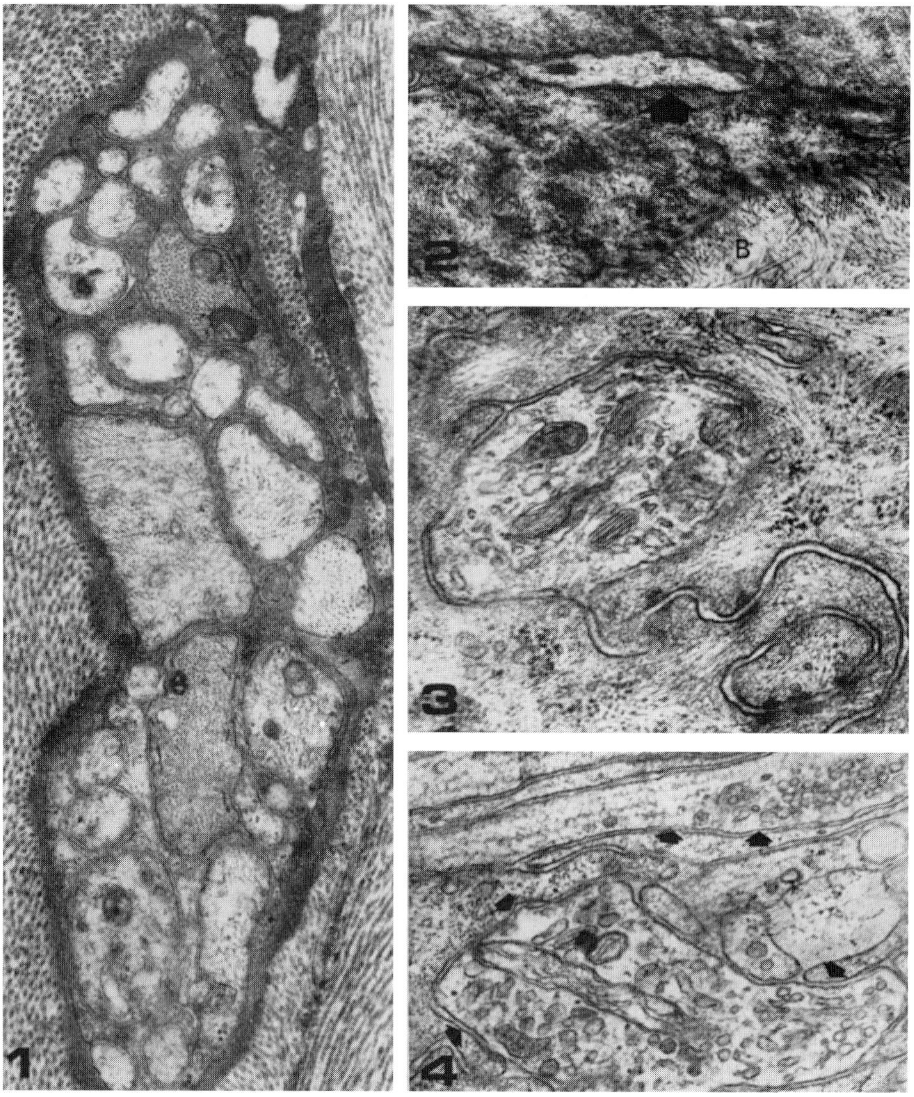

FIG. 24-1. 1. A nerve trunk in the stroma of the rat cornea. Glutaraldehyde-OsO_4 fixation. (Original magnification $\times$32,500) **2.** An axon *(arrow)* penetrating between two basal epithelial cells. B-Bowman's layer. Glutaraldehyde-OsO_4 fixation. (Original magnification $\times$22,000). **3.** An intraepithelial axon profile containing mitochondria and agranular vesicles of varying shapes and sizes. Glutaraldehyde-OsO_4 fixation. (Original magnification $\times$59,100). **4.** Two intraepithelial axons *(arrows)* containing agranular vesicles. Glutaraldehyde-OsO_4 fixation. (Original magnification $\times$ 19,000). (From Lervo, T., Joo, F., Huikuri, K.T., *et al.*: Fine structure of sensory nerves in the rat cornea: An experimental nerve degeneration study. Pain, *6*:57, 1979.)

applied during selective blockade of large-diameter fibers by anoxia, leaving A-delta/C fibers active, produces a short-lasting pain of a pricking nature. The sensation appears similar to that often reported as "first" pain. Activation limited to more slowly conducting fiber populations (C or group IV) has given rise to dull, diffusely localized sensations that were likened to burning or so-called second pain.[351,757–760,762,782]

Afferent Activity Evoked by Stimuli Associated with Behavioral Signs of Pain. Although electrical activation of gross fiber populations may produce pain, it does not necessarily follow that when a high-intensity somatic stimulus is applied, specific afferent populations are activated, or that their specific activation is uniquely correlated with pain sensations. Using single unit recording in human nerve fascicles *in situ*, it has been shown that stimuli that produce sensations of light touch or vibration are accompanied by the activation of rapidly conducting afferents.[409,458–460] Needle pricks associated with verbal reports of marked discomfort evoked rapid firing in C cutaneous afferents (0.5–1.5 m/sec). Chemical (acetic acid or intradermal histamine) or thermal stimuli that produce reports of pain or itch activate populations of slowly conducting fibers.[757,758,760–762,782] An example of such recording and a modality definition of peripheral sensory afferents conducting at a C-fiber velocity are shown in Figure 24-3. Such investigations have provided a number of insights:

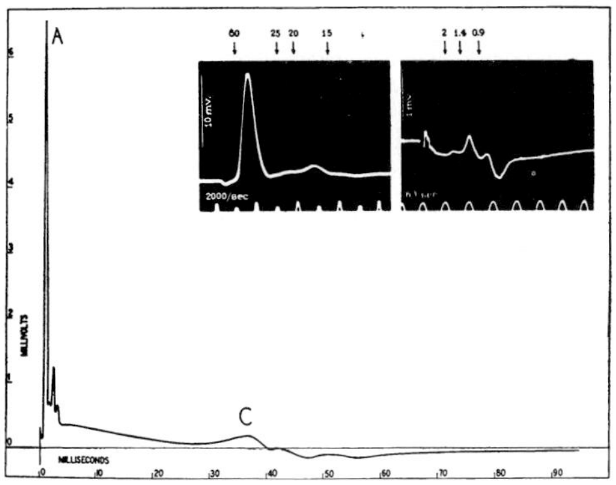

FIG. 24-2. Scale drawing of complete compound action potential of mammalian saphenous nerve. **Left Inset:** Recording of A fiber components. **Right Inset:** Recording of C fiber components. *Numbers* above *arrows* give maximal conduction rates (m/sec) of each component. [From Patton, H.D.: Special properties of nerve trunks and tracts. *In* Ruch, T.C., and Patton, H.D. (eds.): Physiology and Biophysics. pp. 73–94. Philadelphia, W.B. Saunders, 1965.]

1. Activation of only a few C fibers appears not to be sufficient to evoke a pain report.[761,783]

2. Although the activation of fibers conducting at velocities corresponding to A-delta and C fibers is a prerequisite for evoking somatic pain in humans, activity in all slowly conducting fibers is not uniquely associated with a pain event. Populations of slowly conducting afferents communicate information on warmth, cooling, or muscle pressure,[101,389] stimulus conditions that are not normally aversive. This heterogeneity is emphasized in Table 24-2, where the classes of afferents (as defined by conduction velocity) are correlated with the categories of "natural" stimuli that result in their excitation.

3. Electrical or mechanical stimulation sufficient to activate a slowly conducting component of a compound action potential and evoke a pain event will also evoke activity in rapidly conducting afferent fibers. Although the above observations indicate that the pain report may be obtained in the absence of large fibers, they cannot absolutely exclude them from a role in characterizing the pain event. Thus, prolonged intense mechanical stimuli will give rise to an initial burst of activity in low-threshold afferents where, unlike the small-diameter fibers, is not sustained. High-frequency stimulation of the sural nerve, at an intensity where the electrical stimulus was just sufficient to generate a rapidly conducting volley (A-alpha), was adequate to provoke reports of pricking pain.[818] Finally, in Fabry's disease, in which small-diameter fibers are damaged and the largest fibers remain functional, pain sensations remain.[226,227,618]

Factors Influencing Afferent Activity After Tissue Injury

As noted in the preceding section, mechanical stimuli producing extreme distortion of the skin, or thermal stimuli greater than 42° to 48°C, will evoke a stimulus-dependent activation of small sensory afferents and a correlated increase in pain behavior. Although such stimuli constitute an important element in the sensory environment of the organism, it is clear following tissue injury that: (i) there appears a persistent low level of discharge in these small afferents; and (ii) not infrequently, these axons will show an exaggerated response to a subsequent mechanical or thermal stimulus. An example of such an altered stimulus-response relationship is shown in Figure 24-4.[468,670] Of particular interest,

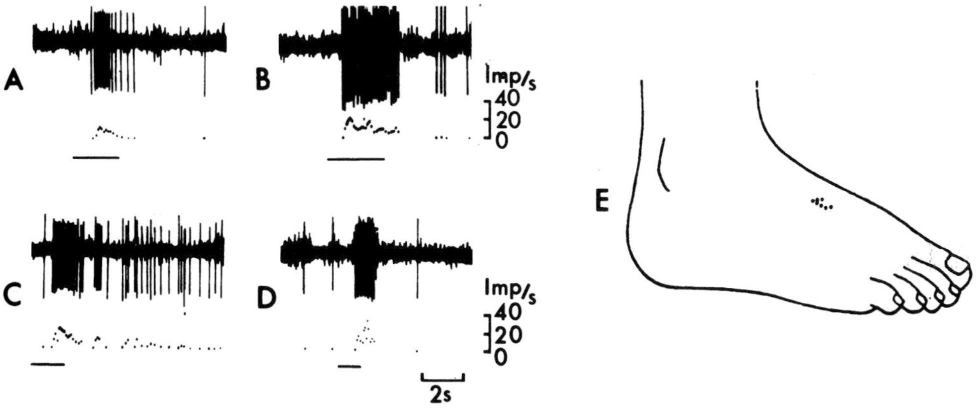

FIG. 24-3. Activity in afferent C unit (conduction velocity 0.64 m/sec) recorded in peroneal nerve at knee level. Various stimuli applied to receptive field on dorsum of big toe are indicated by bars under recordings. **A:** Sustained pressure with Frey hair, 2 g. Sensation: itch after about 2 seconds. **B:** Needle penetration through skin. Sensation: pricking and delayed pain. **C:** Touching skin with nettle leaf. Sensation: pain followed by itch. **D:** Touching skin with glowing match. Sensation: pricking followed by burning pain. **E:** Example of receptive field of C unit, recording being made from superficial peroneal nerve. Field measured 0.6 cm by 1.7 cm and consisted of seven receptive maxima *(dots)* surrounded by unresponsive areas. (From Hagbarth, K.E.: Exteroceptive, proprioceptive, and sympathetic activity recorded with microelectrodes from human peripheral nerves. Mayo. Clin. Proc., *54*:353, 1979.)

TABLE 24-1. *Summary of sensory afferents and their characteristics*

Receptor type	Effective stimulus	Background activity	Range of conduction velocity (m/sec)	Selected references
Cutaneous mechanoreceptors				
Type I	Indentation of dome	0	30–90	460,637
Type II	Skin deformation	+	30–70	460,637
C mechanoreceptors	Skin indentation	0	<1	54
Meissner's corpuscle and Krause's end-bulb	Skin indentation	0	40–80	459,749
Pacinian corpuscle	Vibration	0	50–80	459,637
Cutaneous nociceptors				
A-delta mechanical	Damage	0	5–60	285,637
C mechanical	Damage	0	<1	56,285
A-delta heat	Noxious heat or mechanical damage	0	4–40	285,390
C polymodal	Noxious heat; mechanical algesic agents	0	<1	41,176,782
Warm	Increased temperature	+		
Muscle nociceptors				
Group III	Pressure; damage	+/0	60–90	624
Group IV	Pressure; damage	+/0	<2.5	266
Group III	Pressure; damage	+/0	60–90	624
Group IV	Pressure; damage	+/0	<2.5	266
Joint nociceptors				
A-delta	Extreme bending		<30	151
Visceral mechanoreceptors				
Intestine	Distention, tension on mesentery or blood vessels (intestine)	+/0	<1–30	55,156,575
Bladder	Distention or contraction	+/0	<2–20	156,828
Visceral nociceptors				
Intestine	Intense mechanical, thermal, and chemical stimuli	+/0		156

systematic studies have revealed that it is often possible to identify slowly conducting afferents that have thresholds which exceed the maximum possible mechanical stimulus. In the face of inflammation, however, such axons have been shown to develop spontaneous activity and an exquisite sensitivity to subsequent mechanical stimulation. These axons, frequently found in joint afferents (see following), have been designated as "silent nociceptors."[696] These observations, in conjunction with the observed chemical sensitivity of the small afferent suggests that the contents of the "inflammatory soup"[337] that have been identified in the inflamed tissue may play an important role in the afferent message generated in the post-injury pain state. There are two components to this consideration: (i) the nature of the materials that are elaborated and (ii) the effect of these products on afferent activity and pain behavior.

The Post-Injury State. A common result of a high-intensity thermal or mechanical stimulus is tissue damage and is defined by Lewis[497] as a "triple response": a flush at the site of the stimulus accompanied by a flare resulting from widespread arterial dilation and a local edema secondary to increased vascular permeability (see Chapter 23.1, Figs. 23.1-2 to 23.1-4). This state of inflammation is often accompanied by a local decrease in the magnitude of the stimulus required to elicit a pain response, that is, a primary hyperalgesia,[60,833] referred to by Lewis[497] as "nocifensor tenderness." The region of primary hypersensitivity is often surrounded by a much larger region of secondary hypersensitivity.[497] Evidence that at least a fraction of these phenomena were mediated by a peripheral mechanism derives from the following observations: (i) antidromic electrical activation of sensory afferent fibers produces hypersensitivity and flare in the skin region innervated by the nerve, and (ii) blockade of the nerve central to the site of antidromic stimulation does not block the hypersensitivity evoked by such nerve stimulation.[496] Because the antidromic volley evokes a primary hyperalgesia and vasodilation in the absence of sympathetic innervation and the required stimulation intensities evoke discharges in C fibers, it appears likely that the effects are mediated by unmyelinated somatic afferents.[140,364,496] Lewis[496] presciently suggested that primary hypersensitivity was due to the release of algogenic agents from damaged tissue and from nerve terminals in the skin by means of an axon reflex activated by the proximate tissue damage. In this case, it is suggested that action potentials evoked in the terminals of a sensory fiber which are in the damaged regions travel not only back to the spinal cord, but also antidromically into the surrounding vascular bed by means of axon collaterals. This is associated with the release of a vasodilator agent that increases blood flow (thereby producing the flare), increases vascular permeability (producing edema), and, as a result of either a direct effect or a subsequent release of an intermediate agent, activates or facilitates the activation of peripheral sensory afferent terminals (hypersensitivity). The local release of chemical intermediates, as suggested above, may also explain the occurrence of continued sensation after the primary stimulus (e.g., thermal or mechanical) has been removed. Thus mild heat damage to the receptive fields has been shown to produce significant increases in the excitability of polymodal nociceptors (C fibers, see following)[43,44,56,638] and high-threshold mechanoreceptors.[252] As noted above, the parodoxical discharges of cold receptors to noxious heat also display sensitization.[223] A chemical intermediary with a prolonged half-life that alters the environs of the adjacent nerve terminals and facilitates their activity could explain one component of the accompanying hyperalgesia.

Agents Released After Injury and Their Action on Afferents and Behavior. Endogenous agents that may mediate these algogenic and facilitatory effects can be categorized according to their chemical class and their presumed origin, for example: tissue (serotonin, histamine, potassium, hydrogen ion, members of the arachidonic acid cascade), plasma (kinins, adenosine), or nerve terminals (substance P[SP]; calcitonin gene-related peptide [CGRP]). This listing is meant only to be representative and is neither inclusive nor exclusive.[141] Nevertheless, it provides some sense as to the complexity of the chemical milieu that occurs after a local tissue injury.

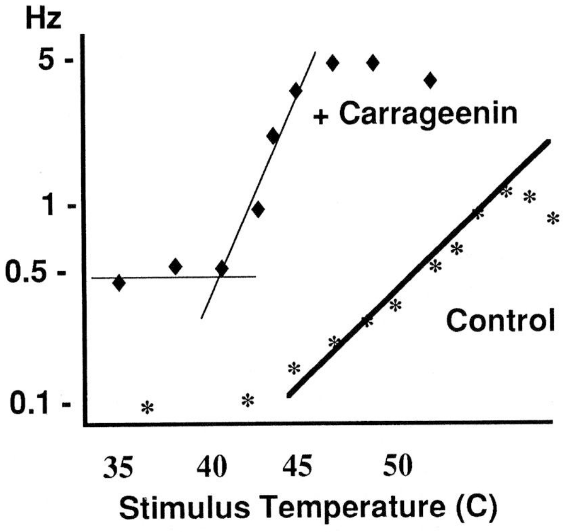

FIG. 24-4. Firing of small afferent in the skin at increasing temperatures. Following the injection of carrageenan into the skin, the afferent shows increasing spontaneous activity, a left shift, and an increase in the slope of the stimulus response curve, indicating a facilitated response to thermal stimuli *(right).* (Data from Reeh, P.W.: Sensory receptors in a mammalian skin-nerve *in vitro* preparation. Progr. Brain Res., *74:*271, 1988.) A similar result is observed if the skin of the receptive field is injured, as with a mild burn yielding an erythema.

Potassium/Hydrogen. Tissue injury results in prominent release of intracellular K^+ and a lowering of tissue pH. Following intense exercise or burns, for example, extracellular K may reach high mM concentrations.[349,506] Blister base fluid may display pH values as low as 4 or 5 in cardiac ischemia, fracture-related hematomas, and exercising muscle.[732] The mechanisms of this increase probably reflect failure of cell membrane integrity and dysfunction of the Na/K pump function.[349]

Amines. Histamine (granules of mast cells, basophils, and platelets)[310] and serotonin (mast cells and platelets)[238] are released by mechanical trauma, heat, radiation, and certain by-products of tissue damage, most notably neutrophil lysosomal materials, certain immunologic processes, thrombin, collagen, and epinephrine, as well as by lipid acids of the arachidonic acid cascade, such as the leukotrienes, and the prostaglandins.[421,574,737,779]

Serotonin, histamine, and acetylcholine have all been shown to excite primary afferents. Close intra-arterial injection of serotonin excites populations of cutaneous mechanoreceptive and high-threshold afferents.[40,41] Similar administration of histamine was shown to excite populations of C fiber/group IV cutaneous mechanoreceptors and nociceptors sensitive to thermal and mechanical stimuli, but not myelinated (presumably nonnoxious) mechanoreceptive afferents.[254,260] Administration of 48/80, which releases histamine from mast cells, activated small-diameter fiber nociceptors.[56] A variety of agents (acetylcholine, histamine, serotonin) injected into the ear of a rabbit isolated from the body except for its nerve supply evoked a reflex depressor response indicative of the activation of small-diameter cutaneous nociceptive afferents.[414] Direct application of histamine or serotonin onto a blister base induced by cantharidin, or the direct injection of these agents into the skin, induced a significant pain response in humans.[29,233,423] In dogs, the intra-arterial but not the intravenous injection of serotonin and histamine induced pseudo-affective responses (barking, efforts to escape, pupil dilatation)[318] (see also Fig. 24-1), the most potent agent being bradykinin.[318]

Kinins. Bradykinin is synthesized by the cascade that is triggered when factor XII is activated by agents such as kallikrein and trypsin. In the course of the cascade, even more kallikrein is produced; this is converted to bradykinin by the enzyme timenogenase.[142,157] Bradykinin is released by noxious insult.[340,677,826]

The local injection of bradykinin has been shown to have potent stimulatory effects in small afferents.[41,345,558,694] After intra-arterial injection in the dog or application in the blister base in humans,[805] bradykinin produces potent pseudo-affective pain behavior. This activity in producing pain behavior and the elaboration of bradykinin during the injury state has led to considerable speculation as to its role in sustaining post-injury evoked activity. Pharmacologic investigations have emphasized the existence of two bradykinin receptors (B1/B2[671]). It appears that under normal circumstances, pharmacologic studies have indicated there is a preponderance of B2 sites which can activate small afferents, whereas in the face of continued inflammation, there appears to be an up-regulation of B1 sites.[219,635]

Lipidic acids. Prostanoids are synthesized upon the release of cell-membrane-derived arachidonic acid by the activation of phospholipase A.[687] Various agents, including norepinephrine and dopamine, stimulate the synthesis of cellular phospholipids by releasing nonesterified free fatty acid precursors.[259,528] Membrane-bound enzymes, lipoxygenase[604] or cyclooxygenase, act on these substrates to synthesize the leukotrienes and the prostanoids. Agents such as acetylsalicylic acid and indomethacin inhibit cyclooxygenase[258,722,784] and prevent the synthesis of these agents. Elevated levels of prostaglandins and leukotrienes are found following local injury and inflammation in joints and damaged skin.[309,826,819] Local intra-arterial bradykinin will enhance the formation and release of prostaglandins.[415,416,490,540]

Prostaglandins (PGs) injected alone evoked little pain response except in high doses.[177,243,378] Although these prostanoids commonly have little evocative effect, they readily facilitate the pseudo-affective and autonomic responses produced by intra-arterial administration of bradykinin in dogs and rabbits.[243,414,570] Thus, in the knee joint, PGI_2 will excite and facilitate the responsiveness of slowly conducting joint afferents.[694] In the behaving animal, intradermal injections of PGE_I augmented the pain evoked by: (i) peripheral injections of bradykinin and histamine,[244] (ii) the writhing response evoked by intraperitoneal phenylbenzylquinone,[165,395] (iii) the response to pressure in the rat's inflamed paw,[242,770] and (iv) on dog's inflamed knee joint.[570] Perfusion of the receptive field of a thermal nociceptive afferent with PGE_2 did not alter its resting discharge. However, PGE_2 produced a dose-dependent increase in the discharge rate of the fiber in response to a stimulus.[336] Similarly, the simultaneous administration of PGE_I and bradykinin, each in a dose that by itself was ineffective, produced significant activity in afferent fibers.[139] That some or all of bradykinin's algogenic effects may be mediated or potentiated by prostaglandins is suggested by a nociceptive response to the kinin being blocked by prior treatment with a cyclooxygenase inhibitor.[243,489,570] If the prostaglandins produce their sensitizing effects by a common biochemical mechanism in a different species and several organ systems, a common order of potency for the lipidic acids should be observed. Where examined, the following rank order has, in fact, been typically observed: $PGE_1 > PGE_2 > PGF_{2a}$, 2 PGF_{2B} 2 $PGA_1 = PGB_2 = PGI_2 = 0$.[243,414,570,770,785]

Adenosine. Adenosine has been shown to be released post-muscle ischemia after exercise, correlating with a reported pain state.[739] Conversely, treatment with a nonselective adenosine receptor antagonist, theophylline, reduced the pain associated with ischemic pain of the forelimb.[413]

Cytokines. Injury and the evolution of the inflammatory state, or local skin injury, will lead to the release into the local extracellular fluid of a number of cytokines such as epidermal growth factor, tumor necrosis factor α (TNF-α), and a number of interleukins, including IL1 and IL8.[240,241,308] Although relatively little work has been done with these agents, it appears certain that their local interactions can lead to the release of prostaglandins, which can subsequently activate small afferents. This interaction provides mechanisms whereby general immune reactions can be affiliated with activity in small afferents (such as, perhaps, the aching sensation associated with influenza, or the reaction to foreign bodies as in chimeric antibody therapy for cancer).

Afferent peptides. Substance P and CGRP are peptides found in peripheral afferent C fiber terminals in the skin,[274,369,370] cortical blood vessels,[533,577] tooth pulp,[614] and eye.[61] Peptide levels in the peripheral tissues are typically elevated in inflamed tissues and joints.[483] Antidromic sensory stimulation has been shown to release SP or CGRP in a variety of peripheral tissues, including tooth pulp,[85] knee joint,[839] skin,[353] and trachea.[385] Importantly, a stimulus that serves to activate the nerve terminal will itself yield the release of the afferent peptide.[385]

With regard to the effects of the afferent peptides, SP has been shown not to be algogenic when administered peripherally,[488] and will not activate peripheral nociceptive afferents.[475] However, it has been shown that conditioning a nerve terminal with SP will result in a facilitation of the response of the terminal to subsequent chemical mediators.[447] Aside from a direct terminal interaction, locally released afferent peptides can serve to alter the local milieu. However, antidromic afferent nerve stimulation will produce flare and sensitization in the region of skin innervated by the stimulated sensory nerve.[741] As exogenously administered, SP has been shown to induce plasma extravasation in both normal and denervated skin,[488] and because other peptides such as vasoactive intestinal peptide (VIP) do not produce such extravasation,[274] SP appears to be a likely mediator for the neurogenically evoked increase in capillary wall permeability. Administration of capsaicin will deplete SP content in skin,[274] and this depletion is accompanied by a loss of the ability of peripheral nerve stimulation to produce extravasation.[396,742] Exogenously administered SP or antidromic stimulation evokes an increase in local blood flow and capillary permeability. The effects of either manipulation are reversed by putative SP antagonists.[171,679] These observations appear to reflect mechanisms that may be quite common. Thus, the SP in plexuses surrounding cerebral vessels and that which originates in the trigeminal ganglion may be released and occasion the vascular syndrome of migraine.[577] Aside from their effects upon the vasculature, the locally released peptides may serve to bring into play a number of systems that may subsequently interact with the afferent terminal. Thus, antidromic stimulation and SP can degranulate mast cells and evoke kinin release.[146]

Sensory Innervation Excited by Natural Stimuli

Table 24-1 presents a summary of the classes of afferents that are activated by various physical stimuli capable of evoking pain behavior. In the following section, characteristics of these afferents as a function of their respective innervated organs are discussed.

Cutaneous Stimuli. The cutaneous input is richly innervated by afferents that transduce a variety of stimulus modalities.

Mechanosensitive afferents. High-threshold mechanoreceptive fibers responding only at pressure sufficient to produce innervating glabrous tissue damage and conducting in the range of A-delta fibers (15–25 m/sec) have been identified.[41,101,102,285,637] These afferents tend to respond with a rate of discharge proportional to the magnitude of the pressure applied. Receptive fields for these mechanoreceptors are large in the trunk (1–8 cm^2) and smaller on the face (1–2 cm^2). While on the limbs, distal receptive fields tend to be smaller than proximal fields. Mechanoreceptors conducting at C fiber velocities have been shown with thresholds requiring von Frey hair stimuli greater than 2 g and with receptive fields ranging from small (5 mm^2) to strips covering several square centimeters. These fibers discharge with a frequency that is monotonically proportional to the stimulus intensity.[56,285]

Thermoreceptive afferents. Warm receptors have been observed that respond to temperature increments of less than 1°C within the range of 30° to 40°C with small peripheral receptive fields (less than 0.5 mm in diameter).[391] These fibers have also been shown to respond to thermal stimuli of noxious intensity with an increasing frequency of discharge. High-intensity stimulation within the range of 47° to 51°C evokes a transient high-frequency discharge. These response characteristics are to be differentiated from those reported for the mechanical-thermal receptive units (see following) in that the response rate commonly is all or none in character.[221,222] Certain afferent cutaneous fibers that respond to decreases in temperature on the order of less than 1°C (i.e., "cold" receptors) may show a paradoxical response to heat. As skin temperature has risen to 45° to 52° C, the fiber's rate of discharge has also increased.[211,223,357,481]

Mechano-Thermoreceptive nociceptive afferents. Afferents have been reported to respond to high-intensity mechanical and thermal stimulation, conduct within an A-delta range (10–40 m/sec), and exhibit a positively accelerating monotonic stimulus response function.[40,101] Activation threshold may lie between 40° and 60°C, and a maximum response is commonly observed at 45° to 53°C.[221,222,285,390] Receptive fields for these units are small (less than 5 mm^2) and frequently occur as several spots, suggesting extensive collateralization of the terminals. These afferents may mediate the "first" pain of heat, for example, the pricking sensation reported immediately after the application of a strong thermal stimulus.[655]

Polymodal C fiber afferents. A major portion of C fiber afferents that respond to nociceptive stimuli are "polymodal" in character. These fibers may constitute 80% to 90% of the primate nociceptive C fiber population.[44] These axons are activated equally well by several classes of stimuli, including mechanical (greater than 1 g), thermal (45°–53°C), and frequently chemical stimuli applied to the characteristically small (< 3 mm^2) receptive field. The response to such ongoing stimuli is a sustained, vigorous discharge, in which the frequency is monotonically related to stimuli intensity.[43,44,56,478]

Recordings in humans from single afferents conducting in the range of 0.5 to 2.0 m/sec have been made from sensory nerves innervating nonglabrous skin. These fibers are activated by strong mechanical stimuli (von Frey hairs of 0.7–13 g; needle pricks; and local compression) and produce an ongoing discharge that adapts slowly in the presence of the sustained stimulus.[757,758,760–762,782,783] (For an example of one such unit, see Fig. 24-8.) Such units are not spontaneously active at temperatures up to 40°C, but temperatures in excess of 45°C evoke activity in an increasing number of units.[761,762,783] Local application of acid, histamine, or potassium chloride evokes a prolonged discharge.[761,762,783] Receptive fields of polymodal C afferents tend to be larger in humans (1 mm^2–1 cm^2) but frequently may also display several sites, suggesting extensive collateralization.[758,761,762,782] These slowly conducting fibers, presumably unmyelinated in character, show clear signs of fatigue and failure of conduction upon repeated high-frequency electrical stimulation.[757,760]

Skeletal Muscle. It has been reported that, excluding the stretch receptors, the principal sensory innervation of the skeletal muscle derives from free nerve endings in fascia and the adventitia of blood vessels that arise from myelinated and nonmyelinated fibers.[730] High threshold groups III and IV mechanoreceptors in muscle activated by intense contraction have been reported.[392,475] Intense thermal stimuli applied to muscle belly evokes monotonically-increasing activity in these afferents.[363] Hypertonic solutions of sodium chloride[624] and close intra-arterial injections of a number of algogenic agents (histamine, bradykinin, and serotonin) evoke significant activity in afferent groups III and IV.[260,266,558] However, the terminals are not functionally homogeneous. At least three groups of afferents have been identified: (i) those activated by algogenic agents but not by muscle activity, (ii) those activated by muscle activity but not by algogenic agents, and (iii) those activated by both sustained muscle activity and algogenic agents.[461] The sensitivity to chemical agents makes it likely that these nociceptive groups III and IV afferents are activated by agents that are released locally during muscle contraction. Extracellular potassium levels double (5–15 mM) during isometric testing in the cat.[366] Failure of nominal concentrations of phosphate and lactate to alter group IV afferent activity suggests that metabolic by-products alone do not constitute a source of muscle pain.[461] The apparent ability of prostaglandins to sensitize algogenic receptors to otherwise inactive concentrations of chemical stimulants in cardiac muscle (see following), and the likelihood of their release during intense skeletal muscle contraction, could be a significant factor in the activation of groups III and IV skeletal muscle afferents by metabolic by-products.

Cardiac Muscle. The heart receives afferents that travel with both the parasympathetic and the sympathetic tree. In the latter, the cell bodies are in the nodose ganglia, and in the former, the cell bodies are in the respective thoracic dorsal root ganglia. Pain arising from the heart appears to be mediated to a significant degree by activity in the sympathetic afferents, but vagal afferents may play an important if undefined role.[548]

Occlusion of the coronary artery leading to ischemia of ventricular muscle produces pain in humans[65,808] and pseudo-affective response in animals.[738] Sensory afferents in the inferior cardiac nerve projecting to the T1–T5 segments of the spinal cord mediate the transmission of such information.[261,264,505,809] Recording single units from the T2–T3 ramus communicans reveals that during coronary occlusions, activity in A-delta/C afferents increases.[92,93,773] The cardiac afferents are activated by moderate- to high-intensity mechanical stimulation,[92,515,771] noxious heating,[601] and several algogenic agents.[99,601,772] The stimulus for angina may be the release from ischemic muscle of humoral factors that sensitize or activate cardiac afferents. Serotonin and histamine stimulate cardiac afferent fibers,[216,601,602] and blood levels of bradykinin in the coronary sinus after occlusion are sufficient to evoke pseudo-affective responses when administered in dogs.[318,453,731,773] In the heart, (i) reflex cardiovascular changes suggestive of angina discomfort occur following the topical application of several algogenic agents to the wall of the left ventricle, and (ii) temporary occlusion of the coronary artery supplying the area of the ventricle under study sensitizes the heart to the algogenic effects of bradykinin.[730] Importantly, co-application of prostaglandins ($PGE_1 > PGE_2 > PGF_{2a}$) with bradykinin has significantly potentiated the algogenic effects of bradykinin. Pretreatment with a prostaglandin synthesis inhibitor reduced the algogenic effects of bradykinin and the sensitizing effects of prior ischemia. The potentiation of bradykinin's algogenic effects by exogenous prostaglandins was evident for as long as 60 minutes and could not be attenuated by indomethacin. This is consistent with the observation that prostaglandins are formed and released in the heart muscle following hypoxia or ischemia.[11,63,803] Thus angina could speculatively result, in part, from the neurohumoral activation of afferent terminals by the joint release of both prostaglandins and bradykinin.

Teeth. Innervation of the teeth occurs both intradentally (within the tooth) and periodontally (within the surrounding connective tissue). Free nerve endings are found within the pulp and the surrounding blood vessels. Fibers that originate in afferent plexuses adjacent to the inner dentinal surface pass through the odontoblasts to the dentinal tubules that run parallel to the odontoblast processes.[265,615] In tooth pulp, the unmyelinated fibers are ensheathed by Schwann cells and interlace with the odontoblast somata. Tooth pulp afferents consist of fibers having diameters and apparent conduction velocities in the A-delta and C fiber range.[20,194,311,875] The periodontal afferents travel through the maxillary and mandibular branches of the trigeminal nerve to terminate within collagen fibers of the alveolar ligament with specializations similar to the Meissner corpuscle. Transdentinal electrical stimulation produces a sharp pain of brief duration,[147] which gives rise to jaw opening and closing reflexes and attempts to escape.[781,791,792] In shock titration paradigms, primates maintain the current intensity of dental stimulation at or immediately above that intensity which, in a single escape paradigm, will support escape behavior.[613] These observations correspond to studies in humans suggesting that the difference between a perceivable threshold stimulus (prepain) and a stimulus sufficient to evoke a pain report is small.[17,18] Conversely, activity in intradentinal sensory nerves has been shown to correlate closely with the sensation of pain.[229] Pressure, touch, or tooth movement is likely to be mediated by afferents from the periodontal and gingival structures in which the tooth is embedded.[80,642]

Thermal stimulation of teeth has been reported to evoke neuronal activity in dental nerves.[270,531] In cats, the frequency of discharge of dental afferents rose when the dentin temperature was elevated from 34° to 37°C within a 10-second period.[704] Slow heating of the cat tooth surface to 47°C failed to elicit such activity.[4] Repeated intense thermal stimulation of the tooth (60°C), however, did evoke a persistent afferent discharge. Pretreatment, but not post-treatment, with prostaglandin synthesis inhibitors reduced the discharge associated with repetitive heating.[5] The generation of cyclooxygenase products may therefore sensitize nerve endings to stimuli originating in the local pulpal environment. Because nerve endings do not penetrate to the enamel dentin interface, the effective stimulus in tooth sensations has been proposed to be the distortion of odontoblasts or alterations in hydraulic flow produced by changes in temperature.[79] Inflammation or edema associated with thermal damage, as described above, or direct pressure could increase pulpal volume and deform the mechanically sensitive nerve terminals that lie between the odontoblasts. That changes in pulpal pressure can evoke activity in tooth afferents is supported by the observations that (1) bursts of 1 to 4 spikes occur in synchrony with the systolic pulse and (ii) pulpal pressure changes as much as 5 mm Hg with the systolic pulse pressure in the normal tooth.[59,704] Presumably, where inflammation has occurred, such changes may be augmented because of the increased pulpal volume in a restricted space.

Synovial Joints. Cutaneous afferents and branches of adjacent muscle afferents innervate the joints.[275] Intense deformation or inflammation-induced expansion within the joint will evoke activity in the group III (A-delta) fibers.[151–153] Urate crystals,[253] carrageenan,[570,780] and endotoxin[362] injected into the synovial joint evokes an acute local inflammation, whereas the intradermal injection of killed bacteria suspended in Freund's adjuvant results in a chronic polyarthritis.[305] A marked sensitivity to stimulation of the affected limbs is observed in animals so treated. Joint pain associated with gout-induced arthritis in humans probably results from urate crystal deposition.[537] Altered sensitivity to mechanical stimulation may be mediated by the generation of chemical intermediaries such as prostaglandins. The ability of cyclooxygenase or phospholipase A inhibitors to reduce the sensitivity associated with the inflamed joints and to reduce the inflammation is consistent with this hypothesis.[96,780] Other inhibitors of cyclo-oxygenase, such as paracetamol, are effective against joint pain but exert no effect on arthritic swelling.[539,830] This has led to the speculation that nonsteroidal anti-inflammatory drugs (NSAIDs) may either work by a separate mechanism[538] or be associated with a central action.[516,517]

Visceral Organs. Information regarding the state of the visceral organs projects to the central nervous system by afferents that travel with both parasympathetic (essentially vagal above the diaphragm and sacral parasympathetics for the abdominal viscera) and sympathetic innervation. For the vagus, the cell body of the afferent lies in the nodose ganglion, while for the sympathetic and the sacral parasympathetic, the afferent cell body lies in the respective dorsal root ganglia. Many of the axons are small and lightly myelinated or unmyelinated.[130,548,595] Manipulation of a number of healthy visceral organs such as the liver, kidney, and spleen does not appear to give rise to reports of pain. However, it appears likely that three conditions are associated with visceral pain.

1. Distention of hollow viscus. Thus, expansion of the gastrointestinal tract (esophagus, stomach duodenum, large and small intestines), smooth muscle organs (gallbladder), and urinary tract (urethra and bladder) will yield short-latency pain behavior in animals and humans.[544,595]
2. Inflammation. Internal body organs clearly become symptomatic in the presence of mechanical distortion and particularly during inflammation. Based on the ability of some of the inflammatory products outlined above, such as bradykinin and prostaglandins, to induce activity in visceral innervation and to induce pain behavior,[47,51,566,567,730] such a correlation appears reasonable.
3. Ischemia. Occlusion of the vasculature is recognized as a potential source of visceral pain. Ischemia induces activity in visceral afferents[343] and results in a septic shock state in which large quantities of active humors are released locally and into the circulation (e.g., heart—coronary; viscera—splanchnic). As in the above comments on inflammation, the presence of these products can both facilitate and activate the transduction properties of the innervating afferent.

Abnormal Origins of Activity in Peripheral Afferents. Commonly, orthodromic discharge of a peripheral afferent originates at the distal terminals secondary to generator potentials induced by the appropriate peripheral stimulus. Pressure briskly applied mid-axon evokes only a transient neural activity (Fig. 24-5).[380,795] Acute nerve compression in humans may be reported as transiently painful, if perceived at all.[228,426] Simple, slow distortion of mid-axon regions, however, is ineffective in generating neural activity.[2,302,307,417,795] Thus chronic pressure alone, such as that generated by benign tumors, is often not reported as painful.[426] However, mechanical insensitivity of the mid-axon region is altered after nerve injury. Upon severance of a nerve, there is a shower of activity that disappears. With time, the cut end reseals and a neuroma develops. Systematic studies in animal models have shown that this neuroma frequently gives rise to ongoing orthodromic activity in the nerve (see Chapter 23.1, Fig. 23.1-7). The activity occurs

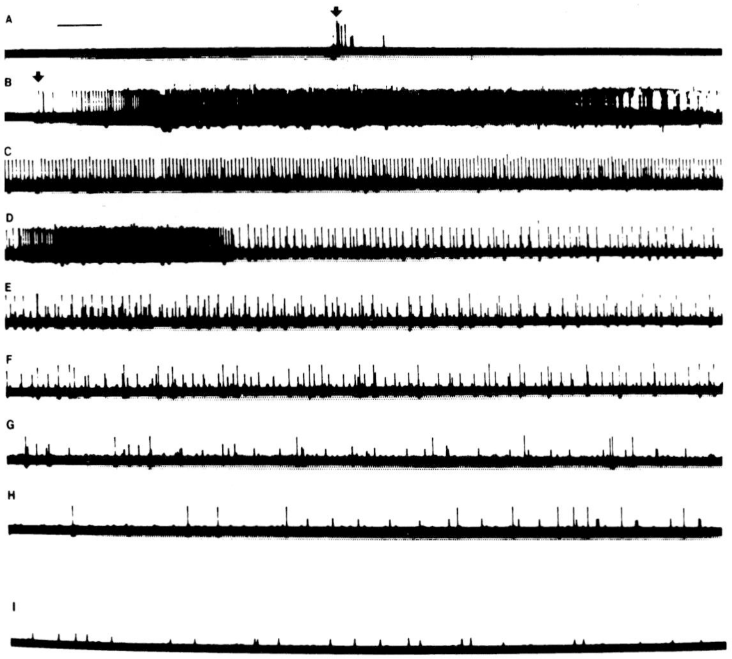

FIG. 24-5. Effects of dorsal root ganglion (DRG) compression. Multiple unit recording from a small filament of dorsal root. **A:** For contrast, the response of the units to dorsal root compression. **B–H:** Response in same filament to maintained DRG compression. Each line represents the first 3 seconds of successive 1-minute intervals. **I:** The first 3 seconds of activity sampled 25 minutes after initiation of DRG compression, showing persistent A-delta activity. Time bar, 200 m/sec. Compression begins at the arrow in **B** and is maintained throughout the recording. (From Howe, J.F., Loeser, J.D., and Calvin, W.H.: Mechanosensitivity of dorsal root ganglia and chronically injured axons: A physiological basis for the radicular pain of nerve root compression. Pain, *3*:25, 1977.)

within fibers having conduction velocities, suggestive of small-diameter myelinated fibers.[795] Small distortions of the cut region now produce long periods (30 seconds) of repetitive discharge. These observations suggested that the local injury had transformed that region of the axon and endowed it with properties of excitability similar to those in the terminal region. Importantly, it has been shown that after such peripheral nerve injury, the dorsal root ganglion cell of the injured nerve also begins to display a spontaneous activity.[201]

Ectopic foci in these injured nerves have been suggested to be the source of the abnormal sensations that occur after amputation.[114,217] Neurotomy in several species, including mice, rats, cats, and rabbits,[37,202,795] gives rise to autotomy of the denervated region, which may result from the abnormal discharges generated by the neuroma formed. The self-mutilation, when and if it does develop, apparently is not due to the anesthetic state, but (i) mutilation begins only after several days,[797] (ii) guanethidine, which suppresses the ectopic discharges associated with neuromas in mice, suppresses the autotomy in neurectomized rats and mice,[633] and (iii) selective spinal tractotomies abolish the autotomy.[37]

Dorsal root ganglion cells are apparent exceptions to the above discussion of nonterminal afferent spike generation. As shown in Figure 24-5, slow, minor distortion of the dorsal root ganglion evokes repetitive firing that lasts minutes. Similar distortion of the dorsal roots was not as effective.[378] It has been proved that this stimulation evoked a pain event by the fact that acute injury to the dorsal root ganglion evokes immediate tachycardia and mass flexion reflexes in the lightly anesthetized animal. These observations support the suggestion that the radicular pain of sciatica might be associated with such a focal distortion of the dorsal root ganglion and not the root or nerve proper. Patients suffering from tic douloureux are often reported to have an artery, a small tumor, or plaque impinging upon the trigeminal root.[399,442,446] Although such mechanical stimulation may not account for the unique sensory barrage associated with tic episodes, the mechanical sensitivity of the dorsal root may provide a background upon which a mechanical stimulus, such as that provided by the adjacent artery, might alter innocuous sensory input and thus generate the pain event.[32,109,110]

Spinal Terminals of Primary Afferents

Dorsal Root Entry Zone

As the dorsal root approaches the spinal cord, small myelinated and unmyelinated fibers tend to aggregate in the lateral aspect of the dorsal root, and larger myelinated fibers aggregate medially (Fig. 24-6).[438,501,665,666,723] Entering the spinal cord, the primary afferents bifurcate into rostrally and caudally projecting branches. Large fibers proceed along the dorsal columns for varying distances; many terminate in the spinal gray matter.[117,734] Large-diameter afferent collaterals exit from the dorsal column axis perpendicularly and pursue a ballistic trajectory, coursing deeply into the gray matter before turning dorsally to terminate in the upper portions of the gray matter.[108] The smaller-caliber fibers project rostrally and caudally one or two segments into the medial portion of the tract of Lissauer. Small-diameter fibers enter the dorsal gray matter directly and terminate dorsally, as will be discussed. Both large- and small-diameter fibers give rise to collaterals that distribute ventrally in the spinal gray matter (see Fig. 24-6).

Although the preponderance of afferents terminate ipsilaterally, there is evidence that a proportion of the afferents also terminate contralaterally.[19,501,502,659,672] These fibers travel dorsal to the central canal to terminate in laminae III and IV of the contralateral dorsal horn, forming a longitudinally ori-

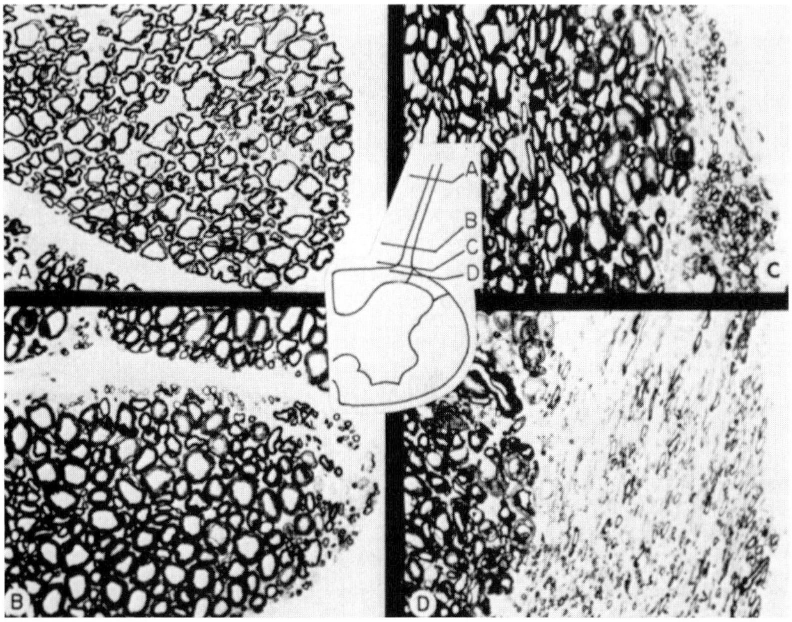

FIG. 24-6. Distribution of large and small fibers in the L7 dorsal root of the cat at selected intervals. **A:** At 5 mm from the root entry zone (REZ) there is no evidence of segregation. **B:** At approximately 1 mm from the REZ, the small fibers are arranged in a peripheral ring. **C:** Just before entering the REZ, the great majority of small fibers are located in the lateral aspect of the rootlet. **D:** The small fibers have merged with the tract of Lissauer. (From Kerr, F.W.L.: Pain: A central inhibitory balance theory. Mayo Clin. Proc., *50*:685, 1975.)

ented plexus one to two segments in length.[180] These contralateral projections occur most commonly at the cervical and sacral levels of the spinal cord, although crossing fibers have been described in the lumbar cord.[501,502] Early work demonstrated the behavioral significance of the medial to lateral distribution of the large and small primary afferents by making discrete lesions in the dorsal root entry zone.[665] Lateral cuts, presumably severing the smaller-caliber myelinated fiber population, produced a significant blockade of the pseudo-affective response of the animal to strong, otherwise aversive, stimuli on the side where the lesions were made. It is likely that such a section also produced local infarcts of the adjacent dorsal gray matter.[350] Discrete surgical lesions directed at the dorsal horn through the dorsal root entry zone have been shown to alleviate pain, particularly that associated with root avulsions.[589,590]

The principal portion of the sensory afferents enters the spinal cord through the dorsal root entry zone, consistent with the "law" of Bell and Magendie. However, a significant number of unmyelinated afferent fibers, which arise from dorsal root ganglion cells, also exist within the ventral roots.[27,155,156,161,162] After the injection of horseradish peroxidase into the spinal gray matter of cats with previously sectioned dorsal roots, reaction products appeared in small dorsal root ganglion cells. Failure to label large dorsal root ganglion neurons is consistent with the observation that the ventral root afferents are largely unmyelinated.[536,863] The relevance of the ventral root afferents in pain transmission remains to be fully defined. This alternate pathway may account for the failure of dorsal rhizotomies to reliably relieve pain.[620] The origin of dorsal and ventral root afferents in dorsal root ganglion neurons would suggest that ganglionectomy would be superior to rhizotomy if afferent input is to be abolished.[621]

Afferent Terminals in Dorsal Horn

The concept that the spinal gray matter of the adult spinal cord may be organized according to a distinctive lamination of cell bodies and terminal regions has been used fruitfully to delimit the anatomy of the spinal gray matter (Fig. 24-7).[673,674]

Organization of Terminals by Fiber Type. Retrograde transport of horseradish peroxidase to the distal cut ends of primary afferent fibers after medial section of the dorsal root revealed that the horseradish peroxidase reaction product was located primarily in the most dorsal laminae of the spinal gray matter. Terminals from smaller myelinated fibers were located in the marginal zone, the ventral portion of lamina II, and throughout lamina III.[501] Fine-caliber unmyelinated fibers largely terminated throughout lamina II. In contrast, the large-caliber fibers passing in the medial portion of the root entry zone terminated largely in the nucleus proprius and in more ventral regions of the dorsal gray matter. These larger fibers made few direct contacts with neurons of the substantia gelatinosa and marginal layer, terminating largely

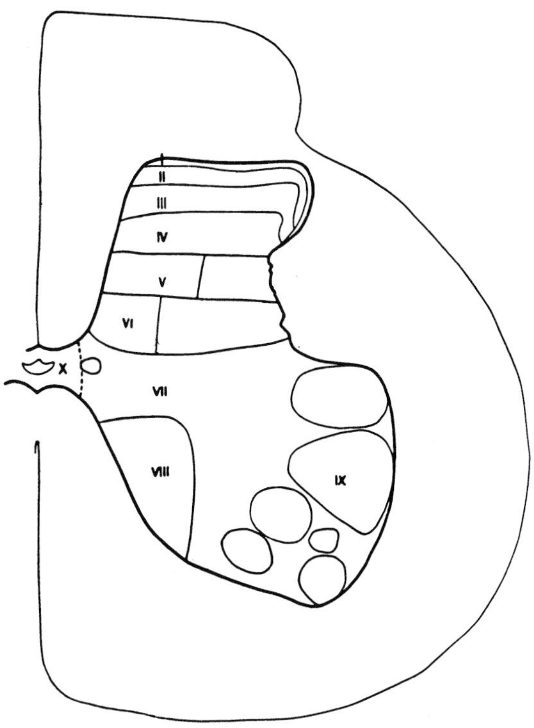

FIG. 24-7. Schematic drawing of the lamination of the ventral cell column of the 7th lumbar spinal cord segment in the full-grown cat. Lamina VIII occupies only the medial part of the ventral horn, lamina IX with its large motor nuclei has swung laterally and dorsally, and lamina VII extends between them both deeply into the horn. (From Rexed, B.: The cytoarchitectonic organization of the spinal cord in the cat. J. Comp. Neurol., *96*:415, 1952.)

below lamina II. Similar results were obtained in studies in which the distribution of functionally defined afferents was examined after intra-axonal application of horseradish peroxidase.[502] Intermediate- to fine-diameter cutaneous nociceptive mechanoreceptors terminated largely in the marginal zone. Terminals of low-threshold mechanoreceptors activated by D-hairtype (down hair) receptors were distributed in the dorsal portion of laminae IV and V as well as in the ventral portions of the substantia gelatinosa. These comments are summarized schematically in Figure 24-8.

After the entry of the axon into the dorsal root entry zone, the axons typically display bifurcations or trifurcations. The large afferents send projections rostrally and caudally within the dorsal columns and directly into the dorsal horn. This is indicated schematically in Figure 24-9. The rostrally projecting collaterals may continue as far forward as the dorsal column nuclei. However, many of the axons send collaterals off into the spinal horn at progressively distal segments. Small axons display a similar collateralization, though the rostrocaudal spread occurs in the lateral tract of Lissauer.[431] Systematic mapping studies have shown that these projections may extend as far as 4 to 11 segments. Thus, in the rat, labeled terminals from the sural nerve were found in the grey matter up to three to four segments caudal to their root entry,

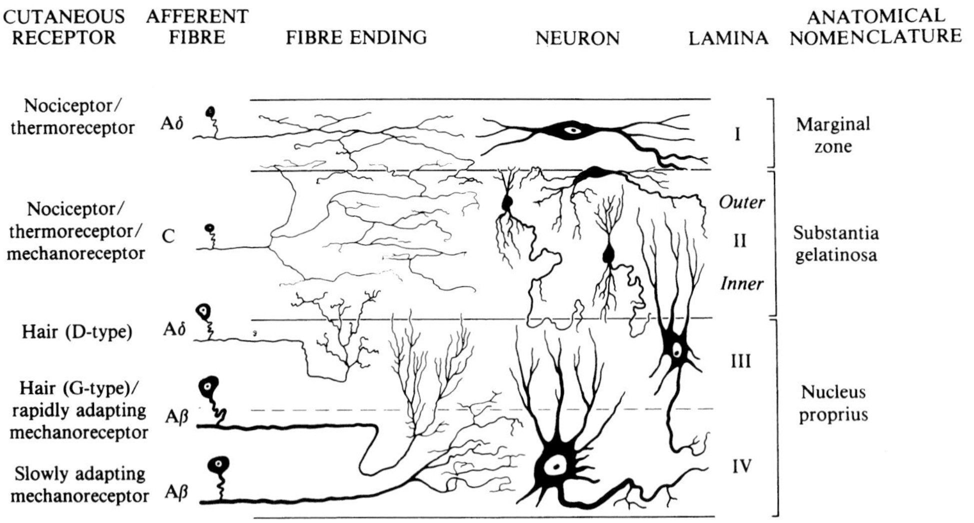

FIG. 24-8. Schematic diagram of the neuronal organization of, and afferent input to, the superficial dorsal horn. The diagram represents an imaginary transverse section of the dorsal horn and illustrates the afferent fiber endings and neuronal elements present in the first four laminae of the dorsal horn. To the left of the diagram the types of afferent fiber and relevant receptor groups associated with them are listed. Fiber endings in the dorsal horn are schematized diagrams taken from published morphologic studies. Neurons in the diagram represent standard types of neuron in the superficial dorsal horn. The following types have been illustrated *(from top to bottom)*: a marginal cell, an SG limiting cell, two SG central cells, and two neurons of the nucleus proprius, the most superficial of which has dendrites penetrating lamina II. Indicated at the right of the diagram are the laminar division of the superficial dorsal horn and corresponding anatomic nomenclature. (From Cervero, F., and Iggo, A.: The substantia gelatinosa of the spinal cord. A critical review. Brain, *103:*717, 1980.)

and for the sciatic nerve in S4, four to six segments caudal to the segment of root entry.[794] Importantly, the strength of the excitatory drive is greatest at the segment of entry and diminishes so that input from distal dermatomes have a progressively decreasing excitatory influence.[555] The significance of this large and small afferent collateralization is that there is an excitatory drive which occurs at spinal segments distal to the segment of entry. Factors that regulate the postsynaptic excitability of the distal cells receiving these projections will serve to define the size of the receptive field of the respective neuron.

PHARMACOLOGY OF PRIMARY AFFERENTS

Spinal Afferent Terminals

The synapse made by primary afferents with neurons of the spinal cord represents the first-order link between the periphery and the central nervous system. Electrophysiologic studies have provided substantial evidence that conducted potentials interact with the second-order neuron by an excitatory synapse. No evidence of a classic monosynaptic inhibitory influence by primary afferents has been hitherto presented.[376] A second property of the neuronal response

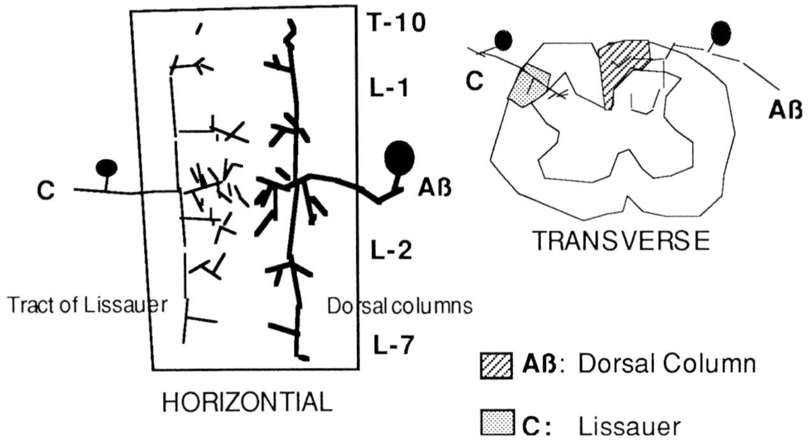

FIG. 24-9. Schematic diagram displaying the ramification of C fibers *(left)* into the dorsal horn and collateralization into the tract of Lissauer and of Aβ fibers *(right)* into the dorsal columns and into the dorsal horn. Note that the greatest density of terminations is within the segment of entry, and that there are less dense collateralizations into the dorsal horns at the more distal spinal segments. This density of collateralization corresponds to the potency of the excitatory drive into these distal segments.

evoked by afferent excitation is that at least two populations of excitatory postsynaptic potentials are seen which are thought to be monosynaptic: (i) fast-onset and short-lasting and (ii) delayed and of a relatively extended duration.[454,777,872] These electrophysiologic findings in concert with the presence of morphologically distinct vesicle populations in the same terminal are interpreted as revealing the presence of at least two classes of neurotransmitters released from the same terminal.

Considerable efforts have been directed at establishing the identity of neuroactive substances in the primary afferent. Several criteria are classically accepted as minimum requirements in the establishment of the correspondence between the endogenous material and a given substance: (i) the material must be found in the terminals of the afferent population in question (and it or its precursor in the respective dorsal root ganglion cell); (ii) the material must be present in a fraction that is released when the appropriate afferents undergo depolarization; (iii) the postsynaptic effects of the exogenously applied materials must mimic the effects that result when the endogenous afferent systems are physiologically activated; and (iv) those physiologic effects that result from the actions of the endogenously released and exogenously administered agents must possess an identical pharmacology (i.e., the characteristics of the receptor acted upon by the endogenous and exogenous agents must be indistinguishable).

Localization of Putative Afferent Neurotransmitters. Currently, excitatory amino acids such as aspartate and glutamate[183] and a number of peptides including SP, VIP, somatostatin, a VIP homologue (peptido-histidine-isoleucine [PHI]), cholecystokinin (CCK), angiotensin II, bombesin, and related peptides have been observed to possess the following characteristics: (i) they have been found in the dorsal horn of the spinal cord (where most primary afferent terminals are found; (ii) the levels in the dorsal horn are reduced by rhizotomy or ganglionectomy, or both; and (iii) the peptides have been shown to exist within subpopulations of small dorsal root ganglion cells (type-B cells) (Table 24-2). This latter observation is of particular importance because it is thought to be small afferents arising from the type-B cells that are perhaps relevant to pain transmission (see also Fig. 24-14). Immunohistochemical studies directed at the dorsal horn have revealed distinguishable differences in the discrete distribution of the several peptides in the dorsal laminae. SP is predominantly located in Rexed lamina I and the outer layer of II; VIP is principally found in lamina I, whereas somatostatin is found in the outer layer of II. Fluoride-resistant acid phosphatase, found in small ganglion cells separate from those containing SP or somatostatin,[586] is distributed primarily in the inner layer of lamina II in regions distinct from those that SP, VIP, or somatostatin project.[587]

Additionally, a decrease in SP levels in the dorsal horn after ventral rhizotomies has been reported.[857] These observations are consistent with findings discussed previously that unmyelinated afferent fibers course in the ventral roots.

Ability of Putative Afferent Neurotransmitters to Be Released. Important considerations are whether the materials present in afferent terminals exist within a releasable fraction and whether the axons from which they derive are relevant to pain transmission. From spinal cord slices, SP and somatostatin levels in the extracellular fluid have been shown to be elevated in a Ca^{2+}-dependent fashion by depolarization.[7,408,623,691,710] *In vivo* studies using a variety of spinal perfusion models[849] have demonstrated the release of materials from primary afferents, including SP,[295,845] CGRP,[166] VIP, CCK,[62,842] and glutamate.[520,721,725] With these peptides, release was produced by stimulation that activated A-delta/C but not A-beta afferents. The release of SP from the spinal cord has been shown to be antagonized by the local application of mu and delta but not kappa opioid agonists and by $alpha_2$ agonists.[745] These observations are consistent with the presence of opioid and alpha-adrenergic receptors on primary afferent terminals and the effects of opiates and adrenergic agonists on afferent terminals.[402,838,840,858]

Postsynaptic Actions. Glutamate and aspartate applied onto dorsal horn neurons result in a powerful, reversible depolarization with rapid onset, accompanied by an increase in membrane conductance.[879] Examination of the subclasses of neurons excited by glutamate or aspartate reveals no functional selectivity. Thus motor horn cells and dorsal horn neurons excited by A-beta, A-delta, and C fibers show a characteristic excitatory response to glutamate administration.[53,879]

Iontophoretic application onto the dorsal horn of several peptides found in primary afferents has been shown to produce excitatory effects. The focal administration of SP onto spinal neurons results in a slow progressive depolarization of the cell.[354,581,880] Substance P will excite cells that are naturally activated by noxious radiant heat,[354] strong mechanical stimuli,[664] and the intra-arterial injection of bradykinin;[643,834] and facilitate responses of cells activated by noxious cutaneous stimuli. Other agents such as glutamate, CCK, and VIP appear somewhat less selective, since they have been shown to produce excitatory and facilitatory effects on neurons that respond to a wide variety of innocuous stimuli (see previous). Thus, there appears to be a significant correlation between the ability of SP to evoke a progressive depolarization in a dorsal horn neuron and the existence of an afferent drive from small fibers.[643] VIP and CCK have been shown to similarly evoke excitation of dorsal horn neurons.[401,403] Somatostatin has been shown to produce an inhibition of the activity of dorsal horn neurons after iontophoretic administration.[664] This finding is somewhat surprising, because a monosynaptic inhibition by primary afferents on second-order neurons has not been described, but reflects the fact that these agents may exist in several systems, not in primary afferents alone.

As noted above, populations of afferents, particularly those of a small diameter, have more than one material in their terminals that can be released. Electron microscopy has long indicated the presence of several morphologically distinct vesicle populations in primary afferent terminals, no-

TABLE 24-2. *Summary of receptor mediated effects of afferent transmitter candidates*

Candidate	Receptor IT antag classes (*in vivo*)[a]	DRG type	Location (binding or membrane immunoreactivity)	Effects[b]		IT agonist (*in vivo*)[c]
Tachykinins BAP[256]	NK1	Small[352]	D>V[352]	SD[190,777]	PB, HY[159,482]	BHY[861]
	NK2	Small[352]	D>V[352]	SD[777]	PB, HY[159,482]	?
	NK3	Small[352]	D>V[352]	?	NE, BAP[482]	?
CGRP		Small & medium[646]	D>V[646]	SD[831]	HY[159]	?
Bombesin		Small[626]	D>V[607,837]	HP[191]	PB[607]	?
Somatostatin	Small[368]	D>V[368]	HP[580]	NE,[281] BAP[569]		BHY[612]
VIP		Small & medium[286]	D>V[837]	SD[401]	NE[708]	?
Glutamate	NMDA	Small[38]	D>V[400,563]	SD[188]	PB,[1] HY[1,159]	BHY[862]
	Kainate		D>V[400,563]	FD[188]	PB,[1] NE[159]	?
	AMPA		D>V[400,563]	FD[188]	PB,[1] NE[159]	BHY[d]
Nitric oxide (NO) (enzyme inhibition)	(activate guanylate cyclase)	Medium[6]	D>V[565] (NO synthase)	?	?	BHY[518,547]

[a] antag, antagonist; BAP, blocks acute pain behavior (e.g., thermal such as hot plate, tail flick); BHY, blocks hyperalgesia as evoked by peripheral injection of irritants (i.e., formalin test, phase 2).
[b] SD, slow depolarization; FD, fast depolarization; HP, hyperpolarization; ?, unknown.
[c] PB, evokes pain behavior (i.e., scratching/biting); HY, evokes hyperalgesia (i.e., reduced nociceptive thresholds or response latencies); NE, produces no effect; ?, unknown.
[d] Malmberg, A.B.: unpublished observation.

tably those that are dense core and now thought to contain peptides and smaller clear vesicles that may contain amino acids.[367] Intracellular recording in rat spinal cord slices has revealed that repetitive stimulation of the dorsal roots results in an initial burst of monosynaptically driven spikes followed by a prolonged, slow hypopolarization.[777] The slow depolarization of dorsal horn neurons evoked by afferent stimulation or focally applied SP (but not VIP) was blocked by co-administration of a putative SP receptor antagonist or by the prior administration of capsaicin, a neurotoxin that results in the depletion of afferent stores of SP and CCK and destroys small afferents marked by the cytosol enzyme fluoride-resistant acid phosphatase, but has no effect on large-diameter afferents.[98,218] The early depolarization was unaffected by these manipulations. These observations suggest that for this particular neuronal population in neonatal rat spinal cord, afferent stimulation results in two events: a delayed depolarization likely to be mediated by a population of SP-containing terminals; and an immediate depolarization mediated by a second neuroactive agent, perhaps an excitatory amino acid.[394,493]

Role of Neurotransmitters in Pain Transmission. In view of the foregoing data, one may tentatively hypothesize that both the excitatory amino acids and one or more peptides may play some role in pain transmission at the level for the primary afferent synapse. As indicated in Table 24-2, the direct application of several of the peptides and glutamate onto the dorsal horn of the spinal cord results in mild scratching behavior and signs of agitation. Importantly, given the co-containment and likely co-release of peptides and glutamate, the effect of the intrathecal agents is translated into a profound increase in behavioral signs of irritation when the peptide is co-administered with glutamate.[568] The potentiating effects are reduced when this is co-administered with low doses of putative SP receptor antagonists. Aside from the direct excitation and behavioral indices of pain, the spinal delivery of several of these peptides and glutamate have been shown to produce a powerful augmentation of the animal's response to an external stimulus. Thus, the iontophoresis of SP and glutamate will increase the size of the receptive field of the cell and enhance its response to light tactile stimulation as well as noxious thermal and mechanical stimuli.[214,215] This increased spinal reactivity after spinal delivery of glutamate is accompanied by behaviorally defined thermal hyperalgesia and tactile allodynia (see Table 24-2). These effects underlie the prominent states of facilitated processing that will be discussed further below.

NOCICEPTIVE ELEMENTS IN THE SPINAL CORD

The differential distribution in the Rexed laminae[674] of terminals associated with fibers that are activated by specific noxious stimuli is consistent with the existence of populations of second-order neurons relevant to the rostrad transmission of nociceptive information (see Figure 24-8).

Marginal Zone (Lamina I)

The superficial layer of the dorsal horn comprises classes of large neurons oriented transversely across the cap of the dorsal gray matter. Some cells project to the thalamus by means of contralateral ascending pathways,[438,657,763,765,822] while others project intrasegmentally and intersegmentally along the dorsal and dorsolateral white matter.[106,693,740] The dendritic plexus of these neurons extends up to several hundred microns along both the transverse and longitudinal axes of the cord, although the dendritic tree is largely confined to the marginal layer.[108,300] As displayed schematically in Figure 24-8, afferent terminals tend to synapse distally in the dendritic tree, whereas non-afferent terminals tend to be proximal on the cell body.[438,444] Lamina I neurons may be divided physiologically into three groups: (i) neurons activated by fibers having A-delta/C fiber conduction velocities that respond to intense mechanical stimulation, (ii) neurons activated by innocuous skin cooling with afferents having a conduction velocity akin to those of an A-delta fiber, and (iii) a small percentage of neurons activated by C fiber polymodal afferents.[132,150,476,657,823] Although initial observations suggested that these neurons of lamina I were specifically sensitive to intense stimuli, a significant proportion of these cells also possess a wide dynamic range, that is, a response frequency proportional to the intensity of the stimulus.[132] Importantly, those neurons responding to A-delta and C fiber input can also be activated by group III and group IV muscle afferents, indicating a convergence of muscle and cutaneous input.

Substantia Gelatinosa (Lamina II)

The clear band of neural tissue lying ventral to the marginal layer and dorsal to a region of coarser texture known as the nucleus proprius was given the name substantia gelatinosa by Rolando.[678] The substantia gelatinosa, defined by gross observation in unfixed or semifixed tissue, corresponds to the laminae II of Rexed. Lamina II is divided into outer and inner layers. The former is characterized by small, densely packed cells and a neuropil made complex by the presence of a larger number of dendrites. The latter zone is similar but has a less coarse texture owing to the relative paucity of terminals. The principal cell type in lamina II is the stalk cell, with cone-shaped dendritic trees arborizing through lamina II into III and axons branching into lamina I.[299,693] The terminals of A-delta afferents that project to this lamina are a likely source of the numerous axodendritic contacts observed in this region.[164,225,298,444,661,804]

A significant proportion of the substantia gelatinosa neurons receive A-delta/C fiber input.[131,477,503,796] Neurons located in lamina II (the outer portion of the substantia gelatinosa) tend to be excited by activation of thermal receptive or mechanical nociceptive afferents.[503] Neurons retrogradely labeled with horseradish peroxidase and activated by nociceptive input display dendritic branching in the outer layer of the substantia gelatinosa, whereas neurons activated by innocuous mechanical stimuli have dendritic trees in the inner layer of the substantia gelatinosa.[502] Receptive fields of gelatinosa neurons responsive to peripheral stimuli are small (less than 2 cm^2). Several properties of gelatinosa neurons have emerged.

1. Unlike those cells lying more deeply (see following), neurons of the substantia gelatinosa commonly exhibit prolonged periods of excitation and inhibition after afferent activation.[358,796].

2. Islet and stalked cells constitute several classes of functionally distinct cells, with variable degrees of background activity, in which afferent input will drive complex "on/off" responses. Significantly, those cells inhibited by non-noxious stimuli were excited by noxious input, whereas cells inhibited by noxious input were excited by non-noxious input.[135,136] Such profiles suggest that the activity of substantia gelatinosa neurons is governed by a convergence of excitation arising from large and small fiber input acting either directly on these neurons or by inhibitory interneurons.

Nucleus Proprius (Laminae III, IV, and V)

Lamina III contains fewer neurons and a less dense neuropil than does lamina II. In addition, the islet neuron[296,301] (Golgi type II) appears in high concentration, in contrast to the stalk cells that occur predominantly in the outer layer of lamina II.

Lamina IV, as defined by Rexed, is composed of a broad layer of relatively large neurons (10 to 15 μm in diameter) that endow this region with their characteristic morphology. The dendritic tree of these neurons transversely and dorsally spreads into laminae II and III. The neuropil of lamina II and IV is characterized by axodendritic and axoaxonic synapses,[443,661] originating from: (i) afferent input of the large diameter fibers that contact the apical portion of the dendritic tree,[662] and (ii) local axonal plexuses derived from intrinsic fibers.[438]

Lamina V, located along the neck of the dorsal horn, displays a dendritic organization that does not differ prominently from that of neurons in lamina IV.

Neurons in both lamina IV and lamina V project to the ventrobasal thalamus, mesencephalon,[290,429,763–765] and the lateral cervical nucleus,[89,131] and provide propriospinal projections within the spinal cord in various species (see following). Cells in the nucleus proprius may be broadly classed as those that respond to low-threshold (A-beta) input and those that respond at a progressively greater frequency as a function of stimulus intensity. This reflects the convergent input from several classes of functionally defined afferent types (e.g., A-beta, A-delta, and C). These dorsal horn cells are referred to as wide dynamic range neurons.[552] The latter class of cells respond to transient brush and touch but show no elevation in activity with prolonged pinch; these cells are referred to as "lamina IV," while the former class of neurons are referred to as lamina V neurons because of the early studies that localized them in that region.[799]

Lamina V neurons have several discrete properties which make them of particular interest to our interpretation of nociceptive mechanisms.

1. In these cells, light innocuous touch evokes activity that increases as the intensity of pressure or pinch is increased. Thermal stimuli applied to the receptive field will similarly evoke a rate of discharge that is proportional to temperature; some units show an exponential increase in discharge rate at temperatures above 45°C.[484,654,656] Because of this characteristic response profile, these cells are referred to as wide dynamic range (WDR) neurons. An acute stimulus applied to a sensory nerve will evoke a characteristic biphasic activation reflecting the excitation evoked first by the rapidly conducting A fibers and then a second phase mediated by the arrival of the more slowly conducting A-delta and C fibers.

2. Repetitive electrical stimulation at a slow rate (<0.1 Hz) results in a stable response. However, at a slightly faster rate (0.5 to 1 Hz), the WDR neurons will show a progressive incrementation in discharge velocity with each subsequent stimulus. This augmentation, referred to as "wind-up," depends upon the activation of C, but not Aβ, fibers and produces a gradual increase in the frequency discharge until the neuron is in a state of virtually continuous discharge.[552]

3. Receptive fields for wide dynamic range neurons are more extensive than those of the primary afferent neurons that impinge upon them, again indicating a convergence of afferent input onto the dendritic tree of this cell. As with marginal neurons (and the primary afferents), receptive field size decreases as one moves distally on the extremities.[95,97,132] Although somatotopically convergent input is the rule for wide dynamic range neurons and the activity of such neurons can be highly influenced by input from several adjacent spinal cord segments, these neurons are activated most effectively by input arriving from the dermatome in which they lie.[658,793] Importantly, many early investigations were carried out in decerebrate or decerebrate/spinal animals to avoid the use of anesthetics. In experiments using intact anesthetized preparations, receptive fields, sometimes including the whole body, have been found in addition to the more restricted ones observed when the spinal cord has been transected. Moreover, the magnitude of the receptive field is under an ongoing modulation by intrinsic systems that can increase and decrease the size of the complex field (see following).

4. Wide dynamic range neurons commonly demonstrate organ convergence as well as somatic convergence. Thus neurons in the nucleus proprius have been observed that are activated by (i) stimulation of sympathetic afferents and by coronary artery occlusion, as well as by noxious pinches applied within the dermatomes that coincided with the segmental location of those cells (T1–T5),[261] (ii) stimulation of the splanchnic nerve and A-beta/A-delta cutaneous input,[335,648,705,706] (iii) distention of the hollow viscera (bladder, small intestine, and gallbladder),[801] (iv) injection of bradykinin into the mesenteric artery and cutaneous input,[315] and close intra-arterial administration of bradykinin or the injection of hypertonic saline into muscle/tendon or group III afferent stimulation from the gastrocnemius,[262,648] and cutaneous input field. Correlation of those areas of the skin (forepaw, hindpaw, hind leg, abdomen, thorax) where stimulation would evoke activity in neurons known to be activated by distention of the gallbladder or the urinary bladder revealed that about one-third of the units examined responded to stimulation of the gallbladder and various cutaneous regions, with the highest percentage associated with the thorax and perineum.[249] Progressive bladder distention activated cells in widespread dermatomal regions, but most effectively activated neurons responsive to cutaneous stimuli applied to the abdomen. These results indicate that the phenomenon of "referred" visceral pain probably has its substrate in viscerosomatic and musculosomatic convergence onto dorsal horn neurons.[681]

Central Canal (Lamina X)

Although the central canal is a parvicellular region, recent studies have demonstrated that branches of small, lightly myelinated fibers were observed to enter the region.[501] Transport studies have further demonstrated that a significant proportion of these neurons projected both ipsilaterally and contralaterally in the ventrolateral tract into the bulbar reticular formation. Electrophysiologic studies in this region have shown that local neurons possess properties similar to those of the marginal cells noted above. Thus cells have been observed that respond primarily to high-threshold temperature and noxious pinch with small receptive fields.[373,375,588]

Ascending Spinal Tracts

Ventral Funicular Systems

Unilateral and ventrolateral tractotomies elevate the threshold for visceral and somatic pain reports on the side contralateral to the lesion.[729,787,790,811] Conversely, stimulation of the ventrolateral tracts in awake subjects undergoing percutaneous cordotomies has resulted in reports of contralateral warmth and pain.[535,811] The analgesia is characterized by a loss or reduction in the response to thermal (heat and cold), mechanical (pinprick), itch,[812] and deep somatic (Achilles tendon) stimuli. Midline myelotomies that destroy fibers crossing the midline at the levels of the cut produce bilateral pain deficits.[365,700] These observations suggest that the relevant pathways for nociception are predominantly crossed. It should be stressed that midline myelotomies are not identical to ventrolateral cordotomies. As summarized by Vierck and colleagues,[787] after midline myelotomy there tends to be (i) an increased incidence of paresthesia, (ii) no decrease in the magnitude of evoked cutaneous pain, (iii) preserved dull–sharp discrimination, and (iv) enduring losses of deep pain. The rostrad transmission of nociceptive information, however, is not unique to the ventrolateral funiculus (VLF). This is evidenced by (i) the anomalous recovery of pain three months to one year after cordotomy, (ii) the persistence of contralateral pain sensations after a unilateral lesion (suggestive of bilateral projections), and (iii) the ability of high-intensity stimulation to produce a "breakthrough" of pain resembling the diffuse, burning pain of C fiber activation.[813]

Cells of Origin. Localization of the cells of origin of this system has been made by (i) examining the chromatolytic reaction after spinal section, (ii) antidromic activation of spinal neurons by brain-stem electrodes, and (iii) labeling of spinal neurons with horseradish peroxidase injected into probable terminal regions of axons projecting in the VLF. Retrograde chromatolytic reactions were observed early in neurons of the marginal zone and of the deeper laminae (IV and V) of the dorsal horn of patients with clinically effective lesions of the VLF. Chromatolytic cell bodies lying more deeply in the ventral horn were also found after ventrolateral cordotomy. Injection of horseradish peroxidase into the lateral thalamic nuclei or into the spinothalamic tract itself resulted in labeled neurons in the marginal zone, the substantia gelatinosa,[822] and laminae IV and V.[764] Stimulating electrodes placed in the contralateral VLF at cervical or mesodiencephalic levels will antidromically activate neurons in the marginal zone, the substantia gelatinosa, and laminae IV and V, as well as in laminae VII and VIII in the cat.[8,10,209,290] Fibers in the ventral funiculi are myelinated with diameters of 1 to 11 μm.[508] Application of the Hurst factor for myelinated fibers estimates conduction velocities that closely correspond to those reported for these fibers by several laboratories (18–58 m/sec in cats,[209] (7–74 m/sec in primates[823]).

Organization. Fibers traveling rostrad in this tract originate in the dorsal horn and cross in the dorsal commissure at levels up to two segments from the point of origin.[812,822] White and associates[810] noted a rostral displacement of the analgesic dermatomes after a ventrolateral cordotomy and suggested that before crossing, these axons may remain medial for one or two segments. A somatotopic arrangement within the VLF has been so described that the fibers arising from the more caudal segments are located laterally, whereas those entering from the more rostral segments lie medially and ventrally in the funiculi.[387] Although it has been suggested that there may also be an anatomically defined organization by modality in the ventrolateral tract (for example, pain and touch), single-unit recording studies in primates have failed to document such modality segregation.[820]

Rostral Terminals. Because spinofugal tracts do not appear to show major or reliable differences with regard to their point of origin within the spinal gray matter (see below), the tracts projecting rostrally within the VLF are commonly classified according to the brain regions in which they terminate. Long tract systems that may be relevant to the rostrad transmission include the spinoreticular, spinomesencephalic, and spinothalamic tracts. The first two have often been referred to as the paleospinothalamic system, and the last as the neospinothalamic system by virtue of the increasing size of the diencephalic projections in phylogenetically advanced species.[546] It should be remembered, however, that up to half of the fibers in the VLF in humans (which are not destined for the cerebellum) terminate caudal to the rostral aspect of the inferior olive.[75]

Spinoreticular Fibers. Spinoreticular axons terminate both ipsilaterally and contralaterally to their site of origin in the spinal cord.[250,878] Entering the medulla, the fibers aggregate laterally, and collaterals of these fibers terminate in the more medially situated brain stem reticular nuclei (the n. reticularis gigantocellularis, the n. reticularis paragigantocellularis, the n. reticularis pontis caudalis, and the n. subcoeruleus).[77,445,545,680,878] Terminals have also been reported in the n. raphe magnus and pallidus,[82,84,545] making both somatic and dendritic contacts.[798] Stimulating electrodes in the reticular formation antidromically activate neurons in laminae V through VIII.[246,247,492] Discrete injections of horseradish peroxidase into the n. reticularis gigantocellularis and the magnocellular part of the lateral reticular nucleus have labeled neurons situated throughout the contralateral spinal cord in laminae IV, V, and VIII, and in the ipsilateral laminae IV and V.[429,448] Lamina I neurons have not been identified as an origin of spinoreticular fibers in the above cited studies. This suggests that marginal zone neurons, some reported to be specifically nociceptive in function, do not contribute a significant projection into the medial medullary region. It is important to remember that although many of the projections to the bulbar reticular formation are ipsilateral, a small contingent of fibers may cross at the medullary level. Degeneration in this bulbar region after extensive midline myelotomies has not been observed.[431] Consistent with these anatomic observations, response latencies of neurons in the n. reticulogigantocellularis to stimulation of the ipsilateral hind paw in the cat were shorter in 60% of the units examined.[72] Using stimulating electrodes placed at several brain stem levels, it has been shown in cats that axons projecting no further than the brain stem reticular formation do exist and possess cell bodies located throughout the n. proprius of the dorsal horn, as well as laminae VI to IX.[246] This suggests that spinoreticular terminals do not represent only the collaterals of fibers in transit to more rostrad sites. Retrograde transport studies have demonstrated, however, that some spinifugal axons do indeed project to both the brain stem and the thalamus.[449,450] With regard to electrophysiologic properties, spinoreticular neurons have been shown to possess receptive fields that may be restricted cutaneous, restricted deep, or complex extensive. Although the receptive fields are predominantly ipsilateral excitatory, bilateral fields and fields with inhibitory components have also been observed. A high proportion of spinoreticular neurons have wide dynamic range response characteristics.[246]

Spinomesencephalic Fibers. Fibers originate from neurons located in the spinal gray matter in regions similar to those reported for spinoreticular fibers. Two spinomesencephalic tracts have been reported. The largest tract crosses within the spinal cord; the lesser tract ascends ipsilaterally and crosses in the tegmentum at the level of the intertectal commissure.[545,878] Degenerating terminals following lesions of the ventrolateral cord have been observed in the midbrain reticular formation, for example, the nucleus cuneiformis, the inferior and superior colliculi, and the periaqueductal gray matter of several species.[26,76,77,445,545,878] In contrast to the spinoreticular projections, midline myelotomies produce extensive signs of degeneration in the mesencephalon.[431] Using retrograde labeling, cells of origin have been demonstrated in laminae I and V.[509,557] Physiologic properties of identified spinomesencephalic neurons have not been examined extensively. Uniformly shorter response latencies of these neurons in the mesencephalon have been reported for contralateral as compared with ipsilateral somatic stimulation, suggesting a largely crossed afferent input.[13,45,73] A population of these cells displays a significant response to noxious stimuli.[866]

Spinothalamic Fibers. The cells of origin of this tract, the most extensively studied of the spinal projection systems, are not limited to the dorsal gray matter. Figure 24-10 presents a summary of the position of cells in three species located by retrograde transport or antidromic activation. The existence of cell systems lying in the dorsal gray matter is expected, but the density around the neck of the proprius and the central canal emphasizes the possible role of this deep system in nociceptive transmission.[588] The tract ascends predominantly in the contralateral ventral quadrant. Crossed fibers predominate, but it is clear that uncrossed fibers represent a significant component of the spinothalamic population. Retrograde labeling studies revealed that following unilateral injection of horseradish peroxidase into the thalamus of the monkey, about 25% of the projections from the sacral cord were ipsilateral.[822]

The spinothalamic system ascends in the medulla, dorsolaterally to the pyramid, and inferiorly to the olivary nucleus. In the rostral mesencephalon, fibers are located ventromedially to the inferior colliculus. The spinothalamic fibers differentiate into a lateral and medial component in the posterior portions of the thalamus. The medial component passes through the internal medullary lamina to terminate in the n. parafascicularis and intralaminar and paralaminar nuclei.[545,571,878] The majority of fibers pass laterally through the external medullary lamina to terminate in small clusters scattered throughout the n. ventralis posterolateralis, the medial aspects of the posterior n. complex, and the intralaminar nuclei.[50,67,174,445,545,641] In primates, thalamic stimulation evokes antidromic activation of neurons located dorsally in the lateral aspect of the nucleus proprius and in the marginal zone.[8,763,823] With horseradish peroxidase studies, neurons in lamina I project uniquely to the region lying between the rostral, ventrolateral, and caudal ventrolateral thalamic nuclei. Spinothalamic neurons lying in laminae IV and V terminate in the posterior nuclei of the thalamus, whereas neurons in laminae VII and VIII are generally labeled after injections of horseradish peroxidase into the intralaminar thalamic nuclei.[119,288,764]

In the primate, a significant proportion of the neurons projecting laterally in the thalamus (ventral posterior lateral complex) also project to the medial (central lateral nucleus or dorsal medial nucleus) portion. In contrast, a second population of neurons appear to project only to the medial thalamus. At least four classes of spinothalamic neurons have been identified: (i) narrow dynamic range neurons that respond only to innocuous tactile stimuli (laminae IV and V); (ii) neurons situated deep that are responsive to proprioceptive input (laminae IV and V); (iii) wide dynamic range neurons that respond in a frequency-dependent fashion to stimuli of increasing intensity receive convergent input from cutaneous, visceral, and muscle sources, respond to thermal and chemical stimuli in the noxious range, and display a sustained discharge to pressure but a rapid adaptation to light tactile input (lamina V); and (iv) neurons that respond uniquely to high-intensity noxious stimuli. These high-threshold units display a slowly adapting response to noxious cutaneous mechanical and thermal stimuli.[289] Lamina I neurons having such properties have been observed.[150,262,263,334,477,823] In the studies noted above, neurons that project to *both* the medial and the lateral thalamus display a significant proportion of wide dynamic-range type cells. In contrast, medially projecting cells have been largely characterized as high-threshold-selective.[289]

With regard to receptive fields, antidromic activation of spinothalamic neurons with electrodes placed in both the medial thalamus and lateral thalamus reveals three types of spinothalamic neurons: (i) those that project only to the lateral thalamus; (ii) those that project only to the medial thalamus; and (iii) those that project to both the medial and the lateral thalamus. Receptive field properties of those neurons that project to the lateral thalamus are conventional (small fields with larger surrounding regions that require more intense stimulation for activation of the neuron), and many neurons have inhibitory fields extending over broad body areas. Neurons projecting to the medial thalamus display large, often whole body receptive fields, although the contralateral field often is most effective in activating the cell. These neurons display discharge patterns that last beyond the stimulus. Severing the cord reduces the receptive field to that observed for spinal animals and abolishes the poststimulus discharge. Thus somatic stimuli gaining access to supraspinal centers can re-address spinal projection neurons in what appears to be a spino (contralateral)-bulbo (crossed)-spinal (ipsilateral) feedback circuit.[824]

Dorsal Funicular Systems

Transections of the dorsal quadrant of the spinal cord in the cat produce significant increases in the nociceptive

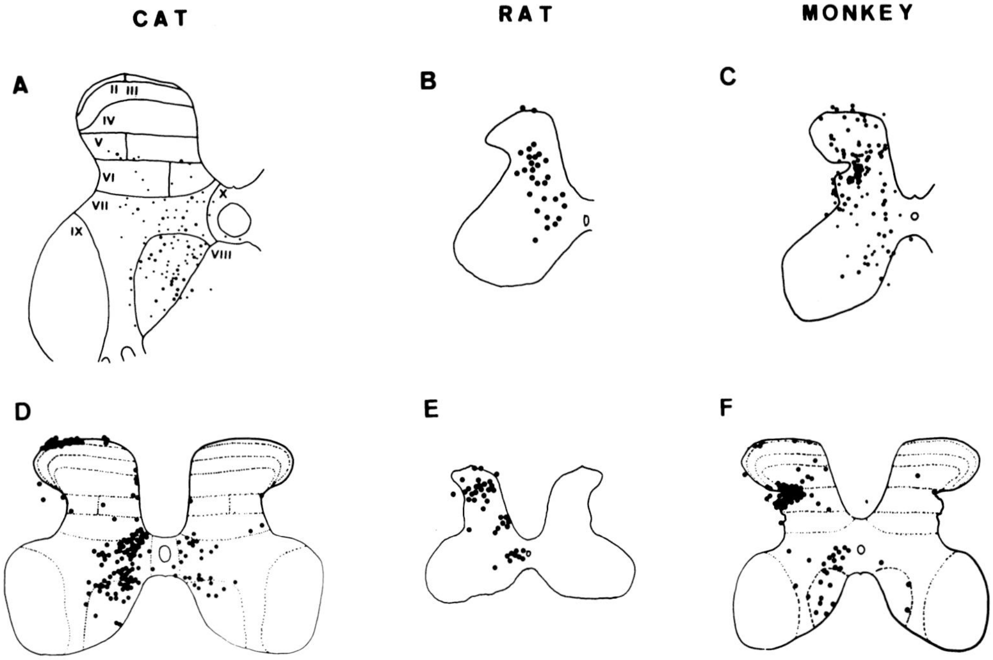

FIG. 24-10. A–C: Recording sites from which antidromic action potentials can be recorded from spinothalamic tract cells in the lumbosacral enlargement of the cat, rat, and monkey following stimulation in the contralateral thalamus. **D–F:** Location of spinothalamic tract cells labeled retrogradely following injection of horseradish peroxidase into the thalamus in cat, rat, and monkey. [From Willis, W.D.: Ascending somatosensory systems. *In* Yaksh, T.L. (ed.): Spinal Afferent Processing. pp. 243–274. New York, Plenum Press, 1986.]

threshold.[427] Severance of the dorsal columns or the spinocervical tract, or both, may account for this elevation. In primates and humans, lesions of the dorsolateral quadrant have been reported to produce a hyperalgesia.[594,788] Although large-diameter afferent fibers, sensitive to light touch and vibration, terminate in the dorsal column nuclei after ascending in the dorsal columns, many nonprimary afferent fibers originating in lamina V also ascend in the dorsal column as well.[682,683] These fibers respond to tactile and noxious mechanical and thermal stimuli.[24] Dorsal column lesions in humans do not alter pain threshold,[169] and stimulation of the dorsal columns in humans often gives rise to sensations of vibration, not of pain.[591] In primates, a slight decrease in pain reactivity has been observed.[788] As noted, a postsynaptic pathway originating from lamina V neurons in the dorsal horn has been shown. The role of this system is not known. Axons of spinocervical neurons project ipsilaterally in the dorsolateral quadrant of the spinal cord to terminate in the lateral cervical nucleus.[89,97] These neurons lie predominantly in the nucleus proprius (laminae III and IV).[89,97] Several types of spinocervical neurons have been identified, and they appear to be activated by tactile (hair movement, pressure), noxious thermal (40°–53° C), and noxious mechanical (pinch) stimuli[90,91,131] and close intra-arterial injection of algogenic agents.[462] The spinocervical tract has been well described in cats,[455] but its presence is much reduced in lower primates[320,321,599] and is practically nonexistent in humans.[766]

Intersegmental Systems

The ability of ventrolateral cordotomies to alter pain illustrates the important role of long tracts in the rostral transmission of nociceptive information. For reasons stated above, the existence of alternate spinal pathways appears certain. Early studies showed that alternating hemisections will abolish neither the behavioral nor the autonomic responses to strong stimuli.[36,81,457] These observations suggest that systems that project for short distances ipsilaterally may contribute to the rostrad transmission of nociceptive information. Kerr[440,441] proposed that selective destruction of the dorsal gray matter, for example, spinonucleolysis, might prove to be a possible method of pain management in light of the relevance of nonfunicular pathways traveling in the spinal gray matter. Subsequent work revealed that such lesions could produce significant and prolonged pain relief associated with nerve avulsions and other chronic, otherwise intractable, somatosensory pain syndromes.[589,701] These results offer support for the proposed relevance in pain transmission of systems traveling within the dorsal gray matter. Alternately, the recent role of cell systems in lamina X and the likelihood of local systems traveling in the dorsal columns indicates the possibility that midline myelotomies may act not only by the severance of crossing fibers, but may also be the cause of damage to relevant midline systems. Early studies suggested that visceral pain was dependent upon the central core.[189,787] Several segmental pathways that may be relevant to the rostrad transmission of nociceptive information include the Lissauer tract, the dorsolateral propriospinal system, and the dorsal intracornual tract.

The tract of Lissauer is divided into medial and lateral components. The medial portion of the tract consists largely of collaterals of the unmyelinated or lightly myelinated primary afferent fibers that travel several segments rostrally and caudally before entering the dorsal horn gray matter.[438,666,667,740] The lateral tract lies in the dorsolateral funiculus immediately lateral to the dorsal root entry zone and consists of myelinated or small myelinated fibers deriving from neurons in the substantia gelatinosa and marginal layers.[673] These fibers may travel only a few millimeters in either direction before disappearing into the dorsal horn.[134,438,796,798] Although the medial and lateral components of Lissauer's tract can be separated at the dorsal root entry zone, they merge at the cervical level and cannot be easily differentiated.[798]

Lesions of the dorsolateral quadrant that destroy Lissauer's tract have been reported to elevate the nociceptive threshold[388,427] and to enlarge the dermatomal fields associated with a given segment of the spinal cord. Tractotomies of the medial Lissauer tract in primates exert the opposite effect and result in shrinkage of the dermatome associated with a given spinal cord root.[196]

The ipsilateral projections of the dorsolateral propriospinal system travel lateral to the axis of the nucleus proprius and contain axons originating from neurons of the substantia gelatinosa and marginal zone.[108] The role of many marginal neurons in pain transmission and the possibility that these neurons may project in this pathway suggest that a certain proportion of nociceptive information may be transmitted by means of the dorsolateral propriospinal tract. The dorsal intracornual tract consists of small-diameter fibers coursing longitudinally through the medial regions of the nucleus proprius. Because rhizotomies do not reduce the number of these fibers, it appears they arise from intrinsic neurons.[438]

Despite corollary evidence suggesting that intrasegmental systems may transmit nociceptive information, the role of these pathways in pain transmission remains speculative. The results of a ventrolateral cordotomy clearly indicate the importance of crossed pathways; the segmental pathways are largely ipsilaterally organized. Yet there is evidence that some primary afferent neurons do terminate contralaterally (see previous), and interneurons do cross the midline along the longitudinal axis of the cord, as evidenced by the existence of crossed reflexes. Crossing fibers may serve to transmit the ipsilateral message to a contralateral projection. Moreover, as noted previously, afferent axons collateralize and may project many segments rostrally, where they would initiate an excitation at levels above the spinal long tract section. The existence of segmental spinal systems might explain the recurrence of pain 3 to 12 months after ventrolateral cordotomy and, particularly, the "breakthrough" mediated by small fibers that occurs when high-intensity stimuli are applied[787] (see previous).

CONSIDERATION OF SPECIAL SENSORY SYSTEMS

In the preceding section, specific interest was directed at general systems whereby sensory information enters the central nervous system. Although the essential characteristics of the afferent input are reasonably uniform across the sensory systems, two systems have special complexities that render particular interest. These are the trigeminal system and the systems whereby visceral information enters the central nervous system.

Trigeminal System

The essential characteristics of afferent input through the trigeminal system are similar to those of the spinal cord. However, certain morphologic and functional considerations make it worth noting this system separately.

Trigeminal Input. The face, head, and buccal regions are innervated by the ophthalmic, mandibular, and maxillary divisions of the trigeminal nerve, the cell bodies of which are located in the ganglion of the 5th nerve (gasserian). The afferents are organized somatotopically in the sensory root in a medial to lateral fashion. The mandibular nerve branch is posterolaterally positioned, the ophthalmic branch anteromedially located, and the maxillary branch situated in an intermediate position.[39,186,442] The more rostral the peripheral terminal fields, the more ventrally and laterally situated are the cell bodies in the ganglia.[39,186,442]

As in the spinal cord, a large proportion of the afferent input enters through the sensory root (the portio major), but sensory fibers may enter also by way of the portio minor or the efferent outflow of the trigeminal system. Because visceral efferent fibers are not thought to course in the portio minor, the observation that about 20% of the axons are unmyelinated suggests a situation analogous to that studied in greater detail in the lumbar and sacral cord.[876] The continued presence of these afferent fibers may be a possible reason for the preservation of tactile sensitivity and of various pathologic facial pains following trigeminal nerve rhizotomy.[197,398]

Brain Stem Organization. The trigeminal sensory nucleus is divided into the main sensory and the more caudally located spinal nucleus (extending as far caudally as the cervical spinal cord). The spinal nucleus is further divided into three subdivisions: the n. oralis, n. interpolaris, and n. caudalis (rostral-caudal presentation).[617] The central processes of the trigeminal afferent neurons enter the brain stem at the level of the pons to terminate in these nuclei.[154] The somatotopic arrangement of the three branches of the trigeminal nerve observed within the ganglion is maintained in the descending trigeminal tract, in the main sensory,[442,473] and in the spinal nuclei.[442,647]

Large-diameter afferents bifurcate within the brain stem, giving rise to ascending and descending branches that terminate in the main sensory and spinal nuclei, respectively.[31,108] Horseradish peroxidase injected into axons of physiologically identified afferents of vibrissae has confirmed the bifurcation of these afferents and their co-innervation of the main sensory and spinal nuclei.[344] A population of large-diameter afferents also exists that does not bifurcate but descends in the spinal tract to innervate the entire rostrocaudal extent of the spinal nucleus, a course similar to that followed by smaller-diameter myelinated and unmyelinated fibers. Physiologic studies have supported the anatomic evidence for widespread termination of trigeminal afferents within the nuclear subdivisions. Neurons responsive to tactile stimuli (subserved by activity in large-diameter afferents) are not localized to any one nucleus. Neurons of the n. oralis,[430,451] the n. interpolaris,[430] and the n. caudalis,[430,474,579,654] and neurons within the main sensory nucleus[430,451,474] are activated by the application of tactile stimuli (light touch, hair movement, brush) to their receptive fields. Neurons responsive to thermal or noxious stimuli have been reported in the n. caudalis.[207,578,579,654,655,867] Significantly, trigeminal neurons may be driven by input from spinal afferent collaterals and other cranial nerves. Thus stimulation as far caudally as the C2 root will produce an excitatory drive of neurons receiving trigeminal input,[433–436] with the likelihood that unusual pain syndromes, such as those seen in atypical facial neuralgias, might reflect the contribution of these collateral projections. The role of the n. caudalis in pain has been emphasized on the basis that trigeminal tractotomy at the level of the medullary obex relieves ipsilateral facial pain with preservation of touch.[718a,812] The nociceptive responses of neurons situated in the n. caudalis reveal two populations of neurons that are remarkably similar to those reported in the spinal cord.[654] Neurons located in the marginal rim of the n. caudalis (corresponding to lamina I of the spinal cord[296]) have been termed "nociceptive specific." The receptive fields of these neurons are predominantly ipsilateral and small in size.[578,579,654,655,867] The second population of nociceptive neurons is "wide dynamic range" and is situated ventrally in the magnocellular portion of the n. caudalis. These neurons receive convergent input from large-diameter afferents being activated by stimulation of low-threshold rapidly conducting fibers, as well as by light touch, hair movement, and vibration.[579,654,655]

Ascending Projections. After the injection of horseradish peroxidase into the ventrobasal thalamus of the rat, retrogradely labeled neurons are found throughout the entire trigeminal sensory complex, with the possible exception of the n. oralis of the spinal nucleus.[103,269] These trigeminothalamic projections are predominantly contralateral, although a small ipsilateral projection from the main sensory nucleus has been described.[103,269] Neurons in the n. caudalis responsive to noxious, or innocuous stimuli, and project to the ventroposterior thalamus[654] and to the adjacent reticular formation.[753] Neurons of the n. caudalis also project within the trigeminal tract to the more rostral sensory nuclei.[297,383,735,753] This intranuclear projection may serve to modulate the activity of neurons in the more rostral trigeminal sensory nuclei and may explain why neurons responsive to noxious stimuli are not localized to the n. caudalis.[451] Neurons of the main sensory nucleus and n. oralis are activated by electrical stimulation of the n. caudalis.[451] Activation of n. caudalis neurons by topical application of strychnine (a glycine receptor antagonist) potentiates the responses of main sensory and n. oralis neurons to both noxious and innocuous stimuli. Conversely, cold block of the n. caudalis decreases the responses of neurons in the n. oralis and main sensory nucleus to peripheral stimuli.[312] Consistent with these observations, electrical stimulation or strychnine on the n. caudalis has been reported to hyperpolarize the preterminal endings of primary afferent neurons in the n. oralis.[703] The application of strychnine to the n. caudalis potentiates the hyperpolarization induced by dental pulp stimulation of primary afferent terminals located in the rostral sensory nuclei.[874] Thus neurons of the n. caudalis may hyperpolarize primary afferent terminals synapsing on neurons in the more rostral sensory trigeminal nuclei. Behavioral evidence for such a facilitatory action of n. caudalis neurons on afferent impulse transmission in the n. oralis and main sensory nucleus has been obtained in the cat. After application of strychnine to the n. caudalis, strong pseudoaffective responses to stroking of the fur have occurred.[455] Clinical observations on patients with syringomyelia progressing to syringobulbia are not in agreement, however, with the proposed role of ipsilateral projections within trigeminal nuclei in pain. Because this lesion normally does not involve the trigeminal nuclei, the loss of pain coincident with the rostral progression of thermalgesia into the facial region in an onion-skin distribution cannot be attributed to severance of rostrocaudal projections within the trigeminal nuclei. Rather, such observations would suggest that fibers decussating within the brain stem have been interrupted.

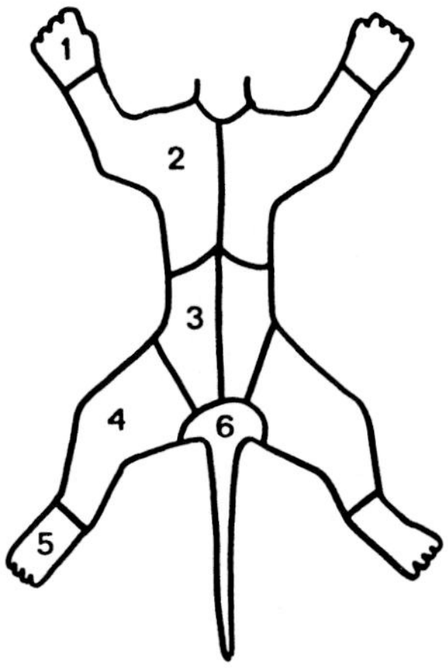

FIG. 24-11. Partitioning of cat's body surface for principal cutaneous receptive fields of spinal neurons. Percentage of cells by region that responds to somatic stimulation and also to gallbladder or urinary bladder stimulation (/) is 1: 40/18; 2: 56/11; 3: 38/44; 4: 33/31; 5: 35/28; 6: 43/25. (Adapted from Fields, H.L., Partridge, L.D., and Winter, D.L.: Somatic and visceral receptive field properties of fibers in ventral quadrant white matter of the cat spinal cord. J. Neurophysiol., *33*:827, 1970.)

Visceral Afferent Organization

Innervation of the visceral organs derives from sensory afferents, the cell bodies of which are in the dorsal root ganglia, and the fibers of which travel with sympathetic and parasympathetic axons. It has been estimated that the visceral afferents account for about 10% of the fibers that run in the dorsal roots. Yet these visceral afferents serve an organ surface area equivalent to about 25% of the body surface, which suggests that visceral sensitivity will be poorly localized. To understand visceral pain, one must recognize that these afferents appear to converge onto somatotopically organized dorsal horn systems, which receive cutaneous input. As shown in Figure 24-11, gallbladder and urinary bladder stimulation serves to excite cells that have a corresponding cutaneous dermatomal field. Thus it is not surprising that certain visceral pains are associated predominantly with certain dermatomal segments. Such segments correspond with the cutaneous innervation of that particular spinal segment. With regard to thoracic input, therefore, sensory information from thoracic viscera will serve to activate sensory afferents traveling with sympathetic fibers that terminate in cord segments T1–T4. Similarly, sensory input that results in activity in visceral sympathetic afferents will enter the spinal cord at segments T5–T12/L1, traveling via the splanchnic nerves through the celiac plexus (see Chapter 23.1, Fig. 23.1-20 and Table 23.1-4). These afferents enter the dorsal horn of the spinal cord to terminate in the dorsal gray matter. At this point, convergence with somatic afferent input onto common postsynaptic neurons occurs. As noted in previous sections, both spinoreticular and spinothalamic projecting neurons showed such viscerosomatic and muscular somatic convergence as a common property. Such neurons will respond not only to noxious events, that is, cardiac ischemia or smooth muscle spasm, but also to more benign input such as distention of the bladder (see previous).

SUPRASPINAL ELEMENTS IN NOCICEPTIVE TRANSMISSION

Supraspinal nuclear groups participating in the processing of pain-relevant information have been tentatively identified on the basis of their connectivity and their response to a peripheral stimulus adequate to evoke pain behavior. The accessibility of the pathways that project in the VLF has facilitated extensive investigations of the supraspinal connections of these pathways. As noted earlier, there are essentially three major sites of termination: the medulla, the mesencephalon, and the diencephalon.

Medullary Reticular Formation

Given the spinopetal projections and the reticulothalamic projections from the medullary reticular neurons to the intralaminar and ventrobasal nuclei of the thalamus, the medullary reticular formation has been suggested as a "relay" station for the rostrad transmission of nociceptive information. Retrogradely labeled neurons have been localized to neurons in the medullary reticular formation following the injection of horseradish peroxidase into the thalamus.[429] Medullary reticular neurons are activated antidromically by stimulation in the thalamus.[523] Conversely, stimulation of the medullary reticular formation has been reported to activate thalamic neurons.[72,424,523] Physiologic studies support the anatomic evidence that medullary reticular neurons receive peripheral input by means of spinal systems that travel in the VLF. Neurons of the lateral reticular nucleus,[13] the n. gigantocellularis,[125,316,485,631,634] the n. raphe magnus and pallidus,[21] and the n. locus coeruleus[129] are activated by noxious or innocuous stimuli, or both, applied to their peripheral receptive fields. These receptive fields, both ipsilateral and contralateral, are large, often including an entire limb or extending over the entire body.[13,21,46,125] Because the spinoreticular fibers that project to these regions do not commonly display such broad receptive fields and project predominantly ipsilaterally (see previous), the existence of extensive receptive fields suggests supraspinal convergence. Many of these neurons that are responsive to somatic input are also activated by auditory and visual stimuli.[72]

A significant proportion of neurons of the various medullary reticular nuclei behave as spinal wide dynamic range neurons.[21,125,129,631] Neurons of the n. gigantocellularis are most effectively activated following electrical stimulation of nerves sufficient to evoke afferent volleys in A-delta and C fibers; volleys in larger diameter A fibers are ineffective or less so.[125,303,485,634] Intra-arterial injection of algogenic agents such as bradykinin or intense stimulation of the splanchnic nerve will alter the discharge of n. gigantocellularis neurons.[316] Although the number of neurons responding to muscle afferents is small, the most effective input has arisen from group II and III fibers.[504,647]

Several lines of evidence may be marshaled to correlate neural activity in the n. gigantocellularis with pain behavior in unanesthetized animals:[121,123,124,424]

1. In unanesthetized cats, as the intensity of an electrical stimulus applied to the radial nerve is elevated (through chronically implanted electrodes), so too is the discharge frequency of single neurons of the n. gigantocellularis. The stimulus intensity that evokes escape behavior is also the minimum intensity that produces a maximum discharge rate in that neuron.
2. The discharge frequency of thalamic neurons has been correlated with the intensity of stimuli delivered to the n. gigantocellularis and the escape threshold in awake animals.
3. Stimulation of n. gigantocellularis may be used to evoke learned escape behavior in rats and cats. Additionally, such stimuli can serve as an unconditioned stimulus in pavlovian conditioning paradigms. In unanesthetized animals, the activity of n. gigantocellularis neurons co-varies with the intensity of somatic stimulation, and stimuli applied to the n. gigantocellularis will drive thalamic neurons, evoke escape behavior, and support pavlovian conditioning.

4. Lesions of the n. gigantocellularis have been shown to attenuate the response to otherwise aversive stimuli in the absence of any significant signs of motor impairment.

Several cautionary notes should be considered in these and other studies in which the behavioral effects of stimulating and lesioning of supraspinal systems are used to examine the involvement of a given structure in a pain event. Electrical stimulation or lesions of nuclei also affect fibers of passage and so may inhibit or activate ascending or descending pathways relevant to the pain event. Thus stimulation of spinothalamic fibers could produce a direct drive of thalamic substrates in a manner independent of the system within the nuclei being stimulated. Within the brain stem, particularly the n. gigantocellularis, there is a preponderance of connections with autonomic nuclei and sensations related to gastric secretion, nausea, or tachycardia that are likely to be stimulated by activation of efferent/autonomic pathways. These syndromes might be unpleasant, and such sensations themselves might underlie the "aversive" characteristics of local stimulation. It is thus possible that the role played by these nuclei is not related to the "conscious" perception of a pain event, but rather they could serve as the mediators of the autonomic sequelae evoked by high-intensity somatic stimulation.

Mesencephalic Reticular Formation and Central Gray Matter

These regions receive crossed/uncrossed projections from spinomesencephalic neurons. Neurons of the central gray project rostrally to terminate in the midline and intralaminar nuclei of the thalamus and the caudal hypothalamus.[74,148,327,523,676] Of particular interest are the massive projections that connect the central gray matter with the subjacent tegmentum.[327]

Units in the mesencephalic central gray matter and in the adjacent mesencephalic reticular formation are differentially responsive to innocuous and noxious cutaneous and electrical stimuli, with units phasically excited by innocuous mechanical stimulation but responding to noxious stimuli (i.e., pinching or heating) with sustained discharges.[34,42,161,168,873] There is a close correlation between the high-frequency discharge of these neurons evoked by noxious natural stimulation and the ability of electrical C fiber activation to drive the unit.[42,168,232] As in other brain stem regions, few if any neurons in this region are uniquely nociceptive. Thus cells that appear to be activated only by noxious tail pinch can be driven by electrical stimulation of the coccygeal nerve at intensities that evoke only a fast-conducting (A-beta) volley.[232] Thus experiments that examine only "natural" input may fail to observe the presence of weak but clearly present connections. Neurons of the mesencephalic reticular formation display a high degree of convergence with bilateral receptive fields that may include the entire body.[34,45,232,873] There is little evidence for a specific somatotopic organization of input to these regions, although there may be a distribution.[313,500] Stimulation of the mesencephalic central gray matter and adjacent mesencephalic reticular formation evoke signs of intense discomfort in the cat as characterized by flattening of the ears, vocalization, pupil dilatation, and attempts to escape. In humans, autonomic responses are elicited along with reports of dysphoria.[195,456,592,720,728]

Although electrolytic lesions of the central gray/mesencephalic reticular nuclei have been reported to alter nociceptive responsiveness,[325,550] a significant portion of the literature suggests little, if any, effects after either lesion or reversible blockade.[58,192,499,853] Observation that activation of these areas has an aversive consequence are consistent with the known projections of these nuclei to the medial and intralaminar nuclei of the thalamus. Yet the failure of lesions to elevate the pain threshold indicates that this region is not essential. It might be argued that lesions failed to affect a sufficient volume of tissue and that total destruction of this complex region would leave the animal moribund. The observation that electrical stimulation of the mesencephalic reticular formation would excite spinothalamic cells suggests that pathways either originating in, or passing through, the mesencephalon may exert an excitatory effect on the activity of spinothalamic neurons otherwise evoked by noxious peripheral stimuli.[824] Such a situation might explain why stimulation in the mesencephalon would be aversive while lesions would fail to block the rostrad transmission of information via the diffuse spinothalamic and mesencephalic system and so would not alter the pain threshold.

Diencephalon

Several nuclear groups of the thalamus receive projections primarily from the spinal cord thought to be associated with the transmission of somatic information evoked by noxious stimuli: the posterior nuclear complex, the ventrobasal complex, and the medial intralaminar nuclear complex. (For further comments, see previous section on ventrolateral tract projections.)

Posterior Nuclear Complex. The posterior nuclear area comprises the suprageniculate limitants and a heterogeneous region of ill-defined cell groups extending rostrally in the medial geniculate toward the caudal pole of the ventromedial group.[105] Input into this region is primarily contributed by the spinothalamic system[67,70,445,513] and lemniscal input from the dorsal column nuclei and the spinocervical tract.[69] Several projections arise from the posterior complex, but of principal interest are the projections to the posterior portion of the somatosensory area (I–II) of the cortex.[105]

Populations of neurons in the posterior nuclear complex respond to noxious stimuli.[126,428,640,644] These neurons display large bilateral receptive fields. A number of the neurons resemble the wide dynamic range neurons in the spinal cord (discharge frequency proportional to the intensity of the applied stimulus). Electrical activation of A-delta afferents from tooth pulp, presumably noxious in nature, also evokes activity in neurons of the posterior thalamic complex.[714] Although these investigations clearly suggest the existence of neurons in the posterior complex that can be activated by nociceptive input, other investigations have failed to observe as large a population of neurons responsive to noxious input.[49,182,605] Lesions of the monkey posterior nuclear complex reduce the responsiveness of animals to maximum mechanical stimuli,[702] but the literature is generally inconclusive concerning the effects of such lesions in humans; at best, the effects are transient.[342]

Ventrobasal Complex. The ventrobasal complex (n. ventralis posterior and n. ventralis lateralis) is situated in the ventrolateral quadrant of the thalamus. Neurons of this region project in a somatotopic manner to SI and SII of the somatosensory cortex. The projection to SI is greater than to SII. The SII receives no independent input, but rather appears innervated by collaterals of the projection to SI.[268,411,412,524,689,815]

The ventrobasal nuclei classically have been thought to receive primarily lemniscal input from the dorsal column nuclei.[68,513,645] The spinothalamic tract is a minor source of input.[67,545,814] After sectioning of the dorsal columns, sparing the VLF, only a small number of neurons in the ventrobasal region are activated by either noxious or non-noxious peripheral stimuli.[636] Most neurons in the ventrobasal complex are responsive to innocuous tactile or thermal stimuli, or to joint movement and aversive visceral stimulation.[104,314,341,472,645,650] The number of neurons responsive to noxious stimuli is much smaller, about 6% to 10% of the sample.[341,606,714] In the ventroposterolateral axis, large populations of neurons responsive to noxious input have been identified.[122,374,463] Lesions in the ventrobasal complex in a variety of species alter somatosensory discrimination. White and Sweet noted in humans that such lesions produce transient analgesia.[812] Similar findings have been reported in cats.[293] Stimulation of the ventrobasal complex in humans commonly produces non-noxious paresthesias and tingling.[747]

Medial and Intralaminar Nuclei. The intralaminar nuclear complex forms a shell around the lateral aspect of the nucleus medialis dorsalis and comprises five nuclear groups: the n. paracentralis, n. centralis medialis, n. centromedian, n. centralis lateralis, and n. parafascicularis. Input to these nuclei is contributed primarily by the spinothalamic tract[67,70,513,545] and the n. reticularis gigantocellularis. These reticulothalamic projections are thought to be a major source of input to the intralaminar complex.[72,522,632] The intralaminar thalamic complex projects diffusely to wide areas of the cerebral cortex, including the frontal, parietal, and limbic regions.[410]

Populations of neurons in the medial and intralaminar nuclei respond to noxious stimuli and encode the stimulus intensity in the duration and frequency of patterned discharges.[192] A proportion of neurons in these regions respond exclusively to innocuous stimuli or responds to both innocuous and noxious stimuli.[9,25,126,212,633,636,775] Consistent with these observations, volleys in A-delta and C fibers produced by electrical stimulation of peripheral nerves evoke activity in neurons of the medial and intralaminar nuclei.[212] The receptive fields of neurons in these regions are large, often bilateral, with little evidence for a somatotopic organization of input.[9,212,633,775] Neurons of the medial and intralaminar nuclei receive convergent input from skin, joints, and muscle.[9,212] In humans, neurons in the centromedian-parafascicular region that possess large receptive fields, occasionally including the contralateral half and ipsilateral upper half of the body, are found to be responsive to noxious stimuli. Two classes of neurons have been described: those activated with a short latency to response and those activated with a long latency. The former category of neurons is found predominantly in the basomedial portions of the parafascicular nucleus, and the latter group is localized to the dorsal centromedian and parafascicular regions.

While the current thinking strongly implicates intralaminar nuclei, particularly the centromedian-parafascicular region, in nociception, lesion studies conducted in rats, cats, and monkeys have, however, failed to report an alteration in the animals' response to noxious stimuli following large lesions.[193,251,852] Such lesions have produced increases in nociceptive threshold as assessed by tooth pulp stimulation in cats[418,564] and operant response to shock in primates.[527,768] In addition, a significant relief of intractable pain arising from neoplastic disease has been reported following lesions of the medial thalamus.[688] The centromedian-parafascicular medialis dorsalis complex appears to be a critical determinant of effectiveness. Conversely, electrical stimulation of these nuclei has commonly elicited sensations of burning pain experienced contralaterally.

Within the medial thalamus, attention has been focused particularly on the n. submedius. This region displays neurons that are primarily nociceptive-selective and receives significant projections from marginal neurons.[64,172,173,789] Electrical stimulation in this region has been shown to evoke pain behaviors in unanesthetized animals[213] from marginal neurons. The n. submedius displays strong ipsilateral projections to the ventrolateral orbital cortex.[870]

Cortical Projections

The somatosensory areas (SI/SII) receive input indirectly from the three major spinal systems through which ascending sensory and noxious information may travel.[66] Investigations have focused attention on the importance of the SII area in the reception and perception of pain information. This area of the cortex may be divided into an anterior and a posterior region.[815] The anterior region is thought to receive input primarily from the ventrobasal thalamic nuclei,[268,411,412,689] and neurons in this region are activated by light tactile stimuli. Input to this region is somatotopically arranged; receptive fields correspond with precise symmetric sites on both sides of the body.[815]

Posterior SII receives input largely from the posterior thalamic complex.[105] Neurons in this region possess receptive fields that encompass large asymmetric areas of the body.[815] These neurons are polysensory, and a number respond to high-intensity mechanical stimuli.[118,815] The responsive properties of these neurons resemble those reported for neurons in the posterior thalamic nuclei.[636,644] Neurons in the posterior thalamic complex are antidromically activated by stimulation of posterior SII and nociresponsive neurons could still be observed in the cortex of cats having lesions of the dorsal funiculus, suggesting that input eventually arriving at the cortex could, in fact, travel over the ventrolateral quadrants.[22,48] It has been observed that bilateral destruction of that area to which the posterior thalamic nuclei project produces an increase in the nociceptive threshold.

In humans, the assessment of blood flow and metabolic activity using positron emission tomography has revealed that aversive thermal stimulation (as compared to non-aversive or vibrotactile stimuli) produces a very consistent increase in activity in the anterior cingulate cortex (area 24).[120,163,198,748]

The role of these higher-order processing systems remains to be elucidated. Clearly, at some point, the information generated by a particular family of stimuli must achieve access to functional systems that lead to the interpretation of that stimulus in the context of past experiences. The observation of a surprisingly selective activation in the anterior cingulate suggests that such a region may play a linking role. Importantly, this region has strong reciprocal connections with the limbic forebrain and could serve in that capacity. As such, this provides a substrate for the functionally defined affective-motivational components of the pain state.[549]

NONICEPTIVE PROCESSING: MODULATORY SUBSTRATES

As noted in the introductory sections of this chapter, the consideration of the afferent limb of the ascending pathways through which pain-related information travels may be thought of not only in terms of the elements through which the information travels, but also in terms of the systems that modulate transmission at each level of the synapse. From a historical perspective the role of modulation has been considered in the context of a suppression of the magnitude of the pain message and the teleology of "endogenous analgesic systems." In the late 1970s and early 1980s, much attention was therefore paid to the role of descending pathways and endogenous, endorphinergic systems (see Chapter 23.1, Figs. 23.1-18 and 23.1-19). These systems clearly continue to play a role, but of greater interest has been the evolving insight that afferent input can serve to drive a *facilitation* in the response evoked by a given stimulus, e.g., tissue injury evokes changes that result in the augmentation of the response evoked by a subsequent stimulus (see Chapter 23.1, Figs. 23.1-2 to 23.1-4). Further, while it has been appreciated since the early prescient writings of Weir-Mitchell and colleagues[802] that there can be a prominent pain state evoked by light touch (allodynia) after nerve injury, the significance of that had been poorly incorporated into theoretic mechanisms until the last several years (see Chapter 23.1, Fig. 23.1-8). As will be discussed, it is clear now that peripheral injury leads to an acute alteration in the response evoked by light touch and to long-term changes in the connectivity of the spinal systems. Accordingly, it is now clear that the encoding of afferent information is much more complex than originally appreciated and that the processing of somatic and visceral information is an extremely dynamic event. Appreciation of these characteristics provides insights into the important principles that define the encoding of information leading to pain behavior.

In the following sections, several of the networks that are believed to play an important role in altering the encoding or afferent transmission along the neuraxis will be considered. After this, current thinking regarding the role played by several of these systems in modifying the response otherwise generated by a given somatic stimulus will be considered, e.g., the substrates that modify the processing of the message generated by high- and low-intensity somatic stimuli.

Brain-Stem–Spinal Linkages

Classic work by Hagbarth and Kerr[322] demonstrated the ability of descending long tract systems to modulate spinal-evoked activity. Early on, Takagi and colleagues[744] pointed to a possible role of descending systems in mediating the effects of morphine. It has long been known that activation of the pathways originating in the brain stem and descending to the spinal cord can inhibit activity evoked in flexor reflex afferents.[236,237,372] Virtually every pathway carrying nociceptive information, including the spinoreticular[371] and spinothalamic,[821] has been shown to be under modulatory control of pathways that originate supraspinally. The classic observation that microinjections of morphine into the brain stem could inhibit spinal reflex activity,[767] and the subsequent demonstration that stimulation in the mesencephalon and medulla will inhibit the discharge of neurons in the spinal cord and trigeminal nucleus[247,512,707,821,867] evoked by nociceptive stimulation, emphasized the likely role of spinopetal systems in controlling spinal processing. In unanesthetized animals, such stimulation has been shown to alter the response to noxious stimuli and inhibit reflex function.[534,616]

The mechanism of this descending inhibition has been a subject of considerable investigation, and it is increasingly apparent that a significant proportion of this modulation is mediated by the activation of descending monaminergic pathways. Evidence for this may be briefly summarized as follows: (i) electrical stimulation or microinjections of opiates at brain stem sites such as the periaqueductal gray or the nucleus gigantocellularis will inhibit nociceptive reflexes, and this effect is antagonized by the intrathecal administration of serotonergic or noradrenergic antagonists, or both;[111,332,854] (ii) microinjections of morphine or focal stimulation in the medulla or periaqueductal gray that alter nociceptive thresholds are associated with an increased release of serotonin or norepinephrine in the spinal cord;[331,849] and (iii) the spinal application of adrenergic or serotonergic agonists either by iontophoresis or by intrathecal administration in the unanesthetized animal will significantly antagonize the A-delta/C-fiber-evoked activity in dorsal horn neurons and is associated with significant analgesia, respectively.[347,669,796] As noted above, both serotonin and norepinephrine are released in the spinal cord by high- but not low-intensity stimulation of afferent input (sciatic nerve).[769] Importantly, spinal transections inhibit this effect, indicating that the release is mediated by a spinobulbospinal loop. Significantly, stimulation of regions remote from the lumbar spinal cord region from which the release has been measured (infra-orbital branch of the trigeminal nerve) also produces release of serotonin and norepinephrine in the lumbar spinal cord region. This suggests that these particular descending systems, the activity of which is manifested by serotonin and norepinephrine release, are globally activated by afferent input. This is in marked contrast to the enkephalin-evoked release from the spinal cord, where such distal stimulation has failed to have any influence on spinal release.[769,844] Although the principal interest thus far has focused largely on spinopetal aminergic pathways, other neurotransmitter systems have been shown to project to the spinal cord, including dopamine,[71,719] substance P,[71] thyrotropin-releasing hormone,[71] and cholecystokinin.[525] The complexity of this system is emphasized further by the fact that a number of these agents may be co-contained, such as SP and serotonin[143] and enkephalin and serotonin. The role of these several systems has yet to be ascertained, but clearly they provide additional substrates whereby brain-stem systems may interact with spinal cord sensorimotor processing.

Brain-Stem–Brain-Stem Linkages

Although most work examining the effects of brain-stem manipulations on nociceptive responsiveness has focused on projections to the spinal cord, significant evidence suggests that supraspinal, brain-stem, and modulatory influences are being exerted by various systems. Thus the nucleus gigantocellularis, as discussed previously, may represent an important supraspinal link in systems through which nociceptive information may travel en route to higher centers. It has been demonstrated that mesencephalic stimulation will inhibit the discharge of neurons in the nucleus gigantocellularis in response to peripheral stimulation.[576]

Thus, although brain-stem manipulations that inhibit spinal reflex functions (such as the tail flick) may indeed alter the rostral transmission of information relevant to pain behavior, it is likely that this is not the only method whereby these supraspinal systems modulate the ascending pain message. Intrathecal administration of aminergic antagonists, therefore, will produce a significant reversal of the effects of these descending systems on spinal reflex function but has a subtotal effect on the supraspinally mediated aspects of the behavior.[111,406,407] This suggests that these supraspinal systems may act at several levels to modulate the animal's processing of nociceptive information.

Brain-Stem—Forebrain Linkages

Several lines of evidence have recently begun to emphasize the role of descending systems in the modulation of the organism's response to noxious stimulus. Current evidence indicates that there are significant projections from the mesencephalic central gray matter into the vicinity of the medial thalamus.[328,526,639] Stimulation in the periaqueductal gray matter has been demonstrated to produce a significant inhibition of the response of these medial thalamic neurons.[14,393] The neurotransmitter mediator of this is not known, although ascending serotonergic projections from the raphe have been well described, and the iontophoretic administration of serotonin will reduce the firing of these thalamic neurons.[15,27] Importantly, stimulation of the dorsal raphe will produce similar effects on the firing of parafascicular neurons.[14] These observations are of particular interest in view of the clinical reports that brain-stem stimulation can produce significant changes in the patient's response in various chronic pain conditions. Although it has been suggested that this is due to the activation of *descending* pathways, such stimulation rarely has any effect on spinal reflex function, even in those limited cases in which analgesia has been reported and documented.[319,379,561,675]

Early studies have demonstrated that stimulation of the caudate nucleus produces significant interaction of the medial thalamic and interlaminar nuclei and that this interaction is largely inhibitory in character.[470] Electrical stimulation of the caudate nucleus in primates has been reported to reduce the affective response to strong cutaneous stimulation.[507]

Corticospinal systems have long been known to have a significant effect on spinal afferent transmission. Thus electrical stimulation of the sensory cortex has been reported to affect afferent transmission and reflex pathways.[322,511] More recently it has been demonstrated that the stimulation of the somatosensory SI region of the cortex can result in a significant reduction in the response of spinothalamic neurons to C-fiber activity evoked by high-intensity thermal mechanical stimuli.[865]

DYNAMIC CHARACTERISTICS OF ENCODING SYSTEMS FOR NOCICEPTION

In the preceding section, it was emphasized that a variety of physiologically defined linkages can influence processing at all levels of the neuraxis. In the present section, we will focus on several aspects of the afferent processing that emphasize the dynamic and "plastic" nature of the encoding process. These directions of research have provided a rich source for practically defining the mechanisms whereby pain information is encoded.

As noted, principal classes of neurons in the dorsal horn

show an excitation evoked by large (low-threshold) and small (high-threshold) primary afferents. Each cell displays a principal excitatory drive from a relatively limited dermatome. However, as noted, afferents display significant extrasegmental projections that exert a progressively smaller postsynaptic effect at the more distal segments. This organization, though simplified, suggests how prominent changes in responsiveness can be induced by a variety of influences at the brain stem and spinal level, which either depress or facilitate the postsynaptic responsiveness of local circuits.

Inhibitory Systems

As indicated previously, dorsal horn neurons typically display an increasing response in the face of an increasing stimulus intensity. It is likely that this reflects an increased release of afferent excitatory transmitter and the subsequent depolarization of the second-order neuron. Factors that diminish that input-output function would predictably change the magnitude of the pain behavior evoked by a given stimulus. A number of physiologic and pharmacologic mechanisms have been shown to reduce the slope of the stimulus-response relationship at the spinal level. These will be considered in the following sections.

Physiologic Components of Inhibition. Activation of a number of physiologically defined elements has been shown to diminish spinal afferent transmission.

1. Dorsal column stimulation activates collaterals of large primary afferents and depresses the evoked discharge of dorsal horn interneuron nociceptors.[40] These results fulfilled one prediction of the gate control theory originally proposed by Melzack and Wall,[551] and led to the clinical use of dorsal column stimulation for the relief of pain.[598,709] The neuronal pathways that mediate the mechanisms of inhibition of the cord are not well understood.

2. Stimulation of the lateral Lissauer tract (a presumed outflow of gelatinosa neurons) results in the development of segmental dorsal root potentials (DRPs)[800] and a concurrent inhibition of the polysynaptic ventral root reflex, as well as the discharge of wide dynamic range neurons evoked by noxious stimulation.[798,850] In contrast, lesion of the Lissauer tract results in an increased receptive field size.[196]

3. Bulbospinal projections will diminish the slope of the response (frequency of discharge) versus stimulus intensity curve of dorsal horn neurons, as well as shift the temperature intercept of the stimulus-response curve to the right, indicating an increase in the threshold stimulus intensity necessary to evoke activity in the cell.[282,283]

Pharmacology of Spinal Inhibitory Receptors. Pharmacologic investigations have revealed that the activation of a variety of spinal receptor systems will depress the discharge of dorsal horn neurons that is evoked by small high-intensity/small afferent-mediated input. As indicated in Table 24-3, certain receptor classes including those for the mu, delta opioid, and alpha$_2$ adrenergic will produce a powerful suppression of the excitation of the activation of dorsal horn neurons produced by the activation of populations of small afferents and yield a selective inhibition of the animal's response to a strong threshold after spinal delivery (see Table 24-3). The mechanisms by which these several modulatory receptor systems exert their surprisingly selective effect upon afferent-evoked excitation and pain behavior are several:

1. *Presynaptic actions.* As indicated in Table 24-3, several of the receptor systems display binding that is presynaptic on primary afferents, and given the selective effects of capsaicin as a C fiber neurotoxin,[218] this appears to be largely on small fibers.[248,600] Consistent with the presynaptic locus of binding, agonist occupancy of these receptors has been shown to diminish the depolarization evoked release of spinal excitatory amino acids (glutamate) and peptide (SP and CGRP).[408,520,845,859]

2. *Postsynaptic actions.* While rhizotomy may diminish significantly the binding for a number of the receptor systems, none has shown a reduction greater than 50%. This suggests that there is additional binding which is not on the primary afferent. A variety of studies has shown that many of these receptors exert their effect by increasing K^+ conduction through a $G_{i/o}$ coupled protein. This results in a hyperpolarization that serves to depress excitability of the respective post-afferent neuron.[603]

It is thus considered that agents that possess a joint pre- and postsynaptic action may exert their powerful modulatory influence by a selective effect upon small fiber input and a coincidental postsynaptic action.[860]

The behavioral relevance of these inhibitory receptor systems via pain is emphasized by the observation that the spinal delivery of the appropriate agonists will serve to regulate the animal's response to mechanical, thermal, and chemical stimuli, which would otherwise evoke indices of pain behavior in animals (e.g., escape, vocalization) and humans. Thus, as summarized in Table 24-4, the spinal delivery of mu, delta opioid, and alpha$_2$ adrenoceptor agonists, neuropeptide Y, and agonists for several 5-HT receptors can produce a powerful antinociceptive effect. Such actions have been substantiated in humans as with the spinal actions of mu, delta, and alpha$_2$ adrenoceptor agonists.[838,840] Such behavioral observations substantiate interneurons the powerful role played by these receptor systems in the regulation of afferent traffic evoked by a high-intensity stimulus.

Endogeneous Inhibitory Systems. The presence of these receptors and the powerful effects of exogenously administered adrenoceptor and opiate agonists on spinal nociceptive functioning lead to the question of what are the *endogenous* systems that normally act on these receptors and what normally activates those systems. As summarized in Table 24-3, the transmitters with which these several receptors are associated are found in descending (bulbospinal pathways), such as those for the amines (noradrenaline, dopamine, and serotonin) and intrinsic interneurons, such as the enkephalins.

TABLE 24-3. *Summary of non afferent spinal receptor systems which can modulate nociceptive processing*

Endogenous ligand/origin	Receptor	Location of spinal binding		Spinal effects SP release	Spinal effects WDR	Prototypical Agonist/Antagonist
Opioid						
Enkephalin	mu	Pre/post[273,481a]	D>V[572a]	↓[295]	↓[255,377]	Morphine/Naloxone
(intrinsic BS						Sufentanil/CTAP
project)	delta	Pre/post[273,481a]	D>V[572a]	↓[295]	↓[255,377]	DPDPE/Naltrindole
						DADL/ICI174816
Dynorphin	kappa	Pre/post[373,481a]	D>V[572a]	Ø[295]	↓[255,377]	U50488H/norBNI
(intrinsic)						
Adrenergic						
Noradrenaline	alpha$_1$	?	?	Ø[295]	Ø[257]	Methoxamine/Prazocin
(BS	alpha$_2$	Pre/post[381]	D>V[627]	↓[295,619]	↓[257]	Medetomidine/Yohimbine
projections)						Clonidine/Atipamezole
						(nonA?) ST-91/Prazocin
Serotonin						
Serotonin	5-HT			Ø[295]	↓[234]	5-HT
(BS project)	5-HT$_{1A}$	Pre/Post[187]	D>V[187,630]	?	↓[234]	8-OH-DPA/Methiothepin
	5-HT$_{1B}$	?	D>V[630]	?	↓[234]	RU-24969, DOI/ketanserin
	5-HT$_2$	?	D>V[630]	?	Ø[234]	a-methyl-5-HT
	5-HT$_3$	Pre/Post[333]	D>V[333]	↑[690]	↓[12]	2-methyl-5-HT
Adenosine						
Adenosine	A$_1$/A$_2$	Post[284]	D>V[78]	Ø[786]	↓[686]	L-PIA/Theophylline
(Intrinsic, PA)						
GABA						
GABA	A	Pre/Post	D>V[754]	↓[295]	↓[12]	Muscimol, THIP/Bicuculine
(Intrinsic)	B	Pre/Post	D>V[653]	Ø[295]	↓[203]	Baclofen/Phaclofen
Cholinergic						
ACh	M$_1$/M$_2$	Pre/Post[292]	D≈V[291]	?	↓[583]	Oxotremorine/Atropine
(BS project)	Nicotinic	?	D≈V[291]			
Neuropeptide Y						
NPY1–36		?	D>V[422]	↓[224]	?	NPY 1–36, NPY 18–36
(BS project; PA)						
Neurotensin						
NT1–13		?	D>V[239]	?	↑[562]	NT 1–13
(Intrinsic)						
Glutamate						
Glutamate	NMDA	? (Post[188])	D>V[271]	?	↑[697]	NMDA/MK-801
(BS project;	non-NMDA					AMPA/CNQX
PA; DH neurons)						Kainate

Origin of ligand: Intrinsic, cell bodies in the spinal cord; PA, primary afferents; BS project, spinopetal pathways originating in the brain stem. *Location of binding in spinal cord*: D, dorsal; V, ventral horn; Pre, binding presynaptic on primary afferent; Post, binding postsynaptic (not on primary afferent). *Spinal effects*: SP release, ↓ depression, ↑ increase or Ø no effect by agonist on the release of substance P from spinal cord; WDR, wide dynamic range neuron in spinal dorsal horn. *Agonist/Antagonist*: representative competitive agonists and antagonists of the receptor.

Several populations of endorphins have been identified, including those derived from the pre/pro hormones of pro-opiomelanocortin, pre/pro-enkephalin, and pre/pro-dynorphin.[855,856] Products of the latter two populations, such as met- and leu- enkephalins, and various extended peptides such as Phe7Arg6-Met5-enkephalin and extended chains of leuenkephalin (yielding dynorphins), have been identified in dorsal horn neurons. Importantly, these classes of opioids have been shown to possess a differential receptor preference.[855,856] These intrinsic systems have been shown to be activated by a variety of conditions. Thus, both the bulbospinal pathways (amines) and the intrinsic spinal neurons (endorphins) are released from the spinal cord in animal models by high, but not low-intensity, stimulation and irritant stimuli.[137,138,769,844,848] It should be stressed that while these systems clearly have the potential of regulating the afferent traffic as indicated by the powerful effects of the exogenously delivered receptor agonists, there is surprisingly

TABLE 24-4. *Antinociceptive effects of spinally delivered receptor selective agents in the rat**

		Antinociceptive measure		
		Formalin test[d]		
	HP[a]/TF[b]	Phase 1	Phase 2	Strychnine[f] (allodynia)
AGONISTS				
Opioid				
mu	+ +[694a,846]	+ +[861,862]	+ +[861,862]	(+)[836]
delta	+ +[694a]	?	+ +[582]	(+)[836]
kappa	(+)[694a]	0[519]	+[519]	0[836]
Alpha Adrenergic				
2 > 1	+ +[668,746]	+ +[519]	+ +[519]	0[836]
Serotonin				
$5\text{-}HT_{1A}$	+[g]	?	?	?
$5\text{-}HT_{1B}$	+[g]	?	?	?
$5\text{-}HT_2$	0/+?[g]	?	?	?
$5\text{-}HT_3$	+[294]	?	?	?
Adenosine				
$A_1 > A_2$	+[726,h]	0[486,519,h]	+[486,519,h]	+ +[727]
GABA				
A	0[329]	+ +[210]	+ +[210]	?
B	+[330]	+[210]	+ +[210]	+[836]
Benzodiazepine	+[230,864]	0[210]	0/+[210]	?
Cholinergic				
$M_1/M_3 > M_2$	+ +[585,i]	?	?	?
Neuropeptide Y	+ +[384]	?	?	?
ANTAGONISTS				
Glutamate				
NMDA	0[593]	(+)[862]	+ +[862]	+ +[836]
non-NMDA	+[593]	+[593,j]	+[593,j]	+[836]
Tachykinin				
NK-1	0[k]	(+)?[861]	+ +[861]	?
NK-2	+[256]	?	?	?
ENZYME INHIBITORS				
Cholinesterase (Muscarinic)	+ +[304,i]	?	?	?
Cyclooxygenase	0[517,835]	(+)[517]	+[517]	?
NO synthase	0[519]	(+)[519]	+[519]	?
Enkephalinase (Opioid)	+[622]	?	?	?

* The confidence with which any receptor is affiliated with the specific changes in pain behavior depends upon the use of receptor preferring agonists and antagonists. For the case of agents such as NPY, specific antagonists do not at present exist, or for the 5-HT antagonists, there is controversy as to the selectivity of the agonists/antagonists and specific receptor designations must be considered as tentative. In the case of agents such as cholinesterase and enkephalinase inhibitors, the use of selective antagonists are used to define the site acted upon by the augmented levels of endogenous transmitter produced by the enzyme inhibitors.

[a] HP: 52.5°C hot plate
[b] TF: tail flick
[c] distention of the bowel with balloon, examination of the behavioral or blood pressure response
[d] Injection of dilute formalin into one hindpaw; assessment of licking/flinching during the first phase 5–10 min or second phase 10–60 min after formalin
[e] Loose or partial compression of the sciatic nerve and examination of the thermal response latency
[f] Intrathecal injection of the glycine antagonist strychnine evoked tactile evoked agitation (allodynia) or increase in blood pressure
[g] Ware, and Yaksh, T.L.: unpublished data
[h] Yaksh, T.L. and Spath,: unpublished data
[i] Naguib, M. and Yaksh, T.L.: unpublished data
[j] Malmberg, A.B. and Yaksh, T.L.: unpublished data
[k] Yamamoto, T. and Yaksh, T.L.: unpublished data

little support for the thesis that these systems play a significant ongoing role in the regulation of C-fiber–evoked activity. Thus, with few exceptions, antagonists for these systems such as naloxone (all opiate receptors) or phentolamine (alpha adrenoceptor antagonist) fail to produce evident hyperalgesia.

Facilitatory Systems

The magnitude of the response to a given noxious stimulus may be enhanced in the absence of change in the magnitude of the stimulus. In contrast to the effects of local inhibition, processes that lead to facilitation of the response to a given input should serve to augment the magnitude of the pain behavior.

Physiologic Components of Spinal Facilitation. The best example of this was first described by Mendell and Wall.[553] They noted that repetitive activation of C fibers, but not A fibers, leads to an augmented response to subsequent C-fiber input, a phenomenon referred to as "wind-up," and an increase in the size of the receptive field of the respective neuron.[205,552] Behavioral correlates of the event have been observed in a number of animal models in which local injury or inflammation have evoked a prolonged burst of afferent activity followed by an ongoing low level of afferent discharge. One example of this is found in the action of formalin injected into the paw of the rat. In this, recording of saphenous nerve output reveals a prominent burst of activity lasting for approximately 10 minutes followed by a protracted ongoing barrage of sensory outflow in the small afferent.[348] Examination of the animals behavior reveals that the injection of the irritant occasions a prominent licking of the paw which lasts for 10 minutes, at which time it subsides. This is followed, approximately 20 minutes later, with a second phase of intense flinching and licking of the injected paw. This second phase occurs in the absence of a significant barrage, and it is believed that this second phase of licking and flinching reflects on a facilitated processing of otherwise modest input (see Fig. 24-12). The parallel to this event in the rat has been observed in humans after the intradermal injection of the C-fiber stimulant capsaicin.[479,756]

Pharmacology of Spinal Inhibitory Receptors. Several lines of evidence indicate that spinal facilitation evoked by repetitive C-fiber activity ("wind-up") is mediated by an SP (neurokinin [NK-1]) site and a glutamate receptor of the N-methyl-D-aspartate (NMDA) subtype: (i) C-fiber–evoked wind-up is blocked or attenuated by the spinal action of NMDA and NK-1 receptor antagonists,[190,204,832] and (ii) direct activation of spinal glutamate and tachykinin receptors with intrathecal agonists will induce an augmented response to a noxious thermal stimulus (i.e., a hyperalgesia[1,175,516]). The relevance of these spinal receptor systems to behavioral indices of a pain state has been well documented. Thus, as described in Figure 24-12, injection of an irritant such as for-

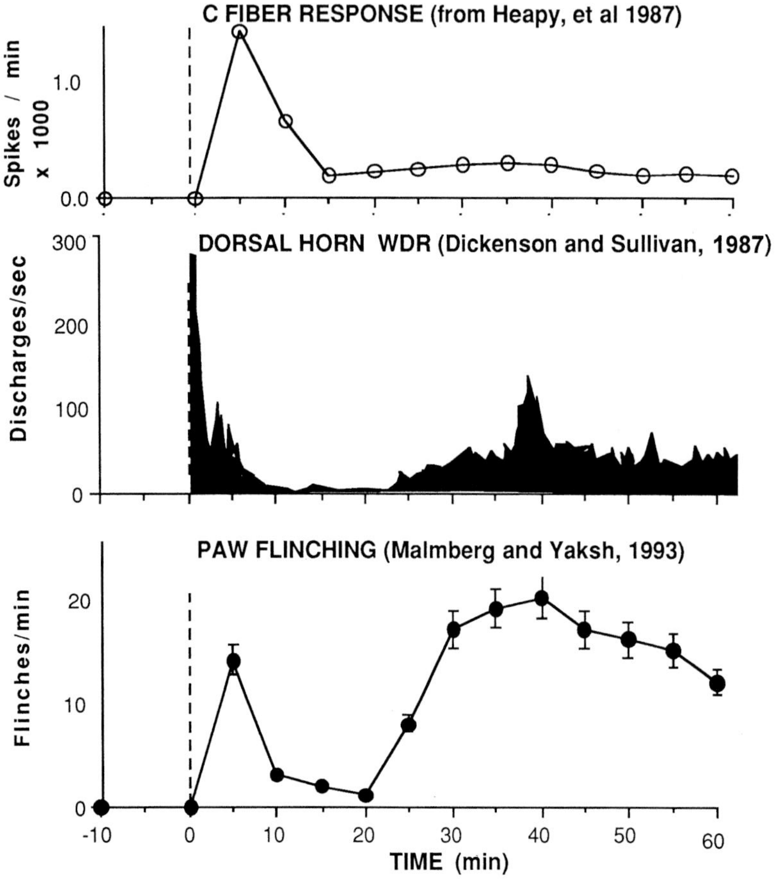

FIG. 24-12. C fiber activity *(top)* measured in the saphenous nerve of the anesthetized rat and number of flinches in the unanesthetized rat measured before and after the ipsilateral subcutaneous injection of formalin (5%/50 μl) into the hind paw at the time indicated by the vertical dashed line. Note the low level of input during the second phase, where behavior suggestive of pain is particularly high. (Afferent recording data adapted from[348]; spinal data adapted from[206]; behavioral data adapted from.[517])

malin into the paw results in a burst of small afferent activity, followed by a prolonged low level of afferent discharge.[348] Behaviorally, the animal displays an initial transient phase of flinching and licking of the injected paw (phase 1), followed after a brief period of quiescence by a second prolonged phase of licking and flinching. Spinal delivery of NMDA and NK-1 antagonists have little effect upon the first phase, but will significantly diminish the magnitude of the second-phase response (see also Table 24-4).[160,861,862] Physiologic parallels to this behavior have been observed in which NMDA antagonists have little effect on acute excitation of dorsal horn neurons,[346,711] but will significantly reduce the elevated, ongoing activity evoked by the induction of a peripheral injury state.[692,711]

Mechanisms of Facilitation. As summarized schematically in Figure 24-13, NK-1 binding sites are believed to be postsynaptic to the primary afferent terminal (see Table 24-3). In contrast, NMDA antagonists do not block monosynaptic afferent-evoked activity in dorsal horn wide dynamic range neurons, and thus do not lie on membranes immediately postsynaptic to the primary afferent.[188] These data thus suggest the role of a glutamatergic interneuron activated by primary afferent input. An important characteristic of this system is that the afferent drive appears to trigger the initiation of temporally defined events. Thus, NMDA and NK-1 antagonists given after the first phase of the formalin test have little effect upon the second-phase response.[160,861,862] The magnitude of the second phase is thus dependent upon processes that are initiated by NMDA and NK-1 activity during the first minutes after the stimulus, but these sites are not required for the sustenance of the second-phase activity and occur independently of these sites.

Several intervening mechanisms, which may account for these sustained states of facilitation, have been identified. Depolarization of neurons or the activation of the NMDA receptor will lead to an increase in intracellular Ca^{2+} [514] (see Chapter 23.1, Figs. 23.1-10 to 23.1-14) which evokes a cascade of biochemical events. The contributions of two elements of this cascade, prostaglandins and nitric oxide, are considered below.

1. *Prostaglandins.* Increased intracellular Ca^{2+} activates phospholipase A_2, leading to the appearance of cytosolic arachidonic acid and formation of cyclooxygenase and lipoxygenase products.[491] Primary afferent stimulation or direct activation of spinal neurons with NMDA evokes the spinal release of prostanoids.[158,663,724] These extracellular lipidic acids can (i) facilitate the depolarization-evoked increases in Ca^{2+} conductance in dorsal root ganglion cells and increase secretion of primary afferent peptides,[597] and (ii) evoke a thermal hyperalgesia after spinal delivery.[743,774,835] Spinal cyclooxygenase inhibitors suppress the thermal hyperalgesia induced by spinally injected SP or NMDA[516] and the behavioral hyperalgesia resulting from peripheral tissue injury.[517]

2. *Nitric oxide synthase.* Nitric oxide (NO) formation is induced by NMDA receptor-mediated increases in Ca^{2+} [279] (see Chapter 23.1, Fig. 23.1-13). The thermal hyperalgesia induced by spinal NMDA[518,547] or the second phase of the formalin test can be blocked by spinal injection of an inhibitor of NO synthesis.[518] NO synthase has been found to occur in the dorsal horn[16,565] and in dorsal root ganglion cells (diaphorase-positive type B ganglion cells[6,573]). Because NO has the ability to readily penetrate cell membranes, it has been proposed as a likely candidate for a retrogradely acting messenger on presynaptic terminals.[699]

While these studies outlined above reflect the probable role of glutamate and substance P, the large number of afferent transmitters strongly suggests that a variety of these candidate transmitters may subserve roles similar to those defined above for excitatory amino acids and SP.

Dynamic Components of Encoding Systems: Low-Intensity Input

An important criterion of the definition of the components of systems that mediate the "pain state" has been the association of activity evoked by small afferent input (Aδ/C) and the lack of association of large afferent (A) input with those conditions.[660] There is, however, an extensive literature in which low-threshold, otherwise nonaversive, stimulation may yield a well-defined pain state. As reviewed in the initial section, the psychophysics of this state clearly emphasize that the pain may be evoked by the activation of low-threshold mechanoreceptors (Aβ afferents).[113] Such states of allodynia are frequently observed after a variety of injuries to the peripheral and central nervous systems.

Gamma-Aminobutyric Acid (GABA)/Glycine Systems. It has been appreciated that low-threshold afferents terminate in Rexed lamina below the substantia gelatinosa but converge upon lamina V wide dynamic range neurons. As noted in the preceding section, these cells are also activated by small afferents and are believed to play a role in the encoding of the pain message. Early studies revealed that the local inhibition of GABA and glycine receptor systems in the vicinity of the primary afferent terminals (using bicuculline or strychnine, respectively) would: (i) significantly enhance the discharge evoked by Aβ afferents, but only modestly the input generated by high-threshold afferents,[451,869] and (ii) permit light tactile stroking of the skin to evoke a well-defined pain state as defined by autonomic and behavioral criteria.[712,836] These simple observations suggest that the encoding of low-intensity mechanical stimuli as innocuous depends upon the presence of a tonic activation of intrinsic glycine and/or GABAergic neurons. Such neurons are found within the dorsal horn,[116,755] and glycine[35,877] and GABA[718] binding in the dorsal horn has been demonstrated. These GABA-containing terminals are frequently presynaptic to the large central afferent terminal complexes and may form reciprocal synapses.[33] GABAergic axosomatic connections on spinothalamic cells have also been identified.[116]

The relevance of these inhibitory amino acid systems in regulating behavior generated by low-threshold afferent transmission is suggested by: (i) mice[807] and bovine [317] dis-

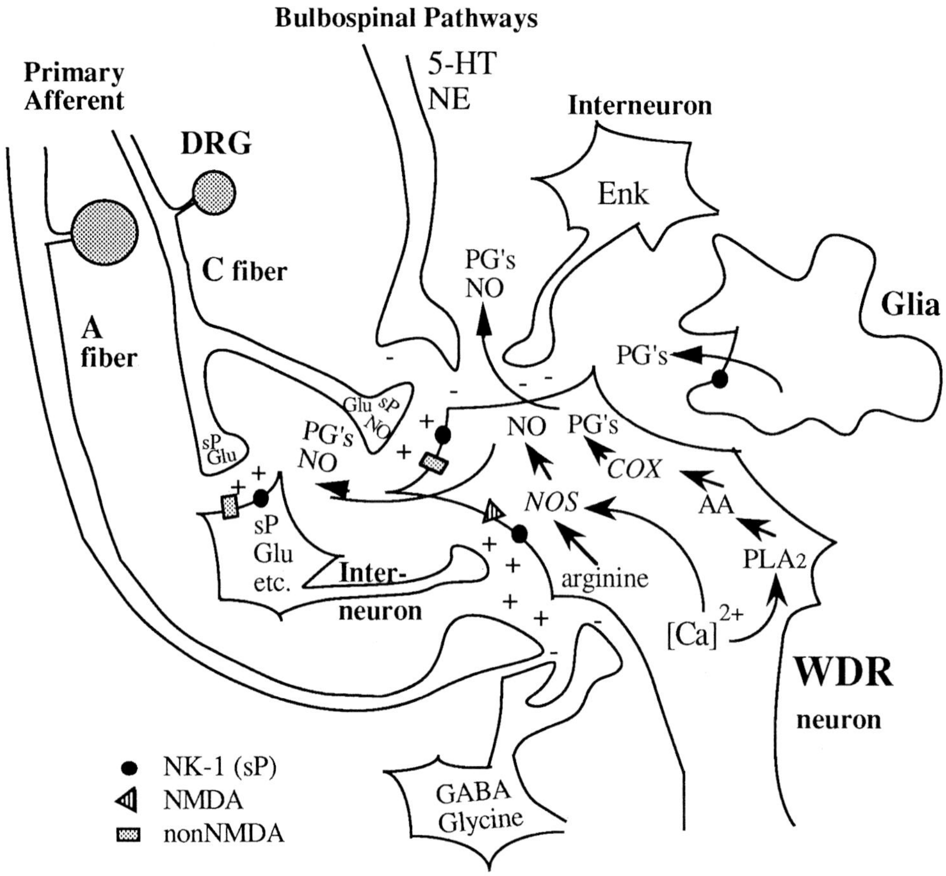

FIG. 24-13. This cartoon presents a schematic summary of the functional organization of elements in the dorsal horn discussed in the text which impact upon the processing of afferent input. Such an organization reflects the response to acute stimulation, development of the hyperalgesic state induced by repetitive small afferent stimulation, and development of anomalous pain states secondary to large afferent stimulation. See text for details and references. (i) The primary afferent C fiber contain and release both peptide (e.g., *SP/CGRP*) and excitatory amino acid *(Glu)* products. Small dorsal root ganglion cells *(DRG)* as well as postsynaptic elements are diaphorase positive, suggesting that they contain nitric oxide *(NO)* synthase *(NOS)* and are thus able, upon depolarization, to synthesize and release NO. (ii) These peptides and excitatory amino acids, acting transynaptically can evoke excitation in second-order neurons. For glutamate, it is believed that the excitation is mediated by non-NMDA receptors. (iii) Under the appropriate circumstances, interneurons excited by the afferent barrage evoke excitation in the second-order neuron by an action mediated by an *NMDA* receptor. This leads to a marked increase in intracellular Ca^{2+} and the activation of a number of kinases and phosphorylating enzymes. In this scenario, based on the effects of various enzyme inhibitors, it is believed that cyclooxygenase *(COX)* products (prostaglandins: *PGs*) and *NO* are formed and released. These agents move extracellularly to subsequently facilitate transmitter release from primary and nonprimary afferent terminals. (iv) Intervening products, such as the prostanoids, may arise from non-neuronal structures, such as glia by the action of SP. [From Marriot, D., Wilkin, G.P., Coote, P.R., and Wood, J.N.: Eicosanoid synthesis by spinal cord astrocytes is evoked by substance P, possible implications for nociception and pain. *In* Samuelsson, B., Dahlen, S-E., Fritsch, J., and Hedqvist, P. (eds.): Trends in Eicosanoid Biology. Advances in Prostaglandin, Thromboxane, and Leukotriene Research. Vol. 20. Philadelphia, Lippincott-Raven, 1990.] (v) In certain instances, second-order neurons also receive excitatory input from large afferents. Based on the effects of various inhibitory amino acid antagonists, it appears that the excitatory effects of large afferents is under a GABA-A/glycine modulatory control, removal of which results in an allodynia. (vi) Interneurons containing peptides such as enkephalin, or bulbospinal pathways containing monoamines (norepinephrine, serotonin) and peptides (enkephalin, neuropeptide Y [NPY]) may be activated by afferent input and "reflexly" exert a modulatory influence upon the release of C fiber peptides and postsynaptically to hyperpolarize projection neurons. [From Yaksh, T.L., and Malmberg, A.B.: Central pharmacology of nociceptive transmission. *In* Wall, P.A., and Melzack, R. (eds.): Textbook of Pain. pp. 165–200. New York, Churchill Livingstone, 1994.]

playing a prominent somatic sensitivity up to a 10-fold decrease in glycine binding, (ii) strychnine intoxication in humans, as characterized by a hypersensitivity to light touch,[28] and (iii) spinal cord ischemia, known to destroy amino acid-containing interneurons and yield a tactile allodynia.[338,339,530]

Post-Nerve Injury Allodynia. In the human state, allodynic conditions are frequently observed after peripheral nerve compression or injury (see Chapter 23.1, Fig. 23.1-8).[629,649] From animal studies, several models have evolved in which peripheral nerve compression will lead to a state of hyperalgesia or tactile allodynia.[452,715] Pursuit of the changes that are induced by such nerve injury has provided some insights into the systems that may be involved in the evolution of the allodynia following nerve injury. Following peripheral nerve ligation or section, several events occur, signaling long-term changes in peripheral and central processing.

1. Persistent small afferent fiber activity originates after an interval of days to weeks from the lesioned site (neuroma) and from the dorsal root ganglion (DRG) of the injured nerve.[100,201]

2. Peripheral changes in terminal sensitivity are noted. The sprouted terminals display a characteristic growth cone, which possesses transduction properties that were not possessed by the original axon. These include significant mechanical and chemical sensitivity. Thus, these sprouted endings may have sensitivity to a number of humoral factors, such as PGs, catecholamines, and cytokines.[201] In addition, it is known that these regenerating terminals have significant densities of various ion channels, notably those for sodium.[199] Increased ionic conductance may result in the increase in spontaneous activity that develops in a sprouting axon.[199,532]

3. Prominent changes in the morphology of the DRG cells are observed. Recent data, for example, have indicated that following peripheral lesion, there is a hyperinnervation of the type A ganglion cells by sympathetic terminals,[543] and cross-talk between A and C fibers develops in the ganglion.[200]

4. Prominent morphologic changes have been identified in the spinal dorsal horn ipsilateral to the ligation. The mechanism of these changes is not clear, but the possibility of persistent changes secondary to the chronic afferent barrage or to a change in factors transported from the lesioned site seem likely. Trans-synaptic changes include the appearance of early immediate gene products such as c-fos; an increase in the message for specific neurotransmitters, such as SP; and "dark staining" neurons in the spinal dorsal horn.[52,112,277,278,361,736] These alterations signal significant changes in dorsal horn function.

5. After peripheral nerve lesions, large primary afferents (Aβ) have been shown to sprout and to send terminals dorsally into the overlying substantia gelatinosa.[833] As previously discussed, small afferents typically project only into the substantia gelatinosa, and there appears to be a fine demarcation into the projection fields of the fiber classes. This sprouting thus places the large afferents in close proximity with systems that were originally only impacted by small afferents. While the precise significance of this is not known, it appears reasonable that such anomalous projections may

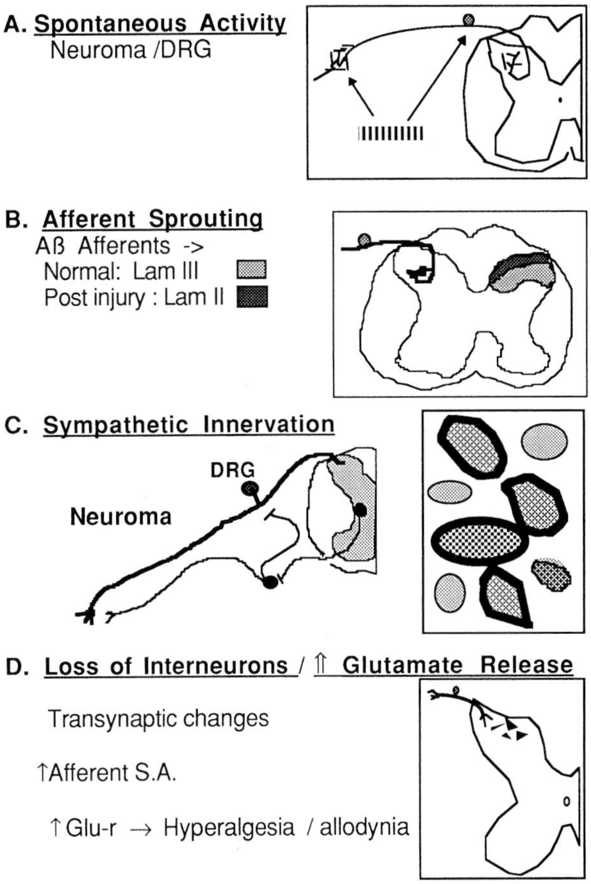

FIG. 24-14. Principal changes in function and connectivity potentially contributing to pain states after peripheral nerve injury. **A:** After nerve injury, spontaneous activity develops in the injured terminal (neuroma), in the dorsal root ganglion cell of the injured axon, *and* in the spinal cord dorsal horn. Sprouted endings may develop sensitivity to a number of humoral factors and display increases in the densities of sodium channel. **B:** Laminae I and II receive smaller, unmyelinated axons that are typically high-threshold in character, while larger low-threshold afferents terminate in lamina III or deeper. After injury, large afferent terminals sprout into lamina II. **C:** After peripheral nerve injury, there is a significant increase in sympathetic innervation at the neuroma of the resprouting axon. Dorsal root ganglia *(DRG)* cells display basket-like projections around dorsal root ganglion cells from proliferating postganglionic sympathetic terminals. These projections have been shown to drive activity in DRG cells. **D:** There is an increased incidence of "dark staining" neurons, suggesting a loss of interneurons (some of which are believed to contain GABA/glycine). In addition, after injury, there is an increased release in spinal glutamate, perhaps secondary to loss of inhibitory interneurons and to increased spontaneous afferent drive. Loss of spinal glycine inhibition and/or increased glutamate receptor activation will lead to hyperalgesia and allodynia.

underlie some of the connectivity required to explain the phenomenon of low-threshold afferents driving a pain state.

Pharmacology of the Allodynic State

The evolution of the preclinical models in which allodynia plays an important role in the behavioral syndrome leads naturally to the question of what regulates this behavior. Table 24-4 summarizes some of the pharmacology that appears to regulate the animal's allodynic response.

A common factor that has permeated the preclinical allodynia studies has been the probable importance of the release of glutamate. Thus, spinal NMDA antagonists appear to be particularly potent in reversing the allodynia observed in a number of nerve injury-allodynia animal models (see Table 24-4). Direct measurement of the release of glutamate from the spinal cord has indicated the appearance of an ongoing elevation in glutamate levels. As noted previously, direct activation of the glutamate receptor by spinal drug delivery will evoke a hyperalgesic/allodynic state. It thus seems probable that at least a component of the allodynia following nerve injury may be the consequence of an increased spontaneous release of glutamate. Importantly, agents thought to regulate glutamate release, such as the adenosine A-1 receptor,[170,267] also display a potent anti-allodynic effect.[486] Importantly, this role of enhanced glutamatergic activity may reflect a change in the postsynaptic coupling (e.g., more receptors) or an enhanced release, perhaps occurring secondary to the spontaneous activity originating from the neuroma or the dorsal root ganglion cell. In this regard, in case reports on human patients suffering from significant allodynia secondary to a presumed nerve injury, allodynia can be blocked by local anesthetic injections into the injured region.[306] This argues that whatever changes may have occurred within the neuraxis, the appearance of the pain state requires the ongoing input from the periphery. Further, it is interesting to note that some allodynic states may be driven. Thus, brushing an area of dysesthesia (e.g., driving large afferent input) may evoke a widespread area of tactile allodynia.[471] The diminished effect of spinal opiates on neuropathic pain in humans[30] and animal models (see above) is consistent with electrophysiologic observations that spontaneous activity generated in dorsal horn neurons following brachial plexus lesion is not very sensitive to opiates, and clinical reports suggest mixed effects of opiates on neuropathic pain states. Alternately, the marginal effect of opiates in the neuropathic pain models as compared to the acute thermal response model (hot plate) is consistent with the probable role of C fibers in the acute pain models and A fibers in the neuropathic models. In recent work, it was shown that spinal alpha$_2$ agonists have a potent anti-allodynic effect in post-nerve injury models.[841] This effect was believed to be mediated in part by the sympatholytic effects of spinal alpha$_2$ agonists.

In conclusion, it appears likely that the allodynic state that follows nerve injury may have several mechanisms. These include (i) changes in spinal cord connectivity after nerve injury (e.g., sprouting of large afferents; sprouting of the sympathetic efferent into the neuroma and dorsal root ganglia), (ii) the loss of intrinsic modulatory systems, which alters the subsequent encoding of afferent-evoked excitation (e.g., dark-staining neurons), (iii) an up-regulation of excitatory processes (e.g., dorsal horn NK receptors, among others), and (iv) dynamic processes that are reflected by tonic afferent input generated by the appearance of spontaneous activity arising from the neuroma and the dorsal root ganglion cell. It is important to appreciate that as acute pain states have many components, it is similarly true that all "neuropathic pain" is not the same and each is likely to display distinct mechanisms. This can be intuited from the simple case report noted above. In a patient suffering from a spontaneous dysesthesia, brushing the dysesthetic region evoked a large area of tactile allodynia. Both sensory signs reflected components of a neuropathic pain state. However, in intrathecal NMDA receptor antagonism, the evoked tactile allodynia was affected, but the area of spontaneous dysesthesia was not.

CONCLUDING COMMENTS

In the preceding sections, an outline has been provided of systems that potentially serve as substrates through which information initiated by high-intensity stimuli may gain access to various regions within the nervous system. The likelihood that "pain-relevant" information passes along a diversity of pathways is clear, even at the level of the spinal cord. Upon reaching the second-order neuron, the most apparent characteristic is that of polymodal convergence. At supraspinal levels the issue becomes predictably more complex.

While considerable advances have been made in our understanding of the connectivity of these afferent linkages, an equally important component has been the appreciation that the information processing is subject to a variety of modulatory influences that govern the encoding of the afferent message. In the period from 1975 through the early 1980s, the emphasis was on the importance of systems that down-regulated the response of the nervous system. The bulbospinal pathways and the endogenous opiates systems were in fact the pre-eminent part of any consideration of afferent processing. While these component remain part of the total system, in the past 10 years there has been a progressive appreciation of the role played by systems that "up-regulate" the response to a given stimulus. The concept of wind-up and facilitated pain states, and the evolution of changes whereby low-threshold afferent input evokes a pain state, clearly occupy an important place in our current appreciation of pain processing. Importantly, these lines of research have led to fundamental insights that have practical implications for the management of anomalous pain states. There is indeed a growing appreciation that the post–nerve-injury pain, far from being a sequelae affecting a small population, may impact on most major pain states such as cancer. Here, tumor compression and the sequelae of chemotherapy and radiation may induce changes that are as florid as those observed after a frank section of the nerve. Accordingly, the pharmacology of nerve injury pain states may have equal significance for chronic pain states in which tissue injury is the obvious companion to the syndrome.

Perhaps the next aspect in the evolution of our understanding of pain is a growth in our understanding of the mechanisms whereby the supraspinal component of the message evoked by a high-intensity stimulus leads to a "consciousness" of the stimulus. It would seem difficult given the convergence of the many systems to achieve a selective alteration in that component without altering all components of our psychological status. However, the observation that specific regions of the limbic system and the cortex show a differential response to a strong stimulus provides some support for selective interventions. Moreover, it is widely appreciated that changes in emotional status, such as depression, can significantly alter the pain report in humans and animals.[860] The pharmacology of those states is now beginning to be addressed with respect to pain. The richness of the pharmacology and the complexity of the connections may serve to be daunting, but that very richness and that complexity provide promise that the system is subject to powerful manipulation and control.

REFERENCES

1. Aanonsen, L.M., and Wilcox, G.L.: Nociceptive action of excitatory amino acids in the mouse: Effects of spinally administered opioids, phencyclidine and sigma agonists. J. Pharmacol. Exp. Ther., *243:*9, 1987.
2. Adrian, E.D.: The effects of injury on mammalian nerve fibers. Proc. R. Soc. Lond. B., *106:*596, 1930.
3. Agudelo, C.A., Schumauser, H.R., and Phelps, P.: Effect of exercise on urate crystal-induced inflammation in canine joints. Arthritis Rheum., *15:*609, 1972.
4. Ahlberg, K.F.: Dose-dependent inhibition of sensory nerve activity in the feline dental pulp by anti-inflammatory drugs. Acta Physiol. Scand., *102:*434, 1978.
5. Ahlberg, K.F.: Influence of local noxious heat stimulation on sensory nerve activity in the feline dental pulp. Acta Physiol. Scand., *103:*71, 1978.
6. Aimi, Y., Fujimura, M., Vincent, S.R., and Kimura, H.: Localization of NADPH-diaphorase-containing neurons in sensory ganglia of the rat. J. Comp. Neurol., *306:*382, 1991.
7. Akagi, H., Otsuka, M., and Yanagisawa, M.: Identification by high-performance liquid chromatography of immunoreactive substance P released from isolated rat spinal cord. Neurosci. Lett., *20:*259, 1980.
8. Albe-Fessard, D., and Kruger, L.: Duality of unit discharges from cat centrum medianum in response to natural and electrical stimulation. J. Neurophysiol., *25:*3, 1962.
9. Albe-Fessard, D., Levante, A., and Lamour, Y.: Origin of spinothalamic tract in monkeys. Brain Res., *65:*503, 1974.
10. Albe-Fessard, D., Levante, A., and Lamour, Y.: Origin of spinothalamic and spinoreticular pathways in cats and monkeys. Adv. Neurol., *4:*157, 1974.
11. Alexander, R.W., Kent, K.M., Pisano, J.J., *et al.*: Regulation of canine coronary blood flow by endogenous synthesized prostaglandins. Circulation, *48*(Suppl. IV):107, 1973.
12. Alhaider, A.A., Lei, S.Z., and Wilcox, G.L.: Spinal 5-HT3 receptor-mediated antinociception: Possible release of GABA. J. Neurosci., *11:*1881, 1991.
13. Amassian, V.E., and Waller, H.J.: Spatiotemporal patterns of activity in individual reticular neurones. *In* Jasper, H.H., Proctor, L.D., Knighton, R.S., and Noshay, W.C. (eds.): Reticular Formation of the Brain. pp. 69–108. Boston, Little, Brown & Co., 1958.
14. Andersen, E., and Dafny, N.: Dorsal raphe stimulation reduces responses of parafasicular neurons to noxious stimulation. Pain, *15:*323, 1983.
15. Andersen, E., and Dafny, N.: Microiontophoretically applied 5-HT reduces responses to noxious stimuli in the thalamus. Brain Res., *241:*176, 1982.
16. Anderson, C.R.: NADPH diaphorase-positive neurons in the rat spinal cord include a subpopulation of autonomic preganglionic neurons. Neurosci. Lett., *139:*280, 1992.
17. Anderson, D.J., Curwen, M.P., and Howard, L.V.: The sensitivity of human dentin. J. Dent. Res., *37:*669, 1958.
18. Anderson, D.J., Hannam, A.G., and Matthews, B.: Sensory mechanisms in mammalian teeth and their supporting structures. Physiol. Rev., *50:*171, 1970.
19. Anderson, F.D.: Distribution of dorsal root fibers in the cat spinal cord. Anat. Rec., *136:*154, 1960.
20. Anderson, K.V., and Perl, G.S.: Conduction velocities in afferent fibers from feline tooth pulp. Exp. Neurol., *43:*281, 1974.
21. Anderson, S.D., Basbaum, A.I., and Fields, H.L.: Response of medullary raphe neurons to peripheral stimulation and to systemic opiates. Brain Res., *123:*363, 1977.
22. Andersson, S.A.: Projection of different spinal pathways to the second somatic sensory area in cat. Acta Physiol. Scand., *56*(Suppl. 194):1, 1962.
23. Andres, K.H.: Untersuchungen uber den Feinbau von Spinalganglien. Z. Zellforsch., *55:*1, 1961.
24. Angaut-Petit, D.: The dorsal column system: Functional properties and bulbar relay of the postsynaptic fibers of the cat's fasciculus gracilis. Exp. Brain Res., *22:*471, 1975.
25. Angel, A.: The effect of peripheral stimulation on units located in the thalamic reticular nuclei. J. Physiol. (Lond.), *171:*42, 1964.
26. Antonetty, C.M., and Webster, K.E.: The organization of the spinotectal projection. An experimental study in the rat. J. Comp. Neurol., *163:*449, 1975.
27. Applebaum, M.L., Clifton, G.L., Coggeshall, R.E., *et al.*: Unmyelinated fibres in the sacral 3 and caudal 1 ventral roots of the cat. J. Physiol. (Lond.), *256:*557, 1976.
28. Arena, J.M.: Poisoning Toxicology, Symptoms, Treatments. 4th Ed. Springfield, IL, Charles C. Thomas, 1970.
29. Armstrong, D., Dry, R., Keele, C.A., and Markham, J.W.: Observations on chemical excitants of cutaneous pain in man. J. Physiol. (Lond.), *120:*326, 1953.
30. Arner, S., and Meyerson, B.A.: Lack of analgesic effect of opioids on neuropathic and idiopathic forms of pain. Pain, *33*(1):11, 1988.
31. Astrom, K.E.: On the central course of afferent fibers in the trigeminal, facial, glossopharyngeal, and vagal nerves and their nuclei in the mouse. Acta Physiol. Scand., *29*(Suppl. 106):209, 1953.
32. Baker, G.S., and Kerr, F.W.L.: Structural changes in the trigeminal system following compression procedures. J. Neurosurg., *20:*181, 1963.
33. Barber, R.P., Vaughn, J.E., Saito, K., McLaughlin, B.J., and Roberts, E.: GABAergic terminals are presynaptic to primary afferent terminals in the substantia gelatinosa of the rat spinal cord. Brain Res., *141:*35, 1978.
34. Barnes, K.L.: A quantitative investigation of somatosensory coding in single cells of the cat mesencephalic reticular formation. Exp. Neurol., *50:*180, 1976.
35. Basbaum, A.I.: Distribution of glycine receptor immunoreactivity in the spinal cord of the rat: Cytochemical evidence for a differential glycinergic control, of lamina I and lamina V neurons. J. Comp. Neurol., *278:*330, 1988.
36. Basbaum, A.I.: Conduction of the effects of noxious stimulation by short-fiber multisynaptic systems of the spinal cord in the rat. Exp. Neurol., *40:*699, 1973.
37. Basbaum, A.I.: Effects of central lesions on disorders produced by multiple dorsal rhizotomy in rats. Exp. Neurol., *42:*490, 1974.
38. Battaglia, G., and Rustioni, A.: Coexistence of glutamate and substance P in dorsal root ganglion neurons of the rat and monkey. J. Comp. Neurol., *277:*302, 1988.
39. Beaudreau, D.E., and Jerge, C.R.: Somatotopic representation in the gasserian ganglion of tactile peripheral fields in the cat. Arch. Oral. Biol., *13:*247, 1968.
40. Beck, P.W., and Handwerker, H.O.: Bradykinin and serotonin effects

on various types of cutaneous nerve fibers. Pflugers Arch., *374:*209, 1974.

41. Beck, P.W., Handwerker, H.O., and Zimmerman, M.: Nervous outflow from the cat's foot during noxious radiant heat stimulation. Brain Res., *67:*373, 1974.
42. Becker, D.P., Gluck, H., Nulsen, F.E., and Jane, J.A.: An inquiry into the neurophysiological basis for pain. J. Neurosurg., *30:*1, 1969.
43. Beitel, R.E., and Dubner, R.: Fatigue and adaptation in unmyelinated (C) polymodal nociceptors to mechanical and thermal stimuli applied to the monkey face. Brain Res., *112:*402, 1976.
44. Beitel, R.E., and Dubner, R.: Response of unmyelinated (C) polymodal nociceptors to thermal stimuli applied to monkey's face. J. Neurophysiol., *39:*1160, 1976.
45. Bell, C., Sierra, G., Buendia, N., and Segundo, J.P.: Sensory properties of neurons in the mesencephalic reticular formation. J. Neurophysiol., *27:*961, 1964.
46. Benjamin, R.M.: Single neurons in the rat medulla responsive to nociceptive stimulation. Brain Res., *24:*525, 1970.
47. Berkley, K.J., Robbins, A., and Sato, Y.: Afferent fibers supplying the uterus in the rat. J. Neurophysiol., *59*(1):142, 1988.
48. Berkley, K.J., and Palmer, R.: Somatosensory cortical involvement in response to noxious stimulation in the cat. Exp. Brain Res., *20:*363, 1974.
49. Berkley, K.J.: Response properties of cells in ventrobasal and posterior group nuclei of the cat. J. Neurophysiol., *36:*940, 1973.
50. Berkley, K.J.: Spatial relationships between the terminations of somatic sensory and motor pathways in the rostral brainstem of cats and monkeys. I. Ascending somatic sensory inputs to lateral diencephalon. J. Comp. Neurol., *193:*283, 1980.
51. Berkley, K.J., Hotta, H., Robbins, A., and Sato, Y.: Functional properties of afferent fibers supplying reproductive and other pelvic organs in pelvic nerve of female rat. J. Neurophysiol., *63:*256, 1990.
52. Besse, D., Lombard, M.C., Perrot, S., and Besson, J.M.: Regulation of opioid binding sites in the superficial dorsal horn of the rat spinal cord following loose ligation of the sciatic nerve: Comparison with sciatic nerve section and lumbar dorsal rhizotomy. Neuroscience, *50:*921, 1992.
53. Besson, J.M., Catchlove, R.F.H., Feltz, P., and Le Bars, D.: Further evidence for postsynaptic inhibitions on lamina V dorsal horn interneurons. Brain Res., *66:*531, 1974.
54. Bessou, P., Burgess, P.R., Perl, E.R., and Taylor, C.B.: Dynamic properties of mechanoreceptors with unmyelinated (C) fibers. J. Neurophysiol., *34:*116, 1971.
55. Bessou, P., and Perl, E.R.: A movement receptor of the small intestine. J. Physiol., *182:*404, 1966.
56. Bessou, P., and Perl, E.R.: Response of cutaneous sensory units with unmyelinated fibers to noxious stimuli. J. Neurophysiol., *32:*1025, 1969.
57. Bevan, S., and Szolcsanyi, J.: Sensory neuron-specific actions of capsaicin: mechanisms and applications. Trends Pharmacol. Sci., *11*(8):330, 1990.
58. Beven, T., and Pert, A.: The effect of midbrain and diencephalic lesions on nociception and morphine induced antinociception in the rat. Fed. Proc., *34:*713, 1975.
59. Bevenridge, E.E., and Brown, A.: The measurement of human dental intrapulpal pressure and its response to clinical variables. Oral Surg., *19:*655, 1965.
60. Bilisaly, F.N., Goodell, H., and Wolff, H.G.: Vasodilatation, lowered pain threshold, and increased tissue vulnerability. Effects dependent upon peripheral nerve function. Arch. Intern. Med., *94:*759, 1954.
61. Bill, A., Stjernschantz, J., Mandahl, A., *et al.*: Substance P: Release on trigeminal nerve stimulation; effects in the eye. Acta Physiol. Scand., *106:*371, 1979.
62. Blank, M.A., Anard, P., Lumb, B.M., *et al.*: Release of vasoactive intestinal polypeptide-like immunoreactivity (VIP) from cat urinary bladder and sacal spinal cord during pelvic nerve stimulation. Dig. Dis. Sci., *27:*115, 1984.
63. Block, A.R., Feinberg, H., Herbaczynska-Cedra, K., and Vane, J.R.: Anoxia-induced release of prostaglandins in rabbit isolated hearts. Circ. Res., *36:*34, 1975.
64. Blomqvist, A., Ericson, A.C., Broman, J., and Craig, A.D.: Electron microscopic identification of lamina I axon terminations in the nucleus submedius of the cat thalamus. Brain Res., *585:*425, 1992.
65. Blumgart, H.L., Schlesinger, M.J., and Davis, D.: Studies on the relation of the clinical manifestations of angina pectoris, coronary thrombosis and myocardial infarction to the pathological findings, with particular reference to the significance of the collateral circulation. Am. Heart J., *19:*1, 1940.
66. Boivie, J., and Perl, E.R.: Neural substrates of somatic sensation. *In* Hunt, C.C. (ed.): MTP International Review of Science, Physiology Series One. Vol. 3. pp. 303–411. Baltimore, University Press, 1975.
67. Boivie, J.: An anatomical reinvestigation of the termination of the spinothalamic tract in the monkey. J. Comp. Neurol., *186:*343, 1979.
68. Boivie, J.: Anatomical observations on the dorsal column nuclei and the cytoarchitecture of some somatosensory thalamic nuclei. J. Comp. Neurol., *178:*17, 1978.
69. Boivie, J.: The termination of the cervicothalamic tract in the cat. An experimental study with silver impregnation methods. Brain Res., *19:*333, 1970.
70. Boivie, J.: The termination of the spinothalamic tract in the cat. An experimental study with silver impregnation methods. Exp. Brain. Res., *12:*331, 1971.
71. Bowker, R.M., Westlund, K.N., Sullivan, M.C., *et al.*: Descending serotonergic, peptidergic and cholinergic pathways from the raphe nuclei: A multiple transmitter complex. Brain Res., *288:*33, 1983.
72. Bowsher, D., Mallart, A., Petit, D., and Albe-Fessard, D.: A bulbar relay to the centromedian. J. Neurophysiol., *31:*288, 1968.
73. Bowsher, D., and Petit, D.: Place and modality analysis in nucleus of posterior commissure. J. Physiol. (Lond.), *206:*663, 1970.
74. Bowsher, D.: Diencephalic projections from the midbrain reticular formation. Brain Res., *95:*211, 1975.
75. Bowsher, D.: Role of the reticular formation in responses to noxious stimulation. Pain, *2:*361, 1976.
76. Bowsher, D.: Termination of the central pathway in man: The conscious appreciation of pain. Brain, *80:*606, 1957.
77. Bowsher, D.: The sub-diencephalic distribution of fibres from the anterolateral quadrant of the spinal cord in man. Mschr. Psychiatr. Neurol., *143:*75, 1962.
78. Braas, K.S., Newby, A.L., Wilson, V.S., and Snyder, S.H.: Adenosine containing neurons in the brain localized by immunocytochemistry. J. Neurosci., *6:*1952, 1986.
79. Brannstrom, M., and Astrom, A.: The hydrodynamics of the dentine; its possible relationship to dentinal pain. Int. Dent. J., *22:*219, 1972.
80. Brashear, A.D.: The innervation of the teeth. An analysis of nerve fiber components of the pulp and peridental tissue and their probable significance. J. Comp. Neurol., *64:*169, 1936.
81. Breazile, J.E., and Kitchell, R.L.: A study of fiber systems within the spinal cord of the domestic pig that subserve pain. J. Comp. Neurol., *133:*373, 1968.
82. Breazile, J.E., and Kitchell, R.L.: Ventrolateral spinal cord afferents to the brain stem in the domestic pig. J. Comp. Neurol., *133:*363, 1968.
83. Brimijoin, S., Lundberg, J.M., Brodin, E., *et al.*: Axonal transport of substance P in the vagus and sciatic nerves of the guinea pig. Brain Res., *191:*443, 1980.
84. Brodal, A., Walberg, F., and Taber, E.: The raphe nuclei of the brain stem in the cat. II. Afferent connections. J. Comp. Neurol., *114:*261, 1960.
85. Brodin, E., Gazelius, B., Olgart, L., and Nilsson, G.: Tissue concentration and release of substance P-like immunoreactivity in the dental pulp. Acta Physiol. Scand., *111:*141, 1981.
86. Brodin, E., Gazelius, B., Panopoulos, P., and Olgart, L.: Morphine inhibits substance P release from peripheral sensory nerve endings. Acta Physiol. Scand., *117:*567, 1983.
87. Bromm, B., and Treede, R.D.: Human cerebral potentials evoked by CO^2 laser stimuli causing pain. Exp. Brain Res., *67*(1):153, 1987.
88. Brown, A.G., and Franz, D.N.: Responses of spinocervical tract neurons to natural stimulation of identified cutaneous receptors. Exp. Brain Res., *7:*231, 1969.
89. Brown, A.G., Fyffe, R.E.W., Noble, R., *et al.*: The density, distribution and topographical organization of spinocervical tract neurones in the cat. J. Physiol. (Lond.), *300:*409, 1980.
90. Brown, A.G.: Ascending and long spinal pathway: Dorsal columns, spinocervical tract and spinothalamic tracting. *In* Iggo, A. (ed.): Handbook of Sensory Physiology. Vol. II. pp. 315–338. New York, Springer-Verlag, 1973.
91. Brown, A.G.: Organization in the Spinal Cord. New York, Springer-Verlag, 1981.
92. Brown, A.M., and Malliani, A.: Spinal sympathetic reflexes initiated by coronary receptors. J. Physiol. (Lond.), *212:*685, 1971.
93. Brown, A.M.: Excitation in afferent cardiac sympathetic nerve fibers during myocardial ischemia. J. Physiol. (Lond.), *190:*35, 1967.

94. Brown, P.B., Fuchs, J.L., and Tapper, D.N.: Parametric studies of dorsal horn neurons responding to tactile stimulation. J. Neurophysiol., *28:*19, 1975.
95. Brown, P.B., and Fuchs, J.L.: Somatotopic representation of hindlimb skin in cat dorsal horn. J. Neurophysiol., *28:*1, 1975.
96. Brune, K., Walz, D., and Bucher, K.: The avian microcrystal arthritis. 1. Simultaneous recording of nociception and temperature effect in the inflamed joint. Agents Actions *4:*21, 1974.
97. Bryan, R.N., Trevino, D.L., Coulter, J.D., and Willis, W.D.: Location and somatotopic organization of the cells of origin of the spinocervical tract. Exp. Brain Res., *17:*177, 1973.
98. Buck, S.H., and Burks, T.F.: The neuropharmacology of capsaicin: Review of some recent observations. Pharmacol. Rev., *38:*179, 1986.
99. Burch, G.E., and DePasquale, N.P.: Bradykinin. Am. Heart J., *65:*116, 1963.
100. Burchiel, K.J.: Spontaneous impulse generation in normal and denervated dorsal root ganglia: Sensitivity to alpha-adrenergic stimulation and hypoxia. Exp. Neurol., *85*(2):257, 1984.
101. Burgess, P.R., and Perl, E.R.: Cutaneous mechanoreceptors and nociceptors. *In* Iggo, A. (ed.): Handbook of Sensory Physiology. Vol. II. pp. 29–78. New York, Springer-Verlag, 1973.
102. Burgess, P.R., and Perl, E.R.: Myelinated afferent fibers responding specifically to noxious stimulation of the skin. J. Physiol. (Lond.), *190:*541, 1967.
103. Burton, H., and Craig, A.D.: Distribution of trigeminothalamic projection cells in cat and monkey. Brain Res., *161:*515, 1976.
104. Burton, H., Forbes, D.J., and Benjamin, R.M.: Thalamic neurons responsive to temperature changes of glabrous hand and foot skin in squirrel monkey. Brain Res., *24:*179, 1970.
105. Burton, H., and Jones, E.G.: The posterior thalamic region and its cortical projection in new world and old world monkeys. J. Comp. Neurol., *168:*249, 1976.
106. Burton, H., and Loewy, A.D.: Descending projections from the marginal cell layer and other regions of the monkey spinal cord. Brain Res., *116:*485, 1976.
107. Byers, M.R., Fink, B.R., Kennedy, R.D., *et al.*: Effects of lidocaine on axonal morphology, microtubules, and rapid transport in rabbit vagus nerve *in vitro.* J. Neurobiol., *4:*125, 1973.
108. Cajal, S.R.: Histologie du Systeme Nerveux del'Hommes et des Vertebres. Madrid, Instituto Ramon y Cajal, 1909 (1952 reprint).
109. Calvin, W.H., Howe, J.F., and Loeser, I.D.: Ectopic repetitive firing in focally demyelinated axons and some implications for trigeminal neuralgia. *In* Anderson, D., and Matthews, B. (eds.): Pain in the Trigeminal Region. pp. 125–136. Amsterdam, Elsevier/North Holland, 1977.
110. Calvin, W.H.: Some design features of axons and how neuralgias may defeat them. *In* Bonica, J.J., Liebeskind, J.C., and Albe-Fessard, D. (eds.): Advances in Pain Research and Therapy. Vol. 3. pp. 297–309. New York, Raven Press, 1979.
111. Camarata, P.J., and Yaksh, T.L.: Characterization of the spinal adrenergic receptors mediating the spinal effects produced by the microinjection of morphine into the periaqueductal gray. Brain Res., *336:*133, 1985.
112. Cameron, A.A., Cliffer, K.D., Dougherty, P.M., *et al.*: Changes in lectin, GAP-43 and neuropeptide staining in the rat superficial dorsal horn following experimental peripheral neuropathy. Neurosci. Lett., *131:*249, 1991.
113. Campbell, J.N., Raja, S.N., Meyer, R.A., and Mackinnon, S.E.: Myelinated afferents signal the hyperalgesia associated with nerve injury. Pain, *32*(1):89, 1988.
114. Carlen, P.L., Wall, P.D., Nadvorna, H., and Steinbach, T.: Phantom limbs and related phenomena in recent traumatic amputations. Neurology, *28:*211, 1978.
115. Carlton, S.M., and Hayes, E.S.: Light microscopic and ultrastructural analysis of GABA immunoreactive profiles in the monkey spinal cord. J. Comp. Neurol., *300:*162, 1990.
116. Carlton, S.M., Westlund, K.N., Zhang, D., and Willis, W.D.: GABA-immunoreactive terminals synapse on primate spinothalamic tract cells. J. Comp. Neurol., *322:*528, 1992.
117. Carpenter, M.D., Stein, B.M., and Shriver, J.E.: Central projections of spinal dorsal roots in the monkey. II. Lower thoracic, lumbosacral and coccygeal dorsal roots. Am. J. Anat., *123:*75, 1968.
118. Carreras, M., and Andersson, S.A.: Functional properties of neurons of the anterior ectosylvian gyrus of the cat. J. Neurophysiol., *26:*100, 1963.
119. Carstens, E., and Trevino, D.L.: Laminar origins of spinothalamic projections in the cat as determined by the retrograde transport of horseradish peroxidase. J. Comp. Neurol., *182:*151, 1978.
120. Casey, K.L., Minoshima, S., Berger, K.L., *et al.*: Positron emission tomographic analysis of cerebral structures activated specifically by repetitive noxious heat stimuli. J. Neurophysiol., *71*(2):802, 1994.
121. Casey, K.L., and Keene, J.J.: Unit analysis of the effects of motivating stimuli in the awake animal: Pain and self stimulation. *In* Phillips, M.I. (ed.): Brain Unit Activity During Behavior. pp. 115–129. Springfield, IL, Charles C. Thomas, 1973.
122. Casey, K.L., and Morrow, T.J.: Ventral posterior thalamic neurons differentially responsive to noxious stimulation of the awake monkey. Science, *221:*675, 1983.
123. Casey, K.L.: Escape elicited by bulboreticular stimulation in the cat. Int. J. Neurosci., *2:*29, 1971.
124. Casey, K.L.: Responses of bulboreticular units to somatic stimuli eliciting escape behavior in the cat. Int. J. Neurosci., *2:*15, 1971.
125. Casey, K.L.: Somatic stimuli, spinal pathways, and size of cutaneous fibers influencing unit activity in the medial medullary reticular formation. Exp. Neurol., *25:*35, 1969.
126. Casey, K.L.: Unit analysis of nociceptive mechanisms in the thalamus of the awake squirrel monkey. J. Neurophysiol., *29:*727, 1966.
127. Cauna, N.: Fine structure of the receptor organ and its probable functional significance. *In* de Reuck, A.V.S., and Knight, J. (eds.): Touch, Heat, and Pain. pp. 117–127. CIBA Symposium. London, Churchill, 1966.
128. Cauna, N.: The fine morphology of the sensory receptor organs in the auricle of the rat. J. Comp. Neurol., *136:*81, 1969.
129. Cedarbaum, J.M., and Aghajanian, G.K.: Activation of locus coeruleus neurons by peripheral stimuli: Modulation by a collateral inhibitory mechanism. Life Sci., *23:*1383, 1978.
130. Cervero, F., and Janig, W.: Visceral nociceptors: A new world order? Trends Neurosci., *15*(10):374, 1992.
131. Cervero, F., Iggo, A., and Molony, V.: Responses of spinocervical tract neurones to noxious stimulation of the skin. J. Physiol. (Lond.), *267:*537, 1977.
132. Cervero, F., Iggo, A., and Ogawa, H.: Nociceptor-driven dorsal horn neurones in the lumbar spinal cord of the cat. Pain, *2:*5, 1976.
133. Cervero, F., and Iggo, A.: The substantia gelatinosa of the spinal cord. A critical review. Brain, *103:*717, 1980.
134. Cervero, F., Molony, V., and Iggo, A.: Extra and intracellular recordings from neurones in the substantia gelatinosa. Brain Res., *136:*565, 1977.
135. Cervero, F., Molony, V., Iggo, A.: Supraspinal linkage of substantia gelatinosa neurones: Effects of descending impulses. Brain Res., *175:*351, 1979.
136. Cervero, F.: Dorsal horn neurons and their sensory inputs. *In* Yaksh, T.L. (ed.): Spinal Afferent Processing. pp. 197–216. New York, Plenum Press, 1986.
137. Cesselin, F., Bourgoin, S., Artaud, F., and Hamon, M.: Basic and regulatory mechanisms of *in vitro* release of metenkephalin from the dorsal zone of the rat spinal cord. J. Neurochem., *43:*763, 1984.
138. Cesselin, F., Oliveras, J.L., Bourgoin, S., *et al.*: Increased levels of metenkephalin-like material in the CSF of anaesthetized cats after tooth pulp stimulation. Brain Res., *237:*325, 1982.
139. Chahl, L.A., and Iggo, A.: The effects of bradykinin and prostaglandin E1 on rat cutaneous afferent nerve activity. Br. J. Pharmacol., *59:*343, 1977.
140. Chahl, L.A., and Ladd, R.J.: Local oedema and general excitation of cutaneous sensory receptors produced by electrical stimulation of the saphenous nerve in the rat. Pain, *2:*25, 1976.
141. Chahl, L.A.: Pain induced by inflammatory mediators. *In* Beers, R.F., Jr., and Bassett, E.G. (eds.): Mechanisms of Pain and Analgesic Compounds. pp. 273–284. New York, Raven Press, 1979.
142. Chan, J.V.C., Burrowes, C.E., and Movat, H.Z.: Surface activation of factor XII (Hageman factor)—Critical role of high molecular weight kininogen and another potentiator. Agents Actions, *8:*65, 1978.
143. Chan-Palay, V.: Combined immunocytochemistry and autoradiography after *in vivo* injections of monoclonal antibody to substance P and 3H-serotonin. Anat. Embryol., *156:*241, 1979.
144. Chapman, C.R., Casey, K.L., Dubner, R., *et al.*: Pain measurement: An overview. Pain, *22*(1):1, 1985.
145. Chapman, C.R., Schimek, F., Colpitts, Y.H., Gerlaeh, R., and Dong, W.K.: Peak latency differences in evoked potentials elicited by painful dental and cutaneous stimulation. Int. J. Neurosci., *27*(1-2):1, 1985.

146. Chapman, L.F., Ramos, A.O., Goodell, H., and Wolff, H.G.: Neurohumoral features of afferent fibers in man. Arch. Neurol., *4:*617, 1961.
147. Chatrain, G.E., Canfield, R.C., Knauss, T.A., and Lettich, E.: Cerebral responses to electrical tooth pulp stimulation in man: An objective correlate of acute experimental pain. Neurology, *25:*745, 1975.
148. Chi, C.C.: An experimental silver study of the ascending projections of the central gray substance and adjacent tegmentum in the rat with observation in the cat. J. Comp. Neurol., *139:*259, 1970.
149. Chouchkov, C.N.: On the fine structure of free nerve endings in human digital skin, oral cavity and rectum. Z. Mikrosk. Anat. Forsch. *86:*273, 1972.
150. Christensen, B.N., and Perl, E.R.: Spinal neurons specifically excited by noxious or thermal stimuli: Marginal zones of the dorsal horn. J. Neurophysiol., *33:*293, 1970.
151. Clark, F.J., and Burgess, P.R.: Slowly adapting receptors in cat knee joint: Can they signal joint angle? J. Neurophysiol., *38:*1448, 1975.
152. Clark, F.J.: Central projection of sensory fibers from the cat knee joint. J. Neurobiol., *3:*101, 1972.
153. Clark, F.J.: Information signaled by sensory fibers in medial articular nerve. J. Neurophysiol., *38:*1464, 1975.
154. Clarke, W.B., and Bowsher, D.: Terminal distribution of primary afferent trigeminal fibers in the rat. Exp. Neurol., *6:*372, 1962.
155. Clifton, G.L., Coggeshall, R.E., Vance, W.H., and Willis, W.D.: Receptive fields of unmyelinated ventral root afferent fibers in the cat. J. Physiol. (Lond.), *256:*573, 1976.
156. Clifton, G.L., Vance, W.H., Applebaum, M.L., *et al.*: Responses of unmyelinated afferents in the mammalian ventral root. Brain Res., *82:*163, 1974.
157. Cochrane, C.G.: The Hageman factor pathways of kinin formation, clotting and fibrinolysis. *In* Beers, R.F., and Bassett, E.G. (eds.): The Role of Immunological Factors in Infectious, Allergic and Autoimmune Processes. pp. 237–245. New York, Raven Press, 1976.
158. Coderre, T.J., Gonzales, R., Goldyne, M.E., West, M.E., and Levine, J.D.: Noxious stimulus-induced increase in spinal prostaglandin E_2 is noradrenergic terminal-dependent. Neurosci. Lett. *115:*253, 1990.
159. Coderre, T.J., and Melzack, R.: Central neural mediators of secondary hyperalgesia following heat injury in rats: Neuropeptides and excitatory amino acids. Neurosci. Lett., *131:*71, 1991.
160. Coderre, T.J., and Melzack, R.: The contribution of excitatory amino acids to central sensitization and persistent nociception after formalin-induced tissue injury. J. Neurosci., *12:*3665, 1992.
161. Coggeshall, R.E., Applebaum, M.L., Fazen, M., *et al.*: Unmyelinated axons in human ventral roots, a possible explanation for the failure of dorsal rhizotomy to relieve pain. Brain, *98:*157, 1975.
162. Coggeshall, R.E., Coulter, J.D., and Willis, W.D., Jr.: Unmyelinated axons in the ventral roots of the cat lumbosacral enlargement. J. Comp. Neurol., *158:*39, 1974.
163. Coghill, R.C., Talbot, J.D., Evans, A.C., *et al.*: Distributed processing of pain and vibration by the human brain. J. Neurosci., *14*(7):4095, 1994.
164. Coimbra, A., Sodre-Borges, B.P., and Magalheas, M.M.: The substantia gelatinosa Rolandi of the rat. Fine structure cytochemistry (acid phosphatase) and changes after dorsal root section. J. Neurocytol., *3:*199, 1974.
165. Collier, J.G., Karim, S.M.M., Robinson, B., and Somers, K.: Action of prostaglandins A_2, B_1, E_2, F_2 on superficial hand veins of man. Br. J. Pharmacol., *44:*374P, 1972.
166. Collin, E., Mantelet, S., Frechilla, D., *et al.*: Increased *in vivo* release of calcitonin gene-related peptide-like material from the spinal cord in arthritic rats. Pain, *54:*(2):203, 1993.
167. Collins, W.F., Nulsen, F.E., and Randt, C.T.: Relation of peripheral nerve fiber size and sensation in man. Arch. Neurol., *3:*381, 1960.
168. Collins, W.F., and Randt, C.T.: Midbrain evoked responses relating to peripheral unmyelinated or "C" fibers in cat. J. Neurophysiol., *23:*47, 1960.
169. Cook, A.W., and Browder, E.: Function of posterior columns in man. Arch. Neurol., *22:*72, 1965.
170. Corradetti, R., Lo Conte, G., Moroni, F., *et al.*: Adenosine decreases aspartate and glutamate release from rat hippocampal slices. Eur. J. Pharmacol., *104*(1-2):19, 1984.
171. Couture, R., and Cuello, A.C.: Studies on the trigeminal antidromic vasodilatation and plasma extravasation in the rat. J. Physiol., *346:*273, 1984.
172. Craig, A.D., Jr., Linington, A.J., and Kniffki, K.D.: Cells of origin of spinothalamic tract projections to the medial and lateral thalamus in the cat. J. Comp. Neurol., *289*(4):568, 1989.
173. Craig, A.D., and Dostrovsky, J.O.: Thermoreceptive lamina I trigeminothalamic neurons project to the nucleussubmedius in the cat. Exp. Brain Res., *85*(2):470, 1991.
174. Craig, A.D., and Burton, H.: Spinal and medullary lamina I projection to nucleus submedius in medial thalamus: A possible pain center. J. Neurophysiol., *45:*443, 1981.
175. Cridland, R.A., and Henry, J.L.: Comparison of the effects of substance P, Neurokinin A, Physalaemin and Eledoisin in facilitating a nociceptive reflex in the rat. Brain Res., *381:*93, 1986.
176. Croze, S., Duclaux, R., and Kenshalo, D.R.: The thermal sensitivity of the polymodal nociceptors in the monkey. J. Physiol., *263:*539, 1976.
177. Crunkchom, P., and Willis, A.L.: Cutaneous reactions to intradermal prostaglandins. Br. J. Pharmacol., *41:*49, 1971.
178. Csillik, B., and Knyihar, E.: Biodynamic plasticity in the Rolando substance. *In* Progress in Neurobiology. Vol. 10. pp. 203-230. Oxford, Pergamon Press, Ltd., 1978.
179. Cuello, A.C., Priestley, J.V., and Matthews, M.R.: Localization of substance P in neuronal pathways. In Ciba Foundation Symposium 91, Substance P in the Nervous System. pp. 55–83. London, Pitman, 1982.
180. Culberson, J.L., Haines, D.E., Kimmel, D.L., and Brown, P.B.: Contralateral projection of primary afferent fibers to mammalian spinal cord. Exp. Neurol., *64:*83, 1979.
181. Curry, M.J.: The effects of stimulating the somatic sensory cortex on single neurones in the posterior group (PO) of the cat. Brain Res., *44:*463, 1972.
182. Curry, M.J.: The exteroceptive properties of neurones in the somatic part of the posterior group (PO). Brain Res., *44:*439, 1972.
183. Curtis, D.R., and Johnston, G.A.R.: Amino acid transmitters in the mammalian central nervous system. Rev. Physiol. Biochem. Pharmacol., *69:*98, 1974.
184. Dale, H.H.: Pharmacology and nerve endings. Proc. R. Soc. Med., *28:*319, 1935.
185. Dalsgaard, C.J., Vincent, S.R., Hokfelt, T., *et al.*: Coexistence of cholecystokinin- and substance P-like peptides in neurons of the dorsal root ganglia of the rat. Neurosci. Lett., *33:*159, 1982.
186. Darian-Smith, I., Mutton, P., and Proctor, R.: Functional organization of tactile cutaneous afferents within the semilunar ganglion and trigeminal spinal tract in the cat. J. Neurophysiol., *28:*682, 1965.
187. Daval, G., Verge, D., Basbaum, A.I., Bouroin, S., and Hamon, M.: Autoradiographic evidence of serotonin-1 binding sites on primary afferent fibers in dorsal horn of the rat spinal cord. Neurosci. Lett. *83:*71, 1987.
188. Davies, J., and Watkins, J.C.: Role of excitatory amino acids receptors in mono- and polysynaptic excitation in the cat spinal cord. Exp. Brain Res., *49:*280, 1983.
189. Davis, L.E., Hart, J.T., and Crain, R.C.: The pathway for visceral afferent impulses within the spinal cord. II. Experimental dilatation of the biliary ducts. Surg. Gynecol. Obstet., *48:*647, 1929.
190. De Koninck, Y., and Henry, J.L.: Substance P-mediated slow excitatory postsynaptic potential elicited in dorsal horn neurons *in vivo* by noxious stimulation. Proc. Natl. Acad. Sci. USA, *88:*11344, 1991.
191. De Koninck, Y., and Henry, J.L.: Bombesin, neuromedin B and neuromedin C selectively depress superficial dorsal horn neurones in the cat spinal cord. Brain Res., *498*(1):105, 1989.
192. Deakin, J.F.W., and Dostrovsky, J.O.: Involvement of the periaqueductal grey matter and spinal 5-hydroxytryptaminergic pathways in morphine analgesia. Effects of lesions and 5-hydroxytryptamine. Br. J. Pharmacol., *63:*159, 1978.
193. Delacour, J., and Borst, A.: Failure to find homology in rat, cat and monkey for functions of a subcortical structure in avoidance conditioning. J. Comp. Physiol. Psychol., *80:*458, 1972.
194. Delange, A., Hannam, A., and Matthews, B.: The diameters and conduction velocities of fibers in the terminal branches of the inferior dental nerve. Arch. Oral Biol., *14:*513, 1969.
195. Delgado, J.M.R., Rosvald, H.E., and Looney, E.: Evoking conditioned fear by electrical stimulation of subcortical structures in the monkey brain. J. Comp. Physiol. Psychol., *49:*373, 1956.
196. Denny-Brown, D., Kirk, E.J., and Yanagisawa, N.: The tract of Lissauer in relation to sensory transmission in the dorsal horn of the spinal cord in the Macaque monkey. J. Comp. Neurol., *151:*175, 1973.
197. Denny-Brown, D., and Yanagisawa, N.: The function of the descending root of the fifth nerve. Brain, *96:*783, 1973.

394. Jahr, C.E., and Jessell, T.: Synaptic transmission between dorsal root ganglion and dorsal horn neurons in culture: Antagonism of monosynaptic excitatory postsynaptic potentials and glutamate excitation by kynurenate. J. Neurosci., *5:*2281, 1985.
395. James, G.W.L., and Church, M.K.: Hyperalgesia after treatment of mice with prostaglandins and arachidonic acid and its antagonism by anti-inflammatory—analgesic compounds. Arzneimittelforsch., *28:*804, 1978.
396. Jancso, N., Jancso-Gabor, A., and Szolcsanyi, J.: Direct evidence for neurogenic inflammation and its prevention by denervation and by pretreatment with capsaicin. Br. J. Pharmacol. Chemother., *31:*138, 1967.
397. Janig, W., and Koltzenburg, M.: On the function of spinal primary afferent fibres supplying colon and urinary bladder. J. Auton. Nerv. Syst., *30*(Suppl.):S89, 1990.
398. Jannetta, P.J., and Rand, R.W.: Transtentorial retrogasserian rhizotomy in trigeminal neuralgia. *In* Rand, R.W. (ed.): Microsurgery. pp. 156–169. St. Louis, C.V. Mosby, 1969.
399. Jannetta, P.J.: Microsurgical approach to the trigeminal nerve for tic douloureux. Prog. Neurol. Surg., *7:*180, 1976.
400. Jansen, K.L.R., Faull, R.L.M., Dragunow, M., and Waldvogel, H.: Autoradiographic localization of NMDA, quisqualate and kainic acid receptors in human spinal cord. Neurosci. Lett., *108:*53, 1990.
401. Jeftinija, S., Murase, K., Nedeljkov, V., and Randic, M.: Vasoactive intestinal polypeptide excites mammalian dorsal horn neurons both *in vivo* and *in vitro.* Brain Res., *243:*158, 1982.
402. Jeftinija, S., Miletic, V., and Randic, M.: Cholecystokinin octapeptide excites dorsal horn neurons both *in vivo* and *in vitro.* Brain Res., *213:*231, 1981.
403. Jeftinija, S., Semba, K., and Randic, M.: Norepinephrine reduces excitability of single cutaneous primary afferent C-fibers in the cat spinal cord. Brain Res., *219:*456, 1981.
404. Jensen, K., Andersen, H.O., Olesen, J., and Lindblom. U.: Pressure-pain threshold in human temporal region. Evaluation of a new pressure algometer. Pain, *25*(3):313, 1986.
405. Jensen, R., Rasmussen, B.K., Pedersen, B., and Olesen, J.: Muscle tenderness and pressure pain thresholds in headache. A population study. Pain, *52*(2):193, 1993.
406. Jensen, T.S., and Yaksh, T.L.: I. Comparison of antinociceptive action of morphine in the periaqueductal gray, medial and paramedial medulla in rat. Brain Res., *363:*99, 1986.
407. Jensen, T.S., and Yaksh, T.L.: II. Examination of spinal monoamine receptors through which brain stem opiate sensitive systems act in the rat. Brain Res., *363:*114, 1986.
408. Jessell, T., and Iversen, L.L.: Opiate analgesics inhibit substance P release from rat trigeminal nucleus. Nature, *268:*549, 1977.
409. Johansson, R.S.: Tactile sensibility in the human hand: Receptive field characteristics of mechanoreceptor units in the glabrous skin area. J. Physiol. (Lond.), *281:*101, 1978.
410. Jones, E.G., and Leavitt, R.Y.: Axonal transport and the demonstration of non-specific projections to the cerebral cortex and striatum from thalamic intralaminar nuclei in the rat, cat and monkey. J. Comp. Neurol., *154:*349, 1974.
411. Jones, E.G., and Powell, T.P.S.: Connexions of the somatic sensory cortex of the rhesus monkey. III. Thalamic connexions. Brain, *93:*37, 1970.
412. Jones, E.G., and Powell, T.P.S.: The cortical projection of the ventroposterior nucleus of the thalamus in the cat. Brain Res., *13:*298, 1969.
413. Jonzon, B., Sylven, C., and Kaijser, L.: Theophylline decreases pain in the ischaemic forearm test. Cardiovasc. Res., *23*(9):807, 1989.
414. Juan, H., and Lembeck, F.: Action of peptides and other algesic agents on paravascular pain receptors of the isolated perfused rabbit ear. Naunyn-Schmiedebergs Arch. Pharmacol., *283:*151, 1974.
415. Juan, H., and Lembeck, F.: Release of prostaglandins from the isolated perfused rabbit ear by bradykinin and acetylcholine. Agents Actions, *6:*642, 1976.
416. Juan, H.: Mechanism of action of bradykinin-induced release of prostaglandin E. Naunyn-Schmiedebergs Arch. Pharmacol., *300:*77, 1977.
417. Julian, F.J., and Goldman, D.D.: The effects of mechanical stimulation on some electrical properties of axons. J. Gen. Physiol., *46:*297, 1962.
418. Kaelber, W.W., Mitchell, C.L., Yarmat, A.J., *et al.*: Centrum medianum-parafasicularis lesions and reactivity to noxious and non-noxious stimuli. Exp. Neurol., *46:*282, 1975.
419. Kalina, M., and Bubis, J.J.: Ultrastructural localization of acetylcholine esterase in neurons of rat trigeminal ganglia. Experientia, *25:*388, 1967.
420. Kalina, M., and Wolman, M.: Correlative histochemical and morphological study on the maturation of sensory ganglion cells in the rat. Histochemie, *22:*100, 1970.
421. Kaliner, M., and Austen, K.F.: Immunological release of chemical mediators from human tissues. Ann. Rev. Pharmacol., *15:*177, 1975.
422. Kar, S., and Quirion, R.: Quantitative autoradiographic localization of [125I]neuropeptide Y receptor binding sites in rat spinal cord and the effects of neonatal capsaicin, dorsal rhizotomy and peripheral axotomy. Brain Res., *574:*333, 1992.
423. Keele, C.A., and Armstrong, D.: Substances producing pain and itch. *In* Baraoft, H., Davson, H., and Paton, W.D.M. (eds.): Monographs of the Physiological Society. Vol. 12. pp. 1–374. London, Edward Arnold, 1964.
424. Keene, J.J., and Casey, K.L.: Rewarding and aversive brain stimulation: Opposite effects on medial thalamic units. Physiol. Behav., *10:*283, 1973.
425. Kelly, J.B., and Payne, R.: Pain syndromes in the cancer patient. Neurol Clin., *9:*937, 1991.
426. Kelly, M.: Is pain due to pressure on nerves? Spinal tumors and the intervertebral dic. Neurology (Minneap.), *6:*32, 1956.
427. Kennard, M.A.: The course of ascending fibers in the spinal cord of the cat essential to the recognition of painful stimuli. J. Comp. Neurol., *100:*511, 1954.
428. Kenshalo, D.R., Jr., Giesler, G.J., Leonard, R.B., and Willis, W.D.: Responses of neurons in primate ventral posterior lateral nucleus to noxious stimuli. J. Neurophysiol., *43:*1594, 1980.
429. Kerr, F.W.L., and Fukushima, T.F.: New observations on the nociceptive pathways in the central nervous system. *In* Bonica, J.J. (ed.): Pain. pp. 47–61. New York, Raven Press, 1980.
430. Kerr, F.W.L., Kruger, L., Schwassmann, H.O., and Stern, R.: Somatotopic organization of mechanoreceptor units in the trigeminal complex of the macaque. J. Comp. Neurol., *34:*127, 1968.
431. Kerr, F.W.L., and Lippman, H.H.: The primate spinothalamic tract as demonstrated by anterolateral cordotomy and commissural myelotomy. Adv. Neurol., *4:*147, 1974.
432. Kerr, F.W.L., and Lysak, W.R.: Somatotopic organization of trigeminal ganglion neurones. Archiv. Neurol., *11:*593, 1964.
433. Kerr, F.W.L., and Olafson, R.A.: Trigeminal and cervical volleys, convergence on single units in the spinal gray at C-1 and C-2. Arch. Neurol., *5:*171, 1961.
434. Kerr, F.W.L.: A mechanism to account for frontal headache in cases of posterior-fossa tumors. J. Neurosurg., *18:*605, 1961.
435. Kerr, F.W.L.: Atypical facial neuralgias, their mechanism as inferred from anatomic and physiologic data. Mayo Clin. Proc., *36:*254, 1961.
436. Kerr, F.W.L.: Central relationships of trigeminal and cervical primary afferents in the spinal cord and medulla. Brain Res., *43:*561, 1972.
437. Kerr, F.W.L.: Craniofacial neuralgias. *In* Bonica, J J., Liebeskind, I.C., and Albe-Fessard, D. (eds.): Advances in Pain Research and Therapy. Vol. 1. pp. 283–295. New York, Raven Press, 1979.
438. Kerr, F.W.L.: Neuroanatomical substrates of nociception in the spinal cord. Pain, *1:*325, 1975.
439. Kerr, F.W.L.: Pain: A central inhibitory balance theory. Mayo Clin. Proc., *50:*685, 1975.
440. Kerr, F.W.L.: Segmental circuitry and ascending pathways of the nociceptive system. *In* Beers, R.F., Jr., and Bassett, E.G. (eds.): Mechanisms of Pain and Analgesic Compounds. pp. 113–141. New York, Raven Press, 1979.
441. Kerr, F.W.L.: Spinal V nucleolysis and intractable craniofacial pain. Surg. Forum, *17:*419, 1966.
442. Kerr, F.W.L.: The divisional organization of afferent fibres of the trigeminal nerve. Brain, *86:*721, 1963.
443. Kerr, F.W.L.: The fine structure of subnucleus caudalis of the trigeminal nerve. Brain Res., *23:*129, 1970.
444. Kerr, F.W.L.: The fine structure of subnucleus caudalis of the trigeminal: A light and electron microscopic study of degeneration. Brain Res., *23:*147, 1970.
445. Kerr, F.W.L.: The ventral spinothalamic tract and other ascending systems of the ventral funiculus of the spinal cord. J. Comp. Neurol., *159:*335, 1975.
446. Kerr, F.W.L.: Trigeminal neuralgia, pathogenesis and description of a possible etiology for the cryptogenic variety. Trans. Am. Neurol. Assoc., *87:*118, 1962.
447. Kessler, W., Kirchhoff, C., Reeh, P.W., and Handwerker, H.O.: Exci-

tation of cutaneous afferent nerve endings *in vitro* by a combination of inflammatory mediators and conditioning effect of substance P. Exp. Brain Res., *91*(3):467, 1992.
448. Kevetter, G.A., Haber, L.H., Yezierski, R.P., *et al.*: Cells of the origin of the spinoreticular tract in the monkey. J. Comp. Neurol., *207:*61, 1982.
449. Kevetter, G.A., and Willis, W.D.: Collaterals of spinothalamic cells in the rat. J. Comp. Neurol., *215:*453, 1983.
450. Kevetter, G.A., and Willis, W.D.: Spinothalamic cells in the rat lumbar cord with collaterals to the medullary reticular formation. Brain Res., *238:*181, 1982.
451. Khayyat, G.F., Yu, Y.J., and King, R.B.: Response patterns to noxious and non-noxious stimuli in rostral trigeminal relay nuclei. Brain Res., *97:*47, 1975.
452. Kim, S.H., and Chung, J.M.: An experimental model for peripheral neuropathy produced by segmental spinal nerve ligation in the rat. Pain, *50:*355, 1992.
453. Kimura, E., Hashimoto, K., Furukawa, S., and Hayakawa, H.: Changes in bradykinin level in coronary sinus blood after the experimental occlusion of a coronary artery. Am. Heart J., *85:*635, 1973.
454. King, A.E., Thompson, S.W., Urban, L., and Woolf, C.J.: An intracellular analysis of amino acid induced excitations of deep dorsal horn neurones in the rat spinal cord slice. Neurosci. Lett., *89:*286, 1980.
455. King, R.B., and Barnett, J.C.: Studies of trigeminal nerve potentials. Over-reaction to tactile facial stimulation in acute laboratory preparations. J. Neurosurg., *14:*617, 1957.
456. Kiser, R.S., Lebovitz, R.M., and German, D.C.: Anatomic and pharmacologic differences between two types of aversive midbrain stimulation. Brain Res., *155:*331, 1978.
457. Kletzin M., and Spiegel, EA. Spinal conduction by chains of short neurons. Fed Proc., *11:*83, 1952.
458. Knibestol, M., and Vallbo, A.B.: Single unit analysis of mechanoreceptor activity from the human glabrous skin. Acta Physiol. Scand., *80:*178, 1970.
459. Knibestol, M.: Stimulus-response functions of rapidly adapting mechanoreceptors in the human glabrous skin area. J. Physiol. (Lond.), *232:*427, 1973.
460. Knibestol, M.: Stimulus-response functions of slowly adapting mechanoreceptors in the human glabrous skin area. J. Physiol. (Lond.), *245:*63, 1975.
461. Kniffki, K.D., Mense, S., and Schmidt, R.F.: Responses of group IV afferent units from skeletal muscle to stretch, contraction and chemical stimulation. Exp. Brain Res., *31:*511, 1978.
462. Kniffki, K.D., Mense, S., and Schmidt, R.F.: Activation of neurones of the spinocervical tract by painful stimulation of skeletal muscle. Proc. Int. Union Physiol. Sci., *13:*393, 1977.
463. Kniffki, K.D., and Mizumura, K.: Responses of neurons in VPL and VPL-VL region of the cat to algesic stimulation of muscle and tendon. J. Neurophysiol., *49:*649, 1983.
464. Knyihar, E., and Csillik, B.: Effect of peripheral axotomy on the fine structure and histochemistry of the Rolando substances: Degenerative atrophy of central processes of pseudounipolar cells. Exp. Brain Res., *26:*73, 1976.
465. Knyihar, E., and Csillik, B.: Representation of cutaneous afferents by fluoride-resistant acid phosphatase (FRAP)-active terminals in the rat substantia gelatinosa Rolandi. Acta Neurol. Scand., *53:*217, 1976.
466. Knyihar, E., and Gerebtzoff, M.A.: Extra-lysosomal localization of acid phosphatase in the spinal cord of the rat. Exp. Brain Res., *18:*383, 1973.
467. Knyihar-Csillik, E., and Csillik, B.: FRAP: Histochemistry of the primary nociceptive neuron. Progr. Histochem. Cytochem., *14:*1, 1981.
468. Kocher, L., Anton, F., Reeh, P.W., and Handwerker, H.O.: The effect of carrageenan-induced inflammation on the sensitivity of unmyelinated skin nociceptors in the rat. Pain, *29*(3):363, 1987.
469. Koltzenburg, M., Lundberg, L.E., and Torebjork, H.E.: Dynamic and static components of mechanical hyperalgesia in human hairy skin. Pain, *51*(2):207, 1992.
470. Krauthamer, G.M., and Albe-Fessard, D.: Inhibition of nonspecific sensory activities following striopallidal and capsular stimulation. J. Neurophysiol., *28:*100, 1965.
471. Kristensen, J.D., Svensson, B., and Gordh, T. Jr.: The NMDA-receptor antagonist CPP abolishes neurogenic 'wind-up pain' after intrathecal administration in humans. Pain, *51*(2):249, 1992.
472. Kruger, L., and Albe-Fessard, D.: Distribution of responses to somatic afferent stimuli in the diencephalon of the cat under chloralose anesthesia. Exp. Neurol., *2:*442, 1960.
473. Kruger, L., and Michel, F.: A morphological and somatotopic analysis of single unit activity in the trigeminal sensory complex of the cat. Exp. Neurol., *5:*139, 1962.
474. Kruger, L., and Michel, F.: Reinterpretation of the representation of pain based on physiological excitation of single neurons in the trigeminal sensory complex. Exp. Neurol., *5:*157, 1962.
475. Kumazawa, T., and Mizumura, K.: Thin-fibre receptors responding to mechanical, chemical, and thermal stimulation in the skeletal muscle of the dog. J. Physiol. (Lond.), *273:*179, 1977.
476. Kumazawa, T., Perl, E.R., Burgess, P.R., and Whitehorn, D.: Ascending projections from marginal zone (lamina I) neurons of the spinal dorsal horn. J. Comp. Neurol., *162:*1, 1975.
477. Kumazawa, T., and Perl, E.R.: Differential excitation of dorsal horn and subsantia gelatinosa marginal neurons by primary afferent units with fine (A-delta and C) fibers. *In* Zotterman, Y. (ed.): Sensory Functions of the Skin in Primates, with Special Reference to Man. pp. 67–88. New York, Pergamon, 1976.
478. Kumazawa, T., and Perl, E.R.: Primate cutaneous sensory units with unmyelinated (C) afferent fibers. J. Neurophysiol., *40:*1325, 1977.
479. LaMotte, R.H., Lundberg, L.E., and Torebjörk, H.E.: Pain, hyperalgesia and activity in nociceptive C units in humans after intradermal injection of capsaicin. J. Physiol., *448:*749, 1992.
480. LaMotte, R.H., Shain, C.N., Simone, D.A., and Tsai, E.F.: Neurogenic hyperalgesia: Psychophysical studies of underlying mechanisms. J. Neurophysiol., *66:*190, 1991.
481. LaMotte, R.H., and Campbell, J.N.: Comparison of responses of warm and nociceptive C-fiber afferents in monkey with human judgments of thermal pain. J. Neurophysiol., *41:*509, 1978.
482. Laneuville, O., Dorais, J., and Couture, R.: Characterization of the effects produced by neurokinins and three agonists selective for neurokinin receptor subtypes in a spinal nociceptive reflex of the rat. Life Sci., *42:*1295, 1988.
483. Larsson, J., Ekblom, A., Henriksson, K., Lundeberg T., and Theodorsson E.: Immunoreactive tachykinins, calcitonin gene-related peptide and neuropeptide Y in human synovial fluid from inflamed knee joints. Neurosci. Lett., *100:*326, 1989.
484. Le Bars, D., Guilbaud, G., Turna, I., and Besson, J.M.: Differential effects of morphine on responses of dorsal horn lamina V type cells elicited by A and C fibre stimulation in the spinal cat. Brain Res., *115:*518, 1976.
485. LeBlanc, H.J.O., and Gatipon, G.B.: Medial bulboreticular response to peripherally applied noxious stimuli. Exp. Neurol., *42:*264, 1974.
486. Lee, Y.W., and Yaksh, T.L.: Pharmacology of the spinal adenosine receptor which mediates the anti-allodynic action of intrathecal adenosine agonists. J. Pharmacol. Exp. Ther., *277:*1642, 1996.
487. Lele, P.P., and Weddell, G.: The relationship between neurohistology and corneal sensibility. Brain, *79:*119, 1956.
488. Lembeck, F., Gamse, R., and Juan, H.: Substance P and sensory nerve endings. *In* Von Euler, U.S., and Pernow, B. (eds.): Substance P. pp. 169–181. New York, Raven Press, 1977.
489. Lembeck, F., and Juan, H.: Interaction of prostaglandins and indomethacin with algesic substances. Naunyn-Schmiedebergs Arch. Pharmacol., *285:*301, 1974.
490. Lembeck, F., Popper, H., and Juan, H.: Release of prostaglandins by bradykinin as an intrinsic mechanism of its algesic effect. Naunyn-Schmiedeberg's Arch. Pharmacol., *294:*69, 1976.
491. Leslie, J.B., and Watkins, W.D.: Eicosanoids in the central nervous system. J. Neurosurg., *63:*659, 1985.
492. Levante, A., and Albe-Fessard, D.: Localisation dans les couches VII and VIII de Resed de cellules d'origine d'un faisceau spinoreticulaire croise. C.R. Acad. Sci. Hebd. Seances. Acad. Sci. D., *274:*3007, 1972.
493. Levine, J.D., Fields, H.L., and Basbaum, A.I.: Peptides and the primary afferent nociceptor. J. Neurosci., *13:*2273, 1993.
494. Lewis, T., and Pochin, E.E.: The double pain response of the human skin to a single stimulus. Clin. Sci., *3:*67, 1937.
495. Lewis, T.: Experiments relating to cutaneous hyperalgesia and its spread though somatic fibers. Clin. Sci., *2:*373, 1935.
496. Lewis, T.: Experiments relating to cutaneous hyperalgesia and its spread through somatic nerves. Clin. Sci., *2:*373, 1936.
497. Lewis, T.: Pain. New York, MacMillan, 1942.
498. Lewis, T.: The nocifensor system of nerves and its reactions. Br. Med. J., *1:*431, 1937.

499. Lewis, V.A., and Gebhart, G.F.: Evaluation of the periaqueductal central gray (PAG) as a morphine-specific locus of action and examination of morphine-induced and stimulation-produced analgesia at coincident PAG loci. Brain Res., *124:*283, 1977.

499a. Lieberman, A.R.: Sensory ganglia. *In* Landon, D.N. (ed.): The Peripheral Nerve. pp. 188–278. London, Chapman and Hall, 1976.

500. Liebeskind, J.C., and Mayer, D.J.: Somatosensory evoked responses in the mesencephalic central gray matter of the rat. Brain Res., *27:*133, 1971.

501. Light, A.R., and Perl, E.R.: Re-examination of the dorsal root projection to the spinal dorsal horn including observations on the differential termination of coarse and fine fibers. J. Comp. Neurol., *186:*117, 1979.

502. Light, A.R., and Perl, E.R.: Spinal termination of functionally identified primary afferent neurons with slowly conducting myelinated fibers. J. Comp. Neurol., *186:*133, 1979.

503. Light, A.R., Trevino, D.L., and Perl, E.R.: Morphological features of functionally defined neurons in the marginal zone and substantia gelatinosa of the spinal dorsal horn. J. Comp. Neurol., *186:*151, 1979.

504. Limansikyi, Y.P.: Response of neurones of the medullary reticular formation to afferent impulses from cutaneous and muscle nerves. Fiziol. Zh., *11:*151, 1965.

505. Lindgren, I., and Olivecrona, H.: Surgical treatment of angina pectoris. J. Neurosurg., *4:*19, 1947.

506. Lindinger, M.I., and Sjogaard, G.: Potassium regulation during exercise and recovery. Sports Med., *11*(6):382, 1991.

507. Lineberry, C., and Vierck, C.: Attenuation of pain reactivity by caudate nucleus stimulation in monkeys. Brain Res., *98:*110, 1975.

508. Lippman, H.H., and Kerr, F.W.L.: Light and electron microscopic study of crossed ascending pathways in the anterolateral funiculus in monkey. Brain Res., *40:*496, 1972.

509. Liu, R.P.C.: Laminar origins of spinal projection neurons to periaqueductal gray of the rat. Brain Res., *264:*118, 1983.

510. Lloyd, D.P.C.: Neuron patterns controlling transmission of ipsilateral hind limb reflexes in cat. J. Neurophysiol., *6:*293, 1943.

511. Lloyd, D.P.C.: The spinal mechanism of the pyramidal system in cats. J. Neurophysiol., *4:*525, 1941.

512. Lovick, T.A., and Wolstencroft, J.H.: Inhibitory effects of nucleus raphe magnus on neuronal responses in the spinal trigeminal nucleus to nociceptive compared with nonnociceptive inputs. Pain, *7:*135, 1979.

513. Lund, R.D., and Webster, K.E.: Thalamic afferents from the spinal cord and trigeminal nuclei. An experimental anatomical study in the rat. J. Comp. Neurol., *130:*313, 1967.

514. MacDermott, A.B., Mayer, M.L., Westbrook, G.L., Smith, S.J., and Barker, J.L.: NMDA-receptor activation increases cytoplasmic calcium concentrations in cultured spinal cord neurones. Nature, *321:*519, 1986.

515. Malliani, A., Recordati, G., and Schwartz, P.J.: Nervous activity of afferent cardiac sympathetic fibres with atrial and ventricular endings. J. Physiol. (Lond.), *229:*457, 1973.

516. Malmberg, A.B., and Yaksh, T.L.: Hyperalgesia mediated by spinal glutamate or SP receptor blocked by spinal cyclooxygenase inhibition. Science, *257:*1276, 1992a.

517. Malmberg, A.B., and Yaksh, T.L.: Antinociceptive actions of spinal nonsteroidal anti-inflammatory agents on the formalin test in the rat. J. Pharmacol. Exp. Ther., *263:*136, 1992b.

518. Malmberg, A.B., and Yaksh, T.L.: Spinal nitric oxide synthesis inhibition blocks NMDA-induced thermal hyperalgesia and produces antinociception in the formalin test in rats. Pain, *54*(3):291, 1993a.

519. Malmberg, A.B., and Yaksh, T.L.: Pharmacology of the spinal action of ketorolac, morphine, ST-91, U50488H, and L-PIA on the formalin test and an isobolographic analysis of the NSAID interaction. Anesthesiology, *79:*270, 1993b.

520. Malmberg, A.B., and Yaksh, T.L.: Concurrent assessment of formalin-evoked behaviour and spinal release of excitatory amino acids and prostaglandin E_2 using microdialysis in awake rats: Effect of systemic morphine. Br. J. Pharmacol., *114:*1069, 1995.

521. Malmberg, A.B., and Yaksh, T.L.: Cyclooxgenase inhibition and the spinal release of prostaglandin E_2 and amino acids evoked by paw formalin injection: A microdialysis study in unanesthetized rats. J. Neurosci., *15:*2768, 1995.

522. Mancia, M., Broggi, G., and Margnelli, M.: Brain stem reticular effects on intralaminar thalamic neurons in the cat. Brain Res., *25:*638, 1971.

523. Mancia, M., Marginelli, M., Mariotti, M., *et al.*: Brain stem thalamus reciprocal influences in the cat. Brain Res., *69:*297, 1974.

524. Manson, J.: The somatosensory cortical projection of single nerve cells in the thalamus of the cat. Brain Res., *12:*489, 1969.

525. Mantyh, P.W., and Hunt, S.P.: Evidence for cholecystokinin-like immunoreactive neurons in the rat medulla oblongata which project to the spinal cord. Brain Res., *291:*49, 1984.

526. Mantyh, P.W.: Connections of midbrain penaqueductal gray in the monkey. I. Ascending efferent projection. J. Neurophysiol., *49:*567, 1983.

527. Marburg, D.J.: The effect on reaction to painful stimuli of lesions in the centromedian nucleus in the thalamus of the monkey. Int. J. Neurosci., *5:*153, 1973.

528. Marcus, A.J.: The role of lipids in platelet function with particular reference to the arachidonic acid pathway. J. Lipid Res., *19:*793, 1978.

529. Marriott, D., Wilkin, G.P., Coote, P.R., and Wood, J.N.: Eicosanoid synthesis by spinal cord astrocytes is evoked by substance P, possible implications for nociception and pain. *In* Samuelsson, B., Dahlen, S-E., Fritsch, J., and Hedqvist, P. (eds.): Trends in Eicosanoid Biology. Advances in Prostaglandin, Thromboxane, and Leukotriene Research. Vol. 20. pp. 739–741. Philadelphia, Lippincott-Raven, 1990.

530. Marsala, M., and Yaksh, T.L.: Reversible aortic occlusion in rats: post-reflow hyperesthesia and motor effects blocked by spinal NMDA antagonism. Anesthesiology., (Suppl.) *77:*A664, 1992.

531. Matthews, B.: The response of pulpal nerves to thermal stimulation of dentine. J. Dent. Res., *46:*1279, 1967.

532. Matzner, O., and Devor, M.: Na^+ conductance and the threshold for repetitive neuronal firing. Brain Res., *597*(1):92, 1992.

533. Mayberg, M., Langer, R.S., Zervas, N.T., and Moskowitz, M.A.: Perivascular meningeal projections from cat trigeminal ganglia: Possible pathway for vascular headaches in man. Science, *3:*228, 1981.

534. Mayer, D.J., and Liebeskind, J.C.: Pain reduction by focal electrical stimulation of the brain: An anatomical and behavioral analysis. Brain Res., *68:*73, 1974.

535. Mayer, D.J., Price, D.D., and Becker, D.P.: Neurophysiological characterization of the anterolateral spinal cord neurons contributing to pain perception in man. Pain, *1:*51, 1975.

536. Maynard, C.W., Leonard, R.B., Coulter, J.D., and Coggeshall, R.E.: Central connections of ventral root afferents as demonstrated by the HRP method. J. Comp. Neurol., *172:*601, 1977.

537. McCarty, D.J., Gatter, R.A., Brill, J.M., and Hogan, J.M.: Crystal deposition disease—sodium urate (gout) and calcium pyrophosphate (chondrocalcinosis, pseudogout). J.A.M.A., *193:*129, 1965.

538. McCormack, K.: Non-steroidal anti-inflammatory drugs and spinal nociceptive processing. Pain, *59:*9, 1994.

539. McCormack, K., and Brune, K.: Dissociation between the antinociceptive and anti-inflammatory effects of the nonsteroidal anti-inflammatory drugs. A survey of their analgesic efficacy. Drugs, *4:*533, 1991.

540. McGiff, J.C., Terragno, N.A., Malik, K.U., and Lonigro, A.J.: Release of a prostaglandin E-like substance from canine kidney by bradykinin. Circ. Res., *31:*36, 1972.

541. MacIver, M.B., and Tanelian, D.L.: Structural and functional specialization of A delta and C fiber free nerve endings innervating rabbit corneal epithelium. J. Neurosci., *13:*4511, 1993.

542. MacIver, M.B., and Tanelian, D.L.: Free nerve ending terminal morphology is fiber type specific for A delta and C fibers innervating rabbit corneal epithelium. J. Neurophysiol., *69:*1779, 1993.

543. McLachlan, E.M., Janig, W., Devor, M., and Michaelis, M.: Peripheral nerve injury triggers noradrenergic sprouting within the dorsal root ganglia. Nature., *363:*543, 1993.

544. McMahon, S.B.: Mechanisms of cutaneous, deep and visceral pain. *In* Melzack, R., and Wall, P.D.: Textbook of Pain. pp. 129–152. New York, Churchill-Livingstone, 1994.

545. Mehler, W.R., Feferman, M.E., and Nauta, W.J.H.: Ascending axon degeneration following anterolateral cordotomy. An experimental study in the monkey. Brain, *83:*718, 1960.

546. Mehler, W.R.: Some neurological species differences—a posteriori. Ann. N. Y. Acad. Sci., *167:*89, 1969.

547. Meller, S.T., Dykstra, C., and Gebhart, G.F.: Production of endogenous nitric oxide and activation of soluble guanylate cyclase are required for N-methyl-D-aspartate-produced facilitation of the nonciceptive tail-flick reflex. Eur. J. Pharmacol., *214:*93, 1992.

548. Meller, S.T., and Gebhart, G.F.: A critical review of the afferent path-

ways and the potential chemical mediators involved in cardiac pain. Neuroscience, *48*(3):501, 1992.

549. Melzack, R., and Casey, K.L.: Sensory, motivational, and central control determinants of pain. A new conceptual model. *In* Kenshalo, D. (ed.): The Skin Senses. pp. 423–443. Springfield, IL, Charles C. Thomas, 1968.
550. Melzack, R., Stotler, W.A., and Livingston, W.K.: Effects of discrete brain stem lesions in cats on perception of noxious stimulation. J. Neurophysiol., *21:*353, 1958.
551. Melzack, R., and Wall, P.D.: Pain mechanisms: A new theory. Science, *150:*971, 1965.
552. Mendell, L.M.: Physiological properties of unmyelinated fiber projections to the spinal cord. Exp. Neurol., *16:*316, 1966.
553. Mendell, L.M., and Wall, P.D.: Responses of single dorsal cord cells to peripheral cutaneous unmyelinated fibers. Nature, *206:*97, 1965.
554. Mendell, L.M.: Physiological properties of unmyelinated fiber projections to the spinal cord. Exp. Neurol., *16:*316, 1966.
555. Mendell, L.M., Sassoon, E.M., and Wall, P.D.: Properties of synaptic linkage from long ranging afferents onto dorsal horn neurones in normal and deafferented cats. J. Physiol., *285:*299, 1978.
556. Mendell, L.M.: Physiological properties of unmyelinated fiber projection to the spinal cord. Exp. Neurol., *16:*316, 1966.
557. Menetrey, D., Chaouch, A., Binder, D., and Besson, J.M.: The origin of the spinomesencephalic tract in the rat: An anatomical study using the retrograde transport of horseradish peroxidase. J. Comp. Neurol., *206:*193, 1982.
558. Mense, S., and Schmidt, R.F.: Activation of group IV afferent units from muscle by algesic agents. Brain Res., *72:*305, 1974.
559. Mense, S.: Nociception from skeletal muscle in relation to clinical muscle pain. Pain, *54:*241, 1993.
560. Meyer, R.A., and Campbell, J.N.: Myelinated nociceptive afferents account for the hyperalgesia that follows a burn to the hand. Science, *213:*1527, 1981.
561. Meyerson, B.A., Boethius, J., and Carlsson, A.M.: Percutaneous central gray stimulation for cancer pain. Applied Neurophysiology, *41:*57, 1978.
562. Miletic, V., and Randic, M.: Neurotensin excites cat spinal neurones located in laminae I-III. Brain Res., *169:*600, 1979.
563. Mitchell, J., and Anderson, K.J.: Quantitative autoradiographic analysis of excitatory amino acid receptors in the cat spinal cord. Neurosci. Lett., *124:*269, 1991.
564. Mitchell, C., and Kaelber, W.: Effect of medial thalamic lesions on responses elicited by tooth pulp stimulation. Am. J. Physiol., *210:*263, 1966.
565. Mizukawa, K., Vincent, S.R., McGeer, P.L., and McGeer, E.G.: Distribution of reduced-nicotinamide-adenine-dinucleotide-phosphate diaphorase-positive cells and fibers in the cat central nervous system. J. Comp. Neurol., *279:*281, 1989.
566. Mizumura, K., Sato, J., and Kumazawa, T.: Strong heat stimulation sensitizes the heat response as well as the bradykinin response of visceral polymodal receptors. J. Neurophysiol., *68*(4):1209, 1992.
567. Mizumura, K., Sato, J., and Kumazawa, T.: Comparison of the effects of prostaglandins E_2 and I_2 on testicular nociceptor activities studied *in vitro.* Naunyn-Schmiedebergs Arch. Pharmacol., *344*(3):368, 1991.
568. Mjellem-Joly, N., Lund, A., Berge, O.G., and Hole, K.: Potentiation of a behavioural response in mice by spinal coadministration of substance P and excitatory amino acid agonists. Neurosci. Lett., *133:*121, 1991.
569. Mollenholt, P., Post, C., Rawal, N., *et al.*: Antinociceptive and "neurotoxic" actions of somatostatin in rat spinal cord after intrathecal administration. Pain, *32:*95, 1988.
570. Moncada, S., Ferreira, S.H., and Vane, J.R.: Inhibition of prostaglandin biosynthesis as the mechanism of analgesia of aspirin-like drugs in the dog knee joint. Eur. J. Pharmacol., *31:*250, 1975.
571. Mori, F.: A new spinal pathway for cutaneous impulses. Am J. Physiol., *183:*245, 1955.
572. Morin, F., Schwartz, H.G., and O'Leary, J.L.: Experimental study of the spinothalamic and related tracts. Arch. Psychol. Neurol. Scand., *26:*371, 1951.
572a. Morris, B.J., and Herz, A.: Distinct distribution of opioid receptor types in rat lumbar spinal cord. Naunyn Schmiedebergs Arch. Pharmacol., *336:*240, 1987.
573. Morris, R., Southam, E., Braid, D.J., and Gathwaite, J.: Nitric oxide may act as a messenger between dorsal root ganglion neurones and their satellite cells. Neurosci. Lett., *137:*29, 1992.
574. Morrison, D.C., and Henson, P.M.: Release of mediators from mast cells and basophils induced by different stimuli. *In* Bach, M.K. (ed.): Immediate Hypersensitivity: Modern Concepts and Developments, pp. 431–502. New York, Marcel Dekker, 1978.
575. Morrison, J.F.B.: The afferent innervation of the gastrointestinal tract. *In* Brooks, F.P., and Evers, P.W., (eds.): Nerves and the Gut. pp. 297–322. Thorofare, N. J., Slack, 1977.
576. Morrow, T.J., and Casey, K.L.: Analgesia produced by mesencephalic stimulation: Effect on bulboreticular neurons. *In* Bonica, J.J., and Albe-Fessard, D. (eds.): Advances in Pain Research and Therapy. Vol. 1. pp. 503–510. New York, Raven Press, 1976.
577. Moskowitz, M.A., Reinhard, J.F., Jr., Romero, J., *et al.*: Neurotransmitters and the fifth cranial nerve: Is there a relation to the headache phase of migraine? Lancet, *1:*883, 1979.
578. Mosso, J.A., and Kruger, L.: Spinal trigeminal neurons excited by noxious and thermal stimuli. Brain Res., *38:*206, 1972.
579. Mosso, J.A., and Kruger, L.: Receptor categories represented in spinal trigeminal nucleus caudalis. J. Neurophysiol., *36:*472, 1973.
580. Murase, K., Nedeljkov, V., and Randic, M.: The actions of neuropeptides on dorsal horn neurons in the rat spinal cord slice preparation: an intracellular study. Brain Res., *234:*170, 1982.
581. Murase, K., and Randic, M.: Actions of substance P on rat spinal dorsal horn neurones. J. Physiol., *346:*203, 1984.
582. Murray, C.W., and Cowan, A.: Tonic pain perception in the mouse: differential modulation by three receptor-selective opioid agonists. J. Pharmacol. Exp. Ther., *257:*335, 1991.
583. Myslinski, N.R., and Randic, M.: Responses of identified spinal neurones to acetylcholine applied by micro-electrophoresis. J. Physiol., *269*(1):195, 1977.
584. Nagasaka, H., and Yaksh, T.L.: Peripheral and spinal actions of opiates in the blockade of the autonomic response evoked by compression of the inflamed knee joint. Anesthesiology, *85:*808, 1996.
585. Naguib, M., and Yaksh, T.L.: Antinociceptive effects of spinal cholinesterase inhibition and isobolographic analysis of the interaction with μ and α_2 receptor systems. Anesthesiology, *80:*1338, 1994.
586. Nagy, J.J., and Hunt, S.P.: Fluoride-resistant acid phosphatase-containing neurones in dorsal root ganglia are separate from those containing substance P or somatostatin. Neuroscience, *7:*89, 1982.
587. Nagy, J.J., and Hunt, S.P.: The termination of primary afferents within the rat dorsal horn—evidence for rearrangement following capsaicin treatment. J. Comp. Neurol., *218:*145, 1983.
588. Nahin, R.L., Madsen, A.M., and Giesler, G.I.: Anatomical and physiological studies of the grey matter surrounding the spinal cord and central canal. J. Comp. Neurol., *220:*321, 1983.
589. Nashold, B., Urban, B., and Zorub, D.S.: Phantom pain relief by focal destruction of the substantia gelatinosa of Rolando. *In* Bonica, J.J., and Albe-Fessard, G. (eds.): Advances in Pain Research and Therapy. Vol. 1. pp. 959–963. New York, Raven Press, 1976.
590. Nashold, B.J., and Ostdahl, R.H.: Dorsal root entry zone lesions for pain relief. J. Neurosurg., *51:*59, 1979.
591. Nashold, B.S., Jr., and Friedman, N.: Dorsal column stimulation for control of pain. Preliminary report on 30 patients. J. Neurosurg., *36:*590, 1972.
592. Nashold, B.S., Jr., Wilson, W.P., and Slaughter, D.: Sensation evoked by stimulation in the hindbrain of man. J. Neurosurg., *30:*14, 1969.
593. Nässtrôm, J, Karlsson, U., and Post, C.: Antinociceptive actions of different classes of excitatory amino acid receptor antagonists in mice. Eur. J. Pharmacol., *212:*21, 1992.
594. Nathan, P.W., and Smith, M.C.: Some tracts of the anterior and lateral columns of the spinal cord. *In* Knighton, R.S., and Dumke, P.R. (eds.): Pain. pp. 47–57. Boston, Little, Brown and Co., 1966.
595. Ness, T.J., and Gebhart, G.F.: Visceral pain: a review of experimental studies. Pain, *41*(2):167, 1990.
596. Ness, T.J., Randich, A., and Gebhart, G.F.: Further behavioral evidence that colorectal distension is a 'noxious' visceral stimulus in rats. Neurosci. Lett., *131*(1):113, 1991.
597. Nicol, G.D., Klingberg, D.K., and Vasko, M.R.: Prostaglandin E_2 increases calcium conductance and stimulates release of substance P in avian sensory neurons. J. Neurosci., *12:*1917, 1992.
598. Nielson, K.P., Adams, J.E., and Hosobuchi, Y.: Phantom limb pain. Treatment with dorsal column stimulation. J. Neurosurg., *42:*301, 1975.
599. Nijensohn, D.E., and Kerr, F.W.L.: The ascending projections of the dorsolateral funiculus of the spinal cord in the primate. J. Comp. Neurol., *161:*459, 1975.

600. Ninkovic, M., Hunt, S.P., and Kelly, J.S.: Effects of dorsal rhizotomy on the autoradiographic distribution of opiate and neurotensin receptors and neurotensin-like immunoreactivity within the rat spinal cord. Brain Res., *230:*111, 1981.
601. Nishi, K., Sakanashi, M., and Takenaka, F.: Activation of afferent cardiac sympathetic nerve fibers of the cat by pain producing substances and by noxious heat. Pflugers Arch., *372:*53, 1977.
602. Nishi, K.: The action of 5-hydroxytryptamine on chemoreceptor discharges of the cat's carotid body. Br. J. Pharmacol., *55:*27, 1975.
603. North, R.A., Williams, J.T., Suprenant, A., and Christie, M.J.: μ and α receptors belong to a family of receptors that are coupled to potassium channels. Proc. Natl. Acad., Sci. USA, *84:*5487, 1987.
604. Nugteren, D.H.: Arachidonate lipoxygenase. *In* Silver, M., Smith, B.J., and Kocsis (eds.): Prostaglandins in Hematology, pp. 11-25. New York, Spectrum Publications, 1977.
605. Nyquist, J.K., and Greenhoot, J.H.: Unit analysis of nonspecific thalamic responses to high-intensity cutaneous input in the cat. Exp. Neurol., *42:*609, 1974.
606. Nyquist, J.K.: Somatosensory properties of neurons of thalamic nucleus ventralis lateralis. Exp. Neurol., *48:*123, 1975.
607. O'Donohue, T.L., Massari, V.J., Pazoles, C.J., *et al.*: A role for bombesin in sensory processing in the spinal cord. J. Neurosci., *4:*2956, 1984.
608. Ochoa, J., and Mair, W.G.: The normal sural nerve in man. I. Ultrastructure and numbers of fibers and cells. Acta Neuropathol. (Berl.), *13:*127, 1967.
609. Ochs, S., and Hollingsworth, D.: Dependence of fast axoplasmic transport in nerve on oxidative metabolism. J. Neurochem., *18:*107, 1971.
610. Ochs, S., and Jersild, R.A., Jr.: Fast axoplasmic transport in unmyelinated nerve fibers shown by electron microscopic radioautography. J. Neurobiol., *5:*373, 1974.
611. Ochs, S.: Energy metabolism and supply of nerve by axoplasmic transport. Fed. Proc., *33:*1049, 1974.
612. Ohkubo, T., Shibata, M., Takahashi, H., and Inoki, R.: Roles of substance P and somatostatin on spinal transmission of nociceptive information induced by formalin in spinal cord. J. Pharmacol. Exp. Ther., *252:*1261, 1990.
613. Oleson, T.D., Kirkpatrick, D.B., and Goodman, S.J.: Elevation of pain threshold to tooth shock by brain stimulation in primates. Brain Res., *194:*79, 1980.
614. Olgart, L., Hokfelt, T., Nilsson, G., and Pernow, B.: Localization of substance P-like immunoreactivity in nerves in the tooth pulp. Pain, *4:*153, 1977.
615. Olgart, L.: Local mechanisms in dental pain. *In* Beers, R.F., and Bassett, E.G. (eds.): Mechanisms of Pain and Analgesic Compounds. pp. 285–294. New York, Raven Press, 1979.
616. Oliveras, J.L., Redjemi, G., Guilbaud, G., and Besson, J.M.: Analgesia induced by electrical stimulation of the inferior centralis nucleus of the raphe in the cat. Pain, *1:*139, 1975.
617. Olszewski, J.: On the anatomical and functional organization of the spinal trigeminal nucleus. J. Comp. Neurol., *92:*401, 1950.
618. Onishi, A., and Dyck, P.J.: Loss of small peripheral sensory neurons in Fabry's disease. Arch. Neurol., *31:*120, 1974.
619. Ono, H., Mishima, A., Ono, S., Fukuda, H., and Vasko, M.R.: Inhibitory effects of clonidine and tizanidine on release of substance P from slices of rat spinal cord and antagonism by alpha-adrenergic receptor antagonists. Neuropharmacology, *30:*585, 1991.
620. Onofrio, B.M., and Campa, H.K.: Evaluabon of rhizotomy: Review of 12 years' experience. J. Neurosurg., *36:*751, 1972.
621. Osgood, C.P., Dujovny, M., Faille, R., and Abassy, M.: Microsurgical ganglionectomy for chronic pain syndromes. J. Neurosurg., *45:*113, 1976.
622. Oshita, S., Yaksh, T.L., and Chipkin, R.: The antinociceptive effects of intrathecally administered SCH32615, an enkephalinase inhibitor in the rat. Brain Res., *515:*143, 1990.
623. Otsuka, M., and Konishi, S.: Release of substances P-like immunoreactivity from isolated spinal cord of newborn rat. Nature, *264:*83, 1976.
624. Paintal, A.S.: Functional analysis of group III afferent fibres of mammalian muscles. J. Physiol. (Lond.), *152:*250, 1960.
625. Panula, P., Hadjiconstantinou, M., Yang, H.Y., and Costa, E.: Immunohistochemical localization of bombesin/gastrin-releasing peptide and substance P in primary sensory neurons. J. Neurosci., *3:*2021, 1993.
626. Panula, P., Hadjiconstantinou, M., Yang, H.Y., and Costa, E.: Immunohistochemical localization of bombesin, substance P and gastrin-releasing peptide in primary sensory neurons. J. Neurosci., *3:*2021, 1983.
627. Pascual, J., del Arco, C., Gonzalez, A.M., and Pazos, A.: Quantitative light microscopic autoradiographic localization of alpha$_2$-receptors in the human brain. Brain Res., *585:*116, 1992.
628. Patton, H.D.: Special properties of nerve trunks and tracts. *In* Ruch, T.C., and Patton, H.D. (eds.): Physiology and Biophysics. pp. 73–94. Philadelphia, W.B. Saunders, 1965.
629. Payne, R.: Neuropathic pain syndromes, with special reference to causalgia and reflex sympathetic dystrophy. Clin. J. Pain, *2:*59, 1986.
630. Pazos, A., Cortés, R., and Palacios, J.M.: Quantitative autoradiographic mapping of serotonin receptors in the rat brain. I & II. Serotonin-2 receptors. Brain Res., *346:*205, 1985.
631. Pearl, G.S., and Anderson, K.V.: Effects of nociceptive and innocuous stimuli on the firing patterns of single neurons in the feline nucleus reticularis gigantocellularis. *In* Bonica, J.J., and Albe-Fessard, D. (eds.): Advances in Pain Research and Therapy. Vol. 1. pp. 498. New York, Raven Press, 1976.
632. Pearl, G.S., and Anderson, K.V.: Interactions between nucleus centrum medianum and gigantocellularis nociceptive neurons. Brain Res. Bull., *5:*203, 1980.
633. Pearl, G.S., and Anderson, K.V.: Response of cells in feline nucleus centrum medianum to tooth pulp stimulation. Brain Res. Bull., *5:*41, 1980.
634. Pearl, G.S., and Anderson, K.V.: Response patterns of cells in the feline caudal nucleus rebcularis gigantocellularis after noxious trigeminal and spinal stimulation. Exp. Neurol., *58:*231, 1978.
635. Perkins, M.N., Campbell, E., and Dray, A.: Antinociceptive activity of the bradykinin B1 and B2 receptor antagonists, des-Arg9, [Leu8]-BK and HOE 140, in two models of persistent hyperalgesia in the rat. Pain, *53*(2):191, 1993.
636. Perl, E.R., and Whitlock, D.C.: Somabc stimuli exciting spinothalamic projections to thalamic neurons in cat and monkey. Exp. Neurol., *3:*256, 1961.
637. Perl, E.R.: Myelinated afferent fibers innervating the primate skin and their response to noxious stimuli. J. Physiol. (Lond.), *197:*593, 1968.
638. Perl, E.R.: Sensitization of nociceptors and its relation to sensation. *In* Bonica, J.J., and Albe-Fessard, D. (eds.): Advances in Pain Research and Therapy. Vol. 1. pp. 17–28. New York, Raven Press, 1976.
639. Peschanski, M., and Besson, J.M.: Diencephalic connections of the raphe nuclei of the rat brainstem: An anatomical study with reference to the somatosensory system. J. Comp. Neurol., *224:*509, 1984.
640. Peschanski, M., Guilbaud, D., and Gautron, M.: Posterior intralaminar region in rat: Neuronal responses to noxious and nonnoxious cutaneous stimuli. Exp. Neurol., *72:*226, 1981.
641. Peschanski, M., Mantyh, P.W., and Besson, J.M.: Spinal afferents to the ventrobasal thalamic complex in the rat: An anatomical study using wheatgerm agglutinin conjugated to horseradish peroxidase. Brain Res., *278:*240, 1983.
642. Pfaffman, C.: Afferent impulses from the teeth due to pressure and noxious stimulation. J. Physiol. (Lond.), *97:*207, 1939.
643. Piercey, M.F., Einspahr, F.J., Dobry, P.G.K., *et al.*: Morphine does not antagonize the substance P mediated excitation of dorsal horn neurons. Brain Res., *186:*421, 1980.
644. Poggio, G.F., and Mountcastle, V.B.: A study of the functional contributions of the lemniscal and spinothalamic systems to somatic sensibility. Bull. Johns Hop. Hosp., *106:*266, 1960.
645. Poggio, G.F., and Mountcastle, V.B.: The functional properties of ventrobasal thalamic neurons studied in unanesthetized monkeys. J. Neurophysiol., *26:*775, 1963.
646. Pohl, M., Benoliel, J.J., Bourgoin, S., *et al.*: Regional distribution of calcitonin gene-related peptide-, substance P-, cholecystokinin-, met5-enkephalin-, and dynorphin A (1-8)-like materials in the spinal cord and dorsal root ganglia of adult rats: Effects of dorsal rhizotomy and neonatal capsaicin. J. Neurochem., *55:*1122, 1990
647. Pomepiano, O., and Swett, J.E.: Actions of graded cutaneous and muscular afferent volleys on brain stem units in the decrebrate, cerebellectomized cat. Arch. Ital. Biol., *101:*552, 1963.
648. Pomeranz, B., Wall, P.D., and Weber, W.V.: Cord cells responding to fine myelinated afferents from viscera, muscle, and skin. J. Physiol. (Lond.), *199:*511, 1968.
649. Portenoy, R.K.: Management of neuropathic pain. *In* Chapman, C.R., and Foley, K.M. (eds.): Current and Emerging Issues in Cancer Pain. pp. 351–369. New York, Raven Press, 1993.

650. Poulos, D.A., and Benjamin, R.M.: Response of thalamic neurons to thermal stimulation of the tongue. J. Neurophysiol., *31:*28, 1968.
651. Preobrazhenskii, N.N., and Limanskyi, Y.P.: Activation of bulbar reticular neurones by visceral afferents. Neirofiziol. (Kiev), *1:*177, 1969.
652. Price, D.D., and McHaffie, J.G.: Effects of heterotopic conditioning stimuli on first and second pain: A psychophysical evaluation in humans. Pain, *34*(3):245, 1988.
653. Price, G.W., Kelly, J.S., and Bowery, N.G.: The location of GABAβ receptor binding sites in mammalian spinal cord. Synapse, *1:*530, 1987.
654. Price, D.D., Dubner, R., and Hu, J.W.: Trigeminothalamic neurons in nucleus caudalis responsive to tactile, thermal, and nociceptive stimulation of monkey's face. J. Neurophysiol., *39:*936, 1976.
655. Price, D.D., Hu, J.W., Dubner, R., and Gracely, R.: Peripheral suppression of first pain and central summation of second pain evoked by noxious heat pulses. Pain, *3:*57, 1977.
656. Price, D.D., Hull, C.D., and Buchwald, N.A.: Intracellular responses of dorsal horn cells to cutaneous and sural nerve A and C fiber stimuli. Exp. Neurol., *33:*291, 1971.
657. Price, D.D., and Mayer, D.J.: Neurophysiological characterization of the anterolateral quadrant neurons subserving pain in M. mulatta. Pain, *1:*59, 1975.
658. Price, D.D., and Mayer, D.J.: Physiological laminar organization of the dorsal horn of M. mulatta. Brain Res., *79:*321, 1974.
659. Proshansky, E., and Egger, M.D.: Dendritic spread of dorsal horn neurons in cats. Exp. Brain Res., *28:*153, 1977.
660. Raja, S.N., Meyer, R.A., and Campbell, J.N.: Peripheral mechanisms of somatic pain. Anesthesiology, *68:*571, 1988.
661. Ralston, H.J.: Dorsal root projection to dorsal horn neurons in the cat spinal cord. J. Comp. Neurol., *132:*303, 1968.
662. Ralston, H.J.: The organization of the substantia gelatinosa Rolandi in the cat lumbosacral spinal cord. Z. Zellforsch., *67:*1, 1965.
663. Ramwell, P.W., Shaw, J.E., and Jessup, R.: Spontaneous and evoked release of prostaglandins from frog spinal cord. Am. J. Physiol., *211:*998, 1966.
664. Randic, M., and Milehc, V.: Effect of substance P on cat dorsal horn neurons activated by noxious stimuli. Brain Res., *128:*164, 1977.
665. Ranson, S.W., and Billingsly, P.R.: The conduction of painful afferent impulses in the spinal nerves. Am. J. Physiol., *40:*571,1916.
666. Ranson, S.W.: An experimental study of Lissauer's tract and the dorsal roots. J. Comp. Neurol., *24:*531, 1914.
667. Ranson, S.W.: The course within the spinal cord of the non-medullated fibers of the dorsal roots: A study of Lissauer's tract in the cat. J. Comp. Neurol., *23:*259, 1913.
668. Reddy, S.V.R., and Yaksh, T.L.: Spinal noradrenergic terminal system mediates antinociception. Brain Res., *189:*391, 1980.
669. Reddy, S.V.R., Maderdrut, J.L., and Yaksh, T.L.: Spinal cord pharmacology of adrenergic agonist - mediated antinociception. J. Pharmacol. Exp. Ther., *213:*525, 1980.
670. Reeh, P.W., Kocher. L., and Jung, S.: Does neurogenic inflammation alter the sensitivity of unmyelinated nociceptors in the rat? Brain Res., *384*(1):42, 1986.
670a. Reeh, P.W.: Sensory receptors in a mammalian skin-nerve *in vitro* preparation. Prog. Brain Res., *74:*271, 1988.
671. Regoli, D., Jukic, D., Gobeil, F., and Rhaleb, N.E.: Receptors for bradykinin and related kinins: A critical analysis. Can. J. Physiol. Pharmacol., *71*(8):556, 1993.
672. Rethelyi, M., Trevino, D.L., and Perl, E.R.: Distribution of primary afferent fibers within the sacrococcygeal dorsal horn: An autoradiographic study. J. Comp. Neurol., *185:*603, 1979.
673. Rexed, B.: A cytoarchitectonic atlas of the spinal cord in the cat. J. Comp. Neurol., *100:*297, 1954.
674. Rexed, B.: The cytoarchitectonic organization of the spinal cord in the cat. J. Comp. Neurol., *96:*415, 1952.
675. Richardson, D.E., and Akil, H.: Pain reduction by electrical brain stimulation in man. J. Neurosurg., *47:*178, 1977.
676. Robertson, R.T., Lynch, G.S., and Thompson, R.F.: Diencephalic distributions of ascending reticular systems. Brain Res., *55:*309, 1973.
677. Roca e Silva, M., and Antonio, A.: Release of bradykinin and the mechanism of production of a thermic edema (45°C) in the rat's paw. Med. Exp. (Basel), *3:*371, 1960.
678. Rolando, L.: Richerche Anatomie Sulla Struttura del Midollo Spinal. pp. 1–118. Torino, Dalla Stamperia Reale, 1824.
679. Rosell, S., Olgart, L., Gazelius, B., *et al.*: Inhibition of anhdromic and substance P-induced vasodilatation by a substance P-antagonist. Acta Physiol. Scand., *111:*381, 1981.
680. Rossi, G.F., and Brodal, A.: Terminal distribution of spinoreticular fibers in the cat. Arch. Neurol. Psychiatr., *78:*439, 1957.
681. Ruch, T.C.: Pathophysiology of pain. *In* Ruch, T.C., Patton, H.D., Woodbury, J.W., and Towe, A.L. (eds.): Neurophysiology. pp. 350–368. Philadelphia, W.B. Saunders, 1961.
682. Rustoni, A.: Nonprimary afferents to the cuneate nucleus in the brachial dorsal funiculus of the cat. Brain Res., *75:*247, 1974.
683. Rustoni, A.: Nonprimary afferents to the nucleus gracilis from the lumbar cord of the cat. Brain Res., *51:*81, 1973.
684. Sabbe, M.B., Grafe, M.R., Mjanger, E., *et al.*: Spinal delivery of sufentanil, alfentanil and morphine in dogs. Physiologic and toxicologic investigations. Anesthesiology, *81:*899, 1994.
685. Saeki, S., and Yaksh, T.L.: Suppression of nociceptive responses by spinal mu opioid agonists: effects of stimulus intensity and agonist efficacy. Anesth. Analg., *77*(2):265, 1993.
686. Salter, M.W., and Henry, J.L.: Evidence that adenosine mediates the depression of spinal dorsal horn induced by peripheral vibration in the cat. Neuroscience, *22:*631, 1987.
687. Samuelsson, B., Goldyne, M., Granstrom, E., *et al.*: Prostaglandins and thromboxanes. Ann. Rev. Biochem., *47:*997, 1978.
688. Sano, K., Yoshioka, M., Ogashiwa, M., *et al.*: Thalamotominotomy: A new operation for relief of intractable pain. Confin. Neurol., *27:*63, 1966.
689. Saporta, S., and Kruger, L.: The organization of projections to selected points of somatosensory cortex from the cat ventrobasal complex. Brain Res., *178:*275, 1979.
690. Saria, A., Javorsky, F., Humpel, C., and Gamse, R.: 5-HT receptor antagonism inhibit sensory neuropeptide release from the rat spinal cord. Neuroreport, *1:*104, 1990.
691. Sawynok, J., Kato, N., Havlicek, V., and Labella, F.S.: Lack of effect of baclofen on substance P and somatostatin release from the spinal cord *in vitro.* Naunyn-Schmiedeberg's Arch. Pharmacol., *319:*78, 1982.
692. Schaible, H.G., Grubb, B.D., Neugebauer, V., and Oppmann, M.: The effects of NMDA antagonists on neuronal activity in cat spinal cord evoked by acute inflammation in the knee joint. Eur. J. Neurosci. *3:*981, 1991.
693. Scheibel, M.E., and Scheibel, A.B.: Terminal axonal patterns in the cat spinal cord. II. The dorsal horn. Brain Res., *9:*32, 1968.
694. Schepelmann, K., Messlinger, K., Schaible, H.G., and Schmidt, R.F.: Inflammatory mediators and nociception in the joint: Excitation and sensitization of slowly conducting afferent fibers of cat's knee by prostaglandin I_2. Neuroscience, *50*(1):237, 1992.
694a. Schmauss, C. and Yaksh, T.L.: *In vivo* studies on spinal opiate receptor systems mediating antinociception. II. Pharmacological profiles suggesting a differential association of mu, delta, and kappa receptors with visceral chemical and cutaneous thermal stimuli in the rat. J. Pharmacol. Exp. Ther., *228:*1, 1984.
695. Schmidt, R.F.: Presynaptic inhibition in the vertebrate central nervous system. Ergebn. Physiol., *63:*21, 1971.
696. Schmidt, R.F., Schaible, H.G., Messlinger, K., *et al.*: Progr. Pain Res. Mgmt., *2:*213, 1994.
697. Schneider, S.P., and Perl, E.R.: Selective excitation of neurones in the mammalian spinal dorsal horn by aspartate and glutamate *in vitro*: Correlation with location and excitatory input. Brain Res., *360:*339, 1985.
698. Schott, E., Berge, O.G. Angeby-Moller, K., *et al.*: Weight bearing as an objective measure of arthritic pain in the rat. J. Pharmacol. Toxicol. Methods, *31*(2):79, 1994.
699. Schuman, E.M., and Madison, D.V.: A requirement for the intracellular messenger nitric oxide in long-term potentiation. Science, *254:*1503, 1991.
700. Schvarcz, J.R.: Spinal cord stereotactic surgery. *In* Sano, K., Ishii, S., and LeVay, D. (eds.): Recent Progress in Neurological Surgery. pp. 234–241. New York, Elsevier, 1974.
701. Schvarcz, J.R.: Stereotaxic spinal trigeminal nucleotomy for dysesthetic facial pain. *In* Bonica, J.J., Liebeskind, J.C., Albe-Fessard, D. (eds.): Advances in Pain Research and Therapy. Vol. 3. pp. 331–336. New York, Raven Press, 1979.
702. Schwartzman, R.J.: Thalamic sensory nuclear ablations in trained monkeys. Arch. Neurol., *23:*419, 1970.
703. Scibetta, C.J., and King, R.B.: Hyperpolarizing influence of trigemi-

nal nucleus caudalis on primary afferent preterminals in trigeminal nucleus oralis. J. Neurophysiol., *32:*229, 1969.

704. Scott, D., Jr., and Maziarz, R.: What is the most unique form of stimulus to evoke dental pain? *In* Bonica, J.J., and Albe-Fessard, D. (eds.): Advances in Pain Research and Therapy. Vol. 1. pp. 205–213. New York, Raven Press, 1976.
705. Selzer, M., and Spencer, W.A.: Convergence of visceral and cutaneous afferent pathways in the lumbar spinal cord. Brain Res., *14:*331, 1969.
706. Selzer, M., and Spencer, W.A.: Interactions between visceral and cutaneous afferents in the spinal cord: Reciprocal primary afferent fiber depolarization. Brain Res., *14:*349, 1969.
707. Sessle, B.J., Dubner, R., Greenwood, L.F., and Lucier, G.E.: Descending influences of periaqueductal gray matter and somatosensory cerebral cortex on neurones in trigeminal brain stem nuclei. Can. J. Physiol. Pharmacol., *54:*66, 1975.
708. Seybold, V.S., Hylden, J.L.K., and Wilcox, G.L.: Intrathecal substance P and somatostatin in rats: behaviors indicative of sensation. Peptides, *3:*49, 1982.
709. Shealy, C.N., Morhmer, J.T., and Hagfors, N.R.: Dorsal column electroanalgesia. J. Neurosurg., *32:*560, 1970.
710. Sheppard, M., Kronheim, S., Adams, C., and Pimstone, B.: Immunoreactive somatostatin release from rat spinal cord *in vitro.* Neurosci. Lett., *15:*65, 1979.
711. Sher, G., and Mitchell, D.: N-methyl-d-aspartate mediates responses of rat dorsal horn neurons to hind limb ischemia. Brain Res., *522:*55, 1990.
712. Sherman, S.E., and Loomis, C.W.: Morphine insensitive allodynia is produced by intrathecal strychnine in the lightly anesthetized rat. Pain, *56*(1):17, 1994.
713. Sherrington, C.: The Integrative Action of the Nervous System. pp. 228. New Haven, Yale University Press, 1947.
714. Shigenaga, Y., Matano, S., Okada, K., and Sohai, A.: The effects of tooth pulp stimulations in the thalamus and hypothalamus of the rat. Brain Res., *63:*402, 1973.
715. Shir, Y., and Seltzer, Z.: A-fibers mediate mechanical hyperesthesia and allodynia and C-fibers mediate thermal hyperalgesia in a new model of causalgia from pain disorders in rats. Neurosci. Lett., *115:*62, 1990.
716. Shortland, P., and Wall, P.D.: Long-range afferents in the rat spinal cord. II. Arborizations that penetrate grey matter. Philosophical Transactions of the Royal Society of London. Series B: Biol. Sci., *337*(1282):445, 1992.
717. Simone, D.A., Baumann, T.K., LaMotte, R.H.: Dose-dependent pain and mechanical hyperalgesia in humans after intradermal injection of capsaicin. Pain, *38:*99, 1989.
718. Singer, E., and Placheta, P.: Reduction of 3H-muscimol binding sites in rat dorsal spinal cord after neonatal capsaicin treatment. Brain Res., *202:*484, 1980.
718a. Sjoqvist, O.: Studies on pain conduction of the trigeminal nerve. Acta Psychiat. Neurol. Scand., *17*(Suppl.):1, 1938.
719. Skagerberg, G., Bjorklund, A., Lindvall, O., and Schmidt, R.H.: Origin and termination of the diencephalo-spinal dopamine system in the rat. Brain Res. Bull., *9:*237, 1982.
720. Skultety, F.M.: Stimulation of periaqueductal gray and hypothalamus. Arch. Neurol., *8:*608, 1963.
721. Sluka, K.A., and Westlund, K.N.: Spinal cord amino acid release and content in an arthritis model: The effects of pretreatment with non-NMDA, NMDA, and NK1 receptor antagonists. Brain Res., *627*(1):89, 1993.
722. Smith, J.B., and Willis, A.L.: Aspirin selectively inhibits prostaglandin production in human platelets. Nature, *231:*235, 1971.
723. Snyder, R.: The organization of the dorsal root entry zone in cats and monkeys. J. Comp. Neurol., *174:*47, 1977.
724. Sorkin, L.S., Westlund, K.N., Sluka, K.A., Dougherty, P.M., and Willis, W.D. Neural changes in acute arthritis in monkeys. IV. Time-course of amino acid release into the lumbar dorsal horn. Brain Res. Brain Res. Rev., *17:*39, 1992.
725. Sorkin, L.S.: NMDA evokes an L-NAME sensitive spinal release of glutamate and citrulline. Neuroreport, *4*(5):479, 1993.
726. Sosnowski, M., Stevens, C.W., and Yaksh, T.L.: Assessment of the role of A1/A2 adenosine receptors mediating the purine antinociception, motor and autonomic function in the rat spinal cord. J. Pharmacol. Exp. Ther., *250:*915, 1989.
727. Sosnowski, M., and Yaksh, T.L.: Role of spinal adenosine receptor in modulating the hyperesthesia produced by spinal receptor antagonism. Anesth. Analg., *69:*587, 1989.
728. Spiegel, E.A., Keltzkin, M., and Szekely, E.G.: Pain reactions upon stimulation of the tectum mesencephali. J. Neuropathol. Exp. Neurol., *13:*212, 1954.
729. Spiller, W.G., and Martin, E.: The treatment of perisistent pain of organic origin in the lower part of the body by division of anterolateral column of the spinal cord. J.A.M.A., *58:*1489, 1912.
730. Stacey, M.J.: Free nerve endings in skeletal muscle of the cat. J. Anat., *105:*231, 1969.
731. Staszewska-Barczak, J., Ferreira, S.H., and Vane, J.R.: An excitatory nociceptive cardiac reflex elicited by bradykinin and potentiated by prostaglandins and myocardial ischaemia. Cardiovasc. Res., *10:*314, 1976.
732. Steen, K.H., Reeh, P.W., Anton, F., and Handwerker, H.O.: Protons selectively induce lasting excitation and sensitization to mechanical stimulation of nociceptors in rat skin, *in vitro.* J. Neurosci., *12*(1):86, 1992.
733. Steinman, J.L., Komisaurak, B.R., Tyce, G.M., and Yaksh, T.L.: Spinal cord monoamines mediate the antinociceptive effects of vaginal stimulation in rats. Pain, *16:*155, 1983.
734. Sterling, P., and Kuypers, H.G.J.M.: Anatomical organization of the brachial spinal cord of the cat. I. The distribution of dorsal root fibers. Brain Res., *4:*1, 1967.
735. Stewart, W., and King, R.B.: Fiber projections from the n. caudalis of the spinal trigeminal nucleus. J. Comp. Neurol., *121:*271, 1963.
736. Sugimoto, T., Bennett, G.J., and Kajander, K.C.: Transsynaptic degeneration in the superficial dorsal horn after sciatic nerve injury: effects of a chronic constriction injury, transection, and strychnine. Pain, *42:*205, 1990.
737. Sulivan, T.J., and Parker, C.W.: Possible role of arachidonic acid and its metabolites in mediator release from rat mast cells. J. Immunol., *122:*431, 1979.
738. Sutton, D.C., and Lueth, H.C.: Experimental production of pain on excitation of the heart and great vessels. Arch. Intern. Med., *45:*827, 1930.
739. Sylven, C., Jonzon, B., Fredholm, B.B., and Kaijser, L.: Adenosine injection into the brachial artery produces ischaemia like pain or discomfort in the forearm. Cardiovasc. Res., *22*(9):674, 1988.
740. Szentagothai, J.: Neuronal and synaptic arrangement in the substantial gelatinosa Rolandi. J. Comp. Neurol, *122:*219, 1964.
741. Szolcsanyi, J.: Antidromic vasodilatation and neurogenic inflammation. Agents Actions, *23*(1–2):4, 1988.
742. Szolcsanyi, J., Jancso-Gabor, A., and Joo, F.: Functional and fine structural characteristics of the sensory neurone blocking effect of capsaicin. Naunyn - Schmiedeberg's Arch. Pharmacol., *287:*157, 1975.
743. Taiwo, Y.O., and Levine, J.D.: Indomethacin blocks central nociceptive effects of PGF_{2a}. Brain Res., *373:*81, 1986.
744. Takagi, H., Matsumura, M., Yanai, A., and Ogui, K.: The effect of analgesics on the spinal reflex activity of the cat. Jpn. J. Pharmacol., *4:*176, 1955.
745. Takano, M., Takano, Y., and Yaksh, T.L.: Release of calcitonin gene-related peptide (CGRP), substance P (SP), and vasoactive intestinal polypeptide (VIP) from rat spinal cord: Modulation by $alpha_2$ agonists. Peptides, *14*(2):371, 1993.
746. Takano, Y., and Yaksh, T.L.: Characterization of the pharmacology of intrathecally administered $alpha_2$ agonists and antagonists in rats. J. Pharmacol. Exp. Ther., *261:*764, 1992.
747. Talairach, J., Hecaen, M., and David, M.: Recherches sur la coagulation therapeuthique des structures sous-carticates chez l'homme. Rev. Neurol., *81:*4, 1949.
748. Talbot, J.D., Marrett, S., Evans, A.C., *et al.*: Multiple representations of pain in human cerebral cortex. Science, *251*(4999):1355, 1991.
749. Talbot, W.H., Darian-Smith, I., Komhuber, H.H., and Mountcastle, V.B.: The sense of flutter-vibration: Comparison of the human capacity with response patterns of mechanoreceptive afferents from the monkey hand. J. Neurophysiol., *31:*301, 1968.
750. Tervo, T., and Palkama, A.: Innervation of the rabbit cornea. A histochemical and electronmicroscopic study. Acta Anat., *102:*164, 1978.
751. Tervo, T., and Palkama, A.: Ultrastructure of the corneal nerves after fixation with potassium permanganate. Anat. Rec., *190:*851, 1978.
752. Tervo, T., Joo, F., Huikuri, K.T., *et al.*: Fine structure of sensory

nerves in the rat cornea: An experimental nerve degeneration study. Pain, *6:*57, 1979.

753. Tiwari, R.K., and King, R.B.: Fiber projections from trigeminal nucleus caudalis in primate (squirrel monkey and baboon). J. Comp. Neurol., *158:*191, 1974.
754. Todd, A.J., and McKenzie, J.: GABA-immunoreactive neurons in the dorsal horn of the spinal cord. Neuroscience, *31:*799, 1989.
755. Todd, A.J., and Sullivan, A.C.: Light microscopic study of the coexistence of GABA-like and glycine-like immunoreactivities in the spinal cord of the rat. J. Comp. Neurol., *296:*496, 1990.
756. Torebjörk, H.E., Lundberg, L.E., and LaMotte, R.H.: Central changes in processing of mechanoreceptive input in capsaicin-induced secondary hyperalgesia in humans. J. Physiol., *448:*765, 1992.
757. Torebjörk, H.E., and Hallin, R.G.: Excitation failure in thin nerve fiber structures and accompanying hypalgesia during repetitive electric skin stimulation. *In* Bonica, J.J. (ed.): Advances in Neurology. Vol. 4, pp. 733–735. New York, Raven Press, 1974.
758. Torebjörk, H.E., and Hallin, R.G.: Identification of afferent C units in intact human skin nerves. Brain Res., *67:*387, 1974.
759. Torebjörk, H.E., and Hallin, R.G.: Perceptual changes accompanying controlled preferential blocking of A and C fibre responses in intact human skin nerves. Exp. Brain Res., *16:*321, 1973.
760. Torebjörk, H.E., and Hallin, R.G.: Responses in human A and C fibers to repeated electrical intradermal stimulation. J. Neurol. Neurosurg. Psychiatry, *37:*653, 1974.
761. Torebjörk, H.E., and Hallin, R.G.: Skin receptors supplied by unmyelinated (C) fibres in man. *In* Zotterman, Y. (ed.): Sensory function of the skin in primates. pp. 475–487. Oxford, Pergamon, 1976.
762. Torebjörk, H.E.: Afferent C units responding to mechanical, thermal and chemical stimuli in human non-glabrous skin. Acta Physiol. Scand., *92:*374, 1974.
763. Trevino, D., Coulter, J.D., and Willis, W.D.: Location of cells of origin of spinothalamic tract in lumbar enlargement of the monkey. J. Neurophysiol., *36:*750, 1973.
764. Trevino, D.L., and Carstens, E.: Confirmation of the location of spinothalamic neurons in the cat and monkey by the retrograde transport of horseradish peroxidase. Brain Res., *98:*177, 1975.
765. Trevino, D.L., Maunz, R.A., Bryan, R.N., and Willis, W.D.: Location of cells of origin of the spinothalamic tract in the lumbar enlargement of cat. Exp. Neurol., *34:*64, 1972.
766. Truex, R.C., Taylor, M.J., Smythe, M.Q., and Gildenberg, P.L.: The lateral cervical nucleus of cat, dog and man. J. Comp. Neurol., *139:*93, 1970.
767. Tsou, K., and Jang, C.S.: Studies on the site of analgesic action of morphine by intracerebral microinjection. Sci. Sin., *13:*1099, 1964.
768. Tsutsumi, H., and Mark, V.H.: Experimental local thalamic application of xylocaine through silicone rubber chemode. J. Neurosurg., *38:*743, 1973.
769. Tyce, G.M., and Yaksh, T.L.: Monoamine release from cat spinal cord by somatic stimuli: An intrinsic modulatory system. J. Physiol. (Lond.), *314:*513, 1981.
770. Tyers, M.B., and Haywood, H.: Effect of prostaglandins on peripheral nociceptors in acute inflammation. Agents Actions, 6 (Suppl.)*:*65, 1979.
771. Uchida, Y., Kamisaka, K., and Ueda, H.: Experimental studies on anginal pain: Mode of excitation of afferent cardiac sympathetic nerve fibers. Jpn. Circulation J., *35:*147, 1971.
772. Uchida, Y., and Murao, S.: Bradykinin-induced excitation of afferent cardiac sympathetic nerve fibers. Jpn. Heart J., *25:*84, 1974.
773. Uchida, Y., and Murao, S.: Excitation of afferent cardiac sympathetic nerve fibers during coronary occlusion. Am. J. Physiol., *226:*1094, 1974.
774. Uda, R., Horiguchi, S., Ito, S.M., and Hayaishi, O.: Nociceptive effects by intrathecal administration of prostaglandin D_2, E_2 or F_{2a} to conscious mice. Brain Res., *510:*26, 1990.
775. Urabe, M., Tsubokawa, T., and Watanabe, Y.: Alteration of activity of single neurons in the nucleus centrum medianum following stimulation of the peripheral nerve and application of noxious stimuli. Jpn. J. Physiol., *16:*421, 1966.
776. Urabe, M., and Tsubokawa, T.: Stereotaxic thalamotomy for the relief of intractable pain. Tohoku J. Exp. Med., *85:*286, 1965.
777. Urban, L., and Randic, M.: Slow excitatory transmission in rat dorsal horn: possible mediation by peptides. Brain Res., *290:*336, 1984.
778. Urban, L., Perkins, M.N., Campbell, E., and Dray, A.: Activity of deep dorsal horn neurons in the anaesthetized rat during hyperalgesia of the hindpaw induced by ultraviolet irradiation. Neuroscience, 57(1): 167, 1993.
779. Uvnas, B.: The mechanism of histamine release from mast cell. *In* Rocha e Silva, M. (ed.): Handbuch der Experimentallelen Pharmacologie. Vol. 18 (part 2). pp. 75–92. New York, Springer-Verlag, 1978.
780. Van Arman, C.G., Carlson, R.P., Risley, E.A., *et al.*: Inhibitor effects of indomethacin, aspirin and certain other drugs on inflammations induced in rat and dog by carrageenan, sodium urate and ellagic acid. J. Pharmacol. Exp. Ther., *175:*459, 1970.
781. Van Hassel, H.J., Biedenback, M.A., and Brown, A.C.: Cortical potentials evoked by tooth pulp stimulation in rhesus monkeys. Arch. Oral Biol., *17:*1059, 1972.
782. Van Hees, J., and Gybels, J.M.: Pain related to single afferent C fibers from human skin. Brain Res., *48:*397, 1972.
783. Van Hees, J.: Human C fiber input during painful and nonpainful skin stimulation with radiant heat. *In* Bonica, J.J., and Albe-Fessard, D. (eds.): Advances in Pain Research and Therapy. Vol. 1. pp. 35–40. New York, Raven Press, 1976.
784. Vane, J.R.: Inhibition of prostaglandins synthesis as a mechanism of action for aspirin-like drugs. Nature: New Biol., *291:*23, 1971.
785. Vane, J.R.: The mode of action of aspirin and similar compounds. J. Allergy Clin. Immunol., *58:*691, 1976.
786. Vasko, M.R., Cartwright, S., and Ono, H.: Adenosine agonists do not inhibit the K^+ stimulated release of substance P from rat spinal cord slices. Soc. Neurosci. Abstracts, *12:*799, 1986.
787. Vierck, C.J., Jr., Greenspan, J.D., Ritz, L.A., and Yeomans, D.C.: The spinal pathways contributing to the ascending conduction and the descending modulation of pain sensations and reactions. *In* Yaksh, T.L. (ed.): Spinal Afferent Processing. pp. 275–329. New York, Plenum, 1986.
788. Vierck, C.J., Jr., Hamilton, D.M., and Thornby, J.J.: Pain reactivity of monkeys after lesions to the dorsal and lateral columns of the spinal cord. Exp. Brain Res., *13:*140, 1971.
789. Vin-Christian, K., Benoist, J.M., Gautron, M. *et al.*: Further evidence for the involvement of SmI cortical neurons in nociception: Modifications of their responsiveness over the early stage of a carrageenin-induced inflammation in the rat. Somatosens. Mot. Res., *9:*245, 1992.
790. Voris, H.C.: Vanations in the spinothalamic tract in man. J. Neurosurg., *14:*55, 1957.
791. Vyklicky, L., Keller, O., Brozek, G., and Butkhuzi, S.M.: Cortical potentials evoked by stimulation of tooth pulp afferents in the cats. Brain Res., *41:*211, 1972.
792. Vyklicky, L., and Keller, O.: Central projection of tooth pulp primary afferents in the cat. Acta Neurobiol. Exp., *33:*803, 1973.
793. Wagman, I.H., and Price, D.D.: Response of dorsal horn cells of Macaca mulatta to cutaneous and sural nerve A and C fiber stimuli. J. Neurophysiol., *32:*803, 1969.
794. Wall, P.D., and Shortland, P.: Long-range afferents in the rat spinal cord. I. Numbers, distances and conduction velocities. Philosophical Transactions of the Royal Society of London. Series B: Biol. Sci., *334*(1269):85, 1991.
795. Wall, P.D., and Gutnick, M.: Ongoing activity in peripheral nerves: The physiology and pharmacology of impulses originating from a neuroma. Exp. Neurol., *43:*580, 1974.
796. Wall, P.D., Merrill, E.G., and Yaksh, T.L.: Responses of single units in laminae II and III of cat spinal cord. Brain Res., *160:*245, 1979.
797. Wall, P.D., Scadding, J.W., and Tomkiewicz, M.M.: The production and prevention of experimental anaesthesia dolorosa. Pain, *6:*175, 1979.
798. Wall, P.D., and Yaksh, T.L.: The effect of Lissauer tract stimulation on activity in dorsal and ventral roots. Exp. Neurol., *60:*570, 1978.
799. Wall, P.D.: The laminar organization of dorsal horn and effects of descending impulses. J. Physiol. (Lond.), *188:*403, 1967.
800. Wall, P.D.: The origin of a spinal cord slow potential. J. Physiol. (Lond.), *164:*508, 1962.
801. Weber, W.V.: Some actions and interactions of visceral and somatic afferents in the thoracic spinal cord. *In* Kornhuber, J.J. (ed.): The Somatosensory System. Thieme Ed. pp. 227–238. Acton, MA, Publishing Sciences Group, 1975.
802. Weir-Mitchell, S., Moorhouse, G.R., and Keen, W.W.: Gunshot Wounds and Other Injuries of Nerves. pp. 164. Philadelphia, Lippincott, 1864.

803. Wennmalm, A., Chanh, P.H., and Junstad, M.: Hypoxia causes prostaglandin release from perfused rabbit hearts. Acta Physiol. Scand., *91:*133, 1974.
804. Westrum, L.E., and Black, R.C.: Fine structural aspects of the synaptic organization of the spinal trigeminal nucleus (pars interpolaris) of the cat. Brain Res., *25:*265, 1971.
805. Whalley, E.T., Clegg, S., Stewart, J.M., and Vavrek, R.J.: Antagonism of the algesic action of bradykinin on the human blister base. Adv. Exp. Med. Biol., *247A:*261, 1989.
806. Wheeler-Aceto, H., Porreca, F., and Cowan, A.: The rat paw formalin test: Comparison of noxious agents. Pain, *40*(2):229, 1990.
807. White, W.F., and Heller, A.H.: Glycine receptor alteration in the mutant mouse spastic. Nature, *298:*655, 1982.
808. White, J.C., and Bland, E.F.: The surgical relief of severe angina pectoris: Methods employed and end results in 83 patients. Medicine (Baltimore), *27:*1, 1948.
809. White, J.C., Garrey, W.E., and Atkins, J.A.: Cardiac innervation: Experimental and clinical studies. Arch. Surg., *26:*765, 1933.
810. White, J.C., Richardson, E.P., and Sweet, W.H.: Upper thoracic cordotomy for relief of pain: Postmortem correlation of spinal incision with analgesic levels in 18 cases. Ann. Surg., *144:*407, 1956.
811. White, J.C., Sweet, W.H., Hawkins, R., and Nilges, R.G.: Anterolateral cordotomy: Results, complications and causes of failure. Brain, *73:*346, 1950.
812. White, J.C., and Sweet, W.H.: Pain and the Neurosurgeon. Springfield, IL, Charles C. Thomas, 1969.
813. White, J.C., and Sweet, W.H.: Pain, Its Mechanisms and Neurosurgical Control. Springfield, IL, Charles C. Thomas, 1955.
814. Whitlock, D.G., and Perl, E.R.: Thalamic projections of spinothalamic pathways in monkeys. Exp. Neurol., *3:*240, 1961.
815. Whitsel, B.L., Petrucelli, L.M., and Wemer, G.: Symmetry and connectively in the map of the body surface in somatosensory area II of primates. J. Neurophysiol., *32:*170, 1969.
816. Whitsel, B.L., Rustioni, A., Dreyer, D.A., *et al.*: Thalamic projections to S 1 in Macaque monkeys. J. Comp. Neurol., *178:*385, 1978.
817. Willer, J.C.: Comparative study of perceived pain and nociceptive flexion reflex in man. Pain, *3*(1):69, 1977.
818. Willer, J.C., Boureaux, F., and Albe-Fessard, D.: Role of large diameter cutaneous afferents in transmission of nociceptive messages: Electrophysiological study in man. Brain Res., *152:*385, 1978.
819. Willis, A.L.: Release of histamine, kinin and prostaglandin during carrageenin-induced inflammation in the rat. *In* Montegazza, P., and Horton, E.W. (eds.): Prostaglandins, Peptides, and Amines. pp. 31–38. London, Academic Press, 1969.
820. Willis, W.D., and Coggeshall, R.E.: Sensory Mechanisms of the Spinal Cord. New York, Plenum Press, 1978.
821. Willis, W.D., Haber, L.H., and Martin, R.F.: Inhibition of spinothalamic tract cells and interneurons by brainstem stimulation in the monkey. J. Neurophysiol., *40:*968, 1977.
822. Willis, W.D., Kenshalo, D.R., Jr., and Leonard, R.B.: The cells of origin of the primate spinothalamic tract. J. Comp. Neurol., *188:*543, 1979.
823. Willis, W.D., Trevino, D.L., Coulter, J.D., and Maunz, R.A.: Responses of primate spinothalamic tract neurons to natural stimulation of hindlimb. J. Neurophysiol., *37:*358, 1974.
824. Willis, W.D.: Ascending somatosensory systems. *In* Yaksh, T.L. (ed.): Spinal Afferent Processing. pp. 243–274. New York, Plenum Press, 1986.
825. Wilson, P.R., and Yaksh, T.L.: Baclofen is antinociceptive in the spinal intrathecal space of animals. Eur. J. Pharmacol., *51:*323, 1978.
826. Winkelmann, R.K.: Kinins from human skin. *In* Kenshalo, D.R. (ed.): The Skin Senses. pp. 499–511. Springfield, IL, Charles C. Thomas, 1968.
827. Winkelmann, R.K.: Sensory receptors of the skin. *In* Yaksh, T.L. (ed.): Spinal Afferent Processing. pp. 19–57. New York, Plenum Press, 1986.
828. Winter, D.L.: Receptor characteristics and conduction velocities in bladder afferents. J. Psychiatr. Res., *8:*225, 1971.
829. Wolff, H.G., (Dalessio, D.J., rev.): Wolff's Headache and Other Head Pain. 3rd Ed. Reviewed by D.J. Dalessio, New York, Oxford University Press, 1972.
830. Woodbury, D.M., and Fingl, E.: Analgesic antipyretics, antiinflammatory agents, and drugs employed in the therapy of gout., *In* Goodman, L.S., and Gilman, E.A. (eds.): The Pharmacological Basis of Therapeutics. 5th Ed. pp. 325–358. New York, MacMillan, 1975.
831. Woodley, S.J., and Kendig, J.J.: Substance P and NMDA receptors mediate a slow nociceptive ventral root potential in neonatal rat spinal cord. Brain Res., *559:*17, 1991.
832. Woolf, C.J., and Thompson, W.N.: The induction and maintenance of central sensitization is dependent on N-methyl D-aspartic acid receptor activation, implications for the treatment of post-injury pain hypersensitivity states. Pain, *44:*293, 1991.
833. Woolf, C.J., Shortland, P., and Coggeshall, R.E.: Peripheral nerve injury triggers central sprouting of myelinated afferents. Nature, *355:*75, 1992.
834. Wright, D.M., and Roberts, M.H.T.: Responses of spinal neurones to a substance P analogue, noxious pinch and bradykinin. Eur. J. Pharmacol., *64:*165, 1980.
835. Yaksh, T.L.: Central and peripheral mechanisms for the analgesic action of acetylsalicylic acid. *In* Barett, H.J.M., Hirsh, J., and Mustard, J.F., (eds.): Acetylsalicylic Acid: New Uses for an Old Drug. pp. 137–151. New York, Raven Press, 1982.
836. Yaksh, T.L.: Behavioral and autonomic correlates of the tactile evoked allodynia produced by spinal glycine inhibition: effects of modulatory receptor systems and excitatory amino acid antagonists. Pain, *37:*111, 1989.
837. Yaksh, T.L., Michener, S.R., Bailey, J.E., *et al.*: Survey of distribution of substance P, vasoactive intestinal polypeptide, cholecystokinin, neurotensin, metenkephalin, bombesin and PHI in the spinal cord of cat, dog, sloth and monkey. Peptides, *9:*357, 1988.
838. Yaksh, T.L., Jage, J., and Takano, Y.: The spinal actions of a_2-adrenergic agonists as analgesics. *In* Aitkenhead, A.R., Benad, G., Brown, B.R., *et al.* (eds.): Baillière's Clinical Anaesthesiology. Vol. 7. No. 3. Bailliere, 1993.
839. Yaksh, T.L.: Substance P release from knee joint afferent terminals: modulation by opioids. Brain Res., *458*(2):319, 1988.
840. Yaksh, T.L.: The spinal actions of opioids. *In* Herz A. (ed.): Handbook of Experimental Pharmacology. Vol. 104. pp. 53–90. Berlin/Heidelberg, Springer-Verlag, 1993.
841. Yaksh, T.L., Pogrel, J.M., Lee, Y. Woo, *et al.*: Reversal of nerve ligation-induced allodynia by spinal $alpha_2$ adrenoceptor agonists. J. Pharmacol. Exp. Ther., *272:*207, 1995.
842. Yaksh, T.L., Abay, E.O., and Go, V.L.W.: Studies on the location and release of cholecystokinin and vasoactive intestinal peptide in rat and cat spinal cord. Brain Res., *242:*279, 1982.
843. Yaksh, T.L., Dirksen, R., and Harty, G.J.: Antinociceptive effects of intrathecally injected cholinomimetic drugs in the rat and cat. Eur. J. Pharmacol., *117:*81, 1985.
844. Yaksh, T.L., and Elde, R.P.: Factors governing the release of methionine-enkephalin-like immunoreactivity from the mesencephalon and spinal cord of the cat *in vivo.* J. Neurophysiol., *46:*1056, 1981.
845. Yaksh, T.L., Jessell, T.M., Gamse, R., *et al.*: Intrathecal morphine inhibits substance P release from mammalian spinal cord *in vivo.* Nature, *286:*155, 1980.
846. Yaksh, T.L., Noueihed, R.Y., and Durant, P.A.C.: Studies of the pharmacology and pathology of intrathecally administered 4-anilinopiperidine analogues and morphine in rat and cat. Anesthesiology, *64:*54, 1986.
847. Yaksh, T.L., Schmauss, C., Micevych, P.E., *et al.*: Pharmacological studies on the application, disposition and release of neurotensin in the spinal cord. Ann. N.Y. Acad. Sci., *400:*228, 1982.
848. Yaksh, T.L., Terenius, L., Nyberg, F., *et al.*: Studies on the release by somatic stimulation from rat and cat spinal cord of active materials which displace dihydromorphine in an opiate-binding assay. Brain Res., *268:*119, 1983.
849. Yaksh, T.L., and Tyce, G.M.: Resting and K^+ evoked release of serotonin and norepinephrine *in vivo* from the cat and rat spinal cord. Brain Res., *192:*133, 1980.
850. Yaksh, T.L., and Wall, P.D.: Activation of a local spinal inhibitory system by focal stimulation of the lateral Lissauer tract in cats. Fed. Proc., *37:*398, 1978.
851. Yaksh, T.L., and Wilson, P.R.: Spinal serotonin terminal system mediates antinociception. J. Pharmacol. Exp. Ther., *208:*446, 1979.
852. Yaksh, T.L., Yeung, J.C., and Rudy, T.A.: Medial thalamic lesions in the rat: Effects on nociceptive threshold and morphine antinociception. Neuropharmacology, *16:*107, 1977.
853. Yaksh, T.L., Yeung, J.C., and Rudy, T.A.: Systematic mapping of the central gray medial thalamic axis of the rat: evidence for a somatotopic distribution of morphine sensitive sites within the penaqueductal gray. (Abstr.) Neuroscience, *1:*283, 1975.

854. Yaksh, T.L.: Inhibition by etorphine of the discharge of dorsal horn neurons: Effects upon the neuronal response to both high- and low-threshold sensory input in the decerebrate spinal cat. Exp. Neurol., *60:*23, 1978.
855. Yaksh, T.L.: Multiple opioid receptor systems in brain and spinal cord. Part 2. Eur. J. Anaesthesiol., *1:*201, 1984.
856. Yaksh, T.L.: Multiple opioid receptor systems in brain and spinal cord: Part 1. Eur. J. Anaesthesiol., *1:*171, 1984.
857. Yaksh, T.L.: Neuropharmacology of the spinal cord reaction to noxious inputs. Proc. Int. Union Physiol. Sci., *14:*283, 1980.
858. Yaksh, T.L.: Pharmacology of spinal adrenergic systems which modulate spinal nociceptive processing. Pharmacol. Biochem. Behav., *22:*845, 1985.
859. Yaksh, T.L.: The effects of intrathecally administered opioid and adrenergic agents on spinal function. *In* Yaksh, T.L. (ed.): Spinal Afferent Processing. pp. 505–539. New York, Plenum Press, 1986.
860. Yaksh, T.L., and Malmberg, A.B.: Central pharmacology of nociceptive transmission. *In* Wall, P.D., and Melzack, R. (eds.): Textbook of Pain. pp. 165–200. New York, Churchill Livingstone, 1994.
861. Yamamoto, T., and Yaksh, T.L.: Stereospecific effects of a nonpeptidic NK1 selective antagonist, CP, 96-345: Antinociception in the absence of motor dysfunction. Life Sci., *49:*1955, 1991.
862. Yamamoto, T., and Yaksh, T.L.: Comparison of the antinociceptive effects of pre- and post-treatment with intrathecal morphine and MK801, an NMDA antagonist on the formalin test in the rat. Anesthesiology, *77:*757, 1992.
863. Yamamoto, T., Takahashi, K., Satomi, H., and Ise, H.: Origins of primary afferent fibers in the spinal ventral roots in the cat as demonstrated by the horseradish peroxidase method. Brain Res., *126:*350, 1977.
864. Yanez, A., Sabbe, M.B., Stevens, C.W., and Yaksh, T.L.: Interaction of midazolam and morphine in the spinal cord of the rat. Neuropharmacology, *29:*359, 1990.
865. Yezierski, R.P., Gerhart, K.D., Schrock, B.J., and Willis, W.D.: A further examination of effects of cortical stimulation on primate spinothalamic tract cells. J. Neurophysiol., *49:*424, 1983.
866. Yezierski, R.P., and Schwartz, R.H.: Receptive field properties of spinomesencephalic tract (SMT) cells. Pain, 2(Suppl.)*:*184, 1984.
867. Yokota, T., and Hashimoto, S.: Periaqueductal gray and tooth pulp afferent interaction on units in caudal medulla oblongata. Brain Res., *117:*508, 1976.
868. Yokota, T.: Excitation of units in marginal rim of trigeminal subnucleus caudalis excited by tooth pulp stimulation. Brain Res., *95:*154, 1975.
869. Yokota, T., Nishikawa, N., and Nishikawa, Y.: Effects of strychnine upon different classes of trigeminal subnucleus caudalis neurons. Brain Res., *168:*430, 1979.
870. Yoshida, A., Dostrovsky, J.O., and Chiang, C.Y.: The afferent and efferent connections of the nucleus submedius in the rat. J. Comp. Neurol., *324:*(1):115, 1992.
871. Yoshida, S., and Matsuda, Y.: Studies on sensory neurons of the mouse with intracellular recording and horseradish peroxidase—injection techniques. J. Neurophysiol., *42:*1134, 1979.
872. Yoshimura, M., and Jessell, T.M.: Primary afferent evoked synaptic response and slow potential generation in rat substantia gelatinosa neurons *in vitro.* J. Neurophysiol., *622:*96, 1989.
873. Young, D.W., and Gottschaldt, R.M.: Neurons in the rostral mesencephalic reticular formation of the cat responding specifically to noxious mechanical stimulation. Exp. Neurol., *51:*628, 1976.
874. Young, R.F., and King, R.B.: Excitability changes in trigeminal primary afferent fibers in response to noxious and nonnoxious stimuli. J. Neurophysiol., *35:*87, 1972.
875. Young, R.F., and King, R.B.: Fiber spectrum of the trigeminal sensory root of the baboon determined by electron microscopy. J. Neurosurg., *38:*65, 1973.
876. Young, R.F.: Unmyelinated fibers in the trigeminal motor root. Possible relationship to the results of trigeminal rhizotomy. J. Neurosurg., *49:*538, 1978.
877. Zarbin, M.A., Wamsley, J.K., and Kuhar, M.J.: Glycine receptor: light microscopic autoradiographic localization with [3H] strychnine. J. Neurosci., *1:*532, 1981.
878. Zemlan, F.P., Leonard, C.M., Kow, L.M., and Pfaff, D.W.: Ascending tracts of the lateral columns of the rat spinal cord: A study using the silver impregnation and horseradish peroxidase techniques. Exp. Neurol., *62:*298, 1978.
879. Zieglgansberger, W., and Phil, E.A.: Actions of glutamic acid on spinal neurons. Exp. Brain Res., *17:*35, 1973.
880. Zieglgansberger, W., and Tulloch, I.F.: Effects of substance P on neurones in the dorsal horn of the spinal cord of the cat. Brain Res., *166:*273, 1979.
881. Zotterman, Y.: Touch, pain, and tickling: An electrophysiological investigation on cutaneous sensory nerves. J. Physiol. (Lond.), *95:*1, 1939.

Neural Blockade in Clinical Anesthesia and Management of Pain, Third Edition,
edited by M.J. Cousins and P.O. Bridenbaugh.
Lippincott–Raven Publishers, Philadelphia © 1998.

CHAPTER 25

Psychological Aspects of Pain

Implications for Neural Blockade

Ronald Melzack

Pain is a personal, subjective experience influenced by cultural learning, the meaning of the situation, attention, and other psychological variables. Pain processes do not begin with the stimulation of receptors. Rather, injury or disease produces neural signals that enter an active nervous system that (in the adult organism) is the substrate of past experience, culture, anxiety, and so forth. These brain processes actively participate in the selection, abstraction, and synthesis of information from the total sensory input. Pain, then, is not simply the end product of a linear sensory transmission system; it is a dynamic process that involves continuous interactions among complex ascending and descending systems.

This chapter will address four areas of interest to anesthesiologists and psychologists: (i) the major psychological contributions to pain, (ii) theories of pain, which are based on psychological assumptions of the nature of perception, (iii) the measurement of pain, and (iv) labor pain, which is influenced by anesthetic blocks as well as by manipulating psychological variables.

PSYCHOLOGICAL CONTRIBUTIONS TO PAIN

When compared with vision or hearing, the perception of pain seems simple, urgent, and primitive. We expect the nerve signals evoked by injury to "get through," unless we are unconscious or anesthetized. But experiments and clinical observations show that pain is much more variable and modifiable than many people have believed in the past. Pain differs from person to person and from culture to culture. Stimuli that produce intolerable pain in one person may be tolerated without a whimper by another. Pain perception, then, cannot be defined simply in terms of particular kinds of stimuli. Rather, it is a highly personal experience that depends in part on psychological factors that are unique to each individual.[40]

Cultural Determinants

It is often asserted that variations in pain experience from person to person are due to different "pain thresholds"; however, there are several thresholds related to pain, and it is important to distinguish among them. Typically, thresholds are measured by applying a stimulus such as electric shock or radiant heat to a small area of skin and gradually increasing the intensity. Four thresholds can be measured by this technique: (i) sensation threshold (or lower threshold)—the lowest stimulus value at which a sensation such as tingling or warmth is first reported; (ii) pain perception threshold—the lowest stimulus value at which the person reports that the stimulation feels painful; (iii) pain tolerance (or upper threshold)—the lowest stimulus level at which the subject withdraws or asks to have the stimulation stopped; and (iv) encouraged pain tolerance—the same as (iii), but the person is encouraged to tolerate higher levels of stimulation.

There is now evidence that all people, regardless of cultural background, have a uniform *sensation threshold.* Sternbach and Tursky[52] made careful measurements of sensation threshold, using electric shock as the stimulus, in American-born women belonging to four different ethnic groups: Italian, Jewish, Irish, and Old American. They found no differences among the groups in the level of shock that was first reported as producing a detectable sensation. The sensory conducting apparatus, in other words, appears to be essentially similar in all people so that a given critical level of input always elicits a sensation.

Cultural background, however, has a powerful effect on

R. Melzack: Department of Psychology, McGill University, Montreal, Quebec H3A 1B1 Canada.

the *pain perception threshold*. For example, levels of radiant heat that are reported as painful by people of Mediterranean origin (such as Italians and Jews) are described merely as warmth by Northern Europeans.[11] Similarly, Nepalese porters on a climbing expedition are much more stoic than the Occidental visitors for whom they work. Even though both groups are equally sensitive to changes in electric shock, the Nepalese porters require much higher intensities before they call them painful.[4]

The most striking effect of cultural background, however, is on *pain tolerance levels*. Sternbach and Tursky[52] report that the levels at which subjects refuse to tolerate electric shock, even when they are encouraged by the experimenters, depend in part on the ethnic origin of the subject. Women of Italian descent tolerate less shock than women of Old American or Jewish origin. In a similar experiment[19] in which Jewish and Protestant women served as subjects, the Jewish, but not the Protestant, women increased their tolerance level after they were told that their religious group tolerated pain more poorly than others.

These differences in pain tolerance reflect different ethnic attitudes toward pain. Zborowski[61] found that Old Americans have an accepting, matter-of-fact attitude toward pain and pain expression. They tend to withdraw when the pain is intense, and cry out or moan only when they are alone. Jews and Italians, on the other hand, tend to be vociferous in their complaints and openly seek support and sympathy. The underlying attitudes of the two groups, however, appear to be different. Jews tend to be concerned about the meaning and implications of the pain, whereas Italians usually express a desire for immediate pain relief.

Meaning of the Pain-Producing Situation

There is considerable evidence to show that people attach variable meaning to pain-producing situations and that the meaning greatly influences the degree and quality of pain they feel. Beecher[1] observed that soldiers wounded in battle rarely complained of pain, whereas civilians with similar surgical wounds usually claimed that they were in severe pain. Beecher[1] concluded the following from his study:

> The common belief that wounds are inevitably associated with pain, and that the more extensive the wound the worse the pain, was not supported by observations made as carefully as possible in the combat zone. . . . The data state in numerical terms what is known to all thoughtful clinical observers: there is no simple direct relationship between the wound *per se* and the pain experienced. The pain is in very large part determined by other factors, and of great importance here is the significance of the wound. . . . In the wounded soldier (the response to injury) was relief, thankfulness at his escape alive from the battlefield, even euphoria; to the civilian, his major surgery was a depressing, calamitous event.

A similar study[3] of Israeli soldiers with traumatic amputations after the Yom Kippur War provided similar observations. Most of the wounded men spoke of their initial injury as painless and used neutral terms such as "bang," "thump," or "blow" to describe their first sensation. They often volunteered their surprise that the injury did not hurt.

Melzack, Wall, and Ty[41] examined the features of acute pain in patients at an emergency clinic. Patients who had severe, life-threatening injuries or who were agitated, drunk, or "in shock" were excluded from the study. Of 138 patients who were alert, rational, and coherent, 51 (37%) stated that they did not feel pain at the time of injury. The majority of these patients reported onset of pain within an hour of injury, although the delays were as long as 9 hours or more in some patients. The predominant emotions of the patients were embarrassment at appearing careless or worry about loss of wages.

The occurrence of delays in pain onset was related to the nature of the injury. Of 46 patients whose injuries were limited to skin (lacerations, cuts, abrasions, burns), 53% had a pain-free period. Of 86 patients with deep-tissue injuries (fractures, sprains, bruises, amputation of a finger, stabs, and crushes), 28% had a pain-free period. The results indicate that the relation between injury and pain is highly variable and complex.

Attention, Anxiety, and Distraction

If a person's attention is focused on a potentially painful experience, he will tend to perceive pain more intensely than he would normally. Hall and Stride[10] found that the simple appearance of the word "pain" in a set of instructions made anxious subjects more likely to report a given level of electric shock as painful; the same level of shock was rarely reported to be painful when the word was absent from the instructions. Thus the mere anticipation of pain is sufficient to raise the level of anxiety and thereby the intensity of perceived pain. Similarly, Hill, Kornetsky, Flanary, and Wikler[14,15] have shown that if anxiety is dispelled (by reassuring the subject that he has control over the pain-producing stimulus), a given level of electric shock or burning heat is perceived as significantly less painful than the same stimulus under conditions of high anxiety.

In contrast to the effects of attention on pain, it is well known that distraction of attention away from pain can diminish or abolish it. Distraction of attention may partly explain why boxers, football players, and other athletes sometimes sustain severe injuries during the excitement of the sport without being aware that they have been hurt.

Distraction of attention, however, is usually effective only when the pain is steady or rises slowly in intensity.[42] If radiant heat is focused on the skin, for example, the pain may rise so suddenly and sharply that subjects are unable to control it by distraction. But when the pain rises slowly, people may use various stratagems to distract their attention from it. They often find that the pain actually levels off or decreases *before* it reaches the anticipated intolerable level. Distraction stratagems are used effectively by some people to control pain produced by dental drilling and extraction.[9]

Feelings of Control Over Pain

It is now apparent that the severity of postsurgical pain is significantly reduced when patients are taught how to cope with their pain. Patients who were scheduled to undergo major surgery to remove the gallbladder, uterus, or portions of the digestive tract were given detailed information about the pain they would feel after the operation and how they could best cope with it. They were told where they would feel pain, how severe it could be, how long it could last, and that such pain is normal after an operation. They were also shown how to relax by using breathing and relaxation stratagems. Finally, they were told that total relaxation is difficult to achieve and that they should request medication if they were uncomfortable. The results showed that patients who received these instructions reported significantly less pain, asked for many fewer medications during recovery, and spent less time in hospital than a similar group of patients who received no instructions.[7]

It was originally thought that the information alone is sufficient psychological preparation to reduce the uncertainty and anxiety associated with major surgery. It is evident, however, that knowledge, in this case, may only increase the anxiety because of the certain expectation of pain and various discomforts. The essential ingredient is providing the patient with skills to cope with the pain and anxiety—at the very least, to provide the patient with a sense of control. Recent studies have shown that simply giving patients information about their pain tends to make them focus on the discomforting aspects of the experience, and their pain is magnified rather than reduced; however, when the patients are taught skills to cope with their pain, such as relaxation or distraction strategies, the pain is less severe.[20] Other studies have shown that the amount of postsurgical pain is directly proportional to the amount of anxiety perceived by the patient.[22] Achieving a sense of control, then, appears to diminish both anxiety and pain.

Suggestion and Placebos

The influence of suggestion on the intensity of perceived pain is clearly demonstrated by studies of the effectiveness of placebos. Clinical investigators[1] have found that severe pain, such as postsurgical pain, can be relieved in some patients by giving them a placebo (usually some nonanalgesic substance such as a sugar or salt solution) in place of morphine or other analgesic drugs. About 35% of the patients report marked relief of pain after being given a placebo. This is a strikingly high proportion because morphine, even in large doses, relieves severe pain in only about 75% of patients.

Another interesting discovery about placebos is that their effectiveness is of the order of 50% that of the drug with which it is being compared, even in double-blind experiments;[8] that is, if the drug is a mild analgesic such as aspirin, the pain relief produced by the placebo is half that of the aspirin. If it is a powerful drug such as morphine, the placebo has greater pain-relieving properties, again about 50% of that of morphine. This indicates that even though the "double-blind" is maintained, the therapist's enthusiasm is conveyed to the patient. However, in a recent analysis of controlled trials, 38% of patients obtained more than 10% of maximum possible pain relief after placebo, while 16% obtained greater than 50% relief (50% of maximum with a potent agent). Thus there was considerable variation among patients in placebo response, within a given study.[8a]

There are large individual differences in susceptibility to placebos, and studies have been done to determine some of the factors involved.[59] These studies have revealed that placebos are more effective for severe pain than for mild pain and are more effective when the patients are under great stress and anxiety than when they are not. McGlashan and co-workers[23] have shown that placebo-induced analgesia is not significantly related to suggestibility, hypnotic susceptibility, or anxiety induced specifically by pain or the therapeutic situation (which is known as "state-anxiety"); however, placebo effects occur more powerfully in people who have chronic generalized anxiety (personality "trait-anxiety").

There are other fascinating factors in the placebo response. Two placebo capsules, for example, are more effective than one capsule, and large capsules are better than small ones. A placebo is more effective when injected than when given by mouth and is more potent when accompanied by strong suggestion that a powerful analgesic has been given. In short, the greater the implicit and explicit suggestion that pain will be relieved, the greater is the relief obtained by the patient. Unfortunately, however, patients tend to get less and less relief from repeated administration of placebos.

Hypnosis

The manipulation of attention together with strong suggestion is part of the phenomenon of hypnosis. The hypnotic state eludes precise definition. Loosely speaking, hypnosis is a trance state in which the subject's attention is focused intensely on the hypnotist while attention to other stimuli is markedly diminished. After people are hypnotized they can, with appropriate suggestion, be cut or burned yet report that they did not feel pain.[50,51] They may say that they felt a sharp tactile sensation or strong heat, but they maintain that the sensations never welled up into pain. Evidently a small percentage of people can be hypnotized deeply enough to undergo major surgery entirely without anesthesia. For a larger number of people, hypnosis reduced the amount of painkilling drug required to produce successful analgesia.

Despite the long history of hypnotism, which goes back hundreds of years under different names such as animal magnetism and mesmerism, very little is known about its mechanisms. Still worse, most of its major features are highly controversial. For example, there is a vigorous debate on the nature of hypnosis. Is it a special state of consciousness known as a "trance state," or is it merely a trait of responsiveness to strong suggestion? There is no resolution yet to this question.[51]

Nevertheless, anyone who has observed the behavior of people who have been hypnotized realizes that this is an especially interesting phenomenon. Under hypnosis, people sustain pain, during demonstrations or experiments, at levels at which they would normally cry out and withdraw. Countless articles describe these procedures, and there are reports that hypnosis is effective in relieving severe clinical pains, such as phantom limb pain. Although excellent studies of hypnotic analgesia have been carried out with experimentally induced pains,[13] there are as yet no convincing studies, using the necessary control groups, of clinical pain. The evidence thus far is observational or "anecdotal."

It is known, however, that not all people can be hypnotized. About 30% of people can reach a state of deep hypnosis, 30% reach a moderate state, and another 30% achieve a drowsy-like state. About 10% of people are not susceptible at all. These figures resemble the proportions of placebo reactors and nonreactors. There is, however, strong evidence that the lack of responsiveness to pain in hypnotized subjects is more than a placebo effect. An elegantly designed experiment[23] has shown that pain perception threshold and pain tolerance level are strikingly increased during hypnosis but that only the pain perception threshold is raised after administration of a placebo. In fact, this study demonstrated that the hypnotic procedure itself has not only a placebo effect, but also an additional effect that raises pain threshold and tolerance still further.

THEORIES OF PAIN

The Gate Control Theory

The traditional specificity theory of pain, which is still widely taught, proposes that pain is a specific sensation and that the intensity of pain is proportional to the extent of tissue damage. The theory implies a fixed, straight-through transmission system from somatic pain receptors to a pain center in the brain. The evidence just reviewed, however, shows that pain not only is a function of injury, but also is influenced by psychological variables.

In 1965, Melzack and Wall[39] proposed the gate control theory of pain. Basically, the theory proposes that neural mechanisms in the dorsal horns of the spinal cord act as a gate that can increase or decrease the flow of nerve impulses from peripheral fibers to the spinal cord cells that project to the brain. Somatic input is therefore subjected to the modulating influence of the gate *before* it evokes pain perception and response. The theory suggests that large-fiber inputs tend to close the gate whereas small-fiber inputs generally open it, and that the gate is also profoundly influenced by descending influences from the brain. It further proposes that the sensory input is modulated at successive synapses throughout its projection from the spinal cord to the brain areas responsible for pain experience and response. Pain occurs when the number of nerve impulses that arrives at these areas exceeds a critical level.

Melzack and Wall[40] have assessed the present-day status of the gate-control theory in light of new physiologic research. Despite considerable controversy and conflicting evidence, the concept of gating (or input modulation) is stronger than ever. A slightly revised model of the gate control theory has been presented (Fig. 25-1).[40]

Dimensions of Pain Experience

Research on pain, since the beginning of this century, has been dominated by the concept that pain is purely a sensory experience. Yet pain also has a distinctly unpleasant, affective quality. It becomes overwhelming, demands immediate

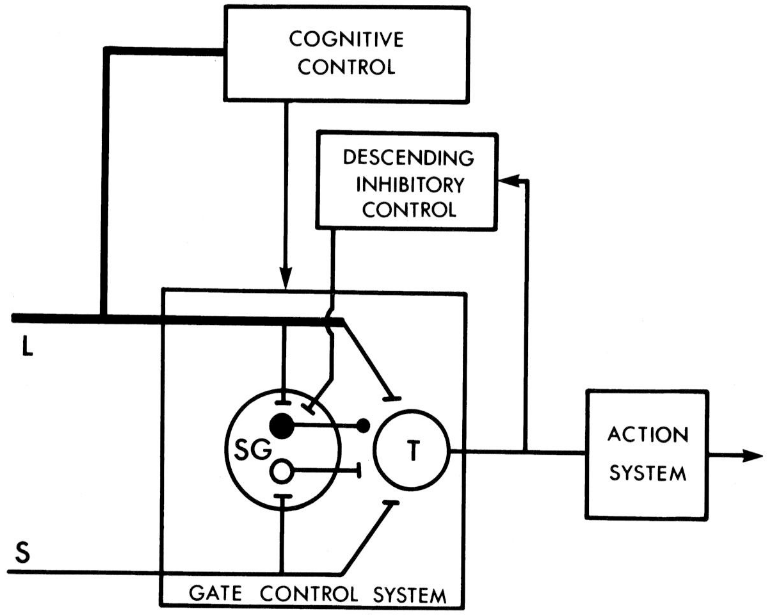

FIG. 25-1. The gate control theory: Mark II. The new model includes excitatory *(white circle)* and inhibitory *(black circle)* links from the substantia gelatinosa *(SG)* to the transmission *(T)* cells, as well as descending inhibitory control from brainstem systems. The round knob at the end of the inhibitory link implies that its action may be presynaptic, postsynaptic, or both. All connections are excitatory, except the inhibitory link from SG to T cell.

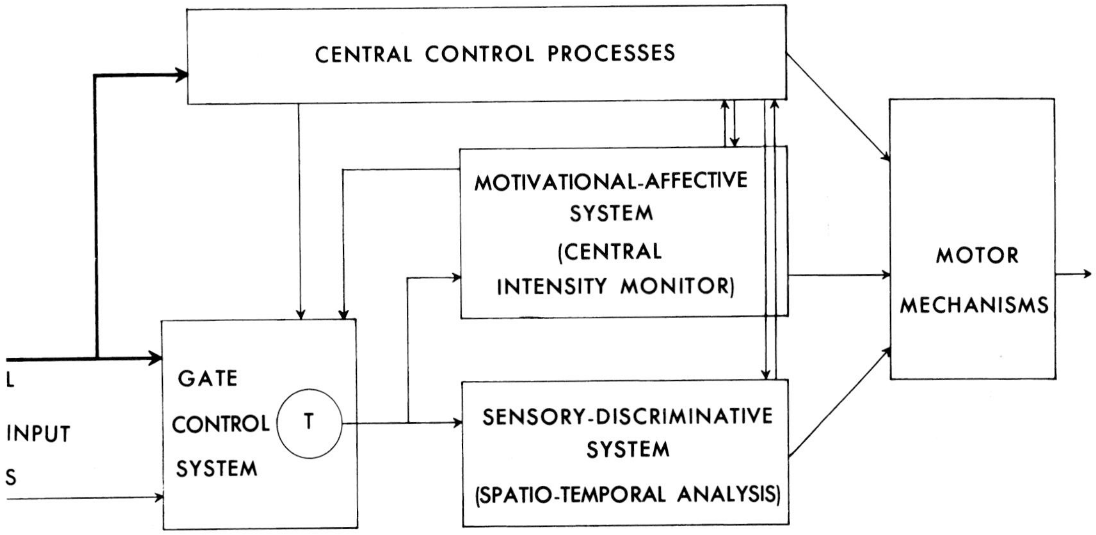

FIG. 25-2. Conceptual model of the sensory, motivational, and central control determinants of pain. The output of the T cells of the gate control system projects to the sensory-discriminative system (via neospinothalamic fibers) and the motivational-affective system (via the paramedial ascending system). The central control trigger is represented by a line running from the larger fiber system to central control processes; these, in turn, project back to the gate control system and to the sensory-discriminative and motivational-affective systems. All three systems interact with one another and project to the motor system.

attention, and disrupts ongoing behavior and thought. It motivates or drives the organism into activity aimed at stopping the pain as quickly as possible. To consider only the sensory features of pain and ignore its motivational-affective properties is to look at only part of the problem. Even the concept of pain as a perception, with full recognition of past experience, attention, and other cognitive influences, still neglects the crucial motivational dimension.

These considerations led Melzack and Casey[32] to suggest that there are three major psychological dimensions of pain: sensory-discriminative, motivational-affective, and cognitive-evaluation. They proposed that they are subserved by physiologically specialized systems in the brain (Fig. 25-2):

1. The sensory-discriminative dimension of pain is influenced primarily by the rapidly conducting spinal systems.
2. The powerful motivational drive and unpleasant affect characteristic of pain are subserved by activities in reticular and limbic structures that are influenced primarily by the slowly conducting spinal systems.
3. Neocortical or higher central nervous system processes, such as evaluation of the input in terms of past experience, exert control over activity in both the discriminative and motivational systems.

It is assumed that these three categories of activity interact with one another to provide *perceptual information* on the location, magnitude, and spatiotemporal properties of the noxious stimuli, *motivational tendency* toward escape or attack, *cognitive information* based on past experience, and probability of outcome of different response strategies. All three forms of activity could then influence motor mechanisms responsible for the complex pattern of overt responses that characterize pain.

Neuromatrix Theory

Melzack[28,29] has recently proposed a new conceptual model, based largely on the properties of phantom limbs, especially the pain that is often felt in them.[35] He summarized the available data on phantoms in the form of four propositions, which derive from the data:

1. The experience of a phantom limb has the quality of reality because it is produced by the same brain processes that underlie the experience of the body when it is intact.
2. Neural networks in the brain generate all the qualities of experience that are felt to originate in the body; inputs from the body may trigger or modulate the output of the networks but are not essential for any of the qualities of experience.
3. The experience of the body has a unitary, integrated quality which includes the quality of the "self"—that the body is uniquely one's own and not that of any other individual.
4. The neural network that underlies the experience of the body-self is genetically determined but can be modified by sensory experience.

The anatomic substrate of the body-self, Melzack[28,29] proposes, is a network of neurons that extends throughout widespread areas of the brain. He has labeled the network, whose spatial distribution and synaptic links are initially determined genetically, and are later sculpted by sensory inputs, as a *"neuromatrix."* Thalamocortical and limbic loops that comprise the neuromatrix diverge to permit parallel processing in different components of the neuromatrix and converge repeatedly to permit interactions between the output products of processing. The repeated cyclical processing and synthesis of nerve impulses in the neuromatrix imparts a characteristic pattern or *"neurosignature."*

The neurosignature of the neuromatrix is imparted on all nerve impulse patterns that flow through it; the neurosignature is produced by the patterns of synaptic connections, which are initially innate and then modified by experience, in the entire neuromatrix. All inputs from the body undergo cyclical processing and synthesis so that characteristic patterns are impressed on them in the neuromatrix. Portions of the neuromatrix are assumed to be specialized to process information related to major sensory events (such as injury) and may be labeled as neuromodules, which impress subsignatures on the larger neurosignature.

About 70% of amputees suffer burning, cramping, and other qualities of pain in the first few weeks after amputation. Even 7 years after amputation, 50% still continue to suffer phantom limb pain.[17] Why is there so much pain in phantom limbs? Melzack[28] proposes that the active neuromatrix, when deprived of modulating inputs from the limbs or body, produces an abnormal signature pattern that subserves the psychological qualities of hot or burning, the most common qualities of phantom limb pain. Cramping pain, however, may be due to messages from the neuromatrix to produce movement. In the absence of the limbs, the messages to move the muscles may become more frequent and "stronger" in the attempt to move a part of the limb. The end result of the output message may be felt as cramping muscle pain. Shooting pains may have a similar origin, in which the neuromatrix attempts to move the whole limb and sends out abnormal patterns that are felt as pain shooting down from the groin to the foot. The origins of these pains, then, lie in the brain. Sensory inputs, however, clearly contribute to the phantom; stimulation of the stump or other body sites often produces sensations referred to the phantom limb.[16]

Surgical removal of the somatosensory areas of the cortex or thalamus generally fails to relieve phantom limb pain.[60] However, the new theory conceives of a neuromatrix that extends throughout selective areas of the whole brain, including the somatic, visual, and limbic systems. Thus, to destroy the neuromatrix for the body-self which generates the neurosignature pattern for pain is impossible. However, if the pattern for pain is generated by cyclical processing and synthesis, it should be possible to block it by injection of a local anesthetic into appropriate discrete areas that are hypothesized to comprise the widespread neuromatrix. Data obtained in rats have shown that localized injections of lidocaine into diverse areas, such as the lateral hypothalamus,[55] the cingulum,[57] and the dentate gyrus,[24] produce striking decreases in experimentally produced pain, including the pain in an animal model of phantom limb pain.[58]

The neuromatrix model has important clinical implications since it searches for brain mechanisms as the causes of pain rather than focusing exclusively on peripheral factors. The fact that the most common kinds of pain—low-back pain and headache (including migraines)—remain a mystery is testimony to the extent of our ignorance. In the case of low-back pain, the majority of patients who suffer this pain have no apparent physical signs. A variety of forms of therapy are tried, including disk surgery, trigger-point injections, physical therapy, and behavior modification techniques. Yet a substantial number of people continue to suffer pain in spite of all these efforts. The search for the causes of low-back pain is usually focused on the periphery: protruding discs, arthritis, pinched sensory roots, stress on ligaments and joints, spasm in muscles. Given the relatively high frequency of failures in the attempt to rectify possible peripheral causes, it is reasonable to begin considering central mechanisms, such as a neuromatrix responsible for the body's actions.

Because the action neuromatrix maintains specific tensions on all muscles at all times, it is possible that sudden minor accidents (such as a fall) may produce stresses and strains on muscles in a localized part of the body, which then send abnormal messages to the body neuromatrix. The action neuromatrix, in order to maintain posture and balance, may then change the tension on more distant muscles and ultimately produce a vicious cycle of abnormal feedback and output for action.

A brief abnormal message, therefore, may produce a prolonged state of abnormal central outflow. The traditional trigger-point and physical therapies could produce changes in inputs which sometimes help, but the major cause may be the abnormal messages from the brain that maintain abnormal tensions on a large part of the body musculature. In the attempt to correct the inappropriate feedback, excessive tension may be put on other, distant muscles to maintain balance and readiness for action. In this way, minor momentary injury of a shoulder may, for example, lead to pain in the upper back and the other shoulder, and eventually in the lower back and legs. In this case, the therapy that is needed may be far more complex, involving the "re-education" of the musculature of a large part of the body in the attempt to adjust the tension on muscles to their normal, appropriate levels.

Myofascial syndromes such as fibrositis also remain a mystery and are difficult to understand. It is well known that fibrositis (which also has many other names) is associated with a characteristic distribution of trigger spots and sleep disorder, and is usually found in tense, hard-working, younger people. Here again, the initiating cause may be peripheral (muscle tension), but the sustaining cause that maintains abnormal tension is now central. The underlying mechanism is usually sought in long-term activities in the spinal cord, but the cause may, in fact, be in the brain, and an abnormal output thus maintains an abnormal pattern of tension on musculature throughout a widespread portion of the body. Once again, therapy may require re-education of the muscles of a large part of the body. Obviously, there are many inputs to the action neuromatrix that may maintain the abnormal activity—such as abnormal muscle feedback, anxiety, depression, and fatigue. All of these provide further avenues for health professionals to attempt to bring about a normal action-neuromatrix output.

MEASUREMENT OF PAIN

Psychophysical Approaches

Until recently, the methods used for pain measurement treated pain as though it were a single, unique quality that varied only in intensity.[1] The most common of these methods is the use of words such as "mild," "moderate," and "severe," and subjects (or patients) are asked to choose the word that best describes the intensity of their pain. Another method consists of a five-point scale that ranges from 1 (mild pain) to 5 (unbearable pain), and subjects are asked to choose the most appropriate number. In this way, some quantitative measure of pain is obtained. Still another method is the use of fractions; subjects who have received injections of analgesic drugs such as morphine are asked whether their pain is a third or a half of what it was before the injection. Yet another method is the "visual analogue scale."[49] The patient or subject is presented with a line 10 cm long and is told that one end represents no pain and the other represents the worst pain imaginable. He is then asked to make a mark on the line that represents the intensity of his pain. A ruler is then used to get a numeric measure of pain intensity such as 7 cm, or units, of pain intensity. These simple methods have all been used effectively in hospital clinics and have provided valuable information about pain and analgesia.

All of these methods specify only intensity. It is now clear, however, that the word "pain" refers to an endless variety of qualities that are categorized under a single linguistic label, not to a specific, single sensation that varies only in intensity. Each pain has unique qualities. The pain of a toothache is obviously different from that of a pinprick, just as the pain of a coronary occlusion is uniquely different from that of a broken leg.

The McGill Pain Questionnaire

Melzack and Torgerson[38] have made a start toward specifying the qualities of pain. In the first part of their study, subjects were asked to classify 102 words, obtained from the clinical literature relating to pain, into smaller groups that describe different aspects of the experience of pain. On the basis of the data, the words are categorized into three major classes and 16 subclasses. The major classes are (i) words that describe the *sensory qualities* of the experience in terms of temporal, spatial, pressure, thermal, and other properties; (ii) words that describe *affective qualities,* in terms of tension, fear, and autonomic properties that are part of the pain experience; and (iii) *evaluative* words that describe the subjective overall intensity of the total pain experience. Each subclass, which was given a descriptive label, consists of a group of words that were considered by most subjects to be qualitatively similar.

The second part of the study was an attempt to determine the pain intensities implied by the words within each subclass. Groups of doctors, patients, and students were asked to assign an intensity value to each word, using a numeric scale ranging from least (or mild) pain to worst (or excruciating) pain. When this was done, it was apparent that several words within each subclass had the same relative intensity relationships in all three sets. For example, in the spatial subclass, "shooting" was found to represent more pain than "flashing," which in turn implied more pain than "jumping." Although the precise intensity values differed for the three groups, all three agreed on the positions of the words relative to each other.

Because of the high degree of agreement on the intensity relationships among pain descriptors by subjects who have different cultural, socioeconomic, and educational backgrounds, it has been possible to develop a questionnaire (Fig. 25-3) for use as a measuring instrument in studies of clinical pain.[25,27,56]

One of the most exciting features of the McGill Pain Questionnaire (MPQ) is its potential value as a diagnostic technique.[6] The questionnaire was administered to 95 patients suffering from one of eight known pain syndromes: postherpetic neuralgia, phantom limb pain, metastatic carcinoma, toothache, degenerative disk disease, rheumatoid arthritis or osteoarthritis, labor pain, and menstrual pain. A multiple group discriminant analysis revealed that each type of pain is characterized by a distinctive constellation of verbal descriptors. Further, when the descriptor set for each patient was classified by the computer program into one of the eight diagnostic categories, a correct classification was made in 77% of cases. It is evident, then, that there are appreciable and quantifiable differences in the way various types of pain are described, and that patients with the same disease or pain syndrome tend to use remarkably similar words to communicate what they feel.

Worker's Compensation and Pain

Patients who receive worker's compensation or are awaiting litigation after an accident have long been regarded as neurotics or malingerers who are exaggerating their pain for financial gain. There is, however, a growing body of evidence, based on pain measurement, that patients who receive worker's compensation are no different from patients who do not. In particular, a recent study[43] found no differences between compensated and noncompensated patients based on pain scores obtained with the MPQ. A subsequent study of 145 patients suffering low-back and musculoskeletal pain also revealed that compensated and noncompensated patients had virtually identical sensory and total pain scores and pain descriptor patterns.[33] They were also similar on the Minnesota Multiphase Personality Inventory (MMPI) pain

McGill Pain Questionnaire

Patient's Name ______________ Date ________ Time ______ am/pm

PRI: S ______ (1-10) A ______ (11-15) E ______ (16) M ______ (17-20) PRI(T) ______ (1-20) PPI ______

1 FLICKERING __ QUIVERING __ PULSING __ THROBBING __ BEATING __ POUNDING __	11 TIRING __ EXHAUSTING __
2 JUMPING __ FLASHING __ SHOOTING __	12 SICKENING __ SUFFOCATING __
3 PRICKING __ BORING __ DRILLING __ STABBING __ LANCINATING __	13 FEARFUL __ FRIGHTFUL __ TERRIFYING __
4 SHARP __ CUTTING __ LACERATING __	14 PUNISHING __ GRUELLING __ CRUEL __ VICIOUS __ KILLING __
5 PINCHING __ PRESSING __ GNAWING __ CRAMPING __ CRUSHING __	15 WRETCHED __ BLINDING __
6 TUGGING __ PULLING __ WRENCHING __	16 ANNOYING __ TROUBLESOME __ MISERABLE __ INTENSE __ UNBEARABLE __
7 HOT __ BURNING __ SCALDING __ SEARING __	17 SPREADING __ RADIATING __ PENETRATING __ PIERCING __
8 TINGLING __ ITCHY __ SMARTING __ STINGING __	18 TIGHT __ NUMB __ DRAWING __ SQUEEZING __ TEARING __
9 DULL __ SORE __ HURTING __ ACHING __ HEAVY __	19 COOL __ COLD __ FREEZING __
10 TENDER __ TAUT __ RASPING __ SPLITTING __	20 NAGGING __ NAUSEATING __ AGONIZING __ DREADFUL __ TORTURING __
	PPI 0 NO PAIN __ 1 MILD __ 2 DISCOMFORTING __ 3 DISTRESSING __ 4 HORRIBLE __ 5 EXCRUCIATING __

BRIEF __	RHYTHMIC __	CONTINUOUS __
MOMENTARY __	PERIODIC __	STEADY __
TRANSIENT __	INTERMITTENT __	CONSTANT __

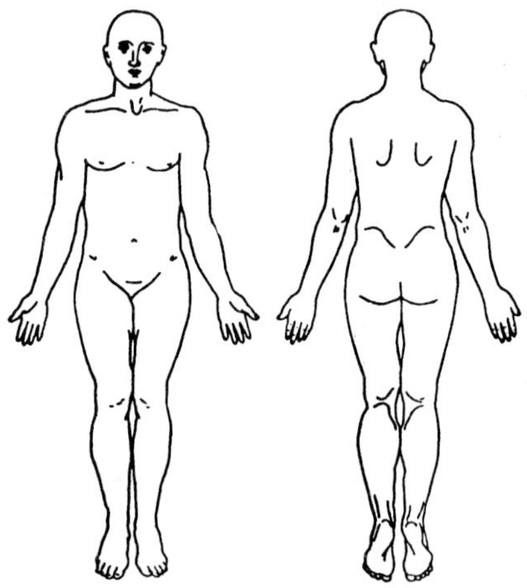

E = EXTERNAL

I = INTERNAL

COMMENTS:

FIG. 25-3. McGill Pain Questionnaire,[25] adapted for a study of narcotic drugs. Descriptors fall into four major groups: sensory, 1 to 10; affective, 11 to 15; evaluative, 16; and miscellaneous, 17 to 20. The rank value for each descriptor is based on its position in the word set. The sum of the rank values is the "pain rating index" *(PRI)*. The "present pain intensity" *(PPI)* is based on a scale of 0 to 5.

triad (depression, hysteria, hypochondriasis) and on several other personal variables that were examined. The only differences were small but significantly lower affective scores in the low-back group and lower evaluative scores in the musculoskeletal group. These results suggest that the financial security provided by compensation decreases anxiety, which is reflected in the lower affective or evaluative ratings but not in the sensory or total MPQ scores. Compensated patients, contrary to traditional opinion, appear not to differ from people who do not receive compensation. Accidents that produce injury and pain should be considered as potentially psychologically traumatic as well as conducive to the development of subtle physiologic changes such as trigger points. Patients on compensation or awaiting litigation deserve the same concern and compassion as all other patients who suffer chronic pain. It is prejudice, not evidence, that underlies the old idea of "the compensation neurotic" and adds insult to the patient's injury.

LABOR PAIN

Labor pain provides an excellent model of acute pain. It is associated with obvious sensory events—uterine contractions and cervical dilation—which can be measured in terms of frequency, intensity, spatial extent, and duration. It begins with contractions and ends with the birth of a baby. Labor pain, then, has a specifiable beginning and end, and should reflect all the variables that contribute to other acute pains. As do all pains, labor pain shows an astonishingly high degree of variability among individuals in its intensity and its spatial and temporal distribution.[26] This variability allows us to search for the underlying determinants and their contributions to the overall acute pain.

Most women suffer intense pain during labor. In a study of women in the first stage of labor at the Montreal General Hospital,[37] using the MPQ, 60% of primiparas had severe or extremely severe pain, 30% had moderate pain, and only 10% had mild pain. Among multiparas, 45% had severe or extremely severe pain, 30% had moderate pain, and 25% had mild pain. Figure 25-4 shows a comparison of labor pain intensities in relation to different kinds of chronic and acute pain. High pain intensities were also found among Scottish women,[45] who are well known for their stoicism; 60% of them reported that labor pain was the most intense pain they had ever experienced.

Although the average labor pain intensity is high, the variability of pain scores is remarkable. While some women had horrendous pain, others had virtually none. There is some evidence[47] that the latter group of women may generally be less sensitive to all kinds of pain. There is also great individ-

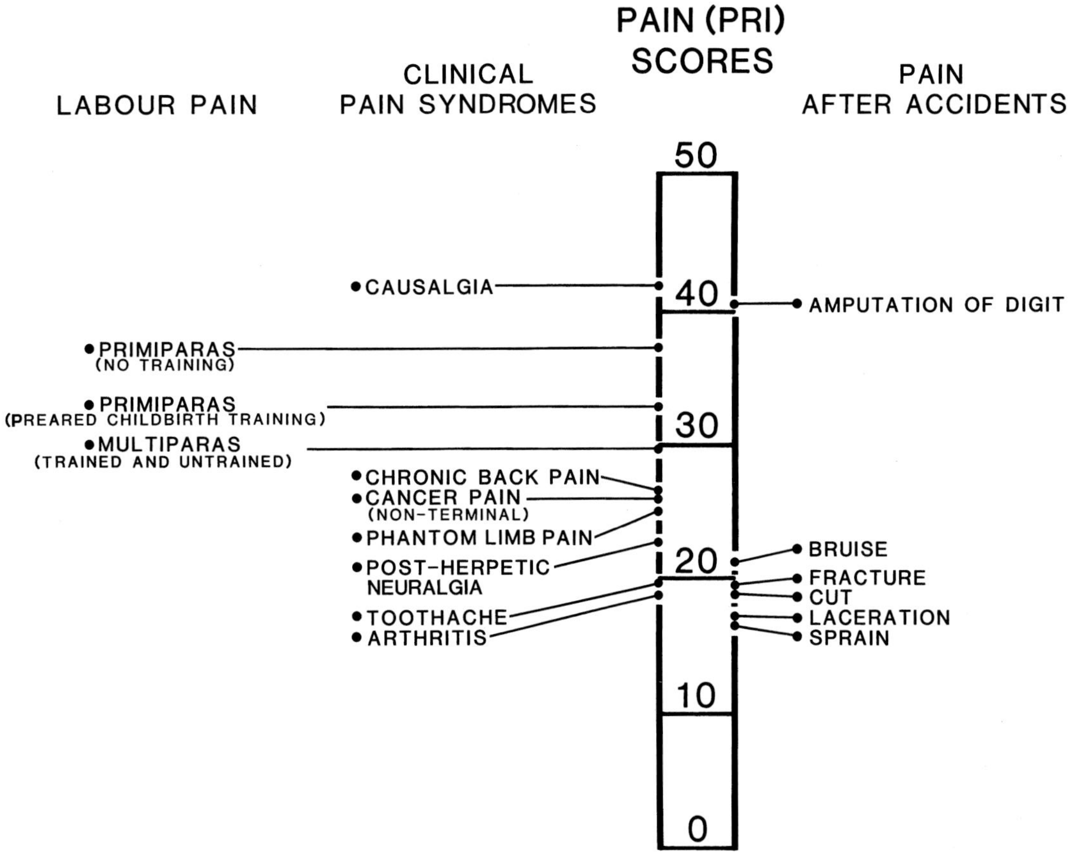

FIG. 25-4. Comparison of pain scores, using the McGill Pain Questionnaire, obtained from women during labor[37] and from patients in a general hospital pain clinic[25] and an emergency department.[41] The pain score for causalgic pain is reported by Tahmoush.[54]

ual variability among women in the spatial distribution of pain in the abdomen, sides, and back.[34]

Several important variables correlate with labor pain.[34,37] The major determinant is parity; primiparous women have more pain than multiparas. Another determinant is prepared childbirth training, which produces a small (about 10%), statistically significant reduction in both the sensory and affective dimensions of pain. Average pain reductions, depending on the trainer, ranged from 0% to 30%. In addition, older women had less pain than younger women, and women of higher socioeconomic status had less pain than women of lower socioeconomic status. Another determinant is the fact that women who have more painful menstrual periods also have higher levels of labor pain. It is possible that some women produce higher levels of prostaglandins during both menstrual cramps and labor contractions.

Physical factors also play a role.[34] Among multiparas, the more the baby weighs, the more pain the mother has, and heavier mothers also tend to have more pain. The pain of primparas is related to their normal weight/height ratio, that is, women who weigh more per unit of height have more pain.

Yet another determinant is the time of day when the baby is born. Harkness and Gijsbers[12] found that most women tend to give birth at night and, moreover, have significantly less pain and stress than women who give birth during daylight hours. Previous experience of pain unrelated to labor also diminishes labor pain,[46] presumably due to the opportunity to develop coping strategies.

Low-back pain during labor has recently been the subject of a series of studies. Severe, continuous low-back pain is reported by about 33% of women during labor.[36] It is described as being qualitatively different from the pains associated with uterine contractions. The pain of contractions felt in the back is often reported as "riding on" the continuous low-back pain, so that both together may reach "horrible" or "excruciating" intensities. Continuous low-back pain is probably caused by the distention and pressure on adjacent visceral and neural structures in the peritoneum, in contrast to the rhythmic pains that are clearly related to contractions of the uterus. It is possible that each of these major kinds of pain may be controlled by different anesthesiologic and psychological procedures.

A further study[30] attempted to determine whether episodes of acute low-back pain prior to pregnancy is a predictor of low-back pain during labor. The results show that episodic low-back pain before pregnancy is not correlated with any aspect of labor pain. However, it is significantly correlated with episodes of low-back pain during pregnancy. In contrast, low-back pain during menstruation is postively correlated with labor pain scores recorded for back and front contraction pain as well as for continuous back pain. The significant correlation of labor pain with back pain during menstruation suggests that both share a common underlying mechanism. The correlation of low-back pain during pregnancy with episodes of acute low-back pain before pregnancy suggests that the strain on back muscles during pregnancy may activate the mechanisms that underlie the usual forms of low-back pain.

Finally, an experiment[31] was carried out to determine whether women in labor report less pain when they are in a vertical (sitting or standing) position than in a horizontal (side-lying or supine) position. Pain scores were obtained from 60 women in early labor (dilation 2 to 5 cm) who alternated between the two positions. The results show that about 35% of women feel less front pain and 50% feel less back pain when they are in a vertical position than in a horizontal position. The amount of decrease in continuous back pain (83%) was particularly impressive, but the front and back pains associated with contractions were significantly diminished as well. These results, together with observations by Roberts et al.,[48] indicate that many women in *early labor* have less pain and are generally more comfortable in a vertical than in a horizontal position. Since early labor comprises a substantial proportion of the entire process of labor and delivery, any simple procedure that alleviates pain without danger to mother or child, such as shifting from a horizontal to a vertical position, should be promoted and employed. During the later stages of labor, however, women prefer to lie down rather than sit because it is more comfortable.[48]

Most of the studies described so far are based on data obtained with the MPQ administered during the first stage of labor. When women receive an MPQ after the birth, they report that the second stage is the most painful part of labor and reaches peak intensity at the emergence of the baby's head.[45]

Epidural blocks are usually administered during the first stage of labor at the request of the mother when the pain approaches intolerable levels. They are highly effective in about 90% of women.[27,34,37] However, the 10% of women who experience a failed epidural block are deeply dissappointed. In some of these cases, the epidural appears to be effective for the first hour or so, but then the pain returns at its previously high intensity or higher, sometimes with an unusual spatial distribution.[34] In one study,[34] the failure rate was about 30%, which is unusually high, and probably was due to the inexperience of incoming residents in anesthesiology. The variability of the effectiveness of anesthesiologists is as distressing as the variability of effectiveness of prepared childbirth trainers to women whose expectations of pain relief are unfulfilled.[21]

As a model of acute pain, labor pain highlights individual differences—extraordinary variability in every aspect of pain. Recent studies have revealed a multitude of factors, both psychological and physical, that contribute to the variability of labor pain. Each makes a small contribution, but no single one of them is prepotent in its contribution to pain. Therefore, the relief of labor pain requires multiple convergent approaches.[40]

It is clear that prepared childbirth training does not produce the large, dramatic effects promised by many of its proponents and by best-selling books with titles like "Painless Childbirth."[18] The intensity of the feelings of guilt, anger, and failure in some women when they anticipate a "natural, painless birth" and are then confronted with such severe pain or complications that they require an epidural or a cesarean section recently has been documented. Stewart[53] reports that some women may become miserable and depressed (even suicidal), may lose interest in sex and in their marriage, and may require psychotherapy. In some cases, the husbands of women who anticipated "natural" births required psychotherapy after intense feelings of nausea at the sight of blood or seeing their wives in such terrible pain. They experienced a profound sense of guilt and helplessness, and needed therapy for impotence, phobias, and depression.

It is now amply clear that there are no panaceas to abolish labor pain. The Dick-Read[5] and Lamaze[18] procedures have limited effectiveness. The Leboyer method to prevent a "violent birth" has no demonstrable effects,[44] and the concept of "early bonding" has fallen by the wayside.[2] The recent enthusiasm for birthing chairs has also begun to wane in light of convincing evidence that women in the later stages of labor actually prefer to lie down rather than sit because it is more comfortable.[48] Even epidural blocks may fail, forcing women to cope with deep disappointment in addition to pain.

The enormous individual differences in every parameter described above lead to the same conclusion reached by Lumley and Astbury: it is absurd to treat all women and all labors in the same way.[21] Women should be informed that the "average" labor is a statistical concept and many women will have patterns of pain that deviate from this concept. In short, any prepared childbirth training course should spend considerable time preparing the prospective mother for possible deviations from the "average"—preparing her for the possibility that she may (or may not) need an epidural block, a forceps delivery, or a cesarean section. Prepared childbirth training and *skillfully* administered epidural analgesia are compatible, complementary procedures that allow recognition of the individuality of each woman (see also Chapter 18).

REFERENCES

1. Beecher, H.K.: Measurement of Subjective Responses. New York, Oxford University Press, 1959.
2. Brody, J.E.: Influential theory of birth "bonding" losing supporters. New York Times, reprinted in The Gazette, Montreal, April 2, 1983.
3. Carlen, P.L., Wall, P.D., Nadvorna, H., and Steinbach, T.: Phantom limbs and related phenomena in recent traumatic amputations. Neurology, *28:*211, 1978.
4. Clark, W.C., and Clark, S.B.: Pain responses in Nepalese porters. Science, *209:*410, 1980.
5. Dick-Read, G.: Childbirth Without Fear. New York, Harper, 1944.
6. Dubuisson, D., and Melzack, R.: Classification of clinical pain descriptions by multiple group discriminant analysis. Exp. Neurol., *51:*480, 1976.
7. Egbert, L.D., Battit, G.E., Welch, C.D., and Bartlett, M.K.: Reduction of post-operative pain by encouragement and instruction of patients. N. Engl. J. Med., *270:*825, 1964.
8. Evans, F.J.: The placebo response in pain reduction. *In* Bonica, J.J. (ed.): Advances in Neurology. Vol. 4. New York, Raven Press, 1974.

8a. McQuay, H., Carroll, D., and Moore, A.: Variation in the placebo effect in randomised controlled trials of analgesics: All is as blind as it seems. Pain, *64:*331, 1995.

9. Gardner, W.J., and Licklider, J.C.R.: Auditory analgesia in dental operations. J. Am. Dent. Assn., *59:*1144, 1959.
10. Hall, K.R.L., and Stride, E.: The varying response to pain in psychiatric disorders: A study in abnormal psychology. Br. J. Med. Psychol., *27:*48, 1954.
11. Hardy, J.D., Wolff, H.G., and Goodell, H.: Pain Sensations and Reactions. Baltimore, Williams & Wilkins, 1952.
12. Harkness, J., and Gijsbers, K.: Pain and stress during childbirth and time of day. Ethol. Sociobiol., *10:*255, 1989.
13. Hilgard, E.R., and Hilgard, J.: Hypnosis in the Relief of Pain. Los Altos, CA, Kaufmann, 1975.
14. Hill, H.E., Kornetsky, C.H., Flanary, H.G., and Wikler, A.: Effects of anxiety and morphine on discrimination of intensities of painful stimuli. J. Clin. Invest., *31:*473, 1952a.
15. Hill, H.E., Kornetsky, C.H., Flanary, H.G., and Wikler, A.: Studies of anxiety associated with anticipation of pain. I. Effects of morphine. Arch. Neurol. Psychiat., *67:*612, 1952b.
16. Katz, J., and Melzack, R.: Referred sensations in chronic pain patients. Pain, *28:*51, 1987.
17. Krebs, B., Jensen, T.S., Kroner, K., *et al.*: Phantom limb phenomena in amputees seven years after limb amputation. *In* Fields, H.L., Dubner, R., and Cervero, F. (eds.): Advances in Pain Research and Therapy. Vol. 9. New York, Raven Press, 1985.
18. Lamaze, F.: Painless Childbirth: Psychoprophylactic Method. Chicago, IL, Regnery, 1970.
19. Lambert, W.E., Libman, E., and Poser, E.G.: Effect of increased salience of membership group on pain tolerance. J. Pers., *28:*350, 1960.
20. Langer, E., Janis, I.L., and Wolfer, J.A.: Reduction of psychological stress in surgical patients. J. Exp. Soc. Psychol., *11:*155, 1975.
21. Lumley, J., and Astbury J.: Birth Rites, Birth Rights. Melbourne, Sphere Books, 1980.
22. Martinez-Urrutia, A.: Anxiety and pain in surgical patients. J. Consult. Clin. Psychol., *43:*437, 1975.
23. McGlashan, T.H., Evans, F.J., and Orne, M.T.: The nature of hypnotic analgesia and placebo response to experimental pain. Psychosom. Med., *31:*227, 1969.
24. McKenna, J.E., and Melzack, R.: Analgesia produced by lidocaine microinjection into the dentate gyrus. Pain, *49:*105, 1992.
25. Melzack, R.: The McGill Pain Questionnaire: Major properties and scoring methods. Pain, *1:*277, 1975.
26. Melzack, R.: The myth of painless childbirth. Pain, *19:*321, 1984.
27. Melzack, R.: The short-form McGill Pain Questionnaire. Pain, *30:*191, 1987.
28. Melzack, R.: Phantom limbs. Reg. Anesth., *14:*208, 1989.
29. Melzack, R.: The gate control theory 25 years later: New perspectives on phantom limb pain. *In* Bond, M.R., Charlton, J.E., and Woolf, C.J. (eds.): Proceedings of the 5th World Congress on Pain. Amsterdam, Elsevier, 1990.
30. Melzack, R., and Bélanger, E.: Labour pain: correlations with menstrual pain and acute low-back pain before and during pregnancy. Pain, *36:*225, 1989.
31. Melzack, R., Bélanger, E., and Lacroix, R.: Labor pain: Effect of maternal position on front and back pain. J. Pain Symptom Manage., *6:*476, 1991.
32. Melzack, R., and Casey, K.L.: Sensory, motivational, and central control determinants of pain: A new conceptual model. *In* Kenshalo, D. (ed.): The Skin Senses. Springfield, IL, Charles C. Thomas, 1968.
33. Melzack, R., Katz, J., and Jeans, M.E.: The role of compensation in chronic pain: Analysis using a new method of scoring the McGill Pain Questionnaire. Pain, *23:*101, 1985.
34. Melzack, R., Kinch, R., Dobkin, P., *et al.*: Severity of labour pain: Influence of physical as well as psychologic variables. Can. Med. Assoc. J., *130:*579, 1984.
35. Melzack, R., and Loeser, J.D.: Phantom body pain in paraplegics: Evidence for a central "pattern generating mechanism" for pain. Pain, *4:*195, 1978.
36. Melzack, R., and Schaffelberg, D.: Low-back pain during labor. Am. J. Obstet. Gyn., *156:*901, 1987.
37. Melzack, R., Taenzer, P., Feldman, P., and Kinch, R.A.: Labour is still painful after prepared childbirth training. Can. Med. Assoc. J., *125:*357, 1981.
38. Melzack, R., and Torgerson, W.S.: On the language of pain. Anesthesiology, *34:*50, 1962.
39. Melzack, R., and Wall, P.D.: Pain Mechanism: A new theory. Science, *150:*971, 1965.

40. Melzack, R., and Wall, P.D.: The Challenge of Pain. 3rd ed. New York, Penguin, 1988.
41. Melzack, R., Wall, P.D., and Ty, T.C.: Acute pain in an emergency clinic: Latency of onset and descriptor patterns. Pain, *14:*33, 1982.
42. Melzack, R., Weisz, A.Z., and Sprague, L.T.: Stratagems for controlling pain: Contributions of auditory stimulation and suggestion. Exp. Neurol., *8:*239, 1963.
43. Mendelson, G.: Chronic pain and compensation issues. *In* Wall, P.D., and Melzack, R. (eds.): Textbook of Pain. 3rd Ed. Edinburgh, Churchill Livingston, 1994.
44. Nelson, N.M., Enkin, M.W., Saigal, S., *et al.*: A randomized clinical trial of the Leboyer approach to childbirth, N. Engl. J. Med., *302:*655, 1980.
45. Niven, C., and Gijsbers, K.: Obstetric and non-obstetric factors related to pain. J. Reprod. Infant Psychol., *2:*61, 1984a.
46. Niven, C., and Gijsbers, K.: A study of labour pain using the McGill Pain Questionnaire. Soc. Sci. Med., *19:*1347, 1984b.
47. Niven, C., and Gijsbers, K.: Do low levels of labour pain reflect low sensitivity to noxious stimulation? Soc. Sci. Med., *29:*585, 1989.
48. Roberts, J., Melasanos, L., and Mendez-Bauer, C.: Maternal positions in labor: Analysis in relation to comfort and efficiency. Birth Defects (Orig. Art. Ser.) *17:*97, 1981.
49. Scott, J., and Huskisson, E.C.: Graphic representation of pain. Pain, *2:*175, 1979.
50. Sheehan, P.W., and Perry, C.W.: Methodologies of Hypnosis: A Critical Appraisal of Contemporary Paradigms of Hypnosis. Hillsdale, NJ, Erlbaum Associates, 1976.
51. Spanos, N.P., Carmanico, S.J., and Ellis, J.A.: Hypnotic analgesia. *In* Wall, P.D., and Melzack, R. (eds.): Textbook of Pain. 3rd ed. Edinburgh, Churchill Livingston, 1994.
52. Sternbach, R.A., and Tursky, B.: Ethnic differences among housewives in psychophysical and skin potential responses to electric shock. Psychophysiology, *1:*73, 1965.
53. Stewart, D.E.: Psychiatric symptoms following attempted natural childbirth, Can. Med. Assoc. J., *127:*713, 1982.
54. Tahmoush, A.J.: Causalgia: Redefinition as a clinical pain syndrome. Pain, *10:*187, 1981.
55. Tasker, R.A.R., Choinière, M., Libman, S.M., and Melzack, R.: Analgesia produced by injection of lidocaine into the lateral hypothalamus. Pain, *31:*237, 1987.
56. Turk, D.C., and Melzack, R.: Handbook of Pain Assessment. New York, Guilford, 1992.
57. Vaccarino, A.L., and Melzack, R.: Analgesia produced by injection of lidocaine into the anterior cingulum bundle of the rat. Pain, *39:*213, 1989.
58. Vaccarino, A.L., and Melzack, R.: The role of the cingulum bundle in self-mutilation following peripheral neurectomy in the rat. Exp. Neurol., *111:*131, 1991.
59. Wall, P.D.: The placebo and the placebo response. *In* Wall, P.D., and Melzack, R. (eds.): Textbook of Pain. 3rd ed. Edinburgh, Churchill Livingston, 1994.
60. White, J.C., and Sweet, W.H.: Pain and the Neurosurgeon. Springfield, IL, Charles C. Thomas, 1969.
61. Zborowski, M.: Cultural components in responses to pain. J. Soc. Issues, *8:*16, 1952.

Neural Blockade in Clinical Anesthesia and Management of Pain, Third Edition,
edited by M.J. Cousins and P.O. Bridenbaugh.
Lippincott–Raven Publishers, Philadelphia © 1998.

CHAPTER 26

Acute Pain Management and Acute Pain Services

Raymond S. Sinatra

Pain is among the most common of patient complaints encountered by health professionals, yet it remains poorly treated. Patients recovering from surgery, invasive medical procedures and major trauma, historically have experienced analgesic under-administration and inadequate pain relief. This chapter describes recent therapeutic breakthroughs, including the development of potent analgesics, more efficient methods of administration, and the introduction of dedicated care teams that have dramatically improved the safety and effectiveness of acute pain management.

THE UNDER TREATMENT OF ACUTE PAIN

The inadequacy of traditional pain management is a world-wide problem brought to the attention of the medical community by numerous editorials and review articles.[10,75,97,190,199,200,204,332] Compelling reasons to provide more effective relief come from the realization that more than 75% of patients treated with on-demand doses of narcotic may experience moderate to severe pain, and that the total dose of analgesic administered may be less than 25% of the amount ordered.[97,199] Similar findings have been reported in pediatric patients.[200,204]

Analgesic under-administration and the "benign neglect" that patients often experience have been related to a variety of factors, including a lack of formal education in pain management, mistaken beliefs, errors in pain assessment, misinterpretation of orders, and the traditional emphasis on "PRN" dosing.[10,39,66,73,75,192,199] Angell[10] noted that certain attitudes and misconceptions of health professionals and patients were responsible for ritualized and inadequate administration of analgesics. These misconceptions included: (i) the belief that pain intensity can be accurately assessed by observation alone; (ii) that analgesic dosage should be restricted and dosing interval prolonged, since risks of physical/psychological dependence and respiratory depression were more likely to have a negative impact upon patient outcome than poorly controlled pain. In this regard, analgesics are restricted and often denied to elderly and debilitated patients because of fears that such therapy may be blamed for complicating or worsening their clinical status. This is unfortunate, since these are often the very patients who have the most to gain from optimal pain relief. An article entitled "Paralyzed with Pain,"[192] highlighted educational deficiencies, including the fact that health professionals could not distinguish differences between opioid analgesics, neuromuscular blocking agents, or sedative hypnotics. Many physicians have little knowledge of opioid pharmacology and commonly underestimate effective dose ranges, while overestimating analgesic duration and potential for overdose.[75,192] In general, analgesic prescriptions are unrealistically low, while poorly written orders are commonly misinterpreted. The fact that nurses generally administer as little as 25% of the dose prescribed further compounds the problem.[75,97,192,199] Nurses frequently err when estimating pain intensity and overestimate analgesic effectiveness,[34,66,73,75,152] leading to the patient's accurate perception that pain medication was not administered in high-enough dose or as frequently as was required. A related factor responsible for undermedication has been the lack of formal assessment and documentation of pain intensity, pain relief, and the satisfaction patients experience with analgesic therapy.[34,79]

PATHOPHYSIOLOGY OF ACUTE PAIN

The International Association for the Study of Pain (IASP) defines pain as ". . . an unpleasant sensory and emotional experience, associated with actual or potential tissue

R.S. Sinatra: Department of Anesthesiology, Yale University School of Medicine, Acute Pain Management Service, Yale-New Haven Hospital, New Haven, Connecticut 06510.

damage or described in terms of such damage."[208] This definition applies to acute pain just as it does to chronic and cancer pain. Nociception reflects activation of nociceptors following thermal, mechanical or chemical injury, afferent transmission to the spinal cord dorsal horn, and relay to supraspinal centers for processing and reaction (see Chapters 23 and 24). Pain perception can be divided into two major components: (i) the sensory discriminative component, which describes the location and quality of the stimulus, is transmitted via myelinated A-delta fibers and relayed to the neothalamus and somatosensory cortex. This component quickly alerts the organism, resulting in prompt withdrawal from the noxious stimulus;[178,183,248] (ii) the affective-protopathic component is more slowly conducted via unmyelinated C fibers, and establishes numerous synaptic contacts within the brain stem, midbrain, and limbic system.[248] This more persistent component underlies the suffering and emotional aspects of pain and is responsible for learned avoidance and other behavioral responses.[177,183,248,343] While alerting and withdrawal behavior serve to limit further tissue injury and promote wound healing, subsequent physiological and emotional responses to poorly controlled pain are less desirable in post-surgical settings (see also Chapter 23.1, Figs. 23.1-18 and 23.1-19).

In addition to the ethical and humanitarian reasons for minimizing pain and suffering, there is the need to appreciate that pain-related anxiety, sleeplessness, and release of stress hormones and catecholamines may have deleterious effects upon postsurgical outcome. This is particularly true in elderly or critically ill populations.[22,38,40,41,51,115,167,168,322,343,352] The following physiological responses may increase pain intensity and associated morbidity following acute injury (see also Chapters 5, 23.1, and 23.2).

1. Peripheral sensitization describes neurohumoral alterations which mediate hyperalgesia; it is an altered state of sensibility in which the intensity of pain is increased following noxious stimulation. Following injury, a local reflex is established whereby bradykinin, prostaglandin, and substance P, sensitize nociceptors immediately adjacent to the site of tissue damage.[77,113,144,177,178,248] Sensitization of peripheral nerve endings results in a heightened inflammatory response, neurogenic edema, and hyperalgesia.[76,113,183] Primary hyperalgesia refers to changes occurring at the site of injury,[144,177,178,183,248] whereas secondary hyperalgesia describes enhanced sensitivity in surrounding, nontraumatized, regions.[177,178,248] The origins and elaboration of secondary hyperalgesia are complex and controversial, involving both peripheral sensitization and changes in the central nervous system (see also Chapter 23.1).[177,248,343,346]

2. Central facilitation (or sensitization) reflects the enhancement of synaptic transmission and nociceptive processing within the dorsal horn. Central facilitation is initiated by the action of neuropeptides and excitatory amino acids (EAA), such as aspartate and glutamate, upon neurokinin (NK), N-methyl-D-aspartate (NMDA) and alpha-amino-3-hydroxy-5-methyl-4-isoxazole propionic acid (AMPA) receptors.[343,344,350] Substance P promotes the release of EAAs and increases the responsiveness of dorsal horn wide dynamic range (WDR) neurons to NMDA.[198,343] The initial phase, termed "wind-up," is characterized by an immediate increase in WDR firing rate and associated behavioral responses, lasting about 5 minutes.[5,93,321] This is followed 15 to 20 minutes later by a second phase, termed "long-term potentiation," in which WDR neurons exhibit enhanced sensitivity for prolonged periods.[321,343,350] This second phase of excitability outlasts the initial barrage of sensory input, does not require further noxious stimulation to be maintained,[343,344,345] and is not antagonized by inhalational anesthetics.[5,345,350] Clinical manifestations associated with central facilitation include secondary hyperalgesia, the elaboration of ipsilateral and contralateral flexion reflexes (splinting), and alterations in regional sympathetic tone.[77,177,324] As a result, pain is perceived in dermatomes above and below the site of injury. This situation is worsened by ambulation or movement and leads to an increase in dynamic or effort dependent pain.

3. Sympathoadrenal activation. Plasma levels of epinephrine and norepinephrine rise during surgical manipulation and remain elevated postoperatively.[40,41,141] The magnitude and duration of this response is directly related to the extent of surgery. Pathophysiologic changes associated with increased sympathetic activity include the following: (i) perioperative ischemia: although this predictor of postsurgical cardiac morbidity may be provoked by hypothermia, anxiety, and tracheal intubation[122] tachycardia and other responses to poorly controlled pain represent important causal factors, particularly in patients with poorly compensated coronary artery disease;[22,40,41,64,109,122] (ii) hypertension: elevations in arterial pressure may increase risks of myocardial infarction and stroke, while vasospasm following peripheral vascular surgery may compromise distal graft patency;[40,41,67,117] (iii) altered perfusion: as blood flow is directed to high-priority organs, perfusion in injured tissues, adjacent musculature, and in the viscera may be diminished. Reductions in circulation have been associated with impaired wound healing, enhanced sensitization of nociceptors, muscle spasm, and visceral-somatic ischemia (see also Chapter 5).[41,77,100,169]

4. Neuroendocrine responses. Severe postsurgical pain may induce significant alterations in hypothalamic-adrenal function.[38,51,64,167,168] This stress response to injury is characterized by elevations in plasma levels of cortisol, glucagon, and epinephrine,[140,167–169] resulting in hyperglycemia and a negative nitrogen balance.[38,140,168] While providing the injured organism with short-term benefits of enhanced energy production, prolonged tissue catabolism may adversely affect post-surgical outcome.[38,100,167] Detailed descriptions of the sympathoadrenal and neuroendocrine response to pain are presented in Chapter 5.

5. Alteration in pulmonary function. Beecher[23] was first to describe pulmonary responses to abdominal surgery,

which included an increase in respiratory rate and diminutions in tidal volume (TV), vital capacity (VC), and forced expiratory volume in one second (FEV_1). The percentage reduction in VC and FEV_1 is highest in patients following upper abdominal and thoracic surgery and lowest in patients recovering from pelvic and extremity procedures.[8,23] Reductions in pulmonary function are the result of poorly controlled effort-dependent pain, reflex spasm of the chest wall and pleuritic irritation. Reductions in FEV_1 and functional residual capacity are most pronounced at 24 hours, and are associated with atelectasis and a reduced ability to cough and to clear secretions.[8,23,53,262] For these reasons, clinically significant hypoxia, hypocapnia (followed by *hyper*capnia), and pneumonia are common postoperative events, particularly in patients with underlying pulmonary disease, where the incidence of such morbidity approaches 70%.[8,53,262]

6. Deep Venous Thrombosis. Poorly controlled effort-dependent pain limits patient ambulation, ending in decreased venous return.[36,210,211] Catecholamines, angiotensin, and factors associated with surgical stress increase platelet adhesiveness and lead to a hypercoagulable state.[36,67,274,322] In addition, surgical manipulation in and around the pelvis may damage venous conduits, diminishing blood return from the lower extremity. This triad of venous stasis, hypercoagulability, and endothelial injury increases the risks of clot formation and deep venous thrombosis.

7. Persistent Pain. Humoral and neurologic alterations at the site of injury may be responsible for increased postoperative discomfort, acute pain disability, and impaired rehabilitation.[77,324,331] Continued sensitization of nociceptors secondary to compression, inflammation, infection, and hematoma may lead to a progressive increase in pain intensity. Muscular, peritoneal, and periosteal irritation may incite reflex muscle spasm and myofascial pain.[76,324] Prolonged nociceptor sensitization has also been related to heightened sympathetic tone and vasoconstriction.[75,343] These alterations may underlie sympathetically maintained pain and persistent pain syndromes.[75,324,343] Physiologic responses to poorly controlled pain are outlined in Figure 26-1 (see also Chapter 23.1, Figs. 23.1-1 to 23.1-16).

Deficiencies Associated with Traditional Analgesic Delivery

On-demand (PRN) administration of intramuscular analgesics represents a simple, inexpensive, and widely employed method of controlling acute pain, however several deficiencies limit its clinical usefulness.[97,111,130,192,199,209,229] Delays in analgesic dosing are common with on-demand regimens, since patients often wait too long to request pain relief and staff may not be able to deliver medication immediately. In a survey of patients receiving intramuscular (IM) narcotics following surgery, the majority expected moderate to severe pain and indicated that they would wait as long as possible before requesting analgesics.[111,229] Un-

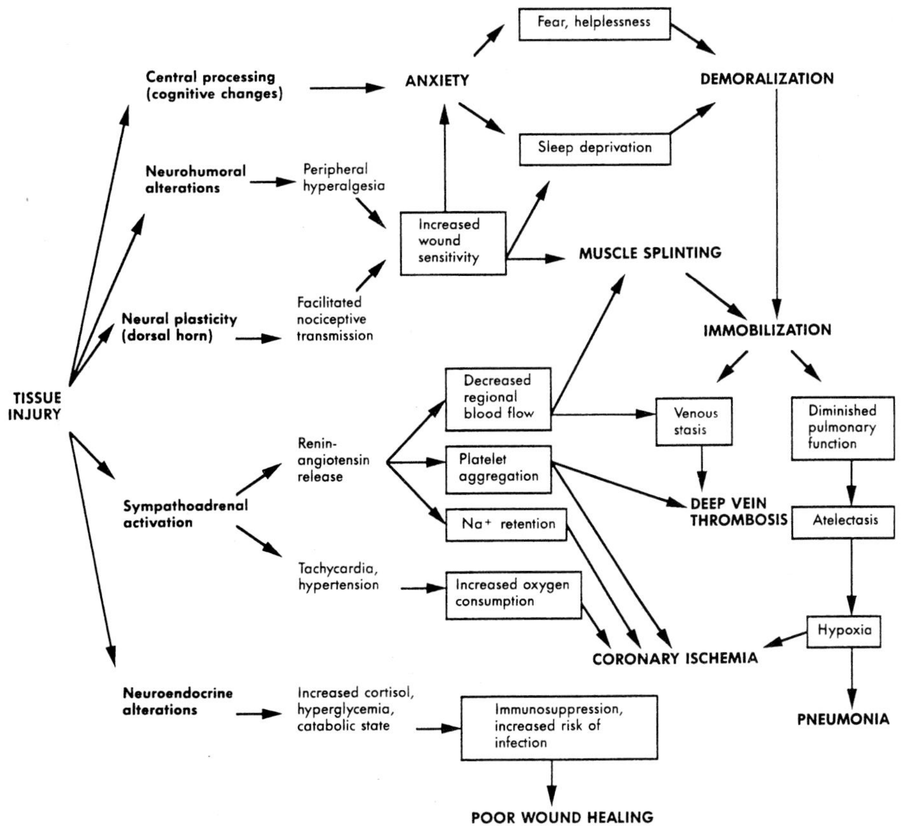

FIG. 26-1. Outline of physiological responses associated with surgical trauma and their impact upon key target organs. [Reproduced with permission from Sinatra, R.S.: The pathophysiology of acute pain. *In* Sinatra, R.S., Hord, A.H., Ginsberg, B., and Preble, L.M. (eds.): Acute Pain Mechanisms and Management. St. Louis, Mosby–Year Book, 1992.]

fortunately, more than 75% expected that pain medication would be delivered immediately upon request, a highly unrealistic expectation on busy postsurgical wards.[229]

A second problem associated with PRN dosing is its inability to maintain therapeutic plasma concentrations. While most physicians are comfortable with the ease and simplicity of PRN and by-the-clock regimens, analgesic onset is often delayed, and effectiveness may be unpredictable. When IM analgesics are administered every 3 to 4 hours, concentrations in plasma may equal or exceed minimal effective analgesic concentration (MEAC) only 30% of this time interval.[14,15,130] Moreover, individual differences between peak plasma concentrations vary 3 to 5 fold, and time to peak activity, 7 to 10 fold.[14,15,130,324] It is apparent that a number of pharmacokinetic variables, site and extent of injury, and coping skills must be accounted for in the algorithm of providing adequate analgesia.[14,15,317,318]

Traditional PRN Q 3 to 4-hour dosing involves an elaborate sequence of events which inevitably delays administration by at least 30 minutes to an hour and results in repetitive cycles of increasing pain [112,130] (Fig. 26-2). Because pain may not be considered an emergency, the length of time patients wait for analgesic is dependent upon the nursing workload at the time of the request. In general, the amount administered is related directly to the number of nurses on duty.[73,130,199] Once the nurse has responded, he or she usually screens the complaint to assess whether the patient really needs additional pain medication. Despite published research indicating that physical dependence occurs in fewer than 0.1% of hospitalized patients, this screening is done presumably in order to avoid opioid abuse.[73,192,199,200,209] When the level of pain is deemed significant to warrant treatment, a long sequence of events occurs before the patient actually achieves relief. The nurse must sign out the medication, prepare an injection, and administer the dose. The drug must then be absorbed from the IM or subcutaneous (SC) site of administration and activate central nervous system (CNS) receptor sites. These steps delay the onset of effective relief and worsen pain induced anxiety, helplessness, and sleep deprivation. Since the dose administered is relatively large and absorption is erratic and prolonged, the initial analgesic effect is often followed by sedation and some degree of respiratory depression.[130]

Recognition of the Problem

Given the fact that nearly 25,000,000 surgeries are performed annually in the United States, and that most require some form of pain management, the Department of Health and Human Services in 1992 introduced the Clinical Practice Guideline entitled "Acute Pain Management: Operative or Medical Procedures and Trauma."[61,155] This initial monograph, and others which followed,[203,257] focused attention upon the under-medication of pain and benefits associated with optimal control. The guidelines' major goals were to: (i) reduce the severity of acute postoperative or post-traumatic pain in both adult and pediatric populations; (ii) introduce more effective methods of providing pain relief; (iii) educate patients to understand that marked increases in pain intensity should not be tolerated, and educate caregivers about the importance of prompt evaluation and treatment; (iv) contribute to fewer complications, improved outcome, and shortened hospital stay. The guidelines emphasized that pain management should be considered an essential part of the physicians' commitment to patient care, and recommended an organized, individualized approach to pain control, with clear lines of responsibility, frequent reassessment of patient comfort, and use of pharmacological and nondrug therapies. Governmental recognition of the problem was followed quickly by reviews in the medical and lay press, which reshaped attitudes about, and expectations of, acute pain control.

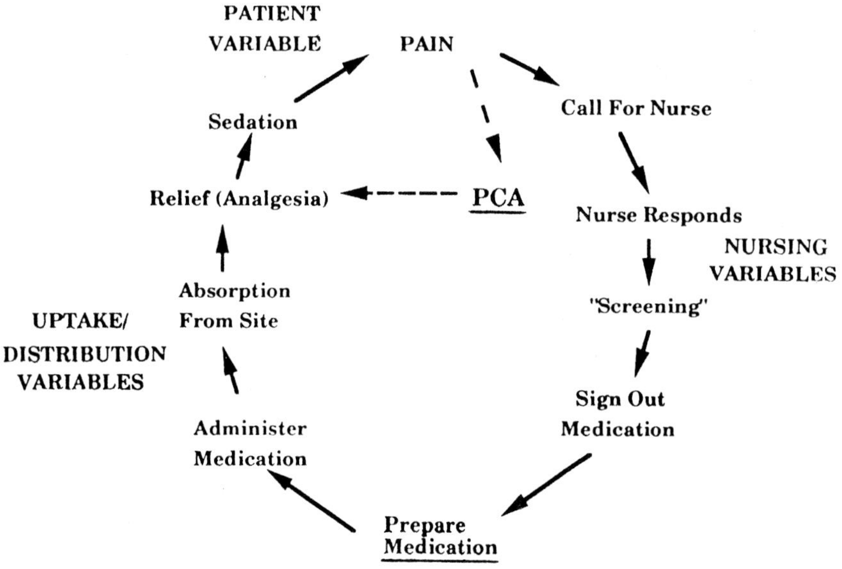

FIG. 26-2. The postoperative pain cycle associated with intramuscular PRN doses of opioid analgesics. Patient-controlled delivery avoids nursing and absorption variables, thereby eliminating the cycle. (Modified from Graves, D., Foster A., Batenhorst, R.L., and Bennett, R.L.: Patient-controlled analgesia. Ann. Intern. Med., *99*:360, 1983.)

UNIT NO.
NAME
ADDRESS

DEPARTMENT OF ANESTHESIOLOGY – PAIN SERVICE CONSULT 161401

LOCATION	PRIMARY PHYSICIAN/REFERRING SURGEON (First and Last Name)				ATTENDING ANESTHESIOLOGIST	
CRNA OR RESIDENT	AGE (YR-MO)	HT.	WT.	ASA	SURGICAL SVC	SEX
DATE OF O.R.:	O.R. ATTENDING ANESTHESIOLOGIST:				DATE OF INITIAL SERVICE:	
DIAGNOSIS/PROCEDURE		EPIDURAL / SPINAL PRIMARY ANESTHETIC ☐ YES ☐ NO			PAIN LOCATION	DIAGNOSIS #

PLAN:
The patient will receive: ☐ **PCA** ☐ **Caudal** ☐ **Epidural** ☐Lumbar ______ ☐Thoracic ______ ☐ **Spinal** ☐ **Regional** ______ ☐ **Consult**

Drug and dosage ______

Patient Clinical Information ______

Medications ______

Allergies ______

24 hour total					
Side Effects Rx					
VAS Rest Movement					
VAS Sat					

Acute Pain #10-55 ☐ Commercial ☐ BC/BS ☐ Medicare ☐ Medicaid ☐ MD Health ☐ PHS

INSURANCE BILLING	*Day 1* ______	*Day 2* ______	*Day 3* ______	*Day 4* ______	*Day 5* ______
	☐ Insert ☐ Mgmt ☐ Re-Insert	☐ Insert ☐ Mgmt ☐ Re-Insert	☐ Insert ☐ Mgmt ☐ Re-Insert	☐ Insert ☐ Mgmt ☐ Re-Insert	☐ Insert ☐ Mgmt ☐ Re-Insert
Cont. Infusions	Epidural ☐	Epidural ☐	Epidural ☐	Epidural ☐	Epidural ☐
Cont. Infusions-Peds	Caudal ☐	Caudal ☐	Caudal ☐	Caudal ☐	Caudal ☐
Continuous Therapy	Regional block ☐	Regional block ☐	Regional block ☐	Regional block ☐	Regional block ☐
Single Dose Therapy	Spinals F/U ☐	Caudals F/U ☐	Epidurals F/U ☐		
Therapy (IV)	PCA ☐	PCA ☐	PCA ☐	PCA ☐	PCA ☐
Consultation ☐	**Other:**				

FIG. 26-3. Standardized pain service consultation form used at Yale-New Haven Hospital.

Development of Dedicated Acute Pain Services

During the last 10 to 15 years, new treatment protocols and more effective methods of drug administration have made optimal pain control and high patient satisfaction a realistic goal in most circumstances. In an effort to ensure further safety and analgesic efficacy, responsibility for drug administration was assigned to interested, highly-trained specialists.[247] These professionals selected the techniques that would be offered and acquired the manpower, certification, and funds to support them.[247,260,279] In their pioneering report which described an anesthesiology-based pain service, Ready and co-workers[260] listed a variety of reasons why this therapist group was prepared to assume a leadership role in management of acute pain: Anesthesiologists have extensive knowledge of pain physiology, analgesic pharmacology, and the anatomic pathways involved in pain transmission and modulation. They routinely provide pain control in the operating theatre, obstetrical wards, and in the chronic pain clinic, and have expertise with regional nerve blockade, and epidural administration of analgesics. Other factors adding to their appropriateness in this role include familiarity with the electromechanical devices used for monitoring and therapy, and ability to interact effectively with primary care providers.[247,260,279] Finally, the report said, anesthesiologists tend to be goal-oriented consultants, who appreciate the importance of minimizing patient discomfort and pain-related morbidity. While the opportunity to manage postsurgical pain was gained largely by default, it has gradually become the natural extension in time and scope of the anesthesiologist's perioperative responsibility.[149,150,247,260,279] In the United States, the vast majority of acute pain services, in academic centers and larger community hospitals, have been developed and are directed by departments of anesthesiology.[255,256] Similar responsibility for acute pain management is evident in major teaching and public hospitals in Canada, Australia, and New Zealand.[255]

YALE-NEW HAVEN HOSPITAL

DOCTOR'S ORDERS

PLEASE USE BALL POINT PEN – BEAR DOWN

INSTRUCTIONS

1. EACH TIME A PHYSICIAN WRITES A MEDICATION ORDER, DETACH TOP COPY AND SEND TO PHARMACY
2. RULE OFF UNUSED LINES AFTER LAST COPY (PINK) HAS BEEN SENT TO PHARMACY. IMPRINT NEW SET AND PLACE IN CHART.

DO NOT USE THIS SHEET UNLESS A NUMBER SHOWS ▶ 3

DATE	TIME	ORDERS	DOCTOR'S SIGNATURE	NURSE'S SIGNATURE
		ACUTE PAIN SERVICE/DEPARTMENT OF ANESTHESIOLOGY		
		CONTINUOUS EPIDURAL/INTRATHECAL INFUSION ORDERS		
	1.	INFUSION: Drug(s) and concentration(s) ___ rate: ___ cc/hr		
	2.	HEAD OF BED greater than ___ degrees. ACTIVITY: per surgeon. VITAL SIGNS per routine, except respiratory rate q _ h x ___ hours, then q _ h x ___ hours, then q4h. MAINTAIN IV access while epidural catheter is in place.		
	3.	PULSE OXIMETRY Yes __; No __. Continuous ___ for ___ hours; Intermittent ___ q __ hours for ___ hours.		
	4.	Naloxone (Narcan) two (2) ampules in patient's unit dose cassette		
	5.	NO SYSTEMIC NARCOTICS/SEDATIVES TO BE GIVEN EXCEPT AS ORDERED BY APS.		
	6.	Treatment of nausea/vomiting: Yes __; No __ droperidol (Inapsine) 0.2ml (0.5mg) IV q2h prn x 2 doses; Yes __; No __ metoclopramide (Reglan) __mg IV q4h prn x 2 doses; Yes __; No __ transderm scopolamine patch (mastoid area) for 72 hours; Yes __; No __ other:		
	7.	Treatment of pruritus (itching): Benadryl 12.5mg IV q30 minutes prn x 2 doses		
	8.	Prophylactic infusion for itching: Yes __; No __. Naloxone __; or Nalbuphine __. Add ___ ampule(s) per liter of maintenance IV fluid x ___ liter(s)		
	9.	Adjuvant therapy: Yes __; No __. Ketorolac, loading dose of ___mg ___(route); then ___mg ___(route) q ___h PRN; or ___mg ___(route) q ___ hours for ___ doses.		
	10.	Notify APS, beeper 128-2154, for: a) somnolence or confusion; b) respiratory rate of 10 or less; c) inadequate analgesia; d) pruritus or nausea/vomiting unresponsive to treatment; e) oxygen saturation less than 90%; f) leakage or redness around insertion site		
		Date: ___________ ___________	MD	

F-854 (Rev. 7/87)

FIG. 26-4. Standardized orders for continuous epidural analgesia used at Yale-New Haven Hospital.

Specialist-Directed Services

Pain services have been categorized by the complexity of therapy provided, whether anesthesia-based, or multi-departmental, and also by whether they are associated with a university medical center or with private practice groups. Each institution should develop the resources necessary to provide effective and appropriate pain control for its patients, and to designate which department or group of caregivers will be responsible for its safe delivery.

University and large academic hospital services tend to be managed by anesthesiologists but may include caregivers with diverse educational and professional backgrounds who help facilitate research and teaching or provide clinical care.[149,327] Members include the pain service director, attending physicians, residents, and fellows, the clinical nurse coordinator (CNC), associate nurse specialists, a research nurse, and a pharmacist. The pharmacist compounds patient-controlled analgesia (PCA) and epidural medications, in preservative-free normal saline, using strict aseptic technique. Utilizing Centers for Disease Control (CDC) sterility guidelines, preservative-free solutions have a refrigerated shelf life of 7 days and a 24 to 36-hour expiration date from the time they are dispensed to the patient. In addition to formulating and dispensing drugs, the pharmacist is responsible for providing drug information and patient education, and for developing a control system to identify potential misuse.

University medical centers have a major obligation to ensure that resident education is provided, that its professionals are actively involved in research, and that flexible pain management protocols are offered.[149,260,327] In this regard, departments of anesthesiology have developed and optimized a variety of analgesic techniques, including neuroaxial opioids, intravenous patient-controlled analgesia (IV-PCA), and neural blockade. Residents are trained to initiate therapy, to provide the follow-up necessary to assess and optimize analgesia effects, and to treat associated side effects.[174,260] In addition to managing postsurgical discomfort, the pain service is responsible for controlling pain secondary to invasive medical procedures, exacerbations of malig-

YALE-NEW HAVEN HOSPITAL

DOCTOR'S ORDERS

PLEASE USE BALL POINT PEN – BEAR DOWN

INSTRUCTIONS

1. EACH TIME A PHYSICIAN WRITES A MEDICATION ORDER, DETACH TOP COPY AND SEND TO PHARMACY.
2. RULE OFF UNUSED LINES AFTER LAST COPY (PINK) HAS BEEN SENT TO PHARMACY. IMPRINT NEW SET AND PLACE IN CHART.

DO NOT USE THIS SHEET UNLESS A NUMBER SHOWS ▶

DATE	TIME	ORDERS	DOCTOR'S SIGNATURE	NURSE'S SIGNATURE
		ACUTE PAIN SERVE/DEPARTMENT OF ANESTHESIOLOGY		
		INTRAVENOUS OR EPIDURAL PATIENT-CONTROLLED		
		ANALGESIA ORDERS		
1.	Drug ___			
	Concentration (mg/ml) ___ (µg/ml) ___			
	PCA dose (ml) ___			
	Continuous infusion rate (ml/hr) ___			
	4 hour limit (ml) ___			
2.	HEAD OF BED greater than ___ degrees. ACTIVITY: per surgeon.			
	VITAL SIGNS per routine, except respiratory rate q___h___ x ___ hours, then q___h___			
	x ___ hours, then q4h. MAINTAIN IV access while epidural catheter is in place.			
3.	PULSE OXIMETRY Yes ___; No ___. Continuous ___ for ___ hours; Intermittent ___ q			
	___ hours for ___ hours.			
4.	Naloxone (Narcan) two (2) ampules in patient's unit dose cassette.			
5.	NO SYSTEMIC NARCOTICS/SEDATIVES TO BE GIVEN EXCEPT AS ORDERED			
	BY APS.			
6.	Treatment of nausea/vomiting:			
	Yes ___; No ___ droperidol (Inapsine) 0.2 ml (0.5 mg) IV q2h PRN x 2 doses			
	Yes ___; No ___ metoclopramide (Reglan) ___ mg IV q4h PRN x 2 doses			
	Yes ___; No ___ other: ___			
7.	Treatment of pruritus (itching):			
	Benadryl 12.5 mg IV q30 minutes PRN x 2 doses			
8.	Prophylactic infusion for itching/sedation: Yes ___; No ___,			
	Naloxone ___; or Nalbuphine ___. Add ___ ampule(s) per liter of maintenance IV fluid x			
	___ liter(s)			
9.	Ketorolac therapy: Yes ___; No ___. Loading dose ___ mg slow IV; then ___ mg q6			
	hours x ___ hours			
10.	Notify APS, beeper ___ for:			
	a) somnolence or confusion			
	b) respiratory rate of 10 or less			
	c) inadequate analgesia			
	d) pruritus or nausea/vomiting unresponsive to treatment			
	e) oxygen saturation less than 90%			
	f) leakage or redness around insertion site			
	Date: ___ ___ M.D.			

F-854 (Rev. 7/87)

1193 DISCHARGE DIAGNOSES IN ORDER OF DECREASING PRIORITY MUST BE SUPPLIED AT TIME OF PATIENT'S DISCHARGE.

FIG. 26-5. Standardized orders for Intravenous and Epidural Patient-Controlled Analgesia, used at Yale-New Haven Hospital.

nancy-related and benign pain, management of sickle cell crisis, and other acute "medical" pain.

Hubbard and co-workers[150] have revealed several inherent common denominators in successful acute pain services. They include the following: (i) appointment of a *director* knowledgeable in pain management and willing to take on a wide range and depth of responsibilities. In this regard, the pain service director must assume the role of clinician, negotiator, educator, and section head.[150,260] The pain service director, together with the CNC, is responsible for introduction and maintenance of specialized therapy, development of standardized protocols, nursing education, and interactions with the pharmacy. (ii) *Pain control is centralized vertically* around the patient, from the time of preadmission screening until discharge.[150,255,260] Surgical consultation for service should be gained well ahead of time, and a standardized consultation request form prepared (Fig. 26-3). A new patient management list is prepared daily and circulated to the pharmacy, postanesthesia care unit (PACU) staff, and to members of the pain service. PCA and epidural pumps are stored in central supply and are delivered to the PACU, where therapy is initiated. At some institutions, epidural infusions are initiated intraoperatively. (iii) *Standardization* is one of the more important components of an effective pain service. A stepwise order sequence will provide nurse professionals with the opportunity to treat inadequate analgesia, as well as side effects associated with pain therapy. The number of analgesics employed, concentration of drug, and devices required for infusion should be limited to minimize confusion and errors in administration. (iv) Effective *nurse education*, continued in-service training, and the use of standardized orders will significantly reduce the number of nurse calls for assistance; nevertheless, a physician contact number must be available for emergent situations (Figs. 26-4 and 26-5). (v) *Quality Improvement*, *procedures* including daily pain rounds, follow-up notes, and charting of pain scores and side effects by the floor nursing staff, help to rate the effectiveness of therapy, as well as the frequency of treatment-related morbidity. When a shortcoming is identified, therapy must be altered quickly to correct the problem, to minimize patient, nursing, and surgical staff dissatisfaction.[150,260] (vi) The pain management service is expected to function as an *institutional resource* so that basic knowledge of pain control can be disseminated to other caregivers within the institution.[75,192]

Nurse-Managed Services

In contrast to the specialist-based model, pain services in smaller community hospitals place less emphasis on physician responsibility, and rely instead upon highly standardized protocols. Many private-practice anesthesiology groups cannot spare a physician during the day to be dedicated to pain service, or to provide immediate "in-house" backup during late-evening shifts. In these settings, simpler, less expensive models, supervised by pharmacy personnel and well-trained nurse professionals, have been developed. A nurse-based service used in 25% of all Swedish hospitals was presented recently by Rawal.[249] In this model, anesthesiologists do not supervise acute pain management, but instead function as teachers, pain experts, and specialists who initiate regional blockade and epidural analgesia. A specially trained Acute Pain Nurse (APN) or CNC is hired by the hospital, and, together with surgeons, anesthesiologists, and ward nurse managers, establishes protocols for patient selection, assessment of pain intensity, monitoring routines, and drug and dosage guidelines. The APN makes daily rounds on all post-surgical patients, interacts with designated pain-representative nurses on each ward, and trouble-shoots technical problems. The pain-representative and ward nurses are responsible for implementing management guidelines, monitoring routines, and for initiation and adjustment of analgesic therapy. Using this model, Rawal[249] estimated that the cost of acute pain control at the Orebro Medical Center Hospital in Sweden averages less than three dollars per day (APN salary divided by 20,000 patient days/year). It should be pointed out, however, that the majority of patients managed by this service would not require follow-up by a specialist and would receive standardized IM or IV doses of pain medication rather than IV-PCA or epidural analgesia. While offering efficient pain control for healthy patients recovering from uncomplicated surgery, the effectiveness of nurse-directed pain management may be compromised in high-risk settings, because nurses are less likely to administer opioid-loading doses, adjust pain medication, or employ adjunctive analgesic therapy than are acute pain specialists.[304]

ROLE OF THE ACUTE PAIN NURSE

In both academic medical centers and smaller community hospitals, the position of acute pain nurse or CNC is second in importance only to the pain service director. In either setting, the clinical and administrative responsibility of this individual will be extensive; therefore, outlining the job description, funding the position, and selecting the most qualified individual becomes key to the success of the service.[238] The APN applicant should be a management-level nurse, preferably with a master's degree, who has worked extensively within the hospital. The applicant's appreciation of the unique political structure of the institution will facilitate working relationships with hospital administrators, primary caregivers, nurse managers, and the nursing staff. In private practice settings, the position generally is funded by the hospital, while in academic centers, the APN may be employed by the department of anesthesiology. As a member of the anesthesiology team, the APN can more readily support departmental interests, including resident education and research, while facilitating introduction and acceptance of new analgesic techniques. When hired by the hospital, the APN provides follow-up and supervision of surgical and nurse-managed patients. Nursing responsibility and patient safety are always given highest priority. Clear policy and procedures, standardized orders, and nursing education must be provided before new forms of therapy are introduced. Nursing in-servicing includes basic overviews of IV-PCA, neuroaxial opioid and local anesthetic pharmacology, knowledge of infusion devices, assessment of analgesia and treatment of side effects. The APN is also expected to provide physician and patient education, coordinate complicated referrals from surgical or nurse-managed services, and to collect data for research, billing, and quality assurance.[150,238]

MULTIDISCIPLINED PAIN SERVICE MODEL

In recent years, many departments of anesthesiology have discarded specialist-based acute pain management, and increasingly support nurse-managed models, employed by countries with nationalized health care.[150,238,249] Others remain convinced that only the most knowledgeable and interested providers can serve their patient needs best, and continue to subsidize specialist-based pain management.[196,255,304]

Acute pain management at Yale-New Haven Hospital employs a multidisciplined approach that combines the best aspects of specialist-based and nurse-directed services.[150,249] Overall responsibility, including policy-procedure, education, and therapeutic expertise, is provided by the Department of Anesthesiology, including the director, APNs, pain service, specialists, and residents. This team has developed a professional collaboration and trust with the nursing staff, surgical specialists, and other primary care physicians and is responsible for their training in acute pain. With appropriate training and APN supervision, unit nurses, and the surgical staff routinely manage healthy patients (The American Society of Anesthesiology [ASA] class 1,2) treated with IM opioids, IV-PCA, and single doses of neuroaxial opioid. High-risk (ASA class 3 and above) and opioid-tolerant individuals who require IV-PCA, as well as all patients treated with continuous epidural analgesia and plexus blockade, are referred to and followed by Anesthesiology Department-based caregivers. This separation in management is in agreement with the U.S. Health Care Financing Administration's (HCFA's) belief that surgeons have historically managed postoperative pain, and should continue to do so, except under special or complicated circumstances.[155,196] Since this system of coverage was initiated, the number of patients receiving IV-PCA and directly managed by the Department of Anesthesiology has decreased by 60%, with a corresponding 50% reduction in personnel requirements. This reduction in daily patient census has allowed the pain service to concentrate on those individuals who have most to gain from optimal acute pain management, and has led to an expansion in the number of patients receiving epidural and continuous regional analgesic therapy.

VARIABLES INFLUENCING ACUTE PAIN MANAGEMENT

Age. Age appears to be the most important variable in determining the degree of pain relief attained following administration of opioid analgesics. Advancing age typically alters opioid dose-response.[25,58,161,180,206] Belville and co-workers[25] observed significant age-related improvements in analgesic response to fixed doses of morphine and pentazocine in male patients aged 30 to 70 years. These differences were not related to pharmacokinetic changes, since the incidence of respiratory depression and other drug-induced side effects did not increase in older individuals. A more recent evaluation,[58] utilizing patient-controlled analgesic delivery, found no correlation between age and the quality of postoperative pain relief, but did observe diminished opioid consumption with increasing age. In contrast, another study of PCA requirements in the 24 hours following surgery found a correlation with age, but not with weight, in adult patients.[206]

Patient Weight. Although opioid analgesics are frequently administered on a mg/kg basis, there is no evidence to link body weight and individual dose requirement. In this regard, Belville et al.[25] was unable to detect relationships between body weight or surface area, and opioid dose necessary, for subjective pain relief. Similar findings were reported by Burns,[58] and Tamsen,[316,317] who failed to detect correlations between body size, opioid consumption, and plasma concentrations in age-matched patients recovering from similar surgical procedures.

Culture. Patients react to pain according to what it means to them emotionally and how they have been taught to respond.[233,244,276,310] Reaction to pain is a conditioned behavior that reflects the values of a given culture. Responses can be divided into 2 broad categories: (i) stoic, where patients express minimal vocal response to discomfort; (ii) emotive, where patients are quite vocal and highly emotional.[244,276,310] While caregivers should never generalize about group reactions, an appreciation of cultural conditioning may help them assess pain-related behavior in selected individuals.

Gender. Studies evaluating whether self-administered opioid dose requirements are influenced by gender have reported conflicting results.[58,233,237,316] Burns, et al.[58] studied 100 patients of similar age recovering from upper abdominal surgery. Male patients self-administered greater amounts of morphine during the first 24 hours to achieve equivalent pain relief. In contrast, Tamsen and co-workers[316] found no gender-related differences in opioid dose requirements in patients recovering from similar procedures.

Psychological Factors. Early evaluations of psychological factors and their influence upon acute pain revealed that anxious patients reported higher pain scores and required greater amounts of pain medication.[83,286] Highly aggressive and angry patients also tend to consume more medication than patients whose coping styles are more passive.[83,119] Locus-of-control testing can be used to predict adaptive responses to acute pain.[119,276] Patients demonstrating an internal locus of control tend to be highly motivated and enjoy self-administration analgesic regimens, which restore some level of control in a setting where most other aspects of care have been taken away from them. Individuals having an external locus of control tend to be poorly motivated, report high pain scores despite appearing fairly comfortable, and tend to fail IV and epidural PCA therapy, because they fear taking control of any aspect of their medical care.[244]

Site and Extent of Surgery. The site, extent, and duration of surgery may influence the intensity of postoperative pain and analgesic requirements.[233,237,244] Patients recovering from thoracotomy, upper abdominal procedures, and nephrectomy experience severe effort-dependent pain, and require significantly greater amounts of analgesic than individuals recovering from hip replacement, herniorraphy, and mastectomy. Patients in community (private) hospitals generally experience less discomfort than individuals in training institutions, because similar surgical procedures are performed faster and with less tissue injury.[244]

Pharmacokinetic Alterations Associated with Major Organ Failure. Decline in cardiac, hepatic, and renal function are often associated with significant alterations in the volume of distribution, clearance, and excretion of most analgesic agents. For analgesics having high hepatic uptake and clearance, reductions in hepatic blood flow are accompanied by proportional decrements in the overall extraction rate and prolonged pharmacological effects.[307,308] Analgesics which are bio-transformed or eliminated by the kidneys may produce CNS toxicity/depression in patients with renal failure, unless dose adjustments are made.[29,307] This can be accomplished by either reducing dose size or by increasing the interval between doses. Dosage adjustment is of critical importance if renal function is less than 50% of normal, and the parent drug and active metabolites are primarily eliminated by the kidney.[245,307] Patients suffering congestive heart failure experience greater reductions in hepatic and renal perfusion than blood flow directed to the heart, lungs, and CNS. As would be expected, both hepatic clearance/biotransformation and renal elimination of drug may be compromised.[244,245]

History of Substance Abuse or Opioid Tolerance. Despite the fact that they experience the same intensity of postsurgical discomfort, caregivers tend to limit opioid administration to patients who have a history of substance abuse.[244] Since self-administered analgesic delivery may reinforce drug-seeking behavior, IV-PCA is often withheld from these individuals and neural blockade or epidural analgesic techniques substituted. More recent thinking allows selected patients presenting with histories of alcohol and cocaine abuse to use PCA in well-supervised settings.[244] Patients with a history of chronic pain and significant opioid tolerance also require increased amounts of drug to compensate for both baseline requirements, as well as that needed to control pain following surgery.

Pharmacodynamics and Other Variables. Alterations in the blood–brain barrier (BBB), up- or downregulation of opioid receptors, cross-tolerance, and levels of endogenous opioids may be responsible for interpatient variabilities in pain perception and analgesic response.[74,244,308,319] Patients presenting with low plasma concentrations of beta-endorphin required significantly greater amounts of morphine following surgery than individuals with higher levels.[74] A similar relationship between PCA meperidine consumption and endogenous opioid levels was reported by Tamsen and coworkers in patients recovering from laparotomy.[319] These investigators observed a linear relationship between analgesic demand and preoperative concentrations of endogenous opioids in cerebrospinal fluid (CSF). Similar correlations have been observed in the pediatric population.[314]

THERAPEUTIC OPTIONS FOR OPTIMAL POSTOPERATIVE ANALGESIA

Selecting the most optimal method to control acute pain is an individualized prescription based upon the physiological status of the patient, the extent of surgical injury, the technical expertise of the caregivers, and the economic resources of the hospital. While most often employed as primary therapy, IV-PCA may be used to supplement regional neural blockade, or to maintain pain relief following single-dose administration of intrathecal or epidural opioids. Intermittent dose and continuous epidural analgesia are offered to adult and pediatric patients recovering from more extensive or painful surgery. Epidural patient-controlled analgesia (Epi-PCA) is used in settings where the combination of patient-controlled delivery plus neuroaxial activity may offer unique advantages. Regional nerve blockade, including local infiltration, peripheral nerve block, continuous plexus block, and intrapleural catheter techniques, may be employed as primary therapy in patients recovering from traumatic injury or orthopedic surgery.

INTRAVENOUS PATIENT-CONTROLLED ANALGESIA

Patient-controlled analgesia is an analgesic modality used to some extent in 96% of larger American hospitals.[255,256] The technique allows patients to titrate small doses of pain medication in amounts proportional to a perceived pain stimulus.[129,287] PCA avoids cycles of excessive sedation and ineffective pain control observed with either on-demand or by-the-clock IM dosing, and limits variabilities related to inappropriate screening, delays in administration and drug absorption.[111,112,129,130,151,171,287,339] Patient-controlled delivery compensates for the fact that pain intensity rarely is constant, is intensified by movement and coughing, and seems to have a circadian rhythm, with increasing pain at night.[15,111,112,316,318]

Commercially developed PCA devices use microprocessors that allow the patient to self-medicate with an infusion pump connected to his/her intravenous line.[234] Patients activate the pump by pressing a button connected to the apparatus. A preprogrammed dose of opioid, termed the incremental bolus, is administered over a 10 to 30 second period. A lockout interval begins, preventing a second dose from being delivered within a pre-set time period.[234,339] Since total opioid dose and dosing interval are titrated by the patient, optimal analgesic concentrations are more likely to be maintained, and individual variations in pharmacokinetics and pain perception are more easily accommodated.[180,230]

An opioid loading dose, which provides baseline plasma levels of analgesic, is administered before PCA is begun. In general, 0.1 to 0.2 mg/kg morphine or 0.5 to 1 mg/kg meperidine, are titrated to the patient's comfort level. Morphine remains the opioid of choice for IV-PCA, despite delays in analgesic onset, progressive sedation, and histamine release that are associated with its use.[18,282,299,300] Other suitable agents include rapid-acting, intermediate duration, opioids such as hydromorphone, meperidine, and oxymorphone.[18,299,326] Opioids with either ultra-short or prolonged durations of activity are less effective in this setting.[339] IV-PCA dosing guidelines are presented in Table 26–1.

The inherent safety of IV-PCA has much to do with the fact that opioid-induced respiratory depression and other side effects occur at higher plasma/brain concentrations than that needed to produce analgesia.[14,129,130,195,287,316,318,340] By adjusting the rate of self-administration, most patients achieve and maintain MEAC. In this regard, the rate of administration required to maintain morphine and meperidine MEAC averaged 2.7 and 26 mg/hr respectively.[88,316] A continuous (basal) opioid infusion may be added to supplement patient controlled delivery. This dual form of administration generally is offered to patients recovering from extremely painful procedures, and to individuals presenting with opioid

TABLE 26-1. *Dosing guidelines for IV-patient-controlled analgesia*

Opioid	Concentration	Loading dose	Incremental bolus dose	Lockout interval	Basal infusion (rate)	Comments
Morphine	1 mg/ml	3–10 mg	0.5–1.5 mg	6–8 min	0.5–1.5 mg/hr	Major abdominal/ orthopedic surgical pain
Meperidine	10 mg/ml	25–50 mg	5–15 mg	6–8 min	not recommended	Useful for visceral pain, limit dose to 600 mg/24 hrs
Hydromorphone	0.2 mg/ml	0.5–1 mg	0.1–0.3 mg	6–8 min	0.1–0.3 mg/hr	Rapid onset, minimal side effects
Oxymorphone	0.1 mg/ml	0.3–1 mg	0.1–0.2 mg	6–8 min	0.1–0.2 mg/hr	Rapid onset, best for severe pain
Fentanyl	20 mcg/ml	30–100 mcg	10–20 mcg	5–6 min	10–20 mcg/hr	Rapid onset, short duration of effect requires basal infusion

tolerance.[339] Studies evaluating the benefits of concurrent basal opioid infusions have provided conflicting results. While patients receiving patient-controlled doses plus a basal infusion of morphine (0.5 to 1 mg/hr) reported lower effort-dependent pain scores, 24-hour dose requirements, and incidences of adverse effects were greater than those observed with PCA alone.[231,236,299] Since machine-controlled opioid delivery may reduce overall safety, patients who receive concurrent basal infusions should be more carefully observed than those treated with PCA.[340]

For patients who use IV-PCA successfully, acceptable pain relief represents a compromise between a tolerable level of discomfort and the appearance of annoying side effects.[174,195,230] A number of adjunctive analgesic and antiemetic agents may be employed to improve pain relief, while reducing dose-dependent side effects, such as nausea/vomiting and excessive sedation.[111,288,339]

Spinal Opioid Analgesia

The identification of specific binding sites and receptor subtypes has helped to clarify how and where opioid analgesics act within the neuroaxis[240,328] (see Chapters 24 and 29 for more detailed discussion). Prior to 1975, investigators favored the view that systemically administered opioid either modulated pain at supraspinal centers or activated descending inhibitory pathways; they did not, it was believed, have a direct effect on spinal activity. Later, Kitahata[173] and others,[99] provided evidence that morphine suppressed nociceptive neurons in laminae II and V of dorsal horn. This activity was quite selective, since laminae IV and VI cells, which respond to non-noxious cutaneous and proprioceptive stimuli, were unaffected. Using animal behavioral models, Yaksh and co-workers[347,348] observed that small doses of intrathecal morphine produced naloxone-reversible analgesia of prolonged duration. These findings, coupled with established techniques for spinal and epidural delivery of analgesics, provided a new and potentially useful method of controlling pain in a variety of clinical settings. In 1979, Wang and colleagues presented the first double-blind, controlled study of neuroaxial opioid use in humans.[334] In 6 out of 8 patients suffering from intractable cancer pain, intrathecal morphine (0.5 to 1.0 mg) produced complete relief for 12 to 24 hours without evidence of significant sedation, respiratory depression, or impaired neuromuscular function. Thousands of literature citations have since confirmed the high analgesic efficacy of neuroaxial opioids, and such therapy has gained considerable popularity for controlling post-operative pain.[80,81,341]

The complex pharmacokinetics associated with intrathecal and epidural opioids are discussed in Chapter 29 and must be appreciated to understand the benefits and potential complications of neuroaxial analgesia. Opioids administered at either site provide effective pain relief; however, epidural dosing is complicated by anatomical and physiological factors, including dural and pial penetration, absorption by epidural fat, and the consequences of vascular uptake.[24,80,81,124,134,218,225,296] A portion of the epidural dose ,crosses the dura, enters the CSF, and penetrates spinal tissue in amounts proportional to the lipid solubility of the agent.[80,124,134,243] A small fraction of drug binds to receptors in dorsal horn, effectively blocking nociceptive input at the first synapse in the CNS. The remainder is absorbed by the vasculature, producing plasma levels comparable to that achieved with intramuscular injections, and providing some degree of supraspinal analgesia.[225] Although opioid dose, volume of injectate, and degree of ionization are considered important variables, lipid solubility appears to play the key role in determining onset of analgesia, dermatomal spread, and duration of activity.[69,80,124,329] Highly lipid-soluble opioids have a more rapid analgesic onset than ionized lipid-insoluble agents such as morphine. Duration of activity is influenced by the rate drugs are removed from sites of activity. Lipid soluble opioids are cleared rapidly by the vasculature, while highly-ionized, lipid insoluble agents remain in CSF and spinal tissues for prolonged periods of time.[57,78,80,134]

Single Bolus or Intermittent Boluses of Epidural Opioids

Intermittent boluses of epidural opioids are commonly utilized for control of pain following trauma and surgery. While this method of administration provides excellent pain relief and does not require sophisticated delivery systems, duration of activity is limited, and abrupt elevations in CSF opioid concentrations which follow each dose may be responsible for annoying and clinically significant side effects.[49,50,134,160,225] The technique limits opioid selection to longer-acting agents such as morphine and generally excludes the use of local anesthetics. Despite these deficiencies, single bolus and intermittent dosing may be safely employed, provided that dose and dosing interval are carefully adjusted in older and high-risk patient populations.[259,261]

Three different classes of opioid analgesics have been advocated for epidural/intrathecal administration; these include the hydrophilic opiate, morphine, moderately lipophilic opioids such as hydromorphone and meperidine, and highly lipophilic agents including fentanyl and sufentanil. Morphine was first to receive Food and Drug Administration (FDA) approval for epidural and intrathecal use and remains the most widely investigated and extensively used spinal opioid. Single epidural doses of morphine effectively relieve visceral pain following abdominal or pelvic surgery, as well as somatic pain associated with orthopedic procedures.[24,50,78,80,145,193,211,252,293] Doses are usually administered via lumbar catheters; however, thoracic administration offers more efficient and effective control of upper abdominal or thoracic pain.[293,294] Onset and duration of analgesia following single-dose administration of morphine varies according to the surgical stimulus, dose, and site of administration. In general, analgesic onset occurs after 30 to 60 minutes, with peak effect at 90 to 120 minutes, and duration ranges from 12 to 24 hours.[78,296,298] Ready and co-workers[261] studied age as a predictor of epidural morphine bolus dose requirements in postsurgical patients. Therapeutic goals of their evaluation were to produce a pain-free or nearly pain-free state, with minimal adverse effects. Despite considerable interpatient variability, a correlation between patient age and effective 24-hour epidural morphine dose was noted (Fig. 26-6). On the other hand, analgesic quality and frequency of morphine-associated side effects did not change in relation to increasing patient age.

The superiority of epidural morphine analgesia, as determined by descriptive and visual analog scores, over pain relief offered by parenteral opioids, has been demonstrated in a variety of postsurgical settings.[32,80,105,145,154,193,254,293] In this regard, the quality and uniformity of postoperative analgesia provided by a single dose of epidural morphine was superior to that offered by IM morphine or patient-controlled analgesia with morphine, while requiring only 1/15 the

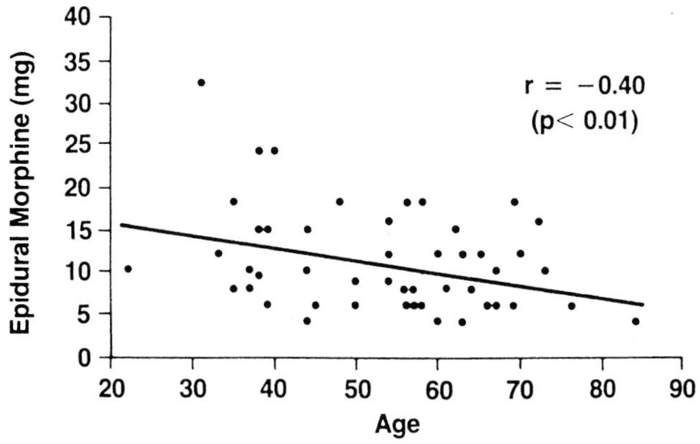

FIG. 26-6. Age versus 24-hour epidural morphine dose requirements in patients recovering from intra-abdominal gynecologic surgery. (Reproduced with permission from Ready, L.B., Chadwick, H.S., and Ross, B.: Age predicts effective epidural morphine dose after abdominal hysterectomy. Anesth. Analg., *66:*1215, 1987.)

parenteral dose over the 24-hour study period (Fig. 26-7).[105,145,193]

The recognition that respiratory depression and other adverse effects observed with epidural morphine were related to its retention and rostral spread in CSF, spurred investigation and clinical utilization of lipid-soluble opioids, which rapidly exit CSF and penetrate spinal tissue.[3,48,121] Moderately lipophilic opioids such as meperidine and hydromorphone provide a more rapid onset but shorter duration of analgesia than morphine. The onset of postsurgical analgesia with epidural meperidine occurred at 5 minutes, peaked at 30 minutes, and lasted 8 hours.[121] Few side effects were noted, but early-onset respiratory depression, occurring within the first hour following administration, was observed in patients receiving more than 75 mg.[121]

Epidural hydromorphone also provides rapid and effective pain relief, with onset of analgesia noted at 15 minutes and peak effect at 30 minutes after administration.[48,49,52,62,65,98,292] Hydromorphone's removal from the epidural space is slower than that of highly lipophilic opioids, while its ability to remain in CSF and spread rostrally is greater.[52,243] This property provides important clinical advantages: (i) Doses administered via lumbar catheters can control pain at higher dermatomal segments; (ii) epidural administration is associated with a greater potency gain than similar amounts given IV. In this regard, equianalgesic doses of epidural hydromorphone are 2 to 4 fold less than intravenous requirements.[235,274] Intermittent doses, ranging from 0.5 to 1 mg, provide 5 to 12 hours of pain relief.[52,65] The safety and side effect profile of epidural hydromorphone is superior to morphine, because equivalent doses are associated with less respiratory depression, pruritus, and excess sedation.[48,62]

Epidural boluses of lipophilic opioids such as fentanyl and sufentanil provide rapid control of postsurgical pain[3,125,154,184,222,270,328] with a lesser incidence of delayed respiratory depression than morphine.[59,120,191,270] Drawbacks associated

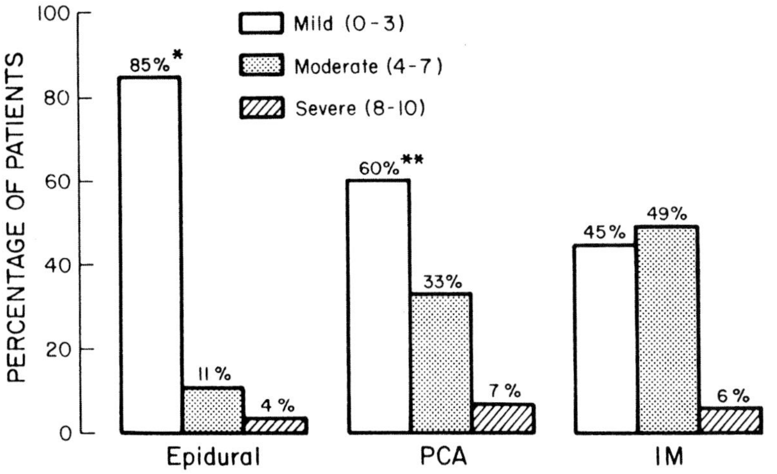

FIG. 26-7. The percentage of patients in each group reporting mild (VAS 0-3), moderate (VAS 4 to 7), or severe (VAS 7-10) pain during the first 24 hours following cesarean section. Epidural = 5 mg epidural morphine; PCA = morphine 1 mg IV every 6 minutes as required; IM = morphine 10 to 15 mg every 4 hours. *P < 0.05 Epidural vs PCA and IM; **P = NS PCA versus IM. (Reproduced with permission from Harrison, D.M., Sinatra, R., and Morgese, L.: Epidural narcotic and patient-controlled analgesia for postcesarean section pain relief. Anesthesiology, *68*:454, 1988.)

with lipophilic opioids include: (i) Epidural doses are surprisingly high, and approach or exceed parenteral requirements.[120,191] (ii) Early-onset ventilatory depression can occur; and (iii) Duration of action, while dose-dependent, is limited.[120,191,290] In a double-blind comparison study,[270] the onset of postoperative analgesia with epidural sufentanil (50 mg) was more rapid than morphine (5 mg); however, the duration of morphine analgesia was twice as long. Fentanyl's short duration of effect and its ability to control pain following upper abdominal surgery may be improved when administered in larger volumes of diluent.[30,294]

Bolus doses of highly lipophilic opioids may be employed in the following settings: (i) augmentation of intraoperative epidural anesthesia; (ii) rapid control of postoperative discomfort in patients experiencing breakthrough pain; (iii) facilitating the transition between regression of epidural anesthesia and the initiation of IV-PCA in settings where postoperative epidural analgesia cannot be provided;[290] (iv) as the rapid-acting component of combination therapy where fentanyl or sufentanil may be combined with morphine in an effort to minimize the delays in analgesic onset.[298]

Continuous Infusion of Epidural Opioids

Continuous infusion of epidural opioids control postoperative pain with fewer adverse effects than intermittent bolus dosing.[107,114,190,336] Infusion techniques allow analgesics to be titrated to patient comfort and rapidly terminated if problems should occur. The high CSF concentrations associated with intermittent epidural boluses are avoided and risk of rostral spread and delayed respiratory depression are reduced.[53,80] Other benefits include decreased time spent administering agents and assessing effect, and a reduced risk of contamination and medication errors. Epidural infusions also provide greater therapeutic versatility, because shorter-acting opioids and dilute local anesthetic solutions may be administered continuously.

Epidural infusions of morphine, meperidine, and hydromorphone offer effective pain relief and uniform analgesia in a variety of settings.[48,107,114,118] El-Baz and colleagues[107,190] evaluated the safety and efficacy of continuous epidural morphine (0.5 mg/hr) infusions versus intermittent doses of morphine or bupivacaine for postthoracotomy analgesia. Patients in the infusion group reported excellent pain relief while experiencing less pruritus, fewer effects from oversedation than patients treated with intermittent doses of morphine, and less urinary retention and hypotension than individuals receiving bupivacaine. In a recent retrospective analysis of over 4,000 patients, de Leon-Casasola and coworkers[90] reported that epidural infusions of morphine-bupivacaine provided excellent analgesia, were associated with an extremely low incidence of serious adverse events, and could be safely administered to patients recovering on routine postsurgical units.

Brodsky and colleagues[48] reported a series of 44 patients receiving continuous lumbar epidural infusions of hydromorphone (0.5%) for post-thoracotomy analgesia. Postsurgical analgesia was excellent, with greater than 90% of patients reporting either no pain or only mild discomfort during the 48-hour study interval. The incidence of hypoventilation, pruritus, and nausea was lower than that observed with equipotent doses of epidural morphine. Chaplan and co-workers[62] compared a 3:1 dose ratio of morphine and hydromorphone for continuous epidural infusions; with patients in the hydromorphone group receiving 0.15 to 0.3 mg/hr. Patients in both groups reported uniform pain relief; however, those receiving morphine infusions were more sedated and had a higher incidence of pruritus and nausea.

Highly lipophilic opioids such as fentanyl and sufentanil are commonly employed as continuous epidural infusions.[17,59,102,116,336] Welchew and Thornton[336] were among the first to evaluate epidural fentanyl infusions, reporting that such therapy offered uniform analgesia and improved pulmonary function following thoracotomy. In subsequent evaluations, patients receiving continuous infusions of fentanyl or sufentanil following upper abdominal surgery or cesarean section benefited from superior pain relief and fewer adverse effects than individuals treated with parenteral opioids.[17,102,116,120,127]

Significant amounts of fentanyl and sufentanil are absorbed by epidural and spinal vasculature, causing progressive increases in plasma concentration that approach or exceed intravenous MEAC.[71,116,120,191] Loper et al.[191] compared epidural versus IV fentanyl infusions in patients recovering from total knee surgery noting equivalent intragroup pain scores at rest and during movement (Fig. 26-8). Similarly, Geller and co-workers[116] were unable to detect differences in dose requirements and pain scores in patients receiving IV and epidural sufentanil infusions following abdominal surgery. These findings have raised questions about the neuroaxial specificity of these agents. High-volume epidural infusions [303] or administration at interspaces adjacent to spinal sites of activity may improve epidural specificity (Fig. 26-9).[132,280] Thoracic epidural infusions of fentanyl were superior to lumbar epidural and intravenous delivery in reducing dose requirements, hormonal responses, and hospital stay in patients recovering from thoracotomy.[132,280,281] In contrast, Swenson and co-workers[312] found no clinical advantage between thoracic versus lumbar administered sufentanil with respect to quality of postthoracotomy analgesia, preservation of pulmonary function, and total dose requirement.

Epidural analgesia may also be improved when lipophilic opioids are combined with dilute solutions of local anesthetic.[17,189,285] In a recent analysis of 1,014 patients recovering in nonintensive care unit (non-ICU) settings, Scott and colleagues[285] reported that infusions of fentanyl plus bupivacaine provided excellent pain control with minimal side effects. Lui and co-workers[189] suggest that 0.05% bupivacaine is the optimal concentration for use with epidural fentanyl for postthoracotomy analgesia. This concentration provided a significant fentanyl dose-sparing effect, while avoiding hypotension and motor weakness observed with 0.1% bupivacaine. Guidelines for single/intermittent epidural dosing and continuous epidural infusions are presented in Table 26-2.

Epidural Patient-Controlled Analgesia

Epi-PCA offers greater reductions in pain intensity with lower opioid dose requirements than IV-PCA, while providing increased control and higher patient satisfaction than either intermittent doses or continuous infusions of epidural opioids.[194,333] Epi-PCA was developed in response to findings that epidural opioids provide the most optimal pain relief, while IV-PCA offered greater patient autonomy, higher satisfaction, and fewer troublesome side effects.[105,145] The technique involves standard placement of an epidural catheter, administration of an analgesic loading dose (opioids, local anesthetic, or both), and initiation of patient-activated epidural boluses alone, or in combination with a continuous epidural infusion. Development of specialized infusion devices that offer precise epidural PCA dosing and 250-500 ml analgesic solution capacity have increased the safety, reliability, and overall acceptance of the technique. The potential advantages of Epi-PCA vs. IV-PCA and con-

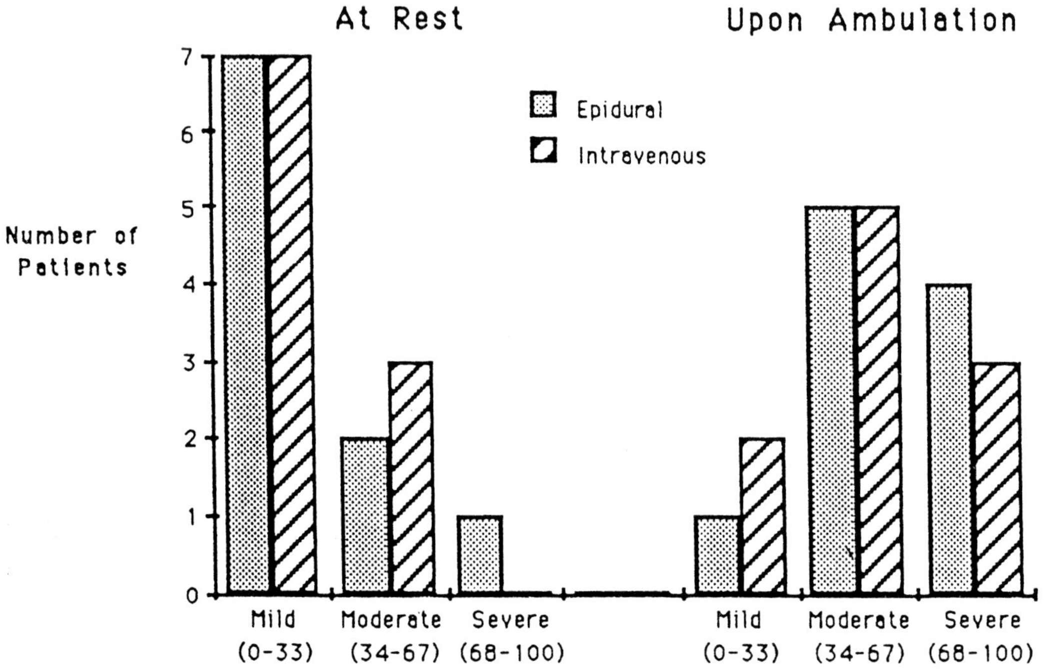

FIG. 26-8. Distribution of rest and ambulation pain scores in patients recovering from orthopedic knee surgery and treated with epidural *(gray bars)* or intravenous *(hatched bars)* infusions of fentanyl. (Reproduced with permission from Loper, K.A., Ready, L.B., Downey, M., *et al.*: Epidural and intravenous fentanyl infusions are clinically equivalent after knee surgery. Anesth. Analg., *70:*72, 1990.)

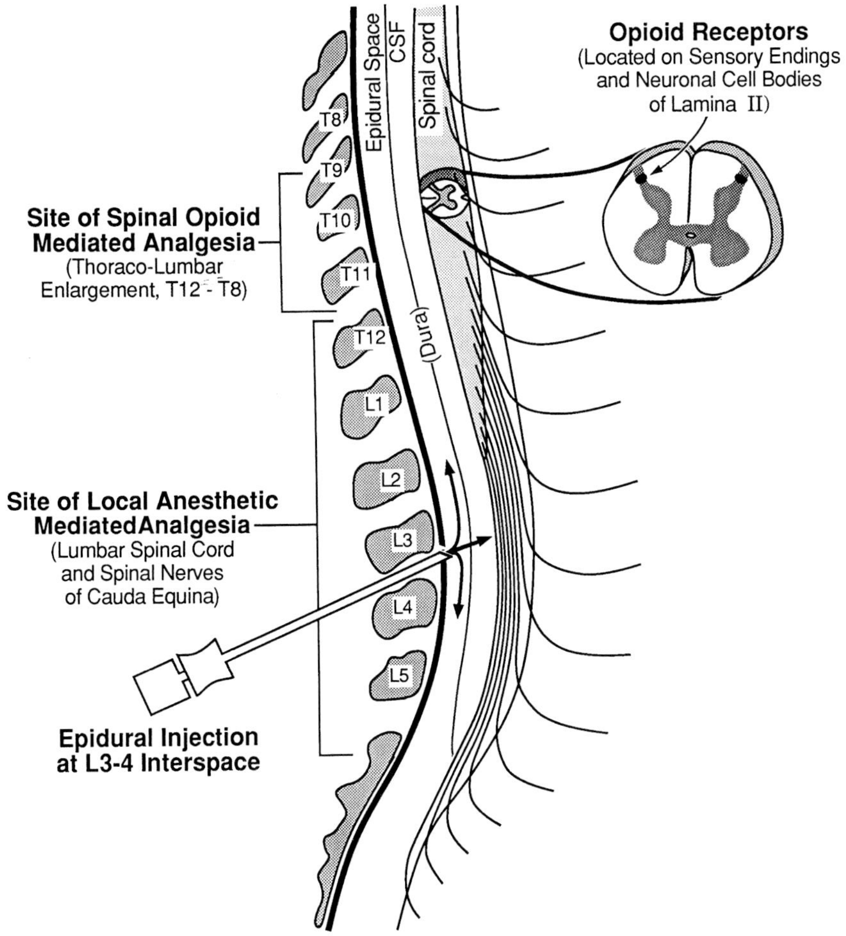

FIG. 26-9. Relationships between epidural deposition of opioid analgesics and local anesthetics in regard to site or sites of activity. [Reproduced with permission from Sinatra, R.: The pharmacology of spinal opioids. *In* Sinatra, R., Hord, A.H., Ginsberg, B., and Premble, L.M. (eds.): Acute Pain Mechanisms and Management. St. Louis, Mosby–Year Book, 1992.]

tinuous epidural opioid infusions are presented in Table 26-3.

Most of the early work describing Epi-PCA were performed in Europe.[68,302] Chrubasik[68] and Sjostrom[302] reported that the amount of morphine self-administered epidurally for postoperative pain relief was significantly lower than that required with IV-PCA or continuous epidural infusion. Investigators at the University of Kentucky evaluated Epi-PCA morphine in over 4,000 patients recovering from a variety of surgical procedures.[333] They noted that total dose requirements and plasma morphine concentrations required for pain control were significantly less than that observed with IV-PCA (Fig. 26-10).[333] According to their protocol, patients are loaded with 2 to 3 mg of epidural morphine. Thereafter, a basal infusion of 0.4 mg/hr is started and patients are allowed to self-administer 0.2 mg morphine every 10 to 15 minutes, with a maximal dose of 1.2 mg/hr.

Lipophilic opioids which offer greater analgesic titratability and fewer adverse effects than morphine also have been evaluated in this setting.[120,126,226,294] Patients treated with Epi-PCA administered less fentanyl following thoracotomy than others utilizing IV-PCA, while achieving equivalent levels of pain relief.[126] Serum fentanyl concentrations were not measured, however. In a well-controlled evaluation of epidural vs. IV-PCA fentanyl, Glass et al.[120] noted no intragroup differences in postoperative pain scores or total fentanyl dose requirements (Fig. 26-11). Grass and co-workers[127] reported that Epi-PCA sufentanil offered more rapid pain relief and superior control of movement-associated pain than did IV-PCA morphine. A major criticism of this investigation was the omission of an IV-sufentanil control group. In a more recent double-blind evaluation of IV and Epi-PCA sufentanil,[295] no differences in postsurgical analgesia, dose requirements, and plasma concentrations were noted; however patients in the IV group experienced a higher incidence of sedation and respiratory depression.

Hydromorphone has also been evaluated for Epi-PCA.[187,235,301] Patients using Epi-PCA following cesarean section required significantly less hydromorphone and benefited from a more rapid return of gastrointestinal function than individuals utilizing IV-PCA (Fig. 26-12).[235] These findings were confirmed in a more recent comparison of IV versus Epi-PCA hydromorphone.[187] Patients in the epidural group achieved equivalent pain relief following radical prostatectomy, while requiring 50% less drug than individuals using IV-PCA.[187] Dosing guidelines for patient controlled epidural analgesia are presented in Table 26-4.

TABLE 26-2. *Dosing guidelines for epidural opioid analgesia*

Opioid	Site of administration	Intermittent bolus technique[a]	Continuous infusion technique[a]	Adjunctive therapy
Morphine	Lumbar catheters for incisions below T8, thoracic catheters for upper abdominal and thoracic surgery	Administer 3–8 mg bolus in 10 ml preservative free saline every 8–24 hrs as clinically indicated	2–4 mg bolus followed by infusion (50 mcg/ml) at 8–15 ml/hr lumbar catheters, 4–8 ml/hr thoracic catheters	IV Ketorolac 15–30 mg q 6 hr, epidural bupivacaine 0.1–0.03%
Hydromorphone	Lumbar catheters for incisions below T8, thoracic catheters for upper abdominal and thoracic surgery	0.5–1.5 mg bolus every 5–10 hrs	0.5–1.5 mg bolus followed by infusion (10 mcg/ml) at 8–15 ml/hr lumbar catheters, 4–8 ml/hr thoracic catheters	IV Ketorolac 15–30 mg q 6 hr, epidural bupivacaine 0.1–0.03%
Meperidine	Lumbar catheters for incisions below T10, thoracic catheters for upper abdominal and thoracic surgery	50–75 mg bolus every 4–8 hrs	50–75 mg bolus followed by infusion (100 mcg/ml) at 8–15 ml/hr lumbar catheters, 4–8 ml/hr-thoracic catheters	IV Ketorolac 15–30 mg q 6 hr, epidural bupivacaine 0.1–0.03%
Fentanyl	Lumbar catheters for incisions below T12, thoracic catheters for almost everything else	50–100 mcg bolus every 2–3 hrs (not recommended)	50–100 mcg bolus followed by infusion (5 mcg/ml) at 8–15 ml/hr lumbar catheters, 4–8 ml/hr-thoracic catheters	IV Ketorolac 15–30 mg q 6 hr, epidural bupivacaine 0.05–0.1% or less
Sufentanil	Lumbar catheters for incisions below T12, thoracic catheters for almost everything else	20–30 mcg bolus every 2–3 hrs (not recommended)	20–30 mcg bolus followed by infusion (1–2 mcg/ml) at 8–15 lumbar catheters, 4–8 ml/hr-thoracic catheters	IV Ketorolac 15–30 mg q 6 hr, epidural bupivacaine 0.05–0.1% or less

[a] Dependent on age, physical status, height, extent of surgical dissection, and so on.

Intrathecal Opioid Analgesia

Intrathecal doses of morphine provide prolonged postsurgical analgesia but share many of the problems associated with single-dose epidural techniques, including limited duration, lack of titratability, and risks of postdural puncture headache and CSF infection. Intrathecal morphine originally was associated with a higher incidence of annoying and potentially serious adverse effects than were doses administered epidurally.[78,132,135] In retrospect, the high frequency of adverse events resulted from the inappropriately large doses employed in preliminary clinical trials.[132] In recent years "mini" and "microdoses" of intrathecal morphine have been advocated to provide safe and effective pain relief in patients recovering from cesarean delivery and orthopedic and upper abdominal surgery.[2,78,132,136,170] Intrathecal morphine was particularly useful in patients recovering from gallbladder surgery, offering up to 24 hours of complete analgesia, with minimal risk of precipitating sphincter of Oddi spasm.[349] Gwirtz and colleagues[136] presented a 5-year evaluation of 4,135 postsurgical patients treated with intrathecal morphine. Morphine dosage ranged from 0.2 to 0.8 mg, depending upon the surgical site, incision size, and patient age. Eighty-five percent of patients experienced good to excellent pain control on postoperative day one, and there were no serious or life-threatening side effects. The major disadvantage of intrathecal morphine is the limited duration of analgesia it provides. Benefits include effective pain control during the immediate postoperative period and a reduction in overall

TABLE 26-3. *Advantages of epidural patient-controlled analgesia (Epi-PCA)*

- Versus intravenous patient-controlled analgesia
  - Superior pain relief
  - Reduced drug requirement
  - Reduction in drug-related side effects
  - Shorter hospitalization
- Versus continuous epidural opioid infusion
  - Patient self-adjustment
  - Reduced hourly infusion requirement
  - Accommodation for changes in pain intensity (i.e. ambulation)
  - Reduced anxiety, increased patient control

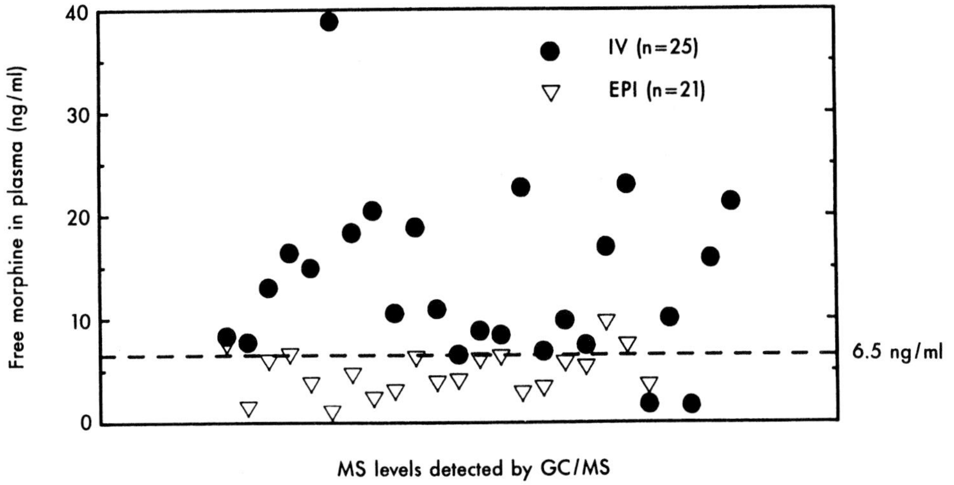

FIG. 26-10. Free, unconjugated morphine serum levels after 24 hours of epidural patient-controlled analgesia *(white triangles)*, and intravenous patient controlled analgesia *(black circles)*, using morphine in 46 patients. Samples were drawn at least 30 minutes after the last PCA bolus. *EPI,* epidural; *IV,* intravenous; *GC/MS,* gas chromatography-mass spectrometry; *MS,* morphine sulfate. [Reproduced with permission from Wamsley, P.N.H.: Patient-controlled epidural analgesia. *In* Sinatra, R., Hord, A.H., Ginsberg, B., and Premble, L.M. (eds.): Acute Pain Mechanisms and Management. St. Louis, Mosby–Year Book, 1992.]

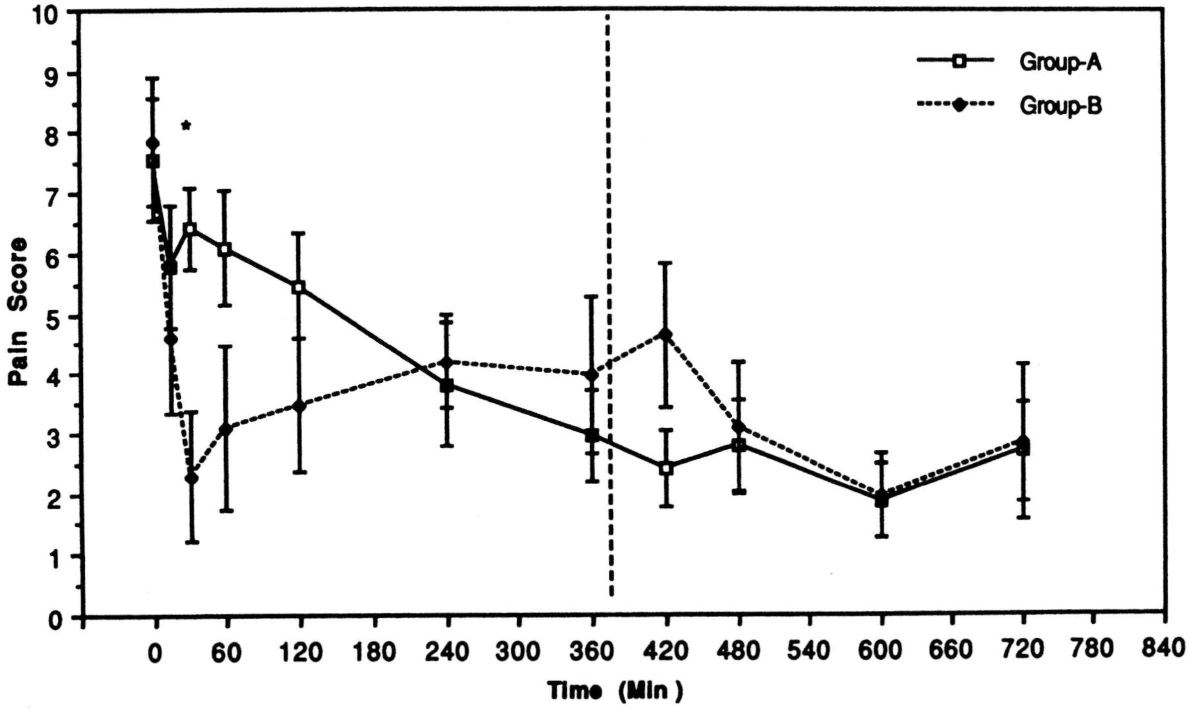

FIG. 26-11. Mean (±SEM) pain scores (as measured by VAS) after patient controlled administration of fentanyl either epidurally *(white boxes)* or intravenously *(black circles)*. Dotted line indicates time of crossover in site of administration. Pain scores after IV fentanyl were statistically lower during the first hour than in the epidural group ($P < 0.05$). Thereafter, there were no pre- or post-crossover differences in pain scores. (Reproduced with permission from Glass, P.S.A., Estok, P., Ginsberg, B., *et al.*: Use of patient-controlled analgesia to compare the efficiency of epidural to intravenous fentanyl administration. Anesth. Analg., *74*:345, 1992.)

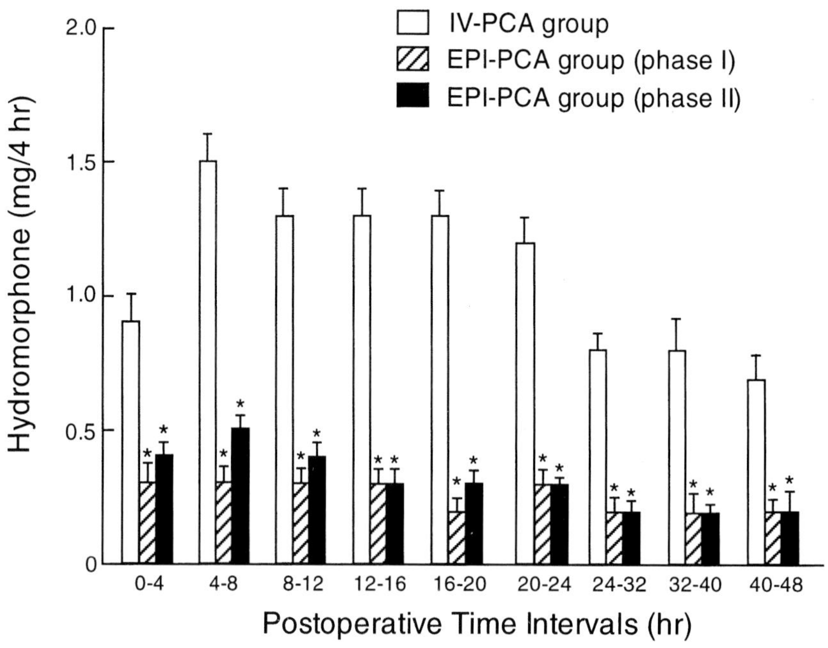

FIG. 26-12. Self-administered hydromorphone dose (mg/4hr) in patients recovering from cesarean section and utilizing either intravenous PCA (*white bar*) or epidural PCA (group I, *light gray bar*; group II, *dark gray bar*). *significant reduction in dose epidural groups I and II versus intravenous group. (Reproduced with permission from Parker R.K., and White, P.F.: Epidural patient-controlled analgesia: An alternative to intravenous patient-controlled analgesia for pain relief after cesarean delivery. Anesth. Analg., *75*:245, 1992.)

TABLE 26-4. *Epidural PCA dosing guidelines*

Opioid	Concentration	Loading dose[a]	EPI-PCA dose[a]	Lockout (min)	Continuous rate[a]	4 hr limit
Morphine	50 mcg/ml	2–4 mg	2–4 ml	10–15	6–12 ml/hr	40–70 ml
Hydromorphone	10 mcg/ml	500–1500 mcg	2–4 ml	6–10	6–12 ml/hr	40–70 ml
Fentanyl	5 mcg/ml	75–100 mcg	2–4 ml	6	6–15 ml/hr	40–70 ml
Sufentanil	2 mcg/ml	0.5 mcg/kg	2–4 ml	6	0.1 mcg/kg/hr	40–70 ml

[a] Dependent upon site of epidural catheter, extent of surgery, patient physical status

TABLE 26-5. *Intrathecal morphine dose guidelines for postoperative analgesia*[a]

Surgical procedure	Intrathecal dose (mg)
Vaginal hysterectomy, cesarean section	0.15–0.2
Hip and knee surgery	0.2–0.3
Lower abdominal surgery	0.2–0.4
Upper abdominal surgery	0.4–0.5
Nephrectomy	0.4–0.5
Cholecystectomy	0.4–0.5
Abdominal aortic aneurysm	0.4–0.6
Whipple procedure	0.5–0.6
Retroperitoneal lymph node dissection	0.5–0.6
Thoracotomy	0.6–0.7

[a] Dependent on age, physical status, height, extent of surgical dissection, and so on. [Modified from Gwirtz, K.H.: Single-dose opioids in the management of acute postoperative pain. *In* Sinatra, R.S., Hord, A.H., Ginsberg, B., and Preble, L.M., (eds.): Acute Pain Mechanisms and Management. St. Louis, Mosby–Yearbook, 1992.]

requirements of IV-PCA or IM narcotics. Intrathecal morphine doses for patients recovering from various surgical procedures are presented in Table 26-5.

Lipophilic opioids are rarely administered intrathecally by themselves since single doses offer only 2 to 4 hours of pain relief.[78,96] Intrathecal combinations of lipophilic opioids such as fentanyl and meperidine plus morphine offer several clinical advantages, including a rapid onset of analgesia and an extended duration of pain relief[76].

Continuous intrathecal administration has been employed to extend the analgesic duration of lipophilic opioids. Domsky and Tarantino[95] described a 70-year-old patient recovering from hip surgery in whom a standard 19-gauge epidural catheter, inserted 2 cm into the subarachnoid space, was utilized, so that the patient could self-administer intrathecal fentanyl. The patient required 2 μg of fentanyl per hour for 48 hours, and experienced excellent pain relief with minimal side effects.

ADVERSE EVENTS ASSOCIATED WITH SPINAL OPIOIDS

Epidural and intrathecal opioids are associated with a number of annoying, and occasionally serious, adverse effects, including pruritus, nausea, urinary retention, somnolence, and respiratory depression.[49,50,78,110,160] Treatment protocols have been developed which decrease the incidence and severity of side effects and improve patient safety while maintaining effective analgesia. The presence of side effects should be assessed frequently and treated quickly, to minimize morbidity and patient dissatisfaction.

Respiratory Depression. Although rare in comparison with other side effects, respiratory depression is the most feared complication associated with epidural and intrathecally administered opioids.[49,110,160,337,338] Respiratory depression following epidural/intrathecal morphine occurs at two different intervals.[49,160,110] An early phase observed soon after administration reflects rapid systemic absorption and is of similar magnitude to that noted following parenteral dosing. A later, more insidious depression occurring over a period of 8 to 12 hours has been related to rostral flow of CSF and delivery of morphine molecules to the brain stem respiratory centers[160] Mild depression of CO_2 responsiveness is common following administration of 3 to 5 mg of epidural and 0.2 mg intrathecal morphine (Fig. 26-13), but the incidence of clinically significant respiratory compromise is very low, ranging between 0.1 and 0.4%.[2,160,250,261] Delayed respiratory depression usually is gradual in onset and generally occurs within the first 12 hours following epidural administration.[110,159] Increasing somnolence, a respiratory rate of less than 10 minutes, or evidence of diminished tidal volume, is treated promptly with naloxone. (40 to 80 mcg IV) followed by a naloxone infusion (300 to 400 mcg/liter of crystalloid every 8 hours). Prophylactic naloxone infusions have been advocated to reduce the risk of opioid induced respiratory depression in elderly or debilitated patients.[158] Risk factors for delayed respiratory depression are outlined in Table 26-6.

Single epidural or intrathecal boluses of lipophilic opioids are not associated with delayed respiratory depression,[78,110,217] but early-onset depression, usually occurring within 30 minutes of administration, has been observed.[6,31,305,338] Early onset respiratory depression is caused by vascular uptake by the epidural or subarachnoid venous plexus and transport via the systemic circulation to brain stem respiratory centers.[6,57] Early-onset depression, while measurable, is usually of lesser significance than delayed-onset respiratory compromise, and is more likely to occur in high visibility, controlled settings (operating room, recovery room, ICU) with the anesthesiologist present or immediately available. The risk of delayed or progressive respiratory depression with epidural infusions of fentanyl and sufentanil appears low,[116,298] however, plasma levels may rise above minimal analgesic concentrations 20 to 30 hours after initiation of therapy.[71] A case report describing late-onset respiratory arrest has been published.[337]

Pruritus. Generalized pruritus is often observed with morphine, and to a lesser extent, with other neuroaxial opioids. Mild pruritus, usually involving the face or chest, occurs even more frequently; however, patients may not complain unless directly questioned. Occasionally, the intensity of itching is so annoying that it interferes with sleep.[49,105,145] Opioid-induced pruritus does not reflect an acute release of histamine, since peak effects are noted 3 to 6 hours following administration.[49,80] Furthermore, pruritus is commonly observed with opioids such as fentanyl and sufentanil that do not release histamine. Changes in spinal outflow may indirectly release small amounts of histamine in tissues adjacent to peripheral nerve endings.[78,354] This finding may explain why antihistamines might provide some relief of symptoms. Pruritus associated with epidural morphine is treated according to its severity. Mild facial pruritus may be relieved with cold compresses, while moderate generalized itching may respond to one or more doses of diphenhydramine, of 12.5 to 25 mg. Patients with moderate to severe pruritus are treated with IV boluses of naloxone (40 to 80 mcg), which generally improves patient comfort without reversing spinal opioid analgesia.[69,251] One may conveniently maintain a continuous IV infusion by adding 1 or 2 ampoules of naloxone (0.4 to 0.8 mg) to each liter of the patient's maintenance intravenous fluid. An infusion rate of 125 ml/hr will deliver 50 to 100 mcg/hr of naloxone. Borgeat and colleagues[37,278] noted that subhypnotic doses (10 mg) of IV propofol provided rapid relief of spinal-morphine-induced pruritus. They proposed that propofol's antipruritic action is not dependent upon specific antagonism of opioid receptor-mediated effects, but rather by nonselective depression of neural transmission in spinal cord.

Nausea and Vomiting. Although nausea and vomiting is commonly observed in patients recovering from abdominal and pelvic surgery, the incidence of symptoms may increase in patients treated with epidural and intrathecal opi-

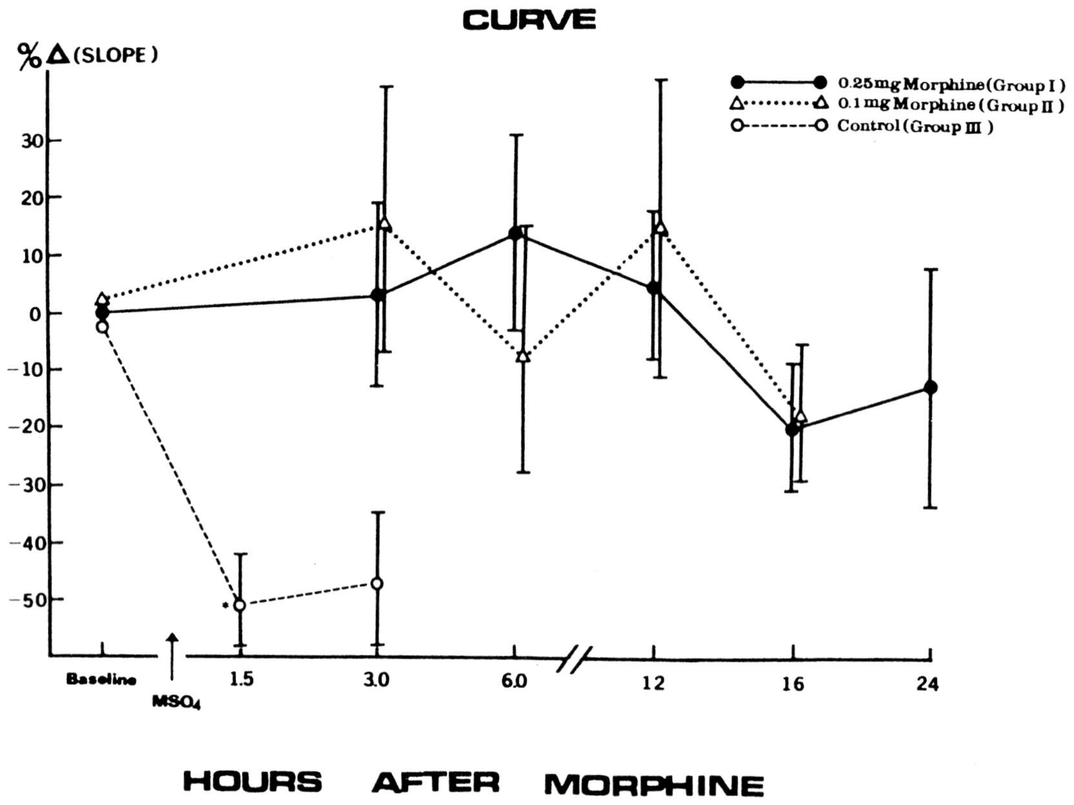

FIG. 26-13. Percent change in CO_2 response slopes (L. min-1 · mm Hg-1) from baseline values after patients received intrathecal *(solid circle, triangle)* or subcutaneous morphine control *(open circle)*. (Reproduced with permission from Abboud, T.K., Dror, A., Mosaad, P., *et al.*: Minidose intrathecal morphine for the relief of postcesarean section pain: Safety and efficiency, and ventilatory responses to carbon dioxide. Anesth. Analg., *67*:137, 1988.)

oids.[49,78,135] Nausea may result either from rostral spread of the drug in spinal fluid to the brain stem, or vascular uptake and delivery to the vomiting center and chemoreceptor trigger zone.[49,78,80] In general, patients treated with intermittent boluses of morphine experience the highest incidence of nausea and vomiting, while patients receiving continuous opioid infusions are affected less often.[114]

A variety of agents have been evaluated for prevention and treatment of opioid-induced emesis. Droperidol (0.625 to 1.25 mg), and metoclopramide (10 mg), administered either as prophylaxis or every 4 to 6 hours have proven to be effective.[69,195] The use of a transdermal scopolamine patch also has been reported to reduce the incidence of nausea and vomiting associated with epidural morphine, particularly during the first 10 hours following administration.[175] This preparation has a latency-to-onset of 3 to 4 hours, and is generally ineffective in treating acute episodes. In the presence of intractable nausea, an intravenous bolus of naloxone, followed by continuous infusion of 0.5 to 1 μg/kg/hr may provide relief.[69] A final antiemetic that may be helpful in cases of intractable nausea is ondansetron. While controlled studies have yet to be completed, doses of between 2 to 4 mg may reduce the incidence and severity of symptoms.[294]

Urinary Retention. A final adverse effect which adds to the morbidity of spinal opioid analgesia is urinary retention. Urinary retention has been related to inhibition of sacral parasympathetic outflow, which results in relaxation of the bladder detrusor muscle, and an inability to relax the sphincter.[253] This complication occurs most often, but not exclusively, in young male patients and is rarely observed in individuals receiving long-term epidural opioid therapy. Urinary retention is disturbing to both patient and surgeon, especially

TABLE 26-6. *Factors which increase the risk of spinal opioid-induced respiratory depression*

Drug-related factors
Hydrophilic opioids
Excessive dose
Large volume of injectate
Excessive dose frequency
Concomitant administration of parenteral opioids
Patient-related factors
Age greater than 60 years
Debilitated individuals
Coexisting respiratory disease
Raised intrathoracic pressure
Shock-wave lithotripsy
Trendelenberg position

when its severity requires frequent urethral catheterization. Intravenous naloxone and urocholine may provide relief in selected patients.[69,253]

INITIATION OF EPIDURAL OPIOID ANALGESIA AND MONITORING GUIDELINES

At Yale-New Haven Hospital, single preoperative doses of epidural and intrathecal morphine are administered routinely for postsurgical analgesia. After 8 to 24 hours, additional pain control is provided by IV-PCA or IM pain medication. IV-PCA has been advocated as a method of augmenting epidural morphine that is comparatively safer than larger "rescue" doses of IM opioids.[170,223,294] In agreement with findings of Kemper and Trieber[170] and Negre et al.[223] we have found that small to moderate doses of intrathecal/epidural morphine reduce IV-PCA requirements by 60% to 70% during the first 24 hours (PCA-sparing effect) in patients recovering from hysterectomy, cesarean section, and major orthopedic surgery (Fig. 26-14).

High-risk patients, and individuals recovering from extensive surgical procedures and major trauma, are treated with continuous epidural infusions or Epi-PCA. Epidural catheters are placed preoperatively at interspaces immediately adjacent to the site of surgery, and an opioid loading dose is administered before surgical incision. Morphine and hydromorphone are used for large, painful procedures, such as nephrectomy, staging laparotomy, upper abdominal surgery, and thoracotomy. Continuous fentanyl infusions generally are reserved for lower extremity procedures, but may be used for pain control following thoracotomy, when administered via thoracic catheters. Continuous epidural opioid infusions and Epi-PCA are supplemented with epidural bupivacaine, and intravenous ketorolac (15 mg q 6 hr) unless medical or surgical contraindications such as hypovolemia or coagulopathy exist. In agreement with previous reports,[194,285] we have observed that dilute high-volume infusions (10 to 12 ml per hour) containing small amounts of bupivacaine (0.02 to 0.03%) improve postsurgical analgesia, without increasing the incidence of orthostatic hypotension or interfering with safe, assisted ambulation. Epi-PCA, with hydromorphone (10 to 20 μg/ml) and 0.03% bupivacaine, has become the epidural analgesic technique employed most commonly at our institution for patients recovering from major surgical procedures. In reviewing records of over 3,000 patients treated with this combination, greater than 90% reported good-to-excellent analgesia.[294] Side effects, such as pruritus, nausea, and sedation are less common than previously

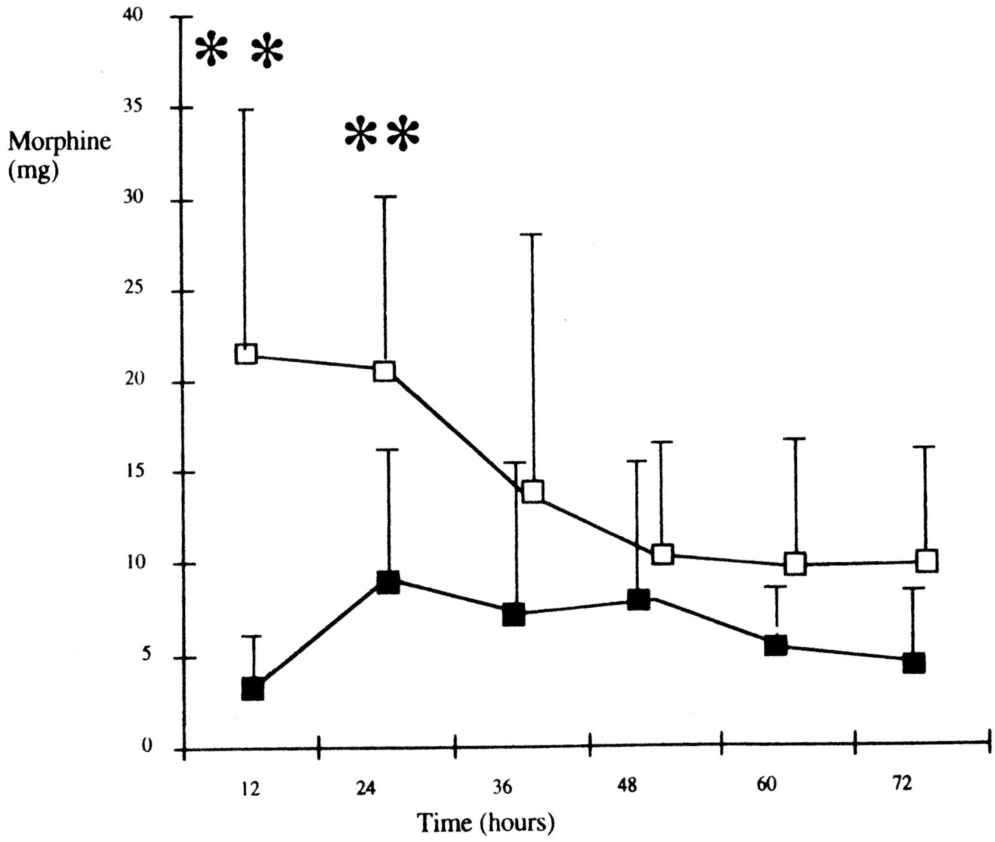

FIG. 26-14. Intravenous PCA morphine requirement per 12 hour period (mean ± SD). *White box*, control group; *black box*, group given 5 mg epidural morphine prior to surgery. **$p < 0.01$ between groups. (Reproduced with permission from Negre, I., Gueneron, J.P., Jamali, S.J., *et al.*: Preoperative analgesia with epidural morphine. Anesth. Analg., *79*:298, 1994.)

observed with epidural morphine or with more concentrated solutions of hydromorphone.[184,235] Patients receive an intraoperative loading dose of 0.5 to 1.0 mg hydromorphone or morphine (2 to 3 mg) with 0.5% bupivacaine or 2% lidocaine. A basal infusion of hydromorphone (10 μg to 20 μg/ml) at a rate of 6 to 12 ml/hr is initiated in the postanesthesia care unit (PACU). Epidural infusion rates are reduced by 1/3 when administered via thoracic catheters. When the patient is alert and oriented, Epi-PCA doses of 3 to 4 ml with a 6 to 8-minute lockout are added. An alternative approach best suited for elderly or debilitated patients, utilizes an intraoperative loading dose of reduced size (hydromorphone 0.25 to 0.5 mg with 0.25 to 0.5% bupivacaine), which is immediately followed by a hydromorphone 10 to 20 μg/ml and 0.03% bupivacaine infusion. This method is useful in prolonged operative procedures, and insures effective pain relief when the patient awakens. Epi-PCA dosing is added in the PACU when the patient is alert and cooperative.

The safety of epidural opioid analgesia in the postoperative period depends upon specific orders and frequent patient

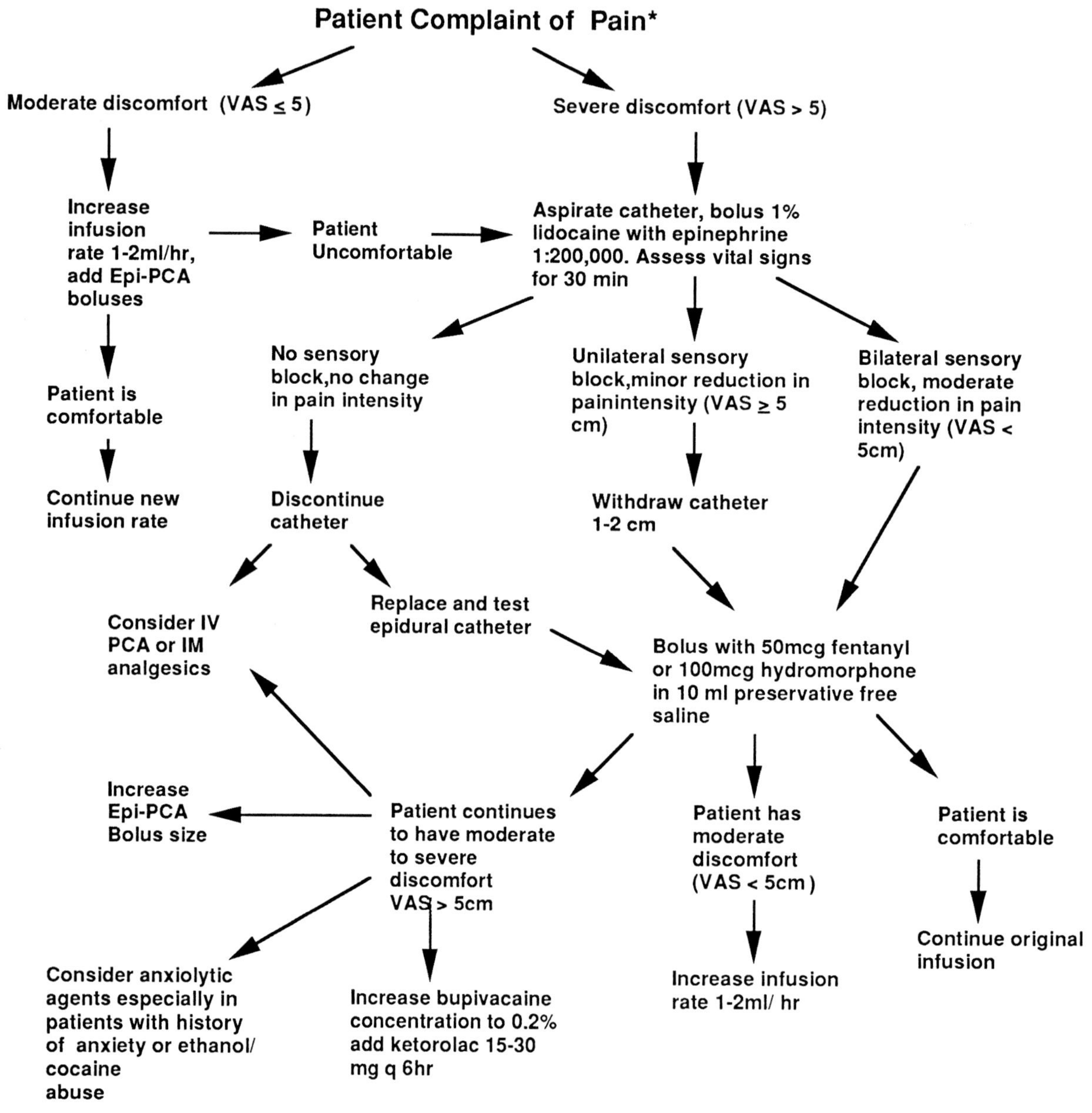

* Initial infusion - Morphine 50mcg/ml- bupivacaine 0.05- 0.1%; Epi- PCA, Epidural patient-controlled analgesia; VAS, visual analog scale score; IV PCA, intravenous patient-controlled analgesia; IM- intramuscular

FIG. 26-15. Algorithm for assessing and treating inadequate epidural analgesia (From the Yale University Department of Anesthesiology, Acute Pain Service, 1992–1996.)

monitoring. Epidural medications, rate of infusion, and patient-controlled dose, must be individualized with regard to individual status and extent of surgery. The adequacy of pain relief, level of sedation, and degree of sensory motor block are assessed and documented in the chart. Side effects including pruritus, nausea/vomiting, and urinary retention are treated by the floor nursing staff who follow standardized orders (see Figs. 26-4 and 26-5).[90,257,259] Inadequate analgesia may be the result of catheter-related problems, undermedication, and patient-related variability. An algorithm used to assess comfort level and to treat breakthrough pain is presented in Figure 26-15. The caregiver must first rule out catheter dislodgment by assessing the site and testing its function with dilute local anesthetic. Patients receiving morphine infusions are treated rapidly with rescue doses of fentanyl to reestablish a state of comfort; then addition of local anesthetic or increased infusion rate are considered. Since hydromorphone has a rapid analgesic onset, fentanyl rescue is not necessary. With functional catheters, 50 to 100 μg bolus of hydromorphone, followed by an increase in infusion rate, usually improves patient comfort within 10 to 15 minutes.[294]

What is the most appropriate method of respiratory monitoring for patients treated with epidural/intrathecal opioids? This question is difficult, and no one solution appears applicable to every institution. The decision of how to monitor patients must be left to the judgment of the acute pain service in conjunction with the nursing staff. Various noninvasive monitors have been advocated, including pulse oximetry, and end-tidal Pco_2 monitoring; however, none of these methods alone has become universally accepted. In most published studies, hourly monitoring of respiratory rate has been the most common method used to detect respiratory compromise. Apnea monitors may be prone to annoying false alarms; they do not detect hypoventilation, and they must be turned off prior to ambulation. Pulse oximeters share the drawbacks of patient inconvenience, frequent motion artifact alarms, and an inability to detect hypercarbia. Epidural opioid-induced respiratory depression does not develop suddenly, but slowly and progressively, and is generally preceded by nausea, vomiting, and increased sedation.[49,78,80,251] Vigilant nursing observation, and documentation of inadequate respiratory effort, slow respiratory rate, or unusual somnolence, represent the best form of monitoring.[259,260] With appropriate staff education, epidural opioids may be administered to most healthy patients recovering on surgical units.[259] Two recent large-scale evaluations noted that intermittent doses and continuous infusions of morphine were provided safely on routine postsurgical units, where nurses were well trained with respect to dose, patient assessment, and treatment of side effects.[90,259] These authors recommend that an acute pain service or in-house anesthesia personnel be available immediately to back up the nursing staff. Elderly individuals and patients with major organ dysfunction are at higher risk for opioid-induced respiratory depression.[78,250] To ensure safety in this population, it is essential that these patients spend the first 24 hours of postsurgical recovery in an intensive care facility. During this time, oxygen saturation should be monitored continuously and respiratory rate and arterial Pco_2 closely followed. Patients with optimal levels of spinal opioid analgesia generally maintain an elevated Pco_2. Unless deemed clinically inappropriate, we set a target at 42 to 44 mm Hg. Progressive increases in sedation and Pco_2 are corrected, either by reducing the infusion rate, or by initiating a low-dose intravenous infusion of naloxone (40 μg to 50 μg/hr).[251]

Contraindications to spinal opioid analgesia include infection at the insertion site, septicemia, epidural mass, or metastases, bleeding diatheses, and anticoagulant therapy. Epidural administration of morphine generally is avoided in patients with documented hypersensitivity and active bronchial asthma. Scopolamine and excessive doses of benzodiazepines should be restricted in elderly patients treated with epidural narcotics to avoid profound sedation, confusion, and airway obstruction.[250,259,294] Patients presenting with a history of ethanol abuse may also pose management challenges. These individuals often appear anxious, highly irritable, and dissatisfied with epidural pain therapy, despite the fact that clinical evidence indicates that they are experiencing highly effective analgesia. In this setting, anxiolytic therapy and ethanol withdrawal prophylaxis may dramatically improve patient cooperation and satisfaction.

NEURAL BLOCKADE FOR ACUTE PAIN MANAGEMENT

Neural blockade may be employed as a sole technique for intraoperative anesthesia, as supplement for general anesthesia, and as a method of maintaining effective postoperative analgesia. Advantages of combined regional/light general anesthesia, followed by continuous neural blockade, include decreased inhalational anesthetic requirements, a pain-free state upon completion of surgery, and a reduced need for postoperative pain medications. The possibility that preincisonal blockade of nociceptive input may also reduce persistent postsurgical pain and the development of neuropathic disorders, offers additional clinical advantages.[16,106,324] Techniques which provide central and peripheral neural blockade minimize exposure to opioids and are ideally suited for patients sensitive to narcotic-induced ileus and bowel obstruction. Other indications include avoidance of respiratory depression, particularly in patients with underlying pulmonary disease.

Epidural administration of local anesthetics or central neural blockade offer reliable, segmental analgesia for patients recovering from general and orthopedic surgery or traumatic injury. However, the technique is associated with sensory/motor, sympathetic, and sacral parasympathetic blockade, and may precipitate cardiovascular instability in hypovolemic patients, urinary retention, and lower extremity weakness. In this regard, hypotension, and impaired micturition occur more frequently with epidural local anesthetics than with morphine.[50,78,107] To ensure patient safety and reduce the incidence and severity of side effects, the catheter tip should be placed at epidural segments immediately adjacent to the surgical injury (i.e. T5–T6 for thoracotomy incision, T8 for upper abdominal, T12 for lower abdominal and L3 for lower extremity procedures). Infusions should contain the lowest concentration of local anesthetic needed to maintain effective analgesia. Solutions of bupivacaine 0.1 to 0.25% are employed for the following reasons: (i) Dilute solutions of bupivacaine offer fairly selective C-fiber blockade, while generally sparing motor fibers; (ii) Tachyphylaxis develops slowly and dose requirements remain fairly constant during short courses of therapy.[294]

Peripheral neural blockade is accomplished by a variety of techniques including local anesthetic infiltration, isolated nerve block, and plexus blockade. Detailed descriptions of each technique are provided in Chapters 11 to 14. Infiltration techniques include: (i) wound injection techniques, which employ undiluted local anesthetic such as 0.25 to 0.5% bupivacaine, infused into skin, subcutaneous tissues, and fascia.[106,157,207,224] These techniques commonly are employed for control of pain following herniorraphy, hysterectomy, cholecystectomy, and varicose vein ligation. (ii) Continuous infiltration techniques employ multihole 19-gauge catheters for continuous infusion of 0.125 or 0.25% bupivacaine under the skin and muscle layers of the incision.[55,320] A modification of this technique, termed iliac crest infiltration, may be used to control pain following iliac crest-spine fusion surgery.[55] A 19-gauge catheter is sutured within the iliac crestbone-graft site, and a solution of 0.125% bupivacaine is continuously infused at a rate of 5 to 8 ml/hr.

Isolated nerve block techniques include iliohypogastric/ilioinguinal nerve block for inguinal hernia and postcesarean analgesia, femoral nerve block, and intercostal nerve block. Femoral nerve block offers effective analgesia for femur fracture and pain following arthroscopic knee surgery.[11,266] Intravenous or oral nonsteroidal anti-inflammatory drugs (NSAIDs) and opioid analgesics may be administered for additional pain relief. Continuous femoral techniques involve placement of 19-gauge catheters into the fascial compartment of the femoral nerve and subsequent infusion of dilute bupivacaine solutions (see Chapter 11).

Blockade of intercostal nerves T5–T11 with 0.5% bupivacaine (3 to 5 ml per nerve) reduce the need for opioid analgesics, and are employed for pain control following upper abdominal and thoracic surgery, traumatic thoracic injury, and cholecystectomy, performed via subcostal incision.[131,212,227,241] Continuous intercostal blockade may be provided by infusions of bupivacaine (0.125 to 0.25%) administered via 19-gauge epidural-type catheter. This technique offers effective pain relief for patients recovering from rib fracture, mini-thoracotomy, and cholecystectomy[131,220] At high rates of infusion (8 to 12 ml/hr), the local anesthetic solution spreads to intercostal and paravertebral spaces above and below the site of administration providing multisegmental blockade.[220] Additional analgesia if required may be provided by IV-PCA morphine or intermittent doses of IV ketorolac.

Plexus blockade techniques offer selective management of acute pain. The lumbar plexus block may be used for pain relief following knee or hip arthroplasty[11] while brachial plexus block is employed for upper extremity procedures.[198,327] Continuous brachial plexus blockade offers an extended duration of postoperative analgesia.[198] The technique employs dilute solutions of bupivacaine 0.125% to 0.25% infused via 20-gauge plastic cannula catheters placed within the neurovascular sheath. Brachial plexus block for shoulder surgery is best accomplished via the interscalene approach, while supraclavicular block is employed for forearm and hand procedures.[198,327] A recent modification of brachial plexus blockade involves the coadministration of local anesthetic plus opioid analgesics. Single injection supraclavicular block with mepivacaine plus small amounts of fentanyl (75 μg) provided more effective pain relief than mepivacaine alone; however, analgesic benefits were limited to the first three hours following surgery.[163] Continuous brachial plexus infusions of fentanyl (2 μg/ml) plus bupivacaine (0.1% or less) offer a more extended duration of pain relief and IV-PCA dose-sparing effect.[294] Similar results have been reported with brachial plexus infusions of mepivacaine (0.5%) plus butorphanol (100 μg/ml): patients recovering from elective upper extremity surgery reported lower pain scores and required less supplementary analgesic than did individuals receiving local anesthetic alone.[331] Whether opioid augmentation of neural blockade is the result of direct activity within the brachial plexus, vascular uptake, and CNS effect, or penetration into the epidural space, providing a limited degree of neuroaxial analgesia, remains to be clarified.

Interpleural Analgesia

Interpleural analgesia provides a therapeutic option in managing acute and chronic pain localized to the thorax and upper abdomen. Since the description of interpleural analgesia by Reiestad and Stromskag,[263] the technique has been employed for pain control following cholecystectomy, thoracic surgery, breast reconstruction, multiple rib fractures, and acute pancreatitis.[4,43,60,101,162,182,267,271,313]

The technique involves insertion of 17-gauge Tuohy epidural needle at the anterior axillary line and placement of a 19-gauge open-tip epidural catheter (see Chapter 14, Fig. 14-10). A distinct click is noted following penetration of the parietal pleura, and is accompanied by a loss of resistance in a saline-filled syringe.[4,263,313] The catheter is advanced carefully 3 to 5 cm towards the shoulder and taped in place. Two ml increments of bupivacaine 0.5% are injected every 2 to 3 minutes, until a total of 15 to 20 ml has been administered. Pain relief is noted within 5 to 10 minutes following administration. Doses are repeated every 4 to 6 hours. Intermittent interpleural dosing is labor-intensive, and each dose is followed by significant elevations in plasma bupivacaine, which may approach toxic levels.[3,4,175,181] Laurito et al.[182] compared the safety and efficacy of continuous interpleural infusions of bupivacaine, versus intermittent bolus injections following cholecystectomy. Patients in the infusion group experienced a more uniform level of pain relief and required less supplementation with IV-PCA morphine. Interpleural analgesia, like other forms of regional analgesia, may be associated with windows, or regions of less effective analgesia. Patients complaining of inadequate pain relief may benefit from concomitant administration of IV-PCA opioids, and ketorolac. An alternative method of improving interpleural analgesia may be achieved by adding fentanyl (1 to 2 μg/ml) to the bupivacaine infusion.[294]

Interpleural catheter placement is associated with a number of minor side effects such as small hematoma, nonleaking lung puncture, or small pneumothoraces. The risk for serious complications, such as tension pneumothorax, is low but exists no matter what technique, needle, or syringe used.[4,263] Contraindications include: positive end expiratory pressure ventilation, pleural fibrosis, pleural adhesions, pleuritis, pleural effusion, and infection at proposed site of insertion.

Other Techniques. Oral transmucosal and transdermal fentanyl delivery systems have been introduced for acute pain management.[183,289,309] Although transdermal fentanyl preparations provide useful postoperative analgesia, a prolonged latency in onset and progressive increases in narcosis and nausea and vomiting limit their overall usefulness in this setting.[289] Oral transmucosal fentanyl is a lozenge-shaped preparation attached to a plastic stick that has been undergoing clinical trials in the United States.[185,309] While originally developed for pediatric premedication, more recent applications include control of acute postoperative pain and breakthrough cancer pain. In a preliminary evaluation, Lind and co-workers[185] reported that transmucosal fentanyl was well tolerated and provided effective analgesia in patients recovering from major orthopedic surgery.

The use of transcutaneous electrical nerve stimulation (TENS) represents a conservative nonpharmacologic method of reducing pain associated with injury or surgery.[54,63] While unable to relieve the most intense aspects of acute pain, TENS provides useful supplementation of analgesia. TENS in combination with low-dose IV-PCA morphine, and IV ketorolac offers effective analgesia with acceptable levels of sedation while reducing self-administered opioid requirements.[63,309]

Pediatric Acute Pain Management

Children recovering from surgery and acute trauma tend to be undermedicated for their pain and generally suffer greater discomfort than do adults.[200,214] Similar complaints of severe pain are observed in children suffering from sickle cell crisis and terminal malignancies.[123,283,291] It is recognized now that children either cannot or will not report inadequate analgesia to their caregivers, and that poorly controlled pain has negative physical and psychosocial effects.[9,21,27,61,204] The Agency for Health Care Policy and Research (AHCPR) pediatric pain guidelines recommend that health care professionals assess pain intensity/pain relief scores frequently and have a high degree of suspicion that the child is experiencing discomfort.[61,155] Children and their parents should be involved actively in pain assessment and management, and taught that optimal relief of pain plays an important role in the recovery period (see also Chapter 20).

A variety of pharmacologic techniques such as IV opioid infusions, IV-PCA, epidural opioids, and neural blockade, and nonpharmacologic techniques, including distraction, hypnosis, and TENS have been advocated for pediatric pain management. Oral administration of analgesics should always be considered the route of choice in children tolerating fluids and food; however, because of nausea, vomiting, and ileus, this form of dosing is unreliable following surgery.[27,297] Although IM injections can provide reliable postoperative analgesia, children are often frightened by such invasive therapy and often deny the presence of pain to avoid the distress associated with injections. In recent years, intramuscular injections have been superseded by the convenience and greater analgesic uniformity provided by continuous intravenous infusions and IV-PCA.[39,269,297] Children and adolescents using IV-PCA experience superior pain relief while requiring less morphine than age-matched controls treated with IM injections.[27,269,283,291,297] At what age children can effectively use IV-PCA remains open to question. At Yale-New Haven Hospital, children eight years and older, capable of making competent decisions about analgesic self-administration, are routinely treated with PCA.[297] With proper selection and training, such therapy may be offered to younger patients. Alternatively, very young children may be treated with "parent and nurse assisted" PCA.[27] With appropriate in-service nursing and standardization of orders, IV-PCA can be provided safely to healthy children and does not require additional nursing care or extensive monitoring.

Neuroaxial opioid techniques provide important therapeutic options for pediatric pain management.[27,139] Single or intermittent boluses of morphine may be administered at intrathecal, caudal, and epidural sites.[44,46,139,176] This therapy is safe and highly effective, provided that doses are adjusted carefully and guidelines for monitoring and treatment of side effects have been formulated. The caudal approach commonly is used in infants and young children and provides effective analgesia following genitourinary, or lower extremity orthopedic surgery. Single-dose caudal morphine (0.05 to 0.1 mg/kg), or "Kiddie caudal," covers pain associated with pelvic through thoracic surgery for periods up to 24 hours.[46,139,176] In children recovering from major surgical procedures, caudal morphine offers more effective analgesia and superior hemodynamic stability than does IV morphine.[25,139,176] Krane et al.[176] compared use of varying doses of caudal morphine (0.03, 0.07 and 0.1 mg/kg) in infants recovering from lower abdominal surgery. While all doses provided excellent pain relief, duration was longest and incidence of adverse events highest in the group receiving 0.1 mg/kg. Caudal administration of ketamine 0.1 mg/kg alone or in combination with bupivacaine also provides safe and effective postoperative analgesia; however, the average duration of pain relief is limited to 4 to 5 hours.[221] Note also that ketamine is not approved for caudal administration by any drug regulatory body.

Intrathecal opioids are used less commonly in pediatric patients and are usually reserved for pain relief following extensive surgical procedures, including open heart surgery. Postoperative analgesia provided by intrathecal morphine was evaluated in 59 children recovering from open heart surgery.[159] Sixty percent of patients noted excellent pain relief for up to 22 hours; 9 children experienced significant respiratory depression. Intrathecal morphine (0.01 to 0.025 mg/kg) provided up to 18 hours of pain control with no evidence of respiratory depression in children recovering from Harrington rod placement and spinal fusion surgery.[44,89]

Epidural opioids alone or in combination with local anesthetics are commonly employed for acute pain control in older children.[13,25,26,139,207] Attia et al.[13] evaluated pharmacokinetic and CO_2 responses in chidren receiving epidural morphine (0.05 mg/kg) following upper abdominal surgery. All patients experienced excellent pain relief, but CO_2 sensitivity was impaired for 22 hours following administration. Because of morphine's association with prolonged and delayed respiratory depression, many pediatric caregivers employ more lipophilic opioids such as hydromorphone, fentanyl, and sufentanil.[25,26,139] Lipophilic opioids may be associated with early onset respiratory depression. In this regard, epidurally administered sufentanil (0.75 mcg/kg) provided analgesia for 200 minutes following urologic surgery, but respiratory depression lasted for more than 240 minutes.[26]

Continuous infusions offer greater safety and a more extended duration of effect than bolus doses.[139] Solutions of fentanyl 2 μg/ml with bupivacaine 0.1% are infused at a rate of 0.1 to 0.5 ml/kg/hr, depending upon the site of incision and physical status of the child.[25,139] Infusions of hydromorphone or morphine are reserved for pain control following upper abdominal or thoracic surgery. Hydromorphone is administered in concentrations of 10 to 20 μg/ml and infused at 0.1 to 0.25 ml/kg/hr.[139,294] Epidural and caudal infusions of dilute bupivacaine (0.125% or lower) provide C-fiber selectivity and a prolonged duration of effect. Bupivacaine infusions are indicated for children intolerant of opioid-induced respiratory depression.[342] Intrathecal, epidural, and caudal doses of opioid analgesics for pediatric patients are presented in Table 26-7.

Local anesthetic infiltration and regional nerve blockade offer significant advantages in pediatric patients[265,351] (see Chapter 20 for a detailed review). Children awaken from surgery with minimal discomfort and without excessive narcosis or other opioid-related side effects. In ambulatory settings, children receiving regional anesthesia required less pain medication and were discharged sooner than untreated controls.[179] These benefits are associated with high patient and parent satisfaction. Of 200 parents interviewed postoperatively, 90% said they would allow their child to have another regional block.[47] Since children fear needle placement and find paresthesias disturbing, neural blockade generally is performed using a nerve stimulator following induction of general anesthesia.[265] Neural blockade can be performed in cooperative well-sedated children and adolescents. The following nerve blocks are of particular use in pediatric patients: (i) Ilioinguinal/Iliohypogastric nerve block with 0.25 to 0.5% bupivacaine (2 mg/kg) offers effective and long-lasting pain relief after hernia repair and orchiopexy.[143,179]

TABLE 26-7. *Recommended agents and rates of infusion for pediatric epidural, caudal, and intrathecal analgesia[a]*

	Surgical site		
Catheter site	Lower extremity Lower abdomen	Upper abdomen	Thoracic
Thoracic catheter		**(1)** 0.1–0.5 ml/kg/hr **(3)** 0.1–0.5 ml/kg/hr	**(1)** 0.1–0.5 ml/kg/hr **(3)** 0.1–0.5 ml/kg/hr **(4)** 0.1–0.5 ml/kg/hr **(5)** 0.05–0.25 ml/kg/hr
Lumbar or caudal catheters	**(1)** 0.1–0.5 ml/kg/hr	**(1)** 0.1–0.5 ml/kg/hr	**(1)** 0.1–0.5 ml/kg/hr
	(3) 0.1–0.5 ml/kg/hr	**(3)** 0.1–0.5 ml/kg/hr **(4)** 0.1–0.5 ml/kg/hr **(6)** 0.1–0.5 ml/kg/hr	**(3)** 0.1–0.5 ml/kg/hr **(5)** 0.1–0.25 ml/kg/hr **(7)** 0.1–0.25 ml/kg/hr
Caudal (single dose)	**(2)** 0.05 ml/kg/segment	**(8)** 0.05–0.10 mg/kg in 3 ml preservative-free normal saline	**(8)** 0.05–0.10 mg/kg in preservative-free normal saline
Intrathecal		**(8)** 0.01–0.02 mg/kg	**(8)** 0.01–0.02 mg/kg

(1), bupivacaine 0.1%; **(2)**, bupivacaine 0.25%; **(3)**, bupivacaine 0.1% and fentanyl 2 mcg/ml; **(4)**, Bupivacaine 0.1% and hydromorphone 10 mcg/ml; **(5)**, bupivacaine 0.1% and hydromorphone 20 mcg/ml; **(6)**, hydromorphone 10 mcg/ml; **(7)**, hydromorphone 20 mcg/ml; **(8)**, morphine, preservative free. (From Haber, D.W., and Berde, C.B.: Spinal opioids for pediatric pain management. *In* Sinatra, R.S., Hord, A.H., Ginsberg, B., and Preble, L.M., (eds): Acute Pain Mechanisms and Management. St. Louis, Mosby–Yearbook, 1992.)

(ii) Block of the dorsal penile nerves with 1 to 2 ml 0.25% bupivacaine provides analgesic benefits for up to 24 hours in neonates recovering from circumcision and hypospadius repair.[45,108,353] Topical anesthesia provided by an eutectic mixture of local anesthetics (EMLA) cream has been used to blunt pain associated with neonatal circumcision.[265] (iii) Femoral nerve block, either by itself or in combination with sciatic nerve block, offers useful anesthesia/analgesia in a variety of lower extremity orthopedic procedures.[28,265] (iv) The axillary approach to blocking the brachial plexus provides effective pain relief following upper extremity procedures and is popular in pediatric patients because of its safety and technical simplicity. Transarterial and nerve stimulator-assisted approaches performed in lightly anesthetized children are associated with an equal rate of success.[265] (v) Intercostal nerve block with 0.5% bupivacaine has been used to control post-thoracotomy pain and severe discomfort following chest injury. Because plasma concentrations rise rapidly following intercostal injection, dosage must be restricted to 2 to 3 mls per nerve, with total dose not to exceed 3 mg/kg.[275] (vi) Continuous interpleural catheter techniques also have been advocated for pediatric patients recovering from thoracotomy.[205]

POST-TRAUMATIC PAIN

Undermedication of severely burned and traumatized patients occurs frequently; caregivers fear that pain medications may mask changes in status and risk patient addiction. However, in a recent survey involving over 10,000 patients in 151 burn centers, no cases of iatrogenic opioid addiction were reported.[239] Pain management in the trauma patient has been divided into three phases: emergent, acute, and rehabilitative.[133,306] During the emergent phase, primary attention must be given to stabilizing the patient's respiratory and cardiovascular status; thereafter, the intensity of pain may be assessed and carefully controlled. Primary analgesic therapy includes intravenous titration of opioids in doses that provide pain relief while not compromising the patient's hemodynamic status or obscuring the diagnostic process.

The acute phase begins with admission to the intensive care facility and continues upon transfer to the medical/surgical ward.[306] Analgesia for unconscious, mechanically ventilated and confused patients is best provided with careful titration of IV opioids, but if the patient is alert and cooperative more advanced techniques such as IV-PCA and epidural analgesia may be utilized. The choice of analgesic is based on the location and severity of pain, as well as individual patient factors. Upper extremity injuries may limit application of IV-PCA, while spinal fractures and anticoagulation may contraindicate placement of an epidural catheter. IV-PCA provides useful pain control following major orthopedic trauma and extensive soft tissue injuries.[306] If there are no contraindications to regional analgesia, IV-PCA may be supplemented with intercostal, brachial plexus, or interpleural blocks.[4,131,272]

Continuous epidural analgesia should be considered the technique of choice in patients recovering from multiple rib fractures and flail chest, where effort-dependent pain associated with cough and deep breathing is poorly tolerated.[325] Whenever possible, the epidural catheter should be placed at the dermatomal level of the injury, reducing overall opioid/local anesthetic dose, and providing a more segmental level of analgesia.[325] In general, epidural morphine may be administered at lumbar sites while hydromorphone and fentanyl are infused via thoracic catheters. Dilute concentrations of bupivacaine (0.1 to 0.03%) are added to the epidural infusate in hemodynamically stable patients.

Manipulative procedures, including external bone fixation, wound debridement, burn eschar excision, and dressing changes, increase pain intensity and generally require greater amounts of analgesia than is routinely prescribed for baseline discomfort.[306] During these procedures, IV-PCA may be supplemented with rapid-acting short-duration opioids (fentanyl 1 to 5 μg/kg or equivalent doses of alfentanil), ketamine (1 to 3 mg/kg), and small doses of midazolam.[142,306] In selected patients, self-administered 50% nitrous oxide in oxygen may be used to supplement analgesia, provided that caregivers skilled in airway maintenance are immediately available.[21]

The rehabilitative phase begins when the patient is transferred from the ICU to the medical/surgical unit, and ends with full recovery.[133] Patients are expected to move out of bed, ambulate with increasing frequency, and participate in physical therapy. As GI function returns and diet is advanced, IV-PCA and epidural analgesia may be discontinued and oral pain medications substituted. Baseline (resting) pain may be relieved with timed-release preparations of morphine (MS contin) and oxycodone (Oxycontin), or methadone elixir. Increases in pain intensity associated with physical therapy may be controlled with morphine or oxycodone elixir given immediately prior to the procedure. During the rehabilitative phase, NSAIDs may be used to augment timed-release oral opioids, while tricyclic antidepressants, clonidine, and sympathetic blockade may be employed to control persistent neuropathic and sympathetically mediated pain.[306]

OPTIMIZING ACUTE PAIN MANAGEMENT: NEW CONCEPTS

Preemptive Analgesia

Recent advances in pain management have resurrected ideas proposed 70 years ago, that blockade of pain transmission prior to the initiation of surgical injury may reduce postoperative morbidity/mortality.[53,82] Crile and Lower[82] suggested that noxious stimuli slowed postoperative recovery and that the CNS could be protected by combining adequate premedication and neural blockade with general anesthesia. In the late 1980s, Wall[382] introduced the concept of preemptive preoperative analgesia, suggesting that analgesic intervention is most effective when made in advance of the pain stimulus rather than in reaction to it. It is recognized now that peripheral injury triggers a state of neuronal excitability in dorsal horn termed central facilitation or wind-up.[5,343,346] Central facilitation may be prevented by preemptive administration of analgesics and peripheral neural blockade, though such therapy becomes less effective following injury.[5,93,197,321,330,344,345]

One of the first clinical trials designed to detect benefits of pre- versus postsurgical neural blockade was performed by Ringnose and Cross.[266] They noted that patients treated with femoral nerve block prior to arthroscopic knee surgery required 50% less opioid analgesic during the first 24 hours of recovery than did individuals receiving a similar block at completion of the procedure. In a study evaluating postinguinal herniorrhaphy pain, patients who received local anesthetic infiltration of the incision and of fascial tissues, before induction of general anesthesia, experienced significant reductions in postoperative discomfort and required lower doses of opioid analgesics than did patients treated with general anesthesia alone or spinal anesthesia (Fig. 26-16).[305] While Ejlersen[106] reported similar preemptive benefits; Dierking and colleagues[94] were unable to discern differences between pre- and postincisional lidocaine infiltration with respect to pain control following herniorraphy. In this study, preemptive benefits may have been obscured by the fact that both treatment groups received continuous infusions of fentanyl during surgery. In a recent editorial, Kissin[172] outlined several reasons why preemptive benefits may not be detected in clinical settings, including insufficient duration or degree of preemptive blockade, a partial preemptive effect in the control group, and the use of surgical models associated with low-intensity noxious stimulation.

Preoperative administration of opioids[223,246,268] NMDA receptor antagonists,[277,323] and nonsteroidal anti-inflammatory drugs[232,288] offer alternative forms of preemptive therapy that may be particularly useful in settings where peripheral neural blockade may be technically difficult or inappropriate. McQuay et al.[207] reported striking variation in requests for pain medication following orthopedic surgery. The median time to first request, which averaged less than 2 hours in untreated controls, was extended to more than 5 hours in patients receiving opioid premedication (Fig. 26-17). Tverskoy noted that patients receiving preincisional doses of fentanyl (5 μg/kg) or the noncompetitive NMDA antagonist, ketamine (2 mg/kg), experienced decreased wound hyperalgesia following abdominal hysterectomy.[323] In a subsequent study, Roytblat and co-workers[277] reported that low-dose ketamine (0.15 mg/kg IV), administered prior to incision, delayed the first request for analgesics, reduced postsurgical pain scores, and decreased IV-PCA morphine dose requirements.

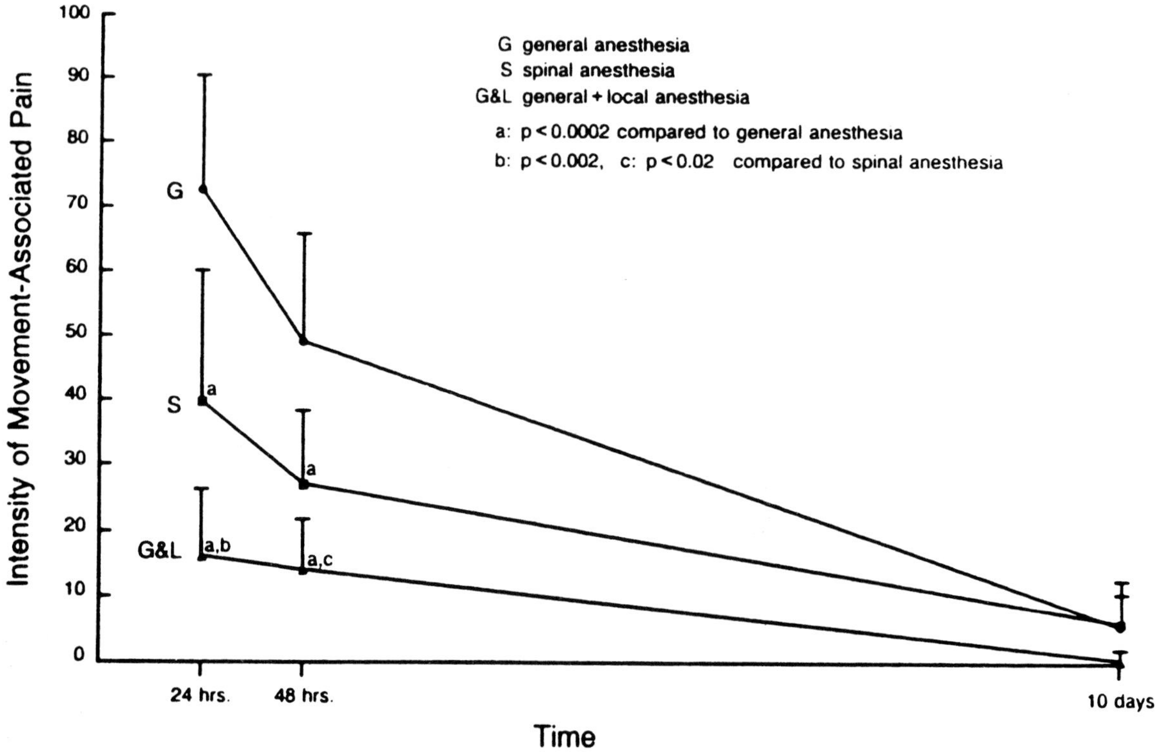

FIG. 26-16. Movement-associated pain scores in patients recovering from inguinal hernia repair during either general anesthesia (*group G*), spinal anesthesia (*group S*), or general anesthesia plus local anesthetic infiltration. (Reproduced with permission from Tverskoy, M., Cozacov, C., Ayache, M., *et al.*: Postoperative pain after inguinal herniorrhaphy with different types of anesthesia. Anesth. Analg., *70*:29, 1990.)

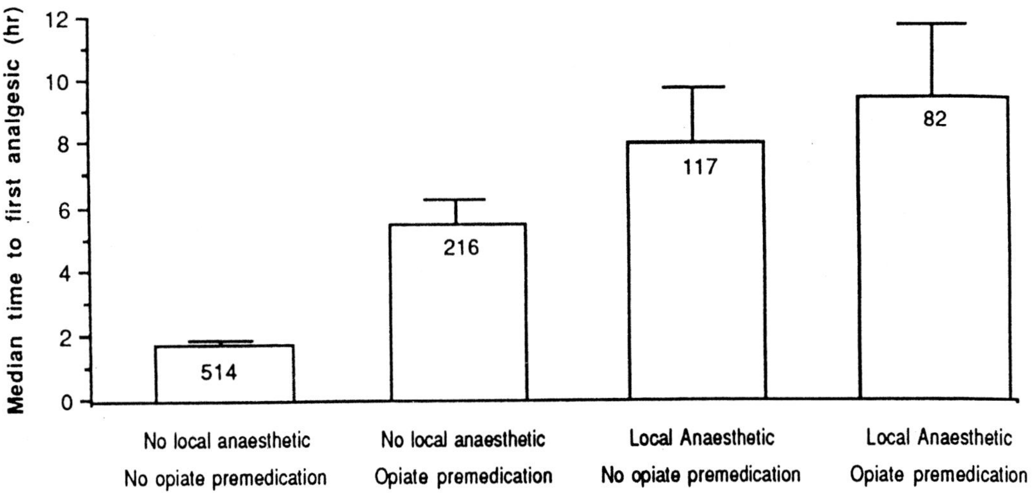

FIG. 26-17. Median time (hour) to first request for postoperative analgesic by treatment category. Bars represent upper 95% confidence interval. (Reproduced with permission from McQuay, H.J., Carrol, D., and Moore, R.A.: Postoperative orthopaedic pain—The effect of opiate premedication and local anesthetic blocks. Pain, *33:*291, 1988.)

Preemptive analgesic benefits also have been observed with epidural opioids. Katz and co-workers[164] reported that epidural fentanyl (4 μg/kg), administered prior to incision, was more effective than postincisional dosing in reducing pain scores and IV-PCA morphine requirements 12 to 24 hours following thoracotomy. In a more recent report,[268] epidural morphine-mepivacaine, administered prior to surgical incision, reduced postsurgical IV-PCA requirements, compared with groups receiving these agents upon completion of surgery, or not at all (Fig. 26-18).

While single doses of epidural opioid/local anesthetic block nociception associated with surgical dissection/manipulation, they may not prevent postsurgical central facilitation resulting from inflammation, movement, and

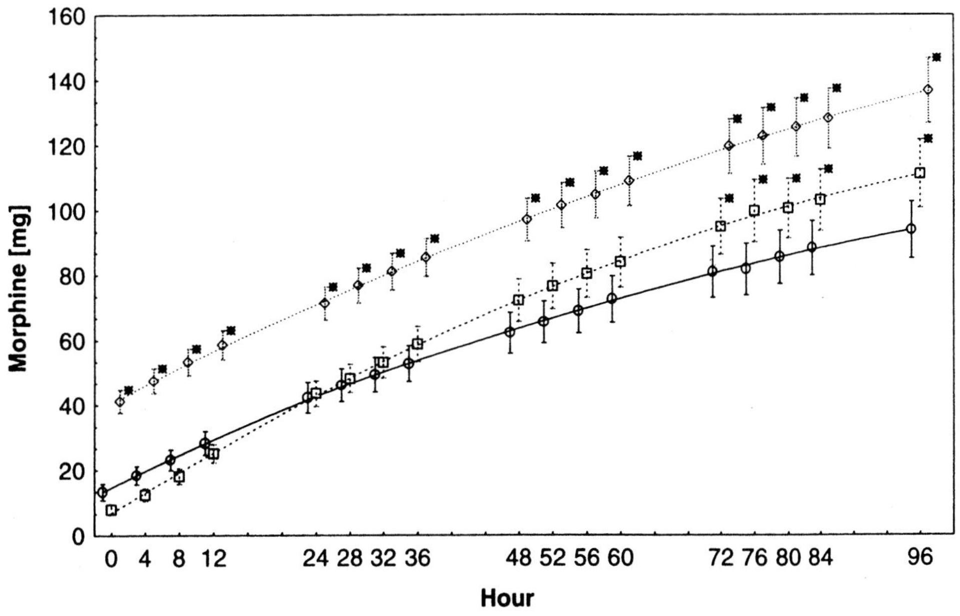

FIG. 26-18. Cumulative morphine consumption on postoperative days 1 to 5, Time 0 = 8 am the morning of the first postoperative day: Group 1 (*circles, solid line*), preincisional morphine/mepivacaine/diclofenac treatment; Group 2 *(squares, dotted line)*, postincisional treatment; Group 3 (*diamonds, dotted line*), no perioperative treatment. Values represent mean ± SEM, *P < 0.05 greater PCA morphine use compared to Group 1. (Reproduced with permission from Rockemann, M.G., Seeling, W., Bishof, C., *et al.*: Prophylactic use of epidural mepivacaine-morphine, systemic diclofenac, and metamizol reduces postoperative morphine consumption after major abdominal surgery. Anesthesiology, *84:*1027, 1996.)

stretching of the injury site. Woolf[343] has proposed that optimal preemptive analgesia should include preoperative initiation, as well as postoperative maintenance of effective therapy. His argument that single-treatment preemptive analgesia may be insufficient for the management of pain beyond the immediate postoperative period is presented in Figure 26-19. To date, only a few studies have compared pre- versus postoperative initiation of continuous analgesic therapy.[84,246] Dahl and co-workers[84] were unable to detect differences in postoperative pain in patients receiving epidural bupivacaine-morphine infusions initiated either before or following completion of colonic surgery. These results have been criticized because the degree of afferent blockade in the preemptive-dosed group was insufficient to prevent central sensitization. Pryl and colleagues[236] evaluated the benefits of preemptive epidural blockade, followed by continuous infusion, in patients recovering from lower abdominal surgery. They reported that the preincisional group experienced lower movement-associated pain scores in the immediate postoperative interval, but in time, no additional benefits could be detected, because both groups reported very low pain scores.

Efforts to lower hospitalization costs have resulted in a large increase in same-day surgical procedures, as well as early patient discharge. These trends underscore the importance of preemptive analgesia, which provides benefits that outlast the pharmacological duration of the therapy employed, minimizing discomfort after the patient is discharged. The anesthesiologist can play a key role by employing preoperative and intraoperative agents and tech-

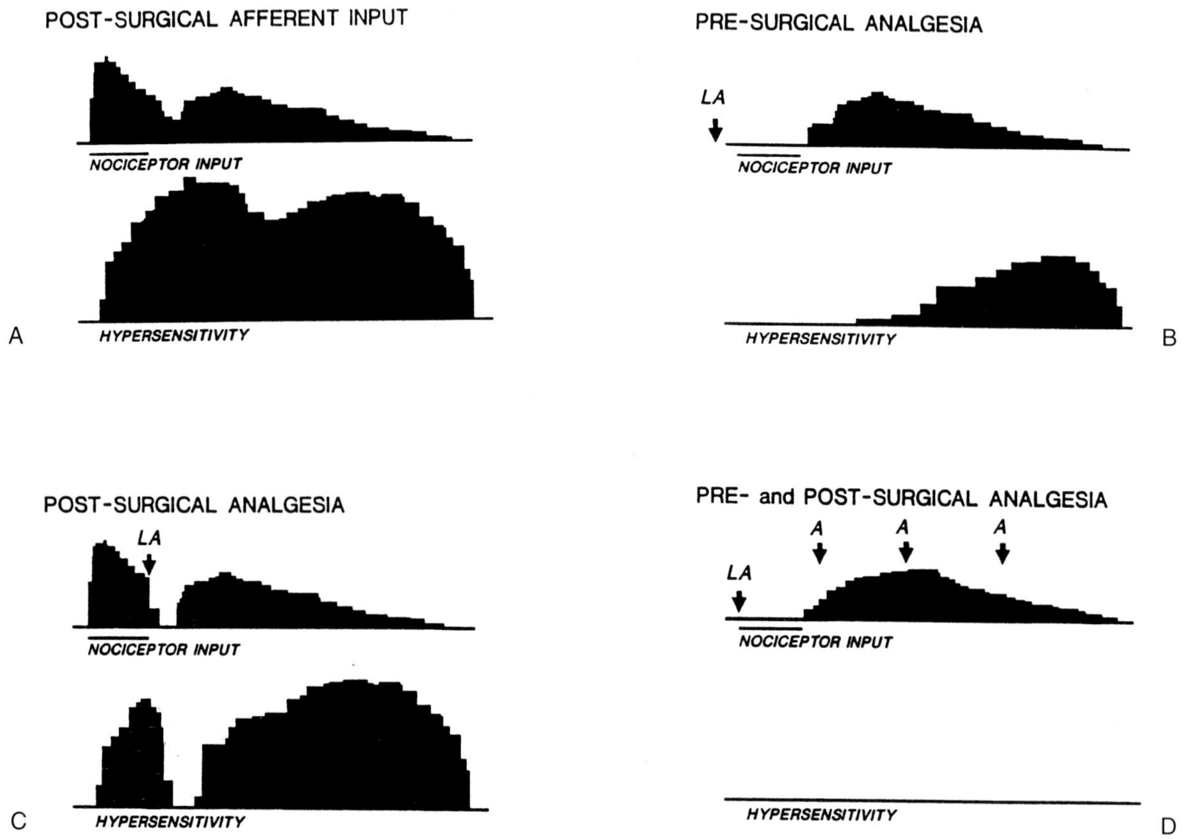

FIG. 26-19. A model illustrating why single-treatment preemptive analgesia may be insufficient for the management of postoperative pain. Surgery leads to a nociceptive input not only during the surgery itself (solid line beneath the drawing of Nociceptor Input represents the duration of surgery), but also postoperatively as a result of the inflammatory response to the damaged tissue. This secondary wave of input can sustain the hypersensitivity state. **(A).** Regional anesthesia administered for the duration of the surgery, although eliminating the first phase of nociceptive input and therefore preempting the first stage of postsurgical hypersensitivity, will not prevent initiation of central sensitization in response to the second inflammatory phase **(B),** although it might have greater relative effect than a single postoperative treatment **(C).** The optimum form of treatment may be one that acts continuously both on the first intraoperative phase (e.g., regional anesthesia or preoperative opioids) and then on the afferent activity generated postoperatively (e.g., nonsteroidal anti-inflammatory drugs, opioids, and continuous epidural/regional blockade) **(D).** *LA,* local anesthesia. (Reproduced with permission from Woolf, C.J., and Chong, M.S.: Pre-emptive analgesia-treating postoperative pain by preventing the establishment of central sensitization. Anesth. Analg., *77*:362, 1993.)

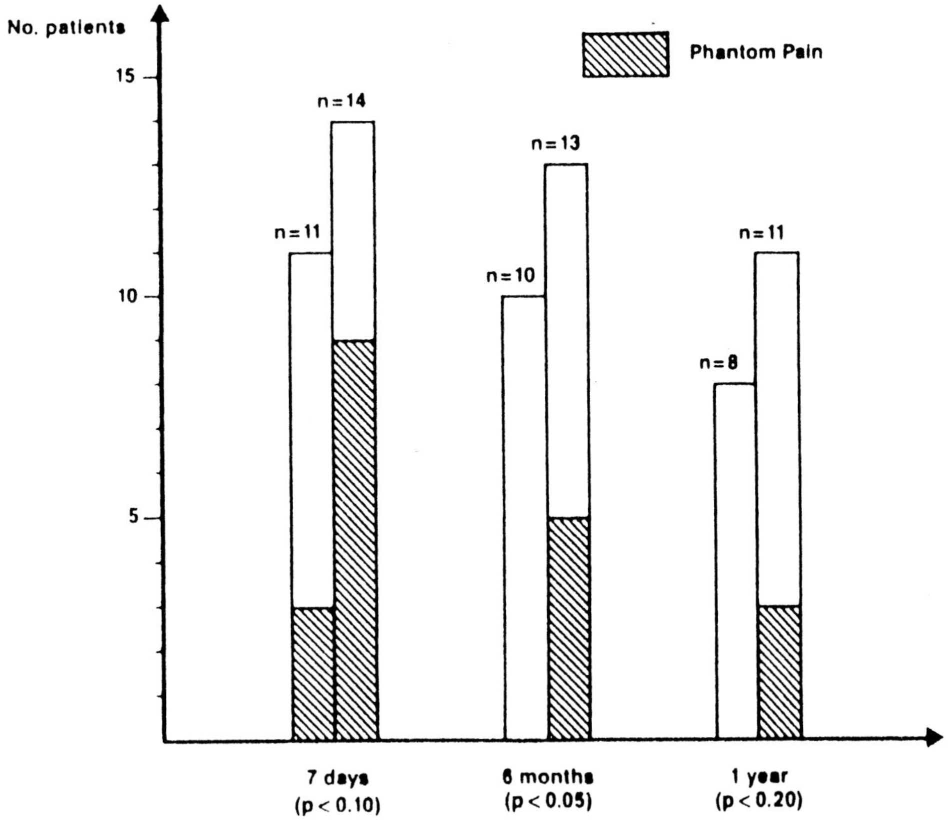

FIG. 26-20. The incidence of phantom limb pain in patients undergoing lower extremity amputation with either general anesthesia (*left side bar* at each time interval) or continuous epidural anesthesia begun preoperatively and continued for postoperative analgesia *(right side bar)*. Hatched segments represent the number of patients experiencing phantom pain. (Reproduced with permission from Bach, N.H., Noreng, M.F., and Tjellden, N.U.: Phantom limb pain in amputees during the first 12 months following limb amputation after preoperative lumbar epidural blockade. Pain, *33*:297, 1988.)

niques that complement postoperative pain management. Leaders in the field of pain management have criticized anesthetic techniques which, in an effort to ensure rapid emergence, employ dense neuromuscular blockade and relatively small amounts of analgesic.[12,42] When surgery is performed in such a lightly anesthetized setting, the neuroaxis is exposed to high levels of nociceptive input[5,338] and postsurgical pain is more difficult to control.[203] Bridenbaugh[42] suggests that practitioners take a step back to the time when most patients were premedicated with opioid analgesics, and that intraoperative management included local anesthetic infiltration and neural blockade. High levels of noxious input are associated with *central* facilitation and activation of NMDA and neurokinin (NK) receptors (see Chapter 23.1). This leads inevitably to "memories of pain" capable of causing persistent pain.[20] Such "memories" begin to be formed in dorsal horn, and move centrally, surprisingly soon after acute injury. Thus, acute, subacute, and chronic pain must be regarded as a continuum. It is likely that new drugs, acting on NMDA and NK receptors and associated mechanisms, may be needed to reliably block central sensitization and memories of pain.[20]

While the majority of clinical studies have concentrated on improving acute pain and disability, preemptive analgesia also may reduce the severity of convalescence pain[324] and provide long-term rehabilitative benefits by preventing or minimizing persistent pain syndromes[16,72,164] Patients recovering from back-fusion surgery, in which donor bone is taken from the iliac crest, may develop chronic periosteal pain that persists for months to years after the operation. Perioperative infusion of bupivacaine via an iliac crest catheter appears to minimize the development of chronic sensitivity.[55] Neuralgias, phantom limb pain, and deafferentation syndromes are common after amputation. Preemptive analgesia provided by perioperative epidural conduction blockade may prevent the development of chronic stump and phantom limb pain in patients recovering from below-the-knee amputation.[16] This is also suggested by a study reporting that degree of acute pain after thoracic surgery predicts long-term postthoracotomy pain[164] (Fig. 26-20). Optimization of rehabilitative/convalescence pain following amputation and other extensive surgical procedures may also require at home IV- or Epi-PCA and a system to monitor patient status away from the hospital.

MULTIMODAL ANALGESIA

Complete abolition of postsurgical pain (pain prevention) is difficult to achieve with a single drug or analgesic technique.[87,166] In an effort to minimize dose requirements and potential toxicity associated with reliance on one agent, balanced, or multimodal, analgesic regimens have been advocated.[87,166,214] Important principles underlying multimodal analgesia include: (i) that effective pain relief may be achieved by the additive or synergistic activity of two or more analgesics,[237] and (ii) that by reducing the amount of each drug administered, the incidence and severity of annoying and potentially serious side effects may be diminished. Multimodal analgesic therapy employs a variety of agents which interfere with noxious transmission and pain perception at different levels within the peripheral and central nervous system. These sites of activity are outlined in Figure 26-21.

In clinical settings, NSAIDs offer useful augmentation of intravenous and neuroaxial opioid-based analgesia without increased risk of sedation, pruritus, and respiratory depression.[86,123,128,137,201,214,258,268,288,311,318] The multimodal combination of epidural fentanyl plus IV ketorolac reduced movement-associated pain, and resulted in a more rapid return of gastrointestinal function than did fentanyl alone (Fig. 26-22).[128] Similar results were noted with epidural hydromorphone plus intravenous ketorolac in patients recovering from thoracotomy.[303]

The combination of neural blockade such as femoral nerve block, and local anesthetic infiltration plus intravenous opioids or NSAIDs offers significant prolongation in the time to first request for postoperative analgesics than either form of therapy alone.[207] In patients recovering from extremely painful procedures, continuous plexus blockade can reduce IM and IV-PCA opioid requirements.[241,243] Analgesic potentiation is also observed with epidural opioid-local anesthetic combinations.[7,85,90,118,147,148,258,284,319] Epidural infusions of morphine plus bupivacaine offer more effective pain relief than administration of local anesthetic alone in patients recovering from abdominal[146,147,284] and thoracic surgery.[118,188] Whether analgesia observed with opioid-local anesthetic combinations is superior to that achieved with epidural opioids alone is less evident.[7,18,84,85]

Neuroaxially administered opioids and alpha-2-adrenergic agonists, and γ-aminobutyric acid-B ($GABA_\beta$) agonists and anticholinergic agents, either mimic or accentuate the activity of endogenous modulators in this region.[1,104,219,242,352] Epidural combinations of opioids plus clonidine or neostigmine offer effective post-surgical pain relief, reductions in analgesic dose requirements and high patient safety.[104,181,214,215,219,228,242,352] Facilitation of pain transmission in dorsal horn is mediated by the activation of NMDA and substance P (NK_1) receptors.[343] Although specific antagonists have yet to be released, ketamine in low doses provides non-specific NMDA receptor blockade and clinically measurable augmentation of opioid analgesia.[153,277,323]

Efferent motor and autonomic responses to noxious stimulation are associated with cardiovascular instability and muscle-splinting, and may increase acute pain-related disability.[87,166,273] Benzodiazepines augment IV-opioid based analgesia by decreasing skeletal muscular spasm and associated discomfort at dermatomes adjacent to the site of injury. Metoclopramide provides useful supplementation of IV-PCA morphine by reducing visceral, spasmodic pain and associated nausea.[273]

Intramuscular, intravenous, and IV-PCA administration of opioid analgesics generally maintain pain localization while diminishing intensity, suffering, and other pain-related behaviors. Emotional responses to pain, including increased anxiety, fear, and helplessness, may be controlled with benzodiazepines. Clonidine, and beta-adrenergic antagonists, have been included within multimodal analgesic regimens to control sympathetic responses accompanying surgical trauma. Epidural opioid-bupivacaine infusions can suppress hormonal responses that follow lower abdominal and extremity procedures, but responses associated with upper abdominal surgery and thoracotomy are more difficult to attenuate.[22,36,41,51,168] Administration of substrate (glucose, branched-chain amino acids) and systemic administration of glucocorticoids, may compensate for catabolic hormonal responses and negative nitrogen balance.[38,168]

While a number of multimodal trials have reported superior postsurgical analgesia, including reductions in effort-dependent pain and total analgesic requirements, it remains unclear whether improvements over single-agent therapy represent additive or synergistic interactions of the combinations employed. Such determinations require strict double-blinded protocols and complex isobolographic analyses that often present ethical dilemmas when designing clinical investigations.[172,315] Factors that remain to be clarified include which analgesic combination, which dose, and which precise timing of administration offer the greatest clinical benefit.[166,343]

PAIN CONTROL AND POSTSURGICAL OUTCOME

An important question raised by clinicians and health care administrators is whether efforts directed to minimize postoperative pain and associated stress responses result in improved postsurgical outcome. Improvements in outcome and length of hospital stay are difficult variables to measure; a variety of factors other than pain control may influence time to discharge. These include hospital census, individual surgeons' criteria for discharge, insurance guidelines, and differences in nursing, physical therapy, and nutritional support (see also Chapter 5).

Although IV-PCA provides uniform pain relief and high patient satisfaction, such therapy cannot eliminate pain perception and associated physiologic responses. Visual analog scale pain scores measured in patients successfully utilizing PCA range from 2 to 4 out of 10, indicating mild to moderate discomfort.[339] This level of pain intensity may be associ-

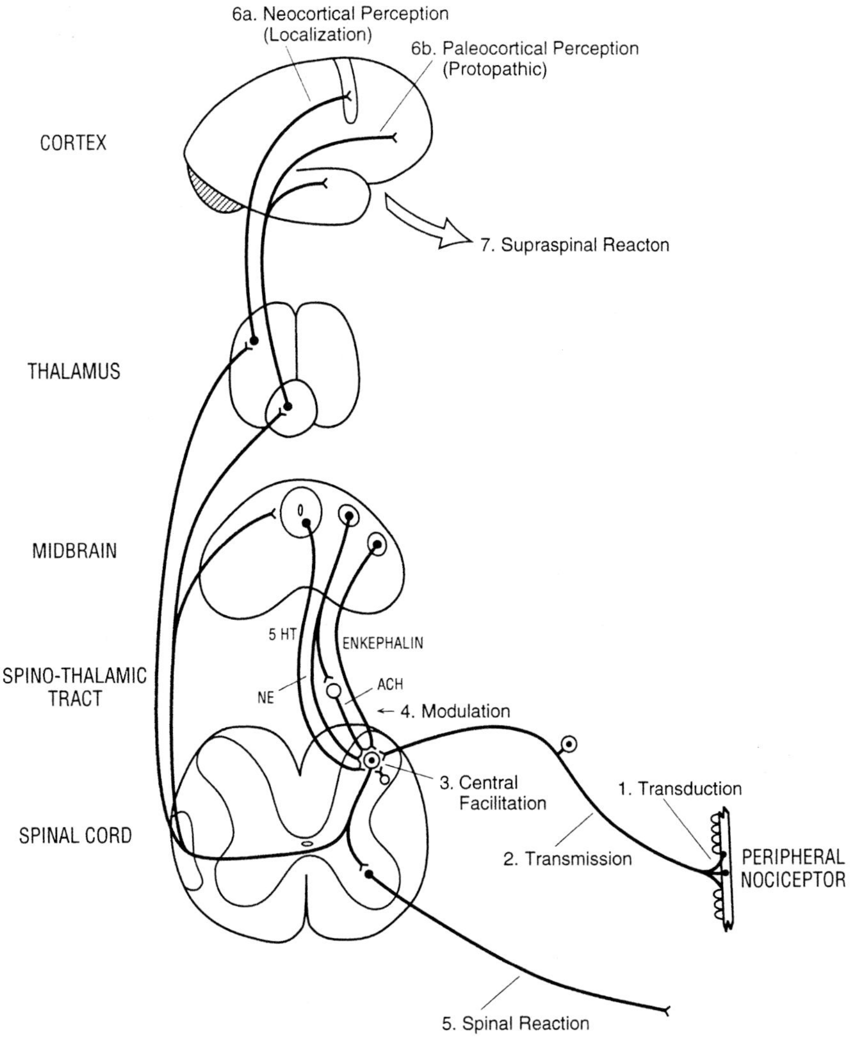

FIG. 26-21. Peripheral, Spinal and Supraspinal Mechanisms Involved in Pain Perception and Reaction—Simplified Version (see also Chapter 23.1, Figs. 23.1–18 and 23.1–19).
1. Transduction: Refers to the activation of peripheral nociceptors. Transduction is inhibited by NSAIDs, antihistamines, and topical local anesthetics.
2. Transmission: Propagation of action potentials from peripheral nociceptive endings to second-order cells in dorsal horn. Nociceptive impulses ascend via the spinothalamic tract to reach supraspinal targets. Transmission is blocked by local anesthetics.
3. Central Facilitation: Activation of N-methyl-D-aspartic acid (NMDA) receptors is associated with increased sensitivity and firing frequency of dorsal horn neurons. Central facilitation is inhibited by NMDA antagonists such as ketamine.
4. Modulation: Modulation is mediated by descending enkephalinergic, adrenergic, and cholinergic nerve fibers, which either inhibit release of nociceptive transmitters from primary afferents or blunt responses of second-order cells. Modulation is enhanced by neuroaxial administration of opioids, clonidine, and neostigmine.
5. Spinal Reaction: Increased motor and sympathetic outflow results in hypertension, tachycardia, adrenal activation, muscle spasm/splinting. Spinal reactions are suppressed by benzodiazepines, beta-adrenergic antagonists, and metaclopramide.
6. Supraspinal Perception: Includes the neocortical epicritic component which is responsible for pain localization, and the paleocortical protopathic component, responsible for the severe discomfort and suffering aspects of pain. Protopathic perception is blunted by opioid analgesics.
7. Supraspinal Reaction: Describes neocortical and paleocortical limbic responses including fear, anxiety, depression, and other pain-related behaviors, and pituitary-hypothalamic responses including release of stress hormones, neuropeptides, and activation of the sympathetic axis. Supraspinal reactions are blunted by regional blockade, beta-adrenergic agonists, and anxiolytics.

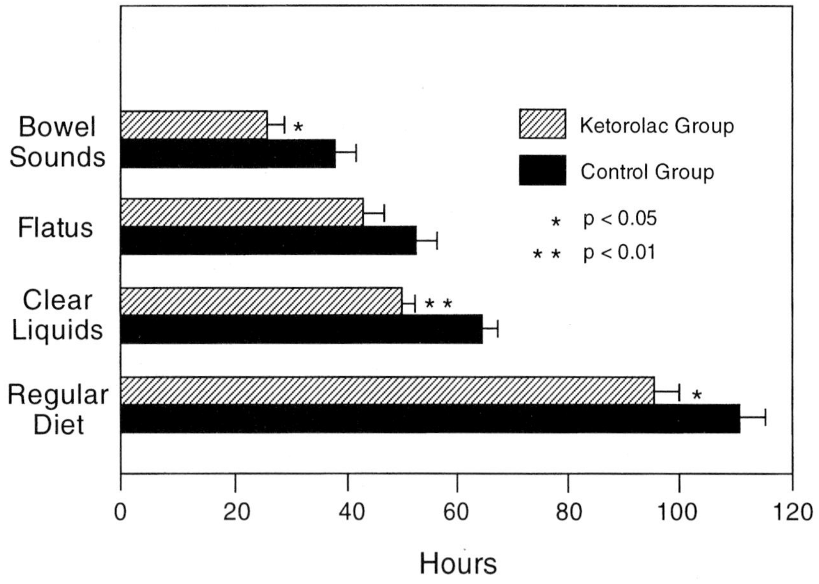

FIG. 26-22. Recovery of gastrointestinal function in patients recovering from radical prostatectomy treated with fentanyl epidural patient-controlled analgesia and either intramuscular ketorolac *(black bars)* or saline *(white bars)*. (Reproduced with permission from Grass, J.D., Sakima, N.T., Valley, M., *et al.*: Assessment of ketorolac as an adjuvant to fentanyl patient-controlled epidural analgesia after radical retropubic prostatectomy. Anesthesiology, *78*:642, 1993.)

ated with hemodynamic instability and some degree of respiratory compromise.[22,56,216] Intravenous PCA was unable to suppress catecholamine and cortisol responses to pain, or to postoperative tachycardia, in high-risk patients recovering from major operative procedures.[22,216] There have been few controlled evaluations of IV-PCA and its effect on postoperative outcome.[103,335,339] In a randomized evaluation of high-risk patients, those utilizing IV-PCA experienced better pain control and less confusion than age-matched controls treated with IM narcotics;[103] duration of hospital stay did not differ, however (see also Chapter 5).

When compared with IV-PCA, epidural administration of local anesthetics, opioid analgesics and their combination offer superior pain control and improvements in postoperative outcome, but these advantages must be carefully balanced on a case-by-case basis against dose-associated side effects, and the greater invasiveness of such therapy. Nevertheless, the higher intensity of analgesia associated with continuous epidural infusions is capable of providing pain prevention,[12,32,87] cardiovascular stability, and improved pulmonary function in the immediate post-surgical period.[33,38,56,92,156,280,281] Therapeutic gains are evident in patients presenting with significant cardiovascular and pulmonary disease, and in individuals recovering from extensive surgical procedures. Advantages are less obvious in healthy individuals recovering from minimally invasive procedures (see also Chapter 5).[284]

Epidural analgesic techniques offer significant reductions in effort dependent pain and greater preservation of preoperative pulmonary function.[50,56,280,292] Using respiratory effort as an index of postsurgical analgesia, Bromage et al.[50] reported that patients receiving epidural morphine maintained 67% of baseline FEV_1. Patients treated with standard doses of IV morphine experienced significantly greater reductions in respiratory effort, maintaining only 45% of baseline FEV_1. Patients randomized to receive epidural morphine following lung resection reported less pain at 2 and 8 hours, and experienced a smaller reduction of baseline FEV_1 and functional residual capacity (FRC) during the first 24 hours, than others treated with IV morphine.[292] Salomaki and colleagues[280,281] compared epidural and IV fentanyl infusions for postthoracotomy analgesia in a randomized double-blind fashion. Patients in the epidural group benefited from improved respiratory function, a lower incidence of oversedation, and reductions in neuroendocrine response. These findings were confirmed by Jayr et al.[156] who noted that postoperative pain scores, forced vital capacity (FVC), and O_2 saturation in patients treated with epidural morphine was superior to that observed with parenteral morphine. Despite these improvements, therapy-related differences in pulmonary morbidity were not observed, possibly because of the low-risk patient population that was evaluated. In this regard, Rawal and co-workers[252] reported that higher-risk morbidly obese patients treated with epidural morphine benefited from earlier ambulation, reduced pulmonary morbidity, and decreased hospital stay.

Epidural infusion of local anesthetics can reduce thromboembolic complications in patients recovering from hip surgery[146,210–212] and radical prostatectomy.[145] In a study employing perfusion lung-scanning, the incidence of pulmonary embolism following hip replacement surgery was reduced from 33% to 10% in patients treated with continuous epidural analgesia.[210,211] Reduction in thromboembolic risk has been attributed to increases in venous blood flow resulting from sympathetic blockade, attenuation of stress-induced hypercoagulability, and the inhibitory effect of[211] absorbed local anesthetics on adenosine diphosphate (ADP)-induced platelet aggregation.[36,211,213] Epidural opioids appear to be less effective than local anesthetics in reducing thromboembolic complications.[211]

Epidural infusions of morphine plus dilute bupivacaine provide a more rapid return of GI function following abdom-

TABLE 26-8. *Perioperative analgesic technique: analgesic consumption, incidence of side effects, and recovery of GI function*

	Epidural morphine bupivacaine (group MB)	Epidural morphine (group M)	Epidural bupivacaine (group B)	Intravenous PCA (group P)
Morphine ($mg \cdot h^{-1}$)	0.027 ± 0.002	0.052 ± 0.003		1.4 ± 0.2
Bupivacaine ($mg \cdot h^{-1}$)	9.0 ± 0.9		21.6 ± 1.5	
Pruritus	21	58[a]	14	125
Nausea	14	17	14	8
Orthostatic hypotension (>20% change in heart rate or blood pressure with change from supine to sitting)	14	17	57[a]	17
Time until first flatus (h)	43 ± 4[b]	71 ± 4	40 ± 2[b]	81 ± 3
Calories consumed on day of discharge ($kcal \cdot kg^{-1}$)	19 ± 1	18 ± 1	20 ± 1	21 ± 2
Oral intake on day of discharge ($ml \cdot kg^{-1}$)	32 ± 2	35 ± 3	36 ± 2	35 ± 2
Time until fulfillment of discharge criteria	68 ± 8[b]	102 ± 13	62 ± 5[b]	96 ± 7

[a] Different from all other groups ($P < 0.05$) as determined by Fisher's exact test
[b] Different from groups M and PCA ($P < 0.005$)

(From: Liu, S., Carpenter, R.L., Mulroy, M.F., *et al.*: Effects of perioperative analgesic technique on rate of recovery after colon surgery. Anesthesiology, *83*:757, 1995.)

inal surgery than IV-PCA morphine, and greater safety than more concentrated infusions of bupivacaine (see Table 26-8).[188] Epidural opioids were more effective than IV-PCA in reducing plasma catecholamine concentrations and hypertensive responses after major vascular surgery.[22,32,49,226,264] Reiz and colleagues[264] observed decreased myocardial ischemia in patients anesthetized with a "light general"-epidural local anesthetic technique. This finding may have particular significance, since ischemia during the first 24 to 48 hours following surgery is the most important predictor of postoperative cardiac outcome.[49,122] In a study of critically ill patients recovering from major surgery, Yeager and colleagues[352] noted that patients treated with epidural anesthetics and postoperative epidural morphine analgesia benefited from reductions in cardiac and respiratory failure and experienced a lower incidence of major infections than others receiving general anesthesia followed by IV opioids. Seventy-six percent of patients in the general anesthetic group developed some form of organ failure versus 32% of those who received epidural analgesia. Perioperative mortality was also higher (four deaths versus zero in the epidural group). While this study has been criticized for its small sample size, several larger follow-up evaluations have confirmed these findings. Tuman and colleagues[322] evaluated the interaction of epidural anesthesia, coagulation status, and outcome following lower extremity revascularization in 80 patients randomized to receive either general anesthesia and postoperative epidural analgesia or general anesthesia plus IV-PCA. The epidural group benefited from a shortened duration of postoperative ICU stay and reductions in significant cardiovascular and infectious complications. Christopherson et al.[67] evaluated 100 patients recovering from elective lower extremity revascularization procedures, and randomized to receive either epidural anesthesia/postoperative epidural analgesia or general anesthesia followed by IV-PCA. The incidence of cardiac morbidity, was similar in both treatment groups, but patients receiving epidural analgesia experienced a lower incidence of a repeated surgery for inadequate tissue perfusion. DeLeon-Cassola and co-workers[92] studied the incidence of myocardial ischemia and infarction in high-risk patients admitted to the intensive care unit after upper abdominal surgery. They noted that patients receiving epidural anesthesia followed by epidural morphine-bupivacaine analgesia experienced significantly less postoperative tachycardia, ischemia, and myocardial infarction than individuals treated with general anesthesia plus IV opioids. In a follow-up investigation,[91] patients receiving either continuous epidural infusions of morphine-bupivacaine or IV-PCA morphine reported effective analgesia following major oncological surgery. Patients in the epidural group benefited from a more rapid postoperative recovery as judged by shortened mechanical ventilation time, decreased ICU and hospital stays, and subsequently lower overall hospitalization cost. Liu and Carpenter, in an extensive review of epidural anesthesia and analgesia and their role in postoperative outcome, conclude that the weight of evidence points to a favorable effect on outcome (see also ref. 355).[186]

FUTURE OF ACUTE PAIN MANAGEMENT

The future of acute pain management is, to a great extent, being dictated by medical economics. Although AHCPR acute pain guidelines underscored the importance of optimal postsurgical analgesia, little was said regarding cost and relative cost-effectiveness of therapy. In most hospitals, expenses associated with IV and epidural infusion devices, drug preparation, and supervision, are higher than traditional forms of analgesia. In an effort to reduce health care costs, the U.S. government and third-party providers have been making negative decisions regarding reimbursement of acute pain management, without factoring in its influence upon postsurgical outcome. In some regions of the United States, reimbursement has declined so precipitously that many practitioners have reluctantly given up or greatly scaled back their involvement. In this regard, both the HCFA and private medical insurers have halted reimbursement to anesthesiologists for IV-PCA and single epidural doses of morphine in uncomplicated postsurgical settings. These decisions have important implications, since IV-PCA reimbursement pays for a major portion of pain service overhead, including personnel costs, pharmacy charges, and equipment expenses.

In an increasingly competitive marketplace, acute pain specialists in both community and academic settings are being asked to provide proof that the services they offer are associated with positive clinical outcome. To satisfy these requests the following issues require attention:

1. During the last 10 years, pain-related research has focused on improving analgesic efficacy. There is a scarcity of data assessing costs associated with specialized therapy and dedicated teams, versus savings provided by decreased postsurgical morbidity. With payment for acute pain management being determined by accountants and medical administrators[196,202] research must be refocused upon documenting improvements in outcome, as well as ways to reduce the cost of pain management while maintaining patient safety. Large-scale multicenter studies are needed to confirm preliminary findings[92,188,322,352] that optimal pain control can reduce morbidity/mortality and overall hospital costs. Reductions in morbidity, and other value-added benefits, including more rapid return of gastrointestinal (GI) function, and decreased ICU and hospital stay, should compensate for costs associated with its delivery. Meta-analysis of controlled randomized clinical trials may also provide the power necessary to demonstrate reductions in perioperative morbidity;[343] but comparisons between clinical trials are difficult to control because of surgical, anesthetic, and hospital-based variability. The Cochrane collaboration, which includes study groups in the United Kingdom, Australia, U.S., and Europe, is developing a series of meta-analyses, in which the efficacy and side effects of various analgesic techniques upon postsurgical outcome may be determined.[70]
2. Large-scale analysis is needed to help formulate guidelines that ensure effective pain control while minimizing therapy-related morbidity. Which agent(s), site of administration, and duration of therapy are most effective in different surgical settings? What forms of monitoring are most often used, and how reliable are they? What group of patients receiving neuroaxial opioids can be sent to the surgical ward, and which ones should be more closely monitored in the ICU? In this regard, a small number of adverse outcomes related to inadequate supervision might erase the analgesic benefits experienced by hundreds of other patients. There have been very few large scale evaluations[90,91,343] and "odds ratio" meta-analyses that answer these questions. Accurate assessment of benefit versus risk will require fully double-blind trials with complete matching of experimental and control groups (see also Chapter 29).[172,343]
3. Pain services must standardize billing codes and charges. Categories of current procedural terminology (CPT) coding should be uniform and related to appropriate diagnostic codes described in the ICD (International Classification of Disease) manual. The cost of acute pain therapy should be realistic and proportional to the service rendered and the duration of treatment. A global fee submitted for the management of high-risk patients should include initial assessment and formal consultation note, initiation of therapy, and up to 3 days treatment, daily follow-up notes, and ongoing quality assurance.
4. Finally, there is an important need to maintain and strengthen formal representation for acute pain. Affiliation with the International Association for the Study of Pain, and national bodies such as the American Society of Anesthesiologists and the American Society of Regional Anesthesia, has led to an improved dialog with government and private health care providers, development of minimum standards of care, and the credentialing of physicians and nurse coordinators in pain management.

REFERENCES

1. Aanonsen, L.M., and Wilcox, G.L.: Muscimol, gamma-aminobutyric acid receptors and excitatory amino acids in the mouse spinal cord. J. Pharmacol. Exp. Ther., *248:*1034, 1989.
2. Abboud, T.K., Dror, A., Mosaad, P., *et al.*: Minidose intrathecal morphine for the relief of postcesarean section pain: Safety and efficacy, and ventilatory responses to carbon dioxide. Anesth. Analg., *67:*137, 1988.
3. Abboud, T.K., Moore, M., Zhu, J., *et al.*: Epidural butorphanol and morphine for relief of postcesarean section pain. Anesth. Analg., *66:*887, 1987.
4. Abraham, Z.A.: Interpleural analgesia. *In* Sinatra, R.S., Hord, A.H., Ginsberg, B., and Preble L.M. (eds.): Acute Pain Mechanisms and Management. St. Louis, Mosby–Year Book, 1992.
5. Abram, S.E., and Yaksh, T.L.: Morphine but not inhalational anesthesia blocks postinjury facilitation: The role of preemptive suppression of afferent transmission. Anesthesiology, *78:*713, 1993.
6. Ahuja, B.R., and Strunin, L.: Respiratory effects of epidural fentanyl. Anaesthesia, *40:*949, 1985.
7. Akerman, B., Arwenstrom, E., and Post, C.: Local anesthetic potentiates spinal morphine antiociception. Anesth. Analg., *67:*943, 1988.
8. Ali, J., Weisel, R.D., Layug, A.B., *et al.*: Consequences of postoperative alterations in respiratory mechanics, Am. J. Surg., *128:*376, 1974.
9. Anand, K.J.S., and Hickey, P.R.: Halothane-morphine compared with high-dose sufentanil for anesthesia and postoperative analgesia in neonatal cardiac surgery. N. Engl. J. Med., *326:*1, 1992.
10. Angell, M.: The quality of mercy. N. Engl. J. Med., *306:*98, 1982.
11. Anker-Moller, E., Spangsberg, N., Dahl, J.B., Christensen, E.F., *et al.*: Continuous blockade of the lumbar plexus after knee surgery. Acta Anaesthsiol. Scand., *34:*468, 1990.
12. Armitage, E.N.: Postoperative pain prevention or relief. Br. J. Anaesth., *63:*136, 1989.
13. Attia, J., Ecoffey, C., Sanddouk, P., *et al.*: Epidural morphine in children: Pharmacokinetics and CO_2 sensitivity. Anesthesiology, *65:*590, 1986.

14. Austin, K.L., Stapleton, J.V., and Mather, L.E.: Relationship between blood meperidine concentrations and analgesic response. Anesthesiology, *53:*460, 1980.
15. Austin, K.L., Stapleton, J.V., and Mather, L.E.: Multiple intramuscular injections: A major source of variability in analgesic response to meperidine. Pain, *8:*47, 1980.
16. Bach, S., Noreng, M.F., and Tjellden, N.U.: Phantom limb pain in amputees during the first 12 months following limb amputation after preoperative lumbar epidural blockade. Pain, *33:*297, 1988.
17. Badner, N.H., Bhandari, R., and Komar, W.E.: Bupivacaine 0.125% improves continuous postoperative epidural fentanyl analgesia after abdominal or thoracic surgery. Can. J. Anesth., *41:*387, 1994.
18. Bahar, M., Rosen, M., and Vickers M.D.: Self-administered nalbuphine, morphine, and pithidine following cholecystectomy. Anaesthesia, *40:*529, 1985.
19. Bailey, P.W., and Smith, B.E.: Continued epidural infusion of fentanyl for postoperative analgesia. Anesthesia, *35:*1002, 1980.
20. Basbaum, A.I.: Memories of Pain. Science and Medicine, *3:*22, 1996.
21. Baskett, P.: Analgesia for the dressing of burns in children: A method using neuroleptanalgesia and Entonox. Medicine, *48:*138, 1972.
22. Beattie, W.S., Buckley, D.N., and Forrest, J.B.: Epidural morphine reduces the risk of postoperative myocardial ischemia in patients with cardiac risk factors. Can. J. Anaesth., *40:*523, 1993.
23. Beecher, H.K.: The measured effect of laparotomy on the respiration. J. Clin. Invest., *12:*639, 1993.
24. Behar, M., Magora, F., Olshwang, D., *et al.*: Epidural morphine in the treatment of pain. Lancet, *1:*527, 1979.
25. Bellville, J.W., Forrest, W.H., Miller, E., *et al.*: Influence of age on pain relief from analgesics. J.A.M.A., *217:*1835, 1971.
26. Benlabed, M., Ecoffey, C., Levron, J.C., *et al.*: Analgesia and ventilatory response to CO_2 following epidural sufentanil in children. Anesthesiology, *67:*948, 1987.
27. Berde, C.B.: Pediatric postoperative pain management. Pediatr. Clin. North Am., *36:*921, 1989.
28. Berkowitz, A.R., and Rosenberg, H.: Safety of femoral and lateral femoral cutaneous nerve block for muscle biopsy for malignant hyperthermia. Reg. Anesth., *9:*32, 1984.
29. Berkowitz, B.A., Nagai, S.H., Yang, J.C., *et al.*: The disposition of morphine in surgical patients. Clin. Pharmacol. Ther., *17:*629, 1975.
30. Birnbach, D.J., Arcurio, T., Johnson, M.D., *et al.*: Effect of diluent volume on analgesia produced by epidural fentanyl. Anesth. Analg., *60:*13, 1988.
31. Blackburn, C.: Respiratory arrest after epidural sufentanil. Anaesthesia, *42:*665, 1987.
32. Blau, W., Dogra, S., Davis, W., and Calhoun, P.: Postoperative analgesia at rest and during motion following laparotomy: Continuous epidural morphine versus IV-PCA morphine, Reg. Anesth., *21*(2S):16, 1996.
33. Blomberg, S., Emanuelsson, H., Kvist, H., *et al.*: Effects of thoracic epidural anesthesia on coronary arteries and arterioles in patients with coronary artery disease. Anesthesiology, *73:*840, 1990.
34. Bond, M.R., and Pilowsky, I.: Subjective assessment of pain and its relationship to the administration of analgesics in patients with advanced cancer. J. Psychsom. Res., *10:*203, 1966.
35. Bonica, J.J.: Definitions and taxonomy of pain. *In* Bonica, J.J. (ed.): Management of Pain. pp. 18–27. Philadelphia, Lea & Febiger, 1990.
36. Borg, T., and Modig, J.: Potential anti-thrombotic effects of local anesthetics due to inhibition of platelet function. Acta Anaesthesiol. Scand., *29:*739, 1985.
37. Borgeat, A., Saiah, M., Wildersmith, O., *et al.*: Subhypnotic doses of propofol relieve pruritus induced by epidural and intrathecal morphine. Anesthesiology, *76:*510, 1992.
38. Brandt, M.R., Fernandes, A., Mondhorst, R., *et al.*: Epidural analgesia improves postoperative nitrogen balance, Br. Med. J., *1:*1106, 1978.
39. Bray, J.: Postoperative analgesia provided by morphine infusion in children. Anaesthesia, *38:*1075, 1983.
40. Breslow, M.J., Jordan, D.A., Christopherson, R., *et al.*: Epidural morphine decreases postoperative hypertension by attenuating sympathetic nervous system hyperactivity. J.A.M.A., *261:*3577, 1989.
41. Breslow, M.J.: Neuroendocrine responses to surgery. *In* Breslow, M.J., Miller, C.F., and Rogers, M.C. (eds.): Perioperative Management. pp. 180–193. St. Louis, Mosby–Year Book, 1990.
42. Bridenbaugh, P.O.: Preemptive analgesia—Is it clinically relevant? (editorial) Anesth. Analg., *78:*203, 1994.
43. Brisman, B., Pettersson, N., Tokies, L., *et al.*: Postoperative analgesia with interpleural administration of bupivacaine. Acta Anaesth Scand., *31:*515, 1987.
44. Broadman, L.M., Higgins, T.T., Hannallah, R.S., *et al.*: Intraoperative subarachnoid morphine for postoperative pain control following Harrington rod instrumentation in children. Can. J. Anaesth., *34:*S96, 1987.
45. Broadman, L.M., Hannallah, R.S., Belman, A.B., *et al.*: Postcircumcision analgesia—A prospective evaluation of subcutaneous ring block of the penis. Anesthesiology, *67:*399, 1987.
46. Broadman, L.M., Hannallah, R.S., Norden, J.M., *et al.*: "Kiddie caudals:" Experience with 1,154 consecutive cases without complications. Anesth. Analg., *66:*S18, 1987.
47. Broadman, L.M., and Hannallah, R.S.: Regional anesthesia in children—an analysis of risk and parental acceptance. Reg. Anesth., *10:*33, 1985.
48. Brodsky, J.B., Chaplan, S.R., Brose, W.G., and Mark, J.B.D.: Continuous epidural hydromorphone for post-thoracotomy pain relief. Ann. Thorac. Surg., *50:*888, 1990.
49. Bromage, P.R., Camporesi, E.M., Durant, P.A.C., *et al.*: Nonrespiratory side effects of epidural morphine. Anesth. Analg., *61:*490, 1982.
50. Bromage, P.R., Camporesi, E., Chestnut, D.: Epidural narcotics for postoperative analgesia. Anesth. Analg., *59:*473, 1980.
51. Bromage, P.R., Shibata, H.R., and Willoughby, H.W.: Influence of prolonged epidural blockade and blood sugar and cortisol responses. Surg. Gynecol. Obstet., *132:*1051, 1971.
52. Brose, W.G., Tanelian, D.L., Brodsky, J.B., Mark, J.B.D., *et al.*: CSF and blood pharmacokinetics of hydromorphone and morphine following lumbar epidural administration. Pain, *45:*11, 1991.
53. Brown, D.L., and Carpenter, R.L.: Perioperative analgesia: A review of risks and benefits. J. Cardiothorac. Anesth., *4:*368, 1990.
54. Brown, R.E.: Transcutaneous electical nerve stimulation for acute and postopertive pain. *In* Sinatra, R.S., Hord, A.H., Ginsberg, B., and Preble, L.M., (eds.): Acute Pain Mechanisms and Management. pp. 379–389. St. Louis, Mosby–Year Book, 1992.
55. Brull, S.J., Lieponis, J., Murphy, M., *et al.*: Acute and long-term benefits of iliac crest donor site perfusion, with local anesthetics. Anesth. Analg., *74:*145, 1992.
56. Buckley, D.N., MacIntosh, J., and Beattie, W.S.: Epidural analgesia prevents loss of lung volume. Anesthesiology, *73:*A764, 1990.
57. Bullingham, R.E.S., McQuay, J.H., and Moore, R.A.: Unexpectedly high plasma fentanyl levels after epidural use. Lancet, *1:*1361, 1980.
58. Burns, J.W., Hodsman, N.B.A., McLintock, T.T., *et al.*: The influence of patient characteristics on the requirements for postoperative analgesia. Anaesthesia, *44:*2, 1989.
59. Camu, F., Verborgh, C., Van der Auwern, A., *et al.*: Pharmacokinetics and analgesic effect of epidural sufentanil. Acta Anaesthesiol. Scand., *80*(Suppl.)*:*82, 1985.
60. Carabine, U.A., Gilliland, H., Johnstone, J.R., and McGuigan, J.: Pain relief for thoracotomy: Comparison of morphine requirements using intrapleural bupivacaine. Reg. Anesth., *20*(5):412, 1995.
61. Carr, D.B., Jacox, A., Chapman, R.C., *et al.*: Acute pain management in infants, children and adolescents: Operative and medical procedures, Department of Health and Human Serv. Pub. No. 92-0032, Agency for Health Care Policy and Research, Public Health Service, US Department of Health and Human Services, Rockville, M.D., 1992.
62. Chaplan, S.R., Duncan, S.R., Brodsky, J.B., and Brose, W.G.: Morphine and hydromorphone epidural analgesia: A prospective, randomized comparison. Anesthesiology, *77:*1090, 1992.
63. Chapman, C.R., and Benedetti, C.: Analgesia following transcutaneous electrical stimulation and its partial reversal by a narcotic antagonist. Life Sci., *21:*1625, 1977.
64. Chernow, B.: Hormonal responses to a graded surgical stress. Arch. Intern. Med., *147:*1273, 1987.
65. Chestnut, D.H., Choi, W.W., and Isbell, T.J.: Epidural hydromorphone for postcesarean analgesia. Obstet. Gynecol., *68:*65, 1986.
66. Choinière, M., Melzack, R., Girard, N., *et al.*: Comparisons between patients' and nurses' assessment of pain and medication efficacy in severe burn injuries. Pain, *40:*143, 1990.
67. Christopherson, R., Beattie, C., Meinert, C.L., *et al.*: Perioperative morbidity in patients randomized to epidural or general anesthesia for lower extremity vascular surgery. Anesthesiology, *79:*1, 1993.
68. Chrubasik, J., and Wiemers, K.: Continuous-plus-on demand epidural infusions of morphine for postoperative pain relief. Anesthesiology, *62:*263, 1985.

69. Chung, J.H.: Spinal opioids: Treatment of side effects. *In* Sinatra, R.S., Hord, A.H., Ginsberg, B., and Preble, L.M. (eds.): Acute Pain Mechanisms and Management. pp. 272–292. St. Louis, Mosby–Year Book, 1992.
70. Cochrane. Collaboration: Pain management metaanalysis (In preparation).
71. Coda, B.A., Kawata, J., and Ross, B.K.: Plasma sufentanil concentration during prolonged epidural infusion for postoperative analgesia. Anesth. Analg., *76:*S49, 1993.
72. Coderre, T.J., Katz, J., Vaccarino, A.L., and Melzack, R.: Contribution of central neuroplasticity on pathological pain: Review of clinical and experimental evidence. Pain, *52:*259, 1993.
73. Cohen, F.L.: Postsurgical pain relief: Patients' status and nurses' medication choices. Pain, *9:*265, 1980.
74. Cohen, M.R., and Pickar, D.: Stress-induced beta-endorphin immunoreactivity may predict postoperative morphine usage. Psychiatry Res., *6:*7, 1982.
75. Collins, J.G.: Historical overview of pain management: From undermedication to state of the art. *In* Sinatra, R.S., Hord, A.H., Ginsberg, B., and Preble, L.M. (eds.): Acute Pain Mechanisms and Management. pp. 1–7. St. Louis, Mosby–Year Book, 1992.
76. Connelly, N.R., Dunn, S.M., Ingold, V., and Villa, E.A.: The use of fentanyl added to morphine-lidocaine-epinephrine spinal solution in patients undergoing cesarean section. Anesth. Analg., *78:*918, 1994.
77. Cousins, M.J.: Acute pain and the injury response: Immediate and prolonged effects. Reg. Anesth., *16:*162, 1989.
78. Cousins, M.J., Cherry, D.A., and Gourlay, G.K.: Acute and chronic pain: Use of spinal opioids. *In* Cousins, M.J., and Bridenbaugh, P.O. Neural Blockade in Clinical Anesthesia and Management of Pain. 2nd ed. pp. 993–996. Philadelphia, JB Lippincott, 1987.
79. Cousins, M.J., and Phillips, G.D.: Acute pain management. *In* Cousins, M.J. and Phillips, G.D. (eds.): Clinics in Critical Care Medicine. New York, Churchill Livingstone, 1986.
80. Cousins, M.J., and Mather, L.E.: Intrathecal and epidural administration of opioids. Anesthesiology, *61:*276, 1984.
81. Cousins, M.J., Mather, L.E., Glynn, C.J., *et al.*: Selective spinal analgesia. Lancet, *1:*1141, 1979.
82. Crile, G.W., and Lower, W.E.: Anoci-association. pp. 223–225. Philadephia, Saunders, 1914.
83. Cronin, M., and Redfern, P.A.: Psychometry and postoperative complaints of pain in surgical patients. Br. J. Anaesth., *45:*879, 1973.
84. Dahl, J.B., Hansen, B.L., Hjortso, N.C., *et al.*: Influence of timing on the effect of continuous extradural analgesia with bupivacaine and morphine after major abdominal surgery. Br. J. Anaesth., *69:*4, 1992.
85. Dahl, J.B., Rosenberg, J., Hansen, B.L., *et al.*: Differential analgesic effects of low-dose epidural morphine and morphine-bupivacaine at rest and during mobilization after major abdominal surgery. Anesth. Analg., *74:*362, 1992.
86. Dahl, J.B., and Kehlet, H.: Nonsteroidal anti-inflammatory drugs: Rational for use in severe postoperative pain. Br. J. Anaesth., *66:*703, 1991.
87. Dahl, J.B., Rosenberg, J., Dirkes, W.E., *et al.*: Prevention of postoperative pain by balanced analgesia. Br. J. Anaesth., *64:*518, 1990.
88. Dahlstrom, B., Tamsen, A., Paalzow, L., *et al.*: PCA therapy-pharmacokinetics and analgesic plasma concentrations of morphine. Clin. Pharmacokinet., *7:*266, 1982.
89. Dalens, B., and Tanguy, A.: Intrathecal morphine for spinal fusion in children. Spine, *13:*494, 1988.
90. de Leon-Casasola, O.A., Parker, B., Lema, M.J., *et al.*: Postoperative epidural-bupivacainemorphine therapy: Experience with 4,227 surgical cancer patients. Anesthesiology, *81:*368, 1994.
91. de Leon-Casasola, O.A., Parker, B.M., Lema, M.J., *et al.*: Epidural analgesia versus intravenous PCA. Reg. Anesth., *19:*307, 1994.
92. de Leon-Casasola, O.A., Karabella, D., Harrison, P., and Lema, M.J.: A decrease in postoperative myocardial ischemia and infarction by epidural bupivacaine-morphine after upper abdominal surgery. Reg. Anesth., *18:*66, 1993.
93. Dickenson, A.H., and Sullivan, A.F.: Subcutaneous formalin-induced activity of dorsal horn neurones in rat: Differential response to an intrathecal opiate administered pre- or postformalin. Pain, *30:*349, 1987.
94. Dierking, G.W., Dahl, J.B., Kanstrup, J., *et al.*: Effect of pre- vs. postoperative inguinal field block on postoperative pain after herniorrhaphy. Br. J. Anaesth., *68:*344, 1992.
95. Domsky, M., and Tarantino, D.: Patient-controlled spinal analgesia for postoperative pain control. Anesth. Analg., *75:*453, 1992.
96. Donadoni, R., Vermeulen, H., Noordwin, H., *et al.*: Intrathecal sufentanil as a supplement to subarachnoid anesthesia with lignocaine. Br. J. Anaesth., *59:*1523, 1987.
97. Donavan, M., Dillon, P., and Mcguire, L.: Incidence and characteristics of pain in a sample of medical-surgical inpatients. Pain, *30:*69, 1987.
98. Dougherty, R.T.B., Baysinger, C.L., Henenberger, D., *et al.*: Epidural hydromorphone for postoperative analgesia. Anesth. Analg., *68:*318, 1989.
99. Duggan, A.W., and Headley, P.M.: Suppression of transmission of nociceptive impulses by morphine. Br. J. Pharmacol., *61:*65, 1977.
100. Duncan, P.G., and Cullen, B.F.: Anesthesia and immunology. Anesthesiology, *45:*522, 1976.
101. Durrani, Z., Winnie, A.P., and Ikuta, P.: Interpleural catheter analgesia for pancreatic pain. Anesth. Analg., *67:*479, 1988.
102. Dyer, R.A., Anderson, B.J., Michell, W.L., and Hall, J.M.: Postoperative pain control with a continuous infusion of epidural sufentanil in the intensive care unit: A comparison with epidural morphine. Anesth. Analg., *71:*130, 1990.
103. Egbert, A.E., Parks, L.H., Short, L.M., and Burnett, M.L.: Randomized trial of postoperative patient controlled analgesia vs. intramuscular narcotics in frail elderly men. Arch. Intern. Med., *150:*1897, 1990.
104. Eisenach, J.C., D'Angelo, R., Taylor, C., and Hood, D.D.: An isobolographic study of epidural clonidine and fentanyl after cesarean section. Anesth. Analg., *79:*285, 1994.
105. Eisenach, J.C., Grice, S.C., Dewan, D.M., *et al.*: PCA following cesarean section: A comparison with intramuscular and epidural narcotics. Anesthesiology, *68:*444, 1988.
106. Ejlersen, E., Andersen, H.B., Eliasen, K., and Mogensen, T.: A comparison between preincisional and postincisional lidocaine infiltration and postoperative pain. Anesth. Analg., *74:*495, 1992.
107. El-Baz, N.M.I., Faber, L.P., and Jensik, R.J.: Continuous epidural infusion of morphine for treatment of pain after thoracic surgery: A new technique. Anesth. Analg., *63:*757, 1984.
108. Elder, P.R.: Post circumcision pain: A prospective evaluation of subcutaneous ring block of the penis. Reg. Anesth., *9:*48, 1984.
109. Ellis, J.E., Busse, J.R., Foss, J.F., *et al.*: Postoperative management of myocardial ischemia. Anesthesiol. Clin., *9:*609, 1991.
110. Etches, R.C., Sandler, A., and Daley, M.D.: Respiratory depression and spinal opioids. Can. J. Anaesth., *36:*165, 1989.
111. Ferrante, F.M., and Covino, B.G.: Patient-controlled analgesia: A historical perspective. *In* Ferrante, F.M., Ostheimer, G.W., and Covino, B.G. (eds.): Patient-controlled Analgesia. Boston, Blackwell Scientific, 1990.
112. Ferrante, F.M., Orav, E.J., Rocco, A.G., *et al.*: A statistical model for pain in PCA and conventional intramuscular opioid regimens. Anesth. Analg., *67:*457, 1988.
113. Ferreira, S.H.: Prostaglandins hyperalgesia and the control of inflammatory pain. *In* Bonta, I.L., Bray, M.A., and Parnham, M.J. (eds.): Handbook of Inflammation. Vol 5. The Pharmacology of Inflammation. pp. 108–116. New York, Elsevier, 1985.
114. Fisher, R.L., Lubenow, T.R., Liceaga, A., *et al.*: Comparison of continuous epidural infusion of fentanyl-bupivacaine and morphine-bupivacaine in management of postoperative pain. Anesth. Analg., *67:*559, 1988.
115. Freeman, L.J., Nixon, P.G., Sallabank, P., *et al.*: Psychological stress and silent myocardial ischemia. Am. Heart J., *114:*477, 1987.
116. Geller, E., Chrubasik, J., Graf, R., *et al.*: A randomized double-blind comparison of epidural sufentanil vs. intravenous sufentanil or epidural fentanyl analgesia after major abdominal surgery. Anesth. Analg., *76:*1243, 1993.
117. Gelman, S.: General vs. regional anesthesia for peripheral vascular surgery: Is the problem solved? (editorial) Anesthesiology, *79:*415, 1993.
118. Geurts, A.M., Jessen, H.J.G., Megans, J.H., *et al.*: Continuous high thoracic epidural administration of morphine with bupivacaine after thoracotomy. Reg. Anesth., *20*(1):27, 1995.
119. Gil, K.M.: Psychologic aspects of acute pain. *In* Sinatra, R.S., Hord, A.H., Ginsberg, B., and Preble, L.M. (eds.): Acute Pain Mechanisms and Management. pp. 58–69. St. Louis, Mosby–Year Book, 1992.
120. Glass, P.S.A., Estok, P., Ginsberg, B., *et al.*: Use of patient-controlled analgesia to compare the efficacy of epidural to intravenous fentanyl administration, Anesth. Analg., *74:*345, 1992.

121. Glynn, C.J., Mather, L.E., and Cousins, M.J.: Peridural meperidine in humans. Anesthesiology, *55:*520, 1981.
122. Goldman, L., Caldera, D.L., Southwick, F.S., *et al.*: Cardiac risk factors and complications in noncardiac surgery. Medicine, *57:*357, 1978.
123. Goodman, E.: Use of ketorolac in sickle-cell disease and vaso-occlusive crisis. Lancet, *338:*641, 1991.
124. Gourlay, G.K., Cherry, D.A., Plummer, J.L., *et al.*: The influence of drug polarity on the absorption of opioid drugs into CSF. Pain, *31:*297, 1987.
125. Graf, G., Frasca, A., Sinatra, R.S., *et al.*: Epidural sufentanil for postoperative analgesia: A dose-response study in patients recovering from abdominal surgery. Anesth. Analg., *73:*405, 1991.
126. Grant, R., Dolman, J., Harper, J., *et al.*: Patient-controlled lumbar epidural fentanyl compared with patient-controlled intravenous fentanyl for post-thoracotomy pain. Can. J. Anaesth., *39:*214, 1992.
127. Grass, J.A., Zuckerman, R.L., Sakima, N.T., and Harris, A.P.: Patient-controlled analgesia after cesarean delivery—Epidural sufentanil versus intravenous morphine. Reg. Anesth., *19:*90, 1994.
128. Grass, J.A., Sakima, N.T., Valley, M., *et al.*: Assessment of ketorolac as an adjuvant to fentanyl patient-controlled epidural analgesia after radical retropubic prostatectomy. Anesthesiology, *78:*642, 1993.
129. Graves, D., Foster, A., Batenhorst, R.L., Bennett, R.L.: Patient-controlled analgesia. Ann. Intern. Med., *99:*360, 1983.
130. Graves, D.A., Arrigo, J.M., Foster, T.S., *et al.*: Relationship between plasma morphine concentrations and pharmacological effects. Clin. Pharm., *4:*41, 1985.
131. Graziotti, P.J., and Smith, G.B.: Multiple rib fractures and head injury—an indication for intercostal catheterization and infusion of local anesthetics. Anaesthesia, *43:*964, 1988.
132. Guinard, J.P., Mavrocordatos, P., Cuttat, J.F., and Carpenter, R.: A randomized comparison of intravenous vs. lumbar and thoracic epidural fentanyl for analgesia after thoracotomy. Anesthesiology, *77:*1108, 1992.
133. Guiliani, C.A., and Perry, G.A.: Factors to consider in the rehabilitation aspect of burn care. Phys. Ther., *65:*619, 1985.
134. Gustafsson, L.L., Grell, A.M., Garle, M., *et al.*: Kinetics of morphine in cerebrospinal fluid after epidural administration. Acta Anaesthesiol. Scand., *28:*535, 1984.
135. Gustafsson, L.L., Schild, B., and Jacobsen, K.: Adverse effects of extradural and intrathecal opiates: Report of a nationwide survey in Sweden. Br. J. Anaesth., *54:*479, 1982.
136. Gwirtz, K.H., Young, J.V., Walker, S.G., *et al.*: Intrathecal opioid analgesia for acute postoperative pain: Experience with 4,134 surgical patients. Anesthesiology, *83:*A780, 1995.
137. Gwirtz, K.H., Helvie, J.E., Young, J.V., and Li, W.: Ketorolac enhances intrathecal analgesia after major surgery. Anesthesiol. Rev., *20:*222, 1993.
138. Gwirtz, K.H.: Single-dose opioids in the management of acute postoperative pain. *In* Sinatra, R.S., Hord, A.H., Ginsberg, B., and Preble, L.M. (eds.): Acute Pain Mechanisms and Management. St. Louis, Mosby–Year Book, 1992.
139. Haber, D.W., and Berde, C.B.: Spinal opioids for pediatric pain management, *In* Sinatra, R.S., Hord, A.H., Ginsberg, B., and Preble, L.M. (eds.): Acute Pain Mechanisms and Management. St. Louis, Mosby–Year Book, 1992.
140. Hagen, C., Brandt, M.R., and Kehlet, H.: Prolactin, LH, FSH, GH, and cortisol response to surgery and the effect of epidural analgesia. Acta Endocrinol., *94:*151, 1980.
141. Halter, J.B., Pflug, A.E., and Porte, D.: Mechanisms of plasma catecholamine increases during surgical stress in man. J. Clin. Endocrinol. Metab., *51:*1093, 1980.
142. Handrop, M., and Spinella, J.: Ketamine: Featured protocol. J. Burn Care Rehabil., *8:*148, 1987.
143. Hannallah, R.S., Broadman, L.M., Belman, A.B., *et al.*: Comparison of ilioinguinal/iliohypogastric block for control of postorchiopexy pain in pediatric ambulatory surgery. Anesthesiology, *66:*832, 1987.
144. Hardy, J.D., Wolff, H.G., and Goodell, H.: Cutaneous hyperalgesia. J. Clin. Invest., *29:*115, 1950.
145. Harrison, D.M., Sinatra, R., and Morgese, L.: Epidural narcotic and patient-controlled analgesia for postcesarean section pain relief. Anesthesiology, *68:*454, 1988.
146. Hendolin, H., Mattila, M., Poikolainen, E.: The effect of lumbar epidural analgesia on the development of deep vein thrombosis after open prostatectomy. Acta Chir. Scand., *147:*425, 1981.
147. Hjortso, N.C., Lund, C., Mogensen, T., *et al.*: Epidural morphine improves pain relief and maintains sensory analgesia during continuous epidural bupivacaine after abdominal surgery, Anesth. Analg., *65:*1033, 1986.
148. Hjortso, N.C., Christensen, N.J., Andersen, T., *et al.*: Effects of extradural local anesthetics and morphine on morbidity after abdominal surgery, Acta Anaesthesiol. Scand., *27:*790, 1985.
149. Hord, A.H., and Kelly, P.M.: University-based acute pain treatment service. *In* Sinatra, R.S., Hord, A.H., Ginsberg, B., and Preble, L.M. (eds.): Acute Pain Mechanisms and Management. pp. 532–538. St. Louis, Mosby–Year Book, 1992.
150. Hubbard L.: Community-based pain service. *In* Sinatra, R.S., Hord, A.H., Ginsberg, B., and Preble, L.M. (eds.): Acute Pain Mechanisms and Management. pp. 7–18. St. Louis, Mosby–Year Book, 1992.
151. Hull, C.J.: Pharmacokinetics of opioid analgesia, PCA. *In* Harmer, M., Rosen, M. (eds.): Patient Controlled Analgesia. Oxford, Blackwell, 1985.
152. Iafrati, N.S.: Pain on the burn unit: Patient vs. nurse perceptions. J. Burn Care Rehabil., *7:*413, 1986.
153. Islas, J.A., Astorga, J., and Laredo, M.: Intrathecal ketamine for control of postoperative pain. Anesth. Analg., *64:*1161, 1985.
154. Jacobson, L., Chabal, C., and Brody, M.C.: Intrathecal methadone, and morphine for postoperative analgesia: A comparison of efficacy, duration, and side effects. Anesth. Analg., *67:*1082, 1989.
155. Jacox, A., Carr, D.B.: Clinical Practice Guideline for Acute Pain Management: Operative or Medical Procedures and Trauma, Department Health Human Services, Pub. No. 91–0046, Agency for Health Care Policy and Research, Public Health Service, US Department of Health and Human Services, Rockville, MD., 1991.
156. Jayr, C., Thomas, H., Rey A., *et al.*: Postoperative pulmonary complications: Epidural analgesia versus parenteral opioids. Anesthesiology, *78:*666, 1993.
157. Johansson, B., Glise, H., Hallerback, B., *et al.*: Preoperative local infiltration with ropivacaine for postoperative pain relief after cholecystectomy. Anesth. Analg., *78:*210, 1994.
158. Johnson, A.: Influence of intrathecal morphine and naloxone intervention on postoperative ventilatory regulation in elderly patients. Acta Anaesthesiol. Scand., *36:*436, 1992.
159. Jones, S.E.F., Beasley, J.M., McFarlane, D., *et al.*: Intrathecal morphine for postoperative pain relief in children. Br. J. Anaesth., *56:*137, 1984.
160. Kafer, E.R., Brown, J., Scott, D., *et al.*: Biphasic depression of ventilatory responses to CO_2 following epidural morphine. Anesthesiology, *58:*418, 1983.
161. Kaiko, R.F.: Age and morphine analgesia in cancer patients with postoperative pain. Clin. Pharmacol. Ther., *28:*823, 1980.
162. Kambam, J.R., Handte, R.E., Parris, W.C., *et al.*: Interpleural anesthesia for post-thoracotomy pain relief. Reg. Anesth., *12:*106, 1987.
163. Kardash, K., Schools, A., Concepcion, M.: Effects of brachial plexus fentanyl on supraclavicular block: A randomized, double-blind study. Reg. Anesth., *20*(4):311, 1995.
164. Katz, J., Kavanaugh, B.P., Sandler, A., *et al.*: Pre-emptive analgesia: Clinical evidence of neuroplasticity contributing to postoperative pain. Anesthesiology, *77:*439, 1992.
165. Katz, J., Jackson, M., Kavanaugh, B.P., and Sandler, A.: Acute pain after thoracic surgery predicts long-term post-thoracotomy pain. Clin. J. Pain, *12:*50, 1996.
166. Kehlet, H., and Dahl, J.B.: The value of "multimodal" or "balanced analgesia" in postoperative pain treatment. Anesth. Analg., *77:*1048, 1993.
167. Kehlet, H.: Surgical stress: The role of pain and analgesia. Br. J. Anaesth., *63:*189, 1989.
168. Kehlet, H.: Modification of responses to surgery by neural blockade: Clinical implications. *In* Cousins, M.J., and Bridenbaugh, P.O. (eds.): Neural Blockade in Clinical Anesthesia and Management of Pain. 2nd ed. pp. 145–188. Philadelphia, Lippincott, 1987.
169. Kehlet, H.: The stress response to anesthesia and surgery: Release mechanisms and modifying factors. Clin. Anesth., *21:*315, 1984.
170. Kemper, P.M., and Treiber, H.: Neuraxial morphine plus PCA: A new method in post-cesarean analgesia. Analg. Anesth., *70:*S198, 1990.
171. Kenady, D.E., Wilson, J.F., Schwartz, R.W., Bannon, C.L., *et al.*: A randomized comparison of patient-controlled analgesia versus standard analgesia requirements in patients undergoing cholecystectomy. Surg. Gynecol. Obstet., *174:*216, 1992.

172. Kissin, I.: Preemptive Analgesia: Why its effect is not always obvious. Anesthesiology, (editorial) *84:*1015, 1996.
173. Kitahata, L.M., and Collins, J.G.: Spinal action of narcotic analgesics. Anesthesiology, *54:*153, 1981.
174. Kluger, M.T., Owen, H., *et al.*: Patients' expectations of patient-controlled analgesia. Anaesthesia, *45:*1072, 1990.
175. Kotelko, D.M., Rottman, R.L., and Wright, W.C., *et al.*: Transdermal scopolamine decreases nausea and vomiting following cesarean section in patients receiving epidural morphine. Anesthesiology, *71:*675, 1989.
176. Krane, E.J., Tyler, D.C., and Jacobson, L.E.: The dose response of caudal morphine in children. Anesthesiology, *71:*48, 1989.
177. LaMotte, R.H., Thalhammer, J.G., and Robinson, C.J.: Peripheral neural correlates of magnitude of cutaneous pain and hyperalgesia. J. Neurophysiol., *50:*1, 1983.
178. LaMotte, R.H., Thalhammer, J.G., Torebjork, H.E., *et al.*: Peripheral neural mechanisms of cutaneous hyperalgesia following mild injury by heat. J. Neurosci., *2:*765, 1982.
179. Langer, J., Shandling, B., and Rosenberg, M.: Intraoperative bupivacaine during outpatient hernia repair in children. J. Pediatr. Surg., *22:*267, 1987.
180. Lasagna, L., and Beecher, H.K.: The optimal dose of morphine. J.A.M.A., *156:*231, 1954.
181. Lauretti, G.R., Reis, M.P., Prado, W.A., and Klamt, J.G.: Dose response study of intrathecal morphine versus intrathecal neostigmine, their combination, or placebo for postoperative analgesia in patients undergoing anterior and posterior vaginoplasty. Anesth. Analg., *82:*1182, 1996.
182. Laurito, C.E., Kirz, L.I., VadeBoncouer, T.R., *et al.*: Continuous infusion of interpleural bupivacaine maintains effective analgesia after colecystectomy. Anesth. Analg., *72:*516, 1991.
183. Lewis, T.: Experiments relating to cutaneous hyperalgesia and its spread through somatic nerves. Clin. Sci., *2:*373, 1936.
184. Leysen, J.E., and Niemegeers, C.J.E.: 3H-sufentanil: A superior ligand for mu-opiate receptors. Eur. J. Pharmacol., *87:*209, 1983.
185. Lind, G., Ashburn, M.A., and Gillie, M.H.: Oral transmucosal fentanyl citrate for the treatment of postoperative pain. Anesthesiology, *73:*783, 1990.
186. Liu, S., and Carpenter, R.L.: Epidural anesthesia and analgesia: Their role in postoperative outcome. Anesthesiology, *82:*1474, 1995.
187. Liu, S., Carpenter, R.L., Mulroy, M.F., *et al.*: Intravenous versus epidural administration of hydromorphone. Anesthesiology, *82:*682, 1995.
188. Liu, S., Carpenter, R.L., Mackey, D.C., Thirlby, R.C., *et al.*: Effects of perioperative analgesic technique on rate of recovery after colon surgery. Anesthesiology, *83:*757, 1995.
189. Liu, S., Angel, J., Owens, B.D., and Carpenter, R.L.: .05% bupivacaine is an optimal concentration for use with fentanyl for post-thoracotomy analgesia. Anesthesiology, *81:*A975, 1994.
190. Logas, W.G., El-Baz, N., El-Ganzouri, A., *et al.*: Continuous thoracic epidural analgesia for postoperative pain relief following thoracotomy: A randomized prospective study, Anesthesiology, *67:*787, 1987.
191. Loper, K.A., Ready, L.B., Downey, M., *et al.*: Epidural and intravenous fentanyl infusions are clinically equivalent after knee surgery. Anesth. Analg., *70:*72, 1990.
192. Loper, K.A., Butler, S., Nessly, M., and Wild, L.: Paralyzed with pain: The need for education. Pain, *37:*315, 1989.
193. Loper, K.A., and Ready, L.B.: Epidural morphine after anterior cruciate ligament repair: A comparison with PCA morphine. Anesth. Analg., *68:*350, 1989.
194. Lubenow, T.R., Tanck, E.N., Hopkins, E.M., McCarthy, R.J., *et al.*: Comparison of patient-assisted epidural analgesia with continuous-infusion epidural analgesia for postoperative patients, Reg. Anesth., *19:*206, 1994.
195. Lussos, S.A., Bader, A.M., Thornhill, M.L., and Datta, S.: The antiemetic efficacy and safety of prophylactic metoclopramide for elective cesarean delivery during spinal anesthesia. Reg. Anesth., *17:*126, 1992.
196. Mackey, D.C., Ebener, M.K., and Howe, B.L.: Patient-controlled analgesia and the acute pain service in the United States: HCFA policy is impeding optimal PCA Management. Anesthesiology, *83:*433, 1995.
197. Malmberg, A.B., and Yaksh, T.L.: Pharmacology of the spinal action of ketorolac, morphine, ST-91, U50488H, and L-PIA on the formalin test. Anesthesiology, *79:*270, 1993.
198. Manriquez, R.G., and Pallares, V.: Continuous brachial plexus block for prolonged sympathectomy and control of pain. Anesth. Analg., *57:*128, 1978.
199. Marks, R.M., and Sachar, E.J.: Undertreatment of medical inpatients with narcotic analgesics. Ann. Intern. Med., *78:*173, 1973.
200. Mather, L.E., and Mackie, J.: The incidence of postoperative pain in children. Pain, *15:*271, 1983.
201. Maves, T.J., Pechman, P.S., Meller, S.T., and Gebhart, G.F.: Ketorolac potentiates morphine antinociception during visceral nociception in the rat. Anesthesiology, *80:*1094, 1994.
202. Max, M.B.: U.S. Government disseminates acute pain treatment guidelines: Will they make a difference? (editorial) Pain, *50:*3, 1992.
203. Max, M.B., Donovan, M., Portenoy, R.K., Cleeland, C.S., Ready, L.B., *et al.*: American Pain Society quality assurance standards for relief of acute pain and cancer pain. Proceedings of the 6th World Congress on Pain. pp. 185–189. Amsterdam, Elsevier Science Publishers, 1991.
204. McGrath, P.A.: Pain in children and adolescents. New York, Elsevier, 1987.
205. McIlvaine, W.B., Knox, R.F., Fennessey, P.V., *et al.*: Continuous infusion of bupivacaine via intrapleural catheter for analgesia after thoracotomy in children. Anesthesiology, *69:*261, 1988.
206. McIntyre, P.F., and Jarvis, D.A.: Age is the best predictor of postoperative morphine requirements. Pain, *64:*357, 1995.
207. McQuay, H.J., Carrol, D., and Moore, R.A.: Postoperative orthopaedic pain—The effect of opiate premedication and local anesthetic blocks. Pain, *33:*291, 1988.
208. Merskey H.: Pain terms: A list with definitions and notes on usage. Recommended by IASP Subcommittee on Taxonomy. Pain, *6:*249, 1979.
209. Melzack, R., Abbott, F.V., Zackon, W., *et al.*: Pain on a surgical ward: A survey of the duration and intensity of pain and the effectiveness of medication. Pain, *29:*67, 1987.
210. Modig, J., Borg, T., Bagge, L., and Saldeen, T.: Role of extradural and general anesthesia in fibrinolysis and coagulation after total hip replacement. Br. J. Anaesth., *55:*625, 1983.
211. Modig, J., and Paalzow, L.: A comparison of epidural morphine and epidural bupivacaine for postoperative pain relief. Acta Anesthesiol. Scand., *25:*437, 1981.
212. Modig, J., Hjelmstedt, A., Sahlstedt, B., and Maripuu, E.: Comparative influences of epidural and general anesthesia on deep vein thrombosis and pulmonary embolism after total hip replacement. Acta Chir. Scand., *147:*125, 1981.
213. Modig, J., Malmberg, P., and Karlstrom, G.: Effect of epidural versus general anesthesia on calf blood flow. Acta Anesthesiol. Scand., *24:*305, 1980.
214. Mogensen, T., Vegger, P., Jonsson, T., *et al.*: Systemic piroxicam as an adjunct to combined epidural bupivacaine and morphine for postoperative pain relief. Anesth. Analg., *74:*366, 1992.
215. Mogensen, T., Eliasen, K., Ejlersen, E., *et al.*: Epidural clonidine enhances postoperative analgesia from a combined low dose epidural bupivacaine morphine regimen. Anesth. Analg., *75:*607, 1992.
216. Moller, I.W., Dinesen, K., Sondergard, S., *et al.*: Effect of patient-controlled analgesia on plasma catecholamine, cortisol and glucose concentrations after cholecystectomy. Br. J. Anaesth., *61:*160, 1988.
217. Moon, R.E., and Clements, F.M.: Accidental epidural overdose of hydromorphone. Anesthesiology, *63:*238, 1985.
218. Moore, R.A., Bullingham, R.E.S., McQuay, J.H., *et al.*: Dural permeability to narcotics: In vitro determination and application to extradural administration. Br. J. Anaesth., *54:*1117, 1982.
219. Motsch, J., Graber, E., and Ludwig, K.: Addition of clonidine enhances postoperative analgesia from epidural morphine. Anesthesiology, *73:*1067, 1990.
220. Murphy, D.F.: Continuous intercostal nerve blockade for pain relief following cholecystectomy. Br. J. Anaesth., *55:*521, 1983.
221. Naguib, M., Sharif, A.M., Seraj, M., *et al.*: Ketamine for caudal analgesia in children: Comparison with caudal bupivacaine. Br. J. Anaesth., *67:*559, 1991.
222. Naulty, J.S., Datta, S., and Ostheimer, G.W.: Epidural fentanyl for post-cesarean delivery pain management. Anesthesiology, *63:*694, 1985.
223. Negre, I., Gueneron, J.P., Jamali, S.J., *et al.*: Preoperative analgesia with epidural morphine. Anesth. Analg., *79:*298, 1994.
224. Nordberg, G.: Pharmacokinetic aspects of spinal morphine analgesia. Acta Anaesthesiol. Scand., *79:*1, 1984.

225. Nordberg, G., Hedner, T., Mellstrand, T., and Dahlstrom, B.: Pharmacokinetic aspects of epidural morphine analgesia. Anesthesiology, *58:*545, 1983.
226. Norris, E., Parker, S., Breslow, M., *et al.*: The endocrine response to surgical stress: A comparison of epidural anesthesia/analgesia vs. general anesthesia/PCA. Anesthesiology, *75:*A696, 1991.
227. Nunn, J.F., and Slavin, G.: Posterior intercostal nerve block for pain relief after cholecystectomy. Br. J. Anaesth., *52:*253, 1980.
228. Ossipov, M.H., Suarez, L.J., and Spaulding, T.C.: Antinociceptive interactions between alpha-2 adrenergic and opiate agonists in rodents. Anesth. Analg., *68:*194, 1989.
229. Owen, H., McMillan, V., and Rogowski, D.: Postoperative pain therapy: A survey of patients' expectations and their experiences. Pain, *41:*303, 1990.
230. Owen, H., Plummer, J.L., Armstrong, I., *et al.*: Variables of PCA: 1. Bolus size. Anaesthesia, *44:*7, 1989.
231. Owen, H., Szekely, S.M., Plummer, J.L., *et al.*: Variables of PCA: 2. Concurrent infusion. Anaesthesia, *44:*11, 1989.
232. Owen, J., Glavin, R.J., and Shaw, N.A.: Ibuprofen in the management of postoperative pain. Br. J. Anaesth., *58:*1371, 1986.
233. Parbrook, G.D., and Steel, D.F.: Factors predisposing to postoperative pain: A study of male patients undergoing elective gastric surgery. Br. J. Anaesth., *45:*21, 1973.
234. Parker, A.J., Sinatra, R.S., and Glass, P.S.A.: Patient-controlled analgesia systems, *In* Sinatra, R.S., Hord, A.H., Ginsberg, B., and Preble, L.M. (eds.): Acute Pain Mechanisms and Management. pp. 205–224. St. Louis, Mosby–Year Book, 1992.
235. Parker, R.K., and White, P.F.: Epidural patient-controlled analgesia: An alternative to intravenous patient-controlled analgesia for pain relief after cesarean delivery. Anesth. Analg., *75:*245, 1992.
236. Parker, R.K., Holtman, B., and White, P.F.: Patient-controlled analgesia—Does a concurrent opioid infusion improve pain management after surgery? J.A.M.A., *266:*1947, 1992.
237. Parker, R.K., Perry, F., Holtman, B., *et al.*: Demographic factors influencing the PCA morphine requirement. Anesthesiology, *73:*A818, 1990.
238. Pasero, C.L., and Preble, L.M.: Role of the clinical coordinator. *In* Sinatra, R.S., Hord, A.H., Ginsberg, B., and Preble, L.M. (eds.): Acute Pain Mechanisms and Management. pp. 552–559. St. Louis, Mosby–Year Book, 1992.
239. Perry, S., and Heidrich, G.: Management of pain during debridement: A survey of U.S. burn units. Pain, *13:*267, 1982.
240. Pert, C.B., Kuhar, M.J., and Snyder, S.H.: Autoradiographic localization of the opiate receptor in rat brain. Life Sci., *16:*1849, 1975.
241. Perttunen, K., Nilsson, E., Heinonen, J., *et al.*: Extradural, paravertebral, and intercostal nerve blocks for post-thoracotomy pain. Br. J. Anaesth., *75:*541, 1995.
242. Plummer, J.L., Cmielewski, P.L., Gourlay, G.K., Owen, H., and Cousins, M.J.: Antinociceptive and motor effects of intrathecal morphine combined with intrathecal clonidine, noradrenaline, carbachol, and midazolam in rats. Pain, *49:*145, 1992.
243. Plummer, J.L., Cmielewski, G.D., Reynolds, G.K., and Gourlay, G.K.: Influence of polarity on dose response relationships of intrathecal opioids in rats. Pain, *40:*339, 1987.
244. Preble, L., and Sinatra, R.S.: Patient characteristics influencing postoperative pain management. *In* Sinatra, R.S., Hord, A.H., Ginsberg, B., and Preble, L.M. (eds.): Acute Pain Mechanisms and Management. pp. 140–150. St. Louis, Mosby–Year Book, 1992.
245. Prescott, L.F., Adejepon-Yamoah, K.K., and Talbot, R.G.: Impaired lignocaine metabolism in patients with myocardial infarction and cardiac failure. Br. J. Med., *1:*939, 1976.
246. Pryl, B.J., Vanner, R.G., Enriquez, N., and Reynolds, F.: Can preemptive lumbar epidural blockade reduce post-operative pain following lower abdominal surgery? Anaesthesia, *48:*120, 1993.
247. Raj, P.P.: The anesthesiologist's role in pain management. *In* Sinatra, R.S., Hord, A.H., Ginsberg, B., and Preble, L.M. (eds.): Acute Pain Mechanisms and Management. pp. 517–520. St. Louis, Mosby–Year Book, 1992.
248. Raja, S.N., Meyer, R.A., and Campbell, J.N.: Peripheral mechanisms of somatic pain. Anesthesiology, *68:*571, 1988.
249. Rawal, N.: Acute pain services: A nurses' job-pro. *In* American Society of Regional Anesthesia, 21st Annual Meeting Syllabus. pp. 235, 1996.
250. Rawal, N., Arner, S., Gustafsson, L.L., *et al.*: Present state of extradural and intrathecal opioid analgesia in Sweden. Br. J. Anaesth., *59:*791, 1987.
251. Rawal, N., Schott, U., Dahlstrom, B., *et al.*: Influence of naloxone infusion on analgesia and respiratory depression following epidural morphine. Anesthesiology, *64:*194, 1986.
252. Rawal, N., Sjostrand, U.H., Christofferson, E.: Comparisons of intramuscular and epidural morphine for postoperative analgesia in the grossly obese: Influence on postoperative ambulation and pulmonary function. Anesth. Analg., *63:*584, 1984.
253. Rawal, N., Mollefors, K., Axelsson, K., *et al.*: An experimental study of urodynamic effects of epidural morphine and naloxone reversal. Anesth. Analg., *62:*641, 1984.
254. Rawal, N., Sjostrand, U.H., Dahlstrom, B., *et al.*: Epidural morphine for postoperative pain relief: A comparative study with intramuscular narcotic and intercostal block. Anesth. Analg., *61:*93, 1982.
255. Ready, L.B.: Acute pain services. *In* American Society of Regional Anesthesia, 21st Annual Meeting Syllabus. pp. 235, 1996.
256. Ready, L.B.: How many acute pain services are there in the United States, and who is managing PCA? Anesthesiology, *82:*322, 1995.
257. Ready, L.B., Ashburn, M., Caplan, R.A., *et al.*: Practice guidelines for acute pain management in the perioperative setting: A report by the American Society of Anesthesiologists Task Force on Acute Pain, Acute Pain Section. Anesthesiology, *82:*1071, 1995.
258. Ready, L.B., Brown, C.R., Stahlgren, L.H., Egan, K.J., *et al.*: Evaluation of intravenous ketorolac administered by bolus or infusion for treatment of postoperative pain, a double-blind, placebo-controlled, multicenter study, Anesthesiology, *80:*1277, 1994.
259. Ready, L.B., Loper, K.A., Nessly, M., and Wild, L.: Postoperative morphine is safe on surgical wards. Anesthesiology, *75:*452, 1991.
260. Ready, L.B., Oden, R., Chadwick, H.S., *et al.*: Development of an anesthesiology-based postoperative pain management service. Anesthesiology, *68:*100, 1988.
261. Ready, L.B., Chadwick, H.S., and Ross, B.: Age predicts effective epidural morphine dose after abdominal hysterectomy. Anesth. Analg., *66:*1215, 1987.
262. Reeder, M.K., Goldman, M.D., Loh, L., *et al.*: Postoperative hypoxaemia after major abdominal vascular surgery. Br. J. Anaesth., *68:*23, 1992.
263. Reiestad, F., and Stromskag, K.E.: Interpleural catheter in management of postoperative pain. Reg. Anesth., *11:*89, 1986.
264. Reiz, S., Balfors, E., and Sorensen, M.B.: Coronary hemodynamic effects of general anesthesia and surgery: Modification by epidural analgesia. Reg. Anesth., *7*(Suppl.):8, 1982.
265. Rice, L.J., and Britton, J.T.: Neural blockade for pediatric pain management. *In* Sinatra, R.S., Hord, A.H., Ginsberg, B., and Preble, L.M. (eds.): Acute Pain Mechanisms and Management. pp. 483–507. St. Louis, Mosby–Year Book, 1992.
266. Ringrose, N.H., and Cross, M.J.: Femoral nerve block in knee joint surgery. Am. J. Sports Med., *12*(5):398, 1984.
267. Rocco, A., Reiestad, F., Gudman, J., *et al.*: Interpleural administration of local anesthetics for pain relief in patient with multiple rib fractures. Reg. Anesth., *12:*10, 1987.
268. Rockemann, M.G., Seeling, W., Bischof, C., *et al.*: Prophylactic use of epidural mepivacaine-morphine, systemic diclofenac, and metamizol reduces postoperative morphine consumption after major abdominal surgery. Anesthesiology, *84:*1027, 1996.
269. Rogers, B.M., Weeb, C.J., Stergios, D., *et al.*: Patient-controlled analgesia in pediatric surgery. J. Pediatr. Surg., *23:*259, 1988.
270. Rosen, M.A., Dailey, P.A., Hughes, S.C., *et al.*: Epidural sufentanil for postoperative analgesia after cesarean section. Anesthesiology, *68:*448, 1988.
271. Rosenberg, P.H., Scheinin, B.A., Lepantale, M.J., *et al.*: Continuous interpleural infusion of bupivacaine for analgesia after thoracotomy. Anesthesiology, *67:*811, 1987.
272. Rosenblatt, R., Pepitone-Rockwell, F., and McKillop, M.J.: Continuous axillary analgesia for traumatic hand injury. Anesthesiology, *51:*565, 1979.
273. Rosenblatt, W., Saberski, L., Sinatra, R.S., *et al.*: Metoclopramide: An analgesic adjunct to patient-controlled analgesia. Anesth. Analg., *73:*553, 1991.
274. Rosenfeld, B.A., Beattie, C., Christopherson, R., *et al.*: The effects of different anesthetic regimens on fibrinolysis and the development of postoperative arterial thrombosis. Anesthesiology, *79:*435, 1993.
275. Rothstein, P., Arthur, G.R., Feldman, H.S., *et al.*: Bupivacaine for intercostal nerve blocks in children: Blood concentrations and pharmacokinetics. Anesthesiology, *65:*625, 1986.

276. Rotter, J.B.: Generalized expectancies for internal versus external control of reinforcement. Psychol. Monogr., *80:*1, 1966.
277. Roytblat, L., Korotkoruchko, A., Katz, J., *et al.*: Postoperative pain: The effect of low-dose ketamine in addition to general anesthesia. Anesth. Analg., *77:*1161, 1993.
278. Saiah, M., Borgeat, A., Wilder-Smith, O.H.G., *et al.*: Epidural-morphine induced pruritus: Propofol versus naloxone. Anesth. Analg., *78:*1110, 1994.
279. Saidman, L.J.: The anesthesiologist outside the operating room: A new and exciting opportunity. Anesthesiology, (editorial) *68:*1, 1988.
280. Salomaki, T.E., Leppaluoto, J., Laitinen, J.O., *et al.*: Epidural versus intravenous fentanyl for reducing hormonal, metabolic, and physiologic responses after thoracotomy. Anesthesiology, *79:*672, 1993.
281. Salomaki, T.E., Laitinen, J.O., and Nuutinen, L.S.: A randomized double-blind comparison of epidural versus intravenous fentanyl infusion for analgesia after thoracotomy. Anesthesiology, *75:*790, 1991.
282. Scalley, R.D., Berquist, K., and Cochran, R.S.: Patient-controlled analgesia in orthopedic procedures. Orthop. Rev. *17*(11):1106, 1988.
283. Schecter, N.L., Berrien, F.B., and Katz, S.M.: The use of patient-controlled analgesia in adolescents with sickle cell crisis: A preliminary report. J. Pain Symptom Manage., *3:*109, 1988.
284. Schulze, S., Roikjaer, O., Hasselstrom, L., *et al.*: Epidural bupivacaine and morphine plus systemic indomethacin eliminates pain, but not the systemic response and convalescence, after cholecystectomy. Surgery, *103:*321, 1988.
285. Scott, D.A., Beilby, D.S., and McClymont, C.: Postoperative analgesia using epidural infusions of fentanyl with bupivacaine. Anesthesiology, *83:*727, 1995.
286. Scott, L.E., Clum, G.A., and Peoples, J.B.: Preoperative predictors of postoperative pain. Pain, *15:*283, 1983.
287. Sechzer, P.H.: Objective measurement of pain. Anesthesiology, *29:*209, 1968.
288. Sevarino, F.B., Sinatra, R.S., Paige, D., *et al.*: The efficacy of intramuscular ketorolac in combination with intravenous PCA morphine for postoperative pain relief. J. Clin. Anesth., *4:*285, 1992.
289. Sevarino, F.B., and Ning, T.: Transdermal fentanyl for acute pain management. *In* Sinatra, R.S., Hord, A.H., Ginsberg, B., and Preble, L.M. (eds.): Acute Pain Mechanisms and Management. St. Louis, Mosby–Year Book, 1992.
290. Sevarino, F.B., Sinatra, R.S., *et al.*: Epidural fentanyl effect on IV PCA requirements. Can. J. Anesth., *38:*450, 1991.
291. Shapiro, B.: The management of pain in sickle cell disease. Pediatr. Clin. North Am., *36:*1029, 1989.
292. Shulman, M.S., Wakerlin, G., Yamaguchi, L., and Brodsky, J.B.: Experience with epidural hydromorphone for post-thoracotomy pain relief. Anesth. Analg., *66:*1331, 1987.
293. Shulman, M., Sandler, A.N., Bradley, J.W., *et al.*: Post-thoracotomy pain and pulmonary function following epidural and systemic morphine. Anesthesiology, *61:*569, 1984.
294. Sinatra, R.S.: Unpublished Observations, 1994–1997, Yale University Acute Pain Service.
295. Sinatra, R.S., Sevarino, F.B., Paige, D., *et al.*: Patient-controlled analgesia with sufentanil: A comparison of epidural versus intravenous administration. J. Clin. Anesth., *8:*123, 1996.
296. Sinatra, R.S.: Pharmacokinetics and pharmacodynamics of spinal opioids. *In* Sinatra, R.S., Hord, A.H., Ginsberg, B., and Preble, L.M. (eds.) Acute Pain Mechanisms and Management. pp. 111–120. St. Louis, Mosby–Year Book, 1992.
297. Sinatra, R.S., and Savarese, A.: Parenteral analgesic therapy and patient-controlled analgesia for pediatric pain management, *In* Sinatra, R.S., Hord, A.H., Ginsberg, B., and Preble, L.M. (eds.): Acute Pain Mechanisms and Management. pp. 453–469. St. Louis, Mosby–Year Book, 1992.
298. Sinatra, R.S., Sevarino, F.B., Chung, J.H., *et al.*: Comparison of epidurally administered sufentanil, morphine and sufentanil-morphine combination for postoperative analgesia. Anesth. Analg., *72:*522, 1991.
299. Sinatra, R.S., Harrison, D.M., Sibert, K., *et al.*: A comparison of meperidine, morphine and oxymorphone for use in PCA following cesarean delivery. Anesthesiology, *70:*585, 1989.
300. Sinatra, R., Chung, K.S., Silverman, D.G., *et al.*: An evaluation of morphine and oxymorphone administered via PCA or PCA plus basal infusion. Anesthesiology, *71:*20, 1989.
301. Singh, H., Bossard, R.F., White, P.F.: Epidural PCA: Effect of ketorolac vs. bupivacaine supplementation on pulmonary functions after thoracotomy. Anesthesiology, *83:*A874, 1995.
302. Sjostrom, S., Hartvig, D., and Tamsen, A.: Patient-controlled analgesia with extradural morphine or pethidine. Br. J. Anaesth. *60:*358, 1988.
303. Snijdelaar, D.G., Hasenbos, M.A., van Egmond, J., Wolff, A.P., *et al.*: High thoracic epidural sufentanil with bupivacaine: Continuous infusion of high-volume versus low-volume. Anesth. Analg., *78:*490, 1994.
304. Stacey, B.R., Rudy, T.E., and Nellhaus, D.: Differences between primary service and acute pain service management of patient-controlled analgesia. Reg. Anesth., *21*(2S):17, 1996.
305. Steinstra, R., and Van Poorten, F.: Immediate respiratory arrest after caudal sufentanil. Anesthesiology, *71:*993, 1989.
306. Stevens, D.S., and Dunn, W.T.: Acute pain management for the trauma patient, *In* Sinatra, R.S., Hord, A.H., Ginsberg, B., and Preble, L.M. (eds.): Acute Pain Mechanisms and Management. pp. 412–422. St. Louis, Mosby–Year Book, 1992.
307. Stoelting, R.K.: Pharmacokinetics and pharmacodynamics of injected and inhaled drugs. *In* Stoelting, R.K. (ed.): Pharmacology and Physiology in Anesthetic Practice. Philadelphia, Lippincott, 1987.
308. Stoelting, R.K.: Opioid agonists and antagonists. *In* Stoelting, R.K., (ed.): Pharmacology and Physiology in Anesthetic Practice. pp. 1–32. Philadelphia, Lippincott, 1987.
309. Streisand, J.: Controlled iontophoretic and transmucosal delivery of opioids. *In* Sinatra, R.S., Hord, A.H., Ginsberg, B., and Preble, L.M. (eds.): Acute Pain Mechanisms and Management. pp. 370–378. St. Louis, Mosby–Year Book, 1992.
310. Streltzer, J., and Wade, T.: The influence of cultural group on the undertreatment of postoperative pain. Psychsom. Med., *43:*397, 1981.
311. Sun, H.L., Wu, C.C., Lin, M.S., and Chang, C.F.: Effects of epidural morphine and intramuscular diclofenac combination in postcesarean analgesia: A dose-range study. Anesth. Analg., *76:*284, 1993.
312. Swenson, J.D., Hullander, M., Bready, R.J., and Leivers, D.: A comparison of patient-controlled epidural analgesia with sufentanil by the lumbar versus thoracic route after thoracotomy. Anesth. Analg., *78:*215, 1994.
313. Symreng, T., Gomez, M.N., Johnson, B., *et al.*: Intrapleural bupivacaine: Technical considerations and intraoperative use. J. Cardiothorac. Anesth., *3:*139, 1989.
314. Szyfelbein, S.K., Osgood, P.F., Murphy, J.L., *et al.*: Comparison of fentanyl plasma levels and pain scores in burned children. Proc. Am. Burn Assoc., *17:*107, 1985.
315. Tallarida, R.: Statistical analysis of drug combinations for synergy. Pain, *49:*93, 1992.
316. Tamsen, A., Hartwig, P., Fagerlund, C., *et al.*: PCA therapy—pharmacokinetics of pithidine in the pre- and postoperative periods. Clin. Pharmacokinet., *7:*266, 1982.
317. Tamsen, A., Sakurada, T., Wahlstrom, A., *et al.*: Postoperative demand for analgesics in relation to individual levels of endorphins and substance P in CSF. Pain *13:*171, 1982.
318. Tamsen, A., Hartwig, P., Dahlstrom, B., *et al.*: Patient-controlled analgesia in the early postoperative period. Acta Anesthesiol. Scand., *23:*462, 1979.
319. Terjani, G.A., Rattan, A.K., and McDonald, J.S.: Role of spinal opioid receptors in the antinociceptive interactions between intrathecal morphine and bupivacaine. Anesth. Analg., *74:*726, 1992.
320. Thomas, D.F.M., Lambert, W.G., and Lloyd-Williams, K.: The direct perfusion of surgical wounds with local anesthetic solutions: An approach to postoperative pain. Ann. R. Coll. Surg. Engl., *65:*226, 1983.
321. Thompson, S.W.D., and Woolf, C.J.: Primary afferent-evoked prolonged potentials in the spinal cord and their central summation: Role of the NMDA receptor. *In* Bond, M.R., Charlton, J.E., and Woolf, C.J. (eds.): Proceedings of the 6th World Congress on Pain. pp. 291–297. Amsterdam, Elsevier, 1991.
322. Tuman, K.J., McCarthy, R.J., March, R.J., *et al.*: Effects of epidural anesthesia and analgesia on coagulation and outcome after major vascular surgery. Anesth. Analg., *73:*696, 1991.
323. Tverskoy, M., Oz, Y., Isakson, A., Finger, J., *et al.*: Pre-emptive effect of fentanyl and ketamine on postoperative pain and wound hyperalgesia. Anesth. Analg., *78:*205, 1994.
324. Tverskoy, M., Cozacov, C., Ayache, M., *et al.*: Postoperative pain after inguinal herniorrhaphy with different types of anesthesia. Anesth. Analg., *70:*29, 1990.
325. Ullman, D., Fortune, S.B., Greenhouse, B.B., *et al.*: The treatment of patients with multiple rib fractures using continuous thoracic epidural narcotic infusion. Reg. Anesth. *14:*43, 1989.

326. Urquhart, M.L., Klapp, K., and White, P.F.: Patient-controlled analgesia: A comparison of intravenous vs. subcutaneous hydromorphone. Anesthesiology, *69:*428, 1988.
327. VadeBoncouer, T.R., and Ferrante, F.M.: Management of a postoperative pain service in a teaching hospital. *In* Ferrante, F.M., and VadeBoncouer, T.R. (eds.): Postoperative Pain Management. pp. 625–639. New York, Churchill Livingstone, 1993.
328. Van der Auwern, A., Verborgh, C., and Camu, F.: Analgesic and cardiorespiratory effects of epidural sufentanil and morphine. Anesth. Analg., *66:*999, 1987.
329. Van den Hoogen, R.H., and Colpaert, F.C.: Epidural and subcutaneous morphine, meperidine, fentanyl, and sufentanil in the rat. Anesthesiology, *66:*186, 1987.
330. Varrassi, G., Panella, L., Piroli, A., *et al.*: The effects of perioperative ketorolac infusion on postoperative pain and endocrine-metabolic response. Anesth. Analg., *78:*514, 1994.
331. Wajima, Z., Nakajima, Y., Kim, C., *et al.*: Comparison of continuous brachial plexus infusion of butorphanol, mepivacaine and mepivacaine-butorphanol for postoperative analgesia. Br. J. Anaesth., *75:*548, 1995.
332. Wall, P.D.: The prevention of postoperative pain. Pain (editorial), *33:*289, 1988.
333. Wamsley, P.N.H.: Patient-controlled epidural analgesia. *In* Sinatra, R.S., Hord, A.H., Ginsberg, B., and Preble, L.M. (eds.): Acute Pain Mechanisms and Management. pp. 312–320. St. Louis, Mosby–Year Book, 1992.
334. Wang, J.K., Nauss, L.A., and Thomas, J.E.: Pain relief by intrathecally applied morphine in man. Anesthesiology, *50:*149, 1979.
335. Wayslak, T.J., English, M.J.M., and Jeans, M.E.: Reduction of postoperative morbidity following patient-controlled morphine. Can. J. Anesth., *37:*726, 1990.
336. Welchew, E.A., and Thornton, J.A.: Continuous thoracic epidural fentanyl. Anaesthesia, *37:*309, 1982.
337. Weightman, W.M.: Respiratory arrest during epidural bupivacaine-fentanyl. Anesth. Intensive Care, *19:*282, 1991.
338. Wells, D.G., and Davies, G.: Profound CNS depression from epidural fentanyl for extracorporeal shock wave lithotripsy. Anesthesiology, *67:*991, 1987.
339. White, P.W.: Use of patient-controlled analgesia for management of acute pain. J.A.M.A., *259:*243, 1988.
340. White, P.F.: Mishaps with patient-controlled analgesia. Anesthesiology, *66:*81, 1987.
341. Winnie, A.P.: New uses for old drugs. Anesthesiol. Rev., *7:*8, 1980.
342. Wolf, A.R., Valley, R.D., Fear, D.W., *et al.*: Bupivacaine for caudal analgesia in infants and children: The optimum effective concentration. Anesthesiology, *69:*102, 1988.
343. Woolf, C.J., and Chong, M.S.: Preemptive analgesia-treating postoperative pain by preventing the establishment of central sensitization. Anesth. Analg., *77:*362, 1993.
344. Woolf, C.J., and Thompson, W.N.: The induction and maintenance of central sensitization is dependent upon N-methyl-D-aspartic acid receptor activation. Pain, *44:*293, 1991.
345. Woolf, C.J., and Wall, P.D.: Morphine-sensitive and morphine-insensitive actions of C-fiber input on the rat spinal cord. Neurosci. Lett., *64:*221, 1986.
346. Woolf, C.J.: Evidence for a central component of post-injury pain hypersensitivity. Nature, *306:*686, 1983.
347. Yaksh, T.L.: Analgetic actions of intrathecal opiates in cat and primates. Brain Res., *153:*205, 1978.
348. Yaksh, T.L., and Rudy, T.A.: Analgesia mediated by a direct spinal action of narcotics. Science, *192:*1357, 1976.
349. Yamaguchi, H., Watanabe, S., Motokawa, K., *et al.*: Intrathecal morphine dose response data for pain relief after cholecystectomy. Anesth. Analg., *70:*168, 1990.
350. Yamamoto, T., and Yaksh, T.L.: Comparisons of the antinociceptive effects of pre- and post-treatment with intrathecal morphine and MK801, an NMDA antagonist, on the formalin test in the rat. Anesthesiology, *77:*757, 1992.
351. Yaster, M., and Maxwell, L.G.: Pediatric regional anesthesia. Anesthesiology, *70:*324, 1989.
352. Yeager, M.P., Glass, D.G., and Neff, R.K.: Epidural anesthesia and analgesia in high-risk surgical patients. Anesthesiology, *66:*729, 1987.
353. Yeoman, P.M., Cooke, R., and Hain, W.R.: Penile block for circumcision? A comparison with caudal blockade. Anesthesia, *38:*862, 1983.
354. Zakowski, M., Ramanathan, S., and Khoo, P., *et al.*: Plasma histamine with intraspinal morphine in cesarean section. Anesth. Analg., *70:*S40, 1990.
[Editor's note: Additional helpful review]
355. Meibner, A., Rolf, N., and Vanaker, H.: Thoracic epidural anesthesia and the patient with heart disease: Benefits, risks and controversies. Anesth. Analg. *85:*1, 1997.

Neural Blockade in Clinical Anesthesia and Management of Pain, Third Edition, edited by M.J. Cousins and P.O. Bridenbaugh. Lippincott–Raven Publishers, Philadelphia © 1998.

CHAPTER 27

Diagnostic and Prognostic Neural Blockade

Quinn H. Hogan and Stephen E. Abram

Use of neural blockade to establish the diagnosis or prognosis of painful conditions is motivated by several compelling characteristics of clinical pain treatment. Pain is an entirely subjective phenomenon with limited means of measurement; painful conditions are inexactly delineated, so that a single descriptive label may be applied to a heterogenous group of maladies, and our understanding of the pathophysiology of pain is poorly developed; and, finally, chronic pain is a complex melange of nociception (the stimulation of pain-sensing pathways) and neuropathy (aberrant neural function), mixed with social, emotional, financial, and legal influences. The ambiguity caused by these factors argues strongly for the use of blocks to gain clear knowledge of the pathophysiology of the pain: the contribution of sympathetic activity, the site of nociception (visceral vs. somatic), or the pathway of afferent neural signals (in an extensively injured limb for example). Information gained from blocks can be useful guides toward choice of medicines, therapeutic blocks, or surgical therapy. Also, blocks may be used to anticipate response to surgical ablation, which rarely produces a more satisfactory response than does the prognostic block. By means of a suitable block, the patient may experience motor and sensory changes on a temporary basis before committing to a long-term or permanent lesion.

However, the same uncertainties surrounding pain treatment that lead clinicians to seek hard data from neural blockade, also cloud the information gained from them. It is rarely simple to interpret even the most meticulously performed procedure; we may unwittingly confirm preconceived expectations or, at worst, respond to the disproportionate remuneration associated with performing procedures. Few blinded and controlled studies exist that test the utility of these alluring methods.

Q.H. Hogan: Department of Anesthesiology, Pain Management Center, Medical College of Wisconsin, Froedtert Memorial Hospital, Milwaukee, Wisconsin 53226-3569.

S.E. Abram: Department of Anesthesiology and Critical Care, University of New Mexico School of Medicine, Albuquerque, New Mexico 87131-5216.

The premise of this chapter is that blocks are informative only in proportion to the care with which they are performed and the thoroughness with which the response is evaluated, and that the findings should be interpreted cautiously. Therefore, we emphasize limitations so that the reader may avoid the pitfalls. Physiologic, anatomic, and psychosocial issues which influence the quality of information from diagnostic blocks are reviewed first, before the various procedures are discussed.

PAIN PHYSIOLOGY

The rationale for performing a diagnostic block often is based upon the same misconception that prompts surgeons to interrupt neural pathways for permanent pain relief: belief that pain is transmitted by a simple and direct "hard-wired" system. This theory, based on the Cartesian model of pain perception conceived in the 17th century dominated thinking about pain sensation through the mid-20th century, and continues to drive much present-day treatment. Use of a nerve block to identify a nerve pathway that is the source of an individual's ongoing pain assumes three potentially false premises: (i) pathology causing pain is located in an exact peripheral location and impulses from this site travel via a unique and consistent neural route, (ii) injection of local anesthetic totally and selectively abolishes sensory function of intended nerves, and (iii) relief of pain following local anesthetic block is due solely to block of the target neural pathway. These assumptions are limited by certain complexities of the anatomy, physiology, and psychology of pain perception, and the effect of local anesthetics on impulse conduction.

Nociceptor Activity (Table 27-1)

Pain that originates in somatic structures is generally associated with activation of nociceptors, sensory receptors that respond to intense, potentially tissue-injuring, stimulation. There is considerable controversy about the existence

TABLE 27-1. *Diagnostic blocks—limitations from variable 1ry afferent nerve activity*

Due to:
- Tissue factors (receptor sensitization)
- Spontaneous discharge (neuroma, dorsal root ganglion)
- Antidromic propagation
- Sympathetic efferent activity (ephapsis, receptor sensitization neuroma stimulation, inflammation)

of visceral receptors that respond solely to pain, and many researchers argue that visceral pain results from high-frequency discharge of visceral afferents that ordinarily subserve other functions.[220,262] In somatic structures, frequency of discharge of nociceptors correlates directly with the intensity of the stimulus. Thermal nociceptors, for instance, increase their discharge frequency in a linear fashion as temperature rises above 43°C.[366] This schema is compatible with the Cartesian "hard-wired" model.

However, receptor performance is not a fixed function of stimulation, but is also sensitive to tissue factors (see Chapter 23.1, Figs. 23.1-2 to 23.1-4). Bradykinin, histamine, and 5–hydroxytryptamine are capable of lowering response thresholds of nociceptors.[325] Several eicosanoids are important in sensitization of nociceptors, and at least two of the prostaglandins (PGE_2 and $PGE_{2\alpha}$) increase nociceptor sensitivity, while prostacyclin potentiates edema induced by bradykinin and histamine.

Peripheral nerve activity associated with pain perception may arise from injured nerves, independent of nociceptor activity. It is now well accepted that spontaneous impulses can be initiated from a neuroma or from an injured nerve segment,[78,323] and there is evidence that dorsal root ganglia proximal to injured or transsected nerves participate in abnormal impulse generation.[78] Blockade of an injured nerve proximal to the injured segment may not provide relief of pain if spontaneous activity continues at the level of the dorsal root ganglion. This may lead to the false assumption that the injured nerve is not responsible for the patient's pain (see Table 27-1).

Nerve blocks usually are interpreted in terms of their effect on afferent neural activity, but important efferent traffic must be considered. Impulse generation arising from an injured nerve fiber is likely to be propagated both orthodromically toward the spinal cord and antidromically toward the innervated tissues. For instance, bursts of sural nerve activity are recorded during straight leg-raising in a patient with S-1 radiculopathy.[251] Antidromic activity from injured sensory nerves (probably only C fibers) is thought to cause release of substance P and perhaps other substances, such as bradykinin, histamine, 5-HT, 2nd prostaglandins, which may produce changes in threshold of nociceptors by direct and indirect means.[71] Therefore, nerve block distal to the primary site of nerve pathology may alter pain perception by interrupting antidromic impulses, contrary to the common assumption that axonal function must be interrupted proximal to the area of injury to provide relief. Peripheral blockade of the sciatic nerve has been shown to provide profound relief of pain for patients with documented lumbosacral radiculopathy,[189,358] perhaps by blocking antidromic impulses which arise from the nerve root or dorsal root ganglion and are propagated to the periphery, producing changes in nociceptor sensitivity[2] (see Table 27-1).

Sympathetic Contributions

Another important type of efferent traffic affected by neural blockade is sympathetic motor activity, which can alter responses in sensory fibers. Receptors at the terminus of C fibers from an injured nerve become excited during sympathetic stimulation or norepinephrine application, and show enhanced responsiveness to irritating stimuli.[294] At the site of the nerve injury, sympathetic efferent impulses may depolarize nociceptive afferent fibers (ephaptic transmission), potentially producing both orthodromic and antidromic activity. Increased sympathetic activity or high levels of norepinephrine have been shown to increase discharge rates of spontaneous impulses arising from neuromas,[26,79] and the injection of epinephrine in the vicinity of neuromas in pain patients is associated with aggravation of pain[327] (Table 27-1).

In uninjured tissues, it is well accepted that sympathetic supply can modulate sensory responses,[286] but the role of the mechanism in producing pain is less certain. Mechanoreceptor sensitivity is heightened by increases in sympathetic discharge rates. Since nociceptors are not excited by sympathetic stimulation, elevated sympathetic efferent activity alone is unlikely to cause pain. However, aberrant central processing of these signals by sensitized wide dynamic range (WDR) neurons in the dorsal horn (see below) may result in the allodynia[286] present in certain cases of "reflex sympathetic dystrophy" (Fig. 27-1). (As described in Chapter 23.1, reflex sympathetic dystrophy is now denoted as "complex regional pain syndrome type I" [Figs. 23.1-8 and 23.1-9]). In addition to actions on sensory fibers, there is growing recognition of a sympathetic component in the inflammatory response, especially in joints.[190] Apart from its obvious peripheral effects, some reports also have documented analgesia by an undefined central mechanism after sympathetic block.[211,270]

Pain reduction following sympathetic blockade cannot be clearly distinguished in these several possible pain mechanisms: irritation of peripheral nociceptor sensitized by sympathetic efferent activity, signal generation in a neuroma induced by normal sympathetic tone, primary pathologic increase in sympathetic activity resulting in abnormally sensitive receptors, and inflammatory or central effects. When local anesthetic blockade of the sympathetic chain produces temporary relief, surgical or neurolytic interruption of the sympathetic pathways can, nonetheless, fail to provide sustained analgesia. Upregulation of adrenergic receptors in the affected limb may lead to such receptor hypersensitivity that

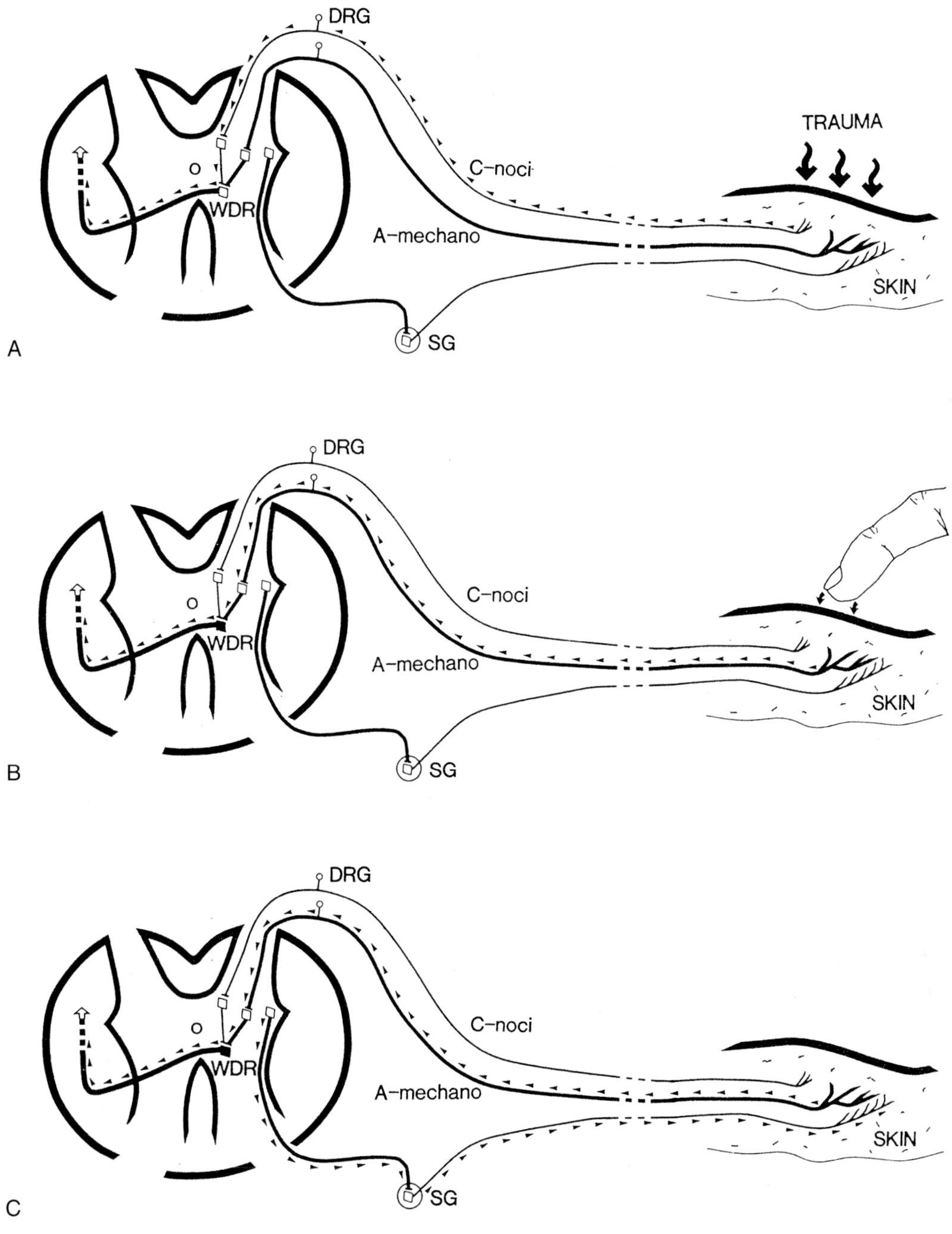

FIG. 27-1. Robert's hypothesis to explain allodynia and spontaneous pain after tissue trauma, for instance in reflex sympathetic dystrophy. **A:** An initiating injury provides a conditioning stimulus via nociceptive C fibers which sensitizes the wide dynamic range (*WDR*) cells in the dorsal horn. **B:** *WDR* cells which transmit to the brain now fire in response to innocuous stimuli conveyed via low threshold A-mechanoreceptor afferents. **C:** Spontaneous pain is produced by sympathetic efferent actions on A-mechanoreceptor afferents. (Reproduced with permission from: Roberts, W.J.: A hypothesis on the physiological basis for causalgia and related pains. Pain, *24*:297, 1986.)

circulating catecholamines may be sufficient to reproduce sympathetically maintained pain.

Spinal Processing (Table 27-2)

Whatever the contribution of receptor, neuropathic, or sympathetic mechanisms, activity in nociceptive afferent fibers is subject to further, variable processing in the spinal cord. The balance between large and small fiber inputs is an important determinant of the response of dorsal horn neurons to noxious stimulation.[236] Conceivably, loss of large fiber activity following peripheral or neuraxial blockade could increase dorsal horn cell activity, particularly if there is preservation of C fiber input (see Chapter 25, Fig. 25-1), producing a paradoxical increase in pain.

In addition to segmental influences on dorsal horn func-

TABLE 27-2. *Diagnostic blocks—limitations from changes in spinal processing*

Via:

- Altered balance between large fiber/small fiber input
- Block of inhibitory descending spinal tracts
- Stress-induced analgesia
- Descending potentiation of nociception
- Convergence (inputs from multiple receptive fields determine 2° neuron activity

tion, descending pathways modulate the response of spinal cord neurons to sensory stimuli (see Chapter 23.1, Figs. 23.1-18 and 23.1-19). Noradrenergic and serotoninergic fibers originate in the medulla and descend via the dorsolateral funiculus of the spinal cord to terminate in the dorsal horn where they inhibit nociceptive traffic.[14] Since these tracts lie superficially in the cord, they are susceptible to blockade by intrathecally administered local anesthetics, possibly leading to disinhibition of nociceptive transmission. The relative effect of the drug on afferent pathways, versus descending inhibitory tracts, would then determine the analgesic effect of a subarachnoid block. Descending cerebral influences may obscure findings during a diagnostic test by producing analgesia in response to stress, independent of the specific nature of the block. Conversely, descending modulation may be stimulatory and produce pain that is independent of sensory input. Dubner[91] has demonstrated in primates that nonpainful signals (flashing light) can be associated with nociceptive stimuli (laser heat) by conditioning with simultaneous presentation. Eventually, the light alone can result in firing of secondary nociceptive neurons and presumably in the sensory experience of pain. The importance of this model is that diagnostic blocks which produce no relief may suggest a diagnosis of malingering or psychiatric disease, when in fact descending influences are generating sensory activity.

Convergence and Referred Pain (Table 27-2)

Another confounding feature of pain perception is the phenomenon of convergence. Many second order neurons in the spinal cord respond to a variety of input from primary afferents with either visceral and somatic receptive fields[269] (see Chapter 23.1, Figs. 23.1-20 to 23.1-22). In other instances, convergence is the result of C fibers which have both visceral and cutaneous collaterals.[246] When afferent input arises from both somatic and visceral structures, or from separate somatic foci, the perception of pain may be dependent on a level of neuronal activity from both components (Chapter 23.1, Fig. 23.1-20). Interruption of one limb of the convergent inputs may be enough to provide complete pain relief, leading to false assumptions about the source of the pain. For instance, a patient with pain of pancreatic cancer may have inputs from splanchnic nerves, as well as from a focus of myofascial pain in the paravertebral muscles. Infiltration of a painful trigger point in the affected muscle may reduce the combined input to a level insufficient to exceed the pain threshold, and the interpretation would be that the pain is entirely somatic. As a further example, a patient may have combined gluteus medius myofascial pain and S-1 radiculopathy, with pain perceived in the distribution of the S-1 root. Infiltration of the gluteal trigger point provides blockade of input from muscle afferents to the S-1 segment, and may provide sufficient decrease in convergent input to relieve the radicular pain completely. This could then be interpreted as providing evidence that the patient's pain is entirely myofascial in origin, and the radicular component may be ignored when therapy is proposed.

Plasticity (Table 27-3)

Sensory processing is not stable but depends on preceding events, a phenomenon called neuronal plasticity. Small fiber (nociceptive) activity initiates a series of events in the dorsal horn that lead to heightened responsiveness of neurons activated by noxious stimuli. A brief noxious stimulus produces activation of the α-amino-3-hydroxy-5-methyl-4-isoxazopropionic acid (AMPA) receptor, which in turn produces a brief postsynaptic potential. Repetitive or prolonged firing of small afferent fibers (conditioning stimuli) releases excitatory amino acids, which in turn activate the N-methyl-D-aspartate (NMDA) receptor, causing prolonged postsynaptic potentials. NMDA activation gives rise to a series of intracellular biochemical events (Fig. 27-2) that produce enhanced neurotransmitter release from primary afferents and heightened sensitivity of postsynaptic neurons lasting many minutes to hours.[352] In certain instances, more prolonged changes in sensory processing, known as long-term potentiation (LTP) may occur[275,352] (see also Chapter 23.1, Figs. 23.1-10 to 23.1-16 and Chapter 24).

Sensitization in response to noxious stimulation is known to affect WDR neurons, which ordinarily respond at very low firing rates to non-noxious (mechanoreceptor, proprioceptor, thermoreceptor) inputs and at high firing rates to nociceptor activity. Following sensitization or LTP, these cells may respond to non-noxious stimuli at sufficiently high firing rates to cause pain perception (allodynia). It is impossible to predict responses to local anesthetic blockade of afferent impulses under conditions of dorsal horn sensitization. Afferent blockade of conditioning stimuli could lead to normalization of dorsal horn responsiveness and profound, prolonged relief. In other circumstances, however, spinal sensitization might persist independent of afferent activity, with little or no change in pain level.

TABLE 27-3. *Diagnostic blocks—limitations from plasticity*

- Sensitization (nociceptive potentiation from previous small fiber conditioning stimuli)
- Deafferentation (new receptive fields for nerves after loss of other input)

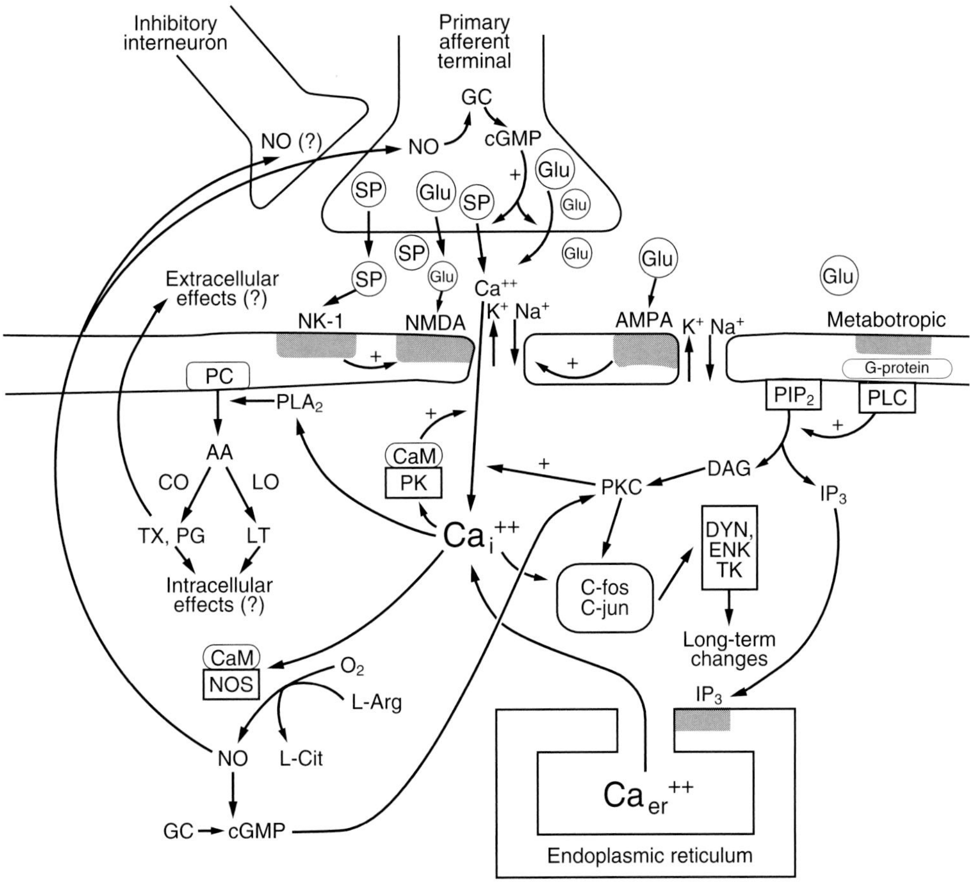

FIG. 27-2. Sequence of events leading to sensitization of dorsal horn neurons following injury and intense nociceptive stimulation. Intense activation of primary afferent neuron stimulates release of glutamate (*Glu*) and substance P (*SP*). The NMDA receptor, at physiologic Mg^{++} levels, is initially unresponsive to Glu, but following depolarization of the AMPA receptor by Glu or the NK-1 receptor by SP, it becomes responsive to Glu, allowing Ca^{++} influx. Action of Glu on the metabotropic receptor stimulates G-protein mediated activation of phospholipase C (*PLC*), which catalyzes hydrolysis of phosphatidylinositol 4,5-biphosphate (*PIP_2*) to produce inositol triphosphate (*IP_3*) and diacylglycerol (*DAG*). DAG stimulates production of protein kinase C (*PKC*), which is activated in the presence of high levels of intracellular Ca^{++} (Ca_i^{++}). IP_3 stimulates release of intracellular Ca^{++} from intracellular stores within the endoplasmic reticulum (*Ca_{er}^{++}*). Increased PKC induces a sustained increase in membrane permeability and, in conjunction with increased intracellular Ca^{++}, leads to increased expression of proto-oncogenes such as *c-fos* and *c-jun*. The proteins produced by these proto-oncogenes encode a number of neuropeptides such as enkephalins (*ENK*), dynorphin (*DYN*), and tachykinins (*TK*). Increased Ca_i^{++} also leads to activation of calcium/calmodulin dependent protein kinase (*CaM PK*), which produces a brief increase in membrane permeability, and to activation of phospholipase A_2 (*PLA_2*) and to activation of nitric oxide synthase (*NOS*) through a calcium/calmodulin mechanism. PLA_2 catalyzes the conversion of phosphatidyl choline (*PC*) to prostaglandins (*PG*) and thromboxanes (*TX*) and by lipoxygenase (*LO*) to produce leucotrienes (*LT*). NOS catalyzes the production of nitric oxide (*NO*) and L-citrulline (*L-Cit*) from L-argenine (*L-Arg*). NO activates soluble guanylate cyclase (*GC*), which increases the intracellular content of cyclic GMP (*cGMP*) and leads to increased production of protein kinases, such as PKC, and alterations in gene expression. NO diffuses out of the cell to the primary afferent terminal, where, through a GC/cGMP mechanism, it increases the release of glutamate. It is speculated that NO may interfere with release of inhibitory neurotransmitters from inhibitory neurons.

Pain and abnormal sensory responses after injury often are found in a distribution inconsistent with any nerve or root, such as an entire limb, or a stocking or glove pattern. This may lead to the diagnosis of psychoneurosis rather than to a neurologic condition. However, injury to a single peripheral nerve may create allodynia in adjacent territories innervated by other nerves, due to altered central processing of afferent signals from the uninjured as well as injured nerve.[322] Blockade of the uninjured nerve will relieve pain within the borders of its innervation. The likely but erroneous interpretation would be that the blocked nerve had been injured, which could lead to injection therapy or surgical neurolysis.

Local anesthetic blockade may outlast the duration of local anesthetic effect by hours or days,[10] leading to speculation that pain is psychosomatic or factitious. However, it is possible that a period of interruption of nociceptor activity may lead to temporary reversal of the sensitization of spinal cord neurons. Once the peripheral generator recommences, hours or days may go by before sufficient dorsal horn sensitization occurs to cause perception of pain.

Conversely, decreases in afferent input can lead to functional changes in the dorsal horn. Following periods of deafferentation, cells that respond to noxious stimulation become hypersensitive to remaining afferent inputs and may develop responsiveness to stimulation of tissues that did not previously produce activation (receptive field expansion).[355] Denervation may also produce sufficient sensitization of WDR neurons that non-noxious stimulation, including stimuli from outside the original receptive field, can produce pain (see Chapter 24). Blockade of such stimulation could cause false indication of the pathology site. Alternatively, blockade of an injured nerve may not provide relief of pain and allodynia if the receptive field of sensitized dorsal horn neurons has spread beyond the distribution of the injured nerve, leading again to the mistaken conclusion that the injured nerve is not involved. Denervation of peripheral afferent fibers has been shown to cause dramatic functional changes in responses of WDR neurons in the dorsal horn.[80]

Summary

These physiologic observations demonstrate that pain is not a process taking place at a single site, is not fixed over time, and is not solely dependent on afferent activity. In addition to the diagnostic implications noted above, short-acting local anesthetic blocks often fail to predict beneficial responses to neurodestructive procedures. Nerve regrowth may lead to pain recurrence, but several other factors also cause failure of peripheral neuroablation despite profound relief from local anesthetic blocks. The nerve injury itself, whether caused by surgical transection, neurolytic block with phenol or alcohol, thermocoagulation, or cryotherapy, may induce spontaneous discharge or increased mechanosensitivity at the site of injury.[26,62,78,323] Successful denervation, even in the absence of increased peripheral inputs, may lead to changes in dorsal horn cell function, with sensitization of WDR neurons and expansion of receptive fields.

LOCAL ANESTHETIC PHYSIOLOGY

Intensity of Blockade (Table 27-4)

Diagnostic and prognostic blocks are accomplished by the action of local anesthetics (and occasionally by neuraxial opioids[64]) upon nerves. It has long been recognized that neural blockade is not an all-or-none response. For instance, analgesia usually is evident earlier and to a greater extent than loss of perception of mechanical stimuli after peripheral neural blockade. This should be recalled when diagnostic sympathetic blocks are performed; the lack of anesthesia to touch in the involved area does not assure that pain relief is accomplished by sympathetic interruption, because a subtle somatic block could produce analgesia without anesthesia, resulting in pain relief independent of a sympathetic mechanism.[73] In the opposite sense, apparent intense blockade with complete insensitivity to touch and pain is nonetheless not a complete afferent blockade; studies of different types of blocks with various agents uniformly demonstrate incomplete elimination of somatosensory potentials evoked by stimulation of the anesthetized region.[214] This may be the mechanism behind tourniquet pain and the humoral response to upper abdominal anesthesia, both of which occur despite apparently adequate blocks. If pain continues after a diagnostic block, one cannot be certain that the injected pathway is not involved, since neural blockade is not absolute.

TABLE 27-4. *Diagnostic blocks—limitations from complexity of local anesthetic effect*

- Blocks rarely complete (afferent sensory, efferent-sympathetic)
- Subtle block without obvious sensory change
- Differential block unpredictable (fiber type, length of exposure)
- Use dependent block (nerve activity influences anesthetic effect)

The variable and partial nature of local anesthetic effects is evident also in blockade of efferent sympathetic activity. Skin conduction responses, a manifestation of sympathetic action at sweat glands, often is present in areas of apparently complete somatic blockade,[221] and skin warming has been noted in the center of a truncal band of segmental epidural anesthesia.[164] During total thoracolumbar epidural anesthesia, norepinephrine levels decrease by only about 60%[318] or not at all,[319] indicating persistent sympathetic synaptic release. These considerations weaken the predictive value of sympathetic blocks, unless monitoring confirms the loss of sympathetic activity concurrent with the onset of relief.

Differential Block (Table 27-4)

The variable effects of local anesthetics upon fibers performing different functions is termed differential block. Were it possible to predict and control the neural modalities that are blocked, diagnostic distinctions could be discerned by selectively interrupting sympathetic or somatic fibers. This goal has proved elusive. The physiologic mechanisms that result in differential effects of local anesthetics are complex and multiple[278] (see also Chapter 2). Most commonly cited is the importance of fiber size. Since fibers of different cross-sectional areas serve different functions (large $A\alpha \rightarrow$ motor, $A\beta$ touch/proprioception; small $A\delta \rightarrow$ cold/hot/pain, $B \rightarrow$ preganglionic sympathetic, $C \rightarrow$ postganglionic sympathetic, pain, temperature), dependence of anesthetic action upon size would explain clinically observed graded blockade of sensory and motor functions by local anesthetics. Erlanger and Gasser formulated this concept in 1929, but despite the appealing simplicity of the model, it has not withstood the test of time. They studied the effects of cocaine upon amphibian nerves, but only examined large myelinated A fibers at room temperature, and not under equilibrium conditions. Further study[110,111] has shown that, contrary to the size principle, the concentrations (C_M) necessary for blockade of A and B fibers are less than those for C fibers. In general, the intrinsic sensitivity of nerve fibers to local anesthetics is probably A<B<C. Problematic for the use of local anesthetics in diagnosis, however, is the great variability of sizes within a fiber type, and the lack of correlation of size and C_M within the group.[110,279] The overlap of C_M between different groups "appears to negate any possibility of obtaining steady state differential interruption" by local anesthetics.[110]

The size principle fails to explain clinically evident (nonsteady state) differential effects, but different diffusion barriers of the various fiber types probably does. The lipid barrier of myelinated A fibers is a greater impediment to ability of local anesthetics to reach the axonal membrane binding site than it is for C fibers, which lack the insulating myelin.[353] Despite the inherent greater resistance of C fibers to blockade, they are exposed to higher local anesthetic concentration early in the onset of the block, because of more rapid diffusion, so the sequence of blockade is usually B first (due to intrinsic sensitivity), then C and Aδ before Aα and Aβ. Using intraneural recording to study conduction in radial nerves of human subjects after injection of 0.25% lidocaine,[326] preferential blockade of C fibers is evident. Full differential block is not possible, however, since completely abolished C fiber activity is accompanied by partial A fiber block. Sensory loss progresses in the order of sensibility for warmth, dull ache, cold, prick and finally touch.[218] The combination of high lipid solubility and low pKa (high non-ionized fraction) for etidocaine accounts for its thorough penetration into well protected Aα (motor) fibers, and therefore minimal differential block, compared to bupivacaine, which has a weak motor block (see Chapter 2).

Even with concentrations of local anesthetic high enough to eliminate sodium conductance completely, an action potential can still "jump" two adjacent totally blocked nodes (about 4 mm for the largest fibers) and excite the nerve beyond the blocked segment. To prevent conduction, at least three nodes in succession must be blocked.[117] If local anesthetic is limited in longitudinal extent, large fibers with long internodal distances may lack exposure to three nodes, while smaller fibers have the necessary three nodes exposed and are blocked (Fig. 27-3). At concentrations that produce less intense sodium channel blockade, the influence of exposure length extends even further, so that a concentration of local anesthetic that blocks conduction in 3 cm of exposed nerve may not block conduction when only 2 cm is exposed.[280] With low concentrations of local anesthetic, not all sodium

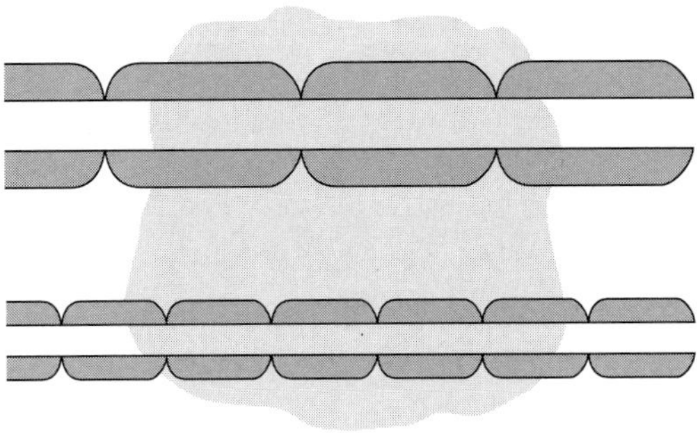

FIG. 27-3. Effect of exposure length in producing differential block. A large axon with long internodal lengths may continue to conduct despite exposure to local anesthetic at concentrations adequate to block the nodes completely if only 2 nodes are exposed to local anesthetic. A smaller axon with closer nodes will have more nodes blocked and not be able to conduct. (Reproduced from DeJong, R.H.: Local Anesthetics. pp. 89. St. Louis, Mosby–Yearbook, 1994.)

channels are inactivated, so a diminished but present action potential results (i.e., the action potential is not "all-or-none"). Less current reaches the adjacent node, causing it to fire but with an even smaller action potential. During this so-called decremental conduction, the action potential may propagate for many nodes before it finally fails to depolarize the next node. The result is that (i) conduction may fail through a segment of exposed nerve even if none of the nodes have been made completely inexcitable (Fig. 27-4), and (ii) C_M is inversely related to exposed nerve length. These phenomena may explain differential blockade that develops with spinal and epidural anesthesia,[112] but also dictate that anesthetic potency and the degree of differential effects varies with the length of nerve exposed, an added variable which is hard to control (see also Chapter 2).

Further subtle influences upon local anesthetic action may cloud the interpretation of diagnostic blocks. Sodium channel closure by local anesthetics depends on nerve use; tonic block in an infrequently firing axon is less intense than the phasic block that develops progressively with higher firing rates. Local anesthetic will affect those fibers more completely that are most active. The ongoing activity of B vasomotor fibers may contribute to their preferential blockade, especially since these fibers show the greatest degree of phasic block. Phasic amplification of blockade may play a minor role for C (pain) fibers because their firing rates are too low. The spectrum of anesthetic effects will depend, therefore, upon the pattern of activity of the subject's various neuron types when the diagnostic block is undertaken, and also will depend upon the choice of anesthetic. Bupivacaine, the agent with the greatest degree of phasic block, also shows a high degree of differential blockade. Since the earliest perturbation of nerve function at very low anesthetic concentrations is the prolongation of the latent interval for refiring,[279] information encoded with bursts will be transformed into a more continuous signal. By this means, sensations can be

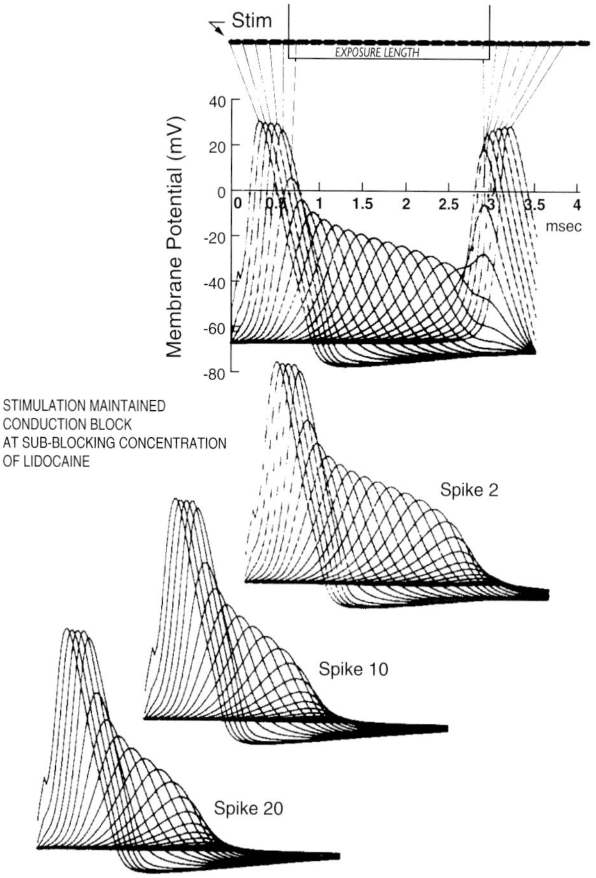

FIG. 27-4. Modeling of conduction in an axon exposed to local anesthetic concentration below the threshold for complete block at a node. Reduced current from a partially blocked axon provides a diminished stimulus to the next node, so amplitude declines along the 15 node exposed segment. Intensified block for subsequent impulses causes the signal to perish before it can reach the unexposed node. There is signal interruption despite the lack of complete blockade of any node. Response will be highly sensitive to slight changes in signal frequency, exposure length, or anesthetic concentration. (Reproduced with permission from Raymond, S.A., and Strichartz, G.R.: The long and short of differential block. Anesthesiology, *70*:725, 1989.)

made to change without any actual termination of transmission (see Chapter 2).

To summarize, it is apparent now that local anesthetic effects are more subtle, complex, and variable than has been realized in the past. This does not invalidate their use for diagnostic exercises, but should inspire caution in the interpretation of blocks.

Systemic Effects (Table 27-5)

When assessing the effect of local anesthetic blocks on pain perception, it is important to consider the systemic effect of the anesthetic as it is absorbed from the site of injection. There is considerable data available on the systemic effect of local anesthetics on neuropathic pain, but relatively little on other types.

TABLE 27-5. *Diagnostic blocks—limitations from local anesthetic systemic effects*

- Suppression of spontaneous neuroma activity
- Depression of spinal nociceptive transmission
- Block of central sensitization (high circulating concentrations)
- Occasional prolonged responses

At local anesthetic blood levels (e.g., 1 to 5 μg/ml lidocaine) insufficient to produce side effects in humans (dizziness, tinnitus, tremor, or paresthesias), there is little or no appreciable effect on impulse conduction in normal peripheral nerves[62,78,323,356] or on cutaneous C fiber terminal function.[356] Local anesthetics also have little or no analgesic effect in animal models of acute nociception.[356] Therefore, possible techniques are likely to include effects of the drug on impulse generation in injured nerves, or on processing of sensory information in the central nervous system.

There is considerable evidence that systemically administered local anesthetics affect spontaneous impulse generation arising from injured nerves. Intravenous lidocaine in subconvulsant doses produces suppression of spontaneously active nerve fibers originating from sciatic neuromas in rats.[62] In addition, lidocaine decreases the sensitivity of these neurons to mechanical stimulation. Tanelian and MacIver[323] evaluated the effect of lidocaine on injury-induced discharge of corneal C and Aδ fibers. At concentrations ranging from 1 to 20 μg/ml, they demonstrated suppression of tonic action potential discharge, but did not block electrically evoked nerve conduction at concentrations below 250 μg/ml. Spontaneous activity arising from neuromas in rats is suppressed with low doses of intravascular lidocaine, and impulse generation in the dorsal root ganglia is suppressed at even lower doses.[78] Electrically evoked peripheral nerve activity remains completely intact at these doses.

Non-toxic doses of systemic local anesthetics also have depressant effects on spinal transmission of nociceptive inputs. Lidocaine significantly suppresses the spinal polysynaptic reflex evoked by stimulation of sural nerve C fibers.[356] An increase in nociceptive flexion reflex thresholds in diabetic patients, and in healthy human subjects, is observed following intravenous infusion of 5 mg/kg lidocaine.[13]

In an effort to determine the relative potency of local anesthetics on spinal versus peripheral mechanisms, Abram and Yaksh[4] assessed the effects of intravenous lidocaine on hyperalgesia induced by sciatic nerve ligation and on hyperalgesia following tissue injury in rats. Intravenous lidocaine at a blood level of 1 μg/ml reversed the thermal hyperalgesia induced by nerve injury (Fig. 27-5). However, spinal sensitization following tissue injury (subcutaneous formalin) was prevented only when lidocaine blood levels exceeded 6 μg/ml. This indicates that the principal effect of systemic local anesthetics on neuropathic pain is peripheral.

There have been several clinical reports of the efficacy of intravenous lidocaine in patients with neuropathic

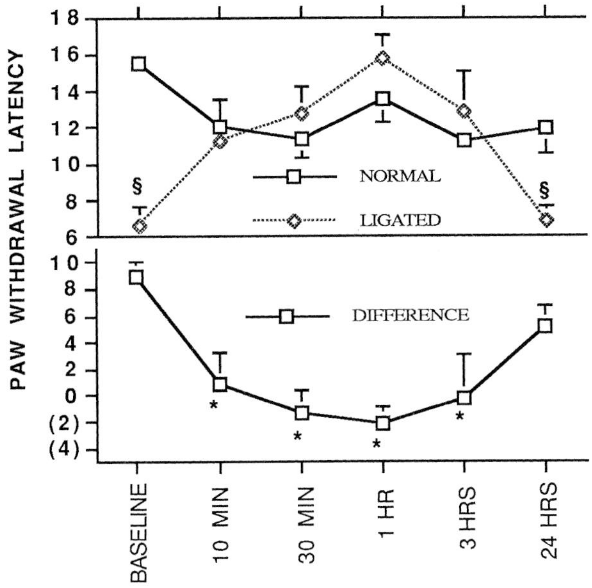

FIG. 27-5. Effect of systemic lidocaine on hyperalgesia after sciatic nerve ligation in rats. The accelerated paw withdrawal (in seconds) on the side of nerve injury compared to the uninjured normal side, is made normal by lidocaine at a blood level of 1 μg/ml.[53]

pain.[13,28,97,181,223,323] While some cite very transient effects,[223,323] others indicate analgesic effects lasting several days or more.[97,181] Doses of local anesthetic required to relieve neuropathic pain are generally 1 to 3 mg/kg. It would be unlikely, therefore, that a selective nerve root block with 3 ml 1% lidocaine would produce pain relief by a systemic effect. On the other hand, a lumbar sympathetic block, using 15 ml 1% lidocaine, might be capable of relieving neuropathic pain at a location distant from the site of injection.

PSYCHOSOCIAL INFLUENCES

Even though the practitioner uses diagnostic blocks to obtain specific, convincing, "hard" data, he or she must still be aware that the procedure is also a social interaction (Table 27-6). While the patient may not seek to deceive the doctor, it is impossible to dissociate the experience of pain from surrounding social and psychological factors. Important aspects to consider include: (i) Communication may be incomplete. Answers are reliable only if the physician is able to enter into the same frame of reference as the patient and to use descriptive terms in the same way.[313] (ii) The clinic is not the patient's home,[265] and unfamiliarity, stress, and anxiety may create an environment dissimilar to that in which the pain usually exists. (iii) The patient and physician may not have the same agenda. Whereas the doctor may seek pathophysiologic information, the patient may be looking for reassurance, confirmation of suspicions or proof to persuade doubting family members, certification of disability for legal and financial reasons, or simply have a wish to please the doctor. Any of these purposes may enter into the patient's reporting.

TABLE 27-6. *Diagnostic blocks—limitations from psychological issues*

- Communication problems
- Evaluation in an unfamiliar environment
- Divergent patient/physician agendas

To diminish the ambiguities created by these psychosocial factors, a physician might choose to inject a placebo (Latin for I please), an inert substance with no known pharmacodynamic effect. Although desirable in many situations, the use of a placebo is an incomplete means of clarification. Problems include ethical considerations[66] of performing an invasive procedure to inject an inactive substance, and the difficulty of obtaining permission while not revealing that the injected substance is a placebo. This may be circumvented by comparing the duration of response to two local anesthetics with different pharmacokinetics (e.g., lidocaine vs. bupivacaine);[15] comparative durations of relief not in keeping with expected durations of local anesthetic effect could be interpreted as a placebo response, but this unproven method requires more subtle distinctions than the clear case of a response to saline injection.

A more limiting uncertainty is what to make of a patient who responds favorably to a placebo (Table 27-7). Patients obtain relief from placebos administered during acute pain about 1/3 of the time,[18] and may be up to twice as likely to obtain relief of chronic pain with a placebo. For example, 82% of patients in a study of chronic arthritis reported definite improvement in pain and function after weekly subcutaneous normal saline.[305] In another study, 59% had relief from a placebo tablet, while 57% of those who didn't respond to a pill had relief from a subsequent placebo injection.[329] In patients with causalgia, 3 ml of subcutaneous normal saline relieved spontaneous pain in 68% of patients, and also relieved mechanically induced pain (allodynia) in 56% and Tinel's sign in 67%.[334] Probability of analgesia from a placebo is proportionate to the intensity of pain.[203] No personality features predict a placebo response.[206] Individuals are not consistent in being responders or nonresponders, and most eventually will respond to a placebo if administered repeatedly.[167] Thus, it is hard to conclude much from identifying a placebo response. Certainly, this is not a way to determine whether the pain is real.

Psychologic theory explaining placebo response focuses on the subject's expectations[195] and on conditioning.[339] In the context of diagnostic blocks, the expectation of a favorable response may make analgesia more likely. By condi-

TABLE 27-7. *Diagnostic blocks—limitations from placebo response*

- Always possible
- Unpredictable
- Frequent in chronic pain
- Potent with injection
- Based on conditioning, endorphins
- Operator-dependent

tioning, a patient's response to an injection is based upon what they experienced after previous similar events. It has been shown that most subjects can be trained to have a placebo response,[340] and that a placebo response is more likely if the test with the active agent precedes the placebo administration.[179] Other implications are that a patient's previous analgesic experiences will condition the potency of a placebo,[202] and that withdrawal of even a pharmacologically inactive therapy may lead to an increase in chronic pain.[339] On a physiologic level, the placebo response is a demonstration of descending modulation of nociception. Evidence of an opioid mechanism includes the antagonism of placebo analgesia with naloxone,[134,204] and the documentation of increased cerebrospinal fluid (CSF) endogenous opioid activity after a placebo response, but this is not so if there was no response.[209] In view of this, placebos can be considered active agents in their own right (see also Chapter 25).

When local anesthetic is injected for diagnostic nerve blockade, it is very difficult to be certain that relief has not occurred by a placebo mechanism rather than by neural interruption. In general terms, placebo responses are incomplete, inconsistently repeatable, and may lack the appropriate time course for the onset or duration of the active agent. These generalizations are impossible to apply in any particular clinical case. Placebo action may be as intense as the active agent, usually will mimic the active agent in dose/response and time/effect relationships,[102] and may develop over as prolonged an interval as 60 minutes (Fig. 27-6).[109,335] Injections, like surgery, are especially potent placebos.[102]

An important component of the placebo event is the practitioner. It has been demonstrated repeatedly[102,131] that even in carefully blinded protocols, unintended communication from the examiner takes place. When placebo is compared to morphine, the placebo responders have analgesia comparable to that induced by morphine, whereas if aspirin is being tested, the placebo response resembles aspirin. Patients told they might receive either a narcotic analgesic or narcotic antagonist for acute pain only developed placebo analgesia (to saline) if they were in a group that the physician knew would receive fentanyl vs. saline, and not if they were in a group which the physician knew would get only naloxone vs. saline. This held true even if the physician knew only which group the patient was in and not whether saline or drug was given (Fig. 27-7). The history of new therapies demonstrates the same phenomenon: Initial reports by enthusiasts are commonly contradicted by subsequent blinded and critical trials.[22,82] It is inescapable that the physician's convictions play a large role in generating placebo responses.

The potency and frequency of the placebo effect is underestimated by the majority of physicians and nurses.[130] Far from being a minor inconvenience, this effect is a central concern in the performance of diagnostic blocks. In a sense, each diagnostic block resembles a clinical study of a drug or procedure, but with a study group of only a single subject; convincing results are elusive without repeated testing with a blinded subject and physician. What can be done to lessen the confusion introduced by placebo responses? Ironically, when an elaborate protocol is used to control for physician and patient bias, and adequate time is allowed for the full development of placebo response, all subjects have placebo analgesia.[109] Our recommendations are to (i) inform the patient that a placebo injection may be used at some point during diagnostic testing; (ii) use more than one trial of a diag-

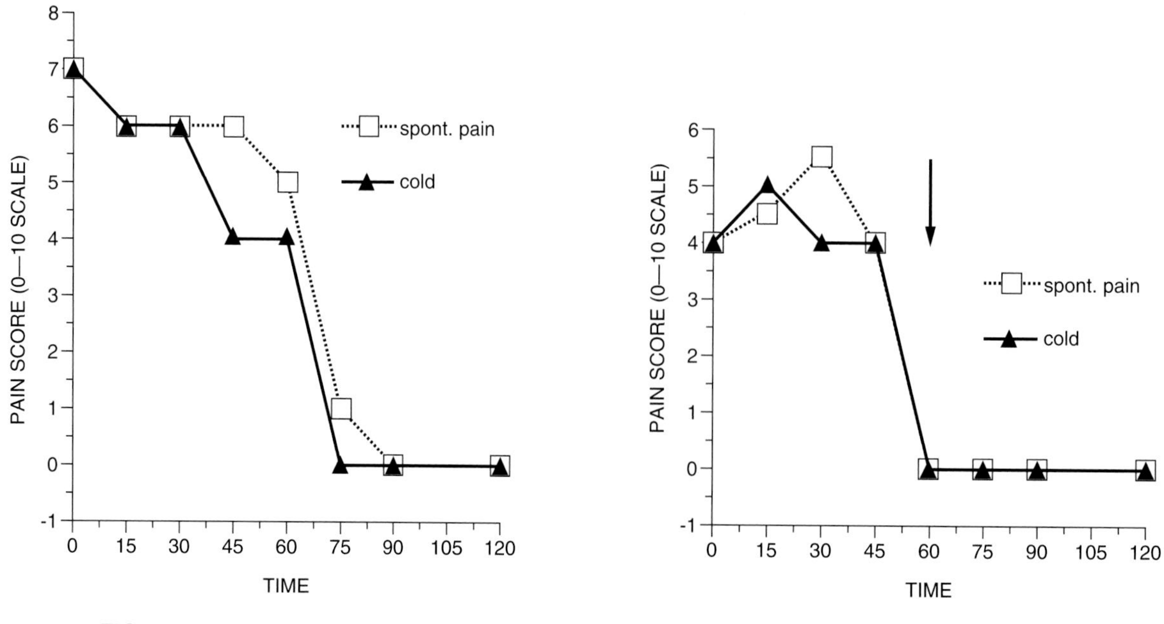

FIG. 27-6. The time course for development of placebo response in a patient with chronic low back pain. Saline is administered at each 15-minute mark and phentolamine is administered IV at the arrow in the right frame, in a carefully constructed double-blind protocol. Placebo analgesia evolves over one hour to both spontaneous and cold-induced pain (*left frame*).[78]

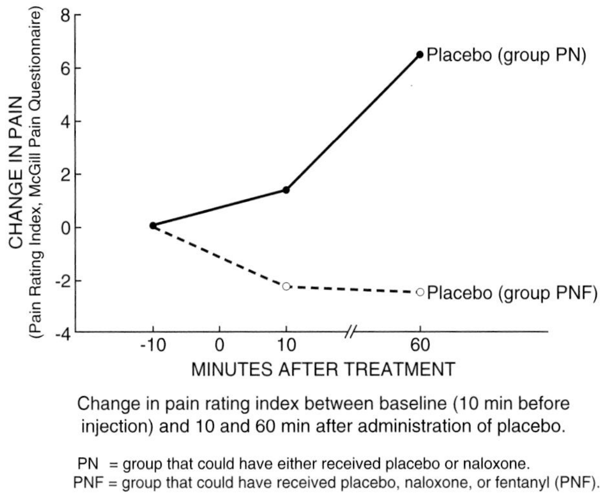

FIG. 27-7. The effect of physician awareness on placebo response. There is no analgesia when placebo is administered to the group PN that the physician knew would receive no opioid, only placebo (saline) or narcan, in a blinded fashion. However, placebo analgesia (downward trend in pain scores) is evident in the group PNF that the physician knew might be given fentanyl as one of the blinded choices.[80]

nostic block; (iii) include a saline injection at least once during a series of blocks, preferably through the same needle that will then be used for the local anesthetic, allowing time between injections for questioning as to relief; (iv) if possible, blind the operator performing the block as to the agent injected; (v) recognize relief from a placebo as a normal and expected event; (vi) consider a response to local anesthetic more persuasive if it differs in quality, intensity, or timing from the saline injection, or if there was no placebo response; and (vii) bear in mind that relief from local anesthetic injection may still be by a placebo mechanism. A final concern is the negative placebo: 28%[288] to 34%[83] of subjects given inactive agents will have side effects such as headache, drowsiness, asthenia, dizziness, nausea, and vomiting.

ANATOMICAL CONSIDERATIONS

The use of blocks for diagnosis and prognosis depends on an assumption of anatomic consistency: we expect nerve structures to be found in predictable places and to have predictable connections. There are important limitations to these expectations. Like any biologic feature, most anatomic parameters show variability about a norm. For example, Tuffier's line between the ilaic crests crosses the vertebral column most often at the L4/L5 disc (perhaps higher on average in men than in women)[98] but the range is from as low as the L5/S1 disc to as high as the L3/L4 disc.[98,217,271] A normal distribution also describes the level of termination of the spinal cord[284] and the termination of the dural sac (Fig. 27-8).[201] This indicates that surface and palpation landmarks are unreliable indicators of deep structures, which is borne out by a 50% accuracy in guessing vertebral level of needle placement without x-ray imaging.[107,123,240,312,331]

Anatomic variability is not limited to relative dimensions and positions of structures, but also includes the number and connections of anatomic items, and idealized textbook descriptions hold in only about 50 to 70% of actual subjects.[25] For instance, even though patterns of vertebral segmentation are stable in the cervical and thoracic levels, lumbar and sacral regions show a marked variety of segmentation. The last lumbar or first sacral vertebra may be indeterminate in configuration, with fusion of L5 to S1 in 6.2% (sacralization of L5), or incomplete fusion of S1 to S2 in 5.3% (lumbarization of S1), and one or more sacral segments may be absent.[354] The distribution of nerve roots to the intervertebral foramina is anomolous in about 8% of subjects[191,249] and in-

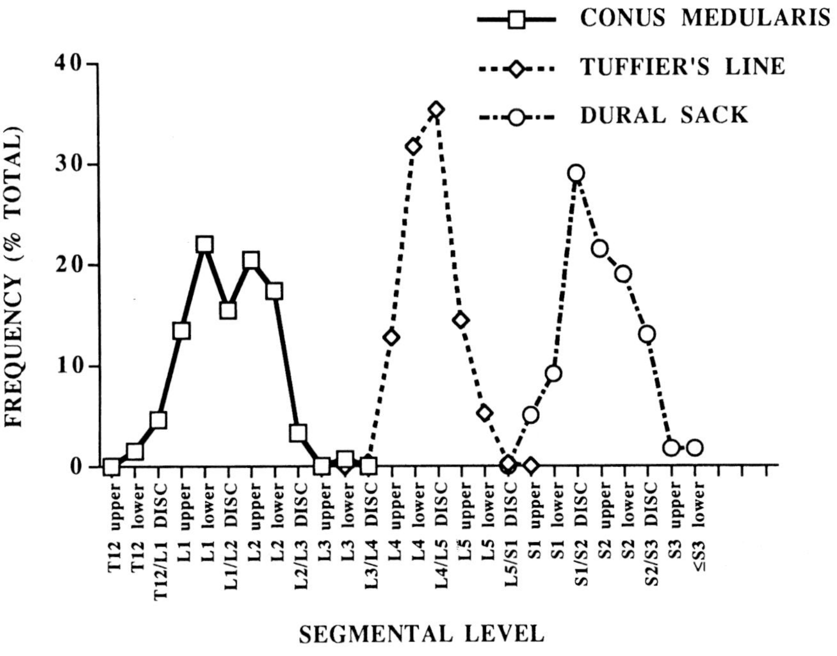

FIG. 27-8. Bony vertebral levels for conus medullaris, Tuffier's line, and dural sac. Anatomic features such as the termination of the spinal cord and dural sac and the point at which the line between the iliac crests (Tuffier's line) crosses the vertebral column are not exact. A normal distribution describes most anatomic measures.

cludes two root pairs exiting at one level with an adjacent empty foramen.[245] These variations occur because the dorsal root ganglia develop from a continuous sheet of neural crest tissue, and separation into segments is imprecise. The clinical consequence of aberrant arrangements is the development of anesthesia in an unexpected distribution following foraminal injection, with resulting diagnostic ambiguity.[249]

Separation of somatic input into a discernible segmental pattern is a fundamental concept underlying many diagnostic blocks. No segmentation is evident upon the surface of the spinal cord or by histologic examination of its substance. It is only by the grouping of rootlets into rootlet bundles bound for a common dorsal root ganglion and intervertebral foramen that a pattern of segments is superimposed upon the otherwise seamless connections of the peripheral system with the central nervous system (CNS). There is, however, variability in the formation of segmental spinal nerves and their peripheral distribution. Multiple interconnections of adjacent rootlets and roots are found within the dural sac in all subjects, with between three and nine such intersegmental anastomoses at the upper cervical region and a similar number at the lumbosacral level.[260,261] The pattern of spinal nerve contributions to the limb is highly inconsistent. For example, 28% of lumbosacral plexuses have central connections shifted proximally ("prefixed") or distally ("postfixed") along the vertebral column compared to the usual pattern.[166] Seven major configurations of the brachial plexus are possible with none having more than 57% representation, and 61% of individuals differing in type between right and left.[185] The resulting distribution of fibers to the skin has been mapped, using zoster eruptions, residual sensation after sectioning the roots on either side of an intact segment, absent sensation after root section or anesthesia, vasodilatation during stimulation of roots, or pain with nerve root compression and visceral disease.[40] The dermatome diagrams these methods produce show considerable disagreement, especially in the extremities. Also, extensive overlap between consecutive peripheral dermatomes is evident, because the division of an individual root rarely produces an appreciable loss of sensibility. As a consequence, the sensory innervation of a particular site cannot be assigned with certainty to any segmental level, and sensory changes after local anesthetic injections about the vertebral column are variable. There is also segmental inconsistency in the motor innervation of the extremities. Marked departure from the usual distribution of L5 and S1 motor fibers is found in 16% of subjects,[364] in whom stimulation of a root produces movement typical of the other root.

Important differences in the peripheral distribution of sympathetic motor fibers are relevant to diagnostic blocks. Preganglionic axons originate only from the T1 through L2 segments. Fibers bound for tissues with cervical or low lumbar and sacral somatic innervation are deployed by the paravertebral chains. Therefore, segmental neuraxial local anesthetic application will block sympathetic innervation to different tissues than are somatically denervated. For instance, a low spinal anesthetic may produce intense sensory block to the feet, ankles, calves, and buttocks (low lumbar and sacral segments) without any sympathetic changes in these areas (derived from L1 and L2). Sympathetic outflow is only weakly segmental, due to the crossing of rami communicates[333] and extensive divergence of sympathetic activity in the ganglia. Efferent sympathetic fibers supplying a cutaneous region do not necessarily arrive by the same peripheral nerve as the sensory afferents supplying that area. For instance,[54] the radial aspect of the dorsum of the hand receives sensory and sudomotor innervation via the radial nerve, but vasomotor innervation from the median nerve. Similarly, the lateral aspect of the foot may receive its sympathetic input from peroneal branches, while transmitting sensory information in the sural nerve.[154] The extent of sympathetic blockade after regional anesthetic is poorly understood and difficult to predict.

Anatomic variability is also evident in the distribution of injected solutions. Spread is guided by the vagaries of tissue pressures and adherence, and may be entirely unidirectional, rather than expanding concentrically from the injection site. The vertebral canal is a common pathway for aberrant injectate flow after injections near the vertebral column. As pressure of the solution rises at the injection site, spread to the canal may occur, because pressure in the canal does not rise above CSF pressure (about 15 cm H_2O), since inflow displaces CSF. Epidural anesthetic effect may be an undesired component of various diagnostic blocks (facet, lumbar sympathetic, stellate, nerve root, and plexus blocks; see following).

Less is known about the patterns of visceral sensory connections. Visceral receptive fields are large and overlapping, and extensive convergence of afferent traffic is evident at many CNS levels.[246] Most visceral pain travels in sympathetic nerves, but afferents from the thoracic organs, the pancreas, and biliary tree ascend in the phrenic nerve and pass to the thoracic cord via medial branches of the sympathetic chain. From the sigmoid colon, rectum, neck of the bladder, prostate, and cervix of the uterus, most visceral afferent fibers retrace the route of parasympathetic efferent neurons, entering the cord in the posterior roots of S2–S4. A few fibers from these organs ascend in the prevertebral plexuses to enter at L1–L2. Pain that is not relieved by blocks of sympathetic pathways may still be visceral in origin but transmitted by these nonsympathetic routes (see Chapter 23.1, Figs. 23.1-20 to 23.1-22).

The role and even presence of nociceptive fibers from the limbs that travel in sympathetic structures has been debated.[176,177] Lumbar sympathetic block prevents the poorly localized dull ache during surgical manipulation of the femoral vein or from lower extremity thrombophlebitis.[76,255] Surgical sympathectomy blocks responses to venous distension in canine lower extremities [118] and almost eliminates the aching and stinging pain from cold exposure of human extremities.[172] Sympathetic block also interrupts pain from mechanical stimulation of the femoral medullary cavity.[188] These observations indicate that afferent sensory impulses travel from vascular structures in the extremities via sympathetic pathways which, when blocked by diagnostic sympathetic blockade, could be interpreted falsely as an indication of an efferent sympathetic pathogenesis of pain. One recent analysis attributes most "sympathetic dependent" pain to visceral afferent activity[297] (see also Chapter 13 and Chapter 23.1, Fig. 23.1-8).

Deep somatic pain from bones, joints, muscles, and fascia shares many features of visceral pain including poor somatotopic localization, referred pain, and a generalized increase in CNS excitability with motor and autonomic reflexes.[176] Additionally, the fibers from many deep somatic elements (costovertebral joint, posterior and anterior longitudinal ligaments, anular ligament of the intervertebral disc, dura) traverse the sympathetic rami and chain.[30,135,136,197] It is likely that some pains relieved by sympathetic blocks are unrelated to sympathetic efferent activity (sympathetically maintained pain) and instead are deep somatic pains transmitted by sympathetic pathways.[297]

METHODOLOGY

Diagnostic blocks should be performed in a manner that yields the most certain information possible, in order not to add to the inherent ambiguity of clinical pain. In many cases, needle position should by confirmed by radiologic imaging. Determination of the segmental level is unreliable without confirmation by x-ray (see previously), and studies of a variety of injection procedures have shown inadequate consistency of needle placement without imaging.[107,175,285,349] Since small volumes of local anesthetic need to be used to minimize spread to undesired nerves, meticulous needle placement is required to assure adequate blockade of the desired nerve. Injection of a small amount of radio-opaque contrast, prior to the anesthetic, can identify passage into an unwanted space (vascular, subarachnoid) or in an ineffective direction. The usefulness of guiding needle insertion by the nature of provoked pain is limited by the lack of specificity of deep sensations.[229,238]

Pain before and after blockade should be evaluated by asking the patient to rate the intensity, between 0 (none) and 10 (worst imaginable), to facilitate communication and documentation. Provocative measures, such as palpation of a tender area or joint movement, may help patient and clinician discern changes in incident pain, when compared before and after the block. For instance, in a patient who has pain only when ambulating, an implanted pump for intrathecal opioid treatment is not indicated in a prognostic trial, after which the patient is kept in bed. Not only may a patient with spontaneous pain respond differently than if he or she has induced pain, but blocks used may act differently upon pain induced by repetitive dynamic mechanical stimulation (dynamic mechanical allodynia) versus steady pressure (static mechanical allodynia).[256] Careful examination is required to discern these subtle block effects. If the patient is not having the usual pain at the time of a diagnostic block, little can be learned about the pain mechanism. When pain is relieved by neural blockade, the duration of analgesia should be determined. Relief lasting only the expected duration of the anesthetic effect suggests an ongoing peripheral focus of nociception. If relief obviously outlasts the anesthetic, a central potentiating process may be involved.

Pain relief, however, cannot be the only measured parameter. Independent confirmation of neural blockade is necessary, because performing the procedure correctly and with care does not guarantee that the intended nerve will be anesthetized and the desired physiologic change achieved. Detailed sensory and motor testing before and after injection can identify somatic nerve block effects. Meticulous care may be necessary to delineate sensory changes. For instance, vibration transmitted through the skin and soft tissue may stimulate receptors at a considerable distance, creating the misimpression that an area is incompletely insensate.[170] Tactile threshold changes can be identified by testing with fibers of different stiffness (von Frey hairs), and fast pain (Aδ) sensation examined by the scratch from the folded corner of a foil alcohol pad wrapper.

More elaborate methods are necessary for an adequate test of C fiber (slow pain) sensation. Stimuli should be performed as consistently as possible since a stimulus that is more intense, more frequently repeated, or more broadly distributed, may be perceived, while weaker stimuli are blocked.[310] Inconsistent stimulation may cause confusion. For instance, a subtle somatic block may be missed during diagnostic sympathetic block, if application of stimuli is more vigorous after the block than during baseline examination.

Many measures have been used to judge the efficacy of sympathetic blockade, although none has become an accepted standard. Horner's syndrome documents only blockade of sympathetic fibers to the head. Skin resistance response (sympathogalvanic response)[19,208] and pulse amplitude changes[192,235] are difficult to quantify. Microneurography[208] is invasive and requires elaborate equipment and expertise, as does laser skin blood flow measurement.[20] Sweat testing[23] is cumbersome, time-consuming, and not well accepted by patients, and therefore not widely used. Most common is the measurement of skin temperature by thermography or contact thermometry. A temperature increase of 1.0 to 3.0°C is typically used[57,145,156] as a threshold for confirming the onset of sympathetic blockade, but the method is ineffective if skin is warm at the outset of a block. Although local anesthetic blockade of sympathetic activity to the extremities produces vasodilatation, vasoconstriction follows segmental block of sympathetic fibers to the trunk,[164] possibly by blockade of sympathetic vasodilator fibers.[182] Skin temperature in pathologic conditions is controlled by a balance between sympathetic vasoconstriction and vasodilatation from release of vasoactive peptides from C nociceptor during antidromic activity.[257] Temperature change in the field of a blocked peripheral nerve will depend on the relative contribution of these opposing systems.

Pain caused by the procedure may result in a confused diagnosis, because relief following the injection may be the relief of the iatrogenic pain and not of the pre-existing pain for which the block was done. Also, intense pain from the procedure may diminish the perceived severity of the original pain (noxious counter-irritation),[306] creating the illusion that neural blockade effects relieved the pain. Judicious use of local anesthetics in the superficial tissues, small needles, and careful needle guidance limit the pain of the procedure.

SPECIFIC PROCEDURES

In the format adopted below, commonly used diagnostic blocks will be considered individually, first with regard to the rationale behind the procedure, including indications for the block. The discussion of technique that follows also addresses methods to monitor response to the block and to possible complications. (Technique of blocks discussed elsewhere in this book are covered briefly.) Limitations are reviewed, focusing on sources of error in interpreting results from the injections. If studies of the diagnostic utility of the procedure are available, these are reviewed with emphasis on documentation of success and measures of the diagnostic value. Finally, an evaluation of the utility of the block is offered.

Clinical studies of the blocks are of variable quality. Important considerations include entrance criteria (type of patients or normal subjects studied), study size, and the use of controls. The prevalence of placebo responses in pain patients greatly weakens the relevance of studies in which no controls or blinding was used. Where possible, neural blockade tests are evaluated numerically, using standard definitions (see table in next column).[234] The importance of false positive rate (how often patients without a condition will nonetheless have a positive test) and false negative rate (how often a patient with disease will have a negative test for it) is evident, because the rates vary inversely with specificity and sensitivity respectively. (Sensitivity = 1 − false negative rate; specificity = 1 − false positive rate.) For many painful conditions, however, a credible standard to document the disease for comparison with test results is unavailable, such as when sympathetic involvement is suspected or with cervicogenic headache. At worst, the block under scrutiny may be the defining gold standard. For these blocks, numerical values for diagnostic efficacy are elusive. Many studies, for obvious ethical reasons, obtain operative confirmation of disease only in patients with positive results from the diagnostic block. A false negative rate is unknown, and the false positive rate, which requires knowledge of true disease incidence in the entire group, also cannot be calculated. From these studies, only the positive predictive value (frequency of confirming disease in those with a positive test) can be derived.

	Disease Present	Disease Absent
Test Positive	a	c
Test Negative	b	d
Sensitivity (true positive rate)	$a/(a + b)$	
False Positive Rate	$c/(c + d)$	
Specificity (true negative rate)	$d/(c + d)$	
False Negative Rate	$b/(a + b)$	
Positive Predictive Value	$a/(a + c)$	
Negative Predictive Value	$d/(b + d)$	

The proper interpretation of a positive test must take into consideration the prevalence of the condition. For example, a test with a 95% sensitivity will have a positive result in 5% of healthy subjects. If the condition being sought is rare (if, for instance, it occurs in only 2% of the test group), false positive responses will outnumber true positive tests, and the majority of positive results will occur in subjects who actually are healthy. This issue is especially relevant to the study of painful conditions by diagnostic blocks, since the incidence of most of these maladies is low or unknown.

TISSUE INFILTRATION

Rationale

If nociceptive impulses are thought to arise from a particular site (for example, from a scar, painful structure in a specific muscle, inflamed joint, bursa, or tendon sheath), then the injection of local anesthetic into that site should be of help in establishing the diagnosis. Failure to relieve tenderness by infiltration of superficial tissues, like skin or muscle, focuses attention on a deeper site (bone, joint, nerve root). Painful scars generally are thought to be caused by the development of small neuromas. While some scars are diffusely tender, most scar pain is associated with very localized areas of tenderness. Some patients who experience relief from local anesthetic will have lasting relief if depot steroids are injected subsequently. When inflammatory processes are the cause of the pain, local anesthetic infiltration may be of prognostic benefit in predicting the response to subsequent steroid injections.

Technique

A skin wheal followed by injection of a small amount of saline in the vicinity of the planned procedure may indicate whether analgesia obtained from local anesthetic injection is due to placebo response. A small amount of local anesthetic is then injected into the affected muscle, joint, tendon sheath, scar, bursa, etc. It is helpful to determine whether needle placement and local anesthetic injection (as well as the placebo injection) reproduce the clinical pain, and whether local anesthetic injection relieves the pain at rest as well as the pain produced by maneuvers that usually aggravate the pain.

Local infiltration techniques are relatively benign in terms of potential for adverse effects. Infection is always a potential problem in immunocompromised patients and bleeding may be troublesome if coagulation function is impaired. Extensive infiltration of painful muscles conceivably could result in local anesthetic toxicity. In general, the occurrence of complications relates to proximity to other structures. Injection of the rhomboids or trapezius muscles could cause pneumothorax. Infiltration of muscles or scars near the neuraxis may allow spread of drug epidurally or intrathecally. Infiltration of occipital scars overlying bony cranial defects, following posterior fossa surgery, could mean that drug might be injected into the intracranial CSF, or even into the brain itself. Careful monitoring of blood pressure should be carried out when neuraxial or intracranial injections are possible.

TRIGGER-POINT INJECTION

Rationale

Myofascial pain syndrome is characterized by pain arising from affected muscles, pain associated with movement of those muscles, and reproduction of pain with palpation of well localized "trigger-points" in the affected muscle.[309] By definition, stimulation or palpation of trigger-points causes referred pain, perceived some distance from the site of palpation. Usually, the involved muscle is felt as a tight palpable band. Myofascial syndrome often is found in association with other painful disorders, such as facet arthropathy or radiculopathy, and it is often helpful to determine whether a patient's pain is predominantly myofascial, because appropriate treatment may be very different if such is the case. Other means of documenting myofascial pain, such as electromyelography (EMG), have not proved reliable.[147,169] Muscle tenderness also is seen in fibromyalgia, which differs from myofascial pain syndrome in that tender points in the muscle are much more diffuse and numerous, and usually symmetrical; palpation generally produces local, but not referred pain.[228] Trigger-point injections, particularly if repeated several times, may have therapeutic benefit for myofascial pain syndrome but not for fibromyalgia.[198]

Technique

The area of maximum tenderness is identified within the affected muscle. It may be helpful to immobilize the muscle between the thumb and forefinger. After antiseptic preparation of the skin, a small gauge needle is introduced into the trigger point. Often a brief twitch of the affected muscle is noted. The patient should be questioned about the location and intensity of the pain evoked by needle placement. Exacerbation of the pain and the presence of referred pain at this time helps confirm the diagnosis of myofascial pain syndrome. Following the injection of several ml of local anesthetic, the degree of pain relief and the presence or absence of tenderness is reassessed. Pressure algometry may be used to determine the degree of tenderness before and after injection.

A variety of local anesthetics have been used for trigger-point injection. From a diagnostic point of view, there is little reason to choose one over another. Some clinicians choose to avoid bupivacaine, because accidental blockade of nearby neural structures results in prolonged effects, toxic local anesthetic reactions are potentially more serious, and bupivacaine produces more muscle degeneration than do other anesthetics.[116] Ironically, the predictable and selective destruction of mature myocytes by local anesthetic infiltration[157] might be the therapeutic mechanism of long-term response to trigger-point injection, because it encourages the growth of a new generation of myocytes, in which case bupivacaine is a suitable agent. Reproduction of pain during injection and relief of pain after injection suggest that myofascial pain is at least partially responsible for the patient's pain.

Limitations

Pain relief after trigger-point injection does not guarantee that myofascial pain is the principle cause of pain. Placebo effect and systemic uptake of local anesthetic, particularly after multiple injections, may be the cause of the improvement, as may be spread to adjacent nerves. For instance, injection of the piriformis muscle is likely to have some effect on the sciatic nerve, which either penetrates or passes in contact with the muscle. Some doubt about the specificity of the technique is raised by reports showing comparable efficacy from less specific techniques, such as dry needling of trigger-points[205] and jet injection of local anesthetic into the skin overlying trigger-points.[282]

Evaluation

Reproduction of pain during injection followed by relief of pain is helpful in confirming the tissue site (scar, muscle, etc.) as the focus of nociceptive activity, if the duration of relief is at least as long as the expected duration of local anesthetic. Controlled studies have not confirmed this belief.

SOMATIC NERVE BLOCK

Rationale

A common reason to perform diagnostic peripheral nerve blocks is to determine the likelihood of success after surgical decompression or neurolysis of a peripheral nerve. Diagnostic blocks may be performed before a planned peripheral nerve section, neurolytic block, or cryoanalgesia lesion. Entrapment neuropathies include digital nerve entrapment (Morton's neuroma), carpal tunnel entrapment of the median nerve, and tarsal tunnel entrapment of the tibial nerve. Posttraumatic neuropathy of the ilioinguinal and iliohypogastric nerves can occur following herniorrhaphy.

Technique

Techniques for specific peripheral nerve blocks are covered in Chapters 10,11, and 14 to 17. When performing diagnostic blocks, it is important to use small volumes of anesthetic solution, to document that appropriate sensory blockade is achieved, and to ensure that the block is limited to the intended nerve distribution. In assessing relief of pain, one should determine the duration of the pain relief and the duration of sensory block. If pain returns long before the return of sensory function, the analgesia may be a placebo response. Use of bupivacaine for peripheral diagnostic blocks may be preferable to the use of shorter-acting agents, because it provides a long interval during which placebo responses may subside, and a prolonged period for patients to experience the effect of the block. In general, diagnostic blocks are performed with relatively small volumes of local anesthetic (usually 2 to 3 ml for small nerves, 5 ml for medium-sized nerves, e.g. median nerve at the wrist and 10 ml for large nerves) and the risk of toxic reactions is small. Intercostal blocks done near the spinal column may be associated with spread of drug to the subarachnoid space, if the needle is placed within the perineurium.

Limitations

It must be kept in mind that relief of pain following blockade of the appropriate nerve does not necessarily confirm the diagnosis of neuropathy at that site. There may be a nociceptive source of pain within the distribution of the blocked nerve, or there may be a neuropathic source of pain proximal to the site of block (e.g., radiculopathy or plexopathy) that may be relieved by the procedure.[2,189,358]

For multiple reasons cited earlier in this chapter, pain relief from local anesthetic block often fails to predict relief of pain from a neuroablative procedure; the local anesthetic block produces profound relief, but the neuroablative procedure fails to provide long-term relief.[250]

Study

The diagnostic utility of injection of lidocaine and steroid has been examined in patients suspected to have carpal tunnel syndrome.[133] The test identified most patients with the disease demonstrated subsequently at surgery (sensitivity 85%), but it indicated lack of carpal tunnel syndrome in only 38% of those surgically negative (specificity).

Evaluation

Relief of pain from a peripheral nerve block, plus diminished sensation in the distribution of the blocked nerve provides additional, although not conclusive, evidence that the nerve is either the source of neuropathic pain or conveys afferent fibers from a source of nociception. Relief following peripheral block may predict response to neural decompression but has little prognostic value in predicting response to neuroablation, which is often ineffective.

VISCERAL NERVE BLOCK

Rationale

It is often helpful to distinguish whether thoracic, abdominal, or pelvic pain is due to pathology of visceral elements or somatic (body wall) structures. If it can be established that pain is visceral in origin, treatment may be directed toward exploration of abdominal or pelvic organs or toward denervation of visceral structures, if untreatable malignancy is the source of the pain.

In addition to chest pain from pulmonary or cardiac sources, there are several common painful somatic conditions, such as costal chondritis, myofascial syndrome, and intercostal neuralgia, which can cause chest pain. These conditions can be relieved either by intercostal blocks or local infiltration. Sensory innervation to much of the heart can be interrupted by left stellate ganglion block. Information about the origin of a given chest pain may be obtained by comparison of placebo injection, left stellate block, and the appropriate somatic block.

Sensory innervation of the upper abdominal viscera can be interrupted by blocking the celiac plexus or the splanchnic nerves proximal to the site where they join the celiac plexus. Such blocks are useful when it is unclear whether abdominal pain is of visceral origin, such as that which occurs with pancreatitis, distension of the hepatic capsule, or cholecystitis, or of somatic origin, as in the case of entrapment of an intercostal nerve or pain of muscular origin. In such cases, it is helpful to compare the response of celiac or splanchnic block to that of intercostal block or local infiltration of the abdominal wall, to that of placebo injection.

It is worthwhile to perform a prognostic celiac or splanchnic block prior to neurolysis for the treatment of pancreatic cancer, since celiac plexus blocks may be relatively ineffective when local tumor spread and resultant inflammation are extensive. In such situations, splanchnic block may still be effective. If tumor spread is extensive enough to involve retroperitoneal somatic structures, both celiac and splanchnic block may be ineffective. This should be tested by the use of local anesthetic blocks. Long-term epidural analgesia may be a preferable technique when cancer is widespread.

Blockade of the afferent innervation of the pelvic viscera can be accomplished by the technique of superior hypogastric plexus block. This relatively new technique has been used mainly to predict the response to neurolytic blockade of the superior hypogastric plexus, a technique that has been developed in lieu of surgical presacral neurectomy for treatment of pain due to pelvic cancer.

Technique

All patients should have an intravenous line placed prior to celiac and splanchnic blocks, and possibly before hypogastric plexus block. Patients with a history of congestive failure, or with suspected hypovolemia, may benefit from placement of a central venous line. Frequent monitoring of blood pressure is essential, and continuous verbal contact is helpful to detect signs of local anesthetic toxicity.

Celiac and Splanchnic Blocks

Technique for celiac and splanchnic blocks are described in Chapter 14, Figs. 14-6. Local anesthetic doses of 20 to 30 ml have been advocated for diagnostic celiac blocks,[266] although some authors use a total dose of 50 ml.[3] A total of 20 ml (10 ml on each side) is adequate for a diagnostic splanchnic block.[3] The use of 0.25% bupivacaine is reasonable in this situation, as it provides fairly prolonged analgesia, allowing the patient to experience the effect on pain of physical activity or eating. It also provides a period of block that is likely to outlast the duration of a placebo response. For instance, if pain recurs within one hour of the block, it is likely to be a placebo reaction, or an effect of absorbed local anesthetics, as opposed to a physiologic response to the block, and recovery from the block.

Diagnostic celiac and splanchnic blocks should be performed with use either of biplane fluoroscopy or computed tomography (CT) scan. Since subsequent treatment is to be determined by response to the block, and there is no sure way to document its success, it is important to ensure that the anesthetic is placed correctly. The use of small quantities of radiographic dye prior to the anesthetic injection further ensures correct needle placement.

Some clinicians advocate using prognostic blocks at least 24 hours before performance of a neurolytic celiac or splanchnic block, arguing that this gives one time to assess thoroughly the analgesic effects and potential side effects, especially hypotension. Others suggest that if the prognostic local anesthetic block is effective, the neurolytic agent should be injected through the same needles, after a short assessment period to evaluate pain relief, vital signs, and possible presence of somatic block. The rationale for doing the neurolysis immediately is that the local anesthetic injection at that exact site has been shown to provide pain relief, and is devoid of somatic blocking effects. In addition, when alcohol is chosen as the neurolytic agent, prior local anesthetic injection will markedly reduce the pain associated with the injection of neurolytic agent.

When the prognostic block is done immediately before neurolysis, a higher concentration of neurolytic agent may be needed. For instance, if 30 ml of local anesthetic is injected initially, one may choose to use absolute alcohol rather than 50% alcohol as the neurolytic agent. It may be unwise to choose phenol as the neurolytic agent when such a technique is used because the use of large amounts of local anesthetic plus phenol may produce systemic toxic reactions (seizures).

Serious complications are unusual following local anesthetic celiac or splanchnic blocks. Hypotension, particularly orthostatic hypotension, is fairly common, so intravenous fluid-loading should be carried out prior to the block, and an attendant should be present if the patient attempts to stand or walk before the block wears off. Toxic reactions to local anesthetic are possible, given the large volumes of local anesthetics used and the proximity of major vessels. Substantial bleeding can occur in patients with coagulopathies. Spread of drug to adjacent nerve roots is possible, particularly with splanchnic blocks. Pneumothorax can occur with either celiac or splanchnic blocks.

Hypogastric Plexus Block

Needles are placed bilaterally at the anterolateral surfaces of the S1 segment of the sacrum.[267] As with celiac plexus and splanchnic block, biplane fluoroscopy or CT scan are essential for documentation of proper needle placement. Radiographic dye injection allows documentation of proper spread of the drug. Relatively small volumes, about 6 to 8 ml on each side, are required (see Chapter 14, Fig. 149).

Hypotension does not appear to be a common problem. Few complications have been reported. Potential problems include intravascular injection or bleeding following puncture of the iliac vessels, ureteral damage, or somatic nerve (especially L5 nerve root) damage.

Limitations

Given the relatively large volumes of anesthetic often used for these blocks, consideration of systemic local anesthetic effects and possible spread to somatic nerves must be included during interpretation of the response.

Evaluation

Despite the lack of studies documenting prognostic benefits of visceral blocks, it would seem prudent not to pursue neuroablative techniques in the absence of relief from local anesthetics. Information obtained from diagnostic visceral blocks may be helpful in confirming clinical impressions.

SACROILIAC INJECTION

Rationale

It is probable that the sacroiliac joint can be the source of acute or chronic pain, because the joint is well innervated.[315] Stimulation by injection of radiographic contrast into the joint, in subjects without complaints of back pain, produces pain in the immediate area, often also in the surrounding gluteal area, and occasionally into the posterior thigh and knee.[115] Diagnostic criteria are uncertain for determining a sacroiliac origin of low back pain. Gaeslen's maneuver, or compression of the apex of the sacrum, with the patient prone on a firm surface, may reproduce the pain, but the specificity of this test is unknown. Other physical exam maneuvers frequently indicate disease in asymptomatic individuals[87] and correlate poorly with diagnoses reached by other means.[291] Typically, there is tenderness over the sacrum just medial to the posterior superior iliac spines. CT scans of the joint may show erosions, narrowing of the cartilagenous portion of the joint, and bony sclerosis of the adjacent ilium. However, the normal anatomy of the joint shows asymmetry of cartilage thickness (thinner on the iliac side), and cartilage-covered irregularities in the bony surfaces, which interlock with reciprocal depressions on the opposite surface, enhancing joint stability.[338] Such changes are more prominent in men, and with age there is a predictable thickening of the capsule, roughening of the cartilage, and growth of marginal osteophytes.[49] For these reasons, it is often difficult to identify pathologic changes in sacroiliac joints and the extent of the sacroiliac contribution to back pain.

Local anesthetic injection of the sacroiliac joint may be helpful in confirming that the joint is a source of low back pain, particularly when diffuse degenerative disease involving the lumbosacral spine is present. A common source of pain and tenderness in the sacroiliac region is myofascial syndrome, involving the sacrospinalis muscle. It is therefore useful to infiltrate the muscle with local anesthetic before sacroiliac joint injection. Lack of relief from that procedure rules out placebo response or myofascial pain. It is thought by some clinicians that local anesthetic injections of the joint may have some value in predicting response to intra-articular steroid injections.

Technique

The method for performing sacroiliac injection is more fully discussed in Chapter 28. It is important to recognize that the common method, using palpable landmarks to guide the needle,[41] cannot assure passage of the needle tip into the joint space, and anatomic considerations make this unlikely, because of the great inter-individual variability in size and contour of sacroiliac joints,[49] and the inaccessibility of the joint line. Under fluoroscopic or CT control, the inferior extent of the joint can be identified, where the space may be entered more easily, and, thus, success confirmed.[115,151] For diagnostic purposes, the patient should be questioned as to whether presence of the needle or injection of the anesthetic reproduces the pain.

Limitations

Without imaging, there is no means to confirm accurate delivery of local anesthetic. When imaging is used to document the intra-articular spread of injectate, intra-articular placement is found to be reliable.[115] It is not clear whether intra-articular spread is needed to achieve efficacy. Pain relief after injection actually may be related to infiltration of sacroiliac ligament or sacrospinalis muscle with anesthetic, and thus gives the incorrect impression that the joint is the pain source. Anesthetic actually injected into the joint may exit the capsule anteriorly and spread along the lumbosacral plexus,[368] conceivably relieving pain from sources other than the joint. The character and distribution of pain evoked by needle contact or contrast injection is of uncertain value because exact reproduction of the pain is not significantly more frequent in patients who obtain relief following anesthetic injection, compared to those with a negative response to anesthetic.[368]

Clinical Studies

Injection with local anesthetic and triamcinolone diacetate performed without fluoroscopy produced transient relief in 28 of 35 patients (Reynolds, A.R., and Abram, S.E., unpublished data, 1984); data showed that 28 patients experienced transient relief. At the end of 6 months, 7 of 20 had persistent improvement in symptoms (relief of 75% of pain or better). A prospective study of x-ray-controlled injection[368] indicated that 30% of patients with chronic low back pain below L5 were relieved by local anesthetic sacroiliac injection, most of whom exhibited a tear in the joint capsule. Most subjects with tears, however, did not get relief from block. Groin pain was a distinguishing complaint of subjects who obtained relief from joint injection. Radiation of pain below the knee was as common in patients relieved by sacroiliac injection as it was in those with no response. No prospective or controlled evaluations of the technique have been published, and no data is available to indicate the sensitivity or specificity of sacroiliac injection as a means of diagnosing the joint as a source of pain.

Evaluation

Analgesia after sacroiliac injection with local anesthetic may be helpful in differentiating sacroiliac arthropathy from facet disease, myofascial pain, or disc disease, although this is unproven. Patients who experience relief from local anesthetic injection may possibly have lasting relief from corticosteroid injection.

FACET INJECTION

Rationale

The zygapophyseal (facet) joints are paired diarthrodial articulations between the posterior elements of adjacent vertebrae. The joint surfaces are midway between the axial and coronal plane in the cervical region and are more vertically inclined at the thoracic levels because the inferior articular processes overlap the superior articular processes like shingles on a roof. Lumbar facet joints are complex and formed into a posteriorly concave surface, the posterior portion of the joint almost parallel to the sagittal plane and the anterior portion in a coronal plane (Fig. 27-9). These arrangements determine the relative motions of sections of the vertebral column. The lumbar articulations prevent rotation but allow flexion. Rotation is maximal in the thoracic column, and the

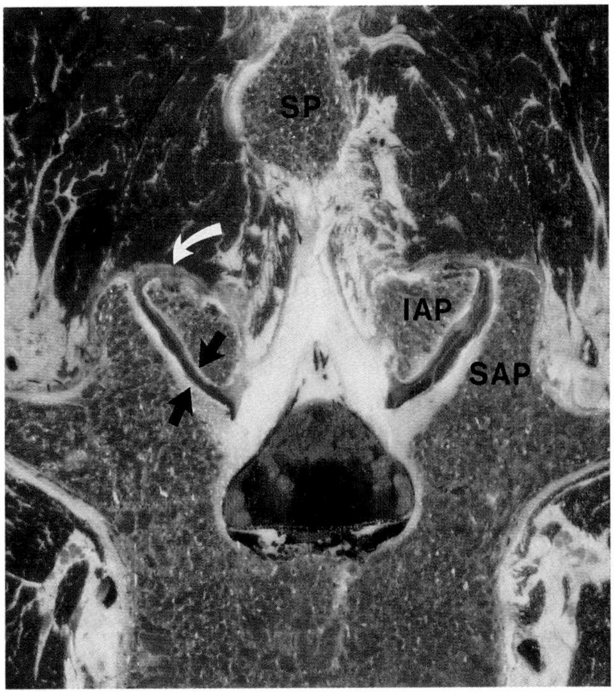

FIG. 27-9. Unstained axial cryomicrotome section through the third lumbar vertebral body, showing facet joints (*straight arrows*). The medial joint capsule is reinforced by the yellow ligamentum flavum, while the posterolateral extent of the joint ends in a redundant pocket (*curved arrows*). Cartilage loss is evident. *IAP*, inferior articular process; *SP*, spinous process; *SAP*, superior articular process.

cervical vertebrae permit both rotation and extensive movement in the sagittal plane. Rudimentary fibroadipose menisci and synovial folds cushion the superior and inferior poles of the lumbar zygapophyseal joints,[31] but with age these typically disappear and the cartilage thins on the joint surfaces.[343]

The median branch of the dorsal primary ramus of the spinal nerve supplies the facet joint as well as the supraspinous and intraspinous ligaments. Of these, only the facet joint consistently is found to be well innervated by nociceptive fibers penetrating the capsule as well, and into the synovial folds.[124,233] Each facet joint receives branches from the spinal nerve exiting the vertebral canal through the adjacent intervertebral foramen and the nerve, one segment above.[32,33] Injection of hypertonic saline into or around the lumbar facet joint capsule produces pain in the back, buttocks, and proximal thigh.[229,238] Physiologic recordings in laboratory animals have documented mechanoreceptive sensory fields in facet joints.[61,360] Distension of normal cervical facet joint capsules produces unilateral pain ranging from occipital and upper neck from atlanto-occipital, atlanto-axial, and C2/C3 joints, to scapular pain from joint C6/C7.[93,88] Immunohistochemical evidence of substance P in facet capsule neurons[99] also supports the concept of the facet joints as a source of nociception. Rotation and extension between two adjacent vertebrae increases facet stress, as does loss of disc height,[92] all of which may be stimuli for facet pain. Facet menisci are innervated by small myelinated nerves,[125] in which substance P is present[126] but rare.[140] An entrapment syndrome involving the facet menisci has been proposed,[31] but there is no clear evidence to implicate this in the production of back pain.

Radicular pain is distinctive (distal radiation and burning, electrical quality), is associated with clear signs of nerve deficit or irritation, correlates fairly well with anatomic defects found on imaging, and usually can be confirmed by electrodiagnostic (EMG, nerve-conduction) studies. Nonradicular back and neck pain is more ambiguous and almost always poses a diagnostic dilemma. In addition to the facet joints, other structures in the vertebral column also are richly innervated, such as the posterior and anterior longitudinal ligaments, anular ligament of the intervertebral disc, anterior dura mater, and the costovertebral joints.[34,35,94,114,135,136,317] Stimulation of these other vertebral elements by injection or during surgery in awake patients with local anesthesia evokes pain in the back, hip, and buttock, indistinguishable from pain produced by facet irritation.[94,106,152,184,200,242,314,350] Clinical features that suggest a facet joint origin include pain into the proximal but not distal ipsilateral limb, localized paraspinal tenderness, and reproduction of pain with extension and rotation.[149] Pain can occur in the absence of changes on plane x-rays of the vertebral column. Computed tomographic imaging is more sensitive, but degenerative facet arthritis is seen in 10.4% of asymptomatic patients.[351] Although the value of bone scan is unproven, a positive finding may support the diagnosis of facet arthropathy and may direct attention to a particular joint. Because there is no specific pathognomonic finding or test, the clinical criteria for making the diagnosis of facet pain remain undefined. Therefore, diagnostic injections often are performed to help indicate the contribution of the facet.

Technique

Local anesthetic can be injected either into the joint space or around the nerves innervating the joint. These procedures are described in Chapter 28. For reliable diagnosis, certainty of successful injection requires fluoroscopic imaging at least. With advanced disease and joint changes, CT imaging may be helpful for injection into the joint space.[244] When intra-articular injection is used for diagnostic purposes, the patient should be asked to compare the distribution of pain created by needle contact with the joint to his or her usual pain. There is no physiological means to test the adequacy of intra-articular anesthesia. When blockade of the posterior primary ramus is performed, two injections are needed to anesthetize a joint because each facet receives terminal fibers from two posterior rami (e.g., the L4/L5 facet is innervated at its upper pole by branches from L3 and at its lower pole by branches from L4). At lumbar levels, there is no cutaneous innervation by these branches, so adequacy of the block cannot be confirmed by superficial examination. Although the medial branches of the 3rd, 4th, and often 5th cervical posterior branches have cutaneous ramifications, they are small areas near the midline and have not been shown to provide accurate evidence of proximal neural blockade. Provocative stimuli of the joint, such as mechanical or chemical irritation, could be performed after the block to check adequacy of denervation, but this has not been investigated. After injection into the joint space or of interruption of the sensory nerves to the joint, the patient's pain can be attributed to the facet if pain relief is noted in response to local anesthetic injection, with attention focused on the maneuvers that provoked the pain prior to injection, and sensory exam shows no evidence of segmental spinal nerve block.

Limitations

The use of facet or medial branch injections for diagnosis rests upon the assumption that facets are a source of pain. This premise is accepted by most authorities, although the frequency of this as the primary element producing a patient's pain is debated. Disc degeneration is present in all cases of lumbar facet disease evident by CT or magnetic resonance (MR) imaging.[51] Disc disease identified by discography was present in 64% of patients with a positive cervical medial branch test for facet joint disease.[36] Pathologic changes in facets are a common cause of injury to nerve roots,[100] and may irritate afferents on the posterolateral aspect of the disc. These other disease processes could, therefore, be the cause of pain in patients with incidental abnormalities of the facet, or at least could contribute to a condition more complex than a facet origin of pain. Since there is no histopathologic or imaging standard,[243] the frequency of pain from the facet *per se* has been estimated only by relief in response to injections. As is discussed below, this inevitably involves circular logic, but gives a positive indication of cervical facet etiology in unselected patients with postraumatic neck pain of about 70% (range 63% to 100%).[9,15,16,36,37,168,290] In subjects clinically suspected of having lumbar facet pain, confirmation by relief after injection ranges from 16% to 94%.[55,56,77,104,149,238,241,244,281] In a noncontrolled and nonblinded study of patients with chronic low back pain without radiculopathy, 25% of those assigned to receive median branch nerve blockade of a randomly chosen joint had immediate relief, and 38% had relief after injection into the suspected joint.[224] These comparable rates are similar to the frequency of placebo response. Total absence of pain after injection of local anesthetic into the lumbar facets is much less common, occurring in only about 7% of back pain patients.[55,173] It is reasonable to conclude that in many study groups the facets are an origin of at least part of the patients' pain, but rarely are the unique or major source.

Mechanical irritation of the joint capsule during facet injection may produce discomfort resembling the patient's typical pain. Since cervical[93,213] and lumbar[213,225,229,238] facet stimulation produces broadly overlapping areas of pain distribution even into the distal extremity (see Chapter 28, Fig. 28-6), this is not a strong indicator of pain origin. Patients whose usual pain is provoked by facet stimulation do not necessarily obtain pain relief by local anesthetic injection in the facet joint,[212,104] and there is a poor correlation between pain provocation and relief from local anesthetic injection.[300] In one study,[241] 31% of patients with a positive response to pain provocation failed to have relief after anesthetic injection into that lumbar facet, and 40% who had relief from injection had not had typical pain during needle stimulation or distension of the facet capsule with contrast.

The specificity of facet denervation depends upon limiting anesthetic spread to the joint or nerves to the joint. Detailed sensory neural testing after these blocks has not been reported. The facet joints are not capacious. Rupture during intra-articular injection has been identified after injection of more than 1 ml into cervical facets,[85] and after most lumbar injections,[77,86] and has been demonstrated in cadaver facet injections.[241] Since this spills local anesthetic into neighboring tissues, pain relieved by facet injection could in fact originate in other structures such as muscle, periosteum, and ligaments. Passage of anesthetic into the epidural space or intervertebral foramen, which occurs routinely with capsule rupture (see Chapter 28),[77,86] could interrupt nociception from sensitive structures in the vertebral canal, such as anterior dura and posterior longitudinal ligament, or from any distal site by effects on afferent fibers in the spinal roots. Of patients with clinical indications of having lumbar facet pain, 18% are found to have spondylolysis,[219] a defect in the vertebral arch due to chronic stress. With this condition, intra-articular facet injection is followed consistently by spread of solution into the epidural space and to adjacent and contralateral facets, and even laterally along a spinal nerve,[121,219,232] limiting the specificity of the test. Injection into the subarachnoid space has been reported.[129]

Blockade of medial branches not only denervates the joints they supply, but also muscles, ligaments, and periosteum. Sources of pain in these alternative sites will be relieved by medial branch block. Fluid distribution during cervical medial branch block is variable, with the area of consistent coverage being a small subset of the area into which spread may be observed. Injectate, however, does not travel to anterior primary rami or to medial branches of adjacent posterior rami.[16] Since each medial branch supplies parts of two facets, complete denervation of one facet requires partial blockade of the one above and below. Therefore, relief from the blocks cannot distinguish between pain originating at any of the three. Since medial branch blockade more accurately simulates the effect of radiofrequency denervation than does intra-articular injection, it is the appropriate diagnostic test before that procedure.

The reproducibility of the test is uncertain. In one study, facet injections in 176 low back pain patients produced relief in 83 (47%), but a repeat injection was positive in only 26 of the 83 (31%).[299] This indicates either a strong placebo component or subtle technical difficulties that cannot be controlled. (The authors of this study claim that the second injection determines which of the responders to the initial injections were true positives, and not placebos. This logic apparently dismisses the more obvious explanation that the two time-positive responders were placebo responders each time.) Even when relief is found during repeated diagnostic injections, there is no feature of the patients' histories or physical exams that correlates with a positive diagnosis by this more demanding criterion,[298] drawing the relevance of blocks into uncertainty.

Studies

Validation of the use of intra-articular and medial branch injections to document facet pain requires demonstration that (i) the injections as described are effective in denervating the joint and (ii) such denervation can be used to distinguish between various sources of back pain. No means has been described to test the adequacy of facet denervation, so success rates have not been determined. Relief of pain in patients with presumed facet arthropathy is not a suitable test of physiologic blockade success. Since the diagnosis of a painful facet relies upon injections for confirmation, evidence for either is circular. No block can be assumed to be effective every time, so inability to confirm directly that the block is successful and that the joint is denervated, weakens the diagnostic utility of facet and medial branch nerve injections. That is, even though the pain has changed after the injection, to attribute this change securely to the block requires independent evidence to confirm that the block actually happened. Inability to enter the joint during attempted intra-articular injection has been reported in 16% to 38% of lumbar injections[55,215] and 44% of cervical facet injections.[290] To a degree, cervical medial branch block has been validated by comparison to intra-articular injection; all of seven patients who were relieved by blockade of the branches innervating a joint had relief after intra-articular injection of that joint on a different occasion, although up to 2 ml of local anesthetic was injected into the joint.[37]

Since no standard to confirm facet pain is available for correlation with block findings, the ability of facet blocks to aid in valid diagnosis of the source of back pain has not been established. However, the clinical utility of facet blocks is drawn into question by several findings. In general, a facet etiology is identified infrequently when small intra-articular injectate volumes are used.[241,279] This means that either larger volumes (more than 1.5 ml) are necessary for adequate intra-articular block, or that large volume injections block pain from sources other than the facet. The only studies done with controls are not optimistic. In one, local anesthetic resulted in relief in 54% of patients with back pain, but 43% of these responders also were relieved by injection of a randomly chosen uninvolved facet joint.[104] A controlled trial which examined improvement one hour after injection found no difference in groups that had had local anesthetic injected into the joints, or outside the joints, or normal saline injected into the joints.[207] In a study comparing duration of analgesia following cervical medial branch blocks on two different occasions in order to determine a false positive rate, 27% either had a duration of analgesia longer for lidocaine than for bupivacaine, or no analgesia at all on the second injection.[17] The only study that was controlled and blinded showed no difference in pain relief between intra-articular lidocaine or saline injection.[173]

Little data is available on the ability of facet blocks to predict the response to more definitive therapy. Radiofrequency facet denervation failed to benefit 36% of patients who had excellent relief from intra-articular injection.[213] In another report,[252] the positive predictive value of relief after local anesthetic block of the lumbar medial branch of the posterior primary ramus was 0.45 in anticipating success from radiofrequency denervation (45% of block successes also were radiofrequency successes). Specificity and sensitivity cannot be determined because radiofrequency surgery was not performed if blocks provided less than moderate relief. Relief after facet injection has been examined as a prognostic indicator for response to posterolateral lumbosacral fusions,[174] but block results did not predict surgical outcome.

Therapeutic responses have been reported following intra-articular zygapophysial joint injection, especially if steroid is included. Steroid injected into the lumbar facet joints results in significant relief, outlasting the local anesthetic in between 30% and 54% of groups of selected patients with back pain.[55,77,149,207,215,244] Response rates are lower for patients with previous lumbar spine surgery,[213] and after extra-articular injection, are less likely to be therapeutic.[215] It is not encouraging to note that the pain returns by six months in many of the steroid responders,[77] and in one report, the results for steroid were no different than those for saline injection.[207] Beneficial effects of cervical facet injection with steroid have been reported in 91% of patients, but recurrence occurred in half.[290] Another study found no benefit from cervical facet steroid injection, even though the same patients had experienced complete relief from local anesthetic.[168] The only blinded trial of facet steroid injection found that saline injected into lumbar joints produced only slightly less improvement than steroid, and that the completeness of response to local anesthetic did not predict the degree of steroid effect.[55] Steroid injection probably is appropriate during a diagnostic injection study, since the additional risk of injecting the steroid after the needle is already in place is minor. However, the efficacy of intra-articular steroid in the facet joint has not been proven.

Evaluation

Injections intended to block afferents from facet joints have been found useful by a number of authors. However, the literature on the topic is from relatively few advocates, sometimes with repeated presentation of data.[15,17] Also, the inability to confirm success of a block and the lack of convincing evidence for efficacy and diagnostic specificity of these techniques dictates that findings should be interpreted cautiously.

INTERVERTEBRAL DISC INJECTION

Rationale

The annular ligament of the intervertebral disc fuses in the midline with the posterior longitudinal ligament. Both these structures are well innervated by sensory fibers, and may provoke pain.[95,106,152,242,314,350] Several methods are available to identify pathologic changes, in order to identify the source of pain in subjects with non-radiating back pain. Because myelography only demonstrates disc abnormalities that deform the dural sac, the injection of radiopaque contrast into the nucleus pulposus of the disc (discography) was developed to reveal the internal details of the disc. More recently, CT and MR have provided sensitive means of identifying changes in disc anatomy. Myelography, CT, and MR imaging all suffer from inadequate specificity, since asymptomatic discs frequently appear abnormal. Myelograms show lumbar nerve root involvement by disc disease in 24% of asymptomatic subjects and cervical involvement in 21%.[153] Herniated nucleus pulposus is evident by CT scan in 19.5% of asymptomatic subjects under 40 years old, and in 26.9% of those over 40.[351] Lumbar disc degeneration is documented by MR in 1/3 to 1/2 of subjects without clinical evidence of back disease between the ages of 21 and 40 years, and in 90% over the age of 60 years.[29,178,268,348] By imaging alone, there is no way to tell painful discs from others, especially if abnormal anatomy is evident at multiple levels.

Identifying a particular disc as the source of pain is challenging because of overlapping patterns of pain between various discs, and similar pain from facets. Therefore, discography has been recommended as an objective method for determining a specific disc as the origin of pain, and for planning discectomy or vertebral fusion. The premise is that a dynamic test, in which the ability of a disc to produce the patient's typical pain, combined with the sensitivity of detailed intradiscal imaging, can most accurately identify the pathogenic site.

Technique

Since the procedure involves both interpretation of radiographic images, as well as clinical pain phenomena, it is ideally performed by a physician treating the patient in conjunction with a radiologist. Typically, two to three consecutive discs are examined as one procedure. An early method involved passage of a needle in the posterior midline through the dural sac, to enter the disc through the posterior longitudinal ligament.[69] Occasionally, this is still necessary for discs that are difficult to enter, especially at L5/S1. A posterolateral approach is used most often (Fig. 27-10).[307] Specially designed needles are available, but a 22-gauge, 5-inch needle is suitable. Sometimes a larger needle is passed first to the disc to guide the needle that actually punctures the anulus. Fluoroscopy is used[328] to determine the disc level and to direct the needle from the skin puncture site about 8 cm from the midline to the posterolateral aspect of the disc, anterior to the spinal nerve. A single needle is placed in each disc, but it must terminate within the nucleus pulposus, which can be assured by placing the tip in the inner 1/3 of the disc, as seen by both lateral and anteroposterior views. As contrast (water soluble, nonionic, e.g., iopamidol) is injected, the patient is asked to compare the sensation created to his or her usual pain, in both distribution and quality. The tension in the disc is estimated by the resistance to injection; this has been formally quantified as an indicator of disc condition.[272] Injection is stopped when resistance to further injection is noted, when pain is created, or when about 3 ml has entered. Images are recorded with high-quality plane radiographs or CT axial scans.

A discogram is positive for disc degeneration if the image reveals altered texture of the nucleus, clefts in the nucleus and anulus, fissures leading to the perimeter of the anulus, or a radial tear that allows contrast to escape (Fig. 27-11).[5] Discomfort that duplicates the patient's typical pain is also necessary for a completely positive test response.

Reported complications are few and include disc space infection[69,307,308] and allergic response to the contrast.

Limitations

Authorities report that the quality of testing by discography depends strongly upon the skill and experience of the operator. Proper placement of the needle tip within the nuclear portion of the disc is imperative. Repeated needle in-

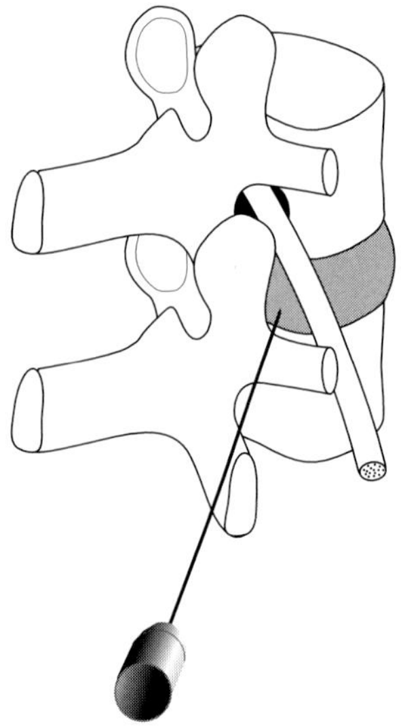

FIG. 27-10. Needle placement for lumbar discography. (From Konings, J.G., and Veldhuizen, A.G.: Topographic anatomical aspects of lumbar disc puncture. Spine, *13*:958, 1988.)

Discogram type		Stage of disc degeneration
1. Cottonball	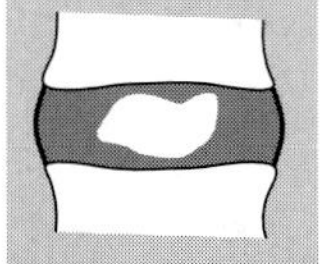	No signs of degeneration. Soft white amorphous nucleus
2. Lobular	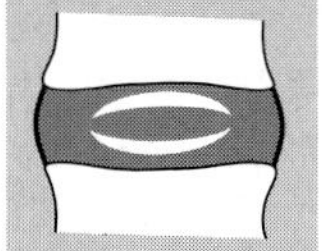	Mature disc with nucleus starting to coalesce into fibrous lumps
3. Irregular	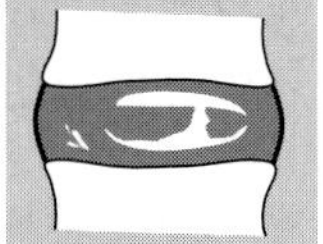	Degenerated disc with fissures and clefts in the nucleus and inner annulus
4. Fissured	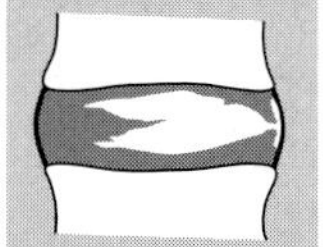	Degenerated disc with radial fissure leading to the outer edge of the annulus
5. Ruptured	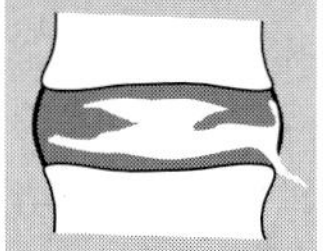	Disc has a complete radial fissure that allows injected fluid to escape. Can be in any state of degeneration

FIG. 27-11. The five types of discogram and the stages of disc degeneration they represent.[245]

sertions or the removal of the needle after injection but prior to imaging may produce artifactual tracks of contrast through the anulus.

Discography is fairly uncomfortable for the subject, but deep sedation should be avoided so that pain provocation can be evaluated. The value of this invasive test compared to CT and MR imaging is the subject of debate and numerous studies.

Studies

The pathoanatomic validity of discography has been established in cadaver studies by comparison of dissection with plane radiographs[5] and CT or MR imaging.[336,365]

Satisfactory discogram testing is impossible to complete in few patients. As with any invasive study, some may find the pain of needle insertion intolerable. Inability to enter the disc and nucleus pulposus occurs in about 4% of discs, often at the L5/S1 level.[119,122] Complete disc collapse was reported to preclude discography in 14% of patients.[68] CT imaging after injection probably improves the sensitivity of the test compared to plane radiographs.[336]

The false positive rate determines the practical utility of the test. Early studies of asymptomatic subjects found positive discograms in 93% of cervical injections[162] and in 37% of lumbar injections in 20- to 40-year-olds.[163] In part because of these findings, cervical disc injections are performed rarely. A recent replication of the study of lumbar injections in asymptomatic subjects also found that discograms were falsely positive in 17% of asymptomatic subjects, but if severe and concordant pain is included as a criterion for a positive test, the false positive rate becomes 0%.[342] Others studying patient groups with back pain have found that subjects with pain during injection are a subset of those with abnormal disc anatomy and that 22% to 40% of discs unresponsive to pain provocation are anatomically abnormal.[141,332] These data point to the conclusion that disc degeneration is a predictable age-related process that inconsistently results in pain. Unexplained are the 2% to 24% of back pain patients with induced pain during discography who have normal disc anatomy.[141,332,367]

Since discography is invasive, indications and utility of the test must be compared to MR. Examination of cadaver material shows that radial tears of the annulus were evident by MR in only 67% of the discs with tears shown by discography and documented by dissection.[365] In clinical comparison, MR and discography may differ in up to 45% of patients with back pain,[308] due to both normal MR with abnormal discography and the reverse. Discography is more prone to operator and interpretation error apparent on reinspection.[122] MR images with clear evidence of either present or absent disc pathology usually agrees with disc injection testing if provoked pain is included in the evaluation,[165] so discography can be reserved safely for determination of the disease state of discs with intermediate MR patterns.

Although discography with evaluation of induced pain can discern structurally abnormal and sensitive discs, this does not establish whether the test identifies the source of the patient's pain. Using local anesthetic injection to stop disc pain has not been evaluated as an additional phase of the test. However, the pressure-sensitive anulus would not necessarily be affected by anesthetic within the nucleus, and leakage through a disrupted disk would distribute anesthetic to multiple potentially painful elements. The only independent means available for determining the nociceptive source is comparison of the test response to the outcome from surgery, with the assumption that if surgery at a particular level relieves the pain, then that was the source of the pain. Simmons et al.[307] reported the diagnostic accuracy in predicting surgical outcome was 91% at cervical levels and 82% for lumbar discs, when discography was used to identify the painful disc. These figures are about twice the accuracy of clinical exam and myelography, but the calculations were not clearly defined. In a prospective study of back pain patients,[68] in which all patients subsequently had an operation regardless of discogram result, 88% of patients with pain on injection and an abnormal discogram had a favorable outcome from surgery at the level indicated by testing (positive predictive value = 88%). However, this seemingly persuasive finding is due partly to the very high prevalence of favorable surgical outcomes in the entire group; 82% of all subjects, regardless of injection test results, had a favorable surgical outcome. About equal numbers of surgical nonresponders had positive and negative tests (false positive rate = 52%), and subjects with a negative discogram image or no pain upon injection (negative test) were equally likely to have surgical success or failure (negative predictive value = 52%).

Evaluation

In settings where MR imaging is ambiguous, discography is a sensitive although invasive means of obtaining additional anatomic detail about disc structure. Provoking a comparable sensory response to injection is a critical component of the test. Statistical documentation of diagnostic validity awaits blinded study of a large group of patients.

SELECTIVE SPINAL NERVE INJECTION

Rationale

Radiculopathy is often obvious in its characteristic burning quality and distal radiation of pain. However, patients with more complicated conditions may present, in whom the contribution of root inflammation to pain may not be certain or in whom the level of the pathology is unclear. Imaging by CT or MR and electrophysiologic evaluation by EMG may be inconsistent or may not fit with clinical findings. Frequent positive findings in imaging of asymptomatic subjects[29,153,268,348,351] demonstrates the inability of abnormal anatomy to indicate a pain source. A further cause of confusion is the presence of pathology at multiple levels, since the origin of pain may be any one or a combination of sites; this is also true when upper lumbar pathology coexists with hip joint disease. Finally, evaluation is especially difficult after laminectomy, since imaging is impeded by scarring in the epidural space.

In these unclear situations, injection of individual spinal nerves by a paravertebral approach (also termed foraminal injection or nerve root injection), usually at lumbar levels, has been used to elucidate the mechanism and source of pain. The premise is that eliciting the patient's characteristic pain through needle contact will identify the pathologic nerve and that local anesthetic delivered to this nerve will be uniquely analgesic. Advocates point out that selective spinal nerve block, as with facet injection and discography, tests pain production mechanisms dynamically rather than simply displaying anatomic abnormalities that may or may not produce pain. Often this method is used for surgical planning, for instance, to determine the site of foramenotomy.

Technique

Technical aspects of this procedure are discussed in detail in Chapter 14 and in Chapter 28.

For diagnostic utility, it is important to obtain a paresthesia by gentle contact with the nerve. At this point, the patient is asked whether the quality and distribution of the provoked sensation is similar to his or her usual pain. Successful blockade is evident if a segmental sensory deficit develops. This may be subtle, so scratch and cold should be tested as well as touch. Since these patients often have neural dysfunction as part of their pathophysiology, a careful examination is necessary for comparison before injection. Maneuvers that produced pain prior to the block, such as straight leg lift or walking, should be repeated afterwards. A test is considered positive for a given nerve if it produced pain similar to the patient's usual pain, and if relief followed local anesthetic injection. Optimal insight into the origin of the pain is gained by testing two or three adjacent nerves on separate occasions.[301]

Block of the first sacral nerve is performed by a transacral approach with the patient prone (Fig. 27-12). Because of the lumbar lordosis, fluoroscopic guidance is improved when the beam is angled caudally, to be perpendicular to the sacrum. With the posterior and anterior sacral foramina superimposed, the needle can be passed to make contact with the spinal nerve in the middle portion of the canal. The rest of the block is done in the same manner as at lumbar levels.

Limitations

The pain provocation portion of the spinal nerve injection test examines pain quality and distribution. Duplication of the typical quality of the pain as a criterion is supported by the demonstration that inflamed nerves are more sensitive to manipulation than are normal nerves.[106,314] Whereas mechanical stimulation of normal nerves produces paresthesias, an inflamed nerve reproduces characteristic sciatica when touched. The distribution of the evoked sensation is less certain to be reliable. Since pain with the stimulation of different roots produces overlapping areas of radiation,[314] these patterns may not distinguish the involved root from adjacent ones.

Confirmation of successful blockade is a desirable step prior to attributing pain and function changes to the block. It is not clear that anesthetizing a single spinal nerve should produce discernible peripheral sensory changes. Isolated monoradiculopathy commonly is associated with numbness, but this pathologic condition is probably more complex than just segmental nerve dysfunction, including changes in central connections.[357] Selective spinal nerve injection reliably produced peripheral sensory changes in dermatome mapping studies, but 2 ml of anesthetic were injected, raising the question of spread to adjacent levels.[183] Since surgical division of a single root produces no loss of cutaneous sensation,[113] it remains uncertain whether cutaneous sensory monitoring can indicate accurately the presence or absence of selective spinal nerve block. No other methods of determining block success, such as thermography or somatosensory-evoked potentials, have been examined.

Pain relief with blockade of a spinal nerve cannot distinguish between pathology of the proximal nerve in the inter-

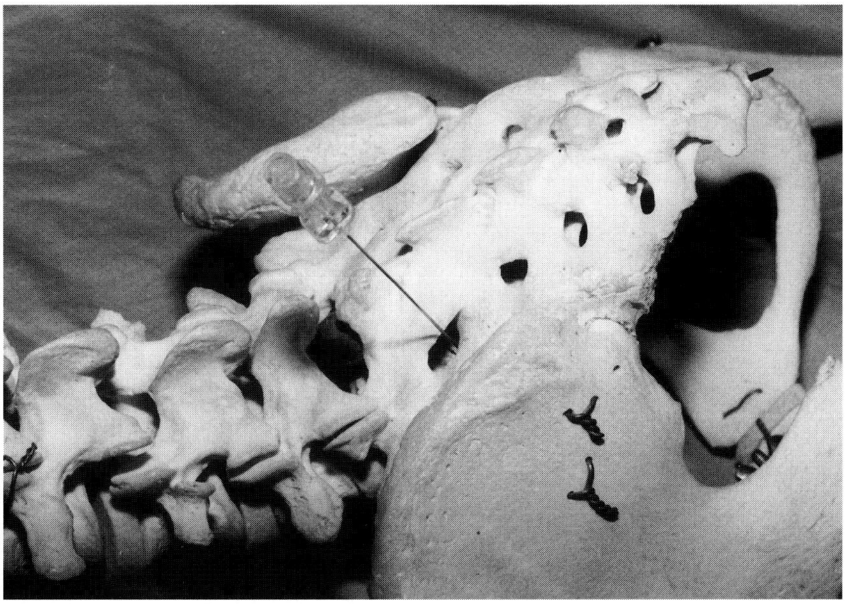

FIG. 27-12. Trans-sacral approach to the first sacral nerve. The needle is guided by x-ray imaging into the first posterior sacral foramen and advanced to the anterior foramen either until a paresthesia is evoked or lateral imaging shows the tip flush with the anterior surface of the sacrum.

vertebral foramen or pain transmitted from distal sites by that nerve. Tissue injury in the nerve's distribution and neuropathic pain alike would be relieved by a proximal block of a nerve. The ability of injection to block vertebral pain, without blocking hip pain, has not been demonstrated. The accuracy of spinal nerve block depends upon limiting spread of anesthetic to the selected nerve alone. Flow into the intervertebral foramen and epidural space is commonly observed (see Chapter 8) and definitely compromises this assumption.[75,84,148,199,321] Not only will this block pain transmitted by the sinuvertebral nerve from the dura, posterior longitudinal ligament, and annular ligament of the disc, but spread via the epidural space to other segmental levels could produce misleading results. For instance, injection of a normal S1 with spread to an inflamed L5 could produce relief, with the guilty nerve assumed to be S1. For this reason, this test should not be used outside the context of thorough overall evaluation.

Studies

The frequency of successful spinal nerve blockade has not been determined. In no studies using spinal nerve block for diagnosis were cutaneous sensory changes examined. Satisfactory needle placement could not be achieved in 10% of patients at L4, 15% at L5, and 30% at S1.[148] In another report, 18% of tests failed because of pain that exceeded the patient's tolerance or failure to stimulate the desired root, most often at S1.[316]

Several retrospective studies have investigated the ability of selective spinal nerve blocks to diagnose disease and predict surgical outcome. The positive predictive value (fraction of patients with injections indicating radiculopathy, in whom surgery confirmed radicular pathology at the level indicated by the test), ranged from 87% to 100%.[84,148,199,301] The negative predictive value (percent of patients with a negative injection test and confirmed at surgery to have normal nerve roots), has been poorly studied because few patients had surgery in the negative test groups; negative predictive values were found in 27% and 38% of the small number of patients operated upon, despite negative tests.[84,148] Only one prospective study has appeared, which showed a positive predictive value of 95% and an untested negative predictive value.[316] Sensitivity and specificity cannot be determined from these studies because of the unknown disease incidence in the full group. In general, the accuracy of nerve blocks was better than imaging or EMG.[148,316] No controls were used in these studies, and the utility of cervical diagnostic spinal nerve injections has not been examined formally.

A recent retrospective report[75] attempted to predict surgical outcome by evaluating pain relief in response to steroid injection at the spinal nerve. Most were tested with selective spinal nerve blocks, but 20% received epidural injection, and patients who were not relieved by local anesthetic were not included in the steroid test. All patients were operated upon regardless of test outcome, so complete outcome data is available. False positive rate (percent of patients with failed surgery who had favorable response to injection) was 5%, and false negative rate (percent of surgical successes who had no response to steroid) was 35%, indicating that patients unlikely to benefit from surgery can be identified reliably by failing to respond to steroid, but some who would benefit from surgery will be missed by this test. In patients with pain lasting longer than one year, however, nearly all patients who would benefit from surgery were identified by their response to steroid (false negative 15%).

Studies have demonstrated repeatedly that pain relief by paravertebral spinal nerve injection does not predict success by neuroablative surgery, either by dorsal rhizotomy[210,259] or dorsal root ganglionectomy.[253]

Therapeutic responses are seen occasionally after selective spinal nerve injection, especially if steroid has been used. No study has been designed with controls to test the value of this treatment.

Evaluation

Even though spinal nerve injection has not been proven to be a valid diagnostic tool by conclusive studies, a broad group of surgical authorities have found benefits in its use for planning decompressive surgery on complicated patients. Controlled and blinded studies are needed to refute or support these beliefs. Its role in evaluating patients for neuroablative procedures is very uncertain.

EPIDURAL STEROID INJECTION

Two studies have used the response to epidural steroids as a prognostic factor. In one,[75] subjects receiving epidural injections were mixed with a larger group tested with spinal nerve injections, so the results cannot be interpreted. In the other report,[344] sciatica patients who did not have satisfactory long-term benefit from lumbar epidural steroids had their initial response to epidural steroid injection compared to the outcome of subsequent chemonucleolysis. In a small group, patients who had some relief from steroids uniformly responded to chemonucleolysis, while only 46% of steroid nonresponders benefited from chemonucleolysis. No correlation was found between steroid response and surgical outcome. The study was uncontrolled.

GREATER OCCIPITAL NERVE BLOCK

Rationale

The greater occipital nerve is the continuation of the median branch of the posterior primary ramus of the C2 spinal nerve (see Chapter 15, Fig. 15-10), which is the only segmental level in the body where the posterior primary ramus exceeds the anterior primary ramus in size. It distributes cutaneous sensory fibers to the scalp as far rostral as the vertex, where it abuts the territory of the supraorbital nerve, lateral to the area of the mastoid innervated by the great auricular and lesser occipital nerves of the cervical plexus (anterior primary rami), and inferior to the area of the third occipital nerve in the upper neck. From its origin at the second posterior root ganglion, it emerges between the atlas and axis (C1 and C2 vertebrae), loops under the inferior oblique capitus muscle, ascends medially under the semispinalis capitus muscle, which it penetrates before turning laterally under the trapezius. Emergence to the subcutaneous tissue occurs through the tendinous portion of the trapezius' insertion into the nuchal ridge of the skull adjacent to the occipital artery.

Several theories have proposed involvement of the C2 spinal and greater occipital nerves in production of headache. Initial analysis suggested that the origin of the spinal nerve or the posterior root ganglion may be pinched between the atlas and axis by extension and rotation.[171] Further research proved that this is mechanically unlikely.[38,347] A more popular theory invokes irritation of the greater occipital nerve as it penetrates the muscle layers. The passage through the muscular portion of the semispinalis capitus rarely is restricted, but the aperture through the trapezius is by a nondistensible channel which typically deforms the nerve.[337] Entrapment here may be the origin of nerve irritation which initiates neuralgic pain.

Greater occipital neuralgia and cervical facet arthropathy are putative sources of cervicogenic headache, which is clinically distinguished from migraine and tension-type headaches by unilateral pain, symptoms and signs of neck involvement (ipsilateral neck, shoulder, or arm pain; tenderness or postural pain in the neck; decreased range of neck motion), nonclustering moderate pain which throbs and spreads forward from the neck, and a history of head or neck trauma.[45,311] Transient elimination of pain by greater occipital nerve block is used as a key criterion in the work-up of cervicogenic headache.[311]

Technique

Although the greater occipital branches to the scalp can be anesthetized by deposition of local anesthetic in a transverse band anywhere rostral to the nuchal ridge (see Chapter 15, Fig. 15-10), selective blockade of the nerve at the proposed pathogenic site requires injection as it penetrates through the trapezius. In two studies, this has been located on average at a point 3.2 cm lateral and 2.2 cm inferior to the external occipital protuberance,[337] or 2.4 cm lateral and 1.2 cm inferior.[46] There is marked interindividual variability, but 3 to 5 ml of anesthetic (lidocaine 1% or bupivacaine 0.5%) injected at 3 cm lateral and 2 cm inferior to the occipital protuberance (approximately midway between the occipital protuberance and the mastoid process) should spread to block most nerves. Bone should be contacted at a depth of no greater than 1 to 2 cm. A rostral angle and aspiration before injection are important to avoid injection into the CSF of the cisterna magna with resulting total spinal anesthesia. Injection should be made upon withdrawal a few mm from the bone.

Anesthesia should be confirmed by sensory examination of the scalp ipsilateral and rostral to the injection. Determination of changes in headache should follow.

Limitations

Cervicogenic headache is a poorly documented entity[96] with no consistent histopathological or radiological findings.[264] The typical lack of sensory deficit in the area of distribution of the greater occipital nerve does not support a neuropathic mechanism.[38] Alternatively, it is possible that pain radiating in the distribution of the greater occipital nerve represents converging deep somatic input from the lateral atlantoaxial joint, which is innervated by the C2 anterior ramus,[38] or from irritation of suboccipital muscles and periosteum, which has been shown to produce ascending headache.[52,72,105]

Since all the proposed pathophysiologies of cervicogenic headache are unproven, the meaning of blockade responses does not rest on a solid mechanistic base. No defined process has been proven when relief follows greater occipital nerve block. Also, the therapeutic plan is not well defined after a favorable response to test injections. There are no data on the use of this block for treatment, and the surgical therapy for presumed greater occipital neuralgia has not been promising.[47,227] Favorable responses to radiofrequency lesions of the greater occipital nerve have been claimed.[27] Patients who had pain relief after bilateral greater occipital nerve block, with 10 to 15 ml of local anesthetic on each side, received heat lesions to the nerves during general anesthesia. Although good to excellent relief was reported in 85% of cases, neural interruption was not documented and there were no controls.

Studies

No information is available regarding rates of successful greater occipital nerve blockade. The ability of the block to identify patients with disease is hampered by inexact definition of cervicogenic headache and no means of certain confirmation. Most studies, as well as the definition of the condition, come from a single group. In one report,[48] patients clinically categorized as having migraine, cervicogenic, or tension-type headaches, were tested with greater occipital and supraorbital nerve blocks, with the latter as control. Cervicogenic headache patients were most relieved by occipital injection. However, supraorbital block also produced relief (about half as much, and not selective for cervicogenic patients), and the two blocks relieved pain at the other poles of the head. Although this calls into question the basis of relief, a mechanism is offered in which sensory tracts converge on common upper cord and brain stem centers.[186,187] In another report,[45] the ability of greater occipital nerve block to provide relief (confirmed as successful by sensory examination) was compared to selective blocks of cervical spinal nerves and the C2/C3 facet in patients with symptoms of cervicogenic headache. The patterns of responses were felt to be discriminatory between various origins of pain, but analgesia followed most blocks, to some degree.

Evaluation

The greater occipital nerve is easily blocked and anesthetic efficacy is readily confirmed, but the diagnostic meaning of a favorable analgesic response is clouded by the lack of pathophysiologic understanding of cervicogenic headache.

SELECTIVE SYMPATHETIC BLOCKADE

Rationale

Sympathetic efferent activity is a suspected pathogenic component in a number of conditions. In some, the participation of sympathetic fibers is well documented, such as in hyperhidrosis. In other diseases, such as sudden sensory-neural hearing loss, peripheral vascular disease, dysrhythmia from long-QT syndrome, central pain,[211] pain following plexus injury, and trigeminal or post-herpetic neuralgia,[158] the diagnosis is clear but the role of sympathetic activity is uncertain and controversial. Finally, in a large category of poorly defined pain states which are grouped under the terms reflex sympathetic dystrophy or causalgia (complex regional pain syndrome Type I and II; see Chapter 23), a sympathetic contribution is suspected, because blood flow and trophic changes are evident, but the pathophysiology is largely obscure. In these settings, selective interruption of sympathetic neural traffic to the involved area may provide diagnostic insight and guidance of future therapy. If sympathetic block relieves pain, indicated therapies might include further local anesthetic blocks, systemic treatment with sympathetically active drugs (e.g., clonidine, prazocin), or destructive therapy with neurolytic injection or surgery. Failure of relief after sympathetic blockade would argue against the use of these treatments.

Peripheral to where the gray rami communicantes deliver postganglionic sympathetic fibers to the spinal nerves, somatic and sympathetic elements are intermixed within nerve trunks, so that both are affected by peripheral neural blockade. (The pathway to a cutaneous destination may not always be the same for sympathetic and sensory fibers, however.[54,154]) In contrast to peripheral nerves, the paravertebral sympathetic structures are separate anatomic routes which provide an opportunity for isolated sympathetic blockade. Diagnostic block seeks to determine the sympathetic contribution to disease by selective sympathetic interruption, while leaving somatic pathways intact (see Chapter 13). Although epidural or brachial plexus blocks, for instance, produce intense sympathetic blockade, changes in disease state during or after these procedures cannot clearly be attributed to somatic or sympathetic effects.

Techniques

The techniques and complications are described in Chapter 13. Several issues are specifically relevant to diagnostic use of the blocks.

Documentation of sympathectomy in the area of disease is essential if diagnostic conclusions are sought regarding sympathetic activity. Block is evident by sudomotor, vasomotor, and ocular changes (see Chapter 13). Since sympathetic activity is most intense in distal portions of the extremity, confirmation of blockade of sympathetic fibers to the arm and leg is best done by examination of sympathetic activity in the hand and foot, even if the symptomatic site is more proximal. The cervical trunk may be blocked independent of the stellate ganglion or fibers to the brachial plexus, so occurrence of ptosis, meiosis, facial anhydrosis, conjunctival hyperemia, or nasal stuffiness does not assure sympathetic block of fibers to the arm. Stellate, thoracic, or lumbar sympathetic injections that produce no measurable evidence of sympathetic blockade, reveal nothing about disease pathophysiology, regardless of the pain response.

Careful sensory examination, including the ability to distinguish nociceptive stimuli (e.g., scratch or pin-point) from touch, should precede and follow diagnostic sympathetic blockade. Otherwise, local anesthetic actions on nociceptive afferents could produce analgesia that is mistakenly viewed as evidence of a sympathetic mechanism.

Limitations

Stellate ganglion injection may fail to produce sympathetic denervation by several causes. Alternative routes allow sympathetic fibers to reach peripheral sites without transit through the stellate ganglion. These include passage in the nerves of Kuntz from the second and third intercostal nerves to the brachial plexus,[139,194] distribution via the carotid, subclavian, and vertebral arteries,[155,193,303] and direct entry to the peripheral nerves after entry into synapses outside the sympathetic chain in intermediate ganglia located in spinal nerve roots.[8] Sympathetic fibers probably can also bypass the sympathetic chain in the sinuvertebral nerve of Luschka.[330] As surgeons learned in previous decades, it is essentially impossible to achieve sympathetic denervation of the upper limb by a single surgical lesion or injection.

The principal reason for failure of injection to produce stellate ganglion blockade is lack of delivery of anesthetic to the ganglion. Whereas the ganglion resides at the lower edge of the head of the first rib,[159] solution injected at cervical levels passes anteriorly into the mediastinum.[142,160]

At lumbar levels, multiple pathways of sympathetic fibers include collateral chains[70,98] and crossover of fibers from the contralateral chain.[196,346,363] These alternative pathways may allow persistent sympathetic innervation to reach the lower extremities, despite a properly performed lumbar sympathetic block. Confusion can result if local anesthetic solution is conveyed to the epidural space through the fibrous tunnel along the waist of the vertebral body (see Chapter 13, Fig. 13–24). The undesired somatic blockade that ensues could produce analgesia, which is then attributed to a sympathetic mechanism.

The diagnostic utility of sympathetic blockade depends upon the ability to interfere selectively with sympathetic activity and to maintain continuity of somatic pathways. The stellate ganglion lies anterior to the anterior primary ramus of the first thoracic spinal nerve at a distance of about 1 cm. Since no fibrous barrier separates these structures, it is likely that local anesthetic delivered to the ganglion would have at least a partial blocking effect on the brachial plexus. Also, injection of solution into the paravertebral space readily enters the epidural space.[103] The only study examining detailed somatic sensory changes following sympathetic blocks found that nociceptive block without anesthesia was common.[74] A subtle somatic block with analgesia but intact sense of touch would create the impression of analgesia from sympathetic blockade if altered pain sensation is not identified specifically.

Blocks of the paravertebral sympathetic chain inevitably interrupt visceral afferent signals, as well as efferent sympathetic activity.[297] This could create a false conclusion about the source and mechanism of pain. For instance, a stellate ganglion block will stop arm pain from myocardial ischemia, but could be credited with identifying a sympathetically dependent pain process.

A fundamental limitation of diagnostic sympathetic blockade is a lack of understanding about the role of the sympathetic nervous system in pain production.[21,296] Evidence now indicates that excessive sympathetic activity almost certainly is not the explanation of pain.[59,65,90,287,327] The enigmatic pathophysiology and ambiguous definitions of reflex sympathetic dystrophy (RSD; complex regional pain syndrome [CRPS] type 1; see Chapter 23.2) and other painful conditions in which the sympathetic nervous system plays a putative role frustrate the interpretation and application of findings from blocks;[258] we really don't know what we are testing for (see Chapter 23.1, Fig. 23.1-8).

Studies

Rates of success in actually interrupting sympathetic activity following injections intended for that purpose are incompletely known. After cervical paratracheal injection, Warrick[345] observed that very few patients had warming of the hand. Carron and Litwiller[57] reported that a 3 ml injection produced a temperature increase of 1.5° C in all of more than 700 blocks. Using 15 ml of an equal mix of 1% lidocaine and 0.5% bupivacaine, Ready et al.[283] had 100% success in producing a Horner's syndrome, but 75% success in warming the ipsilateral hand by 1° C. Malmqvist et al.[222] observed an 87% success rate in producing Horner's syndrome, but 26 of 54 (48%) subjects with initial ipsilateral hand temperature of $\leq$32°C failed to warm to $\geq$34°C within 20 minutes. Only 11.5% of their blocks met five criteria of success; Horner's syndrome, increased hand temperature, $\geq$50% increase in skin blood flow, increased skin resistance ($\geq$13% baseline), and abolished skin resistance response. In 100 consecutive C6 anterior tubercle blocks in our clinic,[156] 84% resulted in a Horner's syndrome, indicative of at least some blockade of sympathetic fibers to the head. Only 60% caused the ipsilateral hand to warm by 1.5° C or more, and because the contra-lateral hand frequently warmed also, in only 27% did the ipsilateral hand warm by 1.5° C more than the contralateral hand. From these studies, it is apparent that sympathetic blockade is a variable result of stellate ganglion injections. There is little difference in the adequacy of sympathetic blockade by paravertebral injection at C7 level, compared with C6.[160,222,226,359] Injection through a needle placed at the head of the first rib requires CT guidance but assures successful blockade.[101]

Success rates for lumbar sympathetic block have not been determined except with use of phenol; with this, success in increasing the skin temperature >1° C was reported in 61 to 68% of patients.[146] Diagnostic sympathetic blocks are used most often to evaluate painful conditions (see Chapter 13). There is no histopathologic or serologic standard to confirm a sympathetic contribution to pain production, so there are few studies measuring the ability of blockade to diagnose accurately a sympathetic role. The reports that are available raise doubt as to whether analgesia after sympathetic blockade indicates a sympathetic contribution to pain. For example, the degree of sympathetic dysfunction does not correlate with the response of pain to sympathetic blockade,[211,320] and the timing of changes in pain do not necessarily match the onset of manifestations of sympathetic block. When sympathetic activity is measured with microelectrode neurography in limbs with pain relieved by local anesthetic sympathetic block, sympathetic efferent traffic is normal.[327] Response of pain to sympathetic blockade does not predict levels of norepinephrine and its metabolite in the venous effluent from limbs with features of reflex sympathetic dystrophy.[90] In fact, catecholamines are consistently fewer on the painful side than on the nonaffected side. These findings make less plausible the belief that sympathetic block analgesia identifies regional sympathetic hyperactivity. The important question of whether the response to sympathetic blockade guides therapy toward a better outcome has not been addressed in any formal way (see also Chapter 13).

Evaluation

Confusion surrounds many aspects of care for patients in whom pain or other dysfunction is suspected to be based in the sympathetic nervous system. Response to a block, therefore, offers an apparently concrete diagnostic insight. Considerations enumerated above, however, suggest that the diagnostic value of sympathetic blockade has been overestimated. Appropriate use calls for care in documenting the desired physiologic response and caution in interpretation of the results. We should avoid the circular logic of defining sympathetically maintained pain as conditions improved by sympathetic blocks, and the blocks defined as successful if they relieve a pain assumed to be sympathetically maintained.

INTRAVENOUS REGIONAL SYMPATHETIC BLOCK

Rationale

Intravenous regional (IVR) injection of both guanethidine[143] and bretylium[144] have been used therapeutically in patients with sympathetically maintained pain (see Chapters 12 and 13). Both drugs inhibit release of norepinephrine from nerve terminals, and guanethidine depletes tissues of norepinephrine. Since there is a period of regional sympathetic block lasting several hours or more following these procedures, the patient's response during the postblock period should be an indicator of the extent to which pain is mediated sympathetically.

Technique

With the patient supine, a tourniquet is placed on the upper arm or thigh, and intravenous catheter is placed in a vein in the hand or foot. The limb is elevated and exsanguinated by wrapping with an Esmarch bandage. The tourniquet is inflated to at least 100 torr above systolic pressure, the Esmarch is removed, and 20 to 30 mg guanethidine or 2 to 3 mg/kg bretylium in 40 ml normal saline is injected into the venous system. The tourniquet remains inflated for 15 to 30 minutes and is then released. Pain relief may occur while the cuff is still inflated or after deflation. Pain scores and sensory changes are noted before and after the block. Guanethidine often causes severe burning pain in patients with allodynia,[212,341] perhaps due to norepinephrine released with the onset of guanethidine action. Itching, piloerection, edema, or engorgement of the tissues in the injected area may also occur. Complications from systemic distribution following release of the cuff have not been observed.

Limitations

The ischemic block produced by the tourniquet may have a profound effect on certain types of pain (see following). It would seem reasonable, therefore, when using this technique diagnostically, to perform the procedure twice: once with guanethidine or bretylium and once with saline alone. A more profound or more prolonged response to the procedure done with the active drug would then indicate a sympathetic component to the pain.

Guanethidine has been demonstrated to affect CNS levels of serotonin and to have anticholinergic effects.[120] Local anesthetic affects are not reported, and local anesthetic IVR blockade has produced only brief relief of pain in patients who had prolonged relief following IVR guanethidine.[212]

Studies

IVR guanethidine predictably eliminates allodynia, but has no effects on other sensory function.[127,212] Increased peripheral temperature and blood flow follows IVR guanethidine but not IVR saline. Vasodilatation may be delayed by hours after cuff deflation, and complete blockade of vascular control is rare.[212] There is no temporal relationship between pain relief and manifestations of sympathetic blockade. This may be due to a vasodilatory action of guanethidine that is independent of effects on norepinephrine release.[1]

Bonelli et al.[39] found that IVR guanethidine was more effective in patients who exhibited dystrophic changes associated with RSD. Loh and Nathan[211] found that pain and sensory response was congruent in 9 of 10 painful limbs when comparing IVR guanethidine and local anesthetic sympathetic chain injections. There is a high correlation between relief of pain from intravenous phentolamine and from IVR guanethidine.[11] These cross-comparisons support the notion that each is producing analgesia by a common sympatholytic mechanism.

There is so far no confirmation of the diagnostic value of IVR sympathetic block for identifying patients who can be expected to have long-term therapeutic benefit from systemic or regional sympatholytic measures.

Evaluation

Analgesia following intravenous regional guanethidine or bretylium may in part confirm a sympathetic component of a given patient's pain, particularly if IVR placebo injection fails to do so. Information obtained from the procedure cannot be the sole means of diagnosis, but should be evaluated together with clinical findings and response to other diagnostic interventions, including paravertebral sympathetic blocks, or the phentolamine test.

PRESSURE AND ISCHEMIC DIFFERENTIAL EXTREMITY BLOCK

Rationale

Different fiber types convey a variety of painful sensations that are to a great degree unique to that neuronal category. First pain, produced by impulses in small myelinated $A\delta$ fibers, is prompt, well localized, and has a pricking and sharp character. Second pain, characteristic of nonmyelinated C fibers, is not felt in an exact location, has gradual onset and offset, and an aching quality. Pain invoked by soft touch of the skin (mechanical allodynia) probably is due to stimulation of fast conducting $A\beta$ fibers with subsequent aberrant central processing (see above). While the current importance of distinguishing fiber types subserving pain in a particular patient is largely academic, advances in the neuropharmacology of pain may produce therapies suitable only for certain pathophysiologic conditions, making distinctions of fiber types important. For example, it is likely that capsaicin, which depletes substance P from the skin terminals of C fibers, is effective only in treating pain due to unmyelinated fibers.

Nerve compression is the oldest reported means of producing differential interruption of sensory function, with initial documentation in 1855.[310] Whereas local anesthetics block peripheral nerve C fibers prior to $A\delta$ and $A\beta$[326] (see above), the reverse can be achieved either by direct focal pressure to the nerve or by a tourniquet which produces both compression of the nerve and ischemia of the limb. Both have a preferential effect upon transmission of myelinated fibers. Direct compression of the nerve is limited to sites in which the nerve can be pressed against bone, such as the superficial radial nerve at the wrist.[218,326] The psychophysical response to direct compression of a nerve is the same as tourniquet compression-ischemia,[67] which is more generally applicable.

The initial sensory event during compression and ischemia of a nerve is intense paresthesiae[237] due to paralysis of the Na^+/K^+ pump and depolarization of the axon. Fasciculations representing spontaneous activity in motor axons accompany only prolonged periods of nerve compression.[44] After about five minutes, conduction in ischemic nerves begins to fail in a decremental fashion, in which impulses travel progressively more slowly, and more limited distances, before failing.[248] Perception of soft touch fails after 5 to 20 minutes, soon followed by loss of sense of cold and first (sharp) pain. These three sensations may be difficult to separate reliably by compression-ischemia.[362] Sense of warmth is inhibited next. Second (aching) pain remains intact after the loss of warmth and may not be completely abolished by compression and ischemia.[218,310,361] Efferent sympathetic impulses persist unimpeded.[60]

Technique

Meticulous sensory testing should precede the block and be charted during the development of blockade. Direct pressure requires special equipment, and is not generally applicable. For compression-ischemia, an inflatable tourniquet is placed proximal to the site of extremity pain and inflated to a pressure 100 mm Hg above systolic arterial pressure after exsanguination of the limb by elevation. Findings usually are complete within 30 to 45 minutes. Complications are few, although ischemia may be uncomfortable and the tourniquet may not be tolerated on a sensitive extremity. Numbness has persisted for as long as one week after blockade.[218]

Studies

Persuasive confirmation of the differential specificity of compression and ischemic blockade has been provided by direct microneurographic recording of neuronal impulses.[67,218,326] These studies document that susceptibility is greatest for $A\beta$ and $A\delta$ fibers, while C fibers are resistant.

Elimination of sensory potentials recorded proximally from electrical stimulation also confirms that $A\beta$ afferents are blocked by ischemia while C fibers remain active.[60] Since the timing of electrophysiologically measured conduction block matches the changes of the particular sensory mode transmitted by each fiber type, standard neurologic testing is adequate to detect deactivation of the various fibers.

Compression-ischemic blockade has been used to identify algogenic impulse transmission by myelinated A fibers[53,132] and nonmyelinated C fibers[67,256] in painful conditions. In these studies, secondary confirmation by other block techniques and psychophysiologic manipulations has supported the accuracy of differential compression-ischemic block for identifying the fiber type conducting pain.

Evaluation

The physiologic accuracy of differential compression-ischemic block is based on thorough basic research. Practical utility of the test requires further developments in the taxonomy and neuropharmacology of pain.

DIFFERENTIAL NEURAXIAL BLOCK

Rationale

The purpose of differential spinal or epidural block is to provide diagnostic information for patients with lower extremity and/or lower trunk pain.[6,230,276] In the classic approach, a placebo is injected first, followed by a local anesthetic solution capable of selectively blocking sympathetic efferents. If no relief is achieved, a concentration capable of producing sensory blockade is injected. If this produces no pain relief, a solution is then injected that will block motor fibers as well. The changes in pain during the different phases of the block indicate whether the pain is labeled as psychogenic, sympathetic, nociceptive (sensory based), or central.

Technique

A subarachnoid site of injection has been used most extensively. The block is performed with the patient in the lateral decubitus position. A spinal needle is placed in lumbar subarachnoid space. Blood pressure and pulse are checked at frequent intervals. Prior to the initial injection and 10 to 15 minutes after each successive injection is performed, the following observations are made in an identical manner:

1. A verbal and/or visual analog pain score is recorded; if possible, mechanical reproduction of pain (passive movement of legs, pressure over tender points) should be done.
2. Skin temperature of the lower extremities is recorded; other measures of sympathetic function, e.g., galvanic skin response, may be done.
3. Sensory and motor testing of the lower extremities is done.

Following placement of the subarachnoid needle, injections are made at 10-minute intervals using the following solutions:

1. Placebo: 5 ml isotonic saline
2. Sympathetic block: 10 ml 0.2% procaine
3. Sensory block: 10 ml 0.5% procaine
4. Motor block: 10 ml 1.0% procaine

If pain relief occurs after placebo injection, this is interpreted as a placebo response. Some authors interpret a placebo response to be evidence of a psychogenic pain mechanism, particularly if relief is prolonged. If the analgesia is brief, it is reasonable to continue on to step 2 (sympathetic blocking anesthetic concentration) and to compare the degree and duration of pain relief to that obtained following saline injection.

Interpretation of response to 0.2% procaine can be made only if there is evidence of sympathetic blockade and no evidence of sensory block (the authors have found this to occur in a relatively small proportion of individuals). If there is indeed pain relief and a differential effect on sympathetic function, this provides evidence of sympathetically maintained pain.

If pain relief occurs following the onset of sensory blockade after injection of 0.5% procaine, this is interpreted as evidence of a somatic mechanism of pain. If pain relief occurs only after the injection of 1% procaine, this again is interpreted as evidence of a somatic mechanism. The higher concentration is thought to be required in some patients because a more complete sensory block is required to relieve the pain, or because motor activity in some way contributes to the clinical pain.

If no relief occurs despite complete motor and sensory blockade, the interpretation is that the pain is of a central mechanism. The possible causes of central pain include:

1. A CNS lesion of the upper spinal cord or brain;
2. Self-sustaining neural activity in the CNS above the level blocked;
3. Psychogenic pain; and
4. Malingering.

A major drawback to the differential spinal block is the prolonged time required to perform and assess the individual steps. In a modified technique,[7] only 2 steps are required. The first is the placebo (saline) injection, as described above. Subsequently, 100 mg procaine (2 ml 5%) is injected intrathecally. Pain relief following placebo response or lack of pain relief from procaine is interpreted as is done in the classical technique. If the patient experiences pain relief after the procaine injection, the timing of the return of sensation is noted. If the return of pain is coincident with the return of sensation to pin prick, the interpretation is that the pain is somatic in origin. If pain relief persists until or beyond the return of sympathetic function, the interpretation is that the pain is sympathetically mediated.

An epidural technique also has been used in a fashion similar to the subarachnoid method.[64] Following a placebo injection of saline, 0.25% lidocaine is injected to block sympathetic fibers, then 0.5% lidocaine to block sensation as well, and finally 1% lidocaine to produce surgical anesthesia.

A preliminary report has suggested the use of opioid instead of local anesthetic as the analgesic agent,[64] arguing that opioid effects are more specific and don't provide a cue of numbness or warmth to trigger placebo or psychogenic responses. Following placebo injections, fentanyl 1 μg/kg in 5 ml normal saline is injected through an epidural catheter. Analgesia indicates a predominantly physical basis for pain, as does reversal of the analgesia by intravenous injection of naloxone 0.4 mg, unobserved by the subject. Finally, local anesthetic blockade with concentrated lidocaine serves the same purpose as that described in the method above.

Limitations

There are a number of possible drawbacks to the traditional technique of differential spinal. Even early descriptions of the technique report that either pain fibers or sympathetic fibers may be blocked first,[293] and that the injected solutions may fail to provide the desired block.[6,230] The entire premise is flawed without the ability to achieve a steady state block of certain fiber types while sparing others in the desired order. As discussed above, lack of obvious sensory changes does not assure that neural processing has not been altered, and a dense block adequate for surgery does not indicate an absence of afferent sensory traffic or efferent sympathetic impulses. Neurophysiologic study of awake humans, and analysis of conduction in various laboratory preparations, consistently point to the impossibility of complete block of one fiber type without at least partial block of others.

Further considerations erode the theoretic plausibility of diagnostic differential blockade. When nociceptive afferent fibers are active, as may occur with spontaneous discharge arising from an injured peripheral nerve or from persistent discharge of a nociceptor by a noxious stimulus, they may be subject to use-dependent block and be more affected by low concentrations of anesthetic than normal afferents that are quiescent. Additionally, sub-blocking concentrations of local anesthetics are capable of reducing the maximum firing rates of axons.[279] Since pain induced by nociceptor activation is proportional to firing frequency, a modest reduction in the firing frequency could result in diminished pain. In both instances, while evidence of sensory block is not detected by sensory testing, pain relief from blockade of nociceptor fibers may be achieved and pain relief may be attributed mistakenly to sympathetic blockade. While the one-shot technique has the advantage that it is not dependent upon achieving a critical concentration of anesthetic in the CSF, it does depend on the premise that both A and C fibers recover function before B fibers, which is probably incorrect (see previously).

Even if a true differential block of sympathetic fibers were documented, there are a number of potential causes for uninterpretable responses or misinterpretation: (i) patients who fail to obtain relief from subarachnoid 0.5% or 1% procaine actually may experience an increase in activity of some spinal cord neurons, because of blockade of certain afferent or spinal cord pathways. For instance, A fibers, including Aβ fibers, may be blocked by a concentration of anesthetic that spares C fibers,[110] reducing the inhibitory effect of large afferent activity on dorsal horn neurons. (ii) Intrathecal local anesthetic may block descending inhibitory fibers lying superficially in the dorsolateral funiculus,[14] again producing disinhibition. (iii) The fact that pain returns after pin-prick sensation does not necessarily imply a sympathetic mechanism. Prolonged pain relief has been described after local anesthetic blocks in conditions other than sympathetic dystrophy.[10] Such prolonged effects may be related to changes in central processing. The temporary reduction in sensory input may allow sensitized dorsal horn neurons to return to more normal function, and it may take considerable time before noxious inputs can re-establish spinal cord sensitization. (iv) There is no way to assess pain in any position other than lateral recumbent, ruling out any diagnostic benefit for patients whose pain improves when lying down or is activity-dependent. (v) Anatomic consideration makes unlikely a uniform progression of block from sympathetic to sensory. Specifically, complete block of roots caudal to L2 will provide sensory interruption but leave sympathetic fibers unaffected,[24] since all white rami communicantes exit the cord between T1 and L2.

Failure of pain to respond to neuraxial opioid does not necessarily indicate that the pain has a psychogenic etiology, since pain with other origins, such as neuropathic and visceral pain or incident pain with movement, may also be resistant to spinal and epidural opioid.[12,161] Additionally, systemic naloxone is not likely to reverse completely the analgesic effects of neuraxial opioids.[277]

Studies

Despite claims that differential spinal block leads to selection of more effective treatment,[276] there have been no outcome studies to document this belief. Specifically, there are no data documenting higher success rates from repeated sympathetic blocks among patients who experienced relief after 0.25% procaine, compared to patients exhibiting other responses. Sanders et al.[292] examined the relationship between the presence of psychopathology and the incidence of inappropriate responses to differential spinal. They concluded that psychopathology was no more likely among inappropriate responders.

Evaluation

There is minimal evidence to support the ability of differential neuraxial blocks to distinguish the pathophysiologic origin of painful conditions. Current concepts of neurophysiology and local anesthetic action make it unlikely that a predictable and truly selective block can be achieved in a clinical setting.

SYSTEMIC MEDICATIONS

Local Anesthetics

Rationale

A selective action of intravenous lidocaine has been proposed because it often provides temporary relief of neuropathic pain, but is generally ineffective for nociceptive pain (see previous). Therefore it could be used as a means of distinguishing the pathophysiology of a painful condition. Since lidocaine is structurally analogous with oral agents tocainide and mexiletine, response to intravenous lidocaine may be helpful also in predicting which patients with neuropathic pain will gain analgesia from a therapeutic course of these oral sodium channel blockers.

Technique

When using intravenous lidocaine to determine possible response to oral mexiletine, a lidocaine infusion is prepared. Initially, pain is assessed using a Visual Analogue Scale (VAS) and sensory testing is carried out to determine the degree of allodynia. A saline infusion is then begun. After five minutes, the VAS and sensory testing is repeated. The placebo testing should be repeated over another 5-to-10-minute interval, then 2 mg/kg lidocaine is infused over a five-minute period. This is followed by a constant infusion of 50 μg/kg/min which is continued for 30 minutes. VAS scores and sensory testing are repeated at the end of the initial bolus dose and several times during the steady-state infusion. If at any time the patient begins to experience symptoms of local anesthetic toxicity (tinnitus, dizziness, tremor, etc.), the infusion is terminated. Blood pressure, heart rate, and electrocardiogram (ECG) are monitored during the infusion. Other authors use as little as 1.5 mg/kg in a single bolus with no infusion,[223] or as much as 5 mg/kg over 30 minutes.[13,97,181] A computer-controlled infusion pump, using pharmacokinetic parameters, has been reported to result in predictable plasma lidocaine concentration for neuropathic pain.[295]

Studies

Systemic lidocaine analgesic effects on pain with different mechanisms was tested in a study of five patients with a variety of central and peripheral neuropathic pain.[28] Ischemic pain of comparable intensity was induced in an uninvolved arm. Both pains responded to the high blood lidocaine concentrations (average 5.6 μg/ml) which immediately followed 3 mg/kg lidocaine IV over three minutes, but the clinical pain showed significantly greater analgesia than did the ischemic pain. The lower concentrations of lidocaine, (1.5 to 2.0 μg/ml), which followed infusions of 4 mg/min relieved only the clinical pain. Mild symptoms of toxicity developed during the infusion in two subjects. Another study[289] similarly found that low concentrations of lidocaine achieved during infusions at a rate of 60 μg/kg/min or less fail to alter perception of experimentally produced pain. These results indicate there is a mild general systemic analgesic effect with high blood concentrations of lidocaine, but selective analgesia of central and peripheral neuropathic pain can be expected with lower lidocaine concentrations.

In another placebo-controlled and blinded study,[223] 10 patients with chronic neuropathic pain were given saline or lidocaine 1.5 mg/kg IV over one minute and sensory changes were evaluated. There were minimal effects after saline but pain relief for 15 to 30 minutes was noted in all subjects after lidocaine, including allodynia to cold and mechanical stimuli, as well as Tinel's sign. Four patients felt lightheaded and dizzy. While this report documents the efficacy of systemic lidocaine in producing analgesia for neuropathic pain, it does not demonstrate a selective effect preferentially upon neuropathic pain, and so does not support a diagnostic use.

Two papers have reported relief from oral mexiletine in patients who previously responded to IV lidocaine.[263,302] Randomized and controlled studies, however, have not been done to test the ability of systemic lidocaine to predict the response to mexiletine.

Evaluation

Intravenous lidocaine may be of some diagnostic value in distinguishing between neuropathic and nociceptive pain, although the therapeutic implications of such a distinction may be quite limited. Intravenous lidocaine may be helpful in predicting response to oral sodium channel blockers, but this remains to be proved by controlled studies.

Phentolamine

Rationale

Action of endogenous catecholamines upon peripheral sensory afferent neurons has been proposed as a mechanism by which sympathetic efferent activity provokes pain.[273] Analgesia which accompanies intravenous infusion of phentolamine, an α adrenergic blocking agent, has been claimed to indicate that a component of a patient's pain is sympathetically mediated. This method has the diagnostic advantage over local anesthetic sympathetic blocks in that it does not interrupt afferent traffic from visceral or somatic structures. Although sudomotor function is mediated by cholinergic transmission and therefore is not affected by adrenergic blockade, sudomotor activity does not play an important role in pain generation.[128] Response to IV phentolamine should identify patients who can expect a beneficial response to intermittent or continuous local anesthetic sympathetic blocks, or to oral or transdermal sympatholytic drugs.

Technique

The patient is placed supine and an intravenous line is placed. Sensory testing is performed to determine the severity and extent of allodynia, and a VAS pain rating is obtained. Sensory testing and VAS ratings are repeated five minutes after each placebo or phentolamine injection. Blood pressure and heart rate are monitored throughout the testing period, and skin temperature of the affected and contralateral extremity are recorded continuously. An infusion of normal saline is begun, and 500 ml is infused over a 30-minute period. Some authors recommend administration of propranolol 1 mg IV if the heart rate is greater than 70 min^{-1}. Bolus injections of saline are given at the beginning of the infusion and 15 and 30 minutes later. At five-minute intervals, the following doses of phentolamine are administered: 1 mg, 2 mg, 3 mg, 5 mg, 7 mg, and 10 mg. Whenever substantial relief of pain is obtained or significant hypotension occurs, the test is terminated.[11,273]

If phentolamine produces evidence of sympathetic block such as nasal congestion, hypotension, or skin warming, absence of concurrent pain relief indicates no sympathetic contribution. If placebo produces no analgesia but phentolamine does, a sympathetic role is suspected. The appearance of an increase in skin temperature coincident with pain relief provides added assurance of the diagnosis. The procedure is safe, with predictable nasal stuffiness and occasional sinus tachycardia, premature ventricular contractions, dizziness, or wheezing.[304] The safety of reduced doses of phentolamine has been confirmed in children.[11] Subjects with advanced cardiovascular disease such as heart block, unstable angina, or congestive heart failure probably are not suitable for the test.

Limitations

Phentolamine has been shown to have local anesthetic properties,[254,274] which raises the question of whether relief could be by pharmacologic mechanisms other than sympathetic block. As with other tests of sympathetic function, a fundamental limitation is the ambiguous role of sympathetic function in pain. The role of α receptors is uncertain.[258] Even though a patient experiences relief from IV phentolamine, oral sympathetic blocking drugs may be ineffective because side effects, particularly orthostatic hypotension, may preclude intense blockade comparable to the potent effect of intravenous phentolamine.

Studies

Raja et al.[273] administered intravenous phentolamine, 25 to 35 mg in incremental bolus doses, and, on another occasion, local anesthetic sympathetic blocks to 20 patients with suspected sympathetically maintained pain. When comparisons were made of the maximum pain relief from the two procedures, they found a high degree of correlation. Patients generally experienced relief of both spontaneous and evoked pain (allodynia). Only three patients had relief from saline, an extraordinarily low incidence of placebo response (see previous). Arner[11] found that 33% of 48 patients tested with intravenous phentolamine (5 to 15 mg) experienced relief of pain. All of the patients who had relief with phentolamine experienced a reduction in pain with intravenous regional guanethidine, while only 1 of 12 patients who failed the phentolamine test had relief from guanethidine. Overall, they found a false positive rate of 0% and a false negative rate of 32% if guanethidine relief is assumed to indicate presence of disease (sympathetically maintained pain).

Shir et al.[304] found relief from phentolamine infusion in 25% of pain patients with clinical evidence of a sympathetic contribution. The low response rates in this and the study by Arner et al.[11] are at or below typical placebo response rates. Several authors[109,335] caution that placebo responses may require 15 to 60 minutes to become evident. If adequate time is allowed, phentolamine-induced analgesia does not differ from placebo response[335] and placebo analgesia is observed in all subjects, making the phentolamine test impossible to administer.[109] No studies have been carried out that determine the relationship of response to IV phentolamine with the response to repeated or continuous local anesthetic blocks or to systemic sympathetic blocking agents.

Studies typically report administration of phentolamine to a predetermined dose, rather than until a physiologic effect (nasal congestion, hypotension, skin warming) is achieved. Without such an end point, it is not possible to distinguish inadequate phentolamine dose from a lack of α receptor involvement in the pain generation.

Evaluation

Intravenous phentolamine appears to correlate well with responses to local anesthetic paravertebral sympathetic blocks and guanethidine intravenous regional sympathetic blocks. It is not clear, however, that either of these are an acceptable standard of pure and complete sympathetic interruption (see sections in this chapter on these blocks). Response to phentolamine should be considered in conjunction with clinical findings and other diagnostic tests. Considered alone, it may not be very sensitive or specific. The ability of the phentolamine response to predict outcome of therapy with sympatholytic treatments has not been tested. It is not clear how using a phentolamine trial would improve upon a simple trial of oral therapy in the first place.

Barbiturates

Rationale

Small intravenous doses of rapidly acting barbiturates have been used in psychiatric practice to promote a state of relaxation to facilitate communication of thoughts.[180] In the diagnosis of pain, a light hypnotic state may be used to discern the contribution of cognitive and emotional issues in pain behavior. For instance, a limb that relaxes or allodynia that dissipates with sedation may be due to psychological factors such as anxiety, hysterical conversion, or malingering. Non-nociceptive pain, such as pain related to CNS injury, often is relieved by subanesthetic barbiturate doses.[42]

Technique

Even if a detailed psychiatric interview is not planned, it probably is wise to perform a barbiturate test with a psychiatrist present who has experience with the technique. Thiopental is injected intravenously in 50 mg increments. The patient is instructed to give a verbal pain score or to relate the degree of pain relief after each dose. Response to provocative stimuli during the hypnotic state are compared to baseline responses. Doses are repeated until there is either an increase or a decrease in pain, or until the patient becomes too drowsy to cooperate.

Limitations

Because of the complex involvement of cerebral activity and the conscious mind in the production and manifestation of pain, and the resulting behavior, changes during barbiturate administration are very difficult to interpret. Small doses of intravenous barbiturates are reported to cause an increase in pain that has a nociceptive basis.[43] This anti-analgesic effect has been demonstrated in pressure algometry studies[50] and may be related to the ability of these drugs to interfere with descending inhibitory mechanisms through a medullary GABA receptor mechanism.[89] The physician should be prepared for the occasional exposure of a distressing, disruptive, and previously unrecognized psychosis during barbiturate administration.

Evaluation

The diagnostic utility of this technique has not been tested. Given its purely empirical basis and the inexact nature of the information obtained, it would seem unwise to attach much significance to data collected from this procedure.

REFERENCES

1. Abboud, F.M., and Eckstein, J.W.: Vasodilator action of guanethidine. Circ. Res., *11:*788, 1962.
2. Abram, S.E.: Pain mechanisms in lumbar radiculopathy. Anesth. Analg., *67:*1135, 1988.
3. Abram, S.E., and Boas, R.A.: Sympathetic and visceral nerve blocks. *In* Benumof, J.L. (ed.): Clin. Proc. Anesth. Intensive Care. pp. 796–805. Philadelphia, J.B. Lippincott, 1992.
4. Abram, S.E., and Yaksh, T.L.: Systemic lidocaine blocks nerve injury-induced hyperalgesia and nociceptor-driven spinal sensitization in the rat. Anesthesiology, *80:*383, 1994.
5. Adams, M.A., Dolan, P., and Hutton, W.C.: The stages of disc degeneration as revealed by discograms. J. Bone Joint Surg., *68*(B):36, 1986.
6. Ahlgren, E.W., Stephen, C.R., Lloyd, E.A.C., and McCollum, D.E.: Diagnosis of pain with a graduated spinal block technique. J.A.M.A., *195:*125, 1966.
7. Akkineni, S.R., and Ramamurthy, S.: Simplified differential spinal block. ASA Ann. Mtg. (Abstr.), 765, 1977.
8. Alexander, W., Kuntz, A., Henderson, W., and Ehrlich, E.: Sympathetic ganglion cells in ventral nerve roots: Their relation to sympathectomy. Science, *109:*484, 1949.
9. Aprill, C., and Bogduk, N.: The prevalence of cervical zygapophyseal joint pain: A first approximation. Spine, *17:*744, 1992.
10. Arner, S., Lindblom, U., Meyerson, B.A., and Molander, C.: Prolonged relief of neuralgia after regional anesthetic blocks: A call for further experimental and systematic clinical studies. Pain, *43:*287, 1990.
11. Arner, S.: Intravenous phentolamine test: Diagnostic and prognostic use in reflex sympathetic dystrophy. Pain, 46:17, 1991.
12. Arner, S., and Arner, B.: Differential effects of epidural morphine in the treatment of cancer related pain, Acta Anaesthsiol. Scand., *29:*32, 1985.
13. Bach, F.W., Jensen, T.S., and Kastrup, J., *et al.*: The effects of intravenous lidocaine on nociceptive processing in diabetic neuropathy. Pain, *40:*29, 1990.
14. Basbaum, A.I., and Fields, H.L.: Endogenous pain control systems: Brainstem spinal pathways and endorphin circuitry. Ann. Rev. Neurosci., *7:*309, 1984.
15. Barnsley, L., Lord, S., and Bogduk, N.: Comparative local anaesthetic blocks in the diagnosis of cervical zygapophysial joint pain. Pain, *55:*99, 1993.
16. Barnsley, L., and Bogduk, N.: Medial branch blocks are specific for the diagnosis of cervical zygapophyseal joint pain. Reg. Anesth., *18:*242, 1993.
17. Barnsley, L., Lord, S., Wallis, B., and Bogduk, N.: False-positive rates of cervical zygapophyseal joint blocks. Clin. J. Pain., *9:*124, 1993.
18. Beecher, H.K.: The powerful placebo. J.A.M.A., *159:*1602, 1955.
19. Bengtsson, M., Löfström, J.B., and Malmqvist, L-Å.: Skin conduction changes during spinal analgesia. Acta Anaesthesiol. Scand., *29:*67, 1985.
20. Bengtsson, M., Nilsson, G.E., and Löfström, J.B.: The effect of spinal analgesia on skin blood flow, evaluated by laser Doppler flowmetry. Acta Anaesthesiol. Scand., *17:*206, 1983.
21. Bennet, G.: The role of the sympathetic nervous system in painful peripheral neruopathy. Pain, *45:*221, 1991.
22. Benson, H., and McCallie, D.P.: Angina pectoris and the placebo effect. N. Engl. J. Med., *300:*1424, 1979.
23. Benzon, H., Cheng, S., Avram, M., and Molloy, R.: Sign of complete sympathetic blockade: Sweat test or sympathogalvanic response. Anesth. Analg., *64:*415, 1985.
24. Benzon, H.T.: Caution in interpreting modified differential spinal anesthesia: Does sympathetic block always persist after recovery of motor and sensory modalities? Reg. Anesth., *9:*156, 1983.
25. Bergman, R.A., Thompson, S.A., Afifi, A., and Saadeh, F.A.: Compendium of Human Anatomic Variation. Baltimore, Urban and Schwarzenberg, 1988.
26. Blumberg, H., and Janig, W.: Discharge pattern of afferent fibers from a neuroma. Pain, *20:*335, 1984.
27. Blume, H., Kakolewski, J., Richardson, R., and Rojas, C.: Radiofrequency denaturation in occipital pain: Results in 450 cases. Appl. Neurophysiol., *45:*543, 1982.
28. Boas, R.A., and Shahnarian, A.: Analgesic responses to IV lidocaine. Br. J. Anaesth., *54:*501, 1982.
29. Boden, S.D., Davis, D.O., Dina, T.S., Patronas, N.J., and Wiesel, S.W.: Abnormal magnetic-resonance scans of the lumbar spine in asymptomatic subjects. J. Bone Joint Surg., *72*(A):403, 1990.
30. Bogduk, N.: The innervation of the lumbar spine. Spine, *8:*286, 1983.
31. Bogduk, N., and Engel, R.: The menisci of the lumbar zygapophyseal joints. Spine, *9:*454, 1984.
32. Bogduk, N., and Long, D.M.: The anatomy of the so-called "articular nerves" and their relationship to facet denervation in the treatment of low-back pain. J. Neurosurg., *51:*172, 1979.
33. Bogduk, N.: The clinical anatomy of cervical dorsal rami. Spine, *4:*319, 1982.
34. Bogduk, N.: The innervation of the lumbar spine. Spine, *8:*286, 1983.
35. Bogduk, N., Tynan, W., and Wilson, A.S.: The nerve supply to the human lumbar intervertebral discs. Acta Anat., *132:*39, 1981.
36. Bogduk, N., and Aprill, C.: On the nature of neck pain, discography, and cervical zygapophyseal joint blocks. Pain, *54:*213, 1993.
37. Bogduk, N., and Marsland, A.: The cervical zygopophysial joints as a source of neck pain. Spine, *13:*610, 1988.
38. Bogduk, N.: The anatomy of occipital neuralgia. Clin. Exp. Neurol., *17:*167, 1981.
39. Bonelli, S., Conoscente, F., Movilia, B.G., Restelli, L., Francucci, B., and Grossi, E.: Regional intravenous guanethidine vs stellate ganglion block in reflex sympathetic dystrophies. A randomized trial. Pain, *16:*297, 1983.
40. Bonica, J.J.: The Management of Pain. 2nd Ed. pp. 133–146. Philadelphia, Lea and Febiger, 1990.
41. Bonica, J.J.: The Management of Pain. pp. 1200. Philadelphia, Lea and Febiger, 1953.
42. Bonica, J.J., and Loeser, J.D.: Pain resulting from central nervous system pathology. *In* Bonica, J.J. (ed.): The Management of Pain. pp. 271–272. Philadelphia, Lea and Febiger, 1990.
43. Bonica, J.J., and Loeser, J.D.: Medical evaluation of the patient with pain. *In* Bonica, J.J. (ed.): The Management of Pain. 2nd Ed., pp. 570–571. Philadelphia, Lea and Febiger, 1990.
44. Bostock, H., Baker, M., Grafe, P., and Reid, G.: Changes in excitability and accommodation of human motor axons following brief periods of ischemia. J. Physiol., (Lond), *441:*537, 1991.
45. Bovim, G., Berg, R., and Dale, L.G.: Cervicogenic headache: Anesthetic blockades of cervical nerves (C2-C5) and facet joint (C2-C3). Pain, *49:*315, 1992.
46. Bovim, G., Bonamico, L., Fredriksen, T.A., *et al.*: Topographic variations in the peripheral course of the greater occipital nerve. Spine, *16:*475, 1991.
47. Bovim, G., Fredriksen, T.A., Stolt-Nielsen, A., and Sjaastad, O.: Neurolysis of the greater occipital nerve in cervicogenic headache: A follow-up study. Headache, *32:*175, 1992.
48. Bovim, G., and Sand, T.: Cervicogenic headache, migraine without aura and tension-type headache: Diagnostic blockade of greater occipital and supraorbital nerves. Pain, *51:*43, 1992.
49. Bowen, V., and Cassidy, J.D.: Macroscopic and microscopic anatomy of the sacroiliac joint from embryonic life until the eighth decade. Spine, *6:*620, 1981.
50. Briggs, L.P., Dundee, J.W., Bahar, M., and Clarke, R.S.J.: Comparison of the effect of diisopropyl phenol (ICI 35868) and thiopentone on response to somatic pain. Br. J. Anaesth., *54:*307, 1982.
51. Butler, D., Trafimow, J.H., Andersson, G.B.J., McNeill, T.W., and Hackman, M.S.: Discs degenerate before facets. Spine, *15:*111, 1990.
52. Campbell, D.G., and Parsons, C.M.: Referred head pain and its concomitants. J. Nerv. Ment. Dis., *99:*544, 1944.
53. Campbell, J.N., Raja, S.N., Meyer, R.A., and Mackinnon, S.E.: Myelinated afferents signal the hyperalgesia associated with nerve injury. Pain, *32:*89, 1988.
54. Campero, M., Verdugo, R.J., and Ochoa, J.L.: Vasomotor innervation of the skin of the hand: A contribution to the study of human anatomy. J. Anat., *182:*361, 1993.
55. Carette, S., Marcoux, S., Truchon, R., *et al.*: A controlled trial of corticosteroid injection into facet joints for chronic low back pain. N. Engl. J. Med., *325:*1002, 1991.
56. Carrera, G.F.: Lumbar facet joint injection in low back pain and sciatica: Preliminary results. Radiology, *137:*665, 1980.
57. Carron, H., and Litwiller, R. Stellate ganglion block. Anesth. Analg., *54:*567, 1975.

59. Casale, R., and Elam, M.: Normal sympathetic nerve activity in a reflex sympathetic dystrophy with marked skin vasoconstriction. Pain, *41:*215, 1992.
60. Casale, R., Glynn, C., and Buonocore, M.: The role of ischaemia in the analgesia which follows Bier's block technique. Pain, *50:*169, 1992.
61. Cavanaugh, J.M., El-Bohy, A, Hardy, W.N., *et al.*: Sensory innervation of soft tissues of the lumbar spine in the rat. J. Orthop. Res., *7:*378, 1989.
62. Chabal, C., Russell, L.C., and Burchiel, K.J.: The effect of intravenous lidocaine, tocainide, and mexilitene on spontaneously active fibers originating in rat sciatic neuromas. Pain, *38:*333, 1989.
64. Cherry, D.A., Gourlay, G.K., McLachlan, M., and Cousins, M.J.: Diagnostic epidural opioid blockade and chronic pain: Preliminary report. Pain, *21:*143, 1985.
65. Christensen, K., and Hendriksen, O.: The reflex sympathetic dystrophy syndrome. Scand. J. Rheumatol., *12:*263, 1983.
66. Citron, M.L.: Placebos and principles: A trial of ondansetron. Ann. Intern. Med., *118:*470, 1993.
67. Cline, M.A., Ochoa, J., and Torebjork, H.E.: Chronic hyperalgesia and skin warming caused by sensitized C-nociceptors. Brain, *112:*621, 1989.
68. Colhoun, E., McCall, I.W., Williams, L., and Cassar Pullicino, V.N.: Provocation discography as a guide to planning operations on the spine. J. Bone Joint Surg., *70*(B):267, 1988.
69. Collis, J.S., and Gardner, W.J.: Lumbar discography: An analysis of one thousand cases. J. Neurosurg., *19:*452, 1962.
70. Cowley, R.A., and Yeager, G.H.: Anatomic observations on the lumbar sympathetic nervous system. Surgery, *25:*880, 1949.
71. Cuello, A.C., and Matthews, M.R.: Peptides in the peripheral sensory nerve fibers. *In* Melzack, R., and Wall, P.D. (eds.): Textbook of Pain. pp. 65. New York, Churchill Livingstone, 1984.
72. Cyriax, J.: Rheumatic headache. Br. Med. J., *2:*1367, 1938.
73. Dellemijn, P.L.I., Fields, H.L., Allen, R.R., McKay, W.R., and Rowbotham, M.C.: The interpretation of pain relief and sensory changes following sympathetic blockade. Brain, *117:*1475, 1994.
74. Dellemijn, P.L.I., Allen, R.R., Rowbotham, M.C., and Fields, H.L.: Modulatory influence of the sympathetic nervous system on thermal thresholds and thermal pain as assessed with quantitative sensory testing. Brain, *117:*1475, 1994.
75. Derby, R., Kine, G., Saal, J.A., *et al.*: Response to steroid and duration of radicular pain as predictors of surgical outcome. Spine, *17:*S176, 1992.
76. de Sousa, P.A.: The innervation of the veins: Its role in pain, venospasm and collateral circulation. Surgery, *19:*731, 1946.
77. Destouet, J.M., Gilula, L.A., Murphey, W.A., and Monsees, B.: Lumbar facet joint injection: Indication, technique, clinical correlation, and preliminary results. Radiology, *145:*321, 1982.
78. Devor, M., Wall, P.D., and Catalan, N.: Systemic lidocaine silences neuroma and DRG discharge without blocking nerve conduction. Pain, *48:*261, 1992.
79. Devor, M., and Janig, W.: Activation of myelinated afferents ending in neuroma by stimulation of the sympathetic supply in the rat. Neurosci. Lett., *24:*43, 1981.
80. Devor, M.: Central changes mediating neuropathic pain. *In* Dubner, R., Gebharrt, G.F., and Bond, M.R. (eds.): Proceedings of the 5th World Congress on Pain. pp. 114–128. Amsterdam, Elsevier, 1988.
82. Devor, M.: What's in a laser beam for pain therapy? Pain, *43:*139, 1990.
83. Dhume, V.G., Agshikar, N.V., and Diniz, R.S.: Placebo-induced side effects in healthy volunteers. Clinician, *39:*289, 1975.
84. Dooley, J.F., McBroom, R.J., Taguchi, T., and MacNab, I.: Nerve root infiltration in the diagnosis of radicular pain. Spine, *13:*79, 1988.
85. Dory, M.A.: Arthrography of the cervical facet joints. Radiology, *148:*379, 1983.
86. Dory, M.A.: Arthrography of the lumbar facet joints. Radiology, *140:*23, 1981.
87. Dreyfuss, P., Dryer, S., Griffin, J., Hoffman, J., and Walsh, N.: Positive sacroiliac screening tests in asymptomatic adults. Spine, *19:*1138, 1994.
88. Dreyfuss, P., Michaelsen, M., and Fletcher, D.: Atlanto-occipital and lateral atlanto-axial joint pain patterns. Spine, *19:*1125, 1994.
89. Drower, E.J., and Hammond, D.L.: GABAergic modulation of nociceptive threshold: Effects of THIP and bicuculline microinjected in the ventral medulla of the rat. Brain Res., *450:*316, 1988.
90. Drummond, P.D., Finch, P.M., and Smythe, G.A.: Reflex sympathetic dystrophy: The significance of differing plasma catecholamine concentrations in affected and unaffected limbs. Brain, *114:*2025, 1991.
91. Dubner, R., Hoffman, D., and Hayes, R.: Neuronal activity in medullary dorsal horn of awake monkeys trained in a thermal discrimination task. III. Task-related responses and their functional role. J. Neurophysiol., *46:*444, 1981.
92. Dunlop, R.B., Adams, M.A., and Hutton, W.S-C.: Disc space narrowing and the lumbar facet joints. J. Bone Joint Surg., *66*(B):706, 1984.
93. Dwyer, A., Aprill, C., and Bogduk, N.: Cervical zygapophyseal joint pain patterns I: A study in normal volunteers. Spine, *15:*453, 1990.
94. Edgar, M.A., and Ghadially, J.A.: Innervation of the lumbar spine. Clin. Orthop., *115:*35, 1976.
96. Edmeads, J.: The cervical spine and headache. Neurology, *38:*1874, 1988.
97. Edwards, W.T., Habib, F., Burney, R.G., and Begin, G.: Intravenous lidocaine in the management of various chronic pain states. Reg. Anesth., *10:*1, 1985.
98. Edwards, E.: Operative anatomy of the lumbar sympathetic chain. Angiology, *2:*184, 1951.
99. El-Bohy, A., Cavanaugh, J.M., Getchell, M.L., *et al.*: Localization of substance P and neurofilament immunoreactive fibers in the lumbar facet joint capsule and supraspinous ligament of the rabbit. Brain Res., *460:*379, 1988.
100. Epstein, J.A., Epstein, B.S., Lavine, L.S., *et al.*: Lumbar nerve root compression at the intervertebral foramina caused by arthritis of the posterior facets. J. Neurosurg., *39:*362, 1973.
101. Erickson, S.J., and Hogan, Q.: CT-guided stellate ganglion injection: Description of technique and efficacy of sympathetic blockade. Radiology, *188:*707, 1993.
102. Evans, F.J.: The placebo response in pain reduction. *In* Bonica, J.J. (ed.): Advances in Neurology. Vol. 4. pp. 289–300. New York, Raven Press, 1984.
103. Evans, J., Dobben, G., and Gay, G.: Peridural effusion of drugs following sympathetic blockade. J.A.M.A., *200:*573, 1967.
104. Fairbank, J.C.T., McCall, I.W., and O'Brian, J.P.: Apophyseal injection of local anesthetic as a diagnostic aid in primary low-back pain syndromes. Spine, *6:*598, 1981.
105. Feinstein, B., Langton, J.N.K., Jameson, R.M., and Schiller, F.: Experiments on pain referred from deep somatic tissues. J. Bone Joint Surg., *36*(A):981, 1954.
106. Fernstrom, U.: A discographical study of ruptured lumbar intervertebral discs. Acta Chir. Scand., *S258:*10, 1960.
107. Ferrer-Brechner, T., and Brechner, V.L.: Accuracy of needle placement during diagnostic and therapeutic nerve blocks. Adv. Pain Res. Ther., *1:*679, 1976.
109. Fine, P.G., Roberts, W.J., Gillette, R.G., and Child, T.R.: Slowly developing placebo responses confound tests of intravenous phentolamine to determine mechanisms underlying idiopathic chronic low back pain. Pain, *56:*235, 1994.
110. Fink, B.R., and Cairns, A.M.: Lack of size-related differential sensitivity to equilibrium conduction block among mammalian myelinated axons exposed to lidocaine. Anesth. Analg., *66:*948, 1987.
111. Fink, B.R., and Cairns, A.M.: Differential use-dependent (frequency-dependent) effects in single mammalian axons: Data and clinical considerations. Anesthesiology, *67:*477, 1987.
112. Fink, B.R.: Mechanisms of differential blockade in epidural and subarachnoid anesthesia. Anesthesiology, *70:*851, 1989.
113. Foerster, O.: The dermatomes in man. Brain, 56:1, 1933.
114. Forsythe, W.B., and Ghoshal, N.G.: Innervation of the canine thoracolumbar vertebral column. Anat. Rec., *208:*57, 1984.
115. Fortin, J.D., Dwyer, A.P., West, S., and Pier, J.: Sacroiliac joint: Pain referral maps upon applying a new injection/arthrography technique. Part I: Asymptomatic volunteers. Spine, *19:*1475, 1994.
116. Foster, A.H., and Carlson, B.M.: Myotoxicity of local anesthetics and regeneration of the damaged muscle fibers. Anesth. Analg., *59:*727, 1980.
117. Franz, D.N., and Perry, R.S.: Mechanisms of differential block among single myelinated and nonmyelinated axons by procaine. J. Physiol., *236:*193, 1974.
118. Freeman, L.W., Shumacker, H.B., and Radigan, L.R.: A functional study of afferent fibers in peripheral sympathetic nerves. Surgery, *28:*274, 1950.
119. Friedman, J., and Goldner, M.Z.: Discography in evaluation of lumbar disk lesions. Radiology, *65:*653, 1955.
120. Furst, C.I.: The biochemistry of guanethidine. Adv. Drug Res., *4:*133, 1967.

121. Ghelman, B., and Doherty, J.H.: Demonstration of spondylolysis by arthrography of the apophyseal joint. Am. J. Roentgenol., *130:*986, 1978.
122. Gibson, M.J., Buckley, J., Mulholland, R.C., and Worthington, B.S.: Magnetic resonance imaging and discography in the diagnosis of disc degeneration. J. Bone Joint. Surg., *68*(B):369, 1986.
123. Gielen, M.J., Slappendel, R., and Merx, J.L.: Asymmetric onset of sympathetic blockade in epidural anesthesia shows no relation to epidural catheter position. Acta Anaesthesiol. Scand., *35:*81, 1991.
124. Giles, L.G.F., and Taylor, J.R.: Human zygapophyseal joint capsule and synovial fold innervation. Br. J. Rheumatol., *26:*93, 1987.
125. Giles, L.G.F., Taylor, J.R., and Cockson, A.: Human zygapophyseal joint synovial folds. Acta Anat., *126:*110, 1986.
126. Giles, L.G.F., and Harvey, A.R.: Immunohistochemical demonstration of nociceptors in the capsule and synovial folds of human zygapophyseal joints. Br. J. Rheumatol., *26:*362, 1987.
127. Glynn, C.J., Basedow, R.W., and Walsh, J.A.: Pain relief following postganglionic sympathetic blockade with I.V. Guanethidine. Br. J. Anaesth., *53:*1297, 1981.
128. Glynn, C.J., Stannard, C., Collins, P.A., and Casale, R.: The role of peripheral sudomotor blockade in the treatment of patients with sympathetically maintained pain. Pain, *53:*39, 1993.
129. Goldstone, J.C., and Pennant, J.H.: Spinal anaesthesia following facet joint injection. Anaesthesia, *42:*754, 1987.
130. Goodwin, J.S., Goodwin, J.M., and Vogel, A.V.: Knowledge and use of placebos by house officers and nurses. Ann. Intern. Med., *91:*106, 1979.
131. Gracely, R.H., Dubner, R., Deeter, W.R., and Wolskee, P.J.: Clinical expectations influence placebo analgesia. Lancet, *1:*43, 1985.
132. Gracely, R.H. Lynch, S.A., and Bennett, G.J.: Painful neuropathy: Altered central processing maintained dynamically by peripheral input. Pain, *51:*175, 1992.
133. Green, D.P.: Diagnostic and therapeutic value of carpal tunnel injection. J. Hand Surg., *9A:*850, 1984.
134. Grevert, P., Albert, L.H., and Goldstein, A.: Partial antagonism of placebo analgesia by naloxone. Pain, *16:*129, 1983.
135. Groen, G.J., Baljet, B., and Drukker, J.: Nerves and nerve plexuses of the human vertebral column. Am. J. Anat., *188:*282, 1990.
136. Groen, G.J., Baljet, B., and Drukker, J.: The innervation of the spinal dura mater: Anatomy and clinical implications. Acta Neurochir., *92:*39, 1988.
139. Groen, G.J., Baljet, B., Boekelaar, A.B., and Drukker, J.: Branches of the thoracic sympathetic trunk in the human fetus. Anat. Embryol., *176:*401, 1987.
140. Gronblad, M., Korkala, O., Konttinen, Y.T., *et al.*: Silver impregnation and immunohistochemical study of nerves in lumbar facet joint plical tissue. Spine, *16:*34, 1991.
141. Grubb, S.A., Lipscomb, H.J., and Guilford, W.B.: The relative value of lumbar roentgenograms, metrizamide myelography, and discography in the assessment of patients with chronic lowback syndrome. Spine, *12:*282, 1987.
142. Guntamukkala, M., and Hardy, P.A.J.: Spread of injectate after stellate ganglion block in man: An anatomical study. Br. J. Anaesth., *66:*643, 1991.
143. Hannington-Kiff, J.G.: Intravenous regional sympathetic block with guanethidine. Lancet, *I:*1019, 1974.
144. Hannington-Kiff, J.G.: Retrograde intravenous sympathetic target blocks in limbs. *In* Stanton Hicks, M. (ed.): Pain and the Sympathetic Nervous System. pp. 191–206. Boston, Klewer Academic Publishers, 1990.
145. Hardy, P.: Stellate ganglion block with bupivacaine: Minimum effective concentration of bupivacaine and the effect of added potassium. Anaesthesia, *44:*398, 1989.
146. Hatangdi, V., and Boas, R.: Lumbar sympathectomy: A single-needle technique. Br. J. Anaesth., *57:*285, 1985.
147. Hatch, J.P., Moore, P.J., Cyr-Provost, M., *et al.*: The use of electromyography and muscle palpation in the diagnosis of tension-type headache with and without pericranial muscle involvement. Pain, *49:*175, 1992.
148. Haueisen, D.C., Smith, B.S., Myers, S.R., and Pryce, M.L.: The diagnostic accuracy of spinal nerve injection studies. Clin. Orthop., *198:*179, 1985.
149. Helbig, T., and Lee, C.K.: The lumbar facet syndrome. Spine, *13:*61, 1988.
151. Hendrix, R.W., Lin, P.P., and Kane, W.J.: Simplified aspiration or injection technique for the sacroiliac joint. J. Bone Joint Surg., *64A:*1249, 1982.
152. Hirsch, C., Ingelmark, B., and Miller, M.: The anatomical basis for low back pain. Acta Orthop., *33:*1, 1963.
153. Hitselberger, W.E., and Witten, R.M.: Abnormal myelograms in asymptomatic patients. J. Neurosurg., *28:*204, 1968.
154. Hoffert, M.J., Greenberg, R.P., Wolskee, P.J., *et al.*: Abnormal and collateral innervations of sympathetic and peripheral sensory fields associated with a case of causalgia. Pain, *20:*1, 1984.
155. Hoffman, H.: An analysis of the sympathetic trunk and rami in the cervical and upper thoracic regions in man. Ann. Surg., *145:*94, 1957.
156. Hogan, Q., Taylor, M.L., Goldstein, M., Stevens, R., and Kettler, R.: Success rates in producing sympathetic blockade by paratracheal injection. Clin. J. Pain., *10:*139, 1994.
157. Hogan, Q., Dotson, R., Erickson, S., Kettler, R., and Hogan, K.: Local anesthetic myotoxicity: A case and review. Anesthesiology, *80:*942, 1994.
158. Hogan, Q.: The sympathetic nervous system in postherpetic neuralgia. Reg. Anesth., *18:*271, 1993.
159. Hogan, Q., and Erickson, S.: MR imaging of the stellate ganglion: Normal appearance. Am. J. Roentgenol., *158:*655, 1992.
160. Hogan, Q., Erickson, S., Haddox, J.D., and Abram, S.: The spread of solutions during "stellate ganglion" blockade. Reg. Anesth., *17:*78, 1992.
161. Hogan, Q., Haddox, J.D., Abram, S., Weissman, D., Taylor, M.L., and Janjan, N.: Epidural opiates and local anesthetics for the management of cancer pain. Pain, *46:*271, 1991.
162. Holt, E.P.: Fallacy of cervical discography. J.A.M.A., *188:*799, 1964.
163. Holt, E.P.: The question of lumbar discography. J. Bone Joint Surg., *50*(A):720, 1968.
164. Hopf, H., Weissbach, B., and Peters, J.: High thoracic segmental epidural anesthesia diminishes sympathetic outflow to the legs, despite restriction of sensory blockade to the upper thorax. Anesthesiology, *73:*882, 1990.
165. Horton, W.C., and Daftari, T.: Which disc as visualized by magnetic resonance imaging is actually a source of pain? Spine, *17:*S164, 1992.
166. Horwitz, M.T.: The anatomy of (A) the lumbosacral nerve plexus—its relation to variations of vertebral segmentation, and (B), the posterior sacral nerve plexus. Anat. Rec., *74:*91, 1939.
167. Houde, R.W., Wallenstein, M.S., and Rogers, A.: Clinical pharmacology of analgesics: A method of assaying analgesic effect. Clin. Pharmacol. Ther., *1:*163, 1966.
168. Hove, B., and Gyldensted, C.: Cervical analgesic facet joint arthrography. Neuroradiology, *32:*456, 1990.
169. Hubbard, D.R., and Berkoff, G.M.: Myofascial trigger points show spontaneous needle EMG activity. Spine, *18:*1803, 1993.
170. Hunt, C.C.: On the nature of vibration receptors in the hind limb of the cat. J. Physiol., *155:*175, 1961.
171. Hunter, C.R., and Mayfield, F.H.: Role of the upper cervical roots in the production of pain in the head. Am. J. Surg., *78:*743, 1949.
172. Hyndman, O.R., and Wolkin, J.: The sympathetic nervous system influence on sensibility to heat and cold and to certain types of pain. Arch. Neurol. Psychiatry, *46:*1006, 1941.
173. Jackson, R.P., Jacobs, R.R., and Montesano, P.X.: Facet joint injection in low-back pain: A prospective statistical study. Spine, *13:*966, 1988.
174. Jackson, R.P.: The facet syndrome. Clin. Orthop., *279:*110, 1992.
175. Jain, S., Shah, N., and Bedford, R.: Needle position for paravertebral and sympathetic nerve blocks: Radiologic confirmation is needed. Anesth. Analg., *72:*S125, 1991.
176. Janig, W.: Neuronal mechanisms of pain with special emphasis on visceral and deep somatic pain. Acta Neurochir., (Suppl.)*385:*16, 1987.
177. Janig, W.: The sympathetic nervous system in pain: Physiology and pathophysiology. *In* Stanton-Hicks, M. (ed.): Pain and the Sympathetic Nervous System. pp. 17–89. Boston, Kluwer Academic Publishers, 1990.
178. Jensen, M.C., Brant-Zawadzki, M.N., Obuchowski, N., *et al.*: Magnetic resonance imaging of the lumbar spine in people without back pain. N. Engl. J. Med., *331:*69, 1994.
179. Kantor, T.G., Sunshine, A., Laska, E., Meisner, M., and Hopper, M.: Oral analgesic studies: Pentazocine hydrochloride, codeine, asparin, and placebo and their influence on response to placebo. Clin. Pharmacol. Ther., *7:*447, 1966.
180. Kaplan, H.I., and Sadock, B.J.: Comprehensive Textbook of Psychiatry. 4th Ed. pp. 1571. Baltimore, Williams and Wilkins, 1985.
181. Kastrup, J., Peterson, P., and Dejgard, A., *et al.*: Intravenous lidocaine

infusion—A new treatment for chronic painful diabetic neuropathy? Pain, *28:*69, 1987.
182. Kawarai, M., and Koss, M.C.: Neurogenic cutaneous vasodilation in the cat forepaw. J. Auton. Nerv. Syst., *37:*39, 1992.
183. Keegan, J.J., and Garrett, F.D.: The segmental distribution of the cutaneous nerves in the limbs of man. Anat. Rec., *102:*409, 1948.
184. Kellgren, J.H.: On the distribution of pain arising from deep somatic structures with charts of segmental pain areas. Clin. Sci., *4:*35, 1939.
185. Kerr, A.T.: The brachial plexus of nerves in man, the variations in its formation and branches. Am. J. Anat., *23:*285, 1918.
186. Kerr, F.W.L.: Structural relation of the trigeminal spinal tract to upper cervical roots and the solitary nucleus in the cat. Exp. Neurol., *4:*134, 1961.
187. Kerr, F.W.L., and Olafson, R.A.: Trigeminal and cervical volleys. Arch. Neurol., *5:*171, 1961.
188. Kiaer, S.: Afferent pain paths in man running from the spongiosa in the femoral head and passing through the lumbar sympathetic ganglia. Acta Orthop. Scand., *19:*383, 1950.
189. Kibler, R.F., and Nathan, P.W.: Relief of pain and paraesthesiae by nerve block distal to a lesion. J. Neurol. Neurosurg. Psychiatry, *23:*91, 1960.
190. Kidd, B.L., Cruwys, S., Mapp, P.I., and Blake, D.R.: Role of the sympathetic nervous system in chronic joint pain and inflammation. Ann. Rheum. Dis., *51:*1188, 1992.
191. Kikuchi, S., Hasue, M., Nishiyama, K., and Ito, T.: Anatomic and clinical studies of radicular symptoms. Spine, *9:*23, 1984.
192. Kim, J.M., Arakawa, K., and VonLintel, T.: Use of pulse-wave monitor as a measurement of diagnostic sympathetic block and of surgical sympathectomy. Anesth. Analg., *54:*289, 1975.
193. Kimmel, D.: Rami communicantes of cervical nerves and the vertebral plexus in the human embryo. Anat. Rec., *121:*321, 1955.
194. Kirgis, H., and Kuntz, A.: Inconstant sympathetic neural pathways. Arch. Surg., *44:*95, 1942.
195. Kirsch, I.: Response expectancy as a determinant of experience and behavior. Am. Psychol., *40:*1189, 1985.
196. Kleiman, A.: Evidence of the existence of crossed sensory sympathetic fibers. Am. J. Surg., *87:*839, 1954.
197. Kojima, Y., Maeda, T., Arai, R., and Shichicawa, K.: Nerve supply to the posterior longitudinal ligament and the intervertebral disc of the rat vertebral column as studied by acetylcholinesterase histochemistry. II. Regional differences in the distribution of the nerve fibers and their origins. Acta Anat., *169:*247, 1990.
198. Kraus, H., and Fischer, A.A.: Diagnosis and treatment of myofascial pain. Mt. Sinai J. Med., *58:*235, 1991.
199. Krempen, J.S., Smith, B., and DeFreest, L.J.: Selective nerve root infiltration for the evaluation of sciatica. Orthop. Clin. North Am., *6:*311, 1975.
200. Kuslich, S.D., and Ulstrom, C.L.: The tissue origin of low back pain and sciatica: A report of pain response to tissue stimulation during operations on the lumbar spine using local anesthesia. Orthop. Clin. North Am., *22:*181, 1991.
201. Larsen, J.L., and Olsen, K.O.: Radiographic anatomy of the distal dural sac. Acta Radiol., *32:*214, 1991.
202. Laska, E., and Sunshine, A: Anticipation of analgesia: A placebo effect. Headache, *13:*1, 1973.
203. Levine, J.D., Gordon, N.C., Bornstein, J.C., and Fields, H.L.: Role of pain in placebo analgesia. Proc. Nat. Acad. Sci., *76:*3528, 1979.
204. Levine, J.D., Gordon, N.C., and Fields, H.L.: The mechanism of placebo analgesia. Lancet, *2:*654, 1978.
205. Lewit, K.: The needle effect in the relief of myofascial pain. Pain, *6:*83, 1979.
206. Liberman, R.: An experimental study of the placebo response under three different situations of pain. J. Psychiatr. Res., *2:*233, 1964.
207. Lilius, G., Laasonen, E.M., Myllynen, P., Harilainen, A., and Gronlund, G.: Lumbar facet joint syndrome: A randomized clinical trial. J. Bone Joint Surg., *71*(B):681, 1989.
208. Lindberg, L., and Wallin, B.G.: Sympathetic skin nerve discharges in relation to amplitude of skin resistance responses. Psychophysiology, *18:*268, 1981.
209. Lipman, J.J., Miller, B.E., Mays, K.S., *et al.*: Peak B endorphin concentration in cerebrospinal fluid: Reduced in chronic pain patients and increased during the placebo response. Psychopharmacology, *102:*112, 1990.
210. Loeser, J.D.: Dorsal rhizotomy for the relief of chronic pain. J. Neurosurg., *36:*745, 1972.
211. Loh, L., and Nathan, P.W.: Painful peripheral states and sympathetic block. J. Neurol. Neurosurg. Psychiatry, *41:*664, 1978.
212. Loh, L., Nathan, P.W., Schott, G.D., and Wilson, P.G.: Effects of regional guanethedine in certain painful states. J. Neurol. Neurosurg. Psychiatry, *43:*446, 1980.
213. Lora, J., and Long, D.: So-called facet denervation in the management of intractable back pain. Spine, *2:*121, 1976.
214. Lund, C., Selmer, P., Hansen, D.B., Hjortso, N-C., and Kehlet, H.: Effects of epidural bupivacaine on somatosensory-evoked potentials after dermatomal stimulation. Anesth. Analg., *66:*34, 1987.
215. Lynch, M.C., and Taylor, J.F.: Facet joint injection for low back pain. J. Bone Joint Surg., *68*(B):138, 1986.
217. MacGibbon, B., and Farfan, H.F.: A radiologic survey of various configurations of the lumbar spine. Spine, *4:*258, 1979.
218. Mackenzie, R.A., Burke, D., Skuse, N.F., and Lethlean, A.K.: Fiber function and perception during cutaneous nerve block. J. Neurol. Neurosurg. Psychiatry, *38:*865, 1975.
219. Maldague, B., Mathurin, P., and Malghem, J.: Facet joint arthrography in lumbar spondylosis. Radiology, *140:*29, 1981.
220. Malliani, A.: Cardiovascular sympathetic afferent fibers. Rev. Physiol. Biochem. Pharmacol., *94:*11, 1982.
221. Malmqvist, L., Tryggvason, B., and Bengtsson, M.: Sympathetic blockade during extradural analgesia with mepivacaine or bupivacaine. Acta Anaesthesiol. Scand., *33:*444, 1989.
222. Malmqvist, E.L., Bengtsson, M., and Sorensen, J.: Efficacy of stellate ganglion block: A clinical study with bupivacaine. Reg. Anesth., *17:*340, 1992.
223. Marchettini, P, Lacerenza, M., and Marangoni, C., *et al.*: Lidocaine test in neuralgia. Pain., *48:*377, 1992.
224. Marks, R.C., Houston, T., and Thulbourne, T.: Facet joint injection and facet nerve block: A randomised comparison in 86 patients with chronic low back pain. Pain, *49:*325, 1992.
225. Marks, R.: Distribution of pain provoked from lumbar facet joints and related structures during diagnostic spinal infiltration. Pain, *39:*37, 1989.
226. Matsumoto, S.: Thermographic assessments of the sympathetic blockade by stellate ganglion block—Comparison between C7-SGB and C6-SGB in 40 patients. Masui., *40:*562, 1991.
227. Mayfield, F.H.: Neurosurgical aspects: Symposium on cervical trauma. Clin. Neurosurg., *2:*83, 1955.
228. McCain, G.A., and Scudds, R.A.: The concept of primary fibromyalgia (fibrositis): Clinical value, relation and significance to other musculoskeletal pain syndromes. Pain, *33:*237, 1988.
229. McCall, I.W., Park, W.M., and O'Brien, J.P.: Induced pain referral from posterior lumbar elements in normal subjects. Spine, *4:*441, 1979.
230. McCollum, D.E., and Stephen, C.R.: The use of graduated spinal anesthesia in the differential diagnosis of pain of the back and lower extremities. South Med. J., *57:*410, 1964.
232. McCormick, C.C., Taylor, J.R., and Twomey, L.T.: Facet joint arthrography in lumbar spondylolysis: Anatomic basis for spread of contrast medium. Radiology, *171:*193, 1989.
233. McLain, R.F.: Mechancoreceptor endings in human cervical facet joints. Spine, *19:*195, 1994.
234. McNeal, B.J., Keeler, E., and Adelstein, S.J.: Primer on certain elements of medical decision-making. N. Engl. J. Med., *293:*211, 1975.
235. Meijer, J., deLange, J., and Ros, H.: Skin pulse-wave monitoring during lumbar epidural and spinal anesthesia. Anesth. Analg., *67:*356, 1988.
236. Melzack, R., and Wall, P.D.: Pain mechanisms: A new theory. Science, *150:*971, 1965.
237. Merington, W.R., and Nathan, P.W.: A study of post-ischemic paresthesiae. J. Neurol. Neurosurg. Psychiatry, *12:*1, 1949.
238. Mooney, V., and Robertson, J.: The facet syndrome. Clin. Orthop., *115:*149, 1976.
240. Moore, D.C.: Guest discussion. Anesth. Analg., *49:*916, 1970.
241. Moran, R., O'Connell, D., and Walsh, M.G.: The diagnostic value of facet joint injections. Spine, *13:*1407, 1988.
242. Murphey, F.: Sources and patterns of pain in disc disease. Clin. Neurosurg., *15:*343, 1968.
243. Murphy, W.A.: The facet syndrome. Radiology, *151:*533, 1984.
244. Murtagh, F.R.: Computed tomography and fluoroscopy-guided anesthesia and steroid injection in facet syndrome. Spine, *13:*686, 1988.
245. Neidre, A., and MacNab, I.: Anomalies of the lumbosacral nerve roots: Review of 16 cases and classification. Spine, *8:*294, 1983.

246. Ness, T., and Gebhart, G.F.: Visceral pain: A review of experimental studies. Pain, *41:*167, 1990.
248. Nielson, V.K., and Kardel, T.: Decremental conduction in normal human nerves subjected to ischemia? Acta Physiol. Scand., *92:*249, 1974.
249. Nitta, H., Tajima, T., Sugiyama, H., and Moriyama, A.: Study of dermatomes by means of selective lumbar spinal nerve block. Spine, *13:*1782, 1993.
250. Noordenbos, W., and Wall, P.D.: Implications of the failure of nerve resection and graft to cure chronic pain produced by nerve lesions. J. Neurol. Neurosurg. Psychiatry, *44:*1068, 1981.
251. Nordin, M., Nystrom, B., Wallin, U., and Hagbarth, K-E.: Ectopic sensory discharges and paresthesiae in patients with disorders of peripheral nerves, dorsal roots and dorsal columns. Pain, *20:*231, 1984.
252. North, R.B., Han, M., Zahurak, M., and Kidd, D.H.: Radiofrequency lumbar facet denervation: Analysis of prognostic factors. Pain, *57:*77, 1994.
253. North, R.B., Kidd, D.H., Campbell, J.N., and Long, D.M.: Dorsal root ganglionectomy for failed back surgery syndrome: A 5-year follow-up study. J. Neurosurg., *74:*236, 1991.
254. Northover, B.J.: A comparison of the electrophysiological actions of phentolamine with those of some other antiarrhythmic drugs on tissues isolated from the rat heart. Br. J. Pharmacol., *80:*85, 1983.
255. Ochsner, A., and DeBakey, M.: Treatment of thrombophlebitis by novacain block of sympathetics. Surgery, *5:*491, 1939.
256. Ochoa, J.L., and Yarnitsky, D.: Mechanical hyperalgesias in neuropathic pain patients: Dynamic and static subtypes. Ann. Neurol., *33:*465, 1993.
257. Ochoa, J.L., Yarnitsky, D., Marchettini, P., Dotson, R., and Cline, M.: Interactions between sympathetic vasoconstrictor outflow and C nociceptor-induced antidromic vasodilatation. Pain, *54:*191, 1993.
258. Ochoa, J., and Verdugo, R.: Reflex sympathetic dystrophy: Definitions and history of the ideas; A critical review of human studies. *In* Low, P.A. (ed.): The Evaluation and Management of Clinical Autonomic Disorders. pp. 473–492. Boston, Little, Brown and Co., 1993.
259. Onofrio, B.M., and Campa, H.K.: Evaluation of rhizotomy: Review of 12 years' experience. J. Neurosurg., *36:*751, 1972.
260. Pallie, W.: The intersegmental anastomoses of posterior spinal rootlets and their significance. J. Neurosurg., *16:*188, 1959.
261. Pallie, W., and Manuel, J.K.: Intersegmental anastomoses between dorsal spinal rootlets in some vertebrates. Acta Anat., *70:*341, 1968.
262. Perl, E.R.: Is pain a specific sensation? J. Psychiatr. Res., *8:*273, 1971.
263. Peterson, P., and Kastrup, J.: Dercum's disease (adiposa dolorosa): Treatment of the severe pain with intravenous lidocaine. Pain, *28:*77, 1987.
264. Pfaffenrath, V., Dandekar, R., Pollmann, W.: Cervicogenic headache—The clinical picture, radiologic findings and hypotheses of its pathophysiology. Headache, *27:*495, 1987.
265. Pickering, T.G., James, G.D., Boddie, C., *et al.*: How common is white coat hypertension? J.A.M.A., *259:*225, 1988.
266. Plancarte, R., Velazquez, R., and Patt, R.B.: Neurolytic blocks of the sympathetic axis. *In* Patt, R.B. (ed.): Cancer Pain. pp. 377–425. Philadelphia, J.B. Lippincott, 1993.
267. Plancarte, R., Amescua, C., Patt, R.B., and Aldrete, J.A.: Superior hypogastric plexus block for pelvic cancer pain. Anesthesiology, *73:*236, 1990.
268. Powel, M.C., Wilson, M., Szypryt, P., Symonds, B.M., and Worthington, B.S.: Prevalence of lumbar disc degeneration observed by magnetic resonance in symptomless women. Lancet, *2:*1366, 1986.
269. Pomeranz, B., Wall, P.D., and Weber, C.V.: Cord cells responding to fine myelinated afferents from viscera, muscle, and skin. J. Physiol., (Lond), *199:*511, 1983.
270. Price, D.D., Bennett, G.J., and Rafii, A.: Psychophysical observations on patients with neuropathic pain relieved by a sympathetic block. Pain, *36:*273, 1989.
271. Quinnell, R.C., and Stockdale, H.R.: The use of in vivo lumbar discography to assess the clinical significance of the position of the intercrestal line. Spine, *8:*305, 1983.
272. Quinnell, R.C., Stockdale, H.R., and Harmon, B.: Pressure standardized lumbar discography. Br. J. Radiol., *53:*1031, 1980.
273. Raja, S.N., Treede, R-D., Davis, K.D., and Campbell, J.N.: Systemic alpha-adrenergic blockade with phentolamine: A diagnostic test for sympathetically maintained pain. Anesthesiology, *74:*691, 1991.
274. Ramirez, J.M., and French, A.S.: Phentolamine selectively affects the fast sodium component of sensory adaptation in an insect mechanoreceptor. J. Neurobiol., *21:*893, 1990.
275. Randic, M., Jiang, M.C., and Cerne, R.: Long-term potentiation and long-term depression of primary afferent neurotransmission in the rat spinal cord. J. Neurosci., *13:*5228, 1993.
276. Ramamurthy, S., and Winnie, A.P.: Diagnostic maneuvers in painful syndromes. Int. Anesthesiol. Clin., *83:*47, 1983.
277. Rawal, N., Schott, U., Dahlstrom, B., *et al.*: Influence of naloxone infusion on analgesia and respiratory depression following epidural morphine. Anesthesiology, *64:*194, 1986.
278. Raymond, S., and Gissen, A.J.: Mechanisms of differential nerve block. *In* Strichartz, G. (ed.): Local Anesthetics. pp. 95–164. Springer-Verlag, 1987.
279. Raymond, S.A.: Subblocking concentrations of local anesthetics: Effects on impulse generation and conduction in single myelinated sciatic nerve axons in frog. Anesth. Analg., *75:*906, 1992.
280. Raymond, S., Steffensen, S.C., Gugino, L.D., and Strichartz, G.R.: The role of length of nerve exposed to local anesthetics in impulse blocking action. Anesth. Analg., *68:*563, 1989.
281. Raymond, J., and Dumas, J-M.: Intra-articular facet block: Diagnostic test or therapeutic procedure? Radiology, *151:*333, 1984.
282. Ready, L.B., Kozody, R., Barsa, J.E., and Murphy, T.M.: Trigger point injections vs. jet injection in the treatment of myofascial pain. Pain, *15:*201, 1989.
283. Ready, L.B., Kozody, R., Barsa, J.E., and Murphy, T.M.: Side-port needles for stellate ganglion block. Reg. Anesth., *7:*160, 1982.
284. Reimann, A.F., and Anson, B.J.: Vertebral level of termination of the spinal cord with report of a case of sacral cord. Anat. Rec., *88:*127, 1944.
285. Renfrew, D., Moore, T., Kathol, M., El-Khoury, G., Lemke, J., and Walker, C.: Correct placement of epidural steroid injections: Fluoroscopic guidance and contrast administration. Am. J. Neuroradiol., *12:*1003, 1991.
286. Roberts, W.J.: A hypothesis on the physiological basis for causalgia and related pains. Pain, *24:*297, 1986.
287. Rosen, L., Ostergren, J., Fagrell, B.F., and Stranden, E.: Skin microcirculation in the sympathetic dystrophies evaluated by videophotometric capillaroscopy and laser Doppler fluxometry. Eur. J. Clin. Invest., *18:*305, 1988.
288. Rosenzweig, P., Brohier, S., and Zipfel, A.: The placebo effect in healthy volunteers: Influence of experimental conditions on the adverse events profile during phase I trials. Clin. Pharmacol. Ther., *54:*578, 1993.
289. Rowlingson, J.C., DiFazio, C.A., Foster, J., and Carron, H.: Lidocaine as an analgesic for experimental pain. Anesthesiology, *52:*20, 1980.
290. Roy, D.F., Fleury, J., Fontaine, S.B., and Dussault, R.: Clinical evaluation of cervical facet joint infiltration. J. Can. Assoc. Radiol., *39:*118, 1988.
291. Russell, A.S., Maksymowych, W., and LeClerq, S.: Clinical examination of the sacroiliac joints: A prospective study. Arthritis Rheum., *24:*1575, 1981.
292. Sanders, S.H., McKeel, N.L., and Hare, B.D.: Relationship between psychopathology and graduated spinal block findings in chronic pain patients. Pain, *19:*367, 1984.
293. Sarnoff, S.J., and Arrowood, J.G.: Differential spinal block. Surgery, *20:*150, 1946.
294. Sato, J., and Perl, E.R.: Adrenergic excitation of cutaneous pain receptors induced by peripheral nerve injury. Science, *251:*1608, 1991.
295. Schnider, T.W., Gaeta, R., Brose, W., Minto, C.F., Gregg, K.M., and Shafer, S.L.: Derivation and cross-validation of pharmacokinetic parameters for computer-controlled infusion of lidocaine in pain therapy. Anesthesiology, *84:*1043, 1996.
296. Schott, G.: Mechanisms of causalgia and related clinical conditions: The role of the central and of the sympathetic nervous systems. Brain, *109:*717, 1986.
297. Schott, G.D.: Visceral afferents: Their contribution to 'sympathetic dependent' pain. Brain, *117:*397, 1994.
298. Schwarzer, A.C., Aprill, C.N., Derby, R., *et al.*: Clinical features of patients with pain stemming from the lumbar zygapophyseal joints. Spine, *19:*1132, 1994.
299. Schwarzer, A.C., Aprill, C.N., Derby, R., Kine, J., and Bogduk, N.: The false-positive rate of uncontrolled diagnostic blocks of the lumbar zygapophysial joints. Pain, *58:*195, 1994.
300. Schwarzer, A.C., Derby, R., Aprill, C.N., *et al.*: The value of the provocation response in lumbar zygapophyseal joint injections. Clin. J. Pain., *10:*309, 1994.
301. Schutz, H., Lougheed, W.M., Wortzman, G., and Awerbuck, B.G.: Intervertebral nerve-root in the investigation of chronic lumbar disc disease. Can. J. Surg., *16:*217, 1973.

302. Scott, R.M.: Mexilitine and vascular headaches. Aust. N. Z. J. Med., *93*:92, 1981.
303. Sheehan, D.: On the innervation of the blood vessels of the upper extremity: Some anatomical considerations. Br. J. Surg., *20*:412, 1932.
304. Shir, Y., Cameron, L.B., Raja, S., and Bourke, D.L.: The safety of intravenous phentolamine administration in patients with neuropathic pain. Anesth. Analg., *76*:1008, 1993.
305. Sidel, N., and Abrams, M.I.: Treatment of chronic arthritis: Results of vaccine therapy with saline injections as controls. J.A.M.A., *114*:1740, 1940.
306. Sigurdsson, A., and Maixner, W.: Effects of experimental and clinical noxious counterirritants on pain perception. Pain, *57*:265, 1994.
307. Simmons, E.H., and Segil, C.: An evaluation of discography in the localization of symptomatic levels in discogenic disease of the spine. Clin. Orthop., *108*:57, 1975.
308. Simmons, J.W., Emery, S.F., McMillin, J.N., Landa, D., and Kimmich, S.J.: Awake discography: A comparison with magnetic resonance imaging. Spine, *16*:S216, 1991.
309. Simons, D.G., and Travell, J.G.: The myofascial genesis of pain. Postgrad. Med., *11*:425, 1952.
310. Sinclair, D.C., and Hinshaw, J.R.: A comparison of the sensory dissociation produced by procaine and by limb compression. Brain, *73*:480, 1950.
311. Sjaastad, O., Fredricksen, T.A., and Pfaffenrath, V.: Cervicogenic headache: Diagnostic criteria. Headache, *30*:725, 1990.
312. Sjogren, P., Gefke, K., Banning, A., Parslov, M., and Olsen, L.B.O.: Lumbar epidurography and epidural analgesia in cancer patients. Pain, *36*:305, 1989.
313. Smith, R.C., and Hoppe, R.B.: The patient's story: Integrating the patient- and physician-centered approaches to interviewing. Ann. Intern. Med., *115*:470, 1991.
314. Smyth, M.J., and Wright, V.: Sciatica and the intervertebral disc. J. Bone Joint Surg., *40*(A):1401, 1958.
315. Solonen, K.A.: The sacroiliac joint in light of anatomical, roentgenological, and clinical studies. Acta Orthop. Scand., *27*(S):1, 1957.
316. Stanley, D., McLaren, M.I, Euinton, H.A., and Getty, C.J.M.: A prospective study of nerve root infiltration in the diagnosis of sciatica. Spine, *15*:540, 1990.
317. Stilwell, D.L.: The nerve supply of the vertebral column and its associated structures in the monkey. Anat. Rec., *125*:139, 1956.
318. Stevens, R., Artuso, J., Kao, T., *et al.*: Changes in human plasma catecholamine concentrations during epidural anesthesia depend on the level of the block. Anesthesiology, *74*:1029, 1991.
319. Stevens, R., Beardsley, D., White, J.L., *et al.*: Does the choice of local anesthetic affect the catecholamine response to stress during epidural anesthesia? Anesthesiology, *79*:1219, 1993.
320. Tahmoush, A.J., Malley, J., and Jennings, J.R.: Skin conductance, temperature, and blood flow in causalgia. Neurology, *33*:1483, 1983.
321. Tajima, T., Furukawa, K., and Kuramochi, E.: Selective lumbosacral radiculography and block. Spine, *5*:68, 1980.
322. Tal, M., and Bennett, G.J.: Extra-territorial pain in rats with a peripheral mononeuropathy: Mechanohyperalgesia and mechano-allodynia in the territory of an uninjured nerve. Pain, *57*:375, 1994.
323. Tanelian, D.L., and MacIver, M.B.: Analgesic concentrations of lidocaine suppress tonic A-delta and C-fiber discharges produced by acute injury. Anesthesiology, *74*:934, 1991.
325. Terenius, L.: Biochemical mediators in pain. Triangle, *20*:19, 1981.
326. Torebjork, H.E., and Hallin, R.G.: Perceptual changes accompanying controlled preferential blocking of A and C fiber responses in intact human skin nerves. Exp. Brain Res., *16*:321, 1973.
327. Torebjork, E.: Clinical and neurophysiological observations relating to pathophysiological mechanisms in reflex sympathetic dystrophy. *In* Stanton-Hicks, M., Janig, W. and Boas, R.A. (eds.): Reflex Sympathetic Dystrophy. pp. 71–80. Boston, Kluwer Academic Publishers, 1990.
328. Troisier, O.: An accurate method for lumbar disc puncture using a single channel intensifier. Spine, *15*:222, 1990.
329. Traut, E.F., and Passarelli, E.W.: Study in the controlled therapy of degenerative arthritis. A.M.A. Arch. Intern. Med., *98*:181, 1956.
330. Van Buskirk, C.: Nerves in the vertebral canal: Their relation to the sympathetic innervation of the upper extremities. Arch. Surg., *43*:427, 1941.
331. Van Gessel, E.F., Forster, A., and Gamulin, Z.: Continuous spinal anesthesia: Where do spinal catheters go? Anesth. Analg., *76*:1004, 1993.
332. Vanharanta, H., Sachs, B.L., Spivey, M.A., *et al.*: The relationship of pain provocation to lumbar disc deterioration as seen by CT/discography. Spine, *12*:295, 1987.
333. Van Rhede van der Kloot, E., Drukker, J., Lemmens, H.A.J., and Greep, J.M.: The high thoracic sympathetic nerve system—Its anatomic variability. J. Surg. Res., *40*:112, 1986.
334. Verdugo, R., and Ochoa, J.L.: High incidence of placebo responders among chronic neuropathic pain patients. Ann. Neurol., *30*:294, 1991.
335. Verdugo, R., Rosenblum, S., and Ochoa, J.: Phentolamine sympathetic blocks mislead diagnosis. Soc. Neurosci., (Abstr.) *17*:107, 1991.
336. Videman, T., Malmivaara, A., and Mooney, V.: The value of the axial view in assessing discograms: An experimental study with cadavers. Spine, *12*:299, 1987.
337. Vital, J.M., Dautheribes, M., Baspeyre, H., Lavignolle, B., and Senegas, J.: An anatomic and dynamic study of the greater occipital nerve (n. of Arnold). Surg. Radiol. Anat., *11*:205, 1989.
338. Vleeming, A., Stoeckart, R., Volkers, A.C.W., and Snijders, C.J.: Relation between form and function in the sacroiliac joint. Part I: Clinical anatomic aspects. Spine, *15*:130, 1990.
339. Voudouris, N.J., Peck, C.L., and Coleman, G.: The role of conditioning and verbal expectancy in the placebo response. Pain, *43*:121, 1990.
340. Voudouris, N.J., Peck, C.L., and Coleman, G.: Conditioned placebo responses. J. Per. Soc. Psychol., *48*:47, 1985.
341. Wahren, L.K., Torebjork, E., and Nystrom, B.: Quantitative sensory testing before and after regional guanethidine block in patients with neuralgia in the hand. Pain, *46*:23, 1991.
342. Walsh, T.R., Weinstein, J.N., Spratt, K.F., *et al.*: Lumbar discography in normal subjects. J. Bone Joint Surg., *72*(A):1081, 1990.
343. Wang, Z.L., Yu, S., and Haughton, V.M.: Age-related changes in the lumbar facet joints. Clin Anat., *2*:55, 1989.
344. Warfield, C.A., and Crews, D.A.: Epidural steroid injection as a predictor of surgical outcome. Surg. Gynecol. Obstet., *164*:457, 1987.
345. Warrick, J.W.: Stellate ganglion block in the treatment of Meniere's disease and in the symptomatic relief of tinnitus. Br. J. Anaesth., *41*:699, 1969.
346. Weber, R.: An analysis of the cross-communications between the sympathetic trunks in the lumbar region in man. Ann. Surg., *145*:365, 1957.
347. Weinberger, L.M.: Cervico-occipital pain and its surgical treatment: The myth of the bony millstones. Am. J. Surg., *135*:243, 1968.
348. Weinreb, J.C., Wolbarsht, L.B., Cohen, J.M., Brown, C.E.L., and Maravilla, K.R.: Prevalence of lumbosacral intervertebral disk abnormalities on MR images in pregnant and asymptomatic nonpregnant women. Radiology, *170*:125, 1989.
349. White, A., Derby, R., and Wynne, G.: Epidural injections for the diagnosis and treatment of low-back pain. Spine, *5*:78, 1980.
350. Wiberg, G.: Back pain in relation to the nerve supply of the intervertebral disc. Acta Orthop., *19*:211, 1949.
351. Wiesel, S.W., Tsourmas, N., Feffer, H.I., Citrin, C.M., and Patronas, N.: A study of computer-assisted tomography. I. The incidence of positive CAT scans in an asymptomatic group of patients. Spine, *9*:549, 1984.
352. Wilcox, G.L.: Excitatory neurotransmitters and pain. *In* Bond, M.R., Charlton, J.E., and Woolf, C.J. (eds.): Proceedings of the 6th World Congress on Pain. pp. 97–117. Amsterdam, Elsevier, 1991.
353. Wildsmith, J.A.W., Gissen, A.J., Gregus, J., and Covino, B.G.: Differential nerve-blocking activity of aminoester local anesthetics. Br. J. Anaesth., *57*:612, 1985.
354. Willis, T.A.: An analysis of vertebral anomalies. Am. J. Surg., *6*:163, 1929.
355. Woolf, C.J.: Central mechanisms of acute pain. *In* Bond, M.R., Charlton, J.E., and Woolf, C.J. (eds.): Proceedings of the 6th World Congress on Pain. pp. 25–34. Amsterdam, Elsevier, 1991.
356. Woolf, C.J., and Wiesenfeld-Hallin, Z.: The systemic administration of local anesthetics produces a selective depression of C-afferent fiber-evoked activity in the spinal cord. Pain, *23*:361, 1985.
357. Woolf, C.J., Shortland, P., and Coggeshall, R.E.: Peripheral nerve injury triggers central sprouting of myelinated afferents. Nature, *355*:75, 1992.
358. Xavier, A.V., McDanal, J., and Kissin, I: Relief of sciatic radicular pain by sciatic nerve block. Anesth. Analg., *67*:1177, 1988.
359. Yamamuro, M., and Kaneko, T.: The comparison of stellate ganglion block at the transverse process of the 7th and the 6th cervical vertebra. Masui., *27*:376, 1978.

360. Yamashita, T., Cavanaugh, J.M., El-Bohy, A.A., Getchell, T.V., and King, A.I.: Mechanosensitive afferent units in the lumbar facet joint. J. Bone Joint Surg., *72*(A):865, 1990.
361. Yarnitsky, D., and Ochoa, J.L.: Differential effect of compression-ischemia block on warm sensation and heat-induced pain. Brain, *114:*907, 1991.
362. Yarnitsky, D., and Ochoa, J.L.: Sensations conducted by large and small myelinated fibers are lost simultaneously under compression-ischemia block. Acta Physiol. Scand., *137:*319, 1989.
363. Yeager, G.H., and Cowley, R.A.: Anatomical observations on the lumbar sympathetics with evaluation of sympathectomies in organic vascular disease. Ann. Surg., *127:*953, 1948.
364. Young, A., Getty, J., Jackson, A., Kirwan, E., Sullivan, M., and Parry, C.W.: Variations in the pattern of muscle innervation by the L5 and S1 nerve roots. Spine, *6:*616, 1983.
365. Yu, S., Haughton, V.M., Sether, L.A., and Wagner, M.: Comparison of MR and discography in detecting radial tears of the anulus: A postmortem study. A.J.N.R., *10:*1077, 1989.
366. Zimermann, M., and Handwerker, H.O.: Total afferent inflow and dorsal horn activity upon radiant heat stimulation of the cat's footpad. *In* Bonica, J.J. (ed.): Advances in Neurology. Vol. 4. pp. 29–38. New York, Raven Press, 1974.
367. Zucherman, J., Derby, R., Hsu, K., *et al.*: Normal magnetic resonance imaging with abnormal discography. Spine, *13:*1355, 1988.
368. Schwarzer, A.C., Aprill, C.N., and Bogduk, N. The sacroiliac joint in chronic low back pain. Spine, *20*:31, 1995.

Neural Blockade in Clinical Anesthesia and Management of Pain, Third Edition,
edited by M.J. Cousins and P.O. Bridenbaugh.
Lippincott–Raven Publishers, Philadelphia © 1998.

CHAPTER 28

Back Pain and the Role of Neural Blockade

Donald C. Manning and John C. Rowlingson

Back pain is a primary cause of disability in the United States. Eighty percent of workers will lose some time from their working lives because of back pain, and few adults escape an active recreational life without a number of episodes.[1] Back pain is the second most frequent chronic pain problem, just behind headache as a reason for patients to seek medical help.[67,85,153,200] The human suffering related to back pain ranges in intensity from transient discomfort to frank incapacitation. There is an inverse relationship between the severity of the back pain and the number of patients who experience it. Yet the financial costs of back pain to society at large are enormous. The nonmonetary costs embody diminished vocational productivity and interference with normal and recreational activities. The billions of dollars spent annually on back pain pay for medical evaluations, diagnostic tests, therapy, compensation to patients who are off work, wages for replacement workers, and disability payments for those whose work capacity is diminished or lost (see also Chapter 33). The Agency for Health Care Policy and Research (AHCPR) recently released clinical practice guidelines for management of acute back pain. They document that 90% of patients with acute back pain are better in one month (better means spontaneous recovery of activity tolerance); but an addendum to the guidelines notes that "more than half the people who recover from a first episode of acute low back pain symptoms will have another episode within a few years."[19]

The 10% to 15% with acute back pain who do not improve account for approximately 85% of the annual expenditures listed above.[187,199] When the pain complaints persist, myriad nonphysical elements intermingle with the physical findings; establishing a diagnosis that respects all the factors contributing to the pain is a difficult task.[47,106,153,188] Back pain is a classic chronic pain problem. It has a vast differential diagnosis; the records that document the patient's previous involvements with the health care system (which must be reviewed) are voluminous, the patient's telling of his/her tale can take an inordinate amount of time, physical examination findings may be inconsistent from one examination to the next, modern diagnostic tests often fail to show a cause for the patient's disabling pain, and the psychosocial, legal, and economic aspects of chronic pain complicate the total problem. Back pain can continue even after the original cause is gone[106,110,188] because:

1. The patient becomes physically deconditioned during the recovery phase and his or her attempts to resume normal activity too quickly result in recurrent pain.
2. The pain provokes changes in the behavior of the patient, some of which are reinforced by beneficial consequences, and these entrenched behaviors are hard to change when the original pain passes.
3. The constant bombardment of the central nervous system (CNS) with nociceptive impulses induces alterations in the neural response. This "neural memory" of pain remains, even though a distinct peripheral source is not there. The obvious clinical corollary is that treatment only of the apparent source of pain will not relieve all of the patient's symptoms. When pain has become chronic, we must deal with the physical, the psychosocial, *and* the neurophysiologic ramifications.

Anesthesiologists have been practicing pain medicine for decades, with the unique application of specific nerve blocks as a highly valued contribution to patient care.[161] Even though the relief may be temporary, the demonstration to the patient that something effective can be done about the pain restores hope and fosters cooperation with other components of the therapeutic program. The fact that the patient also receives another evaluation and an explanation about both the etiology of the pain and the rationale for treatment is an additional benefit.

D. C. Manning and J. C. Rowlingson: Department of Anesthesiology, Pain Management Center, University of Virgina Health Sciences Center, Charlottesville, Virginia 22908.

Assessment of the Patient with Back Pain

The patient with low back pain may be bothered by the symptoms only temporarily or may suffer drastic disruption of his or her lifestyle.[19,85,153] Pain is a subjective complaint and the scientific methods to quantitate it are scarce. Because there can be so much more "wrong" with the patient than the simple complaint of back pain connotes, the *evaluation protocol* must be systematic and meticulous.[47,48,106,110] It must encompass the physical manifestations of the pain as well as the numerous psychosocial consequences that can so markedly compound the patient's life. It must unbundle the various problems, so that treatment can be directed rationally at the cause(s) and can help the clinician determine which patients need aggressive intervention and which need only the "tincture of time" and/or moderate medical support. It must permit the clinician to make an educated choice of those patients for whom neural blockade is appropriate.

The three common sources of information about the patient are history, physical examination and laboratory studies. These data may be enhanced by the routine use of questionnaires, psychological interviews and ergonomic assessment. A questionnaire is a common evaluation tool that definitely improves the efficiency of the medical interview process. Since it reveals the patient's responses to the numerous, but routine, physical symptoms and psychosocial questions about the pain problem, and is available for review prior to the actual appointment, the precious interactive time during the office visit can be devoted to aspects of the back pain that are most important *for the patient* to discuss. This enhances patient satisfaction right from the start and should bode well for his or her cooperation with the recommended therapy.[48,68,200]

Table 28-1 lists historical factors that are significant in the decision process relating to invasive procedures. A history of prior back surgery is likely to result in the creation of scar tissue which may restrict the patient's motion and can possibly hamper the response to therapy.[47,171] Abram stated that there was a twofold increase in treatment failure if the patient's back pain symptoms were present for longer than six months.[1] A number of other authors have shown that the duration of symptoms is also a significant issue.[1,171] Hopwood and Abram have reported a multifactorial study showing that outcome depended upon many factors other than invasive therapy only.[106] They assayed 209 patients who received epidural steroid injection (ESI) therapy (50mg triamcinolone in 3 to 5 ml 1% lidocaine) for 33 possible predictive factors culled from previously published studies or chosen for their clinical importance or their ease of assessment. They showed that patients with higher educational levels and nonsmokers responded better to epidural steroid injections than did those who were hurt on the job, missed work secondary to their pain, had prolonged symptoms, had a nonradicular diagnosis, suffered sleep disturbance or a change in recreational activities secondary to pain, or scored highly on psychological tests. Jamison et al. recently reinforced many of these concepts in a study of 249 patients with chronic low back pain who received ESI therapy.[110] Olmarker et al. proposed that the speed of onset of the symptoms may influence the response to treatment.[151] Sandrock and Warfield stated that the five most important factors that influence the outcome from epidural steroid injections were: accuracy of the diagnosis of (nerve) root inflammation, duration of the symptoms, a history of previous surgery, age of the patient, and placement of the injection at the level of pathology.[171]

TABLE 28-1. *Pertinent features of the back pain history*

A history of previous spinal surgery
The number of previous back pain episodes
Trauma, especially a lifting event, initiating the pain
Being injured on the job
Missing work due to back pain
The speed of onset of the radicular symptoms
Pain radiating into the extremity and below the knee or elbow
The presence of impulse pain (as with coughing or lifting)
The effect of physical activity on the pain
The number of previous treatments for pain and their effectiveness
Receipt of compensation for the original injury
The patient's attitude about who's to blame for the pain

(Modified from Rowlingson, J.C.: Epidural steroids: Do they have a place in pain management? A.P.S. Journal, *3*:20, 1994.)

Prior to using any regional analgesic techniques, a physical examination must be done to establish the patient's neurologic baseline and to document the findings[47,48,153] (see Fig. 28-1). Musculoskeletal structures rarely function alone in producing back pain, and physical dysfunction due to back pain is not the only factor influencing the patient's disability.[153,188] In an ideal world, any practitioner would be able to perform examinations in a serial and comparative fashion to detect the progression or regression of the primary disease, or the presence of a new pathological disorder. Patients with chronic pain do develop other reasons for their pain, and all involved in their care must remain vigilant. Caution must be used early in the physical examination where painful tests may be performed, because reflex muscle spasm and guarding by the patient will influence the rest of the examination. As patients improve symptomatically, the contemporary evaluation of their physical readiness for returning to activities and/or their work may include assessment of aerobic capacity, trunk strength, lifting power, endurance, and functional capacity. Table 28-2 suggests data that are important discriminators from the physical examination when patients are selected for neural blockade. Any of these physical findings may coexist with osteoarthritis, rheumatoid arthritis, zygapophysial arthropathy, spinal stenosis, poor physical condition of the patient, faulty neuromuscular coordination, inflexible connective tissue and fatigue. These factors may contribute to or perpetuate complaints of back pain. Waddell et al. presented several other cautions for the selection of patients for invasive procedures.[203] They noted the importance of such signs as a positive skin roll test, an exaggerated response to spinal/axial loading maneuvers, a discrepancy be-

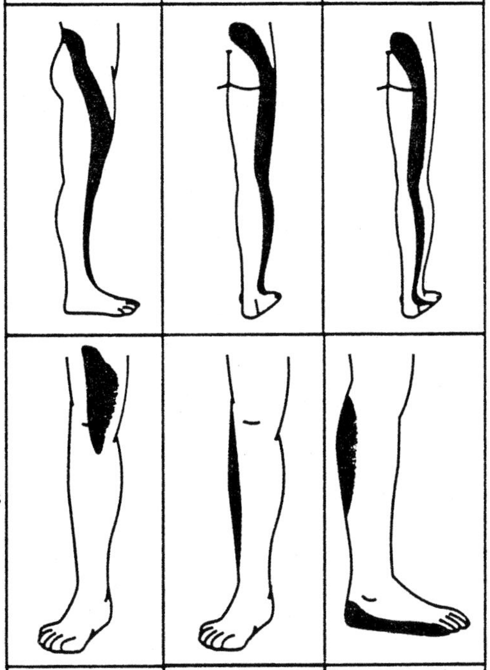

Nerve root	L4	L5	S1
Pain			
Numbness			
Motor weakness	Extension of quadriceps.	Dorsilflexion of great toe and foot.	Plantar flexion of great toe and foot.
Screening exam	Squat & rise.	Heel walking.	Walking on toes.
Reflexes	Knee jerk diminished.	None reliable.	Ankle jerk diminished.

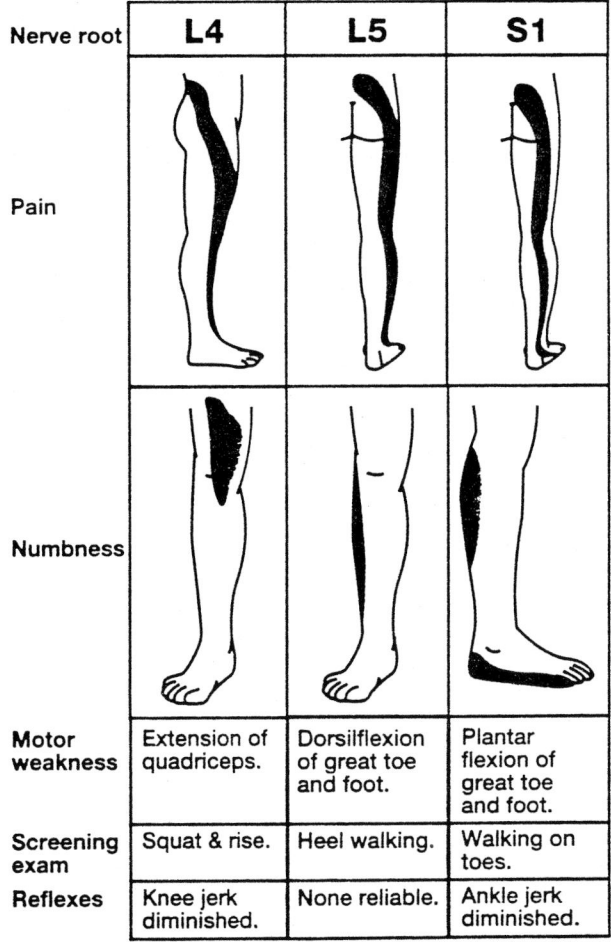

FIG. 28-1. Testing for lumbar nerve root complication. (From: Bigos, S., Bowwyer, O., Braen, G., et al.: Acute Low Back Problems in Adults. Clinical Practice Guideline, Quick Reference Guide Number 14. Rockville, MD, U.S. Department of Health and Human Services. Public Health Service, Agency for Health Care Policy and Research, AHCPR Pub. No. 95-0643, December, 1994.)

tween seated and supine straight-leg-raising (SLR) tests (Figs. 28-2 and 28-3) and nonanatomic motor or sensory testing as being significant indicators of nonorganic pathology in patients with back pain. (These are not, however, signs of malingering).

The hope that sophisticated laboratory tests will show the cause for a given patient's agonizing chronic pain often is not met.[18,22,101,162,205] Negative labs are not usually reassuring to a patient desperate for a diagnosis. Deyo's comment that "...up to 85% of patients with low back pain cannot be given a definitive diagnosis because of the poor association among symptoms, pathologic findings, and imaging results," reflects the reality that the labs often don't contribute greatly to a patient's diagnosis.[69] AHCPR guidelines encourage avoidance of diagnostic tests unless the patient manifests "red flags" (see Table 28-3) with acute back pain or the symptoms exceed four weeks in duration.[19] This should minimize the false association of symptoms with age-related pathology. Labs cannot substitute for taking a history or performing a physical examination. Only those studies that will truly influence the patient's management should be obtained. Plain x-rays are easy to obtain, but may be of limited value, and rarely provide information that changes the approach to (acute) back pain.[19,67] Computed tomography (CT) scans distinguish bony structures from the soft tissues and do so in a noninvasive way. Combined with myelography, this technique can identify the exact level of spinal pathology.[67,23,195] Magnetic resonance imaging (MRI) scans provide the ultimate in contrast between the tissues of the perispinal area. As Thornbury et al. point out, the factors that determine which of these tests is done in patients suspected of having disc-related compression should be cost, the radiation dose to the patient, and the invasiveness of the procedure, because in this population of patients, no one test is more diagnostic than the other.[195] Electromylograms (EMGs) are an extension of the neurologic exam and provide data about the level, duration, and degree of neural involvement. Table 28-4 delineates the ability of different evaluative techniques to identify pathologic causes for back pain complaints.[19] One must not assume that because lab tests are negative, the patient has no "real" or "significant" pain, or that it is only a representation of psychosocial pathology. Equally, an abnormality on a lab test is not necessarily the source of the patient's pain. Trivializing the patient's pain complaints is counterproductive to establishing a diagnosis, and generating a treatment program with which the patient will cooperate.

Chronic pain can adversely affect the patient's attitude and perception about recovering health, willingness to change behavioral responses, motivation, relationships and social integration, self perception, and lifestyle.[2,20,61,67,106,110,137,153,187] What the patient believes about the implications and true causes of the pain are paramount to understanding his or her genuine inclination to make the changes that define successful management of back pain. It is equally important that the patient understand his or her diagnosis and the rationale for each therapeutic option being suggested, because this information will influence markedly compliance and response to treatment. Deyo and Diehl documented that the patient's satisfaction with care for back pain symptoms correlated directly with the explanation given about its cause and management.[68] Most recently, Von Korff et al. showed

TABLE 28-2. *Pertinent features of the examination in back pain*

Dermatomal sensory change
Dermatomal motor findings
Decreased ROM of the cervical or lumbar spine
Sciatic nerve stretch signs (positive SLR, crossed SLR, bowstring sign, Lasegues sign)

ROM, range of motion; SLR, straight-leg raising.

(Modified from Rowlingson, J.C.: Epidural steroids: Do they have a place in pain management? A.P.S. Journal, *3*:20, 1994.)

(1) Ask the patient to lie as straight as possible on a table in the supine position.

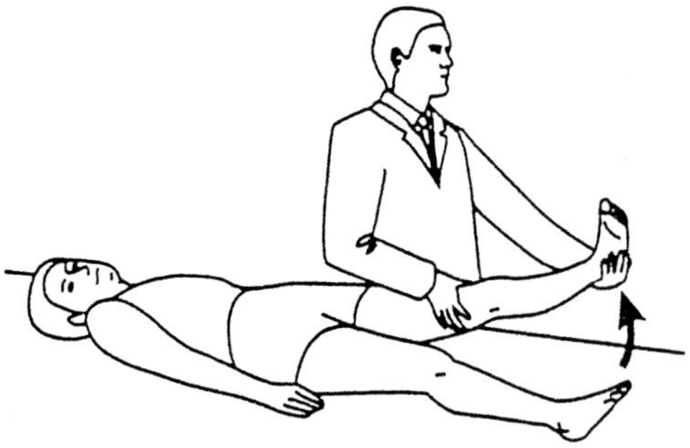

(2) With one hand placed above the knee of the leg being examined, exert enough firm pressure to keep the knee fully extended. Ask the patient to relax.

(3) With the other hand cupped under the heel, slowly raise the straight limb. Tell the patient, "If this bothers you, let me know, and I will stop."

4) Monitor for any movement of the pelvis before complaints are elicited. True sciatic tension should elicit complaints before the hamstrings are stretched enough to move the pelvis.

(5) Estimate the degree of leg elevation that elicits complaint from the patient. Then determine the most distal area of discomfort: back, hip, thigh, knee, or below the knee.

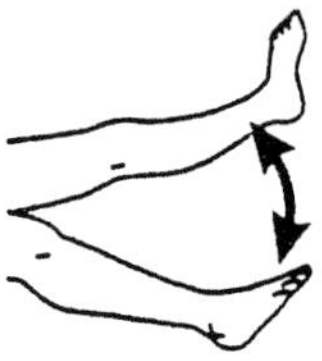

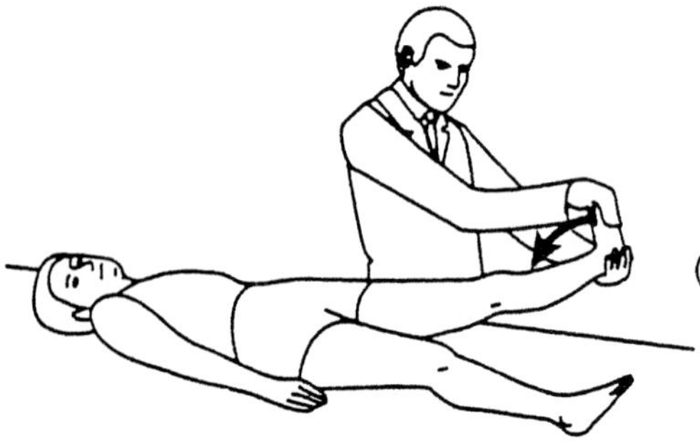

(6) While holding the leg at the limit of straight leg raising, dorsiflex the ankle. Note whether this aggravates the pain. Internal rotation of the limb can also increase the tension on the sciatic nerve roots.

FIG. 28-2. Instructions for the Straight-Leg-Raising (SLR) test. (From: Bigos, S., Bowwyer, O., Braen, G., et al.: Acute Low Back Problems in Adults. Clinical Practice Guideline, Quick Reference Guide Number 14. Rockville, MD, U.S. Department of Health and Human Services. Public Health Service, Agency for Health Care Policy and Research, AHCPR Pub. No. 95-0643, December, 1994.)

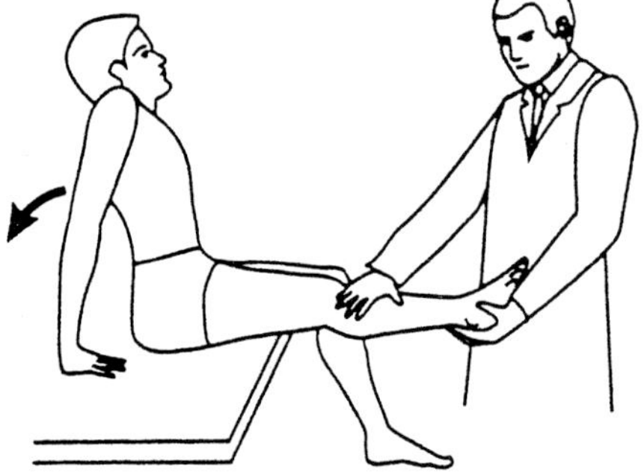

With the patient sitting on a table, both hip and knees flexed at 90 degrees, slowly extend the knee as if evaluating the patella or bottom of the foot. This maneuver stretches nerve roots as much as a moderate degree of supine SLR.

FIG. 28-3. Instructions for sitting knee extension test. (From: Bigos, S., Bowwyer, O., Braen, G., et al.: Acute Low Back Problems in Adults. Clinical Practice Guideline, Quick Reference Guide Number 14. Rockville, MD, U.S. Department of Health and Human Services. Public Health Service, Agency for Health Care Policy and Research, AHCPR Pub. No. 95-0643, December, 1994.)

TABLE 28-3. *Red flags for potentially serious conditions*

	Possible fracture	Possible tumor or infection	Possible cauda equina syndrome
From medical history	Major trauma, such as vehicle accident or fall from height. Minor trauma or even strenuous lifting (in older or potentially osteoporotic patient).	Age over 50 or under 20. History of cancer. Constitutional symptoms, such as recent fever or chills or unexplained weight loss. Risk factors for spinal infection: recent bacterial infection (e.g., urinary tract infection); IV drug abuse; or immune suppression (from steroids, transplant, or HIV). Pain that worsens when supine; severe nighttime pain.	Saddle anesthesia. Recent onset of bladder dysfunction, such as urinary retention, increased frequency, or overflow incontinence. Severe or progressive neurologic deficit in the lower extremity.
From physical examination			Unexpected laxity of the anal sphincter. Perianal/perineal sensory loss. Major motor weakness: quadriceps (knee extension weakness); ankle plantar flexors, evertors, and dorsiflexors (foot drop).

IV, intravenous; HIV, human immunodeficiency virus.

(From Bigos. S, Bowyer O, Braen G, *et al.* Acute Low Back Problems in Adults. Clinical Practice Guideline, Quick Reference Guide Number 14. Rockville, MD: U.S. Department of Health and Human Services. Public Health Service, Agency for Health Care Policy and Research, AHCPR Pub. No. 95-0643. December 1994.)

TABLE 28-4. *Ability of different techniques to identify and define pathology*

Technique	Identify physiologic insult	Define anatomic defect
History	+	+
Physical examination:		
Circumference measurements	+	+
Reflexes	++	++
Straight leg raising (SLR)	++	+
Crossed SLR	+++	++
Motor	++	++
Sensory	++	++
Laboratory studies (ESR, CBC, UA)	++	0
Bone scan[a]	+++	++
EMG/SEP	+++	++
X-ray[a]	0	+
CT[a]	0	++++[b]
MRI	0	++++[b]
Myelo-CT[a]	0	++++[b]
Myelography[a]	0	++++[b]

ESR, erythrocyte sedimentation rate; CBC, complete blood count; UA, urinary analysis; SEP, sensory evoked potentials.

[a] Risk of complications (radiation, infection, etc.): highest for myelo-CT, second highest for myelography, and relatively less risk for bone scan, x-ray, and CT.

[b] False-positive diagnostic findings in up to 30 percent of people without symptoms at age 30.

Note: Number of plus signs indicates relative ability to identify or define.

(From Bigos S, Bowyer O, Braen G, *et al.* Acute Low Back Problems in Adults. Clinical Practice Guideline, Quick Reference Guide Number, 14. Rockville, MD: U.S. Department of Health and Human Services, Public Health Service, Agency for Health Care Policy and Research. AHCPR Pub. No. 95-0643. December 1994.)

that a practice style consistent with back pain self-care, and based upon education of the patient, gave rise to equivalent long-term pain relief and functional outcome *but* at lower costs and with more patient satisfaction, than when more medications and bedrest were prescribed.[200] The expertise of psychologists, psychiatrists, and social workers should be sought, to unravel the complex nonphysical issues that can so complicate the patient's pain complaints. Some patients express psychological turmoil as physical symptoms. Furthermore, all consequences of pain in the patient's life (sympathy, attention, time off from a job he or she doesn't like, financial compensation) may not be bad and an accurate understanding of the "rewards and benefits" for a given patient is necessary to establish realistic expectations about that patient's therapeutic response.

MANAGEMENT OF PATIENTS WITH BACK PAIN

The generic purposes of treating pain, whether acute or chronic, are to relieve the pain and prevent further activity disruption. With the treatment of acute pain, it is expected that pain will disappear, but the realistic goals of managing chronic back pain are:

1. To achieve maximal reduction in the frequency and/or the intensity of the pain in as rapid a time period as possible.
2. To help the patient cope with residual pain and the consequences of the pain that are slower to change or that cannot be altered.
3. To restore the patient's functional ability for vocational and recreational activities.

4. To facilitate the patient's passage through the complex array of legal/social/economic barriers that obstruct recovery.
5. To assess the patient systematically for side effects and complications of therapy.

The AHCPR guidelines, among other sources, stress educating the patient about the problem and providing reassurance about the likelihood of recovery.[3,23,48,200] It is fundamental that the patient's diagnosis and needs will change over time, especially in patients with chronic back pain. Reevaluation by a concerned health care professional and fine-tuning of the treatment program are essential for continued achievement of pain reduction and patient recuperation. The Quebec Task Force on Spinal Disorders recommended that after 3 months of unsuccessful conservative therapy, or accumulated time lost from work due to back pain, the patient should be referred to a multidisciplinary pain clinic.[187] Using meta-analysis, Flor et al. and Cutler et al. recently have shown that treatment at pain centers does restore most patients with chronic low back pain to a greater functional state.[61,80]

In general, when any one therapeutic component is applied in singular fashion and intensely so, there is a lower likelihood of success, than when a program of therapeutic options is crafted for a given patient. The "program of treatment" concept is predicated upon the principle that each element acts on a cause of the pain and contributes to a percentage decrease in the total pain.[23,163,164] Regional analgesic procedures, which are but one method within a treatment program, can have a profound effect, because the benefit, although temporary, may be the first sign to the concerned patient that something really can be done about the pain.[161] A basic challenge in any invasive therapy is the timing of the intervention. The keys for the clinician in providing this potent effect are to: (i) select patients for whom invasive procedures are an appropriate intervention; (ii) explain the rationale for the treatment so that the patient feels more like a partner in the therapy and less like a victim of the system; (iii) perform the procedure with technical expertise; and (iv) use feedback from the patient to guide the provision of *all* subsequent therapy. It is equally fundamental that taking chronic pain away does not instantly solve all of the pain-related problems. Because the clinician is practicing pain medicine in evaluating and treating any patient with back pain, he or she must be aware of other modalities adjunctive to invasive procedures. The following are potential components of a conservative therapy program for patients with back pain.[67,85,150,164,165]

Medications

Patients may need therapeutic doses of nonsteroidal anti-inflammatory drugs (NSAIDs) to treat inflammatory/arthritic pathology or to manage mild to moderate musculoskeletal pain. Acetaminophen will be suitable for the latter purpose, but not the former. The analgesic effect of the NSAIDs and acetaminophen can be potentiated with concurrent use of antidepressant drugs (usually at doses less than those prescribed for depression) and the sedative side-effect of some can be used to advantage in patients who have pain-related insomnia. Drugs that diminish activity-disrupting muscle spasm may be needed on a short-term basis,[200] though the AHCPR guidelines state that there is "no demonstrated benefit" and 30% of patients experience drug-related drowsiness.[19] In patients with neuropathic pain, membrane-stabilizing drugs, such as the anticonvulsants or mexiletine, are useful to decrease the hyper-responsivity induced in the nervous system by the chronic pain. Carefully chosen patients, such as those with "failed back surgery syndrome" or intractable spinal stenosis, clearly benefit from the daily use of opioid medications, and many have shown that they can use these medications responsibly. If this is a mutual choice between the patient and the physician, it is strongly recommended that a signed contract, documenting the agreement and the responsibilities of both parties, be added to the patient's chart. In acute back pain, the AHCPR guidelines state opioids "...appear no more effective than safer analgesics...," and up to 35% of patients using opioids may exhibit poor tolerance of the side effects, which can include nausea, constipation, drowsiness, decreased reaction time, or clouded judgment.[19] The attitude about the chronic use of opioids for patients with noncancer pain problems is swinging from one based on an irrational fear of inducing addiction to viewing this as a reputable and reasonable therapeutic modality. Turk et al. assessed physicians' attitudes and practices concerning long-term prescription of opioids for noncancer pain and found the practice was "relatively widespread."[197]

Physical Therapy (PT)

A prime reason for decreasing a patient's pain is to encourage his or her cooperation with efforts to restore physical capacity for work and recreational activities.[67,48,129] Guided instructions for rehabilitative exercise can follow a professional evaluation by a physical therapist or an exercise physiologist. It is vital, though, that the recovering patient also perform rehabilitative exercises every day at home. The general thrust of such a program is to stretch muscles chronically in spasm, so that they regain their functional length and to restore range of motion (ROM), then to increase overall strength and, ultimately, to build up the patient's endurance for necessary and desired activities. It is fair to say that debate continues over what constitute the best exercises for patients with back pain. Clearly, after the pain begins to recede, management should be focused on improving the patient's physical condition, to overcome physical limitations and increase activity tolerance.[129] It is likely that the patient's back muscles will need to be in better condition than before the original problem developed. Saal et al. demonstrated that a significant portion of their 52 patients with non-operative treatment for lumbar disc disease required up to 12 weeks of exercise to achieve maximal functional outcome.[168] There is no evidence that traction, shoe lifts, corsets, back belts, massage, transcutaneous electrical nervous stimulation (TENS), ultrasound, diathermy, or biofeedback, are of any benefit in acute back pain,[19] but some include these modalities in lists of treatment for chronic back pain.[48] Spinal manipulation in the first month, and that only in patients without radiculopathy, is supported in the AHCPR guidelines for acute back pain, as is heat/cold therapy. Bed rest beyond 4 days, though not infrequently prescribed, is not recommended, but temporary activity alteration is practical to avoid undue irritation of the back.[48,200] Stieg cautions that tests that assess physical function may not accurately predict a patient's true state of disability.[188]

Trigger Points

Trigger-point injections are probably the most common pain-relieving block. It is important that the proposed site for injection be focal, i.e., the size of a nickel or quarter, and not an ill-defined area. Local anesthetics with or without soluble or depot steroids, saline, or neurolytic substances, have all been reported as the injectate.[186] The issues of how many trigger-point injections should be done at any given appointment, or over the course of time, have not been answered scientifically. Basically, to justify the maintenance of this treatment, the patient should manifest obvious and significant benefit from each trigger-point injection, that is recovery of his or her ability to function productively, while continuing other treatment modalities in a pain management program.

Psychology

Because pain is always a combination of somatic and nonphysical input, and because chronic pain precipitates drastic changes in a patient's attitudes, feelings, interactive skills, behavior, and lifestyle, it is reasonable to offer a professional evaluation of these factors. Pain will not respond to even the best treatment program if stress, abuse, or other sources of psychological conflict are rampant, or if the patient continues to feel overwhelmed by pain.[20] The work of Abram, Hopwood and Abram, and Jamison et al. documents the influential nature of psychosocial factors on complaints of back pain and the success of therapy.[1,2,106,110] In summary, important factors include being injured at work and missing work due to pain, low education, being a smoker, lack of response to previous treatment and nonvariation of the pain with activities.

Surgical Procedures

The AHCPR guidelines suggest the use of surgery only in patients with "serious spinal pathology or nerve root dysfunction obviously due to a herniated [lumbar] disc...."[19] They note surgery may hasten recovery in patients with obvious surgical indications but benefits fewer than 40% of patients with questionable physical findings. Calodney notes that more than 300,000 laminectomies are performed annually in the USA.[48] Unfortunately, 15 to 40% of these patients experience persistent pain. Bogduk believes that only 12% of patients with herniated nucleus pulposus require surgery.[23] Saal et al. reported on the use of an aggressive, progressive, conservative, therapy program consisting of physical therapy (PT), selective nerve blocks, and a back school program, in 52 patients with obvious indications for lumbar disc surgery.[168] Fifty of 52 patients had a good to excellent outcome in terms of pain reduction and recovery of activity over the average follow-up period of 3 months. Forty-eight of 50 patients regained function and returned to work. Volinn et al. used the National Hospital Discharge Survey and found a twofold variation among 4 regions of the USA in hospitalization for surgical (discectomy, laminectomy, spinal fusion) and nonsurgical (therapeutic injection, contrast myelography, other diagnostic or nonsurgical procedure) purposes.[200] It is interesting to note that the rate of low back surgery increased over the study period (1979 to 1987) by 49%, whereas the rate for hospitalization for nonsurgical reasons declined by 33%. The average length of a stay decreased for both categories, but, again, varied among the regions. The authors astutely point out that such wide variation in lower back pain (LBP) hospitalization raises the issue of which practices are the most appropriate. As is common now, given the thrust towards health care reform and cost containment, the authors and others urge that outcome analysis should be applied to practice patterns to identify those that are *both* medically and economically effective.[40,199,200] Bush makes the logical case for trying epidural steroid injections (ESIs) in surgical candidates before subjecting them to invasive surgical procedures that in the long run may not be necessary.[44]

Although surgery per se is not considered a conservative therapy, in the contemporary practice of pain medicine, many clinicians are applying percutaneous therapeutic techniques in *appropiate* patients who have been very carefully selected and screened. Components of this growing field are: trials of epidural stimulation preceding implantation of electrodes in the epidural space for dorsal column stimulation; trials, of intrathecal drug administration prior to use of implanted infusion pumps for administration of perispinal opioids. North et al. reported on 50 patients with chronic back pain due to failed back surgery syndrome (average 3.1 prior operations).[149] "Success," defined as at least 50% sustained relief for 2 years or at last follow-up and patient satisfaction with the result, occurred in 53 to 60% at 2.2 years and 47 to 54% at 5 years following spinal cord stimulator implantation. Patients noted improvement in activities of daily living and loss of function was rare.

NERVE BLOCKS FOR PATIENTS WITH BACK PAIN

The potential advantages and disadvantages of using neural blockade (regional analgesic procedures) in patients with back pain are listed in Table 28-5. The actual performance of the procedure is important, but not more so than understand-

TABLE 28-5. *Advantages/disadvantages of neural blockade in pain management*

Advantages
Involves interaction with the patient. The patient must be examined and an explanation about the rationale and risks and benefits of the proposed therapy provided
Can generally be done on an out-patient basis and neural blockade procedures have lower morbidity and shorter convalescence than surgery
The decrease in pain renews the patient's enthusiasm for regaining health
The decrease in pain fosters the use of fewer/less potent analgesics, more cooperation with restorative physical therapy, and a faster recovery of function
Disadvantages
Given the invasive nature of neural blockade, there are risks from the use of needles and the drugs injected
Patients with infection at the proposed site of injection, and perhaps those with systemic infection or taking major anticoagulant drugs, are not candidates for nerve block procedures
The physiologic and/or the pharmacological consequences of the injection may be poorly tolerated by the patient
The expertise for doing the nerve block may not be available
Conscientious follow-up after the neural blockade may not be provided

[Modified from Rowlingson JC. Appropriate use of therapeutic nerve blocks. In Tollison, C.D., Kriegel, M.L. (eds.): Interdisciplinary Rehabilitation of Low Back Pain. pp. 63–73. Baltimore, Williams and Wilkins, 1989.]

ing the importance of the information derived from the evaluation process. Knowing what the pathology is and where it is located is particularly important if diagnostic blocks are to be done appropriately.[87] As with surgery, nerve blocks are generally administered for specific indications in selected patients. The indication for any block must be determined at *every* re-evaluation of the patient. Just being able to provide the procedure is not justification for doing it. The clinician does not want to compromise the advantages of nerve blocks in the total treatment program by unwise patient selection or by an overzealous, aggressive, approach.

INDICATIONS FOR INVASIVE THERAPY

No one invasive procedure will treat all causes for back pain. The basic decisions about whether to offer a procedure, and which procedure is reasonable to offer, are arrived at after distillation of data from the patient's history, physical examination, psychological evaluation and relevant laboratory study results. Patients likely to be considered are:

1. Those with acute, subacute, or chronic, symptoms attributed to a bulging or herniated disc.
2. Patients with back pain related to postural changes (strains/sprains).
3. Patients with postsurgical back pain (so-called failed back surgery syndrome), who often manifest neuropathic pain qualities.
4. Patients with myofascial pain or zygapophysial arthropathy.
5. Patients with tumor cell invasion of the nerve roots that causes radicular pain.[138]

Patients with *classic radicular pain* describe sharp, stabbing pain that radiates from the low back to the buttocks and hips and down the back of the thigh, and extends below the knee (see Fig. 28-1). Patients with cervical discs may not have such specific complaints of pain radiating into the upper extremity. The onset is often associated with a traumatic lifting event.[153] The pain may be dermatomal, increased with activities that increase intradiscal pressure (such as standing, lifting, bending, and sitting), or raise intra-abdominal pressure (as with coughing, sneezing or lifting), and decrease with rest. The majority of disc herniations occur at L4–L5, L5–S1, C5–C6 and C6–C7.[67] There may be dermatomal changes upon sensory, motor, and reflex testing, and with lumbar discs, positive SLR in both the seated and supine positions. The three signs most indicative of lumbar nerve root irritation are positive straight leg raise, crossed straight leg raise, and the bowstring sign.[137] Positive Spurling's maneuver is associated with cervical disc herniation. Perispinal muscle spasm may be marked and range of motion diminished. Bogduk states that the diagnosis of a herniated nucleus pulposus (HNP) can be made solely on clinical grounds 90% of the time.[23] Diagnostic studies may show a bulging or herniated disc, tumor cell infiltration of the nerve roots, hypertrophic changes around the zygapophysial joints, or spinal stenosis.

Postural changes can cause significant back pain.[46] Normally, the weight of the erect spine is borne by the column of bony vertebrae with the interposed fibrocartilaginous discs. This system allows motion, leverage, flexibility, and shock absorption from impacts of various sorts. The bones serve as anchors for muscles and ligaments. The discs have a viscous liquid center, surrounded by circumferential fibrous tissue, forming the annulus. The discs of the lumbar spine account for 1/3 of the spine's height, whereas discs are only 1/5 of the height in other areas. When a patient suffers back pain that provokes muscle spasms (commonly in the semispinalis, multifidus and quadratus lumborum muscles, for low back pain), the normal lordotic curve of the lumbar spine is accentuated because most patients do not have enough abdominal muscle tone to balance this change. This shifts the weight-bearing function to the posterior elements of the spine—the lamina, pedicles and the zygapophysial joints. These structures form a protective arch for the spinal cord emerging nerve roots, serving as anchors for muscles, ligaments, and tendons, and imposing restriction on the motion capacity of the spine. Patients with postural back pain develop the pain because the supportive tissues repeatedly are stressed beyond their tensile strength and shear forces are created on the posterior elements. This results in cumulative musculoskeletal trauma, which persists due to abnormal joint motion and poor distribution of the repetitive mechanical pressures on the spine.[23,24,48,153,169] This repetitive insult contributes to the perpetuation of the smoldering "injury," and these patients ultimately may develop radicular pain. The patients will complain of diffuse pain across the low back or shoulders that is aching and dull in character. Pain may be referred to the hips and buttocks, or to the shoulders and upper arms, depending upon the location of the disc. The physical exam may show muscle spasm, decreased range of motion, and tenderness to palpation over the sacroiliac joints or the posterior superior iliac spine region, in patients with low back pain. Laboratory studies may be unrevealing.

Patients suffering from *postlaminectomy/failed back syndrome* describe pain as constant, dull, and aching, but occasionally as a sharper, almost radicular-like, pain.[47] The pain, which has a number of neuropathic features, is not well localized. Rather, it is felt in the low back, buttocks, hips, posterior thighs and knees, or in the posterior neck, shoulders, and upper extremities. A patient may complain of intermittent numbness and/or weakness of the extremities and state his or her leg can "give out" unexpectedly, or hand-held objects are dropped inexplicably. The patient may have degenerative disc disease plus spinal stenosis, plus a zygapophysial syndrome. Classically, those with a *zygapophysial syndrome* in the lumbar spine complain of unilateral pain that radiates from a site just lateral to the midline, down the thigh and occasionally as far as the back of the knee. Lateral bending with lumbar spinal extension causes intense pain, and one may find tenderness over the zygapophysial joint, paraspinal muscle spasm, and decreased lumbar range of motion. Furthermore, patients with failed back syndrome may have residual neurologic deficits, attributable to scarring from surgical procedures or from irreversible nerve damage from the chronicity of their symptoms. Muscle atrophy may be evident, as well as signs of decreased physical conditioning such as muscle weakness, poor muscle tone and weight gain. Flexibility of the spine usually is diminished, as may be hip or shoulder motion and straight leg raising, due to chronic spasm and lack of physical activity. Laboratory findings in these patients are extremely variable, possibly showing residual scarring from surgery, foraminal narrowing, zygapophysial hypertrophy, or changes suggestive of recurrent or new disc pathology. Past surgery may make accurate interpretation of diagnostic studies extremely difficult(see also Appendix A, Chapter 23.1).

When *myofascial pain* is present, the patient will have musculoskeletal pain from a number of well-recognized musculotendinous locations that are tender to palpation.[150,166,186] Myofascial pain results from direct trauma to muscles, bones, joints, and soft tissue, or can be a secondary result of pain in another part of the body which incited postural changes that chronically stress the musculoskeletal tissues in the painful area. The pain is deep and aching in character, and associated with muscle spasm, stiffness, fatigue, and sleep disturbance. Trigger points in the muscles and their supporting tissues may be found upon examination, as may be muscle spasm and decreased range of motion. Diagnostic studies are likely to be remarkably unrevealing.

PHYSIOLOGY AND ANATOMY

Several areas of the lumbar spine can contribute to painful conditions, either uniquely or in combination, (Table 28-6). These structures include the annulus of the disc, the anterior and posterior longitudinal ligaments, portions of the dura,

TABLE 28-6. *Sources of primary low back pain*

Bones

1. Vertebral bodies: Periosteum pain sensitive (? bone)
   Metabolic Bone Disease (e.g., osteitis fibrosa)
   Primary and Secondary Tumors
   Fractures: ?Pain due to bone or stresses on adjacent joints, muscles, ligaments.
   Osteoporosis: ?Cause of Pain
   Spondylolisthesis: ? Instability irritates nerve roots, ?Ligament strain.
   Infection
2. Other Parts of Vertebrae: e.g., secondary tumors in pedicle and fractures of transverse process.
3. Spinous Processes: 'kissing spines' (Baastrup's disease).
   excessive lordosis or extension injuries.
   periostitis of spinous processes.
4. Inferior Articular Processes
   Impaction of inferior articular process on lamina below in extension injuries.
   Periostitis of lamina.
5. Pars interarticularis
   ?unilateral fracture, a cause of pain
   bilateral fracture causes 'flail segment'.

Muscles

e.g. Quadratus lumborum, psoas (supplied by branches of lumbar ventral rami)
Back muscles (supplied by branches of dorsal rami)
Intertransverse muscles (supplied by dorsal and ventral rami)
Causes of Pain: ?sprain, *strain*, ?imbalance of action, ?trigger points, ?Fibromyalgia.

Thoraco-lumbar Fascia

? compartment syndrome
? herniation of fat

Dura-mater

infection/inflammation
?tethering

Epidural Venous Plexus

? Venous distension due to obstruction by large disc herniation or spinal stenosis

Ligaments: No convincing evidence for ligamentous pain, except in combination, e.g., with annulus fibrosus pathology

Sacro-iliac joints: ? innervation by branches of $L_{4,5}$ $S_{1,2}$ dorsal rami provides a basis for pain

Zygapophysial joints: Innervation by medial branches of dorsal rami.
Causes of Pain: ? osteoarthrosis, fractures of articular processes, subchondral fractures, capsular tears, capsular avulsions and joint space hemorrhage—due to excessive extension or rotation movements of lumbar vertebrae

Discs: extensive innervation by lumbar sinuvertebral nerves and grey rami communicantes and sympathetic trunks.
Causes of Pain: Lesions of pain-sensitive annulus fibrosus (outer third)
torsion injuries cause circumferential tears and an associated inflammatory focus develops
compression injuries cause end-plate fracture and possible inflammatory degradation of disc
degradation isolated disc resorption (painless) or internal disc disruption, radial fissuring of annulus fibrosus and possible disc herniation

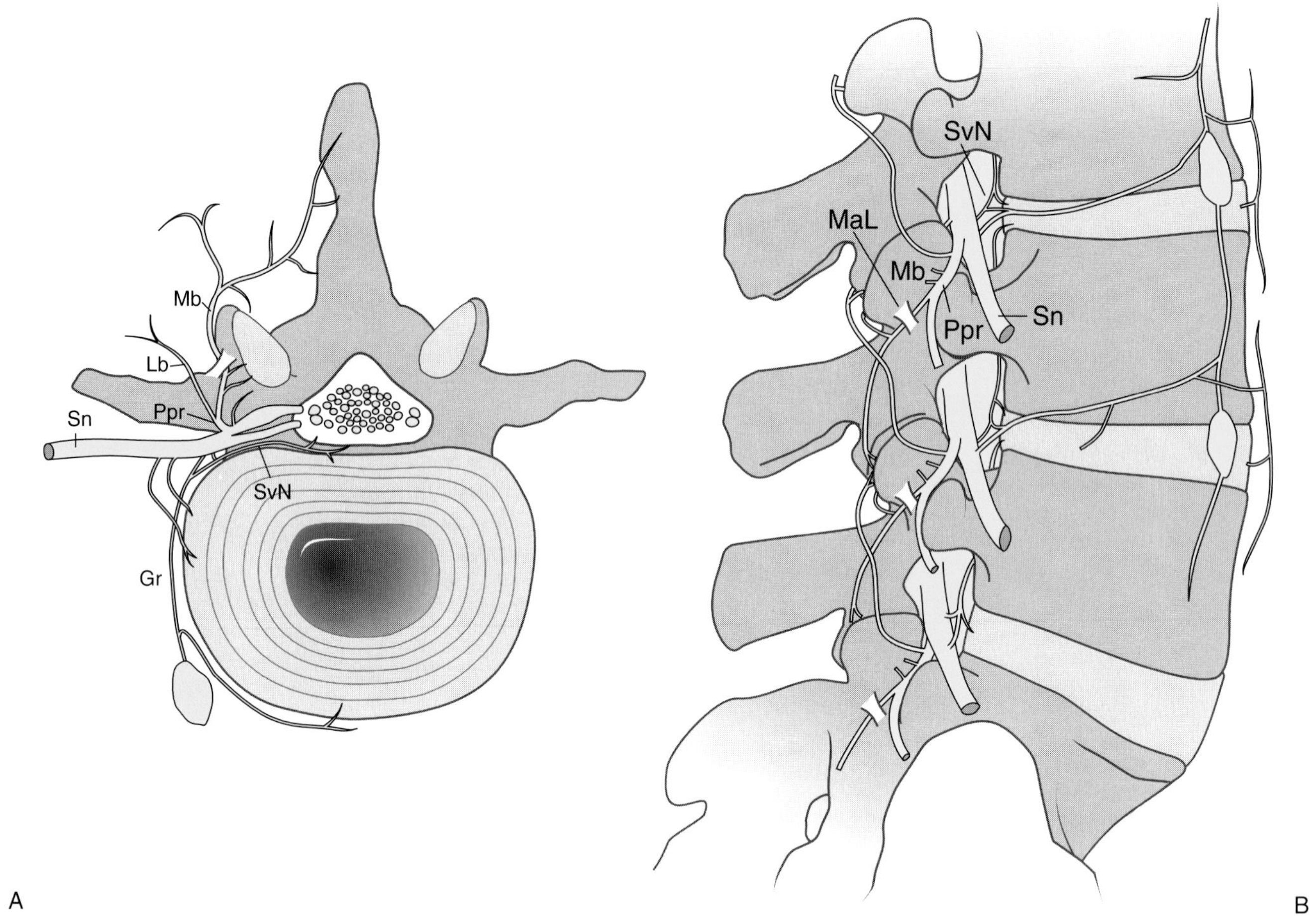

FIG. 28-4. Lumbar spine innervation. Sketch of the innervation of the lumbar spinal structures in transverse **(A)** and lateral **(B)** views. **A:** Note the posterior primary ramus *(Ppr)* leaving the spinal nerve *(Sn)* and splitting into a lateral branch *(Lb)* and a medial branch *(Mb)*. The medial branch passes under the mammillo-accessary ligament *(mal)* to innervate the facet joint and capsule, the spinous process and the multifidus muscles. Sensory fibers traveling with the gray rami *(Gr)* form the sinu-vertebral nerve *(SvN)* and provide sensory function to the disc annulus.

the zygapophysial joints and capsule, the spinal nerve roots, dorsal root ganglia, and, occasionally, the sacroiliac joint[5,25–28,73,122,174] (Fig. 28-4). Bogduk has proposed that the lumbar spine can be divided into dorsal and ventral compartments by a coronal plane through the intervertebral foramina and separated laterally by the transverse processes and the intertransverse ligaments.[27] The ventral compartment then contains the vertebral bodies, discs, anterior and posterior longitudinal ligaments, ventral dura and prevertebral muscles. The ventral compartment is innervated by an interconnected, multisegmental nerve plexus that is derived from the sympathetic chain, communicating rami and perivascular nerves. This multisegmental representation leads to diffuse referral patterns for pain and no discrete site for denervation. The involvement of nerves derived from the sympathetic chain in the innervation of the ventral compartment raises the possibility of sympathetic modulation mechanisms in the generation and maintenance of spinal pain.[93] Recently, the dorsal root ganglion itself has been reported to receive a sympathetic nerve supply.[66,121] The dorsal compartment contains the zygapophysial joints, the dorsal dura, and the intrinsic back muscles and ligaments. Unlike the ventral compartment, the dorsal compartment is predominantly supplied by the lateral and medial branches of the dorsal rami with a variable contribution from the communicating rami (see Fig. 28-4). This innervation pattern is consistent with integration of multiple spinal segments within the connections of the wide dynamic range neurons of the dorsal horn; thus, the need is evident for multiple levels of blockade to address the origin of spinal pain. Innervation of the cervical spine is illustrated in Figure 28-5.

Much of our information about pain-sensitive structures of the back is based upon stimulation studies in normal volunteers[71,73] or from the systematic stimulation of tissue layers of the back during surgery.[122] Stimulation studies in normal volunteers, however, have many limitations, and may have little applicability to the patient with clinical pain. Several neurophysiological studies in animals have demonstrated that a significant proportion of potential nociceptive fibers are silent under normal conditions, meaning that they

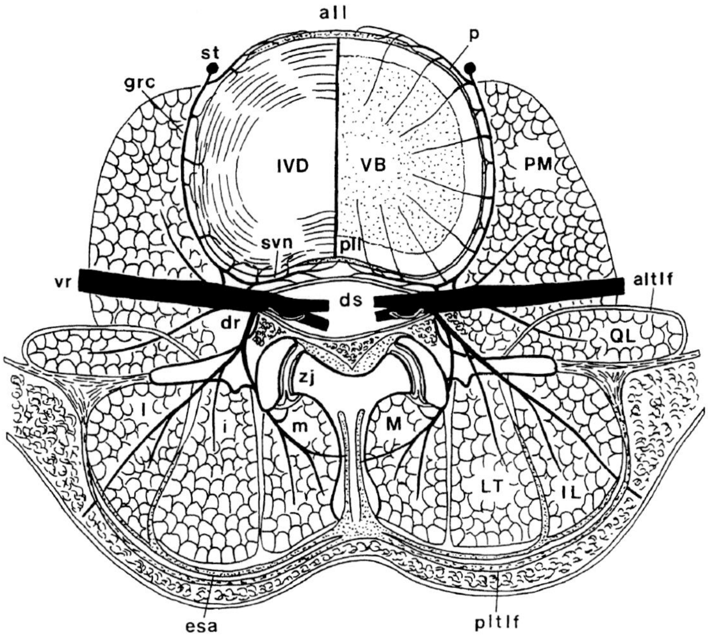

C

FIG. 28-4. *Continued..* **C:** A cross-sectional view incorporating the level of the vertebral body *(VB)* and its periosteium *(p)* on the right of the intervertebral disc *(IVD)* on the left. *PM,* psoas muscle; *QL,* quadratus lumborum; *IL,* iliocostalis lumborum; *LT,* longissimus thoracicus; *M,* mulitfidus; *altf,* anterior layer of thoracolumbar fascia; *pltf,* posterior layer of thoracolumbar fascia; *esa,* erector spinae aponeurosis; *ds,* dural sac; *zj,* zygopophyseal joint; *pll,* posterior longitudinal ligament; *all,* anterior longitudinal ligament; *vr,* ventral ramus; *dr,* dorsal raimus; de, doral sac; *m,* medial branch; *i,* intermediate branch; *svn,* sinu-vertebral nerve; *grc,* gray ramus communicans; *st,* sympathetic trunk. (From Bogduk, N. and Twomey, L. T.: Nerves of the lumbar spine. *In* Clinical Anatomy of the Lumbar Spine. 2nd Ed. pp. 107. Melbourne, Churchill Livingstone 1996.)

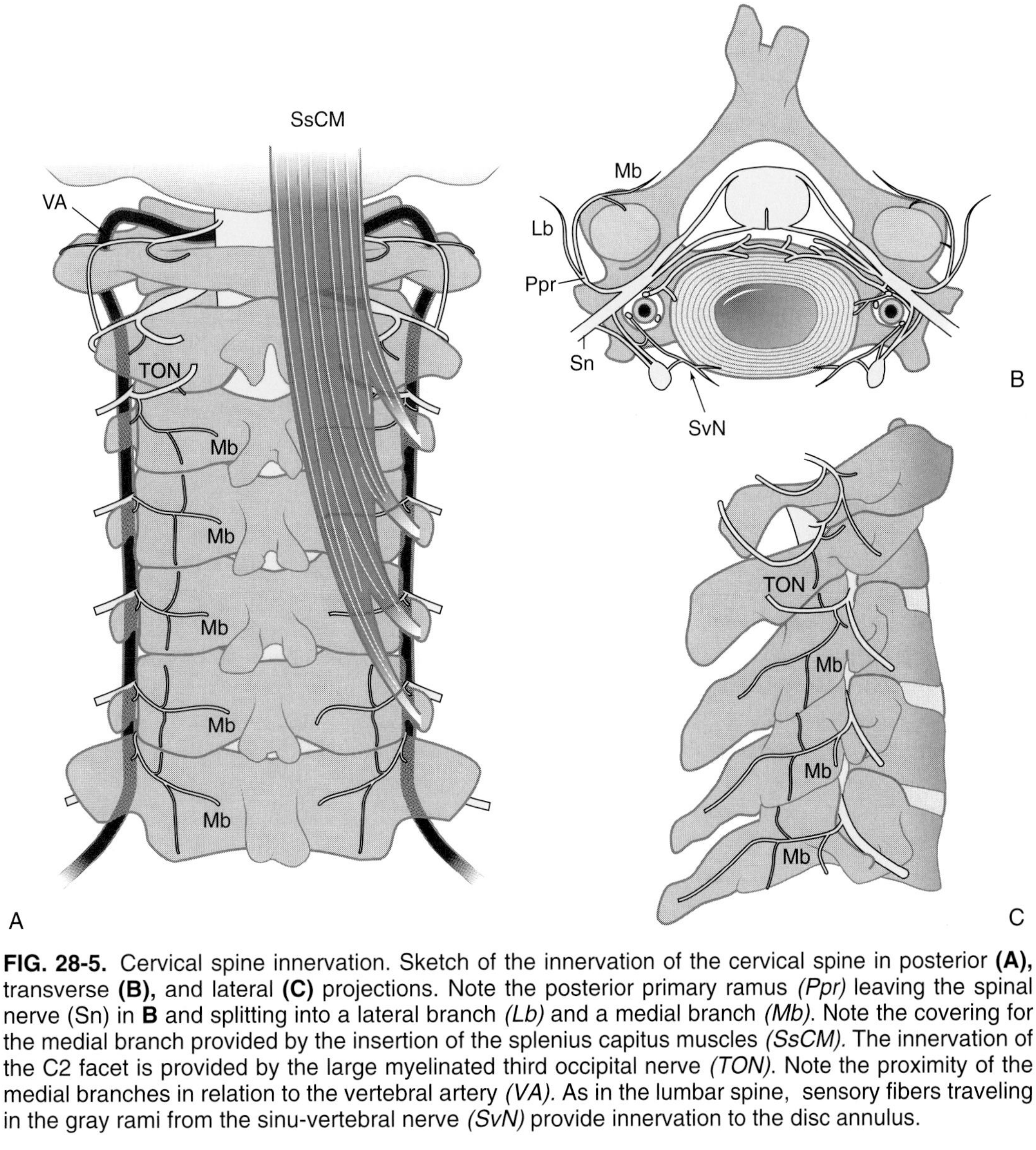

FIG. 28-5. Cervical spine innervation. Sketch of the innervation of the cervical spine in posterior **(A),** transverse **(B),** and lateral **(C)** projections. Note the posterior primary ramus *(Ppr)* leaving the spinal nerve (Sn) in **B** and splitting into a lateral branch *(Lb)* and a medial branch *(Mb)*. Note the covering for the medial branch provided by the insertion of the splenius capitus muscles *(SsCM).* The innervation of the C2 facet is provided by the large myelinated third occipital nerve *(TON).* Note the proximity of the medial branches in relation to the vertebral artery *(VA).* As in the lumbar spine, sensory fibers traveling in the gray rami from the sinu-vertebral nerve *(SvN)* provide innervation to the disc annulus.

are not mechanically responsive.[49,88,141] These fibers, however, can be readily recruited when inflammation or ischemia is present.[62134,] Therefore, structures which are not painful when not inflamed may well become the site of pain in a patient with a relevant back injury or inflammation.[88]

A normal nerve root, when pulled or displaced, does not create sciatic pain, but a compressed or inflamed nerve root will generate the characteristic pain of sciatica when minimal traction is applied.[107] These findings are consistent with development of mechanical sensitivity or hyperalgesia in innervated structures as a response to injury or inflammation.[62,141] These sensitized fibers, as well as many other nonstructural lesions, like edema, inflammation, and dynamic or irritative nerve lesions do not show up as abnormal on any of the conventional imaging techniques; therefore, the true cause for the pain escapes diagnosis.

INJECTION THERAPY AND NEURAL BLOCKADE FOR THE MANAGEMENT OF BACK PAIN

General Considerations

Preparation and Facilities

The neural blockade procedures around the spine discussed below should only be performed by a practitioner familiar with and capable of handling the potential airway and hemodynamic complications of a misplaced injection. Minimum resuscitation equipment would include a bag and mask, oxygen source, suction source, emergency airway equipment (laryngoscope handle, assorted blades and endotracheal tubes), drugs (atropine, ephedrine, epinephrine, lidocaine,) and intravenous fluids and cannulae. During the procedure, the patient should be monitored with at least a blood pressure cuff, pulse oximeter, and possibly an electrocardiogram. In all procedures, the patient should have an intravenous catheter sited, as a precaution for the unlikely event of needing emergency drug administration.

To perform diagnostic and therapeutic spinal blocks in a safe and effective manner, a C-arm fluoroscopy device with a radiolucent table capable of allowing oblique views, is recommended. It is also desirable to have some capability for hard copies of the fluoroscope screen image to document the needle placement, especially if a neurolytic procedure is performed.

Assessment

A pain diary should be used with all diagnostic block procedures. The patient is asked to rate his or her pain on a numerical scale, and to repeat the ratings at defined intervals, i.e., every 30 to 60 minutes. In addition to the pain ratings, the patient should also record the location of the pain and the activity performed at the time. In this way, the patient will be able to give a more accurate and complete picture of the effects of the block. Often, when the pain returns, the patient will forget the short period of relief. The pain diary allows the physician to use local anesthetics of varying duration and establish whether the response is nonspecific, or in keeping with the known kinetics of the drug.[9] Too short a response may be a nonspecific effect as well. Patients will tend to be more objective when they are recording their ratings on their own, rather than doing so under the expectant eye of the treating physician or another observer.

ZYGAPOPHYSIAL JOINT AND MECHANICAL SPINE PAIN

Historical Background

The concept that the zygapophysial joints are involved in the etiology of back pain can be traced to Goldthwaite in 1911.[99] He suggested that an asymmetry of the zygapophysial joints could account for back pain, but that the relationship had never been demonstrated. In 1933, Ghormley[90] proposed that sciatica was due to zygapophysial joint hypertrophy exerting pressure on the nerve root, whereas Badgley in 1941[8] suggested that zygapophysial joints themselves could be a primary source of pain separate from the nerve compression component.

Acceptance of this origin for back pain has been slow, probably due to the strong evidence presented for nerve root compression by a herniated intervertebral disc, as proposed by Mixter and Barr in 1934.[142] This seemed to account for radicular pain, as the pain pattern distribution matched the dermatomal patterns reported by Foerster in 1932.[81] This explanation for radicular pain prevailed for several years until Kellgren in 1938[113] demonstrated that direct stimulation of connective tissue could elicit pain separate from and distal to the dermatomes. This projection pattern was termed a sclerotome pattern. Thus, it has been recognized that many different tissues refer pain to the same location, making the diagnosis of back pain more difficult than previously appreciated. The zygapophysial joint etiology of pain languished for several years until 1963, when Hirsch injected hypertonic saline into the zygapophysial joints.[105] Although the site of the injections were poorly localized, they did initiate pain resembling clinical pain conditions and distributions. Increasingly, practitioners have come to recognize that the zygapophysial (facet) joints are potential sources of mechanical back pain.[159] Zygapophysial joints form a significant portion of the posterior support structure for the spine, and bear most of the shear forces when the spine is flexed.[79] As with any synovial joint degeneration, inflammation and injury can lead to pain upon joint motion. Restriction of motion secondary to pain can lead to overall physical deconditioning, and irritation of the joint innervation can itself lead to secondary muscle spasm.

Although the zygapophysial joints may serve a minimal load-bearing role in the normal spine, degeneration of the intervertebral disc will shift a greater load-bearing role to them. The load transmission and weight-bearing properties of human zygapophysial joints were studied in vitro by Yang and King.[217] They found in a finite element model of the lumbar motion segment that normal zygapophysial joints carried 3 to 25% of the load and arthritic joints could be exposed to as much as 47% of the load. Excessive loads cause the inferior zygapophysial joint to pivot about the pars and stretch the capsule. The zygapophysial joints will assume a greater percentage of the load if the discs are degenerate.[217] Loads are also increased with the spine in an extended position.

Neurophysiological[216] and anatomical[76] studies have found small-diameter, high-threshold fibers in the zygapophysial joint capsules of the rabbit and human. These fibers can subserve nociception—a fact further supported by the finding of substance P (SP) as containing fibers in the zygapophysial joint capsule of rabbit[76] and human.[13] A greater density of potential nociceptive fibers were found in the zygapophysial joint capsule than in the surrounding tissues. These studies may represent an underestimate of the density and sensitivity of the nociceptive fibers. Studies of the innervation of the cat knee joint have demonstrated a significant decrease in the threshold and an increase in the activity of knee joint group IV thinly myelinated fibers in the presence of joint inflammation. This same sensitization of pain-transmitting fibers may explain the back pain in the presence of inflammation or injury to the zygapophysial joints and surrounding tissue. In addition, fibers containing several peptides associated with nociceptive transmission, including SP, calcitonin gene-related peptide (CGRP), vasoactive intestinal polypeptide (VIP), and the autonomic fiber markers neuropeptide Y and tyrosine hydroxylase,[4] have been identified in the synovial folds of the zygapophysial joint, the supraspinous ligament, the posterior longitudinal ligament, and the annulus fibrosus. The SP fibers were found in the subchondral bone, and it can be postulated that intra-articular injections of steroids may not be able to affect the fibers in the deep regions, while blockade of the medial branch would block these fibers easily. This anatomical fact may explain the variable (and mostly poor) results of intra-articular steroids for relief of zygapophysial joint-related mechanical low back pain.[13,10,89]

The zygapophysial joints contain intra-articular synovial inclusions which are very vascular and are altered as the joint moves. These inclusions have been shown to be richly innervated in the human.[91,92] Some forms of back pain have been attributed to the trapping of these inclusions between zygapophysial joint plates. The synovium so trapped becomes inflamed, and eventually develops a fibrotic reaction. The presence of nociceptive nerve fibers within the synovium provides an explanation in support of this mechanism of low back pain. Intra-articular and multifidus muscle injections, with a tracer that is retrogradely transported in nerves to the spinal cord, have revealed specific labeling within dorsal horn nerve terminals.[94] This labeling was consistent with nociceptive input to the superficial layers of the spinal cord. The innervation pattern was diffuse but strictly ipsilateral to the injection. Projections from the zygapophysial joint and the deep muscle are distributed broadly in the dorsal horn of the spinal cord in a diffuse pattern similar to *visceral* projections[94] (see Chapter 23.1, Fig. 23.1-20). This pattern was in direct contrast to the limited and restricted projections of distal extremity tissues. These findings are consistent with the clinical presentation of diffuse, poorly localized pain, with mechanical activation of the zygapophysial joints.

The presence of sympathetic fibers in the zygapophysial joint[4] has several clinical implications. Autonomic innervation to a joint has been implicated in the progression of articular degeneration[123,124] and the presence of sympathetic innervation may explain the occasional report of back pain relief from a sympathetic ganglion block.[41,54]

Indahl and colleagues have demonstrated that stimulation of the articular nerves can produce reflex contraction of the periarticular muscles.[136] In a series of studies, using a unique in vivo system where the spine of a rabbit was subjected to controlled loading in a postero-lateral direction and the afferent fiber activity was measured neurophysiologically, Avramov and colleagues found several classes of mechanoreceptors responding to movement.[7] Three classes of fibers and responses were noted: phasic discharges consistent with velocity detectors, low-threshold group II and III receptors located in the muscles and tendons inserting into the joint (probably serving proprioception) and high-threshold, slowly adapting mechanoreceptors consistent with nociceptive fibers, responding potentially to noxious mechanical stimulation.

The zygapophysial joints are innervated by the medial branches of the dorsal rami of the spinal nerves.[27,29,159] At the L1 through L4 levels, the medial branches cross the transverse process at the medial superior edge and cross the root of the superior articular process. At this point, the medial branch passes medially and is covered by the mammiloaccessory ligament, where it splits into proximal and distal zygapophysial branches. The proximal branch innervates the adjacent zygapophysial joint and capsule and the distal branch innervates the joint and capsule of the next lower level (see Fig. 28-11). The L5 dorsal ramus travels between the ala of the sacrum and its superior articular process. At the caudal edge of the process, the nerve splits into medial and lateral branches. The medial branch continues medially, where it innervates the lumbosacral joint (see Fig. 28-11) and the multifidus muscle. The medial branches also innervate the interspinous ligaments and multifidus muscles. The closely-associated lateral and intermediate branches innervate the iliocostalis and longissimus muscles, respectively. Irritation of the medial branches could thus lead to generalized sensitization of the dorsal rami, with subsequent hyperactivity and spasm of the innervated muscles. In fact, when the medial branch is stimulated electrically in preparation for radiofrequency lesioning, the patients report a deep, boring pain, consistent with their muscle spasm symptoms. Stimulation a short distance away does not elicit this report.

The cervical zygapophysial joints increasingly are impli-

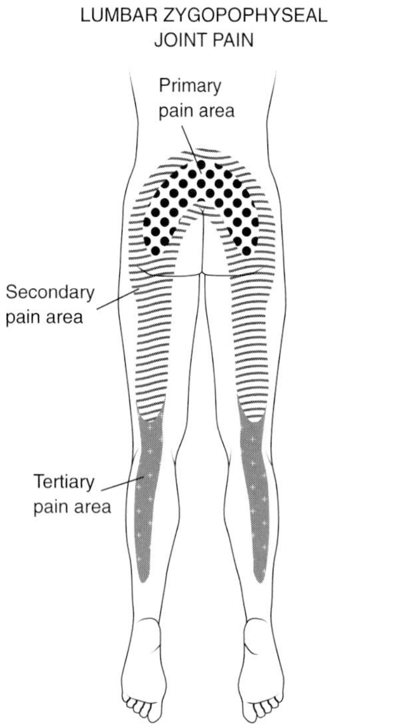

FIG. 28-6. Diagram of the lumbar zygapophysial joint pain distribution.

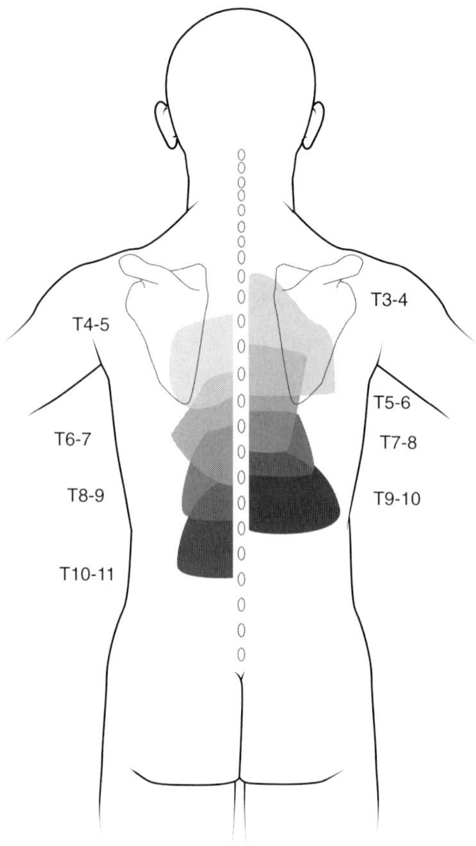

FIG. 28-8. Diagram of thoracic zygapophysial joint pain distribution. Sketch of the average pain referral patterns reported by volunteers subjected to provocative injection into selected thoracic zygapophysial joints as indicated by the labels. (Adapted from Dreyfuss, P., Tibilette, C., and Dreyer, S.J.: Thoracic zygapophysial joint pain patterns: A study in normal volunteers. Spine, *19*:807, 1994.)

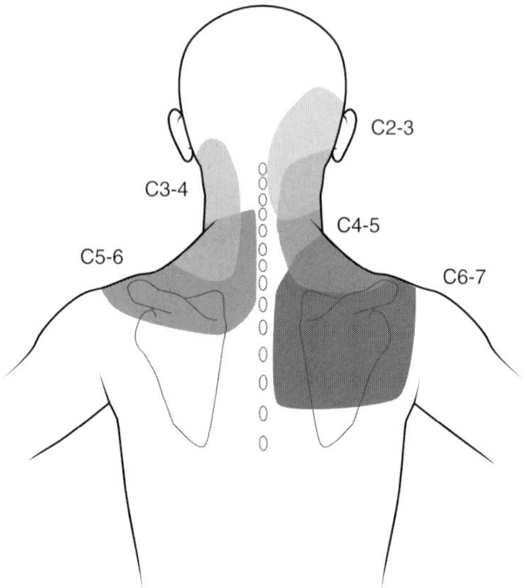

FIG. 28-7. Diagram of cervical zygapophysial joint pain distribution. Sketch of the average pain referral patterns reported by volunteers subjected to provocative injection into selected cervical zygapophysial joints as indicated by the labels. (Adapted from Dwyer, A., Aprill, C., and Bogduk, N.: Cervical zygapophysial joint pain patterns. I. A study in normal volunteers. Spine, *15*:453, 1990.)

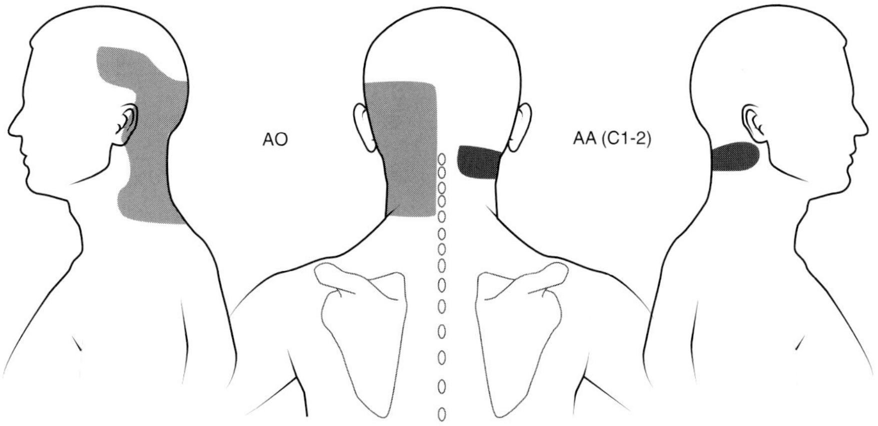

FIG. 28-9. Diagram of atlanto-axial joint pain distribution. Sketch of the average pain referral patterns reported by volunteers subjected to provocative joint injections as indicated. [Adapted from Dreyfus, P., Michaelsen, M., and Fletcher, D.: Atlanto-occipital (*AO*) and lateral atlanto-axial (*AA*) joint pain patterns. Spine, *19:*1125, 1990.]

cated in degenerative and traumatic head, neck, posterior shoulder, and back pain.[9,11,25,26,30,31] Below C2–C3, the cervical zygapophysial joints are supplied by medial branches of the cervical dorsal rami above and below the joint, which also innervate the deep paramedian muscles. The C2–C3 joint is supplied by the third occipital nerve. The medial branches travel across the waist of the articular pillar beneath the tendinous origin of the semispinalis capitis, where local anesthetic can be placed and "contained"[11,32] (see Fig. 28-13).

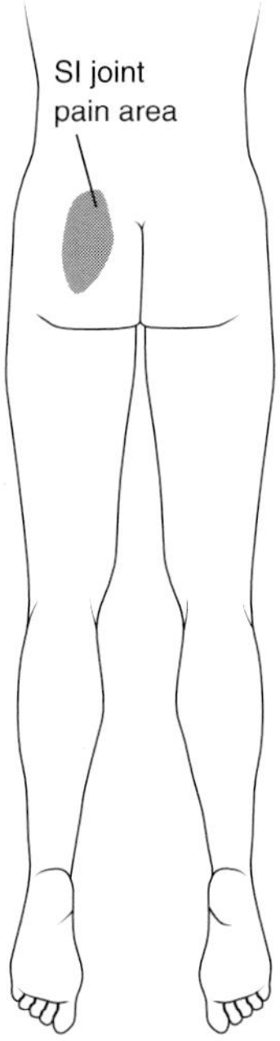

FIG. 28-10. Diagram of sacro-iliac joint pain distribution. Sketch of the average pain referral patterns reported by volunteers subjected to provocative joint injections. Note the overlap in the distribution of the SI joint pain and the primary referral region for the lumbar zygapophysial joints (see Fig. 28-6). (Adapted from Fortin, J.D., Dwyer, A.P., West, S., and Pier, J.: Sacro-iliac joint: Pain referral maps upon applying a new injection/arthrography technique. Part I. Asymptomatic volunteers. Spine, *19:*1475, 1994.)

The lumbar region does not have discrete referral patterns from the zygapophysial joints—the distribution of pain is overlapping from the L1 to S1 levels.[131,159] Referral patterns for zygapophysial joint pain have been mapped for cervical and thoracic regions, as well as for the atlanto-occipital, atlanto-axial and sacroiliac regions, through the use of provocative injections of hypertonic saline,[71–74,84] and confirmed in the cervical region by local anesthetic blocks in patients with neck pain.[6] These various referral maps are presented in Figures 28-6 to 28-10. Based on the clinical presentation and the information from referral maps, the patient is sent for diagnostic local anesthetic blocks, to confirm the diagnosis.

CLINICAL FEATURES OF ZYGAPOPHYSIAL JOINT-RELATED PAIN

The diagnosis of the lumber facet or zygapophysial joint "syndrome" depends on a clinical presentation with mechanical low back pain, described as mainly in the low back with radiation to the buttocks and upper posterior thigh[33,144,159] (Fig. 28-6). The pain typically is brought on or worsened by extension of the back, or lateral loading of the zygapophysial joints, and with prolonged standing or sitting. The pain is typically relieved by bed rest. Radiographic evidence of zygapophysial joint hypertrophy or degeneration may be seen, but often there is either no pathology seen or there is extensive pathology in regions that are not painful. Recently, in a study by Schwarzer et al., 63 patients with low back pain underwent both intra-articular zygapophysial joint blocks and CT scanning.[175] From the results, the authors concluded that CT has no place in the diagnosis of lumbar zygapophysial joint pain.[175] This pain can be present with or without sciatic or radicular symptoms. Given the variable nature of the radiographic presentation and the somewhat nonspecific clinical presentation, the diagnosis of zygapophysial joint syndrome relies on the response to local anesthetic injections into the joint or onto the medial branch of the dorsal ramus innervating the suspected joint. The most frequently involved zygapophysial joints are L5–S1, followed by L4–L5, L3–L4 and L2–L3, respectively.[176] Therefore, the most commonly involved zygapophysial joints, L4–L5 and L5–S1, are tested first in the presence of lumbar pain.

As indicated previously, several structures in the back can be responsible for back and leg pain. In general, the etiologies can be divided into those causing nerve compression or irritation and those with primarily mechanical components. Nerve compression and irritation typically are due to disc pathology such as rupture or herniation, with subsequent nerve root compression. The mechanical pain syndromes can emanate from the posterior elements, such as the zygapophysial joint, the posterior longitudinal ligament, or the back muscles. Stolker et al. argue that the so-called facet or zygapophysial joint syndrome would be better termed the dorsal compartment syndrome, characterized by mechanical pain elicited by hyperextension and rotation, and involving a multisegmental innervation.[189] Schwarzer et al. have challenged the ability to define the zygapophysial joint or dorsal compartment syndrome, based on clinical exam and history, and they advocate the need for differential local anesthetic blocks to assure the diagnosis.[176] There is considerable symptom overlap between myogenic back pain and the dorsal compartment syndrome. The only way to distinguish them is to perform careful medial branch or intra-articular zygapophysial joint blocks. The ventral compartment syndrome commonly is associated with midspinal pain and tenderness, with an increase in pain with flexion and deflexion. Often, the ventral compartment syndrome is associated with MRI findings, and provocative discography can help to make the diagnosis. The ideal therapeutic block for the ventral compartment syndrome is a controversial point. Anatomically, the sinuvertebral nerve would be the best option, but a specific block of this nerve is difficult because the local anesthetic can easily overflow to the communicating ramus and the spinal nerve.[118,189] For the same reasons, creating the radiofrequency lesion is complicated by the possibility of collateral injury to these nerves and to the radicular artery[189] (see Chapter 7, Fig. 7–11).

Upper cervical spine abnormalities can produce both neck pain and cervicogenic headaches.[30,39] All cervical synovial joints can be involved in pain generation. Prediction of affected levels in a given patient is facilitated by the pain maps generated by intra-articular injections in normal individuals (Fig. 28–7). From the C3–C4 joint to the C6–C7 level, the zygapophysial joint is supplied by the medial branches of the dorsal rami above and below the level.[32] In addition to the joint, these nerves supply a portion of the deep paramedian muscles such as multifidus, splenius capitis and splenius cervicis. Despite this stated innervation of these muscles, the total innervation of these muscle groups is so diffuse that it is unlikely that blocking even several of the medial branches would have a significant, direct effect on cervical muscle spasm.[30] The most frequently involved cervical zygapophysial joints in whiplash injury are the C2–C3 and C5–C6 levels.[12] It is not uncommon to have only unilateral involvement of the joints. The C2–C3 level represents a functional transition zone between the rotational segment above and the flexion/extension segments below.[39] This position makes this level more vulnerable to trauma. The C2–C3 joint is supplied by the third occipital nerve and to a variable extent by a branch of the greater occipital nerve.[32] In a manner similar to the lower levels, the third occipital nerve supplies the splenius capitis, but unlike those levels, it also provides a small region of cutaneous innervation in the suboccipital region.[32]

Barnsley et al. have reported that chronic neck pain in up to 54% of patients with whiplash injury may be due to the cervical zygapophysial joints.[12] They reached this conclusion after studying 50 consecutive patients who received lidocaine and bupivacaine in random order, to block the symptomatic joints, on separate occasions. These results are important, because the pain due to whiplash injury is confounded by negative findings on routine diagnostic tests, which lead clinicians to attribute a patient's chronic pain, falsely, to preexisting psychopathology or to secondary gain, thereby complicating the litigation process for patients involved in lawsuits concerning their injuries. In both clinical and experimental studies of human whiplash victims and in animal models, multiple pathologic findings have been observed, including joint capsule tears, hemarthroses and fractures of the articular cartilage and subchondral bone. None of these abnormalities would be discoverable on standard radiologic studies.

The specificity of cervical medial branch blocks has been addressed in an earlier study by Barnsley and Bogduk.[11] These authors injected 0.5 cc of local anesthetic followed by 0.5 cc of radiocontrast dye and documented both the pain relief and spread of the dye. A majority of the patients obtained pain relief, and the dye was noted consistently to be associated only with the course of the medial branch. No other structure was reached reliably by the dye (nor, presumably, by the local anesthetic). The stated objective of the injection was to place the local anesthetic underneath the tendinous origin of the splenus capitis, thus keeping it in specific contact with the medial branch to the zygapophysial joint (Fig. 28-5). The authors concluded that cervical medial branch blocks are target-specific and reliably anesthetize the medial branches of the cervical dorsal rami.

The prevalence of zygapophysial joint-related low back pain has been difficult to determine; there are no absolute screening tests to diagnose such patients by physical exam. The most reliable test is blockade of the joints, either by anesthetizing the joint itself or by blocking the medial branch to the joint. This procedure, however, has been reported to be only 60% to 68% specific when single, uncontrolled, local anesthetic blocks are used. The performance of a second confirmatory block can increase the diagnostic accuracy considerably.[177] Consequently, the incidence of zygapophysial joint-related low back pain may be as low as 4% to 8% of a general population of patients with low back pain who have not had surgery and who are without neurologic symptoms or radiologically identifiable spine disease.[176] This number may be lower than the actual incidence, because a high degree of pain relief was required and many patients may have multiple etiologies for their low back pain. If the zygapophysial joint was only a portion of the patient's pain, it would not have shown up as positive in this restrictive study. In addition, the exclusion of patients who previously had had surgery may have made the study population more uniform, but neglected those patients whose residual pain may have been due to zygapophysial joint disease or spinal fusion, or to instrumentation magnifying shear stress on the adjacent zygapophysial joints.

Schwarzer et al. have shown that no single test, or combination of standard clinical tests, will reliably predict the presence of lumbar zygapophysial joint disease or the response to local anesthetic zygapophysial joint blocks.[176] By the use of contingency tables, they calculated a sensitivity of 95%, specificity of 62%, false positive rate of 38%, positive predictive value of 31% and a negative predictive value of 99%. Sources of false positive results could be spread of local anesthetic to adjacent structures such as the nerve root, and false negative results could be obtained by injection of the local anesthetic into the vasculature, thereby reducing or eliminating the possibility of adequate neural blockade. These authors, however, did show that the presence of midline pain (as opposed to lateral or bilateral pain) was very unlikely to respond to zygapophysial joint blocks. The authors concluded that "the facet (zygapophysial) joint is an important source of pain, but the existence of a facet syndrome must be questioned."[176]

Spread of local anesthetic was shown not to be a problem in the cervical zygapophysial joint blocks by Barnsley et al.[11] The target specificity of medial branch blocks is 90%, making it unlikely that the failure to relieve pain with a second block was due to needle malposition.[11] One caution about using local anesthetics of differing duration in confirmatory blocks is that in up to 30% of patients the local anesthetic can give a prolonged response.[9] This outcome could qualify the patient as a negative responder if the bupivacaine does not outlast that of lidocaine. This, however, may qualify as a false negative if it is due to prolonged reduction in C-fiber input to the spinal cord that reduces a centrally sensitized state, or simply due to the interruption of the vicious cycle of pain and reflex muscle spasm (see Chapter 27).

Incidence

The spine has been described as having a "three-joint complex," referring to the intervertebral joint and the zygapophysial joints as a unit. The assumption had been that degeneration of the disc would lead to associated zygapophysial joint degeneration and the subsequent low back pain would then be multifaceted. This hypothesis was addressed by Schwarzer et al. in a study in which 92 consecutive patients with low back pain were subjected to both provocative discography and either zygapophysial joint or medial branch injections.[174] They concluded that zygapophysial joint pain was unlikely in patients with symptomatic lumbar intervertebral discs and that the incidence of discogenic pain as a unique entity was much greater than the incidence of zygapophysial joint pain. The sample population was somewhat skewed in that these patients with low back pain had been referred for discograms, so that pure zygapophysial joint-related pain probably was under-represented. The study did show, however, that there is not as direct an association between lumbar discogenic pain and zygapophysial joint-related pain as had previously been thought.

The opposite conclusion was reached by Bogduk and Aprill in a study of post-traumatic neck pain.[31] These authors studied 56 patients suffering with neck pain for longer than 6 months, with both provocative discography and zygapophysial joint blocks. Both the disc and the zygapophysial joint were found to be symptomatic in 41% of patients, the disc alone in 20%, and the zygapophysial joints alone in 23%. Only 17% of the sample did not respond to either approach. Barnsley et al. employed a double-blind differential local anesthetic block approach to zygapophysial joint pain associated with whiplash injury, and found a 54% prevalence of symptomatic joints.[12] This qualified as the leading source of pain in this population. Chronic pain following motor vehicle accident trauma, although multifactorial, may involve a higher incidence of zygapophysial joint disease than previously appreciated. As mentioned above, up to 54% of post-whiplash neck pain may be zygapophysial joint-related.[12] Twomey et al. reported 36% of motor vehicle accident (MVA) fatalities examined postmortem had evidence of fracture of a superior articular process or subchondral bone.[198] Seventy-seven percent of fatalities had soft tissue injuries, including capsular and articular cartilage damage. Unsuspected zygapophysial joint damage may therefore be present in MVA trauma survivors. Of note is that none of these lesions would be expected to show up on standard radiological studies.[198]

DIAGNOSTIC BLOCKS

Lumbar Medial Branch Blocks

For lumbar medial branch blocks, the patient is placed prone on the fluoroscopy table with a cushion under the hips to reduce the lumbar lordosis. The targets are localized by anteroposterior fluoroscopy. For the L1–L4 nerves the target is the posterior surface of the most medial end of the transverse process, just below the superior border at the junction with the articular pillar (Fig. 28-11). For the L5 nerve, the target is the medial end of the ala of the sacrum. These targets are constant in the patient who has not had surgery. The back is prepped with an antiseptic solution and draped in a sterile fashion. The skin entry sites are determined and a local anesthetic skin wheal is raised. Several approaches to the target sites have been advanced from a lateral oblique track to a latero-inferior approach. The only approach that is avoided is the direct posterior one, because the superior component of the zygapophysial joint can hang over the target and obstruct the needle placement. A 22- or 25-gauge, 3.5 1/2-inch needle is inserted and advanced, with frequent position checks with the fluoroscope, towards the target site, until bone is encountered. It is recommended that the first encounter be with the transverse process, to determine the depth. The needle is repositioned medially until the lateral edge of the zygapophysial joint is reached and the needle is then moved superiorly until it just "falls" off the superior edge of the transverse process (Fig. 28-12).

Optimum position is regained with the needle moved to the posterior-superior edge of the transverse process. Once in position, the patient may report a reproduction of his or her typical back pain. One to 1.5 cc of 0.5% bupivacaine or 2% lidocaine is injected, which may also elicit the patient's "typical" pain. With this approach, there is little chance of impaling the nerve or injecting into critical structures. As always, one should aspirate before injecting to avoid intravascular injection and a false negative result.

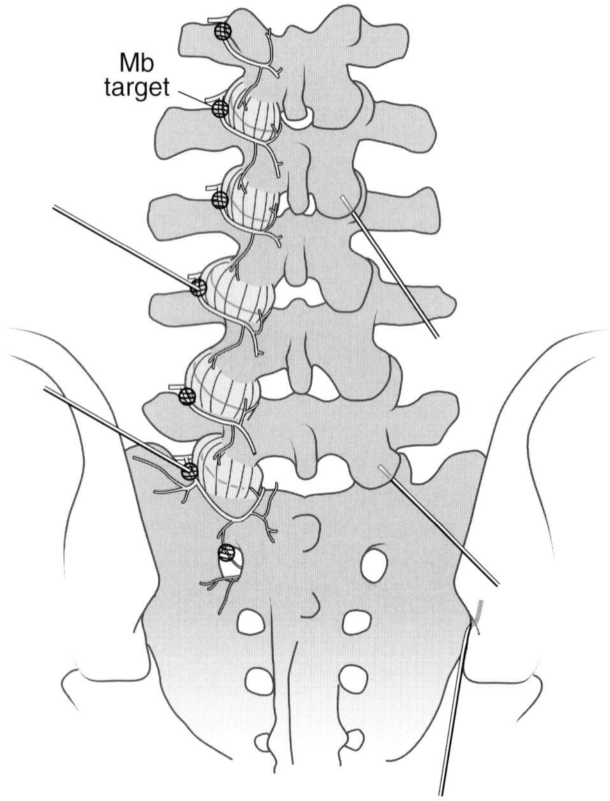

FIG. 28-11. Diagram of lumbar zygapophysial joint blocks (medial branch (M.) and intra-articular). Diagram of needle placements for media branch *(left)* and intra-articular *(right)* injections in the lumbar spine. The joint capsule has been removed to demonstrate the intra-articular entry on the right. The targets for medial branch block are indicated on the left *(hatched circles)*. The sacro-iliac joint is most easily entered from the inferior aspect of the joint as indicated in the diagram. The optimum aperture can be obtained by manipulation of the angle of the fluoroscopic beam as discussed in the text.

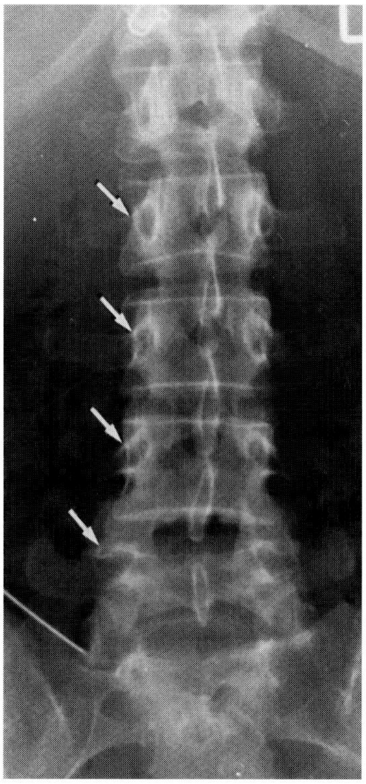

FIG. 28-12. Posteroanterior radiograph of the lumbar spine, showing a needle in position for an L5 medial branch block. Target points for the other lumbar medial branches are indicated by the *arrows*.

To obtain the most accurate information from the patient, little or no sedation is used, and therefore the skill and personality of the operator become key. At the conclusion of the procedure, pain relief is assessed, during spinal extension, and any other motions that have been reported to trigger the pain. Whether or not pain relief is evident, the patient is given a pain diary and is told to keep track of his or her pain over the course of the next 8 hours. A successful block is defined as greater than 50% pain relief for 2 hours after lidocaine or up to 6 hours for bupivacaine. One should also establish that no new sensory deficits have developed, which would indicate spread of the local anesthetic to the spinal root and invalidate the results of the session.

Lumbar Articular Blocks

Lumbar zygapophysial joint blocks are performed with the patient prone on the fluoroscopy table and a pillow placed below the hips, both to reduce the lumbar lordosis, and, potentially, to improve patient comfort. The fluoroscopy beam may have to be angled to achieve a clear view of the targeted articular space. One must be careful not to angle the beam too far or the optimal entry site at the posterior edge will be lost. A local anesthetic skin wheal is placed over the target and a 22- to 25-gauge, 3 1/2-inch needle is inserted and advanced, with frequent imaging, to the middle of the joint cavity. (Fig. 28-11) If bone is contacted, the needle position is adjusted, under fluoroscopic view, to slip into the joint space. Once inside the edge of the joint, a lateral view can be obtained and the needle advanced into the middle of the cavity. The position can be confirmed by the injection of 0.5 cc of radiocontrast dye to produce an arthrogram. The dye is then aspirated and local anesthetic and steroid are injected. The typical dose for the steroid component is 80 mg of methylprednisolone or 50 mg of triamcinolone acetate. The typical volume of a lumbar zygapophysial joint is 1.0 cc, and attempts to inject more than this volume are likely to rupture the joint capsule and deposit the injectate into the epidural or intrathecal space, thereby reducing the specificity of the block. The post-procedure assessment is similar to that outlined above for medial branch blocks.

Cervical Medial Branch Blocks

Several procedures have been proposed for blockade of the cervical medial branches. (Figs. 23-13 to 23-15). Earlier reports described a posterior approach but the passage of a needle through the posterior musculature is often associated with considerable pain, and tends to confound the assessment of pain relief from the block. In addition, the posterior approach requires the patient to lie prone, with the neck flexed, and this is usually reported by the patient to be uncomfortable. We prefer to have the patient placed supine with the neck rotated as much as can be tolerated to the side opposite the one to be blocked. The image intensifier is then rotated obliquely, and the scalloped edge of the ipsilateral articular pillar is observed. This projection has an advantage over the lateral view in that the opposite articular pillar presents less of an interference and the needle can be introduced along the axis of the beam to minimize the number of needle passes required. With the patient in the above-described position, the neck is prepped and draped in a sterile fashion and a local anesthetic skin wheal is raised over the insertion sites. In a normal-to-slightly-obese patient, with an insertion site just posterior to the carotid and jugular vessels, the medial branch can be reached with a 1 1/2-inch, 25-gauge needle. For more obese patients, a 3 1/2-inch spinal needle will be required. In this orientation, the articular pillar presents as a trapezoid, and the target point for C3–C4 and lower levels is the centroid of the pillar (Figs. 28-13 and 28-15). Using this approach the chance of local anesthetic injection onto the cervical nerve root is minimal, as is intravascular injection into the vertebral artery, which is anterior and medial to the needle target. This is not the case in the posterior approach. When the needle position is confirmed, by lateral view if necessary, the patient may report a reproduction of his/her pain but should not report clear radicular symptoms. One half cc of local anesthetic (0.5% bupivacaine or 2% lidocaine) is injected and the needle removed. For the C2–C3 level, the third occipital nerve is blocked at 3 evenly spaced locations along its course, bisecting the C3 articular pillar. Multiple injection sites have been recommended for the third occipital nerve because of its larger size and myelination compared to the other medial branches.

Cervical Articular Blocks[31,73,207]

For injection of the cervical zygapophysial joints at levels C2–C3 and below, the patient is placed prone on a fluoroscope table with a cushion below the upper chest to allow maximal flexion of the neck, and thereby the opening of the zygapophysial joints. The head and/or the fluoroscope may need to be turned to obtain the maximal aperture of the zygapophysial joint of interest. In the upper joints, the mouth may need to be opened to allow joint visualization without interference from the mandible or the teeth (Fig. 28-14). The posterior neck is prepped with an antiseptic wash and draped in a sterile fashion. A 22- to 25-gauge, 3 1/2-inch needle is inserted through a local anesthetic skin wheal at a 45° angle to the skin and advanced to enter the joint or to contact the bony perimeter (Fig. 28-14). The appropriate skin entry site is either 2 to 3 segments below the midpoint of the target joint on antero-posterior (A-P) view (or on lateral views), and can be determined by plotting the extension of the joint cavity plane out to the skin. Adjustments are made under fluoroscopic view until the needle enters the joint capsule.[207] Correct placement is confirmed with the injection of 0.2 cc of radiocontrast dye, which should outline the joint. Position can be confirmed with lateral views. Following confirmation of needle placement, the dye is aspirated if possible, and the joint is injected with a mixture of local anesthetic (0.5% bupivacaine) and depot steroid (25 mg of Triamcinolone, Aristocort [Fujisawa, Deerfield, IL] or 40 mg of methylprednisolone, Depo-Medrol [Upjohn, Kalamazoo, MI]) in a total volume of approximately 1.0 cc.

Atlantoaxial and Atlanto-occipital Joint Blocks

Innervation of the atlanto-occipital (AO) and atlantoaxial (AA) joints is derived from the C1 and C2 roots respectively.[30,33,72] These joints have not been addressed frequently because of the relative risk of injection into or injury to the vertebral or internal carotid arteries, which lie within the usual needle path for zygapophysial joint entry. Both posterior[33] and lateral[72] approaches have been described, but the posterior approach generally is considered safer because of the lateral location of the vertebral artery.

For the posterior approach to the AA joint, the patient is placed in a prone position and the fluoroscopy beam oriented in a posteroanterior orientation.[30,33] The joint space should

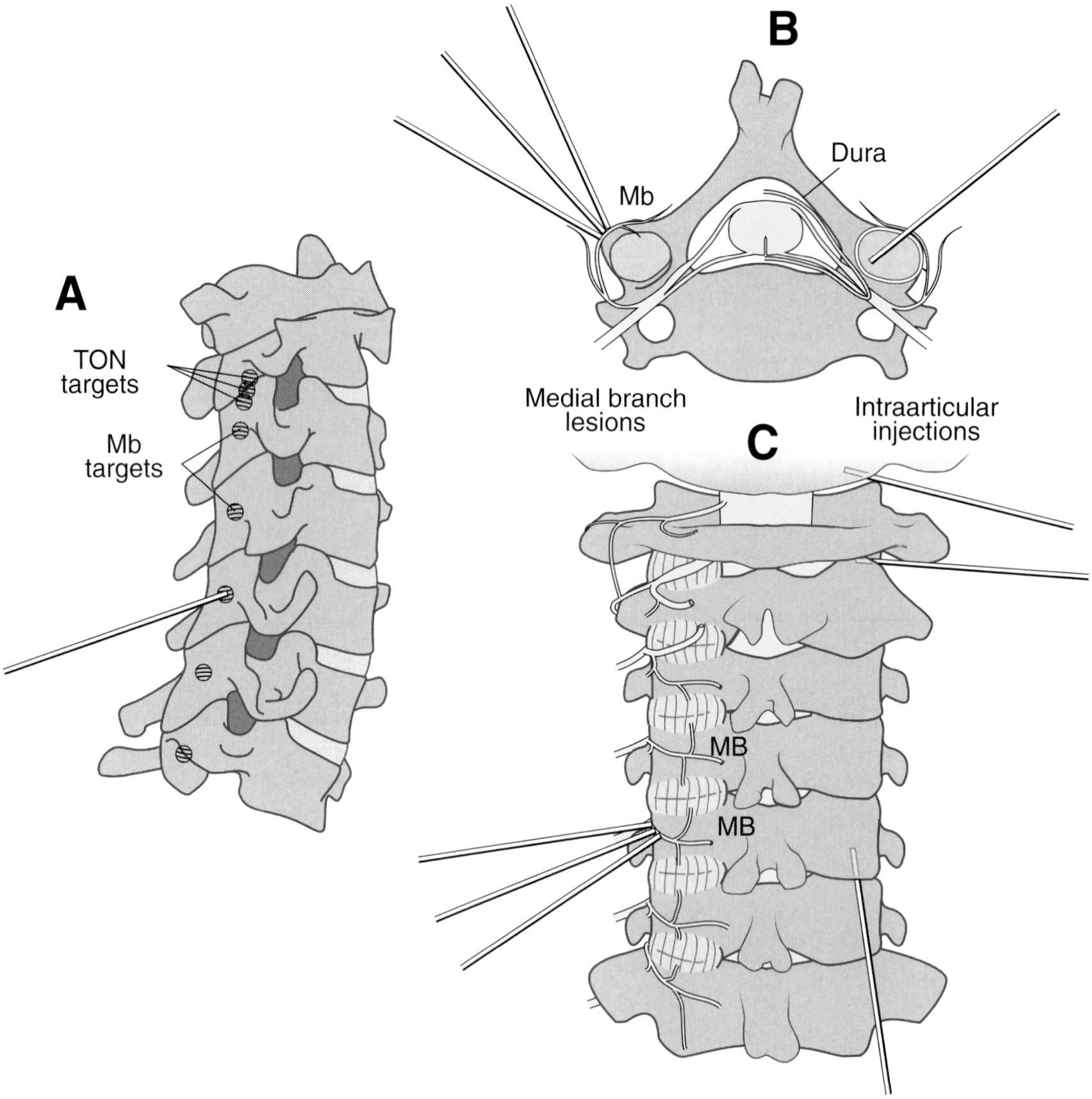

FIG. 28-13. Diagram of cervical zygapophysial joint blocks (medial branch and intra-articular). Diagram of needle placements for cervical medial branch *(MB) B* and *C; left)* and intra-articular *(B* and *C; right)* injections. The joint capsule has been removed on the right to demonstrate the intra-articular entry. Note the proximity of the anterior joint capsule wall and the epidural space. While medial branch blocks can be performed with a single injection, the denervation procedures often require multiple lesions as indicated by the multiple projections on the left. **Panel A** indicates the targets for local anesthetic block in an oblique projection. In **panel C** note the multiple injection sites required for adequate blockade of the third occipital nerve—a larger myelinated nerve. For comparison to lower cervical blocks, the needle placements for atlanto-occipital and atlanto-axial intra-articular blocks are indicated**.**

be clearly seen, but if the mandible or teeth are obstructing the view, the head position should be altered. A 25-gauge needle is introduced from a posterior position to the back of the joint space (Fig. 28-16). Care must be used in needle insertion because the vertebral artery is lateral and the spinal cord and intrathecal space are located in an unprotected site anterior to the joint. At the midpoint of the space lies the C2 ganglion, so the needle should be oriented to a slightly lateral approach. The needle is intentionally directed to the posterior aspect of the joint and the depth carefully noted. From this point the needle is moved in an anterior and medial direction until it enters the joint cavity. Small movements of the needle tip can be accomplished without excessive insertions by altering the orientation of the bevel and letting the tissue direct the needle tip. Once the needle enters the joint, the fluoroscopy unit is rotated to give a lateral view and the needle is inserted to the middle of the joint. Radiocontrast dye is used to confirm the location, then withdrawn. One cc of local anesthetic is injected to anesthesize the joint.

The AO joint poses a more difficult target than does the AA joint.[72] The patient is placed in the lateral decubitus position, but now the head is flexed and rotated 45° toward the table. The mastoid process and the occipital prominence are palpated and a skin mark is placed over the palpable cleft be-

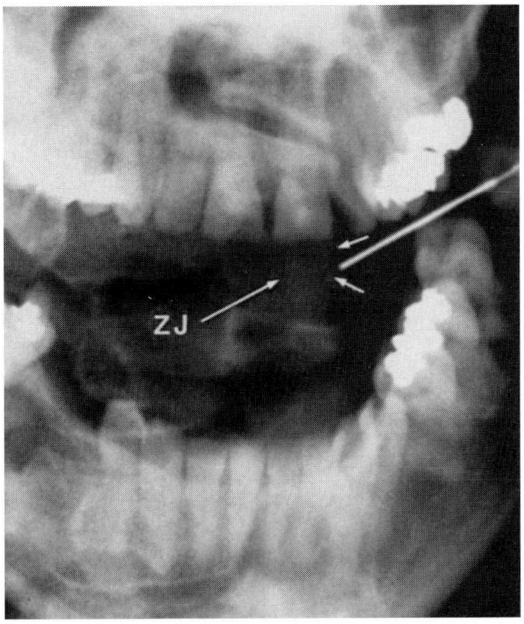

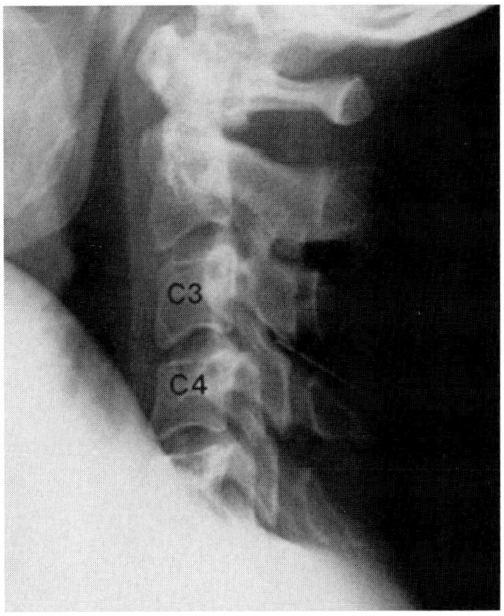

FIG. 28-14. A: Posterior radiograph of the upper cervical spine showing a needle in position at the target-point for a third occipital nerve block. The *arrows* indicate the other sites which should be injected in order to fully block this relatively large nerve. The location of the C2–C3 zygapophysial joint is indicated *(ZJ)*. **B:** Lateral radiograph of the cervical spine showing the appearance of a needle introduced into the C3–C4 zygapophysial joint.

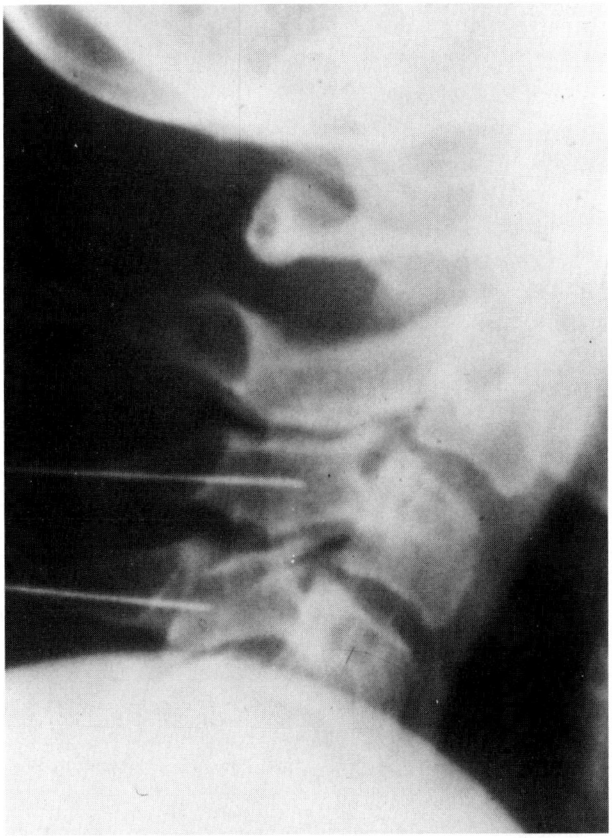

FIG. 28-15. X-ray of cervical zygapophysial joint medial branch nerve block at the C3 and C4 level. Lateral x-ray demonstrating the position of needle tips at the centroid of the trapezoid-shaped articular process in the cervical spine. Injection here would allow minimal diffusion due to insertion of the splenius capitus muscle groups.

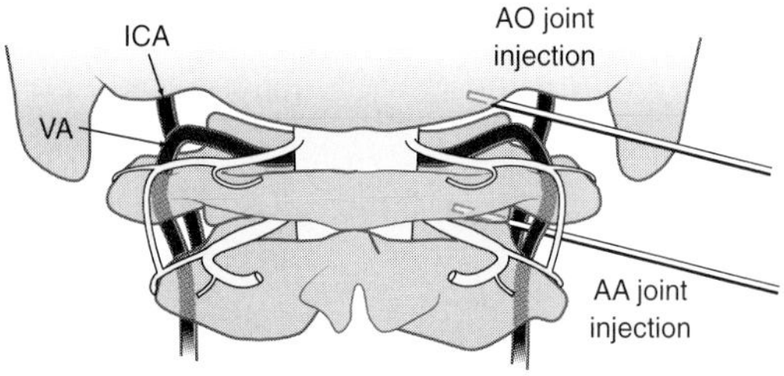

A

FIG. 28-16. A: Diagram of atlanto-axial joint block and atlanto-occipital joint injection. Sketch of needle placements for injections into the AO and AA joints. Note the relation of the vertebral artery *(VA)* posterior to the joints, requiring a lateral approach to the joint between the VA and internal carotid artery *(ICA)*. **B:** Radiographs showing the appearance of a needle introduced into the right lateral atlanto-axial joint. **Left:** posteroanterior view. **Right:** Lateral view.

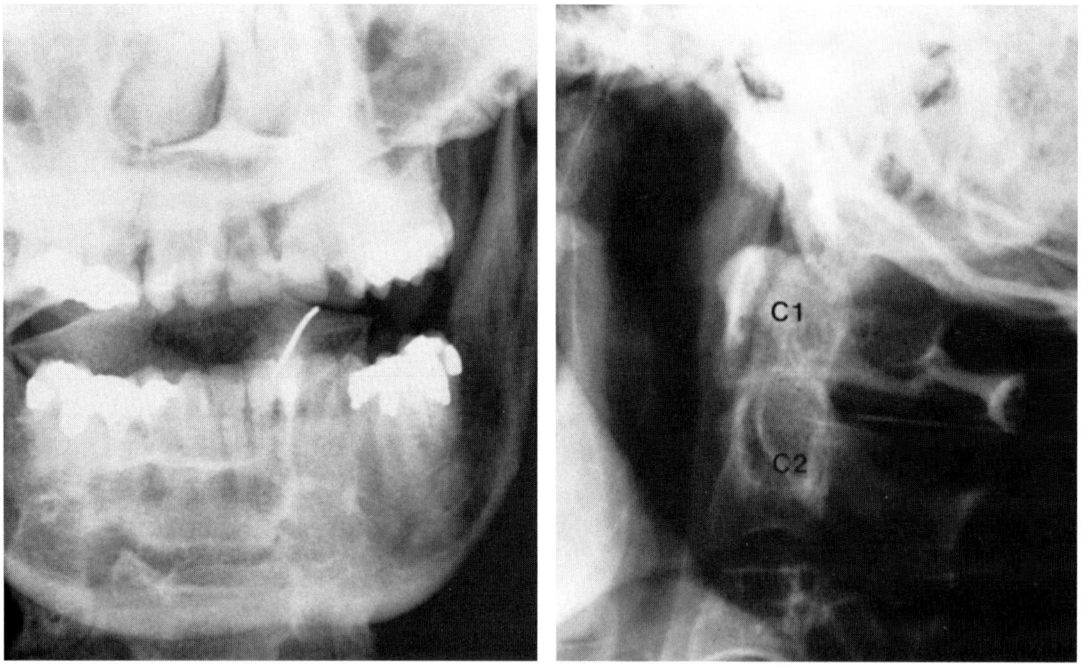

B

tween them and under the occipital brim. This mark is then positioned, through oblique fluoroscopy and head movements, to lie over the superior, lateral, and posterior aspect of the joint. A 25-gauge needle is inserted, through a local anesthetic skin wheal, directly toward the aligned target. Multiple needle repositions through alternating A-P and oblique views may be required before the joint can be entered after contacting bone.

The lateral approach described by Dreyfuss et al. allows access to both the AA and AO joints, although greater skill is required.[72] The patient is positioned in a lateral decubitus position with the symptomatic side up. The C2 and C3 segments are to be aligned perfectly, and then the fluoroscope beam is angled in a cephalad-to-caudad direction to view the greatest articular opening. A 25-gauge needle is inserted through a skin wheal to the juncture of the anterior 1/3 and posterior 2/3 of the joint, to avoid the internal carotid and the vertebral arteries. Appropriate depth is determined by contacting the superior or inferior plate of the joint and carefully repositioning the needle into the joint space under anteroposterior view.

Once the joint cavity is entered, the solution is injected until the patient complains of pain, or the injectionist perceives a firm pressure to injection. The AA joint can accept a mean volume of 0.7 cc, and the AO joint, 1.0 cc.[72] In provocative tests, the AO joint injections produced more intense and diffuse pain than did the AA joint injections. Patients described both injections as producing a dull, deep ache, with heavy pressure, like that of a hangover. The AA joint injections produced ipsilateral pain, lateral and posterior to the C1–C2 segmental level. The AO injections produced more diffuse pain extending from the C5 level almost to the vertex of the skull.

COMPLICATIONS ASSOCIATED WITH CERVICAL ZYGAPOPHYSIAL JOINT BLOCKS

Several complications have been reported following cervical zygapophysial joint blocks. The anterior aspect of the zygapophysial joint capsule is composed of the ligamentum flavum, and reports of spinal blockade occasionally leading to total spinal block have appeared, related to intra-articular zygapophysial joint injections.[98,130] When the C3–C4 through C5–C6 levels are blocked, the phrenic nerve may be compromised if a large volume of local anesthetic is employed. Hematoma formation and infection always are a risk, but should be of low incidence with proper attention to technique. A transient period of disequilibrium has been described rather frequently following third occipital nerve block.[127]

Sacroiliac Joint Blocks

The concept that the sacroiliac (SI) joint is a source of low back pain has been a controversial subject. The clinical tests to diagnose sacroiliac joint pain lack sufficient specificity to diagnose this condition accurately, and independent of other low back disorders that cause pain. Recently, however, there has been increasing evidence presented for a specific role of the SI joint in low back pain.[83,84] Most of our knowledge about the anatomy of the SI joint has been obtained from postmortem studies involving older individuals with significant degenerative joint disease.[201,202] It appears that in younger subjects, the SI joint has more mobility and thus may be more susceptible to weightbearing changes and shear forces. The SI joint receives innervation from the L4–S1

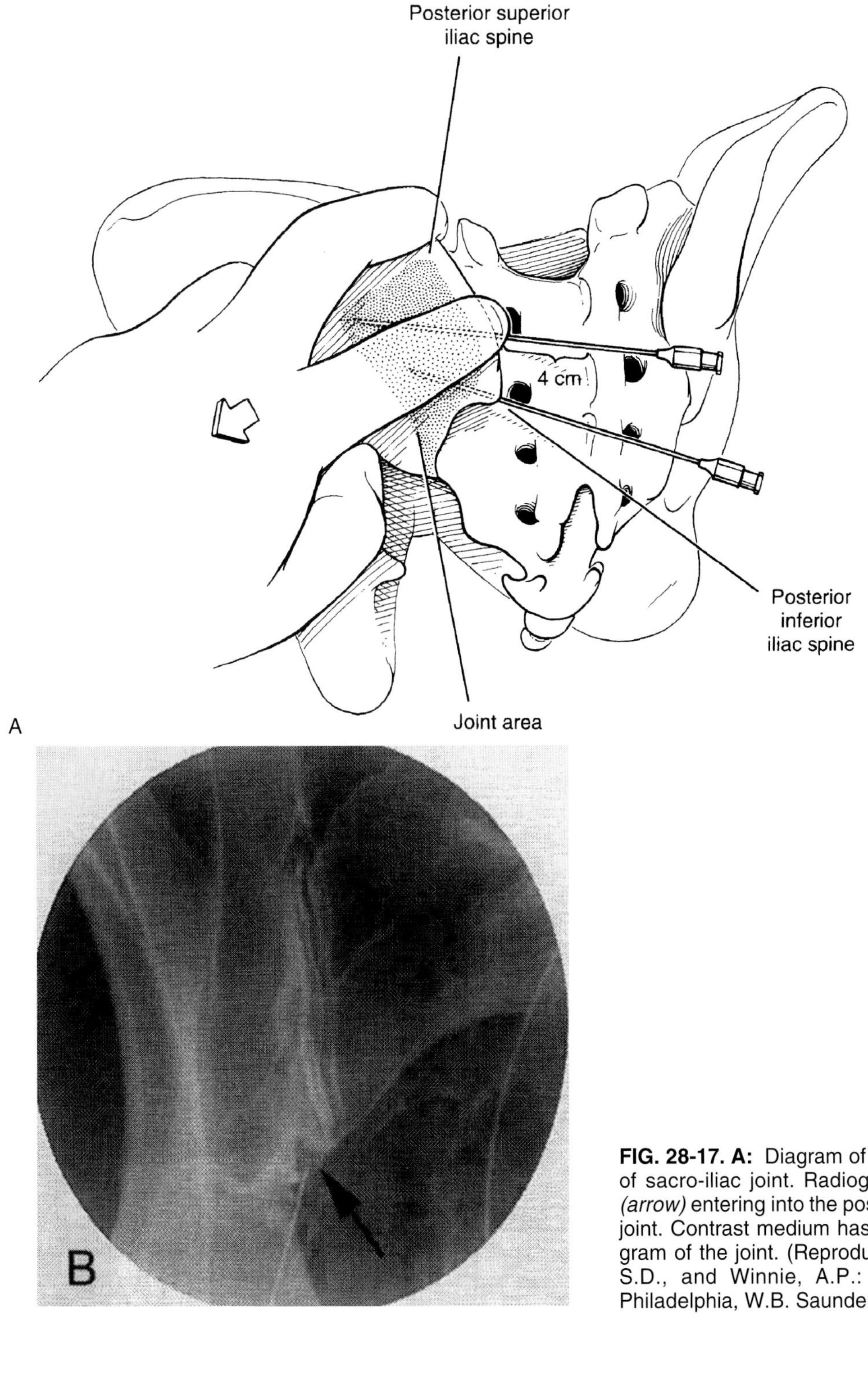

FIG. 28-17. A: Diagram of sacro-iliac joint block. **B:** Arthrogram of sacro-iliac joint. Radiograph demonstrating needle position *(arrow)* entering into the posterio-inferior aspect of the sacro-iliac joint. Contrast medium has been injected to produce an arthrogram of the joint. (Reproduced with permission from Waldman, S.D., and Winnie, A.P.: Interventional Pain Management. Philadelphia, W.B. Saunders, 1996.)

nerve roots, with a contribution from the S2 and possibly the L3 level.[185] Characterizing the pain that emanates exclusively from the SI joint (Fig. 28-10) has been difficult, because most clinical studies have included patients with low back pain, and, presumably, multiple tissue sources for their pain.

The term sacroiliac joint block probably is a misnomer in most cases when injections are performed without the aid of radiologic guidance. The sacroiliac joint is heavily invested externally with ligaments and connective tissue. These tissues have significant innervation and the injection of local anesthetic and/or steroid preparations into this region may give nonspecific, temporary pain relief but should not be referred to as an intra-articular infiltration. Even under radiologic guidance, the entry of the needle into the SI joint can be difficult and certainly makes the patient uncomfortable. Because of the curved nature of the joint, the fluoroscopic beam must be rotated to locate the posterior face of the joint. A strictly posterior or superior approach can be quite difficult. Recently, however, Fortin et al. described a modification of this approach to the sacroiliac joint, involving an inferior-posterior approach[84] (Fig. 28-17). These authors claim that this modified approach is easier to perform and that the patient finds it more comfortable.

Fortin et al. have provided rather convincing pain projection charts for the induction of pain with radiocontrast dye injection into asymptomatic joints.[84] These authors, however, did not obtain consistent relief of SI pain symptoms in patients chosen for intra-articular local anesthetic infiltration. The difficulty in achieving consistent analgesia with SI joint injections may reflect the complex nature of clinical low back pain, or may indicate that the local anesthetic solution did not reach the relevant nerves. This is particularly pertinent if the induced pain was caused by pressurization of the joint capsule. In this case, the relevant nerves would be external to the joint. Obviously further work will be required.

Ray has proposed sites for the radiofrequency denervation of the SI joint and claims good results, but data were not presented.[159] Kline, on the other hand, acknowledges Ray's targets but reports that in his experience the injection of steroid compounds into the joint can give better and more long-lasting results.[118] Again, patient selection and attention to the anatomic detail of the target sites may play a role in the success of this procedure. Further investigations will be needed before this becomes an accepted technique.

TREATMENT OPTIONS FOR ZYGAPOPHYSIAL JOINT PAIN

Zygapophysial joint blocks and other therapeutic procedures are rarely curative. The expectation is that the relief of pain will allow the patient to participate actively in the prescribed rehabilitation program to correct the postural or muscular disorders that contribute to the chronic back pain[140] (see Chapter 33). Zygapophysial joint arthropathy, either degenerative or traumatic, can involve inflammatory mechanisms and sensitization of mechanoreceptors within the joint and the capsule.[4,13,76,91,136,216] As the inflammation progresses, the zygapophysial joints will fuse spontaneously, which produces a reduction of pain at the cost of restricted movement. It is interesting to speculate that zygapophysial joint arthropathy may resemble inflammatory arthropathy in other joints. In animal models, inflammatory joint disease has been proposed to be under the influence of the sensory innervation to that joint.[56,123,124] Selective removal of the joint's sensory input has been shown to slow the progression of the disease.[123] It is possible that zygapophysial joint denervation or prolonged neural suppression may alter the progression of the degeneration, although this has yet to be studied.

Intra-Articular Steroids

Traditionally, facet syndrome has been treated with intraarticular injections of steroid and local anesthetic. The utility of this approach has been questioned in recent studies, suggesting that the injection of steroid is no more effective than placebo injections.[10,89,125] In the study by Carette et al., 95 patients were selected on the basis of greater than 50% pain relief after intra-articular lidocaine zygapophysial joint blocks.[89] At 6-month follow-up, only 20% had sustained improvement, compared to 10% with improvement after placebo injection. Despite the careful selection of patients, the injection of local anesthetic can be associated with nonspecific placebo effects or possible rupture of the joint capsule, with spread of the local anesthetic to the epidural space. These nonspecific effects may have allowed some patients to be entered in the study on the basis of false positive responses to presumed zygapophysial joint blocks. In a similar protocol, Barnsley et al. studied 41 patients with neck pain due to whiplash injury.[10] In this randomized, non-blinded study, a symptomatic cervical zygapophysial joint was identified and a therapeutic trial of intra-articular local anesthetic, or local anesthetic with steroid, was injected into 41 of 42 patients. The authors determined that the time to return to 50% of baseline pain was 3.0 days in the steroid group and 3.5 days in the local anesthetic group. They then concluded that intra-articular injection of steroid was not an effective treatment for cervical joint pain associated with whiplash injuries. In addition, because many of the zygapophysial joint pain syndromes may not be related to inflammation, steroids would have a questionable role in therapy.

Radiofrequency Lesions

An alternate treatment for zygapophysial joint-related pain is the destruction of the medial branches above, at, and below the level of the symptomatic zygapophysial joint. These targets should have been previously established by local anesthetic diagnostic blocks. The interruption of the medial branch has been addressed in several ways, including surgery,[128] as well as cryoanalgesic[174] and radiofrequency lesioning.[34,35,127,159,180] Rees is credited with the first description of the denervation of the zygapophysial joints as a treatment for low back pain. He described a technique that employed a long slender knife to cut the sensory innervation of the joint. In retrospect, it is unlikely that the knife used was long enough to effect an adequate lesion. Subsequent attempts to develop this technique were abandoned due to the unacceptably high morbidity, due to bleeding. Shealy further refined this approach by employing a radiofrequency thermocoagulation probe (see Chapter 32, Figs. 32-1 to 32-4) to create a lesion in the lumbar medial branch nerves to the zygapophysial joints.[181] Subsequently, several groups contributed to the development of the radiofrequency thermocoagulation, by defining the anatomy of the medial branch and describing the physics of the thermal lesion itself (see also Chapter 32).

Once the practitioner is satisfied that the patient has pain related to the zygapophysial joints, as determined by the response to diagnostic blocks, he or she is scheduled for radiofrequency denervation of the medial branches to the joint. The patient is prepared as described above for the diagnostic blocks, except that sedation often is used to increase patient comfort and cooperation. Heavy sedation or general anesthesia is avoided, because the patient still needs to provide feedback to the operator to help prevent inadvertent spinal root injury. The radiofrequency system allows for stimulation, via an insulated needle, to confirm placement, and then the production of a lesion by raising the probe tip temperature to 80°C for 90 seconds.[35,150,159] These settings will create a lesion with approximately a 2 mm radius.[35] The design of the radiofrequency needle is such that the energy field is lateral to the tip of the probe, so that the needle must be placed parallel to the nerve course, unlike the local anesthetic block, where the needle could be perpendicular.[35] Because of this restriction, many practitioners prefer to approach the medial branch from a lateral direction. Depending on patient response to the stimulation, local anesthetic can be placed prior to lesioning, for patient comfort. Following the procedure, the patient is instructed to restrict activities for approximately 2 weeks. If, at the end of this period, the patient has continued relief of mechanical low back pain, then he or she is started on a physical therapy (back-strengthening) program. The medial branch lesion is not considered permanent, because the coagulated nerve fibers will regenerate. In most practitioners' hands, the benefit can be expected to last from 6 to 12 months,[33] during which time the patient can improve his or her back strength and mobility. The procedure can be repeated because the nerves regenerate and the pain returns. The expected success rate for lesioning can be between 50% to 60%.[150] Earlier reports of lower success rates most likely can be attributed to inaccurate needle placement.[33–35]

North et al. recently published a report on a series of patients who had had lumbar zygapophysial joint denervation, with a mean follow-up period of 3.2 years.[150] Although the study was not controlled or blinded, bias was minimized because a disinterested third party conducted the follow-up interviews. Eighty-two patients were selected for diagnostic local anesthetic injections of the medial branch. Forty-two went on to radiofrequency lesioning, based on greater than 50% pain relief from the local anesthetic blocks. Forty-five percent of the denervation patients retained at least 50% pain relief at long-term follow-up. These results led the authors to conclude that this is a useful technique in properly selected patients. They also concluded that the response to diagnostic blocks may lack specificity in predicting long-term response to denervation. At this time, local anesthetic blocks are still the best screening test for selecting patients for denervation procedures. This position has been justified by the near absence of morbidity. To date, no reports of Charcot-type joints have been published. Complications germane to all zygapophysial joint denervation procedures include infection and bleeding, but the incidence of either should be low with proper technique. Deafferentation pain is rare or nonexistent, because the dorsal root ganglion (DRG) is left intact. Neuroma formation is very unlikely and thus far unreported. Radiofrequency thermal lesions coagulate neural and perineural proteins but preserve axonal and nerve sheath integrity.[127]

At least one recent study of thoracic zygapophysial joint denervation has reported good long-term results.[191] Forty patients with mechanical thoracic pain were selected, based on clinical criteria and transient response to prognostic local anesthetic blockade of the thoracic medial branches. Fifty-one radiofrequency lesions were performed in the 40 patients. On long-term follow-up of 36 patients for 18 to 54 months, 83% were either pain-free, or had greater than 50% pain relief. Intra-articular injections in the thoracic region are impractical, because of the risk of pneumothorax.

Lord, Barnsley, and Bogduk recently reported on an uncontolled study of radiofrequency denervation of cervical zygapophysial joints for chronic mechanical neck pain.[127] These authors studied 19 patients selected for denervation based on response to multiple diagnostic local anesthetic blocks of the medial branch of the cervical dorsal ramus. A posterior approach to the cervical articular pillar was used, with one lesion placed on the far lateral edge of the pillar and a second one placed just anterior to the first, via a 30° oblique electrode path. Complications were confined to postoperative pain that persisted for up to 10 days. Only 4 out of 10 patients undergoing third occipital nerve coagulation obtained longlasting relief in contrast to 7 out of 10 patients who obtained complete relief with lower cervical medial branch neurotomy. The authors argue against the use of third occipital neurotomy, given the high failure rate, but encourage further studies of the apparently effective lower cervical medial branch neurotomies.[127]

Cryolesions

Cryoanalgesia has been used extensively for zygapophysial joint denervations, in addition to peripheral nerve lesions.[173] Cryolesions are induced by rapidly cooling the end of a probe inserted percutaneously under fluoroscopic guidance to the target tissue, and then alternating several freeze-thaw cycles[78] (see Chapter 31, Fig. 31-15). The subsequent lesion is a function of the size of the ice-ball produced. Slow freezing will create extracellular ice crystals, which will draw water out of the cells and lead to cellular dehydration. Dehydration will block the nerve only for a temporary period and does not destroy the nerve. More rapid cooling methods will lead to large intracellular crystal formation and destruction of the cell. Unfortunately, most available systems will not be able to freeze at the speed required for creating predictable nerve lesions. Therefore, the cryolesions usually are considered to be temporary. At this time, a major disadvantage of the technique is the lack of disposable tips for the cryoprobes.

RADICULAR PAIN

Mechanisms of Radicular and Non-Radicular Low Back Pain

Direct compression of a nerve root is neither sufficient nor necessary for the development of radiculopathy symptoms.[23,24,46,48,67,101,114,132,145,169,193] Rather, inflammation of the root and/or dorsal root ganglia appears to be the critical feature of acute and subacute radiculopathy.[167] In patients with sudden impact to the spine, or with repetitive microtrauma, the viscoelastic disc is subjected to pressure that is inadequately distributed.[46] Whereas the posterior longitudinal ligament (PLL) may help hold a bulging disc out of the spinal canal in the cervical spine, the PLL thins from L2-L5 and may "permit" disc dislocation in the lumbar region.[46] When the integrity of the annulus is exceeded by too great a pressure, phospholipase A2 (PLA2), among other enzymes, can be leaked from the disc.[133,147,167,169,170] Sciatic pain can result from the liberation of inflammatory mediators, including PLA2 from a herniated nucleus pulposus.[135,170] PLA2 and other enzymes found in high concentration in the intervertebral discs, are capable of liberating arachidonic acid from cell membranes, and thus can provoke an intense inflammatory reaction in surrounding neural tissues.[135] This inflammatory response is capable of sensitizing nerve roots and the dorsal root ganglia, which brings about the clinical signs and symptoms of radiculopathy.[103,136,170,208] Lindahl and Rexed validated that inflammation was present by demonstrating in 1950 that patients with sciatica who presented to surgery had histologic evidence of inflammation.[126] This finding was duplicated in studies by Marshall, Trethwie, and Murphy in the 1970s, with the correlation of clinical symptoms experienced by operative patients with histologic evidence of inflammation in the clinically relevant spinal nerve roots.[132,147] The concept that even an immunologic reaction might be part of the pathologic findings was raised by a number of authors.[21,133,147,154,155] Pankovitch et al. showed that the proteoglycan component of the nucleus pulposus can be antigenic.[155] Another relationship to an immune and/or a chronic inflammation model was provided by Pountain et al.[154] Patients with chronic low back pain who were compared to matched controls were found to have an aberration in fibrinolysis; fibrin deposition occurred and chronic inflammation was evident. The exact correlation of this finding to the patient's clinical complaints was not discussed.

A dog model created by McCarron et al. is the basis for our modern understanding of radiculopathy and disclosed significant revelations about the inflammatory basis for the pathophysiology in patients with extra-discal nucleus pulposus.[135] Autologous nucleus pulposus material injected over 5 to 7 days into the epidural space in dogs provoked an intense inflammatory reaction in the spinal cord, dural sac and nerves adjacent to the level of injection, as measured by biochemical and histological indices. Clinical correlation was not possible in this model, but the data of Saal et al. showed that the concentration of PLA2 was 20 to 10,000 times that of normal tissue when samples were obtained from patients at the time of disc surgery.[170] A key point in acknowledging the significance of PLA2 is that steroids are needed to prevent its action on cell membranes—that of releasing arachidonic acid, which leads to the presence of additional mediators of the inflammatory cascade.

Compression of a nerve root becomes significant when one considers that the nerve root depends on the cerebrospinal fluid (CSF) for its nutrition, and is therefore susceptible to conditions that block CSF flow, such as adhesive arachnoiditis. Sustained pressure on a nerve root will alter the axonal transport efficiency, so that nutrients cannot be delivered to the axonal terminals and neuronotropic agents cannot be transported back to the cell body.[82,103,152] In this way, a focal herniation of a disc can lead to structural and functional changes, both central and distal to the site of compression.

Clinically, nerve root compression alone does not seem to induce pain. Compression will lead to findings such as numbness and weakness, but one needs to have chemical irritation of the root before pain occurs. In the presence of inflammation, relatively low pressures applied to the nerve root, or especially to the dorsal root ganglion, will induce the generation of prolonged neural discharges. It appears that the nerve root and the dorsal root ganglion normally are only marginally sensitive mechanically,[107] but that there is a dramatic increase in mechanical hyperalgesia(or sensitization) in the presence of inflammatory mediators or low pH.[152,167] If the nerve root is tethered in any way, such as with disc herniation or fibrotic compression, then the small movements induced by leg flexion (i.e., straight-leg raise) will give rise to vigorous neural discharges from the dorsal root.[95,107] When the spine flexes, the mechanical stress is most prominent in the lumbar root segments. When the straight-leg raise maneuver is performed, the stress is predominantly at the L5 and S1 roots.[95] The pain of radiculopathy therefore begins with nerve root compression and inflammation, which, when present over a prolonged period of time, lead to nerve root injury, constriction, or irreversible fibrosis.[103,167]

Selective Nerve Root Blockade

Clinically, radiculopathic pain can be relieved by the direct application of local anesthetic and/or steroid preparation to the nerve root. The mechanism(s) for the prolonged analgesia from these blocks are only starting to be understood. A recent animal study has demonstrated that a vascular connection exists between the epidural space and the nerve root.[45] This vascular connection can help to explain the transfer of inflammatory nucleus pulposus materials from the epidural space, selectively, to the nerve root. The therapeutic effectiveness of nerve root injection with local anesthetic and/or steroid may be explained by the transfer of these drugs via this vascular connection to the epidural space.

Alternate explanations can be offered for the response to nerve root injection. Compression or manipulation of nerve root, during retraction in surgery, or tethering in disc herniation, can cause nerve root ischemia and subsequent injury.[95,167,158] Yabuki and Kikuchi, in a recent study of nerve root compression, have demonstrated increased nerve root blood flow in an animal model, by applying local anesthetic either to the nerve root itself or to the adjacent sympathetic ganglion.[215] Thus the therapeutic effect of somatic or sympathetic block may be related to increased radicular blood flow, improved nutrition, or, potentially, to the "washout" of inflammatory or irritative substances. Other animal studies have suggested that nociceptive fibers supplying the lumbar paravertebral muscles may be responsive to sympathetic neural input.[93] These findings suggest a role, although undefined, for the sympathetic nervous system in low back and radicular pain. The blood flow to the nerve root itself is predominantly from the periphery.[146,219] Pain relief with sciatic[116,214] or sympathetic[54] blockade distal to the root lesion may therefore be explained, partially, by the increased blood flow and resolution of ischemia present in root compression. In addition to the alterations in blood flow, other mechanisms may account for the pain following nerve root compression. Experimental chronic nerve root compression can produce specific changes in neuropeptide levels within the peripheral nerve[57] and dorsal horn.[51] The clinical and therapeutic significance of these findings is just starting to be appreciated.

Selective nerve root blocks can have a predictive value for lumbar spine surgery. Derby et al. have reported on 78 subjects who underwent selective nerve root blockade prior to surgery.[63] As expected, those patients with radicular symptoms of less than a year in duration had a good surgical result (89%), regardless of their response to the block. For those patients with a duration of symptoms longer than one year, the analgesic response to steroid applied to the nerve root was a good predictor of positive surgical outcome (85%), and those with little or no response to the steroid and with pain for greater than 1 year had a poor response to surgery (95%). Optimal contact with nerve root is obtained by inserting the needle in the "nerve root sleeve."

When nerve root blocks are used to facilitate surgical decisions, it is best to limit the number of levels blocked to one or two.[194] This restricted blockade will allow more precise localization of the pain source(s) and the use of long-acting local anesthetics. However, a limited number of root levels blocked may also obligate the patient to agree to multiple procedure sessions, to focus attention on the most symptomatic level. Blockade of multiple levels with long-acting agents may lead to unacceptable and potentially dangerous weakness and numbness in the extremity. In the cervical spine, multiple level or bilateral root blocks may lead to phrenic nerve block and respiratory compromise. Specificity in diagnostic root blocks will be improved with the use of fluoroscopic guidance for needle placement and radiopaque dye to identify the penetration of a root sleeve[194] (Fig. 28-18).

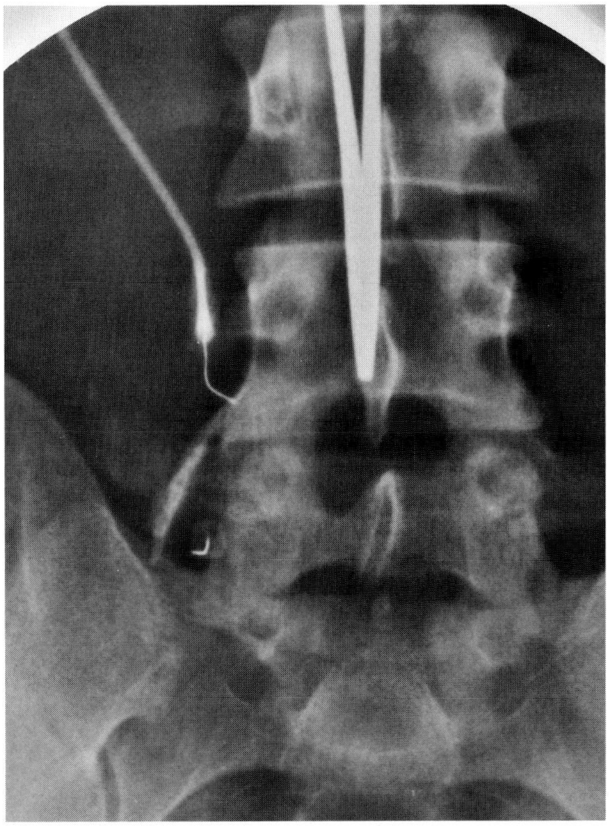

FIG. 28-18. X-ray of lumbar nerve root injection. X-ray demonstrating radio-opaque dye injection around the root sleeve of the left L4 spinal root in a patient undergoing therapeutic lumbar root injections. The needle has a slight curvature and is connected to extension tubing filled with contrast dye. A surface marker is placed over the spinous process of L4.

Provocative Discography

Not all disc-related pain involves herniation of the disc with compression of the spinal root. The outer 1/3 of the annulus fibrosus is innervated by mechanosensitive primary afferent fibers.[28,100] These fibers contain neuropeptides (SP, VIP and CGRP) commonly associated with nociceptive fibers. In fact, in a dog model, disc manipulation led to an increase in the dorsal root ganglion contents of SP and VIP. In the situation of an annular tear, the leakage of nucleus pulposus material not only will irritate the adjacent nerve root, but can also sensitize the annular fibers. In the presence of annular hyperalgesia, any motion which increases pressure within the disc will provoke pain. It is interesting that this can only occur with discs that are intact externally, because only an unimpaired disc will allow the intradiscal pressure to increase. This condition is associated with back pain with or without leg pain, straight-leg raising that causes more back than leg pain, no neurologic deficits, and reproduction of pain by discography. As with several other spine-related pain syndromes, the diagnosis depends on the combination of history, physical examination, and diagnostic blocks. The externally intact discs responsible for this pain would not be identified easily on conventional scans and only intact discs would elicit pain upon injection during provocative discography. Purely descriptive radiologic discography would of course not be able to diagnose this condition either. Discography is a physiological test for identifying symptomatic discs with outer annular ruptures.[143] Schwarzer et al. showed that the presence of a high-grade lumbar disc fissure on CT scan assessment followed by pain provoked by discography indicated that discogenic pain can be the explanation for back pain in as many as 39% of patients in a tertiary care referral population.[174]

That intervertebral discs are one of the main causes of low back and cervical radicular pain seems well documented. However, with the advent of sophisticated and sensitive imaging techniques such as magnetic resonance imaging, the frequency of diagnosis of discs which merely look abnormal, and disc bulges, has increased. The practitioner is left to determine which, if any, of these "abnormal" discs may be causing the patient's symptoms. As an aid to history and physical examination, the techniques of provocative and anesthetic discography were developed.[5,22,31,36,117,160] Simply put, the procedure involves the placement of a needle into the intervertebral disc and the subsequent injection of a small volume of radiocontrast dye, followed by local anesthetic (Fig. 28-19). The patient is sedated only lightly so that he or she can report whether or not the injection reproduces his or her usual pain. As a further confirmation, the presence of the local anesthetic will reduce the pain, and the patient may receive several hours of relief.[209] The combination of an abnormal disc pattern on x-ray (see Chapter 27, Fig. 27–11), provocation of the patient's usual pain and the relief of pain from the injected local anesthetic, gives strong evidence that the injected disc is responsible for the patient's pain.[204,210] Unfortunately, the interpretation of the test is very operator- and patient-dependent.[5,22] Much of the controversy over the utility of provocative discography rests on this relationship. Because of the unresolved issues surrounding discography, Burchiel et al. have stated that "discography should be reserved for patients enrolled in an institutionally approved research protocol.[43] This sentiment was echoed by Esses.[77] The anatomical and clinical justification for discography is

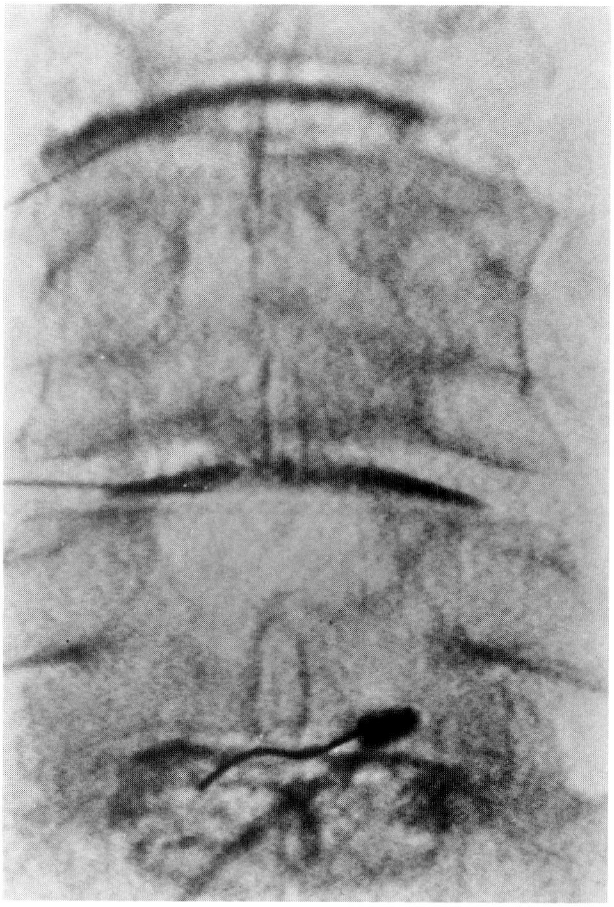

FIG. 28-19. X-ray of lumbar discography. X-ray of lumbar discography performed at the L3, L4, and L5 levels. Note the posterior lateral approach for L3 and L4, and the midline approach for L5. The L3 disc shows lateral dye leakage, indicating a disc disruption compared to the tight uniform intact disc pattern in the L4 disc. L5 shows a diffuse homogeneous distribution of dye without leakage. The L5 disc proved to reproduce this patients, pain pattern while the L3 and L4 levels were asymptomatic.

much better established for lumbar discs than for those in the cervical and thoracic regions.[172] Studies to determine the utility of discography in assessing the surgical outcome from discectomy are sorely lacking. Until these studies are performed, this technique will remain controversial.[212] An unanswered question is what to do with the disc that cannot be distended due to extensive disruption.[50] Presumably, this disc would not produce a positive result with provocative discography, but it still could be contributing to radicular pain secondary to root compression or irritation. Does a negative discogram constitute a reason not to operate on such a patient?

Once one or more symptomatic discs are identified by provocative discography, therapy usually is directed toward surgical excision of the disc; but other analgesic procedures have been developed, based on our emerging knowledge of the innervation of the intervertebral disc.[28,36] The source of contained discogenic pain is the highly innervated annulus itself. Inflammation and pressure within the disc can lead to mechanical low back pain, which can be confused with zygapophysial joint pain that is referred to the buttock, thigh, knee, and, occasionally, the calf. These symptoms can also be accompanied by intermittent paresthesias and back pain with straight-leg raising. Very often, the most symptomatic discs are radiographically intact. Partial discectomy in these cases will not be very effective, as the entire annulus can be involved. The innervation of the disc derives from the lumbar sinuvertebral nerves, branches of the lumbar ventral rami, and the gray rami communicantes of the sympathetic chain.[58,59,118] Currently, the gray ramus communicans is the most commonly lesioned structure. This procedure can relieve pain from the anterior and lateral segments of the disc to such a degree that the patient can avoid surgery.[118,182,183] Great care should be exerted to avoid injury to the lumbar plexus. Because of the pattern of multiple innervation of each spinal level, 3 levels of rami communicantes must be lesioned to address pain from each positive disc identified on discography. Bogduk[37] states that discography has its greatest potential utility in patients with clinical features of disc prolapse. When a needle is placed correctly in the center of the intact, asymptomatic, intervertebral disc, the inner annulus buffers the outer annulus from distending pressure. False positive discograms in normal discs may be a result of inaccurate needle placement and injection into or near the outer annulus. An appropriate protocol for provocative discography involves needle placement into the presumed symptomatic disc as well as 2 adjacent discs. The intact discs would then serve as controls. The most useful result is the finding of a single symptomatic disc, which, when injected, reproduces that patient's pain. Upon injection of adjacent normal (uninvolved) discs, the patient reports either no pain or pain that is dissimilar to his or her usual pain. Caution should be used in interpreting discography procedures where the patient is positive at 2 or 3 levels.

THE RATIONALE FOR THE USE OF STEROIDS IN BACK PAIN

Through the mechanisms outlined above, one can see that steroids, given their capacity to interfere with the inflammation from phospholipase A2, will have analgesic effects. In addition, the ability of steroids to decrease the inflammation-induced increase in capillary permeability will serve to reduce both the intraneural edema and the "internal" compression of the nerve root.[65] The dorsal root ganglion has only a minimal blood-nerve barrier and is, therefore, very sensitive to the influence of inflammatory mediators.[168] The dorsal root ganglion also has a low compliance membrane surrounding it, so any degree of edema will exert significant pressure within the ganglion and lead to cell body damage.[103,167] The portion of the nerve root central to the dorsal root ganglion is surrounded by CSF, and any edema will exert little pressure. The edema fluid will be rapidly cleared within the intrathecal space.

Steroids placed in the epidural space are believed to work by several mechanisms. Steroids suppress both the early and late inflammatory changes in the nerve root.[111] Application of steroids in the epidural space has been shown to inhibit transmission in normal nociceptive C fibers.[111] In a preparation of rat plantar nerve, methylprednisolone acetate suppressed transmission in unmyelinated C fibers, but not in A-B fibers. This effect was reversed when the corticosteroid was removed, suggesting a direct membrane effect.[111] Glucocorticoid binding in the spinal cord has been identified in another rat model.[86] Immunocytochemical studies, using an immunoperoxidase method, have located glucocorticoid receptor sites that were strongly immunopositive on the norepinephrine (NE), epinephrine (E) and 5-hydroxytryptamine (5-HT) neurons located in the lower brainstem, nucleus of the spinal tract of the trigeminal nerve, and the dorsal horn substantia gelatinosa. Thus, glucocorticoids may act to modulate neural responsiveness to nociceptive input from peripheral nociceptors.[85,108]

Traditionally, steroids are believed to act on the cell nucleus to influence gene transcription and to inhibit the development of inflammation. There have been recent reports that suggest a direct membrane receptor-mediated effect of glucocorticoids.[109] This mechanism is thought to account for the rapid actions displayed by steroids on neurons. In a model of guinea pig celiac ganglion neurons in vitro, glucocorticoids caused hyperpolarization of the neurons.[109] This action suppressed those neurons with spontaneous discharges. The same effect was observed when the steroid was attached to a large molecule, thereby restricting access to the cell interior. The actions were prevented by a specific glucocorticoid antagonist, further supporting the concept that steroid actions are occurring via a specific cell surface receptor.

EPIDURAL STEROID INJECTIONS

ESI is time-honored, having been performed for at least 40 years. Definitive outcome studies are lacking,[14,15,42,55,70,97,184,192,213,218] and the debate continues as to the efficacy of this treatment, although its safety has been well-documented.[3,15–17,38,52,64] When the contemporary principles of the practice of pain medicine are applied to the use of ESIs in patients with acute and chronic back pain, a reasonable position for such treatment can be established in the algorithm of patient management.[15,17,38,63,163,171,191] What has changed over the years is the understanding as to why steroids are an appropriate drug in *selected* patients with back pain.

Clinical Studies Regarding Epidural Steroid Injections

High-volume injections of local anesthetics and/or saline was used to treat sciatica until the development of exogenous corticosteroid drugs in the 1940s, which was coupled with the evolving likelihood that sciatica was caused by inflammatory changes in nerve roots.[114] Goebert et al. prospectively showed that 66% of 113 patients with sciatica given (mostly) caudal epidural hydrocortisone (125 mg) improved, and did so at a higher rate than patients given only a local anesthetic.[97] That local anesthetic alone could be of benefit was also shown by Breivik et al., but the rate of improvement again proved to be lower than when corticosteroids were administered concurrently.[42] Coomes reported that the caudal injection of 20 to 50 ml 0.5% procaine in 20 patients with sciatica contributed to their recovery (relief of pain when active and normal SLR) in 11 days, whereas traditional bedrest took 31 days in another 20 patients, further documenting that local anesthetic injections have a salutory effect.[55]

The debate over the true pathophysiologic cause of sciatica, as well as the safety and efficacy of ESI, continues to unfold, though literature keeps appearing that addresses the issues. Winnie et al. published data urging the placement of the drugs at the level of pathology, rather than using high volume injectates.[213] Because at least 80% of their patients with sciatica improved when given only depomedrol (washed in with 4 to 6 cc of local anesthetic) at the level of pathology, they concluded that sciatica was not relieved because the large volume injectates broke up adhesions nor because of the interruption of a reflex sympathetic dystrophy (RSD)-like phenomenon as was previously thought. Breivik et al. reported that 63% of 35 patients with chronic low back pain and sciatica (11 of whom had had past lumbar surgery), studied with a prospective and randomized approach, improved with ESI (20 ml 0.25% bupivacaine and 80 mg methylprednisolone) to such an extent that they were able to return to work.[42] Only 25% of those patients given 20 ml 0.25% bupivacaine and 100 ml saline improved to that same degree. Swerdlow and Sayle-Creer reported that 67% of their 325 patients with lumbosciatic syndrome were improved and added the caveat that their patients were "selected."[193] Hickey made an important addition to clinical practice by demonstrating that only 17% of his 250 patients noted benefit with the first ESI (120 mg methylprednisolone and 7 ml saline at the level of spinal pathology), yet a second injection 2 weeks later added 44% more patients to the improved category, and a third ESI the remaining 39%.[104] The concept of additive benefit from serial ESIs is also supported by Warr, who suggests trying alternately the caudal and the lumbar approach in patients who are referred for ESI due to post-laminectomy changes.[207]

Beliveau provoked discussion when he alternately assigned 48 patients with moderate to severe unilateral sciatica into groups to receive 42 ml 0.5% procaine and saline or 40 ml 0.5% procaine and 80 mg depomedrol into the caudal epidural space.[14] Approximately 70% of patients in *both* groups improved, yet those with symptoms of longer duration did better if given the depomedrol. Dilke et al. compared the clinical effect of 80 mg methylprednisolone in 10ml saline given epidurally to patients, to a control group who received an interspinous ligament injection. The study group was comprised of 100 patients with complaints of unilateral sciatica who also received rehabilitative physical therapy and analgesics.[70] The ESI-treated patients showed more improvement when assessed for use of analgesics, complaints of severe pain at scheduled post-injection evaluation times, referrals for surgery and percentage of return to work. This study is one of only a few that has attempted to use a control group—this flaw in scientific design being a major criticism of the epidural steroid clinical research literature. Parenthetically, the numerous studies are extremely difficult to compare because of the small number of patients included, the tremendous variation in inclusion criteria, the lack of standardization of diagnosis and diagnostic tests, the lack of uniform data, the lack of adequate control groups, differences in the extent and timing of follow-up, and inadequate outcome assessment.[1,101,102] One must respect the natural history of the disease to prevent a false association of benefit with treatment. Abram points out, furthermore, that research on ESIs is difficult because referring physicians want active treatment for their patients and not placebo therapy, and, given the many causes of back pain, a large number of patients would have to be very carefully stratified to do the definitive study.[1] Based upon the Quebec Task Force's thorough review of the available literature, ESI was listed in the category of "...usefulness demonstrated by non-randomized trials..." for patients with "radicular compression presumed."[188] A meta-analysis of the ESI literature from 1966 to 1993 showed that ESI produced a 14% treatment effect, but only a few studies met the established criteria for meta-analysis.[157] A systematic review failed to demonstrate any benefit.[120]

As one might expect, not all studies of ESI show benefits. Snoek et al. reviewed 51 patients with lumbar nerve root compression syndrome.[184] The diagnosis in these patients was based upon their physical signs, symptoms and myelographic findings. A randomization procedure placed patients into either: a group receiving 2 ml saline epidurally or a group receiving 80 mg Depo-Medrol at the level of known disc lesion. At 48 hours, both groups manifested equal improvement and no differences were revealed with longer follow-up. Criticism of this study is based upon its lack of relevance to routine clinical practice because the corticosteroid effect may take as long as 4 to 6 days to become evident,[15] and because of the small injection volume. The same claim about correlation to clinical practice was raised in response to the study by Cuckler et al.[60] They used a prospective, randomized, double-blind protocol with 73 patients who had either well-defined unilateral sciatica or spinal stenosis. All patients received epidural injections at the L3-4 level with either 2 ml water, 80 mg methylprednisolone and 5 ml 1% procaine or 5 ml 1% procaine and 2 ml saline. No statistically significant differences were revealed with short-term (24 hours) or long-term follow-up. Hammonds recently expressed his views that chronic pain patients presenting for ESI may be more vulnerable to the placebo response and that the literature does not support their widespread use.[102] On the other hand, a meta-analysis by Merry et al. found that patients were 2/3 more likely to achieve pain control with epidural steroids than with placebo.[140]

The Safety of Epidural Steroid Injections

The issue of the safety of ESIs is a valid one. The chemical composition of the two most commonly used deposteroids is shown in Table 28-7. One must consider the effects of these compounds on the tissues adjacent to the injection site, as well as the physiologic consequences of the injected drug. Early work by Seghal et al. revealed that the subarachnoid placement of 80 mg methylprednisolone caused a transient increase in CSF protein and a pleocytosis that persisted for a few weeks.[178] When epidural injection became predominant, the matter of tissue safety went unanswered until Delaney et al. showed in a cat model that a single ESI with Aristocort did not produce evidence of tissue damage when compared to matched controls.[64] Ten years later Cicala et al. noted that a single ESI with depomedrol in a rabbit did not result in tissue reaction significantly different from a control group.[52] These studies did not address the clinical scenario in which serial ESIs commonly are given. Abram et al. recently reported on this issue from an experimental design using rats.[3] Their animals were given intrathecal Aristocort for 5 consecutive days and, when sacrificed, no evidence of tissue toxicity or a spinal analgesic effect could be found.

The most consistent protest about the neurotoxic effects of ESIs is raised by Nelson.[144] His primary concern has been that the polyethylene glycol (PEG) in both Aristocort and Depo-Medrol (see Table 28-7) causes arachnoiditis, sterile meningitis and pachymeningitis; this being so, he asks whether the primary injection destination is the subarachnoid or the epidural space. This important clinical question was addressed directly by Benzon et al.[16] Isolated nerves were bathed in graduated concentrations of PEG (from 3% to 40%) and the effect on the compound action potential was used as evidence of toxicity. Only at concentrations of 20% or greater was the compound action potential slowed, but even the effect of 40% was reversible when PEG was washed away. The significance of this finding in clinical practice is based in the reality that the commercial preparations of Aristocort and Depo-Medrol contain only 3% PEG. This is usually diluted by the concurrent use of saline or local anesthetic. A remaining question, then, is, what are the consequences of depositing some or all of a dose of deposteroid unexpectedly into the CSF? The subarachnoid use of deposteroids had been reviewed previously and condemned by Kepes and Duncalf,[115] yet Wilkinson reviewed the extensive literature on intrathecal Depomedrol in 1992 and concluded that the intentional intrathecal placement was safe and even useful.[211] In making these claims, he added the essential advice that the patients must be carefully selected, be given a thorough and balanced explanation of the risks and benefits of the treatment and that conscientious follow-up be provided.

TABLE 28-7. *The ingredients of Depo-Medrol and Aristocort*

Depo-Medrol (single-dose vials)	40 mg/ml	80 mg/ml
methylprednisolone	40 mg	80 mg
PEG 3350	29 mg	28 mg
myristyl-gamma-picolinium	0.195 mg	0.189 mg
pH adjusted to 3.5 to 7.0 with NaOH or HCL)		
Aristocort		
triamcinolone	25 mg/ml	
polysorbate 80 NF	0.20%	(2 mg/ml)
PEG 3350	3.0%	(3 mg/ml)
benzyl alcohol	0.9%	(9 mg/ml)
NaCl	0.85%	(8.5 mg/ml)

Given the invasive nature of regional analgesia procedures, there are always the theoretic risks of inducing bleeding or creating infection.[102] Pertinent to ESIs are the common risks of epidural placement: backache, postdural puncture headache and vasovagal reaction. Case reports have brought to light incidences of nausea, dizziness, nerve root injury, durocutaneous fistula, and meningitis.[18,101,102,164] Also of interest and not solely of theoretic concern is the systemic effect of the corticosteroid injected. Abram recommended not using more than 50 mg triamcinolone or 80 mg methyprednisolone.[1]

These medications are not inert in the body. Goebert et al. reported patients given ESIs who developed congestive heart failure.[97] The question about the exact risk of the injected steroids in at-risk patients, such as those with ulcers or diabetes, or a history of these conditions, or tuberculosis, acquired immunodeficiency syndrome (AIDS), bacterial infections, or psychiatric disorders, are not answered at the present time.[1] In spite of Knight's and Burrell's recommendation that not more than 3 mg per kg methylprednisolone should be used, case reports detail the development of adrenal suppression or Cushing syndrome in patients who have received perispinal steroid injections.[75,119,196] With the advent of long-duration steroid preparations, cumulative effects after repeated dosing can be manifest. Kay et al. have shown both acute and chronic suppression of the hypothalamic-pituitary-adrenal (HPA) axis in a clinically relevant study of 14 patients who received a total of three ESIs (once weekly) with 80 mg of Aristocort in 7 ml of 1% lidocaine.[112] Within 15 minutes of injection there was evidence of the suppression of endogenous corticosteroids, manifested by a significant decrease in both adrenocorticotropic hormone (ACTH) and cortisol. The median duration of the effect was 1 month but 5/14 patients showed suppression for up to 3 months. Kay et al. raise the possibility that patients who have received deposteroids epidurally within 3 months of an operative procedure should be considered as candidates for receiving steroid replacement therapy preoperatively.[112]

An additional finding of interest from the Kay et al. study was that patients given midazolam as a premedication had more pronounced suppression of the HPA axis than those patients who received just the ESI.[112] This isn't all that unexpected since benzodiazepines are known to have a suppressive effect on the HPA axis, as well as a direct inhibitory effect on the adrenal cortex. These data would seem to portend the potential detriment of using such drugs in patients with low back pain who receive ESI.

In contrast, Serrao et al. studied 28 patients with chronic mechanical low back pain.[179] Patients were given either 80 mg methylprednisolone in 10 ml saline epidurally and 3 ml of 5% dextrose intrathecally or 2 mg midazolam in 3 ml 5% dextrose intrathecally and 10 ml saline epidurally and assessed every 2 months with Visual Analogue Scale (VAS), verbal pain scales, the short-form McGill Pain Questionnaire and pain diaries. One-half to 3/4 of each group was improved at 2 months as to activity level, sleep, and the affective and sensory components of the pain. It is interesting that the intrathecal midazolam group manifested more benefit at 3 months' follow-up, as shown by the lower use of medications for pain, than did the group given only the ESI.

Epidural Steroid Injections in Spinal Stenosis

Another area of contention concerning the clinical application of ESI is in patients with spinal stenosis. This is a condition in which the bony frame surrounding the spinal cord and the exiting nerve roots become functionally narrowed by mild vertebral collapse, osteophyte formation, and chronic malalignment of the zygapophysial joints. The question that is raised frequently, is, how efficacious are ESIs in this condition? Benzon's review indicated at least a transient effect.[17] Ciocon et al. found a definite benefit in their elderly population of 30 patients (76 years ± 6.7) who met diagnostic criteria for spinal stenosis on MRI.[53] They were given 80 mg Depo-Medrol in 0.5% lidocaine weekly, times 3, via a caudal technique, because they were poor operative candidates. The pain ratings dropped from 3.4 to 1.5, and the patients were followed for 10 months. The range of benefit of caudal ESI in cases of lumbar canal stenosis was from 4 to 10 months.

Benzon accurately pointed out in 1986 that we still need to define the ideal number of injections, the ideal volume and content (local anesthetic versus saline) of the injectate, the differences related to the level of injection, and the distribution effectiveness of the injected medications, in patients with previous lumbar surgery.[15] The number of ESIs a patient can receive over any specific period of time or a lifetime is not known. Applying medical prudence will assure that ESIs will not be done repetitiously without conscientious regard to both the positive *and* the potentially adverse effects. ESIs can help patients use fewer analgesic medications, increase function, minimize hospital stay, cooperate with rehabilitative PT and return to work.[17,23,40,44,163,168] A treatment protocol will foster a re-evaluation of the patient, so that therapy that is truly helping will be continued and that which is not will be replaced and/or stopped.

REFERENCES

1. Abram, S.E.: Risk versus benefit of epidural steroids: Let's remain objective. APS Journal, *3:*28, 1994.
2. Abram, S.E., Anderson, R.A., and Maitra-D'Cruze, A.M.: Factors predicting short-term outcome of nerve blocks in the management of chronic pain. Pain, *10:*323, 1981.
3. Abram, S.E., Marsala, M., and Yaksh, T.L.: Analgesic and neurotoxic effects of intrathecal corticosteroids in rats. Anesthesiology, *81:*1198, 1994.
4. Ahmed, M., Bjurholm, A., Kreicbergs, A., and Schultzberg, M.: Sensory and autonomic innervation of the facet joint in the rat lumbar spine. Spine, *18:*2121, 1993.
5. April, C.N., III.: Diagnostic disc injection. *In* Frymoyer, J.W. (ed.): The Adult Spine: Principles and Practice. pp. 403. New York, Raven Press, 1991.
6. Aprill, C., Dwyer, A., and Bogduk, N.: Cervical zygapophysial joint pain patterns. II: A clinical evaluation. Spine., *15:*458, 1990.
7. Avramov, A.I., Cavanaugh, J.M. Ozaktay, C.A., Getchell, T.V., and King, A.L.: The effects of controlled mechanical loading on group-II, III, and IV afferent units from the lumbar facet joint and surrounding tissue. An in vitro study. J. Bone Joint Surg., *74:*1464, 1992.
8. Badgley, C.E.: The articular facets in relation to low back pain and sciatic radiation. J. Bone Joint Surg., *23:*481, 1941.
9. Barnsley, L., Lord, S., and Bogduk, N.: Comparative local anaesthetic blocks in the diagnosis of cervical zygapophysial joint pain. Pain, *55:*99, 1993.
10. Barnsley, L., Lord, S.M., Wallis, B.J., and Bogduk, N.: Lack of effect of intra-articular corticosteroids for chronic pain in the cervical zygapophysal joints. N. Engl. J. Med., *330:*1047, 1994.
11. Barnsley, L., and Bogduk, N.: Medical branch blocks are specific for the diagnosis of cervical zygapophyseal joint pain. Reg. Anesth., *18:*343, 1993.
12. Barnsley, L., Lord, S.M., Wallis, B.J., and Bogduk, N.: The prevalence of chronic cervical zygapophysial joint pain after whiplash. Spine, *20:*20, 1995.
13. Beaman, D.N., Graziano, G.P., Glover, R.A., Wojtys, E.M., and Chang, V.: Substance P innervation of lumbar spine facet joints. Spine., *18:*1044, 1993.
14. Beliveau, P. A comparison between epidural anaesthesia with and without corticosteroid in the treatment of sciatica. Rheumatol. Phys. Med., *11:*40, 1971.
15. Benzon, H.T.: Epidural steroid injections for low back pain and lumbosacral radiculopathy. Pain, *24:*277, 1986.
16. Benzon, H.T., Gissen, A.J., Strichartz, G.R., Avram, M.J., and Covino, B.G.: The effect of polyethylene glycol on mammalian nerve impulses. Anesth. Analg., *66:*553, 1987.
17. Benzon, H.T.: Epidural steroids. *In* Raj, P.P. (ed.): Practical Management of Pain. pp. 818. St. Louis, Mosby-Year Book, 1992.
18. Berman, A.T., Garbarino, J.L., Fisher, S.M., and Bosacco, S.J.: The effects of epidural injection of local anesthetics and corticosteroids on patients with lumbosciatic pain. Clin. Orthop., *188:*144, 1984.
19. Bigos, S., Bowyer, O., Braen, G. et al.: Acute Low Back Pain Problems in Adults. Clinical Practice Guideline, Quick Reference Guide Number 14. U.S. Department of Health and Human Services, Public Health Service, Agency for Health Care Policy and Research. AHCPR Pub. No. 95-0643 December 1994.
20. Blair, J.A., Blair, R.S., and Rueckert, P.: Pre-injury emotional trauma and chronic back pain. Spine, *19:*1144, 1994.
21. Bobechko, W.P., and Hirsch, C.: Autoimmune response to nucleus pulposus in the rabbit. J. Bone Joint Surg., *47B:*574, 1965.
22. Bogduk, N.: Diskography. APS Journal, *3:*149, 1994.
23. Bogduk, N.: The lumbar disc and low back pain. Neurosurg. Clin. N. Am., *2:*791, 1991.
24. Bogduk, N., and Twomey, LT. Clinical anatomy of the lumbar spine 2nd Ed. Churchill Livingstone, Melbourne, Austria, 1991.
25. Bogduk, N.: Neck pain. [Review]. Aust. Fam. Physician., *13:*26, 1984.
26. Bogduk, N.: Neck pain: An update. Aust. Fam. Physician., *17:*75, 1988.
27. Bogduk, N.: The innervation of the lumbar spine. Spine., *8:*286, 1983.
28. Bogduk, N., Tynan, W., and Wilson, A.S.: The nerve supply to the human lumbar intervertebral discs. J. Anat., *132:*39, 1981.
29. Bogduk, N., and Long, D.M.: The anatomy of the so-called "articular nerves" and their relationship to facet denervation in the treatment of low-back pain. J. Neurosurg., *51:*172, 1979.
30. Bogduk, N., Marsland, A.: The cervical zygapophysial joints as a source of neck pain. Spine, *13:*610, 1988.
31. Bogduk, N.A., and April, C.: On the nature of neck pain, discography and cervical zygapophysial joint blocks. Pain, *54:*213, 1993.

32. Bogduk, N.: The clinical anatomy of the cervical dorsal rami. Spine, *7:*319, 1982.
33. Bogduk, N.: Back Pain: Zygapophysial Blocks and Epidural Steroids. *In* Cousins, M.J., and Bridenbaugh, P.O. (eds.): Neural Blockade in Clinical Anesthesia and Management of Pain. pp. 935. Philadelphia, J. B. Lippincott, 1988.
34. Bogduk, N., and Long, D.M.: Percutaneous lumbar medial branch neurotomy: A modification of facet denervation. Spine., *5:*193, 1980.
35. Bogduk, N., Macintosh, J., and Marsland, A.: Technical limitations to the efficacy of radiofrequency neurotomy for spinal pain. Neurosurgery, *20:*529, 1987.
36. Bogduk, N., Windsor, M., and Inglis, A.: The innervation of the cervical intervertebral discs. Spine, *13:*2, 1988.
37. Bogduk, N.: Rebuttal. APS Journal, *3:*166, 1994.
38. Bogduk, N., and Cherry, D.: Epidural corticosteroid agents for sciatica. Med. J. Aust., *143:*402, 1985.
39. Bovim, G., Berg, R., and Dale, J.G.: Cervicogenic headache: Anesthetic blockades of cervical nerves (C2–C5) and facet joint (C2–C3). Pain, *49:*315, 1992.
40. Bowman, S.J., Wedderburn, L., Whaley, A., Grahame, R., and Newman, S.: Outcome assessment after epidural corticosteroid injection for low back pain and sciatica. Spine., *18:*1345, 1993.
41. Brena, S.F., Wolf, S.L., Chapman, S.L., and Hammonds, W.D.: Chronic back pain: Electromyographic, motion and behavioral assessments following sympathetic nerve blocks and placebos. Pain. *8:*1, 1980.
42. Breivik, H., Hesla, P.E., Molnar, I., and Lind, B.: Treatment of chronic low back pain and sciatica: Comparison of caudal epidural injections of bupivacaine and methylprednisolone with bupivacaine followed by saline. *In* Bonica, J.J., and Albe-Fessard, D. (eds.): Advances in Pain Research and Therapy. pp. 927. New York, Raven Press, 1976.
43. Burchiel, K.J., Frank, E.H., and Keenen, T.L.: A plea for prospective studies on diskography. APS Journal, *3:*160, 1994.
44. Bush, K.: Lower back pain and sciatica: How best to manage them. Br. J. Hosp. Med., *51:*216, 1994.
45. Byrod, G., Olmarker, K., Konno, S., et al.: A rapid transport route between the epidural space and the intraneural capillaries of the nerve roots. Spine, *20:*138, 1995.
46. Cailliet, R.: Low back pain. *In* Cailliet, R. (ed.): Soft Tissue Pain and Disability. pp. 41. Philadelphia, F.A. Davis, 1977.
47. Calodney, A.: Failed back surgery syndrome. Pain Digest *2:*300, 1992.
48. Calodney, A., and Lorren, T.: Functional management of degenerative spine disease. Pain Digest, *2:*295, 1992.
49. Campbell, J.N., Raja, S.N., Cohen, R.H., et al.: Peripheral neural mechanisms of nociception. *In* Wall, P.D., and Melzack, R. (eds.): Textbook of Pain. pp. 22. New York, Churchill Livingstone, 1989.
50. Campbell, J.N., and Belzberg, A.J.: Use of disk distension to diagnose pain of spinal origin. A.P.S. Journal, *3:*157, 1994.
51. Chatani, K., Kawakami, M., Weinstein, J.N., Meller, S.T., and Gebhart, G.F.: Characterization of thermal hyperalgesia, c-fos expression, and alternations in neuropeptides after mechanical irritation of the dorsal root ganglion. Spine, *20:*277, 1995.
52. Cicala, R.S., Turner, R., Moran, E., et al.: Methylprednisolone acetate does not cause inflammatory changes in the epidural space. Anesthesiology, *72:*556, 1990.
53. Ciocon, J.O., Galindo-Ciocon, D., Amaranath, L., and Galindo, D.: Caudal epidural blocks for elderly patients with lumbar canal stenosis. J. Am. Geriatr. Soc., *42:*593, 1994.
54. Connally, G.H., and Sanders, S.H.: Predicting low-back-pain patients' response to lumbar sympathetic nerve blocks and interdisciplinary rehabilitation: The role of pretreatment overt pain behavior and cognitive coping strategies. Pain, *44:*139, 1991.
55. Coomes, E.N.: A comparison between epidural anaesthesia and bedrest in sciatica. Br. Med. J., *1:*20, 1961.
56. Coderre, T.J., Chan, A.K., Helms, C., Basbaum, A.L., and Levine, J.D.: Increasing sympathetic nerve terminal dependent plasma extravasation correlates with decreased arthritic joint injury in rats. Neuroscience, *40:*185, 1991.
57. Cornefjord, M., Olmarker, K., Farley, D.B., Weinstein, J.N. and Rydevik, B.: Neuropeptide changes in compressed spinal nerve roots. Spine, *20:*670, 1995.
58. Coventry, M.B.: Anatomy of the intervertebral disc. Clin. Orthop., *67:*9, 1969.
59. Coventry, M.B., Ghormley, R.K., and Kernohan, J.W.: The intervertebral disc: Its microscopic anatomy and pathology; Part I. Anatomy, development and physiology. J.B. Joint Surg., *27:*105, 1945.
60. Cuckler, J.M., Bernini, P.A., Wiesel, S.W., et al.: The use of epidural steroids in the treatment of lumbar radicular pain. J. Bone Joint Surg., *67A:*63, 1985.
61. Cutler, R.B., Fishbain, D.A., Rosomoff, H.L., et al.: Does nonsurgical pain center treatment of chronic pain return patients to work? Spine, *19:*643, 1994.
62. Davis, K.D., Meyer, R.A., Treede, R-D., Cohen, R.H., and Campbell, J.N.: Chemosensitivity and sensitization of mechanically insensitive afferents in the primate. Soc. for Neuroscience Abstracts. 6:415, 1991.
63. Davis, R., and Emmons, S.B. Benefits of epidural methylprednisolone in a unilateral lumbar discectomy. J. Spinal Disord. *3:*299, 1990.
64. Delaney, T.J., Rowlingson, J.C., Carron, H., and Butler, A.: Epidural steroid effects on the nerves and meninges. Anesth. Analg., *59:*610, 1980.
65. Derby, R., Kine, G., Saal, J.A., et al.: Response to steroid and duration of radicular pain as predictors of surgical outcome. Spine, *17:*S176, 1992.
66. Devor, M., Jang, W., and Michaelis, M.: Modulation of activity in dorsal root ganglion neurons by sympathetic activation in nerve-injured rats. J. Neurophysiol., *71:*38, 1994.
67. Deyo, R.A., Loeser, J.D., and Bigos, S.J.: Herniated lumbar intervertebral disk. Ann. Intern. Med., *112:*598, 1990.
68. Deyo, R.A., and Diehl, A.K.: Patient satisfaction with medical care in low-back pain. Spine, *11:*28, 1986.
69. Deyo, R.A.: Fads in the treatment of low back pain. N. Engl. J. Med., *325:*1039, 1991.
70. Dilke, T.F.W., Burry, H.C., and Grahame, R.: Extradural corticosteroid injection in management of lumbar nerve root compression. Br. Med. J., *2:*635, 1973.
71. Dreyfuss, P., Tibiletti, C., and Dreyer, S.J.: Thoracic zygapophysial joint pain patterns: A study in normal volunteers. Spine., *19:*807, 1994.
72. Dreyfuss, P., Michaelsen, M., and Fletcher, D.: Atlanto-occipital and lateral atlanto-axial joint pain patterns. Spine., *19:*1125, 1994.
73. Dwyer, A., April, C., and Bogduk, N.: Cervical zygapophysial joint pain patterns I: A study in normal volunteers. Spine., *15:*453, 1990.
74. Dwyer, A., Aprill, C., and Bogduk, N.: Cervical zygapophysial joint pain patterns. I: A study in normal volunteers. Spine., *15:*453, 1990.
75. Edmonds, L.C., Vance, M.L., and Hughes, J.M.: Morbidity from paraspinal depo-corticosteroid injections for analgesia: Cushing's syndrome and adrenal suppression. Anesth. Analg., *72:*820, 1991.
76. El-Bohy, A., Cavanaugh, J.M., Getchell, M.L., et al.: Localization of substance P and neurofilament immunoreactive fibers in the lumbar facet joint capsule and supraspinous ligament of the rabbit. Brain Res. *460:*379, 1988.
77. Esses, S.I.: The diskography dilemma. A.P.S. Journal, *3:*155, 1994.
78. Evans, P.J.D.: Cryoanalgesia: The application of low temperatures to nerves to produce anaesthesia or analgesia. Anaesthesia, *36:*1003, 1981.
79. Farfan, H.F.: Biomechanics of the human spine. *In* Kirkaldy-Willis, W.H., (ed.): Managing Low Back Pain. pp. 9 New York, Churchill Livingstone, 1983.
80. Flor, H., Fydrich, T., and Turk, D.C.: Efficacy of multidisciplinary pain treatment centers: A meta-analytic review. Pain, *49:*221, 1992.
81. Foerster, O.: The dermatomes in man. Brain, *56:*1, 1933.
82. Foley, K.M.: The treatment of cancer pain. N. Engl. J. Med., *313:*84, 1985.
83. Fortin, J.D., Aprill, C.N., Ponthieux, B., and Pier, J.: Sacroiliac joint: Pain referral maps upon applying a new injection/arthrography technique: Part II. Clinical evaluation. Spine., *19:*1483, 1994.
84. Fortin, J.D., Dwyer, A.P., West, S., and Pier, J.: Sacroiliac joint: Pain referral maps upon applying a new injection/arthrography technique. Part I. Asymptomatic volunteers. Spine, *19:*1475, 1994.
85. Frymoyer, J.W.: Back pain and sciatica. N. Engl. J. Med., *318:*291, 1988.
86. Fuxe, K., Harfstrand, A.,Agnati, L.F., et al.: Immunocytochemical studies on the localization of glucocorticoid receptor immunoreactive nerve cells in the lower brain stem and spinal cord of the male rat using a monoclonal antibody against rat liver glucocorticoid receptor. Neurosci. Lett. *60:*1, 1985.
87. Gamburd, R.S.: The use of selective injections in the lumbar spine. Phys. Med. Rehab. Clin. N. Am., *2:*79, 1991.

88. Gamburd, R.S.: The use of selective injections in the lumbar spine. Phys. Med. Rehab. Clin. North Am. *2:*79, 1991.
89. Garette, S., Marcoux, S., Truchon, R. et al.: A controlled trial of corticosteroid injections into facet joints for chronic low back pain. N. Engl. J. Med., *325:*1002, 1991.
90. Ghormley, R.K.: Low back pain, with special reference to the articular facets, with presentation of an operative procedure. J.A.M.A., *101*:1773, 1933.
91. Giles, L.G.F., and Harvey, A.R.: Immunohistochemical demonstration of nociceptors in the capsule and synovial folds of human zygapophysial joints. Br. J. Rheumatol. *26:*362, 1987.
92. Giles, L.G.F., and Taylor, J.R.: Innervation of lumbar zygapophysial joint synovial folds. Acta Orthop. Scand., *58:*43, 1987.
93. Gillette, R.G., Kramis, R.C., and Roberts, W.J.: Sympathetic activation of cat spinal neurons responsive to noxious stimulation of deep tissues in the low back. Pain, *56:*31, 1994.
94. Gillette, R.G., Kramis, R.C., and Roberts, W.J.: Spinal projections of cat primary afferent fibers innervating lumbar facet joints and multifidus muscle. Neurosci. Let., *157:*67, 1993.
95. Goddard, M.D., and Reid, J.D.: Movements induced by straight leg raising in the lumbo-sacral roots, nerves and plexus, and in the intrapelvic section of the sciatic nerve. J. Neurol. Neurosurg. Psychiatry., *28:*12, 1965.
96. Goddard, M.D., and Reid, J.D.: Movements induced by straight leg raising in the lumbo-sacral roots, nerves and plexus, and in the intrapelvic section of the sciatic nerve. J. Neurosurg. Psych., *28:*12. 1965.
97. Goebert, H.W., Jallo, S.J., Gardner, W.J., and Wasmuth, C.E.: Painful radiculopathy treated with epidural injections of procaine and hydrocortisone acetate: Results in 113 patients. Anesth. Analg., *40:*130, 1961.
98. Goldstone, J.C., and Pennant, J.H.: Spinal anaesthesia following facet joint injection: A report of two cases. Anaesthesia, *42:*754, 1987.
99. Goldthwait, J.E.: The lumbosacral articulation: An explanation of many cases of lumbago, sciatica and paraplegia. Boston Medical and Surgical Journal *164*:356, 1911.
100. Groen, G.J., Baljet, B., and Drukker, J.: Nerves and nerve plexuses of the human vertebral column. Am. J. Anat., *188:*282, 1990.
101. Haddox, J.D.: Lumbar and cervical epidural steroid therapy. Anesth. Clin. N. Am., *10:*179, 1992.
102. Hammonds, W.D.: Epidural steroid injections—An unproven therapy for pain. A.P.S. Journal, *3:*31, 1994.
103. Hasue, M.: Pain and the nerve root: An interdisciplinary approach. Spine, *18:*2053, 1993.
104. Hickey, R.F.: Outpatient epidural steroid injections for low back pain and lumbosacral radiculopathy. N. Z. Med. J., *100:*594, 1987.
105. Hirsch, D., Inglemark, B., and Miller, M.: The anatomical basis for low back pain. Acta Orthop. Scand., *33:*1, 1963.
106. Hopwood, M.B., and Abram, S.E.: Factors associated with failure of lumbar epidural steroids. Reg. Anesth., *18:*238, 1993.
107. Howe, J.F., Loeser, J.D., and Calvin, W.H.: Mechanosensitivity of dorsal root ganglia and chronically injured axons: A physiological basis for the radicular pain of nerve root compression. Pain, *3:*25, 1977.
108. Hua, S.Y., and Chen, Y.Z. Membrane receptor-mediated electrophysiological effects of glucocorticoid on mammalian neurons. Endocrinology, *124:*687, 1989.
109. Hua, S-Y, and Chen, Y-Z.: Membrane receptor-mediated electrophysiological effects of glucocorticoid on mammalian neurons. Endocrinology, *124:*687, 1989.
109a. Indahl, A., Kaigle, A., Reikeras, O., and Holm, S.: Electromyographic response of the porcine multifidus musculature after nerve stimulation. Spine, *20*:2652, 1995.
110. Jamison, R.N., VadeBoncouer, T., and Ferrante, F.M.: Low back pain patients unresponsive to an epidural steroid injection: Identifying predictive factors. Clin. J. Pain., *7:*311, 1991.
111. Johansson, A., Hao, J., and Sjolund, B.: Local corticosteroid application blocks transmission in normal nociceptive c-fibres. Acta Anaesthesiol., Scand., *34:*335, 1990.
112. Kay, J., Findling, J.W., and Raff, H.: Epidural triamcinolone suppresses the pituitary-adrenal axis in human subjects. Anesth. Analg., *78:*501, 1994.
113. Kellergren, J.H.: Observations on referred pain arising from muscle p. 175. *In* 1938.
114. Kelley, M.: Pain due to pressure on nerves? Spinal tumors and the intervertebral disc. Neurology, *6:*32, 1956.
115. Kepes, E.R., and Duncalf, D.: Treatment of backache with spinal injection of local anesthetics, spinal and systemic steroids: A review. Pain., *22:*33, 1985.
116. Kibler, R.F., and Nathan, P.W.: Relief of pain and paresthesiae by nerve block distal to a lesion. J. Neurol. Neurosurg. Psychiatry, *23:*91, 1960.
117. Kikuchi, S., Macnab, I., and Moreau, P.: Localization of the level of symptomatic cervical disc degeneration. J. Bone Joint Surg., *63-B:*272, 1981.
118. Kline, M.T.: Stereotactic Radiofrequency Lesions as Part of the Management of Pain. Orlando, Paul M. Deutsch Press, Inc, 1992.
119. Knight, C.L., and Burnell, J.C.: Systemic side effects of extradural steroids. Anaesthesia, *35:*593, 1980.
120. Koes, B.W., Scholtren, R.J., Mens, J., and Bouter, L.M. Efficacy of epidural steroid injections for low-back pain and sciatica: A systematic review of randomized clinical trials. Pain, *63:*279, 1995.
121. Kummer, W.: Sensory ganglia as a target of autonomic and sensory nerve fibres in the guinea-pig. Neuroscience, *59:*739, 1994.
122. Kuslich, S.D., Ulstrom, C.L., and Michael, C.J.: The tissue origin of low back pain and sciatica: A report of pain response to tissue stimulation during operations on the lumbar spine using local anesthesia. Ortho. Clin. North Am., *22:*181, 1991.
123. Levine, J.D., Dardick, S.J., Roizen, M.F., Helms, C., and Basbaum, B.L.: Contribution of sensory afferents and sympathetic efferents to joint injury in experimental arthritis. J. Neurosci., *6:*3423, 1986.
124. Levine, J.D., and Basbaum, A.I.: Neurogenic mechanism for symmetrical arthritis. Lancet, *335:*795, 1990.
125. Lilius, G., Laasonen, E.M., Myllynen, P., Harilainen, A., and Gronlund, G.: Lumbar facet joint syndrome: A randomised clinical trial. J. Bone Joint Surg., Br. Vol., *71:*681, 1989.
126. Lindahl, O., and Rexed, B.: Histologic changes in spinal nerve roots of operated cases of sciatica. Acta Orthop., Scand., *20:*215, 1951.
127. Lord, S.M., Barnsley, L., and Bogduk, N.: Percutaneous radiofrequency neurotomy in the treatment of cervical zygapophysial joint pain: A caution. Neurosurgery *36:*732, 1995.
128. Maigne, R., LeCorre, F., and Judet, H.: Lombalgies basses d'origine dorso-lombaire: Traitment chirurgical par excision des capsules articulaires posterieures. Nouv., Presse. Med., *7:*565, 1978.
129. Malmivaara, A., Hakkinen, U., and Aro, T.: The treatment of acute low back pain—bed rest, exercises, or ordinary activity? N. Engl. J. Med., *332:*351, 1995.
130. Marks, R., and Semple, A.J.: Spinal anaesthesia after facet joint injection [letter]. Anaesthesia, *43:*65, 1988.
131. Marks, R.: Distribution of pain provoked from lumbar facet joints and related structures during diagnostic spinal infiltration. Pain, *39:*37, 1989.
132. Marshall, L.L., and Trethwie, E.R.: Chemical irritation of nerve root in disc prolapse. Lancet, *2:*230, 1973.
133. Marshall, L.L., Trethwie, E.R., and Curtain, C.C.: Chemical radiculitis: A clinical, physiological, and immunological study. Clin. Orthop., *129:*61, 1987.
134. Martin, H.A., Basbaum, A.L., Kwiat, G.C., Goetzl, E.J., and Levine, J.D.: Leukotriene and prostaglandin sensitization of cutaneous high-threshold C- and A-delta mechanonociceptors in the hairy skin of rat hindlimbs. Neuroscience, *22:*651, 1987.
135. McCarron, R.F., Wimpee, M.W., Hudkins, P.G., and Laros, G.S.: The inflammatory effect of nucleus pulposus: A possible element in the pathogenesis of low-back pain. Spine, *12:*760, 1987.
136. McLain, R.F.: Mechanoreceptor endings in human cervical facet joints. Spine, *19:*495, 1994.
137. McCulloch, J.A.: Differential diagnosis of low back pain. *In* Tollison, C.D. (ed.): Handbook of Chronic Pain Management pp. 335. Baltimore, Williams and Wilkins, 1989.
138. Mehta, M.: Intractable pain. *In* Mehta, M., (ed.): The nature of cancer pain. pp. 129. London. W. B. Saunders, 1973.
139. Mehta, M., and Parry, C.B.W.: Mechanical back pain and the facet joint syndrome: Disabil. Rehabil., *16:*2, 1994.
140. Merry, A., Schug, S.A., and Rogers, A.: Epidural steroid injections for sciatica and back pain: A meta-analysis of controlled clinical trials. Reg. Anesth., *21(2S):*64, 1996.
141. Meyer, R.A., Davis, K.D., Cohen, R.H., Treede, R-D., and Campbell, J.N.: Mechanically insensitive afferents (MIAs) in cutaneous nerves of monkey. Brain Res., *561:*252, 1991.
142. Mixter, W.J. and Barr, J.S.: Rupture of the intervertebral disc with involvement of the spinal cord. N. Engl. J. Med., *211:*210, 1934.

143. Moneta, G.B., Videman, T., Kaivanto, K., et al.: Reported pain during lumbar discography as a function of anular ruptures and disc degeneration: A re-analysis of 833 discograms. Spine, *19:*1968, 1994.
144. Mooney, V.: Facet joint syndrome. *In* Jayson, M.I.V., and Dixon, A., (eds.): The Lumbar Spine and Back Pain. pp. 291. New York, Churchill Livingstone, 1992.
144a.Nelson, D.A. Intraspinal therapy using methylprednisolone acetate. Twenty-three years of clinical controversy. Spine, *18:*278, 1993.
145. Murphy, R.W.: Nerve roots and spinal nerves in degenerated disc disease. Clin. Orthop., *129:*46, 1977.
146. Naito, M., Owen, J.H., Birdwell, K.H., and Oakey, D.M.: Blood flow direction in the lumbar nerve root. Spine, *15:*966, 1990.
147. Naylor, A.: Enzymic and immunological activity in the intervertebral disc. Orthop. Clin. North Am., *6:*51, 1975.
148. Nelson, D.A.: Intraspinal therapy using methylprednisolone acetate: Twenty-three years of clinical controversy. Spine, *18:*278, 1993.
149. North, R.B., Ewend, M.G., Lawton, M.T., Kidd, D.H., and Piantadosi, S.: Failed back surgery syndrome: Five-year follow-up after spinal cord stimulator implantation. Neurosurgery, *28:*692, 1991.
150. North, R.B., Han, M., Zahurak, M., and Kidd, D.H.: Radiofrequency lumnbar facet denervation: Analysis of prognostic factors. Pain, *57:*77, 1994.
150a.Raj, P.P. Tutorial 13: Management of low back pPain Digest, 4:55, 1994.
151. Olmarker, K., Rydevik, B., and Holm, S.: Edema formation in spinal nerve roots induced by experimental, graded compression. Spine, *14:*569, 1989.
152. Olmarker, K., and Rydevik, B.: Pathophysiology of sciatica. Orthop Clin North Am., *22:*223, 1991.
153. Osti, O.L., and Cullum, D.E.: Occupational low back pain and intervertebral disc degeneration: Epidemiology, imaging and pathology. Clin. J. Pain., *10:*331, 1994.
154. Pountain, G.D., Keegan, A.L., and Jayson, M.I.V.: Impaired fibrinolytic activity in defined chronic back pain syndromes. Spine, *12:*83, 1987.
155. Pankovitch, A.M., and Korngold, L.: A comparison of the antigenic properties of nucleus pulposus and cartilage protein polysaccharide complexes. J Immunol., *99:*431, 1967.
156. Raj, P.P.: Tutorial 13: Management of low back pain. Pain Digest, *4:*55, 1994.
157. Rapp, S.E., et al.: Epidural steroid injection in the treatment of low back pain: A meta-analysis. Anesthesiology, *81:*A923, 1994.
158. Rasminsky, M.: Ectopic generation of impulses in pathological nerve fibers. *In* Jewett, D.L., McCarroll, H.R., Jr., (eds.): Nerve Repair and Regeneration–Its Clinical and Experimental Basis. pp. 178. St. Louis: C.V. Mosby, 1980.
159. Ray, C.D.: Percutaneous radio-frequency facet nerve blocks: Treatment of the mechanical low-back syndrome. Radionics, *1:*1, 1982.
160. Roth, D.A.: Cervical analgesic discography: A new test for the definitive diagnosis of the painful-disk syndrome. J.A.M.A., *235:*1713, 1995.
161. Rowlingson, J.C.: Appropriate use of therapeutic nerve blocks. *In* Tollison, C.D., and Kriegel, M.D., (eds.): Interdisciplinary rehabilitation of low back pain. pp. 63. Baltimore, Williams & Wilkins, 1989.
162. Rowlingson, J.C., and Kirschenbaum, L.P.: Epidural analgesic techniques in the management of cervical pain. Anesth. Analg., *65:*938, 1986.
163. Rowlingson, J.C.: Epidural steroids: Do they have a place in pain management? APS Journal, *3:*20, 1994.
164. Rowlingson, J.C., and Hamill, R.J.: Treatment of low back pain. Int. Anesthesiol. Clin., *29:*57, 1991.
165. Rowlingson, J.C.: Low back pain. *In* Warfield, C.A. (ed.): Principles and Practice of Pain Management. pp. 129. New York, McGraw-Hill, 1993.
166. Rowlingson, J.C.: Low back pain and pain in the lower extremity. *In* Raj, P.P. (ed.): Practical Management of Pain. pp. 396. St. Louis, Mosby–Year Book, 1992.
167. Rydevik, B., Brown, M.D., and Lundborg, G.: Pathoanatomy and pathophysiology of nerve root compression. Spine, *9:*7, 1984.
168. Saal, J.A., and Saal, J.S.: Nonoperative treatment of herniated lumbar intervertebral disc with radiculopathy: An outcome study. Spine, *14:*431, 1989.
169. Saal, J.S.: The role of inflammation in lumbar pain. Phys. Med. Rehab., *4:*191, 1990.
170. Saal, J.S., Franson, R.C., Dobrow, R., et al.: High levels of inflammatory phospholipase A2 activity in lumbar disc herniations. Spine, *15:*674, 1990.
171. Sandrock, N.J.G., and Warfield, C.A.: Epidural steroids and facet injections. *In* Warfield, C.A., (ed.). Principles and practice of pain management. pp. 410. New York, McGraw-Hill, 1993.
172. Schellhas, K.P., Pollei, S.R., and Dorwart, R.H.: Thoracic discography: A safe and reliable technique. Spine, *19:*2103, 1994.
173. Schuster, G.D.: The use of cryoanalgesia in the painful facet syndrome. J Neurol. Orthop. Surg., *3:*271, 1982.
174. Schwarzer, A.C., Aprill, C.N., Derby, R., et al.: The relative contributions of the disc and zygapophyseal joint in chronic low back pain. Spine, *19:*801, 1994.
175. Schwarzer, A.C., Wang, S., O'Driscoll, D., Harrington, T., Bogduk, N., and Laurent, R.: The ability of computed tomography to identify a painful zygapophysial joint in patients with chronic low back pain. Spine, *20:*907, 1995.
176. Schwarzer, A.C., Aprill, C.N., Derby, R., et al.: Clinical features of patients with pain stemming from the lumbar zygapophysial joints: Is the lumbar facet syndrome a clinical entity? Spine, *19:*1132, 1994.
177. Schwarzer, A.C., Aprill, C.N., Derby, R., et al.: The false-positive rate of uncontrolled diagnostic blocks of the lumbar zygapophysial joints. Pain, *58:*195, 1994.
178. Seghal, A.D., Tweed, D.C., Gardner, W.L., and Foote, M.K.: Laboratory studies after intrathecal steroids. Arch. Neurol., *9:*64, 1963.
179. Serrao, J.M., Marks, R.L., Morley, S.J., and Goodchild, C.S.: Intrathecal midazolam for the treatment of chronic mechanical low back pain: A controlled comparison with epidural steroid in a pilot study. Pain, *48:*5, 1992.
180. Shealy, C.N.: Facet denervation in the management of back and sciatic pain. Clin. Orthop., 157, 1976.
181. Shealy, C.N.: Percutaneous radiofrequency denervation of spinal facets: Treatment for chronic back pain and sciatica. J. Neurosurg., *43:*448, 1975.
182. Sluyter, M.E.: Techniques of neurolysis: The Use of Radiofrequency Lesions of the Communicating Ramus in the Treatment of Low Back Pain. Boston, Kluwer Academic Publishers, 1989.
183. Sluyter, M.E.: The use of radiofrequency lesions for pain relief in failed back patients: International disability studies. Basel, Eular Publishers, 1989.
184. Snoek, W., Weber, H., and Jorgensen, B.: Double-blind evaluation of extradural methyl prednisolone for herniated lumbar discs. Acta Orthop. Scand., *48:*635, 1977.
185. Solonen, K.A.: The sacroiliac joint in the light of anatomical, roentgenological and clinical studies. Acta Orthop. Scand., *27:*1, 1957.
186. Sola, A.E., and Bonica, J.J.: Myofascial pain syndromes. *In* Bonica, J.J., (ed.): The Management of Pain. pp. 352. Philadelphia, Lea and Febiger, 1990.
187. Spitzer, W.O., LeBlanc, F.E., and Dupuis, M.: Scientific approach to the assessment and management of activity-related spinal disorders: A monograph for clinicians. Report of the Quebec Task Force on spinal disorders. Spine, *12:*[suppl]:S1, 1987.
188. Stieg, R.L.: The futility of physical testing in the assessment of disability. APS Journal, *3:*187, 1994.
189. Stolker, R.J., Vervest, A.C.M., and Groen, G.J.: The management of chronic spinal pain by blockades: A review. Pain, *58:*1, 1994.
190. Stolker, R.J., Vervest, A.C., and Groen, G.J.: Percutaneous facet denervation in chronic thoracic spinal pain. Acta Neurochir., *122:*82, 1993.
191. Strong, W.E., Wesley, R., and Winnie, A.P.: Epidural steroids are safe and effective when given appropriately. Arch. Neurol., *48:*1012, 1991.
192. Swerdlow, M., and Sayle-Creer, W.: A study of extradural medication in the relief of the lumbosciatic syndrome. Anaesthesia., *25:*341, 1970.
193. Takata, K., Inoue, S., Takahashi, K., and Ohtsuka, Y.: Swelling of the cauda equina in patients who have herniation of a lumbar disc: A possible pathogenesis of sciatica. J. Bone Joint Surg., *70A:*361, 1988.
194. Tajima, T., Furukawa, K., and Kuramochi, E.: Selective lumbosacral radiculopathy and block. Spine, *5:*68, 1980.
195. Thornbury, J.R., Fryback, D.G., and Turski, P.A.: Disk-caused nerve compression in patients with acute low back pain: Diagnosis with MR, CT myelography, and plain CT. Radiology, *186:*731, 1993.
196. Tuel, S.M., Meythaler, J.M., and Cross, L.L.: Cushing's syndrome from epidural methylprednisolone. Pain, *40:*81, 1990.

197. Turk, D.C., Brody, M.C., and Okifuji, E.A.: Physicians' attitudes and practices regarding the long-term prescribing of opioids for noncancer pain. Pain, *59:*201, 1994.
198. Twomey, L.T., Taylor, J.R., and Taylor, M.M.: Unsuspected damage to lumbar zygapophyseal (facet) joints after motor-vehicle accidents Med. J. Aust., *151:*210, 1989.
199. Volinn, E., Turczyn, K.M., and Loeser, J.D.: Patterns in low back pain hospitalizations: Implications for the treatment of low back pain in an era of health care reform. Clin. J. Pain., *10:*64, 1994.
200. von Korff, M., Barlow, W., Cherkin, D., and Deyo, R.A.: Effects of practice style in managing back pain. Ann. Intern. Med., *121:*187, 1994.
201. Vleeming, A., Stoeckart, R., Volkers, A.C.W., and Snidjers, C.J.: Relation between form and function in the sacroiliac joint; Part I. Clinical anatomical aspects. Spine, *15:*130, 1990.
202. Vleeming, A., Volkers, A.C.W., Snidjers, C.J., and Stoeckart, R.: Relation between form and function in the sacroiliac joint; Part II. Biomechanical aspects. Spine, *15:*133, 1990.
203. Waddell, G., McCulloch, J.A., Kummel, E.D., and Venner, R.M.: Nonorganic physical signs in low-back pain. Spine, *5:*117, 1980.
204. Walsh, T.R., Weinstein, J.N., Spratt, K.F., et al.: Lumbar discography in normal subjects: A controlled prospective study. J. Bone Joint Surg., *72A:*1081, 1990.
205. Warfield, C.A., Biber, M.P., Crews, D.A., and Dwarakanath, G.K.: Epidural steroid injection as a treatment for cervical radiculitis. Clin. J. Pain., *4:*201, 1988.
206. Warr, A.C., Wilkinson, J.A., Burn, J.M.B., and Langdon, L.: Chronic lumbosciatic syndrome treated by epidural injection and manipulation. Practitioner., *209:*53, 1972.
207. Wedel, D.J., and Wilson, P.R.: Cervical facet arthrography. Reg. Anesth., *10:*7, 1985.
208. Weinstein, J.: Neurogenic and nonneurogenic pain and inflammatory mediators. Orthop. Clin. North Am. *22:*235, 1991.
209. Weinstein, J., Claverie, W., and Gibson, S.: The pain of discography. Spine, *13:*1344, 1988.
210. Wiley, J.J., MacNab, I., and Wortzman, G.: Lumbar discography and its clinical applications. Can. J. Surg., *11:*280, 1968.
211. Wilkinson, H.A. Intrathecal Depo-Medrol: A literature review. Clin. J. Pain., *8:*49, 1992.
212. Wilson, P.R.: Diskography is still investigational. APS Journal, *3:*163, 1994.
213. Winnie, A.P., Hartman, J.T., Meyers, H.L., Ramamurthy, S., and Barangan, V.: Pain clinic II: Intradural and extradural corticosteroiuds for sciatica. Anesth. Analg., *51:*990, 1972.
214. Xavier, A.V., McDanal, J., and Kissin, L.: Relief of sciatic radicular pain by sciatic nerve block. Anesth. Analg., *67:*1177, 1988.
215. Yabuki, S., and Kikuchi, S.: Nerve root infiltration and sympathetic block: An experimental study of intraradicular blood flow. Spine, *20:*901, 1995.
216. Yamashita, T., Cavanaugh, J.M., El-Bohy, A.A., Getchell, T.V., and King, A.L.: Mechanosensitive afferent units in the lumbar facet joint. Surgery, *72A:*865, 1990.
217. Yang, K.H., and King, A.L.: Mechanism of facet-load transmission as a hypothesis for low-back pain. Spine, *9:*557, 1984.
218. Yates, D.W.: A comparison of the types of epidural injection commonly used in the treatment of low back pain and sciatica. Rheum Rehabil., *17:*181, 1978.
219. Yoshizawa, H., Kobayashi, S., and Kubota, K.: Effects of compression on intraradicular blood flow in dogs. Spine, *14:*1220, 1989.

Neural Blockade in Clinical Anesthesia and Management of Pain, Third Edition,
edited by M.J. Cousins and P.O. Bridenbaugh.
Lippincott–Raven Publishers, Philadelphia © 1998.

CHAPTER 29

Spinal Route of Analgesia

Opioids and Future Options

Daniel B. Carr and Michael J. Cousins

Ignored until the late 20th century as a substrate for analgesia, the spinal cord has now emerged as one—if not *the*—key target for pain control in clinical anesthesiology. More and more anesthesiologists now give drugs spinally to provide intraoperative[1,79] anesthesia and persistent postoperative analgesia after procedures as diverse as knee arthroscopy, inguinal hernia repair, or even (with a "light" general anesthetic) laparascopic colectomy, thoracoscopy or coronary artery bypass grafting.[77] Such operations used to require extensive incisions under general anesthesia, with prolonged and painful hospital stays.[78] Today, the combination of minimally invasive surgical techniques and spinal analgesia allows these same procedures to be performed on a "fast-track," and often on an out-patient, basis[84,255] Outpatient management of refractory cancer pain is now accomplished routinely by implantation of pumps for spinal drug delivery.[21,31,117,539] Some centers insert chromaffin secretory cells[420] into the intrathecal space to serve as biological pumps, for the same purpose.[69,520] Soon, clinicians may employ cells genetically altered to secrete mixtures of analgesic molecules,[39] that clinical trials registries[240] indicate are optimal for pain due to the individual patient's tumor type and stage. These exciting advances harness sophisticated technologies to enhance patients' clinical outcomes and quality of life while lowering the cost[89,192,238] and burden of care. Such progress reflects the rapid acquisition and application of new knowledge of spinal analgesia since the previous edition of this volume.

D.B. Carr: Departments of Anesthesia and Medicine, Tufts University School of Medicine, New England Medical Center, Boston, Massachusetts 02111.

M.J. Cousins: Department of Anaesthesia and Pain Management, Royal North Shore Hospital, University of Sydney, St. Leonards, New South Wales 2065 Australia.

Only recently has the spinal cord taken "center stage" in analgesia practice and research. For thousands of years, pain relief could be secured only at the expense of central nervous system depression, as with the use of Mandragora, wine, and opium in ancient China; Mandragora and "poppy" in ancient Egypt, Rome, and Greece; and atropine, opium, cocaine, and hallucinogens, by the Incas and ancient Peruvians. Thus, until Koller's daring introduction of local anesthetic blockade in 1884, the major site for pain control was thought to be the brain. Brain and axon continued to be the major options for analgesia[136] until the mid-1970s, when preclinical studies proved[538] that the spinal cord can be a target for selective opioid analgesia. By the early 1980s, with speed unprecedented since Koller's time, these basic observations were harnessed in daily clinical practice worldwide.[31,57,128,135,383] Insight into the chain of events precipitated in the spinal cord by painful peripheral stimuli has spurred novel drug discovery and rekindled interest in spinal delivery of established drugs[182] alone or in combination.[163] This progress, milestones of which are summarized in Table 29-1 (see also Chapter 23.1), has been accelerated by the shared excitement of clinicians and investigators as they participated in a revolution of applied pharmacology. Patient-controlled analgesia,[23] first applied to the intravenous route in the 1960s, also was extended to spinal analgesia and by the 1980s was in wide use for epidural drug delivery.

Brain, spinal cord, axon and periphery, once viewed as distinct sites for the actions of different analgesics, are now known to participate jointly as targets for pain control.[246,387,483] Local anesthetics block axons of sensory (superficial) and motor tracts (deep) in the spinal cord.[136] Systemically applied opioids and nonopioid compounds such as nonsteroidal anti-inflammatory drugs (NSAIDs) or clonidine, have antinociceptive effects at the spinal cord level in animal studies and in humans[244,264] (see Chapter 24). Opi-

TABLE 29-1. *Milestones in spinal analgesic (particularly opioid) research*

- Synthesis of naloxone (1961) and other selective opioid antagonists for in vivo and in vitro studies.
- Melzack and Wall's "gate theory" (1965) suggests nociception is modulated in spinal cord.
- Proposals by Martin (1960s to 1970s) of distinct opioid receptors to explain animal and clinical observations of diverse syndromes of addiction and abstinence for different opioids, and to predict the possibility of analgesia without respiratory depression.
- Demonstrations that electrical stimulation (1969) or microinjection of morphine into periaqueductal gray elicit naloxone-reversible analgesia mediated by monoaminergic systems descending to the dorsal horn of spinal cord.
- Identification in 1973 of saturable, stereoselective receptors for opioids and naloxone independently by Pert and Synder, Terenius, and Simon and co-workers.
- Isolation and characterization (1975) of endogenous opioids, the enkephalins, by Hughes and others.
- Autoradiographic mapping of opioid receptor distribution (1977 on) showing highest densities in substantia gelatinosa of spinal cord, medullary dorsal horn, periaqueductal gray matter, and other brain sites.
- Dose-dependent, stereospecific, naloxone-reversible analgesia demonstrated by Yaksh and Rudy (1977) after intrathecal morphine administration or local, iontophoretic dorsal horn morphine application in the rat.[538] Numerous subsequent studies by Yaksh and others applying spinal catheterization techniques in animal models to elucidate dose-response relationships, potencies, receptors, and mechanisms of opioid analgesia, toxicity, tolerance, and opioid-nonopioid interactions.
- Synthesis of selective opioid ligands for investigative and therapeutic purposes (Hruby, Porreca, Schiller, Lipkowski, Portoghese, et al.).
- Elucidation of anti-opioid systems including hyperalgesic peptides such as substance P or cholecystokinin, excitatory amino acids such as glutamate, and intracellular mediators such as protein kinase C and nitric oxide that act in aggregate to mediate sensitization by nociceptive input, as well as opioid tolerance and latent hyperglesia during continued opioid use.
- Refinement of animal models for evaluation of analgesics for nociceptive and neuropathic (Bennett, Chung) pain.
- Recognition of genes expressed immediately after neuronal activation (e.g., *c-fos*) or in the process of programmed cell death, and their application to elucidate dynamic processes within nociceptive pathways (Basbaum, Besson).
- Clinical application of nonopioid analgesic systems for exploitation singly or in combination with opioids (e.g., alpha-2, cholinergic).
- Cloning of receptors for the endogenous opioids, synthesis of antisense DNA to evaluate receptor function in vivo, and analysis of subregions' functions by site-specific mutation methods.
- Application of novel drug delivery methods (polymers, liposomes, chromaffin cell implants as "biological pumps" for intrathecal analgesic delivery).

oids also act to reduce pain and inflammation through direct effects upon peripheral tissue[464,465] (Table 29-2).

Epidural opioids can be absorbed rapidly into the circulation, producing early effects on the brain (see below). Particularly hydrophilic (e.g., morphine) but also lipophilic opioids migrate in cerebrospinal fluid (CSF) to the brain, producing analgesia along with side-effects such as sedation, dysphoria, nausea and vomiting, and respiratory depression. Very hydrophilic drugs, such as morphine and glucuronide metabolites, accumulate in the brain to produce effects such as "delayed respiratory depression." Indeed, it is now clear that spinal administration of all opioids generates appreciable plasma concentrations that for many drugs approach the analgesic range.[118,120,415] Only small amounts of opioid need reach supraspinal sites to augment spinal opioid analgesia.[282,365,461] Hence, attempts to isolate the relative contributions of spinal, supraspinal,[158,208] and systemic drug (and metabolite) actions during opioid therapy by any route may be irrelevant because all three sites of action are likely involved during all but the lowest doses and briefest courses.

Understanding of the spinal cord's unique importance as a target for regional and systemic analgesics, reviewed in the prior edition of this text, has progressed considerably in the past decade[64,166,539] Interim preclinical and clinical advances allow us now to assess the effects of spinal analgesics, across many scales of space and time, from interactions of ligand molecules and binding sites on specific

TABLE 29-2. *Opioid analgesia: sites and processes*

Site	Processes
At site of tissue injury and inflammation	Decrease peptide mediator (bradykinin, substance P) release Reduce prostaglandin-induced hyperalgesia Reduce edema Influence white cell processes (?) Directly act on opioid receptors in peripheral nerve
At spinal segment	Decrease substance P-mediated neurotransmission from C (± A delta) fiber to second-order neuron Block summation of excitatory postsynaptic potentials in second-order neuron Prevent expansion of receptive fields and reduction of excitatory thresholds of second-order neurons Prevent neuronal gene expression (*c-fos*, opioid precursor molecules)
Supraspinally	Augment endogenous, descending, opioid-sensitive suppression of spinal pain signal transmission ([?] reduce DNIC or augment descending inhibition) Alter (mostly reduce) neuroendocrine and autonomic "stress" responses by acting on brainstem-limbic and hypothalamic opioid receptors Alter cognitive and emotional processing of painful input by acting on limbic and cortical opioid receptors

From Carr, D. B. and Lipkowski, A. W.: Mechanisms of opioid analgetic actions. *In* Rogers, M., Tinker, J. H., Covino, B. J., and Longnecker, D. E. (eds.): Principles and Practice of Anesthesiology. Vol. 1. pp. 1105–1130. St. Louis, Mosby–Year Book, 1993.

DNIC, diffuse noxious inhibitory control.

receptors in dorsal horn neurons, to clinical outcomes that include patient satisfaction and cost of care. Without exaggeration, one may say that spinal cord sensitization has now replaced pituitary-adrenal activation[373] as the principal undesirable "stress response," whose suppression (or better, pre-emption) guides the clinical practice of regional anesthesia and analgesia (see Chapter 5). In contrast to classical stress responses quantitated as blood hormone levels,[254] dorsal horn stress responses are intraneuronal and manifest as long-term structural and functional changes after noxious input[92,173] Thus, current preclinical advances depend upon increasingly sophisticated research methods, whose findings may lack an obvious link to clinical outcomes.

Ironically, the rise of enthusiasm for the spinal route of analgesia has engendered recent negative reaction to its use from two distinct points of view. The first camp is sceptical of the broad application of new medical technologies in advance of proof that they are safe, effective, and cost-effective. Its proponents seek to curb rising costs of health care by reliance upon "low-tech" methods until "high-tech" methods are proven to warrant the increased effort (and usually higher cost) of routine clinical application. They argue with some merit that few randomized, controlled, clinical trials have established conclusively the superiority of epidural analgesia over systemic or infiltration analgesia—at least not for the broad range of patients, drugs delivered, settings of care, and types of pain for which epidural or intrathecal analgesia are now practiced routinely. In contrast, the second group embraces new technologies to improve outcomes and reduce risks and costs of care. Those in the latter group look to novel systemic agents, such as selective inhibitors of inducible cyclo-oxygenase or peripherally active opioids, controlled-release formulations of local anesthetics or opioids, or "single-shot" instillations of chromaffin cells intrathecally, to render obsolete the need for conventional epidural or intrathecal access and drug delivery. In the late 1980s, surveying the field of spinal opioid analgesia in the previous edition of this volume, Cousins and colleagues outlined a substantial number of key questions that required answers for the safe and effective use of spinal opioids[134] and observed that many were unanswered.[133] As pressures increase from many quarters to justify continued, even expanded, reliance upon the spinal route of analgesia, it is sobering to consider how many of these questions remain open. Lack of a firm grounding in clinical evidence parallels much of medical practice and is certainly true of therapies for pain. Faced with mounting pressures for cost containment[80] throughout the industrialized world, and limited health care resources[89] in the developing nations, clinicians and basic scientists must work jointly, not only to develop the treatments of the future, but also to provide pharmacoeconomic data to prove that these innovative therapies lead to outcomes that equal or outweigh their costs[78,216,414,447,505]

To explore the above issues the present chapter will:

- Present succinctly the preclinical basis for desired effects, side effects and tolerance during spinal administration of opioids and nonopioid analgesics (detailed descriptions of the physiology and pharmacology of spinal mechanisms of pain and analgesia are found in Chapters 23.1 and 24);
- Describe the clinical pharmacokinetics and pharmacodynamics of commonly used spinal opioids;
- Review innovations likely to influence the future clinical practice of spinal analgesic therapy with opioids and other agents, singly or in combination;
- Describe the application of spinal opioid analgesia for acute pain and chronic pain due to cancer or nonmalignant conditions;
- Raise again a group of key questions, along with new ones that concern cost, benefit, and outcomes, that now must be confronted by scientists and clinicians if they are to advance the still young and promising field of spinal opioid analgesia.

Our starting point in this discussion will be to present relevant vocabulary and terminology.

OPIOIDS AND RECEPTORS: TERMINOLOGY

The term *narcotic*, ("narco" in Greek means to numb or deaden), is applicable to many drugs and is so vague that it is of little use except as a pejorative term in legal and regulatory contexts. The term *opiate* refers to morphine and related alkaloids derived from the poppy (some reports indicate that opiates are synthesized *de novo* in mammals, possibly by intestinal flora). *Opioid*, a broader term, includes *exogenous* substances with morphine-like properties as well as *endogenous* peptides.[311] Endogenous opioid peptides or *endorphins* all have the aromatic amino acid tyrosine at the initial (i.e., amino or N-terminus) position; all opioids share this tyramine structural motif. Opioid peptides that lack this tyramine moiety do not exert morphine-like effects, but still may have other "nonopioid" biological actions, such as enhancement of memory or immune modulation.

Full opioid agonists at the morphine or mu receptor include morphine, hydromorphone, meperidine and fentanyl. These agents bind to mu opioid receptors and activate them to produce dose-dependent analgesia and other effects[551] that are reversed by the opioid antagonist naloxone. As dose increases, there results a maximum or plateau of full efficacy. Some opioid agonists have less attraction to ("affinity" for) the binding site and require higher concentrations to achieve these effects. For other opioids termed *partial opioid agonists* this plateau is submaximal; buprenorphine is one example (Fig. 29-1). Opioids that are agonists at one opioid receptor type and antagonists at a different opioid receptor type are termed, somewhat confusingly, "mixed agonist-antagonists." Nalbuphine or butorphanol fall in this group; both are antagonists at the mu receptor and agonists at the kappa receptor. Naloxone, a pure opioid antagonist, has high affinity and zero efficacy. The rate of dissociation of opioids from their receptors influences their duration of action. For example, buprenorphine has a slow rate of dissociation from the mu receptor and a long duration of action. For other drugs with a rapid rate of receptor dissociation, the concentration of opioid in the bloodstream or CSF, and drug redis-

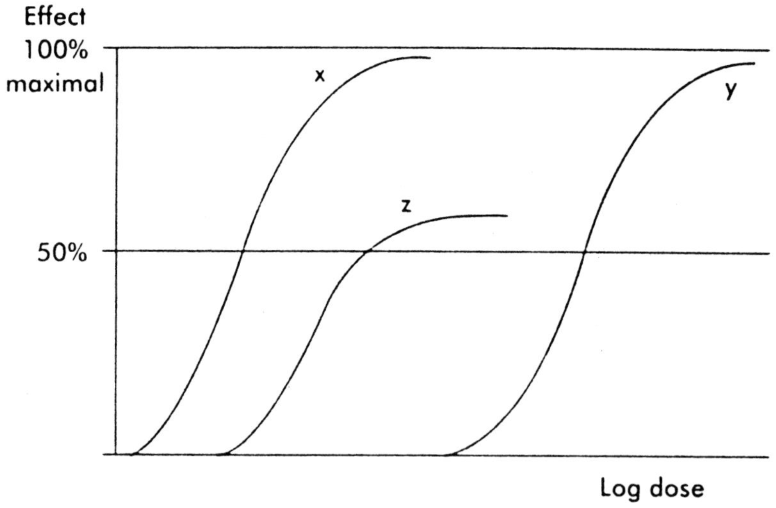

FIG. 29-1. Distinctions between potency and agonism. Drug **x** is more potent than drug **y** but both are "full agonists" that have the capacity to evoke a full biologic effect as dose is increased. Drug **z** produces a half-maximal biological effect at a dose intermediate between that of drugs **x** and **y**, but is a "partial agonist," because increasing doses still produce a submaximal response. [From Carr, D. B. and Lipkowski, A. W.: Mechanisms of opioid analgetic actions. *In* Rogers, M., Tinker, J. H., Covino, B. G., and Longnecker, D. E. (eds.): Principles and Practice of Anesthesiology. Vol. 1. pp. 1105–1130. St. Louis, Mosby–Year Book, 1993.]

tribution and rate of clearance (e.g., by liver), govern duration of action.[311]

The concept that cell membrane *receptors* mediate drug action arose in the nineteenth century. Descriptions of opioid structure-activity relationships presumed to reflect drug-receptor interactions appeared in the 1950s. Different types of opioid receptors were postulated in the 1960s by Martin, who by the mid-1970s had painstakingly catalogued heterogeneous profiles of physiological effects in dogs exposed to or withdrawn from a variety of opioids.[82] Martin discerned three major patterns of in vivo response to all opioids he evaluated, and attributed these three profiles to selective activation of three distinct opioid receptor types. The first he termed "mu," for morphine; the second, "kappa," for ketocyclazocine; and the third, "sigma," for the proprietary drug SKF-10,047. The sigma receptor is no longer considered as an opioid receptor; it is activated by phencyclidine. Soon after Martin published his results, Lord[297] and colleagues from the Kosterlitz group in Aberdeen postulated the existence of another opioid receptor type that they termed "delta," because of its identification in mouse vas deferens. An unusually long interval elapsed between pharmacological identification of opioid receptor types in vivo and their cloning, reflecting technical obstacles such as the lack of a specific gene product to serve as a marker of opioid receptor activation, and the typically inhibitory effect of such activation. Finally, all three types of opioid receptors—mu, kappa and delta—were cloned within a relatively short interval in the early 1990s.[334] Table 29-3 summarizes the properties of the three cloned opioid receptors; sequence differences have not yet been established between subtypes of the same opioid receptor.

Cloning of the opioid receptors has confirmed and extended much information previously gleaned indirectly from pharmacological studies.[161] All three opioid receptor types are "metabotropic," i.e., coupled to guanyl nucleotide-bind-

TABLE 29-3. *Characteristics of the cloned opioid receptors*

	Mu	Delta	$Kappa_1$
Gene family	7 TM G-protein coupled	7 TM G-protein coupled	7 TM G-protein coupled
Gene organization	Intronic	Intronic	Intronic
mRNA Size	10–16 kb	4.5 kb 11.0 kg	5.2 kb
Amino acid length	398	372	380
Binding characteristics[a]	DAMGO Morphine CTOP	DPDPE DSLET Naltrindole	US0488 DYNA(1-17) nBNI
Signal transduction	Coupled to inhibitory G protein: ↓cAMP	Coupled to inhibitory G protein: ↓cAMP	Coupled to inhibitory G protein: ↓cAMP
Number of glycosylation sites	5	2	2
mRNA distribution	Thalamus Striatum Locus coeruleus Nucleus of the solitary tract	Cortex Striatum Lateral reticular	Hypothalamus Nucleus accumbens Substantia nigra Ventral tegmental area Nucleus of the solitary tract

TM, transmembrane.

[a] See references 267 and 291 for discussion of these selective opioid receptor ligands.

From Mansour, A., Fox, C.A., Akil, H., and Watson, S.J.: Opioid receptor mRNA expression in the rat CNS: Anatomical and functional implications. T.I.N.S., *18*:22, 1995.

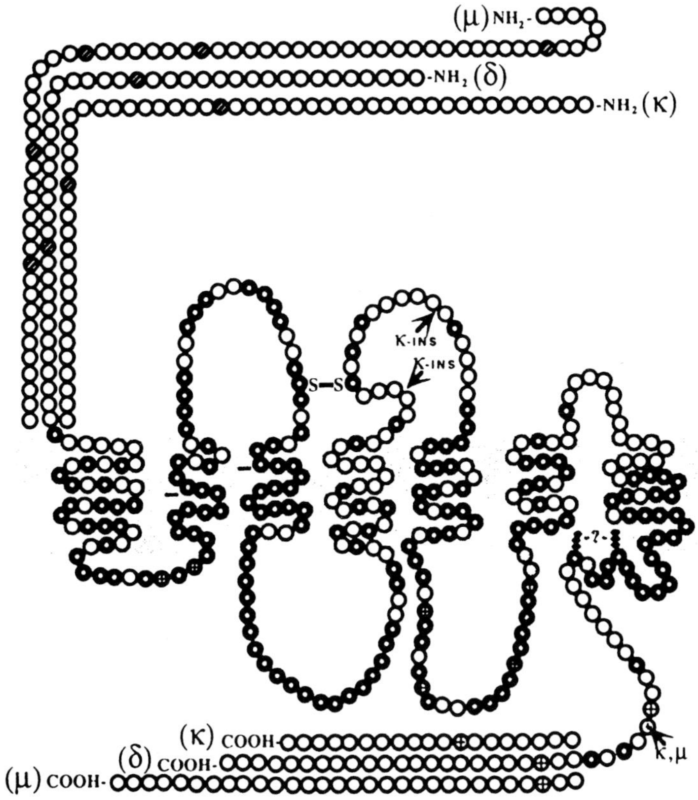

FIG. 29-2. Structural homology among the cloned delta, mu, and kappa opioid receptors (from Reference 334). Each circle indicates one amino acid residue. Black circles with white central dot are identical for mouse delta, rat mu, and mouse kappa opioid receptors. Other shadings within circles indicate sites of possible glycosylation, phosphorylation, or (next to "?") palmitylation. Arrows indicate sites of additional amino acid insertion in kappa or mu receptors. Note sulfhydryl bridge linking amino acid residues adjoining two of the seven membrane-spanning regions. [From Miotto, K., Nagendzo, K., and Evans, C. J.: Molecular characterization of opioid peptides. *In* Tseng, L. F. (ed.): The Pharmacology of Opioid Peptides. pp. 57–71. Langhorn, PA., Harwood Academic Publishers, 1995.]

ing regulatory proteins (G-proteins).[198] They share structural features with other G-protein coupled receptors, including seven conserved hydrophobic domains that span the cell membrane, disulfide bonds between cysteine residues, glycosylation near the amino terminus, and phosphorylation by protein kinase A (PKA) in the first and third cytoplasmic loops as well as near the carboxy (C) terminus.[376] Sequencing of deoxyribonucleic acid (DNA) encoding these three receptors in rat and mouse reveals that each contains nearly 400 amino acids, and that all three types share substantial sequence homology, not only with each other (Fig. 29-2) but also with receptors for somatostatin, angiotensin and certain chemotactic factors.

Messenger RNA for all three types of opioid receptors is present in dorsal root ganglia and superficial layers of the dorsal horn.[305] Opioid binding to the mu receptor activates

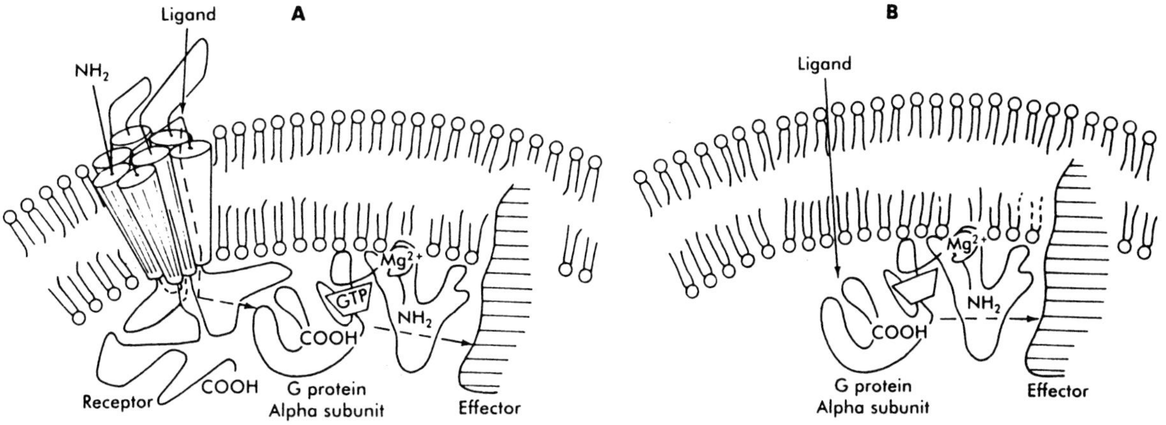

FIG. 29-3. A: Opioid ligand binds to the opioid receptor, changing the conformation of its membrane spanning domain, and thereby activating an intracellular G-protein. **B:** A ligand that can enter the membrane by means of an amphiphilic interaction can activate an intracellular G protein without binding to cell membrane receptor. [From Carr, D. B., and Lipkowski, A. W.: Mechanisms of opioid analgetic actions. *In* Rogers, M., Tinker, J. H., Covino, B. G., and Longnecker, D. E. (eds.): Principles and Practice of Anesthesiology. Vol. 1. pp. 1105–1130. St. Louis, Mosby–Year Book, 1993.]

an intracellular G-protein, G_i, that inhibits guanyl triphosphate formation.[281] Pertussis toxin prevents G_i activation and is useful as a probe of G_i mediation of opioid effects in vivo and in vitro.[121] The common mechanism of ligand, i.e., opioid binding to the receptor and linkage through a G-protein to an effector mechanism, is schematized in Figure 29-3.

The schematic figure of opioid receptor linkage to a G-protein, and thence to intracellular effector mechanisms such as ion channels, does not do justice to the complexity and ongoing controversy as to precise mechanisms by which opioids or other ligands interact with receptors in the cell membrane.[162] For example, opioids and other peptides that bind to cell membranes contain helical regions that are "amphipathic," that is, in which hydrophobic and hydrophilic amino acids are grouped on opposite faces of the helix. This structure positions the ligand, detergent-like, at the surface of the cell membrane.[185] Partial immersion of the ligand's amphipathic helical regions within the cell membrane can stabilize or destabilize the membrane, independent of any specific ligand-receptor interaction.[150] Of relevance to opioid pharmacology also is the recent recognition that activation of G-protein-coupled receptors results from a change in conformation from resting to active states, a two-state model first developed to describe the opening of transmitter-gated membrane ion channels.[284] If a compound has a higher affinity for the conformation of the receptor in its active state, it is an agonist; if its affinity is equal for resting and active states, then it is an antagonist devoid of intrinsic activity; if its affinity is higher for the resting state, then it is an inverse agonist capable of producing effects opposite from those of agonists. The relative affinity of a drug for active and resting states of the receptor also determines whether it will behave as a full or partial agonist. The two-state model not only has advanced understanding of drug-receptor binding but currently influences the design of new compounds and the study of opioid tolerance—two important topics surveyed below.

OPIOID RECEPTOR ACTIVATION: ANALGESIC EFFECTS IN VIVO

Martin's definition of opioid receptor types, that employed *in vivo* animal studies to extend and refine clinical observations, has remained the foundation for all subsequent preclinical and clinical studies in this area.[91] During this time, efforts to characterize receptor-type selectivity of new opioids have shifted from whole-body pharmacological studies towards *in vitro* methods that rely on mathematical analysis of drug-receptor affinity and drug displacement from receptor by highly selective reference opioids. At present, molecular methods to determine the primary sequence of opioid and other receptors, their chemical modification (e.g., glycosylation, phosphorylation, disulfide bridging) at specific sites, and the functions of particular subunits are well established. It is likely that the future literature on opioid receptors will continue this progressive shift in focus from bedside, to animal laboratory, to ligand-receptor binding, to molecular analysis of receptors and genes.

Unfortunately for clinicians practicing opioid analgesia, this paradigm shift has taken place unannounced,[85] making the research literature often confusing because different reports use distinct criteria to determine receptor selectivity of opioids.[356,384] These diverse criteria include behavioral observation (e.g., animal performance in a Y-maze or lever-pressing as an index of subjective similarity between a test drug and a reference opioid); relative efficacy against experimental pain of different origins (e.g., heat versus pressure); potency compared with reference drugs in standardized *in vitro* bioassays (e.g., inhibition of electrical contraction of guinea pig ileum); comparison of dosage of nonselective (pA_2) or selective antagonists to reverse a drug's effects *in vivo* compared to effects of reference drugs; or quantitation of in vitro displacement of radiolabelled tracer amounts of test drug from receptor preparations, or from thin slices of tissue by increasing concentrations of unlabelled drug (Scatchard plot) or selective antagonists.

The above methods have now made it clear that all 3 major types of opioid receptor—mu, kappa and delta—have subtypes, although information about subtype diversity has not yet had clinical application and so will not be covered further in this chapter. Currently, preclinical determinations of novel opioids' receptor selectivity rely upon *in vitro* measurements of their binding affinities for purified opioid receptors, concentrations of selective reference opioids necessary to displace them from defined receptors, and the effect of selective receptor alkylating agents in blocking their binding to receptors. On the other hand, the two-state (see earlier) and earlier models of ligand-receptor interaction dictate caution in extrapolating from binding data to inferences about receptor activation. For example, bremazocine binds equally to mu and kappa receptors, but is selective in activating kappa receptors. Therefore, at present, initial pharmacological screening and characterization *in vitro* must be confirmed by testing in vivo of potency (e.g., ED_{50} for analgesia) and reversal of effect by selective opioid antagonists.[267] This complementary approach preserves the authenticity of *in vivo* observation yet spares much of its associated imprecision, and minimizes animal use. Through this approach, considerable information has emerged on the opioid receptor modulation of analgesia, and of other clinically important processes, such as cardiorespiratory, gastrointestinal, endocrine, and immune function.

Analgesia follows systemic or spinal administration of opioids that act upon mu, delta, or kappa receptors.[162,166] The rare exceptions to this general rule are scattered reports of opioid-induced hyperalgesia[151] or allodynia in animal models or case reports, attributed to algesic metabolites such as morphine-3-glucuronide, inhibition of spinal interneurons that are themselves inhibitory, or stimulation of the excitatory G-protein G_s, in preference to G_i, by low concentrations of an opioid.[232] The recent observation in "knockout" mice who lack the mu receptor, that high doses of morphine sufficient to activate delta receptors do not produce analgesia on tail-flick testing, suggests a unique role for the mu receptor in analgesia.[314] Enhancement of analgesia ("cooperativity"), and, in some reports, synergy, occur when more than one type of opioid receptor is activated simultaneously, such as mu plus delta. Analgesic enhancement may also be achieved by coadministration of an opioid with other analgesics that act on nonopioid receptors as agonists (adrenergic, cholinergic, etc.) or antagonists (to substance P, cholecystokinin, N-methyl-D-aspartate [NMDA], cytokines, etc.)[258–260,382,511,512] that block ion channels (calcium, sodium, etc.) or that inhibit algesic enzyme systems (cyclo-oxygenase, nitric oxide synthase)[424] (see Chapter 24). Cooperativity between opioids active upon distinct receptors, or opioids together with nonopioid analgesic molecules, is evident in natural processes of endogenous analgesia. For example, there is a well-described mismatch between receptor selectivity of the opioid molecules released within the spinal cord or into the peripheral circulation, and the opioid receptors that are occupied by these endorphins both adjacent (paracrine effect) and distal (endocrine effect) to their sites of release. Anatomic sites of opioid analgesic actions are likewise multiple, and include

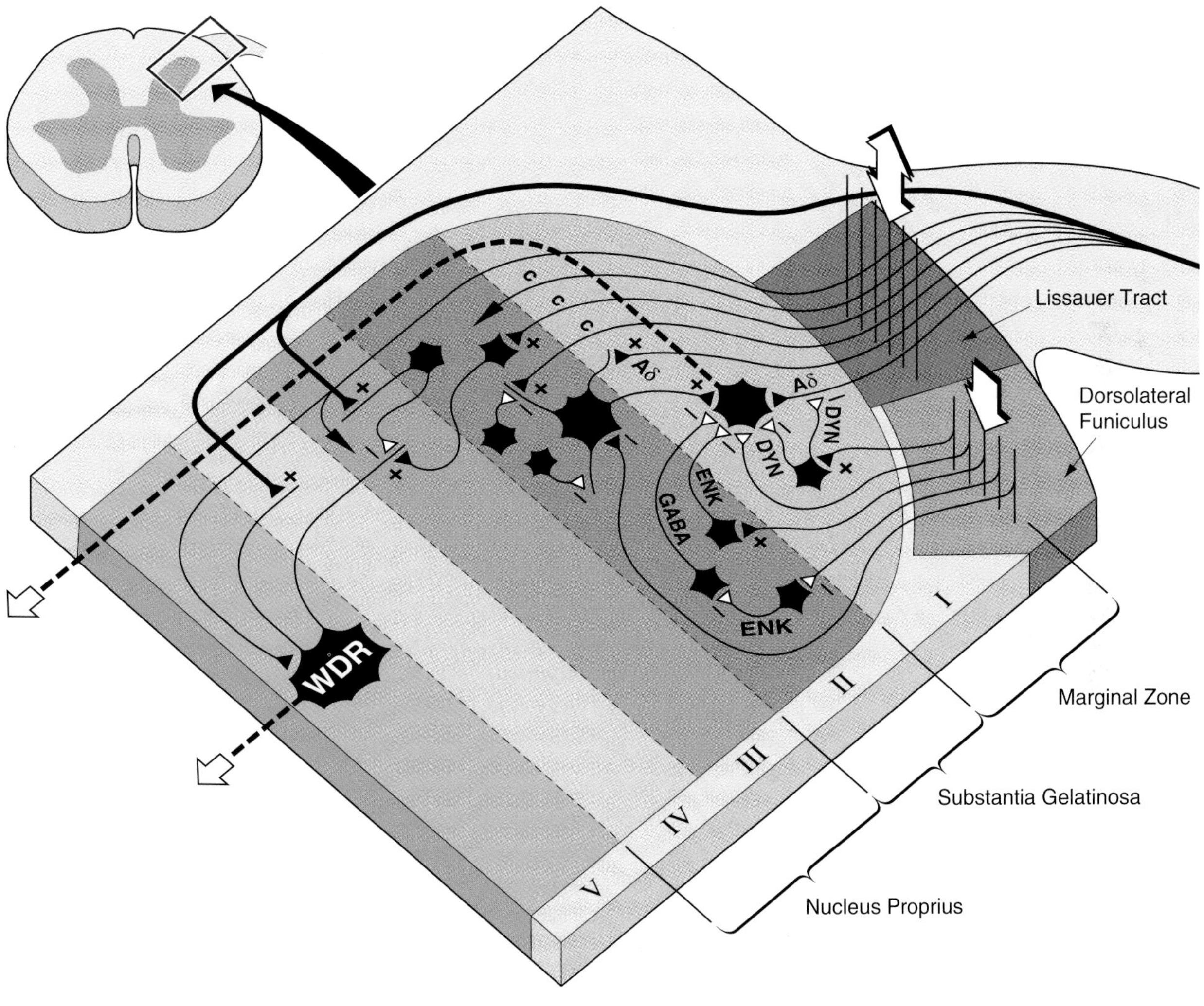

FIG. 29-4. Oblique view of synapses in layers I–V of dorsal horn. Diagrammatic representation of primary afferent nociceptor inputs and connections within the dorsal horn of the spinal cord. Large and small diameter primary afferent neurons have their cell bodies in the dorsal root ganglia. On entry to the dorsal horn, large diameter afferent fibers (shown as a *thickened solid line*) travel medially and small diameter afferent fibers (*thin solid lines* marked Aδ and C) travel in the lateral portion of the entry zone. The spinal terminals of the small fibers enter the cord and have collateral branches which may ascend and descend the spinal cord for several segments in Lissauer's tract before synapsing in the dorsal horn. Aδ fiber afferents terminate in lamina I (marginal zone) and C fiber afferents terminate in lamina II (substantia gelatinosa). Local interneurons may produce synaptic inhibition of small diameter afferents and post synaptic inhibition of projection neurons. Interneurons may have an excitatory action. Modulation also occurs as a result of descending influences arising from fibers in the dorsolateral funiculus. These descending fibers make contact with either projection neurons or interneurons. Neurotransmitters released from interneurons include gamma aminobutyric acid *(GABA)*, leu- or met-enkephalins *(ENK)* and dynorphin *(DYN)*. (see also Chapter 23.1, Figs. 23.1-10 to 23.1-13 and Fig. 23.1-18.)

supraspinal areas, the spinal cord, and injured tissue in the periphery (Table 29-2). Therapeutic benefits therefore follow coadministration not only of different classes of analgesic to the same site (e.g., spinal cord) but also of analgesics to multiple sites at once.

We are not accustomed to viewing our daily clinical practice of spinal opioid analgesia as involving coadministration of opioids to several sites simultaneously, but this undoubtedly occurs within hours of beginning such therapy. Clearly, systemically administered opioids rapidly reach spinal cord, brainstem, and brain. Epidural opioids are distributed into the bloodstream and reach periphery, brainstem, and brain in addition to their spinal target; intrathecal opioids also are carried rostrally in cerebrospinal fluid and, to a lesser degree, the peripheral circulation. Brief courses of clinical opioid therapy for routine postoperative pain control by any route last at least a few days, allowing ample time for equilibration and access to multiple anatomic sites rich in opioid receptors. Yet in contrast to many preclinical reports describing *in vivo* responses to single doses of spinal or systemic opioids or nonopioid analgesics, relatively few studies detail the analgesic effects of repeated, yet short-term, opioid administration.

The physiology of nociception and analgesia resulting from actions of spinally (or systemically) administered opioids upon the dorsal horn has been presented in overview in the introductory section and in greater detail in Chapters 24 and 26. Of special relevance to current and future options for spinal opioid and nonopioid analgesia, Figure 29-4 illustrates targets for opioid actions in the dorsal horn. C fibers, small unmyelinated nociceptive afferents from neurons whose cell bodies are in the dorsal root ganglia, project directly or via interneurons originating in substantia gelatinosa to second-order, wide dynamic range WDR neurons. Classic work by LeBars, Jurna, Yaksh, and others in the 1970s established that systemic or spinal opioid administration greatly inhibits postsynaptic summation in WDR neurons of afferent input from C fibers, while affecting postsynaptic summation of A fiber afferent input to a much lesser degree (Fig. 29-5). Opioid suppression of excitatory neurotransmitter release (substance P, calcitonin gene-related peptide, neurokinin A, etc.) from C but not A fibers reflects mu, delta, or kappa opioid inhibition of calcium channels on the former but not the latter neurons. In particular, opioids act selectively upon small C fibers.[471] By contrast, analgesic concentrations of the analgesic peptide somatostatin inhibit calcium channels on large, but not on small, nociceptive afferents. Postsynaptic effects of mu and delta opioids upon WDR neurons are both direct (those that result from occupancy of postsynaptic opioid receptors coupled through G_i to potassium channels), and indirect, (those that are due to activation of inhibitory pathways that descend from the brainstem to the spinal level). Dual pre- and postsynaptic effects also result from activation of alpha-2 and GABA receptors, respectively, by selective agonists such as clonidine or baclofen. Additional opioid analgesic effects at the spinal level include stimulation of adenosine release and activation (i.e., disinhibition) of spinal interneurons, the latter contributing to opioid-induced pruritus. Despite similarities of receptor pharmacology in synapses within distinct nociceptive pathways of the dorsal horn, (shown in Fig. 29-6) important preclinical and clinical differences exist between analgesic efficacy of

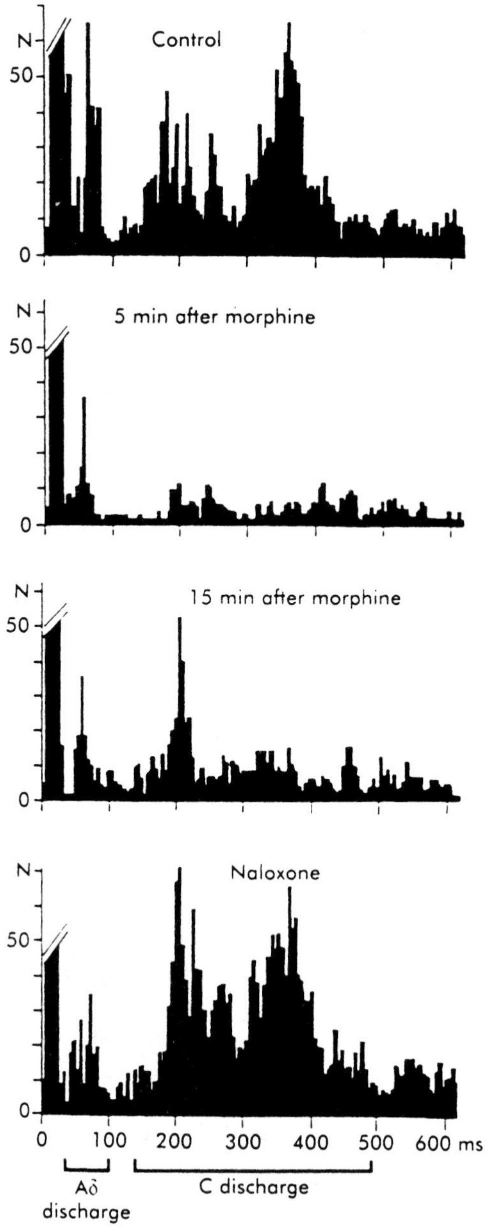

FIG. 29-5. Effect of morphine given systemically or spinally upon dorsal horn summation of excitatory postsynaptic potentials after brief electrical stimulation of peripheral afferent. Morphine inhibits summation more effectively for late (C-fiber dependent) than early (A-delta fiber dependent) responses. Note millisecond scale. The inhibitory effect starts to subside by 15 minutes after morphine administration, or can be quickly reversed by systemic naloxone. (From LeBars, D., Guilbaud, G., Jurna, I., *et al.*: Differential effects of morphine on responses of dorsal horn lamina V type cells elicited by A and C fibre stimulation in the spinal cat. Brain Res., *115*:518, 1976.)

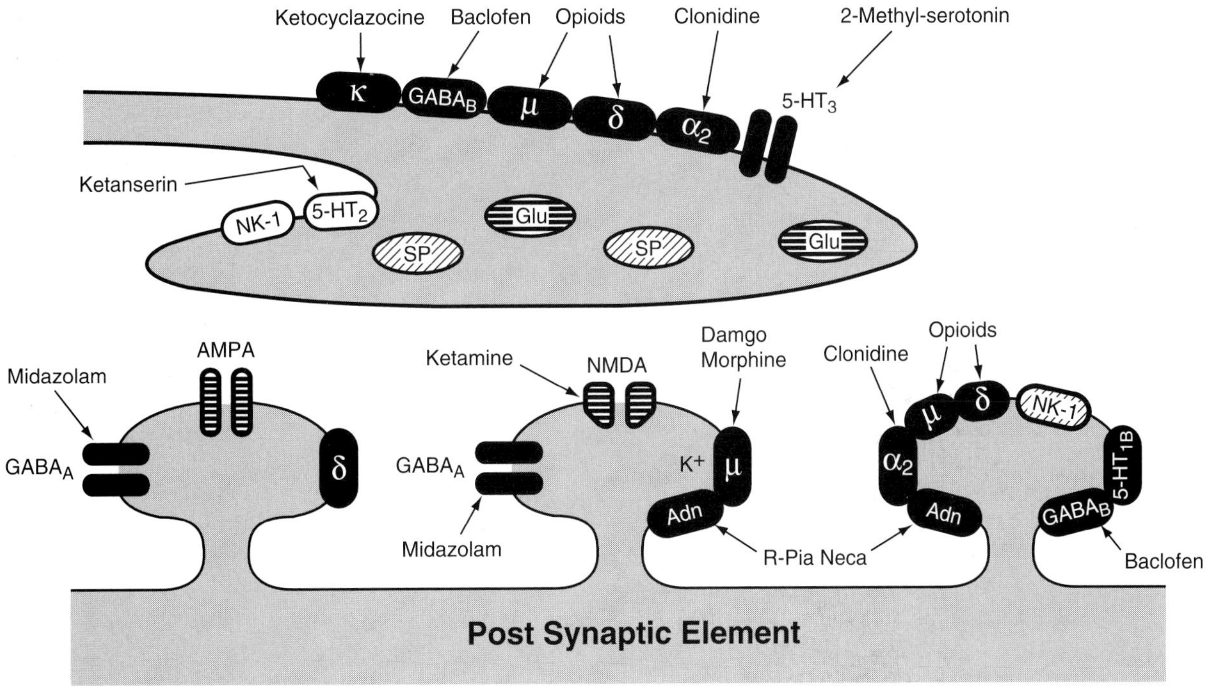

FIG. 29-6. Schematic of pre- and post-synaptic dorsal horn receptors and transmitters. (See Chapter 23.1, Fig. 23.1-11 for details.)

specific drugs applied to treat pain of different origins. By the early 1980s, it was clear that mu opioids are more potent than kappa opioids against thermal pain, and that the reverse is true for pain of mechanical origin, e.g., pressure.[386] (Fig. 29-7) Since then, considerable evidence has accumulated that thermal hyperalgesia at the spinal level is mediated principally by activation of NMDA receptors, activation of protein kinase C (PKC), and generation of nitric oxide and cyclic GMP.[224] Mechanical hyperalgesia relies principally on coactivation of spinal AMPA and metabotropic glutamate

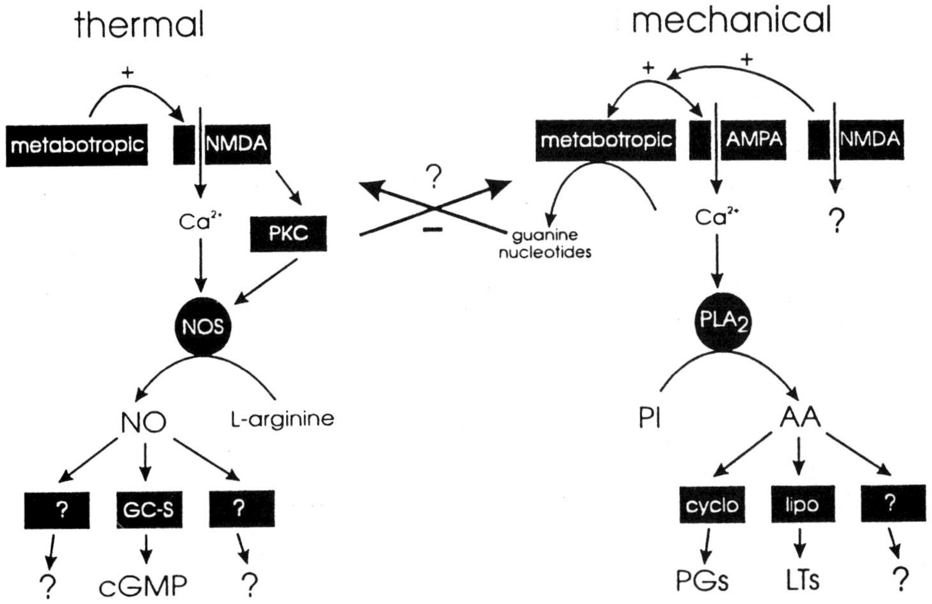

FIG. 29-7. Thermal versus mechanical hyperalgesia may be mediated by distinct receptor-mediated and intracellular events. One or both cascades may occur within the same neuron. *PKC,* protein kinase C; *NOS,* nitric oxide synthase; *PLA$_2$*, phospholipase A$_2$, *GC-S,* soluble guanylate cyclase; *cGMP,* cyclic guanyl monophosphate; *PI,* phosphoinositol; *AA,* arachidonic acid; *cyclo,* cyclo-oxygenase; *lipo,* lipo-oxygenase; *PGs,* prostaglandins; *LTs,* leukotrienes. (From Meller, S. T.: Thermal and mechanical hyperalgesia: A distinct role for different excitatory amino acid receptors and signal transduction pathways. A.P.S. Journal, *3*: 215, 1994.) (see also Chapter 23.1, Figs. 23.1-12, 23.1-13, 23.1-16.)

receptors, activation of phospholipase A2, and the cyclooxygenase cascade.[328]

Other models of nociception, such as peripheral nerve injury, inflammation from infectious or chemical agents, electrical shock, or application of toxins or irritants to the central nervous system, each produce distinct pathophysiologies and display distinct dose-response profiles in potency testing of various opioid and nonopioid compounds. None of these models exactly duplicates common clinical pain problems—such as acute postoperative pain, postcesarean pain, headache, low back pain or cancer pain—syndromes that each involve multiple known and unknown pain mechanisms acting in concert.[4]

Tolerance to opioid analgesic effects refers to a decline in analgesic effect and/or the need to escalate opioid dosage during ongoing therapy.[28] Opioid tolerance occurs in many preclinical pain models, most reliably in normal animals without pain that begin opioid treatment well before challenge with a nociceptive stimulus. This simple yet important phenomenon is complemented by an equally commonplace occurrence that animals or patients predictably experience when they have chronically received an opioid to control pain: "rebound" hyperalgesia when challenged with an opioid antagonist. Both observations imply that opioid tolerance is not—as believed for years and described in the prior edition of this volume—simply a passive consequence of loss of opioid receptors and/or decoupling of opioid-receptor binding from G_i activation.[138] If these were all that happened, then challenge with an opioid antagonist might have little effect. Instead, the occurrence of these phenomena implies that opioid tolerance involves mobilization of active processes, whose potential to produce latent hyperalgesia is masked so long as opioid dosing is maintained. The presence of these active processes does not mean that downregulation (decreased receptor number) and desensitization (decreased receptor-effector coupling) do not take place: they do.[193] However, they cannot by themselves explain the everyday occurrences just mentioned. Thus, our view of opioid tolerance has changed during the past 5 years from an analogy with passive muffling of an ongoing signal, to one of active cancellation of the signal, followed by rebound of the now-unopposed countersignal when the original signal ceases.[307]

Mechanisms of active cancellation of the ongoing opioid signal involve processes ranging from intracellular and organ-level metabolic adaptations such as enhanced glucuronidation of morphine, to activation of anti-opioid, hyperalgesic, peptide systems. Within the neuron, activation of the mu opioid receptor results in translocation of intracellular PKC and phosphorylation of the calcium channel within the NMDA receptor complex.[307] Phosphorylation of this channel removes its magnesium block and allows calcium entry just as after a nociceptive stimulus, even though nociception per se need not have occurred.[319] Activation of nitric oxide synthase (NOS) also mediates NMDA receptor effects, and coadministration of either a NOS inhibitor or an NMDA antagonist, along with a mu opioid, retards development of tolerance.[173] Interestingly, tachyphylaxis to local anesthetic effects is also inhibited in a dose-dependent fashion by a NOS inhibitor or an NMDA antagonist.[513] Animal studies have demonstrated further that tolerance develops more slowly when opioids with high intrinsic activity are administered, compared with equianalgesic doses of opioids with low intrinsic activity. Opioids of higher intrinsic activity require fewer receptors to be occupied to produce a response such as analgesia, thereby leaving their target cells with relatively more unoccupied reserve or spare receptors. Previously, the slower rate of tolerance developed during exposure to opioids of high intrinsic activity was identified with a higher number of remaining spare receptors. However, in light of the recently recognized connection[28,307] between mu receptor activation and intracellular NO and NMDA effects, a more plausible explanation of the slower development of tolerance during treatment with opioids of high intrinsic activity is that binding and activation of fewer mu receptors yields relatively less stimulation of intracellular NOS and PKC. Phosphorylation of the mu opioid receptor itself during prolonged activation has been proposed as an additional mechanism of opioid tolerance.[198,416] In addition to intracellular mechanisms, anti-opioid peptides participate in opioid tolerance. In particular, activation of cholecystokinin and substance P synthesis and release oppose the effect of opioid analgesics, as inferred from augmentation of opioid analgesia after administration of antagonists to either hyperalgesic peptide[201,209] (see Chapter 23.1, Fig. 23.1-16).

The contrast between the ease with which profound opioid tolerance can be induced during spinal or systemic infusions in many species of intact animals, and the sustained therapeutic value during chronic use of opioids in most clinical settings,[385] is still not well understood. In the cat, tolerance to systemic administration of morphine can be demonstrated in dorsal horn neurons after three days.[243] In the primate, daily intrathecal administration of morphine, beta-endorphin, or metkephamid, at doses producing a "just maximum effect" causes a daily reduction in analgesic efficacy. Responsiveness in the primate declines most rapidly for agents having the longest duration of action after each fixed dose. In mice, once-daily doses of opioids of differing intrinsic activity produce tolerance at the same rate although continuous infusions elicit tolerance more quickly with opioids of low intrinsic activity.[178] The latter result is also found during long-term spinal delivery of morphine, sufentanil and alfentanil in dogs.[415] Results from several species indicate that tolerance develops more quickly when a greater proportion of mu receptors is activated by ligand during a greater proportion of each day. Primates made tolerant to intrathecal opioids began to recover opioid responsivity seven days after the last intrathecal administration, and had near-complete recovery by two weeks, indicating that tolerance is reversible.[537] This supports clinicians' common practice of managing tolerance to spinal opioid administration by switching temporarily to an alternative agent such as spinal local anesthetic. It should be emphasized that tolerance is a greater issue in intact animals, or normal volunteers, than during opioid therapy of chronic experimental or clinical pain. Colpaert found that animals exposed to acute pain (mechanical pinch) or chronic pain (intra-articular *Mycobacterium butyricum*) failed to show tolerance to systemically administered opioids when compared with normal controls.[123] Similarly, Glynn and Mather[204] reported that tolerance was not an inevitable consequence of prolonged (one year) treatment of chronic pain in patients receiving systemically administered meperidine. Many observations by practitioners caring for patients with chronic pain from cancer or nonmalignant conditions confirm that systemic or spinal opioid dosage escalation is generally modest and therapeutic effectiveness is sustained, unless the underlying medical condition progresses.[363,380]

In the authors' view, rapid dosage escalation early during opioid therapy of a chronic pain condition is evidence less of tolerance than of either a behavioral/psychological issue, or of pain mechanism(s) that are intrinsically insensitive to opioid analgesia. In such cases, switching to a different opioid or nonopioid, or coadministering opioid plus nonopioid, are supported both by preclinical and clinical observations. Animals rendered tolerant to morphine by daily intrathecal injections showed no loss of sensitivity to the delta opioid DADLE, and only partial loss of effect of the kappa opioid ethylketocyclazocine (EKC).[485] Other studies have reported spinal analgesic effects with the kappa agonist U 50 488H[74] and a loss of effect of the endogenous kappa opioid dynorphin (a kappa opioid) in animals made tolerant to EKC. The prospect of maintaining spinal opioid analgesia for prolonged periods, by rotating opioid agonists of different receptor selectivity as tolerance develops, has clinical potential and is supported by preclinical and limited clinical studies. Some agents that act both at mu and delta receptors, such as metkephamid[534] or biphalin, are effective as analgesics in morphine-tolerant animals.

Nonopiate spinal analgesia has been investigated extensively in both animal and human studies. In particular, the α-agonists (e.g., clonidine) have been shown to have powerful antinociceptive effects, which show no cross tolerance with opioid agonists.[536,537,543] Intrathecal and epidural clonidine have been used successfully in humans tolerant to spinal morphine.[129] and the combination of clonidine and morphine is associated with sustained analgesic efficacy. In patients with "below level" neuropathic pain after spinal injury, spinal morphine is ineffective.[445] However, in a rat model of spinal injury pain, coadministration of intrathecal morphine and clonidine does provide analgesia,[446] and an initial report supports the clinical value of this drug combination for this purpose.[447] Co-administration of catecholamines and enkephalin pentapeptides, secreted together from adrenal, chromaffin cells implanted intraspinally, also appears promising for prolonged analgesia, i.e., to avert tolerance. Similarly, concurrent infusion of spinal local anesthetic plus opioid retains analgesic effectiveness for prolonged periods of time. Although the precise explanations for retarding tolerance by pairing opioid and nonopioid analgesic agents may vary, two common factors probably underlie this therapeutic advantage. First, addition of a second class of analgesic to an opioid reduces dorsal horn neuronal responsivity to afferent nociceptive input; this lessens calcium influx, NOS activation, and PKC translocation. Second, insofar as coadministration of a second agent reduces the fraction of opioid receptors necessary to be activated to achieve analgesia, one would likewise expect tolerance to be retarded for reasons outlined above. Thus, coadministration of opioids with other drugs, or administration of single molecules engineered to act upon opioid plus other pathways (e.g., antagonists to cyclo-oxygenase, substance P, NMDA or NOS, or local anesthetics) is a powerful therapeutic strategy for achieving prolonged analgesia. Spinal antinociceptive systems that are potential targets for nonopioid analgesic molecules are summarized in Chapters 23.1 and 24. Their clinical relevance is discussed below.

NON-ANALGESIC EFFECTS OF SPINAL OPIOID ADMINISTRATION

The following summary describes physiological effects other than analgesia that are the direct result of spinal application of opioids. Accordingly, relationships between spinal opioid administration and alterations of respiratory, gastrointestinal, cardiac, bladder, and sensorimotor function (the latter including neurotoxic potential and pruritus) are surveyed here. Potential side effects of intrathecal and epidural opioid treatment are summarized in Table 29-4 and contrasted with those of local anesthetics.

The present section is intended to complement the above discussion of the pharmacology of spinally administered opioid analgesics in preclinical and clinical settings, rather than to provide a comprehensive review of clinical effects, side effects, and outcomes other than analgesia, during spinal opioid use. Such outcomes, that involve pulmonary or immune status,[428] morbidity, or length of hospital stay, depend upon multiple processes, including many not directly related to spinal opioid actions *per se,* and are covered in Chapters 5 and 26.

Respiratory Depression

Respiratory depression although infrequent is always a concern after spinal opioid administration, particularly in opioid-naive subjects treated for acute pain. Prompt (less than two hours) versus delayed onsets of this side effect have been attributed, respectively, to blood-borne drug reaching the brain quickly, such as after rapid absorption into the circulation of lipophilic opioid given epidurally, versus slow rostral migration of hydrophilic drug, such as morphine deposited within the CSF (see Fig. 29-8). These two mechanisms are not mutually exclusive, however. Sufentanil and meperidine have been detected in cisternal CSF within minutes after epidural or intrathecal administration, respectively.

TABLE 29-4. *Effects and side effects*

Effects and side effects	Spinal opioids	Spinal local anesthetics
Respiratory	Early depression[a,b] (0.1–1 h); systemically absorbed drug and ? CSF-borne drug Late depression[a,b] (6–24 h); opioid in CSF migrating to brain (see Figs. 29-8, 29-13)	Usually unimpaired unless cardiovascular collapse
Gastrointestinal	Prolongs intestinal transit time Nausea common postoperatively	Transit time unchanged Nausea less common
Cardiovascular	Minor heart rate changes	Low-block (below T10) sympathetic blockade: postural hypotension
	Usually no postural hypotension	High-block (above T4) sympathetic blockade: postural hypotension
	Vasoconstrictor response intact	Cardio-accelerator block: ↓ HR, ↓ inotropic drive (see Chapter 8)
Urinary retention	Yes[a,b]	Yes
CNS		
Sedation	May be marked[a]	Mild or absent, depending on agent
Convulsions	Usually not seen with clinical doses; theoretical possibility at high doses	Expected toxicity from two times overdose or with rapid vascular absorption
Other neurologic abnormalities	Confusion, amnesia, catalepsy, hallucinations (reported with high doses intrathecally)	Not usually seen
Opioid withdrawal	If rapid discontinuation of systemic opioids	
Nausea	Yes[a]	Yes—low incidence
Vomiting	Yes[a]	Yes—low incidence
Pruritis	Yes[a]	No
Miosis	Yes[a,b]	No (unless Horner's syndrome)

[a] Antagonized by naloxone, but repeated doses may be required.
[b] Prevented by naloxone infusion 5–10 μg/kg/h without reversal of analgesic effects.[304,307]

Respiratory depression was not a strong focus of initial animal experiments on opioid receptors or on their endogenous ligands, following the birth of this field in the early to mid-1970s. The great importance of this and other side effects was soon appreciated once spinal opioid analgesia came into common clinical use in the late 1970s, and stimulated detailed animal studies.

Animal studies provide strong evidence to connect respiratory depression to CSF concentrations of opioids. Data in baboons and in humans after epidural morphine administration indicate peak levels in CSF near the brain at about three hours.[113,213,467] Studies in other species of cephalad migration of morphine after intrathecal administration indicate a more rapid time course, with drug reaching the ventral brain after only 15 to 30 minutes, and the respiratory center regions by 60 minutes.[219] Opioid traveling cephalad in CSF also may stream against the intracranial CSF circulation to gain retrograde access to the fourth ventricle, with subsequent rapid access to respiratory centers. An alternative site of respiratory depression is a group of cells in the ventrolateral medulla, the nucleus ambiguus, and retroambigualis. These loci are involved in control of both inspiratory and expiratory motor output, but are less dense in opioid receptors, than the subependymal nuclei in the floor of the fourth ventricle. In animal studies, direct injection of opioids into the fourth ventricle or into CSF of the ventral brain stem region results in a rapid (3 to 5 minutes) onset of respiratory depression, which is similar for both sites of injection.[195] Thus, diffusion of the drug through the brain tissue to the respiratory centers in the brain stem appears to be rapid, once the drug reaches this area in sufficient concentration. Once in the intracranial CSF, opioid removal may occur with great efficiency at the choroid plexus,[190] which appears to act as a "cerebral kidney" for these substances (Fig. 29-8). On the other hand, evidence in animals and humans indicates that morphine may be biotransformed within the central nervous system (CNS) to active metabolites such as morphine-6-glucuronide, which can have potent and prolonged respiratory-depressant, as well as analgesic, effects. It is evident from animal and human studies that mu receptors have a predominant role in opioid-induced respiratory depression, although in some species such as dog, delta receptors are also prominent in this regard. Central injection of mu-selective opioids in animals reduces ventilation by slowing respiratory rate. Feurstein and colleagues have attributed the paradoxical effects of a variety of mu-selective opioids, some of which stimulate, and others of which depress, ventilation, to opposite effects of activation of mu-1 and mu-2 receptor subtypes. Activation of high-affinity mu-1 receptors, either by low doses of opioids such as morphine, or by selective mu-1 agonists, appears to stimulate ventilation, while activation of low-affinity mu-2 receptors by higher opioid doses depresses ventilation. It is interesting that in animal species such as rat, mu-1 receptors develop later than mu-2 recep-

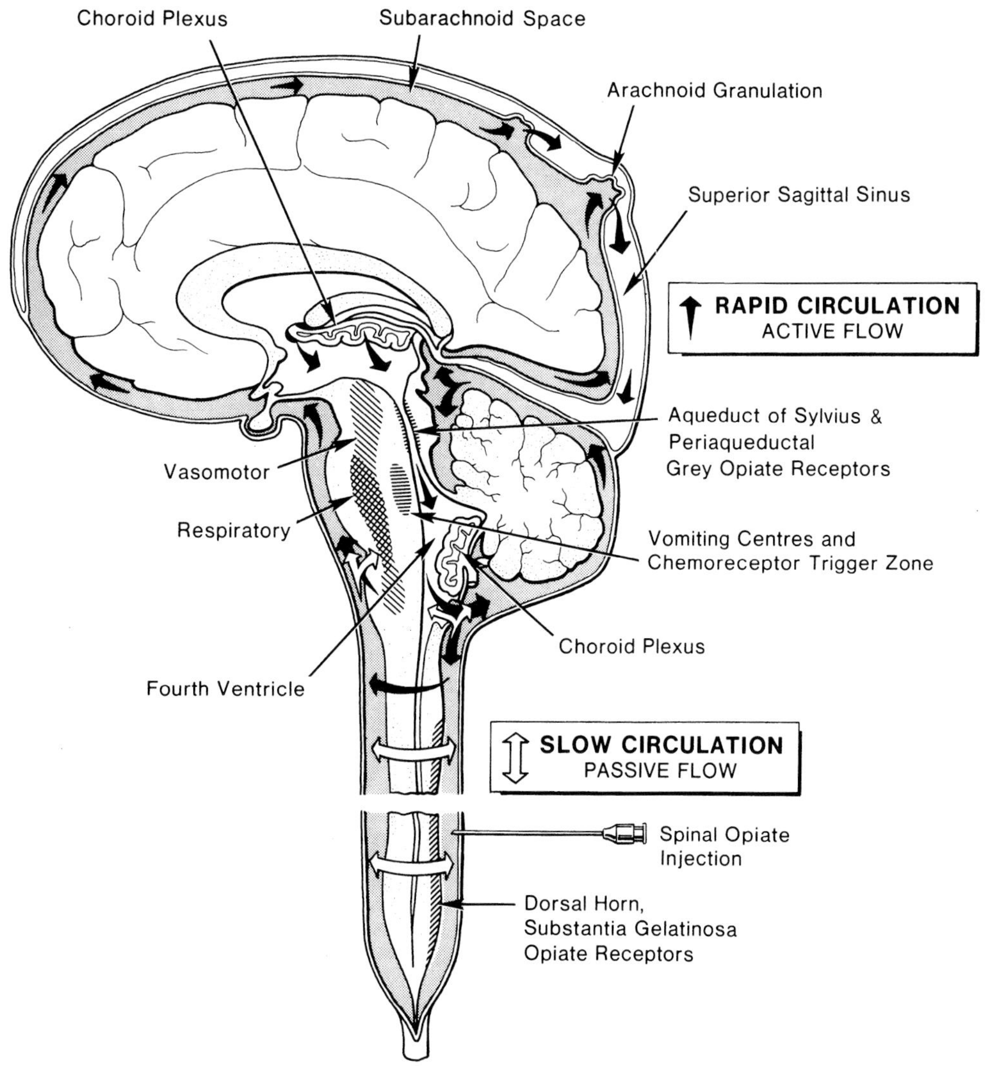

FIG. 29-8. Model of CSF-flow and spread of opioid in CSF. After lumbar intrathecal injection, opioid is carried in the passive flow of CSF to reach peak concentrations in brain after about 3 hours for morphine and 0.5 to 1 hour for meperidine (Demerol). Rapid spread ensues when the opioid mixes with the active flow of the rapid circulation of intracranial CSF. Spinal and brain stem opioid receptors are shown. The latter are seen to be in proximity to cardiorespiratory and vomiting control centers.

tors, raising the possibility that relatively depressed numbers of mu-1 receptors may underlie neonatal sensitivity to opioid-induced respiratory depression (see also Chapter 23.2).

Intrathecal opioid, if given clinically as a single excessive dose or supplemented with intravenous opioid, may result in sudden apnea, necessitating rapid treatment. Onset of respiratory depression after intrathecal morphine administration is variable,[145,146,202,206,219,248,290,359,372] but usually is evident within 6 to 10 hours after the opioid injection. Return of normal respiration has required up to 23 hours afterwards. Therefore, case reports of respiratory depression when opioids were injected in usual doses intramuscularly, within 24 hours of intrathecal opioid,[359] are not unexpected. Usually the progression of respiratory depression and hypercarbia is gradual after intrathecal morphine, allowing time for diagnosis and treatment to avert respiratory arrest. This slow, insidious, depression of ventilatory response to carbon dioxide may be followed by sudden apnea particularly when other risk factors are present, such as concomitant use of CNS depressants. In contrast, local anesthetic-induced convulsions or circulatory depression are usually rapid in onset and mandate urgent treatment.

Delayed respiratory depression after intrathecal morphine for postoperative pain, was first reported toward the end of 1979 independently by Glynn and associates,[206] and by Liolios and Anderson.[290] Glynn and colleagues[206] described two cases of respiratory depression, persisting up to 18 hours after single doses of 3 mg and 5 mg of morphine, respectively. The patients were admitted to an intensive care unit and treated with repeated doses of naloxone. High doses of morphine (20 mg) were injected in a hyperbaric solution of dextrose by Samii and co-workers,[425] with a similar duration of analgesia to that reported by Wang and others.[498] Samii's patients were nursed in semi-sitting positions and side effects were not noted. However, Liolios and Anderson,[290] using a hyperbaric solution of 15 mg of morphine, did observe respiratory depression. Early in 1980, Davies and colleagues reported delayed and prolonged postoperative respiratory depression in three patients who received 1 mg of morphine in an isobaric solution.[145,146] All three patients had been premedicated with a long half-life sedative, diazepam, and remained supine postoperatively. In retrospect, it seems likely that the lack of respiratory depression in initial clinical reports by Cousins and others,[135,206] Wang and others,[498] and Sammi and others,[425] reflected opioid tolerance, since their patients all had had prolonged prior treatment with opioids for cancer pain. In contrast, the cases reported by Glynn and others[206] and Davies and others,[145,146] were postoperative and opioid-naive. Lumbar intrathecal injection of radionuclides,[164,165] or water-soluble contrast media[170] (metrizamide), is followed by a gradual movement of these substances rostrally to reach the fourth and lateral ventricles after 3 to 6 hours. Contrast media can be demonstrated in the fourth and lateral ventricles 6 hours after lumbar injection, indicating major reflux into the ventricles by way of the foramina of Luschka. Gustafsson and associates found that (^{11}C)-morphine appeared at a high cervical level after 60 to 170 minutes.[219] Contrast also appears 6 hours after lumbar injection in the intrathecal space over the entire surface of the brain, and shows significant penetration of brain tissue.[417,418] In summary, small volumes of opioid injected slowly into the intrathecal space are likely to follow the passive circulation of CSF, to reach the cisterns of the brain and then to reach the respiratory center by way of the ventral pons.

Risk factors for respiratory depression after intrathecal opioid administration include advanced age;[202] poor general

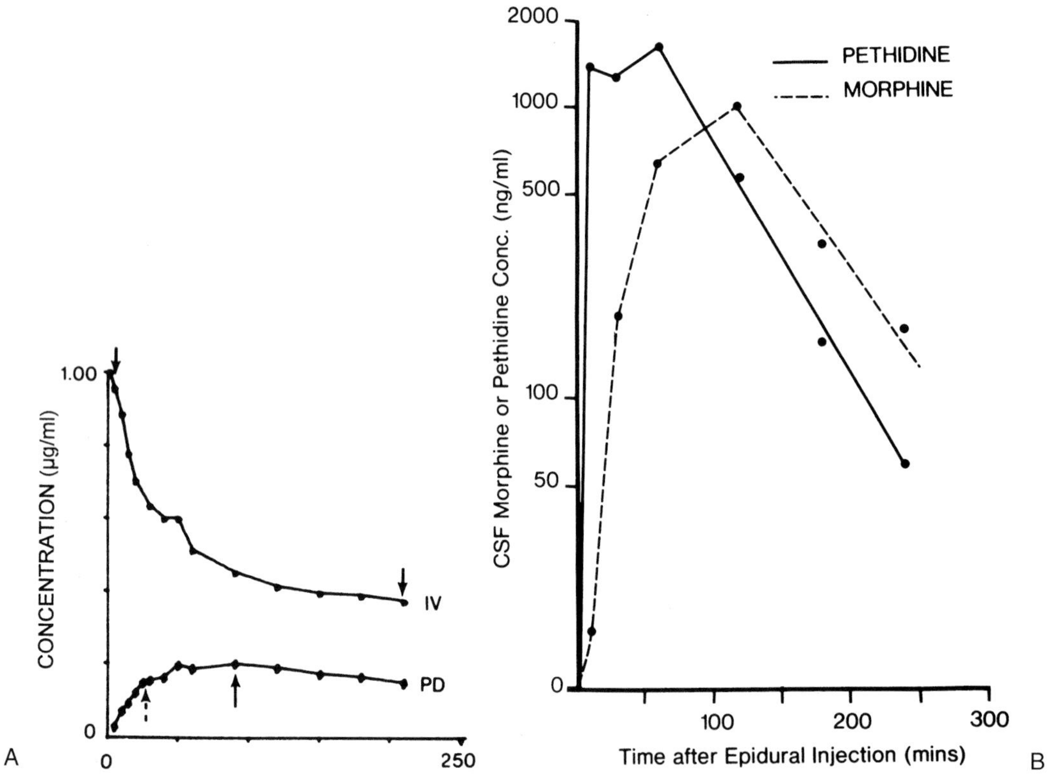

FIG. 29-9. A: Blood concentrations after intravenous *(IV)* and epidural *(PD)* administration of 100 mg and 50 mg meperidine, respectively. *Downward arrows* (↓) indicate onset and regression of analgesia for IV meperidine. *Upward arrows* (↑ ↑) indicate onset of partial and complete analgesia for PD meperidine. (Reprinted from Glynn, C. J., Mather, L. E., Cousins, M. J., *et al.*: Peridural meperidine in humans: Analgetic response, pharmacokinetics, and transmission into CSF. Anesthesiology, *55:*520, 1981, with permission of the publisher.) Pharmacokinetic data after epidural administration of meperidine are also cited in Reference 453. **B: Cervical CSF concentrations** of morphine and pethidine (meperidine) as a function of time following lumbar epidural administration. Morphine (10 mg) and pethidine (50 mg) in 10 ml of normal saline were administered simultaneously by means of a lumbar epidural catheter at L2-L3 interspace, and CSF samples were collected from the C7–T1 interspace at the times shown on the graph. Peak cervical CSF concentrations of pethidine were achieved earlier and declined sooner in comparison to those of morphine. Also, the peak concentrations of pethidine were lower than those of morphine, considering the doses of the two drugs injected. The rapid appearance of pethidine in CSF is in keeping with rapid diffusion through the dura. (Reproduced with permission from Gourlay, G. K., Cherry, D.A., Armstrong, P.A., Plummer, J.L., and Cousins, M.J.: Pain, *31:*297–305, 1987.)

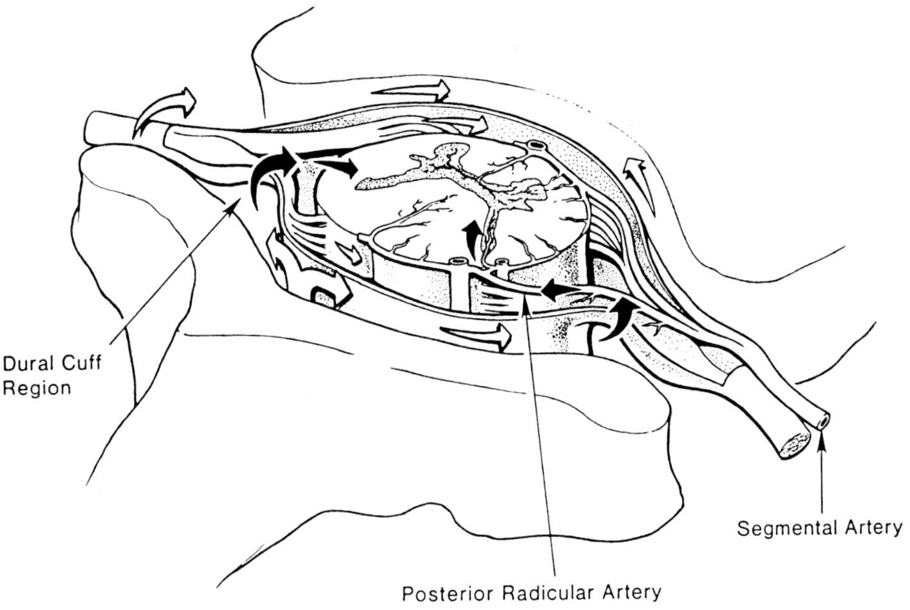

FIG. 29-10. Cross-section of spinal cord and epidural space. Opioid spread in epidural space is depicted by *white arrows,* and spread into CSF, and spinal cord, is depicted by *black arrows.* In dural cuff region, posterior radicular spinal artery is readily accessible to opioid, and this artery directly supplies the dorsal horn region of the spinal cord. Its role is currently speculative (see Chapter 8, pp. 282.)

condition;[399] use of water-soluble opioid, i.e., morphine;[219] high doses;[206] marked changes in thoracoabdominal pressure, including artificial ventilation;[202] lack of tolerance to opioids;[206] and concomitant administration by other routes of opioids or other CNS-depressant drugs.[146,359] Patients with respiratory disease would be expected to be at risk, as they are with the use of opioids by any route. Age may influence spinal fluid volume and pressure, and the brains of elderly patients may be more susceptible to respiratory depression by opioids.[220] The onset and offset of respiratory depression are in agreement with the time courses of minute volume and carbon dioxide response after epidural morphine in volunteers (see following). In many case reports, antagonism of respiratory depression by naloxone has been confirmed and often several doses or an infusion of naloxone have been required.[145,206] Analgesia can be preserved during reversal of spinal opioid induced respiratory depression by titrated doses or infusions of naloxone.[248,399] It has been claimed that the use of the sitting position and a hyperbaric solution of morphine protects against respiratory depression.[425] However, respiratory depression has been reported with such maneuvers and so it seems wiser to limit the dose of drug rather than to rely on the sitting position.[399]

Epidural opioid administration may also produce early or delayed respiratory depression. Compared with the intrathecal route, epidural administration is complicated by pharmacokinetic aspects related to dural penetration, fat deposition, and systemic absorption (Figure 29-2, 29-10). Pharmacodynamic aspects become complicated, since the larger doses of opioid used result in blood concentrations that cannot be ignored (Fig. 29-9A). Simultaneous lumbar epidural injection of morphine and meperidine in patients resulted in detectable levels of both drugs in cervical CSF at about 30 minutes after injection (Fig. 29-9B). Thereafter, CSF meperidine concentrations in cervical CSF decline rapidly.

Most reports of early respiratory depression after epidural meperidine have been in postoperative patients within 1 hour of injection,[218,439] and probably reflect vascular absorption by way of epidural veins, or possibly rapid redirection to brain by way of the basivertebral venous system (see Chapter 8, Fig. 8-15). Thus, it is plausible that lipid-soluble drugs may cause early respiratory depression at least partly as a result of rapid access to the brain, to achieve peak concentrations near the brain stem at about 30 minutes. This concept is supported by studies of plasma concentrations and respiratory effects of fentanyl. Plasma fentanyl concentrations peak after 5 minutes and then decline rapidly, whereas respiratory depression is seen between 15 and 60 minutes.[9,296] These pharmacokinetic considerations (see following) are consistent with clinical observations that delayed respiratory depression is most common with epidural morphine[40,111,347,404,504] and absent with epidural fentanyl.[9,275] As in the case with intrathecal opioid administration, old age, poor general condition, and respiratory disease, probably predispose to respiratory depression.[41,111,266,399] Patients subject to Stokes-Adams attacks also must be treated cautiously.[110] Finally, postoperative patients have a number of potential factors that place them at risk for this complication. (Table 29-5).

Studies in volunteers by Bromage and others[59,60,73] suggested that changes in CO_2 responsivity after epidural morphine paralleled its rostral spread, as judged by the cephalad progression of analgesia to ice and pin scratch (Fig. 29-11).

The concurrence of trigeminal analgesia, nausea, and peak respiratory depression between 6 to 9 hours after epidural drug administration is strong evidence that significant brain opioid concentrations are reached during this interval. There appears to be a relatively slow progression of analgesia, as morphine is carried in the passive flow of the slow circulation of spinal CSF and then merges with the active intracerebral CSF circulation (Fig. 29-8). This time course is in keep-

TABLE 29-5. *Factors potentially contributing to delayed respiratory depression during postoperative epidural opioid analgesia*

Residual effects of parenteral opioids given before, during, or after surgery. In a number of cases, sizeable doses of intramuscular opioid were given either shortly before or after epidural opioid, when it now is known that significant respiratory interactions are possible.
Residual effects of other CNS-depressant drugs used perioperatively (e.g., anti-emetics).
Lack of tolerance to opioid effects or side effects. Most operative patients have not received opioids for prolonged periods before surgery.
Raised intrathoracic pressure, from mechanical ventilation or "grunting" respiration associated with pain.
Raised intra-abdominal pressure and obstruction of inferior vena cava with increased blood flow through azygos system.
Inadvertent dural puncture by needle or delayed catheter penetration.
Large doses (10 mg) of epidural morphine sometimes required for pain relief after major surgery are associated with a higher incidence of respiratory depression that is persistent and prolonged, than lower doses of epidural morphine (2–4 mg).

ing with studies by Gourlay and associates,[213] who reported peak morphine concentrations in cervical CSF 3 hours after lumbar epidural administration, as well as animal pharmacokinetic data,[219] as noted previously.

Studies by Bromage and others[59,60,73] and Gourlay and others[213] help in understanding the time delay of approximately 3 to 12 hours in clinical case reports of delayed respiratory depression after epidural morphine.[268,347,404,504] From this work it may be surmised that further systemic injection of "usual" doses of opioid would be dangerous for up to a day after epidural morphine. Indeed, this risk can be gauged from the 40% reduction in slope and ventilation after 10 mg of morphine intravenously, which would occur beyond the residual 20% reduction in slope and 40% reduction in ventilation remaining at 22 hours after epidural morphine.[60] It is significant that a similar delay in onset of respiratory depression is seen after intrathecal morphine,[145,206,290,399] supporting the importance of rostral spread of morphine in CSF. In an effort to exploit the effect of posture to inhibit rostral morphine spread, a "between-patient" study found the sitting position to be associated with less respiratory depression than the supine position after epidural morphine.[321] However, a controlled study showed no effect of 45-degree elevated posture in protecting against respiratory depression.[340] Using a minimal effective dose of morphine is a more practical approach to achieving safety, since respiratory depression is dose-related.[9,398] Doses of 2 to 4 mg morphine result in much milder and briefer depression of respiration than a dose of 10 mg morphine,[9,398] which continues to depress respiration for more than 17 hours.[398] Fortunately, 2 to 4 mg of epidural morphine often is adequate for peripheral surgery, and 4 to 6 mg is adequate for more extensive surgery, provided sufficient time is allowed for onset.[9,278,466] A wider therapeutic window can be obtained between analgesia and respiratory depression by using low-dose epidural morphine infusion, preceded by a bolus dose in a *low* volume (1 ml), so that peak concentrations of morphine in brain stem regions are decreased and incidence of respiratory depression is low.[112,116,179] Respiratory depression can be prevented, or antagonized when it occurs by naloxone infusion at a dose of 5 μg/kg/hr, without antagonizing analgesia.[394] *The moral is clear*: respiration must be carefully assessed if parenteral opioid is to be given within 24 hours of epidural morphine, and parenteral dosage must be kept as low as feasible, preferably through cautious intravenous titration while an antagonist (naloxone, nalbuphine or butorphanol) is nearby.

All of the lipophilic opioids are reported to induce a brief period of *early* respiratory depression after epidural administration, [67,100,502] possibly from blood-borne access to the brain but more likely as a result of transient peak concentration of drug in cisternal CSF[218,219] (Fig. 29-9B). Because most lipophilic opioids move rapidly into and out of neural tissue, delayed respiratory depression is exceedingly rare.[296,167] These theoretical considerations are borne out clinically, provided the dose of fentanyl or analogue is kept within the therapeutic margin of about two, between safe epidural dose and analgesic intramuscular dose. Ventilatory effects of analgesic epidural doses of fentanyl, alfentanil and sufentanil given to normal volunteers in a dose-ranging study resolved approximately three hours after drug administration.[120] Also in volunteers, epidural fentanyl did not alter CO_2 response curves over a 24-hour period of study, apart from a brief early depression.[275] Low-dose epidural fentanyl infusion (0.5 mcg/kg/h), after a bolus of 1.5 mcg/kg, was not associated with changes in continuously monitored end-tidal CO_2 or respiratory rate, over an 18-hour monitoring period in 21 postoperative patients.[9] On the other hand, epidural infusion of 1 mcg/kg/hr fentanyl, after a bolus dose of 1 mcg/kg, did depress CO_2 responsivity throughout an 18-hour study period in patients after orthopedic surgery. A question that remains is how to approach clinically the relative resistance of sufentanil and lofentanil to antagonism by naloxone; much higher doses are needed, reflecting greater affinity of these opioids for mu receptors.[14,536] Presumably this high affinity dictates using a higher initial naloxone dose and continuing a naloxone infusion for a substantial period of time. If an inadvertently high dose of either sufentanil or lofentanil were given intrathecally, a large amount of drug would reach the brain and produce both early and *prolonged* respiratory depression, rather than delayed depression. Moreover, it is theoretically possible for a small amount of residual lofentanil in the brain to produce delayed depression if a usual analgesic dose of parenteral opioid is given many hours after an epidural dose. Further, epidural application of the partial mu agonist buprenorphine, and the mixed kappa agonist-mu

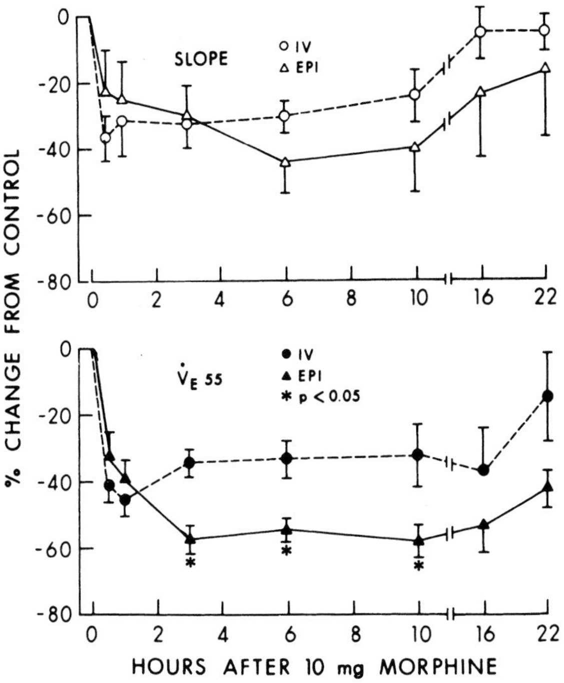

A

DELAYED RESPIRATORY DEPRESSION

HOURS	+0.5	+3	+4.5	+5	+6-9	+16-22
ANALGETIC LEVEL	0	T_{9-11}	T_5	C_{7-8}/T_1	V_1-V_3	
					URINE RETENTION	
				PRURITIS	NAUSEA	
CO_2 RESPONSE	BRIEF↓	SUSTAINED↓ ⟶			PEAK↓	RESIDUAL↓

B

FIG. 29-11. A: Ventilatory response to endogenous CO_2 after epidural *(Epi)* and IV morphine 10 mg by separate injections 2 to 4 weeks apart in 6 subjects. Mean ± SEM percentage change in slope and ventilation at end-tidal P_{CO2} of 55 mm Hg (V_E 55). (Reprinted from Neilsen, C. H., Camporesi, E. M., Bromage, P. R., *et al.*: CO_2 sensitivity after epidural and IV morphine. Anesthesiology, *55*:A372, 1981, with permission of the publisher.) **B:** Respiratory and other side-effects following epidural morphine.

antagonist butorphanol, have both been reported to induce respiratory depression for 12 hours after administration.[134,392]

Extensive preclinical and clinical attention to spinal opioid-induced respiratory depression is offset by voluminous surveillance data attesting to the low incidence of this complication in tens of thousands of patients treated with intrathecal and epidural opioids. Large-scale surveys in Sweden and elsewhere[92,399,405] have enrolled nearly 30,000 patients and yield incidence estimates of respiratory depression, after epidural morphine, that range from 0.09 to 0.25%. These estimates compare favorably with incidences of 1% for respiratory depression after parenteral morphine, whether given by conventional injection or patient-controlled analgesia. Such surveillance also identified the rarity of respiratory depression occurring more than 12 hours after single doses of epidural morphine, and led the Swedish Society of Anesthesiology and Intensive Care to endorse routine observation for only 12 hours. While few would question multiple experimental demonstrations of respiratory effects persisting beyond 12 hours in volunteers given epidural morphine, the interpretation of such responses to exogenous CO_2, and their generalization to patient care, is not straightforward. For example, a variety of studies have found benefits of epidural opioid analgesia upon postoperative pulmonary function and oxygenation, presumably derived from enhanced pain control during deep breathing or coughing. Moreover, respiratory depression is recognized to be uncommon in patients who already are opioid-tolerant,[126,205,363,539] and there have been few reports of this in patients with chronic cancer-related or nonmalignant pain treated with long-term spinal opioids.[106,126,127,141,548] An unusual hazard of epidural opioid use occurs in patients with known or undiagnosed sleep apnea syndrome—in which a small epidural dose of morphine can result in severe sedation and respiratory depression.[276]

Gastrointestinal Function

Most preclinical studies of the gastrointestinal effects of opioids *in vivo* have employed transit (propulsion) as an endpoint, although some have examined mucosal transport of fluid and ions. These two physiological effects are clearly separable: In some models, the antidiarrheal effects of opioids occur principally from antisecretory rather than antipropulsive effects. The relationship between opioid (or other drug) effects upon gastrointestinal contractions, i.e., motility, versus propulsion, i.e., transit, is not a simple one nor is it the same at different sites along the gut. For example, opioids delay propulsion in species in which they inhibit contractions; in other species, opioids increase contractions but delay propulsion. Opioids can affect intestinal function (including gastric acid secretion) by actions in the brain, spinal cord, and periphery. Mu opioid agonists given in analgesic doses at any of these three sites inhibit propulsion, gastric acid secretion, and diarrhea. Analgesic doses of kappa opioid agonists administered at any of these three sites have little effect upon propulsion or gastric acid secretion, and may even stimulate the latter process when given intravenously. Analgesic doses of delta opioid agonists given intracerebroventricularly or systemically do not affect propulsion or gastric acid secretion, but do inhibit diarrhea. Spinally administered delta opioid agonists, however, do inhibit propulsion in preclinical models. In patients followed postoperatively, gastrointestinal motility normally decreases, particularly after abdominal surgery. In normal volunteers, opioids given systemically or epidurally delay gastric emptying and decrease gastrointestinal motility. However, one controlled trial in obese patients found a decrease in times to pass flatus and feces postoperatively, along with a shortened hospital stay, in those given epidural morphine, compared with those given systemic (intramuscular) morphine.[392] Gastrointestinal effects of postoperative epidural local anesthetics alone are minimal; the benefits of their use postoperatively are described in Chapter 5. Thus one may conclude provisionally that clinical findings during application of spinal mu opioid agonists are consistent with preclinical effects, in particular that epidural mu opioid administration results in a slowing of postoperative recovery of gastrointestinal function, intermediate between systemic opioid administration and spinal analgesia with local anesthetics. A comprehensive picture of the gastrointestinal effects of acute and chronic spinal opioid use in humans, that encompasses non-mu opioids, and coadministration of opioid-sparing analgesics such as local anesthetics or nonsteroidals,[377] has not yet emerged.

Nausea and vomiting occur in approximately 1/4 of postoperative patients treated with spinal opioids, although pain itself has been implicated as a cause of postoperative nausea.[466] In a prospective study of 1,085 postoperative patients, Stenseth and associates[466] reported that epidural morphine (dose 4 to 6 mg) was associated with nausea or vomiting in 34% of patients. In a series of 1,200 postoperative patients, nausea and vomiting were present in 17% of the patients,[405] while in another series nausea was present alone in 12%, and with vomiting in 24%.[278] In the latter series, the incidence of nausea and vomiting was similar whether morphine was used intramuscularly or epidurally, or whether saline was injected epidurally. Others, too, have reported a low incidence of nausea and vomiting after epidural morphine in the postoperative period.[480] In labor, the incidence of nausea and vomiting has been reported to be low with epidural opioid,[67,379] in contrast to a high incidence with intrathecal opioid.[26,440] Epidural use of lipid-soluble opioids such as meperidine, fentanyl, and sufentanil,[65,167,507] may be associated with the lowest incidence of nausea and vomiting. In a cross-over study in volunteers, Bromage and colleagues[58] observed nausea and vomiting in 50% of subjects approximately 6 hours after epidural morphine, which coincided with other evidence of rostral spread of morphine in CSF to intracerebral structures, including the vomiting center and the chemoreceptor trigger zone (Fig. 29-11). In contrast, after intravenous morphine only 1 out of 10 subjects had nausea lasting 2 hours. Nausea and vomiting in the postoperative setting are antagonized by intravenous naloxone, without diminishing analgesia, at titrated doses of up to 5 mcg/kg/h.[396] Fortunately, the incidence of nausea and vomiting seems to be much less with repeated epidural dosing, and is low in patients with cancer or nonmalignant pain who require long-term spinal opioid therapy.[126,205,231,548]

Cardiovascular Function

Cardiovascular and pain regulatory systems are closely coupled. Activation or inhibition of one system produces changes in the other, often through overlapping anatomic and neurochemical pathways.[369] Just as analgesia has multiple components such as sensory processing or emotion, key aspects of global cardiovascular status—myocardial contractile state, blood pressure, heart rate, and vascular resistance—although linked, are independently regulated. Cardiovascular effects of opioids differ between basal, pain-free subjects and those studied perioperatively or while in pain. Also, central injections of receptor-selective opioids in animals may elicit different, even opposite, effects upon heart rate and blood pressure if given into nearby sites, or at the same site in low versus high doses. One explanation for dual excitatory and inhibitory effects parallels the explanation for biphasic opioid ventilatory effects, namely, that high-affinity mu-1 receptors mediate excitatory effects, and low-affinity mu-2 receptors mediate inhibitory effects.[369] Analgesic doses of spinal morphine do not change blood pressure or heart rate in animals and in humans, studied under basal conditions in the awake or the anesthetized state.[18,174] In halothane-anesthetized or unanesthetized dogs, intrathecal morphine or fentanyl analogs do not change cardiac output or peripheral resistance.[18,536] A recent study in awake dogs reported dose-dependent reductions in heart rate after either epidural or intrathecal administration of bolus doses of sufentanil, alfentanil or morphine, with tolerance to these effects, during repetitive epidural or intrathecal drug dosing.[415] In resting humans, changes in skin temperature, blood pressure, and heart rate are absent with spinal opioids. Both sudomotor and vasomotor activity (e.g., responses to cold pressor testing or Valsalva maneuver) remain intact.[58,60,135,205] The latter is important because of its homeostatic role during upright posture or blood loss.

During noxious stimulation in awake or anesthetized animals and humans, parasympathetic outflow decreases and sympathetic activity increases, as do levels of circulating catecholamines[137,179,254] (see Chapters 5 and 8). Heart rate, blood pressure, myocardial oxygen consumption, systemic vascular resistance, and ventricular vulnerability to fibrillation, all increase in this situation. Opioid analgesia by spinal or systemic routes decreases all these parameters.[139] One study in dogs reported an increase in cardiac vagal activity after thoracic epidural morphine,[230] consistent with previous findings that systemic opioids stimulate both the central baroceptor reflex and vagal afferent activity. Clinical effects of spinal analgesia upon myocardial function have been most evident when local anesthetics, alone or supplemented with opioids, are administered via the thoracic epidural space.[403] The greater effect of spinal local anesthetics than opioids upon cardiovascular function during pain or stress probably reflects the more complete sympathetic ablation possible with the former class of agents.[95] However, in both experimental and clinical studies, spinal opioid analgesia has not yet been clearly proven to benefit cardiovascular morbidity and mortality, beyond what might be attributed to effective analgesia alone.[43] Attempts to draw conclusions from published clinical series have been impeded by the small numbers of patients studied, and the likelihood that advances in perioperative monitoring and treatment of myocardial ischemia have progressed sufficiently that it may be necessary to study thousands of patients, in order to demonstrate further decrements in cardiovascular complications.[43,207] Thus, identification of the impact, if any, of spinal opioid analgesia upon such complications may require pooling of results from studies of high-risk patients undergoing highly invasive procedures—a synthesis that is not yet possible.

Bladder Function

Spinal morphine in humans produces a naloxone-reversible inhibition of the volume evoked micturition reflex[405] to a greater degree than is seen after systemic administration of equianalgesic doses. This effect seems to be most marked in young males, but demographics are unreliable because many patients treated acutely with spinal opioids are high-risk older patients undergoing major operations, after which they are routinely catheterized.[96] Whether the incidence varies with the opioid used, the duration of treatment, or between males and females is not yet proven. That these factors may be important is suggested by a series of 40,000 injections of epidural meperidine (50 mg) for pain, after cesarean section, in which catheterization of the bladder was not necessary.[65] In this large series, patients routinely had bladder catheterization intraoperatively and for the first 12 hours postoperatively, and then did not require recatheterization. The apparently prophylactic effect of this approach is of interest, since another study reported a low incidence of urinary retention using this method, compared with a high incidence with "in, out" catheterization intraoperatively, followed by epidural morphine.[261]

Urinary retention is a more frequently reported complication[57,393,478,479,496] of spinal opioids administered to volunteer subjects than spinal opioids administered to patients. Current evidence from volunteer studies indicates that urodynamic effects of epidural morphine are not dose-related within a range of clinically relevant doses, but that they are reversed by naloxone.[393] In a dose-response study of epidural morphine for postoperative pain relief, Martin and associates found that the incidence of urinary retention was the same for doses of morphine of 0.5, 1.0, 2.0, 4.0, and 8.0 mg.[392] This was consistent with a urodynamic study in 30 volunteers in whom increased bladder capacity and relaxation of detrusor muscle was similar for epidural doses of morphine of 2, 4, and 10 mg.[393] In a study of postoperative patients using CO_2 cystometry, a great variation in bladder response to epidural morphine was found on the day after surgery. Intravenous naloxone reversed bladder effects in those patients who developed urinary retention.[235] Naloxone infusion of 5 μg/kg/hr in postoperative patients in 1 study reversed urinary retention with only minimal effects on analgesia,[395] but others have reported that naloxone doses large enough to reverse urodynamic changes consistently after epidural morphine (e.g., 10 mcg/kg/hr) may interfere with analgesia. Anecdotal reports suggest that the incidence of bladder dysfunction may be less with spinal fentanyl,[348] meperidine,[65,66] and methadone,[186] than with morphine, but conclusive comparative studies are not available.

The precise mechanism of spinal opioid interference with bladder function has not been elucidated although it is clear that mu opioid receptors are implicated. In humans, cystometrograms show increased bladder capacity owing to decreased detrusor muscle tone,[393] with a slight increase in the urethral sphincter tone.[543] Vesicosphincter dysynergia develops, and this points to inhibition of postganglionic nerves to the urinary bladder.[152] Such inhibition probably results from opioid action at the spinal cord, to diminish sacral parasympathetic outflow and thereby induce detrusor muscle relaxation. Similar spinal opioid effects upon detrusor relaxation are seen in animals.[53,152] In the rat, the rank order of potency for receptor-selective opioids is: β-endorphin $\geqslant$ DADL $\geqslant$ morphine $>$ EKC $>>$ SKF 10047.[543] Consistent with this ranking of receptor-selective opioid agonists is the finding from animal studies that kappa agonists may be devoid of this urinary effect. Other than case reports of minimal interference of epidural buprenorphine or pentazocine with voiding, systematic studies of analgesic efficacy and side effects in humans are not available. For patients with chronic pain, long-term epidural opioid use appears not to obligate bladder catheterization.[106,205,539] Studies to determine whether pre-existing prostatism places patients at prolonged risk of urinary retention during chronic spinal opioid therapy have not been reported.

Unexpected benefits have emerged from these insights into spinal mechanisms of bladder function. Spinal morphine has been used as a treatment in patients with bladder spasm.[29] Naloxone augments the micturition reflex in spinal-transected animals.[543] There are also anecdotal reports of short-term benefits of spinal morphine for enuresis.

Sensorimotor Function, Neurotoxic Potential and Pruritus

In contrast to many clinical reports of rigidity following systemic administration of lipophilic opioids, such as fentanyl or sufentanil, spinal opioids at antinociceptive doses lack measurable effects on motor function.[536,542] Monosynaptic stretch reflexes are unaffected, but spinal opioids do suppress polysynaptic flexion reflexes.[507,515] Clinically, spinal morphine given to subjects with paraplegia blocks the polysynaptic flexion reflex elicited by sural nerve stimulation, but has little effect on the monosynaptic H reflex.[514] Spinal morphine has also been used successfully for treatment of painful muscle spasms associated with spasticity[184] and multiple sclerosis.[469] This benefit is reversible with naloxone.

Neurotoxicity of spinal opioids has been evaluated extensively in both preclinical and clinical settings.[2] High doses of intrathecal morphine in rats may produce two alarming syndromes: (i) convulsive seizures of the hind limbs and hyperreflexia in response to cutaneous stimuli, and (ii) intense motor rigidity. Neither of these are antagonized by naloxone, implying mediation by nonopioids such as the algesic metabolite morphine-3-glucuronide or the inhibitory neurotransmitter glycine. This cautionary note is not paralleled by clinical reports of hyper- and dysesthesia, that are rare[413] and not clearly distinguishable from pruritus (see following). Similar contrast exists between sobering preclinical evidence (including histopathology) of neurotoxicity and motor paralysis after intrathecal administration of peptides, including somatostatin, dynorphin, or delta-selective enkephalin analogs in the rat or dog, and the rarity of corresponding symptoms in clinical trials of these agents. Explanations for this dichotomy include species differences as well as inclusion criteria in clinical trials that select patients who may already be bed-ridden or inactive.

Apart from potential neurotoxicity of spinally administered compounds themselves, other factors relevant to the safety of spinal opioid administration are the compatibility of solutions of such agents with CSF and neural tissue, and inflammatory reactions provoked by intraspinal catheters. Solutions of opioids used in spinal injections (morphine, methadone, meperidine, fentanyl, alfentanil, lofentanil, and buprenorphine), and local anesthetics in normal saline have pH values that range from 4.52 to 6.85. When mixed with CSF, all lowered pH of the CSF by 0.3 or less, but etidocaine lowered pH by 0.82, with clouding of CSF.[50] High concentrations of local anesthetics alone, such as 5% lidocaine given intrathecally, are recognized in animal models and clinical reports to have the potential for irreversible neurotoxicity. Histologic examination of spinal cords of cancer patients who had epidural administration of bupivacaine-morphine mixture for three weeks,[5] or morphine for up to six months,[128] revealed no abnormality attributable to morphine. Two of seven patients had posterior column degeneration consistent with myelopathy of malignancy.[125] Further studies of spinal cord pathology after prolonged spinal administration of opioids, in combination with other agents, are required to define the risks of neurotoxicity as a function of foreign body (i.e., catheter) present in the epidural space versus drug infused through the catheter. A finding of practical significance was focal thickening of the dura in the vicinity of epidural catheters of four patients, with fibrous tissue cocoons surrounding the catheters. Animal studies of the potential damage to the spinal cord of epidural catheters, and repeated injection of opioids, have revealed histologic changes in some but not in all studies. Yaksh reported that 14 macaque monkeys with epidural catheters *in situ* for 4 to 16 months, and receiving 15 to 122 injections of morphine, had no abnormal neurologic signs. Three of the monkeys were sacrificed for autopsy after 6, 8, and 9 months and after 44, 68, and 72 intrathecal injections of a variety of opioids and peptides. No histologic evidence of cord pathology was found.[529,543] Similar findings of safety during chronic epidural or intrathecal infusions of sufentanil, alfentanil, morphine, or saline in the dog were later reported by Yaksh and colleagues.[539] In that study, every animal had fibrosis around its infusion catheter, whether intrathecal or epidural, and many had histological evidence of acute and chronic inflammation in the epidural space. Animals with intrathecal catheters, but not epidural catheters, also had acute and chronic inflammation in the meninges. The incidences of all these histological changes were independent of the dose of opioid used, and were likely to occur equally in animals infused with saline alone. Abouleish and co-workers[5] found no immediate or chronic (42 days) changes in spinal cord histology attributable to a single intrathecal injection of a large dose of morphine (0.07 mg/kg). Coombs and co-workers, however, reported extensive pericatheter reactions in sheep after chronic epidural infusions of high concentrations of hydromorphone and morphine, but not of saline. These reactions were sufficient to produce spinal cord compression, parenchymal damage, and hind limb weakness.

In cats with *intrathecally* implanted catheters, receiving only intrathecal saline and killed 19 to 21 days after implantation, an inflammatory response developed, with a thin fibrotic sleeve surrounding the catheter, with no obstruction to the tip. Where the catheter lay in contact with the spinal cord, mild deformation and local demyelination were present. Animals that received the ED_{100} for alfentanil or sufentanil daily for 5 days, showed spinal cord pathology indistinguishable from those receiving saline. Animals receiving 10 times the ED_{100} of either drug showed results similar to controls.[536] Chronically implanted *epidural* catheters in rats resulted in the rapid development of a fibrotic reaction in 36 of 43 rats after only one day. After 10 days of catheterization, a thick fibrotic reaction, obstructing the catheter tip, was observed in 31 of 33 rats. Injection of methylene blue showed no spread into the epidural space; the dye filled the lumen of the catheter and then the sheath, making a blue spot on the skin if the injection was continued. A mild deformation of the dura was observed in all animals.[176]

Consideration of the above animal studies, particularly those designed to distinguish catheter-related effects from opioid toxicity, and published results of over 1,000 patients treated for pain of malignant and nonmalignant origin by chronic infusions of intrathecal or epidural opioid, indicates that opioids are not neurotoxic at clinical doses and concentrations. However, fibrotic reactions to intrathecal and epidural catheters made of inert polyethylene occasionally may produce clinical symptoms. Symptoms of cord compression and myelopathy have been reported with equal rarity, during chronic spinal cord stimulation. The use of more inert materials for chronically implanted intrathecal and epidural catheters should be investigated. Neuropathology due to long-term administration of local anesthetics, epidurally and intrathecally, has been investigated only recently, as discussed in Chapter 30. Here, too, the growing number of published series of patients treated with spinal infusions of mixtures of local anesthetics and opioids, without evidence of drug-related neurotoxicity or spinal cord dysfunction, attest to the neurotoxicological safety of these combinations.

Pruritus is common during spinal opioid therapy, but incidence estimates vary widely, because its presence (especially if mild) may be revealed only on direct questioning. It seems likely that generalized pruritus associated with spinal opioids is due to widespread alteration in sensory modulation, since it occurs when there is evidence of opioid migration over the entire spinal cord to the brain. Sensory modulatory mechanisms in the upper cervical spinal cord and trigeminal system may be involved, since the onset coincides with the spread of hypalgesia to this region.[58] The facial pruritus that often is reported may be explained by rapid penetration of opioid to the superficially placed caudal portions of the nucleus of the spinal tract of the trigeminal nerve.[219] Pruritus is not due to preservatives, since it occurs with preservative-free opioids, nor is it likely to be due to histamine release,[20] since its onset is approximately 3 hours after epidural or spinal opioid administration[58,59,60] and it occurs with fentanyl, which does not cause histamine release, as well as with morphine.[412] Such benefits as clinicians have observed with anithistamines given for pruritus due to spinal opioid therapy may well derive from their nonspecific sedating actions.

Putative mechanisms of pruritus after spinal opioid therapy include some that involve mu opioid receptor activation, such as stimulation of neuronal G_s (see page 919) or inhibition of inhibitory interneurons in the spinal cord, or stimulation of an itch reflex localized in the trigeminal nucleus. Mechanisms dependent upon the mu receptor underlie successful therapy of spinal opioid-induced pruritus by naloxone,[58,395] or other agents with mu antagonist properties, such as butorphanol or nalbuphine. Indeed, in one obstetric series, the incidence of pruritus was minimal with epidural buprenorphine or butorphanol, but 50 to 60% with epidural morphine or fentanyl.[392] In volunteer studies of epidural morphine, 10 mg, pruritus occurred in 100% of subjects in one study[57] and in three of four subjects in another study.[479] In postoperative patients, pruritus was present in 28% of patients receiving epidural morphine (10 mg) in one study,[278] but in only 1% of patients in studies of morphine (5 mg)[57] and morphine (2 mg),[404] respectively. Pruritus also has been reported with epidural meperidine, fentanyl, alfentanil, sufentanil, and diamorphine, but few comparative data are available. After meperidine (50 mg) was given epidurally for postcesarean section pain, Brownridge reported that 50% of 2,000 patients admitted to pruritus (but only on direct questioning) yet only one patient found it troublesome.[65] In contrast, in some series, epidural morphine resulted in pruritus in up to 70% of patients, but there was no relationship between incidence of pruritus and dose.[20] However, the incidence of severe pruritus that troubles the patient appears to be close to 1%.[57] Other putative mechanisms of spinal opioid-induced pruritus that are independent of the mu receptor include the formation of hyperalgesic metabolites such as morphine-3-glucuronide. This metabolite produces scratching behavior and hyperalgesia, not reversed by naloxone, after injection into monkeys. Further evidence that pruritus need not follow activation of spinal mu-opioid receptors is the absence of pruritus after intrathecal administration of β-endorphin.[367,368] Hyperesthesia of unclear etiology but not reversible by naloxone has been observed after high doses of spinal morphine given to patients with cancer pain.[313,533] Fortunately, even high doses of sufentanil and alfentanil do not appear to be associated with this side effect.[533] It has been reported that prior or concomitant use of bupivacaine epidurally reduces the incidence of pruritus with epidural opioids.[441] The results of one recent trial suggest that subhypnotic doses of propofol may be an attractive, novel, means of treating pruritus.[64] Pruritus often subsides, as does bladder dysfunction, with continuing doses of opioid.

SPINAL OPIOID PHARMACOLOGY

The term *selective spinal analgesia* was suggested by Cousins and associates[135] in 1979 (see following) to emphasize the distinction between spinal opioid analgesia versus analgesia achieved by relatively nonselective blockade of axonal conduction by local anesthetics. From the prior section, it is clear that spinal opioids have many effects other than antinociception. However, animal and human studies have amply validated the concept of selective spinal analgesia mediated by multiple opioid and nonopioid spinal antinociceptive systems. Accumulating evidence points to the feasibility of achieving the ideal of analgesia without unwanted side effects by coadministering two or more agents, such as opioids and local anesthetics, that act upon different antinociceptive targets. This section summarizes preclinical and clinical data that model the pharmacokinetics and pharmacodynamics of intrathecal and epidural opioids, given as sole agents or in combination with other opioid and nonopioid compounds.

Physicochemical Properties

Local anesthetics[322] and nonpeptidic opioids have similar molecular weights and pKa values; partition coefficients for individual agents within both drug classes overlap but vary widely (Table 29-6).

Phenylpiperidine derivatives (meperidine, fentanyl, lofentanil) are highly lipid-soluble and closest in structure to local anesthetics. In contrast, morphine has low lipid solubility. Morphine's slow onset of action after epidural dosing coincides with delayed peak morphine concentrations in CSF[357,453] and its relative hydrophilicity results in slower efflux from spinal cord and CSF, and greater migration to the brain.[213,318] The rate of absorption of meperidine from the epidural space is similar to that of lidocaine. Like lidocaine, meperidine has a rapid onset of analgesia after epidural dosing that coincides with an early peak drug concentration in CSF.[135,205,453] High local concentrations of meperidine can produce peripheral nerve block,[503] a property that is shared to an extent by other opioids, particularly nonalkaloids, along with many other classes of drugs used in anesthesia. Such high concentrations are unlikely to be infused spinally, and meperidine is the only opioid that has significant local anesthetic actions when applied to individual dorsal root axons, or that is effective when used as a sole intrathecal agent for surgery.[335,429] At physiological pH (7.4), the tertiary amine group in each of the nonpeptide opioids is mostly ionized, making them water-soluble. Hydroxyl groups on the morphine molecule increase its water solubility beyond that of any other opioid in clinical use except hydromorphone.

Onset of analgesia after spinal opioid administration is earlier with more lipid-soluble agents. Other factors such as molecular size and shape also contribute to a degree.[341] Morphine, an extreme example of low lipid-solubility and high water-solubility, has the slowest onset of action. This relationship has been confirmed in rats,[536,538] cats,[536] primates,[529,532,535] and humans (see following). A somewhat quicker onset of clinical analgesia for hydromorphone than for morphine, after lumbar epidural administration, despite comparable lipophilicity and similar blood and CSF pharmacokinetics[381] may reflect more rapid supraspinal action of the former compound.[63] Many studies in animals[536,539,529] and humans,[110,220,317,318] indicate the importance of lipid solubility for dural transfer.[452,453] For *intrathecal opioids*, well-controlled studies in the primate measured the time to rise to half maximum shock titration threshold as an index of onset of analgesia: β-endorphin, 1.6 hours; morphine, 1.4 hours, DADL, 0.7 hour; metkephamid, 0.6 hour; meperidine, 0.5 hour; methadone, 0.4 hour; and lofentanil, 0.1 hour. For *epidural opioids*, primate studies found similar onset times

TABLE 29-6. *Physicochemical properties of opioids and local anesthetics*

	Molecular weight[a]	pK_a (25° C)	Partition coefficient[b]
Local anesthetics[c]			
Procaine hydrochloride	236	8.9	0.02[c]
Lidocaine hydrochloride	234	7.9	2.9[d]
Bupivacaine hydrocholoride	288	8.1	27.5[d]
Etidocaine hydrochloride	276	7.7	141[c]
Ropivacaine hydrochloride	329	8.1	141[f]
Opioids[c]			
Hydromorphone hydrochloride	322	8.1	1.23[f]
Morphine sulfate	285	7.9[a]	1.42[f]
Meperidine hydrochloride	247	8.5	38.8[f]
Methadone hydrochloride	309	9.3	116[f]
Fentanyl citrate	336	8.4	813[f]
Sufentanil citrate	386	8.0	1,788[f]
(−)Lofentanil cis-oxalate	408	7.8	1,450[f]

[a] Base.
[b] *n*-Heptane and octanol partition coefficients are strongly correlated for similar compounds in a log–log relationship.
[c] Commonly used forms (see Mather,[250] Tucker and Mather[363]).
[d] *n*-Heptane/pH 7.4 buffer, partition coefficient.
[e] Tertiary amino group.
[f] Octanol/pH 7.4 buffer partition coefficient.

to those for intrathecal opioids: morphine, 2.9 hours; meperidine, 0.7 hour; and lofentanil, 0.2 hour.[529] Metkephamid and β-endorphin were inefficient epidurally in this primate preparation at doses several times those that were analgesic by intrathecal administration.[529,535] In rats the ED_{50} of epidural DADL is 30 to 50 times intrathecal values. Studies in humans confirm that analgesia can be obtained by intrathecal DADL administration[343,364] in patients tolerant to the mu-agonist morphine.

Duration of analgesia is inversely related to lipid solubility, but also influenced by rate of dissociation from receptors and accumulation within epidural fat. An index of duration of analgesia is the time it takes to fall to half maximum threshold in the above primate shock titration model.[529] For intrathecal opioids tested in this model, β-endorphin gave a value of 22 hours; morphine, 16 hours; lofentanil, 7.6 hours; methadone, 6.8 hours; metkephamid, 6.1 hours; DADL, 5.2 hours; and meperidine, 5.1 hours. In rats, the duration of analgesia for fentanyl analogs and morphine in hot-plate and tail-flick tests was dose-dependent.[536] At doses producing an equal magnitude of peak analgesia, the duration of action was in the order: lofentanil > morphine > sufentanil > alfentanil ≥ fentanyl. Intravenous naloxone produced dose-dependent antagonism of antinociception except for lofentanil, that required very high doses of naloxone. Resistance to naloxone antagonism and long duration of action probably reflect lofentanil's high affinity for, and slow dissociation from, mu opioid receptors.

Preclinical Pharmacokinetic Observations

Gustafsson and co-workers performed lumbar intrathecal injections of (^{14}C)-morphine and (^{3}H)-meperidine in rats.[131] Fourteen minutes after injection, lumbar spinal cord radioactivity was 215 times higher for morphine and 75 times higher for meperidine than if distribution in the body were homogeneous. Whole-body autoradiography revealed that 15 minutes after (^{14}C)-morphine injection, the entire spinal cord and ventral parts of the brain contained high levels of radioactivity. At 60 minutes, parts of the brain, including respiratory and vomiting centers and trigeminal nucleus, contained radioactivity that remained detectable at two but not four hours after injection. Only the caudal part of the spinal cord contained radioactivity at four hours. Spinal cord radioactivity as a percentage of dose injected was 26% at 14 minutes, 20% at 44 minutes, 4.5% at 180 minutes. For meperidine, this figure was 7% at 14 minutes and 2% at 44 minutes. These results indicate that the more lipophilic drug meperidine is rapidly taken up and eliminated from the spinal cord, whereas the hydrophilic drug morphine persists in the spinal cord for much longer. Also, morphine spreads rapidly into basal cisterns and later penetrates into brain.

The same group applied positron emission tomography to study kinetics of (^{14}C)-labeled morphine and meperidine after lumbar epidural and intrathecal administration in monkeys.[219] The technique could differentiate between whole body versus spinal canal uptake, but not between epidural, intrathecal, or spinal cord uptake. For meperidine, high activity was observed only in the lumbar spinal region. For morphine, radioactivity was fairly constant along the spinal canal up to C4, where it was low. Cervical CSF showed peak radioactivity about 60 minutes after injection of morphine or meperidine. Injection rapidly or in a large volume increased cephalad spread. Peak concentrations of both drugs in blood occurred five minutes after spinal injection.[219] The terminal half-lives of disposition at the lumbar level were 47 and 60 minutes, respectively, for intrathecal and epidural administration.

Strube and associates injected (^{3}H)-morphine in the lumbar epidural space of anesthetized baboons and tracked cisternal CSF radioactivity for 22 hours. Morphine was detected in cisternal CSF one hour after administration, reached a peak at three hours, then declined with a half-life of eight hours.[468] Chrubasik and others measured morphine in cisternal CSF of dogs after epidural administration of a 2 mg bolus in either 1 or 10 ml saline, followed by an infusion of 0.16 mg per hour. Morphine was detectable near the brain stem after only 10 to 13 minutes. Peak morphine concentrations in cisternal CSF were reached later (2 to 3 hours) after the 1 ml than the 10 ml bolus (0.5 hour) and were much lower (100 ng/ml) after the low-volume bolus than the high-volume bolus (4000 ng/ml).[113]

After epidural injection of (^{3}H)-morphine and inulin in dogs, Durant and Yaksh studied distribution in lumbar CSF, azygos venous and femoral arterial blood, and lymph.[177] During the first 20 minutes, morphine levels in the azygos blood were 3 and 10-fold higher, respectively, than in arterial blood and lymph. By one hour, half the morphine had passed into the azygos system. The elimination phase from CSF was about 106 minutes. Comparison of blood and lymph values indicated that morphine in lymph was derived from systemic distribution. Morphine appeared to be cleared from CSF through the azygos venous system at a similar rate as inulin. The fraction of morphine crossing the dura after epidural injection (0.3%) was half that for inulin (0.6%). Surprisingly, the heavier molecule inulin (MW 5175) was better able to penetrate dura than the lighter molecule morphine (MW 334). A later toxicologic screening study from the same laboratory[415] confirmed rapid systemic redistribution of bolus doses of lumbar epidural or intrathecal sufentanil, alfentanil, and morphine, before and after a 15- or 25-day continuous drug infusion.

Colpaert and co-workers studied opiate receptor binding and drug concentrations in plasma and brain after epidural and intravenous sufentanil in the rat.[123] Epidural sufentanil inhibited (^{3}H)-sufentanil binding throughout brain and spinal cord, but more so in thalamus and lumbar spinal cord. Intravenous sufentanil at an analgesic dose inhibited (^{3}H)-sufentanil binding in brain. The epidural dose to inhibit binding in the lumbar spinal cord was half the intravenous dose. With intravenous sufentanil, more mu opiate receptor binding occurred in the brain. However, the epidural route was only half as potent as the intravenous route in producing detectable levels of sufentanil in plasma and brain. Hence, analgesia with optimal epidural doses of sufentanil probably is due to a spinal action, with a contribution from brain sufentanil action during early stages of analgesia. Increasing epidural doses of sufentanil progressively resemble intravenous administration, as the amount of drug in the brain increases.

The valveless internal vertebral venous plexus communicates with intracranial venous sinuses. Under conditions of increased epidural pressure, venous blood flow may be cephalad, carrying drug absorbed from the epidural space up to the brain. The observation that rapid epidural injection of a small dose of morphine in the cat may provoke retching, yet the same dose given in the femoral vein is without effect[533] suggested that epidural opioids may reach the brain rapidly via a direct vascular channel, in addition to transport in CSF. To test this hypothesis, (^{3}H)-naloxone or (^{14}C)-morphine was injected epidurally, and plasma concentrations of tracer measured in the azygos vein (representing epidural venous drainage to superior vena cava) and in internal jugular vein (representing passage of the drug via the internal vertebral venous plexus to intracranial venous sinuses and then to brain). Vena caval compression decreased radioactivity in the azygos outflow but increased radioactivity in jugular blood.[536]

Clinical Pharmacokinetics and Pharmacodynamics

In 1979, Wang et al.[498] reported the first use of spinal intrathecal opioids in humans conducted as a double-blind, placebo-controlled, crossover study approved by a human studies committee. Eight patients suffering from cancer pain despite chronic systemic opioid therapy received lumbar intrathecal morphine (0.5 or 1.0 mg) or physiologic saline to a total of 17 and 12 injections, respectively. Two patients reported pain relief after both morphine and saline; morphine provided 15 hours of pain relief compared to seven hours after saline. This incidence (two of eight subjects) and duration of placebo response is consistent with many analgesic trials. In the other 6 patients, saline injections were ineffective, while morphine injections were followed by pain relief in 15 to 45 minutes, lasting 12 to 24 hours. The authors reported no sedation, respiratory depression, or neurological deterioration.[498] Also in 1979, Cousins and colleagues reported that 1 to 2 mg of morphine injected in the thoracic intrathecal region relieved the pain of breast or lung cancer for 24 to 48 hours.[206] These patients, who had been treated chronically with systemic opioids, did not experience respiratory depression. Chauvin and associates reported that plasma morphine concentrations were low after 0.02 mg/kg of morphine intrathecally, and thus vascular absorption of morphine was unlikely to contribute to analgesia.[101] Relief of acute or chronic pain after intrathecal opioid administration has now been documented thoroughly in postoperative and cancer pain, as well as in chronic pain not due to malignancy (see following).

Epidural opioid therapy was likewise reported in 1979 by Behar and associates.[31] The same year, Cousins and colleagues described pharmacokinetic and neurologic findings during epidural meperidine administration.[135] Their initial pharmacokinetic study found that epidural meperidine rapidly reaches CSF to produce analgesia, while opioid blood concentrations are below analgesic levels (Fig. 29-12). Because other neurologic functions such as sympathetic vasoconstrictor responses were intact, the term "selective spinal analgesia" was advanced to distinguish analgesia achieved with spinal opioids from that accomplished using spinal local anesthetics.[135] Since then, most clinical pharmacokinetic research on spinal opioids has been based upon epidural, rather than intrathecal, drug administration, because the former technique is better suited for serial and/or multi-site sampling in relatively healthy patients or volunteers.

Epidural meperidine pharmacokinetics in blood and CSF after epidural or intravenous drug administration in the same patients were the subject of the earliest studies in this field.[545] Multi-site sampling permitted calculation, for example, of the rate of absorption of meperidine from the epidural space into the systemic circulation.[135,205] Blood and CSF meperidine concentrations and analgesic responses varied greatly between patients, but patients having a high CSF-to-blood concentration ratio had complete analgesia. A rapid increase in CSF meperidine concentrations in the first 5 minutes after injection coincided with the onset of analgesia (Fig. 29-12A). The observation that epidural meperidine rapidly produced high CSF concentrations[205,312] suggests that lipid-soluble epidural opioids may readily enter spinal fluid and gain access to the superficial dorsal horn by way of the arachnoid granulations in the dural cuff region (Fig. 29-10), in addition to diffusion across the dura.[342] It is also possible that lipid-soluble drugs such as meperidine may reach the spinal cord by rapid uptake into the posterior radicular branch of spinal segmental arteries, which run close to the dural cuff region, but the importance of this route has not been confirmed. The majority of patients who received 100 mg of meperidine epidurally had blood concentrations of 0.2 to 0.7 μg per ml within 20 minutes of epidural injection. Earlier, these blood concentrations had been found to produce analgesia in a separate study in the same patients. However, two patients who failed to achieve minimally effective analgesic blood concentrations still had the rapid onset of analgesia. The residual (i.e., still unabsorbed) epidural dose declined exponentially with a half-life of 15 to 30 minutes. Analgesia after epidural drug administration lasted well beyond the time when blood concentrations declined below minimally effective levels (Fig. 29-12B). These findings have been confirmed by others.[134] However, if similar doses of meperidine are given intramuscularly and epidurally, blood concentrations are similar. Analgesia was significantly greater for epidural than for intramuscular meperidine between 0.25 and 1 hour, in one controlled study.[218,220] Also, some patients had evidence of hypalgesia, indicating a weak local anesthetic effect.[220] The fact that an effective epidural

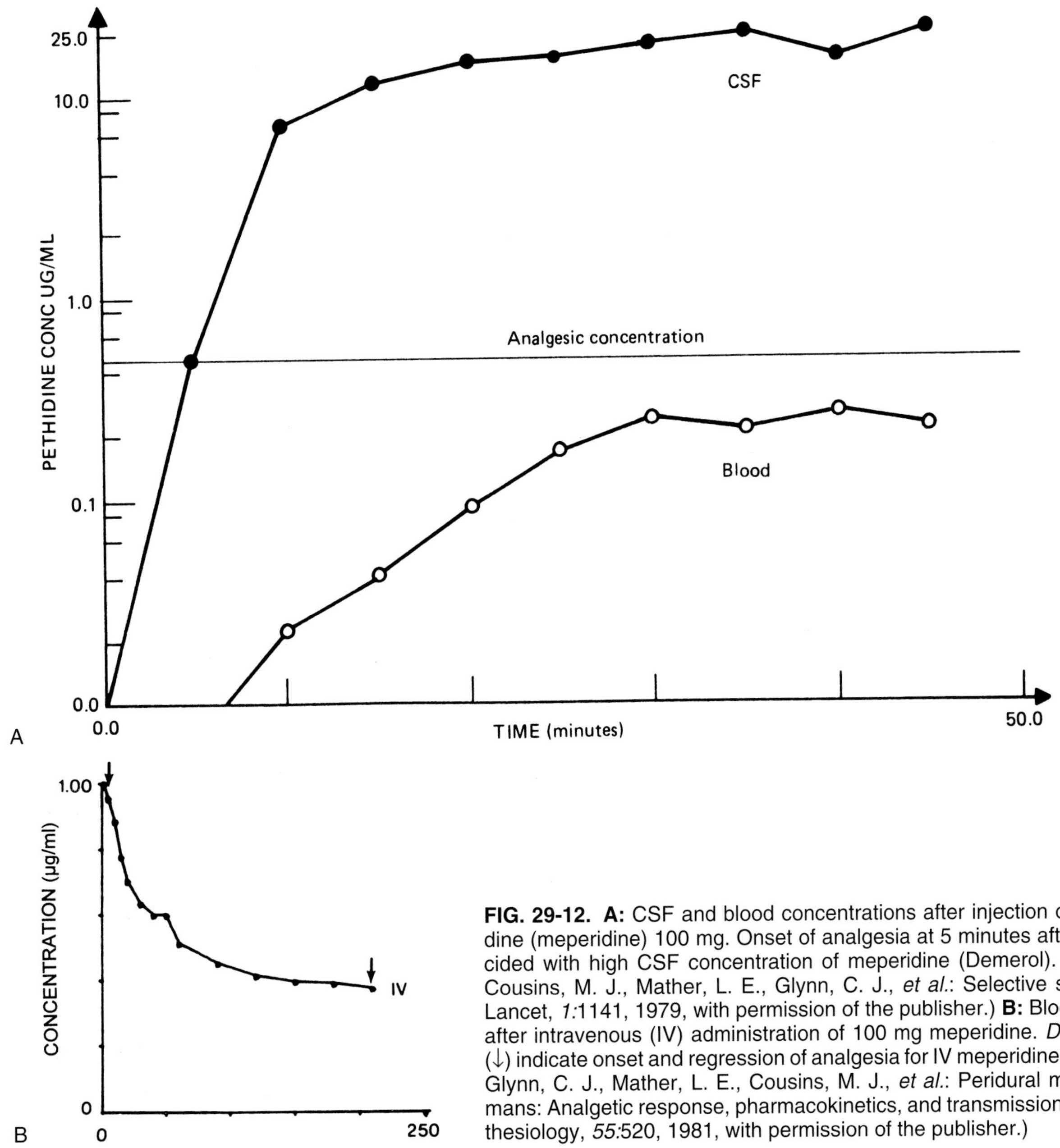

FIG. 29-12. A: CSF and blood concentrations after injection of epidural pethidine (meperidine) 100 mg. Onset of analgesia at 5 minutes after injection coincided with high CSF concentration of meperidine (Demerol). (Reprinted from Cousins, M. J., Mather, L. E., Glynn, C. J., *et al.*: Selective spinal analgesia. Lancet, *1:*1141, 1979, with permission of the publisher.) **B:** Blood concentration after intravenous (IV) administration of 100 mg meperidine. *Downward arrows* (↓) indicate onset and regression of analgesia for IV meperidine. (Reprinted from Glynn, C. J., Mather, L. E., Cousins, M. J., *et al.*: Peridural meperidine in humans: Analgetic response, pharmacokinetics, and transmission into CSF. Anesthesiology, *55:*520, 1981, with permission of the publisher.)

meperidine dose (e.g., 50 mg) is lower than an effective intramuscular dose (e.g., 100 mg) is consistent with a predominantly spinal action.[66,453] During repeated dosing with epidural meperidine at short intervals, vascular absorption inevitably will lead to systemic drug accumulation and redistribution centrally, since the elimination half-life of meperidine is reported to be 5 to 7 hours.[218] On the other hand, only the unbound fraction of intravenously administered meperidine is available to diffuse from the blood, and so the action of systemically administered drug is not reinforced by partitioning of drug into CSF.[49,312]

Epidural morphine pharmacokinetics and pharmacodynamics are well characterized and consistent with a spinal site of action after epidural drug administration.[58,217,341,357,358,397,478,504] Of all opioids studied in the postoperative period, morphine has the greatest dosage-sparing effect for epidural versus intravenous administration.[118] Average postoperative opioid doses and relative dosage requirements for morphine and other opioids given via the intravenous or epidural routes are shown in Table 29-7. The quality of morphine analgesia is superior when this drug is given epidurally than when it is given systemically,[64] and the analgesic effect of epidural morphine correlates poorly with blood morphine concentration. After epidural morphine, some patients report analgesia in the presence of extremely low serum morphine concentrations,[217,358] while others fail to achieve analgesia in the presence of typically analgesic blood concentrations.[102,144,397,504] A cross-over study in vol-

TABLE 29-7. *Relative analgesic potencies*

Postoperative intravenous (IV) and epidural (EPID) opioid dose requirements (ODR) over 17 h and relative ODR ratios of various opioids. IV ODR data corrected (corr) for elimination rate are also listed.

			Relative ODR ratios		
Opioid	(mg) IV	ODR (mg) EPID	IV vs EPID	EPID MOR vs EPID opioid	IV corr vs EPID
Morphine	45.9	5.0	9.2	1.0	35.0
Tramadol	455.0	180.0	2.5	0.03	18.0
Meperidine[a]	442.0	182.0	2.4	0.03	8.1
Methadone	13.0	10.3	1.3	0.5	29.0
Alfentanil	9.1	4.5	2.0	1.1	2.2
Fentanyl	1.2	0.4	3.0	12.5	27.0
Sufentanil	0.152	0.113	1.4	44.0	13.0
Buprenorphine	0.78	0.52	1.5	9.2	3.2

[a] Based upon the "active" R (-)-methadone enantiomer as used in Germany.

From Chrubasik, J., and Chrubasik, S.: Meta-analysis in the efficacy of intrathecal and epidural infusions of morphine for postoperative pain relief by means of a small, externally worn, infusion device. Anesthesiology. *62:* 263, 1985.

unteers found similar blood morphine levels 1 hour after 10 mg epidural or intravenous morphine, but subjects who received intravenous morphine did not experience analgesia. Six hours after epidural morphine, analgesia persisted despite low serum drug concentrations.[58,57] Because morphine metabolites appear in plasma shortly after morphine administration, studies based upon radioimmunoassays that detect morphine and its metabolites concurrently are suspect, e.g., in falsely depicting persistence of morphine or underestimating concentration–analgesia relationships. Nordberg and co-workers[358] used gas chromatography to avoid such analytic pitfalls and found that absorption of epidural morphine into the vascular system occurred rapidly, with peak arterial plasma concentrations occurring within 15 minutes. They reported that the ratio of lumbar CSF:plasma morphine concentrations increased with time after injection, and ranged from 45 to 100:1 at 1 hour to 125 to 175:1 at 5 hours. This increase appeared to be caused by dysequilibrium between plasma and tissue concentrations, since elimination half-lives of morphine in plasma and CSF compartments were similar (approximately four hours). Gustafsson and colleagues[217] and others[134] confirmed the rapid systemic absorption of epidural morphine and reported that peak plasma morphine concentrations occurred earlier, and were also higher (relative to dose) than after intramuscular morphine. It is likely that the hydrophilic nature of morphine minimizes uptake into epidural fat, that otherwise might serve to buffer venous absorption of more lipophilic opioids.[452] Based upon their re-evaluation of the octanol buffer partition coefficient for hydromorphone[381] which revealed it to be closer to that of morphine than previously reported, Cousins and colleagues examined CSF and blood pharmacokinetics of this drug, administered together with morphine, and found striking similarity between these two agents.[63]

Epidural fentanyl yields a quality of analgesia similar to that produced by epidural morphine, and is second only to morphine in the degree of dosage-sparing achieved by epidural versus intravenous drug delivery.[118] Again, in a manner similar to morphine, postoperative analgesia from epidural fentanyl and sufentanil is evident in patients whose plasma opioid concentrations are below analgesic levels.[473,521] Further, analgesia lasted longer and was more profound when the same dose of fentanyl was given epidurally, compared with intramuscularly.[249,296] Fentanyl blood concentrations in patients were reported to be lower for epidural than for intramuscular administration,[249,296] possibly due to fentanyl deposition in epidural fat.[12] A careful experimental study in healthy volunteers by Coda and colleagues[120] demonstrated that lumbar epidural fentanyl, alfentanil, and sufentanil, all produced selective lower extremity analgesia. For each of these 3 agents, low epidural doses yielded plasma levels well below their established minimally effective analgesic concentrations, but higher doses resulted in plasma concentrations that nearly reached minimally effective plasma opioid concentrations. Further support for a segmental action of sufentanil comes from the observation by Hansdottir and colleagues that concentrations of sufentanil are high in CSF near the site of epidural sufentanil administration, and exceed plasma concentrations. However, plasma drug levels during epidural infusion reached or exceeded minimally effective analgesic concentrations during postoperative infusions of fentanyl or sufentanil.[64]

Coda and colleagues concluded that while morphine produces supraspinal effects on the basis of rostral spread in CSF, lipophilic epidural opioids produce supraspinal effects through systemic redistribution. Although one must always be cautious about extrapolating from volunteers (or unstressed animals) to patients, because the blood–brain barrier becomes more permeable during environmental stress,[197] Coda's conclusion reinforces growing clinical experience that epidural administration of lipophilic opioids alone may offer little advantage over the intravenous route.[103,118,120] However, it is clinically valuable to coadminister epidural hydro- or lipophilic opioids and drugs, such as local anesthetics, whose systemic use is not feasible.[93] Hence, although it is now standard practice to employ opioid–local anesthetic mixtures of drugs for epidural analgesia, it is also appropriate to infuse epidural opioids alone for initial postoperative pain management in unstable patients not yet able to tolerate epidural local anesthetics. Upon stabilization (e.g., intravascular volume repletion) such patients can be switched to an epidural infusion containing opioid with local anesthetic. Moreover, when faced with inadequate analgesia cephalad to the epidural catheter tip during a postoperative epidural infusion of fentanyl (with or without local anesthetic), it is helpful first to change the infusate to epidural morphine to increase cephalad coverage and avoid having to reinsert a catheter at a more cephalad level. Such clinical strategies simplify anesthetic and analgesic management by employing the same epidural catheter for intra- and postoperative management while matching agent(s) infused, and the delivery rate, to a changing clinical status. Supplemental, patient-controlled epidural bolus doses to refine analgesic titration further are discussed in Chapter 26.

Pharmacokinetic Models of Intrathecal and Epidural Opioids

The above studies of spinal opioid analgesia have identified a number of factors that affect pharmacokinetics, and hence analgesic effects of such drugs. These factors, principally lipophilicity, dose, delivery mode (bolus vs. infusion), injectate volume, and addition of epinephrine, are summarized for the epidural route in Table 29-8. Pharmacokinetic models of spinal opioid distribution and clearance after intrathecal or epidural injection provide a coherent framework to consolidate preclinical and clinical observations. Classical compartmental descriptions are somewhat oversimplified, however, because the idealized notion of a solute being cleared with a particular rate constant applies only for a stirred pool.

Intrathecal injection of a highly ionized and hydrophilic drug such as morphine produces extremely high CSF concentrations.[280,342,257,486] The comparable onset times for

TABLE 29-8. *Epidural opioids and analgesia: summary of clinical factors affecting use*

Factor	Effect
Drug	
High hydrophilicity, e.g., morphine	Slow onset Long duration Extensive dermatomal spread Late onset respiratory depression
High lipid solubility, moderate receptor affinity, e.g., fentanyl, sufentanil	Rapid onset Duration only slightly longer than IM Very rare late onset respiratory depression
High lipid solubility, high receptor affinity, e.g. buprenorphine, lofentanil	Rapid onset Medium to long duration Very rare late onset respiratory depression
Dose	
Correlates with efficacy up to a plateau	
Large interindividual differences	
Increasing dose hastens onset, prolongs duration but increases risk of complications	
Suggested initial doses of morphine by lumbar epidural catheter:	
Thoracic, upper abdominal surgery	
<65 yrs: 4–6 mg	
>65 yrs: 2–4 mg	
Lower abdominal, hip surgery	
<65 yrs: 2–5 mg	
>65 yrs: 1–3 mg	
Lower limb surgery	
<65 yrs: 2 mg	
>65 yrs: 1–2 mg	
Dose reduced with thoracic catheter for thoracic and upper abdominal surgery	

From Cousins, M.J., Cherry, D.A., and Gourlay, G.K.: Acute and Chronic Pain: Use of spinal opioids. *In* Cousins, M.J. and Bridenbaugh, P.O. (eds.): Neural Blockade. pp. 955–1029. Philadelphia, J.B. Lippincott Publishers, 1988.

analgesia after intrathecal and epidural administration of morphine or other opioids has raised the still-unconfirmed possibility that vascular transport (e.g., via the posterior radicular artery,[133] Fig. 29-10) supplements diffusion from CSF as a mode of drug entry into the cord after either site of drug administration. Because it has low lipid solubility, morphine diffuses slowly from CSF to opioid receptors,[342] nonspecific binding sites and clearance sites (arachnoid granulations) of the spinal cord. Once in the spinal cord, morphine's slow egress produces a long duration of action.[452] Cephalad flow carries drug remaining in CSF[431] upwards toward the brain (Fig. 29-8). Spinal CSF flow to the brain may be hastened by Valsalva maneuver or intermittent positive-pressure ventilation. Morphine also is taken up into the systemic circulation, but plasma concentrations are subanalgesic.[101,357] Lazorthes and co-workers[280] measured morphine concentrations in lumbar spinal fluid after intrathecal administration of morphine (5 mg) in a hyperbaric solution. They found a distribution half-life of 22 minutes and elimination half-life of 4 hours, the latter value being similar to those reported after intrathecal[357] and epidural[358] administration. By comparison, radiolabeled albumin (which stays in the CSF) passes cephalad, so that 20% to 30% of a lumbar intrathecal dose moves intracranially within 12 hours and almost 100% within 24 hours.[164]

Intrathecal injection of an ionized, lipid soluble drug results in low residual concentrations in CSF[205,233] owing to rapid systemic uptake. Hence, less drug is carried in CSF to the brain. High lipid solubility facilitates access via the arterial route into the spinal cord, where drug enters rapidly and binds to opioid receptors and nonspecific binding sites. Unless a particular drug has high affinity for lipid or opioid receptor, however, egress is also rapid. Analgesia therefore tends to remain segmental. Fentanyl, which is over 90% ionized[310] at pH 7.4, has a more rapid onset and shorter duration of analgesia than morphine. Both lofentanil, which has lipid solubility similar to that of fentanyl but has a lower ionized fraction, and sufentanil, have prolonged durations of action, probably because of the persistence of both agents in lipid-binding sites in the spinal cord, and their high affinity for mu opioid receptors.[310,536] Diacetylmorphine (heroin), because of its higher lipid solubility, disappears from CSF much more rapidly than does morphine: minimal or no metabolism of heroin was detected in the spinal cord.[341]

Pharmacokinetic models of **epidural drug injection** are identical to those for intrathecal injection, but must in addition take into account drug equilibration and clearance from the epidural space.[452] (Fig. 29-13) After *epidural injection of a highly ionized and hydrophilic drug* such as morphine, (Fig. 29-13A) epidural concentrations of nonionized, lipid-soluble drug will be low. Transfer of morphine across arachnoid granulations is correspondingly slow, with a peak at 90 minutes,[134] and may rely partly on retrograde transport via cyclic vacuolation within epithelial cells of the arachnoid granulations. For the same reason, direct passage to spinal cord by way of spinal arteries (Fig. 29-10) may be limited. Absorption from the epidural space into the venous system is rapid and peak blood levels occur early,[213] achieving serial plasma morphine values close to those for the same dose given intramuscularly.[101] Because most of the drug present in CSF is ionized, only a small concentration gradient drives diffusion of un-ionized drug from CSF into the spinal cord receptors. For the same reason, later egress of drug from spinal cord to spinal fluid will be equally slow. High concentrations of ionized drug in spinal fluid will be carried rostrally with the CSF flow, extending the level of analgesia as well as migrating to supraspinal structures (Fig. 29-8). For morphine, the foregoing model is consistent with its slow onset and long duration of analgesia, and its potential for delayed respiratory depression—effects that correlate well with delayed peak CSF concentrations and prolonged, high, levels of morphine in cervical CSF after lumbar administration[213,357,453] (Figs. 29-9B ad 29-11).

Epidural injection of a mostly ionized lipophilic drug such as meperidine (Fig. 29-13B) will produce low concentrations of lipid-soluble, un-ionized drug in the epidural space. Un-ionized drug will rapidly be transferred from CSF, into spinal radicular arteries, and into epidural veins. In the presence of brisk spinal artery blood flow and slow epidural venous flow, transfer of the drug to the spinal cord will predominate while the concentration gradient is high. However, drug absorption into epidural veins will reduce the concentration gradient promptly. Egress from spinal cord receptors will be equally rapid, hastened by rapid uptake into epidural veins at the level of arachnoid granulations. Thus, analgesia will be rapid in onset and of moderate duration, fairly independent of the lipid solubility of the agent. Clinical observations confirm that the durations of epidural meperidine and fentanyl do not differ widely.[66,249]

Blood concentrations of epidurally administered opioids are influenced greatly by the dynamics of vertebral venous and arterial blood flow. Rapid absorption of meperidine into the systemic circulation after epidural dosing (Fig. 29-9) undoubtedly occurs via the extensive epidural venous plexus that feeds into the azygos vein. When intrathoracic pressure is high, venous (and drug) flow will be redirected through the basivertebral system up to the brain. Obstruction of the inferior vena cava, as happens in pregnancy, causes distention of epidural veins and increased flow through the azygos vein, which increases systemic absorption of epidural opioid and leaves less drug available for transfer across the dura to the spinal cord. Meperidine carried in the azygos vein to the superior vena cava is distributed to the general circulation and cleared rapidly in the liver. Studies of patients during labor confirm more rapid absorption of epidural meperidine than in nonpregnant women.[218,233,234] Also in pregnancy, epidural absorption is even more rapid than after intramuscular injection.[233] However, analgesia obtained from epidural meperidine during labor was transient (90 minutes) and appeared to correlate with plasma meperidine concentration.[378]

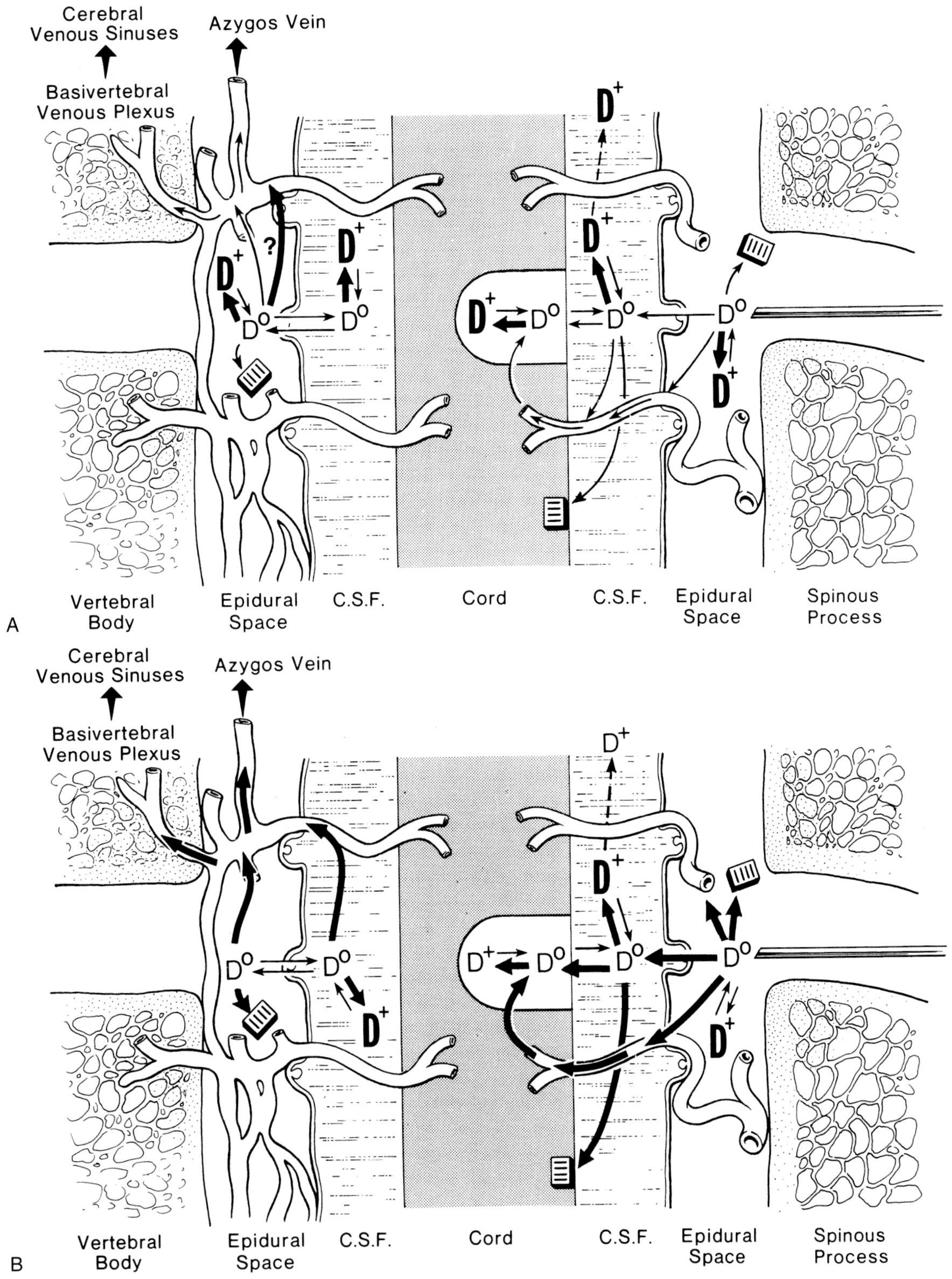

FIG. 29-13. **A:** Pharmacokinetic model: Epidural injection of a hydrophilic opioid such as morphine. *D*°, un-ionized drug; *D*⁺, ionized hydrophilic drug. Major route of clearance is through CSF. Shaded squares are nonspecific lipid binding sites. Role of radicular arteries in drug absorption remains unproven. **B:** Epidural injection of a lipophilic opioid such as meperidine or fentanyl. Note rapid passage of un-ionized species *(D°)* via CSF into cord and then clearance by epidural veins, leaving less ionized species *(D⁺)* remaining in CSF to migrate to brain.

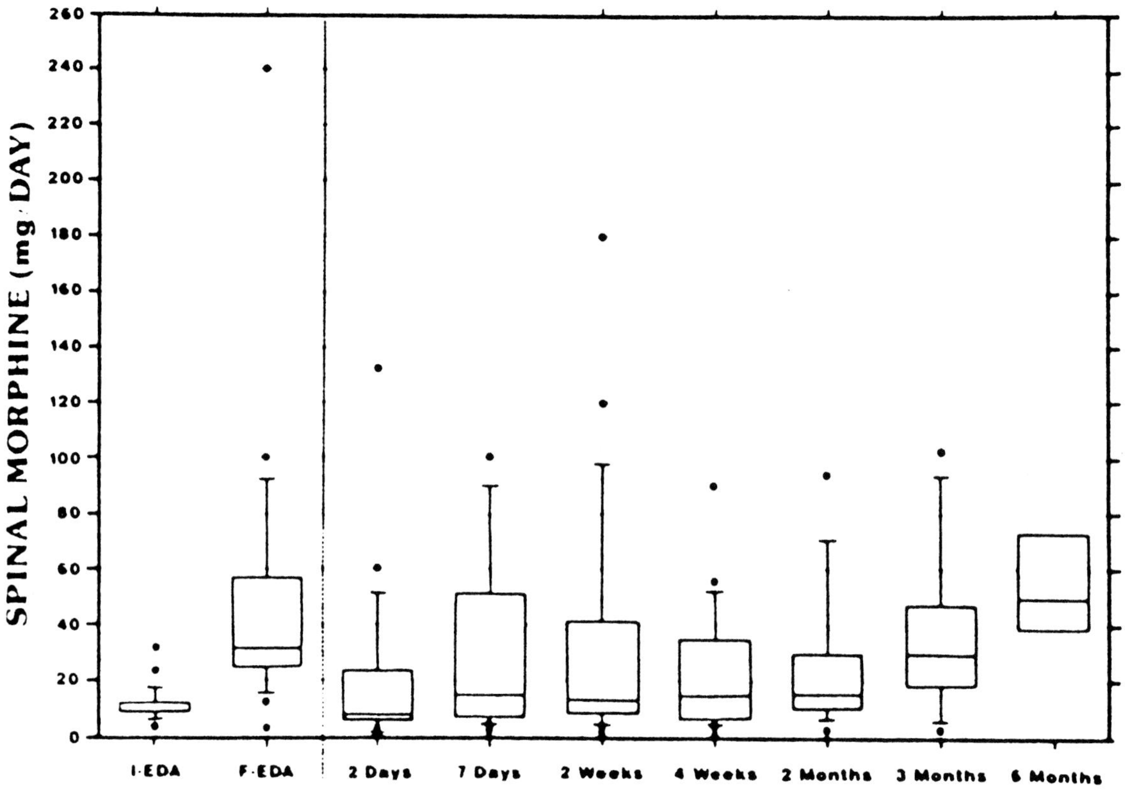

FIG. 29-14. Daily spinal doses of morphine during epidural (*initial* and *final, left of vertical line*) followed by chronic intrathecal (*right of vertical line*) co-infusion of morphine with bupivacaine for cancer pain. Lower and upper edges of boxes show 25th and 75th percentiles; 50th percentile shown by horizontal line within each box. Lower and upper "error bars" indicate 10th and 90th percentiles and dots indicate remaining outliers. Change over from epidural to intrathecal morphine was followed by two months of dose stability, after the first week of treatment. (From Nitescu, P., Appelgren, L., Linder, L. E., *et al.*: Epidural versus intrathecal morphine-bupivicaine: Assessment of consecutive treatments in advanced cancer pain. J. Pain Symptom Manage., *5:*18, 1990.)

It seems probable that early respiratory depression after epidural opioid (see earlier) is due to rapid, early vascular absorption together with transient increases in CSF drug concentrations at the base of the brain. For lipid-soluble opioids, such increases are smaller and briefer than for morphine (Fig. 29-9).[213,219,318] Late respiratory depression is less likely after lipid-soluble than after water-soluble opioids, but both early and late respiratory depression have been described after epidural fentanyl, meperidine, diamorphine, methadone, and sufentanil.[392] In such cases, one cannot exclude sudden redirection of blood flow through basivertebral veins to the brain, as a result of increased intrathoracic pressure, or inadvertent injection of a portion of the epidural dose into the subarachnoid space. Redistribution, rather than systemic clearance, probably is more important in reducing the risk of respiratory depression from blood-borne drug, since dosing intervals for most epidural opioids will be greater than plasma half-lives. An exception is methadone, which has an epidural dosing interval of approximately 4 to 8 hours but a plasma half-life of 24 to 48 hours.[214] Thus, repeated doses of epidural methadone at 8-hour intervals can produce systemic accumulation and an increased risk of delayed (and prolonged) respiratory depression.

SPINAL ANALGESIA: CLINICAL OPTIONS

A recent 17-nation survey by Rawal[392] suggests that the abundant preclinical and clinical research on novel agents for spinal analgesia, performed since the second edition of this text appeared a decade ago, has had little influence upon daily anesthesia practice. The only opioids given epidurally or intrathecally by 10 percent or more of the respondents were morphine (Fig. 29-14), fentanyl, sufentanil, buprenorphine, and meperidine (Table 29-9). Of nonopioids given spinally, excluding local anesthetics, only clonidine crossed the same threshold. Each of these opioids and clonidine, in addition to other agents acting through different mechanisms to achieve spinal analgesia, were described in the prior edition of this text. On the other hand, clonidine was just approved in 1997 by the U.S. Food and Drug Administration for epidural co-administration with opioids for refractory cancer pain,[80] and a variety of different spinal analgesics are now in Phase 1 and 2 clinical trials around the world.[81,434,489,539] It is possible, therefore, that the apparently slow pace of innovation in spinal analgesia may reflect several factors, not all of which are cause for pessimism. First, patient, surgeon, and anesthesiologist satis-

TABLE 29-9. *Choice of opioids for epidural of intrathecal administration in Europe*

	Choice, %			
	Epidural		Intrathecal	
Opioid	Mean	Range	Mean	Range
Morphine	81.2	20–100	54.9	20–100
Fentanyl	59.5	0–100	14.7	0–57
Sufentanil	22.2	0–80	7.1	0–40
Buprenorphine	14.9	0–71.4	1.7	0–28[a]
Meperidine	9.6	0–33	2.3	0–20[a]
Diacetylmorphine	4.7	0–80[b]	2.3	0–20[a]
Alfentanil	3.5	0–20[b]		
Nicomorphine	2.3	0–40[b]		
Piritramide	1.8	0–20[b]	1.2	0–20[a]
Oxycodone	1.2	0–20[b]		
Methadone	1.0	0–16.7[b]		

[a] These opioids are used intrathecally in only the following countries: buprenorphine (Italy), pethidine (France, Portugal), diamorphine (Ireland, United Kingdom), and piritramide (Austria).

[b] These opioids are used epidurally in only the following countries: diamorphine (United Kingdom), alfentanil (Belgium, Ireland, Norway), nicomorphine (Netherlands), piritramide (Austria, Germany), oxycodone (Finland), and methadone (Spain, United Kingdom).

From Rawal, N.: Neuraxial administration of opioids and opioids. *In* Brown, D.L. (ed.): Regional Anesthesia and Analgesia. pp. 208–231. Philadelphia, W.B. Saunders Company, 1996.

faction with currently available agents has remained fairly high since the second edition,[131] that appeared at the close of the initial decade of clinical spinal analgesia, after intense clinical experimentation and refinement around the world. Second, the message that effective analgesia not only improves quality of life but also can reduce short- and long-term cost and burden of care for patients with acute or chronic pain has emerged only recently from basic and clinical research (see below). Given the normally long time lag for novel clinical research findings to exert an impact upon practitioners, policy-makers, and regulators in any area of medicine,[82] years of delay are not unusual. Finally, increasing public demand for better pain control in acute and chronic illness, as well as at the end of life, has reinforced medical motives to optimize pain control and fostered a momentum of rising expectations for clinical analgesia among society at large. For these reasons, it is more appropriate than ever to review current and emerging analgesics and delivery methods, because it is likely that the pace of their clinical adoption will quicken during the next decade. Moreover, the trend to use of spinal drug combinations that target multiple mechanisms of analgesia (or single agents that act upon multiple pathways) mirrors multidrug therapy in many medical disciplines, and provides another reason to describe multiple classes of drugs in this section. Because the preclinical pharmacology of nociception has already been described in Chapter 23.1 and reviewed in detail in Chapter 24, the present description will not be comprehensive, but instead will focus upon agents that practicing anesthesiologists can now (or are likely soon to be able to) obtain. We will omit discussion of local anesthetics, whose basic and clinical features have already been surveyed in several earlier chapters (see Chapters 2–4, 8).

Opioids

Postoperative analgesia is the most common indication for spinal opioid use but long term spinal opioid infusion is being applied with increasing frequency for cancer-related, and also for chronic nonmalignant pain (see below). In the perioperative context, the practical choice between intrathecal versus epidural drug delivery is dictated by the operative procedure and projected duration of the need for optimal postoperative analgesia.[188,189,401] Because of the risk of post dural puncture headache and CSF leakage when conventional epidural catheters are placed intrathecally, and following withdrawal from the market of microcatheters that allowed continuous perioperative subarachnoid drug delivery, the epidural route remains the choice for all but one-shot analgesics.[203] As described in Chapter 24, in preclinical studies selective opioid agonists possess different selectivity against different types of pain. Mu opioid agonists are effective against thermal pain, while kappa opioid agonists are more effective against pressure or visceral pain models (e.g., formalin). On the other hand, clinically available kappa agonists such as butorphanol or nalbuphine are hardly used for spinal application and buprenorphine, which is used in a minority of cases, is a partial mu opioid agonist of low intrinsic efficacy. In fact, good models of postoperative and cancer pain do not yet exist[1,87,547] and so it is not clear how to extrapolate from available animal data to the bedside. The reality at present is that virtually all acute and chronic opioid analgesia is accomplished using mu opioid agonists that are phenylpiperidines or alkaloids (Table 29-10). In the near term, researchers in clinical trials are likely to re-explore promising pilot work since the 1970s that suggested a role for delta opioid peptides[13,343] as alternatives to mu agonists, but now using more selective and potent delta opioids than were earlier available.[168,302,433,448] Despite the increased potency of the newer delta-selective opioids, they remain relatively costly and require high doses for epidural or systemic use; their clinical application will be for intrathecal use. Sex differences in the response to systemic kappa opioid agonists may reflect estrogen-opioid interactions in the dorsal horn.[11]

Alpha-2 Agonists

Spinally applied epinephrine was observed to produce analgesia in animals a century ago, and in humans more than 50 years ago. For decades, veterinary experience with xylazine and other alpha-2 adrenergic agonists has provided convincing evidence that systemic administration of these

TABLE 29-10. *Intraspinal opioids for the treatment of acute pain*

Drug	Single dose[a] (mg)	Infusion rate[b] (mg/hr)	Onset (min)	Duration of single dose[c] (hours)
Epidural				
Morphine	1–6	0.1–1.0	30	6–24
Meperidine	20–150	5–20	5	4–8
Methadone	1–10	0.3–0.5	10	6–10
Hydromorphone	1–2	0.1–0.2	15	10–16
Diamorphine	4–6	?	5	12
Fentanyl	0.025–01	0.025–0.10	5	2–4
Sufentanil	0.01–0.06	0.01–0.05	5	2–4
Alfentanil	0.5–1	0.2	15	1–3
Subarachnoid				
Morphine	0.1–0.3		15	8–24+
Meperidine	10–30		?	10–24+
Diamorphine	1–2		?	20
Fentanyl	0.005–0.25		5	3–6

[a] Low doses may be effective when administered to the elderly or when injected in the cervical or thoracic region.
[b] If combining with a local anesthetic, consider using 0.0625% bupivacaine.
[c] Duration of analgesia varies widely; higher doses produce longer duration.

From Cousins, M.J., Cherry, D.A., and Gourlay, G.K.: Acute and chronic pain: Use of spinal opioids. *In* Cousins, M.J., and Bridenbaugh, P.O. (eds.): Neural Blockade. 2nd ed. pp. 955–1029. Philadelphia, J.B. Lippincott Publishers, 1988; and Ready, L.B., and Edwards, W.T. (eds.): Management of Acute Pain: A Practical Guide. Seattle, IASP Publications, 1992.

agents produces anesthesia. Unfortunately, these and other veterinary anesthetics that act upon adrenergic pathways are unsuitable for use in humans because they produce unpleasant psychological effects. The present era of integrated preclinical and clinical pharmacologic and toxicologic research dates from the 1980s. Prompted by emerging animal data,[537] Tamsen and Gordh administered epidural clonidine to 2 patients with chronic pain, with encouraging results. Since then, the presence of separate opioid and monoaminergic analgesic systems in the spinal cord has been well defined in a number of basic histological and pharmacological studies.[528,530] Of the latter, norepinephrine, acetylcholine (see following) and serotonin, are the principal, clinically relevant, mediators.[212] Because of its dose-dependent anxiolytic, sedative, sympatholytic, and anesthetic-sparing actions, clonidine has enjoyed popularity as a premedication, particularly before cardiovascular surgery.[147] Its propensity to cause hypotension limits systemic dosing, a side effect that is less prominent with the recently introduced and more potent alpha-2 agonist dexmedetomidine. Clonidine given systemically has an opioid-sparing effect. Gordh in his M.D. thesis further demonstrated in a controlled clinical trial the value of clonidine for epidural analgesia, and others, notably Eisenach[182] and the group of Filos, Goudas and colleagues,[191] carried this work further to show that intrathecal clonidine is nontoxic and can be effective as the sole postoperative spinal analgesic after general or obstetric surgery. More than 2,000 patients have now received epidural or intrathecal clonidine safely in published clinical trials. On the basis of this experience, one may prepare an aggregate figure, (Fig. 29-15) summarizing the fraction of patients achieving satisfactory analgesia after clonidine given as the sole analgesic, at various doses, by different routes[212] (Fig. 29-15). As with opioids, clonidine is active as an analgesic when administered systemically or centrally,[35] and in addition has been reported to augment the quality and duration of peripheral neural blockade with local anesthetic. Several pieces of evidence, parallel to those presented above for opioids, indicate that clonidine acts spinally to produce analgesia. Low doses of clonidine infused in the lumbar epidural space produce lower but not upper extremity analgesia, and this analgesia spreads to the upper extremity after prolonged infusion. Clonidine is more potent after epidural than systemic administration, and in volunteers as well as patients, CSF levels of clonidine predict pain relief with much greater accuracy than do blood levels.

Cholinomimetics and Cholinesterase Inhibitors

Spinal acetylcholine release occurs with acute pain in animals and (based upon weaker data) may also occur in clinical settings such as childbirth.[1,166,182] These data, along with the observation that alpha-2 adrenergic analgesia provokes release of acetylcholine from the dorsal horn, suggest that activation of cholinergic receptors is a mechanism of endogenous analgesia. Accordingly, following the same logic as outlined above for alpha-2 adrenergic spinal analgesia, many of the same preclinical and clinical investigators who advanced clonidine from laboratory into clinical practice also have undertaken studies to clarify and exploit cholinergic mechanisms in clinical spinal analgesia. Preclinical studies employing selective nicotinic and muscarinic agonists reveal a role for the latter, but not the former, acetylcholine receptor subtype in mediating spinal analgesic effects. The cholinesterase inhibitor neostigmine also has spinal analgesic properties in preclinical models, that result from increasing acetylcholine effects upon muscarinic receptors. Because preservative-free neostigmine is readily available, Phase 1 clinical safety testing began with this agent. Although neurotoxicity of spinal neostigmine was not apparent in animals, in Phase 1 clinical testing in volunteers, this agent had a poor effect-to-side-effect ratio. Minimal analgesic intrathecal doses (100 mg) produced nausea, vomiting, and transient lower extremity weakness. Initial dose-ranging studies by Lauretti and colleagues[279] in surgical patients confirmed a high incidence of nausea and vomiting at analgesic doses of neostigmine administered as a single intrathecal agent. However, subanalgesic doses of neostigmine had a substantial (30% to 70%) dosage-sparing effect upon supplemental opioid analgesia, while producing minimal nausea. Newer cholinomimetic compounds that enjoy a more favorable effect-to-side-effect ratio are reported now to be entering clinical trials.

Benzodiazepines

Animal studies have demonstrated that muscimol and baclofen, agonists at GABA-A and GABA-B receptors, respectively, produce analgesia upon intrathecal administration. Although baclofen is the sole GABA-ergic agent that has been approved by the U.S. Food and Drug Administration for intrathecal use, this approval is limited to therapy of spasticity, for which extensive post-approval clinical data attest to its efficacy and safety. Its analgesic potency in animal models[517,537] has not yet been evaluated in human trials. On the other hand, benzodiazepines, which enhance the effect of endogenous GABA upon GABA-A receptors, also produce analgesia when administered into the subarachnoid space in rats.[510] This analgesia is reversed by the benzodiazepine antagonist flumazenil as well as the GABA-A antagonist bicuculline. Limited clinical data on intrathecal and epidural administration of midazolam suggest a potential for neurotoxicity based upon prolonged (24 hours) effects after a single dose.

Ion Channel Blockers

Because spinal nociception depends upon ion flux to trigger postsynaptic depolarization in dorsal horn neurons, it is not surprising that all clinically useful spinal analgesics impede this process. Mu or delta opioid agonists inhibit potassium flux, kappa agonists inhibit calcium flux, and local anesthetics inhibit (principally) sodium flux. The paramount importance of calcium influx to initiate the intracellular cascade of genetic and biochemical responses to nociception is indisputable. For more than a decade, preclinical investigators have known that calcium channel blockade potentiates opioid analgesia produced by drugs or environmental stress, and suppresses the opioid abstinence syndrome. Clinical studies have not established an important analgesic effect for any of the previously available, L-type voltage-sensitive calcium channel (VSCC) blockers given as sole agents, although many such as nimodipine potentiate morphine analgesia.[190,430] Recently, however, progress in molecular cloning and electrophysiology has revealed numerous VSCCs with different locations and functional properties.[51]

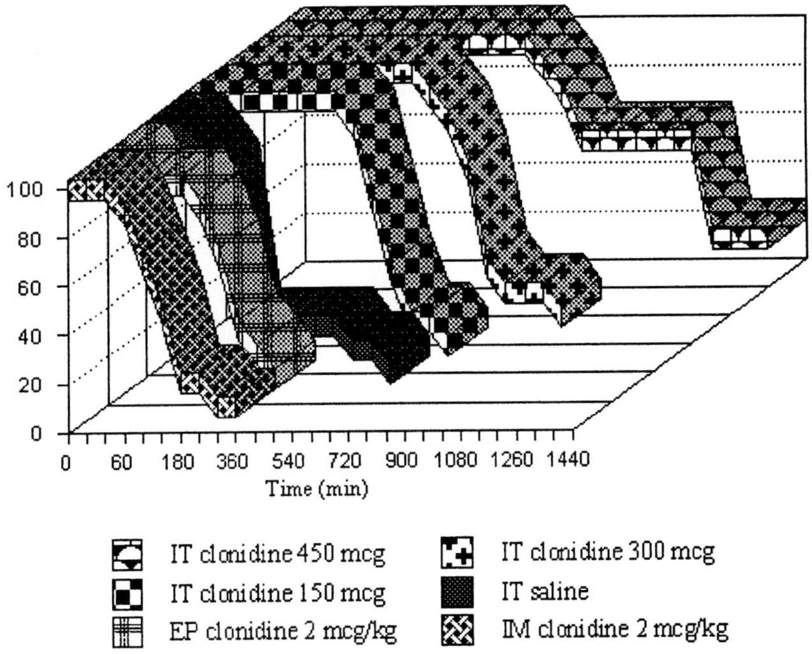

FIG. 29-15. Percentage of patients with satisfactory analgesia after single doses of clonidine. Doses and route (from front to rear of figure): 2 mcg/kg clonidine intramuscular; 2 mcg/kg clonidine epidural; saline intrathecal controls; clonidine 150 mcg intrathecal; clonidine 300 mcg intrathecal; clonidine 450 mcg intrathecal. Pooled data from systematic review: Goudas, L. C., Carr, D. B., Lau, J. *et al.*: The spinal clonidine-opioid analgesic interaction: From laboratory animals to the operating room: A systematic analysis of preclinical and clinical evidence. Analgesia, [In Press].

N-type VSCCs are located almost exclusively on neurons, and are particularly abundant in regions rich in synaptic connections.[491] N-type VSCCs regulate calcium flux across presynaptic neurons that release neurotransmitters during depolarization. In the mid-1980s, peptide "conotoxins" were isolated from the venom of fish-hunting cone snails that capture their prey by paralyzing them. Some omega-conopeptides, the synthetic analogs of these so-called omega-conotoxins, selectively blocked N-type VSCCs but had little effect upon mammalian neuromuscular transmission. After preclinical testing revealed one of these conopeptides (SNX-111) to be particularly potent as a spinal analgesic in animal models of acute and chronic pain, Phase 1 and 2 clinical trials were accomplished. To date, favorable analgesic responses have been reported in multicenter, unblinded, trials of intrathecal SNX-111, administered as a sole agent for as long as 9 months to treat morphine-resistant, refractory pain due to malignancy or neuropathy. Side effects included nausea, lightheadedness (presumably from orthostatic hypotension), headache, constipation, and confusion. Larger scale, controlled trials are now under way. Preclinical data on potassium channel openers administered intrathecally also point towards a similar analgesic potential but clinical trials are not yet under way.

NMDA Antagonists

The importance of excitatory amino acids as mediators of the transition from immediate to prolonged pain has been summarized in Chapter 23.1 and earlier in this chapter, and reviewed in detail in Chapter 24. Insight into the role of these mediators is a key advance in understanding pain physiology since the prior edition of this text a decade ago.[160,523] Although ketamine acts at several sites, it is readily available to clinicians and is known to block the open calcium channel on the NMDA receptor complex. Hence, a profusion of studies have been carried out with ketamine in the brief time since its potential clinical value as an NMDA receptor blocker has become appreciated.[540] Given systemically, ketamine appears to block central summation of experimental second pain, and to reduce pain intensity in instances of neurogenic pain, as in postherpetic neuralgia or phantom limb pain.[269] Postoperative clinical studies usually have employed it as an adjunctive intravenous medication, although a few clinicians have co-administered it in a pre-emptive fashion at the time of initial epidural analgesia.[109] Choe and colleagues, for example, found a greater duration of analgesia, and reduction in supplemental postoperative analgesic requirements, when ketamine (60 mg) was added to morphine (2 mg) given epidurally before induction of anesthesia. On the other hand, results from clinical trials in which ketamine was administered postoperatively as the sole epidural agent have been unimpressive. Cousins and colleagues have found that subcutaneous infusion of ketamine is a valuable adjunct to permit tapering of intrathecal morphine in patients with opioid tolerance after chronic intrathecal infusion.[494] In this context, addition of ketamine prevents rebound hyperalgesia when the intrathecal infusate is switched from morphine to local anesthetic. The other NMDA open-channel blocker in common clinical use is dextromethorphan, an inactive opioid isomer long used as an antitussive. However, dextromethorphan is not formulated for spinal use and clinical trials have administered it orally instead, also (as with ketamine as a sole agent) with unimpressive results. Other agents that act upon the open calcium channel of the NMDA receptor complex, such as MK-801 or phencyclidine, produce unacceptable dysphoria and related psychological side-effects, and so are unsuitable for systemic administration. Phencyclidine, given intrathecally in a pilot clinical study, abolished allodynia and hyperpathia due to chronic neurogenic pain. More selective or better tolerated agents that act upon other sites on the NMDA receptor complex, such as its glycine binding site, are now under development. Intriguingly, the venerable antidepressant amitriptyline, used orally for decades to treat neuropathic pain,[238] recently has been found to bind with high affinity to the NMDA receptor and to suppress NMDA-induced hyperalgesia after intrathecal administration in animals. As a monoamine uptake inhibitor, amitriptyline also enhances analgesia at the spinal level by augmenting the actions of norepinephrine and serotonin (paralleling the above-described effect of intrathecal neostigmine to augment spinal acetylcholine analgesia). Preclinical and Phase 1 clinical studies of safety and efficacy of amitriptyline for intrathecal use are now under way, raising the interesting prospect that both old and new drugs will soon be in clinical trials as intrathecal agents directed against NMDA-induced hyperalgesia.[182]

NSAIDs and Nitric Oxide Synthase Inhibitors

As described above, co-release of substance P and glutamate from presynaptic neurons of the dorsal horn evokes prolonged postsynaptic depolarization and intense calcium influx through the NMDA receptor complex.[470] While NMDA receptor antagonism is one promising strategy to develop novel spinal analgesics, an alternative approach is to inhibit key intracellular enzymes activated by calcium entry into the postsynaptic cell (or experimentally by intrathecal application of NMDA.) Two such intraneuronal enzymes, both known to play a role in wind-up and hyperalgesia, are nitric oxide synthase (NOS) and phospholipase A2.[22] These generate, respectively, nitric oxide[265] from arginine, and arachidonic acid from membrane phospholipid. Arachidonic acid is a substrate for cyclo-oxygenase (COX) isozymes, COX-1 and COX-2, that act upon it to produce a variety of prostanoids. COX-1 is constitutively active in platelets, gastric mucosa, and kidney; inhibition of COX-1 by nonselective NSAIDs correlates with side effects at these sites. COX-2 is induced by inflammation and pain, and is the target of pharmaceutical development to produce new, selective NSAIDs that have a lower side-effect liability.[475] Interestingly, nitric oxide activates COX-1 and COX-2. Preclinical data[303,544] indicate that spinal administration of the NOS inhibitor L-NAME blocks thermal hyperalgesia as well as NMDA-induced hyperalgesia, but little work has been done to harness this effect clinically. In contrast, spinal application of NSAIDs dates back to the 1970s, when Devulder administered lysine salicylate intrathecally to provide analgesia for a patient with refractory cancer pain. Other scattered case reports followed, and in the early to mid-1990s were augmented by a number of preclinical observations of spinal cord release of prostanoids along with excitatory amino acids during nociception from peripheral nerve injury or inflammation.[333,457] Brune, McCormack,[324] Yaksh,[304] and others[487] described antinociception and reversal of hyperalgesia by small doses of centrally administered NSAIDs (including acetaminophen) and distinguished between anti-inflammatory and analgesic mechanisms of NSAIDs.[98] A variety of possible mechanisms for the central analgesic effects of NSAIDs are now under preclinical study; prominent among these are inhibition of presynaptic neurotransmitter release in the dorsal horn through inhibition of presynaptic adenyl cyclase and interference with postsynaptic, NMDA-evoked gene expression. The next generation of clinical administration of spinal NSAIDs, encompassing Phase 1 safety assessment and later controlled clinical trials, is likely to commence shortly.

Adenosine and Nonopioid Peptides

Adenosine receptors are expressed on the surface of nearly all cells. Five adenosine receptors have been identified through pharmacological and cloning techniques, of which the A1 receptor appears most closely linked to analgesia, although a delayed analgesic effect, mediated through the A2 receptor, has been reported.[154] The affinity of a number of adenosine analogs for the A1 receptor appears to correlate well with their in vivo analgesic potency. Indirect evidence suggests that analgesia from central administration of opioids[153] or serotonin is mediated by spinal cord adenosine release.[155] However, although a number of adenosine analogs produce analgesia when given intrathecally in animals,[156] and blockade of endogenous adenosine by spinal application of theophylline produces hyperalgesia,[157] clinical trials of the possible analgesic effects of spinal A1 or A2 activation have not been reported. To date, a single pilot study of intrathecal A1 antagonism in the human has described touch- or vibration-induced allodynia.[292]

A host of peptide systems modulate nociceptive transmission,[291] but studies of their value as targets of intrathecal or epidural analgesia have lagged. The inflammatory and nociceptive effects of substance P and related tachykinins are mediated through receptors termed NK1, NK2, and NK3. Intrathecal injection of NK1 antagonists blocks hyperalgesia in animal models of formalin injection or sciatic nerve ligature.[36] Clinical trials of substance P antagonism have been limited to topical application of a substance P antagonist, and have not included spinal administration despite encouraging data from animal studies (see following). Very low doses of substance P itself potentiate opioid analgesia,[273] perhaps by presynaptic inhibition of substance P release, but clinical trials have not yet been conducted to exploit the therapeutic potential of this paradoxical observation. Cholecystokinin (CCK) and neuropeptide FF appear to function as anti-opioid peptides, particularly as active mediators of opioid tolerance at the spinal level.[329,462] Given intrathecally along with morphine in animals, antagonists to the CCK-B receptor avert morphine tolerance and augment analgesia but have little effect when used as sole agents.[169] Clinical trials of CCK-B receptor antagonists employing the spinal route appear warranted. Of the analgesic peptides employed for spinal administration, the inhibitory peptide somatostatin stands alone in its mixture of success and controversy.[541] Initially reported as effective against postoperative as well as refractory cancer pain, its use was clouded by animal data that disclosed substantial neurotoxicity upon intrathecal administration. Its use was abandoned, until the stable somatostatin analog octreotide was introduced. Thus far, as with somatostatin itself, there has been no documented clinical neurotoxicity, despite analgesia for up to 3 months of intrathecal infusion for opioid-resistant cancer pain. Calcitonin has also been administered epidurally with favorable, if anecdotal, results.

Combination Analgesic Chemotherapy

Aggressive treatment of serious conditions throughout current medical practice typically relies upon multiple forms of therapy delivered simultaneously. Examples of this multimodal approach are easy to come by, whether one considers infection such as tuberculosis, sepsis or human immunodeficiency virus/acquired immunodeficiency syndrome (HIV/AIDS), neoplastic disease; or refractory instances of everyday disorders, such as hypertension, cardiac arrhythmias, or depression. The broad power of such an approach no doubt reflects the multivariate nature of these clinical conditions, and the utility of attacking as many variables as feasible to bring such disorders decisively under control. If one considers that the spinal cord has evolved as an organ of programmed instability (see page 971), poised to become sensitized even after brief exposure to moderate nociceptive input, then the merit of suppressing many elements within this process is apparent.[458] The profound influence of classical pharmacology upon present-day analgesia research and practice probably accounts for a preoccupation with synergy in discussions about the merits of drug combinations to control pain. Preclinical evaluation of synergy may provide important leads to guide exploratory clinical trials, or insight into the mechanisms underlying drug-drug interactions. Solmon and Gephart,[456] and Yaksh and Malmberg,[543] have surveyed such interactions at the spinal level (Table 29-11), thereby providing a useful framework to survey current and future practice. Yet in daily clinical practice, Dickenson[163] has pointed out that "the seeking of synergy could be an un-

TABLE 29-11. *Interaction of different pairs of receptor agonists following intrathecal delivery in the rat*

Spinal agonist pairing	Test	Interaction	Fractional dose
Mu-delta	Hot plate	Synergistic	0.30–0.50
	Tail flick	Synergistic	0.34
Mu-alpha-2	Hot plate	Synergistic	0.10
	Hot plate	Additive	1.10
	Tail flick	Synergistic	0.10–0.70
Mu-local anesthetics	Hot plate	Synergistic	0.70
	Hot plate	Synergistic	0.15
Mu-cycloox. inhib.	Formalin test, phase 1	Synergistic	0.08
	Formalin test, phase 2	Synergistic	0.14
Mu-neostigmine	Hargreaves thermal stimulation	Additive	0.80
Alpha-2-delta	Tail flick	Synergistic	0.06
Alpha-2-adenosine	Hot plate	Synergistic	0.55
	Tail flick	Synergistic	0.60
Alpha-2-cycloox. inhib.	Formalin test, phase 1	Synergistic	0.33
	Formalin test, phase 2	Synergistic	0.52
Alpha-2-neostigmine	Hargreaves thermal stimulation	Synergistic	0.56
Alpha-2-kappa	Tail flick	Synergistic	0.60
Kappa-cycloox. inhib.	Formalin test, phase 1	Additive	1.50
Adenosine-cycloox. inhib.	Formalin test, phase 2	Additive	0.90
NMDA antag-cycloox. inhib.	Formalin test, phase 2	Additive	>1

From Yaksh, T.L., and Malmberg, A.B.: Interaction of spinal modulatory receptor systems, *In* Fields, H.L. and Liebeskind, J.C. (eds.): Pharmacological Approaches to the Treatment of Chronic Pain: New Concepts and Critical Issues. pp. 151–171. Seattle, IASP Press, 1994.

necessary Holy Grail" because all that matters is whether the therapeutic benefit of a combination exceeds that of each component. Beyond this, "synergism. . . is the icing on the cake." Such a point of view avoids complex, often unresolvable, debates as to how best to reconcile animal studies that disclose one pattern of drug-drug interaction such as synergy, and clinical findings of a somewhat different pattern, such as additivity. It also fits well with the current worldwide trend in all areas of medicine to let assessment of practical clinical outcomes guide medical practice (see following). From this standpoint, we will describe several drug combinations whose application to clinical spinal analgesia offers advantages beyond those achieved with single agents, without regard to whether in clinical practice the dosage-sparing interaction is synergistic, additive, or subadditive.

Opioid-opioid interactions have been investigated in several respects, varying from the simultaneous administration of the same opioid spinally plus peripherally[547], to mixing of different opioids spinally.[474] The rationale for the latter approach is twofold. First, animal studies clearly show that combination of spinal opioids gives rise to an extremely powerful dosage-sparing effect.[543] This dosage-sparing effect has been most clearly shown for mu- plus delta-selective opioids,[6,481] a combination that is not yet able to be employed clinically because the latter agents are still in safety testing. A similar statement may be made concerning enkephalin dimers, that typify the design of single molecules with the capacity to act upon multiple receptors simultaneously (see following). Second, owing to the distinct pharmacodynamic properties of lipo- versus hydrophilic opioids that were described above, single spinal doses of the former agents have a rapid onset but also a rapid offset, while the latter offer long duration but slow onset. For this reason, fentanyl has been added to morphine,[474] in an effort to overcome the early analgesic trough. Interestingly, the clearest benefit of this combination is evident when epidural morphine is given before epidural fentanyl. Not unexpectedly, combination of mu opioid agonists with clinically available kappa opioid agonists (that also have mu antagonist actions) has led to results that are difficult to consolidate owing to biphasic responses to different dosage ratios or frankly conflicting results.

Opioid-local anesthetic interactions at the spinal level are now a cornerstone of daily clinical practice.[55] Attempts to demonstrate postoperative benefits from systemic co-infusion of these agents have not succeeded,[93] although in animals systemic lidocaine infusion relieves tactile allodynia for prolonged intervals.[97,468] Based upon compelling preclinical data,[196,476] local anesthetics to provide single-dose spinal anesthesia for surgery are supplemented with small doses of intrathecal opioid such as meperidine,[315] fentanyl, or morphine, to secure postoperative analgesia in patients at many medical centers worldwide. Sameridine, a novel molecule with both local anesthetic and opioid properties, is being tested in clinical trials as a new spinal anesthetic that offers prolonged postoperative pain control.[79] After major surgery or trauma, epidural infusion of a combination of local anesthetic plus opioid is now the worldwide standard by which other methods of acute pain management are judged.[188,283,490] Many clinical reports attest to the safety and efficacy—particularly for movement-related pain[225,388]—of such combinations in thousands of patients, and indicate a reduction of side effects that would be expected if comparable degrees of analgesia were attained through application of each agent alone.[10,149,251] These reports are surveyed in Chapter 26, along with some examples of typical doses for opioids, alone and mixed with local anesthetics. These examples are supplemented by Table 29-12, which describes typical concentrations of each component, infusion rates of the mixture, and incremental dosing to manage breakthrough pain.[148] The value of such mixtures, particularly in managing incident or movement-related pain,[492] has led to their adoption outside the acute care setting, for chronic management of cancer-related and nonmalignant pain. Keeping the concentration of bupivacaine below 0.1% minimizes the incidence of sensorimotor block during both acute and chronic infusion. An earlier section of this chapter describes mechanisms by which the spinal application of nonopioid plus opioid analgesics may have not only a dosage-sparing, but also a tolerance-impeding, effect. Indeed, Nitescu,[352] Sjoberg,[450] and others have documented modest, easily managed dosage escalations of a morphine-bupivacaine mixture during chronic intrathecal infusion for cancer pain (Fig. 29-14). In the rare event that opioid tolerance should develop, based upon the experience of Lema and colleagues[148] it is likely that analgesia can be re-established by substituting sufentanil for morphine. In the settings of both acute[339,410] and chronic pain management, a third component—a systemic NSAID—increasingly is added to the opioid-local anesthetic combination to control breakthrough pain, or as a multimodal strategy to optimize analgesia during activity, and to minimize doses required of each individual agent.

Opioid-alpha 2 interactions underlie the dosage-sparing (or analgesia-potentiating) effects of adrenergic agonists upon spinal opioids in preclinical studies that use behavioral or electrophysiological endpoints.[212] In humans, clonidine augments opioid-induced sedation but not respiratory depression; hypotension is not a common side-effect of opioids, but is frequent with clonidine. Clinical studies of opioid-clonidine combinations for spinal analgesia do not show as dramatic a dosage reduction as animal data (that clearly demonstrate synergy), but are distinctly promising. A valuable complementary effect of intrathecal coadministration of opioids with clonidine is the benefit of the latter agent for neuropathic pain, that in general is less sensitive to opioids.[366] Clonidine also can benefit sympathetically maintained pain that is often a component of chronic neuropathic pain due to cancer or nonmalignant causes. The approval in the U.S. of clonidine as an adjunct to epidural opioids for opioid-resistant cancer pain, based upon its efficacy in controlled clinical trials, will encourage spinal coadministration of these two drug classes to treat other refractory pain, such as from spinal cord injury.[445,447] Dexmedetomidine, a second-generation alpha-2 agonist, produces hypotension less frequently than does clonidine, and currently is in clinical trials as a preoperative medication for perioperative sympatholysis and analgesia.[210] It is likely that this newer agent will prove better tolerated and equally analgesic as clonidine; if so, then it is expected that clinical trials of its spinal application will soon follow.

Apart from the above major interactions that are now part of everyday anesthetic and analgesic practice, a number of other favorable preclinical interactions are under evaluation in clinical trials. Opioid-NMDA interactions, exemplified by coadministration of the currently available NMDA antagonists dextromethorphan or ketamine, are under intense study in many trials currently under way. Already, it is clear that clinically available NMDA antagonists, such as ketamine given spinally, have an analgesia-augmenting and dosage-sparing interaction with spinal opioids.[109] Preclinical studies demonstrate suppression of spinal *c-fos*[99,228] expression or delaying of opioid tolerance by coadministration of morphine and an NMDA antagonist. Most, but not all investigators, have reported that addition of clonidine to local anesthetic intensifies and prolongs anesthesia for peripheral nerve block as it does for intrathecal/epidural block. The combination of intrathecal neostigmine and epidural clonidine has been found to produce additive analgesia in a clinical volunteer study, without adding side effects. Indeed, neostigmine antagonizes the hypotension otherwise seen when intrathecal clonidine is administered as a single agent. Novel analgesic approaches based upon concurrent opioid receptor activation and neurokinin receptor blockade[336], in-

TABLE 29-12. *Epidural opioid/bupivacaine combinations administered by continuous infusion*

Drug combinations	Solution	Bolus dose of bupivacaine (%)	Basal infusion rate	Rescue doses	Increments in serial rescue doses
Morphine	0.01%		6–8 mL/h	1–2 mL every 10–15 min	1 mL of the solution
+ Bupivacaine	0.05–0.01%	0.5–0.25%			
Hydromorphone	0.0025–0.005%		6–8 mL/h	1–3 mL every 10–15 min	1 mL of the solution
+ Bupivacaine	0.05–0.1%	0.5–0.25%			
Fentanyl	0.001%		0.1–0.15 mL kg^{-1} h^{-1}	1–1.5 mL every 10–15 min	1 mL of the solution
+ Bupivacaine	0.05–0.1%	0.5–0.25%			
Sufentanil	0.0001%		0.1–0.2 mL kg^{-1} h^{-1}	1–1.5 mL every 10–15 min	1 mL of the solution
+ Bupivacaine	0.05–0.1%	0.5–0.25%			

From de Leon-Casasola, O.A., and Lema M.J.: Postoperative epidural opioid analgesia: What are the choices? Anesth. Analg. *83*:867, 1996.

cluding the prospect of accomplishing these dual goals with a single molecule,[309] have shown promise in preclinical testing (Fig. 29-16) and are under toxicological evaluation prior to planned clinical trials. As described above, clinical trials with triads of agents such as local anesthetic, opioid and NSAID have reinforced the attractiveness of multimodal analgesia.[256,339] Preclinical stability testing indicates that the triad of morphine, clonidine, and bupivacaine is feasible to employ for long-term use in an implanted pump device.[526] Considering that the number of possible combinations of different analgesics rises as a factorial function of the number of available choices, clinical investigators around the world for some years to come will be occupied in determining the optimum selection and ratios of agents to apply to different patient populations with different origins of pain.

Prolonged Spinal Drug Delivery: Butamben, Depot Preparations, Chromaffin Cell Implants and Gene Therapy

Development of long-acting anesthetic or analgesic agents[406] to secure days or weeks of analgesia after operations or during the course of chronic, painful, conditions such as cancer, has been a goal of anesthesiologists for more

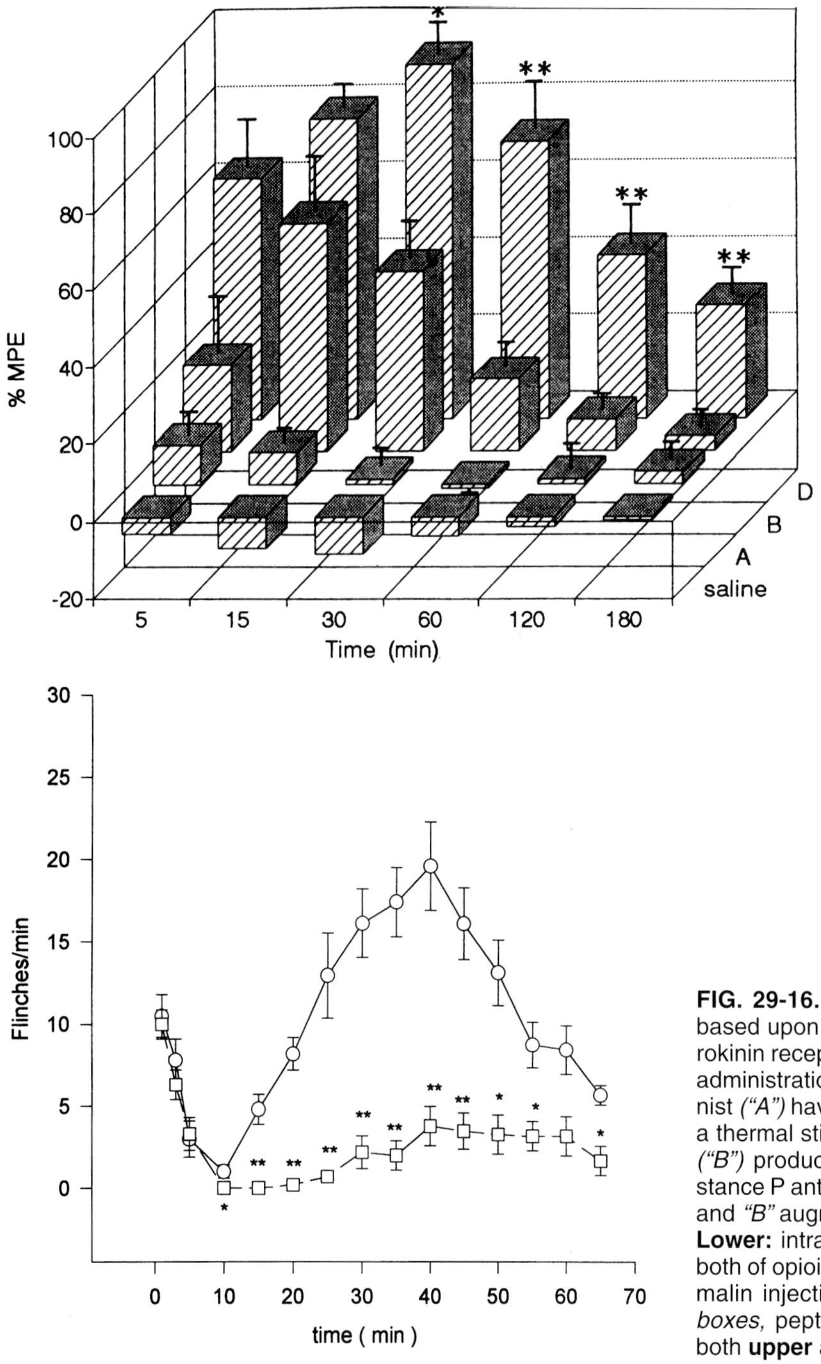

FIG. 29-16. Combination intrathecal analgesic therapies based upon concurrent opioid receptor activation and neurokinin receptor blockade in preclinical (rat) models. **Upper:** administration of intrathecal saline or substance P antagonist *("A")* have little effect upon tail flick latency testing using a thermal stimulus. The opioid peptide biphalin given alone *("B")* produces analgesia. Co-administration *("D")* of substance P antagonist plus biphalin at same doses given in *"A"* and *"B"* augments and prolongs the analgesic response.[336] **Lower:** intrathecal injection of a peptide having properties both of opioid agonist and substance P antagonist, after formalin injection, suppresses tail flinch response.[309] *Open boxes,* peptide; *open circles,* saline control injection. For both **upper** and **lower** figures: *, $P < 0.05$; **, $P < 0.01$.

than 70 years. Butamben (or n-butyl-p-aminobenzoate, an ester of para-aminobenzoic acid and butyl alcohol) is nearly insoluble in water, and for this reason, was employed topically for decades. Beginning in the mid-1980s, Shulman and colleagues,[444] as well as Korsten, Grouls, and co-workers[215] prepared aqueous suspensions of 5% to 10% butamben and observed months of selective analgesia (i.e., without motor block or impaired bladder/bowel function) after epidural application of such suspensions in animals, and humans with refractory cancer pain. In animal studies, the suspension behaved like a low-potency local anesthetic, whose prolonged action resulted from slow dissolution of solid, particulate, compound in the epidural space.[215] The mode of action of butamben may be distinct from that of traditional local anesthetics in that it appears to act upon tetrodotoxin insensitive sodium channels (see Chapter 3). It is plausible that the selectivity of neural blockade exhibited by butamben reflects its access to and action upon nodes of Ranvier in the dorsal epidural space, because motor and large sensory fibers within this space contain an insufficient number of nodes of Ranvier to render them susceptible to blockade. The suspension's very high viscosity has discouraged its widespread clinical use, but recent advances in formulation address this problem and have rekindled interest in clinical trials of this agent. The strategy of deliberately increasing the viscosity of local anesthetic solutions by mixing them with macromolecular compounds is nearly as old as butamben. High molecular weight dextrans were used in the 1930s for this purpose, to prolong the duration of local anesthetics and restrict their spread. More recently, gels such as substituted celluloses or polymers have been used to achieve this objective, but only with moderate prolongation to date. Another simple approach reported to prolong postoperative epidural analgesia is for the surgeon to place an absorbable sponge soaked with morphine and methylprednisolone at the operative site during lumbar discectomy. However, this method obviously is suitable only for open spinal procedures, is not titratable, and the amount of drugs delivered cannot be controlled.[406]

Physicochemical properties of local anesthetics and opioids have been exploited to form a complex of such agents with charged, high, molecular weight molecules such as hyaluronic acid, or to trap them within hydrophobic domains of polymers such as cyclodextrin. Both approaches have achieved slow release of local anesthetic or opioid in preclinical models of epidural or intrathecal injection, while at the same time decreasing systemic uptake of such agents.[406]

Polymer chemistry has created diverse approaches to drug incorporation in a variety of matrices that are engineered to degrade and deliver drug for a number of days to weeks *in situ*. Microspheres containing bupivacine within a polylactic acid matrix have, in preclinical studies employing the epidural route, produced only modest, dose-dependent prolongation of anesthesia compared to bupivacaine in solution, in contrast to the clear lengthening of duration of nerve block when microspheres containing bupivacaine or tetracaine are given peripherally. For this reason, clinical trials of these microspheres for peripheral nerve block are taking place with higher priority than are trials of their use in spinal analgesia. Similarly encouraging preclinical data for peripheral or spinal drug administration has been obtained with polyanhydride polymers as well as copolymers in which local anesthetic or opioid is incorporated for peripheral or spinal administration. Another broad strategy with substantial promise is based upon incorporation of local anesthetics or opioids into lipid carriers.[262] Simply dissolving local anesthetic or opioid in hyperbaric radiography contrast medium (iophendylate) produces a lipid solution that provides longer-lasting epidural anesthesia or analgesia than aqueous administration of these respective agents. However, iophendylate is not approved for intraspinal use, and given the potential for toxicity, application of such preclinical findings must be approached slowly and with caution. Lecithin-coated microcrystals, microemulsions and liquid crystals have been constructed to incorporate local anesthetics, but little work has been done so far to apply these technologies *in vivo*. Liposomes are vesicles that consist of phospholipid bilayers separated by an aqueous phase; depending upon the pK of the drug to be incorporated (i.e., base or hydrochloride) it will be trapped in one or the other phase.[344] In addition to possible local inflammatory effects induced by liposomes (that can also occur with polymers) chemical integrity of carrier phospholipids is a safety issue: lecithin oxidation may produce rapid drug leakage. However, studies of liposome administration intrathecally in animals and epidurally in humans provide no evidence for "burst release" of drug. Instead, paralleling results with polymer microspheres, liposomes containing local anesthetic or opioid given spinally produce higher intrathecal and lower systemic concentrations than aqueous solutions of these drugs. In aggregate, slow-release formulations of such agents show promise, but their routine clinical application will probably be first for peripheral neural blockade. Because of one's inability to reverse persistent effects (e.g., sensorimotor block) of doses after they are injected, their initial spinal application is likely to involve epidural administration, at low concentrations, to patients such as those with refractory cancer pain in whom close monitoring of cord function is not a pressing issue.

Still another approach to spinal drug delivery involves the use of mammalian cells as self-powered units that synthesize and secrete biomolecules[286]—essentially their natural role! Initially, such methods were applied to replenish pathologically low levels of neurotransmitters or hormones in neurodegenerative[8] or endocrine deficiency diseases.[108] Fetal cells, for example, were transplanted into the basal ganglia to serve as a source of dopamine in patients afflicted with Parkinson's disease, with clinical success. Polymer encapsulation was applied during the early 1980s to shield transplanted differentiated cells, such as pancreatic islet cells, from attack by the host immune system, in efforts to normalize glucose homeostasis through replenishment of insulin.[288] Microencapsulation technology also was applied early on to protect transplanted foreign cells ("xenografts") that synthesize and secrete other therapeutic molecules such as neurotrophic factors[226] for motor neuron disease,[422] or clotting factors for hemophilia.[293] Beginning in the mid-1980s, Sagen, Pappas and co-workers reported that chromaffin cells harvested from the adrenal medulla—previously known to secrete both catecholamines and enkephalins—produced long-lasting,[497] potent analgesia when transplanted into rat spinal cord.[419,421] In the 1990s, as microencapsulation technology matured,[299] they applied it to encapsulate bovine chromaffin cells in semipermeable, immunoisolating membranes, to avoid the need for systemic immunosuppression in patients receiving cadaver allografts of human adrenal chromaffin cells. Their technique also permitted implantation and later retrieval of immunoisolated cells by minimally invasive surgery. An initial Phase 1 (unblinded) trial in seven patients with neuropathic and/or nociceptive pain, four of whom were receiving epidural morphine prior to cell implantation, produced sufficiently encouraging results that Phase 2 trials are now under way. This technology, in the future, may be extended further by implanting neoplastic[525,423] or experimentally transformed cells that produce and secrete non-native compounds. Indeed, Porreca, Yaksh and colleagues have infected mouse fibroblasts with a retrovirus containing a hybrid construct of the DNA sequences for the precursor to nerve growth factor, and that for human beta-endorphin,[482] and demonstrated expression of the latter analgesic peptide.[39] Porreca, Lai and co-workers[384] have also administered intrathecal doses of "antisense" oligomers of DNA that enter the cytosol to block expression (i.e., intracellular synthesis) of specific opioid receptors. Although antisense oligomers have to date been applied only as physiological probes in opioid receptor research, there is much interest in applying this novel pharmacotherapeutic technique to block excitatory neurotransmitter actions upon their receptors by preventing expression of the latter. The ingenuity of the above chemical[389] and biological approaches to spinal analgesia is ample evidence of the importance that biotechnologists and clinicians place upon this organ as a target for their best creative effort—an importance and effort not likely to diminish in years to come.[38]

SPINAL OPIOID THERAPY: AN OVERVIEW

In the prior edition of this book a decade ago, considerable text was devoted to presenting evidence that opioids administered intrathecally or epidurally act primarily upon the spinal cord rather than through systemic absorption and delivery to supraspinal sites. Equal, if not more, effort was expended to survey emerging clinical experience with spinal (especially epidural) opioid analgesia, to justify its safety and efficacy in the management of severe pain. In the present edition, for different reasons, neither item warrants detailed reanalysis. First, as emphasized throughout this and other chapters (Chapters 23.1 and 24, for example) efficacy of a spinal site of action for intrathecal and epidural opioids is now proven beyond a reasonable doubt. Second, the safety and efficacy of spinal opioid analgesia are fully accepted, although questions appropriately continue to arise concerning selection of this technique versus systemic medication. Hence, this section will survey evidence that spinal analgesia for control of acute pain has short- and long-term benefits, will review indications for introducing spinal analgesia during the course of chronic pain due to malignancy or nonmalignant conditions, and will present clinical guidelines for implantation and management of spinal catheters and infusion systems, to alleviate such chronic pain. Selection of medication options, already presented above, will not be repeated, although the value of combination drug therapy will be reinforced.

Postoperative Pain

Postsurgery pain is consistently relieved by intrathecal morphine, and many investigators have documented a better quality of pain relief with epidural than with systemic morphine.[402] Kehlet (Chapter 5), Sinatra (Chapter 26), Liu and Carpenter,[294] and others[17,24,90,117,237] have reviewed the benefits of epidural analgesia upon a variety of outcomes. However, all who attempt to synthesize the relevant research literature and apply it clinically are faced with several problems.[222] First, clinical practice evolves more rapidly than do controlled clinical trials of efficacy. As a consequence, the most rigorous analyses can be performed on techniques that have been the subject of numerous trials, but they may not reflect current practice.[83] For example, coadministration of opioid and local anesthetic is now virtually a standard for epidural drug therapy, but historically the largest numbers of published controlled trials have evaluated epidural administration of opioids alone or local anesthetics alone. Kehlet and Dahl[143,257] have pointed out that controlled clinical trials of the analgesic effects of epidural therapy with local anesthetic plus opioid, versus opioid alone, often show little difference. However, if one restricts attention to those few studies that have assessed pain not just at rest but also during cough, mobilization, or exercise, the superiority of the combined epidural analgesic is clear.[437,438] Hence, a second problem—failure to assess pain during activities required during postoperative rehabilitation—renders many otherwise carefully performed studies irrelevant to clinical practice. A third major problem was pointed out by Bromage,[56] who examined all recently (1993 to 1995) published trials in five major English-language anesthesia journals, as a means of sampling the literature as a whole. He found that the majority of recent, peer-reviewed, clinical trials of epidural anesthesia and analgesia for postoperative pain failed to document that perioperative sensory block was achieved and hence "failed. . .to verify the integrity of the therapeutic procedure under investigation." Bromage likened the subsequent impact of uncritical citations of such studies, which frequently found no benefit to the technique, to a "misinformation virus." Finally, synthesis of the literature is problematic, because studies employ diverse epidural infusates at different rates and locations,[471] frequently with inconclusive findings due to enrollment of small numbers of patients.[338] A rigorous means to deal with the inadequate statistical power of individual trials employs meta-analysis, i.e., pooling of published data according to well-defined statistical methods[239,242] An example of the usefulness of this method is shown in Figure 29-17, which reveals a clear benefit of epidural over systemic opioid analgesia in decreasing postoperative pulmonary complications, even though individual trials are conflicting and often fall short of statistical significance. Intriguingly, these clinical benefits were evident despite a lack of significant improvements in pooled physiologic measures of pulmonary function (forced vital capacity [FVC], forced expiratory volume in one second [FEV_1]), suggesting that as yet unidentified effects of postoperative epidural analgesia underlie these positive outcomes.[76]

Pre-emptive analgesia has been observed in animal studies[194,522] but attempts to confirm its clinical relevance have yielded mixed results to date.[52,54,70,130,374] Given the difficulties in evaluating the impact of epidural analgesia upon well-defined postoperative measures (e.g., FEV_1) it is not surprising that controversy surrounds interpretations of clinical trials that examine pre-emptive analgesia when there has been disagreement on the very meaning of this term in the clinical context. Some authors have used the adjective "pre-emptive" simply to mean that an intervention is performed preoperatively or pre-incision.[327] However, extensive animal work during the 1980s and earlier made it clear that hyperalgesia after peripheral tissue injury to a great extent is centrally mediated, and that suppression of the cascade of changes triggered by tissue injury is much more difficult than is preventing such changes from taking place in the first place. Such prevention depends first upon keeping afferent impulses that arise in injured tissue from arriving at the dorsal horn. Because total afferent blockade with epidural anesthesia is difficult to achieve in clinical settings, especially for operations in the upper abdomen and higher, prevention of spinal cord sensitization may in addition require aggressive antagonism of one or more components of the algesic cascade using combinations of agents outlined in prior sections. Trials which compare effects of pre- versus postoperative administration of a small dose of an opioid or NSAID—agents and doses that could not possibly prevent spinal cord sensitization—do not evaluate the concept of pre-emptive analgesia and simply miss the point.[81] Further, to describe as "analgesia" the administration of pharmacologic agents when pain is not present also is confusing; "antinociception"

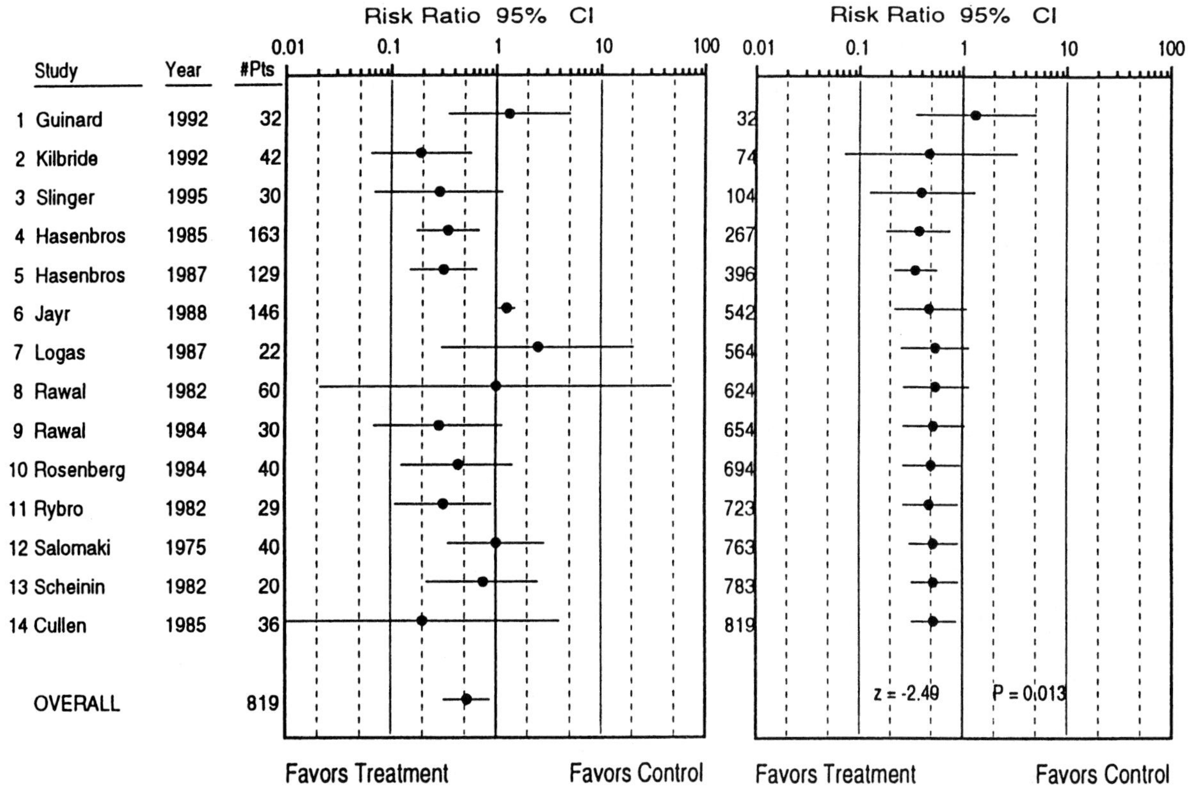

FIG. 29-17. Risk ratios and confidence intervals (CI) for postoperative pulmonary dysfunction in randomized controlled trials of epidural opioid versus intramuscular as-needed opioid, intravenous opioid by continuous infusion, or patient-controlled intravenous opioid bolus doses. **Left:** Results from individual trials. **Right:** Estimates obtained by stepwise accumulation of results from successive trials. (From Ballantyne, J. C., Carr, D. B., Chalmers, T. C., *et al.*: Comparative effects of postoperative analgesic therapies upon respiratory function: meta-analyses of initial randomized control trials. Anesth. Analg. [In Press] 1997.)

is the proper term. Dahl,[143] Kissin,[263] and Niv,[354] separately reviewed the small number of clinical trials in this young area, that document different outcomes, at different time points, using different measures, after different regimens. Outcomes frequently employed in such studies, such as early postoperative opioid consumption, are incomplete and subject to many confounding factors. Instead, one should ask whether aggressive, effective, antinociception in the perioperative interval (including the early postoperative phase) produces longterm reductions in pain, preserves normal (i.e., nonsensitized) sensory function, or decreases the time required to leave the hospital and resume normal function. As more and more carefully designed trials are carried out, which effectively achieve afferent blockade and document doing so during the entire perioperative interval, the existence of pre-emptive analgesia in the clinical arena—already well accepted in animal studies—is becoming harder to refute, as Dahl, Kissin, Bromage, and Gottschalk recently have shown. The next phase of clinical research on this phenomenon must address whether and for which patients and procedures, effective pre-emptive analgesia is achievable in daily practice. Even if it is achievable, economic pressures on anesthesia practice (see following) will mandate demonstration that the cost of such efforts is outweighed by savings from shortened length of hospital stay, fewer complications, and speedier rehabilitation.[391]

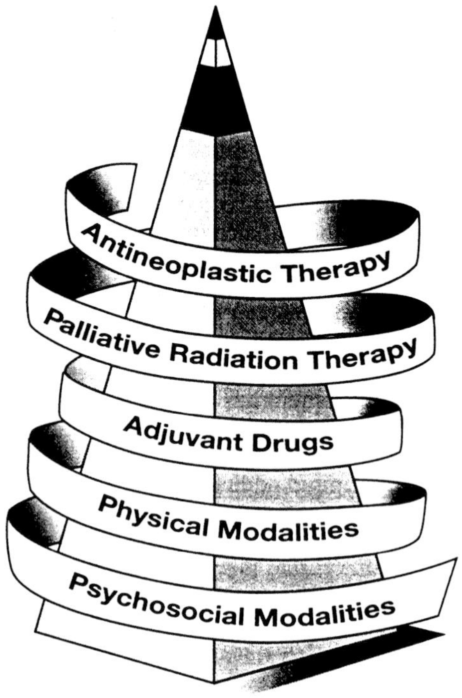

FIG. 29-18. Stratified approach to cancer pain management employs techniques of increasing invasiveness, depicted as a pyramid, along with other modes of antitumor and palliative treatment that may be applied at any time. The latter are shown as a ribbon. Literature and consultant estimates indicate that most patients (lowest layer) have pain that responds to oral, transdermal, or rectal drugs; a smaller number require intravenous or subcutaneous drugs (next layer up); fewer require epidural or intrathecal analgesics (next to top layer) and fewest require lytic blocks, ablative or palliative operations (apex). (From Jacox, A. K., Carr, D. B., Payne, R., *et al.*: Management of Cancer Pain. Clinical Practice Guidelines No. 9. Agency for Health Care Policy and Research. Rockville, Md. US Department of Health and Human Services, 1994.)

Chronic Pain Due to Cancer or Nonmalignant Disease

Endpoints of therapy in trials of cancer pain relief are somewhat different from those in studies of postoperative analgesia. As the number of elderly people has increased throughout the industrialized world, to form an increasing proportion of the entire population, so has recognition on the part of policy makers, health professionals and the populace at large that efforts to prolong life at any cost are becoming harder to justify and support. Accordingly, intense interest has arisen from these same quarters for promotion of palliative care, which in essence seeks to promote quality of life when medical cure is not possible, practical, or desired by the patient and family. Quality of life assessment—in which pain assessment is always an important component—has therefore become a virtual requirement in clinical trials, not only of cancer pain relief, but also of primary anticancer therapies.[460] Development and validation of context- and condition-specific instruments to assess quality of life in clinical trials is a substantial discipline, whose importance will continue to increase as medical practice worldwide shifts to a patient-centered (rather than disease-centered) focus. Already, the World Health Organization (WHO) advocates as policy that palliative care is always cost-effective in contrast to efforts at prevention, early detection, or even cure for many common cancers, whose natural history and public health impact will hardly be influenced by expenditures in the latter directions.[72] Examples of commonly assessed dimensions of quality of life[119] are provided in Table 29-13.

TABLE 29-13. *Commonly identified dimensions of quality of life*

Physical concerns (symptoms; pain)
Treatment satisfaction (including financial concerns)
Functional ability (activity)
Family well-being
Emotional well-being
Social functioning
Occupational functioning
Spirituality
Sexuality/intimacy (including body image)
Future orientation (planning; hope)

From Clinch, J.J., and Schipper, H.: Quality of life assessment in palliative care. *In* Doyle, D., Hanks, G.W.C., and MacDonald, N. (eds.): Oxford Textbook of Palliative Medicine. pp. 61–70. Oxford, Oxford University Press, 1993.

The increased emphasis that patients and health care systems now place on quality of life throughout all of medical care has fostered the application of aggressive or invasive pain control methods to treat chronic pain from nonmalignant conditions. Many object to the use of the word "nonmalignant" to describe pain that is not due to cancer, because noncancer pain can still be malignant in its corrosive effect upon quality of life.[289] Accordingly, analgesic techniques applied to treat cancer-related versus non-cancer-related pain (e.g., the use of opioid medication[390,436]) show less and less difference. Guidelines as to when to employ neuraxial drug delivery[187,270,271] are increasingly framed as applying for "refractory pain" regardless of origin, and typically describe a therapeutic trial of such delivery as appropriate when severe pain cannot be controlled with systemic drugs because of dose-limiting side-effects or toxicity.[370,519] Clinical series that demonstrate how common it is for patients with cancer to have several sites and mechanisms (i.e., neuropathic[223] plus nociceptive) of pain reinforce the view that pain severity and its resistance to less invasive measures, rather than its etiology, should determine the invasiveness of treatment. If one examines, for example, the stratified approach to drug delivery for *cancer pain* advocated in the U.S. federal guidelines for cancer pain treatment (Fig. 29-18), there is hardly any difference from a hierarchical approach to increasingly invasive therapy of severe *chronic pain* not due to malignancy.[237] In this section we will survey the use of spinal opioid therapy for chronic refractory pain without excluding pain from any specific disorder.

The site, nature, and stage of the underlying condition (such as end-stage vascular disease with gangrene, or metastatic spread of cancer), the character of the pain, and the life expectancy and therapeutic preferences of the patient are important factors to consider in deciding whether to commence spinal opioid therapy.[221] Neuropathic or deafferentation pain generally is resistant to opioids given by any route, as is incident or movement-related pain; but deep, constant, somatic pain usually is more responsive.[426] Some types of cancer pain respond variably: cutaneous pain, intermittent somatic pain (e.g., pathologic fracture), intermittent visceral pain[326] (e.g., intestinal obstruction), and coexistent malignant or nonmalignant pain.[15] Because individual patients vary greatly in their response to spinal opioid therapy after failure of systemic medication,[151] it is always desirable to carry out a trial of epidural opioid through a standard percutaneous catheter[107,527] before embarking on more invasive implantation of an epidural or intrathecal system for long-term therapy. Indeed, as summarized in Table 29-14, for patients in the terminal phase a percutaneous "temporary" epidural catheter may be all that is required.

In parallel to growing insight into the merits and mechanisms of spinal opioid therapy for acute pain,[132] clinical trials of opioids as single agents for neuraxial delivery in chronic refractory pain have questioned whether this technique offers advantages over systemic infusion.[68] A small but rigorous double-blinded, cross-over study by Kalso and colleagues[250] found subcutaneous and epidural morphine to be equally valuable in alleviating pain in patients with can-

TABLE 29-14. *Intraspinal drug delivery systems*

System	Advantages	Disadvantages
Percutaneous temporary catheter	Used extensively both intraoperatively and postoperatively, Useful when prognosis is limited (<1 month).	Mechanical problems include catheter dislodgement, obstruction,[a] kinking, or migration. Infection risk with prolonged use.
Permanent silicone-rubber percutaneous epidural catheter	Catheter implantation is a minor procedure. Can deliver bolus injections, continuous infusions, or PCEA (with or without continuous delivery).	Dislodgement, obstruction,[a] infection (but less common than with temporary catheters).
Subcutaneous implanted injection port	Increased stability, less risk of dislodgement. Can deliver bolus injections or continuous infusions (with or without PCA). Potentially, reduced infection in comparison to external system.	Implantation more invasive than external catheters. Approved only for epidural catheter in U.S. Potential for infection increases with frequent injections (may obstruct[a]).
Subcutaneous reservoir	Extends duration of therapy without pump implantation.	Difficult to access, and fibrosis may occur after repeated injection.
Implanted pumps (continuous or programmable)	Potentially, decreased risk of infection. Ease of programming. Complex infusion regimens.	Need for more extensive operative procedure. Need for specialized, costly equipment with programmable systems.

[a] A common cause of obstruction is formation of a fibrous sheath around the epidural catheter.

From Cousins, M.J., Cherry, D.A., and Gourlay, G.K.: Acute and Chronic pain: Use of spinal opioids, *In* Cousins, M.J., and Bridenbaugh, P.O. (eds.): Neural Blockade. 2nd ed. pp. 955–1029. Philadelphia, J.B. Lippincott, 1988; and Jacox, A.K., Carr, D.B., Payne, R., *et al.*: Management of Cancer Pain. Clinical Practice Guideline no. 9. Agency for Health Care Policy and Research. Rockville, Md., US Department of Health and Human Services, 1994.

cer, although these patients had not yet failed oral morphine therapy. Further, Paix and colleagues[371] have reported case series of 11 patients who required cessation of morphine because of intolerable side effects; 10 of these patients received adequate pain relief without unacceptable side effects when treated with subcutaneous fentanyl or sufentanil infusion. The single patient who did not respond to this measure had pelvic visceral and neuropathic pain that responded well to placement of an epidural catheter and infusion of local anesthetic plus opioid. Because oral morphine is recognized to accumulate metabolites such as morphine-6-glucuronide which contribute to nausea or sedation, as well as to analgesia, a possible advantage in switching from the oral to the subcutaneous route is reduction in such metabolites due to avoidance of first-pass hepatic metabolism. Also in well documented case series, changing from one mu opioid agonist to another mu opioid agonist relieved pain that appeared to be opioid-insensitive. Thus one must be sure that alternative opioids are tested before deciding to advance to more invasive therapies. On the other hand, if one considers that drug dosages and costs are much higher during chronic systemic opioid therapy than during chronic intrathecal opioid therapy, and that the cost of subcutaneous infusion pump purchase or long-term rental differ little from those for an implanted device, the latter technique may well be preferable. Further, the second case series cited above illustrates that access to the intrathecal or epidural space is desirable for the patient likely to require multidrug neuraxial infusion (because of neuropathic or incident pain). As is the case for literature reviews of acute pain control with spinal opioids, outcomes associated with current clinical practices are less well documented than those associated with practices that may no longer be current.[183] Thirteen of 18 long-term studies of spinal opioid administration reviewed by Yaksh[539] in 1996 involved use of morphine alone, yet current practice employs combination therapy, such as with local anesthetic or with clonidine, quite liberally. Both local anesthetic and clonidine, when added to morphine, reduce neuropathic pain, the control of which was early recognized to be suboptimal when morphine is given as the sole spinal agent. Efforts by Ballantyne, Carr, and colleagues[24] to combine data from multiple trials of neuraxial opioid delivery were frustrated by the many different drug regimens employed, their (understandable) evaluation of case series, rather than controlled trials, and paucity of detailed information about patient characteristics and analgesic responses. Nevertheless, pooling of data into crude categories of analgesic efficacy and complication rates was accomplished, and this revealed no significant difference in the analgesic success rates between drug delivery accomplished via the epidural, intrathecal, or intracerebroventricular[301] routes (all were around 70%). Catheter and system problems such as pump failure, leakage, or infection, were greatest in the epidural group and significantly lower during intracerebroventricular therapy.[295] Although this last technique is promising,[140] it requires neurosurgical intervention, is not suited to preimplantation therapeutic trials, and certainly cannot be recommended at this time for drug mixtures such as opioid plus local anesthetic or clonidine.

Contraindications

The same contraindications apply to the insertion of a spinal catheter for chronic pain control as for acute pain management, e.g., in obstetrics or general surgery (see Chapters 18 and 26). These include:

1. *Bleeding diathesis.* Hemorrhagic conditions may result in long-term neurologic deficit secondary to the development of an epidural hematoma[19] (see Chapter 21).
2. *Sepsis.* Local superficial infection does not preclude insertion of a spinal catheter at another level because the segmental level chosen is not usually critical, as explained earlier in this chapter. Septicemia is an absolute contraindication because the presence of a foreign body in the epidural space predisposes to formation of an epidural abscess, and its sequelae such as cord compression. If a patient with an implanted epidural catheter subsequently becomes septicemic (e.g., after chemotherapy), then antibiotic therapy combined with prophylactic removal of the catheter generally is indicated.[435]
3. *Insulin-dependent diabetics* have proved to be susceptible to infection at the portal site with potentially serious effects,[252] so this condition is regarded by some as a contraindication to spinal catheter placement.[106]
4. *Immunosuppression* must be weighed on an individual basis with respect to its magnitude (e.g., CD4 cell count in HIV/AIDS) and likely reversibility.
5. *Epidural metastases* are a relative contraindication. Unless the catheter can be positioned away from such lesions, it is probably wise to avoid spinal catheterization in such cases. The possibility of a needle or catheter penetrating a friable epidural mass, with consequent development of paraplegia, is a risk that must always be considered. The potential for eventual distal loculation of CSF, because of pressure on the subarachnoid space by an epidural mass, should encourage placement of catheters cephalad to known or suspected spinal metastases.[105]
6. *Unmotivated, noncompliant or cognitively impaired patients* are in general not good candidates for neuraxial opioid therapy, although each case must be approached individually. In some circumstances, placement of an intrathecal catheter for medication infusion, via programmable implanted pump, offers a simpler and more reliable means to provide analgesia than attempting to follow a complicated oral regimen or maintain a subcutaneous infusion. Indeed, opioid side-effects such as cognitive impairment may be dramatically reduced by a switch from systemic to spinal drug administration and coinfusion of a nonopioid to minimize opioid requirement.

LONG-TERM INTRATHECAL AND EPIDURAL SYSTEMS

Long-term access for spinal administration of opioids in practice means the use of an intrathecal or epidural catheter system connected to an injection system with or without a reservoir.[104,124,126,127,383] Although the dura-arachnoid membrane offers a significant barrier to infection, and therefore the incidence of meningitis should in theory be lower with epidural catheterization, meta-analysis of the relative rates of infection during chronic intrathecal versus epidural catherization does not support this view. The suggestion from such an analysis that repeated refilling of pump or reservoir may predispose to infectious complications further undermines the intuitive view that the epidural route is the safer of the two. Considering that dosage requirements are lower and therefore refilling intervals longer when the intrathecal route is used, one can argue that the intrathecal route may carry a slightly lower (statistically insignificant) infection risk. The impact of a high standard of specialized care upon complication rates is emphasized by the report of Nitescu, Sjoberg, and colleagues on 200 patients with cancer, treated for a total of 14,485 patient days with externalized, tunneled, intrathecal catheters for cancer pain control.[353] Their protocolized approach involved close follow-up with skilled nursing care to assure sterility during dressing changes, medication refills, and antibacterial filter replacement. Two infections (i.e., rate of 1/7,242 treatment days) occurred—an enviable figure but one not likely to be equalled in settings where close follow-up with skilled nursing is not feasible. In this exemplary series, 3.5% of patients had CSF leakage, 1.5% had CSF hygroma and 15.5% had postdural puncture headache, although none of the latter persisted. Of practical significance is clear evidence in animal studies (presented earlier) of rapid formation of a fibrous tissue sheath around epidural catheters, eventually preventing diffusion of drug into the epidural space[128,176] and in one patient causing spinal cord compression.[411] Fibrosis around the epidural catheter tip may partly explain dosage escalation, pain with injection, and high failure rate in follow-up studies at about three months.[126] Whether such a reaction occurs in the subarachnoid space has not been determined but the fluid environment may make it less likely; clinical experience supports a reduced likelihood of fibrosis and pain on injection when the intrathecal route is used. Also of growing clinical importance is the need for subarachnoid access to deliver drugs such as neostigmine or SNX-111, which are ineffective epidurally. Although large molecules such as peptides have been shown to produce some analgesic effects with epidural administration in humans, in animals they are ineffective when given epidurally and highly potent by the intrathecal route.[176,532,539] Thus, lower clinical doses of peptide molecules such as DPDPE, biphalin, metkephamid, somatostatin, and calcitonin, may well have greater effect when given intrathecally than higher doses given epidurally; clinical trials are needed to determine dosage ratios for the 2 routes.

Externalized Catheter Insertion

This method is effective, inexpensive, and potentially available worldwide, although some find it inconvenient to wear and it interferes to an extent with routine daily activities such as washing, dressing, and sleeping. It is well suited for intermittent spinal drug injection, but opioid infusion can be provided readily by connecting the externalized catheter to a small portable pump, such as the Fresenius (Injection MS26), Travenol Infusor and Patient Control Module, Abbott PCA-II, Graseby Dynamics Portable Infusion Pump (with self-administration option), Deltec Cadd-Pac, or an equivalent. External infusion can be effective for bedridden as well as ambulatory patients, who can wear the pump in a shoulder holster and use it for many hours to a day or more before refilling.

Three to 7 days after a percutaneous catheter is placed, the skin at the catheter exit site can become erythematous, or even frankly infected. One means to prevent organisms tracking from skin to the epidural space is to tunnel the catheter laterally from the lumbar interspace, to a percutaneous exit site on the lateral or anterolateral chest wall (Fig. 29-19). A chronic inflammatory response may occur in the skin at the catheter exit site, but in the absence of obstruction, seropurulent material can drain superficially to create a (desirable) sinus. To minimize further opportunistic infection at the exit site one may apply an airtight, waterproof adhesive dressing, with the epidural catheter running under the dressing to its edge. The safety of this technique is documented in thousands of patient-years, as is a very low incidence of CSF fistula formation,[499] or epidural abscess,[124,351] despite the immunologically depressed state of many of these pa-

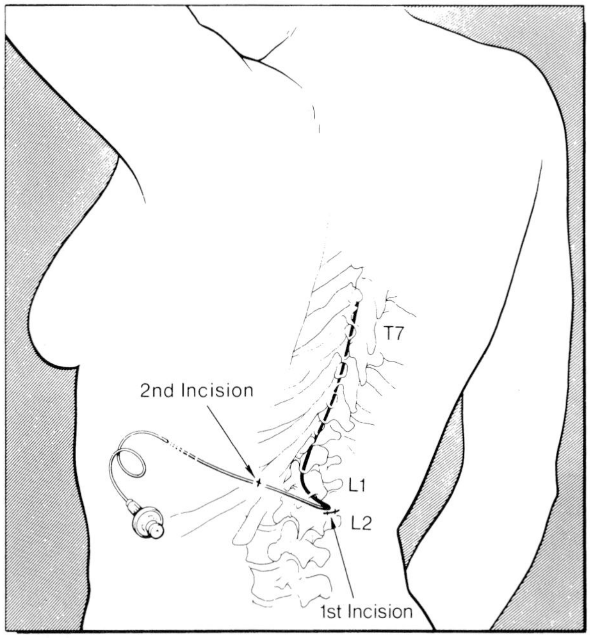

FIG. 29-19. Percutaneous epidural catheter tunneled to exit at the lateral chest wall (see Figs. 29-20 and 29-25 for details of tunneling technique).

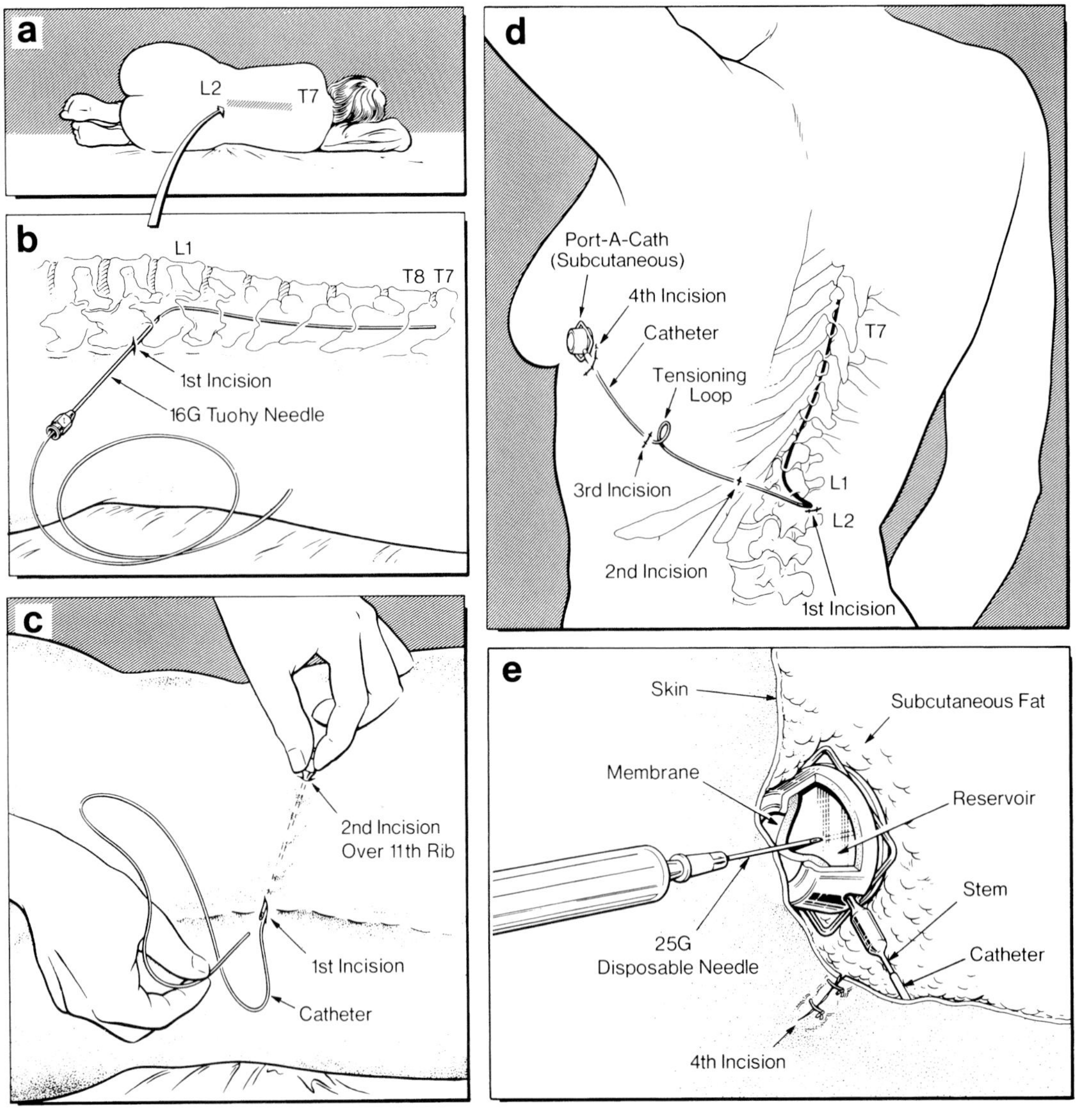

FIG. 29-20. Implantation of the epidural portal system. **a:** Position of patient before implantation. **b:** Insertion of 16-gauge epidural catheter through a Tuohy needle. **c:** Tunneling technique used to relocate the end of the epidural catheter to the anterior chest wall. **d:** Portal attached to the inserted epidural catheter. **e:** Injection technique and exposed view of the epidural portal.

tients.[346,548,549] Relatively inexpensive, easy-to-insert polyethylene (nylon) catheters are well suited for this application. They do not require a stylet for insertion, nor (contrary to some opinion) do they become excessively brittle and break. Such catheters have been used in patients with cancer pain for periods in excess of one year, without apparent undue sequelae. Some centers employ softer and more pliable polyurethane and Silastic catheters, because these catheters are believed to induce less tissue reaction in the epidural space and hence to carry a lower likelihood of epidural fibrosis.[411] Comparative studies are required. Catheter migration from the epidural space into the subdural or subarachnoid space, or even intravascularly, can occur, but is uncommon.[142] Allowing for the pressure changes due to cardiovascular and respiratory pulsations, and motion of the catheter tip in response to vertebral column movement by the patient, one still expects the dura-arachnoid membrane to prevent significant migration. Unrecognized migration into the subarachnoid space may lead to profound respiratory depression,[65,67] although patients who have spinal catheters in place usually are tolerant of the respiratory effects of opioids. Hypotension and/or paralysis are theoretical possibilities if the catheter migrates to deliver local anesthetic intrathecally, but this risk is minimal for chronic catheters in which fibrosis (see earlier) is the prime concern. Bacterial filters (see Fig. 29-19) can be fitted to the end of the catheter to prevent bacteria from entering the catheter lumen. The need to change filters regularly is a component of cost of this form of therapy.

Totally Implanted Systems

Systems that are implanted subcutaneously have obvious advantages in terms of sterility, comfort, and freedom of movement for the patient. Such implanted systems employ either a portal for percutaneous access and bolus injection, or an implanted, pump-driven, percutaneously refillable reservoir system. The portal or reservoir is connected to an epidural or intrathecal catheter and positioned on the anterior chest or abdominal wall for convenient access.

Portal systems should have the following characteristics:

- Easily palpable percutaneously;
- Self-sealing membrane capable of withstanding 1,000 injections at the pressure required to deliver drug solution through a standard epidural or intrathecal catheter;
- Easily discernible end point to injection;
- Ability to maintain patency;
- Injectable by nonmedically trained personnel;
- Inexpensive;
- Simple to implant under local anesthesia; and
- Filter to prevent unwanted particulate matter from reaching the epidural or intrathecal space.

Implantation of a portal system (Portacath) is shown in Figure 29-20. Our experience with insertion of hundreds of these devices for relief of cancer pain previously uncontrolled by oral opioids is that the portal has not been subject to leaking, the membrane has been robust, and staff and patients have found it easy to inject. An early problem of portal outlet obstruction[106] was overcome by moving the inner end of the outlet tube further into its interior (i.e., so as no longer to be flush with the inner surface of the reservoir), thus avoiding the funneling of debris: bits of silicone released from membrane puncture sites, plugs of dermal layers, and skin-swab fibers. Another early problem of catheter blockage is now prevented by a filter in the port, to prevent particulate material from making its way into the catheter.

Implanted Pumps

Pumps designed for subcutaneous implantation must incorporate a drug reservoir as well as some form of powered pump.[274] Morphine for intraspinal use is available commercially at concentrations of 60 mg/ml or higher, implying that a patient who requires a high intrathecal or epidural dose such as 120 mg per 24 hour must receive 2 ml per 24 hours. To make the device a practical alternative to the portal/bolus devices, the reservoir capacity must be at least 20 ml. Together, the reservoir plus pump present a certain minimum volume that in a cachectic patient may have an impact upon the feasibility of pump implantation. A current system for this application, the Infusaid 550, is quite compact, (Fig. 29-21) as are comparable systems such as the Isomed (Fig. 29-22).[124] A different type of system, the Synchromed (Fig. 29-23), is programmable externally allowing flexibility in adjustment of delivered dose.[375] Another system, the Algomed (Fig. 29-24), is powered by the patient, who must depress the activation valve and the pumping chamber simultaneously. Although the Algomed is an "on-demand" system, it is designed so that 1 hour must elapse for the pumping chamber to refill completely after each use. This long lockout interval provides substantial safety.

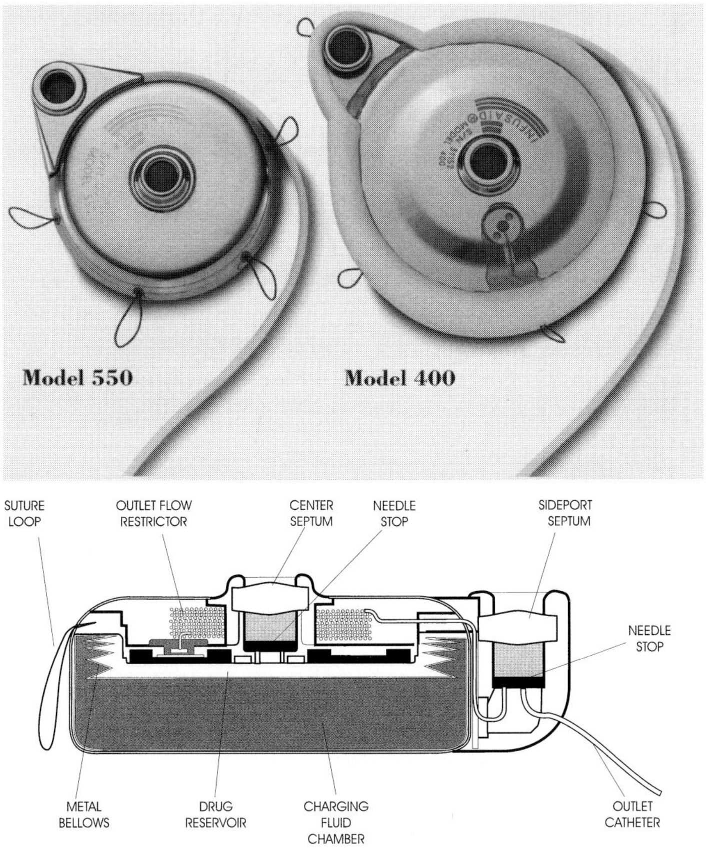

FIG. 29-21. "INFUSAID" Constant Infusion Implantable Pump for continuous intrathecal (or epidural) administration of opioid and nonopioid drugs. **Top:** The central port is for filling the drug chamber. The side port is connected directly to the intrathecal catheter and is used to check catheter placement and patency (by aspiration of CSF and/or injection of contrast medium) and to administer bolus doses. The new model 550 is shown to contrast size with the older model 400. **Bottom:** Cross-section of pump. Note: the drug chamber communicating with the outlet catheter via an "outlet flow restrictor." When the drug chamber is filled a metal bellows permits expansion of the size of the drug chamber; in the "charging fluid chamber," a volatile liquid expands at body temperature and compresses the metal bellows, thus driving drug into the outlet catheter. In the model 550, a silicone rubber coating of the pump is no longer used. (Courtesy of Infusaid Corp. USA).

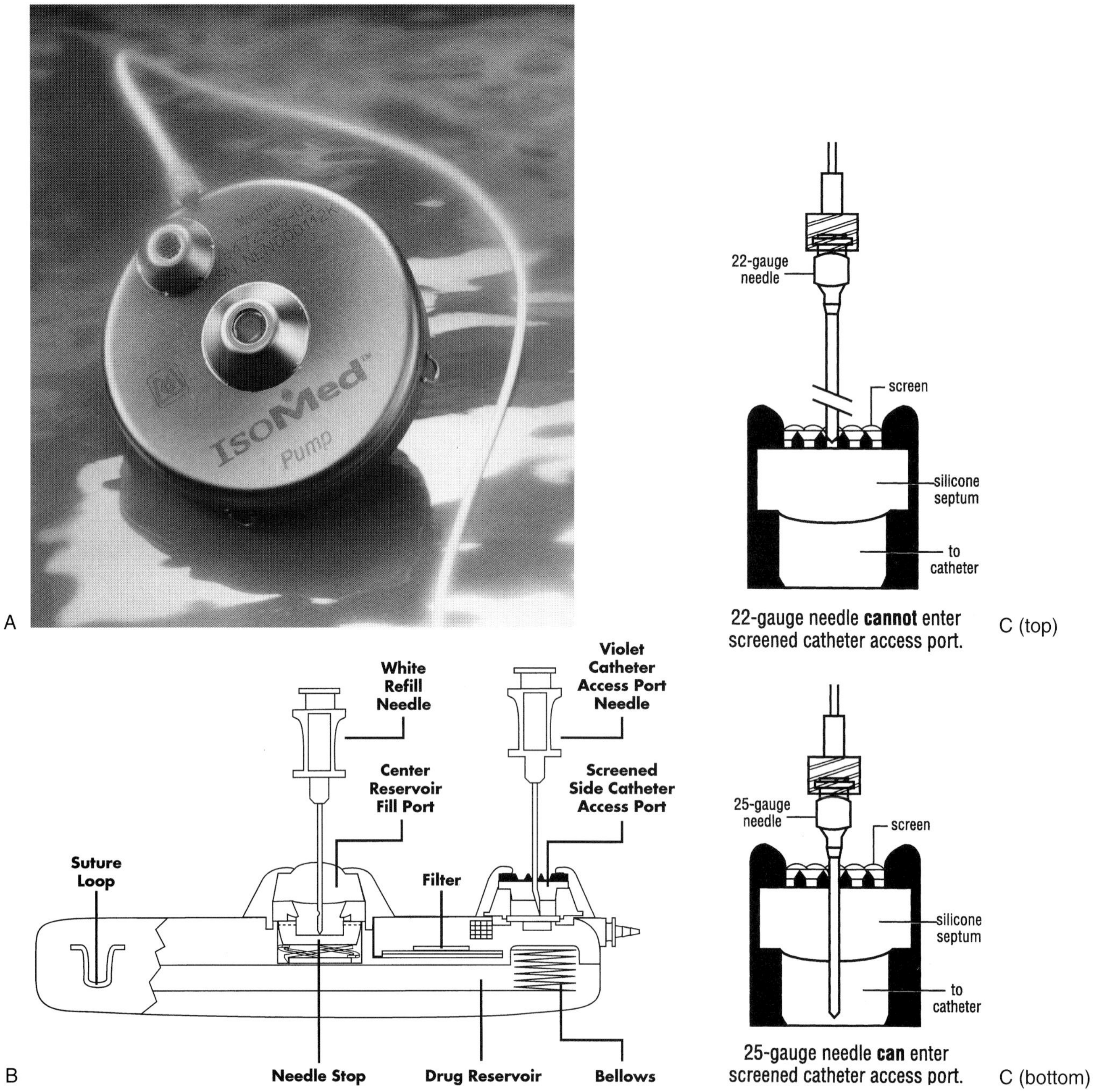

FIG. 29-22. "ISOMED," Medtronic Constant Infusion Implantable Pump, for continuous intrathecal (or epidural) administration of opioid and nonopioid drugs. **A:** External appearance of pump: central port and side port serve a similar role to the INFUSAID. **B:** Cross-section of pump components similar to INFUSAID except that drug reservoir is driven by an inert gas which compresses the "bellows" when the reservoir is filled. Note also the different needle for "central reservoir fill port" and spinal "catheter access port" which is screened to only accept the "access port needle." **C:** *Cross section of catheter Access Port:* **Top:** A 22-gauge needle (as used for central reservoir fill port) is barred entry by the screen. **Bottom:** A 25-gauge needle (supplied in catheter access port kit) can enter. Courtesy of Medtronic Neurological Division, Minneapolis MN, USA.

Regardless of the specific choice of implanted pump type or spinal access (intrathecal or epidural) the procedures of catheter placement and tunneling, pump implantation, and linking of catheter and pump, follow the same general sequence of steps. Figure 29-25 illustrates these steps for the placement of an intrathecal catheter via the lumbar route for drug delivery through a Synchromed pump. Ideally, a pain management unit should work in close harmony with a palliative care team, and this is especially true when sophisticated pain treatment technologies are implanted in patients who receive terminal care in the home. This alliance supplies a powerful, hospital-based focus that can then act as a re-

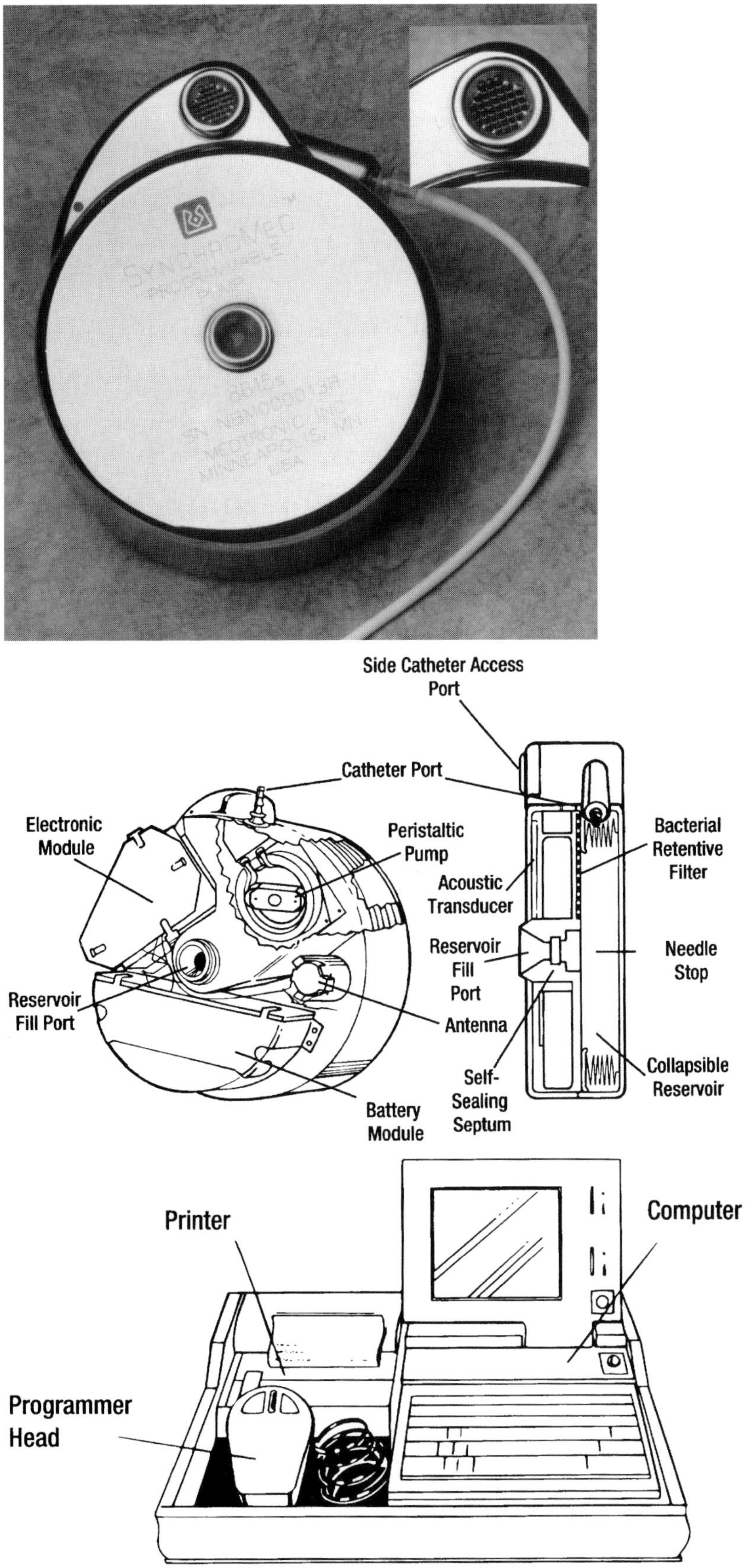

FIG. 29-23. Medtronic "SYNCHROMED" Programmable, Implantable Pump, for intrathecal (or epidural) administration of opioid and non-opioid drugs. **A:** External appearance of the pump: central and side ports serve a similar role to the ISOMED. Note the screen in the side port. **B:** The Synchromed consists of a lithium battery-driven, **peristaltic infusion pump** with a collapsible **drug reservoir**, and **electronic module** with microprocessor-based circuitry and an acoustic transducer attached to an **antenna**. An external programmer **(C)** operates via a programming head which communicates information between the pump (via antenna) and programmer using coded radio-frequency signals. **C:** Synchromed Programmer and Synchromed programmer head: The programmer can be programmed to deliver timed boli, continuous infusions, complex infusions or any combination of these. The programmer head is placed over the pump to obtain information that has been recorded in the pump's electronic module. Then the new programming information is transmitted to the electronic module, which also monitors low reservoir volume and low battery voltage (triggering an alarm). Courtesy of Medtronic Neurological Division, Minneapolis MN, USA.

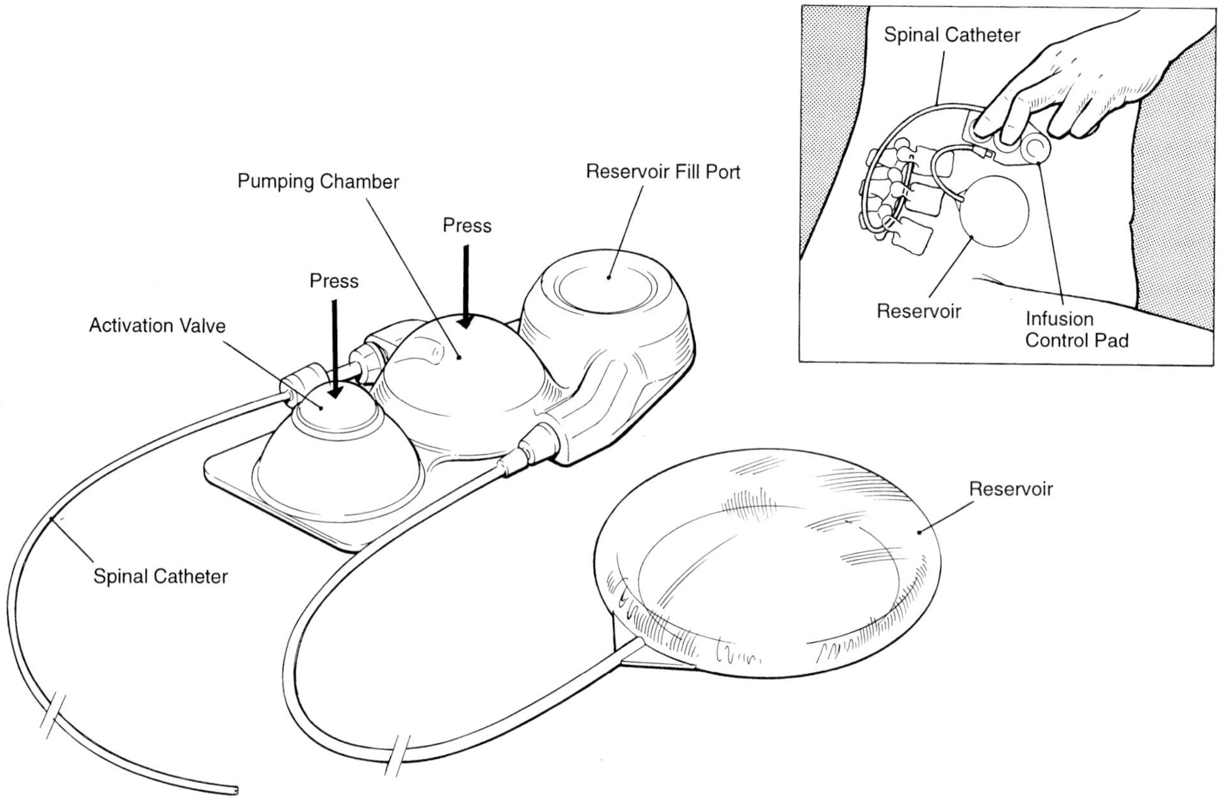

FIG. 29-24. ALGOMED Implantable Patient-Activated Device, for intermittent intrathecal (or epidural) administration of opioid and nonopioid drugs. **Left:** Components of the device. Drugs are loaded into the **reservoir** via the **reservoir fill port.** It is also necessary to use a precise procedure to expel air, and prime with drug, the **pumping chamber** and the spinal catheter. To deliver a dose of drug, (1ml), the patient must simultaneously depress the activation valve and the pumping chamber. Following successful delivery of a dose, the pumping chamber refills over the next 60 minutes (a "lock-out") interval). **Top, right:** Infusion control pad in situ over lower thoracic area, reservoir in adjacent upper abdominal area (via a single incision) and spinal catheter in intrathecal space. (Algomed Medtronic Neurological Division Minneapolis MN, USA.)

source for the home care team of home care nurse, volunteers, general practitioners, and other home care professionals. It is essential to conduct a training program for home care nurses and to have a well-organized system for regular communication with them.

Reasons for Lack of Efficacy

Obstruction to CSF Flow As mentioned previously in this chapter, epidural opioids act by passive diffusion from the epidural space through the dura and subarachnoid membranes into the CSF. Depending upon the lipophilicity of the agent applied, the importance of redistribution to supraspinal sites during chronic infusion may vary. Intrathecally applied opioids also vary in their relative persistence in CSF, and morphine in particular spreads widely cephalad. Occasional case reports describe occlusion of the epidural and subarachnoid spaces by an extradural mass. In such cases, the effective loculation of CSF caudal to the mass has prevented spread of opioid within the CSF and resulted in inadequate pain relief.[105,411] If not contraindicated, (see earlier) the catheter may be repositioned cephalad to the mass; however, in practice such blockage of CSF heralds spinal cord compression whose emergent treatment takes priority. *Tolerance* may reflect a loss of drug effect due to physiological adaptation as described above, or alternatively could indicate progression of the underlying condition or catheter tip encasement by fibrous tissue. Drug switching between opioids (e.g., from epidural morphine to epidural buprenorphine,[75] or intrathecal morphine to intrathecal DADL[129,272,343]) and addition of or switching to agents from other drug categories are clinically validated strategies involving various drugs described previously. Changing from intrathecal to intraventricular morphine[129] also has been reported to restore morphine responsiveness. The best approach to the problem of tolerance would seem to be based upon proactive, preventive use of drug combinations from the outset, to avoid activating the opioid tolerance/hyperalgesia pathway described above. Such regimens are possible, but suitable clinical trials to evaluate whether their use early on could preclude pharmacologic tolerance have not yet been reported. *Pain on injection* most commonly is experienced as a burning pressure sensation in one or other hip during epidural injection of morphine in saline. This pain is surmised to be an effect of concentrated morphine upon a nerve root, but there are no data to prove or disprove this. Such pain can be reduced by administering the injection over 5 to 10 minutes, by pretreating with a small dose of local anesthetic before the morphine injection, or by injecting glucocorticoid through the catheter. Since neuropathological data now suggest that pain may be due to distention of the fibrous sheath that forms around epidural catheters,[177] it is conceivable that glucocorticoid applied locally at this sheath may cause involution, as it does in other fibrous tissue. Despite these measures, some patients still experience significant pain on injection. Should this occur, the catheter must be repositioned, and if, despite repositioning, pain still occurs with injections, then the catheter should be resited in the subarachnoid space. In a series of 200 patients with long-term epidural catheters, this has been found to be necessary on four occasions.[104]

Outcomes of Spinal Opioid Treatment

A number of long-term follow-up series have been reported from around the world since the prior edition of this chapter. Benedetti,[34] for example, presented results from a 16-center trial in which 179 patients with cancer pain were treated for an average of 109 days with morphine delivered to the epidural space via an implanted subcutaneous portal. Pain relief on a 0 to 10 scale rose from 3.8 at the start of therapy to 7.8 after a month and remained stable for the next year. Samuelsson[427] reported a 9-year experience from his institution, involving 146 patients, 70% of whom were able to achieve good pain relief and half of whom could be cared for at home. Samuelsson's report is revealing because during his 9 years of data collection, the use of oral and other (e.g., transdermal) opioids became more aggressive, and combination spinal therapies, such as morphine plus bupivacaine, were introduced. The complexities associated with synthesizing data from even a single institution when its threshold for referral to a specialist (i.e., failure of systemic opioid therapy) has been raised continuously are apparent. Overshadowing the entire field is the fact that very few trials (see previous) have compared costs, effects and outcomes, during prospective trials of alternative routes of opioid therapy. Instead, as remarked earlier, nearly all large-scale published data on chronic spinal opioid therapy are descriptive case series focused on analgesic effects, side effects and complications during the use of morphine alone. Abram and Hopwood[3] recently discussed whether meta-analysis of invasive techniques for neuraxial opioid therapy can "rescue knowledge from a sea of unintelligible data." Their experience accords with that of Benedetti, Samuelsson and many others in the past decade: as oncologists have become more comfortable with managing cancer pain using high doses of oral and parenteral opioids, more and more patients referred for consideration of epidural or intrathecal opioids now have severe pain despite high doses of systemic opioids, and very short life expectancies. These opioid-tolerant patients are likely to receive combinations of opioids plus agents such as local anesthetics or clonidine early in the course of spinal analgesic therapy.[175] Therefore, the relevance of yesterday's studies to today's practice in this rapidly evolving field is suspect. Abram, Hopwood, Ballantyne, and Carr, and Liu and Carpenter (in their review of postoperative epidural analgesia[294]) have voiced reservations about consolidating weak data from multiple uncontrolled trials enrolling mixed patient populations in diverse contexts. The latter authors have pointed out that "epidural analgesia is not a generic term" and the same is true of intrathecal analgesia. All of these authors have urged improvement in the design, execution, and reporting of relevant clinical trials.[241]

CONCLUSION AND FUTURE DIRECTIONS

Jeanne Stover, a patient who participated in the drafting of U.S. clinical practice guidelines on cancer pain, succumbed to her long-term malignancy while that document was in press. She had written: "My dream is for a medication that can relieve my pain while leaving me alert and with no side effects."[237] We are unquestionably closer to attaining this vision—shared by so many other patients with acute, cancer-related, or chronic pain—than a decade ago when this text last appeared.

Acute Pain Treatment

Treatment of acute pain has been changed forever by the application of spinal analgesia to relieve pain after operation or trauma. Early randomized prospective studies[337] provided clear evidence of superiority of epidural opioids as well as of local anesthetics over opioids given intramuscularly, and of patient preference for epidural opioids. However, pain relief with spinal opioids as single agents is similar, in a small number of studies, to carefully tuned intravenous infusion of opioids or meticulously maintained somatic nerve blocks,[199] such as intercostal block.[400] Yet clinical trials of single opioids given spinally or systematically have diminishing relevance to today's practice of spinal analgesia,[149] that relies increasingly upon drug combinations to suppress activity-related pain and to hasten postoperative rehabilitation (see Chapter 5). Recent preclinical studies suggest that high doses of systemic morphine may induce glutathione depletion, oxidative stress, and tissue injury in vulnerable organs such as kidney, liver and portions of the CNS—another potential reason to employ smaller doses of opioids and other nonopioid analgesics administered centrally rather than higher systemic doses of opioids alone.[211] Further, a number of novel potent nonopioid analgesics now in preclinical and clinical evaluation require spinal administration. The importance of spinal analgesia in acute pain management therefore

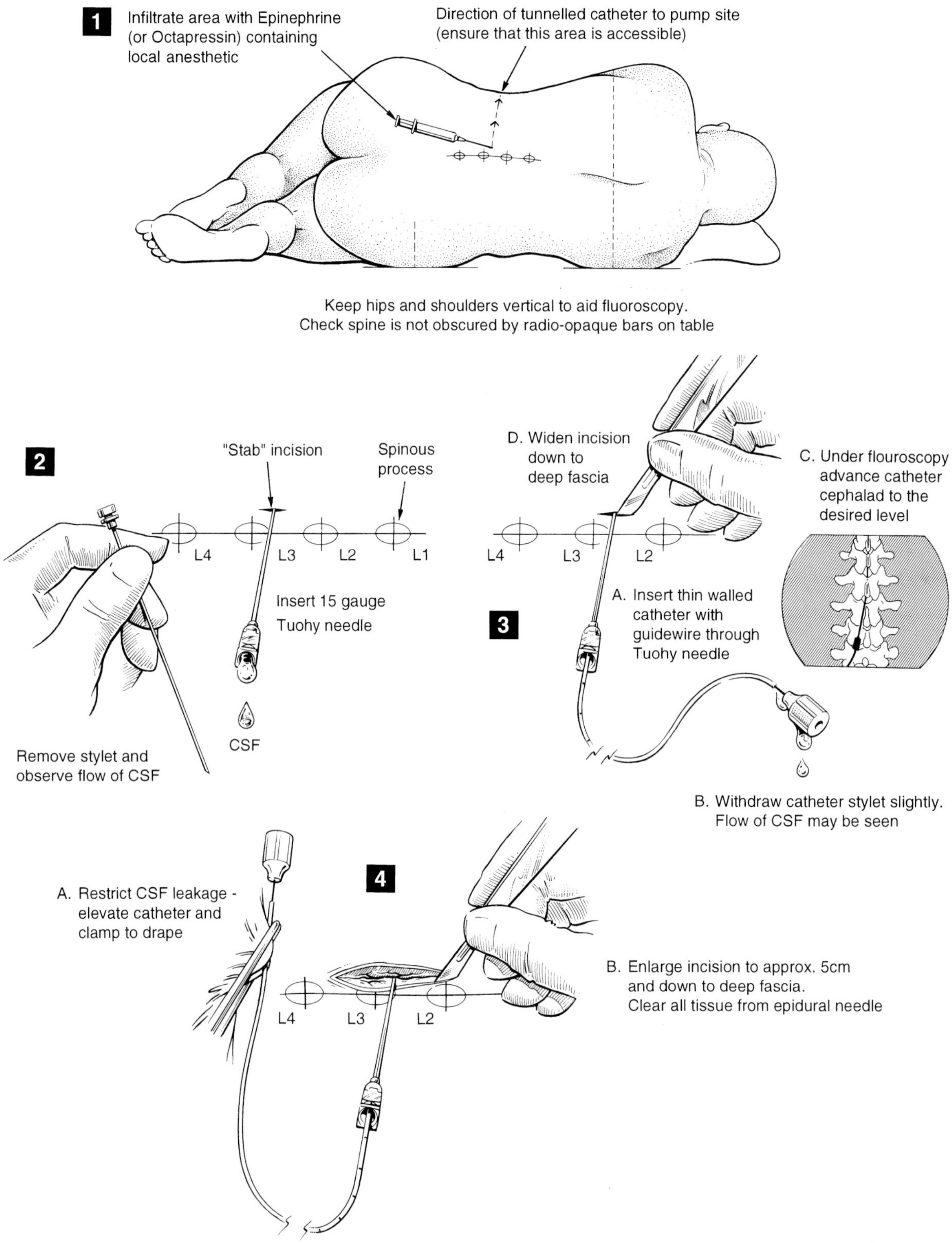

FIG. 29-25. Intrathecal pump implantation. *1* Infiltration of spinal incision area and tunnelling path with local anesthetic and vasoconstrictor solution. Note the careful positioning of the spine to permit a true lateral view with fluoroscopy. *2* Insertion of Tuohy needle. Note that the "stab" incision is not enlarged until a CSF flow is obtained via the needle and the catheter is successfully threaded, and if necessary, checked under fluoroscopy. *4* CSF leakage can be restricted by clamping the catheter, or applying a suture to the catheter. Note that the incision is enlarged only down to the deep fascia.

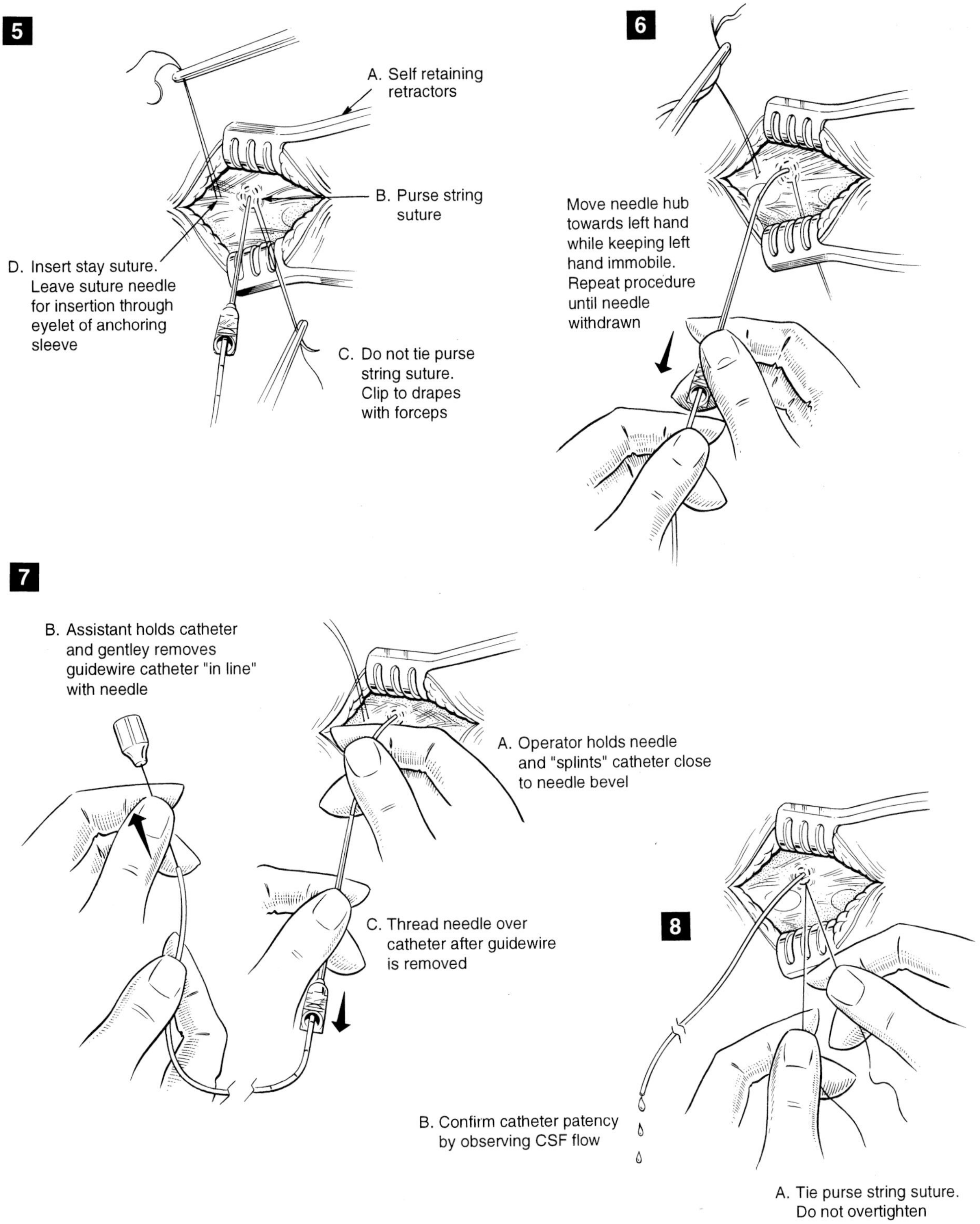
5
A. Self retaining retractors
B. Purse string suture
D. Insert stay suture. Leave suture needle for insertion through eyelet of anchoring sleeve
C. Do not tie purse string suture. Clip to drapes with forceps
6
Move needle hub towards left hand while keeping left hand immobile. Repeat procedure until needle withdrawn
7
B. Assistant holds catheter and gentley removes guidewire catheter "in line" with needle
A. Operator holds needle and "splints" catheter close to needle bevel
C. Thread needle over catheter after guidewire is removed
8
B. Confirm catheter patency by observing CSF flow
A. Tie purse string suture. Do not overtighten

FIG. 29-25. *Continued. 5* Placement of **purse string suture** and **stay sutures.** Note that these sutures must be placed before the Tuohy needle is removed. The use of a self-retaining retractor greatly facilitates this step. *6* **Removal of epidural needle.** Note the measures to avoid retraction of the spinal catheter. *7* **Removal of guidewire.** Note that the guidewire must be removed slowly and carefully to avoid any tendency for the intrathecal catheter to "roll up." *8* **Trying of purse string suture.** Note the suture is tightened sufficiently to grip the intrathecal catheter but not tightly enough to restrict the flow of CSF.

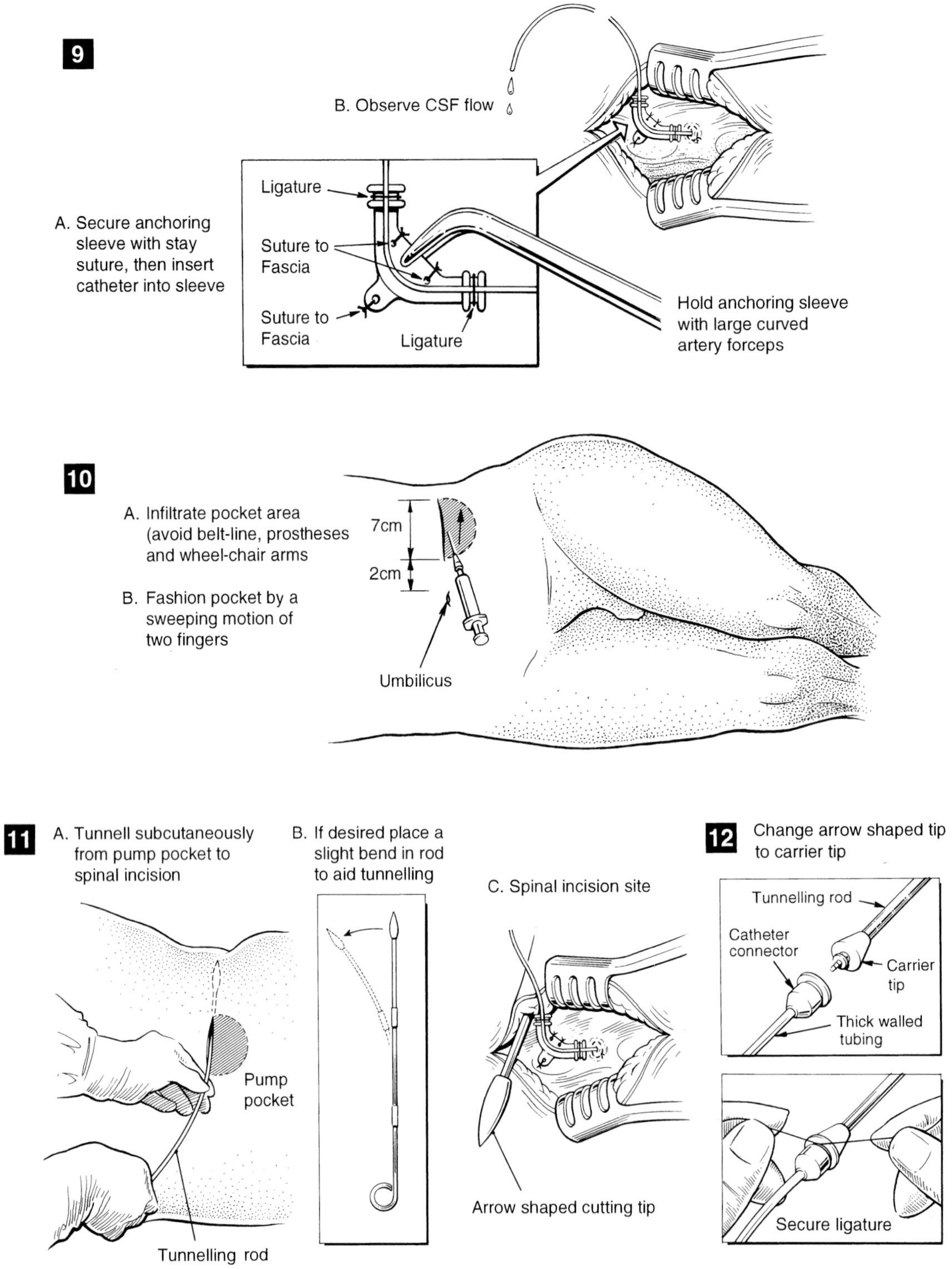
9
B. Observe CSF flow
A. Secure anchoring sleeve with stay suture, then insert catheter into sleeve
Ligature
Suture to Fascia
Suture to Fascia
Ligature
Hold anchoring sleeve with large curved artery forceps
10
A. Infiltrate pocket area (avoid belt-line, prostheses and wheel-chair arms
B. Fashion pocket by a sweeping motion of two fingers
7cm
2cm
Umbilicus
11
A. Tunnell subcutaneously from pump pocket to spinal incision
B. If desired place a slight bend in rod to aid tunnelling
C. Spinal incision site
Pump pocket
Tunnelling rod
Arrow shaped cutting tip
12
Change arrow shaped tip to carrier tip
Tunnelling rod
Catheter connector
Carrier tip
Thick walled tubing
Secure ligature

FIG. 29-25. *Continued. 9* **Placement of anchoring device.** Note the use of a large curved artery forceps to hold the anchoring device in place, while securing it to the fascia, using the previously placed stay suture. Then the spinal catheter is placed in the anchoring device, still holding the device in place with the curved forceps. Finally, ligatures are placed on the anchoring device to hold the spinal catheter. *10* Infiltration of pump pocket area and preparation of pocket. *11* Procedure for tunnelling from pump pocket to spinal area. *12* Securing of catheter connector to tunnelling rod.

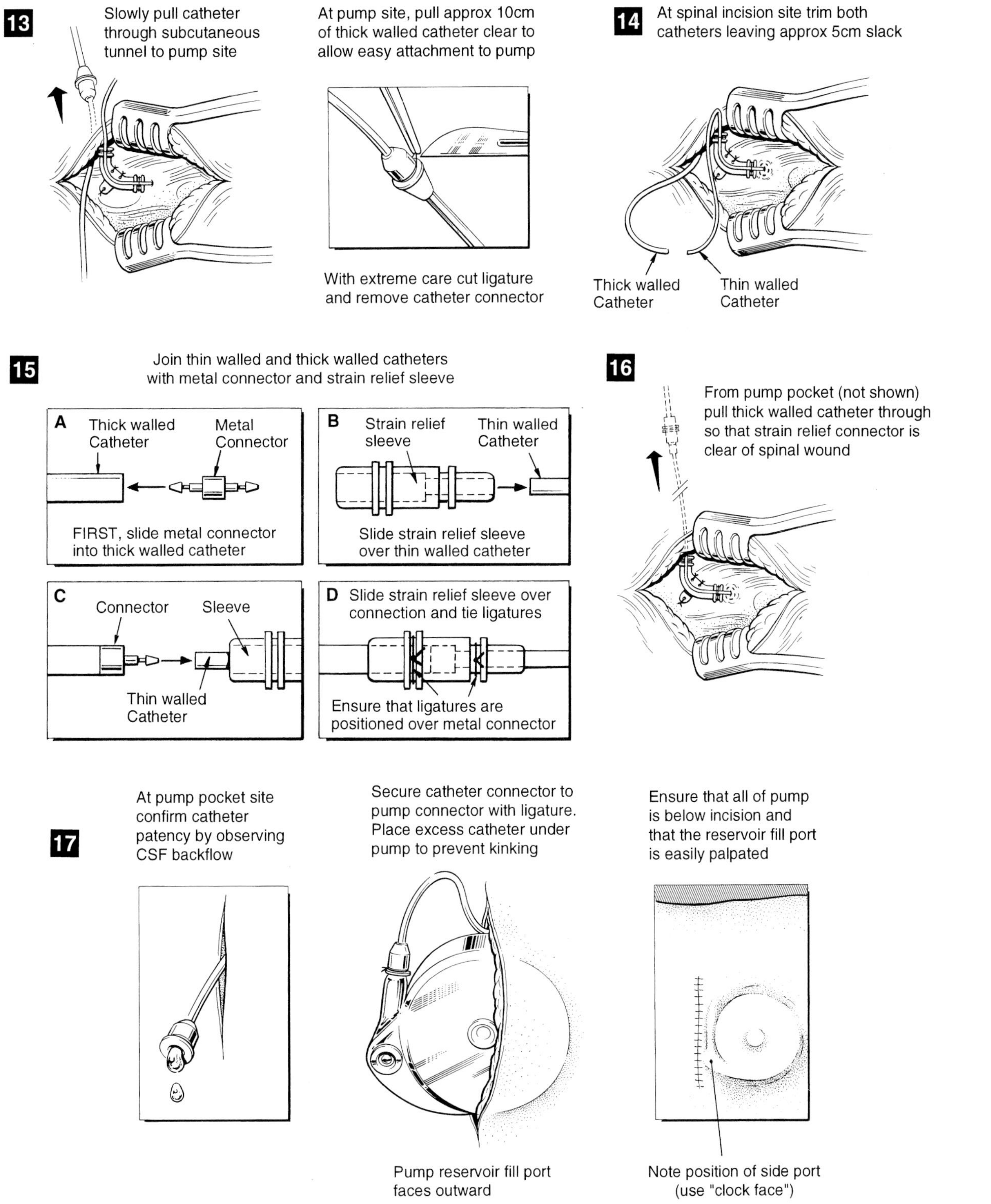

13
Slowly pull catheter through subcutaneous tunnel to pump site
At pump site, pull approx 10cm of thick walled catheter clear to allow easy attachment to pump
With extreme care cut ligature and remove catheter connector
14
At spinal incision site trim both catheters leaving approx 5cm slack
Thick walled Catheter
Thin walled Catheter
15
Join thin walled and thick walled catheters with metal connector and strain relief sleeve
A
Thick walled Catheter
Metal Connector
FIRST, slide metal connector into thick walled catheter
B
Strain relief sleeve
Thin walled Catheter
Slide strain relief sleeve over thin walled catheter
C
Connector
Sleeve
Thin walled Catheter
D
Slide strain relief sleeve over connection and tie ligatures
Ensure that ligatures are positioned over metal connector
16
From pump pocket (not shown) pull thick walled catheter through so that strain relief connector is clear of spinal wound
17
At pump pocket site confirm catheter patency by observing CSF backflow
Secure catheter connector to pump connector with ligature. Place excess catheter under pump to prevent kinking
Ensure that all of pump is below incision and that the reservoir fill port is easily palpated
Pump reservoir fill port faces outward
Note position of side port (use "clock face")

FIG. 29-25. *Continued. 13* Pulling connecting catheter through subcutaneous tissue to pump site. Note that the passage of the connector is greatly facilitated by first dissecting laterally from the spinal site with blunt dissecting scissors. Otherwise, subsequent steps may be more difficult. *14* Spinal site initial steps. *15* Joining of thick-walled and thin-walled spinal catheters. *16* Pulling thick-walled catheter (from pump pocket, not shown) to take up slack in spinal site. Note that as above, the catheter track has been prepared to enable the connector to pass laterally easily. *17* Connecting catheter to intrathecal pump and placement of pump in pocket. Note the check for CSF flow prior to connecting thick-walled catheter to pump.

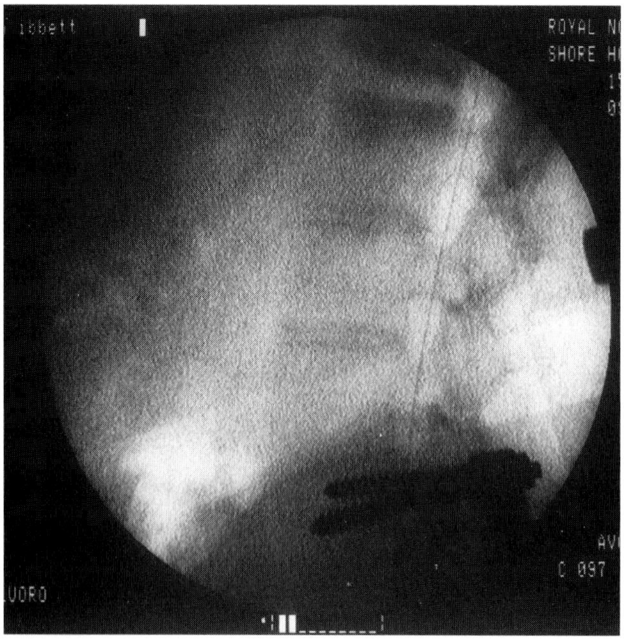

FIG. 29-25. *Continued. 18* X-ray showing intrathecal catheter correctly placed in spinal canal.

is no less today than a decade ago, and trials to compare current practice with systemic infusion of various drug combinations are crucial.[81,316]

Economic pressures on medical practice in every setting, particularly for inpatient care, have increased beyond what could have been anticipated a decade ago. These pressures have in part allowed innovations in pain management to be viewed favorably by insurers and policymakers, who see potential cost-savings from rapid return to normal function after operation, or from care at home rather than in hospital during chronic or terminal illness. "Nocio-economics"—the economics of pain control—has a less sympathetic side, however, manifest as insistence that expenditure of resources for analgesia be linked with demonstrable benefit upon clinical outcomes or cost of care.[62] Payer frugality and patient demands to sustain quality of life are not at odds, however, because both sides benefit when needless and costly pain, impairment, and disability are avoided. Patient satisfaction also has an economic as well as a humanistic dimension, since dissatisfied patients are more likely to change insurance plans and cause revenue loss to those organizations.

Pharmacoeconomics connotes analyses of the incremental improvement in patient outcome that results from an incremental increase in resources expended upon drug therapy, including drug delivery.[48] Australia, New Zealand, the United Kingdom, and parts of Canada now require pharmacoeconomic justification for approval of new drugs. In the U.S., formulary committees of most health maintenance organizations include new drugs (or not) based upon such assessment.[277] Clinical trials with a pharmacoeconomic orientation differ from traditional trials in that the former place greater emphasis on determining effectiveness (what happens under actual conditions of use) than efficacy (what occurs under ideal conditions). Outcomes examined in newer studies go beyond traditional biological or physiological measures, to include measures of quality of life, productivity, and resource consumption. A variety of instruments have been evolved to assess health-related quality of life generically and in specialized fashion for clinical trials, such as analgesic trials, in specific populations or health conditions.[460] Pharmacoeconomics is an evolving and complex discipline that is conducted by individuals with diverse perspectives and agendas. For example, cost analyses[27] can be conducted in terms of cost versus benefit; cost-effectiveness (the latter defined with respect to a specific objective); cost-utility (in which benefit is defined as quality of life, willingness to pay, and patient preference for one intervention over another); cost-minimization; or cost of illness (that includes both direct and indirect measures such as work days lost).[172] Key variables that must be considered in pharmacoeconomic studies of postoperative analgesia include effectiveness, a reduction of pain intensity at rest or with activity;[23] patient-centered outcomes such as acceptance of and satisfaction with devices and care;[83,500] costs of drugs, staff time and effort to perform blocks or place catheters; operating room time, and associated fees; pump purchase and maintenance, and disposable supplies;[245,300,508] risks and expense of potential side effects (nausea, sedation) and complications (respiratory depression, ileus); and finally, cost savings associated with reduced length of stay, fewer complications, earlier return to work (after operation) or less staff time required for care. Surprisingly few studies come close to reporting on all these variables, even for a straightforward analgesic technique such as intravenous patient-controlled analgesia,[27,236,550] but anesthesiologists have awakened to their importance for the continued health of the specialty.[298, 300,459, 501]

Evidence-based practice guidelines are the next step towards data-driven codification of medical practice.[88] Practice guidelines are "systematically developed recommendations that assist the practitioner and patient in making decisions about health care."[323] Strictly speaking, practice guidelines are not mandatory, but pressures to reduce costs and increase quality of care have led health system administrators, insurers, and governmental agencies increasingly to encourage clinicians to follow such guidelines. The past 10 years have been termed "a decade of guidelines in pain management" because of numerous such documents issued by organizations and governments throughout the world.[332] Some of these reports urge incorporation of pain assessment and treatment into quality assurance/improvement procedures so that inadequately treated pain is identified routinely and its cause corrected. In response to this lag, leading medical editors soon will require standardized performance and reporting of clinical trials.[30] Jadad, McQuay, and many others around the world have also begun to apply established methods of meta-analysis to the area of pain control. As described in the preceding section, this last task is far from simple and will require sustained effort internationally, ideally coordinated by groups such as the International Association for the Study of Pain and the Cochrane Collaboration for clinical trials registries.

Chronic Pain from Cancer and Nonmalignant Disease

Continuation of established trends to consider pain control an integral part of medical care in general, and to allocate increasing resources to palliative care, will help those with chronic pain from cancer and nonmalignant disease. Since the initial application of spinal analgesia to patients with cancer pain, broad consensus has existed that this intervention is necessary only for the minority of patients whose pain cannot be relieved by less invasive measures. Yet harnessing the power of spinal analgesia to relieve refractory cancer pain has advanced the field as a whole, not to speak of its benefit upon the quality of life of patients and families who have benefitted from this therapy. A further parallel to the history of postoperative spinal analgesia is that initial enthusiasm for epidural or intrathecal morphine to treat cancer pain[493] has been tempered by subsequent awareness that these techniques may not always be superior to parenteral opioid administration. Recent success with spinal drug combinations[352,353,450] and novel intrathecal analgesics (in patients who tend to have increasingly advanced disease at the point of referral to pain clinics) and wider use of spinal analgesia in patients' homes,[451,455] have altered the context and results of therapy. Current debates concerning patient, device, and infusate selection will not be settled until trials are conducted to compare outcomes carefully during optimal current practice, both within and outside[330] of the hospital, of intrathecal combination therapy versus systemic analgesics and adjuvant medications. In light of growing numbers of patients receiving opioids systematically or by neuraxial infusion for chronic severe pain not due to cancer, separate trials that assess somewhat different outcomes are needed.

Dorsal Horn Amnesia—The Goal of Spinal Analgesia?

The spinal cord is not only a stress-responsive organ but also the site of uniquely adaptive forms of short- and long-term memory.[200] One may distill the above survey of spinal analgesic pharmacology into a simple statement that the sole property common to every current and future spinal analgesic drug is to interfere with one or both types of memory. To understand this view and its implications, it is helpful to recall the four modes of dorsal horn function proposed by Woolf[524] (see Chapters 23.1 and 24), (Table 29-15). In its basal state (Mode 1) a brief volley of afferent nociceptive impulses elicits a somewhat longer response. Local anesthetics applied intrathecally or epidurally suppress this prompt response to afferent impulses by blocking both afferent impulses and dorsal horn responsivity. Spinal or systemic opioids interfere (as depicted in Figure 29-5) with the

TABLE 29-15. *State-dependent processing in the dorsal horn (clinical syndromes)*

Mode	Name	Syndrome
1	Control state	Physiological sensitivity
2	Suppressed state	Hyposensitivity
3	Sensitized state	Postinjury hypersensitivity Inflammatory pain Peripheral neuropathic pain
4	Reorganized state	Peripheral neuropathic pain Central neuropathic pain

From Woolf, C.J., and Chong, M.-S.: Preemptive analgesia: treating postoperative pain by preventing the establishment of central sensitization. Anesth. Analg., *77:* 362, 1993; and Woolf, C.F.: The dorsal horn: State-dependent sensory processing and the generation of pain. *In* Wall, P., Melzack, R. (eds.) Textbook of Pain. 3rd Ed. pp. 110–112. New York, Churchill Livingstone, 1994.

postsynaptic summation of this excitatory volley. Both opioids and local anesthetics impair prolongation and amplification of presynaptic impulses by the postsynaptic cell, that one may identify with "short-term memory" at this site. Continued nociceptive input evokes stimulation produced analgesia for several hours due to release of peptide and monoamine, e.g., acetylcholine and epinephrine, neurotransmitters in endogenous inhibitory pathways.[320] During stimulation-produced analgesia, brief inputs have little effect (Mode 2) and if afferent stimulation ceases, dorsal horn neuronal properties (e.g., firing rates and receptive fields) revert to baseline, much like a spring or pendulum that returns to an initial, stable, state after transient perturbation.[350]

Biochemical mechanisms surveyed earlier and summarized in Figure 29-26 allow persistent noxious input to transform the responses of the dorsal horn from damped and stable (Mode 1) to overdamped (Mode 2), then underdamped (Mode 3), and finally unstable (Mode 4). Sustained nociceptive input into the Mode 2 dorsal horn shifts the pattern of its response: small inputs now evoke large outputs (Mode 3). In shifting from Mode 2 to Mode 3, the dorsal horn changes from a system that attenuates noxious input to one that exaggerates and prolongs it, and develops long-term memory characterized by synaptic reorganization[306] and self-sustaining discharge (Mode 4). In mathematical parlance, the transition from Mode 2 to Mode 3 corresponds to one in which the coefficient that governs the motion of a weight on a spring, or of a pendulum, changes sign. In Modes 3 or 4, brief pertubations are not merely preserved but amplified, and can persist indefinitely. Much theoretical and experimental biology[477] is devoted to understanding such genetically programmed switching between operating modes.[495] The graphical depiction of a stable underlying relationship between all possible inputs and outputs of such dynamic systems is called an "attractor."[442] Replacement of one attractor by another is termed (in a mathematical sense) a "catastrophe," manifest as the system's prompt evolution into a different input-output mode. Genetically programmed catastrophes dictate the abrupt evolution of biological systems from

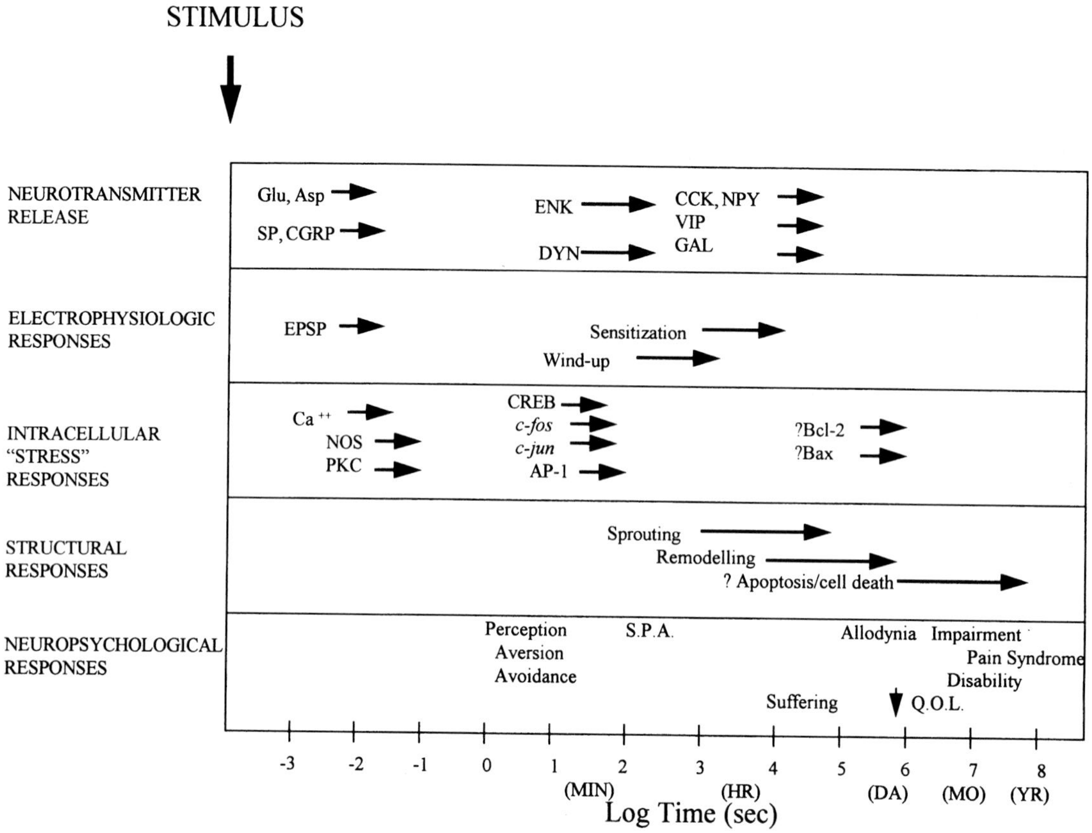

FIG. 29-26. Pain stimulus triggers a cascade of events across many orders of magnitude on the time axis. Peptide, enzyme and gene abbreviations are as in chapter text; S.P.A., stimulation-produced analgesia; Q.O.L., quality of life [From Jones, J.G.: The future of anaesthesia. *In* Keneally, J.P., and Jones, M.R. (eds.): 150 Years On. A Selection of Papers Presented at the 11th World Congress of Anaesthesiologists. pp. 15–21. London, The World Federation of Societies of Anesthesiologists, 1996; and Munglani, R., and Hunt, S.P.: Molecular biology of pain, Br. J. Anaesth., *75*:186, 1995.]

one state to another, such as during normal growth or embryogenesis.[477,518]

Sudden, persistent transitions between dorsal horn modes provoked by nociceptive stimulation correspond to replacement of one attractor by that for the next mode.[477] Every present and future spinal analgesic agent must function to alter the operating characteristics of the dorsal horn neural network, so that the thresholds for these transitions are raised, their onsets delayed, or both. Reversal of such transitions—relevant to reports of cures of acute phantom pain after ketamine[269] or chronic phantom pain after spinal analgesia—is more challenging but not impossible.[350] The present model also suggests that the Mode 4 clinical syndrome of sputtering, sometimes periodic, lancinating neuropathic pain after peripheral nerve injury, corresponds to a complex chaotic output[37] from a coupled array of sensitized dorsal horn neurons originally driven by peripheral input from damaged nerve.[518,432] Pre-emptive analgesia, known to block evolution of the spinal cord dorsal horn beyond Mode 1, therefore may prevent the emergence of such irregular bursts of neuropathic pain, as well as phantom pain long afterwards. Low doses of spinal analgesics, sufficient to diminish slightly the excitability of dorsal horn and impede intercommunication between dorsal horn cells but insufficient to cause sensorimotor block, should also (and do) alleviate such symptoms. It will be helpful to our knowledge of dynamic behavior of the dorsal horn in all its modes if investigations of collective, coupled, aggregates of its cells emerge to supplement the present descriptions based upon single-cell recordings.

Concluding the prior edition of this chapter a decade ago, the authors declared that "Spinal administration of opioids has proved beyond doubt to produce a powerful antinociceptive action that is substantially due to a spinal action. As with many new techniques, spinal opioids have suffered from too much enthusiasm and too little careful documentation of efficacy, safety, indications, and contraindications in the clinical setting. This is a pity, since the animal studies forming the basis of the technique have been meticulous and clear in their implications for the clinician. Further development of spinal opioids must continue to be based on relevant pharmacologic and neuropathologic studies in animals before use in humans. Widespread clinical applications of any further agents or techniques should be preceded by controlled clinical studies." These words still apply today, but the substantial interim advances in preclinical knowledge since they were written,[345] the profusion of new and exciting spinal analgesics now under clinical evaluation or soon to be studied,[454,489,542] and the elevation of standards for clinical trials and their synthesis, make one optimistic for continued progress in, and benefits from, spinal opioid and nonopioid analgesia well into the next millenium.[247]

ACKNOWLEDGMENTS

Support to D.B.C. during preparation of this chapter was provided by the Saltonstall Fund for Pain Research, as well as grants from the National Cancer Institute and the National Institute for Drug Abuse. W. Heinrich Wurm, MD, Chair of the Department of Anesthesia at Tufts University School of Medicine and New England Medical Center, gave ongoing support and encouragement for these and related efforts. Miss Evelyn Hall provided excellent secretarial assistance and John Murray, Charles Fezzie, Iwona Maszczynska, and Dr. Leo Goudas all participated in organizing references and figures. Craig Percy of Lippincott–Raven monitored the preparation of this chapter with grace and forebearance.

REFERENCES

1. Abram, S.E.: Alternative neuraxial pain management techniques. Reg. Anesth., *21:*129, 1996.
2. Abram, S.E.: Spinal cord toxicity of epidural and subarachnoid analgesics. Reg. Anesth., *21:*84, 1996.
3. Abram, S.E., and Hopwood, M.: Can meta-analysis rescue knowledge from a sea of unintelligible data? Reg. Anesth., *21:*514, 1996.
4. Abram, S.E.: Necessity for an animal model of postoperative pain. Anesthesiology, *86:*1015, 1997.
5. Abouleish, E., Barmada, M.A., Nemoto, E.M., Tung, A., and Winter, P.: Acute and chronic effects of intrathecal morphine in monkeys. Br. J. Anaesth., *53:*1027, 1981.
6. Adams, J., Tallarida, R., Geller, E., and Adler, M.: Isobolographic superadditivity between delta and mu opioid agonists in the rat depends on the ratio of compounds, the mu agonist and the analgesic assay used. J. Pharmacol. Exp. Ther., *266:*1261, 1993.
7. Aebischer, P., Tresco, P.A., Winn, S.R., *et al.*: Long term cross-species brain transplantation of a polymer-encapsulated dopamine-secreting cell line. Exp. Neurol., *111:*269, 1991.
8. Aebischer, P., Goddard, M., Signore, A.P., and Timpson, R.L.: Functional recovery in hemiparkinsonian primates transplanted with polymer-encapsulated PC12 Cells. Exp. Neurol., *126:*151, 1994.
9. Ahuja, B.R., and Strunin, L.: Respiratory effects of epidural fentanyl. Anaesthesia, *40:*949, 1985.
10. Åkerman, B., and Arweström, E.: Post C. Local anesthetics potentiate spinal morphine antinociception. Anesth. Analg., *67:*943, 1988.
11. Amandusson, A., Hermanson, O., and Blomquist, A.: Estrogen receptor-like immunoreactivity in the medullary and spinal dorsal horn of the female rat. Neurosci. Lett., *196:*25, 1995.
12. Andersen, H.B., Christensen, C.B., Findlay, J.W., and Janssen, J.A.: Pharmacokinetics of epidural morphine and fentanyl in the goat. Pain, *19*(Suppl.):A564, 1984.
13. Anderson, H.B., Jorgensen, B.C., and Engquist, A.: Epidural met-enkephalin (FK 33-824). A dose-effect study. Acta Anaesthesiol. Scand., *26:*69, 1982.
14. Aoki, M., Senami, M., Kitahata, L., and Collins, J.: Spinal sufentanil effects on spinal pain transmission neurons in cats. Anesthesiology. *64:*225, 1986.
15. Arner, S., and Arner, B.: Differential effects of epidural morphine in the treatment of cancer-related pain. Acta Anaesthesiol. Scand., *29:*32, 1985.
16. Asari, H., Inove, K., Shibata, T., and Soga, T.: Segmental effect of morphine injected into the epidural space in man. Anesthesiology, *54:*75, 1981.
17. Atanassoff, P.G.: Effects of regional anesthesia on perioperative outcome. J. Clin. Anesth., *8:*446, 1996.
18. Atchison, S.R., Durant, P., and Yaksh, T.L.: Cardiorespiratory effects and kinetics of intrathecally injected DADLE and morphine in unanesthetized dogs. Anesthesiology, *65:*609, 1986.
19. Badner, N.H., Reimer, E.J., Komar, W.E., and Moote, C.A.: Low-dose bupivacaine does not improve postoperative epidural fentanyl analgesia in orthopedic patients. Anesth. Analg., *72:*337, 1991.
20. Ballantyne, J.C., Loach, A.B., and Carr, D.B.: Itching after epidural and spinal opiates. Pain, *33:*149, 1988.
21. Ballantyne, J.C., Carr, D.B., Berkey, C.S., *et al.*: Comparative efficacy of epidural, subarachnoid, and intracerebroventricular opioids in patients with pain due to cancer. Reg. Anesth. *21:*542, 1996.
22. Ballantyne, J.C., and Dershwitz, M.: The pharmacology of nonsteroidal anti-inflammatory drugs for acute pain. Curr. Opin. Anesth., *8:*461, 1995.
23. Ballantyne, J.C., Carr, D.B., Chalmers, T.C., *et al.*: Patient-controlled analgesia in the postoperative patient: Meta-analyses of initial randomized control trials. J. Clin. Anesth., *5:*182, 1993.
24. Ballantyne, J.C., Carr, D.B., Chalmers, T.C., *et al.*: Comparative effects of postoperative analgesic therapies upon respiratory function: Meta-analyses of initial randomized control trials. Anesth. Analg. In Press, 1997.
25. Banning, A.M., Schmidt, J.F., Chraemmer, J., *et al.*: Comparison of oral controlled release morphine and epidural morphine in the management of postoperative pain. Anesth. Analg., *65:*385, 1986.
26. Baraka, A., Noueihed, R., and Hajj, S.: Intrathecal injection of morphine for obstetric analgesia. Anesthesiology, *54:*136, 1981.
27. Barbarash, R.A. and Wellman, G.S.: Considerations in the cost analysis of patient-controlled analgesia, Postgrad. Med., 47–50 1986.
28. Basbaum, A.: Insights into the development of opioid tolerance. Pain, *61:*349, 1995.
29. Baxter, A.D., and Kiruluta, G.: Detrusor tone after epidural morphine. Anesth. Analg., *63:*464, 1984.
30. Begg, C., Cho, M., Eastwood, S., *et al.*: Improving the quality of reporting of randomized controlled trials: the CONSORT statement. J.A.M.A., *276:*637, 1996.
31. Behar, M., Olshwang, D., Magora, F., and Davidson, J.T.: Epidural morphine in treatment of pain. Lancet., *1:*527, 1979.
32. Behar, M., Orr, I.A., and Dundee, J.W.: Central action of spinal opiates. Anesthesiology, *55:*334, 1981.
33. Behar, M., Orr, I.A., and Dundee, J.W.: Shrinking pupils is a warning of respiratory depression after spinal morphine. Lancet., *1:*893, 1981.
34. Benedetti, C., McDonald, J.S., Lingam, R., and Seitz, M.: Efficacy of a Port-A-Cath epidural system for cancer pain management. Anesthesiology, *77:*A841, 1992.
35. Bernard, J., Kick, O., and Bonnet, F.: Comparison of intravenous and epidural clonidine for postoperative patient-controlled analgesia. Anesth. Analg, *81:*706, 1995.
36. Bernstein, J.E.: Substance P and substance P antagonists. Curr. Opin. Anesth., *7:*462, 1994.
37. Berry, M.V., Percival, I.C., and Weiss, N.O. (eds): Dynamical Chaos. Princeton, NJ, Princeton University Press, 1987.
38. Besson, J-M.: The pharmacology of pain: Twenty-five years of hope, despair and hope. *In* Gebhart, G.F., Hammond, D.L., Jensen, T.S. (eds.): Proceedings of the 7th World Congress on Pain. Progress in pain research and management. Vol. 2. pp. 23–39. Seattle, IASP Press, 1992.
39. Beutler, A.S., Banck, M.S., Bach, F.W., *et al.*: Retrovirus-mediated expression of an artificial β-endorphin precursor in primary fibroblasts. J. Neurochem., *64:*475, 1995.
40. Bilsback, P., Rolly, G., and Tampubolon, O.: Efficacy of the extradural administration of lofentanil, buprenorphine or saline in the management of postoperative pain: A double-blind study. Br. J. Anaesth., *57:*943, 1985.
41. Boas, R.A.: Hazards of epidural morphine. Anaesth. Intensive Care, *8:*377, 1980.
42. Boas, R.A., and Villiger, J.W.: Clinical actions of fentanyl and buprenorphine: The significance of receptor binding. Br. J. Anaesth., *57:*192, 1985.
43. Bode, R.H., Lewis, K.P., Zarich, S.W., *et al.*: Cardiac outcome after peripheral vascular surgery: Comparison of general and regional anesthesia. Anesthesiology, *84:*3, 1996.
44. Bonnardot, J.P., Maillet, M., Calou, J.C., *et al.*: Maternal and fetal concentrations of morphine after intrathecal administration during labor. Br. J. Anaesth., *54:*487, 1982.

45. Bonnet, F., Blery, C., Zatan, M., *et al.*: Effect of epidural morphine on post-operative pulmonary dysfunction. Acta Anaesthesiol. Scand., *28:*147, 1984.
46. Bonnet, F., Harari, A., and Thibonnier, M.: Suppression of antidiuretic hormone hypersecretion during surgery by extradural anaesthesia. Br. J. Anaesth., *54:*29, 1982.
47. Booker, P.D., Wilkes, R.G., Bryson, T.H.L., and Beddard, J.: Obstetric pain relief using epidural morphine. Anaesthesia, *35:*377, 1980.
48. Bootman, L.J., Townsend, R.J. and McGhan, W.F. (eds.): Principles of Pharmacoeconomics, 2nd ed. Cincinnati, Whitney, 1995.
49. Boreus, L.O., Skoldefors, E., and Ehrnebo, M.: Appearance of pethidine and nor-pethidine in cerebrospinal fluid of man following intramuscular injection of pethidine. Acta Anaesthesiol. Scand., *27:*222, 1983.
50. Borrier, U., Muller, H., Stoyanov, M., and Hempelmann, G.: Epidural opiate analgesia: Compatibility of opiates with tissue and CSF. Anaesthesist, *29:*570, 1980.
51. Bowersox, S.S., Miljanich, G.P., Sugiura, Y., *et al.*: Differential blockade of voltage-sensitive calcium channels at the mouse neuromuscular junction by novel ω-concopeptides and ω-agatoxin-IVA. J. Pharmacol. Exp. Ther., *273:*248, 1995.
52. Breivik, H.: Pre-emptive analgesia. Curr. Opin. Anesth., *7:*458, 1994.
53. Brent, C.R., Harty, G., and Yaksh, T.L.: The effects of spinal opiates on micturation in unanesthesized animals. Soc. Neurosci., *9:*743, 1983.
54. Bridenbaugh, P.O.: Preemptive analgesia—Is it clinically relevant? Anesth. Analg., *78:*203, 1994.
55. Broekema, A.A., Gielen, M.J.M., and Hennis, P.J.: Postoperative analgesia with continuous epidural sufentanil and bupivacaine: A prospective study in 614 patients. Anesth. Analg., *82:*754, 1996.
56. Bromage, P.R.: 50 Years on the wrong side of the reflex arc. Reg. Anesth., *21:*1, 1996.
57. Bromage, P.R., Camporesi, E., and Chestnut, D.: Epidural narcotics for postoperative analgesia. Anesth. Analg., *59:*473, 1980.
58. Bromage, P.R., Camporesi, E.M., Durant, P.A.C., and Niel, C.H.: Nonrespiratory side-effects of epidural morphine. Anesth. Analg., *61:*490, 1982.
59. Bromage, P.R., Camporesi, E.M., Durant, P.A.C., and Niel, C.H.: Rostral spread of epidural morphine. Anesthesiology, *56:*431, 1982.
60. Bromage, P.R., Camporesi, E., and Leslie, J.: Epidural narcotics in volunteers: Sensitivity to pain and to carbon dioxide. Pain, *9:*145, 1980.
61. Bromage, P.R., Joyal, A.C., and Binney, J.C.: Local anesthetic drugs: Penetration from the spinal extradural space into the neuroaxis. Science, *140:*392, 1963.
62. Brose, W.G.: Outcomes and informatics in pain therapy. Curr. Opin. Anesth., *9:*421, 1996.
63. Brose, W.G., Tanelian, D.L., Brodsky, J.B., *et al.*: CSF and blood pharmakokinetics of hydromorphone and morphine following lumbar epidural administration. Pain, *45:*11, 1991.
64. Brown, D.V. and McCarthy, R.J.: Epidural and spinal opioids. Curr. Opin. Anesth., *8:*337, 1995.
65. Brownridge, P.: Epidural and intrathecal opiates for postoperative pain relief. Anaesthesia., *38:*74, 1983.
66. Brownridge, P., and Frewin, D.B.: A comparative study of techniques of postoperative analgesia following cesarean section and lower abdominal surgery. Anaesth. Intensive Care, *13:*123, 1985.
67. Brownridge, P., Wrobel, J., and Watt-Smith, J.: Respiratory depression following accidental subarachnoid pethidine. Anaesth. Intensive Care, *11:*237, 1983.
68. Bruera, E., Brennis, C., Michaud, M., *et al.*: Use of the subcutaneous route for the administration of narcotics in patients with cancer pain. Cancer, *62:*407, 1988.
69. Buchser, E., Goddard, M., Heyd, B., *et al.*: Immunoisolated xenogeneic chromaffin cell therapy for chronic pain: Initial clinical experience. Anesthesiology, *85:*1005, 1996.
70. Budd K: Prevention or cure? Editorial review. Curr. Opin. Anesth., *7:*453, 1994.
71. Burks, T.F.: Opioid peptides in gastrointestinal functions. *In* Tseng, L.F. (ed.): The Pharmacology of Opioid Peptides. pp. 397–410. Langhorn, PA, Harwood Academic Press, 1995.
72. Calman, K.C., Hanks G.: Clinical and health services research in palliative care. *In* Doyle, D., Hanks G, and MacDonald, N. (eds.): Oxford Textbook of Palliative Medicine. pp. 73–77. Oxford, Oxford University Press, 1993.
73. Camporesi, E.M., Nielsen, C.H., Bromage, P.R., and Durant, P.A.: Ventilatory CO_2 sensitivity after intravenous and epidural morphine in volunteers. Anesth. Analg., *62:*633, 1983.
74. Cardan, E.: Spinal morphine in enuresis. Br. J. Anaesth., *57:*354, 1985.
75. Carl, P., Crawford, M.E., Ravlo, O., and Bach, V.: Long-term treatment with epidural opioids: A retrospective study comprising 150 patients treated with morphine chloride and buprenorphine. Anaesthesia, *41:*32, 1986.
76. Carli, F., and Halliday, D.: Continuous epidural blockade arrests the postoperative decrease in muscle protein fractional synthetic rate in surgical patients. Anesthesiology, *86:*1033, 1997.
77. Carpenter, R.L., Abram, S.E., Bromage, P.R., and Rauk, R.L.: Consensus statement on acute pain management. Reg. Anesth., *21:*152, 1996.
78. Carpenter, R.L.: Future directions for outcome research in acute pain management: Design of clinical trials. Reg. Anesth., *21:*137, 1996.
79. Carpenter, R.L.: Future epidural or subarachnoid analgesics: Local anesthetics. Reg. Anesth., *21*(6S):75, 1996.
80. Carr, D.B.: Economics of patient-controlled analgesia: An annotated bibliography. *In* Campbell, J.N. (ed.): Pain 1996: An Updated Review. pp. 437–439. Seattle, IASP Press, 1996.
81. Carr, D.B.: Preemptive analgesia implies prevention. Anesthesiology. *85:*1498, 1996.
82. Carr, D.B., and Lipkowski, A.W.: Today's versus tomorrow's opioids for cancer pain: Who will close the gap? Analgesia, *2:*1, 1996.
83. Carr, D.B., Miaskowski, C., Dedrick, S.C., Williams, G.R.: Management of perioperative pain in hospitalized patients: A national survey. J. Clin. Anesth., In press.
84. Carr, D.B.: The evolving practice of regional anesthesia. Curr. Opin. Anesth., *7:*427, 1994.
85. Carr, D.B.: Opioids. Int. Anesthesiol. Clin., *26:*283, 1988.
86. Carr, D.B.: Evidence, explanation-or "the power of myth"? Curr. Opin. Anesth., *9:*415, 1996.
87. Carr, D.B.: Spinal opioid and nonopioid analgesia. Anesth. Analg., (Suppl.) 19–25, 1997.
88. Carr, D.B., and Aronoff, G.M.: The future of pain management. *In* Aronoff, G.M. (ed.): Evaluation and Treatment of Chronic Pain. pp. 507–521. Baltimore, Williams & Wilkins, 1995.
89. Carr, D.B., and Goudas, L.C.: Postoperative pain control: A survey of promising drugs and pharmacoeconomic criteria for purchasing them. *In* Campbell, J.N. (ed): Pain 1996: An Updated Review. pp. 189–194. Seattle, IASP Press, 1996.
90. Carr, D.B., Jacox, A.K., Chapman, C.R., *et al.*: Acute pain management: Operative or medical procedures and trauma. Clinical Practice Guidelines No. 1. Rockville, MD. U.S. Department of Health and Human Services, 1992.
91. Carr, D.B., and Lipkowski, A.W.: Mechanisms of opioid analgetic actions. *In* Rogers, M., Tinker, J.H., Covino, B.G., and Longnecker, D.E. (eds.): Principles and Practice of Anesthesiology. Vol 1. pp. 1105–1130. St. Louis, Mosby–Year Book, 1993.
92. Cepeda, M.S., and Carr, D.B.: The stress response and regional anesthesia. *In*: Brown, D.L. (ed.): Regional Anesthesia and Analgesia. pp. 108–123. Philadelphia, W.B. Saunders Company, 1996.
93. Cepeda, M.S., Delgado, M., Ponce, M., *et al.*: Equivalent outcomes during postoperative patient-controlled intravenous analgesia with lidocaine plus morphine versus morphine alone. Anesth. Analg., *83:*102, 1996.
94. Chakravarty, K., Tucker, W., Rosen, M., and Vickers, M.D.: Comparison of buprenorphine and pethidine given intravenously on demand to relieve post-operative pain. Br. Med. J., *2:*895, 1979.
95. Chaney, M.A.: Intrathecal and epidural anesthesia for cardiac surgery. Anesth. Analg., *84:*1211, 1997.
96. Chaney, M.A.: Side effects of intrathecal and epidural opioids. Can. J. Anaesth., *42:*891, 1995.
97. Chaplan, S.R., Bach, F.W., Shafer, S.L., and Yaksh, T.L.: Prolonged alleviation of tactile allodynia by intravenous lidocaine in neuropathic rats. Anesthesiology, *83:*775, 1995.
98. Chapman, V., and Dickensen, A.H.: The spinal and peripheral roles of bradykinin and prostaglandins in nociceptive processing in the rat. Eur. J. Pharmacol., *219:*427, 1992.
99. Chapman, V., Haley, J., and Dickenson, A.H.: Electrophysiologic analysis of preemptive effects of spinal opioids on N-methyl-D-aspartate receptor-mediated events. Anesthesiology, *81:*1429, 1994.
100. Chauvin, M., Salbaing, J., Perrin, D., *et al.*: Clinical assessment and

plasma pharmacokinetics associated with intramuscular or extradural alfentanil. Br. J. Anaesth., *57:*886, 1985.
101. Chauvin, M., Samii, K., Schermann, J.M., *et al.*: Plasma morphine concentration after intrathecal administration of low doses of morphine. Br. J. Anaesth., *53:*1065, 1981.
102. Chauvin, M., Samii, K., Schermann, J.M., *et al.*: Plasma pharmacokinetics of morphine after I.M. extradural and intrathecal administration. Br. J. Anaesth., *54:*843, 1981.
103. Cheam, E.W.S., and Morgan, M.: The superiority of epidural opioids for postoperative analgesia—fact or fantasy? Anaesthesia, *49:*1019, 1994.
104. Cherry, D.A.: Drug delivery systems for epidural administration of opioids. Acta Anaesthesiol. Scand. Suppl., *85:*54, 1987.
105. Cherry, D.A., Gourlay, G.K., and Cousins, M.J.: Extradural mass associated with lack of efficacy of epidural morphine, and undetectable CSF morphine concentrations. Pain, *25:*69, 1986.
106. Cherry, D.A., Gourlay, G.K., Cousins, M.J., and Gannon, B.J.: A technique for the insertion of an implantable portal system for the long-term epidural administration of opioids in the treatment of cancer pain. Anaesth. Intensive Care, *13:*145, 1985.
107. Cherry, D.A., Gourlay, G.K., McLachlan, M., and Cousins, M.J.: Diagnostic epidural opioid blockade and chronic pain: Preliminary report. Pain, *21:*143, 1985.
108. Chick, W.L., Perna, J.J., Lauris, V., *et al.*: Artificial pancreas using living beta cells: Effects on glucose homeostasis in diabetic rats. Science, *197:*780, 1977.
109. Choe, H., Choi, Y-S., Kim, Y-H., *et al.*: Epidural morphine plus ketamine for upper abdominal surgery: Improved analgesia from preincisional versus postincisional administration. Anesth. Analg. *84:*560, 1997.
110. Christensen, P., and Brandt, M.R.: Extradural morphine and Stokes-Adams attacks. Br. J. Anaesth., *54:*363, 1982.
111. Christensen, V.: Respiratory depression after extradural morphine. Br. J. Anaesth., *52:*841, 1980.
112. Chrubasik, J., Meynadier, J., Blond, S., *et al.*: Somatostatin, a potent analgesic. Lancet. *2:*1208, 1984.
113. Chrubasik, J., Scholler, K., and Bammert, J.: Epidural morphine injection and cisternal cerebellomedullary CSF bioavailability of morphine in dogs. *In* Erdmann, W., Oyama, T., and Pernak, M. (eds.): The Pain Clinic. pp. 47–49. Utrecht, UNU Science Press, 1985.
114. Chrubasik, J., Meynadier, J., Scherperell, P., *et al.*: The effect of epidural somatostatin on postoperative pain. Anesth. Analg., *64:*1085, 1985.
115. Chrubasik, J., Volk, J., Meynadier, J., *et al.*: Observations in dogs receiving chronic spinal somatostatin and calcitonin. Schmerz. Pain Douleur, *1:*10, 1986.
116. Chrubasik, J., and Wiebers, K.: Continuous-plus-on-demand epidural infusions of morphine for postoperative pain relief by means of a small, externally worn infusion device. Anesthesiology, *62:*263, 1985.
117. Chrubasik, J., and Chrubasik, S.: Meta-analysis in the efficacy of intrathecal and epidural opiates. *In* Parris, W. (ed.): Cancer Pain Management. pp. 207–214. Boston, Butterworth-Heinemann, 1997.
118. Chrubasik, J., Chrubasik, S., and Mather, L. (eds.): Postoperative Epidural Opioids, Germany, Springer-Verlag, 1993.
119. Clinch, J.J., and Schipper, H.: Quality of life assessment in palliative care. *In* Doyle, D., Hanks, G.W.C., and MacDonald, N. (eds.): Oxford Textbook of Palliative Medicine. pp. 61–70. Oxford, Oxford University Press, 1993.
120. Coda, B.A., Brown, M.C., Schaffer, R., *et al.*: Pharmacology of epidural fentanyl, alfentanil, and sufentanil in volunteers. Anesthesiology, *81:*1149, 1994.
121. Coleman, D.E., Berghuis, A.M., Lee, E., *et al.*: Structures of active conformations of $G_I\alpha_1$ and the mechanism of GTP Hydrolysis. Science, *265:*1405, 1994.
122. Colpaert, F.C.: Can chronic pain be suppressed despite purported tolerance to narcotic analgesia? Life Sci., *24:*1201, 1979.
123. Colpaert, F.C., Leysen, L.E., Michiels, M., and Van den Hoogen, R.: Epidural and intravenous sufentanil in the rat: Analgesia, opiate receptor binding, and drug concentrations in plasma and brain. Anesthesiology, *65:*41, 1986.
124. Coombs, D.W.: Management of chronic pain by epidural and intrathecal opioids: Newer drugs and delivery systems. *In* Sjostrand, U.H., and Rawal, N. (eds.): Regional Opioids in Anesthesiology and Pain Management. Int. Anesthesiol. Clin., *24:*58, 1986.
125. Coombs, D.W., Fratkin, J.D., Meier, F.A., *et al.*: Neuropathologic lesions and CSF morphine concentrations during chronic continuous intraspinal morphine infusion. Pain, *22:*337, 1985.
126. Coombs, D.W., Maurer, L.H., Saunders, R.L., and Gaylor, M.: Outcomes and complications of continuous intraspinal narcotic analgesia for cancer pain control. J. Clin. Oncol., *2:*1414, 1984.
127. Coombs, D.W., Sanders, R.L., Gaylor, M., and Pageau, M.G.: Epidural narcotic infusion: Implantation technique and efficacy. Anesthesiology, *55:*469, 1981.
128. Coombs, D.W., Saunders, R.L., Harbaugh, R., *et al.*: Relief of continuous chronic pain by intraspinal narcotics infusion via an implanted reservoir. J.A.M.A., *250:*2336, 1983.
129. Coombs, D.W., Saunders, R.L., LaChance, D., *et al.*: Intrathecal morphine tolerance: Use of intrathecal clonidine, DADLE, and intraventricular morphine. Anesthesiology, *62:*358, 1985.
130. Cousins, M.J. Prevention of postoperative pain. *In* Bond, M.R., Charlton, J.E., and Woolf, J. (eds.): Proceedings of the 7th World Congress on Pain. pp. 41–52. London, Elsevier Science Publishers, 1991.
131. Cousins, M.J., Cherry, D.A., and Gourlay, G.K.: Acute and chronic pain: Use of spinal opioids. *In* Cousins, M.J., and Bridenbaugh, P.O. (eds.): Neural Blockade. pp. 955–1029. Philadelphia, J.B. Lippincott, 1988.
132. Cousins, M.J. and Plummer, J.L.: Spinal opioids in acute and chronic pain. *In* Max, M.B., Pourtenoy, R.K., and Laska, E.M. (eds.): Advances in Pain Research and Therapy. pp. 457–479. New York, Raven Press, 1991.
133. Cousins, M.J., and Bridenbaugh, P.O.: Spinal opioids and pain relief in acute care. In Cousins, M.J., and Phillips, G.D. (eds.): Acute Pain Management. pp. 151–185. New York, Churchill-Livingstone, 1986.
134. Cousins, M.J., and Mather, L.E.: Intrathecal and epidural administration of opioids. Anesthesiology, *61:*276, 1984.
135. Cousins, M.J., Mather, L.E., Glynn, C.J., *et al.*: Selective spinal analgesia. Lancet, *1:*1141, 1979.
136. Cousins, M.J., Mather, L.E., and Gourlay, G.K.: Axon, spinal cord and brain: Targets for acute pain control. *In* Scott, D.B., McClure, J., and Wildsmith, J.A. (eds.): Regional Anaesthesia 1884–1984. Denmark, J.H. Schultz, 1984.
137. Cowen, M.J., Bullingham, R.E.S., Paterson, G.M.C., *et al.*: A controlled comparison of the effects of extradural diamorphine and bupivacaine on plasma glucose and plasma cortisol in postoperative patients. Anesth. Analg., *61:*15, 1982.
138. Cox, B.M.: Molecular and cellular mechanisms in opioid tolerance. *In* Basbaum, A.I., and Besson, J.M. (eds): Towards a New Pharmacotherapy of Pain. pp. 137–156. New York, A Wiley-Interscience Publication, 1991.
139. Cozian, A., Pinaud, M., Lapage, *et al.*: Effects of meperidine spinal anesthesia on hemodynamics, plasma catecholamines, angiotensin I, aldosterone, and histamine concentrations in elderly men. Anesthesiology, *64:*815, 1986.
140. Cramond, T., and Stuart, G.: Intraventricular morphine for intractable pain of advanced cancer. J. Pain Symptom Manage., *8:* 465, 1993.
141. Crawford, M.E., Andersen, H.B., *et al.*: Pain treatment on outpatient basis utilizing extradural opiates: A Danish multicentive study comprising 105 patients. Pain, *16:*41, 1983.
142. Crul, B., and Delhass, E.: Technical complications during long-term subarachnoid or epidural administration of morphine in terminally ill cancer patients: A review of 140 cases. Reg. Anesth., *16:*209, 1991.
143. Dahl, J.B.: The status of pre-emptive analgesia. Curr. Opin. Anaesth. *8:*323, 1995.
144. Dailey, P.A., Brookshire, G.L., Shnider, S.M., *et al.*: The effects of naloxone associated with the intrathecal use of morphine in labor. Anesth. Analg., *64:*658, 1985.
145. Davies, G.K., Tolhurst-Cleaver, C.L., and James, T.L.: CNS depression from intrathecal morphine. Anesthesiology, *52:*280, 1980.
146. Davies, G.K., Tolhurst-Cleaver, C.L., and James, T.L.: Respiratory depression after intrathecal narcotics. Anaesthesia, *35:*1080, 1980.
147. De Kock, M.: Alpha-2 adrenoceptor agonists: Clonidine, dexmedetomidine, mivazerol. Curr. Opin. Anesth., *9:*295, 1996.
148. de Leon-Casasola, O.A., and Lema, M.J.: Postoperative epidural opioid analgesia: What are the choices? Anesth. Analg. *83:*867, 1996.
149. de Leon-Casasola, O.A.: Clinical outcome after epidural anesthesia and analgesia in high-risk surgical patients. Reg. Anesth., *21:*144, 1996.

150. Deber, C.M., and Li, S.: Peptides in membranes: Helicity and hydrophobicity. Biopolymers., (Peptide Science), *37:*295, 1995.
151. DeConno, F., Caraceni, A., Martini C., *et al.*: Hyperalgesia and myoclonus with intrathecal infusion of high-dose morphine. Pain, *47:*337, 1991.
152. DeGroat, W.C., Kawatani, M., *et al.*: The role of neuropeptides in the sacral autonomic reflex pathways of the cat. J. Auton. Nerv. Syst., *7:*339, 1983.
153. DeLander, G.E., and Hopkins, C.J.: Spinal adenosine modulates descending antinociceptive pathways stimulated by morphine. J. Pharmacol. Exp. Ther., *239:*88, 1986.
154. DeLander, G.E., and Hopkins, C.J.: Involvement of A_2 adenosine receptors in spinal mechanisms of antinociception. Eur. J. Pharmacol., *139:*215, 1987.
155. DeLander, G.E., and Hopkins, C.J.: Interdependence of spinal adenosinergic, serotonergic and noradrenergic systems mediating antinociception. Neuropharmacology, *26:*1791, 1987.
156. DeLander, G.E., and Keil II, G.J.: Antinociception induced by intrathecal coadministration of selective adenosine receptor and selective opioid receptor agonists in mice. J. Pharmacol. Exp. Ther., *268:*943, 1993.
157. DeLander, G.E., and Wahl, J.J.: Behavior induced by putative nociceptive neurotransmitters is inhibited by adenosine or adenosine analogs coadministered intrathecally. J. Pharmacol. Exp. Ther. *246:*565, 1988.
158. DeLander, G.E. and Wahl, J.J.: Morphine (intracerebroventricular) activates spinal systems to inhibit behavior induced by putative pain neurotransmitters. J. Pharmacol. Exp. Ther. *251:*1090, 1989.
159. Denson, D.D., Raj, P.P., Joyce, T.H., *et al.*: Kinetics of continuous epidural bupivacaine infusions. Anesthesiology, *55:*A159, 1981.
160. Dickenson, A.H.: NMDA receptor antagonists as analgesics. *In* Fields, H.L., and Liebeskind, J.C. (eds.): Pharmacological Approaches to the Treatment of Chronic Pain: New Concepts and Critical Issues. pp. 173–187. Seattle, IASP Press, 1994.
161. Dickenson, A.H.: Where and how do opioids act? *In* Gebhart, G.F., Hammond D.L. and Jensen, T.S. (eds.): Proceedings of the 7th World Congress on Pain. pp. 525–552. Seattle, IASP Press, 1994.
162. Dickenson, A.H.: Spinal cord pharmacology of pain. Br. J. Anaesth., *75:*193, 1995.
163. Dickenson, A.H., and Sullivan, A.F.: Combination therapy in analgesia; Seeking synergy. Curr. Opin. Anesth., *6:*86, 1993.
164. DiChiro, G.: Movement of the cerebrospinal fluid in human beings. Nature, *204:*290, 1964.
165. DiChiro, G.: Observations on the circulation of the cerebrospinal fluid. Acta Radiol. [Diagn.] (Stockh.), *5:*988, 1966.
166. Dohi, S: Spinal antinociception. Curr. Opin. Anesth., *9:*404, 1996.
167. Donadoni, R., Rolly, G., Noorduin, H., and Vanden Bussche, G.: Epidural sufentanil for postoperative pain relief. Anaesthesia, *40:*634, 1985.
168. Dooley, C.T., Chung, N.N., Wilkes, B.C., *et al.*: An all D-amino acid opioid peptide with central analgesic activity from a combinatorial library. Science, *266:*2019, 1994.
169. Dourish, C.T., O'Neil, M.F., Schaffer, L.W., *et al.*: The cholecystokinin receptor antagonist devazepide enhances morphine-induced analgesia but not morphine-induced respiratory depression in the squirrel monkey. J. Pharmacol. Exp. Ther., *255:*1158, 1990.
170. Drayer, B.P., and Rosenbaum, A.E.: Studies of the third circulation: Amipaque CT cisternography and ventriculography. J. Neurosurg., *48:*946, 1978.
171. Drower, E.J., Stapelfeld, A., Rafferty, M.F., *et al.*: Selective antagonism by naltrindole of the antinociceptive effects of the delta opioid agonist cyclic [D-Penicillamine^2-D-Penicillamine^5] enkephalin in the rat. J. Pharmacol. Exp. Ther., *259:*725, 1991.
172. Drummond, M.F.: Cost-of-illness studies: A major headache. Pharmacoeconomics., *2:*1, 1992.
173. Dubner, R., and Ren, K.: Central mechanisms of thermal and mechanical hyperalgesia following tissue inflammation. *In* Boivie, J., Hansson, P. and Lindblom, U. (eds.): Touch, Temperature, and Pain in Health and Disease: Mechanisms and Assessments. pp. 267–277. Seattle: IASP Press, 1993.
174. Duggan, A.W., Morton, C.R., Johnson, S.M., and Zhao, Z.Q.: Opioid antagonists and spinal reflexes in the anaesthestized cat. Brain Res., *297:*33, 1984.
175. DuPen, S.I., Kharasch, E.D., Williams, A., *et al.*: Chronic bupivacaine-opioid infusion in intractable cancer pain. Pain, *49:*293, 1992.
176. Durant, P.A., and Yaksh, T.L.: Epidural injections of bupivacaine, morphine, fentanyl, lofentanil and DADL in chronically implanted rats: A pharmacologic and pathologic study. Anesthesiology, *64:*43, 1986.
177. Durant, P.A., and Yaksh, T.L.: Distribution in cerebrospinal fluid, blood and lymph of epidurally injected morphine and insulin in dogs. Anesth. Analg., *65:*583, 1986.
178. Duttaroy, A., Pharm, B.S., Byron, M.S., and Yoburn, C.: The effect of intrinsic efficacy on opioid tolerance. Anesthesiology, *82:*1226, 1995.
179. El-Baz, N.M., Faber, L.P., and Jensik, R.J.: Continuous epidural infusion of morphine for treatment of pain after thoracic surgery: A new technique. Anesth. Analg., *63:*757, 1984.
180. Eisenach, J.C., DuPen, S., Dubois, M., *et al.*: Epidural clonidine analgesia for intractable cancer pain. Pain, *61:*391, 1995.
181. Eisenach, J.C.: New agents to clinical practice: Introduction to clinical trials. Reg. Anesth., *21:*135, 1996.
182. Eisenach, J.C.: Three novel spinal analgesics: Clonidine, neostigmine, amitriptyline. Reg. Anesth., *21:*81, 1996.
183. Erdine S, and Aldemir T: Long-term results of peridural morphine in 225 patients. Pain, *45:*155, 1991.
184. Erickson, D.L., Blacklock, J.B., Michaelson, M., *et al.*: Control of spasticity by implantable continuous flow morphine pump. Neurosurgery., *16:*215, 1985.
185. Epand, R.M., Shai, Y., Segrest, J.P., and Anantharamaiah, G.M.: Mechanisms for the modulation of membrane bilayer properties by amphipathic helical peptides. Biopolymers (Peptide Science), *37:*319, 1995.
186. Evron, S., Samueloff, A., Simon, A., *et al.*: Urinary function during epidural analgesia with methadone and morphine in post-cesarean section patients. Pain, *23:*135, 1985.
187. Ferrante, F.M., Bedder, M., Caplan, R.A., *et al.*: Practice guidelines for cancer pain management. Anesthesiology., *84:*1243, 1996.
188. Ferrante, F.M. and VadeBoncouer, T.R.: Epidural analgesia with combinations of local anesthetics and opioids. *In* Ferrante, F.N., and VadeBoncouer, T.R. (eds.): Postoperative Pain Management. pp. 305–333. New York: Churchill-Livingstone, 1993.
189. Fields, H.L. (ed.): Core Curriculum for Professional Education in Pain. 2nd ed. Seattle, IASP Press, 1995.
190. Filos, K.S., Goudas, L.C., Patroni, O., and Tassoudis, V.: Analgesia with epidural nimodipine. Lancet, *342:*1047, 1993.
191. Filos, K.S., Goudas, L.C., Patroni, O., and Polyzou, V.: Intrathecal clonidine as a sole analgesic for pain relief after cesarean section. Anesthesiology, *77:*267, 1992.
192. Fisher, D.M., and Marcario, A.: Economics of anesthesia care: A call to arms! Anesthesiology, *86:*1018, 1997.
193. Fleming, W.W., and Taylor, D.A.: Cellular mechanisms of opioid tolerance and dependence. *In* Tseng, L.F. (ed.): The Pharmacology of Opioid Peptides. pp. 463. Langhorn, PA, Harwood Academic Press, 1995.
194. Fletcher, D., Kayser, V., and Guilbaud, G.: Influence of timing of administration on the analgesic effect of bupivacaine infiltration in carageenin-injected rats. Anesthesiology, *84:*1129, 1996.
195. Florez, J., McCarty, L.E., and Borison, H.L.: A comparative study in the cat of the respiratory effects of morphine injected intravenously and into the cerebrospinal fluid. J. Pharmacol. Exp. Ther., *163:*448, 1968.
196. Fraser, H.M., Chapman, V., and Dickenson, A.H.: Spinal local anesthetic actions on afferent-evoked responses and wind-up nociceptive neurones in the rat spinal cord: Combination with morphine produces marked potentiation of antinociception. Pain, *49:*33, 1992.
197. Freidman, A., Kaufer, D., Shemer, J., *et al.*: Pyridostigmine brain penetration under stress enhances neuronal excitability and induces early immediate transcriptional response. Nat. Med. *12:*1382, 1996.
198. Garzon, J.: Cellular transduction regulated by μ and δ-opioid receptors in supraspinal analgesia: GTP binding regulatory proteins as pharmacological targets. Analgesia, *1:*131, 1995.
199. Gauthier-Lafaye, P., and Muller, A.: (eds.): Anesthésie loco-régionale et traîtement de la douleur. 3rd Ed. Paris, Masson, 1996.
200. Gebhart, G.F., Hammond, D.L., Jensen, T.S. (eds.): Proceedings of the 7th World Congress on Pain. Vol 2. Seattle, IASP Press, 1994.
201. Gericke, M., Morgenstern, R., and Ott, T.: The influence of tifluadom on cholecystokinin-induced antinociception. Eur. J. Pharmacol., *180:*187, 1990.
202. Gjessing, J., and Tomlin, P.J.: Postoperative pain control with intrathecal morphine. Anaesthesia, *36:*268, 1981.

203. Glass, P.S. and Grichnik, K.P.: The role of opioids for epidural analgesia. Curr. Opin. Anesth., *8:*283, 1993.
204. Glynn, C.J., and Mather, L.E.: Clinical pharmacokinetics applied to patients with intractable pain: Studies with pethidine. Pain, *13:*237, 1982.
205. Glynn, C.J., Mather, L.E., Cousins, M.J., *et al.*: Peridural meperidine in humans: Analgetic response, pharmacokinetics and transmission into CSF. Anesthesiology, *55:*520, 1981.
206. Glynn, C.J., Mather, L.E., Cousins, M.J., *et al.*: Spinal narcotics and respiratory depression. Lancet, *2:*356, 1979.
207. Go, A.S., and Browner, W.S.: Cardiac outcomes after regional or general anesthesia: Do we have the answer? Anesthesiology, *84:*1, 1996.
208. Gogas, K.R., Presley, R.W., *et al.*: The antinociceptive action of supraspinal opioids results from an increase in descending inhibitory control: Correlation of nociceptive behavior and cfos expression. Neuroscience, *42:*617, 1991.
209. Goodman, C.B., Elmer, G.I., Yang, H.T., *et al.*: Modulation of opioid receptors by anti-opioid peptides. *In* Tseng, L.F. (ed.): The Pharmacology of Opioid Peptides. pp. 303–320. Philadelphia, Harwood Academic Press, 1995.
210. Goudas, L.C.: Clonidine. Curr. Opin. Anesth., *8:*455, 1995.
211. Goudas, L.C., Hassan, W.N., Carr, D.B., *et al.*: Renal oxidative stress induced by central morphine administration: Uncoupled regulation of JNK/p38 MAP kinases. J. Biol. Chem. (submitted).
212. Goudas, L.C., Carr, D.B., Lau, J., *et al.*: The spinal clonidine—opioid analgesic interaction: From laboratory animals to the operating room: A systematic analysis of preclinical and clinical evidence. Analgesia., In press.
213. Gourlay, G.K., Cherry, D.A., and Cousins, M.J.: Cephalad migration of morphine in CSF following lumbar epidural administration in patients with cancer pain. Pain, *23:*317, 1985.
214. Gourlay, G.K., Wilson, P.R., and Glynn, C.J.: Pharmacodynamics and pharmacokinetics of methadone during the perioperative period. Anesthesiology, *57:*458, 1982.
215. Grouls, R.J.E., Meert, T.F., Korsten, H.H.M., *et al.*: Epidural and intrathecal n-Butyl-p-Aminobenzoate solution in the rat—Comparison with bupivacaine. Anesthesiology, *86:*181, 1997.
216. Gouveia, W.A.: Applying patient outcomes and pharmacoeconomics in patient care; Executive summary. Am. J. Health Syst. Pharm., *52:*[s]3, 1995.
217. Gustafsson, L.L., Friberg-Nielsen, S., and Garle, M.: Extradural and parenteral morphine: Kinetics and effects in postoperative pain: A controlled clinical study. Br. J. Anaesth., *54:*1167, 1982.
218. Gustafsson, L.L., Garle, M., Johannisson, J., *et al.*: Regional epidural analgesia: Kinetics of pethidine. Acta Anaesthesiol. Scand., *74*(Suppl.):165, 1982.
219. Gustafsson, L.L., Hartvig, P., Bergstrom, K., *et al.*: Distribution of ^{11}C-labelled morphine and pethidine after spinal administration to Rhesus monkey. Acta Anaesth. Scand., *33:*105, 1989.
220. Gustafsson, L.L., Johannisson, J., and Garle, M.: Extradural and parenteral pethidine as analgesia after total hip replacement: Effects and kinetics. A controlled clinical study. Eur. J. Clin. Pharmacol., *29:*529, 1986.
221. Hanks, G.W., DeConno, F., Ripamonti, C., *et al.*: Morphine in cancer pain: Modes of administration. Br. Med. J., *312:*823, 1996.
222. Hasselblad, V., Mosteller, F., Littenberg, B., *et al.*: A survey of current problems in metaanalysis. Discussion from the Agency for Health Care Policy and Research Inter-PORT Work Group on Literature. Med. Care., *33:*202, 1995.
223. Hassenbusch, S.J., Stanton-Hicks, M., Covington, E.C., *et al.*: Long-term intraspinal infusions of opioids in the treatment of neuropathic pain. J. Pain Symptom. Manage., *10:*527, 1995.
224. Henry, J.L. and Radhakrishnan, V.: Hyperalgesia following noxious thermal, mechanical, or chemical stimulation involves overlapping spinal mechanisms and interactive participation of excitatory amino acids and neuropeptides. A.P.S. J., *3:*249, 1994.
225. Hjortsø. N.-C., Lund, C., Mogensen, T., *et al.*: Epidural morphine improves pain relief and maintains sensory analgesia during continuous epidural bupivacaine after abdominal surgery. Anesth. Analg., *65:*1033, 1986.
226. Hoffman, D., Breakfield, X.O., Short, P., and Aebischer, P.: Transplantation of a polymer-encapsulated cell line genetically engineered to release NGF. Exp. Neurol., *122:*100, 1993.
227. Hogan, Q., Haddoz, J.D., Abram, S., *et al.*: Epidural opiates and local anesthetics for the management of cancer pain. Pain, *46:*271, 1991.
228. Honore, P., Chapman, V., Buritova, J., and Besson, J.M.: Concomitant administration of morphine and an N-methyl-D-aspartate receptor antagonist profoundly reduces inflammatory evoked spinal c-fos expression. Anesthesiology, *85:*150, 1996.
229. Horan, P.J., Mattia, A., Bilsky, E.J., *et al.*: Antinociceptive profile of biphalin, a dimeric enkephalin analog. J. Pharmacol. Exp. Ther. *265:*1446, 1993.
230. Hotvedt, R., and Refsum, H.: Cardiac effects of thoracic epidural morphine caused by increased vagal activity in the dog. Acta Anaesthesiol. Scand., *30:*76, 1986.
231. Howard, R.P., Milne, L.A., and Williams, N.E.: Epidural morphine in terminal care. Anaesthesia, *36:*51, 1981.
232. Huang, L.M.: Cellular mechanisms of excitatory and inhibitory actions of opioids. *In* Tseng, L.F. (ed.): The Pharmacology of Opioid Peptides. pp. 131–150. Langhorn, PA, Harwood Academic Press, 1995.
233. Husemeyer, R.P., Cummings, A.J., Rosankiewicz, J.R., and Davenport, H.T.: A study of pethidine kinetics and analgesia in women in labour following intravenous, intramuscular and epidural administration. Br. J. Clin. Pharmacol., *13:*171, 1982.
234. Husemeyer, R.P., Davenport, H.T., Cummings, A.J., and Rosankiewicz, J.R.: Comparison of epidural and intramuscular pethidine for analgesia in labour. Br. J. Obstet. Gynecol., *88:*711, 1981.
235. Husted, S., Djurhuus, J.C., Husegaard, H.C., *et al.*: Effect of postoperative extradural morphine on lower urinary tract function. Acta Anaesthesiol. Scand., *29:*183, 1985.
236. Jacox, A.K., Carr, D.B., Mahrenholz, D.M., and Ferrell, B.R.: Cost considerations in patient- controlled analgesia. Pharmacoeconomics *12:*109, 1977.
237. Jacox, A.K., Carr, D.B., Payne, R., *et al.*: Management of cancer pain. Clinical Practice Guidelines No. 9. Agency for Health Care Policy and Research. Rockville, MD, US Department of Health and Human Services, 1994.
238. Jadad, A.R.: Opioids in the treatment of neuropathic pain: A systematic review of controlled clinical trials. *In* Portenoy, R.K., and Bruera, E. (eds.): Supportive Care Medicine. Oxford, Oxford University Press, 1996.
239. Jadad, A.R., and McQuay, H.J.: Meta-analysis to evaluate analgesic interventions: A systematic qualitative review of their methodology. J. Clin. Epidemiol., *49:*235, 1996.
240. Jadad, A.R., Carroll, D., Moore, R.A., and McQuay, H.J.: Developing a database of published randomized clinical trials in pain research. Pain, *66:*239, 1996.
241. Jadad, A.R., Moore, R.A., Carroll, D., *et al.*: Assessing the quality of reports of randomized clinical trials: Is blinding necessary? Control. Clin. Trials, *17:*1, 1996.
242. Jadad, A.R.: Meta-analysis in pain relief: A valuable but easily misused tool. Curr. Opin. Anesth., *9:*426, 1996.
243. Johnson, S.M., and Duggan, A.W.: Tolerance and dependence of dorsal horn neurones of the cat: The role of the opiate receptors of the substantia gelatinosa. Neuropharmacology. *20:*1033, 1981.
244. Johnson, S.M., and Duggan, A.W.: Evidence that opiate receptors of the substantia gelatinosa contribute to the depression by intravenous morphine of the spinal transmission of impulses in the unmyelinated primary afferents. Brain Res., *207:*223, 1981.
245. Johnstone, R.E., and Martinec, C.L.: Costs of anesthesia. Anesth. Analg., *76:*840, 1993.
246. Jones, A.K.P., and Derbyshire, S.W.G.: Positron emission tomography as a tool of understanding the cerebral processing of pain. *In* Boivie, J., Hansson, P., and Lindblom, U., (eds.). Touch, Temperature, and Pain in Health and Disease: Mechanisms and Assessments. pp. 491–520. Seattle, IASP Press, 1993.
247. Jones, J.G.: The future of anesthesia. *In* Keneally, J.P., and Jones, M.R. (eds.): 150 Years On. A Selection of Papers Presented at the 11th World Congress of Anaesthesiologists. pp. 15. London, The World Federation of Societies of Anesthesiologists, 1996.
248. Jones, R.D.M., and Jones, J.G.: Intrathecal morphine: Naloxone reverses respiratory depression but not analgesia. Br. Med. J., *281:*645, 1980.
249. Justins, D.M., Knott, C., Luthman, J., and Reynolds, F.: Epidural versus intramuscular fentanyl: Analgesia and pharmacokinebcs in labor. Anaesthesia, *38:*937, 1983.
250. Kalso, E., Heiskanen, T., Rantio, M., *et al.*: Epidural and subcutaneous morphine in the management of cancer pain: A double-blind cross-over study. Pain, *67:*443, 1996.

251. Kalso, E.: Effects of intrathecal morphine, injected with bupivacaine, on pain after orthopaedic surgery. Br. J. Anaesth., *55:*415, 1983.
252. Kamei, J., and Kasuya, Y.: The effects of diabetes on opioid-induced antinociception. *In* Tseng, L.F. (ed.): The Pharmacology of Opioid Peptides. pp. 271. Langhorn, PA, Harwood Academic Press, 1995.
253. Kaufman, J.J., Semo, N.M., and Koski, W.S.: Microelectrometric titration measurements of the pkas and partition and drug distribution coefficients of narcotics and narcotic antagonists and their pH temperature dependence. J. Med. Chem., *18:*647, 1975.
254. Kehlet, H.: The modifying effect of general and regional anaesthesia on the endocrine metabolic response to surgery. Reg. Anaesth., *7*(Suppl.):538, 1982.
255. Kehlet, H.: Organizing postoperative accelerated recovery programs. Reg. Anesth., *21*(6S):149, 1996.
256. Kehlet, H.: Postoperative pain relief: A look from the other side. Reg. Anesth., *19:*369, 1994.
257. Kehlet, H. Postoperative pain relief—What is the issue? Br. J. Anaesth., *72:*375, 1994.
258. Kellstein, D.E., and Mayer, D.J.: Chronic administration of cholecystokinin antagonists reverses the enhancement of spinal morphine analgesia induced by acute pretreatment. Brain Res. *516:*263, 1990.
259. Kellstein, D.E., and Mayer, D.J.: Spinal coadministration of cholecystokinin antagonists with morphine prevents the development of opioid tolerance. Pain, *47:*221, 1991.
260. Kellstein, D.E., Price, D.D., and Mayer, D.J.: Cholecystokinin and its antagonist lorglumide respectively attenuate and facilitate morphine-induced inhibition of C-fiber evoked discharges of dorsal horn nociceptive neurons. Brain Res., *540:*302, 1991.
261. Kerr-Wilson, R.H., and McNally, S.: Bladder drainage for caesarean section under epidural analgesia. Br. J. Obstet. Gynaecol., *93:*28, 1986.
262. Kim, T., Murdande, S., Gruber, A., and Kim, S.: Sustained-release morphine for epidural analgesia in rats. Anesthesiology, *85:*331, 1996.
263. Kissin, I.: Preemptive Analgesia: Why its effect is not always obvious. Anesthesiology *84:*1015, 1996.
264. Kitahata, L.M., and Collins, J.G.: Spinal action of narcotic analgesics. Anesthesiology, *54:*153, 1981.
265. Kitto, K.F., Haley, J.E., and Wilcox, G.L.: Involvement of nitric oxide in spinally mediated hyperalgesia in the mouse. Neurosci. Lett., *148:*1, 1992.
266. Klinck, J.R., and Lindop, M.J.: Epidural morphine in the elderly: A controlled trial after upper abdominal surgery. Anaesthesia., *37:*907, 1982.
267. Knapp, R.J., Vaughn, L.K., and Yamamura, H.I.: Selective ligands for μ and σ opioid receptors. *In* Tseng, L.F. (ed.): The Pharmacology of Opioid Peptides. pp. 1–28. Langhorn, PA, Harwood Academic Publishers, 1995.
268. Knill, R.L., Clement, J.L., and Thompson, W.R.: Epidural morphine causes delayed and prolonged ventilatory depression. Can. Anaesth. Soc. J., *28:*537, 1981.
269. Knox, D.J., McLeod, B.J., and Goucke, C.R.: Acute phantom limb pain controlled by ketamine. Anaesth. Intensive Care, *23:*620, 1995.
270. Krames, E.S.: Intraspinal opioid therapy for chronic nonmalignant pain: Current practice and clinical guidelines. J. Pain Symptom Manage., *11:*333, 1996.
271. Krames, E.S.: Intrathecal infusional therapies for intractable pain: Patient management guidelines. J. Pain Symptom. Manage., *8:*36, 1993.
272. Krames, E.S., Wilkie, D.J., and Gershow, J.: Intrathecal d-Ala2-d-Leu5-enkephalin (DADL) restores analgesia in a patient analgetically tolerant to intrathecal morphine sulphate. Pain, *24:*205, 1986.
273. Kream, R.M., Kato, T., Shimonaka, H., *et al.*: Substance P markedly potentiates the antinociceptive effects of morphine sulfate administered at the spinal level. Proc. Natl. Acad. Sci., *90:*3564, 1993.
274. Laffer, U., Bachmann-Mettler, I., and Metzger, U. (eds.): Implantable Drug Delivery Systems. Switzerland, S. Karger, A.G., 1991.
275. Lam, A.M., Knill, R.L., Thompson, W.R., *et al.*: Epidural fentanyl does not cause delayed respiratory depression. Can. Anaesth. Soc. J., *30:*578, 1983.
276. Lamarche, Y., Martin, R., Reiher, Y., and Blaise, G.: The sleep apnea syndrome and epidural morphine. Can. Anaesth. Soc. J., *33:*231, 1986.
277. Langley, P.C.: Pharmacoeconomics and the quality of decision-making by pharmacy and therapeutics committees. Am. J. Health Syst. Pharm., *52:*S24, 1995.
278. Lanz, E., Kehrberger, E., and Theiss, D.: Epidural morphine: A clinical double-blind study of dosage. Anesth. Analg., *64:*786, 1985.
279. Lauretti, G.R., Reis, M.P., Prado, W.A., and Klamt, J.G.: Dose response study of intrathecal morphine versus intrathecal neostigmine, their combination, or placebo for postoperative analgesia in patients undergoing anterior and posterior vaginoplasty. Anesth. Analg., *82:*1182, 1996.
280. Lazorthes, Y., Gouarderes, C.H., Verdie, J.C., *et al.*: Analgésie par injection intrathecale de morphine: Etude pharmacocinetique et application aux douleurs irréducibles. Neurochirurgie, *26:*159, 1980.
281. Law, P.: G-proteins and opioid receptors' functions. *In* Tseng, L.F. (ed.): The Pharmacology of Opioid Peptides. pp. 109–130. Langhorn, PA, Harwood Academic Press, 1995.
282. Le Bars, D., Bouhassira, D., and Villanueva, L.: Opioids and diffuse noxious inhibitory control (DNIC) in the rat. *In* Bromm, B., and Desmedt, J.E. (eds.): Advances in Pain Research and Therapy. Vol. 22. pp. 517–539. New York, Raven Press, 1995.
283. Lee, A., Simpson, D., Whitfield, A., and Scott, D.B.: Postoperative analgesia by continuous extradural infusion of bupivacaine and diamorphine. Br. J. Anaesth., *60:*845, 1988.
284. Leff, P.: The two-state model of receptor activation. Trends Pharmacol. Sci., *16:*89, 1995.
285. Lenzi, A., Gali, G., Gandolfini, M., and Marini, G.: Intraventricular morphine in paraneoplastic painful syndrome of the cervicofacial region: Experience in thirty-eight cases. Neurosurgery, *17:*6, 1985.
286. Levitan, I.B., and Kaczmarek, L.K.: The neuron. *In* Cell and Molecular Biology, 2nd ed. Oxford, Oxford University Press, 1997.
287. Liao, J., Harrison, P., Buckley, J.J., and Takemori, A.: Sympathetic reflexes in morphine vs lidocaine spinal block. Anesthesiology, *55:*A148, 1981.
288. Lim, F., and Sun, A.M.: Microencapsulated islets as bioartificial endocrine pancreas. Science, *210:*908, 1980.
289. Lindblom, U.: Analysis of abnormal touch, pain, and temperature sensation in patients. *In* Boivie, J., Hansson, P., Lingblom, U., (eds.): Touch, Temperature, and Pain in Health and Disease: Mechanisms and Assessments pp. 63–84. Seattle, IASP Press, 1993.
290. Liolios, A., and Anderson, F.H.: Selective spinal analgesia. Lancet, *2:*357, 1979.
291. Lipkowski, A., Carr, D.B.: Neuropeptides: Peptide and nonpeptide analogs. *In* Gutte, B. (ed.): Peptides: Synthesis, Structures and Applications. pp. 287–320. San Diego, Academic Press, 1995.
292. Lipkowski, A.W. and Maszczynska, I.: Peptide, N-methyl-D-aspartate and adenosine receptors as analgesic targets. Curr. Opin. Anesth., *9:*443, 1996.
293. Liu, H.W., Ofosu, F.A., and Chang, P.L.: Expression of human factor IX by microencapsulated recombinant fibroblasts. Hum. Gene. Ther., *4:*291, 1993.
294. Liu, S., Carpenter, R.L., and Neal, J.M.: Epidural anesthesia and analgesia, their role in postoperative outcome. Anesthesiology, *82:*1474, 1995.
295. Lobato, R.D., Madrid, J.L., Fatela, L.V., *et al.*: Intraventricular morphine for intractable cancer pain: Rationale, methods, clinical results. Acta Anaesthesiol. Scand., *31*, (Suppl.)*85:*68, 1987.
296. Lomessy, A., Magnin, C., Viale, J- P., *et al.*: Clinical advantages of fentanyl given epidurally for post-operative analgesia. Anesthesiology, *61:*466, 1984.
297. Lord, J.A., Waterfield, A.A., Hughes, J., and Kosterlitz, H.: Endogenous opioid peptides: Multiple agonists and receptors. Nature, *267:*495, 1977.
298. Lubarsky, D.A., Glass, P.S., Ginsberg, B., *et al.*: The successful implementation of pharmaceutical practice guidelines: Analysis of associated outcomes and cost savings. Anesthesiology, *86:*1145, 1997.
299. Lysaght, M.J., Frydel, B., Gentile, F., Emerich, D., and Winn, S.: Recent progress in immunoisolated cell therapy. J. Cell. Biochem., *56:*196, 1994.
300. Macario, A., Vitez, T.S., Dun, B., and McDonald, T.: Where are the costs in perioperative care? Analysis of hospital costs and charges for inpatient surgical care. Anesthesiology, *83:*1138, 1995.
301. Madrid, J.L., Fatela, L.V., Lobato, R.D., and Gozalo, A.: Intrathecal therapy: Rationale, technique, clinical results. Acta Anaethesiol. Scand., *85:*60, 1987.
302. Malmberg, A.B., Grafe, M.R., Haaseth, R.C., *et al.*: Spinal toxicology of [D-Pen^2, D-Pen^5] Enkephalin (DPDPE) after multiple lumbar intrathecal injections in the rat. Neurotoxicology., submitted: 1995.

303. Malmberg, A.B., and Yaksh, T.L.: Spinal nitric oxide synthase inhibition blocks NMDA induced thermal hyperalgesia and produces antinociception in the formalin test in rats. Pain *54:*291, 1993.
304. Malmberg, A.B., and Yaksh, T.L.: Antinociceptive actions of spinal non-steroidal antiinflammatory agents on the formalin test in the rat. J. Pharmacol. Exp. Ther. *163:*136, 1992.
305. Mansour, A., Fox, C.A., Akil, H., and Watson, S.J.: Opioid-receptor mRNA expression in the rat CNS: Anatomical and functional implications. T.I.N.S., *18:*22, 1995.
306. Mantyh, P.W., DeMaster, E., Malhotra, A., *et al.*: Receptor endocytosis and dendrite reshaping in spinal neurons after somatosensory stimulation. Science *268:*1629, 1995.
307. Mao, J., Price, D.D., and Mayer, D.J.: Mechanisms of hyperalgesia and morphine tolerance: A current view of their possible interactions. Pain., *62:*259, 1995.
308. Masters, T.: Neural, Novel and Hybrid Algorithms for Time Series Prediction. New York, John Wiley and Sons, Inc., 1995.
309. Maszczynska, I., Goudas, L., Lipkowski, A.W., *et al.*: Spinal antinociceptive effects of AA 501: A novel putative opioid agonist and neurokinin antagonist in rats. Anesth. Analg., *84:*S523, 1997.
310. Mather, L.E.: Clinical pharmacokinetics of fentanyl and its newer derivatives. Clin. Pharmacokinet., *8:*422, 1983.
311. Mather, L.E., and Cousins, M.J.: Pharmacology of opioids: Basic and clinical aspects. Med. J. Aust., *144:*424, 1986.
312. Mather, L.E., and Pavlin, E.G.: Transfer of pethidine to CSF following intravenous administration. Anaesth. Intensive Care, *9:*205, 1981.
313. Mathews, E.: Epidural morphine. Lancet, *1:*673, 1979.
314. Matthes, H.W., Maldonado, R., Simonin, F., *et al.*: Loss of morphine-induced analgesia, reward effect and withdrawal symptoms in mice lacking the mu-opioid-receptor gene. Nature, *383:*819, 1996.
315. Maurette, P., Bonada, G., Djiane, V., and Erny, P.: A comparison between lidocaine alone and lidocaine with meperidine for continuous spinal anesthesia. Reg. Anesth., *18:*290, 1993.
316. Max, M.B.: Combining opioids with other drugs: Challenges in clinical trial design. *In* Gebhart, G.F., Hammond, D.L., and Jensen, T.S. (eds.): Proceedings of the 7th World Congress on Pain. pp. 569–586. Seattle, IASP Press, 1994.
317. Max, M., Inturrisi, C.E., Grabrinsh, P., *et al.*: Epidural opiates: Plasma and cerebrospinal fluid (CSF) pharmacokinetics of morphine, methadone and beta-endorphin. Pain, *1*(Suppl.):S122, 1981.
318. Max, M.B., Inturrisi, C.E., Kaiko, R.F., *et al.*: Epidural and intrathecal opiates: Cerebrospinal fluid and plasma profiles in patients with chronic cancer pain. Clin. Pharmacol. Ther., *38:*631, 1985.
319. Mayer, D., Mao, J., and Price, D.: The development of morphine tolerance and dependence is associated with translocation of protein kinase C. Pain, *61:*365, 1995.
320. Mayer, D.J., and Manning, B.H.: The role of opioid peptides in environmentally-induced analgesia. *In* Tseng, L.F. (ed.): The Pharmacology of Opioid Peptides. pp. 345–396. Langhorn, PA, Harwood Academic Press, 1995.
321. McCaughey, W., and Graham, J.L.: The respiratory depression of epidural morphine: Time course and effect of posture. Anaesthesia, *37:*990, 1982.
322. McClure, J.H.: Ropivacaine. Br. J. Anaesth., *76:*300, 1996.
323. McCormick, K.A., Moore, S.R., and Siegel, R.A. (eds.): Clinical Practice Guideline Development: Methodology Perspectives. Agency for Health Care Policy and Research, Rockville, MD, U.S. Department of Health and Human Services., 1994.
324. McCormack, K.: Non-steroidal anti-inflammatory drugs and spinal nociceptive processing. Pain, *59:*9, 1994.
325. McDonald, A.M.: Complication of epidural morphine. Anaesth. Intensive Care, *8:*490, 1980.
326. McMahon, S.B., Dmitrieva, N., and Klotzenburg, M.: Visceral pain. Br. J. Anaesth., *75:*132, 1995.
327. McQuay, H.J.: Pre-emptive analgesia: A systematic review of clinical studies. Ann. Med., *27:*249, 1995.
328. Meller, S.T.: Thermal and mechanical hyperalgesia: A distinct role for different excitatory amino acid receptors and signal transduction pathways? A.P.S. J., *3:*215, 1994.
329. Melton, P.M. and Riley, A.L.: An assessment of the interaction between cholecystokinin and the opiates within a drug discrimination procedure. Pharmacol. Biochem. Behav., *46:*237, 1993.
330. Mercadante, S.: Intrathecal morphine and bupivacaine in advanced cancer pain patients implanted at home. J. Pain Symptom. Manage., *9:*201, 1994.
331. Messahel, F.M., and Tomlin, P.J.: Narcotic withdrawal syndrome after intrathecal administration of morphine. Br. Med. J., *283:*471, 1981.
332. Miaskowski, C.: Effective cancer pain management: From guidelines to quality improvement. Pain., *2*(2), 1994.
333. Minami, T., Uda, R., Horiguchi, S., *et al.*: Allodynia evoked by intrathecal administration of prostaglandin F2a to conscious mice. Pain, *50:*223, 1992.
334. Miotto, K., Magendzo, K., and Evans, C.J.: Molecular characterization of opioid receptors. *In* Tseng, L.F. (ed.): The Pharmacology of Opioid Peptides pp. 57–71. Langhorn, PA, Harwood Academic Publishers, 1995.
335. Mirceau, N., Constaninescu, C., Jianu, C., *et al.*: Anesthesie sous-arachnoidienne par la pethidine. Ann. Fr. Anesth. Reanim., *1:*167, 1982.
336. Misterek, K., Maszczynska, I., Dorociak, A., *et al.*: Spinal coadministration of peptide substance P antagonist increases antinociceptive effect of the opioid peptide biphalin. Life Sci., *54:*939, 1994.
337. Modig, J., Paalzow, L.: A comparison of epidural morphine and epidural bupivacaine for postoperative pain relief. Acta Anaesthesiol. Scand., *25:*437, 1981.
338. Moher, D., and Olkin, I.: Meta-analysis of randomized clinical trials: A concern for standards. Commentary. J.A.M.A. *274:*1962, 1995.
339. Moiniche, S., Dahl, J.B., Rosenberg, J., and Kehlet, H.: Colonic resection with early discharge after combined subarachnoid-epidural analgesia, preoperative glucocorticoids, and early postoperative mobilization and feeding in a pulmonary high-risk patient. Reg. Anesth., *19:*352, 1994.
340. Molke-Jensen, F., Madsen, J.B., Guldager, H., *et al.*: Respiratory depression after epidural morphine in the postoperative period: Influence of posture. Acta Anaesthesiol. Scand., *28:*600, 1984.
341. Moore, R.A., Bullingham, R.S.J., McQuay, H.J., *et al.*: Spinal fluid kinetics of morphine and heroin in man. Clin. Pharmacol. Ther., *35:*40, 1984.
342. Moore, R.A., Bullingham, R.S.J., McQuay, H.J., *et al.*: Dural permeability to narcotics: In vitro determination and application to extra-dural administration. Br. J. Anaesth., *54:*1117, 1982.
343. Moulin, D.E., Max, M.B., Kaiko, R.F., *et al.*: The analgesic efficacy of intrathecal D-Ala^2-D-Leu^5-enkephalin in cancer patients with chronic pain. Pain, *23:*213, 1985.
344. Movat, J.J., Mok, M.J., MacLeod, B.A., and Madden, T.D.: Liposomal bupivacaine. Anesthesiology, *85:*635, 1996.
345. Munglani, R., and Hunt, S.P.: Molecular biology of pain. Br. J. Anaesth., *75:*186, 1995.
346. Muller, H., Borner, U., Stoyanov, M., *et al.*: Peridurale opiatapplikation bie malignombedingten chronischen schmerzen. Anesth. Intensivther. Notfallmed., *16:*251, 1981.
347. Muller, H., Borner, U., Stoyanov, M., and Hempelmann, G.: Intraoperative peridural opiate analgesia. Anaesthesist, *12:*656, 1980.
348. Naulty, J.S., Johnson, M., Burger, G.A., *et al.*: Epidural fentanyl for post-cesarean delivery pain management. Anesthesiology, *59:*A415, 1983.
349. Ni, Q., Xu, H., Partilla, J.S., *et al.*: Opioid peptide receptor studies 2. [^{3}H]SNC-121, a novel, selective, and high-affinity ligand for opioid delta receptors. Analgesia, *1:*185, 1995.
350. Nicolis, G., and Prigogine, I.: Self-organization in Equilibrium Systems pp. 68–69. New York, John Wiley, 1977.
351. Nielson, T.H., Husegaard, H.C., and Joensen, F.: Tunnel-leret spiduralkateter og infektion. Ugeskr. Laeger, *147:*1548, 1985.
352. Nitescu, P., Appelgren, L., Linder, L.E., *et al.*: Epidural versus intrathecal morphine/bupivacaine: Assessment of consecutive treatments in advanced cancer pain. J. Pain Symptom Manage., *5:*18, 1990.
353. Nitescu, P., Sjoberg, M., Appelgren, L., and Curelaru, I.: Complications of intrathecal opioids and bupivacaine in the treatment of "refractor" cancer pain. Clin. J. Pain, *11:*45, 1995.
354. Niv, D.: Intraoperative treatment of postoperative pain. *In* Campbell, J.N. (ed.): Pain 1996: An Updated Review. pp. 173–187. Seatle, IASP Press, 1996.
355. Niv, D., Rudick, V., Golan, A., and Chayen, M.S.: Augmentation of bupivacaine analgesia in labor by epidural morphine. Obstet. Gynecol., *67:*206, 1986.
356. Nock, B; κ and ϵ opioid receptor binding. *In* Tseng, L.F. (ed.): The Pharmacology of Opioid Peptides. pp. 29. Langhorn, PA, Harwood Academic Press, 1995.

357. Nordberg, G.: Pharmacokinetic aspects of spinal morphine analgesia. Acta Anaesthesiol. Scand., *79:*1, 1984.
358. Nordberg, G., Hedner, T., Mellstrand, T., and Dahlstrom, B.: Pharmacokinetic aspects of epidural morphine analgesia. Anesthesiology, *58:*545, 1983.
359. Odoom, J.A.: Respiratory depression after intrathecal morphine. Anesth. Analg. *61:*70, 1982.
360. Oldendorf, W.H., Hyman, S., Braun, L., and Oldendorf, S.Z.: Blood—brain barrier: Penetration of morphine, codeine, heroin and methadone after carotid injection. Science, *178:*984, 1972.
361. Olshwang, D., Shapiro, A., Perlberg, S., and Magora, F.: The effect of epidural morphine on ureteral colic and spasm of the bladder. Pain, *18:*97, 1984.
362. Onofrio, B.M., Yaksh, T.L., and Arnold, P.G.: Continuous low-dose intrathecal morphine administration in the treatment of chronic pain of malignant origin. Mayo Clin. Proc., *56:*516, 1981.
363. Onofrio, B.M., and Yaksh, T.L.: Long-term pain relief produced by intrathecal morphine infusion in 53 patients. J. Neurosurg., *27:*200, 1990.
364. Onofrio, B.M., and Yaksh, T.L.: Intrathecal delta-receptor ligand produces analgesia in man. Lancet, *1:*1386, 1993.
365. Ossipov, M., Kovelowski, C., Nichols, M., Hruby, V., and Porreca, F.: Characterization of supraspinal antinociceptive actions of opioid delta agonists in the rat. Pain, *62:*287, 1995.
366. Ossipov, M.H., Lopez, Y., Bian, D., *et al.*: Synergistic antinociceptive interactions of morphine and clonidine in rats with nerve ligation injury. Anesthesiology, *86:*196, 1997.
367. Oyama, T., Matsuki, A., Taneichi, T., *et al.*: Beta-endorphin in obstetric analgesia. Am. J. Obstet. Gynecol., *137:*613, 1980.
368. Oyama, T., Toshiro, J.I.N., and Yamaya, R.: Profound analgesic effects of beta-endorphin in man. Lancet *1:*122, 1980.
369. Paakkari, P., and Feuerstein, G.: Opioid peptides in cardiovascular and respiratory regulation. *In* Tseng, L.F., (ed.): The Pharmacology of Opioid Peptides. pp.425–444. Langhorn, PA, Harwood Academic Press, 1995.
370. Paice, J.A., Penn, R.D., and Shott, S.: Intraspinal morphine for chronic pain. A retrospective, multicenter study. J Pain Symptom Mange., *11:*71, 1996.
371. Paix, A., Coleman, A., Lees, J., *et al.*: Subcutaneous fentanyl and sufentanil infusion for morphine intolerance in cancer pain mangement. Pain, *63:*263, 1995.
372. Paulus, D.A., Paul, W., and Munson, E.S.: Neurologic depression after intrathecal morphine. Anesthesiology, *54:*517, 1981.
373. Pechnick, R.N.: Effects of opioid on the hypothalamo-pituitary-adrenal axis. Annu. Rev. Pharmacol. Toxicol., *32:*353, 1993.
374. Pedersen, J.L., Crawford, M.E., Dahl, J.B., *et al.*: Effect of pre-emptive nerve block on inflammation and hyperalgesia after human thermal injury. Anesthesiology, *84:*1010, 1996.
375. Penn, R.D., Paice, J.A., Gottschalk, W., and Ivankovich, A.D.: Cancer pain relief using chronic morphine infusion. Early experience with a programmable implanted drug pump. J. Neurosurg., *61:*302, 1984.
376. Pennypacker, K.R.: Pharmacological regulation of opioid peptide gene expression: Second and third messenger systems. *In* Tseng, L.F.(ed.): The Pharmacology of Opioid Peptides. pp.73–86. Langhorn, PA, Harwood Academic Press, 1995.
377. Petring, O.U., Dawson, P.J., Blake, D.W. *et al.*: Normal postoperative gastric emptying after orthopaedic surgery with spinal anesthesia and i.m. ketorolac as the first postoperative analgesic. Br. J. Anaesth., *74:*257, 1995.
378. Perriss, B.W.: Epidural pethidine in labour: A study of dose requirements. Anaesthesia, *35:*380, 1980.
379. Perriss, B.W., and Malins, A.F.: Pain relief in labour using epidural pethidine with adrenaline. Anaesthesia, *36:*631, 1981.
380. Plummer, J.L., Cherry, D.A., Cousins, M.J., *et al.*: Long-term spinal administration of morphine in cancer and non-cancer pain; a retrospective study. Pain, *44:*215, 1991.
381. Plummer, J.L., Cmielewski, P.L., Reynolds, G.D., *et al.*: Influence of polarity on dose response relationships of intrathecal opioids in rats. Pain, *40:*339, 1990.
382. Poggioli, R., Vergoni, A.V., Sandrini, M., *et al.*: Influence of the selective cholecystokinin antagonist L-364,718 on pain threshold and morphine analgesia. Pharmacology, *42:*197, 1991.
383. Poletti, C.E., Cohen, A.M., Todd, D.P., *et al.*: Cancer pain relieved by long-term epidural morphine with permanent indwelling systems for self-administration. J. Neurosurg., *55:*581, 1981.
384. Porreca, F., Bilsky, E.J., and Lai, J.: Pharmacological characterization of opioid σ- and κ-receptors. *In* Tseng, L.F. (ed.): The Pharmacology of Opioid Peptides. pp. 219–248. Langhorn, PA, Harwood Academic Publishers, 1995.
385. Portenoy, R.R.: Opioid tolerance and responsiveness: Research findings and clinical observations. *In* Gebhart, G.F., Hammond, D.L., and Jensen, T.S.(eds.): Proceedings of the 7th World Congress on Pain. pp. 595–619. Seatle, IASP Press, 1995.
386. Price, D.D.: Psychophysical measurement of normal and abnormal pain processing. *In* Boivie, J., Hansson, P., and Lindblom, U. (eds.): Touch, Temperature, and Pain in Health and Disease: Mechanisms and Assessments. pp. 3–26. Seattle, IASP Press, 1993.
387. Proudfit, H.K., and Yeomans, D.C.: The modulation of nociception by enkephalin-containing neurons in the brainstem. *In* Tseng, L.F. (ed.): The Pharmacology of Opioid Peptides. pp. 197–218. Langhorn, PA, Harwood Academic Press, 1995.
388. Raj, P.P., Knarr, D.C., Vigdorth, E., *et al.*: Comparison of continuous epidural infusion of a local anesthetic and administration of systemic narcotics in the management of pain after total knee replacement surgery. Anesth. Analg., *66:*401, 1987.
389. Rang, H.P. and Urban, L.: New molecules in analgesia. Br. J. Anaesth., *75:*145, 1995.
390. Rathmell, J.P., and Jamison, R.N.: Opioid therapy for chronic noncancer pain. Curr. Opin. Anesth., *9:*436, 1996.
391. Rauk, R.: Cost-Effectiveness and cost/benefit ratio of acute pain management. Reg. Anesth., *21*[6S]:139, 1996.
392. Rawal, N.: Neuraxial administration of opioids and nonopioids. *In* Brown, D.L. (ed.): Regional Anesthesia and Analgesia. pp. 208–231. Philadelphia, W.B. Saunders Company, 1996.
393. Rawal, N., Mollefors, K., Axelsson, K., *et al.*: An experimental study of urodynamic effects of epidural morphine and of naloxone reversal. Anesth. Analg., *62:*641, 1983.
394. Rawal, N., Schott, U., Dahlstrom, B., Inturrisi, C.E., Tandon, B., Sjostrand, U., and Wennhager, M.: Influence of naloxone on analgesia and respiratory depression following epidural morphine. Anesthesiology, *64:*194, 1986.
395. Rawal, N., Schott, U., Tandon, B., *et al.*: Influence of intravenous naloxone infusion on analgesia and untoward effects of epidural morphine. Anesth. Analg., *64:*270, 1985.
396. Rawal, N., Sjostrand, U., Christoffersson, E., *et al.*: Comparison of intramuscular and epidural morphine for postoperative analgesia in the grossly obese: Influence on postoperative ambulation and pulmonary function. Anesth. Analg., *63:*583, 1984.
397. Rawal, N., Sjostrand, U.H., and Dahlstrom, B.: Postoperative pain relief by epidural morphine. Anesth. Analg., *60:*726, 1981.
398. Rawal, N., and Wattwil, M.: Respiratory depression following epidural morphine: An experimental and clinical study. Anesth. Analg., *63:*8, 1984.
399. Rawal, N., Arner, S., Gustaffson, L.L., and Allvin, R.: Present state of extradural and intrathecal opioid analgesia in Sweden. A nationwide follow-up survey. Br. J. Anaesth., *59:*791, 1987.
400. Rawal, N., Sjostrand, U.H., Dahlstrom, B., *et al.*: Epidural morphine for postoperative pain relief: A comparative study with intramuscular narcotic and intercostal nerve block. Anesth. Analg., *61:*93, 1982.
401. Ready, L.B., Ashburn, M., Caplan, M., *et al.*: Practice guidelines for acute pain management in the perioperative setting. Anesthesiology, *82:*1071, 1995.
402. Ready, L.B., and Edwards, W.T. (eds.): Management of Acute Pain: A Practical Guide Seattle, IASP Press, 1992.
403. Reiz, S. and Bennett, S.: Cardiovascular effects of epidural anaesthesia. Curr. Opin. Anaesth., *6:*813, 1993.
404. Reiz, S., Ahlin, J., Ahrenfeld, B., *et al.*: Epidural morphine for postoperative pain relief. Acta Anaesthesiol. Scand., 25:111, 1981.
405. Reiz, S., Westberg, M.: Side effects of epidural morphine. Lancet, *2:*203, 1980.
406. Renck, H., and Wallin, R.: Slow-release formulations of local anaesthetics and opioids. Curr. Opin. Anesth., *9:*399, 1996.
407. Richelson, E.: Spinal opiate administration for chronic pain: A major advance in therapy. Mayo Clin. Proc., *56:*523, 1981.
408. Rigg, J.R.A., Ilsley, A.H., and Vedig, A.E.: Relationship of ventilatory depression to steady state blood pethidine concentrations. Br. J. Anaesth., *56:*613, 1981.
409. Robinson, J.O., Rosen, M., Evans, J.M., *et al.*: Self-administered intravenous and intramuscular pethidine: A controlled trial in labour. Anaesthesia., *35:*763, 1980.

410. Rockemann, M.G., Seeling, W., Bischof, C., *et al.*: Prophylactic use of epidural mepivacaine/morphine, systemic diclofenac, and metamizole reduces postoperative morphine consumption after major abdominal surgery. Anesthesiology, *84:*1027, 1996.
411. Rodan, B.A., Cohen, F.L., Bean, W.J., and Martyar, S.N.: Fibrous mass complicating epidural morphine infusion. Neurosurgery, *16:*68, 1985.
412. Rosow, C.E., Moss, J., Philbin, D.M., and Savarese, J.J.: Histamine release during morphine and fentanyl anesthesia. Anesthesiology, *56:*93, 1982.
413. Rozan, J.P., Kahn, C.H., and Warfield, C.A.: Epidural and intravenous opioid-induced neuroexcitation. Anesthesiology, *83:*860, 1995.
414. Russell, L.B., Gold, M.R., Siegel, J.E., *et al.*: The role of cost-effectiveness analysis in health and medicine: J.A.M.A., *276:*1170, 1996.
415. Sabbe, M.B., Grafe, M.R., Mjanger, E., *et al.*: Spinal delivery of sufentanil, alfentanil, and morphine in dogs: Physiologic and toxicologic investigations. Anesthesiology, *81:*899, 1994.
416. Sadee, W., Wang, Z., Arden, J.R., and Segredo, V.: Constitutive activation of the μ-opioid receptor: A novel paradigm of receptor regulation in narcotic analgesia, tolerance, and dependence. Analgesia, *1:*11, 1994.
417. Sage, M.R.: Kinetics of water-soluble contrast media in the central nervous system. A.J.R., *141:*815, 1983.
418. Sage, M., Kilpatrick, C., Fon, G.T., Wilcox, J., and Burns, R.J.: Brain parenchyma penetration by metrizamide following lumbar myelography. Austalas. Radiol., *28:*90, 1984.
419. Sagen, J., Hama, A.T., Winn, S.R., *et al.*: Pain reduction by spinal implantation isolated in polymer capsules. Soc. Neurosci. (Abstr.) *19:*234, 1993.
420. Sagen, J., Pappas, G.D., and Pollard, H.B.: Analgesia induced by isolated bovine chromaffin cells implanted in rat spinal cord. Proc. Natl. Acad. Sci. U.S.A., *83:*7522, 1986.
421. Sagen, J., and Pappas, G.D.: Morphological and functional correlates of chromaffin cell transplants in CNS pain modulatory regions. Ann. N.Y. Acad. Sci., *495:*306, 1987.
422. Sagot, Y., Tan, S.A., Baetge, E., *et al.*: Polymer encapsulated cell lines genetically engineered to release ciliary neurotrophic factor can slow down progressive motor neuropathy in the mouse. Eur. J. Neurosci., *7:*1313, 1995.
423. Saitoh, Y., Taki, T., Arita, N., *et al.*: Analgesia induced by transplantation of encapsulated tumor cells secreting beta-endorphin. J. Neurosurg., *82:*630, 1995.
424. Salvemini, D., Misko, T.P., Maferrer, J.L., *et al.*: Nitric oxide, an inhibitor of lipid oxidation by lipoxygenase, cyclooxygenase and hemoglobin. Lipids, *27:*46, 1992.
425. Samii, K., Feret, J., Haran, A., and Viars, P.: Selective spinal analgesia. Lancet, *1:*1142, 1979.
426. Samuelsson, H., and Hedner, T.: Pain characterization in cancer patients and the analgesic response to epidural morphine. Pain, *46:*3, 1991.
427. Samuelsson, H., Malmberg, F., Eriksson, M., and Hedner, T.: Outcomes of epidural morphine treatment in cancer pain: Nine years of clinical experience. J. Pain Symptom Manage, *10:*105, 1995.
428. Sanders, V.M.: The role of opioid peptides in immune function. *In* Tseng, L.F. (ed.): The Pharmacology of Opioid Peptides. pp. 411–424. Langhorn, PA, Harwood Academic Press, 1995.
429. Sangarlangkarn, S., Klaewtanong, V., Jonglerttrakool, P., and Khankaew, V.: Meperidine as a spinal anesthetic agent: A comparison with lidocaine-glucose. Anesth. Analg., *666:*235, 1987.
430. Santillan, R., Maestre, J.M., Hurle, M.A., and Florez, J.: Nimodipine, a calcium channel blocker, enhances opiate analgesia in patients with cancer pain tolerant to morphine. *In* Gebhart, G.F., Hammond, D.L., and Jensen, T.S. (eds.): Proceedings of the 7th World Congress on Pain. pp.587–594. Seattle, IASP Press, 1994.
431. Sato, O., Asai, T, Amaro, Y., *et al.*: Formation of cerebrospinal fluid in spinal sub-arachnoid space. Nature, *233:*129, 1971.
432. Scheinerman, E.R.: Invitation to Dynamical Systems. pp. 153–230. Upper Saddle River, N.J., Prentice-Hall, 1996.
433. Schmauss, C., Shimohigashi, Y., Jensen, T.S., *et al.*: Studies on spinal opiate receptor pharmacology. III. Analgetic effects of enkephalin dimers as measured by cutaneous-thermal and visceral-chemical evoked responses. Brain Res., *337:*209, 1985.
434. Schmidt, W.K.: Survey of current and investigational drugs for the treatment of acute and chronic pain. American Pain Society Annual Meeting, 1995.
435. Schneider, M.C., and Hampl, K.F.: Complications of epidural and spinal anesthesia in adults. Curr. Opin. Anaesth., *8:*414, 1995.
436. Schug, S.A., and Large, R.G.: Opioids for chronic noncancer pain. Pain: Clin. Updates, *3*(3), 1995.
437. Scott, D.A., Beilby, D.S.N., and McClymont, C.: Postoperative analgesia using epidural infusions of fentanyl with bupivacaine. Anesthesiology, *83:*727, 1995.
438. Scott, N.B., Mogensen, T., Bigler, D., *et al.*: Continuous thoracic extradural 0.5% bupivacaine with or without morphine: Effect on quality of blockade, lung function, and the surgical stress response. Br. J. Anaesth., *62:*253, 1989.
439. Scott, D.B., and McClure, J.: Selective epidural analgesia. Lancet, *1:*1410, 1979.
440. Scott, P.V., Bowen, F.E., Cartwright, P., *et al.*: Intrathecal morphine as sole analgesic during labour. Br. Med. J., *281:*351, 1980.
441. Scott, P.V., and Fisher, H.B.: Intraspinal opiates and itching: A new reflex? Br. Med. J., *284:*1015, 1982.
442. Segel, L.: Modeling Dynamic Phenomena in Molecular and Cellular Biology. Cambridge, U.K., Cambridge University Press, 1984.
443. Shapiro, B.A.: Why must the practice of anesthesiology change? It's economics, doctor! Anesthesiology, *86:*1020, 1997.
444. Shulman, M., Joseph, N.J., and Haller, C.A.: Effect of epidural and subarachnoid injections of a 10% butamben suspension. Reg. Anesth., *15:*142, 1990.
445. Siddall, P.J., Grat, M., Rutkowski, S., and Cousins, M.J.: Intrathecal morphine and clonidine in the management of spinal cord injury pain: A case report. Pain, *59:*147, 1994.
446. Siddall, P.J., Xu, C.L., and Cousins, M.J.: Allodynia following traumatic spinal injury in the rat. Neuroreport, *6:*1241, 1995.
447. Siddall, P.J., Taylor, D.A., and Cousins, M.J.: Classification of pain following spinal cord injury. Spinal Cord, *35:*69, 1997.
448. Siegel, J.E., Weinstein, M.C., Russell, L.B., and Gold, M.R.: Recommendations for reporting cost-effective analyses. J.A.M.A., *276:*1339, 1996.
449. Silbert, B.S., Lipkowski, A.W., Cepeda, M.S., *et al.*: Analgesic activity of a novel bivalent opioid peptide compared to morphine via different routes of administration. Agents Actions, *33:*3, 1991.
450. Sjoberg, M., Applegren, L., Einarsson, S., and Hultman, E.: Long-term intrathecal morphine and bupivacaine in 'refractory' cancer patients: Results from the first series of 52 patients. Acta Anaesthesiol. Scand., *35:*30, 1991.
451. Sjogren, P., and Banning, A.: Pain, sedation, and reaction time during long-term treatment of cancer pain with oral and epidural opioids. Pain, *39:*5, 1989.
452. Sjostrom, S., Tamsen, A., Persson, P., and Hartvig, P.: Pharmacokinetics of intrathecal morphine and meperidine in man. Anesthesiology, *67:*889, 1987.
453. Sjostrom, S., Hartvig, P., Persson, P., and Tamsen, A.: Pharmacokinetics of epidural morphine and meperidine in man. Anesthesiology., *67:*877, 1987.
454. Smart, N.G., Cousins, M.J., and Mather, L.E.: The spinal route of analgesia: Opioids and future options. *In* Stanley, T.H., and Ashburn, M. (eds.): Anesthesiology and Pain Management. pp. 195–226. *Amsterdam,* Kluwer Medicine, 1994.
455. Smith, D.E.: Spinal opioids in the home and hospice setting. J. Pain Symptom. Manage., *5:*175, 1990.
456. Solomon, R.E., and Gebhart, G.F.: Synergistic antinociceptive interactions among drugs administered to the spinal cord. Anesth. Analg., *78:*1164, 1994.
457. Sorkin, L.S., and Moore, J.H.: Evoked release of amino acids and prostanoids in spinal cords of anesthetized rats: Changes during peripheral inflammation and hyperalgesia. Am. J. Ther., *3:*268, 1996.
458. Sosnowski, M., and Yaksh, T.L.: Spinal administration of receptor-selective drugs as analgesics: New horizons. J. Pain Symptom Manage., *5:*204, 1990.
459. Sperry, R.J.: Principles of economic analysis. Anesthesiology, *86:*1197, 1997.
460. Spilker, B. (ed.): Quality of Life in Clinical Trials. New York, Raven Press, 1990.
461. Stamford, J.A.: Descending control of pain. Br. J. Anaesth. *75:*217, 1995.
462. Stanfa, L.C. and Dickenson, A.H.: Cholecystokinin as a factor in the enhanced potency of spinal morphine following carrageenin inflammation. Br. J. Pharmacol., *180* (4):967, 1993.
463. Stapleton, J.V., Aushn, K.L., and Mather, L.E.: A pharmacokinetic

approach to pain control: Continuous infusion of pethidine. Anaesth. Intensive Care., *7:*25, 1979.
464. Stein, C.: Peripheral and non-neuronal opioid effects. Curr. Opin. Anaesth., *7:*347, 1994.
465. Stein, C.: The control of pain in peripheral tissue by opioids. N. Engl. J. Med., *332:*1685, 1995.
466. Stenseth, R., Sellevold, O., and Breivik, H.: Epidural morphine for postoperative pain: Experience with 1,095 patients. Acta Anaesthesiol. Scand., *29:*148, 1985.
467. Strichartz, G.: Protracted relief of experimental neuropathic pain by systemic local anesthetics. Anesthesiology *83:*864, 1995.
468. Strube, P.J., Downing, J.W., and Brock-Utne, J.G.: CSF pharmacokinetics of extradural morphine. Br. J. Anaesth, *56:*921, 1984.
469. Struppler, A., Burgmayer, B., Ochs, G., *et al.*: The effect of epidural application of opioids on spasticity of spinal origin. Life Sci., *33:*607, 1983.
470. Sukiennik, A.W., and Kream, R.M.: N-methyl-D-aspartate receptors and pain. Curr. Opin. Anesth., *8:*445, 1995.
471. Taddese, A., Nah, S-Y., and McCleskey, E.W.: Selective opioid inhibition of small nociceptive neurons. Science, *270:*1366, 1995.
472. Tamsen, A., Sakuroda, T., Wahlstrom, A., *et al.*: postoperative demand for analgesics in relation to individual levels of endorphins and substance P in cerebrospinal fluid. Pain, *13:*171, 1982.
473. Tan, S., Cohen, S.E., and White, P.F.: Sufentanil for analgesia after cesarean section: Intravenous versus epidural administration. Anesth. Analg., *65*(Suppl.):1, 1986.
474. Tanaka, M., Watanabe, S., Ashimura, H., *et al.*: Minimum effective combination dose of epidural morphine and fentanyl for posthysterectomy analgesia: A randomized, prospective, double-blind study. Anesth. Analg., *77:*942, 1993.
475. Taniguchi, Y., Ikesue, A., Noda, K., *et al.*: Selective inhibition by nimesulide, a novel nonsteroidal anti-inflammatory drug, with prostaglandin endoperoxide synthase-2 activity in vitro. Pharm. Sci., *1:*173, 1995.
476. Tejwani, G.A., Rattan, A.K., and McDonald, J.S.: Role of spinal opioid receptors in the antinociceptive interactions between intrathecal morphine and bupivacaine. Anesth. Analg., *74:*726, 1992.
477. Thom, R.: Structural Stability and Morphogenesis. Reading, Massachusetts, Benjamin/Cummings, 1975.
478. Thompson, W.R., Smith, P.T., Hirst, M., *et al.*: Regional analgesic effect of epidural morphine in volunteers. Can. Anaesth. Soc. J., *28:*530, 1981.
479. Torda, T.A., Pybus, D.A., Liberman, H., *et al.*: Experimental comparison of extradural and I.M. morphine. Br. J. Anaesth., *52:*939, 1980.
480. Torda, T.A., and Pybus, D.A.: Clinical experience with epidural morphine. Anaesth. Intensive Care, *9:*129, 1981.
481. Traynor, J.R, and Elliot, J.: Opioid receptor subtypes and cross-talk with mu receptors. T.I.P.S., *14:*84, 1993.
482. Tseng, L.F.: Mechanisms of β-endorphin-induced antinociception. *In* Tseng, L.F. (ed.): The Pharmacology of Opioid Peptides. pp. 249–271. Langhorn, PA, Harwood Academic Press, 1995.
483. Tseng, L.F., Tsai, J.H.H., Collins, K.A., and Portoghese, P.S.: Spinal delta$_2$-, but not delta$_1$-, μ-, or κ-opioid receptors are involved in the tail-flick inhibition induced by β-endorphin from nucleus raphe obscurus in the pentobarbital-anesthetized rat. Eur. J. Pharmacol., *277:*251, 1995.
484. Tung, A.S., Tenicela, R., and Winter, P.M.: Opiate withdrawal syndrome following intrathecal administration of morphine. Anesthesiology, *53:*340, 1980.
485. Tung, A.S., and Yaksh, T.L.: In vivo evidence for multiple opiate receptors mediating analgesia in the rat spinal cord. Brain Res., *247:*75, 1982.
486. Tung, A., Maliniak, K., Tenicela, R., and Winter, P.M.: Intrathecal morphine for intraoperative and postoperative analgesia. J.A.M.A., *244:*2637, 1980.
487. Uda, R., Horiguchi, S., Ito, S., *et al.*: Nociceptive effects induced by intrathecal administration of prostaglandin D2, E2, or F2alpha to conscious mice. Brain Res., *510:*26, 1990.
488. U.S. Department of Health and Human Services—Agency for Health Care Policy and Research: Using Clinical Practice Guidelines to Evaluate Quality of Care. Vol. 2: Methods. AHCPR, 1995.
489. U.S.F.D.A.: Guidelines for the clinical evaluation of analgesic drugs. Docket Number 91D 0425. Group for analgesic drugs pilot drug evaluation staff (HFD-007) F.D.A. December 1992.
490. VadeBoncouer, T.R., and Ferrante, F.M.: Epidural and subarachnoid opioids. *In* Ferrante, F.M., and VadeBoncouer T.R. (eds.): Postoperative Pain Management pp. 279–303. New York, Churchill Livingstone, 1993.
491. Valentino, K., Newcomb, R., Gadbois, T., *et al.*: A selective N-type calcium channel antagonist protects against neuronal loss after global cerebral ischemia. Proc. Natl. Acad. Sci., U.S.A., *90:*7894, 1993.
492. Van Dongen, R.T.M., Crul, B.J.P, and de Bock, M.: Long-term intrathecal infusion of morphine/bupivacaine mixtures in the treatment of cancer pain: A retrospective analysis of 51 cases. Pain, *55:*119, 1993.
493. Ventafridda, V., Spoldi, E., Caraceni, A., and DeConno, F.: Intraspinal morphine for cancer pain. Acta Anaesthesiol. Scand., *31:*47, 1987.
494. Walker, S.M., and Cousins, M.J.: Reduction in hyperalgesia and intrathecal morphine requirements by low-dose ketamine infusion. J. Pain Symptom Manage. Sept., 1997.
495. Walters, E.T.: Possible clues about the evolution of hyperalgesia from mechanisms of nociceptive sensitization in aplysia. *In* Willis, W. (ed.): Hyperalgesia and Allodynia. pp. 45–58. New York, Raven Press, 1992.
496. Walts, L.F., Kaufman, R.D., Moreland, J.R., and Weiskopf, M.: Total hip arthroplasty: An investigation of factors related to postoperative urinary retention. Clin. Orthop., *194:*280, 1985.
497. Wang, H. and Sagen, J.: Absence of appreciable tolerance and morphine cross-tolerance in rats with adrenal medullary transplants in the spinal cord. Neuropharmacology, *33:*681, 1994.
498. Wang, J.K., Nauss, L.E., and Thomas, J.E.: Pain relief by intrathecally applied morphine in man. Anesthesiology, *50:*149, 1979.
499. Wanscher, M., Riishede, L., and Krogh, B.: Fistula formation following epidural catheter: A case report. Acta Anaesthesiol. Scand., *29:*552, 1985.
500. Warfield, C.A., and Kahn, C.H.: Acute pain management: Programs in U.S. hospitals and experiences and attitudes among U.S. adults. Anesthesiology, *83:*1090, 1995.
501. Watcha, M.F., and White, P.F.: Economics of anesthetic practice. Anesthesiology, *86:*1170, 1997.
502. Watson, J., Moore, A., McQuay, H., *et al.*: Plasma morphine concentrations and analgesic effects of lumbar extradural morphine and heroin. Anesth. Analg., *63:*629, 1984.
503. Way, E.L.: Studies on the local anesthetic properties of isonipecaine. J. Am. Pharm. Assoc., *35:*44, 1946.
504. Wedel, S.J., and Ritter, R.R.: Serum levels following epidural administration of morphine and correlation with relief of post surgical pain. Anesthesiology, *54:*210, 1981.
505. Weinstein, M.C., Siegel, J.E., Gold, M.R., *et al.*: Recommendations of the panel on cost-effectiveness in health and medicine. J.A.M.A., *26:*1253, 1996.
506. Weinstock, M., Davidson, J.T., Rosin, A.J., and Schnieden, H.: Effect of physostigmine on morphine-induced postoperative pain and somnolence. Br. J. Anaesth., *54:*429, 1982.
507. Welchew, E.A.: The optimum concentration for epidural fentanyl. Anaesthesia, *38:*1037, 1983.
508. Wetchler, B.V.: Economic impact of anesthesia decision-making, J. Clin. Anesth., *4*(Suppl 1.) 20S, 1992.
509. White, W.D., Pearce, D.J., and Norman, J.: Postoperative analgesia: A comparison of intravenous on-demand fentanyl with epidural bupivacaine. Br. Med. J., *2:*166, 1979.
510. Whitwam, J.G.: Benzodiazepine receptors. Anaesthesia, *38:*93, 1983.
511. Wiertelak, E.P., Maier, S.F., and Watkins, L.R.: Cholecystokinin antianalgesia: Safety cues abolish morphine analgesia. Science, *256:*830, 1992.
512. Wiesenfeld-Hallin, Z., Xu, X., Hughes, J., *et al.*: PD134308, a selective antagonist of cholecystokinin type B receptor, enhances the analgesic effect of morphine and synergistically interacts with intrathecal galanin to depress spinal nociceptive reflexes. Proc. Natl. Acad. Sci. *87:*7105, 1990.
513. Wilder, R.T., Shoales, M.G., and Berde, C.B.: N^G-Nitro-L-arginine methyl esther (L-NAME) prevents tachyphylaxis to local anesthetics in a dose-dependent manner. Anesth. Analg., *83:*1251, 1996.
514. Willer, J.C., Bergeret, S., and Gaudy, J.H.: Epidural morphine strongly depresses nociceptive flexion reflexes in patients with postoperative pain. Anesthesiology, *63:*675, 1985.
515. Willer, J.C., and Bussel, B.: Evidence for a direct spinal mechanism in

morphine-induced inhibition of nociceptive reflexes in humans. Brain Res., *187:*212, 1980.

516. Willis, W. (ed.): Hyperalgesia and Allodynia. New York, Raven Press, 1992.
517. Wilson, P.R., and Yaksh, T.L.: Baclofen is antinociceptive in the spinal intrathecal space of animals. Eur. J. Pharmacol., *51:*323, 1978.
518. Winfree, A.T.: The Geometry of Biological Time. pp. 317–336. New York, Springer-Verlag, 1980.
519. Winkelmuller, M., Winkelmuller, W.: Long-term effects of continuous intrathecal opioid treatment in chronic pain of nonmalignant etiology. J. Neurosurg. *85:*458, 1996.
520. Winnie, A.P., Pappas, G.D., Das Gupta, T.K, *et al.*: Subarachnoid adrenal medullary transplants for terminal cancer pain: A report of preliminary studies. Anesthesiology, *79:*644, 1993.
521. Wolfe, M.J., and Davies, G.K.: Analgesic action of extradural fentanyl. Br. J. Anaesth., *52:*357, 1980.
522. Woolf, C.J., and Chong, M.-S.: Preemptive analgesia—Treating postoperative pain by preventing the establishment of central sensitization. Anesth. Analg., *77:*362, 1993.
523. Woolf, C.J., and Thompson, S.W.N.: The induction and maintenance of central sensitization is dependent on N-methyl-D-aspartic acid receptor activation: Implications for the treatment of post-injury pain hypersensitivity states. Pain., *44:*293, 1991.
524. Woolf, C.F.: The dorsal horn: State-dependent sensory processing and the generation of pain. *In* Wall, P., Melzack, R. (eds.): Textbook of Pain. 3rd Ed. pp. 101–112. New York, Churchill Livingstone, 1994.
525. Wu, H.H., Wilcox, G.L., and McLoon, S.C.: Implantation of AtT-20 or genetically modified AtT-20/hENK cells in mouse spinal cord induced antinociception and opioid tolerance. J. Neurosci., *14:*4806, 1994.
526. Wulf, H., Gleim, M., and Mignat, C.: The stability of mixtures of morphine hydrochloride, bupivacaine hydrochloride, and clonidine hydrochloride in portable pump reservoirs for the management of chronic pain syndromes. J. Pain Symptom Manage., *9:*308, 1994.
527. Yablonski-Peretz, T., Klin, B., Beilin, Y., *et al.*: Continuous epidural narcotic analgesia for intractable pain due to malignancy. J. Surg. Oncol., *29:*8, 1985.
528. Yaksh, T.L.: Direct evidence that spinal serotonin and noradrenaline terminals mediate the spinal antinociceptive effects of morphine in the periaqueductal gray. Brain Res., *160:*180, 1978.
529. Yaksh, T.L.: In vivo studies on spinal opiate receptor systems mediating antinociception. I. Mu and delta receptor profiles in the primate. J. Pharmacol. Exp. Ther., *226:*303, 1983.
530. Yaksh, T.L.: (ed.): Spinal Afferent Processing. New York, Plenum Press, 1986.
531. Yaksh, T.L., Abay, E.O., and Go, V.L.: Studies on the location and release of cholecystokinin and vaso-active intestinal peptide in rat and cat spinal cord. Brain Res., *242:*279, 1982.
532. Yaksh, T.L., Gross, K.E., and Li, C.H.: Studies on the intrathecal effects of beta-endorphin in the primate. Brain Res., *241:*261, 1982.
533. Yaksh, T.L., Harty, G.J., and Onofrio, B.M.: High doses of spinal morphine produce a nonopiate receptor mediated hyperesthesia. Practical and theoretical implications. Anesthesiology. *64*(5):590, 1986.
534. Yaksh, T.L., Huang, S.P., Rudy, R.T., and Fredenckson, R.C.: The direct and specific opiate-like effect of met^5-enkephalin and analogues on the spinal cord. Neuroscience, *2:*593, 1977.
535. Yaksh, T.L., and Li, C.H.: Studies on the intrathecal effects of beta-endorphin in primate. Brain Res., *241:*261, 1982.
536. Yaksh, T.L., Noueihed, R.Y., and Durant, A.C.: Studies of the pharmacology and pathology of intrathecally administered 4-aminopiperidine analogues and morphine in the rat and cat. Anesthesiology, *64:*54, 1986.
537. Yaksh, T.L., and Reddy, S.V.: Studies on the primate on the analgetic effects associated with intrathecal actions of opiate alpha-adrenergic agonists and baclofen. Anesthesiology, *54:*451, 1981.
538. Yaksh, T.L., and Rudy, T.A.: Studies on the direct spinal action of narcotics in the production of spinal analgesia in the rat. J. Pharmacol. Exp. Ther., *202:*411, 1977.
539. Yaksh, T.L.: Intrathecal and epidural opiates: A review. *In* Campbell, J.N. (ed.): Pain 1996: An Updated Review. pp. 381–393. Seattle, IASP Press, 1996.
540. Yaksh, T.L.: Epidural ketamine: A useful, mechanistically novel adjuvant for epidural morphine? Reg. Anesth., *21:*508, 1996.
541. Yaksh, T.L.: Spinal somatostatin for patients with cancer. Risk-benefit assessment of an analgesic. Anesthesiology, *81:*531, 1994.
542. Yaksh, T.L., and Collins, J.G.: Studies in animals should precede human use of spinally administered drugs. Anesthesiology, *70:*4, 1989.
543. Yaksh, T.L., and Malmberg, A.B.: Interaction of spinal modulatory receptor systems. *In* Fields, H.L. and Liebeskind, J.C. (eds.): Pharmacological Approaches to the Treatment of Chronic Pain: New Concepts and Critical Issues. pp. 151–171. Seattle, IASP Press, 1994.
544. Yamamoto, T. and Shimoyama, N.: Role of nitric oxide in the development of thermal hyperesthesia induced by sciatic nerve constriction injury in the rat. Anesthesiology, *82:*1266, 1995.
545. Yarnell, R.W., Polis T., Reid, G.N., *et al.*: Patient-controlled analgesia with epidural meperidine after elective cesarean section. Reg. Anesth., *17:*329, 1992.
546. Yeung, J.C., and Rudy, T.A.: Multiplicative interaction between narcotic agonism expressed at spinal and supraspinal sites of antinociceptive action as revealed by concurrent intrathecal and intracerebroventricular injections of morphine. J. Pharmacol. Exp. Ther., *215:*633, 1980.
547. Zahn, P.K., Gysbers, D., and Brennen, T.J.: Effect of systemic and intrathecal morphine in a rat model of postoperative pain. Anesthesiology, *86:*1066, 1997.
548. Zenz, M.: Epidural opiates: Long-term experiences in cancer pain. Klin. Wochenschr., *63:*225, 1985.
549. Zenz, M., Schappler-Scheele, B., Neuhans, R., *et al.*: Long-term peridural morphine analgesia in cancer pain. Lancet, *1:*91, 1981.
550. Zenz, M.W., and Tryba, M.: Economic aspects of pain therapy. Curr. Opin. Anesth., *9:*430, 1996.
551. Zieglgansberger, W., Tolle, T.R., Zimprich, A., *et al.*: Endorphins, pain relief, and euphoria. *In* Bromm, B., Desmedt, J.E. (eds.): Advances In Pain Research and Therapy, Vol. 22. pp. 439–457. New York, Raven Press, 1995.

Neural Blockade in Clinical Anesthesia and Management of Pain, Third Edition,
edited by M.J. Cousins and P.O. Bridenbaugh.
Lippincott–Raven Publishers, Philadelphia © 1998.

CHAPTER 30
Neuropathology of Neurolytic Agents

Robert R. Myers

The specialized structure of a peripheral nerve bundle is essential to its normal sensory and motor functions. Pathologic alterations in the structure of nerve fibers or changes in the biochemistry and biophysics of their environment are associated with abnormal function. While these changes usually are caused by diseases or injuries to nerves, it may be therapeutically desirable to induce temporary nerve injury with neurolytic agents or mechanical devices for the clinical purpose of interrupting nerve sensory function. This chapter will review the important neuropathologic features of peripheral nerves relevant to the neurolytic management of pain, highlighting both the factors needed for nerve regeneration, and the causes of failed neurolytic procedures as indicated by behavioral studies and neuropathologic evaluation of experimental tissue. As the development of intrathecal pharmacology and pain management techniques improve, it is argued that the need for local neurolytic interventions will diminish.[46] Incentive for this transition is fostered in part by the non-selective nature of many neurolytic agents, which increases the risk when they are used. Development of more selective neurolytic agents, targeted at sensory systems, holds promise for long-term pain management. For this reason, several of these experimental agents are presented in this chapter, even though they have not yet been used clinically. Lastly, the effect of specific neurolytic and semi-destructive agents and techniques used clinically will be discussed with respect to their capacity to relieve pain by altering the structure and function of peripheral nerves and their associated support cells.

NERVE STRUCTURE AND NORMAL FUNCTION

Peripheral nerve fibers are processes of cell bodies located in the spinal cord of the central nervous system or the dorsal roots of the peripheral nervous system. As such, they are conduits for the axonal transport of structural proteins and organelles needed for the metabolic activity and growth of these fibers. Interruption or compression of the axon results in axonal swelling of the proximal portion, due to accumulation of transport particles and degeneration in the distal portion, as shall be discussed later.

The axonal particles include mitochondria, endoplasmic reticula, neurofilaments, microtubules, and dense particles (Fig. 30-1). The mitochondria are 0.1 to 0.3 microns in diameter, 0.5 to 0.8 microns in length and are divided into outer and inner compartments. The outer compartment contains monoamine oxidase, which is responsible for degradation of catecholamines; the inner compartment, bounded by highly infolded membranes called cristae, contains the respiratory electron transport and energy transport enzymes and coenzymes involved in the Krebs cycle. The nucleotides ATP and ADP are also contained in the intracellular compartment. The concentration of mitochondria is greater in smaller axons, which probably are formed in the cell body and then slowly transported down the axon, where they are usually located randomly throughout the peripheral nerve; their movement seems to be dictated by the location of microtubules and neurofilaments.

The smooth endoplasmic reticulum (SER) is generally an agranular, irregular structure in the peripheral axon. With electron microscopy, SER may appear as vesicles, tubules, or cisternae, generally arranged in rows parallel to the length of the axon. The wall of the endoplasmic reticulum has a trilaminar appearance, containing none of the ribosomes observed in the rough (granular) endoplasmic reticulum (RER). The RER takes part in protein synthesis, while the SER probably does not.

The neurofilament is a tubular structure 100 Å in diameter, with a single wall approximately 30 Å thick. The wall seems to be a helically-coiled thread composed of globular protein. The function of neurofilaments is thought to be related to the intracellular transport of ions and metabolites, and to skeletal support of the cell.

The microtubules are composed of tubules that measure approximately 250 Å in diameter, with walls 60 Å thick. The center may contain a thin central filament or row of granules. Microtubules seem to be most prevalent in unmyelinated ax-

R. R. Myers: Department of Anesthesiology Research, University of California at San Diego, La Jolla, California 92093-0629.

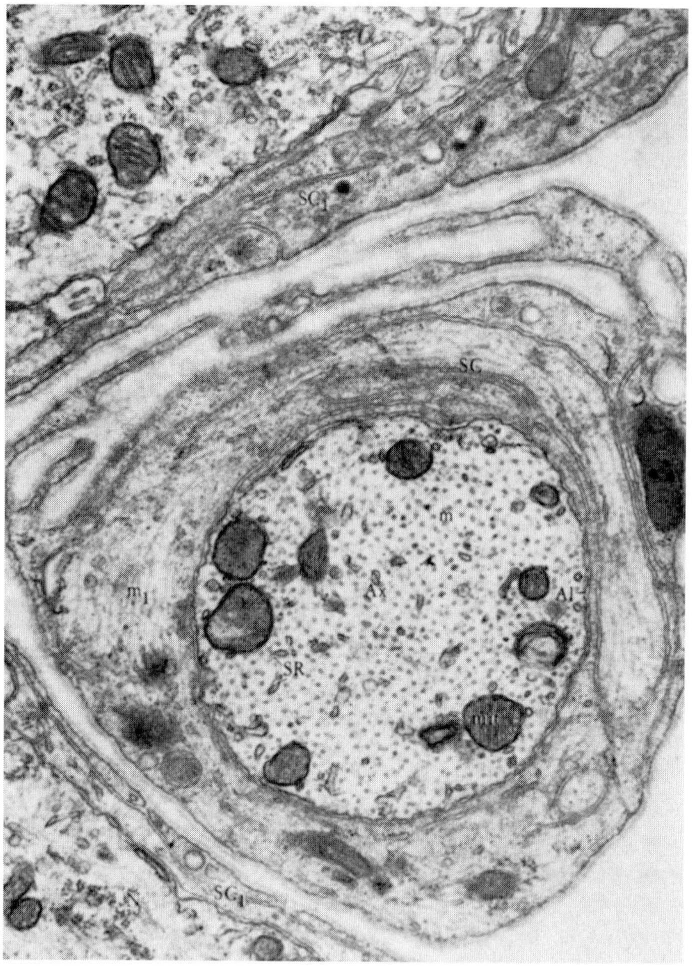

FIG. 30-1. Electron micrograph of transverse section from mouse ganglion cell axon. The axolemma *(Al)* is the boundary of the axoplasm and is surrounded by Schwann cell processes *(Sc)* containing microtubules *(ml)*. Within the axoplasm, microtubules *(m)* are homogeneously dispersed. Mitochondria *(mit)* and tubular profiles of smooth endoplasmic reticulum *(SR)* are also seen in this section. Original magnification ×26,000. (From Peters, A, Palay, S.L., and deF. Webster, H.: The Fine Structure of the Nervous System. pp. 103. New York, Oxford University Press, 1991.)

ons where neurofilaments are rare. Their function is thought to be similar to that of the neurofilaments.

Dense particles often are aligned in the cytoplasm, next to the plasma membrane adjacent to the axolemma. Groups of dense particles sometimes are seen in the cytoplasm near the node of Ranvier. Function of the dense particles is unknown, but they may be lysomal in nature, and indicate a normal turnover of axonal organelles.

These are the major particles in the axoplasm, which, together with its cytoplasmic fluid, displays a viscosity approximately 5 times that of water.[28] The basic properties of axoplasmic transport and the role of axonal transport in disease have been reviewed recently.[8,76]

An important concept in this regard, with respect to toxic agents, is their ability to inhibit one or more factors contributing to axonal transport, because this ultimately results in neuropathic injury to the nerve, and to altered neuronal function. Figure 30-2 illustrates the sites at which interruption of axonal transport affects the replenishment of structural proteins and neurotransmitters at the axonal terminals. Interruption of the viability of these processes leads directly to nerve damage. Additionally, vesicular retrograde axonal transport of compounds, taken up at the axonal terminal, can influence neuronal function in the dorsal root ganglia. For example, tetanus toxin and herpes simplex virus are taken up at the peripheral terminal and transported retrogradely to the cell body.[43,88] Other neuronal-specific toxins, like ricin and capsaicin, which may eventually have therapeutic value in pain management, also gain entry to the cell body via retrograde axonal transport.

Unmyelinated Fibers

The axon is bounded by a surface membrane, the axolemma, which is approximately 8 nm thick. Internal to the axolemma is the axoplasm, which contains the neurofilaments, neurotubules, vesicles, and organelles discussed previously. The Schwann cell encompasses a variable number of unmyelinated axons in a common compartment separating them by Schwann cell tongues. Thin septa also prevent axon–axon contact. Collagen pockets are included in the Schwann cell tubes and help separate axons. Finally, a basal lamina contains the packet of axons and Schwann cell. Some concern has existed about electrical "cross-talk" between unmyelinated axons, but the variable longitudinal course of axons within unmyelinated nerve fibers reduces the impact of this hypothesized artifact. Unmyelinated and myelinated

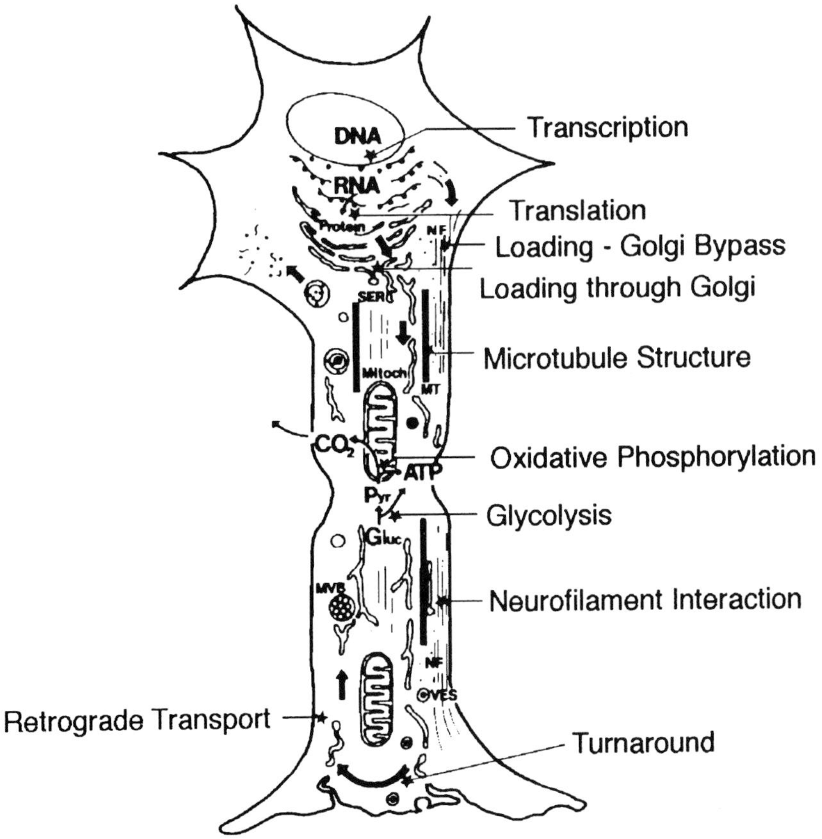

FIG. 30-2. Diagram of the stages in rapid axonal transport and sites at which interruption of transport can take place. The stages include transcription, translation, and loading of transported proteins in the cell body and then their energy-dependent movement along the axon. Turnaround of proteins and retrograde transport of proteins and other substances, including neurotoxins, at the axon terminal play important roles in regulating neuronal protein production. DNA, deoxyribonucleic acid; RNA, ribonucleic acid; SER, smooth endoplasmic reticulum. [Modified from Ochs, S. and Brimijoin, W.S.: Axonal transport. *In* Dyck, P.J., *et al.* (eds.): Peripheral Neuropathy. p. 331. Philadelphia, W.B. Saunders Company, 1993.]

fibers are not distributed randomly and groups of unmyelinated fibers cluster together (Fig. 30-3).

Myelinated Fibers

The chief morphologic difference in myelinated and unmyelinated fibers is the lack of myelin lamellae in unmyelinated fibers. The axoplasms are qualitatively similar in their constituents, although the surface distribution of ionic channels is not uniform, and in myelinated fibers, the axoplasm is constricted at the nodes of Ranvier. Peripheral myelinated axons are surrounded by a tubular myelin sheath derived from Schwann cells. The Schwann cell insulation permits increased conduction velocity that enhances the direct relationship between axonal diameter and the velocity of impulse conduction. The Schwann cell is of trapezoid shape and wrapped spirally around the axon and axolemma. The number of concentric layers of wrapped myelin is directly proportional to the diameter of the axon. Myelin completely covers the axon, except at the axon terminal, where there is usually a 1 to 2 micron gap and at the nodes of Ranvier, the sites between adjacent Schwann cells. At a node of Ranvier, the axolemma is exposed for 1 to 1.5 microns. On either side of the gap, the total myelin thickness is somewhat less than average, owing to a progressive reduction in the number of lamellae and their terminal myelin loops. The axoplasm is also reduced in volume and cross-sectional area in the nodal and paranodal spaces. However, the nodal region is critical to proper nerve function, since it is the site of sodium channels between the axoplasm and endoneurial environment that are responsible for the saltatory conduction of nerve impulses. The paranodal region contains potassium channels[10]

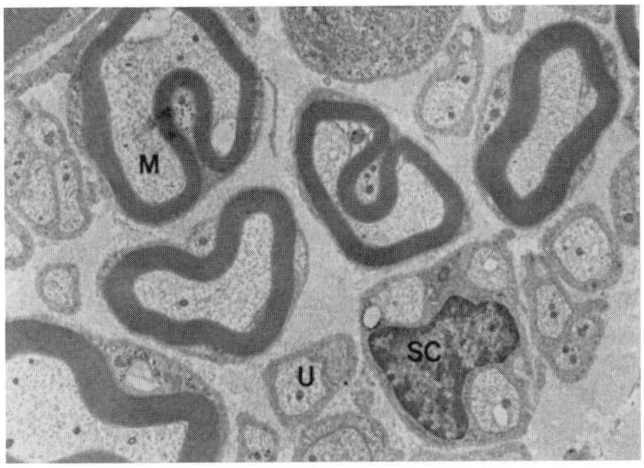

FIG. 30-3. Electron micrograph of normal human peripheral nerve illustrating coexistence of myelinated (with dark staining myelin sheaths) *(M)* and unmyelinated *(U)* fibers. A Schwann cell nucleus *(SC)* is seen in the lower right associated with a group of 3 unmyelinated fibers. Mitochondria and smaller organelle can be seen in the axoplasm of both myelinated and unmyelinated fibers. Stained with uranyl acetate and lead citrate. (Provided through the courtesy of Dr. Henry C. Powell, University of California, San Diego.)

not normally observed except during fiber injury; paranodal demyelination is an early pathologic change. The Schwann cell is contained by a continuous basal lamina that extends across the node of Ranvier, forming a tubular scaffolding that is important in nerve regeneration.

Connective Tissue

Peripheral nerve fibers are maintained in a specialized environment created by the selective permeability of the connective tissue elements of nerve bundles and the blood–nerve barrier of the vasa nervorum.

The epineurium is the outermost covering of the nerve, and has numerous blood vessels of arteriolar and venular size, running longitudinally along its axis, as well as fat cells which help cushion the nerve against compression injury.[113] (Figs. 30-4, 30-5). The epineurium may also contain fibroblasts, and a variable number of mast cells. Epineurial vessels have a fenestrated endothelium that permits the extravasation of macromolecules such as Evans blue-albumin or horseradish peroxidase.[77] Epineurial vessels are adrenergically innervated and constrict in the presence of epinephrine.[60] The epineurial tissue itself consists of areolar connective tissue that is loosely attached to the perineurium which it surrounds. Collagen bundles are oriented primarily in the longitudinal axis, giving the epineurium high-yield strength when pulled along this axis.[29] Lundborg reports that small segments of the epineurium can be removed without affecting peripheral nerve function because of an extensive anastomosis of the extrinsic epineurial circulation with the intrinsic vasa nervorum[54] (Figs. 30-5, 30-6). The radicular epineurial vessels pass through the epineurium and perineurium, at an acute angle, to anastomose with the intrinsic nerve circulation where capillary exchange occurs (Fig. 30-5). We have shown that extensive removal of the epineurium, a surgical procedure called external neurolysis, which is sometimes useful in freeing a nerve from fibrotic attachments to surrounding tissue,[56] can interfere with nutritive blood flow to nerve fibers. The resulting ischemic insults produce demyelinating or axonal neuropathies, depending on the magnitude and duration of ischemia.[61] Axonal neuropathies have been associated with significant hyperalgesia to mechanical and thermal stimuli of the associated dermatome.[74]

The perineurium is an especially important tissue, both because of the vessels that pass through it, and because of its functions as a semielastic and semipermeable membrane that organizes nerve fibers into fascicles and helps to regulate their interstitial fluid environment. The perineurium consists of a laminated arrangement of flattened polygonal cells, up to 15 layers thick, bounded by a basal lamina.[113] The junctions between perineurial cells are tight and normally do not permit the free entry of macromolecules. Vesicular transport does occur, however, and is a route for macromolecular exchange between the epineurial and endoneurial spaces. Collagen fibrils are oriented primarily in the longitudinal axis; their relative lack in the circumferential axis contributes to the ballooning or stretching of the perineurium when edema occurs in the endoneurial space of the nerve.

Finally, the endoneurium comprises the intrafascicular connective tissue. While the endoneurium is defined as a connective tissue element of nerve, the term generally is

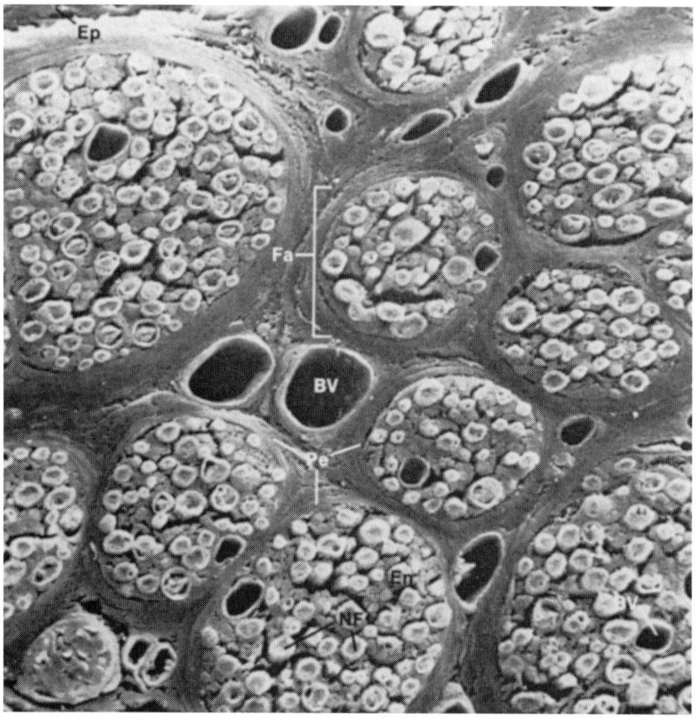

FIG. 30-4. Scanning electron micrograph of a peripheral nerve in cross-section. Nerve fibers *(NF)* are organized in bundles called fascicles *(Fa)*, each of which is surrounded by a collagen-rich sheath, the perineurium *(Pe)*. Loose connective tissue forms the epineurium *(Ep)* which encircles groups of fascicles. The endoneurium *(En)* is a division of the perineurium forming thin layers of connective tissue surrounding nerve fibers. In practice, the entire space bounded by the perineurium is referred to as endoneurial space. Blood vessels *(BV)*, with fenestrated endothelial cells, are numerous in the epineurial space. Somewhat smaller vessels within the endoneurium form the vasa nervorum with tight endothelial cell junctions. These two circulations communicate via vessels that pass obliquely through the perineurium. (From Ressel, R.G., and Rardon, R.H.: Tissue and Organs. pp. 79. W.H. Freeman, 1979.)

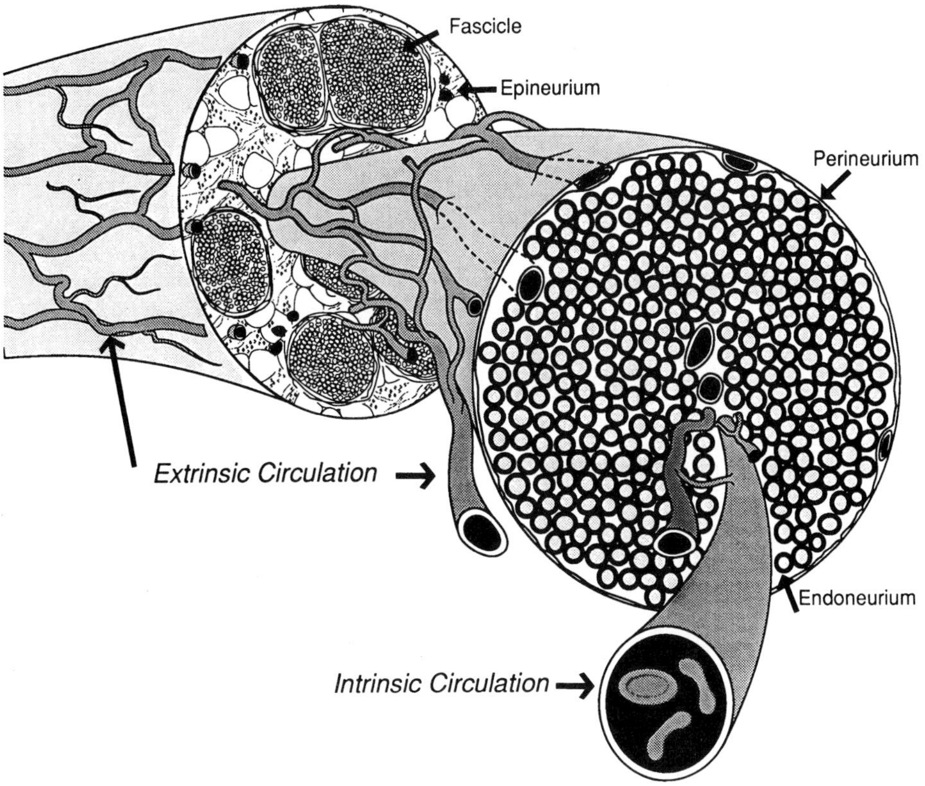

FIG. 30-5. Schematic illustration of the circulation in peripheral nerve. The relationship between the extrinsic epineurial vessels and the intrinsic endoneurial vessels is emphasized. Numerous branching vessels form a rich anastomotic network on the surface of the fascicles. These vessels are connected to the intrinsic vasculature by transperineurial vessels, which are vulnerable to compressive forces acting from within or on the external surface of the nerve sheath. Vessels in the extrinsic circulation are adrenergically innervated; those within the endoneurium lack innervation. (From Myers, R.R., Heckman, H.M., Galbraith, J.A., and Powell, H.C.: Subperineurial demyelination associated with reduced nerve blood flow and oxygen tension after epineural vascular stripping. Lab. Invest., *65*:41, 1991.)

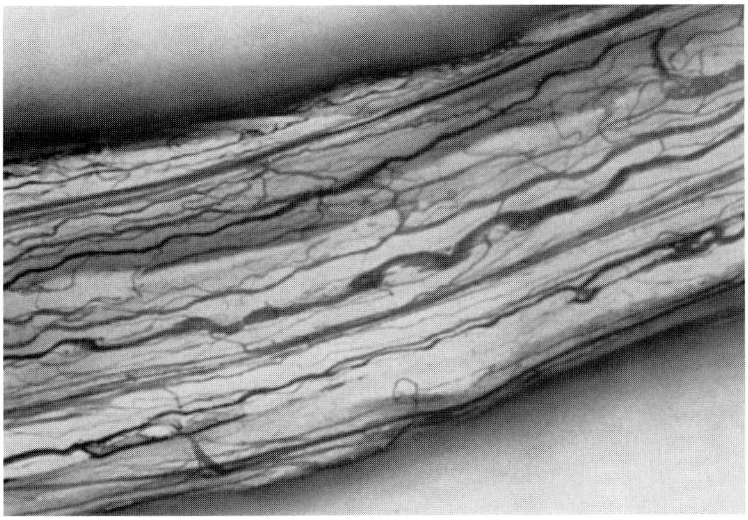

FIG. 30-6. Gelatin cast of rat sciatic nerve illustrating the extrinsic epineurial circulation. The cast was made by injecting a gelatin mass into the vasculature at systolic pressure. After the gelatin hardened, the tissue was cleared with methyl methacrylate. Note sinusoidal course of vessels to allow for stretching, and the extensive anastomoses between vessels.

used to identify the space and tissue surrounded by the perineurium. Thus, the endoneurium contains the individual myelinated and unmyelinated nerve fibers, their Schwann cells, the capillaries of the intrinsic vasa nervorum, collagen, and an interstitial fluid environment that promotes conduction of electrical nerve impulses.

Endoneurial Environment

The endoneurial environment is a delicately balanced fluid space that serves as a sink for electrolyte exchange with nerve fibers, making possible the propagation of action potentials. While the unique characteristics of this space had been hypothesized for some time, it was not until the introduction of quantitative neuropathological and bioengineering techniques that the pathogenic significance of the endoneurial environment became apparent. Using an indirect technique, involving the drying and ashing of whole nerves, Krnjevic[44] predicted elevated concentrations of electrolytes in endoneurial (interstitial) fluid. Modern techniques using 100 picoliter volumes of endoneurial fluid aspirated directly from rat sciatic nerve have confirmed that endoneurial fluid electrolyte concentrations are hypertonic with respect to serum.[62] In studies of lead neuropathy, it has been observed that when the blood–nerve barrier was damaged by the ingestion of lead, the endoneurial fluid electrolyte concentrations asymptomatically approached serum levels. This occurred early in the course of the neuropathy, when there was electrophysiologic dysfunction but no demyelination.[62,87] Mizisin et al.[57] have shown that endoneurial sodium concentrations in galactosemic neuropathy are nearly double the control value of 152 mEq/l. In this neuropathy, the blood-nerve barrier is not damaged, but there is significant endoneurial edema. This finding may help explain the source of the osmotic force responsible for endoneurial hydration, and the edema that is a nearly ubiquitous finding in neuropathy.

There are no lymphatic channels in peripheral nerve and normal endoneurial hydration produces a slightly positive endoneurial fluid pressure of 2.0 $\pm$ 1.0 cm H_2O.[52,70] In galactosemic neuropathy and in many of the neuropathies caused by neurolytic agents, endoneurial fluid pressure can be significantly elevated.[52,68] The removal of endoneurial fluid occurs at the nerve terminals where the perineurium is absent. This process is thought to be driven by a gradient in endoneurial fluid pressure distally from the dorsal rool ganglion (DRG).

ABNORMAL STRUCTURE AND PATHOPHYSIOLOGIC FUNCTION

Wallerian Degeneration

Wallerian degeneration is the term used to describe the complex series of events associated with nerve fiber degeneration in the distal stump of a transected nerve. These events were originally described by Augustus Waller in 1850.[118] The term also applies to the pathological events following crush injury, and other injuries to nerve bundles that produce focal axonopathy,[85] including reduced nerve blood supply.[81] Initially, swelling occurs at the proximal stump, due chiefly to accumulation of mitochondria and lysosomes. The axolemma fragments and the axoplasm undergo granular dissolution. These primary events are followed by the collapse and digestion of the myelin sheath, as a secondary change of Wallerian degeneration. However, Schwann cells react within minutes of an injury to the nerve fiber. The myelin sheath retracts from the node of Ranvier and exposes the potassium channels. Eventually, the myelin sheath collapses, forming darkly staining myelin ovoids (Fig. 30-7). Macrophages and Schwann cells, which also have a phagocytic role, are active during this time, and assist in the removal of disintegrating material. Schwann cells proliferate within the confines of the old basal lamina vacated by degenerating nerve fibers that create the bands of Bungner, important to the successful regeneration of nerve fibers (Fig. 30-8). When nerves are transected, the basal lamina is interrupted, which makes it considerably more difficult for regenerating nerve fibers to find their appropriate end-organs.[108]

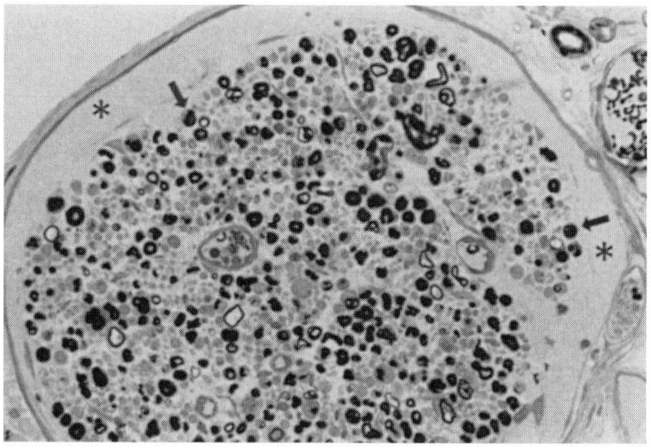

FIG. 30-7. Transverse section of rat sciatic nerve fascicle 6 days following crush injury. Note extensive endoneurial edema (*). Endoneurial fluid pressure was elevated approximately 3 times normal. Following axonal injury, Wallerian degeneration is characterized by collapse of the myelin sheath and accumulation of osmiophilic debris into myelin ovoids, as is seen extensively here *(arrows)*. Stained with paraphenylene diamine.

Wallerian degeneration is a fundamentally basic neuropathological event about which there is still much to learn. Recent work on the pathogenesis of neuropathic pain following experimental nerve injury highlights the importance of immunological events mediated by activated macrophages and their relationship to Wallerian degeneration.[74] This process involves all classes of endoneurial cells and their complex mechanisms of communication.[27] The role of

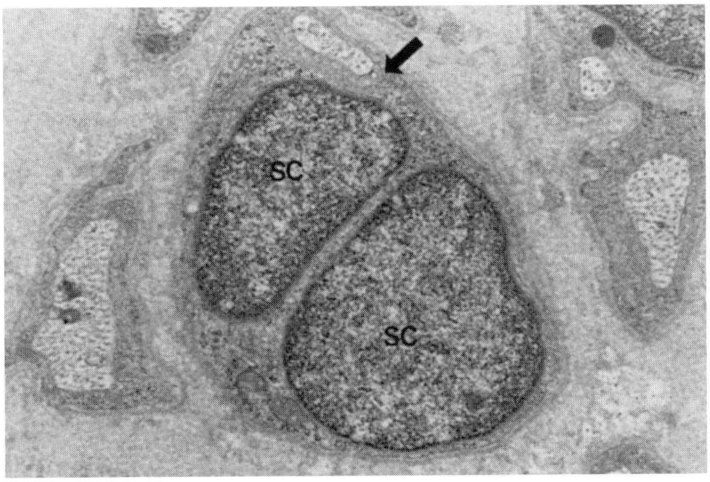

FIG. 30-8. Electron micrograph from human nerve showing the proliferation of Schwann cells *(SC)* within the existing basal lamina structure of a previous Schwann cell, creating a band of Bungner. Note 2 Schwann cell nuclei in the center and duplicate basal lamina surrounding them *(arrows)*. Stained with uranyl acetate and lead citrate. (Provided through the courtesy of Dr. Henry C. Powell, University of California, San Diego.)

cytokines in the process of Wallerian degeneration is especially important, because production of interleukin-I and other cytokine factors at the site of nerve injury is necessary for the recruitment of hematogeneous macrophages responsible for production of most of the chemical factors causing axonal lysis, and the subsequent phagocytosis of debris that precedes regeneration. Other, unknown, signals are required to initiate Wallerian degeneration. This finding is best demonstrated in the genetic mouse strain C57BL/WLD (formally called C57BL/O1a), in which Wallerian degeneration is delayed significantly after nerve injury, even though hematogeneous macrophage function is normal.[83]

In pain studies, it has been suggested that cytokines or secondary cytokine events at the lesion site are part of the signaling mechanism, from the periphery to central neurons that lead to changes in neuronal function associated with neuropathic pain states.[74] The communication may occur via retrograde axonal transport. In support of this hypothesis is the well-known relationship between increases in interleukin (IL)-1, Schwann cell expression of nerve growth factor and receptor, and their retrograde transport to the cell body, which switches DRG neuronal function from production of neurotransmitters to production of axonal skeletal proteins.[78] It has been shown, also, that blockade of axonal transport with colchicine, applied topically to the nerve and proximal to an injury site, eliminates the hyperalgesia that otherwise would be expected to occur.[128]

Regeneration Process

The regeneration of the proximal portion of the axon usually is marked by the formation of an axoplasmic mass with filopodia at the end of the severed axon. Inside this growth cone can be seen increased mitochondria, dense bodies, vesicular elements, neurofilaments, and smooth endoplasmic reticulum (Fig. 30-9). Variation in mitochondrial shape and size may also be noted.

Accompanying the development of the growth cone, the Schwann cells undergo mitotic activity, forming a framework for developing fibers (Fig. 30-10). One axon actually may send out many growth cones. It is at this point, typically 7 to 14 days after injury, that ectopic electrophysiologic activity develops,[126] which can be painful. If all regenerating growth cones reach the end organ, there may actually be more fibers distally than proximally. Many of these additional fibers degenerate over the course of 1 year. The growth of the regenerating axon is occasionally blocked by glial scars and cystic spaces that develop from lysis of neural debris. If a sensory fiber reaches a motor endplate, or a motor fiber reaches a sensory terminal, the fiber eventually will degenerate.[47]

Regeneration occurs at the rate of approximately 1 mm per day, so that reinnervation of a structure 5 cm away would take approximately 50 days. However, recovery of function may not always depend upon regeneration, because alternative pathways may take over the impulse route. For example, after thoracic neurolytic subarachnoid block of posterior roots, pain conduction may reroute by way of the anterior roots that are known to possess about 10% to 12% afferent C fibers. Alternatively, overlapping innervation from adjacent dermatomes may compensate for denervated axons.

Clinically, after simple injuries, the ulnar nerve requires approximately 8 weeks for recovery to begin. However, healing after a major injury, such as one caused by gunshot, requires a minimum of 4 months. Return of voluntary muscle action after brachial plexus injury may be as early as 3 months, or it may be delayed for 2 or more years, depending on the severity of injury.[108]

Endoneurial Fluid Pressure

Increased endoneurial fluid pressure (EFP) is a frequent finding in neuropathies caused by toxic, metabolic, or traumatic insult to nerve fibers, their supporting cells, or their en-

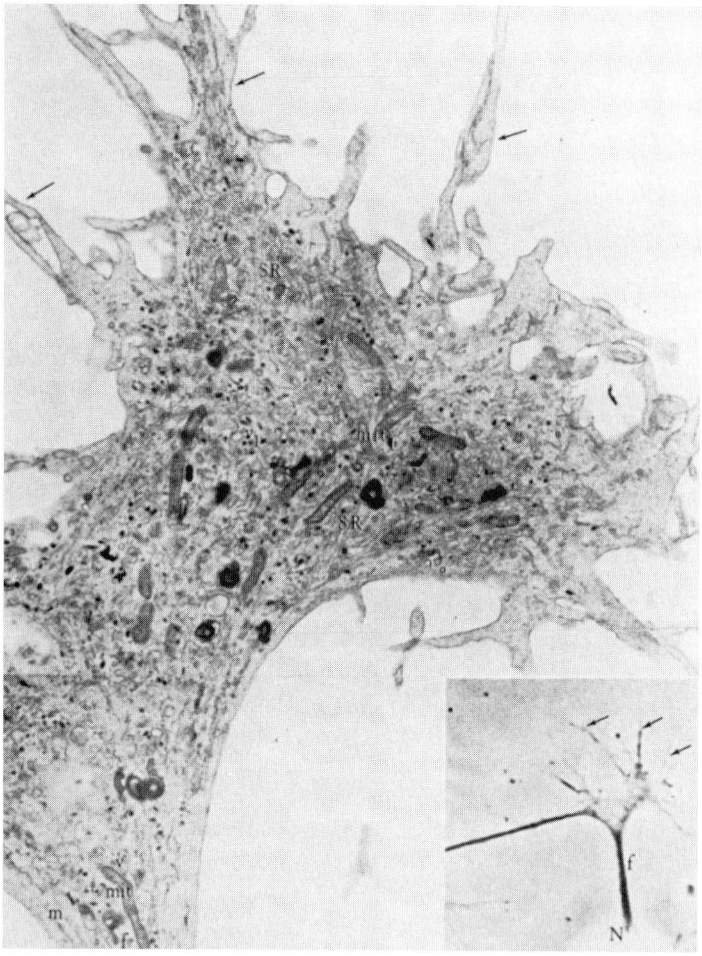

FIG. 30-9. Growth cone from sympathetic neuron in tissue culture. Insert is phase contrast micrograph showing fibers *(f)* extending from perikaryon *(N)* of a neuron. Filopodia *(arrows)* extend from growth cone. The electron micrograph from the same growth cone shows filopodia *(arrows)* and numerous cytoplasmic particles, including elongated mitochondria *(mit)*, smooth endoplasmic reticulum *(SR)*, vesicles *(v)*, vesicles with dense contents *(vl)*, and microtubules *(m)*. Original magnification ×1400 for EM; ×1350 for phase contrast. (From Peters, A., Parlay, S.L., and Webster, H. de F.: The Fine Structure of the Nervous System. New York, Oxford University Press, 1991.)

vironment.[68] Several different etiological mechanisms are revealed in the process of Wallerian degeneration, following crush injury, where there is a complex series of changes in nerve hydration, producing elevated EFP (Fig. 30-11). EFP initially is elevated due to damage of the blood–nerve barrier, but peaks approximately 6 to 7 days after the injury[86] and corresponds to the time of greatest discomfort in patients. The peak in EFP is due to a summation of events, in each the result is increased endoneurial volume. Mast cells degranulate, releasing vasoactive chemicals that increase the permeability of the blood–nerve barrier, Schwann cells proliferate, and phagocytic cells are active. EFP gradually declines and is normal 1 month following injury, when regeneration is nearly complete.

Abnormal Nerve Blood Flow

Nerve blood flow (NBF) has been measured with quantitative methods.[66,69,104,114] Normal NBF is approximately 16 ml/100g tissue/min and is thus slightly less than the blood flow value for cerebral white matter. In edematous neuropathies with increased endoneurial fluid pressure, it has been shown that NBF is decreased significantly. Morphologic evidence supports ischemia as a pathogenic mechanism causing nerve fiber injury.[69,85] Researchers are working earnestly to discover the pathogenic mechanism for reduced nerve blood flow in the presence of elevated EFP. Current hypotheses include a theory that endoneurial capillaries are separated by edema[114] and a view, based on the apparent susceptibility of transperineurial vessels to occlusion when the perineurium is stretched by increased EFP, that there is a pathologic valve mechanism in perineurial vessels.[53] The argument in support of the reduced capillary density hypothesis is based on blood flow per unit weight of tissue and an increased weight of edematous nerve. However, blood flow is still less than normal if the tissue weight is normalized by subtracting the excess water weight from the wet-weight of the nerve.[66] The existence of a pathologic valve mechanism in vessels traversing the perineurium is supported by both morphologic and theoretical evidence.[67] Morphologic evidence comes from serial sections of tissue that are reconstructed to follow the course of transperineurial vessels (Fig. 30-12). In the illustration, a sciatic nerve with increased EFP 48 hours following topical application of the clinical preparation of 2-chloroprocaine local anesthetic,

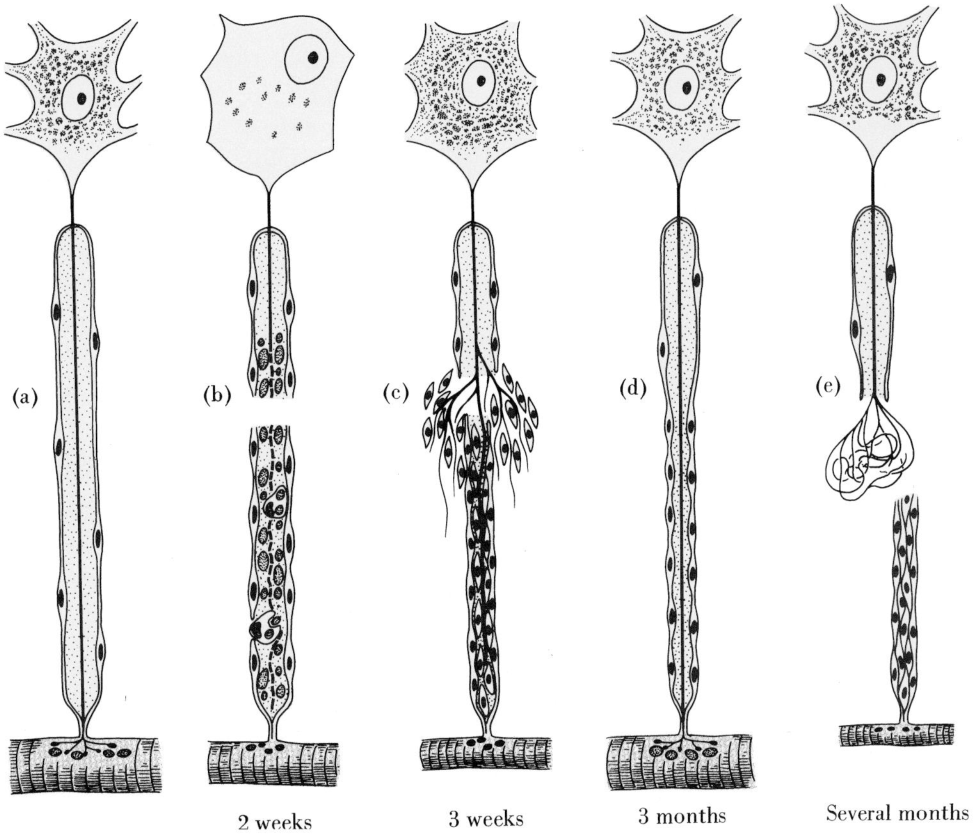

FIG. 30-10. Major changes associated with nerve fiber regeneration. **A:** Normal nerve fiber with its perikaryon and its effector cell (striated skeletal muscle). The axon is surrounded by myelin generated by Schwann cells. **B:** When the fiber is injured, the neuronal nucleus moves to the periphery and Nissel bodies in the perikaryon become greatly reduced in number. The nerve fiber distal to the injury degenerates along with its myelin sheath—Wallerian degeneration. The blood–nerve barrier is damaged and debris is phagocytized by macrophages. **C:** By 3 weeks, the muscle fiber shows a pronounced disuse atrophy. Schwann cells proliferate, forming a compact cord through which an axon may grow. The axon grows at a rate of approximately 1 mm/day. **D:** In this example, the nerve fiber has generated successfully 3 months after injury. **E:** In other cases, however, the axon may not find its original end-organ successfully, if growth is impeded by mechanical obstacles or is unorganized for other reasons. [From Willis, R.A., and Willis, A.T.: The Principles of Pathology and Bacteriology. Butterworths, 1972; redrawn for Ross, M.H., Reith, E.J., Moss, M.H., et al. (eds.): Histology: A Text and Atlas. Reading, MA, Addison-Wesley, 1985.]

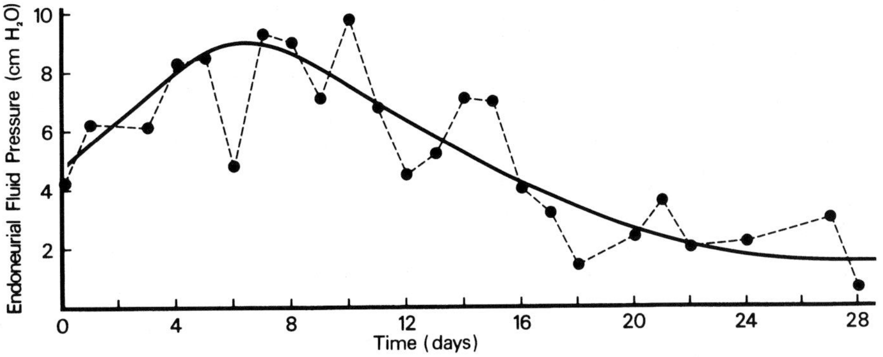

FIG. 30-11. Progressive changes in endoneurial fluid pressure (EFP) following proximal crush injury to rat sciatic nerve. Initially, EFP is elevated due to vascular damage associated with the crush. A peak in EFP is reached between the 6 to 7 day post-compression and represents a summation of events explained in the text. EFP gradually declines during the course of regeneration. (From Powell, H.C., Myers, R.R., Costello, M.L., and Lampert, P.W.: Endoneurial fluid pressure in Wallerian degeneration. Ann. Neurol., *5*:550, 1979.)

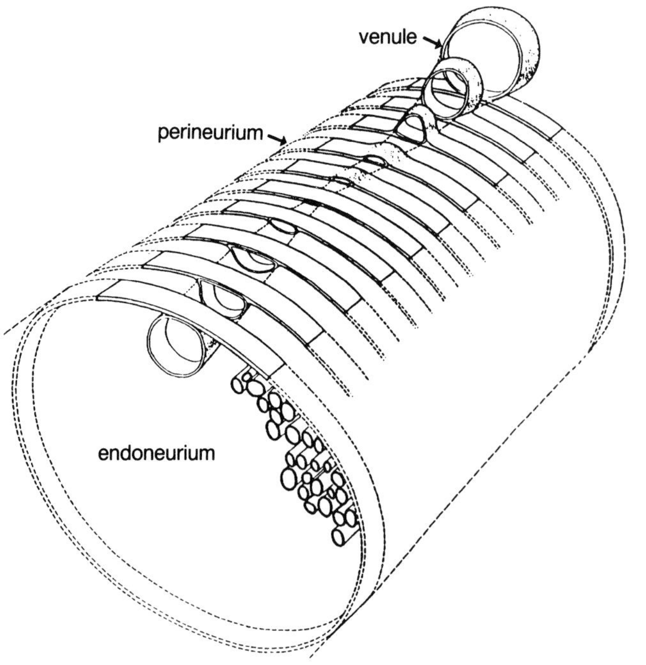

FIG. 30-12. Serial, transverse sections of nerve reconstructed to illustrate the passage of an epineurial vessel through the perineurium. Note: In this actual example from an edematous nerve 48 hours following topical application of 3% 2-chloroprocaine, the lumen of the venous vessel is reduced in cross-sectional area when it traverses the perineurium. (From Myers, R.R., Murakami, A.P., and Powell, H.C.: Reduced nerve blood flow in edematous neuropathies—A biochemical mechanism. Microvasc. Res., *32*:145, 1986.)

was fixed in phosphate-buffered glutaraldehyde and serially sectioned at 1-micron intervals. The reconstructed sections cover a distance of approximately 1.5 mm and show a venule traversing the perineurium. The segment surrounded by perineurium is reduced greatly in cross-sectional area, and stasis is seen in the epineurial segment. This can be explained by a biomechanical model studied by computer. EFP is the force that stretches the perineurium and closes vessels, even though the EFP values are less than capillary closing pressures—the pathologic valve mechanism. This occurs because of the unequal stretching of the perineurium, in the longitudinal and circumferential directions, when subjected to a distending pressure in the endoneurial compartment.

Additionally, anesthetics have a direct effect on reductions in nerve blood flow, and this effect is enhanced by epinephrine.[38,60,82] The common mechanism may involve nitric oxide.[37]

Summary: Neuropathological Processes Producing Analgesia

We have seen in the preceding discussion the sensitive relationship between neuronal structure and function and the many mechanisms by which the nerve can be injured. Because partial nerve injuries can give rise to chronic debilitating pain conditions, neurolytic techniques carry the added risk that failed procedures can be more painful than the conditions for which they were used.

Experimental knowledge of this sort, however, can provide insight into basic mechanisms of pain. Toward that end, we have performed partial freeze lesions of rat sciatic nerve and correlated behavioral measures of pain with neuropathologic evaluation of the injured nerve.[73] If all nerve fibers are injured, the nerve is anesthetic to peripheral stimuli—the intended neurolytic effect (Fig. 30-13). However, if there are surviving myelinated fibers traversing the injury site, the animal becomes allodynic and has a hyperalgesic response to peripheral stimuli proportional to the magnitude of the Wallerian degeneration-like response resulting from axonal injury (Fig. 30-14).

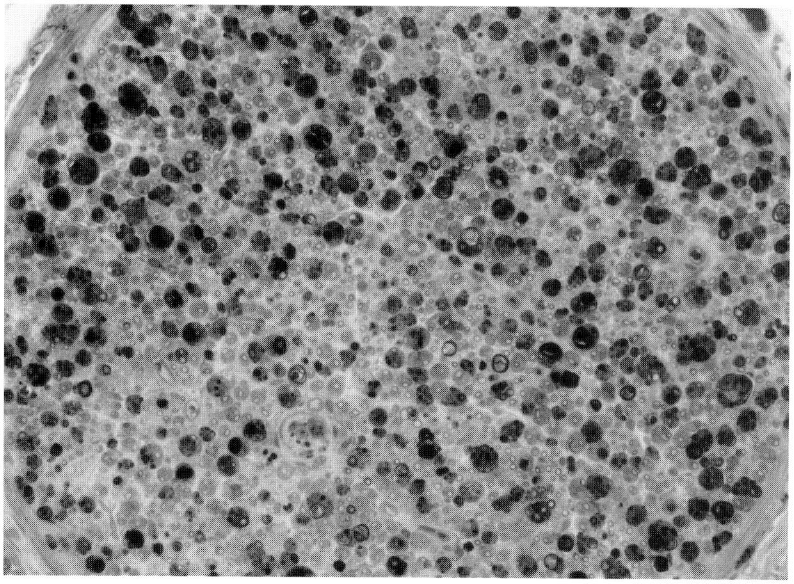

FIG. 30-13. Cryogenic nerve lesion, rat sciatic nerve. Nerve was frozen for 30 seconds, followed by a 5-second thaw, then by another 30-second freeze. This procedure injures all myelinated nerve fibers, resulting in extensive Wallerian degeneration and anesthesia to peripheral stimuli. Photomicrograph taken 14 days after lesion. Note extensive, early remyelination, evidenced by numerous small-diameter axons that are thinly myelinated. Wallerian degeneration is still ongoing, with numerous dark-staining lipid debris being taken up by macrophages.

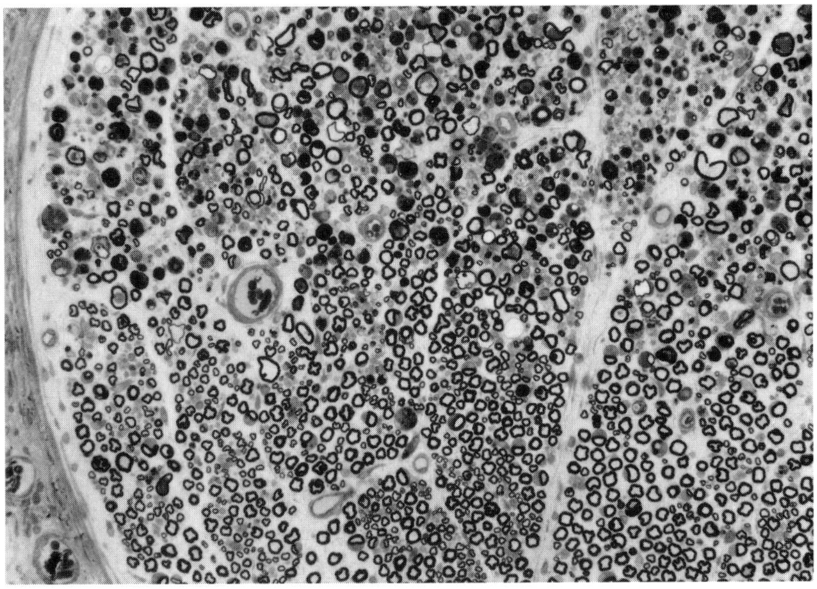

FIG. 30-14. 2-second cryogenic nerve lesion in rat sciatic nerve 3 days postinjury. Note endoneurial edema in subperineurial and perivascular spaces as an early manifestation of nerve injury. Only the upper half of fascicle is significantly injured and will undergo Wallerian degeneration. Myelin ovoids are evident throughout this area. Dark-staining axoplasm indicates accumulated organelles and impending degeneration. Animals with partial nerve injury involving Wallerian degeneration are likely to have abnormal behaviors, suggestive of neuropathic pain syndromes seen in humans.

AGENTS AND TECHNIQUES

Hypertonic and Hypotonic Solutions

Subarachnoid injection of hypertonic and hypotonic solutions produce pathologic change in nervous system tissue,[35,42,95] and have been used to treat pain.[32] The clinical impression that pain fibers are affected preferentially is not corroborated by histological evidence.[75,95] Physiologically, it has been noted that osmotic swelling of the nerve bundle is associated with a deficit in nerve conduction.[17] Fink proposed a mechanism of hypo-osmotic conduction block, based on the development of endoneurial edema in isolated peripheral nerves.[17] The presence of the perineurium was an essential factor in the conduction block, suggesting that the mechanism was a compression block caused by osmotic swelling of the fascicle, affecting nerve metabolism. Structural change to myelin and axon are not seen unless nerves are soaked for at least 1 hour in distilled water or solutions of osmolality of greater than 1,000 mmol/l. In this case, the myelin lamellae separate, and unmyelinated fibers may show total destruction. Thus, the early functional change observed clinically apparently is not caused by acute structural damage, but rather by a change in the endoneurial environment, which may later affect nerve structure and prolong the functional deficit.

Hypothermia and Freeze Lesions

Hypothermia can produce either transient or long-lasting damage to peripheral nerves, depending on the degree to which temperature is lowered. In 1945, Denny-Brown et al.[12] reported on the pathology of nerves subjected to cold, noting the sensitivity of A-delta and C sensory fibers to damage. Subsequent studies have attempted to define the pathophysiologic changes of hypothermia and to provide a theoretical rationale for its use on the spinal cord to relieve pain.[3,19,80] A physiologic effect, manifested as a prolonged axon potential, is seen in all fibers when cooled to 5°C. It is generally agreed now that unmyelinated axons are blocked at a lower temperature than myelinated axons,[14] and that conduction is blocked in all myelinated fibers at approximately the same temperature.[80] Early cytopathology showed abnormalities of Schwann cells and endoneurial capillaries. This was thought to be due to accelerated enzyme production affecting Schwann cell metabolism. The pathogenic role of edema was not considered, however, even though Schwann cells are sensitive to ischemia and are easily damaged by elevated EFP.

Although the mechanisms of injury involving cooling are complex, it is clear that freezing results in formation of ice crystals, causing necrosis of all tissue elements.[112] Freezing produces a longer-lasting clinical deficit, and has become an attractive method of neurolysis of intercostal nerves following thoracotomy; it reduces the need for narcotic analgesia.[41] In this technique, a small nerve segment is frozen, with a 2-mm diameter cryoprobe cooled to approximately −60°C, by the rapid expansion of pressurized nitrous oxide from its tip. When left in contact with the nerve for 60 seconds, a 2 to 4 mm diameter ice ball is formed that freezes the nerve and completely damages the nerve fibers.[71] Initially, this produces severe vascular injury and edema, with diapedesis of polymorphonuclear cells through vessel walls (Fig. 30-15). Endoneurial fluid pressure is elevated within 90 minutes of creation of the lesion, obtaining a level of approximately 20 cm H_2O, or twice that observed in edematous neuropathies developing more slowly. EFP is reduced, however, over the next 24 hours, presumably due to changes in the elastic characteristics of the perineurium. EFP then increases again, to reach a plateau at 6 days, that is associated with Wallerian degeneration of the distal fibers. Wallerian degeneration is the prominent pathologic feature in these nerves and affects the entire nerve. While freezing causes complete damage to

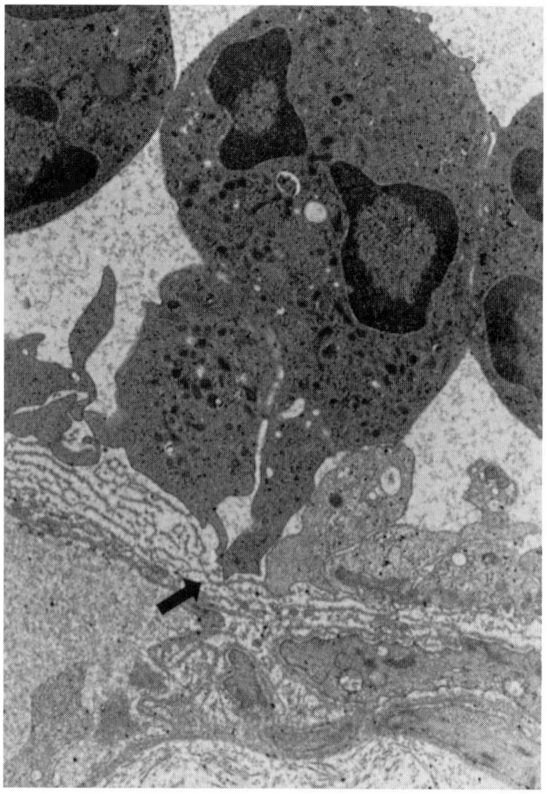

FIG. 30-15. Damage to the vasa nervorum following cryoprobe freeze lesion to peripheral nerve. Electron micrograph showing polymorphonuclear cells with filopodia adjacent to exposed endothelial cell basement membrane *(arrow)* which also appears fragmented and shows reduplication. Stained with uranyl acetate and lead citrate. (From Myers, R.R., Powell, H.C., Heckman, M.M., Costello, M.L., and Katz, J.: Biophysical and pathological effects of cryogenic nerve lesions. Ann. Neurol., *10*:478, 1981.)

nerve fibers, the basal lamina fortunately, is spared and provides a conduit for nerve fiber regeneration. Thus, freezing causes an acute, severe injury to all nerve fibers which will persist for approximately 1 month. Regeneration is aided by presence of Schwann cell basal lamina, making possible the complete and appropriate reinnervation of distal structures.

DeLeo et al. have used a modification of cryogenic nerve injury as a model of allodynia and autotomy.[11] In their model, the addition of moderate stretch injury to the nerve at the time of complete cryoneurolysis ends in pain behaviors. While the pathogenesis of these behaviors is not entirely clear, it should serve as a warning to the clinician not to manipulate the nerve too aggressively before freezing.

Hyperthermia and Laser Lesions

Heating of peripheral nerves with ultrasonic energy can produce 3 levels of nerve conduction effects: enhancement, reversible depression, and irreversible depression.[48] In Lele's study[48], nerves that were damaged irreversibly by heat, in a situation where "irreversible" implies a functional deficit lasting more than 18 hours, there was nodularity and fragmentation of axis cylinders, with the perineurium apparently being unaffected. These nerves also showed poor staining in osmium tetroxide and vacuolation of myelin sheaths. While these effects were largely dose-dependent, there was wide variability in the results that could not be completely ascribed to biological variability in the subjects. Temperatures in the vicinity of the nerve never exceeded 42°C.

A better control for heating peripheral nerve is produced with a laser, because the energy output heats the nerve directly, and does not heat the surrounding tissue, and the output of the laser is controllable, both in magnitude and duration. Thus, the severity of the lesion is influenced by the frequency, energy density, and duration of the irradiation as well as the absorption coefficients of the tissue. Laser irradiation of peripheral nerve produces localized lesions characterized histologically by a concentric zone of coagulation necrosis, surrounded by persistent nerve edema. The perineurium is not damaged and the resulting edema increases endoneurial fluid pressure.[64] In nerves irradiated for 0.5 seconds with 5 watts of energy from a carbon dioxide laser, there was considerable damage to nerve fibers and endoneurial edema that affected adjacent fascicles (Fig. 30-16). Sections of laser-injured nerves showed discrete endoneurial lesions characterized by nerve fibers undergoing Wallerian degeneration. Electron microscopy showed greatly swollen axons packed with organelles, changes characteristic of axonal dystrophy during acute Wallerian degeneration. Because laser injury produces Wallerian degeneration and can be finely controlled and focused, it could be a useful neurolytic technique, providing there is direct visual access to the nerve.

Local Anesthetic Solutions

In an animal model, pure local anesthetic solutions alter the endoneurial environment and can produce nerve fiber injury when in prolonged contact with peripheral nerves.[39] The use of modern neuropathological techniques has demonstrated that local anesthetic solutions administered to laboratory animals can cause nerve fiber injury, and that the recently reported neurotoxic effects of antioxidants and pH[22] may be in addition to the direct effect of the local anesthetic itself.[39,65] In the late 1930s and early 1940s, anesthetic-oil mixtures were used for long-term nerve blockade; it was thought that oil suppressed absorption of the anesthetic and prolonged the effect. It was subsequently shown in 1943 that benzyl alcohol, a component common to all mixtures, was the likely cause of long-term neurologic dysfunction.[16]

In 1984, it was reported that bisulfite in "Nesacaine-CE" chloroprocaine solution could produce irreversible changes in neural function, which was dose- and pH-related.[22,117] Also, in epidural block, it was postulated that large volume injection may increase cerebrospinal fluid (CSF) pressure. This may decrease spinal cord perfusion, if combined with hypotension due to a high level of blockade, or the direct

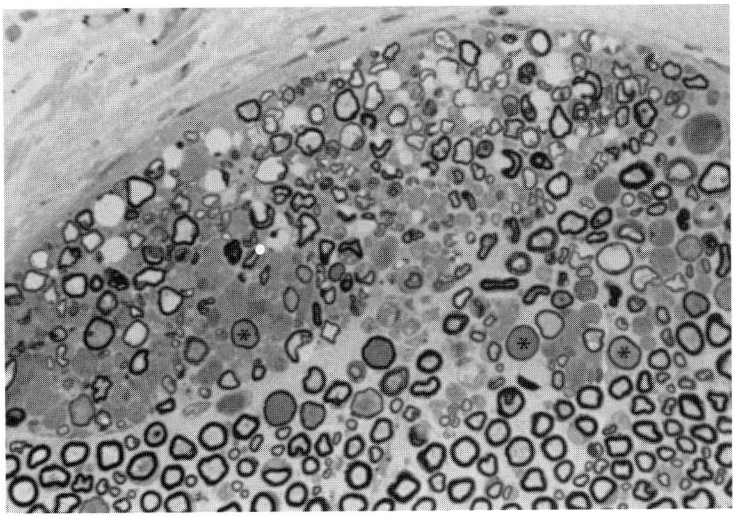

FIG. 30-16. Light micrograph of localized lesion caused by laser irradiation with a 5-watt carbon dioxide laser for 0.5 seconds. Note Wallerian degeneration in this tissue 48 hours after irradiation. There is massive swelling of affected fibers with darkly stained axoplasm and attenuated myelin sheaths (*). Stained with paraphenylene diamine. (From Myers, R.R., James, H.E., and Powell, H.C.: Laser injury of peripheral nerve: A model for focal endoneurial damage. J. Neurol. Neurosurg. Psychiatry, *48*:1265, 1985.)

effect of anesthetics on the local vasculature. This low level of spinal cord perfusion may increase susceptibility of the spinal cord to neurotoxicity.[22] In studies of neural function where pH, bisulfite content, and volume of local anesthetic solution were controlled, the local anesthetic in itself was not neurotoxic after short-term application.[22,90,117]

Other work, however, indicates that local anesthetics may cause endoneurial edema and Wallerian degeneration. It is important to assess the results of these animal studies with respect to mode of application, volume, concentration of local anesthetic, and presence of adjuvants. For example, when local anesthetics are injected intrafascicularly, there are changes in the permeability of the blood–nerve barrier associated with edema and nerve fiber injury.[24,39,40,101] It has been reported that osmotic swelling, due to application of hypo-osmotic solutions, results in a deficit of nerve conduction.[18] Injury can occur even though the solutions are not injected into the endoneurial compartment. Recent, unpublished, results indicate that the endoneurial fluid in edematous nerves, following exposure to local anesthetics, is hypotonic to normal endoneurial fluid and may affect nerve conduction. When peripheral nerves are bathed in high concentrations of local anesthetics such as 3% 2-chloroprocaine, 1% tetracaine, or 10% procaine, the permeability of the perineurium is altered and endoneurial edema is striking 48 hours later (Fig. 30-17). Increased EFP is a consequence of this treatment, as is perineurial fibrosis.[65] Electron microscopy reveals abnormal mast cells and proliferation of endoneurial fibroblasts, in addition to Schwann cell injury and axonal dystrophy. Schwann cell necrosis was characterized by cytoplasmic accumulation of myelin debris and lipid droplets (Fig. 30-18). Lipid droplets also were seen in the perineurium and in fibroblasts. At low concentration, local anesthetic induced pathology was limited to changes in nerve hydration, seen as subperineurial edema and mild structural damage to myelin and Schwann cells, that rapidly resolved. These changes are dose-dependent, and are observed with local anesthetics not containing antioxidants or preservatives.[39,40] More severe Wallerian degeneration was observed at higher concentrations and was associated with abnormal function during the period of nerve regeneration.

Single lumbar subarachnoid injection in rabbits of a low volume of pure solutions of tetracaine, bupivacaine, lidocaine, and 2-chloroprocaine, did not produce neural damage at usual clinical concentrations. Lidocaine and tetracaine could be prepared in high concentrations (16% to 32% and 4% to 8%, respectively) and these produced neurologic deficits at 48 hours that persisted until animals were killed at 5 to 7 days. This was also the case for bisulfite in concentrations of 0.4 to 0.8%, but not 0.2%. These effects were accompanied by histologic evidence of damage to spinal cord

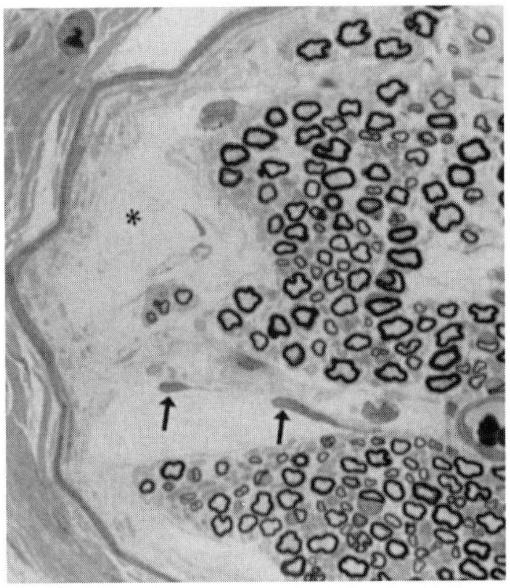

FIG. 30-17. Transverse section from rat sciatic nerve 48 hours following topical application of 2-chloroprocaine. Note extensive subperineurial edema (*) and fibroblasts *(arrows)*. Endoneurial fluid pressure was approximately 3 times the normal value. Stained with paraphenylene diamine.

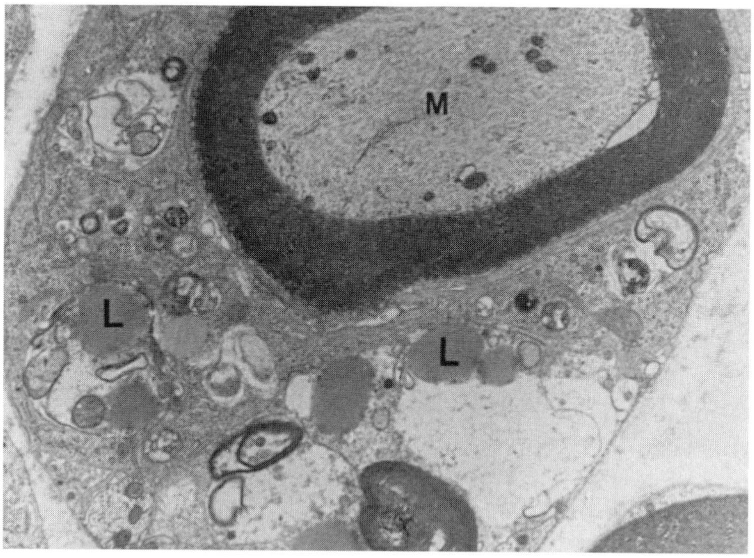

FIG. 30-18. Electron micrograph of lipid inclusions 48 hours following topical application of 2-chloroprocaine. Intact myelinated fiber *(M)* surrounded by disintegrating Schwann cell and macrophage. Note numerous lipid inclusions *(L)*. Stained with uranyl acetate and lead citrate.

and nerve roots. However, there was not a good correlation between functional loss and histologic findings.[90]

Prolonged lumbar subarachnoid infusion of local anesthetic solutions in the rat resulted in spinal cord neurotoxicity and residual paralysis, in over half the rats studied. Bupivacaine 0.5% (pH 5.6), lidocaine 1.5% (pH 5.2) and chloroprocaine (pH 3.0 plus 0.2% bisulfite) all produced intra- and perineuronal vacuolation in spinal cord grey matter. The neurotoxic effects were dose-related: 13 of 15 receiving the infusion for 24 hours, 10 of 15 of which received 6 hours, and 4 of 15 of which received 3 hours, had residual paralysis. No control animals receiving Hartman's solution were paralyzed. There was a poor correlation between neuropathology and clinical findings. It was of interest that the damage with lidocaine and chloroprocaine was more severe than it was with bupivacaine.[50] Since lidocaine and bupivacaine did not contain bisulfite, neurotoxicity with these solutions could be explained only by a neurotoxic effect of prolonged exposure to these drugs.

While local anesthetic neurotoxic injuries are rare, the problem is persistent. Several recent instances of neurotoxic injury following continuous spinal anesthesia in humans, with microbore catheter delivery of 5% lidocaine, have reinforced the hypothesis that local anesthetics are neurotoxic in high concentrations. This issue, which has led to Food and Drug Administration (FDA) withdrawal of the technique, has been reviewed recently.[58] The causes of these injuries are not entirely clear, but the consenses of investigators studying the problem is that drug delivery through intrathecal microbore catheters does not allow for adequate CSF dilution, and that concentrated depots of 5% lidocaine are neurotoxic to nerve roots in the cauda equina, where barrier systems are less substantial than in peripheral nerves.[15,45,58,96,100]

In summary, it seems that the following circumstances may pose a potential for neurotoxicity: high concentrations of local anesthetics; prolonged subarachnoid infusion of local anesthetics; perhaps high CSF pressure and low spinal cord perfusion due to hypotension in combination with local anesthetic effects; and excessive concentrations of bisulfite and low pH. Many of these factors can be guarded against: bisulfite can be kept to low concentrations or even eliminated from epinephrine-free local anesthetics; pH can be adjusted to above 5; high local anesthetic concentrations are unnecessary on peripheral nerves; large volumes should not be injected rapidly into the epidural space; and accidental subarachnoid placement can be detected clinically. The safety of long-term epidural infusion of local anesthetics remains to be examined by studies of neural function and neuropathology (Fig. 30-19). To understand local anesthetic neurotoxicity fully, it will be necessary to document further the sequence of pathologic events, because structural abnormalities are the basis for persistent functional deficit.[72]

Alcohol

Alcohol is the classic neurolytic agent and has been used extensively as such in concentrations from 50% to 95%. Due to its hypobaric nature (specific gravity = 0.80) with respect to CSF (specific gravity = 1.01), special positioning of the intended lesion site is required, and it is not recommended for use by the unskilled.[123] When alcohol is injected into the CSF, it will rise, and can diffuse quite rapidly from the injection site. After a slow injection, the highest concentration of alcohol will be at the top of the fluid space in contact with the injection site. Because of its nonselective action, it can cause serious damage to neurologic tissue remote from the injection site if proper precautions are not exercised. Ethyl alcohol acts on nervous system tissue by extraction of cholesterol, phospholipid, and cerebroside, and also causes precipitation of lipoproteins and mucoproteins.[97] Its widest application has been in central nervous system, where it has been injected into the trigeminal ganglion, subarachnoid space, and into the celiac plexus and lumbar and abdominal sympathetic chains.[20] The effective duration of intrathecal alcohol is approximately 4 months or less. A disadvantage of this technique is that often only partial relief is seen, or that relief only lasts for a short period. Histologic sections of these tissues show spotty areas of demyelination and mild, focal, inflammatory changes in the meninges.[21] With subarachnoid injection, the injury often is confined to the posterior portion of the cord and involves Lissauer's tract. Remote degeneration of the spinal cord can be seen, and is probably due to Wallerian degeneration of the distal fibers.

Alcohol applied topically to peripheral nerves produces damage to both the Schwann cell and axon. Schwann cell cytoplasm has swollen mitochondria and the myelin sheath is disrupted. Dilated vesicles can be seen in the dystrophic axons and Wallerian degeneration is a prominent feature[125] (Fig. 30-20). In vivo electrophysiologic investigation of peripheral nerves of cats revealed significant depression of compound action potentials (CAP), when tested 8 weeks after injection of alcohol close to the nerve. There was a small increase in effect on CAP as alcohol concentration increased from 50% to 100%. However, the 100% solution caused marked skin slough.[25]

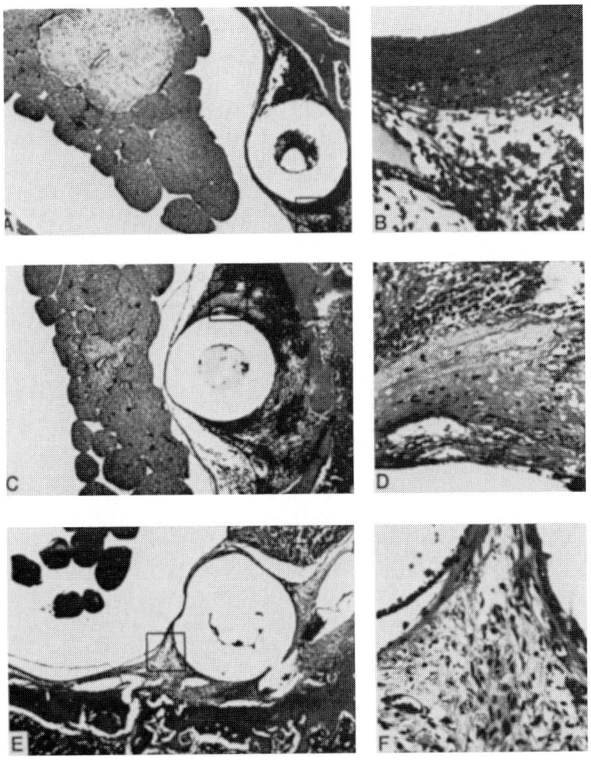

FIG. 30-19. Neuropathology of epidural catheter. Histologic sections of vertebral columns of 3 epidurally implanted rats that did not receive any drug. After 1 day of catheterization, the epidural catheter is essentially surrounded by red blood cells (**A** and **B**, *L3 section*), after 2 days by edema (**C** and **D**, *L4 section*) and after 10 days by connective tissue (**E** and **F**, *L4 section*). The areas in the black squares on **A, C,** and **E** (original magnification, ×50) are shown on **B, D,** and **F** (original magnification, ×300). Granulomas, giant cells, and fat are not present. (From Durant, P.A.C., and Yaksh, T.L.: Epidural injections of bupivacaine, morphine, fentanyl, lofentanil, and DADL in chronically implanted rats: A pharmacologic and pathologic study. Anesthesiology, *64*:43, 1986.)

Phenol

Phenol has been used extensively as a neurolytic agent.[79,124] Its primary effect is to coagulate proteins[84] and is similar to alcohol in its potency and nonselective damage to nervous system tissue. Phenol is distributed diffusely throughout the endoneurium; autoradiography of labeled phenol gives no clear indication of its localization.[84] Subarachnoid injection of 5% to 8% phenol produces a mild meningeal reaction, although larger concentrations cause extensive fibrosis and thickening of the arachnoid. The histological findings following phenol injection are similar to those for ethyl alcohol and include degeneration of fibers in the posterior columns and posterior nerve roots (Fig. 30-21). Both segmental demyelination and Wallerian degeneration are characteristic of phenol injury. The specific neurotoxic reaction is related to the concentration of phenol, with Wallerian degeneration owing to exposure to a higher concentration; Schaumburg reports that the amount of Wallerian degeneration increases in proportion to the strength and duration of phenol application.[99] Axonal pathology is apparent only with high concentrations or long exposure to phenol. This finding is similar to that of Denny-Brown and Brenner, who found that mild trauma damages the myelin sheath, while more severe injury involves the axon as well, in experiments of ischemia of peripheral nerve.[13] Another analogy can be made with nerve entrapment.[84] Mild compression causes a transient conduction block, while more severe or longer duration compression causes an irreversible block by damaging axons. Such findings contribute to the controversy about the capability of phenol to produce a differential block of nerve fibers. However, a combined electrophysiological and histological study of the effect of phenol on peripheral nerve by Schaumburg et al. concluded that phenol's neurotoxic effect is dose-related and that there is no differential effect on nerve fibers.[99] Finally, in a series of experiments reviewed by Wood,[124] it was seen that the overall destructive effect of phenol contributed to its neurolytic effect. The affinity of phenol was greater for vascular tissue than for brain neurophospholipid, suggesting that injury to blood vessels may be an important pathogenic factor contributing to the observed neuropathology. This raises a concern about the use of large amounts of phenol near major blood vessels. This is the reason some specialists prefer alcohol to phenol for celiac plexus block. Electrophysiologic and histopathologic investigation of phenol in Renografin injected close to peripheral nerves of cats in vivo revealed a highly significant, concentration-related, depression of CAP at 1 and 2 weeks after injection. Maximum effect required 12% phenol. By 8 weeks, remyelination was clearly evident and CAPs had returned to normal.[26]

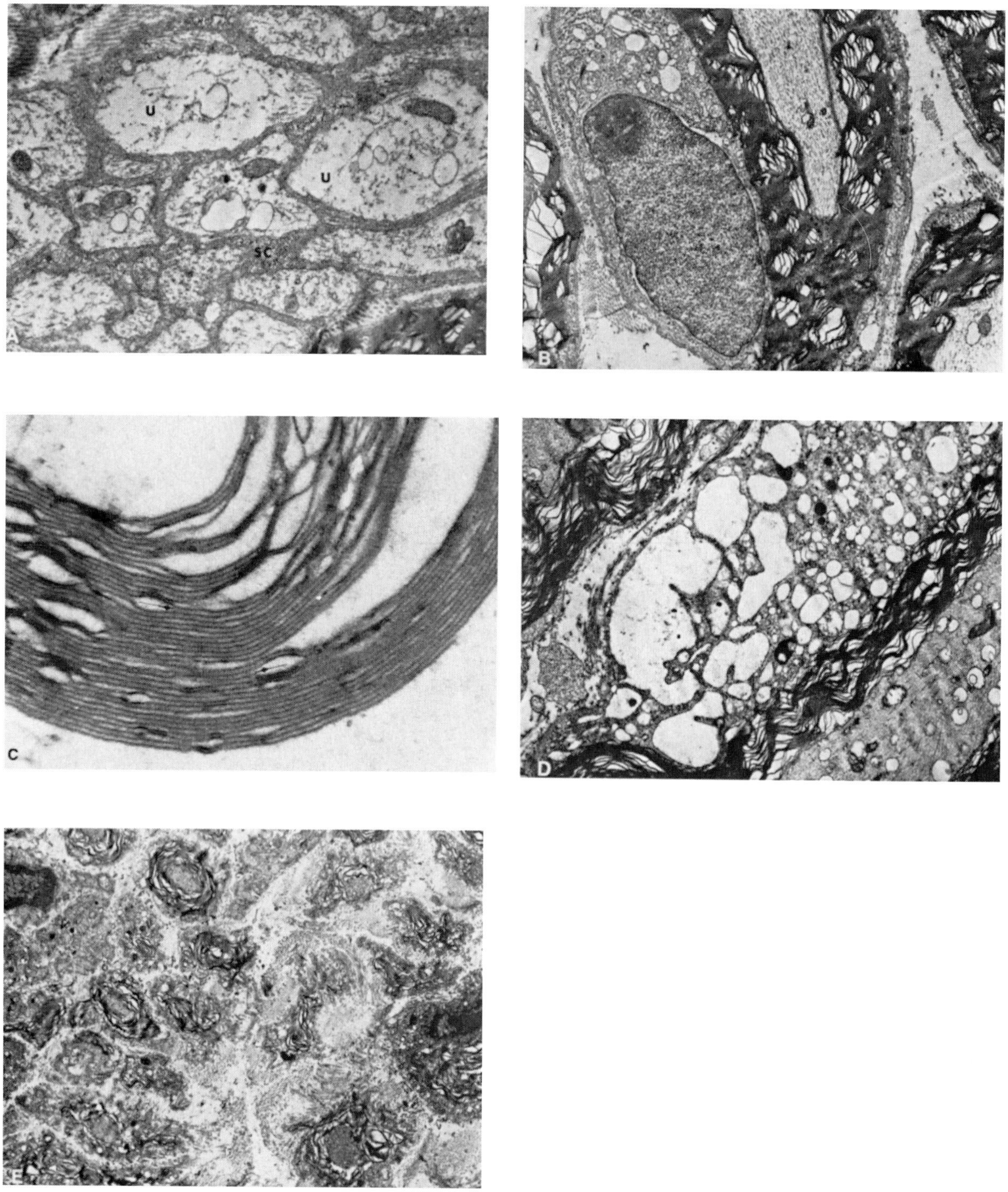

FIG. 30-20. **A:** Effect of alcohol on peripheral nerve, 15 seconds after topical application of 100% alcohol. This electron micrograph shows the sciatic nerve of a mouse after alcohol application. The arrows denote swelling of unmyelinated nerve fibers *(U)*; S denotes Schwann cell cytoplasm that is clumped and granular—Schwann cell destruction (×5,000). **B:** This electron micrograph shows the Schwann cell after alcohol exposure. Note splitting of myelin sheath *(MS)* and dilated endoplasmic reticulum *(ER)*, indicating acute injury to Schwann cell and myelin sheath (×4,300). **C:** Effect of alcohol on peripheral nerve, 1 minute after application. This electron micrograph shows splitting of myelin sheath after exposure to topical 100% alcohol (×9,600). **D:** Effect of alcohol on peripheral nerve, 24 hours after a 15-second exposure to 100% alcohol. Note degenerating axons *(A)*, splitting myelin lamellae *(M)*, and beginning of connective tissue reaction (×2,200). **E:** Effect of alcohol on peripheral nerve, 4 hours after a 15-second exposure. This electron micrograph shows vacuolization in Schwann cell after 100% alcohol exposure. (From Woolsey, R.M., Taylor, J.J., and Nagel, J.H.: Acute effects of topical ethyl alcohol on the sciatic nerve of the mouse. Arch. Phys. Med. Rehabil., *53*:410, 1972.)

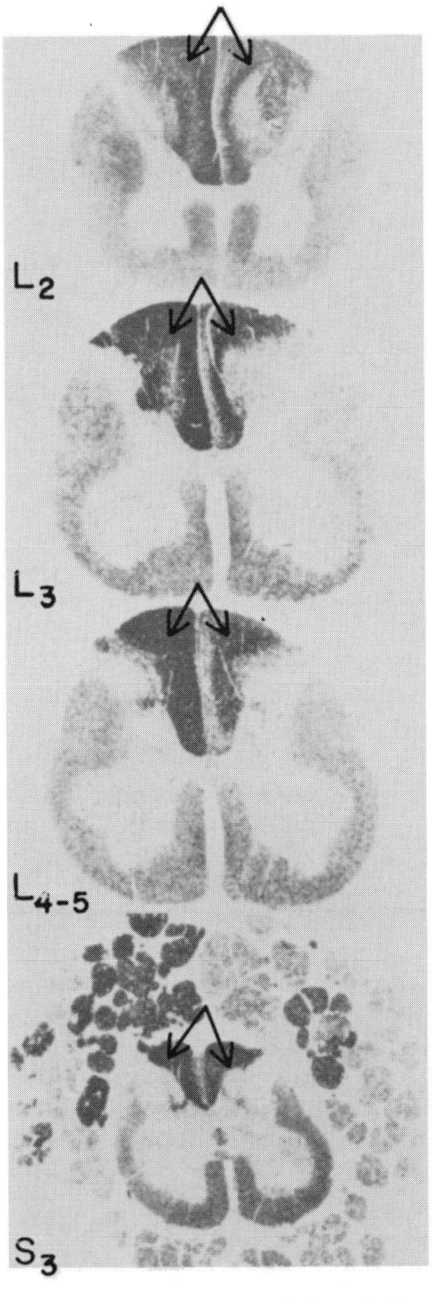

FIG. 30-21. Effect of phenol on spinal cord. These micrographs show transverse sections through a patient's spinal cord. Note posterior column degeneration *(arrows)*, following subarachnoid injection of phenol. These sections were taken at the levels of spinal cord indicated adjacent to the section. Injection was made at bony spine level L3-4. (From Smith, M.C.: Histological findings following intrathecal injections of phenol solutions for relief of pain. Br. J. Anaesth., *36*:387, 1964.)

Glycerol

The neurolytic effect of glycerol was discovered accidentally[30] and rapidly led to use of the agent in the treatment of facial pain.[55,98,109] The technique of percutaneous retrogasserian glycerol rhizotomy for the treatment of tic douloureux is reported to be far superior to radiofrequency rhizotomy,[24] since no permanent injury to surrounding structures occurs, and there is preservation of facial sensation in most patients.[55] The histological study of experimental material shows that intraneural injection of glycerol is more damaging than topical application, although significant, localized, subperineurial damage is seen following topical application of a 50% glycerol solution.[92] The histologic changes include the presence of numerous inflammatory cells, extensive myelin swelling and axonolysis. Myelin disintegration occurs weeks after the injury, along with ongoing axonolysis during periods of myelin restitution,[92] indicating an ongoing nerve fiber injury, possibly caused by secondary events such as compression of transperineurial vessels and ischemia. Electron microscopy shows evidence of Wallerian degeneration; with intraneurial injection, essentially all nerve fibers are destroyed. Lipid droplets are seen in Schwann cells and phagocytic cells (Fig. 30-22) and there is mast cell degranulation. The molecular basis of the toxic effects is unknown, but Rengachary suggests that it might be similar to that of ethanol, because both compounds are structurally related.[92] In spite of evidence for the differential effect of glycerol on the electrophysiologic function of peripheral nerves,[9] histologic data are lacking.

Ammonium Salts

The first reported use of salts for long-term relief of pain was in 1935, when Judovich used pitcher plant distillate (Sarracenia purpnea) for certain forms of neuralgia. It was later reported that the ammonium ion in the form of ammonium chloride or ammonium hydroxide, (depending on the pH of the distillate), was the active 25 component.

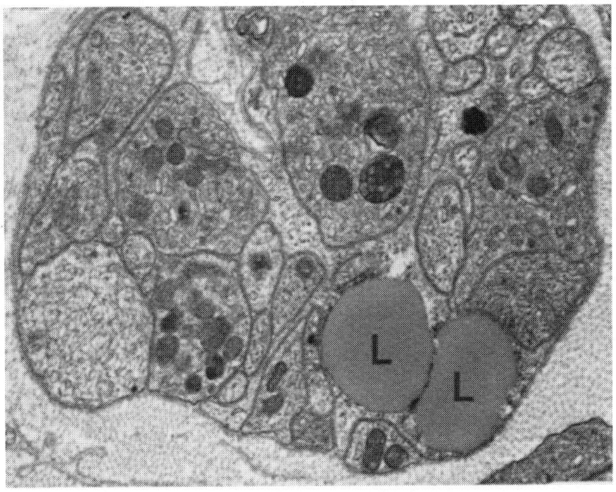

FIG. 30-22. Electron micrograph of glycerol-treated nerves. Lipid droplets *(L)* are seen in the cytoplasm of a Schwann cell in an unmyelinated nerve fiber. Increased numbers of organelles are present in some axons. They include mitochondria and electron-dense, membrane-enveloped structures resembling lysosomes and vesicular inclusions. These changes are consistent with axonal degeneration. Stained with uranyl acetate and lead citrate.

In 1942, a report on the use of ammonium salts for nerve pain stated the following:[2]

> "... In no instance has there been any motor weakness, following injection of peripheral nerves, nor loss of touch, pressure, pinprick, and temperature sensibility. In some instances, 1 infiltration of the distillate is sufficient to provide permanent relief of pain, even in cases of long duration ..."
>
> "... In man, perineural infiltration of 0.5 to 1% solutions of ammonium chloride produces the same effects as does the filtration of pitcher plant extract. The immediate effect of the injection is an increased intensity of the pain, which then subsides during the first 30 minutes after injection. The neuralgic pain is relieved, the zone of hyperesthesia contracts and disappears, and when injected around the sciatic nerve, there results no weakness and the sensations of touch, pressure, pinprick, and temperature on the outer aspect of the leg, are unimpaired ..."

The action of ammonium salts on nerve impulses produces obliteration of C fiber potentials with only a small effect on A fibers. Subsequent clinical information has shown that with concentrations of 10% of ammonium salts, motor function can be retained despite good analgesia. Limited pathologic studies suggest that injection of ammonium salts around a peripheral nerve causes an acute degenerative neuropathy, affecting all fibers.

Experimental Agents

The continuing study of basic neuropathologic mechanisms of nerve injury holds promise that new and more effective agents and techniques will be developed to manage chronic pain clinically. The ideal agent would be given peripherally and would target the afflicted sensory system selectively, without risk of systemic toxic injury.

When capsaicin was described in 1981 as a sensory neurotoxin, clinicians hoped that it would be an agent with these properties.[34] Indeed, given to neonatal animals, this component of hot peppers causes degeneration of mitochondria in DRG primary sensory neurons. The result is rapid degeneration of the neurons, with accumulation of neurofilaments and secondary fissures of the cytoplasm, and cell fragmentation.[33] The primary target is small diameter DRG neurons, although larger A-type neurons may also be injured. Unfortunately, capsaicin is not as effective in adult animals.

Ricin is another agent with selective neurotoxic effects.[31] Ricinus communis agglutins (RCA 60 and RCA 120) are highly toxic lectins from caster beans that have been used to produce experimental sensory ganglionectomy.[128] Given directly into peripheral nerves, they result in DRG degeneration by way of "suicide transport."[122] Within 24 hours, there is evidence of chromatolysis, with disintegration of the endoplasmic reticulum and dispersion of free ribosomes.[128] Mitochondria are affected, and Wallerian degeneration of the fiber ensues. The exploitation of ricin and other toxic lectins may be limited by several problems, including hepatocellular necrosis, and degeneration of motor neurons.

Conclusions

Neurotoxic agents can produce neurolysis of nerve fibers, depending on the concentration of agent in direct contact with the tissue. Agents applied topically can alter perineurial permeability to gain access to nerve fibers, but their effects may be diluted. Intraneural injection of neurotoxic agents produces the most severe damage, almost always resulting in significant axonal pathology and Wallerian degeneration. Techniques that physically damage the nerve with heat or cold produce similar results. There appears to be no differential effect of these agents or techniques on electrophysiologic function; rather, variations in concentration produce different clinical findings, suggesting a dose-related response. When nerve fibers are damaged, Wallerian degeneration is often the major finding, and accounts for the desirable, long-lasting, clinical effect; but it is important that all nerve fibers be injured, because the presence of patent fibers traversing the lesion site may give rise to pain syndromes. The persistence of the basal lamina around the Schwann cell tube (the bands of Bungner) permit the successful and appropriate regeneration of nerve fibers, eliminating the formation of painful neuromas, and justifying the use of neurolytic agents over surgical interruption of nerve fibers in the treatment of chronic pain.

Changes in the endoneurial environment are thought to affect electrophysiologic function by altering the electrolyte concentration of endoneurial fluid. Local anesthetic-induced edema reduces endoneurial electrolyte concentration and increases endoneurial fluid pressure, which may lead to ischemia by compressing transperineurial blood vessels. These subtle pathogenic factors may exacerbate the principal neuropathological effect of neurolytic agents which is Wallerian degeneration.

Lastly, continued laboratory work should identify agents that are selectively neurotoxic and that can be used clinically with improved success and reduced risk.

NEW HORIZONS IN THE NEUROPATHOLOGY OF PAINFUL NERVE INJURIES

The relationship between nerve injury and pain has been a major theme of this chapter, with the point taken that incomplete nerve injuries can set the stage for the development of a chronic neuropathic pain state. This brief supplement to the chapter focuses on the role of cytokines produced by Schwann cells, macrophages, and other endoneurial cells in causing nerve injury and pain. Based on electron microscopy studies of nerve fibers, we have argued that edema, Schwann cell abnormalities, demyelination, and axonal injury, are progressive parts of a continuous neuropathologic spectrum that reflects the initiation of the neuropathic pain state.[74,105] We now suggest that both the abnormal structure and function of nerve can be linked to cytokine actions. Thus, it may be useful, for purposes of further research, to speculate that cytokines represent a generic link between pathology and pain.

It has been shown that there are changes in plasma cytokines associated with peripheral nerve injury,[121] and these circulating factors may influence neuronal function directly.[120] It is more likely, however, that there may be a more targeted effect, mediated by retrograde axonal transport of higher concentrations of cytokines from the nerve injury site, or by retrograde transport of other factors stimulated by local cytokine release.[59] In this regard, it is known that tumor necrosis factor (TNF)-α and IL-1 stimulate Schwann cells to express nerve growth factor (NG-F) on their surfaces, and that regrograde transport of NG-F and its receptor from the injury site is an important signal affecting the function of dorsal root ganglia neurons.[36] Some authors have suggested that NG-F or an octapeptide of NG-F is painful when injected peripherally, but it is not clear by what mechanism this may be mediated.[49,111] However, recent work by the Koltzenburg group[111] suggests that recruitment of nociceptive units, rather than sensitization of fibers, could account for the observed hyperalgesia following the NG-F administered in their experiments.

Recent investigations have identified cytokines directly as neuroactive substances[127] that may be involved in the pathogenesis of pain. Cytokines are soluble peptide mediators, classically identified by their production in immune cells such as macrophages, and for their role in inflammation. Our attention initially was drawn to the possible involvement of cytokines in neuropathic pain by the observation that nerve injury produces substantial inflammation.[74] Macrophages are present in large numbers in the injured endoneurium[4,106] and the percentage of macrophages was correlated directly with the expression of neuropathic behavior.[63]

We hypothesized that macrophages and other cells contributed to neuropathic behaviors through the secretion of cytokines in the injured endoneurium, which then chemically altered the activity of sensory fibers and resulted in a behavioral pain response.

One well-understood pro-inflammatory cytokine produced and secreted by activated macrophages is TNF-α. TNF-α is a small (17kD) pluripotent peptide best known as the primary mediator of septic shock resulting from endotoxin,[6] although TNF-α also is responsible in part for the neurotoxic damage found in Guillain-Barré syndrome,[103] experimental allergic encephalitis,[93] multiple sclerosis,[94] and rheumatoid arthritis.[7] In particular, TNF-α production is concurrent with ischemia-produced neuronal pathology,[51] and this may be mediated in part by tissue macrophages.[1] Thus, increased TNF-α levels are common to painful experimental and clinical neuropathies, and may mediate "illness-induced hyperalgesia.[120] Further support for TNF-α in painful peripheral neuropathies stems from the observation that the proinflammatory actions of TNF-α are strikingly consistent with the endoneurial pathology that follows nerve injury. TNF disrupts endothelial adhesion and facilitates edema,[5] causes glial cell damage and demyelination[89,91,102] and induces macrophages to release other inflammatory cytokines[119] also associated with the pathological process of nerve fiber degeneration. Taken together, these considerations support an active role for TNF in the ultimate expression of pain behaviors, perhaps mediated through neurotoxic actions involving edema and the resulting ischemia, and glial pathology. Recent studies in our laboratory have demonstrated Schwann cell production of TNF-α following peripheral nerve injury,[115] and the development of hyperalgesia and nerve fiber injury following injection of TNF-α in normal nerves.[116] Lastly, spontaneous firing has been observed in isolated afferent pain fibers following topical application of TNF-α.[107] This effect may be important in establishing the continuing, low-level, peripheral electrophysiologic activity associated with chronic hyperalgesic states.

The importance of this work with respect to neurolytic techniques lies in its insight into the molecular mechanisms by which nerve function is interrupted and the parallel understanding and development of new therapies to control pain.

ACKNOWLEDGMENTS

The authors thank Drs. Henry C. Powell and Tony L. Yaksh for their collaboration in some of these studies.

REFERENCES

1. Albina, J.E., Henry, W.L., Mastrofrancesco, B., Martin, B.A., and Reichner, J.S.: Macrophage activation by culture in an anoxic environment. J. Immunol., *155:*4391, 1995.
2. Bates, W. and Judovich, B.D.: Intractable pain. Anesthesiology, *3:*663, 1942.
3. Basbaum, C.B.: Electrophysiological observations. J. Neurocytol., *2:*171, 1973.
4. Beuche, W., and Friede, R.L.: The role of nonresident cells in Wallerian degeneration. J. Neurocytol., *13:*767, 1984.
5. Beutler, B., and Cerami, A.: The biology of cachectin/TNF—A primary mediator of the host response. Ann. Rev. Immunol., *7:*625, 1898.
6. Beutler, B., Milsark, I.W., and Cerami, A.C.: Passive immunization against cachectin/tumor necrosis factor protects mice from lethal effect of endotoxin. Science, *229:*869, 1985.
7. Brennan, F.M., Cope, A.P., Katsikis, P., *et al.*: Selective immunosuppression of tumour necrosis factor-alpha in rheumatoid arthritis. Chem. Immunol., *60:*48, 1995.
8. Brimijoin, S.: The role of axonal transport in nerve disease. *In* Dyck, P.J., Thomas, P.K., Lambert, E.H., and Bunge, R. (eds.): Peripheral Neuropathy. pp. 477. W.B. Saunders, Philadelphia, 1984.
9. Burchiel, K.J., and Russell, L.C.: Glycerol neurolysis: Neurophysiologic effects of topical glycerol application on rat saphenous nerve. J. Neurosurg., *63:*784, 1985.
10. Chiu, S.Y., and Richie, J.M.: Potassium channels in nodal and internodal axonal membrane of mammalian myelinated fibers. Nature, *284:*170, 1980.
11. DeLeo, J.A., Coombs, D.W., Willenbring, S., *et al.*: Characterization of a neuropathic pain model: Sciatic cryoneurolysis in the rat. Pain, *56:*9, 1994.
12. Denny-Brown, D., Adams, R., Brenner, C., and Doherty, M.M.: The pathology of injury to nerve induced by cold. J. Neuropathol. Exp. Neurol., *4:*305, 1945.
13. Denny-Brown, D., and Brenner, C.: The effect of percussion of nerve. J. Neurol. Neurosurg. Psychiatry., *7:*76, 1944.
14. Douglas, W.W., and Malcolm, J.L.: Effect of localized cooling on conduction in cat nerves. J. Physiol. (Lond.), *130:*63, 1955.

15. Drasner, K.: Models for local anesthetic toxicity from continuous spinal anesthesia. Reg. Anesth., *18:*434, 1993.
16. Duncan, D., and Jarvis, W.H.: A comparison of the actions on nerve fibers of certain anesthetic mixtures and substances in oil. Anesthesiology, *4:*465, 1943.
17. Fink, B.R.: Mechanism of hypo-osmotic conduction block. Reg. Anesth., *5:*7, 1980.
18. Fink, B.R., Barsa, J., and Calkins, D.F.: Osmotic swelling effects on neural conduction. Anesthesiology, *51:*418, 1979.
19. Franz, D.N., and Iggo, A.: Conduction failure in myelinated and non-myelinated axons at low temperatures. J. Physiol., *199:*319, 1968.
20. Fujita, Y.: CT-guided neurolytic splanchnic nerve block with alcohol. Pain *55:*363, 1993.
21. Gallager, H.S., Yonezawa, T., Hay, R.C., and Derrick, W.S.: Subarachnoid alcohol block II: Histologic changes in the central nervous system. Am. J. Pathol., *35:*679, 1961.
22. Gissen, A.J., Datta, S., and Lambert, D.: The chloroprocaine controversy. Reg. Anesth., *9:*124, 1984.
23. Deleted in proof.
24. Gentilli, F., Hudson, A.R., Hunter, D., and Kline, D.G.: Nerve injection injury with local anesthetic agents: A light and electron microscopic, fluorescent microscopic, and horseradish peroxidase study. Neurosurgery, *6:*263, 1980.
25. Gregg, R.V., Costantini, C.H., Ford, D.J., and Raj, P.P.: Electrophysiologic investigation of alcohol as a neurolytic agent. Anesthesiology, *63:*A250, 1985.
26. Gregg, R.V., Costantini, C.H., Ford, D.J., and Raj, P.P.: Electrophysiologic and histopathologic investigation of phenol in Renographin as a neurolytic agent. Anesthesiology, *63:*A239, 1985.
27. Griffin, J.W., George, R., and Ho, T.: Macrophage systems in peripheral nerves: A review. J. Neuropath. Exp. Neurol., *52:*553, 1993.
28. Haak, R.A., Kleinhauns, F.W., and Ochs, S.: The viscosity of mammalian nerve axoplasm measured by electron spin resonance. J. Physiol. (Lond.), *263:*115, 1976.
29. Haftek, J.: Stretch injury of peripheral nerve. Acute effects of stretching on rabbit peripheral nerve. J Bone Joint Surg. (Br.), *52B:*354, 1970.
30. Hakanson, S.: Trigeminal neuralgia treated by the injection of glycerol into the trigeminal cistern. Neurosurgery, *9:*638, 1981.
31. Harper, C.G., Gonatas, J.O., Mizutani, T., *et al.*: Retrograde transport and effects of toxic ricin in the autonomic nervous system. Lab. Invest., *42:*396, 1980.
32. Hitchcock, E.: Osmolytic neurolysis for intractable facial pain. Lancet, *1:*434, 1969.
33. Hiura, A., and Ishizuka, H.: Changes in features of degenerating primary sensory neurons with time after capsaicin treatment. Acta Neuropathol., *78:*35, 1989.
34. Jancsó, G., and Király, E.: Sensory neurotoxins: Chemically induced selective destruction of primary sensory neurons. Brain Res., *210:*83, 1981.
35. Jewett, D.L., and King, J.S.: Conduction block of monkey dorsal rootlets by water and hypertonic saline solutions. Exp. Neurol., *33:*225, 1971.
36. Johanson, S.O., Crouch, M.F., and Hendry, I.A.: Retrograde axonal transport of signal transduction proteins in rat sciatic nerve. Brain Res., *690:*55, 1995.
37. Johns, R.A.: Local anesthetics inhibit endothelium-dependent vasodilation. Anesthesiology, *70:*805, 1989.
38. Kalichman, M.W., and Lalonde, A.W.: Experimental nerve ischemia and injury produced by cocaine and procaine. Brain Res., *565:*34, 1991.
39. Kalichman, M.W., Powell, H.C., Reisner, L.S., and Myers, R.R.: The role of 2-chloroprocaine and sodium bisulfite in rat sciatic nerve edema. J. Neuropath. Exp. Neurol., *45:*566, 1986.
40. Kalichman, M.W., Powell, H.C., and Myers, R.R.: Quantitative histologic analysis of local anesthetic-induced injury to rat sciatic nerve. J. Pharmacol. Exp. Ther., *250:*406, 1989.
41. Katz, J., Nelson, W., Forest, R., and Bruce, D.L.: Cryoanalgesia for post-thoracotomy pain. Lancet, *1:*512, 1980.
42. King, J.S., Jewett, D.L., Phil, D., and Sundberg, H.R.: Differential blockade of cat dorsal root C fibers by various chloride solutions. J. Neurosurg., *36:*569, 1972.
43. Kristensson, K., Lycke, E., and Sjöstrand J. Spread of herpes simplex virus in peripheral nerves. Acta Neuropathol. (Berl.), *19:*44, 1971.
44. Krnjevic, K.: The distribution of Na and K in cat nerves. J. Physiol. (Lond.), *128:*473, 1955.
45. Lambert, D.H., and Hurley, R.F.: Cauda equina syndrome and continuous spinal anesthesia. Anesth. Analg., *72:*817, 1991.
46. Lamer, T.J.: Treatment of cancer-related pain: When orally administered medications fail. Mayo Clin. Proc., *69:*473, 1994.
47. Lampert, P.W.: A comparative electron microscopic study of reactive, degenerating, regenerating, and dystrophic axons. J. Neuropathol. Exp. Neurol., *26:*345, 1967.
48. Lele, P.P.: Effects of focused ultrasound radiation on peripheral nerves, with observations on local heating. Exp. Neurol., *8:*47, 1963.
49. Lewin, G.R., Ritter, A.M., and Mendell, L.M.: Nerve growth factor-induced hyperalgesia in the neonatal and adult rat. J. Neurosci., *13:*2136, 1993.
50. Li, D.F., Bahar, M., Cole, G., and Rosen, M.: Neurological toxicity of the subarachnoid infusion of bupivacaine, lignocaine, or 2-chloroprocaine in the rat. Br. J. Anaesth., *57:*424, 1985.
51. Liu, T., Clark, R.K., McDonnell, P.C., *et al.*: Tumor necrosis factor-alpha expression in ischemic neurons. Stroke., *25:*1481, 1993.
52. Low, P.A.: Endoneurial fluid pressure and microenvironment of nerve. *In* Dyck, P.J., Thomas, P.K., Lambert, E.H., and Bunge. R., (eds.): Peripheral Neuropathy. pp. 599. W.B. Saunders, 1984.
53. Lundborg, G.: Structure and function of intraneural microvessels as related to trauma, edema formation, and nerve function. J. Bone Joint Surg., *57A:*938, 1975.
54. Lundborg, G., and Branemark, P.-L.: Microvascular structure and function of peripheral nerves: Vital microscopic studies of the tibial nerve in the rabbit. Adv. Microcirc., *1:*66, 1968.
55. Lunsford, L.D., and Bennett, M.H.: Percutaneous retrogasserian glycerol rhizotomy for tic douloreux: Part 1, Technique and results in 112 patients. Neurosurgery, *14:*424, 1984.
56. Millisi, H., Rath, T.H., Reihsner, R, and Zoch, G.: Microsurgical neurolysis: Its anatomical and physiological basis and its classification. Microsurgery, *14:*430, 1993.
57. Mizisin, A.P., Myers, R.R., and Powell, H.C.: Endoneurial sodium accumulation in galactosemic rat nerves. Muscle Nerve, *9:*440, 1986.
58. Möllmann, M., Holst, D., Lübbesmeyer, H., and Lawin, P.: Continuous spinal anesthesia: Mechanical and technical problems of catheter placement. Reg. Anesth. *18:*469, 1993.
59. Myers, R.R.: The pathogenesis of neuropathic pain—The 1994 ASRA lecture. Reg. Anesth., *20:*173, 1995.
60. Myers, R.R., and Heckman, H.M.: Effects of local anesthesia on nerve blood flow: Studies using lidocaine with and without epinephrine. Anesthesiology, *71:*757, 1989.
61. Myers, R.R., Heckman, H.M., Galbraith, J.A., and Powell, H.C.: Subperineurial demyelination associated with reduced nerve blood flow and oxygen tension after epineurial vascular stripping. Lab. Invest., *65:*41, 1991.
62. Myers, R.R., Heckman, H.M., and Powell, H.C.: Endoneurial fluid is hypertonic: Results of microanalysis and significance in neuropathy. J. Neuropathol. Exp. Neurol., *42:*217, 1983.
63. Myers, R.R., Heckman, H.M., and Rodriguez, M.: Reduced hyperalgesia in nerve injured WLD mice: Relationship to nerve fiber phagocytosis, axonal degeneration, and regeneration in normal mice. Exp. Neurol., *141:*94, 1996.
64. Myers, R.R., James, H.E., and Powell, H.C.: Laser injury of peripheral nerve: A model for focal endoneurial damage. J. Neurol. Neurosurg. Psychiatry, *48:*1265, 1985.
65. Myers, R.R., Kalichman, M.W., Reisner, L.S., and Powell, H.C.: Neurotoxicity of local anesthesia: Altered perineurial permeability, edema, and nerve fiber injury. Anesthesiology, *64:*29, 1986.
66. Myers, R.R., Mizisin, A.P., Powell, H.C., and Lampert, P.W.: Reduced nerve blood flow in hexachlorophene neuropathy. J Neuropathol. Exp. Neurol., *41:*391, 1982.
67. Myers, R.R., Murakami, H., and Powell, H.C.: Reduced nerve blood flow in edematous neuropathies—A biomechanical mechanism. Microvasc. Res., *32:*145, 1986.
68. Myers, R.R., and Powell, H.C.: Endoneurial fluid pressure in peripheral neuropathies. *In* Hargens, A. (ed.): Interstitial Fluid Pressure and Composition. pp. 193. Williams and Wilkins, Baltimore, 1981.
69. Myers, R.R., and Powell, H.C.: Galactose neuropathy: Impact of chronic endoneurial edema on nerve blood flow. Ann Neurol., *16:*587, 1984.
70. Myers, R.R., Powell, H.C., Costello, M.L., Lampert, P.W., and Zweifach, B.W.: Endoneurial fluid pressure: Direct measurement with micropipettes. Brain Res., *148:*510, 1978.
71. Myers, R.R., Powell, H.C., Heckman, H.M., Costello, M.L., and Katz,

J.: Biophysical and pathological effects of cryogenic nerve lesions. Ann. Neurol., *10:*478, 1981.

72. Myers, R.R., and Sommer, C.: Methodology for spinal neurotoxicity studies. Reg. Anesth. *18:*439, 1993.
73. Myers, R.R., and Sommers, C.: Focal freeze injury of peripheral nerves: A reproducible model of neuropathic pain. Soc. Neurosci. (Abstr.)*20:*125, 1994.
74. Myers, R.R., Yamamoto T., Yaksh T.L., and Powell H.C.: The role of focal nerve ischemia and Wallerian degeneration in peripheral nerve injury producing hyperesthesia. Anesthesiology, *78:*308, 1993.
75. Nicholson, M.F., and Roberts, F.W.: Relief of pain by intrathecal injection of hypothermic saline. Med. J. Aust., *1:*61, 1968.
76. Ochs, S.: Basic properties of axoplasmic transport. *In* Dyck, P.J., Thomas, P.K., Lambert, E.H., and Bunge, R., (eds.): Peripheral Neuropathy. pp. 453. W.B. Saunders, Philadelphia, 1984. (180 refs.)
77. Olsson, Y., and Kristensson, K.: Recent applications of tracer techniques to neuropathology, with particular reference to vascular permeability and axonal flow. *In* Smith, W.T., and Cavanagh, J.B., (eds.): Recent Advances in Neuropathology. pp. 1. Edinburgh, Churchill-Livingstone, 1979.
78. Paravicini, U., Stoeckel, K., and Thoenen, H.: Biological importance of retrograde axonal transport of nerve growth factors in adrenergic neurons. Brain Res. *84:*279, 1975.
79. Parkhouse, H.F., Gilpin, S.A., Gosling, J.A., and Turner-Warwick, R.T.,: Quantitative study of phenol as a neurolytic agent in the urinary bladder. Br. J. Urol. *60:*410, 1987.
80. Paintal, A.S.: Block of conduction in mammalian myelinated nerve fibers by low temperatures. J. Physiol., *180:*1, 1965.
81. Parry, G.J., and Brown, M.J.: Arachidonate-induced experimental nerve infarction. J. Neurol. Sci., *50:*123, 1981.
82. Partridge, B.L.: The effects of local anesthetics and epinephrine on rat nerve blood flow. Anesthesiology, *75:*243, 1991.
83. Perry, V.H., Brown, M.C., Lunn, E.R., Tree, P., and Gordon, S.: Evidence that very slow Wallerian degeneration in C57BL/Ola mice is an intrinsic property of the peripheral nerve. Eur. J. Neurosci. *2:*802, 1990.
84. Politis, M.J., Schaumburg, H.H., and Spencer, P.S.: Neurotoxicity of selected chemicals. *In* P.S., Spencer, and Schaumburg, H.H. (eds.): Experimental and Chemical Neurotoxicity. pp. 613. Williams and Wilkins, Baltimore, 1980.
85. Powell, H.C., and Myers, R.R.: Pathology of the peripheral myelinated axon. *In* Adachi, M. (Ed.): Current Trends in the Neurosciences. Vol. 3. pp. 96. Igaku-Shoin, New York, 1985.
86. Powell, H.C., Myers, R.R., Costello, M.L., and Lampert, P.W.: Endoneurial fluid pressure in Wallerian degeneration. Ann. Neurol., *5:*550, 1979.
87. Powell, H.C., Myers, R.R., and Lampert, P.W.: Changes in Schwann cells and vessels in lead neuropathy. Am. J. Pathol., *109:*193, 1982.
88. Price, D.L., Griffin J., Young A., Peck K., and Stocks, A.: Tetanus toxin: Direct evidence for retrograde intraaxonal transport. Science. *88:*945, 1975.
89. Probert, L., Akassoglou, K., Pasparakis, M., Kontogeorgos, G., and Kollias, G.: Spontaneous inflammatory demyelinating disease in transgenic mice showing central nervous system-specific expression of tumor necrosis factor alpha. Proc. Natl. Acad. Sci. USA *92:*11294, 1995.
90. Ready, B.L., Plumer, M.H., Haschke, R.H., Austin, E., and Sumi, M.: Neurotoxicity of intrathecal local anesthetics in rabbits. Anesthesiology, *63:*364, 1985.
91. Redford, E.J., Hall, S.M., and Smith, K.J.: Vascular changes and demyelination induced by the intraneural injection of tumour necrosis factor. Brain, *118:*869, 1995.
92. Rengachary, S.S., Watanabe, I.S., Singer, P., and Bopp, W.J.: Effect of glycerol on peripheral nerve: An experimental study. Neurosurgery, *13:*681, 1983.
93. Renno, T., Krakowski, M., Piccirillo, C., Lin, J-Y., and Owens, T.: TNF expression by resident microglia and infiltrating leukocytes in the central nervous system of mice with experimental allergic encephalomyelitis. J. Immunol., *154:*944, 1995.
94. Rentzos, M., Nikolaou, C., Rombos, A., *et al.*: Tumour necrosis factor alpha is elevated in serum and cerebrospinal fluid in multiple sclerosis and inflammatory neuropathies. J. Neurol., *243:*165, 1996.
95. Robertson, J.D.: Structural alterations in nerve fibers produced by hypotonic and hypertonic solutions. J. Biophysic. Biochem. Cytol., *4:*349, 1958.
96. Ross, B.K., Coda, B., and Health, C.H.: Local anesthetic distribution in a spinal model: A possible mechanism of neurologic injury after continuous spinal anesthesia. Reg. Anesth., *17:*69–77, 1992.
97. Rumbsy, M.G., and Finean, J.B.: The action of organic solvents on the myelin sheath of peripheral nerve tissue—II (short-chain aliphatic alcohols). J. Neurochem., *13:*1509, 1966.
98. Saini, S.S.: Retrogasserian anhydrous glycerol injection therapy in trigeminal neuralgia: Observations in 552 patients. J. Neurol. Neurosurg. Psychiatry. *50:*1536, 1987.
99. Schaumburg, H.H., Byck, R., and Weller, R.O.: The effect of phenol on peripheral nerve: A histological and electrophysiological study. J. Neuropathol. Exp. Neurol., *29:*615, 1970.
100. Selander, D.: Neurotoxicity of local anesthetics: Animal data. Reg. Anesth. *18:*461, 1993.
101. Selander, D., Brattsand, R., Lundborg, G., Nordborg, C., and Olsson, Y.: Local anesthetics: Importance of mode of application, concentration and adrenaline for the appearance of nerve lesions. Acta Anaesthesiol. Scand., *23:*127, 1979.
102. Selmaj, K.W., and Raine, C.S.: Tumor necrosis factor mediates myelin and oligodendrocyte damage in vitro. Ann. Neurol., *23:*339, 1988.
103. Sharief, M., McLean, B., and Thompson, E.J.: Elevated serum levels of tumor necrosis factor-alpha in Guillain-Barré syndrome. Ann. Neurol., *33:*591, 1993.
104. Sladky, J.T., Greenberg, H.H., and Brown, M.J.: Regional perfusion in normal and ischemic rat sciatic nerves. Ann. Neurol., *17:*191, 1985.
105. Sommer, C., Galbraith, J.A., Heckman, H.M., and Myers, R.R.: Pathology of experimental compression neuropathy-producing hyperesthesia. J. Neuropathol. Exp. Neurol., *52:*223, 1993.
106. Sommer, C., Lalonde, A., Heckman, H.M., Rodriguez, M., and Myers, R.R.: Quantitative neuropathology of a focal nerve injury causing hyperalgesia. J. Neuropathol. Exp. Neurol., *54:*635, 1995.
107. Sorkin, L.S., Xiao, W-H., Wagner, R., and Myers, R.R.: Tumor necrosis factor-α induces ectopic activity in nociceptive primary afferent fibers. Neuroscience, *81*:255, 1997.
108. Sunderland, S.: The anatomical basis of nerve repair. *In* Jewett, D.L., and McCarroll, Jr. H.R. (eds.): Nerve Repair and Regeneration. pp. 14. C.V. Mosby, St. Louis, 1980.
109. Sweet, W.H., Poletti, C.E., and Macon, J.B.: Treatment of trigeminal neuralgia and other facial pain by retrogasserian injection of glycerol. Neurosurgery., *9:*647, 1981.
110. Taiwo, Y.O., Levine, J.D., Burch, R.M., Woo, J.E., and Mobley, W.C.: Hyperalgesia induced in the rat by the amino-terminal octapeptide of nerve growth factor. Proc. Natl. Acad. Sci., *88:*5144, 1991.
111. Tal, M., Schneider, M., Toyka, K.V., and Koltzenburg, M.: Heat hyperalgesia and nociceptor excitation after application of nerve growth factor (NGF) or inflammatory mediators. [Abst], 8th World Congress of Pain. pp. 119. Vancouver, IASP Press, 1996.
112. Thomas, P.K., and Holdroff, B.: Neuropathy due to physical agents. *In* Dyck, P.J., and Thomas, P.K. (Eds.): Peripheral Neuropathy. p. 990. W.B. Saunders, Philadelphia, 1993.
113. Thomas, P.K., Ochoa, J., Berthold, C.-H., Carlstedt, T., and Corneliuson, O.: Microscopic anatomy of the peripheral nervous system. *In* Dyck, P.J., and Thomas, P.K. (eds.): Peripheral Neuropathy. pp. 28, W.B. Saunders, Philadelphia, 1993.
114. Tuck, R.R., Schmelzer, J.D., and Low, P.A.: Endoneurial blood flow and oxygen tension in the sciatic nerves of rats with experimental 37 diabetic neuropathy. Brain., *107:*935, 1984.
115. Wagner, R., and Myers, R.R.: Schwann cells produce tumor necrosis factor alpha: Expression in injured and noninjured nerves. Neuroscience, *73:*625, 1996.
116. Wagner, R., and Myers, R.R.: Endoneurial injection of TNF-alpha produces nociceptive behaviors. Neuroreport *7:*2897, 1996.
117. Wang, B.C., Hillman, D.E., Spielholz, N.I., and Turndorf, H.: Chronic neurologic deficits and Nesacaine-CE. Anesth. Analg., *63:*445, 1984.
118. Waller, A.: Experiments on the section of the glossopharyngeal and hypoglossal nerves of the frog and observations of the alterations produced thereby in the structure of their primitive fibers. Philos. Trans. R. Soc., *140:*423, 1850.
119. Warren, J.S.: Interleukins and tumor necrosis factor in inflammation. Crit. Rev. Clin. Lab. Sci., *28:*37, 1990.
120. Watkins, L.R., Wietelak, E.P., Goehler, L.E., *et al.*: Characterization of cytokine-induced hyperalgesia. Brain Res., *654:*15, 1996.
121. Wells, M.R., Racis, S.P. Jr., and Vaidya, U.: Changes in plasma cytokines associated with peripheral nerve injury. J. Neuroimmunol., *39:*261, 1992.

122. Wiley, R.G., Blessing, W.W., and Reis, D.J.: Suicide transport: Destruction of neurons by retrograde transport of ricin, abrin, and modeccin. Science, *216:*889, 1982.
123. Wilson, F.: Neurolytic and other locally acting drugs in the management of pain. Pharmacol. Ther., *12:*599, 1981.
124. Wood, K.M.: The use of phenol as a neurolytic agent: A review. Pain, *5:*205, 1978.
125. Woolsey, R.M., Taylor, J.J., and Nagel, H.H.: Acute effects of topical ethyl alcohol on the sciatic nerve of the mouse. Arch. Phys. Med. Rehabil., *53:*410, 1972.
126. Xie, Y.K., and Xiao, W.H.: Electrophysiologic evidence for hyperalgesia in the peripheral nerve. Sci. China (B) *33:*663, 1990.
127. Xu, X.J., Hao, J.X., Olsson, T., *et al.*: Intrathecal interferon gamma facilitates the spinal nociceptive flexor reflex in the rat. Neurosci. Lett., *182:*263, 1994.
128. Yamamoto, T., Iwasaki Y., and Konno, H.: Experimental sensory ganglionectomy by way of suicide asoplasmic transport. J. Neurosurg. *60:*108, 1984.
129. Yamamoto T., and Yaksh, T.L.: Effects of colchicine applied to the peripheral nerve on the thermal hyperalgesia evoked with chronic nerve constriction. Pain, *55:*227, 1993.

Neural Blockade in Clinical Anesthesia and Management of Pain, Third Edition,
edited by M.J. Cousins and P.O. Bridenbaugh.
Lippincott–Raven Publishers, Philadelphia © 1998.

CHAPTER 31

Techniques for Neurolytic Neural Blockade

Richard B. Patt and Michael J. Cousins

INTRODUCTION

Neurolytic blockade is an important therapeutic alternative for well-selected patients with severe pain,[27,55,255] and thus it has long been an important focus for the anesthesiologist with specialized training in pain management.[19,341] Neurolysis is most often considered in the setting of advanced cancer,[55,334] but may also be applicable for pain due to other irreversible conditions,[77] such as occlusive vascular disease (see Chapter 13) and acquired immunodeficiency virus (AIDS). Once it has been established that satisfactory pain relief cannot be achieved by less invasive methods, techniques such as lumbar sympathetic,[274] subarachnoid,[269] celiac,[31] and superior hypogastric plexus[275] block are associated with a high degree of success and only a modest level of side effects. With a few important exceptions, neurolytic blockade generally is not suited for patients with undiagnosed medical problems or long life expectancies.

Multidisciplinary Management

Neural blockade is best regarded as only one component of a therapeutic matrix that includes antitumor therapy, pharmacologic strategies, and behavioral and psychiatric approaches, ideally implemented in a multidisciplinary setting.[5,87,146,265,385] In general, a multimodal approach is most likely to accurately determine the cause of pain and establish a management plan that takes into account all of its determinants.[18,215] Such an approach is particularly important when a neurolytic block is being considered, both to establish contingency plans should treatment prove ineffective and to provide support should a complication occur. If a multidisciplinary approach is impractical because resources are limited, the clinician needs to ensure availability of appropriate specialty consultation should it be required. In addition, the sole practitioner must possess expertise in pharmacologic management,[262,263] since careful titration of baseline opioid therapy is generally required once a block has been performed (see Chapters 23.1 and 23.2).

Integration of Pharmacologic and Interventional Treatments

Scientific Foundations and Research Needs

Prospective research on the outcomes and indications for neurolysis has been limited by logistical, scientific, and ethical constraints.[38,307] Problems include accurately characterizing pain, accurately distinguishing among subtly distinct pathologies that elicit similar complaints, variable temporal and anatomic patterns of disease spread, insufficient sample sizes, variability in technique (between practitioners and even, for the same practitioner, from patient to patient), and ethical and logistical constraints on blinding, randomization, and the use of placebo. As a result, much of what is known about neurolysis is garnered from case reports, clinical series, observations of experienced clinicians, and extrapolations from limited basic science investigations. The relative lack of data from controlled studies on neurolysis is a major barrier to the development of scientifically supported algorithmic approaches to decision making that attempt to integrate a full range of treatment approaches. Although such schemata have been proposed,[48,87,146] their utility is limited by the anecdotal nature of available source documents. There is a critical need to more accurately characterize the role of neurolysis with respect to that of pharmacologic approaches, which have been better studied. Progress in reconciling these issues will require discrete controlled comparisons among different treatment techniques for a variety of clinical syndromes. The recent surge of interest in pain management offers promise that neurolysis will not become a lost art of mostly histori-

R. B. Patt: Anesthesia Pain Programs, Pain and Symptom Management Section, University of Texas, M.D. Anderson Cancer Center, Houston, Texas 77030.

M. J. Cousins: Department of Anaesthesia and Pain Management, Royal North Shore Hospital, University of Sydney, St. Leonards, New South Wales 2065 Australia.

cal significance and is expected to stimulate further basic and clinical research.

History and Advances

The history of neural blockade, neurolytic blockade, and intraspinal opioid analgesia has been amply annotated by Fink,[84] Swerdlow[34] and Benedetti,[12] respectively (see Chapter 1). From a technical standpoint, there have been relatively few major advances in neurolysis since these techniques were popularized by Dogliotti,[67,68] Maher,[204] and others.[341] Such technical advances include increased reliance on radiologic guidance, the development of radiofrequency thermocoagulation and cryoablation, modifications of conventional techniques (especially celiac plexus block), and the introduction of several new ones (e.g., superior hypogastric plexus block). Nevertheless, over the years, neither the methods nor the chemical agents used to induce neurolysis have changed dramatically.

Conceptual advances have had more profound effects on how neurolysis is practiced and regarded. These relate primarily to more sophisticated integration of neurolytic techniques within a multidisciplinary framework of treatment options. That decision making has matured remarkably is highlighted by contrasting the contemporary wisdom of careful patient selection with that advanced by an authority of the 1930s who listed 244 indications for subarachnoid alcohol injection, including gout, cystic breast disease, occupational neurosis, painful menstruation, heartburn, and pyelonephritis.[328]

Factors and trends that have influenced the contemporary role of neurolysis include: (i) progress in general medicine, which has established more acceptable options for many chronic illnesses; (ii) increased cumulative experience with conventional neurolytic techniques, their modifications, and new approaches, which has refined the process of screening patients and selecting the optimal procedure; (iii) the evolution of multidisciplinary pain treatment and the recognition that "total pain" is a complex and multiply determined experience; (iv) a growing recognition of the imperative to treat pain aggressively; (v) an upsurge of interest in pain management and attendant dissemination of knowledge, and (vi) profound changes in the medical establishment's attitude toward opioid use.

Current Status of Neurolysis

Status of Opioid Therapy

Owing to cultural bias and scientific misinformation, opioids were not widely advocated for the treatment of cancer pain until the experience gleaned from the British hospice movement in the 1960s[355] exerted its influence during the 1970s and 1980s.[103] A better understanding of the pharmacology of chronically administered opioids, combined with controlled trials demonstrating efficacy and safety, have led cancer pain experts from multiple disciplines to advocate the use of oral opioids as the treatment of first choice for cancer pain that has not responded to antitumor therapy.[5,87,146,257,385] Properties of opioid therapy that support a fundamental role in cancer pain management are listed in Table 31-1.

TABLE 31-1. *Factors supporting opioids as the primary therapy for cancer pain*

Reversibility
Titratability
Suitability for bilateral and midline pains
Suitability for multiple and generalized pains
Lack of long-term organ damage
Relative simplicity
Limited need for specialized training, technical support, and equipment
Rapid development of tolerance to most adverse effects
Applicability across different age groups, cultures, and special populations

New evidence supporting the use of oral opioids as the mainstay of therapy for patients with cancer pain has refined the indications for nerve blocks and other invasive procedures considerably. The application of interventional approaches has come to be regarded as being best confined to those 10% to 30% of cases in which pain or side effects persist despite the judicious use of opioids and other pharmacologic aids. The introduction of intraspinal opioids and the development of microprocessor technology have further reduced the indications for neurolytic blockade by providing more acceptable options for diffuse pain. Though the role of neurolytic procedures is certainly more circumscribed, there remains a large population of patients who are potential candidates for such procedures.

Clinical Integration of Pharmacotherapy and Neurolysis

In the context of a view that considered the use of opioids as being *prima facie* undesirable, there was a tendency to correlate the outcome of nerve blocks with whether opioid use could subsequently be discontinued or dramatically curtailed. With the current emphasis on quality of life independent of opioid doses *per se*, nerve blocks are more appropriately viewed as occupying a role that complements rather than replaces that of opioids. Reductions in opioid use are often still sought as a means to reduce drug side effects and as indirect evidence that the correct procedure has been properly executed. Nevertheless, efficacy is not generally judged directly in light of changes in dose requirements, but instead on clinical reports of pain and toxicity.

Most patients undergoing neurolysis will be receiving concurrent treatment with opioids, usually chronically and often in relatively high doses. Accordingly, consideration of modifying opioid therapy after neurolysis is an important part of planning. Pain is a functional antagonist to opioid effects, and reduction in nociception consequent to successful neurolysis may place patients at risk for *relative* opioid overdose. Previously well-tolerated doses may result in obtundation and even respiratory depression if nociception is suddenly and profoundly interrupted, and consequently it is important to employ early dose reduction in the presence of signs of a successful procedure. Abrupt discontinuation of opioids may induce physical withdrawal (abstinence syndrome). As a rule of thumb, following signs suggestive of efficacy, neurolysis may be followed by a reduction in basal opioids of 25% to 50%, after which close observation, with consideration of further upward or downward dose adjustments, is needed.

Regardless of the technical success of a nerve block, most patients taking opioids chronically will require continued maintenance, albeit at lower doses. Continued opioid requirements may be due to a variety of factors including pain from other sites, incomplete neurolysis, salutary effects on anxiety and dyspnea, and rarely, psychological dependence. The likelihood that most patients will continue to utilize opioid analgesics even after treatment with an invasive procedure makes it imperative that the anesthesiologist pain specialist be facile in prescribing opioids.

ASSESSMENT

The mandate that any medical intervention be preceded by careful assessment is heightened in the case of neurolytic blocks because of their lasting effects. The likelihood of successful treatment hinges on careful consideration of all of the elements gleaned from this assessment, with particular attention to establishing shared goals and expectations that are realistic and specific. Assessment can be accomplished according to a variety of models.[256,299] For an intervention like neurolysis, consideration should be given to extending the assessment over time to help establish a therapeutic alliance, thus enhancing the patient's confidence in the treatment team.

The assessment should be comprehensive in depth and breadth, endeavoring to evaluate the pain, the underlying disease, and the person. The pain history[256,299] focuses on the development and nature of the pain, with the intention of establishing its cause and devising potential therapies. The pathologic process responsible for the pain needs to be carefully characterized, especially as regards its extent, treatability, tempo of progression, likely pattern of spread, and prognosis. Evaluation of the patient's personal, social, and domestic situation is often best aided by consultation from a mental health professional. Such inquiry should seek to identify depression or anxiety which, if managed aggressively, may help to modify pain complaints. The patient and family's understanding of the seriousness of the underlying illness should be cautiously explored, so that informed consent can be assured. Psychological support by means of reassurance, encouragement, and the demonstration of personal interest is an integral part of management. Establishing a relationship founded on trust is therapeutic and may minimize recriminations and the likelihood of medicolegal action, should the outcome of treatment be less favorable than anticipated.

In the setting of advanced irreversible illness, it is essential that pain is not treated in isolation, but instead is viewed as a single though important determinant of quality of life.[320] Thus, when considering pain management options, the potential effects of each intervention on overall function and other symptoms must also be appraised. In general, treatment is geared to both reducing (rarely eliminating) pain and (when possible) restoring function.

General Indications and Patient Selection

Local anesthetic blocks have important but relatively narrow indications for treating pain in patients with cancer and other irreversible medical conditions (Table 31-2). In general when neural blockade is indicated, neurolysis is most often considered, since pain is usually due to ongoing tissue injury and is expected to persist. However, continuous local anesthetic infusions may have a minor role in short-term management of chronic cancer pain.[304] Although exceptions exist, neurolysis is most applicable for pain that is (i) well characterized, (ii) well localized, (iii) somatic or visceral in origin, and (iv) does not comprise a component of a pain syndrome characterized by multifocal aches and pains (Table 31-3) (see also Chapters 23, 26, 27, and 29).

Portrayal of Pain

Patients with vague complaints may be poor candidates for neurolysis simply because their clinical presentation confounds the selection of the optimal intervention. Furthermore, patients who "feel bad all over," or who volunteer that "I can't describe it, it just hurts" may be indirectly communicating a global experience of pain that includes prominent spiritual, psychological, and/or social components (suffering versus nociception). Other clues that expressions of pain reflect global malaise may be gleaned from a structured interview performed by a mental health consultant.[225] Such concerns may be amplified in patients who subscribe to all the descriptors offered by assessment tools like the McGill Pain Questionnaire[107] or Brief Pain Inventory,[47] or predominantly to affective descriptors (e.g., wretched, cruel, agoniz-

TABLE 31-2. *Indications for local anesthetic blocks for cancer pain*

Diagnostic block
Prognostic block
Pain emergency
Muscle spasm
Vertebral compression fracture
Premorbid chronic pain
Treatment-related pain
Tumor-induced reflex sympathetic dystrophy

ing, miserable). Even with expert consultation it is difficult to determine to what degree psychological disturbances are a primary problem or are secondary to unrelieved pain. Although the presence of coexisting psychological conditions does not reduce the imperative to control pain, when they are prominent, if pharmacologic control is feasible it is preferred to neurolysis because of its reversibility and titratability (see also Chapters 23, 25, and 33).

Pain Localization

Well-selected neurolytic procedures tend to be relatively efficacious for pain that is well localized. When extended to provide coverage for pain that is distributed more extensively, the same procedures are more prone to failure and are associated with increased risks of undesired neurologic deficit. However, several important exceptions exist. Sympathetic blockade (stellate ganglion, celiac, lumbar sympathetic, and superior hypogastric block) often provides topographic analgesia that is ample for visceral pain syndromes, most of which tend to be vague in character and relatively diffuse. Epidural neurolysis, although currently performed in a limited number of centers, can often be successfully employed to manage segmental pain in a relatively broad topography without unwanted neurologic deficit, although this remains a risk. Finally, although availability is even more restricted, transnasal alcohol neurolysis of the pituitary gland and various neurosurgical options are applicable for widely disseminated pain in selected cases.

Multiplicity of Pains

Surveys of patients with advanced cancer have determined that pain is present in more than one body part simultaneously in up to 60% of patients.[355] The gate control theory of pain[219] helps to explain why patients may complain of a single predominant source of pain despite multiple pathologic foci. Employing a neurolytic procedure in patients with multiple lesions or multiple distinct foci of pain is therefore associated with the risk that a "new" pain will be unmasked once the primary complaint is eliminated. When feasible, a preliminary local anesthetic block may help to exclude this possibility. Even in patients with multiple sources of pain, however, a localized procedure that effectively reduces the foremost pain complaint may be of value by facilitating control of secondary pains with conservative treatment.

Tempo of Disease Progression

Even when pain is well localized, the aggressiveness of the underlying condition and its tempo of progression should be considered. It is disappointing when the provision of analgesia is followed by the emergence of refractory pain secondary to new or progressive spread of an underlying malignancy. The likelihood of rapid spread is estimated on the basis of the customary biologic behavior of the underlying malignancy, the patient's history, and consultation with an oncologist, but unfortunately cannot be predicted in individual cases with complete accuracy.

Predicted Life Expectancy

Although no reliable guidelines exist to govern decision making at either extreme, predicted life expectancy is an important factor when neurolysis is being considered. Clinicians are often reluctant to estimate the life expectancy of cancer patients, and when predictions are mandated, they are often inaccurate. For example, of a group of 37 patients refused admission to hospice because of a predicted life expectancy of more than 6 months, predictions were inaccurate in 78.4% of cases,[89] and of the 71 patients accepted into hospice, physician and nurse experts overestimated life expectancy by an average of 3.4 weeks.[88]

Upper Limits of Life Expectancy

Although controlled trials are lacking, there is consensus that the effects of neurolytic blocks endure an average of 3 to 6 months. Most large series describe a proportion of cases in which much shorter and longer durations of relief are achieved. Unfortunately, denervation may be followed not just by return of baseline pain, but also by the onset of new pain of neuropathic origin. The optimal time for performing procedures associated with a relatively high incidence of postneurolysis pain (e.g., peripheral neurolysis) therefore is within 6 to at most 12 months of predicted demise. Cryoanalgesia or radiofrequency thermoablation is probably more appropriate in patients with extended life expectancies. Sympatholysis and, to a lesser degree, subarachnoid neurolysis are less frequently implicated as causes of deafferentation pain. As a result, these procedures may be considered more liberally in patients with longer life expectancies, with the expectation that repetition may be required.

Lower Limits of Life Expectancy

Consideration of neurolysis in patients in whom death is imminent must be carefully individualized based on the nature and severity of pain, the likelihood of efficacy relative to more conservative measures, and the goals and expectations of the patient and family members.

When death is imminent, the provision of comfort is obviously the guiding therapeutic principle.[87,343] The risk:benefit ratio in this setting involves weighing the likelihood of pain relief against attendant discomfort, inconvenience, and risk. Procedures that are associated with extensive preparation, discomfort, or recuperation or are otherwise demanding of patients' limited resources should be avoided. In contrast, procedures that are not so arduous may be strongly considered. Even those associated with a significant degree of inherent risk may be considered in the preterminal patient when other more conservative measures have proved unsuccessful. In some settings, for example, subarachnoid neurolysis (Patt, R. B., Unpublished data)[331] or epidural analgesia[259] may be undertaken at the bedside with gratifying results. In contrast, procedures that require radiographic guidance are less often undertaken in this setting.

Pain Mechanism

Pain that is due to somatic or visceral injury is more likely to respond favorably to neurolytic blockade than is neuropathic pain. Although neuropathic pain is often relieved with a local anesthetic block, these results are not often durably reproduced with neurolysis.[347] Although it is still reasonable to consider neurolysis at a level proximal to the presumed neural pain generator, careful local anesthetic blockade is warranted to determine the likelihood of efficacy.

NEUROLYTIC AGENTS

Alcohol and phenol are almost invariably employed when chemical neurolysis is undertaken in contemporary practice. Glycerol (see Retrogasserian Glycerol Gangliolysis) is reserved almost exclusively for trigeminal gangliolysis, although its successful use for peripheral blocks in cancer patients has recently been reported.[43] Although of historical interest, chlorocescol, ammonium salts, iced saline, and hypertonic saline (see Hypertonic and Iced Saline, below) are infrequently utilized in contemporary practice. Radiofrequency thermoablation and cryoneurolysis (see Radiofrequency Thermocoagulation, below, and Cryoablation) however, have been employed with increasing frequency over the last decade as alternatives to chemical neurolysis.

Alcohol

Ethyl alcohol, also referred to as absolute or dehydrated alcohol, is formulated specifically for therapeutic neurolysis in concentrations that near 100%. It is typically available commercially in 1- and 5-ml glass ampuls and can be manufactured by a compounding pharmacist in larger volumes. It is colorless, has a characteristic pungent smell, and unlike preparations of phenol and glycerine, which are viscous, it can easily be injected through small-bore needles. Its specific gravity is 0.789 to 0.807, rendering undiluted concentrations hypobaric when mixed with human cerebrospinal fluid (CSF) (SG = 1.07 − 1.08). Specific gravity is irrelevant, however, for applications outside the theca, which take place in nonfluid mediums. When stored in a closed container, ethyl alcohol has a long shelf life, but once opened, exposure to the atmosphere should be avoided to prevent dilution from absorbed humidity.

Alcohol is generally used undiluted in the subarachnoid space and near peripheral nerves, and in concentrations of 50% to 100% near sympathetic nerves. Although irritating when applied to mucosal surfaces, alcohol has no effect on intact skin. Subcutaneous injection is painful and induces topical anesthesia. Perineural administration is characteristically followed immediately by severe burning pain along the targeted nerve's distribution, which usually lasts moments before yielding to a warm, numb sensation. Pain on injection may be blunted or eliminated by first injecting a small volume of local anesthetic, and residual burning pain is usually well tolerated when patients are forewarned. Denervation and pain relief sometimes accrue over a few days following alcohol injection.

Direct contact between alcohol and neuronal tissue produces dehydration and precipitation, which underlie the mechanism of nerve injury (see Chapter 30). Neuritis occurs more commonly after peripheral blocks than after sympathetic or subarachnoid blocks, and may be more frequent than after phenol. The reported incidence of new pain is variable and has not been thoroughly studied (see Peripheral Neurolysis). Alcohol's systemic toxicity is discussed elsewhere (see Celiac Plexus Neurolysis).

Phenol (Carbolic Acid)

Phenol (carbolic acid) has been used extensively for neurolysis since the 1950s,[204] and because of an apparent lower incidence of neuritis, has to some degree supplanted alcohol. Preparations of phenol in water, saline, glycerine, and contrast medium have been used clinically in concentrations ranging from 3% to 15%. Injectable phenol is not available commercially and requires preparation by a compounding pharmacist.[283,336] Solutions of phenol and water (aqueous phenol) or phenol in glycerine (hyperbaric phenol) are used most commonly.

Phenol is poorly soluble in water, and as a result, stable concentrations in excess of 6.7% cannot be obtained at room temperature. However, phenol is readily soluble in glycerine. Higher concentrations of aqueous phenol may be achieved by the addition of small volumes of glycerine, yielding a final solution that consists of (i) mostly water, (ii) 10% to 15% glycerine, and (iii) the desired concentration of phenol. Shelf life is said to exceed one year when preparations are refrigerated and are not exposed to light. Over time, stored solutions may develop a pink tinge, which does not appear to influence potency.

Aqueous preparations of phenol are used in most clinical settings except for subarachnoid administration, in which case glycerine-based solutions are absolutely indicated. Phenol mixed with glycerine is hyberbaric with respect to CSF, a property that is essential for controlling its spread in the subarachnoid space. Preparations of phenol and glycerine are thick and viscid, and so it is difficult to force them through small-caliber needles. Even with a 20-gauge needle, care must be taken to seat the needle on the syringe firmly, lest the force required to inject the phenol break the seal and spill drug on the patient or care provider. Hyperbaric phenol can be aspirated and injected more easily when it is rendered less viscid by heat. This can be accomplished by immersing the container of phenol water heated in a microwave just prior to use, being careful to maintain sterility. Handling can be rendered even more manageable by using 1-ml syringes. Even with these precautions, the syringe may still be dislodged from the needle, and as a result, care providers should guard their eyes carefully and must be prepared to rinse any skin or mucosal surfaces that are accidentally exposed to phenol.

In the past, phenol was mixed with other substances, including the contrast dye myodil (ethyl iodophenylundeclate) and silver nitrate. Silver nitrate was used when phenol alone produced inadequate relief, as it was believed to act as a mordant, helping to "fix" the phenol to resistant or sheltered nerve roots.[204] Silver nitrate is rarely used in contemporary practice, and myodil is no longer commercially available.

Perineural injection of phenol is less commonly associated with the burning pain observed after alcohol injection. Phenol produces a biphasic response characterized by an initial local anesthetic effect, producing subjective warmth and numbness that gives way to chronic denervation. The hypalgesia that follows may not be as dense as after alcohol, and quality and extent of analgesia may fade slightly within the first 24 hours of administration. Systemic toxicity is discussed elsewhere (see Celiac Plexus Neurolysis).

Butyl Aminobenzoate (Butamben)

Butyl aminobenzoate (Butamben) is an extremely hydrophobic/lipophilic ester local anesthetic used occasionally for topical wound anesthesia because it is too slowly absorbed to be very toxic.[294] Owing mostly to the investigative work of Shulman and also Korsten, butamben appears to have a potential role in the management of chronic pain, although it is not yet widely used.[170,308–311] While considerable controversy exists as to whether butamben is truly neurolytic,[170,311] its effects seem to be relatively selective and lasting. Shulman and Korsten have administered suspensions of 2.5% to 10% butamben for epidural, subarachnoid, and peripheral nerve blocks in patients with pain of malignant and nonmalignant etiology.[308–310] Although repeated injections are often needed, they have been able to demonstrate moderate-duration analgesia with few serious side effects.[170,308–311]

PERIPHERAL NEUROLYSIS

Although peripheral neurolysis is described primarily in case reports, uncontrolled clinical series, and reviews,[2,44,260] when applied selectively it has a definite and important, though circumscribed, therapeutic role.[20,318,342] Controversy exists surrounding the specific indications and exact nature of the role of peripheral neurolysis, which, as is the case for other neuroablative procedures, is most heated regarding the management of refractory pain of non-neoplastic etiology.[44,318] Peripheral neurolysis is carried out relatively infrequently because of concerns about impermanence, the development of neuritis and deafferentation pain, failure due to overlapping sensory innervation, and the potential for motor deficit and unintended damage to adjacent tissues. The impact of each of these potential problems, however, can be minimized by careful patient selection and attention to technique (see also Chapter 27).

Local Anesthetic versus Neurolytic Peripheral Blocks

Techniques for performing peripheral neurolytic blocks are relatively similar to those described for analogous local anesthetic blocks (see Chapters 10, 11, and 14 through 20). The important differences between local anesthetic and destructive blocks of the peripheral nerves lie in their (i) respective indications, (ii) potential complications, (iii) necessity for preliminary diagnostic/prognostic blocks, and (iv) relative need for precise localization, often necessitating radiologic guidance.[271] Local anesthetics are often administered in volumes in excess of that which is actually required to produce anesthesia, based on the principle that these agents spread relatively freely in biologic tissue, especially when injected between tissue planes.[388] For neurolysis, the localization of needles must be undertaken with greater precision and certainty. Because of the propensity of neuroablative techniques to produce nonselective, indiscriminate tissue damage, smaller volumes are generally utilized in order to minimize spread to adjacent structures. In addition, because neurolytic agents are viewed as spreading less freely and predictably in tissue than local anesthetic agents,[17] precise localization is a critical determinant of efficacy, especially given the customary use of modest volumes for chemical neurolysis. The most important distinctions between destructive and local anesthetic peripheral blocks, however, relate to patient selection, since the consequences of the former are often lasting.

Patient Selection

The important features of patient selection are listed in Table 31-3 and include (i) pain that is amenable to peripheral neurolysis (localized, somatically mediated pain), (ii) severe pain that is expected to persist and cannot be modified by less invasive measures, and (iii) limited life expectancy. The latter requirement is debatable, especially as regards the application of less destructive or more discrete methods such as radiofrequency or cryoablation. Peripheral neurolysis of mixed (sensorimotor) nerves should be avoided unless weakness is already present, unless pain is so severe that the risk of motor weakness is acceptable, or unless the resultant weakness would be unlikely to produce significant impairment (e.g., intercostal or masseter weakness). The significance of impermanence of effect, a feature common to most neuroablative procedures, can be minimized by limiting patient selection to those in whom life expectancy is unlikely to exceed the duration of pain relief (1–12 months). In the event that a favorable outcome is more short-lived than anticipated, the peripheral block can often be repeated at the

TABLE 31-3. *Indications for neurolysis*

Pain is severe
Pain is expected to persist
Pain cannot be modified by less invasive means
Pain is well localized[a]
Pain is well characterized[b]
Pain is not multifocal[c]
Pain is of somatic or visceral origin[d]
Limited life expectancy[e]

[a] Blocks are usually most effective when the topographic extent of pain is limited. The main exceptions are sympathetic blocks, which typically provide relief for relatively diffuse visceral pain. In addition, epidural neurolysis may be considered for segmental pain distributed over several dermatomes. Pituitary ablation also has potential applications for disseminated pain emanating from osseous metastases, especially in patients with breast or prostate cancer.

[b] The main exception is visceral pain, which is often vague in nature and difficult for patients to define clearly.

[c] Pituitary destruction may be considered for disseminated pain due to osseous metastases, especially in patients with breast or prostate cancer. Other forms of neurolysis may be cautiously considered with the goal of eliminating the most severe pain and controlling secondary pain with opioids.

[d] Although temporary pain relief can often be achieved with local anesthetic blocks, in general, neuropathic pain is less likely to respond favorably to neurolysis. (Not an absolute contraindication.)

[e] Requires carefully individualized decision making. In general, problems such as deafferentation pain and transience are minimized when selection is limited to patients with predicted life expectancy of less than one year. Less destructive or more discrete techniques (cryoablation, radiofrequency thermoablation) can be considered more liberally in patients with long life expectancies.

same site or more proximally. Transient pain relief after neurolysis is sufficiently common that it is prudent to advise patients to expect repetition at least once.[267] Similarly, problems related to postinjection dysesthesia will be minimized by selecting patients who are likely to succumb to their primary disease prior to the development of these sequelae and in whom the original pain is so severe that, by comparison, dysesthesias are unlikely to be distressing.

Assessment of the effects of preliminary diagnostic/prognostic local anesthetic blockade helps to evaluate the potential for overlap of sensory fields to interfere with outcome. The information obtained serves as a guide to planning a more definitive therapeutic neurolytic block. Likewise, the potential for motor weakness and impairment can be assessed in advance with local anesthetic blockade. Careful assessment will identify patients in whom motor weakness is likely to be well tolerated, e.g., patients already confined to bed, patients with pre-existing motor deficit, and individuals with pain sufficiently severe to render a painful limb already useless. The potential for damage to adjacent nontargeted tissues is less for blocks of superficial peripheral nerves than for blocks of deeper structures, and may be further minimized when localization is facilitated by electrical stimulation, radiographic guidance, and the administration of test doses of local anesthetic.

Technical Aspects

A thorough knowledge and careful review of the pertinent anatomy form the basis for the technical aspects of peripheral neurolytic blockade. These include careful selection of the procedure with consideration of blocking neighboring nerves, attention to the position of the patient, proper selection of drug and drug dosage, and verification of needle placement by aspiration, local anesthetic test doses, electrical stimulation,[284,285,288] and/or radiologic guidance.[271]

The basis for the limited duration of analgesia that is often observed after peripheral neurolysis and the development of new pain (neuritis, deafferentation pain) in a proportion of patients is uncertain, but probably relates to the creation of an incomplete lesion.[17,230,290] As a result, it is essential to achieve as complete and accurate a block as possible. Strict standards for accurately localizing the targeted nerve are essential. Although a sufficient volume of local anesthetic injected into the same or an adjacent tissue plane as a nerve trunk may diffuse through neighboring soft tissue and produce an effective block, neurolytics spread less well and, as a result, must be deposited directly on the nerve to achieve an optimal effect.

In order to avoid complications yet maximize efficacy, the volume and the concentration of the neurolytic agent must be selected carefully. Unfortunately, controlled comparisons among different concentrations and volumes of alcohol and phenol have not been carried out, and as a result, selection ultimately depends on clinical judgment. Most early investigators advocated either absolute alcohol or 5% to 7% aqueous phenol. Today, concentrations of phenol in the 10% to 12% range are commonly employed with the intention of producing more complete neurolysis and improving long-term efficacy.[1,44,142,266,343,345] With respect to complications, it is probably more important to limit volume, which is more likely to correlate with aberrant spread, than concentration, which should correlate better with density of the block. Although authorities have expressed concern that the use of higher concentrations of phenol might predispose to vascular injury,[339] this contention remains unproven.

Selection of Technique and Agent

Surgical Neurectomy

Surgical interruption of peripheral nerves is rarely undertaken,[153,247] fundamentally because durability and efficacy are generally insufficient to warrant its invasiveness *vis-à-vis* percutaneous approaches, and in part because referral patterns tend to direct patients to anesthesiologists who are facile with the latter approaches. Though more conservative options can usually be identified, multiple-level surgical rhizotomies are still occasionally performed.[302]

Radiofrequency Thermocoagulation

Radiofrequency thermocoagulation (thermal ablation) has numerous potential advantages, and since the 1950s has been used with increasing frequency. Underlying principles and the nuances of various techniques have recently been described in an excellent monograph.[167] Contemporary systems are sophisticated and consist of an electrical generator equipped to allow (i) impedance measurement, (ii) stimulation over a wide range of frequencies, (iii) accurate measurement of the lesion's temperature, (iv) measurement of the duration of lesion generation, (v) accurate measurement of amperage and voltage, and (vi) the ability to gradually increase temperature over time.[167] In addition, specialized probes have been designed to facilitate specific procedures such as cordotomy and rhizotomy. Insulated probes are introduced based on anatomic principles and fluoroscopic or computed tomography (CT) guidance, and low-current stimulation is applied to their uninsulated tips to confirm their position. Current flowing through the electrode generates heat in adjacent tissue based on its resistance or impedance until the temperature of the probe and that of the surrounding tissue reach equilibrium. The size of the lesion is controlled by the temperature at the probe's tip, which is monitored by a thermocouple mechanism. Thermal equilibrium is usually established by the application of current for 60-second cycles.[54] Effect can be intensified by re-lesioning at gradually increasing temperatures or by repositioning the probe (see also Chapter 32).

Thermal lesions can be localized more predictably than chemical lesions, since the latter are associated with the potential for aberrant spread and, in addition, the intensity of a thermal lesion can be readily monitored and controlled. Overall, probes are superior to those utilized for cryogenic lesioning, and effects are more lasting. A radiofrequency lesion is produced within seconds, and so great care must be taken to assure that the probe is positioned properly, and overzealous lesioning should be avoided. As with other neuroablative techniques, pain relief is often, but not always, achieved at the expense of numbness; dysesthesias may arise over time, and the potential for motor weakness exists when sensorimotor units are targeted. Unfortunately, contemporary equipment is costly both to procure (upwards of $25,000) and to maintain, owing to the need for careful sterilization. Until recently, anesthesiologists were less likely than neurosurgeons to be exposed to this technique during their training. Radiofrequency lesioning has been advocated for a wide array of procedures (Table 31-4).

TABLE 31-4. *Partial list of potential applications of radiofrequency thermocoagulation*

Percutaneous cordotomy
Trigeminal ganglion lesions
Spinal nerve rhizotomy/ganglionectomy
Facet denervation
Sphenopalatine ganglion lesions
Stellate ganglion lesions
Thoracic sympathetic chain lesions
Lumbar sympathetic chain lesions

Cryotherapy

The application of low temperatures to provide analgesia, a method that dates back to Hippocrates, was used as a means of providing intraoperative analgesia for amputation (refrigeration anesthesia) as recently as 1941.[74] The first practical devices for creating localized cold-induced lesions were developed in the 1960s for ophthalmologic surgery and led to Lloyd's introduction of cryoanalgesia in 1976.[191] Contemporary apparatus consists of a source of compressed nitrous oxide (or carbon dioxide), a probe, and, between the two, a sophisticated unit that houses mechanisms that regulate gas intake and exhaust, electrical stimulation, a timer, and thermocouple. Gas is forced through a conduit within the probe's shaft that ends in a narrow orifice, and as a consequence of the Joule Thompson or Kelvin effect, the expansion of the escaping gas cools the surrounding tissue to $-50°$ to $-70°$. The shaft also contains a larger tube that acts as an exhaust conduit and is connected to a scavenging system. Units generally cost between $15,000 and $25,000 and can be fitted with a variety of sterilizable probes.

The discrete application of low temperatures produces variable degrees of nerve injury that are classically described according to a classification suggested by Sunderland and others.[293,332] First-degree injuries, referred to as neuropraxia, are associated with few histologic changes, interfere with function for days to weeks, and tend to selectively block motor and proprioceptive impulses. Second-degree injuries (axonotmesis) induce a loss of axonal continuity but preserve the architecture of the endoneurium, perineurium, and ectoneurium, which is the goal of therapeutic cryoneurolysis. Axons and their myelin sheaths degenerate distal to the lesion (Wallerian degeneration), and regeneration commences from the proximal stump at a rate of 1 to 1.5 mm/day. Second-degree injuries occur with the application of temperatures below $-20°$, as well as after a nerve is crushed with a hemostat. Third-, fourth-, and fifth-degree injuries, referred to as neurotmesis, involve progressively greater disruption of neural integrity and are associated with erratic, disorganized, or failed regeneration. These injuries are more likely to be produced by radiofrequency thermocoagulation or chemical neurolysis.

The main advantage of cryoablation is that nerve injury is typically reversible, and regeneration is more likely to occur without attendant neuritis or dysesthesias than when other techniques are used. The most extensive experience with cryoanalgesia is with its intraoperative application to prevent post-thoracotomy pain.[155,205] Recently, its use has been ad-

TABLE 31-5. *Partial list of potential applications of cryoablation*

Intercostal neuralgia
Post-thoracotomy pain
Trigeminal neuralgia
Facet arthropathy
Sacral root block for sciatica and perineal pain
Coccydynia
Pituitary ablation

vocated for a variety of chronic pain syndromes (Table 31-5).[72,312,367,389] In view of the likelihood of reversibility without morbidity, many authorities prefer cryotherapy for the management of nonmalignant pain. Newer, less bulky probes have been developed that facilitate percutaneous lesioning, although some authorities advocate creating lesions under direct vision to ensure maximum contact between the probe and the targeted nerve. The main disadvantage of cryolesioning is that pain relief is often evanescent. This is probably often due to failure to accurately localize the targeted nerve, since although an ice ball of 1 to 2 cm is typically formed; only the few millimeters surrounding the probe's tip reach the desired temperatures indicated by the thermocouple.[74] Although a variety of temperatures and freeze/thaw cycles have been advocated to enhance reliability and extend duration,[75] because of its association with relatively short and often unpredictable intervals of denervation, cryotherapy is not generally preferred to treat cancer pain that is expected to persist. However, cryoanalgesia is an important option in noncancer patients with refractory pain.

Chemical Lesions

Alcohol and phenol are commonly used for peripheral neurolysis, although ammonium sulfate and chlorocrescol are occasionally advocated (see Chlorocrescol and Ammonium Salts). Neuritis follows peripheral neurolysis more commonly than it follows lytic blocks of the sympathetic chain or spinal axis, but its incidence is uncertain, with estimates ranging between 2% and 28%.[17,206] Neuritis is held to be more commonly associated with the use of alcohol,[3] although this finding has not been documented in controlled studies.[162] In an unrandomized trial of 57 cancer patients administered peripheral blocks with absolute alcohol or 6% aqueous phenol, Jain et al.[151] achieved equal pain relief and an equal incidence of dysesthesias, although systemic side effects were more common after phenol. Although many authorities state that alcohol and phenol are essentially interchangeable, phenol is typically preferred for noncancer pain. Alcohol appears to produce more intense nerve destruction and sensory blockade than phenol, and thus may be preferred in patients with predictably short life expectancies. In addition, it is often used for cranial nerve blocks based, presumably, on tradition.

Management of Head and Neck Pain with Peripheral Neurolytic Blocks

For decades, neurolytic blocks of the pertinent cranial nerves and their branches have been used successfully to treat intractable pain.[19,108] Recent modifications to established techniques include the use of radiofrequency thermocoagulation,[26,248,313] cryoanalgesia,[389] and topical laser[365] to produce lesions, novel approaches to trigeminal neuralgia, including microvascular decompression,[34] retrogasserian glycerol injection,[388] balloon rhizolysis[237] and the use of CT[6,147] and ultrasound[10] guidance.

Indications: Cranial Neuralgias versus Neoplastic Pain

Invasive procedures such as neurolysis are considered primarily for pain due to malignancy and trigeminal neuralgia and its variants (glossopharyngeal neuralgia, intermedius neuralgia),[164] the contemporary treatment of which differs considerably. Gasserian ganglion neurolysis, once used liberally to treat trigeminal neuralgia,[17] has largely been supplanted, first by the realization that anticonvulsants and other adjuvants could usually control such pain,[335] and later by the introduction of alternate invasive techniques generally associated with a more favorable risk:benefit ratio. The situation for cancer pain differs. Although the need for invasive procedures has been reduced as global expertise in pharmacologic management has improved, when an invasive approach is needed, chemical or thermal neurolysis is often elected because these techniques are straightforward and less demanding than newer innovative options.

Cranial Neuralgias

Radiofrequency Thermogangliolysis

Radiofrequency thermocoagulation of the gasserian ganglion is regarded by many as the optimal procedure for trigeminal neuralgia that is refractory to pharmacologic management.[194] The resultant lesion is more easily controlled than that resulting from chemical neurolysis, and complications such as corneal anesthesia, masseter weakness, and anesthesia dolorosa are infrequent. Technical aspects are similar to those pertinent to chemical neurolysis. After an insulated 22-gauge probe is introduced into the foramen ovale under fluoroscopic guidance, 0.1 to 0.3 volts of current at 50 to 60 Hz is applied until the patient's pain is reproduced, thus confirming that the probe is accurately localized. The administration of atropine or glycopyrrolate is recommended to reduce the likelihood of vasovagal attacks when the foramen is entered. Patients are briefly anesthesized during lesion generation, which commences with a 1-minute cycle at 60° to 80° C; after the patient awakens, sensory testing is performed. Most clinicians aim to produce slight hypalgesia of the trigger zone and maintenance of corneal sensation by repeating lesion generation at successively higher temperatures.[194,301] In one large series with a

2-year follow-up, 28.3% of patients had a recurrence of symptoms after one treatment and 8.3% after multiple treatments. Other than corneal anesthesia in 3.7% of patients, no serious complications occurred. Other groups have reported troublesome dysesthesias in up to 24% of patients[216] (see also Chapter 32).

Retrogasserian Glycerol Gangliolysis

Håkanson introduced retrogasserian glycerol injection after serendipitously observing pain relief during the application of glycerol to facilitate imaging.[117] The foramen ovale is penetrated with an 18- to 20-gauge spinal needle by the usual method, following which the patient is moved to a sitting position and the needle is advanced until CSF is obtained.[78] The needle's tip should be visualized at the trigeminal impression of the petrous apex on AP views, at the middle third of the clival edge on lateral views, and in the center of the foramen on submental vertex views. The head may be flexed 40° for V1 lesions, 25° for V2 lesions, and maintained almost erect for V3 lesions.[78] Alternatively, the needle may be advanced slightly further to treat V2 and V1 pain.[388] Glycerol which, like hyperbaric phenol, is viscous and therefore difficult to infuse, is injected in 0.05-ml increments through a 1-ml syringe until mild sensory changes are appreciated, or a total of 0.1 ml, 0.25 ml, or 0.4 ml is administered for pain involving the V1, V2, and V3 distributions, respectively.[78] Patients are maintained seated with the head flexed for 1 to 2 hours. Pain relief may develop immediately or over the course of days, and treatment is only infrequently associated with corneal anesthesia. In a series of 162 patients, Young[388] reported immediate relief in 90.1% of patients, of whom 18.5% had recurrent pain on long-term follow-up. Corneal reflexes were impaired or absent in 3.1% and 1.8% of patients, respectively, and anesthesia dolorosa was not observed. Recurrence and failure tend to be more common in previously operated patients, and pain relief is often re-established with repetition. In a report on their experience with retrogasserian injection for trigeminal neuralgia in patients with multiple sclerosis, Linderoth et al. reported early relief in over 90% of patients, but a high rate of recurrence at one year[87] (see also Chapter 15 and Fig. 15-5 A–C).

Trigeminal (Balloon) Compression

An alternative approach, described initially by Mullan and Lichtor in 1983,[237] involves penetration of the foramen ovale with a 14-gauge needle through which a No. 4 Fogarty balloon catheter is passed into Meckel's cave and is then inflated with contrast medium for 1 to 10 minutes. General anesthesia is utilized, which capitalizes on one of this technique's advantages: no need for patient cooperation. Meglio and Cioni[216] reported immediate and complete relief in 93.2% of 74 patients. They noted recurrence in 32%, 56%, and 77% of patients at 1, 2, and 3 years, respectively, with an average recurrence time of 6.5 months. They reported three cases of hemorrhage and encountered troublesome dysesthesias in 7% and 24% patients with compression and thermocoagulation, respectively. Their results caused them to conclude that 4 to 6 minutes was the optimum compression time, and that if patients treated in this fashion were separated out, efficacy was similar to that of thermocoagulation at the expense of less dysesthesia.

Microvascular Decompression

Microvascular decompression, also referred to as the Janetta procedure (after the neurosurgeon who popularized it), is based on Dandy's observation of the close juxtaposition of a tortuous vessel and the trigeminal nerve in patients with tic douloureux.[57] The procedure involves a suboccipital craniotomy, microsurgical exploration of the trigeminal nerve at its course between Meckel's cave and the pons, and insertion of a prosthetic sponge between the nerve and adjacent aberrant vessels, which are presumed to produce pain on the basis of nerve compression. More than 90% of patients are said to have evidence of nerve impingement by an artery, vein, or bony prominence. Sustained pain relief (5 years) is estimated at 90%,[194] although, in following patients for an average of 8 1/2 years, Burchiel reported a 47% recurrence rate (31% major recurrence, 17% minor recurrence), with mild sensory loss in 25% of patients, and no corneal anesthesia or anesthesia dolorosa.[104] Mortality and serious morbidity typically occur in 0.5% to 1% of operated patients, and as a result, treatment usually is not offered for medically ill patients or those over the age of 50.[213]

Summary and Conclusions: Trigeminal Neuralgias

There is little consensus regarding the optimum treatment for refractory trigeminal neuralgia, and outcome appears to be predicated in large part on clinician expertise. In view of the low incidences of anesthesia dolorosa and corneal anesthesia reported with newer treatment methods, alcohol and phenol injections of the trigeminal nerve and its branches should probably be avoided unless life expectancy is limited. All procedures are associated with a modest incidence of early failures and recurrence over time. Microvascular decompression is preferred by some, in part because it is presumed to correct the underlying pathology, but it is associated with the mortality and morbidity of a craniotomy and is not generally recommended in frail individuals or those over the age of 50. Although mild sensory loss occurs in up to 20% of patients, anesthesia dolorosa and corneal anesthesia are uncharacteristic.[34] Percutaneous radiofrequency thermocoagulation, by far the most commonly applied invasive therapy (over 14,000 cases documented in 33 reports),[213] involves the generation of a lesion, the extent of which is subject to operator control. Its disadvantages include requirements for a cooperative patient and access to radiofrequency equipment. Its merits include high initial success rates (usually greater than 90%) and only a modest rate of recurrence (20%–30%).[213] Despite some reports to the contrary, corneal anesthesia and anesthesia dolorosa appear to occur in a small proportion of patients. Retrogasserian glycerol injection also has a high initial success rate (75%–90%), but probably a higher rate of recurrence than with thermal lesioning. It requires less patient cooperation and minimal equipment, and appears to be associated with very low incidences of corneal anesthesia and anesthesia dolorosa. Percutaneous balloon microcompression is relatively simple, requiring little specialized equipment and no patient cooperation. Like retrogasserian glycerol, the incidence of initial success is high, but so is recurrence. Dysesthesias and corneal anesthesia appear to be less frequent than after thermocoagulation. The interested reader is referred to a recent comprehensive review of the spectrum of available treatment options for trigeminal neuralgia.[113]

Cancer Pain

Although neoplastic head and neck pain is often responsive to a combination of analgesics and radiotherapy, several factors predispose to pain that is refractory to conservative treatment. Neuropathic pain is relatively common owing to the face's rich innervation, the erosive behavior of many tumors, and injury from surgery and radiotherapy. Pain is often aggravated by simple, relatively involuntary movements related to swallowing, eating, coughing, and talking. The newer alternatives outlined above are more often considered for cranial neuralgias in part because of predicted longevity, while cancer pain usually can be more reasonably managed with more straightforward chemical or radiofrequency neuroablation, techniques that generally require less preparation and patient cooperation.

The craniofacial region is innervated by cranial nerves V, VII, IX, X, and contributions from branches of the second and third cervical nerves. Most of the face is innervated by the trigeminal nerve; exceptions include parts of the ear (VII, IX and X), the posterior third of the tongue and upper pharynx (IX), the larynx and lower pharynx (X), and the angle of the jaw and upper neck (second and third cervical nerves).[379]

Potential problems to be considered when planning ablative therapies in this setting include overlapping innervation; anatomic distortion due to tumor infiltration, surgery, or radiotherapy; and the potential for tumor invasion or radiation fibrosis to reduce contact between the neurolytic and targeted nervous tissue ("sheltering"). In addition, to avoid impairment of swallowing and ventilatory control, neurolytic blocks, especially involving cranial nerves IX or X, should usually be preceded by diagnostic/prognostic local anesthetic injections. Despite these considerations, blockade of the cranial and/or upper cervical nerves is of great value in selected patients.

Pain that is localized to the distribution of the second or third branch of the trigeminal nerve can often be managed with a discrete block of the maxillary or mandibular nerve.[231] Consideration should be given to blocking the gasserian ganglion if there is pain in the distribution of the ophthalmic nerve (V1), if pain involves the receptive field of more than one branch or is likely to extend beyond V2 or V3, or when anatomic considerations prevent a more peripheral approach.[224] Since head and neck neoplasms do not confine themselves to neurologic boundaries, ninth or even tenth cranial nerve destruction is sometimes also required, especially for pain arising from the floor of the mouth or pharynx.[224] The sensory field of the glossopharyngeal nerve includes the nasopharynx, eustachian tube, soft palate, uvula, tonsil, base of the tongue, and part of the external auditory canal. The vagus nerve subserves the larynx and contributes fibers to the ear, external auditory canal, and tympanic membrane. Bilateral blocks of the ninth or tenth cranial nerves are not recommended in order to avoid impairment of swallowing, phonation, and protective airway reflexes.[17,201]

When intractable craniocervical pain is not amenable to nerve block therapy, intraspinal opioid therapy by means of an implanted cervical epidural catheter[361] or intraventricular opioid therapy may be considered.[193] Numerous neurosurgical procedures have been devised to manage rostral pain but are of limited practical value because of their invasive nature and high morbidity and mortality.[259]

Mandibular, Maxillary, Trigeminal, Glossopharyngeal, and Vagus Nerve Blocks

Lysis of the second division (maxillary nerve) or third division (mandibular nerve) is usually performed by an extraoral approach,[231] most commonly with absolute alcohol or radiofrequency thermocoagulation. Mandibular block is indicated for pain involving the jaw, buccal mucosa, and anterior two-thirds of the tongue. Maxillary block is indicated for pain involving the middle third of the face, i.e., the maxilla, cheek, nasal cavity, hard palate, nasal cavity, and tonsilar fossa.[379] If tumor progression is anticipated, it is preferable to prophylactically extend the field of analgesia by blocking the Gasserian ganglion in its entirety.[201,124] Although blockade of the first division (ophthalmic nerve) is well described in the older literature,[324] Gasserian ganglion block is preferred in contemporary practice. However, retrobulbar block with alcohol[212] or phenol[14] is occasionally carried out as an alternative to enucleation in patients with blind, chronically painful eyes, especially due to glaucoma. Neurolytic blockade of the smaller branches of the trigeminal nerve (e.g., mental, inferior alveolar, supraorbital, infraorbital) has been described for cancer pain management.[17] This approach may be undertaken for well-localized pain in a confined distribution, particularly due to an endophytic lesion that is more likely to erode than spread or when anatomic distortion precludes access to the parent nerves. In general, however, because of overlapping innervation and the likelihood of progression, blockade of the major branches of the trigeminal nerve is preferred.

A lateral extraoral approach to V2 and V3 can usually be

implemented without radiographic guidance in cooperative patients. The pterygoid fossa is accessed through the mandibular notch (between the coronoid and condylar process of the mandible), which is appreciated as a slight concavity at the superior aspect of the mandibular ramus just beneath the zygomatic process. Identification of the notch is facilitated by placing a finger beneath the midpoint of the zygomatic process with the mouth closed. When the mouth is opened, the condylar process can be felt to roll anteriorly beneath the palpating finger, and when the mouth is again closed, the finger usually rolls into the notch. As described in Chapter 15, after infiltration with a local anesthetic, a 20- to 22-gauge spinal needle is introduced perpendicularly until a paresthesia is obtained or the pterygoid plate of the sphenoid bone is contacted at a depth of 1.5 to 2 inches, after which the needle is withdrawn and redirected to walk off the bone either posteriorly or anteriorly for block of the mandibular or maxillary nerve, respectively (see Chapter 15, Fig. 15-6). Localization is verified with a paresthesia and/or the application of electrical stimulation, and after careful aspiration, 2 to 4 ml of a local anesthetic or 1 to 2 ml of absolute alcohol is usually administered. Care should be taken that contact with the periosteum is not mistaken for a paresthesia, and a local anesthetic should be administered prior to the neurolytic to confirm the needle's location and to blunt the transient but severe pain that usually follows alcoholization. When pain extends into the cervical region or angle of the jaw, paravertebral blockade of the second or third cervical nerve root may be needed in addition to mandibular block.[264] Alcohol block of the mandibular nerve has been occasionally associated with localized gangrene and skin slough,[231] presumably due to vascular thrombosis. A similar case of slough following one of several supraorbital alcohol nerve blocks was reported in a patient with painful multiple sclerosis.[189]

Although entire textbooks have been written describing various approaches to blocking the trigeminal nerve,[319] a modified Härtel's approach, as described in Chapter 15, is usually used in contemporary practice. This involves local anesthetic infiltration 1 to 2 fingerbreaths lateral to the labial commisure, just medial to the masseter muscle, and introduction of a 20- to 22-gauge spinal needle directed toward the ipsilateral pupil and second molar under fluoroscopic or even CT guidance (see Fig. 15-5). The greater wing of the sphenoid bone is usually first encountered at a depth of 4.5 to 6 cm, following which the needle is withdrawn and walked off the bone into the foramen ovale, which usually lies at a depth of 6 to 7 cm.[30] Paresthesias of V2 or V3 are sought, since a V1 paresthesia may occur outside the foramen. It is essential that the needle's position be verified with radiologic guidance, which should demonstrate impingement of the foramen ovale on submental vertex views and passage just beyond the clivus on lateral films. In addition, scrupulous aspiration and the administration of a test dose of local anesthetic are essential to exclude subarachnoid placement (see Chapter 15, Fig. 15-5A–C).

Ninth and tenth cranial nerve blocks are typically undertaken via an extraoral approach through a skin wheal raised at a point midway between the angle of the mandible and the tip of the mastoid process (see Chapter 15, Fig. 15-7). Under radiologic guidance, a standard spinal needle is inserted perpendicular in all planes until the styloid process is encountered. For glossopharyngeal block, the needle is withdrawn and advanced just beyond the bone either posteriorly[201] or anteriorly,[30] where a paresthesia should be elicited. For vagus nerve block, the needle is positioned posteriorly and about 1 cm deep to the styloid process. After careful aspiration and a test dose of local anesthetic, 1 to 4 ml of neurolytic solution is typically injected. When available, radiofrequency coagulation is the preferred means of lesion generation. Although infrequently performed in contemporary practice, neurolytic blockade of the superior laryngeal nerves (see Fig. 15-8) has been described for laryngeal pain of tabetic, tuberculous, and malignant origin.[20,44]

In 1954, Bonica described the use of neurolytic cranial nerve blocks in a series of 70 patients with cancer pain.[19] Forty-four (62.9%) patients achieved complete relief of pain, 22 (31.4%) moderate relief, and in 4 (5.7%), pain relief was slight or absent. These results are comparable to those published in an earlier series by Grant.[108] Bonica reported complications of a "serious" and "not serious" nature in 4 (5.7%) and 22 (30%) patients, respectively, which in all cases were predictable, i.e., corneal ulceration after trigeminal block in a small proportion of patients, unilateral masticatory paresis in a larger proportion of patients after mandibular block, and one case of unilateral dysphagia after glossopharyngeal block. In another study, McEwen et al.[215] reported achieving good or fair relief in 70% of cancer patients treated with gasserian ganglion block. Siegfried and Broggi have reported achieving lasting comfort in about half of 20 patients treated with percutaneous thermal ablation of the trigeminal ganglion.[313] Of two other patients treated with glossopharyngeal thermoablation, one underwent a repeat procedure at 6 months for recurrence of pain and the other had temporary dysphagia and permanent twelfth nerve palsy, but ultimately both patients were pleased with their outcomes.[26] Using an anterior approach, Pagura et al.[248] reported good to excellent results in 15 cancer patients treated with thermocoagulation of the glossopharyngeal nerve. Treatment was supplemented by trigeminal thermoablation in eight patients because of overlapping pain, and other than transient vagal stimulation, no adverse effects were encountered.

Treatment of Hiccoughs with Phrenic Nerve Block

Unilateral phrenic nerve block is occasionally undertaken to treat intractable hiccoughs (singultus) with good results,[17] although efforts to reverse the underlying cause and treatment with conservative symptomatic measures[355] should first be exhausted. Fluoroscopy is utilized to determine whether one hemidiaphragm is predominantly in spasm and should consequently be blocked. Prior to performing a neurolytic phrenic nerve block, the results of a prognostic block with local anesthetic are evaluated to determine that ventilatory function will not be compromised by a more lasting procedure. Resuscitation equipment should be immediately available.

Upper Extremity. Because the fibers that govern somatically mediated upper extremity pain are closely associated with those subserving limb function (proprioception, tactile sensation, and motor power), peripheral neuroablative procedures are rarely undertaken for nonmalignant pain. Even in oncology patients, iatrogenic loss of motor strength and dexterity must be carefully avoided so as not to add to other cancer-related impairment and losses. Patients will often gratefully exchange unremitting pain for numbness, but loss of function is typically poorly tolerated. In view of the indiscriminate nature of neural injury produced by therapeutic concentrations of alcohol and phenol, motor and mixed sensorimotor nerves should not be targeted for injection unless movement and function are already significantly compromised. A significant proportion of patients, however, present with an essentially useless limb due to neurologic sequelae of tumor invasion, radiation or surgical fibrosis, pathologic fractures, or splinting.

A variety of neurolytic procedures have the potential to relieve upper extremity pain, but all are associated with some risk of limb weakness, and none relieve pain with complete reliability.[21] Stellate ganglion block (see Chapter 13, Figs. 13-18 to 13-20) is only applicable just for sympathetically mediated pain. Cervical subarachnoid neurolysis, while ineffective in up to half of patients,[339] is probably least likely to affect motor function because drug is deposited preferentially on sensory rootlets; thus it should be considered for patients with brachialgia and unimpaired function. Paravertebral block (see Chapter 13, Fig. 13-21) is applicable for well-localized pain, and even then, because of sensory overlap, multiple nerves usually need to be blocked and some degree of motor dysfunction should be anticipated. Radiologic guidance is strongly recommended for neurolytic paravertebral block, as well as careful observation of the effects of preneurolytic test doses of local anesthetic and fractionated administration to avoid subarachnoid or epidural spread. Brachial plexus neurolysis has been used in specific settings with some success, but because of the plexus's large motor component, it should not generally be considered unless motor strength is already deficient. Although neurolysis of the plexus's peripheral branches has important indications for the treatment of spasticity (see Neurolysis for Spasticity), relatively little experience has been reported for carcinomatous upper limb pain. With the exception of suprascapular block, which can often be undertaken for localized shoulder pain with little morbidity, neurolysis of the plexus's peripheral branches should generally be avoided because of the potential for weakness, dysesthesias, and failure due to overlapping innervations. A recent report of the successful management for two weeks of pain from Pancoast's syndrome suggests a possible role for short-term local anesthetic brachial plexus infusions, as well.[340]

Bonica[20] described the treatment of "several" cancer patients who presented with pain and edema sufficient to render their involved upper limb useless. After observing good preliminary results with tetracaine injections, he reported infiltrating the brachial plexus with 20 ml of 95% alcohol, resulting in paralysis but relief of pain until death (duration unspecified). He also mentions having achieved pain relief of 3 1/2 weeks to 3 1/2 months duration with injections of 5% aqueous phenol in the vicinity of the brachial plexus. Kaplan et al.[159] reported on a single but well-documented case of phenol brachial plexus block performed in a patient with recurrent sarcoma involving the humeral head. After a successful prognostic local anesthetic block, 12.5 ml of 6% phenol in water was injected by the supraclavicular route (see Chapter 10, Fig. 10-5), resulting in significant but incomplete pain relief. Residual pain was managed by supplementary paravertebral phenol blocks of C5 and C6 and later, in response to tumor extension, T1–T3 paravertebral blocks (0.5–1.0 ml 6% aqueous phenol/segment). In a report of a single case, Neill[242] achieved excellent palliation of pain secondary to a pathologic humerus fracture in a man with multiple myeloma with two successive interscalene injections (see Chapter 10, Fig. 10-6) of 20 ml of 50% alcohol. Mullin et al.[238] utilized interscalene injections of 3% aqueous phenol to manage pain in five patients with Pancoast's syndrome. Although all patients achieved excellent short-term pain relief, which was sustained for up to 7 months in three patients, repetition at 3- to 6-week intervals was required. Neurologic sequelae were not observed, suggesting that, while the effects of dilute phenol are short in duration, treatment may be relatively safe in patients with normal motor function. In order to achieve a greater duration of response, higher concentrations of phenol have been used in patients in whom limb function is already absent. Patt et al.[266] treated four patients with injections of 10 to 20 ml of 10% to 12% phenol administered by the axillary and/or interscalene approach, with good to excellent pain relief in all cases until death (12 weeks × 2, 8 weeks, and 5 weeks). Although increased motor weakness was observed in all cases, it was well tolerated, and no unexpected complications occurred. In three of the four cases, pain relief accrued gradually over several days. Several other patients referred for brachial plexus block who had relatively intact limb function and predominant shoulder pain were managed effectively with suprascapular neurolysis using 4 to 5 ml of 10% phenol or absolute alcohol.[260]

Non-neurolytic invasive options for managing upper extremity pain include epidural, subarachnoid, or intraventricular administration of opioids, as well as epidural, peripheral, and deep brain stimulation[193,259,361] (see Chapters 23, 29, and 32).

Thoracic and Abdominal Wall. Pain originating in the parietal peritoneum or in the thoracic or abdominal wall can be treated with multiple intercostal[44,70,228,230] or paravertebral blocks,[17,358] as well as subarachnoid neurolysis (see

Subarachnoid Neurolysis). The potential advantages of subarachnoid block include low neurologic morbidity (in the thoracic region), the presence of a reliable end point (CSF), no need to localize multiple individual nerves, and fewer problems related to overlapping distribution, neuritis, and pneumothorax. The shortcomings of subarachnoid neurolysis are discussed below. Clinicians may prefer peripheral blocks because of greater familiarity and easier applicability of prognostic local anesthetic blocks.

Intercostal Blocks

Intercostal block is usually performed posteriorly near the angle of the rib just lateral to the sacrospinalis muscle. The ribs are usually easily palpable here; the nerve is still contained within the costal groove where drug tends to spread more predictably,[230] and failures may be fewer than with anterior approaches because the nerve has not yet given off its lateral cutaneous branch near the midaxillary line. While the use of radiologic guidance has been reported for intercostal block,[230] "walking the needle off" the rib and paresthesias are usually relied on to confirm needle location (see Chapter 14, Figs. 14-2 to 14-4). Except after pneumonectomy, pneumothorax can occur, although with proper technique, the incidence of symptomatic pneumothorax may be as low as 0.092%, as was demonstrated in a series of 50,097 intercostal blocks performed, mostly by residents, in 4333 patients.[228]

There are surprisingly few reports on treatment with intercostal neurolysis. Doyle[70] reported on a series of 46 hospice patients treated with multiple phenol intercostal blocks. He utilized 1.0 to 1.5 ml 5% phenol "in oil" per segment and obtained total relief of pain for a mean duration of 3 weeks (range 1 to 6 weeks). Radiologic guidance was not utilized and no complications were reported. Intercostal cryoneurolysis has been conducted according to a variety of protocols. For example, one group[110] reported on percutaneous freezing (single cycle of four minutes) through a 14-gauge cannula in patients with intercostal neuralgia after thoracotomy (91%) and zoster (9%), who had experienced transient pain relief after local anesthetic blockade. All patients experienced initial pain relief that deteriorated over 2 to 3 weeks, and ultimately one-half and one-quarter of patients reported significant pain relief at 3 and 6 months, respectively. Although three cases of pneumothorax occurred, no patients experienced post-treatment neuritis. That additional caution is advisable when blocking the intercostal nerves of patients who have undergone complicated lung resection is suggested by a case report of a patient with adhesions who experienced acute bronchospasm following an unintentional presumed intrabronchial or intrapulmonary injection of a small amount (0.5 ml) of 8% phenol in saline.[7]

Paravertebral Blocks

Paravertebral neurolytic blocks of the somatic roots just outside the intervertebral formina are infrequently undertaken.[350] The usual technique, which relies on paresthesias and bony landmarks such as the transverse process, is described in Chapter 14 (see Fig. 14-12). For neurolytic block, radiologic guidance, careful observation of the effects of preneurolytic test doses of local anesthetic, and fractionated administration to avoid subarachnoid, epidural, or intrapleural spread, all of which have been documented,[49] are indicated.

Bonica[17] mentions favorable results subsequent to the paravertebral injection of 1 ml alcohol per involved segment in patients with abdominal and chest wall pain secondary to vertebral, paravertebral, and visceral neoplasms associated with peritoneal invasion. Jain[151] mentions performing 39 paravertebral alcohol and phenol injections under radiologic guidance without serious complications. In a brief report, Vernon[358] noted good relief of back pain of metastatic origin and no untoward effects after paravertebral injection of alcohol in two patients.

Other Peripheral Blocks for Parietal Pain

An alternative approach to localized bony pain due to rib metastases or pathologic fractures involves periosteal infiltration with local anesthetic and steroids and even dilute phenol.[261,342] In a partially controlled series of patients with pain due to rib metastases, the outcome of periosteal injections of corticosteroids compared favorably with the results of external beam radiotherapy.[249] A report by Mehta and Ranger,[218] of superficial neurolytic blocks of the individual peripheral branches of the lumbar plexus in 103 patients with abdominal pain of unknown etiology raises the question whether blockade of the peripheral nerves within the parieties abdominal wall might be feasible. They describe having blocked the iliohypogastric (65), ilio-inguinal (10), and upper and lower intercostal (28) nerves within the rectus sheath with 2 to 3 ml of aqueous phenol (see Fig. 14-13). Follow-up at 3 weeks revealed complete and partial relief of pain in 58% and 32% of patients, respectively, with no recurrence in 70% of respondents at 3-year follow-up. Despite their use of a primitive nerve stimulator in some cases, however, their description suggests that trigger point injections (see following) rather than true peripheral nerve blocks may have been administered.

Pelvis, Perineum, and Lower Extremities

Treatment of intractable perineal and lower limb pain is problematic because pain is often bilateral or midline in distribution, and the relevant neuroanatomy predisposes to risks of muscular paresis and incontinence when neurolytic techniques are applied. When bowel and bladder function are not of concern because of pre-existing dysfunction and/or surgical diversions, neurolytic subarachnoid saddle block (see Subarachnoid Neurolysis) is simple and effective, but decision making is more complex in the continent, ambulatory patient with intractable pain. The recent introduction of superior hypogastric plexus and ganglion impar block (see Sympathetic Neurolysis), which are not associated with incontinence, are important options for sympathetically mediated pelvic or rectal pain.[274,275]

Sacral Nerve Root Block

Selective blockade of the sacral roots (see Chapter 11, Fig. 11-4) is a useful approach when it is important to preserve urinary continence[296] in the presence of perineal, rectal, or posterior thigh pain. The sacral roots are readily accessed as they emerge from the posterior plate of the sacrum. A single sacral nerve, most often one of the third[45] or sometimes fourth[297] sacral nerves, usually exerts a dominant influence on bladder tone, and as a result, blockade of nondominant nerves, based on trials of local anesthetic injections, have little urodynamic effect. Diagnostic local anesthetic block is strongly recommended prior to neurolysis to "map out" the nerves that should be targeted for therapeutic blockade. Radiologic guidance is a useful adjunct to confirm placement and exclude caudal spread. While the foramina are not usually well visualized on AP views, penetration of the posterior sacral plate is readily apparent on lateral views. The technique is elegantly described by Moore,[231] and elsewhere in this text (see Chapter 11, Fig. 11-4).

Robertson[296] described a series of nine patients with intractable perineal pain secondary to carcinoma of the rectum whom he treated with sacral root neurolysis. Following successful local anesthetic block, he injected 2.5 ml 6.66% aqueous phenol at the S4 foramen on the predominantly painful side. Satisfactory analgesia was obtained in all cases, and persisted in two cases for 202 and 414 days after a single block. Duration was inadequate in the other cases, but pain relief was uniformly maintained until death by a second or third block. In seven of the nine patients, duration of relief from the first block was under 10 days, suggesting that most patients will require repeated treatment, but this limitation was mitigated by ease of repetition. Motor and autonomic function were unaffected, and no other complications occurred. In a similar study on patients with bladder pain secondary to spasticity, Simon et al.[314] obtained an average of 26.5 months of pain relief in responders after sacral injections of 2 ml of 6% aqueous phenol. Most patients obtained relief with unilateral blockade of the third sacral nerve, although preliminary local anesthetic blocks identified some patients whose pain was mediated by S2 and S4. Several patients required repeat treatment, and no lasting complications were observed.

An isolated report of bladder atony following otherwise successful S3 and S4 alcohol block[106] emphasizes the need for careful observation of the results of preneurolytic prognostic blocks with local anesthetic. A recent well-designed study[46] assessed the spread of a mixture of contrast medium and local anesthetic injected in 1- and 2-ml alliquots for sacral block. The authors demonstrated a wider spread of solution in the latter group and concluded that 1 ml of anesthetic is sufficient to produce a selective sacral nerve root block and, moreover, may be safer. They were also able to demonstrate that reflux into the sacral canal was much less likely when the needle tip was positioned at the anterior border of the sacrum rather than in the midportion of the sacral foramen. It is uncertain how these results apply to the spread of neurolytic solutions.

Psoas Compartment and Psoas Sheath Block

The psoas sheath refers to the potential space between the psoas muscle and its posterior fascia, which contains the lumbar plexus (L1–L4), while the psoas compartment refers to the potential space between the posterior fascia of the psoas muscle and the anterior fascia of the quadratus lumborum, which contains the lower part of the plexus, including the lumbosacral trunk (L4–S1). While these blocks are frequently elected for lower extremity surgery,[40,254] they would seem to be ill-advised for chronic pain because the plexus contains so many motor fibers. Preliminary evidence, however, suggests that psoas compartment or sheath neurolysis may be undertaken with few risks of motor paresis, although the explanation for this observation is unclear.

Two anatomic techniques for psoas block have been described.[254] The lower (psoas compartment) approach involves placing a needle over the fifth lumbar transverse process and advancing it using a loss or resistance technique through the quadratus muscle. Drug is deposited into the psoas compartment, and tracks upward to cover the plexus. The upper (psoas sheath) block is achieved by advancing a needle below and about 1.5 cm beyond the third lumbar transverse process, often with the aid of a nerve stimulator. (see Chapter 13, Figs. 13-22 and 13-23.)

Feldman and Yeung[77] treated 26 patients for intractable claudication with 39 paravertebral injections of 5 to 10 ml of 7.5% phenol in myodil into the psoas sheath between the first and second lumbar transverse processes. Over 90% of patients experienced sustained improvement in their walking ability by 1.5 to 9 times. Hypalgesia to pinprick in the L1–S2 distribution was noted in 25% of patients, but there was neither subjective numbness nor clinical weakness. Two patients experienced transient dysesthesias. Jack[144] reported on the successful management of claudication in two patients with repeated bilateral injections of 5 ml of 10% phenol in iophendylate. In both patients, pain and ambulatory status improved, and neither developed motor or sensory deficit. That 5 to 10 ml of 7.5% phenol and 5 ml of 10% phenol dissolved in contrast medium produced no significant neurologic sequelae is surprising, although it may relate to the large caliber of the plexus. Intrigued by these reports, our group has performed six neurolytic psoas blocks with 10% to 12% aqueous phenol with good analgesia and similar sparing of motor fibers. We have utilized a combined L2 or L3 and L5 approach using two needles.[331]

Other Peripheral Blocks

Neurolytic injections of other peripheral nerves subserving the lower extremity are rarely undertaken, and then only after local anesthetic injection has confirmed that the resulting numbness is well tolerated and that reduction in pain is not accompanied by motor weakness. Doyle[70] mentions performing two femoral nerve blocks (see Chapter 11, Fig. 11-3) with phenol in a patient with invasion of the femoral sheath area, but provides no other details. Our group performed an alcohol injection of the sciatic nerve (see Chapter 11, Fig. 11-5) in a patient with pre-existing motor weakness from invasion of the sciatic nerve by pelvic tumor with good short-term results.[266] However, we also observed heightened distress and poor tolerance of resulting foot drop in other patients with less complete motor deficit exposed to trials of prognostic local anesthetic sciatic blockade. Rastogi and Kumar briefly mention "successful" alcohol block of the sciatic nerve in three patients with cancer.[288] Successful treatment of penile pain and malignant priapism secondary to venous obstruction from bladder cancer has been reported anecdotally with injections of 5% aqueous phenol near the dorsal nerves of the penis close to the symphysis pubis[376] (see Chapter 20, Fig. 20-18).

SUBARACHNOID NEUROLYSIS

Thirty years after the first description of subarachnoid anesthesia,[53] the first neurolytic subarachnoid block (with alcohol) was reported by Dogliotti (1931).[67,68] Although Suvansa first described the use of intrathecal phenol for the treatment of tetanus in 1931,[333] it became a commonplace treatment for pain only after Maher reported on its use as an alternative to alcohol in 1955.[204] Following its introduction, subarachnoid neurolysis was used to treat pain due to a variety of diseases, with mixed results.[327] With refinements in pharmacologic management and the development of other therapeutic alternatives,[146] indications have narrowed, and as a consequence, these techniques are used more sparingly in contemporary practice, but with results that are generally more often favorable than in the past.[267]

Although indications are limited, subarachnoid neurolysis is a valuable technique in carefully selected patients with refractory cancer pain and life expectancy that is unlikely to exceed one year. The most suitable pain problems involve only a few dermatomes, and are ideally unilateral. Intrathecal neurolysis is intended to produce discrete lesions at the level of the cord's posterior roots within the dural sac (chemical rhizolysis). Rather than the extensive anesthesia that accompanies perioperative local anesthetic spinal anesthesia, subarachnoid neurolysis endeavors to produce a band of analgesia that corresponds to or slightly overlaps the boundaries of the patient's pain. Coupled with prudent patient selection, complications are few and favorable results are common. Difficulties, however, are more likely to arise when its use is extended for pain that is bilateral or diffuse, and in the presence of neurologic or undiagnosed disease.[130,338]

Although chlorocresol, cold or hypertonic saline, and ammonium salts are occasionally used, concentrated solutions of alcohol or phenol are preferred. Since the neurolytic effects of these agents are not selective, patients are exposed to risks that include motor weakness and incontinence. These risks can be minimized (though not entirely eliminated) by careful patient selection and by combining the use of hyperbaric or hypobaric solutions with careful positioning of the patient and strict attention to protocol.

Considerations Common to Subarachnoid Alcohol and Phenol Neurolysis

A number of factors need to be considered prior to commencing treatment (Table 31-6). There is an absence of controlled studies comparing outcomes for alcohol versus phenol, and these agents are used almost interchangeably. Despite early suggestions that phenol was associated with preferential effects on small fibers subserving pain,[136,204] subsequent animal and autopsy studies have confirmed that the effects of alcohol and phenol are nonselective, resulting in indiscriminate damage to nerve fibers, the extent of which is dependent on volume and concentration.[241,356] Pathologic findings and mechanisms have been amply reviewed by Papo and Visca[251] and are discussed in Chapter 30. Expert opinion suggests that hyperbaric phenol may be more controllable than hypobaric alcohol (easier to paint the floor than paper the ceiling),[264] but that the neurolytic effects of alcohol may be more potent and lasting.[329] Alcohol is preferred to phenol when the patient cannot lie on his or her painful side. In addition, failed neurolysis with one agent may be best followed with a trial of treatment with another.

In general, subarachnoid neurolysis should not be undertaken if more than six spinal segments are involved, especially since treatment usually aims to block one dermatome above and below the boundaries of the painful region. There is some controversy surrounding the treatment of bilateral symptoms. Some authorities recommend unilateral neurolysis of the more painful side first, followed a few days later by treatment of the contralateral side.[162] However, intrathecal

TABLE 31-6. *Considerations for subarachnoid neurolysis*

Patient education and consent
Consideration of periprocedural sedation
Selection of neurolytic agent (alcohol or phenol)
Selection of concentration (absolute alcohol, 5%–15% phenol in glycerine)
Determination of targeted dermatomes and roots
Determination of injection site
Need for single-versus-multiple needles
Upper and lower volume limits
Positioning of patient
Adjustment of opioid dose and follow-up

and epidural opioid and non-opioid drugs are now better alternatives (see Chapter 29). The patient's overall condition is an important factor in making such decisions. Epidural neurolysis may also be considered for pain that is bilateral or more widely distributed.

The topographic distribution of pain is determined through a careful history, following which anatomic charts are consulted to confirm which spinal nerve roots innervate the painful region. Owing to differential growth, the length of the adult vertebral column exceeds that of the spinal cord; along the caudal half of the axis, nerve roots emerge from the cord a variable number of spinal segments above the level from which they exit the vertebral column through their intervertebral foramen. The targeted roots may be approached either at the interspace where they arise from the cord or somewhat lower, where they exit the bony canal. This controversy relates only to lumbar and low thoracic blocks, since more proximal roots have a shorter, more horizontal intradural course. Based on the view that the effects of alcohol are most profound at the level that the fine rootlets (fila radicularia) arise from the cord, most authorities[121,338] recommend that the roots be targeted at the level where they arise from the cord. A chart depicting the relationship between the spinal nerve roots and the vertebral column is consulted to determine the appropriate interspace for needle placement (Fig. 31-1).

In general, both therapeutic and toxic effects correlate with the volume and concentration of neurolytic used. Owing to the absence of controlled comparative studies among treatment protocols, arbitrary though reasonable upper limits have been proposed by various authors based on their clinical experience. Although limits customarily regarded as safe are exceeded at the peril of increased risk of serious neurologic morbidity, the treatment protocol that is ultimately applied must, to a degree, be individualized. For example, upper volume limits may be reasonably amplified in the mid-thoracic region, which is distant from the outflow to the brachial and lumbosacral plexus, and likewise, volume limits are less critical in preterminal patients who are already confined to bed and in whom continence is not an issue.

The administration of small volumes of drug through multiple needles placed in neighboring interspaces is preferable to using larger volumes through a single needle.[20,251] All aspects of the injection technique should be designed to minimize turbulence that might produce aberrant flow and untoward neurologic changes.

Patient Preparation

The need to remain immobile during and immediately after the injection must be explained. Patients should be led to expect little discomfort during needle placement, but need to be warned of the necessity for assuming an uncomfortable position during and just after the injection. They are coached regarding the need to provide real time feedback regarding the development of new sensations, especially burning, tingling, warmth, numbness, or pain relief. Ideally, premedication is omitted or used sparingly to preserve patient cooperation. The blood pressure cuff is placed on the uppermost arm and used infrequently during the procedure to avoid artefactual numbness from decreased circulation. Finally, it is essential that a careful preprocedural neurologic assessment be performed to familiarize patients with the intraprocedural routine and document pre-existing deficits.

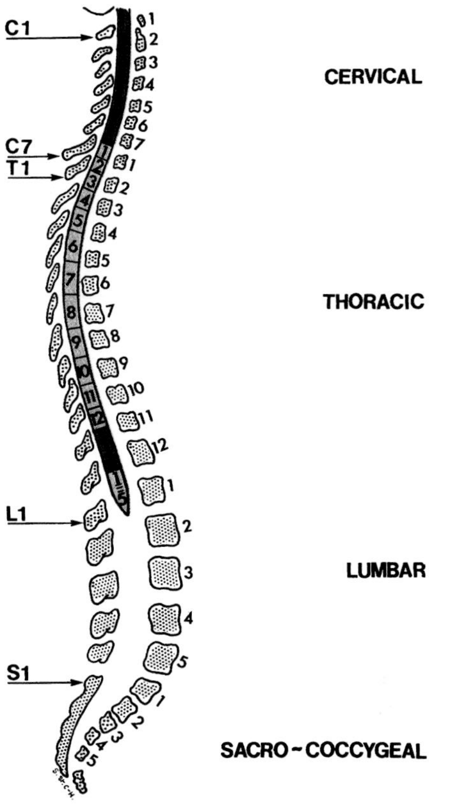

FIG. 31-1. This drawing of the vertebral column and spinal cord indicates their segmental relationships. Significant difference between the vertebral and cord levels occurs only in the lower thoracic and lumbosacral regions.

Subarachnoid Alcohol Neurolysis

For alcohol injection, the patient lies with the painful side uppermost on an adjustable bed, of the type that is typically used for surgery. The patient is positioned so that after needle placement, the injection site can be elevated above the neighboring spinal segments by means of table adjustments and support provided by padding. A firm bolster comprised of folded sheets is preferable to bulky pillows.

The theca can be accessed through a midline or paravertebral approach, although ideally the needle tip should ultimately rest at the superior (uppermost) aspect of the subarachnoid space near the targeted roots. A 22-gauge needle should be utilized to facilitate placement, ensure easy detection of CSF, and minimize any jet effects during injection. The bevel is oriented toward the ceiling to maximize the migration of hypobaric alcohol toward the targeted roots. Free flow of CSF is obtained, following which a 1-ml syringe is firmly connected to the needle's hub, taking care not to alter the needle's depth. The table is adjusted to ensure that the injection site is the least dependent (highest) portion of the vertebral column, and the patient is rolled 45 degrees forward to direct the hypobaric alcohol toward the posterior (sensory) roots (see Fig. 31-4). Alcohol is instilled slowly and steadily in aliquots of 0.1 to 0.2 ml per minute. The patient is coached to report new sensations, especially burning, tingling, warmth, or pain relief. Between injections, a brief neurologic examination is serially performed. If paresthesias or numbness are encountered just above or below the targeted dermatomes, the table's tilt is modified away from the direction in which further spread is desired. If altered sensation occurs distant from the targeted dermatomes, treatment should be halted the needle is repositioned in an alternate interspace.

Subarachnoid Phenol Neurolysis

The technique for subarachnoid neurolysis with phenol is similar to that which has been described for alcohol except insofar as the use of a hyperbaric as opposed to hypobaric solution mandates different positioning of the patient. The patient is positioned laterally with the painful side dependent, and provisions are made for adjusting the table and inserting pads so that the injection site is rendered lower than the adjacent vertebral segments. Because the patient will ultimately be tilted 45 degrees posteriorly (toward the operator) to maximize the spread of hyperbaric phenol to the posterior roots (see Fig. 31-5), he or she must initially be positioned near the edge of the bed to avoid contact between the bed and needle/syringe. A 20- to 22-gauge spinal needle is required because of the viscosity of phenol and glycerine formulations. The needle bevel is directed downward, and whether introduced in a midline or paramedian trajectory, its tip should ultimately lie near the lower portion of the spinal axis.

When using hyperbaric phenol, it is critical that utmost care be exercised in creating a firm seal between the syringe and the needle's hub. Phenol in glycerine is so viscous that even when injected through a 1-ml syringe, the pressure required to advance the plunger often breaks the seal, introducing the risk that the neurolytic solution will spill on the patient's skin or injure the clinician's eyes. Ease of injection can be facilitated by immersing the ampul containing the phenol solution in hot water before aspirating it into the syringe.

In contrast to the transient, or burning pain that may immediately follow subarachnoid alcohol injection, intrathecal phenol characteristically produces relatively mild feelings of warmth, tingling, or prickling, in affected dermatomes, presumably owing to its initial local anesthetic effects.

Other Considerations Common to Subarachnoid Alcohol and Phenol Neurolysis

Brief but careful serial neurologic examinations are performed throughout the procedure to determine the extent of ongoing neural blockade and to detect early signs of motor weakness. Documentation of baseline neurologic function is essential, and patients should be cautioned to move as little as possible during motor and sensory testing. Prolonged maintenance of the lateral decubitus position and frequent blood pressure checks occasionally produce artefactual numbness of the dependent limb(s), which may be mistaken for denervation.

Once the predetermined volume of neurolytic has been injected, the needle(s) stylet should be replaced and the needle tip is allowed to be washed by CSF, to minimize the potential for sinus formation and backache due to the escape of residual drug from the needle as it is withdrawn. The patient's position should be maintained for about 15 minutes following the injection (see below).

Matsuki and co-workers carried out a series of investigations in humans and dogs to determine the rapidity with which CSF concentrations of absolute alcohol[211] and 7% phenol in glycerine[135] decline following therapeutic neurolysis. They determined that the neurolytic solution is rapidly diluted by CSF, which is a reasonable explanation for the inadequate results often observed clinically. Immediately after the completion of incremental injections of 1.0 ml of each agent, the CSF alcohol concentration was only 25.6%, and phenol and glycerine concentrations were, respectively, 30% and 40% of their original concentrations. Ten minutes following the completion of injection, CSF alcohol concentrations had fallen to 3.1%, and 15 minutes after phenol injection, the mean CSF concentrations of phenol and glycerine were 0.1% and 3% respectively.

Several important conclusions can be drawn from these experiments. Rapid decline in CSF levels of the agents studied suggest that patients can be safely repositioned 15 minutes after the spinal injection is complete. In addition, the nearly immediate reduction in concentrations support the need for carefully positioning needles near the targeted roots rather than relying on modifications of the table to affect precise localization of effect. Finally, rapid decline of CSF levels of both phenol and glycerine argues against Maher's[204] contention that glycerine acts as a mordant or carrying agent, releasing phenol slowly.

Cervical Subarachnoid Neurolysis

Typically only a moderate proportion of patients experience lasting pain relief after cervical subarachnoid neurolysis,[339] as is exemplified by a large series that reported excellent-to-good results in 77% of patients overall, but in only 50% of patients treated with cervical block. This has been suggested to be due to anatomic factors that limit contact between the neurolytic and the targeted roots, including the relatively short intradural course of the cervical roots, the narrower caliber of the cervical canal, and rapid dissipation of the lytic agent due to brisk CSF flow. Subdural block, though once advocated as an alternative to cervical subarachnoid neurolysis, is not now commonly used, and experience with cervical epidural neurolysis is meager.

Puncturing the dura at the cervical level is not technically difficult. The cervical column's spinous processes are relatively blunt, and when the neck is flexed, they usually do not overlap. The cervical interspaces can usually be easily palpated, and the theca accessed in the midline from a nearly perpendicular trajectory (see Fig. 8-11). Obviously, the needle needs initially to be advanced cautiously to avoid spinal cord injury. Notwithstanding this important consideration, the cord is routinely penetrated during cordotomy,[188] and workers have reported accidentally piercing the cord with no complications other than transient pain.[272,289] Cervical CSF pressure may be low in the patient in the prone position. If free flow of CSF is not easily established, localization can be aided by gentle aspiration, or alternatively the puncture can be performed with the patient sitting, provided that the return to the decubitus position is undertaken carefully.

The most important potential complications of cervical subarachnoid neurolysis are cranial nerve dysfunction and upper extremity weakness. Cranial nerve palsy is unlikely when proper technique is followed, and few reports are encountered in the literature. Perese[272] described one patient with diplopia of two months' duration after C1–C2 alcohol block. Careful positioning, scrupulous attention to technique, and serial neurologic assessment are employed to minimize the risk of limb paresis, except when the limb has already been rendered useless, in which case ipsilateral motor weakness is not a concern and slightly more liberal volumes can be used. When performing high cervical blocks or attempting to block pain distributed over more than one or two dermatomes, one should consider inserting multiple spinal needles into the two or three neighboring relevant interspaces and injecting smaller increments of absolute alcohol through each needle.[62,169] It may be best to initially exaggerate the head-up and head-down position for hyperbaric and hypobaric techniques, respectively, after which the table can be gently readjusted (see Fig. 31-2).

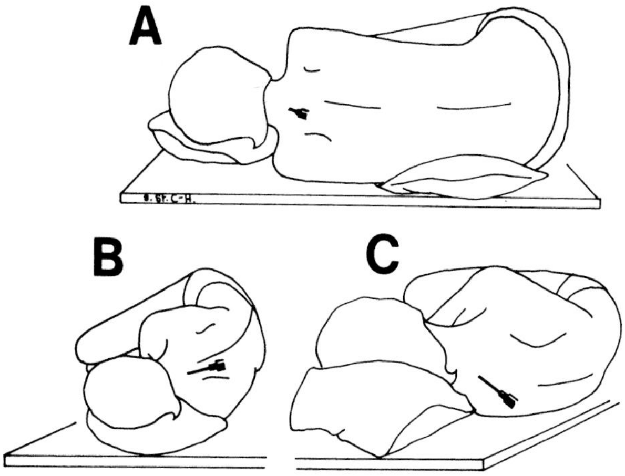

FIG. 31-2. Positioning of the patient for a cervical subarachnoid injection. **A:** Posterior view. **B:** Lateral-prone position used for the injection of absolute alcohol. **C:** Lateral-supine position used for the injection of hyperbaric solutions.

Thoracic Subarachnoid Neurolysis

The approaches to high and low thoracic intraspinal injections are relatively straightforward and are similar to those employed for cervical and lumbar puncture, respectively. The architecture of the midthoracic spine's posterior elements often renders access to the theca difficult at this level. The thoracic spinous processes are elongated and project from the column at an acute angle (see Chapter 8, Fig. 8-13), and as a result, overlapping adjacent processes may render it difficult to introduce a needle into the subarachnoid space. This difficulty may be obviated by adopting a paramedian approach (see Chapter 8, Fig. 8-30). If the desired interspace still cannot be accessed, an attempt may be made one to two segments above or below. If successful, the table is tilted to direct the injectate toward the roots subserving the painful region, and neurolysis can be cautiously initiated.

Relative to the rest of the cord, the midthoracic region is relatively distant from the fibers that subserve limb, bowel, and bladder function, and as a result neurolysis is, overall, safest in this region (Figs. 31-1 and 31-3 to 31-5). Although selective sensory effects are never guaranteed owing to the potential for drug spilling onto anterior motor roots, if segmental unilateral paresis of the intercostal muscles occurs, it rarely embarasses ventilation. Occasionally, a functional hernia develops which, though inconvenient, can be managed with an abdominal binder. Greater caution should be exercised when the upper or lower thoracic roots are targeted.

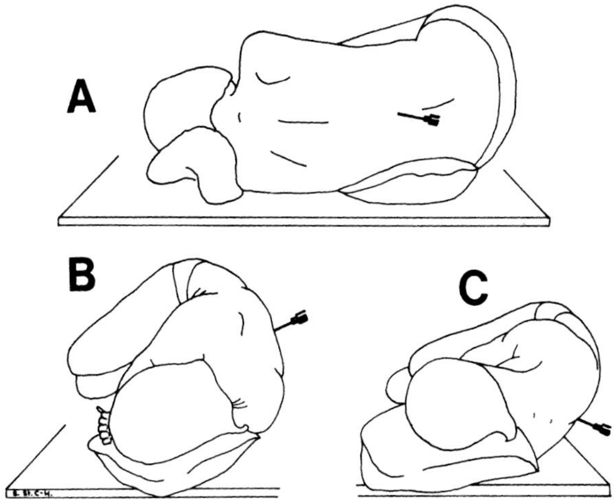

FIG. 31-3. Positioning for the patient for subarachnoid injection in the thoracolumbar region **A:** Posterior view. **B:** Lateral-prone position used for the injection of absolute alcohol. **C:** Lateral-supine position used for the injection of hyperbaric solutions.

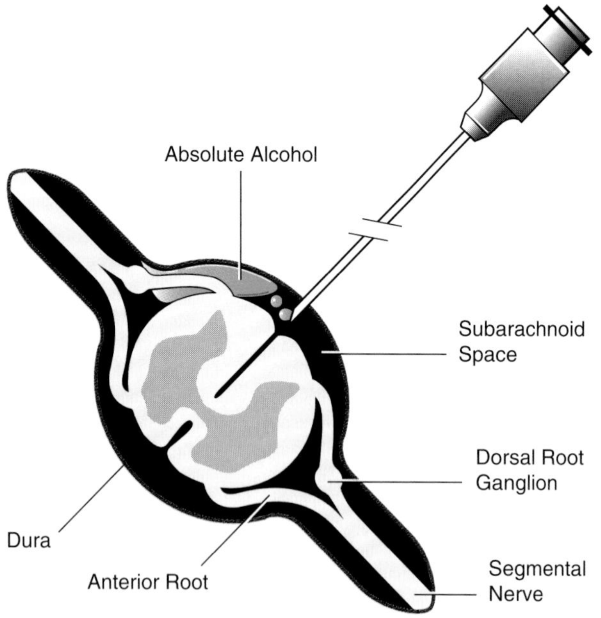

FIG. 31-4. Lateral prone position used for intrathecal injection of absolute alcohol.

Lumbar Subarachnoid Neurolysis

Because of the proximity of fibers subserving pain and lower limb, bowel, and bladder function, lumbar subarachnoid neurolysis is ill-advised except in carefully selected circumstances. In patients with unilateral limb pain, normal strength, and intact bowel and bladder function, percutaneous cordotomy is preferred. If cordotomy is not feasible and lower extremity strength is already compromised, lumbar neurolysis may be carried out cautiously, albeit with a risk of increased weakness of the affected extremity, contralateral weakness, and sphincter disturbances. Incontinence usually, though not consistently, can be avoided by combining careful positioning and modest volumes. In patients with normal strength but impaired ambulation secondary to intractable pain, function may improve even if motor weakness ensues, although this outcome cannot be predicted with certainty. In patients already confined to bed owing to neurologic or systemic effects of cancer, lumbar neurolysis can be performed more freely. The bedbound patient with a urinary diversion and colostomy is subject to insignificant risks. Bedbound patients with intact sphincter function are more likely to accept the modest risk of incontinence than their ambulatory counterparts. In most series, urinary difficulties occur infrequently, and usually are transient, while incontinence of stool is even more rare.

Lumbosacral Neurolysis (Saddle Block)

Perineal hypalgesia can be produced reliably and easily with phenol saddle block, making it an excellent option for midline pain due to rectal and pelvic malignancies in selected patients. Incontinence is relatively common, and as is the case after lumbar block, the incidence of urinary dysfunction exceeds bowel problems, and effects are usually but not always transient. Nevertheless, saddle block is usually avoided in patients with normal sphincters. Superior hypogastric plexus or ganglion impar blocks can be considered when pain is of sympathetic origin, and blocks of the individual sacral nerve roots as they emerge from their foramina are preferred for somatic pain.

Lumbosacral Subarachnoid Phenol Injection (Saddle Block)

The technique is fairly simple, but can be made even more so with adequate preparation. The block is performed with the patient seated and simply requires lumbar puncture at the L5–S1 (or L4–L5) interspace (Fig. 31-6). The bevel of the needle is directed downward, and the needle's caliber must be sufficient to allow easy passage of hyperbaric phenol (20- or 22-gauge). Ultimately, before commencing phenol administration, the patient is inclined 45 degrees backward, a position that is nearly impossible to maintain without support. This difficulty can be overcome by positioning the patient backward on a stool so that its back rest can be held by the patient with both arms. Once the needle is in place, the stool can be moved toward a wall equipped with a safety railing; the railing supports the upper part of the patient's back, while the space between the railing and wall leaves room to connect a syringe and perform the injection. This position is intended to ensure that the hyperbaric phenol is deposited preferentially on the posterior (sensory) roots, and must be

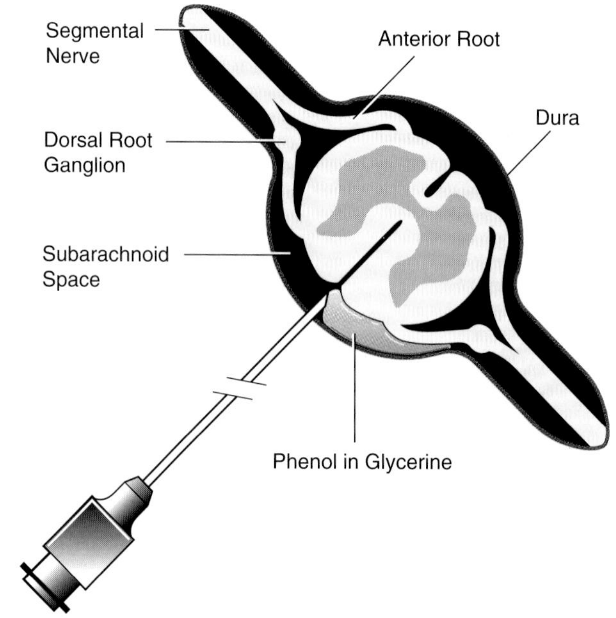

FIG. 31-5. Lateral supine position used for intrathecal injection of phenol.

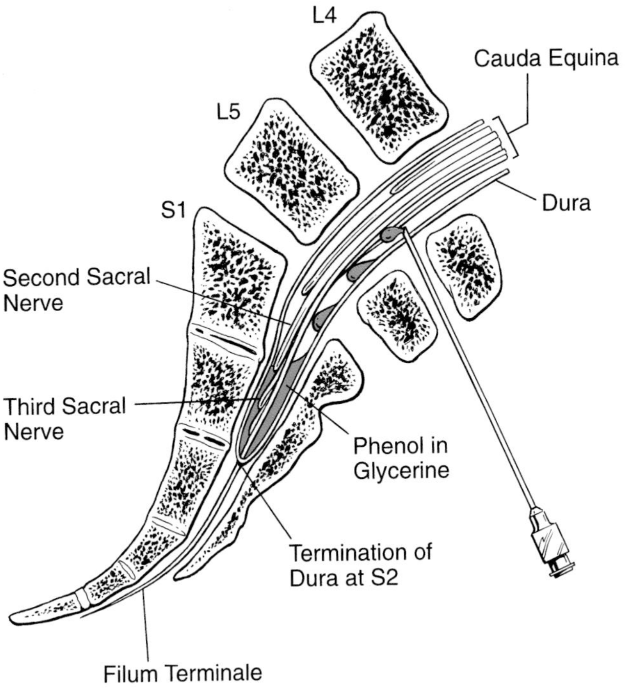

FIG. 31-6. Saddle block with phenol and other hyperbaric solutions is used in the treatment of midline perineal pain of malignant origin.

maintained for about 15 minutes after the injection is complete. Patients usually begin to experience pain relief after the first drops of drug is administered. Sensory testing of the perineum is somewhat difficult because of the patient's seated position, but still must be performed serially, along with tests of lower extremity strength. Administering up to 1.2 ml of 5% phenol, Stovner and Endressen[331] encountered six cases of urinary incontinence and two of bowel incontinence, none of which persisted beyond 10 days. In another series that used 1 ml of 10% phenol,[185] urinary incontinence occurred after 22% of 133 blocks, but resolved within 3 to 7 days in all but two patients. Using 0.8 ml of 5%, 10%, or 15% phenol, Ischia et al.[143] observed both progressively better pain relief and higher incidences of incontinence with stronger solutions. In a subsequent series,[142] utilizing 0.6 to 1 ml of 7.5%, 10%, and 15% phenol, better efficacy was again observed with more concentrated formulations, and one-third of patients with intact urinary function experienced incontinence. Urinary incontinence was observed only in males in the latter series, and neither fecal incontinence nor leg weakness occurred in either series. Their recommendation is to use stronger concentrations, especially when urinary diversion is already present.

In patients with normal bladder and bowel function in whom alternate procedures are inappropriate, the position may be modified by placing padding beneath the buttock that corresponds to the least painful side. Although perineal pain usually crosses the midline, it is often vague, and "bilateral" pain is sometimes eliminated with a predominantly unilateral block on the most affected side. If pain persists, the alternate side can be blocked after an interval of a few days.

Lumbosacral Subarachnoid Alcohol Injection

Because it is so straightforward, phenol saddle block is preferred for perineal pain, although alcohol can be used for the rare patient who cannot sit because of severe pain. The considerations for using alcohol are similar to those described for phenol. Because patients must assume a "jacknife position" (buttocks elevated), difficulty in obtaining a free flow of CSF sometimes arises. Bilateral pain can be treated by having the patient adopt a prone position or, if sphincter function is a concern, padding can be placed beneath the most painful side, and a contralateral injection can be performed on another occasion, if it is still indicated.

"Chemical Cordectomy"

In their classic treatises on regional block, Moore[231] and Bonica[17] refer to so-called alcohol "cordectomy," induced by injecting large volumes (10 ml) of absolute alcohol intrathecally, but little detail or outcome data are provided. This technique has been used mostly to treat refractory severe muscle spasm after spinal cord injury, but occasionally to treat pain of malignant origin. Autopsies performed on patients treated with 4 to 8 ml of intrathecal alcohol for spasticity, though, suggest that results are due to lesions involving the spinal roots rather than the cord.[133] Posterior nerve root degeneration, which was present in all cases, exceeded more limited effects observed on the anterior roots. Evidence of myelitis was limited to a characteristic zone of myelination and gliosis rimming the cord's periphery. Leptomeningeal changes were manifest as fibrosis of the pia and arachnoid, but the dura and major blood vessels were unaffected. Their observation that pathology was similar in patients administered 4 and 8 ml of alcohol led them to conclude that further benefit was unlikely to accompany the administration of larger volumes.

Bruno[33] administered 10 to 12 ml of absolute alcohol intrathecally to 42 paraplegic patients with good results, overall. He injected 2 ml per minute at or below the L1 level in patients positioned with the targeted roots uppermost, but tilted backwards to maximize motor effects. He reported considerable functional improvement, with easier positioning, mobilization, facilitation of physical therapy, and decreased bladder spasm. Complications were limited to three cases of immediate flushing, dizziness and nausea, and occasional postural headache. The authors have utilized injections of large volumes of subarachnoid alcohol (so-called "cordectomy") on six occasions with excellent results (unpublished data). Each patient was already bedbound and incontinent, and suffered from extensive lower extremity and back pain due to malignancy. The administration of 10 ml of alcohol was well tolerated in all cases, and reduced pain and spasm considerably without affecting upper extremity function.

Overall Results for Subarachnoid Neurolysis

Interpretation of the results of the clinical series published over the last few decades is difficult due to variations in investigators' techniques, a lack of uniformity in methods of reporting outcome, and highly varied provision of detail. Notwithstanding these difficulties, Table 31-7 summarizes the pertinent details of several important studies. Studies have not thoroughly evaluated the influence of mechanistic or pathologic factors on efficacy, although a few general statements may be made. Investigators have reported inadequate results in pain due to herpes zoster, lymphedema, and phantom limb pain.[331] Some early investigators reported that patients with longstanding pain were less likely to achieve favorable results, postulating failure due to sheltering of the targeted roots by tumor or inflammation.[203,204,331] This finding has not been uniformly recognized,[76] suggesting that these outcomes may also be due to a failure to address prolonged suffering or recognize physical dependency on opioids. Papo and Visca[252] noted early recurrences to be more common in patients treated for upper limb pain, high rates of failure for abdominal visceral pain, and especially favorable results for pelvic and saddle pain. In a careful review of the published experience with nonmalignant pain, Papo and Visca[251] conclude "... the results are not encouraging, and the indications, if any, for the method in this area are extremely limited."

Pain Relief

While subarachnoid neurolysis is not technically difficult, attention to detail and experience undoubtedly influence outcome. In the hands of experts, results for alcohol and phenol neurolysis seem to be similar,[337] with excellent-to-good results typically reported in 1/2 to 2/3 of patients.[121,142,143,185,203,207,232,252,331] In a literature review of over 2000 cases of subarachnoid alcohol neurolysis, Gerbershagen[99] reported good results in 60%, fair results in 21%, and poor results in 19%. Similarly, in a review of 2500 cases from 13 published seriesof intrathecal phenol neurolysis, Swerdlow noted good relief in 58%, fair relief in 21%, and little or no relief in 20%.[340]

Duration

Unfortunately, though not well characterized by all investigators, duration of relief is highly variable. Although there is no evidence from controlled trials that duration of relief differs for alcohol or phenol, clinical experience suggests that the effects of the former are often more lasting.[46] Using alcohol, Perese[272] reported greater than 6 months' duration in half of 57 patients who obtained initial relief. Using phenol, Lifschitz[185] documented 1 to 2 months' relief in 52%, greater than 2 months' duration in 27%, and less than 2 weeks in 14%. Based on their review of large numbers of reports, Hay[121] and Gerbershagen[99] suggest that, overall, the average duration of relief is 4 months.

Most studies report a moderate proportion of patients who experience excellent relief of just a few days duration, a phenomenon that is most likely due to technical failure from ei-

TABLE 31-7. *Results and technical details from selected case series on subarachnoid neurolysis[a]*

		Drug			Root/	No.	No.	Region				Results		
Ref[b]	Yr[c]	A/P	Conc	Vol (ml)	Vert	Pts	Blks	C	Th	L	LS	Exc	Fair	Poor
173	1958	Alc	100%	1	R	70	119	16	43	60	—	59%	37%	4%
179	1972	Ph	5%	1–1.5		49	73		12	37		37%	10%	54%
168	1962	Alc	100%	1–3	R	252	407	27	75	150	—	46%	32%	22%
183	1984	Ph	5%	.8		20	29	—	—	—	29	35%		65%
		Ph	10%	.8	n/a	15	16	—	—	—	16	80%		20%
		Ph	12%	.8		11	11	—	—	—	11	82%		18%
75	1984	Ph	7.5%	.6–1		8	9	—	—	—	9	25%	13%	62%
		Ph	10%	.6–1	n/a	10	12	—	—	—	12	50%	30%	20%
		Ph	15%	.6–1		15	19	—	—	—	19	60%	20%	20%
176	1976	Ph	10%	1	R	90	133	—	—	133		43%	47%	10%
181	1962	Ph	5%	1	R	30	30	—	6	24	—	30%	40%	30%
182	1979	Ph	5%	—	—	290	—	21	138	52	49	40%	35%	25%
175	1972	Ph	5%	.3–2	R	151	313	5	116	18	12	77%		23%

Ref, reference number; Yr, year of publication; A/P, alcohol or phenol; Alc, alcohol; Ph, phenol (phenol + glycerine); Root/Vert (R/V), injection performed at root or vertebral level; No. Pts, number of patients treated; No. Blks, number of blocks performed; Region: C, cervical, T, thoracic, L, lumbar, LS, lumbosacral.

[a] Due to use of varied terminology in referenced articles, some interpretation was necessary (*e.g.*, authors' reference to " moderate" and "fair" results assumed to connote similar meaning). Refer to references for details.

[b] Despite publication dates, reports necessarily reflect practice patterns of at least several years prior to publication, especially for large case series.

[c] Shaded areas indicate either absent data or unclear explanation of parameters.

ther blockade of too few segments or the use of a neurolytic agent of insufficient strength. The preliminary local anesthetic effect of phenol, which quickly fades, may initially suggest a slightly more ample extension of effect than ultimately encountered. If clinically indicated, it is reasonable, especially when using phenol, to treat initially with the intent of extending the upper and lower limits of hypalgesia one segment beyond the targeted dermatomes. In a comparison of the results of subarachnoid neurolysis with 5% to 15% phenol, Ischia et al.[142,143] noted better outcomes and longer durations of relief in patients treated with more concentrated solutions. It is reasonable to consider repetition in cases of early failure, with consideration for modifying the agent, its concentration, and/or its volume. Although it is atypical, most studies also report a small proportion of patients who experience relief of greater than one year's duration.[99,252]

Complications

Complications vary according to a variety of factors, but especially patient selection, the site that is blocked, and technical aspects. Although some older literature reports high rates, in recent series significant complications present at 1 month follow-up can be found in about 2% of patients.[99] In a review of 1478 subarachnoid alcohol blocks, Gerbeshagen[99] reported transient complications in 12% of patients and permanent complications in 2%. In 2125 alcohol blocks performed in 1478 patients, of 232 complications, the duration was as follows: 28% resolved within 3 days, 23% within 1 week, 21% within 1 month, 9% within 4 months, and only 18% lasted longer than 4 months.[99]

Other than self-limited back pain, the most significant minor complication is postdural puncture headache, which seems to occur less frequently than with local anesthetic blocks, despite the use of large-bore needles.[269] Major complications are mostly neurologic, and depending on their severity and duration and the patient's overall condition, these can range from annoying to devastating in effect (see also Chapter 22).

Unanticipated Complications. When providing informed consent, it is perhaps most useful to refer to significant complications as either expected or unexpected. A modest incidence of regional neurologic complications that varies with the site of injection (see following) is anticipated, but in addition, in a minute proportion of patients, devastating neurologic deterioration may occur from unexpected complications due to spinal artery injury, herniation, or injection near a metastasis.[189,268,338] Citing two cases of paraparesis after cervicothoracic subarachnoid neurolysis, Lipton recommends ensuring free flow of CSF before commencing neurolysis, and warns of increased risks in patients with superior sulcus (Pancoast) tumor, which often extends into the contiguous epidural space.[189] Patients with complete obstruction of the subarachnoid space are at risk for neurologic deterioration if dural puncture and removal of CSF is undertaken distal to the obstruction, due to downward traction on the medulla. The phenomena is refelected in a review of 100 patients with complete spinal block: no morbidity occurred in 50 patients undergoing C1–C2 myelography, whereas 7 of 50 patients deteriorated after a lumbar approach was undertaken.[130]

Anticipated Complications. All patients should be warned of the potential for numbness in the painful dermatomes, although this is usually gratefully accepted in exchange for pain. Most often, however, pain relief is accompanied by a mildly dull sensation (hypalgesia) and only rarely, complete anesthesia or anesthesia dolorosa (painful dysesthesia) ensues. Although attention to careful positioning, titration to effect, and respect for upper dose limits limits spread of the neurolytic agent to anterior motor roots, a small proportion of patients will experience regional, usually unilateral, motor weakness. The true incidence of weakness is often difficult to determine since pretreatment pain often interferes with the accuracy of neurologic testing. Even in the presence of weakness, patients may report increased functional capacity, since splinting due to pain may diminish.

Thoracic subarachnoid neurolysis is associated with a low incidence of complications since the site of injection is distant from the outflow of motor fibers to the limbs and sphincters, and intercostal weakness, should it occur, is usually well tolerated. A single case of a severe pneumothorax has recently been reported.[268]

Subarachnoid neurolysis undertaken in the cervical and lumbar regions is associated with moderate risks of limb paresis. The risk seems to be greater in the lumbar region, perhaps because nerve roots are grouped closely between the levels of T11 and L1 spinous processes (Fig. 31-1). Lumbar neurolysis should be carried out cautiously, if at all, in patients with intact lower extremity strength, but it is generally well tolerated in patients who are bedbound. Bowel and bladder complications are infrequent when leg pain is being treated, especially if the injection is undertaken at the low thoracic level where the lumbar roots exit the cord. Lumbosacral neurolysis, whether performed as a saddle block or in the jacknife position, is associated with significant risks of bowel and bladder difficulties. Bladder function is more commonly affected,[331] and although incontinence is usually transient it is often demoralizing, and so normal urinary function is usually regarded a relative contraindication to lumbosacral neurolysis.

Hypertonic and Isotonic Saline

Subarachnoid Saline

This technique, which was introduced in the 1960s by Hitchcock, enjoyed transient popularity and subsequently has been almost entirely abandoned. The original technique involved the removal of large volumes of CSF, which were replaced by similar volumes of iced isotonic saline.[126] Observations that thawing isotonic saline produced a hypertonic supernatant led to the development of a more accepted modification that substituted normothermic hypertonic (12%–15%) saline and did not involve removal of significant volumes of CSF.[127] Although the mechanisms of pain relief are unclear, postmortem studies after iced saline infusion have demonstrated areas of peripheral demyelination in the cord and brain stem.[190]

General anesthesia is required to ameliorate the severe pain that follows injection and to facilitate safe recovery. Treatment is frequently followed by fasciculations, piloerection, venostasis, and cyanosis of the lower limbs. Tachypnea and hypertension are common responses, and the use of potent antihypertensives has been advocated to limit morbidity.[126] Although Hitchcock[127] and others have reported favorable results, morbidity is significant.[197,349] A survey reporting on 2105 patients treated with normothermic hypertonic saline or iced isotonic saline injection revealed a 10.6% incidence of adverse outcomes, of which muscle spasm, blood pressure changes, and seizure were most prominent, but which also included para- or quadriplegia in 22 patients and two deaths from myocardial infarction.

Epidural Hypertonic Saline

The epidural administration of hypertonic saline is used as a component of a procedure advocated by Racz and others for the relief of back and radicular pain due to epidural fibrosis and scarring.[280] The procedure involves placement of a specialized epidural catheter (Racz catheter) near the site of scarring and serial injections of contrast dye, local anesthetic, corticosteroid, and 10% saline, often on a daily basis. Although widespread trials have not been carried out, treatment seems to be relatively safe and effective. In this setting, hypertonic saline is postulated to act not as a neurolytic agent, but as an osmotic means to reduce local swelling and pressure by driving water out of cells.

Epidural Neurolysis

Given that the epidural route is in such wide use by contemporary anesthesiologists, it is surprising that there have been relatively few reports on epidural neurolysis. After numerous anecdotal reports, early investigators became disenchanted with epidural neurolysis owing either to pain on injection (alcohol) or to disappointing results (phenol).[340] Lack of efficacy of early "single shot" techniques relative to subarachnoid injections presumably relates to reduced contact of the neurolytic with the targeted nerves due to the barrier to diffusion presented by the dura.

There has been a resurgence of interest in epidural neurolysis over the last decade, primarily related to technical modifications that appear to be associated with improved results. The main change has been to substitute serial instillations of dilute phenol through a percutaneous catheter for a single-shot injection. Although treatment has been associated with few adverse neurologic sequelae, a recent study of 6% to 12% epidural phenol in monkeys suggests the potential for considerable damage to the posterior and anterior roots, as well as parts of the cord.[109] In light of these findings, repeated treatments with dilute concentrations would seem to be most prudent.

Brechner[80] reported on 12 cancer patients treated with single-shot epidural injections of 10% phenol. Volumes were based on the volume requirement for analgesia with epidural lidocaine to a maximum of 8 ml. Results were good and fair in one-third and one-half of patients, respectively, and one case each of urinary incontinence and leg weakness occurred. These disappointing results emphasize the rationale for consideration of serial injections of low volumes of dilute phenol. Korevaar[169] administered alcohol to 36 patients on three successive days via an indwelling catheter and reported an 89% incidence of greater than 70% relief, averaging a mean of 3.3 months and until death in 20 patients. Few serious side effects were reported. Racz[279,282] employs a specially designed catheter formulated from spiraled stainless steel coils coated with fluoropolymers designed to facilitate radiologic localization, aspiration, and repositioning. The catheter is advanced through a specially designed nonshearing needle under fluoroscopy until the desired spinal level is reached, and doses of 2.5 to 5.0 ml of 5.5% phenol in saline are injected daily until complete or nearly complete relief is obtained for 24 hours. The procedure is halted if signs of motor involvement appear at any stage. He reported significant benefit in 70% of a mixed population of 60 patients that lasted less than one month in about 50% and 2 to 6 months in the remainder. Best results were achieved in patients with cancer pain or spasticity, and no complications were reported. Using a similar technique (2–6 daily injections of 2 to 4 ml 5% phenol and glycerine), Salmon et al.[300] obtained good relief in 93% of 16 patients (duration unspecified) with no serious complications. Jain and co-workers[149] employed three daily 5-ml transcatheter injections of 5% epidural phenol in water to relieve extensive neoplastic chest wall pain, and in a preliminary report, three of seven patients experienced complete relief and four moderate relief. As an alternative to daily injections, others have successfully performed serial epidural neurolysis after allowing an interval of hours to elapse (Plancarte, R., personal communication, 1994).[357] A special use of epidural neurolysis has been recommended by Doughty.[381] He administers 10% phenol in glycerine epidurally at the level of T12 to L1 to relieve attacks of tenesmus and burning pain in rectal cancer.

Epidural Neurolysis: Technique

The patient is positioned on the painful side in a 45-degree posterior tilt, as for intrathecal phenol block. After antiseptic skin preparation and infiltration of the skin and pertinent interspace with local anesthesia, an epidural needle is introduced into the epidural space and an epidural catheter is threaded under image-intensifier control to the level of the middle of the painful dermatomes. Because of the relatively large volume of solution that is employed, accidental intrathecal injection must be carefully excluded, ideally with the injection of a small amount of nonionic contrast medium to confirm appropriate spread in the epidural space. Some workers recommend use of a small volume of local anesthetic test dose such as 2.0 ml 1% lidocaine, in which case a period of 2 hours or more should be allowed for its effects to dissipate before administering phenol. On the basis of nuclear medicine studies[300] that suggest that the spread of epidural phenol and glycerine may be extensive and variable (mean of 13 segments/3 ml with a range of 6–23), volumes larger than 3.0 ml should probably be avoided. This study suggested that distribution was unaffected by position, and that the extent of spread was less robust with repeat injections. Volumes of up to 5 ml of phenol in water[149] or saline[340] have, however, been used safely.

If a standard catheter is being used, difficulties may be encountered if a standard viscous glycerine-phenol preparation is employed, even when warmed and administered through a 1-ml syringe. This problem may be overcome by using aqueous phenol or phenol dissolved in a combination of water and glycerine. Because of the vascularity of the epidural space, intravascular placement or migration of the catheter tip should be excluded before each neurolytic injection. Although the influence of gravity is uncertain, if a unilateral block is desired, the patient should be kept on his side for about 40 minutes following completion of the injection. In contrast to subarachnoid injection, the patient usually cannot immediately verify the anatomic localization of the neurolytic solution relative to the affected nerve roots. Pain usually disappears about 10 to 15 minutes after each administration.

Complications of Epidural Neurolysis

Epidural neurolysis is rarely followed by complications other than backache and, after the administration of alcohol, occasionally neuritis. However, both urinary incontinence[80,111] and muscle paresis[80] have been reported. In addition, animal studies[109] suggest the potential for anterior root and cord injury with concentrations of 6% and greater. It is inadvisable to administer epidural injections to patients who are anticoagulated because of the risk of epidural hemorrhage if a vein is injured. Cousins[56] recommends that CT or magnetic resonance imaging (MRI) scan be carried out before performing epidural block to exclude local tumor invasion and the potential for hemorrhage, spinal cord compression, and neurologic injury. Furthermore, distortion of the epidural space by tumor may cause the neurolytic solution to spread unpredictably.

As noted, radiographic confirmation of both the integrity of the catheter, which may be chemically or physically damaged,[51] and the position of its tip in the epidural space is recommended before each neurolytic injection. In addition, owing to anecdotal reports of transient widespread anesthesia when neurolytic injection immediately follows a local anesthetic test dose,[169] it is suggested that a reasonable interval be allowed to elapse between injections, and that the neurolytic agent should be injected slowly.

Advantages Vis-a-Vis Subarachnoid Neurolysis

Theoretically, epidural neurolytic injection has potential advantages over subarachnoid block, particularly for pain with an extensive anatomic/topographic distribution. Risks of spread to the cranial cavity and meningeal irritation are fewer, and the incidence of sphincter dysfunction, motor weakness, and headache may be less, especially when incremental treatment using dilute phenol is administered serially.

Disadvantages Vis-a-Vis Subarachnoid Neurolysis

The above advantages are offset by historical impressions of inferior results for single shot injections. Although further work is needed to characterize the efficacy of serial epidural neurolysis, certain technical aspects favor subarachnoid neurolysis, at least in certain settings.

The main advantage of subarachnoid neurolysis is that it is a relatively simple procedure that can usually be performed on an outpatient basis. While subarachnoid puncture is easily verified by the return of CSF, localization of the epidural space must be inferred from the results of epidurograms or test doses of local anesthetic. Although serial epidural neurolysis appears to be efficacious, it is time consuming, mandates inpatient hospitalization, and requires serial epidurograms. Also, although reports suggest that gravity and position can be partially relied on to control the spread of epidural hyperbaric phenol,[80] these factors can be utilized to exert more precise control for subarachnoid injection. A graded intensity of lesioning may perhaps be accomplished with repeat epidural phenol injections, but localization is better assured with subarachnoid administration.

Further trials of serial epidural neurolysis are indicated before it can be determined that it is reliably associated with actual advantages over intrathecal neurolysis. Meanwhile it is reasonable to employ these methods in suitable cases of malignant pain arising from several dermatomes,[66] particularly if other relevant therapies have been unsuccessful.

Subdural (Interarachnoid) Block

Subdural block, usually regarded as a complication of attempted subarachnoid or epidural block, in which case it is usually manifest as diffuse, spotty anesthesia, is occasionally intentionally sought to relieve cancer pain.[204] Subdural block has been proposed as an alternative to cervical subarachnoid neurolysis, because access is purportedly easier in the cervical region and because it presents dilution from rapidly circulating cranial CSF. As a consequence of its disposition between the dura and arachnoid membranes, subdural injection is undertaken deep to the epidural space, after dural puncture has occurred, but before the return of CSF is noted. The subdural space differs from the epidural space in that anatomic studies suggest that it is not a true potential space and only exists as a consequence of iatrogenic cleaving by injection or bleeding, hence the suggestion that it be referred to as the inter-arachnoid space.[116,306] This combined with its small caliber make intentional subdural injection difficult, and sometimes impossible, and has probably contributed to the infrequent use of blocks in this region. The dura and arachnoid appear to be separated by a thin fluid film and, once injection occurs, by strands of connective tissue, which are responsible for the "honeycombed" appearance of AP contrast studies (see Chapter 7, Figs. 7-6 and 7-8 and Figs. 31-7 and 31-8, this Chapter).

Mehta and Maher[217] advocated locating the cervical epidural space with a short-beveled needle introduced through the midline with a loss of resistance technique. The needle is then slightly advanced and rotated 180° until a sudden increase in resistance heralds subdural placement, which is subsequently confirmed radiologically. Swerdlow recommended the instillation of no more than 3 ml of 5% phenol in glycerine, but noted that relief is usually short-lived.[77] Although the older literature proposes subdural neurolysis as a reasonable option for cervicothoracic pain, its viability in contemporary practice is questionable.

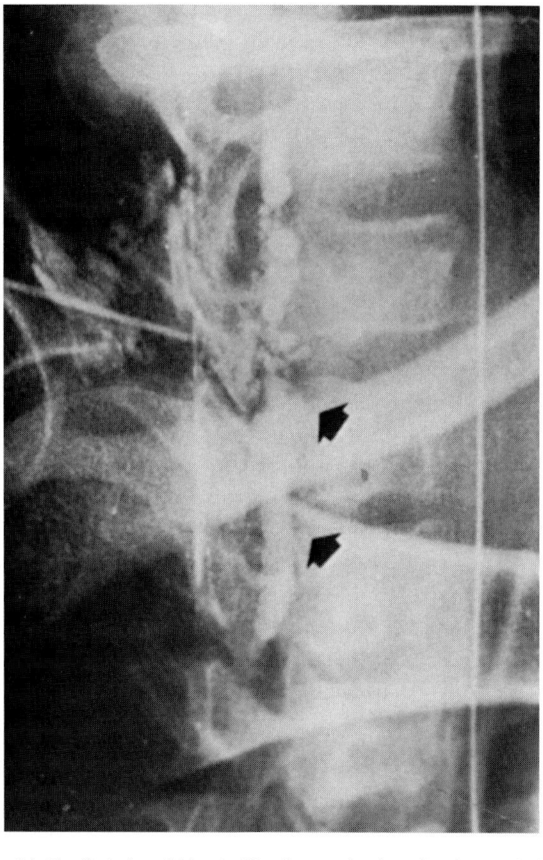

FIG. 31-7. Subdural block. Radiograph showing lateral view. Needletip has been placed in the subdural space and 0.5 ml of iophendylate (Myodil) has been injected. Note the fine line extending up and down from needletip. Also, there is a second broader line *(arrows)* in which contrast medium tends to arrange itself like a "rosary." (From Ischia, S., Maffezzoli, G.F., Luzzani, A., and Pacini, L.: Subdural extra-arachnoid neurolytic block in cervical pain. Pain, *14*:347, 1982)

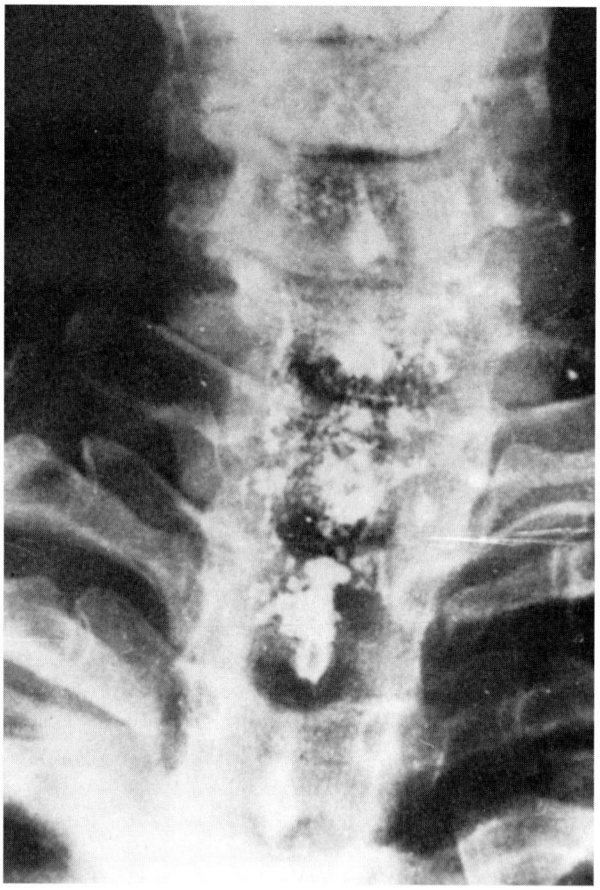

FIG. 31-8. Subdural block. Radiograph showing anteroposterior view after injection of 0.5 ml of Myodil. Note the bilateral spread confined to the interior of the canal, over several segments. The appearance of the contrast medium is like a "nail scratch" shape. (From Ischia, S., Maffezzoli, G.F., Luzzani, A., and Pacini, L.: Subdural extra-arachnoid neurolytic block in cervical pain. Pain, *14*:347, 1982)

Chlorocresol

Chlorocresol (parachlormetacresol), a phenol derivative, was introduced by Maher,[202] in an effort to identify an agent that would selectively damage pain fibers and would more effectively penetrate nerve roots sheltered by tumor or inflammation. Neither property has been confirmed, and although it is occasionally advocated when phenol has failed, contemporary use is infrequent. In an uncontrolled comparison, Swerdlow[341] found both the efficacy and complication rate slightly higher with chlorocresol than with phenol, but concluded that it offered no significant advantage over phenol. The administration of 2% chlorocresol in glycerine is not immediately followed by analgesia, sensory changes, warmth, or numbness, and thus it must be used cautiously, usually in volumes less than 0.5 to 1.0 ml. Treatment is characteristically followed by aching pain for 1 to 2 days, which yields to numbness and hypalgesia that are often more marked than after phenol.

Ammonium Salts

Ammonium salts (ammonium sulfate, ammonium chloride) enjoyed frequent use as neurolytic agents for a time, mostly due to the work of Judovich and Bates.[9,157] These substances were determined to be the active ingredients of the distillate of the carnivorous plant saraccenia purpruea (pitcher plant), and remain available today, formulated as Serapin. Their purported advantages were a selective action on sensory fibers and an absence of post-treatment neuritis. However, since both motor weakness and neuritis have been observed following their use, these properties are doubtful. Both ammonium sulfate and ammonium chloride were used with relative safety and good short-term efficacy for peripheral blocks in 10% concentrations,[226] and, mixed with varying volumes of CSF, in the subarachnoid space. Its proponents claim that when it is used peripherally, neuritis is relatively infrequent. Duration of pain relief, though, is relatively short (days to weeks), and as a result, it is infrequently used to treat cancer pain.[162]

SYMPATHETIC NEUROLYSIS

The sympathetic nervous system is unique in several ways. First, lasting benefit is more likely to be derived from a series of local anesthetic injections than is the case for serial somatic nerve blocks,[98,270,370] often eliminating the need for subsequent neurolysis. Second, because sympathetic nerves do not subserve motor power or sensory innervation of the skin, numbness and weakness do not follow neurolysis which, as a result, tends to be better tolerated than somatic blockade. Finally, although new pain (sympathalgia) may occur after sympathetic neurolysis,[295,354] it is less common and typically less troublesome than after somatic nerve ablation. These factors make sympathetic neurolysis a relatively attractive alternative for patients with pain that is amenable to such procedures (see Chapter 13).

Evolving Targets of Neurolysis

The targets of sympathetic neural blockade classically have tended to include the stellate (cervicothoracic) ganglion, celiac plexus, and lumbar sympathetic chain. Thoracic sympathetic ganglion blocks are less commonly undertaken because of the risks of pneumothorax and injury to adjacent somatic nerve roots, combined with the ease with which similar analgesia can be achieved with stellate ganglion or epidural block. Stellate ganglion neurolysis, once uniformly avoided due to concerns regarding the spread of neurolytic drugs to neighboring structures, has recently been advocated by means of radiofrequency thermocoagulation[100,316] and a modified chemical approach.[281] In addition, over the last decade, percutaneous approaches to the superior hypogastric plexus[63,275] and ganglion impar,[273,276] the most caudad portion of the sympathetic chain, have been introduced.

Stellate Ganglion Neurolysis

Stellate ganglion block with local anesthetics may provide meaningful, though usually temporary, relief from sympathetically mediated pain in the head, neck and upper extremity. If a diagnostic block reduces pain, persistent relief can often be achieved from administering a series of local anesthetic injections which, because of documented ease and safety, is preferred to neurolysis.[270] Successful relief of brachialgia with a single local anesthetic stellate injection in three of 15 patients with lung cancer has been reported by Warfield.[370] The cervical sympathetic chain is not closely confined within a fascial space, and as a result, neurolysis is associated with the potential for injury to adjacent structures (e.g., brachial plexus, superior laryngeal nerve, epidural and subarachnoid nerves, vertebral artery). MRI has demonstrated aberrant and unpredictable spread with routine techniques,[128] and reports of bilateral superior laryngeal block[366] and Horner's syndrome[322] after unilateral injections provide support for these concerns. However, if local anesthetic injections have been documented to provide temporary relief of pain, surgical extirpation of the ganglia may be considered or neurolysis may be performed cautiously, using radiofrequency thermocoagulation or small volumes of dilute phenol injected under fluoroscopic[281] or even CT[129] guidance (see Chapter 13, Figs. 13-18 to 13-20).

Chemical Neurolysis

A variety of techniques have been advocated for stellate ganglion block, of which the anterior paratracheal approach, introduced by LeRiche in 1934[180] (see Chapter 13), is used almost universally. This approach has been modified by Racz and co-workers,[281] who have reported on its successful application with phenol in over 100 patients without serious complications. His group utilizes 3% phenol administered via a modified anterolateral approach under fluoroscopic guidance. Needle entry is at the C7 level, but instead of targeting the transverse process, the ventrolateral aspect of the C7 vertebral body is targeted, purportedly to decrease the risk of injury to pleura, adjacent nerve roots, a dural cuff, or the vertebral artery. This is accomplished by orienting the needle 15 to 30 degrees toward the midline and observing its passage with fluroscopy. Bony contact should occur just medial rather than anterior to the insertion of the longus colli muscle, and the needle is eased back 1 to 2 mm to free its tip from the substance of the anterior longitudinal ligament. The needle is stabilized with a hemostat, and 1 ml of nonionic contrast medium is injected. Racz recommends the injection of 5 ml of phenol, saline, local anesthetic, and steroid mixed to achieve an ultimate concentration of 3% phenol (2.5 ml 6% phenol in saline, 1.5 ml 0.5% bupivicaine, 1 ml 40 mg/ml triamcinalone). Injection should meet minimal resistance, and the margins of the displaced contrast medium should correspond roughly to the extent that the phenol solution has spread. Patients are maintained in the supine position with the head slightly elevated for 30 minutes. In a series of over 100 patients, pain relief and alteration in vasomotor changes accrued rapidly and were relatively long-lasting, although repeated injections (1 to 4, mean of 1.6) were needed, probably because the phenol solution used was relatively dilute. The only adverse sequelae were transient chest wall pain in one patient, transient dysphagia in another, and hoarseness of moderate duration (4 months) in a third.

Radiofrequency Thermocoagulation

This is a relatively new approach to stellate ganglion block that has been described by two investigators for the treatment of reflex sympathetic dystrophy. One group[316] treated nine patients with a 21-volt lesion applied for 60 seconds, rendered with a 23-gauge probe configured with a 5-mm bare tip. Although all patients experienced initial pain relief, in no case was relief maintained beyond 4 months. Of another group of 27 patients who underwent lesioning at the C7 level, 21 experienced complete relief of pain and four partial relief.[100] Although 10 patients required a second treatment, of the 25 responders, 16 were pain-free and 9 were improved one year after their last treatment. Unspecified minor complications occurred, as well as one case of phrenic nerve irritation lasting 2 weeks,[100] and one case of Horner's syndrome of 4 months duration.[316] This would appear to be a valuable technique that requires further investigation.

Thoracic Paravertebral Sympatholysis

Indications

Neural blockade of the thoracic sympathetic ganglia is seldom undertaken because of the potential to achieve pain relief with alternate, safer procedures.[326] Significant hazards include pneumothorax[69] and, due to the absence of an effective fascial barrier between the sympathetic chain and somatic nerve roots, nerve root injury and epidural or subarachnoid injection. Rauck[289] recently reported accidental placement of a 22-gauge needle into the thoracic spinal cord which, though heralded by paresthesias to the leg and chest, was not accompanied by neurologic morbidity. Although stellate ganglion block may provide complete interruption of the sympathetic outflow to the upper limb, the failure of thermographic studies to demonstrate thoracic block after injections of the stellate with up to 20 ml of bupivacaine[120] suggests a continued, though circumscribed, role for thoracic sympathetic block, especially when permanent interruption is indicated, in which case epidural block is insufficiently selective. Thoracic sympathectomy (T2–T4) may be considered for non-bypassable painful circulatory insufficiency and sympathetically maintained upper extremity pain, as well as hyperhidrosis.[289] The thoracic chain may be approached surgically by a dorsal approach (with removal of the heads of the pertinent ribs), by an axillary approach, by a supraclavicular approach (with dissection around the large vessels), and by thoracoscopy.[375] A less invasive approach involves percutaneous radiofrequency lesioning of the thoracic ganglia. Wilkinson[375] describes a technique involving the creation of multiple rostrocaudad lesions per ganglia. Recurrence of pain after one year is not uncommon, however, and pneumothorax may occur.

In a brief report on 30 neurolytic thoracic sympathectomies performed in 20 patients, Ogawa[246] confirmed efficacy for painful circulatory insufficiency (thromboangiitis obliterans, Raynaud's syndrome) and concluded that it was futile for neuropathic disorders, such as brachial plexus avulsion, phantom limb pain, and postherpetic neuralgia. His group blocked the second and third ganglia, from needle insertion sites 4 to 5 cm from the midline at the level of the midportion of the corresponding spinous process. They recommend a loss of resistance technique and the use of fluoroscopy to ensure that contrast spreads neither to the region corresponding to somatic roots nor to the first thoracic vertebra.

Anatomy and Technique

The thoracic sympathetic chain lies posterolateral to the vertebral bodies and anterior to the neck of the ribs. Unlike the sympathetic chain in the cervical and lumbar regions, which is isolated from neighboring somatic roots by the longus colli and psoas muscles, respectively, no effective anatomic barrier exists between the sympathetic and somatic nerves in the thoracic region (see Chapter 13, Fig. 13-21). As a result, extremely precise needle localization and careful limitation of volume is essential to avoid spread to somatic roots and consequent risks of segmental numbness, motor weakness, and dysesthesia. In addition, the thoracic sympathetic chain is related laterally to the pleura and medially to the intervertebral foramina, introducing risks of pneumothorax or accidental subarachnoid or epidural anesthesia from aberrant needle placement.

The posterior, paravertebral approach introduced by Kappis in 1912[161] and modified by Labat,[173] Adriani[4] and Bonica[20] is commonly advocated. The prone position is preferred, but alternatively the lateral decubitus position may be utilized if necessary for comfort. Radiologic guidance is essential, especially for neurolysis. Skin wheals are raised 3 cm lateral to the cephalad aspect of the spinous process of the targeted segment. A 22-gauge 8- to 10-cm needle is initially inserted perpendicular to the skin in all planes until rib or transverse process is contacted, usually at a depth of 2.5 to 3.5 cm. The needle is withdrawn until its tip lies just beneath the skin and is redirected slightly cephalad (see Chapter 13, Fig. 13-21). A saline-filled syringe is attached to the needle's hub, and gentle unremitting or intermittent pressure is applied to its barrel as the needle is reintroduced until its tip impinges on the superior border of the rib. As the needle is slowly advanced beyond the depth at which osseous contact was noted, increased resistance to its passage and attempted injection is noted, corresponding to the superior costotransverse ligament, following which a decrease in resistance indicates that the paravertebral space containing the sympathetic chain has been entered. Passage through the ligament may be heralded by the transmission of a palpable "click," which is amplified by the use of a blunt-tipped or larger-gauge needle. The needle tip lies anterior and inferior to the exiting somatic nerve root. Injected contrast medium should spread freely in the craniocaudad axis and be confined to the paramedian region. After careful aspiration, a test dose of 1 to 3 ml of local anesthetic is administered to exclude subarachnoid, epidural, and somatic nerve root involvement.

Chemical Neurolysis

For chemical neurolysis, 2 to 3 ml of 6% to 10% aqueous phenol is recommended,[289] after which the needle is cleared with air or saline to prevent spillage along its track during removal. In a brief report on 30 neurolytic thoracic sympathectomies performed in 20 patients, Ogawa[246] confirmed efficacy for painful circulatory insufficiency (thromboangiitis obliterans, Raynaud's syndrome), but found the procedure to be futile for neuropathic disorders such as brachial plexus avulsion, phantom limb pain, and postherpetic neuralgia. His group blocked the second and third ganglia, from needle insertion sites 4 to 5 cm from the midline at the level of the midportion of the corresponding spinous process.

Alternatives: Radiofrequency Thermocoagulation and Surgery

Wilkinson[374] describes a radiofrequency technique involving placement of up to six lesions per ganglion. He recommends initially creating a "reversible" block by heating the electrode tip to 60°C for 60 seconds, checking for an absence of Horner's syndrome and the presence of denervation, followed by a 3-minute cycle at 90°C. He achieved good to excellent results in 18 of 19 patients at 22 months' follow-up.

Surgical sympathectomy can be carried out by a dorsal approach (with removal of the heads of the pertinent ribs), an axillary approach, a supraclavicular approach (with dissection around the large vessels), and by thoracoscopy.[374,375]

CELIAC PLEXUS NEUROLYSIS

Celiac plexus block is among the most effective and most commonly utilized nerve blocks performed to provide prolonged relief of cancer pain. Despite its many historical applications,[56] in contemporary practice it is most often used to treat abdominal and referred back pain secondary to pancreatic[28,85,140,168,325] and other intra-abdominal malignancies.[29,154] Most clinical series describe the role of celiac block in patients with pain due to a variety of upper abdominal malignancies.[112,125,171,177,185,229,236,305,359] Fewer series include patients with chronic disorders such as pancreatitis,[15,35,82,102,105,122,123,132,181,351] almost invariably with inferior results; thus its role in such conditions is less certain.[31] The use of local anesthetic and/or steroid celiac blocks is discussed in Chapter 14 (see also Figs. 14-5 to 14-7).

Despite its anatomic disposition—virtually in the body's epicenter, surrounded by major organs such as the aorta, vena cava, kidneys, and pleura—and the customary use of large volumes of potent neurolytic solutions, complications are infrequent (Table 31-8). Widespread acceptance of the need for radiologic guidance and modifications of classic techniques have contributed to celiac block's safety. Despite well-founded criticism that early studies lacked adequate detail and suffered from design problems, there is no question that celiac axis neurolysis is effective in a high proportion of patients (Table 31-8). Though controlled trials are indicated to better determine the optimal timing and technique for celiac block, ample clinical experience and a decidedly favorable risk:benefit ratio support a more prominent role early in the course of treatment (Table 31-9).

Choice of Agent, Volume, Needle, Technique, and Radiographic Guidance

Authorities recommend different anatomic approaches to celiac block (e.g., retrocrural, transcrural, transaortic, transdiscal, splanchnic, anterior, intraoperative), various techniques (e.g., one to four needles positioned based on anatomic landmarks alone, plain radiography, fluoroscopy, sonography, and CT), and the use of various volumes and agents (e.g., 15 to 50 ml of 50% to 100% alcohol or 6% to 8% phenol) (Table 31-8). Studies comparing the efficacy of these alternatives are unavailable, or poorly controlled, or inconclusive, and as a result the choice of technique ultimately should be individualized based on available resources, the patient's physical status, the pattern of tumor spread, and the clinician's experience.

Following a general discussion of the indications, efficacy, and safety of celiac neurolysis, a detailed description of each technique is provided that includes reference to its advantages and disadvantages. The outcomes of clinical series and controlled trials are summarized in Table 31-8, which, given the few controlled trials that exist, is necessarily extensive in order to summarize the plethora of anecdotal data in the literature. This section concludes with a summary of factors pertinent to the selection of a technique.

Indications

The celiac plexus contributes to the innervation of all the intra-abdominal viscera derived from embryonic foregut, in-

TABLE 31-8. *Results and technical details from selected case series on celiac plexus neurolysis*[a]

Ref No.	No. pts	No. blks	Indication	Results (expressed as number/percent)[b] Good	Fair	Poor	Technique[c,d]	Design[e]	Complications
229	87	87	Mixed ca. Pancreatitis	54/62%	21/24%	12/14%		Abstract	hypotension "most common;" diarrhea–10; ileus–4; convulsion–1; local spinal–1
236	44	44	Mixed cancer	Immediate–95%; 30 d–85%; 90 d–50%; 120 d–20%			No guidance; 30–50 ml; 8 unilateral	Abstract	dural puncture-1; arterial puncture–4; transient neuralgia–1; renal puncture–1
112	21		Mixed cancer	18/86%; 25/50 PF until death	9/18%	1/2%	40 ml	Abstract	
	29	57		22/79%; 25/50 PF until death			20 ml 8% aqueous phenol		
					recurrence–10/50 at 107 d (mean); repeated in 7/50–all PF until death				
171	69	72	Mixed cancer	58/84%; 34/69 PF until death	28/41%	7/10%		Abstract	1 permanent paraplegia after repeat–(? cord infarct)
186	20	20	Pancreas cancer	20/100% PF × 3.3 mos (mean), recurrence of pain before death in 13 (65%)			Intraoperative; 20 ml 50% alcohol	Placebo control	2 transient hypertension; no ileus, gastroparesis or hypotension
	45			prophylactic		mean PF period of 7.2 mos compared to 3 mos in placebo group			Double-blind
229	168	186	Mixed ca.	157/94%		11/6%			dural puncture in 18/3000 (.006%)
29	66	75	Nonpanc cancer	48/73%		18/17%			1 permanent foot drop 2 temporary neurologic (local)
177	67	67	Mixed ca. outpatients				12–20 ml 100% alcohol	Abstract	3 orthostasis; 3 nausea; 2 lightheaded; 1 chest pain/SOB; 1 diarrhea
28	136	156	Pancreas cancer	116/85%–(75% until death, 12.5%–½ survival time)		20/15%	39% plain films 1% fluoro, 6% CT, 40% no guidance		2 pneumothorax, 1 dural puncture, 1 congestive heart failure, 1 epidural anesthesia, 10 orthostasis
168	3	3	Pancreas cancer	3/100% complete			bilat transdiscal 20–40 ml 100%	Abstract	
359	33	37	Mixed ca	31; 30 PF until death	0	2	CT	Prosp	49% backache; 24% orthostasis; 18% diarrhea; 1 L 1 neuralgia
351	100	114	Mixed	94/94% (60/100 "lasting")	poor-6/6% (all pancreatitis, n = 3)		no guidance		1 unilateral paraplegia-obese patient in lateral position
220	10	10	Pancreas ca	10/100% (until death)		0	75% alcohol	Comp	1 diarrhea, 2 orthostasis, 1 back pain
90	21	30	Mixed ca	18 (3–5 d)	2	1	CT, 30 ml 100%	Comp	Hypotension ×3; transient sweating, burning & shoulder pain common
	3			2 (3–5 d)	1 (3–5 d)	0 (3–5 d)	CT, TC, 30 ml 100%		
	3			1 (3–5 d)	2 (3–5 d)	0 (3–5 d)	TC/RC, 30 ml 100%		
	3 rpt			2 (3–5 d)	1 (3–5 d)	0 (3–5 d)	CT, unilat, 15 ml 100%		
105	8	8	Mixed ca	8	1		transcatheter		3 back & 1 thigh pain, 2 hypotension
102	38	38	Mixed	1 wk 23/61% 6 mos 23/61% 1 yr 12/39%	1 wk 12/32% 6 m 12/32% 1 yr 16/52%	3/8% 3/8% 3/10%	anterior, US, 30–40 ml 50%, 1 needle	Prosp	5 mild diarrhea 1 "retroperitoneal" pain
123	25		Mixed ca	2 wk–15/60% 8 wk–5/60%	2 wk–7/28% 8 wk–10/40%	2 wk–3/12% 8 wk–10/40%	all CT guided 15–ant-up to		
	3	38	Pancreatitis	2 wk–2/66% 8 wk–1/33%	2 wk–1/33% 8 wk–2/66%	2 wk–0 8 wk–0	80 ml 100% 5–splanchnic-		1 persistent disabling diarrhea
			Unknown	2 wk–1/50% 8 wk–1/50%	2 wk–0 8 wk–0	2 wk–1/50% 8 wk–1/50%	50 ml 80%		
122	36	36	Pancreas ca	16/44%	16/44%	4/11%	80 ml 25%		
	9	9	Pancreatitis	3 mo–3/33%	3 mo–2/22%	3 mo–4/44%			4-transient hypotension

(continued)

TABLE 31-8. *Continued.*

Ref No.	No. pts	No. blks	Indication	Results (expressed as number/percent)[b] Good	Fair	Poor	Technique[c,d]	Design[e]	Complications
35	11	14	Mixed	2 wk–5/36%	2 wk–8/57%	2 wk–2/14%	CT, retro & transcrural 40–50 ml 90%		
82	12	15	Mixed	5/42%	4/33%	3/25%	unilateral, CT, 40–50 ml	Prosp	1 transient shoulder pain 1 transient pleuritic pain
15	100	113	Mixed	PVD 7/36%; pancreatitis 10/64%; pancreas ca 13/70%; other ca 25/70%; misc 2/15%	6/31% 1/4% 5/30% 6/17% 4/31%	7/33% 5/32% 0 5/13% 6/54%	40–45 ml 100%		8 lumbar neuralgia; 3 chest pain; 2 othostassis; 2 ejaculatory failure; 1 urinary difficulty; 1 warmth & fullness of leg
114	7	7	Mixed ca	2 wk–7/100% longer–7/100%	0 0	0 0	CT, trans-catheter, bilat, transcrural, 50 ml 95%		
	6	7	Pancreatitis	2 wk–5/66% longer–2/33%	2 wk–0 longer–1/17%	2 wk–2/33% longer/3/50%			2 temporary hypotension 1 transient hematuria
351	15	15	Mixed	10/67%	3/20%	2/13%	ultrasound; 1 anterior needle 15 ml 100%	Abstract	4 shoulder pain 2 rectal bleeding
315	5	5	Mixed	3 (carcinoma)	1–pancreatitis	1–pancreatitis	bilat, CT, transcrural, 20–40 ml 50%		
	6	6	Mixed	4 (2 carcinoma, 1 pancreatitis, 1 diabetes)	0	2: Crohn's carcinomatosis			
152	50	50	Mixed primaries	32/80%	11/22%	7/14%	CT or fluoro	Abstract	
	14	14	Metastatic cancer	0	3/21% 1 pancreas, 2 peritoneal	11/79% 6 pancreas, 5 peritoneal			
125	35	35	Mixed cancer	25/72% at 3 mo f/u			CT/fluoro, lateral, left trans-crurual, 40 ml 60%	Prosp uncontr	5 diarrhea 2 arterial puncture
184	124	124	Mixed cancer	immediate: 53/43% 6 wk: 44/39%	immediate: 60/48% 6 wk: 56/50%	5/4% 6 wk: 12/11%	CT, transaortic unilateral, 15 ml 100%		67 transient diarrhea 10 transient hypotension
85	41	41	Pancreatic cancer	25/78%; 84% died pf; mean duration 4.3 mos; mean survival 5 mos	3/9.5%	4/12.5%	intraop; 15–20 ml 6% phenol		6/15% perioperative mortality (unrelated to block)
181	23	23	Pancreatitis	12	6	5	general anesthesia 50–75% alcohol		26 orthostasis, 1 urinary incontinence 1 monoparesis, 2 transient root pain
	13	17	Pancreas ca	11–7 PF at death	2	0			
325	11	11	Pancreas ca	9/82%	1/9%	1/9%	CT	Abstract comp	1 perirenal spread
	4	4		3/75%	1/25%	0	transaortic, CT		"thoracic" spread
	3	3		1/33%	2/67%	0	anterior, CT		retrogastric spread
152	12	12	Pancrea ca–no mets	12	0	0			
	45	45	Panc + liver mets only	17	28	0			
	15	15	Widespread abd mets	0	6	0		Abstract	

[a] Shaded areas indicate either absent data or unclear explanation of parameters.
[b] Due to use of varied terminology in referenced articles, some interpretation was necessary (*e.g.,* authors' reference to "moderate" and "fair" results assumed to connote similar meaning). Refer to references for details.
[c] Technique: Unless otherwise noted = "Classic" (Kappis-Moore) technique using total of 50 ml 50% alcohol by fluoroscopically guided percutaneous posterior bilateral paravertebral injection.
[d] Studies comparing multiple techniques appear as consecutive listings with data analyzed separately where possible. Check denominator when assessing results.
[e] Design: assumed to be retrospective and unrandomized unless otherwise stated.
Ref No., reference number; No. pts., number of patients treated; No. blks., number of blocks performed; PF, pain free; ca, carcinoma; wk, week; d, day; mo, month; TC, transcural; RC, retrocrural; ant, anterior approach.

TABLE 31-9. *Potential advantages of early implementation of neural blockade for abdominopelvic cancer pain*

Overall favorable risk:benefit ratio
Better efficacy before extensive perineural infiltration shelters targeted nerves
Increased ease and safety prior to development of massive organomegaly and anatomic distortion
Interventions generally better tolerated in less medically ill patients
May forestall development of chronic pain behavior
Improvements in performance status more likely to meaningfully increase activity and function
May improve compliance with antitumor therapy
Improved performance status may enhance candidacy for investigational therapy
Collateral effects may result in improved gastrointestinal motility
Preliminary evidence of improved survival

cluding much of the gastrointestinal tract (distal esophagus, stomach, duodenum, small bowel, ascending and proximal transverse colon), pancreas, adrenal glands, spleen, liver, and biliary system. Thus, celiac block has potential utility for treating pain emanating from a variety of intra-abdominal structures, although its most important indication is pain due to pancreatic cancer. Though efficacy is less than for pancreatic pain,[148,152] painful hepatic metastases may respond to celiac block, unless referred right shoulder pain is prominent. Diffuse abdominal pain due to disseminated peritoneal implants is unlikely to be relieved after celiac block.[148,152] In one study, inadequate outcomes approached statistical significance in obese patients, but age, gender, weight loss, and prior surgery, chemotherapy, or radiotherapy appear not to affect efficacy.[28] As noted, short- and long-term outcomes for pain of non-neoplastic origin are often disappointing.

Neoplastic Pancreatic Pain

Visceral pain is characteristically vague in distribution and quality and, as a result may be difficult for patients to localize. When chronic, it is characteristically described as a deep, dull, aching, dragging, boring, squeezing, or pressure-like sensation, and when acute or obstructive, it may be paroxysmal, colicky, and associated with nausea, vomiting, diaphoresis, and alterations in blood pressure and heart rate.[243] Visceral pain may be accompanied by referred pain and hyperalgesia in superficial and/or deep tissues, often distant to the source of pathology. Events that elicit visceral pain include abnormal distention or contraction of the smooth muscle of the walls of hollow viscera, rapid stretch of capsular tissue around solid viscera, ischemia, necrosis, chemical irritation of serosal and mucosal surfaces, and distention, traction, or torsion of mesenteric attachments and vasculature.[278]

Pancreatic cancer[86,291] and other retroperitoneal pathology[36] classically present as relentless mid-epigastric pain radiating through or around to the back. An association between retroperitoneal disease and back pain is supported by findings of a 21% incidence of back pain in a series of patients with testicular germ cell tumors and periaortic nodal metastases.[36] Patients often find it difficult to lie flat and may unconsciously seek relief by assuming a modified fetal position, often giving a history of preferring to sleep in a lounge chair or slumped over a table. The mechanism of such pain is presumed to be due to pressure and invasion of retroperitoneal nerves and traction associated with postural changes. While a common presentation, other patterns of pain may be present due to related pathology such as bowel obstruction, portal vein obstruction, cholangitis, ductal obstruction, peripancreatic neuritis, hepatic metastases, peritoneal invasion, and ascites.[86,137] The classic presentation referred to above is most consistent with the likelihood of good outcome after celiac block, whereas alternate symptoms suggest the need for other treatments or diagnostic studies. The identification of obstruction or infection may suggest a role for surgery or antibiotic therapy. Careful attention to bowel management and proper anti-emetic therapy are often indicated.

Efficacy

In addition to the difficulties inherent in evaluating treatment outcomes for pain in general and specific methodologic obstacles for designing controlled trials of interventional techniques, historical studies have often lacked important detail.[307] A trend toward a more critical appraisal of outcome is suggested by a decline in favorable results reported from one large center from 98% (1948–1964) to 80% (1978–1985).[31] As a result of these shortcomings, careful analysis of available clinical data is warranted to make even limited conclusions (see Table 31-8). A recent meta-analysis of 23 studies reviewed data on 1126 patients with either pancreatic cancer pain (64%) or pain due to other intra-abdominal malignancies (36%).[37] Good-to-excellent pain relief was achieved in 90% of evaluable patients during the first 2 weeks after neurolytic celiac block; only 6% of these required a repeat procedure for inadequate analgesia. Partial or complete pain relief was observed in 95% of patients alive at the time of last follow-up, and 87% of patients at the time of death. Significant relief of pain and persistence of effect until death is reported in 62% to 100% and 35% to 100%, respectively, with most studies reporting favorable outcomes in the higher ranges (see Table 31-8). Pain relief is often reestablished with repetition. Time to maximal pain relief is variable, but comfort is usually either immediate or forthcoming within 24 hours.[154]

Rationale for Early Intervention

Despite limited outcome data from controlled trials, the global clinical experience with celiac plexus block performed for oncologic abdominal pain demonstrates safety and efficacy that are sufficient to warrant strong consideration for its application early in the course of treatment (Table 31-9). Dose-limiting side effects of opioids are the most accepted indications for consideration of invasive modalities of pain relief in general.[5,146] However, a number of factors, both generally applicable to medically ill populations and specific to patients with abdominal pain, reduce the likelihood of attaining adequate pain control with systemic analgesics alone (Table 31-10). Nonsteroidal anti-inflammatory drugs may be poorly tolerated or contraindicated due to gastropathy, renal insufficiency, coagulopathy, bone marrow suppression, and masking of fever. The oral route may be unreliable in the presence of gastrointestinal dysfunction, especially due to dysphagia, malabsorption, intestinal obstruction, nausea and vomiting, xerostomia, and coma. Reduced gastrointestinal motility, ileus, and obstruction—common features in this population owing to tumor encroachment, previous surgery, or radiation therapy—are commonly exacerbated by opioids, even with careful bowel management protocols, and as a result the use of opioids in other than low doses may be viewed as undesirable. While a high proportion of patients with intra-abdominal malignancies are not candidates for curative therapy, the application of life-extending palliative treatments may render pharmacologic-based pain control more difficult to achieve as concomitant asthenia and cachexia increase the likelihood of side effects from opioids titrated to therapeutic effect. Although visceral pain tends to be relatively opioid-responsive, neoplastic abdominal pain is often due to a mixed etiology. Neurophatic pain, which may be associated with reduced opioid responsivity,[277] is probably relatively common in pancreatic cancer owing to occult microscopic perineural tumor invasion,[58,137] a contention supported by findings of direct invasion of peripancreatic nerves in 84% of patients with pancreatic cancer at autopsy.[71]

The factors limiting the applicability of purely pharmacologic management (see Table 31-10), combined with historical and contemporary demonstrations of safety and efficacy for the application of celiac block, are compelling arguments for its use in appropriate populations. Celiac block should ideally be applied early, both to maximize potential benefits and minimize difficulties due to disease-related and patient-related factors. Early implementation may result in better pain control and, in addition, may improve overall ease of management by increasing performance status. Reduced sympathetic tone (and unopposed parasympathetic activity) may enhance GI motility, often with improvement of ileus, constipation, and anorexia, effects that are in stark contrast to the obstipating effects of opioids. A recent randomized study of early alcohol-versus-placebo celiac block, demonstrating statistically significant improved survival rates in treated patients,[186] is another exciting consideration that demands further study.

TABLE 31-10. *Factors limiting pharmacotherapy for neoplastic abdominal pain*

Modality	Limitations
NSAIDs	Gastropathy, renal dysfunction, bone marrow depletion, or concerns of masking fever
Oral analgesics	Xerostomia, dysphagia, malabsorption, obstruction, nausea, vomiting, coma
Transdermal analgesics	Dose requirements for opioids that exceed limitations of dose form
Parenteral analgesics	Inadequate household or community support to manage infusions
Opioids	Ileus, partial obstruction, intractable constipation
Opioids	Reduced responsivity due to neuropathic component of pain
Opioids	Dose-limiting side effects due to asthenia and cachexia

NSAIDs, nonsteroidal anti-inflammatory drugs.

Complications

In the hands of skilled clinicians, serious complications are infrequent and, moreover, idiosyncratic in that their incidence does not appear to correlate strongly with a single technique. Nevertheless, since a variety of serious complications have been reported, radiologic guidance is, under ordinary circumstances, mandatory when neurolysis is undertaken (see also Chapter 22).

Minor Complications: Hypotension, Altered Gastrointestinal Motility, Pain

Hypotension[239] and diarrhea are the most common complications of celiac block, but are usually transient, and when anticipated and recognized are usually innocuous. Orthostatic hypotension, which occurs as a result of regional vasodilation and pooling of blood within the splanchnic vessels, can usually be prevented by the IV administration of 500 to 1000 ml of balanced salt solution. Monitoring of blood pressure during the procedure and recovery is mandatory, and small increments of intravenous ephedrine are occasionally required. Preadministration of oral ephedrine (50 mg) and postprocedural use of support hose and abdominal binders, though mentioned in the older literature,[105] are rarely prescribed in contemporary practice. Particular vigilance should be maintained in elderly, debilitated, and chronically or acutely dehydrated patients to avoid hypotension and iatrogenic congestive heart failure.[28] Although it has not been thoroughly investigated, hypotension may be a reliable marker of successful celiac block (Patt, R.B., unpublished data).

Gastrointestinal hypermotility results from unopposed parasympathetic activity. Due to the high incidence of opioid-mediated constipation in treated populations, this phenomenon is usually manifest simply as slightly improved bowel habit, which is usually welcomed. Diarrhea, reported in up to 60% of patients, is usually transient (36 to 48 hours) and self-limited, but is occasionally severe and persistent[348] and, if unrecognized, may even be life-threatening.[210] Patients occasionally void spontaneously at the conclusion of neurolysis, which may signal successful neural blockade.

Patients commonly experience new, usually self-limited pain after neurolysis, frequently manifest as dull back or pleuritic pain after celiac and splanchnic block, respectively. While intraprocedural pain and failure to relieve pain are not true complications, they are sufficiently common to warrant their inclusion in informed consent. Time to maximal pain relief is variable. In the majority of patients, relief will be immediate and complete; in others, it will accrue over a few days.[154]

Neurologic Complications

The most common neurologic complication of celiac neurolysis is somatic nerve injury, which was documented as numbness and/or weakness in the T10–L2 dermatomes in 8% of patients in one large series.[15] Even after confirmation of accurate needle placement, drug may conceivably track backward between the attachments of the psoas muscle or defects in the crura,[240] resulting in deposition near somatic nerves and consequent neurologic injury, most commonly manifest as numbness or dysesthetic pain over the anterior thigh and lower abdominal wall and/or quadriceps weakness.[11] This outcome has been postulated to be more likely when retrocrural techniques are utilized.[315]

Of over 3000 cases (most without radiographic guidance), Moore[229] reported 18 episodes of dural puncture (0.006%) which, in all but one case, was heralded by the spontaneous appearance of CSF. Other possible anomalous modes of entry to the spinal canal include retrograde spread via an elongated dural cuff near a nerve root, and through annular tears after accidental disk penetration.[377] Although well-controlled comparisons between guided and blind procedures are unavailable, radiographic assistance is likely to help one avoid and detect subarachnoid and epidural placement. A case of unilateral paraplegia,[351] presumably due to accidental psoas compartment block, was reported after a celiac block was performed without radiologic guidance in a patient positioned laterally due to obesity and ascites.

An important mechanism of potential neurologic injury is spasm, disruption, or accidental injection into one of the spinal cord's small nutrient vessels, which may result in ischemic injury, typically to the pyramidal and spinothalamic tracts, with relative sparing of proprioception. The artery of Adamkievicz (arteria radicularis magna), the largest of the cord's ventral radicular arteries, provides nutrient blood flow to the lower two-thirds of the spinal cord. After leaving the aorta, it runs laterally, about 80% of the time on the left, and typically reaches the cord between T8 and L4, making it vulnerable to injury during celiac block (Fig. 7-11). This mechanism has been postulated to be responsible for at least five episodes of serious neurologic morbidity after celiac block. De Conno and colleagues[60] reported a case of flaccid paraplegia, after an otherwise uneventful fluoroscopically guided celiac plexus block undertaken by Moore's technique. Despite clinical demonstration of a T8 sensory motor and sensory level that persisted despite corticosteroids, MRI examinations were normal one day and one week after the block. However, the patient did achieve complete pain relief, which was maintained for 5 months until death. In another case, which utilized neither radiologic guidance nor test doses of local anesthetic, rapid onset of persistent paraplegia followed celiac neurolysis with 6 ml of 6% aqueous phenol in a patient with pancreatic carcinoma.[94] The onset of paraplegia was delayed for 2 hours in a third case, which was performed under general anesthesia with the patient in the lateral position, using a single needle and 25 ml of absolute alcohol.[41] Arterial blood had been obtained prior to repositioning the needle for subsequent neurolysis.

A survey of pain clinics performing celiac neurolysis in England and Wales during the 5-year interval between 1986 and 1990 elicited 160 responses (73% response rate), and disclosed four instances of permanent paraplegia, accompanied in three cases by urinary and fecal incontinence.[59] An aggregate of 2730 neurolytic blocks had been performed, representing an unsettling 1/683 incidence of serious neurologic morbidity. Only one of the cases had previously been reported in the literature, and results were verified by a survey of three medical defense societies. The techniques used were not detailed, though it was reported that alcohol was used in varied concentrations (50%, 66%, 90%, 100%), and the blocks were performed for cancer (n=1), pancreatitis (n=2), and an unknown indication. Radiologic imaging was utilized in all cases, making direct neuraxial injection less likely an explanation than indirect ischemic medullary injury. Two of the four cases were performed under general anesthesia, a fact that eliminates the opportunity to detect potential difficulties with test doses of local anesthetic. A third, performed for pancreatitic pain, represented the eighth in a series of blocks, suggesting that repeated neurolysis might produce anatomic abnormalities that predispose to a poor outcome.

Vascular Complications

Although it is an essential safeguard, intermittent aspiration may be inadequate to identify intravascular placement and should be augmented by the preliminary injection of a local anesthetic coupled with a neurologic examination and the use of fluoroscopy to detect "vascular run-off." The use of general anesthesia, which limits the value of test doses, should be discouraged except when specifically indicated (e.g., in pediatric patients[346]). Large vessels may be punctured accidentally[125] or intentionally[145,184] but, if recognized, the puncture is usually innocuous. Although clinically significant bleeding and hematoma have not been reported, even after transaortic blocks, pretreatment coagulation status should be investigated and, if necessary, optimized.

A generalized seizure accompanied by transient loss of consciousness was reported following an apparent accidental intravascular injection of phenol.[13] French investigators[97] described a case of severe cardiac dysrrhythmia followed by circulatory arrest after celiac neurolysis performed under general anesthesia with 30 ml of 6.6% phenol. These cases underscore the need for concern related to the potential for systemic toxicity with large volumes of phenol.

Visceral Injury

Perforation of adjacent viscera, especially the kidney, probably occurs more frequently than is appreciated clinically[115] and is a more significant risk in patients who are obese or have altered anatomy due to tumor compression, organomegaly, or surgery.[233] Although renal puncture and attendant hematuria are characteristically self-limited, the accidental injection of an appreciable volume of neurolytic drug may produce injury and infarction. Based on cadaver studies, Moore[233] states that renal puncture is more likely when needles are inserted more than 7.5 cm lateral to the midline, when needle tips lie excessively lateral to the vertebral body, and when a higher vertebral body (T11) is targeted. With careful attention to technique, perforation of the viscera should not occur; an obvious advantage of CT guidance, however, is direct visualization of viscera, particularly in patients in whom normal anatomy is distorted by the presence of massive tumor.

Pneumothorax has been reported in a patient treated without radiologic guidance, and in another after a block that relied on just plain films for guidance.[28] Based on this experience, chest tube drainage may not be required. Two cases of self-limited pleural effusion were reported after posterior block with 90% alcohol despite CT confirmation of accurate placement.[92] Diaphragmatic irritation from overflow of alcohol into the left subdiaphragmatic space was proposed to explain these complications. Chylothorax, an occasional complication of high translumbar aortography,[50] has been reported after fluoroscopically guided phenol celiac plexus block.[83] In a study of nonradiologically guided paravertebral celiac block (10 cm from the midline) on 20 cadavers, the only cases of visceral injury documented were three instances of pleural puncture.[42] Ejaculatory failure occurred in 2% of one large series[15] but is otherwise rarely reported, presumably because patients needing treatment are rarely sexually active. This complication should be borne in mind when treating nonmalignant pain, but is rarely of concern in medically ill cancer patients.

Wilson[377] recently documented two instances of accidental intravertebral disk penetration, in one case with epidural spread through an annular defect, during attempted celiac block. Disk penetration is usually heralded by increased resistance to needle passage and pain, especially on injection, both of which were absent in these cases, presumably due to disk degeneration. Disk penetration *per se* is usually innocuous and is even deliberately undertaken with modified transdiskal approaches to splanchnic[208] and celiac[168] block, but if unrecognized may produce disastrous complications.

Metabolic and Chemical Complications

Alcohol Intoxication. Serum ethanol levels after celiac block have been documented to range between 21 and 54 mg/dl, values well below legal levels of intoxication, and thus ordinarily insufficient to produce systemic effects.[150,196,303] One study demonstrated significantly higher serum alcohol levels in patients with gastric as opposed to pancreatic cancer, due presumably to surgical changes.[303] Consideration should still be given to the potential interactions of even low serum alcohol levels and the effects of other concurrently administered CNS depressants. Accidental intravascular injection of large volumes of alcohol may induce intoxication, seizures, and unconsciousness.

Acetaldehyde Syndrome. Occasional systemic reactions consisting of facial flushing, palpitations, and diaphoresis observed after alcohol celiac plexus block have been suggested to represent acetaldehyde syndrome.[304] This phenomenon has been postulated to be due to abnormal metabolism of alcohol and high levels of acetaldehyde in individuals with an atypical phenotype for the enzyme aldehyde dehydrogenase (ALDH-1 deficiency). Up to 38% of Japanese possess this phenotype.[244] In addition, susceptible patients may give a history of facial flushing after social consumption of small amounts of alcohol. In one study, blood levels of acetaldehyde were 20 times normal in "flushers."[244] This syndrome is probably underdiagnosed because it is relatively innocuous. A similar but more serious reaction—consisting of flushing, diaphoresis, dizziness, nausea, vomiting, hypotension, and tachycardia—which resolved only after 4 to 8 hours, was observed in a patient taking a β-lactam antibiotic, moxolactam.[356] Alcohol neurolysis should be undertaken only cautiously in patients on Antabuse (disulfiram) therapy for alcohol abuse, and who provide a history of taking other drugs with the capacity to inhibit ALDH such as β-lactam antibiotics (including moxalactam), metronidazole (Flagyl), chloramphenicol (Chloromycetin), tolbutamide (Orinase), and chlorpropramide (Diabinase).[189]

Other Metabolic Complications. Unchanged levels of serum amylase in 20 patients who underwent celiac plexus neurolysis suggested that pancreatic injury is unusual.[150] Alterations in serum CPK levels occasionally occur, but typically are minimal, suggesting that skeletal muscle injury is infrequent. Interestingly, in one series,[196] the two of 20 patients with significantly elevated CPKs (4242 and 1640 IU/L) experienced side effects consistent with muscle injury (bilateral L1 neuritis and back pain).

Phenol. Intravascular injection or absorption of phenol may produce transient tinnitus and flushing.[306] Higher doses may produce CNS stimulation, myoclonus, seizures, unconsciousness, hypotension, cardiac arrhythmias, hepatic and renal insufficiency.[44] Patients may experience malaise for 24 hours after the administration of doses near the upper recommended limits (600-2000 mg).[1,320] Owing to the potential for systemic toxicity, especially given trends toward the use of higher concentrations, Boas recommends that phenol be avoided for celiac block and reserved for splanchnic block, which is usually accomplished with lower volumes.[1] In an unrandomized trial of alcohol and phenol blocks, Jain[151] demonstrated a higher incidence of untoward effects in the latter group.

History

Early History

Kappis first described paravertebral splanchnic block in 1914 as a component of surgical anesthesia.[160] Around the same time, Wendling[372] introduced an anterior percutaneous approach that was soon abandoned due to concerns about safety.[24] Seventy years later, a similar approach guided by computerized tomography was re-introduced[209] and accepted into clinical practice. Other important historical developments include Braun's[23] first application of splanchnic/celiac block during laparotomy (1919), modifications by Labat[172,174] (1920, 1924), Roussiel[298] (who introduced the term "paravertebral block" in 1923), De Takats,[65] and Gage (1947).[93] It was only in 1959 that a technique for neurolytic injection (with alcohol) was first described.[156] In a report on 41 patients, Bridenbaugh and Moore were the first to document the efficacy of celiac axis neurolysis in a large series of patients with pain due to upper abdominal cancer.[25]

Recent History

Although a technique for intraoperative neurolysis was described in the 1960s,[52,85] clinicians usually relied on various minor modifications of Kappis' original posterior paravertebral technique until the 1980s. Over the last two decades several new alternatives have been introduced, many of which are now accepted as being safe and efficacious. In 1969, localization of the celiac trunk with angiography was described in a case report,[145] a technique that did not, however, gain popularity. In 1978, Boas[16] differentiated between the retrocrural and transcrural approach, a distinction that was further refined by Singler's[315] CT-guided approach (1982). Also in 1982, Ischia[141] described a transaortic method of celiac block, and 6 years later a CT-guided anterior approach was introduced by Matamala.[209] Finally, in the context of clinical practice having been guided predominantly by data derived from uncontrolled clinical series[307] and expert opinion, the recent publication of several partially controlled trials[140,141,220] and a meta-analysis[37] is especially noteworthy.

Anatomy and Technique

The regional anatomy pertinent to celiac plexus neurolysis is described in detail in Chapter 14. The plexus is probably best conceived of as a dense, relatively diffuse network or reticulum of fibers embedded in loose areolar tissue, generally comprised of paired ganglia (celiac, superior mesenteric, and aorticorenal, named for adjacent arteries) and their interconnections. The plexus, which measures around 3 cm in length and 4 cm in width, typically encircles the aorta, coalescing along its anterior and anterolateral aspects. While its location and configuration are subject to considerable variation, the plexus is located in the retroperitoneum, behind the stomach and pancreas, and in front of the diaphragmatic crura and vertebral column, extending variably from between the T12 and L1 intravertebral disk and the L2 body.[369] Other important anatomic relations include the inferior vena cava, pancreas, duodenum, kidneys, adrenals, portal vein, and the splenic, phrenic, celiac, superior mesenteric, renal, and suprarenal vessels (see Chapter 14, Figs. 14-5 to 14-7).

"Classic" Retrocrural (Deep Splanchnic) Approach

The most frequently applied approach to celiac plexus block was described by Kappis in 1919[160] and subsequently modified by Moore[229] and others. This approach, described in detail in Chapter 14, involves localizing needles with their tips 1.5 to 3 cm beyond the L1 vertebral body, often using transmitted aortic pulsations as a landmark on the left.[132] This technique is referred to as retrocrural based on CT determinations that needles do not pierce the diaphragmatic crura and ultimately lie with their tips just posterior and cephalad to its crura. The diaphragm, which separates the thoracic and abdominal cavities, is anchored bilaterally by muscular attachments (crura) that arise from the anterolateral surfaces of the upper two or three lumbar vertebrae and disks. In light of recent investigations,[233] it is apparent that the classic approach to celiac plexus block does not deposit drug directly on to the celiac plexus, as was previously thought. Instead, the injectate tends to concentrate posterior to the aorta and along the sides of the L1 vertebral body (see Figs. 14-6 and 14-7), suggesting that pain relief is achieved by blockade of retroaortic fibers, by deep splanchnic nerve block, or, if sufficient volume is administered, by caudal diffusion of drug through the diaphragm's aortic hiatus or defects in the crura,[240] and subsequent celiac block. When needles are placed according to the classic description, injectate often fails to extend to the anterior aspect of the aorta, where the plexus' fibers are concentrated. In view of these findings, Moore has revised his recommendations to include (i) advancing the left-sided needle an additional 1.5 to 2 cm (total of 3 to 4 cm beyond the vertebral body) or until (a) aortic pulsations are appreciated, (b) increased resistance consistent with the aortic wall is encountered, or (c) arterial blood is obtained, and (ii) advancing the right-sided needle a total of 3 to 4 cm beyond the vertebral body. As a result of these modifications, the tip of the left- and right-sided needles should lie just posterior and anterolateral to the aorta, respectively, and 25 ml of solution injected through each needle should encircle the aorta. Using CT scanning and 15-ml volumes injected bilaterally, Fujita has documented spread from the retroaortic to transcrural space in 48% of 28 cases.[90] He went on to measure pre- and postinjection pressures in the retro- and precrural spaces in 12 patients after the injection of 15 ml, and found that mean pressures rose from 14 to 33 and 11 to 19 mm Hg, respectively.

Transcrural Celiac Block

Using fluoroscopy, Boas[16] first distinguished between retrocrural and transcrural celiac block. Transcrural block was further investigated by Singler as a means to minimize the likelihood of posterior spread of drug toward the lumbar plexus.[232,315] Ultimately, needles are positioned with their tips on each side of the aorta near its anterior aspect. Using CT guidance and targeting the region near the celiac arterial trunk (near L1 or T12), Singler plotted a needle trajectory that avoided the vertebral bodies, kidneys, and major vessels. Needles entered the skin in most cases at L1 (occasionally higher), 4 cm from the midline on the left and 5 to 10 cm on the right, and pierced the diaphragmatic crura below the pulmonary parenchyma in all cases. The variable point of entry on the right was required to introduce the needle between kidney and vertebral body so that its tip came to lie between the walls of the aorta and vena cava. In a series of retrocrural blocks, CT-derived entry sites were similar.[90] With transcrural block, the disposition of the needle tips and injectate are below and anterior to the diaphragm, and the likelihood that spread will occur anterior to the aorta where the celiac plexus is most concentrated is increased compared to retrocrural injections. Singler injected 10 to 20 ml of 50% alcohol bilaterally. Most authorities recommend CT guidance for the performance of transcrural block because of the greater risks of puncturing large vessels. Ischia's transaortic technique (see following) is essentially an alternate means of accomplishing left-sided transcrural placement and can be performed with either fluoroscopic or CT guidance.

A single-needle transcrural approach performed with the patient in the right lateral decubitus position has recently been described in a series of 35 patients.[125] After preliminary CT-guided studies on cadavers, the investigators arrived at a technique that targeted the L1 vertebral body from a left-sided entry point below the twelfth rib and 4 to 6 cm from the midline. They walked a blunt-tipped needle off the vertebral body at 9 to 10 cm from the skin, described transiently increased resistance corresponding to the needle's passage through the diaphragmatic crus, and finally arterial pulsations at the needle's final destination anterolateral to the aorta, at a depth of about 15 cm from the skin. After confirming the needle's position with CT or fluoroscopy, 40 ml of 60% alcohol was injected. This technique offers the potential advantage of less tissue trauma due to reliance on a single needle.

Transaortic Celiac Neurolysis

In 1983, Ischia and colleagues[141] introduced the concept of deliberately transgressing the abdominal aorta with a single, posteriorly placed needle in order to ensure preaortic spread of injected solutions. Obviously, this technique results in a transcrural block. A strength of this method, like that of the transaxillary approach to brachial plexus block, is its reliance on the predictable juxtaposition of the targeted nerve and an easily identified vessel. The likelihood of its safety is suggested by previous experience with both transarterial axillary blocks and translumbar aortograms. The latter procedure is associated with a low incidence of clinically significant hemorrage (0.1% to 0.5%) despite the routine use of 14- to 18-gauge needles.[24,214] Despite the potential for aortic tears and subsequent occult retroperitoneal hemorrhage, the transortic approach has been demonstrated to be safe in several clinical series,[79,141,184] including one which measured serial hematocrits[141] and another in which selected patients underwent postprocedural CT scans.[141] Factors that mitigate against hemorrhagic complications include the thick, muscular character of the aortic wall, strong support of the aorta in this region by the diaphragmatic crura and prevertebral fascia, and the use of relatively small-caliber (20- to 22-gauge) needles. Potential advantages of the transaortic method include reliance on a single needle, applicability under fluoroscopy, and assurance that drug is injected near where the plexus is concentrated and distant from the spinal axis.

Though a left-sided transaortic injection may be used as a component of a bilateral block and with CT guidance, it was originally described as a fluoroscopically guided, left-sided paravertebral approach. The technique is similar to those previously described except that the needle is gradually advanced beyond the vertebral body until its tip rests in the preaortic fat. If the needle is in the proper plane, penetration of the posterior aortic wall is heralded by transmitted pulsations to the needle and increased resistance, following which freely aspirated arterial blood signals that the needle is intraluminal, and finally there is increased resistance that yields to a new loss of resistance once the anterior arterial wall is breeched (see Chapter 14, Fig. 14-6C). Lieberman and Waldman[255] modified Ischia's technique by instituting a loss of resistance to the continuous instillation of saline maneuver as the needle is advanced beyond the lumen of the aorta, to more accurately ascertain that its tip has traversed its anterior wall. They further recommend consideration of an alternate approach if CT screening detects significant aortic aneurysm, mural thrombus, or calcifications. On PA views, contrast medium should be confined to the midline with a tendency toward greater concentration around the lateral margins of the aorta. Lateral views should demonstrate a predominantly preaortic orientation extending from around T12–L2, sometimes accompanied by pulsations, and the absence of a narrow longitudinal "line image," which is suggestive of incomplete penetration of the anterior wall and dissection. Contrast dye may not consolidate in the presence of extensive preaortic tumor infiltration. Ischia's group utilized 30 ml of 75% alcohol and fluoroscopic guidance,[141] whereas Lieberman advocates 15 ml of absolute alcohol and CT guidance.[184]

Anterior Approaches

Intraoperative Celiac Neurolysis

Celiac block at the time of laparotomy, popularized in the United Kingdom,[52,85] appears to be as efficacious as percutaneous approaches (see Table 31-8), but nevertheless is infrequently employed. Advances in noninvasive diagnostic techniques, which reduce the incidence of laparotomy, are partially responsible. Other reasons may include the failure of many surgeons to assign pain management a high priority, unfamiliarity with the regional anatomy or technique, poor access to the injection site due to bulky tumor or phlegmon, and concerns about safety. The main disadvantages of intraoperative treatment relate to theoretic concerns that neurologic injury may be masked by general anesthesia[41] and that the localization and spread of injections may be unreliable when tissue planes are disrupted by surgical trauma. The main advantage is that patients are exposed to one less procedure and are spared discomfort during the block. In addition, the potential for intraoperative block as a prophylactic measure has recently been successfully explored by Lillimoe et al.[186] If intraoperative block is declined, the surgeon may consider placing surgical clips in the vicinity of the celiac trunk to facilitate postoperative treatment.[39]

An intraoperative approach was first advocated by Braun[23] as a means to provide anesthesia in combination with field block of the abdominal wall. This approach involved gentle retraction of the stomach and left lobe of the liver to expose the lesser omentum, and placement of a digit between the aorta and vena cava to serve as a guide to injection over the ventral surface of the first lumbar vertebral body. In 1969, Copping et al.[52] described a similar technique using phenol to treat pain in patients undergoing laparotomy for pancreatic cancer, and in addition reported on its histopathologic correlates in canines. Their method, which targets the area between the splanchnic nerves and the plexus—slightly lateral, posterior, and cephalad to the origin of the celiac artery—involves advancing a 20-gauge spinal needle over a digit and injecting 15 to 20 ml of 6% phenol. Lillimoe's[186] recent series employed 20 ml of 50% alcohol injected on each side of the aorta near the L1 vertebral body. A recent report documents postoperative neurolysis through a percutaneously tunneled epidural catheter placed during surgery.[138]

Percutaneous Anterior Celiac Neurolysis

An anterior approach to the celiac plexus block, initially advocated in 1918 (for surgical anesthesia)[372] was resurrected in 1988 by Matamala et al.[209] (for neurolysis) and Lieberman and colleagues[183] (for interventional radiology). The safety of the CT-guided technique, and subsequent sonographically guided modifications,[102,351] is supported by extensive experience with transabdominal fine-needle aspiration biopsy, which—despite frequent passage through liver, stomach, small and large bowel, vessels, and the pancreas—is associated with a very low complication rate.[165,182,360] Disadvantages of the anterior percutaneous approach include the need for CT or sonographic guidance and, though bleeding and infection have not been reported,[183,221] requisite passage of the block needle through bowel and sometimes liver. The potential advantages of anterior techniques are numerous. Targeting the preaortic space where the plexus's fibers are concentrated may enhance efficacy, and because this region is distant from the spinal axis and the usual course of its nutrient vessels, the risk of neurologic injury may be reduced. Periprocedural discomfort and the need for sedation are usually less, since patients do not need to lie prone and only a single needle is used, the trajectory of which does not impinge on periosteum or nerve roots.

The anterior approach involves targeting either the L1 vertebral body[183] or root of the celiac artery[102,132,221] with CT scout films or sonography and, for the former, plotting coordinates to determine the optimal point of insertion, needle trajectory, and depth. These techniques necessarily involve the close cooperation of an experienced radiologist. In Matamala's technique,[209] the abdominal wall is infiltrated with local anesthetic and a 22-gauge 7-inch needle is introduced to the predetermined depth, usually in a roughly perpendicular direction. Up to 10 ml of contrast medium is injected, which should remain within the confines of the preaortic space. For neurolytic block, a preliminary injection of local anesthetic further verifies placement, following which 35 ml of 50% alcohol is administered. An alternate technique utilizes fluoroscopy to guide the passage of a single needle just to the right of the center of the L1 vertebral body, after which it is withdrawn 1 to 3 cm.[183] Precautions that have been recommended include the administration of IV antibiotics and the use of no larger than a 22-gauge needle to minimize the risks of infection and trauma.[102]

Transcatheter Neurolysis

Isolated reports have documented the feasibility of placement of a temporary catheter to facilitate repeat periceliac injections.[8,105,134,138,373] An early series used bilateral over-the-needle catheters for neurolysis.[105] Haaga[114] has reported the use of CT-guided bilateral transcatheter neurolysis in 13 patients, using a posterior transcrural approach, 18-gauge catheters, 19-gauge needles, and 50 ml 95% alcohol. In another report,[134] serial injections of local anesthetic were performed for 14 days in a patient with pancreatitis, following which a neurolytic solution was injected. Fluoroscopy and CT scan performed 13 days after placement revealed an absence of catheter migration, and no perivascular erosion or pleural reaction. Another report describes the intraoperative placement of a percutaneously tunneled epidural catheter, which was used postoperatively to produce neurolysis.[138] When considering catheter placement from a posterior percutaneous approach, CT should be utilized to ensure that the kidney has not accidentally been penetrated.[259]

Splanchnic Nerve Block

Based on evidence from cadaver dissections[233] and tomography,[90] it is now clear that Kappis's "classic" technique of celiac plexus block and most of its modifications actually result in a retrocrural, deep splanchnic nerve block. Alternatively, the splanchnic nerves can be blocked higher and more dorsally at the anterolateral margins of the T12 or T11 vertebral bodies. The classic technique for splanchnic nerve block involves bilateral needle placement from skin sites 7 to 8 cm from the midline, and advancement of needle tips within 1 cm of the anterolateral margin of the T12 or T11 vertebral body[16,24,350] (see Chapter 14, Fig. 14-8A,B). Needles should closely hug the vertebral body to reduce the risk of pneumothorax, which, together with thoracic duct injury, is probably more common when the splanchnic nerves are targeted at this level.[1,350] Needles should not be advanced beyond the anterolateral margins of the vertebra where the splanchnic nerves are located. Generally, lesser volumes are needed to produce complete blockade at this level. Six to 15 ml of 10% phenol has been recommended.[16,350] Splanchnic nerve block may be particularly useful when the retroperitoneum is widely infiltrated by tumor or after failed celiac block.

Boas has presented preliminary data on a more straightforward "transthoracic" approach to splanchnic nerve block, which he used successfully and without complications in ten patients.[1] Standard 22-gauge spinal needles are introduced 6 cm from the midline through the 11th intercostal space, which provides an easy means to reach the anterolateral aspect of the T11 body where 10 ml of 12% phenol is deposited bilaterally. Precautions include attendance to a medial entry point and fluoroscopic observation of the lower limits of the lung parenchyma which, during quiet breathing, usually lie one space higher in the costophrenic angle. Preliminary studies in cadavers and experience with 13 blocks in six patients formed the basis for a report on another new approach to splanchnic nerve block that utilizes 3 1/2 inch needles inserted 3 to 4 cm lateral to the midline at the T12 or T12–L1 level.[253] Needles are angled slightly mesiad and are directed so that their tips come to rest at the anterolateral margin of the T12 body where 10 ml of 50% alcohol are injected bilaterally. Good results were obtained in all cases and no complications occurred. Though limited details were provided, a transdiskal approach to splanchnic nerve block has also recently been described.[208]

Therapeutic Options

Based on available data, it is difficult to recommend one technique of celiac neurolysis over another. Most approaches appear to have similar efficacy and are infrequently associated with significant or lasting side effects. As noted, the choice of technique ultimately should be individualized based on available resources, the patient's physical status, pattern of tumor spread, and the clinician's experience.

Radiologic Guidance

While radiographic guidance does not prevent complications, some form of radiographic guidance would seem to be indicated whenever neurolytic block is undertaken because of the serious nature of potential complications. A 1992 survey[131] completed by 130 U.S. pain programs determined that only 3.4% of neurolytic celiac blocks were performed without radiologic guidance, and that 75% and 21.5% were performed with the aid of fluoroscopy and CT, respectively. Thirty-six percent of respondents used CT occasionally, and an additional 25% would if facilities were available. Of centers using CT guidance, blocks were performed exclusively by a radiologist in 4% of cases, an anesthesiologist in 87% of cases, and as a collaborative effort in the remaining 9%.

Though inexpensive and usually accessible, plain radiography is least preferred because it is time consuming and cannot provide real time information. The obvious advantage of CT scanning relates to its capacity to directly demonstrate tumor spread and details of visceral and vascular anatomy, thus minimizing the likelihood of injury to these structures. These advantages are, to some extent, offset by the limited availability of CT, its cost, the requirement for cooperation from a knowledgeable radiologist, time required, and limited acceptance in claustrophobic patients. Fluoroscopy is an adequate alternative,[195] especially when anatomy is not grossly abnormal and when special techniques are not undertaken. CT is advisable after failed attempts at fluoroscopically guided neurolysis, when prior studies have demonstrated distortion of normal anatomy (e.g., massive ascites, large pleural effusions, hepato- or splenomegaly, displaced kidneys), and when a transcrural or anterior approach is undertaken.[91] Ultrasonography appears to be a reasonable alternative when an anterior approach is planned. Regardless of which anatomic approach or type of guidance is selected, the routine application of fundamental precautions (attention to topographic landmarks, observation for paresthesias, serial aspiration and the use of a local anesthetic test dose) is essential.

Anatomic Approach

The bulk of experience is with the classic retrocrural approach, and thus it can be regarded as being an extremely reliable and overall acceptable approach. Its main advantages are that it is familiar to clinicians and that, except when anatomy is distorted, it can be performed safely under fluoroscopic guidance. Its theoretic disadvantages relate to the requirement for large volumes of neurolytics administered in the retroaortic region. The thrust of most newer techniques involves ensuring maximal spread of drug to the preaortic space, where the celiac plexus tends to be most concentrated. The classic retrocrural technique has recently been demonstrated to actually block the splanchnic nerves directly and less reliably to block the celiac plexus, since in order to do so, drug must traverse the diaphragm through the aortic hiatus or through crural defects.[240] While preaortic spread often occurs with retrocrural approaches, it is inconstant and seems to depend on the administration of large volumes of drug. While the retrocrural approach is preferred by some,[232] advocates of alternate approaches cite the theoretic advantages of depositing drug more directly in the preaortic region, which may result in more profound analgesia despite the routine use of lower volumes and may reduce complications because drug is deposited further from the spinal axis.[232]

Each variant has features that recommend its use, as well as potential drawbacks. Although it is often combined with a classic right-sided block, the transaortic approach requires only a single needle. The aorta serves as a reliable landmark, ensuring anterior deposition of drug. Although it has been described alternately with fluoroscopic and CT guidance, with the former the aorta will not always be encountered. It should probably be avoided in the presence of recent coagulopathy, significant aneurysm, and mural thrombus. Although they have not emerged as clinically significant problems, hemorrhage, hematoma, and aortic dissection are possible. Although CT or sonographic guidance and attendant expertise are required, the anterior approach has several practical advantages. It, too, requires only a single needle and maximizes preaortic spread, and in addition is quick and relatively painless. Anterior approaches are unique in that they are extremely well tolerated in patients who cannot lie prone, and thus general anesthesia or deep sedation may be avoided. Although they have not been reported, hemorrhage, infection, and visceral injury are conceivable risks. The posterior transcrural approach resembles the classic approach, but with the aid of CT scanning, preaortic spread is enhanced and a lower volume of drug can be utilized. High splanchnic block is relatively simple to perform since needles do not need to be advanced beyond the vertebral body, and CT scanning is not ordinarily required. The incidence of pneumothorax is low, and this approach is particularly advantageous in the presence of extensive subdiaphragmatic tumor and lymphadenopathy, which may inhibit the spread of drug with other techniques. Despite the potential that neurologic injury might be masked by general anesthesia, intraoperative therapeutic or prophylactic neurolysis is a reasonable option for patients with pancreatic cancer undergoing laparotomy. No particular advantage seems to be associated with transdiskal and transcatheter approaches, although they may emerge as experience accrues.

Choice of Drug and Needle

Diagnostic blockade is typically achieved with a total of 20 to 50 ml of 0.25% bupivacaine or a similar agent (1% lidocaine, 2% 2-chloroprocaine, 1% etidocaine) injected through one or two needles. Smaller volumes are often used for local anesthetic as opposed to neurolytic block based on the view that the former spreads more readily in tissue. For therapeutic blockade, 25 ml of 50% alcohol and 0.125% bupivacaine or saline is most often administered bilaterally. Moore's experience and anatomic investigations have led him to advocate the use of a total 50-ml volume administered through two needles for retrocrural block. Phenol and other strengths of alcohol (25% to 100%) have been utilized in volumes ranging from 20 to 80 ml without apparent differences.

Although controlled trials of alcohol versus phenol are lacking, alcohol (50% to 100%) would seem to be the agent of choice based on global experience. Alcohol, however, has the disadvantage of producing severe, though transient, pain on injection and is less miscible with contrast medium than is phenol. Intoxication is unlikely, except in the case of accidental intravascular injection, but occasionally an acetaldehyde syndrome is encountered, though it is usually (not always) innocuous. Phenol (6% to 10%) mixes readily with contrast medium, but must be prepared by a compounding pharmacist.[283,336] The apparently greater affinity of phenol for vascular tissue[245] has been cited as a theoretic disadvantage,[339] since this might be predicted to correlate with higher incidences of injury to the spinal cord's nutrient vessels, but the actual clinical significance is unknown. Large volumes of phenol may be associated with systemic and cardiac toxicity,[97] and accidental intravascular injection has been reported to produce seizures.[13] Phenol may be best reserved for (lower volume) splanchnic block, especially if high concentrations are used, due to potential systemic toxicity.[1]

Both 20- and 22-gauge needles are advocated. Although it is more difficult to maintain a straight trajectory with a 22-gauge needle and higher intraluminal pressures interfere with the manual appreciation of differences in tissue compliance, it is reasonable to utilize 22-gauge needles to minimize pain and tissue trauma.[28] as long as radiologic guidance is employed to offset disadvantages. The use of a 22-gauge needle is recommended for anterior[209] and transaortic approaches.[141]

Changing Trends in Practice

Diagnostic/Prognostic Block

Early series advocating the routine performance of a local anesthetic and neurolytic block on separate occasions[28,29,105,351] have given way to a trend toward performing both together, especially for radiographically guided procedures in patients with cancer pain.[140,184] Performing a local anesthetic and neurolytic block on separate days is stressful to patients who are debilitated, utilizes more resources, and in straightforward cases may not be associated with sufficient benefit to justify these disadvantages. Jain's[148] demonstration that successful local anesthetic celiac block did not predict pain relief after neurolysis in 28% of patients suggests that preliminary blockade lacks sensitivity. In addition, when blocks are performed with radiologic guidance and careful attention to technical details, including the use of test doses, the risk of serious complications is low, and in well-selected patients, the likelihood of efficacy is high. Finally, when separate blocks are performed, predictive power and therapeutic results may be affected adversely because needles will ultimately be positioned in slightly different tissue planes, even when the same technique is used. Separate performance of diagnostic and therapeutic blocks is more strongly indicated when the diagnosis is uncertain, and when pain is due to a non-neoplastic process.

Outpatient Celiac Neurolysis

The infrequent occurrence of serious or persistent side effects and complications of celiac neurolysis combined with contemporary fiscal pressures that discourage inpatient hospitalization have resulted in a trend toward outpatient treatment. Although most studies do not discuss patients' residential status, in one review of 67 outpatient procedures,[177] only one patient required hospital admission, and no difficulties occurred in discharged patients. Routine outpatient celiac neurolysis would seem to be warranted for relatively fit patients as long as they are prehydrated, observed for several hours, and provided discharge instructions that include information on contacting a responsible physician.

BLOCKADE OF THE SUPERIOR HYPOGASTRIC PLEXUS AND GANGLION IMPAR

The pelvis contains diverse, multiply and complexly innervated structures (see Chapter 23.1, Fig. 23.1-22) that are potential sources of pain, particularly when the etiologic process is gynecologic or rectal cancer, which tend to spread locally either by direct invasion or metastases to regional lymph nodes. Pelvic pain may be difficult to manage because it is often vague and poorly localized and tends to be bilateral or to cross the midline. One-sided cordotomy, which produces strictly unilateral analgesia, usually represents a poor choice for the treatment of pelvic pain, and bilateral cordotomy is rarely elected because of high associated risks of fatal sleep apnea (Ondine's curse) and bladder dysfunction. In selected patients, midline myelotomy may be applicable, though results vary and surgical recuperation is required.[250] The proximity of the nerves that govern bladder, bowel, and lower extremity function and those that subserve pelvic sensation make subarachnoid and epidural neurolytic injections hazardous in this region. Except in patients with pre-existing colostomy and urinary diversions, neuroaxial blocks should be considered only as a last resort, and even then great care must be taken to avoid limb paresis. Of note is one study that combined unilateral cordotomy with contralateral subarachnoid neurolysis with relatively good results.[142] Intraspinal opioid therapy is an important option for selected patients with pelvic pain that is refractory to conventional pharmacologic management.[368] The utility of chronic intraspinal opioid therapy, though, is potentially limited by factors that include uneven availability of resources for maintenance of therapy, cost, the likelihood of tolerance, and ineffectiveness in a proportion of patients.

Although no published studies exist, bilateral lumbar sympathetic block (see Chapter 13 and Figs. 13-22 to 13-31) has been reported anecdotally to be an effective management tool for some patients with pelvic pain.[20,55] The lumbar sympathetic chain does not directly innervate pelvic structures, but owing to its continuity with the superior hypogastric plexus (see Chapter 13, Fig. 13-2) large volumes of injected solutions probably diffuse caudally. As noted, however, lumbar sympathetic block has yet to be studied systematically for this indication and may be subject to a high rate of failure in patients with large masses or retroperitoneal invasion that restrict the caudal flow of neurolytic solution.

Superior Hypogastric Plexus Block

Despite the existence of a surgical technique for interrupting the superior hypogastric plexus (to treat pelvic pain),[176] it was only recently that a parallel anesthetic approach was described.

Investigations

In the first published study on superior hypogastric block, Plancarte and co-workers[275] reported on 28 patients with intractable pelvic pain secondary to neoplastic disease (cervical cancer, 20; prostate cancer, 4; testicular cancer, 1; radiation enteritis, 3). After treatment, all patients experienced significant reduction or elimination in pain, and no complications occurred. A mean reduction in pain of 70% was observed after neurolysis, and residual pain appeared to be predominantly somatically based. The application of other treatments resulted in a global reduction in pain scores by 90%, and in all but two patients with tumor-mediated pain, there was no return of sympathetically mediated symptoms until their demise (3–12 months). In another study of cancer patients with intractable pelvic pain, de Leon-Casasola and colleagues[63] achieved similar results. Of 26 patients with 10/10 pain, 70% experienced satisfactory relief (<4/10 intensity), and the remaining patients, moderate relief (4–7/10). Complications were not observed, and no patients with satisfactory relief required repetition at 6 months. Both groups of investigators used similar anesthetic techniques.

Anatomy

The superior hypogastric plexus is a retroperitoneal structure located bilaterally at the level of the lower third of the fifth lumbar vertebral body and upper third of the first sacral vertebral body at the sacral promontory and in proximity to the bifurcation of the common iliac vessels[22,323,324,382] (see Chapter 14, Fig. 14-9A). This plexus (sometimes referred to as the presacral nerve) is formed by the confluence of the lumbar sympathetic chains and branches of the aortic plexus, which contains fibers that have traversed the celiac and inferior mesenteric plexuses. In addition, it usually contains parasympathetic fibers that originate in the ventral roots of S2–S4 and travel as slender nervi erigentes (pelvic splanchnic nerves) through the inferior hypogastric plexus to the superior hypogastric plexus.

The superior hypogastric plexus divides into the right and left hypogastric nerves, which descend lateral to the sigmoid colon and rectosigmoid junction to reach the two inferior hypogastric plexuses. The superior plexus gives off branches to the ureteric and testicular (or ovarian) plexuses, to the sigmoid colon, and to the plexus that surrounds the common and internal iliac arteries. The inferior hypogastric plexus is a bilateral structure situated on each side of the rectum, lower part of the bladder, and (in the male) prostate and seminal vesicles, or (in the female) cervix of the uterus and vaginal fornices. In contrast to the superior hypogastric plexus, which is situated in a predominantly longitudinal plane, the configuration of the inferior hypogastric plexus is oriented more transversely, extending posteroanteriorly parallel to the pelvic floor. The location and configuration of the inferior hypogastric plexus does not lend itself to surgical or chemical extirpation.

Technique

The patient assumes the prone position with padding placed beneath the pelvis to flatten the lumbar lordosis. The lumbosacral region is cleansed aseptically. The location of the L4–L5 interspace is approximated by palpation of the iliac crests and spinous processes and is then verified by fluoroscopy. Skin wheals are raised 5 to 7 cm bilateral to the midline at the level of the L4–L5 interspace (or where the pelvis is narrow L3–L4). A 7-inch, 22-gauge short-beveled needle with a depth marker placed 5 to 7 cm along the shaft is inserted through one of the skin wheals with the needle bevel directed toward the midline. From a position perpendicular in all planes to the skin, the needle is oriented about 30 degrees caudad and 45 degrees mesiad so that its tip is directed toward the anterolateral aspect of the bottom of the L5 vertebral body. The iliac crest and the transverse process of L5, which is sometimes enlarged, are potential barriers to needle passage, and necessitate the use of the cephalo-lateral entrance site and oblique trajectory described. If the transverse process of L5 is encountered during advancement of the needle, the needle is withdrawn to the subcutaneous tissue and is redirected slightly caudad or cephalad. The needle is readvanced until the body of the L5 vertebra is encountered or until its tip is observed fluoroscopically to lie at its anterolateral aspect. If the vertebral body is encountered, gentle effort may be made to further advance the needle. If this is unsuccessful, the needle is withdrawn and, without altering its cephalocaudal orientation, is redirected in a slightly less mesiad plane so that its tip is "walked off" the vertebral body. The needle tip is advanced about 1 cm past the depth at which contact with the body occurred, at which point a loss of resistance or "pop" may be felt, indicating that the needle tip has traversed the anterior fascial boundary of the ipsilateral psoas muscle and lies in the retroperitoneal space. At this point the depth marker should, depending on the patient's body habitus, lie close to the level of the skin. The contralateral needle is inserted in a similar manner, using the trajectory and the depth of the first needle as a rough guide (see Chapter 14, Fig. 14-9A).

Biplanar fluoroscopy is utilized during needle passage and to verify needle placement. Anterior-posterior views should demonstrate the needle tip's location at the level of the junction of the L5 and S1 vertebral bodies, and lateral views confirm placement of the needle tip just beyond the vertebral body's anterolateral margin. The injection of 2 to 4 ml of water-soluble contrast medium through each needle is performed to further verify accuracy of placement. In the AP view, the spread of the contrast media should be confined to the midline or paramedian region, and in the lateral view, a smooth posterior contour corresponding to the anterior psoas fascia indicates appropriate needle depth (see Chapter 14, Fig. 14-9B). Alternatively, computerized axial tomography may be utilized, permitting visualization of vascular structures and viscera.

Additional precautions include careful aspiration prior to injection and the use of test doses of local anesthetic. Vascular puncture, with a risk of subsequent hemorrhage and hematoma formation, is possible because of the close proximity of the bifurcation of the common iliac vessels. Intramuscular or intraperitoneal injection may result from an improper estimate of needle depth. These and less likely complications (subarachnoid and epidural injection, somatic nerve injury, renal or ureteral puncture) can be avoided by careful observation of technique. For diagnostic blocks, 8 ml of 0.25% bupivacaine or 1% lidocaine is injected through each needle, and for neurolysis 8 ml of 10% aqueous phenol is utilized bilaterally.

Modifications

Waldman et al.[363] observed bilateral spread of contrast medium injected through a single needle and recommended CT-guided placement of a single needle, through which 10 ml of solution is injected. In a letter to the editor, De Leon-Casasola, Plancarte, Patt, and Lema[64] suggested avoiding a unilateral approach in patients with cancer, since the spread of injectate may be impeded and unpredictable owing to retroperitoneal infiltration by tumor. Ina and colleagues[139] advocate the deliberate passage of needles through the L5–S1 disk for patients with difficult anatomy, and have reported on the safe and successful use of this technique in eight patients. Our group has had good preliminary success with a transvascular approach (Plancarte, R. et al, unpublished data) and in addition, a gynecologist/anesthesiologist investigator has successfully used a transvaginal approach for local anesthetic blocks (MacDonald, J., personal communication, 1994).

Block of the Ganglion Impar

The perineum, which refers to the anatomic area immediately below the pelvis, is comprised of diverse anatomic structures with mixed sympathetic and somatic innervation. Although various interventions have been proposed for the management of intractable perineal pain, their efficacy and applications are limited by the same factors that complicate the management of pelvic pain. In addition, the target of nerve blocks in this region has historically focused on somatic rather than sympathetic components. Recently, blockade of the ganglion impar (ganglion of Walther) has been introduced as an alternative means of managing intractable neoplastic perineal pain of sympathetic origin.[273,276]

Characteristically, sympathetic pain in the perineal region has distinct qualities, *i.e.*, it tends to be vague and poorly localized and is frequently accompanied by sensations of burning and urgency. Although the anatomic interconnections of the ganglion impar are rarely described in any detail in even the anatomic literature, it is probable that the sympathetic component of these pain syndromes derives, at least in part, from this structure. The ganglion impar is a solitary retroperitoneal structure located at the level of the sacrococcygeal junction that marks the termination of the paired paravertebral sympathetic chains (Fig. 31-9).

The first report of interruption of the ganglion impar for relief of perineal pain appeared in 1990.[273] Sixteen patients were studied (13 female, 3 male), ranging in age from 24 to 87 (median = 48). All patients had advanced cancer (cervix, 9; colon, 2; bladder, 2; rectum, 1; endometrium, 2), and pain had persisted in all cases despite surgery and/or chemotherapy and radiation, analgesics, and psychological support. Localized perineal pain was present in all cases, and was characterized as burning and urgent in eight patients and of a mixed character in eight patients. Pain was referred to the rectum (7), perineum (6), or vagina (3). Following preliminary local anesthetic blockade and subsequent neurolytic block, eight patients experienced complete (100%) relief of pain, and the remainder experienced significant reduction in pain (1, 90%; 2, 80%; 1, 70%; 4, 60%) as determined with a visual analogue scale (VAS). Blocks were repeated in two patients with further improvement. Follow-up depended on survival and was carried out for 14 to 120 days. In patients with incomplete relief of pain, residual somatic symptoms were treated with either epidural injections of steroid or sacral nerve blocks.

Technique

The patient is positioned in the lateral decubitus position, and a skin wheal is raised in the midline at the superior aspect of the intergluteal crease, over the anococcygeal ligament, and just above the anus. The stylet is removed from a standard 22-gauge 3 1/2-inch spinal needle, which is then manually bent about one inch from its hub to form a 25 to 30-degree angle. The maneuver facilitates positioning of the needle tip anterior to the concave curvature of the sacrum and coccyx. The needle is inserted through the skin wheal with its concavity oriented posteriorly and, under fluoroscopic guidance, is directed anterior to the coccyx, closely approximating the anterior surface of the bone, until its tip is observed to have reached the sacrococcygeal junction (Fig. 31-9). Retroperitoneal location of the needle is verified by observation of the spread of 2 cc of water-soluble contrast medium, which typically assumes a smooth-margined configuration resembling an apostrophe. Four milliliters of 1%

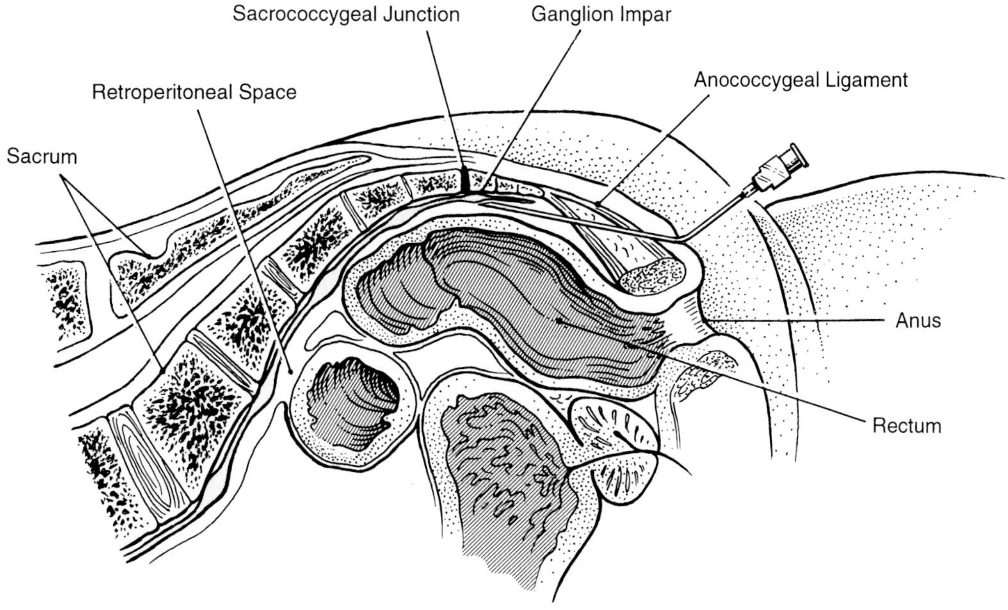

FIG. 31-9. Ganglion Impar block.

lidocaine or 0.25% bupivacaine is injected for diagnostic and prognostic purposes, or alternatively, 4 to 6 ml of 10% phenol is injected for therapeutic neurolytic blockade.

Under most circumstances, needle placement is relatively straightforward. Local tumor invasion, particularly from rectal cancer, may prohibit the spread of injected solutions. Observation that the spread of contrast material is restricted to the retroperitoneum is essential, as we have had experience with one case in which epidural spread within the caudal canal was evident. Also, unless care is taken to confirm the needle's postero-anterior orientation, perforation of the rectum or periosteal injection is possible. In addition, anatomic abnormalities of the sacrococcygeal vertebral column, specifically exaggerated anterior curvature, may inhibit access, in which case the needle may be further modified with an additional bend.

Future Directions

Cancer Pain

Superior hypogastric plexus and ganglion impar block have proven utility, respectively, for sympathetically mediated pelvic and perineal pain due to neoplasm that is refractory to more conservative management. Given the absence of reported complications, further studies are indicated in this population to determine whether earlier institution may permit more rapid and complete pain control than with standard pharmacotherapy. Success may improve further if neurolysis is performed before extensive tumor infiltration shelters the targeted structures. Likewise, trials of surgical or chemical interruption of the plexus at the time of laparotomy are warranted.

Nonmalignant Pain

Chronic pelvic pain of nononcologic origin is a common problem that is often refractory to even comprehensive multidisciplinary treatment.[158,317] Although up to half of patients probably have non-nociceptive determinants of pain,[222,287,353,364] a variety of non-neoplastic conditions (e.g., endometriosis, pelvic inflammatory disease, adhesions) may be amenable to treatment with superior hypogastric plexus block. Trials of superior hypogastric plexus block in this population should include careful stratification of patients as well as measurement of distress, sexual performance, and functional capacity.

PITUITARY ABLATION

Pituitary ablation (neuroadenolysis of the pituitary, chemical hypophysectomy) is performed in a limited number of centers to treat intractable pain due to disseminated bone metastases, especially in patients with primary breast or prostate cancer.

Surgical hypophysectomy was first advocated to reduce tumor spread in 1953.[198] The observation that some patients experienced postsurgical pain relief led Greco[224] and later Moricca[234] and others to suggest pituitary destruction by percutaneous injection of absolute alcohol as a primary treatment for oncogenic pain. When indicated, a needle-based technique with alcohol, less commonly cryogenic lesions[73] and even electrical stimulation,[387] is preferred to surgical extirpation because the former approaches are comparatively simple, safe, and inexpensive, and entail only a brief hospitalization. It is curious that pituitary ablation has not secured a more uniform place in the cancer pain specialist's armamentarium since, although its conduct is technically demanding, there is considerable published experience that reflects favorably on its efficacy and safety.[73,163,175,179,192,387] Although experience is greatest in patients with breast and prostate cancer, recent reports suggest efficacy in patients with other malignant neoplasms, especially if the presenting complaint is head or neck pain.[163,175,179] Chief among pituitary ablation's merits is its applicability for bilateral and disseminated pain. Onset of relief is typically rapid and often complete, but like most ablative procedures, efficacy tends to deteriorate beyond 6 to 12 months.

Mechanism

The mechanism underlying the action of pituitary ablation remains obscure[178], although authorities favor theories that involve activation of a pituitary inhibitory system,[387] alterations in hormonal feedback, and suppression of the hypothalamic axis.[56] It has been further postulated that the capacity for pituitary procedures to relieve pain may involve a stress response similar to that which is observed in animal models, after battle injuries, and in athletes.[179] Although there are some conflicting data, activation of endogenous opioids seems unlikely based on reports that analgesia is not reliably reversed by naloxone administration.[227] Although observations of the spread of contrast medium near the third ventricle led to theories of hypothalamic injury, this mechanism is inconsistent with reports of pain relief after more discrete procedures (cryolesioning and electrical stimulation). Evidence suggests that pituitary destruction, in and of itself, is unlikely to be causal: primate research has demonstrated that neither complete destruction of the gland nor even significant injury is required to achieve pain relief.[386] Similar outcomes in humans treated with alcohol injection and stimulation,[387] and an absence of correlation between the degree of injury observed at autopsy and clinical outcomes, further argue against such a mechanism. Neither is tumor regression a likely explanation, since pituitary injections, oophorectomy, adrenalectomy, and orchidectomy all may produce almost immediate pain relief in appropriate patients. Finally, there is little evidence that hypofunction of the pituitary or the anterior hypothalamus, or straightforward hormonal changes underlie pain relief, in that outcome does not correlate with measurable changes in circulating levels of hormones. In addition, the presence and severity of diabetes insipidus, one marker for glandular injury, does not correlate with pain relief.[179]

Technique

Pituitary ablation has been carried out variously by neurosurgical or anesthesiology teams, or in collaboration, with apparently similar results.[20,223] Both radiologically guided "freehand" and stereotactic techniques have been advocated.[56] Plain radiographs of the skull are reviewed to survey the size and position of the sella turcica, as well as to identify any bony abnormalities. Typically, light general endotracheal anesthesia is induced, and a topical vasoconstrictive anesthetic (4% cocaine paste or 7.5% to 20% cocaine-impregnated packs) is applied to the nasal mucosa of the most patent nostril, which is then cleansed with an organic iodine solution.

Modified Moricca ("Freehand") Technique

For the "freehand" or (modified) Moricca approach, with the patient positioned supine and the head semiflexed, a specially designed "Moricca" needle or 17-gauge styletted spinal needle is passed through one nostril toward the pituitary fossa by the transphenoidal route (Fig. 31-10). Under fluoroscopic guidance the needle is directed posteriorly, superiorly, and slightly medially toward the glabella (from the frontal plane) and zygomatic arch (viewed laterally). The needle is passed through the posterior nasal mucosa until resistance is encountered, which correlates to the skull base, and it is then advanced incrementally by means of gently tapping its hub with a small metal hammer. The position of the needle tip within the anterior bony margins of the pituitary fossa is confirmed with anterior and posterior radiographs (Fig. 31-11 and 31-12), and the Queckenstedt maneuver is performed to exclude extrusion of CSF or blood. A smaller (20-gauge) needle may be introduced through the original needle and advanced a few millimeters into the substance of the gland, after which the spread of the injection of a minute quantity of contrast medium is monitored. Moricca's original technique, which employed the administration 2 to 6 ml of absolute alcohol, has yielded to protocols that call for the injection of a total of 0.8 to 1.0 ml of absolute alcohol in 0.1-ml increments over 10 to 15 minutes. During the injection, anesthesia is lightened to facilitate detection of pupillary movement or dilation that may signal damage to the optic chiasm. If pupillary changes occur, some clinicians advocate discontinuing the injection, turning the patient laterally, and administering corticosteroids

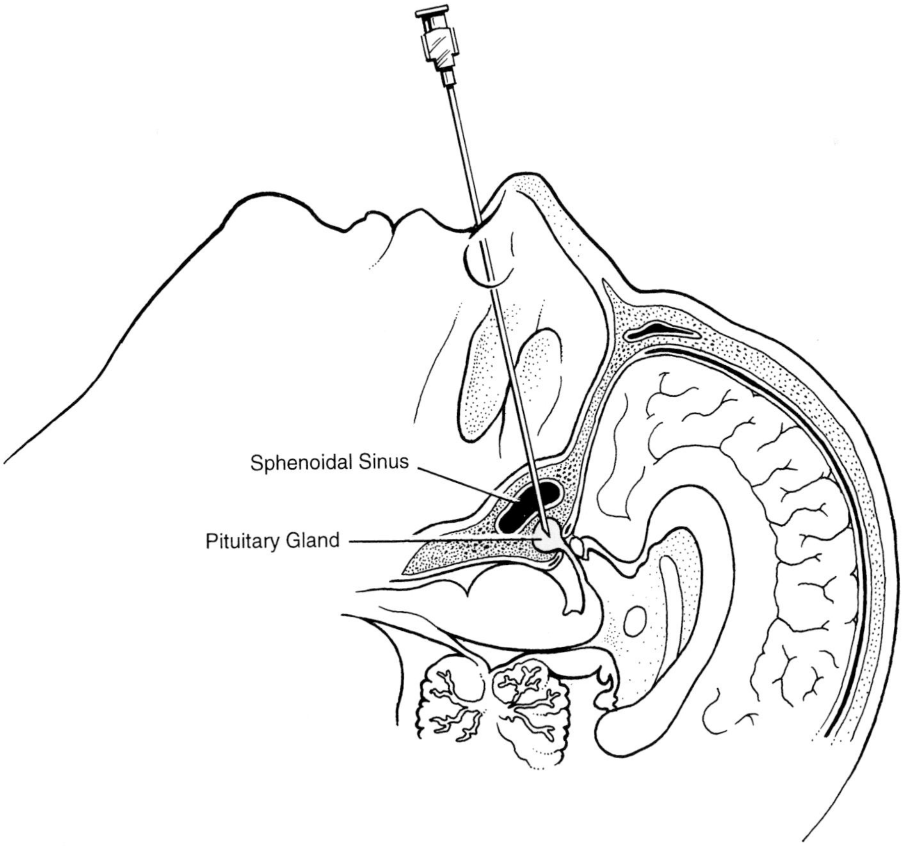

FIG. 31-10. Technique for pituitary ablation (see text).

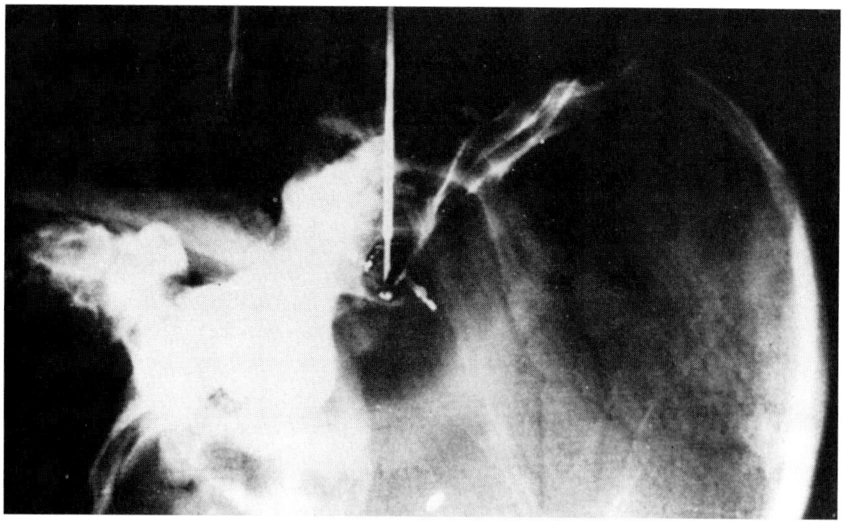

FIG. 31-11. Chemical hypophysectomy. Radiograph, lateral view, showing needle passing through sphenoid sinus and floor of sella turcica. Tip of needle is immediately below level of posterior clinoid processes. Some injected Myodil can be seen moving up the pituitary stalk.

intracisternally. When the injection is complete, after withdrawing the needle to the sella's anterior border, many advocate the injection of 0.5 ml of cyanomethacralate resin as a sealant to prevent CSF leakage.[362]

Stereotactic Technique

A stereotactic approach, pioneered by Levin,[179] differs in just a few important ways from Moricca's technique. It involves positioning the patient in a Todd-Wells head holder equipped with a transverse quadrant assembly (Fig. 31-13). The unit's needle holder is advanced through the prepared nostril and, with fluoroscopic guidance, the posterosuperior aspect of the sella, just below the posterior clinoid processes in the midline, is targeted using a trajectory that maximizes glandular penetration. After additional infiltration, a 6-inch 18-gauge spinal needle is used to penetrate the floor of the sphenoid sinus, where bacitracin is administered. The 18-gauge needle is replaced with a 6-inch 20-gauge spinal needle, which is gently inserted until its tip is radiographically confirmed to have reached the target region. One to 2 ml of absolute alcohol is slowly injected, following which the needle is withdrawn to a point halfway between the target and the sella's floor where a second 1- to 2-ml injection is made, and finally, after further withdrawal, a third 1 to 2-ml injection is performed distally. Anesthesia is lightened and the eyes are monitored during injections so that the procedure can be discontinued should pupillary changes occur.

In addition to visual impairment, postoperative problems may include CSF leak and diabetes or Addisonism, which may require hormone replacement. Monitoring of blood sugar and urine volume is instituted to detect hormonal insufficiency and diabetes insipidus. Typically, patients are given oral hydrocortisone and, if necessary, vasopressin and/or thyroid supplementation.

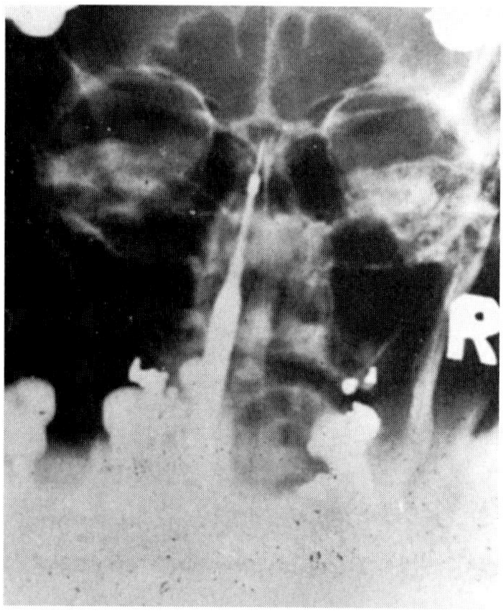

FIG. 31-12. Anteroposterior view showing needle in midline at target. [From Levin A.B., and Ramidel, L.L.: Treatment of cancer pain with hypophysectomy: Surgical and chemical. *In* Benedetti, C., *et al.* (eds.): Advances in Pain Research and Therapy. Vol. 7. pp. 631–645. New York, Raven Press, 1984.]

Results

Results vary among studies owing in part to differences in patient selection and technique. Bonica et al. reviewed the results of 15 clinical series that reported good or complete pain relief in 39% to 87% of patients, and calculated a mean incidence of 86% fair-good results (63% complete or good, 23% fair). In at least one case, analgesia was so profound as to allow a patient previously immobile from pain to return to work for an extended period.[200] Some patients remained free of pain for up to 2 years, and a significant number of patients died painlessly. Pain relief usually develops gradually over the first 24 to 48 hours following the procedure, but in some cases is immediate and in others accrues over more prolonged periods.

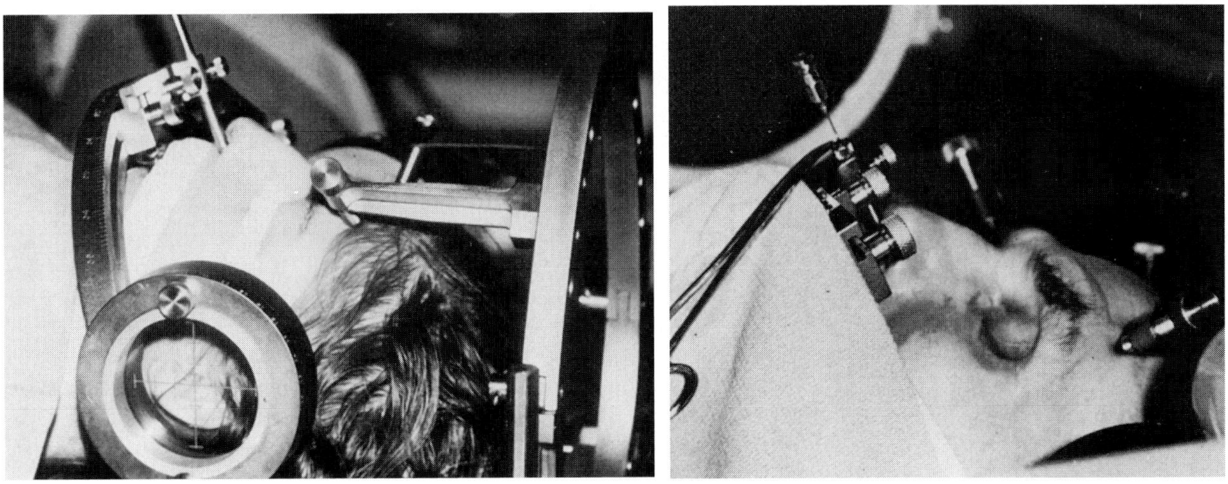

FIG. 31-13. Chemical hypophysectomy. **A:** Stereotaxic apparatus in place on patient's head. Note needle guide inserted into the nostril. **B:** Spinal needle (20-gauge) inserted into needle guide and then passed into sella turcica. [From Levin, A.B., and Ramidel, L.L.: Treatment of cancer pain with hypophysectomy: Surgical and chemical. *In* Benedetti, C., *et al.* (eds.): Advances in Pain Research and Therapy, vol. 7, pp. 631–645. New York, Raven Press, 1984.]

Miles reported six procedure-related deaths in an early series of 250 patients,[223] but in recent, more representative studies there is typically no mortality attributed to the procedure.[175] The most frequent complications in a large series were self-limited headache (17%), diabetes insipidus (17%), and nausea (9%).[73] Visual disturbance, a potentially serious complication, occurs infrequently.

NEUROLYSIS FOR SPASTICITY

In addition to their role in managing pain, neurolytic blocks are commonly used to treat spasticity of various etiologies in adults and children.[104,238,251] Techniques in common use include peripheral and subarachnoid neurolysis, as well as injections directly into spastic muscles, referred to variously as intramuscular neurolysis, motor point blocks, and motor end plate blocks. In the setting of spasticity, neurolysis is intended to interrupt the stretch reflex arc at various levels, and although skeletal muscle is usually targeted, bladder spasm is amenable as well.[378] The goals of neurolysis in spastic patients include improvements in balance, gait, self care and global rehabilitation, as well as in pain. Observers have noted rapid and sustained elimination of clonus, and increased strength and speed of active voluntary motion in antagonists of muscles blocked and occasionally in the blocked muscle itself.[104] Although alcohol is used occasionally, especially for subarachnoid neurolysis, most commonly phenol in concentrations of 2% to 5% and occasionally 7% is used for peripheral and motor point blocks.

Peripheral Blocks

The main distinction between peripheral neurolytic blocks for pain versus spasticity is that, in the latter, motor or mixed nerves are preferentially targeted. Open phenol neurectomy may even be performed to isolate sensory components of mixed nerves.[96] For percutaneous procedures, a nerve stimulator and insulated needle are typically utilized. Moritz[235] reported on a series of 50 spastic patients who received a total of 90 peripheral nerve blocks (musculocutaneous, median, ulnar, tibial, obturator, femoral, and superior gluteal nerves) performed with either 2% phenol in saline or 3% aqueous phenol. Focal motor weakness lasted only about one week in 15% of patients, but the average duration of effect was 8 months. He noted a low incidence of transient dysesthesias (10%), which usually resolved in days or weeks, and no sensory disturbances, findings that are not surprising given the dilute solutions utilized. Reporting on 521 blocks of peripheral nerves performed with 6% aqueous phenol, Gibson[101] noted one serious complication in a 69-year-old hemiplegic patient who, after five successful blocks, underwent a brachioradialis and musculotaneous block and developed an arterial occlusion that required upper limb amputation. Another method of peripheral blockade is the use of the cryoprobe (Figs. 31-14 and 31-15).

Intramuscular Injection of Neurolytics for Spasticity (and Pain)

Although injection takes place directly into the muscle, the intention is to target specific electrosensitive sites (motor points or motor end plates) that are thought to correspond to the site at which the nerve enters the muscle or where motor end plates cluster.[104] These points can often be identified by surface stimulation, nerve stimulation, or electromyography, and in addition the characteristic locations of commonly sought motor points have been published in chart form.[371]

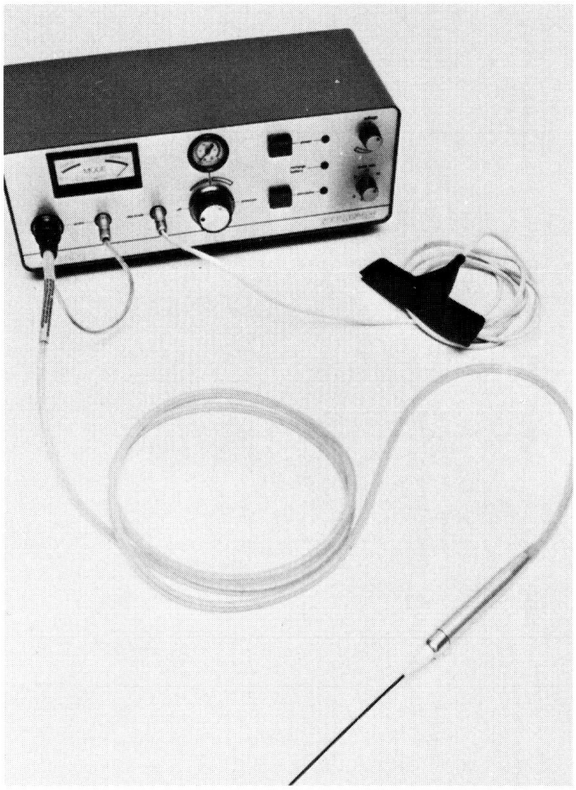

FIG. 31-14. Cryoanalgesia apparatus.

Local (Intramuscular, Periosteal) Neurolysis for Pain

Serial injection of "trigger points" with local anesthetics and/or steroids is a well-accepted means of managing chronic myofascial pain. The clinical and histologic sequelae of locally injected neurolytics are less certain; thus local infiltration is generally avoided because of concerns about skin slough and worsening of pain due to local ischemia or necrosis. Modest experience with the management of localized pain and itch and more extensive experience from the spasticity literature, however, suggests that the creation of discrete local lesions may have limited value in circumscribed settings, and merits further research.

Cousins[56] refers to injecting persistent trigger points with 5% to 6% aqueous phenol but indicates the need for further research. Ramamurthy et al.[286] mention having performed three "myoneural" blocks with 6% aqueous phenol, but provide no further detail. Local injections of 0.1 to 0.5 ml of 5% phenol in glycerine were performed in a study of patients with painful palpable peripheral neuromas.[62,166] Fifteen neuromas were treated in 10 patients with a total of 20 blocks. Complete relief was obtained and maintained in all but one patient for the 8- to 22-month follow-up period, and there were no reports of complications or neuritis. In another series of patients with poststernotomy pain presumably due to scar neuroma,[61,352] seven patients were treated with multiple, serial, local neurolytic injections of 2 to 3 ml of 6% aqueous phenol or 1.5 to 2.0 ml of absolute alcohol. Complete relief was obtained in most patients, and no complications referable to neurolysis were observed. Finally, Defalque[61] obtained complete relief in 63 of 69 patients by performing repeated trigger point injections near surgical scars with 1.0 ml of absolute alcohol, and noted no complications other than localized numbness. Although there is little published clinical experience, periosteal injections of dilute aqueous phenol (3% to 5%) may be effective for refractory bone pain.[261,342]

Subcutaneous infiltration of absolute alcohol for intractable anal and vulvar pruritus has been reported by several authors.[330,383,384] While relevance to the treatment of pain is uncertain, this technique is apparently safe and effective for patients with localized pain associated with itch. In a representative series, over two-thirds of patients experienced complete symptomatic relief that persisted for 1 to 5 years. Complications were limited to local skin reactions that, although initially distressing, subsided over 2 to 3 weeks. Likewise, the extensive experience with intramuscular injections of phenol (i.e., motor point blocks, see Neurolysis for Spasticity) for spasticity suggests reasonable safety, at least for dilute formulations of phenol. Although clinicians have observed local pain, swelling, and induration of a few days' duration, and tender nodules within muscles 1 to 3 weeks following treatment, serious long-term sequelae have not been reported.[95,119] After administering intramuscular phenol to dogs and rats, Halpern[118] observed local necrosis and inflammation within days after treatment, which intensified by 2 weeks and then resolved.

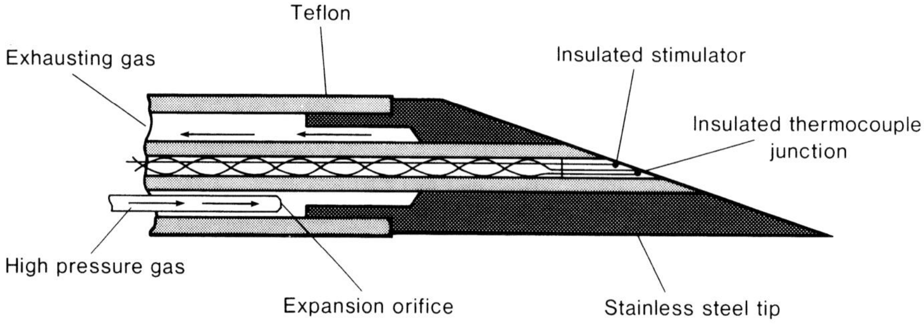

FIG. 31-15. Details of cryoprobe tip [From Lloyd, J.W., Barnard, J.D., and Glynn, C.J.: Cryoanalgesia. A new approach to pain relief. Lancet, *2*:933, 1976.]

CONCLUSION

Neurolysis has specific, compelling indications in the management of intractable cancer pain and similar conditions, as well as other less certain indications for refractory pain states in patients with normal life expectancies. Like all invasive procedures with potential utility for improving intractable pain, careful attention must be paid to the applicability of more conservative alternatives, patient selection, technical aspects, and their complementary role with pharmacologic, physical, and psychological treatment modalities. It is essential that additional carefully controlled studies be designed to better characterize the role of various neurolytic techniques in specific settings.

REFERENCES:

1. Abram, S.E., and Boas, R.A.: Sympathetic and visceral nerve blocks. *In* Benumof, J.L. (ed.): Clinical Procedures in Anesthesia and Intensive Care. pp. 787–805. Philadelphia, J.B. Lippincott, 1993.
2. Abrams, S.: Neurolytic blocks of peripheral nerves. *In* Racz, G.B. (ed.): Techniques of Neurolysis. pp. 185–192. Boston, Kluwer, 1989.
3. Adriani, J.: Labat's Regional Anesthesia. 3rd ed. Philadelphia, W.B. Saunders, 1967.
4. Adriani, J.: Thoracic sympathetic block. *In* Adriani, J. (ed.): Nerve Blocks: A Manual of Regional Anesthesia for Practitioners of Medicine. 1st Ed. pp. 47. Springfield, Ill., Charles C. Thomas, 1954.
5. American Pain Society: Principles of Analgesic Use in the Treatment of Acute Pain and Chronic Cancer Pain. 3rd Ed. Skokie, IL, American Pain Society, 1992.
6. Arbit, E., and Krol, G.: Percutaneous radiofrequency neurolysis guided by computed tomography for the treatment of glossopharyngeal neuralgia. Neurosurgery, *29:*580, 1991.
7. Atkinson, G.L., and Shupack, R.C.: Acute bronchospasm complicating intercostal nerve block with phenol. Anesth. Analg., *68:*1, 1989.
8. Balamoutsos, N.G.: Infiltration block of the coeliac plexus using plastic catheter. Reg. Anaesth., *5:*64, 1982.
9. Bates, W., and Judovich, B.D.: Intractable pain. Anesthesiology, *3:*663, 1942.
10. Bedder, M.D., and Lindsay, D.: Glossopharyngeal nerve block using ultrasound guidance: A case report of a new technique. Reg. Anesth. *14:*304, 1989.
11. Bell, S.N., Cole, R., and Roberts-Thomson, I.C.: Coeliac plexus block for control of pain in chronic pancreatitis. Br. Med. J., *281:*1604, 1980.
12. Benedetti, C.: Intraspinal analgesia: An historical overview. Acta Anaesthesiol. Scand. *85:*17, 1987.
13. Benzon, H.T.: Convulsions secondary to intravascular phenol: A hazard of celiac plexus block. Anesth. Analg., *58:*150, 1979.
14. Birch, M., Strong, N., Brittain, F., and Sanford-Smith, J.: Retrobulbar phenol injection in blind painful eyes. Ann. Ophthalmol., *25:*267, 1993.
15. Black, A., and Dwyer, B.: Coeliac plexus block. Anaesth. Intensive Care, *1:*315, 1973.
16. Boas, R.A.: Sympathetic blocks in clinical practice. Int. Anesthesiol. Clin., *16:*149, 1978.
17. Bonica, J.J., Management of Pain. 1st Ed. Philadelphia, Lea & Febiger, 1953.
18. Bonica, J.J.: Multidisciplinary/interdisciplinary pain programs. *In* Bonica, J.J. (ed.): The Management of Pain. 2nd Ed. pp. 197–208. Philadelphia, Lea & Febiger, 1990.
19. Bonica, J.J.: The management of pain of malignant disease with nerve blocks. Anesthesiology, *15:*134, 1954.
20. Bonica, J.J., Buckley, F.P., Moricca, G., *et al.*: Neurolytic blockade and hypophysectomy. *In* Bonica, J.J. (ed.): Management of Pain. 2nd Ed. pp. 1980. Philadelphia, Lea & Febiger, 1990.
21. Bonica, J.J., Ventafridda, V., and Pagni, C.A. (eds.): Management of superior pulmonary sulcus syndrome (Pancoast syndrome). Adv. Pain Res. Ther. *4:*1, 1982.
22. Brass, A.: Anatomy and physiology: Autonomic nerves and ganglia in pelvis. *In* Netter, F.H. (ed.): The Ciba Collection of Medical Illustrations. Vol. 1. Nervous System. pp. 85. Summit, NJ, U.S.A., Ciba Pharmaceutical Co., 1983.
23. Braun, H.: Ein hilfsinstrument zur ausführung der splanchnicusanästhesie. Zentralbl. Chir., *48:*1544, 1921.
24. Braun, H.: Local Anesthesia: Its Scientific Basis and Practical Use. pp. 311–313. Philadelphia, Lea & Febiger, 1924.
25. Bridenbaugh, L.D., Moore, D.C., and Campbell, D.D.: Management of upper abdominal cancer pain: Treatment with celiac plexus block with alcohol. J.A.M.A., *190:*877, 1964.
26. Broggi, G., and Siegfried, J.: Percutaneous differential radiofrequency rhizotomy of glossopharyngeal nerve in facial pain due to cancer. Adv. Pain Res. Ther. *2:*469, 1979.
27. Brown, A.S.: Current views on the use of nerve blocking in the relief of chronic pain. *In* Swerdlow, M. (ed.): The Therapy of Pain. Philadelphia, J.B. Lippincott, 1981.
28. Brown, B.L., Bulley, C.K., and Quiel, E.C.: Neurolytic celiac plexus block for pancreatic cancer pain. Anesth. Analg., *66:*869, 1987.
29. Brown, D.L.: A retrospective analysis of neurolytic celiac plexus block for nonpancreatic intra-abdominal cancer pain. Reg. Anesth., *14:*63, 1989.
30. Brown, D.L.: Atlas of Regional Anesthesia. Philadelphia, W.B. Saunders, 1992.
31. Brown, D.L.: Neurolytic celiac plexus block: Its place in your practice. Probl. Anesth., *1:*612, 1987.
32. Bryce-Smith, R.: Local and regional anaesthesia. Postgrad. Med. J., *42:*367, 1966.
33. Bruno, G.: Intrathecal alcohol block: Experiences on 41 cases. Paraplegia, *12:*305, 1975.
34. Burcheil, K.J., Clarke, H., Haglund, M., and Loeser, J.D.: Long-term efficacy of microvascular decompression in trigeminal neuralgia. J. Neurosurg. *69:*35, 1988.
35. Buy, J.N., Moss, A.A., and Singler, R.C.: CT guided celiac plexus and splanchnic nerve neurolysis. J. Comput. Assist. Tomogr., *6:*315, 1982.
36. Cantwell, B.M.K., Mannix, K.A., and Harris, A.L.: Back pain: A presentation of metastatic testicular germ cell tumours. Lancet, *i:*262, 1987.
37. Carr, D., Eisenberg, E., and Chalmers, T.C.: Neurolytic celiac plexus block for cancer pain: A meta-analysis. Abstracts. pp. 338. 7th World Congress on Pain, Paris, 1993.
38. Chapman, C.R., and Donaldson, G.W.: Issues in designing trials of nonpharmacologic treatments for pain. Adv. Pain Res. Ther., *18:*699, 1991.
39. Charlton, J.E.: Relief of the pain of unresectable carcinoma of the pancreas by chemical splanchnicectomy during laparotomy. Ann. Roy. Coll. Surg., *67:*136, 1985.
40. Chayen, D., Nathan, H., and Chayne, M.: The psoas compartment block. Anesthesiology, *45:*95, 1976.
41. Cherry, D.A., and Lamberty, J.: Paraplegia following coeliac plexus block. Anaesth. Intens. Care, *12:*59, 1984.
42. Cherry, D.A., and Rao, D.M.: Lumbar sympathetic and coeliac plexus blocks: An anatomical study in cadavers. Br. J. Anaesth., *54:*1037, 1982.
43. Christie, J.M., and Hranowsky, N.: Glycerol application of peripheral nerves for the pain of advanced malignancy. Reg. Anesth., 15(Suppl.):87, 1990.
44. Churcher, M.: Peripheral nerve blocks in the relief of intractable pain. *In* Swerdlow M., and Charlton, J.E.: Relief of Intractable Pain. 4th Ed. pp. 195. Amsterdam, Elsevier, 1989.
45. Clark, A.J., and Awad, S.A.: Selective transsacral nerve root blocks. Reg. Anesth., *15:*125, 1990.
46. Clark, A.J., and Said, A.A.: Selective transsacral nerve root blocks. Reg. Anesth., *15:*125, 1990.
47. Cleeland, C.S.: Assessment of pain in cancer. *In* Foley, K.M., Bonica, J.J., Ventafridda, V., *et al.* (eds.): Second International Congress on Cancer. Advances in Pain Research and Therapy. Vol. 16. pp. 47. Philadelphia, Lippincott–Raven, 1990.
48. Cleeland, C.S., Rotondi, A., Brechner, T., *et al.*: A model for the treatment of cancer pain. J. Pain Symptom Manage., *1:*209, 1986.
49. Conacher, I.D., and Kokri, M.: Postoperative paravertebral blocks for thoracic surgery: A radiological appraisal. Br. J. Anaesth., *59:*155, 1987.

50. Cook, E.E., Flaherty, R.A., Willmarth, C.L., *et al.*: Chylothorax: A complication of translumbar aortography. Radiology, *75:*251, 1960.
51. Coombs, D.W.: Potential hazards of transcatheter serial epidural phenol neurolysis. Anesth. Analg., *64:*1205, 1985.
52. Copping, J., Willix, R., and Kraft, R.O.: Palliative chemical splanchnicectomy. Arch. Surg., *98:*418, 1969.
53. Corning, J.L.: Pain. p. 247. Philadelphia, J.B. Lippincott, 1894.
54. Cosman, E.R., Nahold, B.S., and Bedenbaugh, P.: Stereotactic radiofrequency lesion making. Appl. Neurophys. *46:*160, 1983.
55. Cousins, M.J.: Anesthetic approaches in cancer pain. Adv. Pain Res. Ther., *16:*249, 1990.
56. Cousins, M.J., Dwyer, B., and Gibb, D.: Chronic pain and neurolytic neural blockade. *In* Cousins, M.J., and Bridenbaugh, P.O.: Neural Blockade. 2nd Ed. pp. 1053–1084. Philadelphia, J.B. Lippincott, 1988.
57. Dandy, W.E.: Concerning the cause of trigeminal neuralgia. Am. J. Surg., *24:*447, 1934.
58. Dargent, M.: Role of sympathetic nerve in cancerous pain. Br. Med. J., *1:*440, 1948.
59. Davies, D.D.: Incidence of major complications of neurolytic coeliac plexus block. J. R. Soc. Med., *86:*264, 1993.
60. De Conno, F., Caraceni, A., Aldrighetti, L., *et al.*: Paraplegia following coeliac plexus block. Pain, *55:*383, 1993.
61. Defalque, R.J.: Painful trigger points in surgical scars. Anesth. Analg., *61:*518, 1982.
62. Defalque, R.J., and Bromley, J.J.: Poststernotomy neuralgia: A new pain syndrome. Anesth. Analg., *69:*81, 1989.
63. De Leon-Casasola, O.A., Kent, E., and Lema, M.J. Neurolytic superior hypogastric plexus block for chronic pelvic pain associated with cancer. Pain, *54:*145, 1993.
64. De Leon-Casasola, O.A., Plancarte-Sanchez, R., Patt, R.B., and Lema, M.J.: Superior hypogastric plexus block using a single needle and computed tomography guidance. Reg. Anesth., *18:*63, 1993.
65. De Takats, G.: Splanchnic anesthesia: A critical review of the theory and practice of this method. Surg. Gynec. Obstet., *44:*501, 1927.
66. Dobrogowski, J., and Marian, K.: Epidural neurolytic block in cancer patients. *In* Erdmann, W., Oyama, T., Pernack, M.J. (eds.): Pain Clinic I. pp. 51–54. Utrecht, Netherlands, VNU Science Press, 1985.
67. Dogliotti, A.M.: A new therapeutic method for peripheral neuralgias. Injection of alcohol into the subarachnoid space. Pain Clinic, *1:*197, 1987.
68. Dogliotti, A.M.: Traitement des syndromes douloureux de la peripherie par l'alcoolisation subarachnoidienne. Presse Med., *67:*11, 1931.
69. Dondelinger, R.F., and Kurdziel, J.C.: Percutaneous phenol block of the upper thoracic sympathetic chain with computed tomography guidance. Acta Radiol., *28:*511, 1987.
70. Doyle, D.: Nerve blocks in advanced cancer. Practitioner, *226:*539, 1982.
71. Drapiewski, J.R.: Carcinoma of the pancreas: A study of neoplastic invasion of nerves and its possible clinical significance. Am. J. Clin. Path., *15:*549, 1944.
72. Duthie, A.M.: Pituitary cryoablation. Anaesthesia, *38:*495, 1983.
73. Duthie, A.M., Ingham, V., Dell, A.E., *et al.*: Results of treatment using a transphenoidal cryoprobe. Anaesthesia, *38:*448, 1983.
74. Evans, P.J.D.: Cryoanalgesia. Anesthaesia *36:*1003, 1981.
75. Evans, P.J.D., Lloyd, J.W., and Green, C.J.: Cryoanalgesia: The response to alternations in freeze cycle and temperature. Br. J. Anaesth., *53:*1121, 1981.
76. Evans, R.J., and MacKay, I.M.: Subarachnoid phenol blocks for relief of pain in advanced malignancy. Can. J. Surg., *15:*50, 1972.
77. Feldman, S.A., and Yeung, M.L.: Treatment of intermittent claudication: Lumbar paravertebral somatic block with phenol. Anaesthesia, *30:*174, 1975.
78. Feldstein, G.S.: Percutaneous retrogasserian glycerol rhizotomy in the treatment of trigeminal neuralgia. *In* Racz, G.B. (ed.): Techniques of Neurolysis. pp. 125–132. Boston, Kluwer Academic Publishers, 1989.
79. Feldstein, G.S., and Waldman, S.D.: Loss of resistance technique for transaortic celiac plexus block. Anesth. Analg., *65:*1092, 1986.
80. Ferrer-Brechner, T.: Epidural and intrathecal phenol neurolysis for cancer pain. Anesthesiol. Rev., *8:*14, 1981.
81. Ferrer-Brechner, T.: Neurolytic blocks for cancer pain. *In* Abrams, S. (ed.): Cancer Pain. pp. 111. Boston, Kluwer Academic, 1988.
82. Filshie, J., Golding, S., Robbie, D.S., and Husband, J.E.: Unilateral computerised tomography guided coeliac plexus block: A technique for pain relief. Anaesthesia, *38:*498, 1983.
83. Fine, P.G., and Bubela, C.: Chylothorax following celiac plexus block. Anesthesiology, *63:*454, 1985.
84. Fink, B.R.: History of neural blockade. *In* Cousins, M.J., and Bridenbaugh, P.O. (eds.): Neural Blockade. 2nd Ed. pp. 3–21. Philadelphia, J.B. Lippincott, 1988.
85. Flanigan, D.P., and Kraft, R.O.: Continuing experience with palliative chemical splanchnicectomy. Arch. Surg., *113:*509, 1978.
86. Foley, K.M.: Pain syndromes and pharmacologic management of pancreatic cancer pain. J. Pain Symptom Manage., *3:*176, 1988.
87. Foley, K.M.: Treatment of cancer pain. N. Engl. J. Med., *313:*84, 1985.
88. Forster, L.E., and Lynn, J.: Predicting life-spans for applicants to inpatient hospice. Arch. Int. Med., *148:*2540, 1988.
89. Forster, L.E., and Lynn, J.: The use of physiologic measures and demographic variables to predict longevity among inpatient hospice admissions. Am. J. Hospice Care, *6:*31, 1989.
90. Fujita, Y.: CT-guided neurolytic splanchnic block with alcohol. Pain, *55:*363, 1993.
91. Fujita, Y., Oshumi, A., and Takaori, M.: CT scan and celiac plexus block. Anesthesiology, *68:*968, 1988.
92. Fujita, Y., and Takaori, M.: Pleural effusion after CT-guided alcohol celiac plexus block. Anesth. Analg., *66:*911, 1987.
93. Gage, M., and Floyd, J.B.: The treatment of acute pancreatitis: With discussion of mechanism of production, clinical manifestations and diagnosis and report of four cases. Tr. South S.A., *59:*415, 1947.
94. Galizia, E.J., and Lahiri, S.K.: Paraplegia following coeliac plexus block with phenol. Br. J. Anaesth., *46:*539, 1974.
95. Garland, D.E., Lilling, M., and Keenan, M.A.: Percutaneous phenol blocks to motor points of spastic forearm muscles in head-injured adults. Arch. Phys. Med. Rehabil., *65:*243, 1984.
96. Garland, D.E., Lucie, R.S., and Waters, R.L.: Current uses open phenol nerve block for adult aquired spasticity. Clin. Orthop. Rel. Res., *165:*217, 1982.
97. Gaudy, J.H., Tricot, C., and Sezeur, A.: Troubles du rhythme cardiaque graves apres phénolisation splanchnique peroperatoire. Can. J. Anaesth., *40:*357, 1993.
98. Gerbershagen, H.U.: Blocks with local anesthetics in the treatment of cancer pain. In: Bonica, J. J., and Vertafridda, V. (eds.) International Symposium on Pain of Advanced Cancer. Advances in Pain Research and Therapy. Vol. 2. pp. 11–23. New York, Raven Press, 1979.
99. Gerbershagen, H.U.: Neurolysis: Subarachnoid neurolytic blockade. Acta Anœsth. Belg., *1:*45, 1981.
100. Geurts, J.W.M., and Stolker, R.J.: Relief of pain in upper extremity sympathetic dystrophy by radiofrequency lesions in the stellate ganglion. Reg. Anesth., *17*(3S):63, 1992.
101. Gibson, I.J.M.: Phenol block in the treatment of spasticity. Gerontology, *33:*327, 1987.
102. Giménez, A., Martinez-Noguera, A., Donoso, L., *et al.*: Percutaneous neurolysis of the celiac plexus via the anterior approach with sonographic guidance. Am. J. Radiol., *161:*1061, 1993.
103. Giron, G.P., and Vincenti, E.: Oral morphine. Adv. Pain Res. Ther., *14:*221, 1990.
104. Glenn, M.B.: Nerve blocks for the treatment of spasticity. Arch. Phys. Med. Rehabil., *8:*481, 1994.
105. Gorbitz, C., and Leavens, E.: Alcohol block of the celiac plexus for control of upper abdominal pain caused by cancer and pancreatitis. J. Neurosurg., *34:*575, 1971.
106. Goffen, B.S.: Transsacral block. Anesth. Analg., *61:*623, 1982.
107. Graham, C., Bond, S.S., Gerkovich, M.M., *et al.*: Use of the McGill pain questionnaire in the assessment of cancer pain: Replicability and consistency. Pain, *8:*377, 1980.
108. Grant, F.C.: Surgical methods for relief of pain. Bull. N.Y. Acad. Med., *19:*373, 1943.
109. Gregg, R.V., Sehlhorst, C.S., and Liwnicz, B.H.: Histopathology of epidural phenol in the monkey. pp. 93. Abstracts. 7th World Congress on Pain, Paris, 1993.
110. Green, C.R., deRosayro, A.M., Tait, A.R., *et al.*: Long-term follow-up of cryoanalgesia for chronic thoracic pain. Reg. Anesth., *18:*46, 1993.
111. Grunwald, I.: Neurlise com fenol: Uso de via peridural no tratemonto da dolor de cancer. Rev. Brasil de Anest., *26:*628, 1976.
112. Guerts, J.M.W., Zwart, S.J., van Eys, F., *et al.*: Percutaneous neurolytic coeliac plexus block: A comparison between alcohol 48% and phenol 8%. Abstracts. pp. 565. 7th World Congress on Pain, Paris, 1993.
113. Gybels, J.M., and Sweet, W.H.: Neurosurgical treatment of persisting pain. Physiological and pathological mechanisms of human pain. Pain Headache, *11:*442, 1989.

114. Haaga, J.R., Kori, S.H., Eastwood, D.W., and Borkowski, G.P.: Improved technique for CT-guided celiac ganglia block. Am. J. Radiol., *142:*1201, 1984.
115. Haaga, J.R., Reich, N.E., Havrilla, T.R., and Alfidi, R.J.: Interventional CT scanning. Radiol. Clin. North Am., *15:*456, 1977.
116. Haines, D.E.: On the question of a subdural space. Anat. Rec., *230:*3, 1991.
117. Håkanson, S.: Trigeminal neuralgia treated by the injection of glycerol into the trigeminal cistern. Neurosurgery, *9:*638, 1981.
118. Halpern, D.: Histologic studies in animals after intramuscular neurolysis with phenol. J.A.M.A., *200:*1152, 1967.
119. Halpern, D., and Meelhuysen, F.E.: Phenol motor point block in the management of muscular hypertonia. Arch. Phys. Med. Rehabil., *47:*659, 1966.
120. Hardy, P.A.J., and Wells, J.C.D.: Extent of sympathetic blockade after stellate ganglion block with bupivacaine. Pain, *36:*193, 1989.
121. Hay, R.C.: Subarachnoid alcohol block in the control of intractable pain: Report of results in 252 patients. Anesth. Analg., *41:*12, 1962.
122. Hegedüs, V.: Relief of pancreatic pain by radiography-guided block. Am. J. Radiol., *133:*1101, 1979.
123. Herpels, V., Kurdziel, J.C., and Dondelinger, R.F.: Percutaneous CT guided nerve block of the coeliac plexus and splanchnic nerves. Ann. Radiol., *31:*291, 1988.
124. Hessel, S.J., Adams, D.F., and Abrams, H.L.: Complications of angiography. Radiology, *138:*273, 1981.
125. Hilgier, M., and Rykowski, J.: One needle transcrural celiac plexus block. Reg. Anesth., *19:*277, 1994.
126. Hitchcock, E.: Hypothermic subarachnoid irrigation for intractable pain. Lancet, *i:*1133, 1967.
127. Hitchcock, E: Subarachnoid saline infusion. *In* Morley, T.P. (ed.): Current Controversies in Neurosurgery. pp. 515. Philadelphia, W.B. Saunders, 1976.
128. Hogan, Q.H., Erikson, S.J., Haddox, J.D., and Abrams, S.E.: The spread of solutions during stellate ganglion block. Reg. Anesth., *17:*78, 1992.
129. Hogan, Q.H., Erikson, S.J., and Abrams, S.E.: Computerized tomography-guided stellate ganglion block. Anesthesiology, *77:*596, 1992.
130. Hollis, P.H., Malis, L., and Zappulla, R.A.: Neurological deterioration after lumbar puncture below complete spinal subarachnoid block. J. Neurosurg., *64:*253, 1986.
131. Honet, J.E., Shea, K.L., and Seltzer, J.L.: Celiac plexus neurolytic block: Survey of pain programs. Reg. Anesth., *18*(Suppl.):45, 1993.
132. Hughes, G., Michel, L., and Andree, N.: Celiac plexus neurolysis: Anterior approach guided by echography and pulsed doppler echography. Reg. Anesth., *13*(Suppl.):61, 1988.
133. Hughes, J.T.: Pathological findings following the intrathecal injection of ethyl alcohol in man. Paraplegia, 167.
134. Humbles, F.H., and Mahaffey, J.E.: Teflon epidural catheter placement for intermittent celiac plexus blockade and celiac plexus neurolytic blockade. Reg. Anesth., *15:*103, 1990.
135. Ichiyanagi, K., Matsuki, M., Kinefuchi, S., and Kato, Y.: Progressive changes in the concentrations of phenol and glycerine in the human subarachnoid space. Anesthesiology, *42:*622, 1975.
136. Iggo, A., and Walsh, E.G.: Selective block of small fibers in the spinal roots by phenol. Brain, *83:*701, 1960.
137. Ihse, I: Pancreatic pain. Br. J. Surg., *77:*121, 1990.
138. Illuminati, M., Kizelshteyn, G., Ackert, M., *et al.*: Neurolytic celiac plexus block: Intraoperative catheter technique. Reg. Anesth., *14*(Suppl.):90, 1989.
139. Ina, H., Kobyashi, M.D., Imai, S., *et al.*: A new approach to the superior hypogastric plexus block: Trans-vertebral disc (L5–S1) technique. Reg. Anesth., *17*(Suppl.):123, 1992.
140. Ischia, S., Ischia, A., Polati, E., and Finco, G.: Three posterior percutaneous celiac plexus block techniques: A prospective, randomized study in 61 patients with pancreatic cancer pain. Pain, *76:*534, 1992.
141. Ischia, S., Luzzani, A., Ischia, A., *et al.*: A new approach to neurolytic block of the celiac plexus: The transaortic technique. Pain, *16:*333, 1983.
142. Ischia, S., Luzzani, A., Ischia, A., *et al.*: Subarachnoid neurolytic block (L5–S1) and unilateral percutaneous cervical cordotomy in the treatment of pain secondary to pelvic malignant disease. Pain, *20:*139, 1984.
143. Ischia, S., Luzzani, A., Pacini, L., and Maffezzoli, G.F.: Lytic saddle block: Clinical comparison of the results, using phenol at 5, 10, and 15 percent. Adv. Pain Res. Ther., *7:*339, 1984.
144. Jack, E.D.: Regional anaesthesia for pain relief. Br. J. Anaesth., *47:*278, 1975.
145. Jackson, S.H., Jacobs, J.B., and Epstein, R.A.: A radiographic approach to celiac plexus block. Anesthesiology, *31:*373, 1969.
146. Jacox, A., Carr, D.B., Payne, R., *et al.*: Management of cancer pain: Clinical practice guideline No 9. Rockville, MD, AHCPR Publication No. 94-0592, March, 1994.
147. Jain, S., Alagesan, R., Harris, A., and Chaing, J.: Selective neurolysis of cranial nerve using computerized tomography. Anesthesiology, *75:*A748, 1991.
148. Jain, S., Chiang, J., and Vanderslice, T.: Is diagnostic block necessary prior to neurolytic celiac plexus block? Anesthesiology, *75*(Suppl.):A749, 1991.
149. Jain, S., Foley, K., Thomas, J., *et al.*: Factors influencing efficacy of epidural neurolysis therapy for intractable cancer pain. Suppl. 4. Proc. 5th World Congress I.A.S.P., 1987.
150. Jain, S., Hirsh, R., Shah, N., *et al.*: Blood ethanol levels following celiac plexus block with 50% ethanol. Anesth. Analg., *68:*S135, 1989.
151. Jain, S., Kestenbaum, A., and Khan, Y.: Ethanol or phenol for peripheral neurolysis? Does it make a difference? Pain, *5*(Suppl.):S92, 1990.
152. Jain, S., Shah, N., Rubin, L., *et al.*: Efficacy of celiac plexus block for upper abdominal pain due to malignancy. Proc. Ann. Mtg. Am. Soc. Clin. Oncol., *8:*A1267, 1989.
153. Johans, T.J., and Burchiel, K.J.: Neurectomy, rhizotomy, ganglionectomy for cancer-related pain. *In* Arbit, E. (ed.): Management of Cancer-Related Pain. pp. 333–340. New York, Futura, 1993.
154. Jones, J., and Gough, D.: Coeliac plexus block with alcohol for relief of upper abdominal pain due to cancer. Ann. Reg. Coll. Surg. Engl., *59:*46, 1977.
155. Jones, M.J.T., and Murrin, K.R.: Intercostal block with cryotherapy. Ann. Roy. Coll. Surg. Engl. *69:*261, 1987.
156. Jones, R.R.: A technique of injection of the splanchnic nerves with alcohol. Anesth. Analg., *36:*75, 1957.
157. Judovich, B.D., Bates, W., and Bishop, K.: Intraspinal ammonium salts for the intractable pain of malignancy. Anesthesiology, *5:*341, 1944.
158. Kames, L.D., Rapkin, A.J., Naliboff, B.D., *et al.*: Effectiveness of an interdisciplinary pain management program for the treatment of chronic pelvic pain. Pain, *41:*41, 1990.
159. Kaplan, R., Aurellano, Z., and Pfisterer, W.: Phenol brachial plexus block for upper extremity cancer pain. Reg. Anesth. *13:*58, 1988.
160. Kappis, M.: Erfahrungen mit lokalanästhesia bei bauchoperationen. Verh. Dtsch. Ges. Chir., *43:*87, 1914.
161. Kappis, M.: Sensibilität and local anästhesie in chirurgischen gebiet der bauchhohle mit besonderen berücksichtigung der Splanchnichus-anästhesie. Bruns Beitr. Klin. Chir., *15:*161, 1919.
162. Katz, J.: Current role of neurolytic agents. Adv. Neurol. *4:*471, 1974.
163. Katz, J., and Levin, A.B.: Treatment of diffuse metastatic cancer pain by instillation of alcohol into the sella turcica. Anesthesiology, *46:*115, 1977.
164. Kessler, J.T.: Neurologic causes of head and face pain. *In* Cooper, B.C., and Lucente, F.E. (eds.): Management of Facial, Head and Neck Pain. pp. 23–52. Philadelphia, W.B. Saunders, 1989.
165. Kidd, R., Crane, R.D., and Dail, D.H.: Lymphangiography and fine needle aspiration biopsy: Ineffectiveness for staging early prostate cancer. Am. J. Roentgenol., *141:*1007, 1984.
166. Kirvelä, N.S.: Treatment of painful neuromas with neurolytic blockade. Pain, *41:*161, 1990.
167. Kline, M.T.: Stereotactic Radiofrequency Lesions as Part of the Management of Pain. Orlando, Paul M. Deutsch Press, 1992.
168. Koboyashi, M., Ina, H., Imai, S., *et al.*: Under CT guided celiac plexus block: Trans-intravertebral disc approach. Reg. Anesth., *17*(Suppl.):122, 1992.
169. Korevaar, W.C.: Transcatheter thoracic epidural neurolysis using ethyl alcohol. Anesthesiology, *69:*989, 1988.
170. Korsten, H.H.M., Hellebrekers, L.J., Grouls, R.J.E., *et al.*: Long-lasting epidural sensory blockade by n-Butyl p-Aminobenzoate in the dog: Neurotoxic or local anesthetic effect? Anesthesiology, *73:*491, 1990.
171. Kulichova, M., and Fabus, S.: Neurolytic celiac plexus block for control of intractable abdominal visceral pain. Abstracts. pp. 566. 7th World Congress on Pain, Paris, 1993.
172. Labat, G.: L'anesthesie splanchnique dans les interventions chirurgicales et dans les affections douloureuses de la cavite abdominale. Gaz. d'Hop., *93:*662, 1920.

173. Labat, G.: Paravertebral and dorsal block: Blocking of the dorsal or thoracic nerves. *In* Labat, G. (ed.): Regional Anesthesia: Its Technique and Clinical Application. 1st Ed. pp. 255. Philadelphia, W.B. Saunders, 1924.
174. Labat, G.: Splanchnic analgesia. *In* Labat, G. (ed.): Regional Anesthesia: Its Technique and Clinical Application. 2nd Ed. p. 398. Philadelphia; W.B. Saunders Company, 1928.
175. Lahuerta, J., Lipton, S., Miles, J., *et al.*: Update on percutaneous cervical cordotomy and pituitary alcohol neuroadenolysis: An audit of our recent results and complications. *In* Lipton, S., and Miles, J. (eds.): Persistent Pain. Vol 5. pp. 197–223. New York, Grune and Stratton, 1985.
176. Lee, R.B., Stone, K., Magelssen, D., *et al.*: Presacral neurotomy for chronic pelvic pain. Obstet. Gynecol., *68:*517, 1986.
177. Lee, T.L., and Lamer, T.J.: Outpatient alcohol celiac plexus block for chronic pain patients. Reg. Anesth., *15*(Suppl.):66, 1991.
178. Levin, A.B., Katz, J., Benson, R.C., and Jones, A.G.: Treatment of pain of diffuse metastatic cancer by stereotactic chemical hypophysectomy: Long-term results and observations on mechanism of action. Neurosurgery, *6:*258, 1980.
179. Levin, A.B., and Ramirez, L.L.: Treatment of cancer pain with hypophysectomy: Surgical and chemical. *In* Advances in Pain Research and Therapy. Vol. 7. pp. 631–646. 1984.
180. LeRiche, R., and Fontain, R.: L'anesthesie isolee du ganglion etoile: Sa technique ses indications ses resultas. Presse Med., *42:*849, 1934.
181. Leung, J.W.C., Bowen-Wright, M., Aveling, W., *et al.*: Celiac plexus block in pancreatic cancer and chronic pancreatitis. Br. J. Surg., *70:*730, 1983.
182. Lieberman, R.P., Crummy, A.B., and Matallana, R.H.: Invasive procedures in pancreatic disease.
183. Lieberman, R.P., Nance, P.N., and Cuka, D.J.: Anterior approach to the celiac plexus during interventional biliary procedures. Radiology, *167:*562, 1988.
184. Lieberman, R.P., and Waldman, S.D.: Celiac plexus neurolysis with modified transaortic approach. Radiology, *175:*274, 1990.
185. Lifshitz, S., Debacker, L.J., and Buchsbaum, H.J.: Subarachnoid phenol block for pain relief in gynecologic malignancy. Obstet. Gynec., *48:*316, 1976.
186. Lillemoe, K.D., Cameron, J.L., Kaufman, H.S., *et al.*: Chemical splanchnicectomy in patients with unresectable pancreatic cancer: A prospective randomized trial. Ann. Surg., *217:*447, 1993.
187. Linderoth, B., and Håkanson, S.: Paroxysmal facial pain in disseminated sclerosis treated by retrogasserian glycerol injection. Acta Neurol. Scand., *80:*341, 1989.
188. Lipton, S.: Neurodestructive procedures in the management of cancer pain. J. Pain Symptom Manage., *2:*219, 1987.
189. Lipton, S.: Neurolysis: Pharmacology and drug selection. *In* Patt, R.B. (ed.): Cancer Pain, pp. 343–358. Philadelphia, J.B. Lippincott, 1993.
190. Lloyd, J.W.: Treatment of intractable pain with cerebrospinal fluid barbotage. *In* Morley, T.P. (ed.): Current Controversies in Neurosurgery. pp. 520. Philadelphia, W.B. Saunders, 1976.
191. Lloyd, J.W., Barnard, J.D.W., and Glynn, C.J.: Cryoanalgesia: A new approach to pain relief. Lancet, *ii:*932, 1976.
192. Lloyd, J.W., Rawlinson, W.A.L., and Evans, P.J.D.: Selective hypophysectomy for metastatic pain: A review of ethyl alcohol ablation of the anterior pituitary in a regional pain relief unit. Br. J. Anaesth., *53:*1129, 1981.
193. Lobato, R.D., Madrid, J.L., Fatela, L.V., *et al.*: Intraventricular morphine for intractable cancer pain: Rationale, methods, clinical results. Acta Anaesthesiol. Scand., *31:*68, 1987.
194. Loeser, J.D.: Tic douloureux and atypical facial pain. *In* Wall, P.D., Melzack, R. (eds.): Textbook of Pain. 3rd Ed. pp. 699–710. Edinburgh, Churchill Livingstone, 1994.
195. Lu, G., Frost, E.A.M., and Goldiner, P.L.: Another aspect of celiac plexus block. Anesthesiology, *67:*1017, 1987.
196. Lubenow, T.R., and Ivankovich, A.D.: Serum alcohol, CPK and amylase levels following celiac plexus block with alcohol. Reg. Anesth., *13*(Suppl.):64, 1988.
197. Lucas, J.T., Ducker, T.B., and Perot, P.L., Jr.: Adverse reactions to intrathecal saline injection for control of pain. J. Neurosurg., *42:*557, 1975.
198. Luft, R., and Olivecrona, H.: Experiences with hypophysectomy. J. Neurosurg., *10:*301, 1952.
199. Deleted in proof.
200. Madrid, J.L.: Chemical hypophysectomy. Adv. Pain Res. Ther., *2:*381, 1979.
201. Madrid, J.L., and Bonica, J.J.: Cranial nerve blocks. Adv. Pain Res. Ther., *2:*347, 1979.
202. Maher, R.M.: Intrathecal chlorocrescol in the treatment of pain in cancer. Lancet, *i:*965, 1963.
203. Maher, R.M.: Neurone selection in relief of pain: Further experiences with intrathecal injections. Lancet, *i:*16, 1957.
204. Maher, R.M.: Relief of pain in incurable cancer. Lancet, *i:*18, 1955.
205. Maiwand, M.O., Makey, A.R., and Rees, A.: Cryoanalgesia after thoracotomy. J. Thorac. Cardiovasc. Surg., *92:*291, 1986.
206. Mandl, F.: Paravertebral Block. New York, Grune and Stratton, 1947.
207. Mark, V.H., White, J.C., Zervas, N.T., *et al.*: Intrathecal use of phenol for the relief of chronic severe pain. N. Engl. J. Med., *267:*589, 1962.
208. Masadu, R., and Yokoyama, K.: Study of needle placement for sympathetic blocks under computed tomography (paravertebral approach in thoracic sympathetic block and transdisc approach in splanchnic nerve block. Abstracts. pp. 342. 7th World Congress on Pain, Paris, 1993.
209. Matamala, A.M., Lopez, F.V., and Martinez, L.I.: Percutaneous approach to the celiac plexus using CT guidance. Pain, *34:*285, 1988.
210. Matson, J.A., Ghia, J.N., and Levy, J.H.: A case report of a potentially fatal complication associated with Ischia's transaortic method of celiac plexus block. Reg. Anesth., *10:*193, 1985.
211. Matsuki, M., Kato, Y., and Ichiyanagi, K.: Progressive changes in the concentration of ethyl alcohol in the human and canine subarachnoid spaces. Anesthesiology, *36:*617, 1972.
212. Maumenee, A.E.: Retrobulbar alcohol injections: Relief of pain in eyes with and without vision. Am. J. Opthalmol., *32:*1502, 1949.
213. Mauskop, A.: Trigeminal neuralgia (tic douloureux). J. Pain Symptom Manage. *8:*148, 1993.
214. McAfee, J.G.: A survey of complications of abdominal aortography. Radiology, *68:*825, 1957.
215. McEwen, B.W., DeWilde, F.W., Dwyer, B., *et al.*: The pain clinic: A clinic for the management of intractable pain. Med. J. Aust., *1:*676, 1965.
216. Meglio, M., and Cioni, B.: Percutaneous procedures for trigeminal neuralgia: Microcompression versus radiofrequency thermocoagulation. Personal experience. Pain, *38:*9, 1989.
217. Mehta, M., and Maher, R.: Injection into the extra-arachnoid subdural space. Anaesthesia, *32:*76, 1977.
218. Mehta, M., and Ranger, I: Persistent abdominal pain. Anaesthesia, *26:*330, 1971.
219. Melzack, R.: The gate control theory 25 years later: New perspectives on phantom limb pain. Pain, *5*(Suppl.):S254, 1990.
220. Mercandante, S.: Celiac plexus block versus analgesics in pancreatic cancer pain. Pain, *52:*187, 1993.
221. Mueller, P.R., vanSonnenberg, E., and Casola, G.: Radiographically guided alcohol block of the celiac ganglion. Semin. Intervent. Radiol., *14:*195, 1987.
222. Milano, R.: Pelvic pain: Problems in diagnosis and treatment. *In* Bond, M.R., Charlton, J.E., and Woolf, C.J. (eds.): Proceedings of the VI World Congress on Pain. pp. 453–458. Amsterdam, Elsevier, 1991.
223. Miles, J.: Pituitary destruction. *In* Wall, P.D., and Melzack, R. (eds.): Textbook of Pain. pp. 656–665. New York, Churchill Livingstone, 1984.
224. Miles, J.: Treatment of malignant pain of the head and neck. Appl. Neurophysiol. *47:*223, 1984.
225. Millard, R.W.: Behavioral assessment of pain and behavioral pain management. *In* Patt, R.B. (ed.): Cancer Pain. pp. 85–98. Philadelphia, J.B. Lippincott, 1993.
226. Miller, R.D., Johnston, R.R., and Hosobuchi, Y.: Treatment of intercostal neuralgia with 10% ammonium sulfate. J. Thorac. Surg., *69:*476, 1975.
227. Misfeldt, D.S., and Goldstein, A.: Hypophysectomy relieves pain not via endorphins. N. Engl. J. Med., *297:*1236, 1977.
228. Moore, D., and Bridenbaugh, D.L.: Intercostal nerve block in 4333 patients: Indications, techniques, complications. Anesth. Analg., *41:*1, 1962.
229. Moore, D.C.: Celiac (splanchnic) plexus block with alcohol for cancer pain of the upper intra-abdominal viscera. Adv. Pain Res. Ther., *2:*357, 1979.
230. Moore, D.C.: Intercostal nerve block and celiac plexus block for pain therapy. Adv. Pain Res. Ther., *7:*309, 1984.
231. Moore, D.C.: Regional Block. 4th Ed. Springfield, Ill., Charles C Thomas, 1965.

232. Moore, D.C., Bush, W.H., and Burnett, L.L.: An improved technique for celiac plexus block may be more theoretical than real. Anesthesiology, *57*:347, 1982.
233. Moore, D.C., Bush, W.H., and Burnett, L.L.: Celiac plexus block: A roentgenographic, anatomic study of technique and spread of solution in patients and corpses. Anesth. Analg., *60*:369, 1981.
234. Morrica, G.: Pituitary neuroadenolysis in the treatment of intractable pain from cancer, *In* Lipton, S. (ed.): Persistent Pain: Modern Methods of Treatment. Vol 1. pp. 149–173. New York, Academic Press, 1977.
235. Moritz, U.: Phenol block of peripheral nerves. Scand. J. Rehab. Med., *5*:160, 1973.
236. Moyano, R., Linares, R., Sarmiento, A., and Trujillo, J.: Celiac plexus neurolytic block: Percutaneous technique without radiologic help and with alcohol at 50%. Abstracts. pp. 565. 7th World Congress on Pain, Paris, 1993.
237. Mullan, S., and Lichtor, T.: Percutaneous microcompression of the trigeminal ganglion for trigeminal neuralgia. J. Neurosurg. *59*:1007, 1983.
238. Mullin, V.: Brachial plexus block with phenol for painful arm associated with Pancoast's syndrome. Anesthesiology, *53*:431, 1980.
239. Myhre, J., Hilsted, J., Tronier, B., *et al.*: Monitoring of celiac plexus block in chronic pancreatitis. Pain, *38*:269, 1989.
240. Naidich, D.P., Megibow, A.J., Ross, C.R., *et al.*: Computed tomography of the diaphragm: Normal anatomy and variants. J. Comput. Assist. Tomogr., *7*:633, 1983.
241. Nathan, P.W., Sears, T.A., and Smith, M.C.: Effects of phenol solutions on the nerve roots of the cat: An electrophysiological and histological study. J. Neurol. Sci., *2*:7, 1965.
242. Neill, R.S.: Ablation of the brachial plexus. Anaesthesia, *34*:1024, 1979.
243. Ness, T.J., and Gebhart, G.F.: Visceral pain: A review of experimental studies. Pain, *41*:167, 1990.
244. Noda, J., Umeda, S., Mori, K., *et al.*: Acetaldehyde syndrome after celiac plexus block. Anesth. Analg., *65*:1300, 1986.
245. Nour-Eldin, F.: Preliminary report: Uptake of phenol by vascular and brain tissue. Microvasc. Res., *2*:224, 1970.
246. Ogawa, S.: Neurolytic sympathectomy. *In* Hyodo, M., Oyama, T., and Swerdlow, M. (eds.): The Pain Clinic IV. pp. 139–146. Utrecht, VSP, 1992.
247. Pagni, C.A.: Role of neurosurgery in cancer pain: Reevaluation of old methods and new trends. Adv. Pain Res. Ther., *7*:603, 1984.
248. Pagura, J.R., Schnapp, M., and Passarelli, P.: Percutaneous radiofrequency glossopharyngeal rhizotomy for cancer pain. Appl. Neurophys., *46*:154, 1983.
249. Rowell, N.P.: Intralesional methylprednisolone for rib metastases: An alternative to radiotherapy? *15*:153, 1988.
250. Papo, I.: Spinal posterior rhizotomy and commisural myelotomy in the treatment of cancer pain. Adv. Pain Res. Ther., *2*:439, 1979.
251. Papo, I., and Visca, A.: Intrathecal phenol in the treatment of pain and spasticity. Proc. Neurol. Surg., *7*:56, 1976.
252. Papo, I., and Visca, A.: Phenol subarachnoid rhizotomy for the treatment of cancer pain: A personal account on 290 cases. Adv. Pain Res. Ther., *2*:339, 1979.
253. Parkinson, S.K., Mueller, J.B., and Little, W.L.: A new and simple technique for splanchnic nerve block using a paramedian approach and 3 1/2 inch needles. Reg. Anesth., *14*(Suppl.):41, 1989.
254. Parkinson, S.K., Mueller, J.B., Little, W.L., and Bailey, S.L.: Extent of blockade with various approaches to the lumbar plexus. Anesth. Analg., *68*:243, 1989.
255. Patt, R.B.: Anesthetic procedures for the control of cancer pain. *In* Arbit, E. (ed.): Management of Cancer Related Pain. pp. 381–407. New York, Futura, 1993.
256. Patt, R.B.: Classification of cancer pain and cancer pain syndromes. *In* Patt, R.B. (ed.): Cancer Pain. pp. 3–22. Philadelphia, J.B. Lippincott, 1993.
257. Patt, R.B.: General principles of pharmacotherapy for oncologic pain. *In* Patt, R.B. (ed.): Cancer Pain. pp. 101–103. Philadelphia, J.B. Lippincott, 1993.
258. Patt, R.B.: Neurosurgical interventions for chronic pain problems. Anesth. Clin. North Am., *5*:609, 1987.
259. Patt, R.B.: Interventional analgesia: Epidural and subarachnoid therapy. Am. J. Hospice Care, *6*:18, 1989.
260. Patt, R.B.: Peripheral neurolysis. *In* Patt, R.B. (ed.): Cancer Pain. pp. 359–376. Philadelphia, J.B. Lippincott, 1993.
261. Patt, R.B.: Peripheral neurolysis and the management of cancer pain. Pain Digest, *2*:30, 1992.
262. Patt, R.B.: Pharmacotherapy for cancer pain: An anaesthesiologist's viewpoint. Ann. Acad. Med. Singapore, *23*:598, 1994.
263. Patt, R.B.: Pharmacotherapy: The cornerstone of the anesthesiologist's continued role in the treatment of cancer pain. Probl. Anesth., *7*:486, 1993.
264. Patt, R., and Jain, S.: Management of a patient with osteoradionecrosis of the mandible with nerve blocks. J. Pain Symptom Manage., *5*:59, 1990.
265. Patt, R.B., and Jain, S.: Therapeutic decision making for procedure-based pain. *In* Patt, R.B. (ed.): Cancer Pain. pp. 275–283. Philadelphia, J.B. Lippincott, 1993.
266. Patt, R.B., and Millard, R.: A role for peripheral neurolysis in the management of intractable cancer pain. Pain, *5*(Suppl.):S358, 1990.
267. Patt, R.B., and Reddy, S.: Spinal neurolysis for cancer pain: Indications and recent results. Ann. Acad. Med., Singapore, *23*:2, 1994.
268. Patt, R.B., Reddy, S., Wu, C.L., and Catania, J.A.: Pneumothorax as a consequence of thoracic subarachnoid block. Anesth. Analg., *78*:160, 1994.
269. Patt, R.B., Wu, C.L., Reddy, S., *et al.*: Incidence of postdural puncture headache following intrathecal neurolysis with large caliber needles. Reg. Anesth., *19*(Suppl 2):86, 1994.
270. Payne, R.: Neuropathic pain syndromes, with special reference to causalgia and reflex sympathetic dystrophy. Clin. J. Pain, *2*:59, 1986.
271. Pender, J.W., and Pugh, D.G.: Diagnostic and therapeutic nerve blocks: Necessity for roentgenograms. J.A.M.A., *146*:798, 1951.
272. Perese, D.M.: Subarachnoid alcohol block in the management of pain of malignant disease. Arch. Surg., *76*:347, 1958.
273. Plancarte, R., Amescua, C., and Patt, R.B.: Presacral blockade of the ganglion impar (ganglion of Walther). Anesthesiology, *73*:A751, 1990.
274. Plancarte, R., Amescua, C., and Patt, R.B.: Sympathetic neurolytic blockade. *In* Patt, R.B. (ed.): Cancer Pain. pp. 377–425. Philadelphia, J.B. Lippincott, 1993.
275. Plancarte, R., Amescua, C., Patt, R.B., and Aldrete, J.A.: Superior hypogastric plexus block for pelvic cancer pain. Anesthesiology, *73*:236, 1990.
276. Plancarte, R., Patt, R.B., Allende, S., *et al.*: Treatment of neoplastic perineal pain by presacral chemical blockade of the ganglion impar (ganglion of Walther). Reg. Anesth., In press.
277. Portenoy, R.K., Foley, K.M., and Inturissi, C.: The nature of opioid responsiveness and its implications for neuropathic pain: New hypothesis derived from studies of opioid infusions. Pain, *43*:273, 1990.
278. Procacci, P., and Maresca, M.: Pathophysiology of visceral pain. Adv. Pain Res. Ther. *13*:123, 1990.
279. Racz, G.B., Heavner, J., and Haynsworth, R.: Repeat epidural phenol injections in chronic pain and spasticity. *In* Lipton, S., and Miles, J. (eds.): Persistent Pain. Vol 5. pp. 157. Orlando, Grune & Stratton, 1985.
280. Racz, G.B., Heavner, J.E., Singleton, W., and Carline, M.: Hypertonic saline and corticosteroid injected epidurally for pain control. *In* Racz, G.B. (ed.): Techniques of Neurolysis. pp. 73–86. Boston, Kluwer Academic Publichers, 1989.
281. Racz, G.B., and Holubec, J.T.: Stellate ganglion phenol neurolysis. *In* Racz, G.B. (ed.): Techniques of Neurolysis. pp. 133. Boston, Kluwer Academic Publishers 1989.
282. Racz, G.B., Sabonghy, M., Gintautas, J., and Kline, W.M.: Intractable pain therapy using a new epidural catheter. J.A.M.A. *248*:579, 1982.
283. Raj, P.P.: Practical Management of Pain. 2nd ed. St Louis, Mosby Year Book, 1992, pp. 1021–1022.
284. Raj, P.P., Montgomery, S.J., Nettles, D., *et al.*: The use of the nerve stimulator with standard unsheathed needles in nerve blockade. Anesth. Analg. *53*:827, 1973.
285. Raj, P.P., Rosenblatt, R., and Montgomery, S.: Uses of the nerve stimulator for peripheral blocks. Reg. Anesth. *5*:14, 1980.
286. Ramamurthy, S., Walsh, N.E., Schoenfeld, L.S., *et al.*: Evaluation of neurolytic blocks using phenol and croygenic block in the management of chronic pain. J. Pain Symptom Manage. *4*:72, 1989.
287. Rapkin, A.J., Kames, L.D., Darke, L.L., *et al.*: History of physical and sexual abuse in women with chronic pelvic pain. Obstet. Gynecol., *76*:92, 1990.
288. Rastogi, V., and Kumar, R.: Peripheral nerve stimulator as an aid for therapeutic alcohol blocks. Anaesthesiology, *38*:163, 1983.
289. Rauck, R.: Sympathetic nerve blocks. *In* Raj, P.P. (ed.): Practical Management of Pain. 2nd Ed. pp. 778–812. St Louis, Mosby–Year Book, 1992.

290. Raymond, S.A., Steffensen, S.C., Gugion, L.D., and Strichartz, G.R.: Critical exposure length for nerve block of myelinated fibers with lidocaine exceeds 3 nodes. Reg. Anesth., *13*(Suppl.):46, 1988.
291. Reber, H.A., and Foley, K.M.: Pancreatic cancer pain: Presentation, pathogenesis and management. J. Pain Symptom Manage., *3:*163, 1988.
292. Reid, W., Watt, J.K., and Gray, T.G.: Phenol injection of the sympathetic chain. Br. J. Surg., *47:*45, 1970.
293. Riopelle, J.M., Everson, C., Moustoukus, N., *et al.*: Cryoanalgesia: Present day status. Semin. Anesth. *4:*305, 1985.
294. Ritchie, J.M., and Greene, N.M.: Local anesthetics. *In* Gilman, A.G., Goodman, L.S., and Gilman, A. (eds.): The Pharmacologic Basis of Therapeutics. pp. 300–320. 6th Ed. New York, MacMillan, 1980.
295. Roberts, W.J., Kramis, R.C., and Dow, R.S.: Post-sympathectomy neuralgia: A deafferentatation syndrome? Pain, *5*(Suppl.):S420, 1990.
296. Robertson, D.H.: Transsacral neurolytic nerve block: An alternative approach to intractable perineal pain. Br. J. Anaesth., *55:*873, 1983.
297. Rockswold, G.L., Bradley, W.E., and Chou, S.N.: Effect of sacral nerve blocks on the function of the urinary bladder in humans. J. Neurosurg., *40:*83, 1974.
298. Roussiel, M.: Anesthesie des nerfs splanchniques et des plexus mesenteriques spurior et inferieurs en chirurgie abdominal. Presse Med., *31:*4, 1923.
299. Rowlingson, J., Hammill, R.J., and Patt, R.B.: Assessment of the patient with oncologic pain. *In* Patt, R.B. (ed.): Cancer Pain. pp. 23–39. Philadelphia, J.B. Lippincott, 1993.
300. Salmon, J.B., Finch, P.M., Lovegrove, F.T.A., and Warwick, A.: Mapping the spread of epidural phenol in cancer pain patients by radionuclide admixture and epidural scintigraphy. Clin. J. Pain, *8:*18, 1992.
301. Sanders, M., and Henny, C.H.P.: Results of selective percutaneous controlled radiofrequency lesion for treatment of trigeminal neuralgia in 240 patients. Clin. J. Pain, *8:*23, 1992.
302. Saris, S.C., Silver, J.M., Vieira, J.F., *et al.*: Sacrococcygeal rhizotomy for perineal pain. Neurosurgery, *5:*789, 1986.
303. Sato, S., Okubu, N., Tajima, K., *et al.*: Plasma alcohol concentrations after celiac plexus block in gastric and pancreatic cancer. Reg. Anesth., *18:*366, 1993.
304. Sato, S., Yamashita, S., Iwai, M., *et al.*: Continuous interscalene block for cancer pain. Reg. Anesth., *19:*73, 1994.
305. Shah, S., and Sharma, K.: Coeliac plexus block for upper abdominal malignancies. Abstracts. pp. 338. 7th World Congress on Pain, Paris, 1993.
306. Shantha, T.R.: Subdural space: What is it? Does it exist? Reg. Anesth., *17*(Suppl.):85, 1992.
307. Sharfman, W.H., and Walsh, T.D.: Has the efficacy of celiac plexus block been demonstrated in pancreatic cancer pain? Pain, *41:*267, 1990.
308. Shulman, M.: Epidural butamben for the treatment of metastatic cancer pain. Anesthesiology, *67:*A245, 1987.
309. Shulman, M.: Intercostal nerve block with 10% butamben suspension for the treatment of chronic noncancer pain. Anesthesiology, *71:*A737, 1989.
310. Shulman, M.: Treatment of cancer pain with epidural butyl-amino-benzoate suspension. Reg. Anesth., *12:*1, 1987.
311. Shulman, M., Joseph, N.J., and Haller, C.A.: Local effects of epidural and subarachnoid injections of butyl-amino-benzoate suspension. Reg. Anesth., *12*(Suppl.):23, 1987.
312. Schuster, G.D.: The use of cryoanalgesia in the painful facet syndrome. J. Neurol. Orthopaed. Surg., *3:*271, 1982.
313. Siegfried, J., and Broggi, G.: Percutaneous thermocoagulation of the Gasserian ganglion in the treatment of pain in advanced cancer. Adv. Pain Res. Ther. *2:*463, 1979.
314. Simon, D.I., Carron, H., and Rowlingson, J.C.: Treatment of bladder pain with transsacral nerve block. Anesth. Analg., *61:*46, 1982.
315. Singler, R.C.: An improved technique for alcohol neurolysis of the celiac plexus. Anesthesiology, *56:*137, 1982.
316. Slappendel, R., Crul, B.J.P., and van Dongen, R.T.M.: Radiofrequent lesioning of the stellate ganglion. Reg. Anesth., *17*(3S):62, 1992.
317. Slocumb, J.C.: Neurologic factors in chronic pelvic pain. Trigger points and the abdominal pelvic pain syndrome. Am. J. Obstet. Gyn. *149:*543, 1984.
318. Sluijter, M.E.: Interruption of nerve pathways in the treatment of non-malignant pain. Appl. Neurophys., *47:*195, 1984.
319. Smith, A.E.: Block Anesthesia and Allied Subjects. St Louis, C.V. Mosby, 1920.
320. Smith, J.L.: Care of people who are dying. The hospice approach. *In* Patt, R.B. (ed.): Cancer Pain. pp. 543–552. Philadelphia, J.B. Lippincott, 1993.
321. Smith, M.C.: Histological findings following intrathecal injections of phenol solutions for relief of pain. Br. J. Anaesth., *36:*387, 1964.
322. Smyth, R.J., Evans, D., and Shumka, D.: Bilateral Horner's syndrome following unilateral stellate ganglion block. Pain Digest, *2:*218, 1992.
323. Snell, R.S., and Katz, J.: Clinical anatomy for anesthesiologists. Norwalk, Conn., Appleton and Lange, 1988, p. 271.
324. Southworth, J.L., Hingson, R.A., Pitkin, W.M. (eds.): Conduction Anesthesia, 2nd ed. Philadelphia, J.B. Lippincott, 1953.
325. Solar-Labastida, C., Whizar-Lugo, V., and Rodriguez-Cesena, A.: CT scan guided neurolytic celiac plexus block for pancreatic cancer pain. Pain, *5*(Suppl.):S360, 1990.
326. Stanton-Hicks, M., Abram, S.E., and Nolte, H.: Sympathetic blocks. *In* Raj, P.P. (ed.): Practical Management of Pain. pp. 661. Chicago, Yearbook, 1986.
327. Stern, E.L.: Dangers of intraspinal (subarachnoid) injection of alcohol: Their avoidance and contraindications. Am. J. Surg., *35:*99, 1937.
328. Stern, E.L.: Chronic painful conditions amenable to relief by intraspinal (subarachnoid) injection of alcohol. Am. J. Surg., *36:*509, 1937.
329. Stewart, W.A., and Lourie, H.: An experimental evaluation of the effects of subarachnoid injections of phenol-pantopaque in cats: A histological study. J. Neurosurg., *20:*64, 1963.
330. Stone, H.B.: A treatment for pruritus ani. Bull. Johns Hopkins Hosp., *27:*242, 1916.
331. Stovner, J., and Endressen, R.: Intrathecal phenol for cancer pain. Acta Anaesth. Scand., *16:*17, 1972.
332. Sunderland, S.: Nerves and Nerve Injuries. 2nd Ed. London, Churchill Livingstone, 1978.
333. Suvansa, S.: Treatment of tetanus by intrathecal injections of carbolic acid. Lancet, *i:*1075, 1931.
334. Swarm, R.A., and Cousins, M.J.: Anaesthetic techniques for pain control. *In* Doyle, D., Hanks, G.W.C., and MacDonald, N. (eds.): Oxford Textbook of Palliative Medicine. pp. 204–220. Oxford, Oxford University Press, 1993.
335. Sweet, W.H.: Treatment of trigeminal neuralgia (tic douloureux). N. Engl. J. Med., *315:*174, 1986.
336. Swenson, C., and Patt, R.B.: Manufacturing processes. *In* Patt, R.B. (ed.): Cancer Pain. pp. 612–615. Philadelphia, J.B. Lippincott, 1993.
337. Swerdlow, M.: Neurolytic blocks of the neuroaxis. *In* Patt, R.B. (ed.): Cancer Pain. pp. 427–442. Philadelphia, J.B. Lippincott, 1993.
338. Swerdlow, M. (ed.): Relief of Intractable Pain. 3rd Ed. Amsterdam, Excerpta Medica, 1983.
339. Swerdlow, M.: Spinal and peripheral neurolysis for managing Pancoast syndrome. Adv. Pain Res. Ther. *4:*135, 1982.
340. Swerdlow, M.: Subarachnoid and extradural blocks. Adv. Pain Res. Ther., *2:*325, 1979.
341. Swerdlow, M.: The history of neurolytic blockade. *In* Racz, G.B. (ed.): Techniques of Neurolysis. pp. 1–11. Boston, Kluwer Academic, 1989.
342. Swerdlow, M.: Role of chemical neurolysis and local anesthetic infiltration. *In* Swerdlow, M., and Ventafridda, V. (eds.): Cancer Pain. pp. 105–128. Lancaster, England, MTP Press, 1986.
343. Szalados, J., and Patt, R.B.: Management of a patient with displaced orthopedic hardware. J. Pain Symptom Manage., *6:*394, 1991.
344. Deleted in proof.
345. Takagi, Y., Koyama, T., and Yamamoto, Y.: Subarachnoid neurolytic block with 15% phenol glycerine in the treatment of cancer pain. Pain, *4:*(Suppl.)133, 1987.
346. Tanelian, D., and Cousins, M.J.: Celiac plexus block following high dose opiates in a four-year-old child. J. Pain Symptom Manage., *4:*82, 1989.
347. Tasker, R.R., and Dostrovsky, J.O.: Deafferentation and central pain. *In* Wall, P.D., and Melzack, R. (eds.): Textbook of Pain. pp. 154. 2nd Ed. Edinburgh, Churchill Livingstone, 1989.
348. Teeple, E., and Ghia, J.N.: Problems with neurolytic blocks for cancer pain in patients receiving narcotics and psychoactive drugs. Reg. Anesth., *6:*152, 1981.
349. Thompson, G.E.: Pulmonary edema complicating intrathecal hypertonic saline injection for intractable pain. Anesthesiology, *35:*425, 1971.
350. Thompson, G.E., and Moore, D.C.: Celiac plexus, intercostal, and minor peripheral blockade. *In* Cousins, M.J., and Bridenbaugh, P.O.

(eds.): Neural Blockade. 2nd Ed. pp. 503–530. Philadelphia, J.B. Lippincott, 1988.
351. Thompson, G.E., Moore, D.C., Bridenbaugh, P.O., *et al.*: Abdominal pain and celiac plexus nerve block. Anesth. Analg., *56:*1, 1977.
352. Todd, D.P.: Poststernotomy neuralgia: A new pain syndrome. Anesth. Analg., *69:*691, 1989.
353. Toomey, T.C., Hernandez, J.T., Gittelman, D.F., and Hulka, J.F.: Relationship of sexual and physical abuse to pain and psychological assessment variables in chronic pelvic pain patients. Pain, *53:*105, 1993.
354. Tracy, G.D., and Cockett, F.B.: Pain in the lower limb after sympathectomy. Lancet, *i:*12, 1957.
355. Twycross, R.G.: Pain Relief in Advanced Cancer. Edinburgh, Churchill Livingstone, 1994.
356. Umeda, S.: Disulfiram-like reaction to moxolactam after celiac plexus block. Anesth. Analg., *64:*377, 1985.
357. Valley, M.A., and Raja, S.N.: Relief of intractable pain from metastatic multiple myeloma using epidural phenol injections. J. Pain Symptom Manage., *7:*179, 1992.
358. Vernon, S.: Paralgesia: Paravertebral block for pain relief. Am. J. Surg., *21:*416, 1930.
359. Vijayaram, S., Chandrashekar, N.S., Ramamani, P.V., *et al.*: CT-guided coeliac neurolysis for upper abdominal cancer. The Pain Clinic, *5:*165, 1992.
360. Wajsman, Z., Gamarra, M., Park, J.J., *et al.*: Transabdominal fine needle aspiration of retroperitoneal lymph nodes in staging of genitourinary tract cancer. J. Urol., *128:*1238, 1982.
361. Waldman, S.D., Feldstein, G.S., Allen, M.L., *et al.*: Cervical epidural implantable narcotic delivery systems in the management of upper body pain. Anesth. Analg. *66:*780, 1987.
362. Waldman, S.D., Feldstein, G.S., and Allen, M.L.: Neuroadenolysis of the pituitary: Description of a modified technique. J. Pain Symptom Manage., *2:*45, 1987.
363. Waldman, S.D., Wilson, W.L., and Kreps, R.D.: Superior hypogastric plexus block using a single needle and computed tomography guidance: Description of a modified technique. Reg. Anesth. *16:*286, 1991.
364. Walker, E., Katon, W., Harrop-Griffiths, J., *et al.*: Relationship of chronic pelvic pain to psychiatric diagnoses and childhood sexual abuse. Am. J. Psychiatry, *145:*75, 1988.
365. Walker, J.B., Akhanjee, L.K., Cooney, M.M., *et al.*: Laser therapy for pain of trigeminal neuralgia. Clin. J. Pain, *3:*183, 1988.
366. Wallace, M.S., and Milholland, A.V.: Contralateral spread of local anesthetic with stellate ganglion block. Reg. Anesth., *18:*55, 1993.
367. Wang, J.K.: Cryoanalgesia for painful peripheral nerve lesions. Pain, *22:*191, 1985.
368. Wang, J.K.: Intrathecal morphine for intractable pain secondary to pelvic cancer of pelvic organs. Pain, *21:*99, 1985.
369. Ward, E.M., Rorie, D.K., Nauss, L.A., *et al.*: The celiac ganglion in man: Normal and anatomic variations. Anesth. Analg. *58:*461, 1979.
370. Warfield, C.A., and Crews, D.A.: Use of stellate ganglion blocks in the treatment of intractable limb pain in lung cancer. Clin. J. Pain, *3:*13, 1987.
371. Walthard, K.M., and Tchicaloff, M.: Motor points. *In* Licht, S. (ed.): Electrodiagnosis and Electromyography. 3rd Ed. pp. 153–170. New Haven, Licht, 1971.
372. Wendling, H.: Ausschaltung der nervi splanchnici durch leitungsanästhesie bei magenoperationen und andern eingriffen in der oberen bauchhöhle. Beitr. Klin. Chir., *110:*517, 1918.
373. Whiteman, M.S., Rosenberg, H., Haskin, P.H., and Teplick, S.K.: Celiac plexus block for interventional radiology. Radiology, *161:*836, 1986.
374. Wilkinson, H.A.: Radiofrequency percutaneous upper thoracic sympathectomy: Technique and review of indications. N. Engl. J. Med., *311:*34, 1984.
375. Wilkinson, H.A.: Stereotactic percutaneous upper thoracic sympathectomy. *In* Hyodo, M., Oyama, T., and Swerdlow, M. (eds.): The Pain Clinic IV. pp. 149–151. Utrecht, VSP, 1992.
376. Wilson, F.: Neurolytic and other locally acting drugs in the management of pain. Pharm. Ther., *12:*599, 1981.
377. Wilson, P.R.: Incidental discography during celiac plexus block. Anesthesiology, *76:*314, 1992.
378. Wilson, P.R., Lilley, J.P., and Wang, J.K.: Intrathecal neurolysis may reduce bladder spasm in paraplegia. Reg. Anesth., *13*(Suppl.):35, 1988.
379. Wilson-Pauwels, L., Akesson, E.J., and Stewart, P.A.: Cranial Nerves: Anatomy and Clinical Comments. Toronto, B.C. Decker, Inc, 1988.
380. Winnie, A.P.: Plexus Anesthesia. Vol. 1. Philadelphia, W.B. Saunders, 1983.
381. Wise, R.P.: Treatment of pain. *In* Wiley, W.D., and Churchill-Davidson, H. (eds.): A Practice of Anaesthesia. 4th Ed. pp. 1085. Philadelphia, W.B. Saunders, 1979.
382. Woodburne, R.T., and Burkel, W.E.: Essentials of Human Anatomy. New York, Oxford Press, 1988, p. 552.
383. Woodruff, J.D., and Babkinia, A.: Local alcohol injection of the vulva: Discussion of 35 cases. Obstet. Gynecol., *54:*512, 1979.
384. Woodruff, J.D., and Thompson, B.: Local alcohol injection in the treatment of vulvar pruritus. Obstet. Gynecol., *40:*18, 1972.
385. World Health Organization: Cancer Pain Relief. Geneva, WHO, 1986.
386. Yanagida H., Corssen, G., Ceballos, R., and Strong, G.: Alcohol-induced pituitary adenolysis: How does it control intractable pain? An experimental study using tooth pulp-evoked potentials in rhesus monkeys. Anesth. Analg., *58:*279, 1979.
387. Yanagida, H., Corssen, G., Trouwborst, A., and Erdmann, W.: Relief of cancer pain in man: Alcohol-induced neuroadenolysis vs electrical stimulation of the pituitary gland. Pain, *19:*133, 1984.
388. Young, R.F.: Glycerol rhizolysis for treatment of trigeminal neuralgia. J. Neurosurg. *69:*39, 1988.
389. Zakrzewska, J.M.: Cryotherapy in the management of paroxysmal trigeminal neuralgia. J. Neurol., Neurosurg., Psychiatry *50:*485, 1987.

Neural Blockade in Clinical Anesthesia and Management of Pain, Third Edition,
edited by M.J. Cousins and P.O. Bridenbaugh.
Lippincott–Raven Publishers, Philadelphia © 1998.

CHAPTER 32

Neurostimulation and Percutaneous Neural Destructive Techniques

Ronald R. Tasker

Percutaneous neurosurgical techniques are part of a continuous strategy of reducing the impact and, usually, increasing the precision of surgical procedures. They have become increasingly practical with the development of modern imaging, clinical neurophysiology, and radiofrequency lesion-making, as well as the increased understanding of neuroactive chemicals (see Chapter 23.1) and of modern electronics. Whereas they have been used largely for the treatment of intractable pain, they are also potentially applicable to the problems of epilepsy, motor control, and vascular disease.

CLASSIFICATION OF PERCUTANEOUS TECHNIQUES

Percutaneous neurosurgical techniques can be classified according to application and methodology (Table 32-1). This chapter will be concerned with procedures for the relief of intractable pain. Facet so-called rhizotomy and other percutaneous procedures for the relief of low back pain and the intravenous and/or intrathecal infusion of morphine and other drugs are dealt with in Chapters 26 to 31.

TREATMENT OF INTRACTABLE PAIN

Percutaneous neurosurgical techniques can be used in several ways to treat intractable pain. Most obvious are the destructive techniques that interrupt transmission in pain pathways such as neurectomy, rhizotomy, and destructive lesions in the spinal cord. However, percutaneous modulatory techniques are also available. Most widely used is the instillation of morphine intravenously or intrathecally, which blocks the entry of nociceptive signals into the spinothalamic tract, as discussed in Chapter 29.

R. R. Tasker: Department of Surgery, Division of Neurosurgery, The University of Toronto, The Toronto Hospital, Western Division, Toronto, Ontario M5T 2S8 Canada.

The other type of modulatory surgery is the use of chronic stimulation. Originally employed as prescribed by the Gate Control Theory[185] to suppress activity in small-diameter (pain-conducting) fibers by stimulation of the lower threshold large-diameter (non-pain-conducting) fibers to treat nociceptive pain,[286,344] chronic stimulation was soon found in practice to be more effective in treating neuropathic pain,[307] though there is renewed interest in its use in the form of dorsal column stimulation to treat (nociceptive) low back pain.[7]

CLASSIFICATION OF INTRACTABLE PAIN AND SELECTION OF APPROPRIATE THERAPEUTIC STRATEGY

Before discussing percutaneous techniques for treating intractable pain it is necessary to realize that not all pain syndromes share the same pathophysiology[353] (Table 32-2). There is still a tendency to regard all pain as being the result of transmission in those pain pathways that serve the part of the body where pain is being experienced. For example, the patient who suffers a malar fracture may develop steady burning, dysesthetic pain in infraorbital nerve distribution in an area rendered hypesthetic after the fracture because the latter has damaged the infraorbital nerve. Local anesthetic blockade temporarily alleviates that pain; even blockade distal to the causative lesion does so.[117] However, cutting the infraorbital nerve does not, because the pathophysiology does not depend on transmission in the infraorbital nerve.[40,155,160,307,311,317,343] After all, partial damage to the nerve created the pain in the first place—pain which appears to depend on some unknown central process set in motion by the deafferentation.

Though it has become popular to refer to such pain as "neuropathic," I find this term unsuitable. All chronic pain is neuropathic, and even in a more restricted sense, "neuropathic" includes tic douloureux, which is unique and requires distinc-

TABLE 32-1. *Classification of percutaneous neurosurgical procedures*

Treatment of intractable pain
- 1. Destructive
  - (a) RF lesion-making
  - (b) Injection of destructive substances
  - (c) Use of cryoprobe
  - Nerves: V, occipital; intercostal, facet
  - Roots
  - Cord: V tract
    - myelotomy
    - cordotomy
  - Intrathecal alcohol, phenol
  - Percutaneous sympathectomy
  - Percutaneous hypophysectomy
- 2. Modulatory
  - (a) Chronic stimulation
    - trigeminal nerve
    - other peripheral nerves
    - spinal cord
  - (b) Treatment of vascular disease
    - dorsal column stimulation for angina and PVD
  - (c) Intravenous, intrathecal morphine/nonopioids

Treatment of disorders of motor control
- Spasticity
  - Destructive
    - Neurectomy—obturator neurectomy
  - Modulatory
    - Intrathecal baclofen
    - Dorsal column stimulation

Treatment of epilepsy
- Vagal stimulation

PVD, peripheral vascular disease; RF, radiofrequency.

tive attention. The older term "deafferentation" pain still seems more appropriate, even to describe "central" pain (isn't all pain "central?"), though it came to apply to neural damage pain caused only by peripheral lesions. The fact that neural injury pain can occur in the absence of total or even partial deafferentation and the notion that a stroke does not deafferent tended to discourage use of the term "deafferentation" pain.

Table 32-2 represents an attempt to classify pain on a pathophysiologic basis so that the different techniques of pain surgery can be better tailored to the appropriate pain syndrome with a greater chance of success than would otherwise be possible. Nevertheless, the exercise is far from perfect because of continuing ignorance about many types of pain (see also Chapters 23.1, 23.2 and 24, 25).

The best-understood type of pain is that caused by activation of nociceptors and transmission in pain pathways as detailed in the review by Willis[349] (1a in Table 32-2: nociceptive pain). This is what happens when a patient has pain due to an expanding tumor in a long bone, or suffers from osteoarthritis. Treatment consists of denervating the area of damage that generates the pain, selectively interrupting the pain pathways serving the area (as with cordotomy), or modulating pain transmission from the area by the use of either morphine or periventricular grey (PVG) stimulation (which activates a descending pathway that inhibits the entry of nociceptive messages into the spinothalamic tract).[177] Such types of pain are not the only ones dependent on nociceptor activation. Hyperesthesia and hyperpathia (1b in Table 32-2) share similar pathophysiology except that the noxious stimulus applied is appreciated as excessively noxious by the patient, often with additional features of spatial or temporal spread or dysesthesia. Hyperpathia is often a feature of neuropathic pain syndromes (see Chapter 23.1).

More curious is allodynia (2 in Table 32-2). This too is a feature of neuropathic pain, including sympathetically maintained pain,[15] the patient experiencing as painful a stimulus, that is normally non-noxious, and has been applied to an area of the body that has been partially deafferented. In the case of neuropathic pain from peripheral lesions, allodynia is known to be the result of activation of the spinothalamic tract at the dorsal horn level by abnormal processing of the incoming normally non-noxious signal.[351] Allodynia can be triggered by a variety of stimuli—touch, hair bending, deep pressure, joint or muscle stimulation, hot or cold—all causing the patient to have a sometimes agonizing, spreading, unusually persistent, dysesthetic experience. In the case of central pain from cord or brain lesions, the mechanism is unclear, but clinical experience suggests that it is still dependent on stimulation of spinothalamic pathways. When the results of surgery for the relief of the three common characteristics of cord central pain—steady, neuralgic, evoked (allodynia and hyperpathia)—were reviewed, it was found that surgery that interrupted pain pathways (cordotomy, cordectomy, dorsal root entry zone [DREZ]) was statistically significantly more effective for relieving the evoked and neuralgic aspects than for the steady element.[316] Moreover, when treating central pain of brain origin with chronic deep brain stimulation, it was found that the evoked element was

TABLE 32-2. *Suggested classification of pain (Tasker)*

Dependent on transmission in pain pathways
- 1. Stimulation of nociceptors
  - (a) Acute pain
    - Postoperative pain
    - Cancer in a bone
    - Osteoarthritis including low back pain
  - (b) Hyperpathia and hyperesthesia
- 2. Stimulation of non-nociceptor receptors
  - Allodynia
- 3. Direct stimulation of nerve fibers
  - (a) Tinel's and Lhermitte's signs
  - (b) Stimulation of nerve root by ruptured disk
  - (c) Stimulation of lumbosacral plexus by cancer
  - (d) Ectopic impulses set up proximal to nerve injury site in neuralgic element of neuropathic pain
  - (e) Ephaptic stimulation

Apparently not dependent on transmission in pain pathways
- 4. Psychogenic pain
- 5. ?Steady element of neuropathic pain

better relieved by PVG than by paresthesia-producing stimulation.[229,306,312]

It may come as a surprise to realize that two common pain syndromes, usually considered as nociceptive, which result from root irritation in disk disease (3b in Table 32-2) and from cancerous compression of nerve plexuses (3c in Table 32-2), do not obviously result from nociceptor activation, unless those in nervi nervorum and arteriorum are involved, but rather from direct stimulation of nerve fibers. Nevertheless, once stimulation is established in these conditions, the physiology is the same as if nociceptors were actually activated (see also Chapters 27 and 28).

More obscure is the neuralgic, intermittent, lancinating element of neuropathic pain (3d in Table 32-2). Most prevalent in central pain of cord origin arising from thoracolumbar lesions, it was found to respond preferentially, like evoked pain, to interruption of pain pathways, suggesting that it arose from activation of the spinothalamic tract, possibly because it is dependent on ectopic impulse generation at the injury site or at a synapse proximal to the injury.[307] The role of ephapses remains unclear, but evidence that they contribute to chronic pain syndromes has been published.[307]

Thus far, all the pain syndromes considered depend upon transmission of signals in pain pathways. Thus they should be expected to respond to interruption or modulation of that transmission at any level above the site of activation. However, the remaining groups of syndromes (4, 5 in Table 32-2) are different. Obviously they result in activation of the final common path for pain, presumably cerebral cortex, but, based on clinical experience, not as a result of spinothalamic tract input. Surgery is not knowingly applied for the treatment of one of these, psychogenic pain, but the surgeon often is called upon to treat the other, the steady, often burning (causalgic) aching or dysesthetic element of neuropathic pain, and may all too often, as in the case of infraorbital nerve deafferentation mentioned above, use inappropriate techniques. A confusing feature of neuropathic pain that may contribute to the false opinion that it is psychogenic in origin is the fact that it is idiosyncratic;[311] it does not appear in every individual who suffers a particular neural lesion but only in those who may have a (genetically determined?)[103,142] predisposition to develop neuropathic pain. In my experience, such pain responds poorly to interruption of pain pathways or to attempts at modulation with morphine or PVG stimulation; chronic stimulation that produces paresthesia in the area of the pain appears to be the only reliable surgical modality, and even that is effective in only half the patients that might be expected to respond[306,307,311,312,316,317] (see also Chapter 23.1).

There has been much recent interest in the treatment of noncancerous pain syndromes with morphine.[232] Success should not be entirely surprising, however. Not all noncancerous pain syndromes are of a neuropathic nature; low back pain and pain related to chronic disk disease are multifactorial in origin and contain nociceptive elements while, as has been described, neuropathic pain has different components of which the evoked and neuralgic ones appear to be caused by mechanisms capable of relief by modulation with morphine. Nevertheless, steady burning dysesthetic pain arising from nerve damage does not, in my opinion, respond to treatment with morphine. A similar discussion, which will not be addressed in this chapter,[312] has evolved concerning the role of PVG stimulation which, for practical purposes, can be considered to achieve the same end result as that obtained by morphine therapy. In my experience, paresthesia-producing brain stimulation is effective only for the treatment of the steady element of neuropathic pain (for which it may be the only surgical option), whereas PVG stimulation is effective for nociceptive pain whether or not of malignant origin and for the evoked (and presumably the neuralgic) element of neuropathic pain.

On the other hand, not all pain caused by cancer is dependent on transmission in pain pathways and therefore amenable to treatment with morphine, interruption of pain paths, or PVG stimulation. Cancerous invasion of plexuses causes nociceptive pain, as discussed above, but ongoing invasion eventually causes neural destruction and, as a result, neuropathic pain with all the characteristics of neuropathic pain from other causes of neural damage, including resistance to surgical treatment with neural interruption, morphine, or PVG stimulation[303] (see also Chapter 23.1).

The surgeon must listen to what the patient says. If the patient describes steady burning pain, he is telling us that the mechanism of his pain is different from that producing intermittent shooting neuralgic or evoked pain.[21]

Some guidelines for the selection of surgical procedures are:

1. *For nociceptive, and the neuralgic and evoked elements of neuropathic pain*: interrupt pain pathway or modulate it with morphine (see Chapter 29) or PVG stimulation.

2. *For steady causalgic dysesthetic element of neuropathic pain*: treat by induction of paresthesia in the area of pain (see also Chapter 29).

SELECTION OF PATIENTS FOR SURGERY

The selection of patients for procedures for the relief of pain, disorders of motor control, or epilepsy is a complex process consisting of assessment of cost-effectiveness. First, all simpler methods of treatment must have been tried and found lacking. Second, the proposed surgical procedure should have a reasonable chance of relieving the problem for which it is proposed, commensurate with the severity of the symptoms it is intended to relieve, the impact of the procedure, and the likely complications. Third, the patient and family should understand that the procedure is intended to control specific symptoms, not the underlying disease and other problems related to it. A procedure for pain caused by spinal cord injury does not affect the paraplegia. Fourth, it should be clearly recognized that procedures for pain relief have a relatively low success rate and seldom give permanent relief. Pain usually recurs in time no matter what operation is done[310] quite apart from early failure which may reflect waning of an initial placebo effect, which is usually more transient than a procedure-specific effect.[342] Pain may be looked upon as a signal of actual or impending tissue damage; relief of this pain in the face of ongoing pathology is unnatural. Finally, destructive procedures for pain relief may give rise in themselves to iatrogenic neuropathic or deafferentation pain syndromes[36] (see Chapters 23.1, 23.2 and 24).

OUTCOME EVALUATION

One of the greatest deficiencies in present-day medicine is the lack of accurate outcome data, nowhere more apparent than in the treatment of chronic pain.[81] It is obvious enough what the reasons for this deficiency are, but more difficult to correct them. Ideally, outcome of methods of treatment should be analyzed statistically, using, as far as possible, double-blind crossover studies with controls, looking at individual features capable of quantitative analysis. Unfortunately, no two pain syndromes are identical, pain is multifactorial, quantitative evaluation is impossible, no two observers can usually gather sufficient numbers of sufficiently similar cases and evaluate them identically, there are bound to be differences in technique between surgeons in the extent and site of nervous system affected by identical operations performed in different patients, and eventual recurrence makes the length of follow-up critical.[310] In conclusion, it is impossible to compare the outcomes of two surgeons each claiming, say, 50% significant reduction in the pain of "failed back" syndrome after dorsal column stimulation. However, we can do better than we do now, and the following principles appear to be important:

1. Accurately list the numbers of patients accepted for consideration of treatment and not the final number arrived at after certain exclusions, which may differ among series.
2. Define precisely the pain syndrome addressed and its location. All patients reviewed should suffer from the same syndrome. (see International Association for the Study of Pain [IASP] Subcommittee on Taxonomy, Classification of Descriptions of Pain Terms. Pain, [Suppl. 13], 1986; Appendix A, Chapter 23.1.)
3. Define pain severity in as quantitative terms as possible, at the very least by assessment on a visual analogue scale.
4. Employ precisely described identical treatment strategies in each patient.
5. Review outcomes after the same time interval in each patient.
6. Follow outcomes for as long as possible; short follow-ups are meaningless.
7. Accurately document the nature *and severity* of any complications.
8. If possible, use a control series.
9. Use as quantitatively meaningful evaluations of success as possible.
10. Have evaluations done blindly, if possible, or at least by a disinterested third party.

Admitting that my own evaluation of my work falls short of these guidelines, I strongly advocate international acceptance of an effective *yet still practical* protocol for the evaluation of pain surgery. Clearly, it is not cost-effective to carry out as rigorous studies of every pain operation, in each condition for which it is used, as that recently applied to the study of carotid endarterectomy.

TREATMENT OF INTRACTABLE PAIN—DESTRUCTIVE PROCEDURES

Technique

Many neurodestructive techniques have been proposed for use in association with percutaneous neurosurgical techniques. Wherever possible, radiofrequency (RF) lesion-making is to be preferred because of the ease of making a graded lesion of planned reproducible size.[247,284,287,288] This is accomplished by controlling the diameter and length of the bare tip of the lesion-making electrode and the duration and level of current flow and tip temperature during lesion-making, all easily possible with the electrical back-up provided by systems such as the OWL (Diros Technology, Toronto, Canada; or Radionics Corp., Burlington, MA). In addition, RF lesion-making is easily combined with physiologic localization techniques including recording, stimulation, and impedance measurement to sharpen the control of the percutaneous procedure. RF lesion-making also allows an initial test lesion before a permanent one is made.

The use of a cryoprobe also provides satisfactory lesion-making with some of the same advantages, but requires a rather larger probe that is easily damaged, a supply of liquid nitrogen at the time of surgery, and a delivery system that, in my experience, is prone to blockage and other problems. Furthermore, cryosurgery is not as easily married to physiologic localization (see Chapter 31).

Destructive chemicals have also been extensively used,[27,116,196,228,289,336–338] including absolute alcohol, phenol, and glycerol; also, hypertonic and cold saline have been used intrathecally (see Chapters 30 and 31). The introduction of chemicals has the advantage of applying a destructive agent that diffuses widely beyond the tip of the introductory needle, particularly useful when introduced into the cerebrospinal fluid (CSF), say, in Meckel's cave or the spinal canal. However, all these techniques have the disadvantage of erratic unpredictable spread and variable degrees of penetration of nervous tissue; none is selective for pain fibers. They tend to produce incomplete and nonpermanent lesions. The danger of tracking is also significant; for example, alcohol injected into the infraorbital nerve may leak into the orbit, causing oculomotor palsy or blindness.

The technique of RF lesion-making is similar wherever applied, and details will be given here only for selected procedures. Most RF procedures are performed under local anesthesia with intravenous sedation. Care is taken to provide the necessary analgesia for the patient's ongoing pain, but not sufficient sedation to cloud the patient's ability to cooperate for physiologic testing. The lesion-making electrode is introduced toward the intended target using surface landmarks, plain films (especially image intensification), or even CT guidance. When it appears to be in the correct anatomic location, this fact can be further corroborated in a number of ways. Contrast medium can be injected, monitored by image intensification. Impedance monitoring is helpful, levels of 400 ohms or W being typical of CSF, 800 to 1200 ohms or W of spinal cord. Recording is also useful; microelectrode recording is probably limited to lesion-making in the brain or perhaps the spinal cord, but recording of evoked potentials is much more generally applicable. However, macrostimulation is most often applied for physiologic corroboration. Usually threshold stimulation is applied at low (2 Hz for motor) and high (60–100 Hz for motor and sensory) frequencies, and the responses are compared with ideal findings expected in the procedure at hand. Once localization is deemed satisfactory, a reversible RF lesion is made with parameters appropriate to the procedure being done. If the effects are satisfactory, a gradually larger lesion is made until the desired effect has been achieved.

Percutaneous Neurectomy and Rhizotomy

Conceptually, the simplest technique for treating pain syndromes dependent on pain transmission is percutaneous neurectomy or rhizotomy. Unfortunately, such procedures are not often useful either because pain is seldom restricted to the domain of one or a few nerves or roots or because the inevitable concomitant loss of proprioception and/or motor function is not acceptable.[302,308]

Occipital Neurectomy

For pain syndromes amenable to treatment by denervation that are located in occipital nerve distribution, occipital neurectomy is commonly advocated. A number of techniques are available: percutaneous RF neurectomy, open neurectomy, and ganglionectomy. The latter is often preferred because postoperative regeneration is unlikely, and any sensory fibers traversing the ventral roots will also be interrupted; conveniently the C2 ganglion lies outside the spinal canal. Only the first technique is of interest here. There is poor consensus on indications for occipital neurectomy, the procedure being advocated for diverse pain syndromes in occipital territory including occipital neuralgia, postherpetic neuralgia, and muscle tension pain. According to the guidelines discussed above, the procedure should not be expected to relieve steady neuropathic pain, and conceptually it would not seem useful for the relief of pain caused by lesions proximal to the site of the RF denervation. It may be, however, that denervation of the projected field of the pain would prove effective treatment regardless of the site of the causative lesion; there appears to have been no study of this issue. In a study of C2 ganglionectomy, Lozano[167] found the procedure useful only in patients with truly intermittent neuralgic pain, a restriction that should also apply to percutaneous denervation. Though occipital neurectomy should eliminate the allodynia and hyperpathia of postherpetic neuralgia in C2–C3 territory by denervating the responsible receptors, this strategy is seldom worthwhile since the steady element of the pain persists.

Another condition in which occipital neurectomy may be considered is vascular headache in occipital territory. Patients with recurrent attacks of head pain located consistently in the same territory with the features of vascular headache—drooping of the eyelid and tearing, stuffiness of the nose, nasal discharge, redness of the affected skin, clustering of attacks—sometimes gain temporary relief from division of the peripheral nerves and/or arteries that supply the region of the head involved in the pain, including the occipital region.

The technique of percutaneous RF occipital neurectomy consists of introducing a relatively stiff insulated needle with a bare tip 2 to 4 mm in length (that used for RF coagulation of the trigeminal nerve is satisfactory) (Fig. 32-1) through

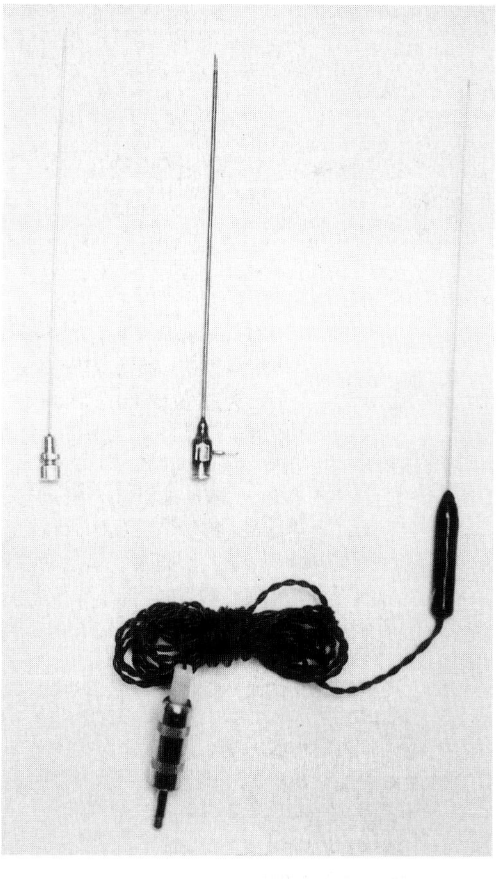

FIG. 32-1. Electrodes for percutaneous surgery. Stylet, electrode, and thermistor for conventional RF trigeminal coagulation. (Manufactured by Diros Technology.)

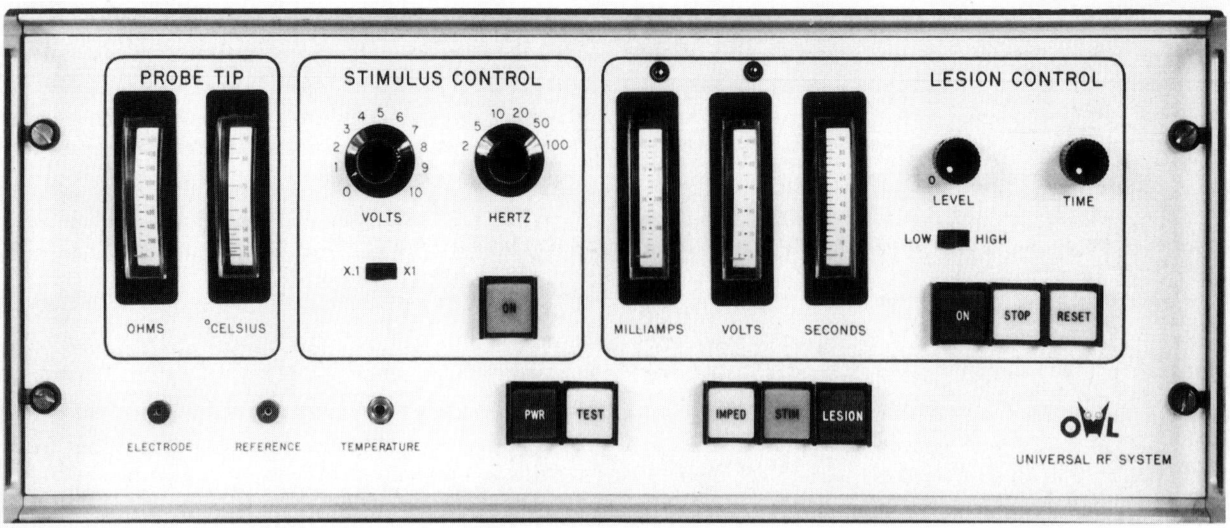

FIG. 32-2. Electronic back-up for impedance monitoring, stimulation, and radiofrequency lesion-making with current, voltage, and temperature monitoring capabilities. (Manufactured by Diros Technology.)

the scalp to the expected location of the greater and/or lesser occipital nerves on the affected side at the base of the skull, using surface landmarks. Then 100 Hz stimulation is applied and the needle moved about between periosteum and scalp until paresthesias are produced in occipital nerve territory at the lowest threshold; an RF lesion is then made and the degree of sensory loss verified. Usually a maximal lesion is required, achieved by gradually increasing current and electrode tip temperature until current "falloff" occurs. "Falloff" signals boiling and gas formation around the electrode tip, which is then insulated from producing further heating and enlargement of the lesion. "Falloff" occurring too early, before adequate temperature has been applied long enough, results in an inadequate lesion. Stimulation and lesion-making are facilitated by the use of an electronic back-up such as the OWL Cordotomy System (Fig. 32-2) available from Diros Technology, Toronto or that provided by Radionics Corp. (Fig. 32-3)(see also Chapter 15, Fig. 15-10).

It is difficult to present outcome data because these depend on the syndrome treated and the nature of the pain; reports fail to distinguish these matters. Published data suggest that 75% of patients enjoy amelioration of occipital pain generally over a 1- to 4-year follow-up.[19,20]

Complications are few, neuropathic pain in the denervated area being an ever-present concern. Recurrence after nerve regeneration is to be expected (see Chapter 23.1).

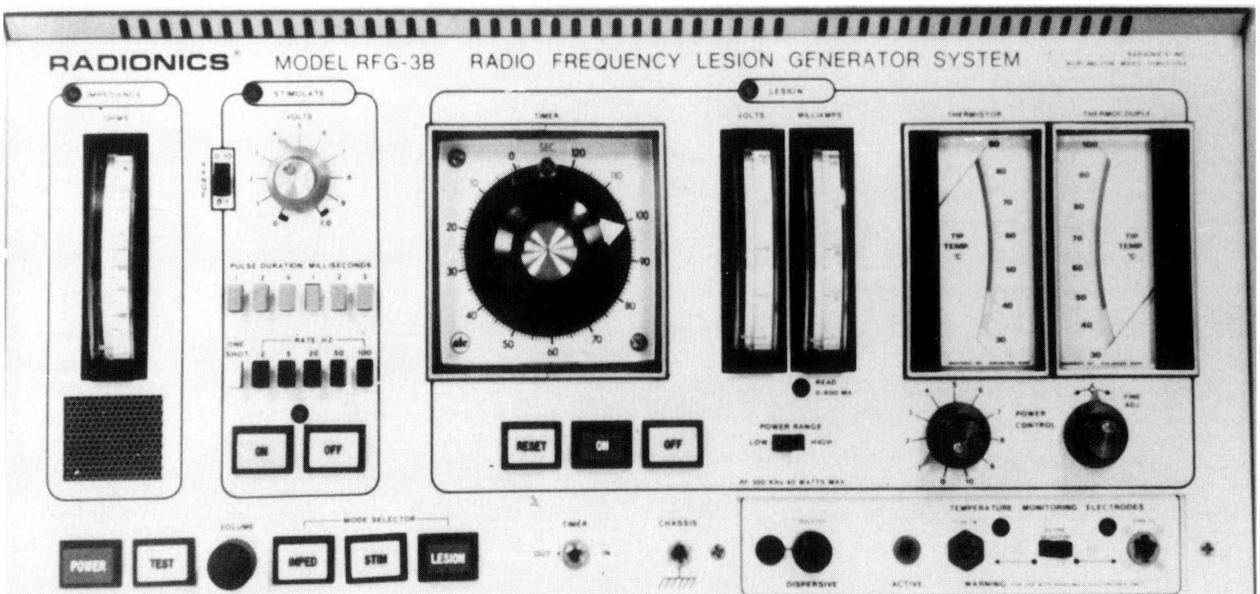

FIG. 32-3. Electronic back-up, as in Figure 32-2. (Manufactured by Radionics Corporation.)

Intercostal Neurectomy

Various pain syndromes such as postherpetic neuralgia, post-thoracotomy pain, intercostal neuralgia, and the pain of cancer affect the chest wall for which percutaneous RF intercostal neurectomy, first employed by us in 1972, may seem a promising procedure since it is not followed by significant functional deficit.[300] However, comments made regarding occipital postherpetic neuralgia also apply to intercostal postherpetic neuralgia, while for obscure reasons, intercostal neurectomy is useless in post-thoracotomy syndrome,[300] only 25% of our 44 patients reporting useful relief. Intercostal neuralgia usually results from compression of a thoracic root by a thoracic disk or foraminal stenosis, though sometimes no cause can be found. Intercostal nerve section distal to a site of irritation is all that can be accomplished in intercostal neuralgia from disk or stenosis and appears to be ineffective. Open section of the root proximal to the lesion site usually is necessary. It is chiefly in pain caused by cancer of the chest wall where intercostal neurectomy is useful, all of our eight patients being relieved when denervation of the painful area was possible and when the pain did not incorporate an old thoracotomy incision.

The procedure is usually performed under general anesthesia. A sturdy insulated needle with a curved 10-mm bare tip (Fig. 32-4) is "walked down" and slid under the inferior margin of the rib related to the nerve to be sectioned, proximal to the expected site of nerve involvement, until it enters or lies alongside the neurovascular bundle. Then 2 Hz stimulation at 10 volts is performed as the needle tip is moved about, and contractions in the appropriate intercostal muscles are monitored until a site is found where the latter occur below 3 v. A graded RF lesion is then made and maximized until "falloff" occurs (usually 90 seconds with 175–250 mA and temperature over 90° C). It is wise to make a second lesion adjacent to the first to ensure adequate denervation. Efficacy is checked by ensuring that appropriate anesthesia has been achieved and/or by demonstrating increased threshold for motor response. An upright chest x-ray is performed immediately postoperatively to identify the chief complication, pneumothorax, which occurred in 6% of patients in my series and required chest drainage in 2% (see also Chapter 14, Figs. 14-1, 14-3).

Dorsal Rhizotomy

According to Gybels and Sweet[82], Uematsu and his colleagues[330–332] were the first to report percutaneous RF dorsal rhizotomy. Though percutaneous RF dorsal rhizotomy has the advantage over neurectomy of not inducing motor deficits unless electrode positioning is faulty and of usually denervating a larger area of the body, it still results in proprioceptive loss, a serious problem if roots supplying limbs are sectioned. The fact that radicular arteries that accompany roots may be end arteries for the spinal cord—especially at the C1, T1–T4, and T11–L1 levels—means that their accidental occlusion with a "blind" percutaneous RF rhizotomy may result in cord infarction and paraplegia (see Chapter 7, Figs. 7-10, 7-11).

Though experience with open rhizotomy has been extensively published, outcome data for the percutaneous technique are limited. In general, the pain syndromes for which dorsal rhizotomy should be considered are nociceptive pain caused by cancer or by spinal pathology that compresses nerve roots and the evoked or neuralgic elements of neuropathic pain. Control of cancerous pain is limited to cases in which the entire area involved can be denervated by rhizotomy lesions that lie proximal to the site of cancerous interference.

More often, pain from irritation or compression of roots by bony abnormalities, disk disease, foraminal stenosis, or fibrosis will be encountered. Even when a single root can be incriminated by careful selective local anesthetic root

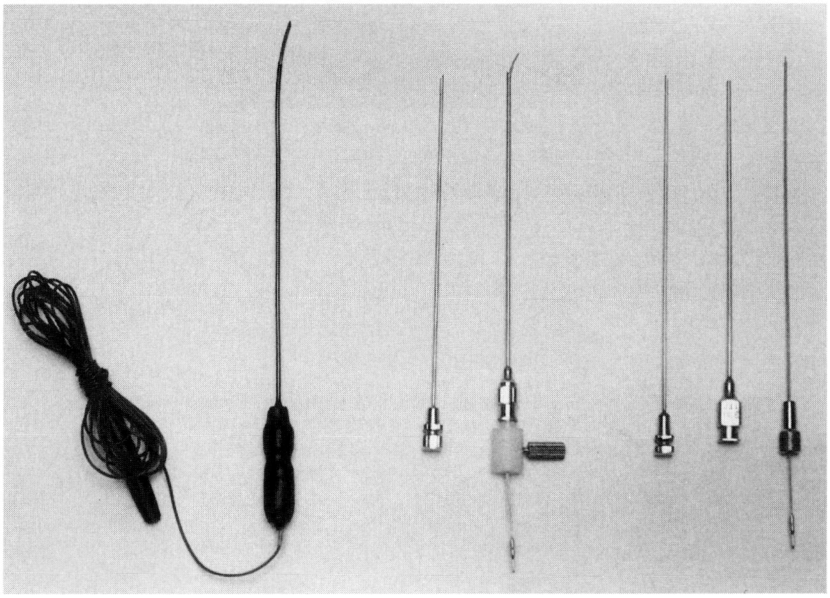

FIG. 32-4. Electrodes for percutaneous surgery. **Left:** Electrode for intercostal neurectomy. **Center:** Stylet, and curved electrode inserted in guide needle, for selective trigeminal thermocoagulation. **Right:** Stylet, guide needle, and conventional electrode for percutaneous cordotomy. A temperature-monitored model is also available. (Manufactured by Diros Technology.)

blocks, the permanent rhizotomy may fail because the lesion cannot be made proximal to the site of entrapment or irritation. Also, because of overlap of innervation of somatic areas, a lesion of a single nerve root may only produce temporary denervation (see Chapter 27). In patients with neuropathic pain in whom allodynia or hyperpathia are prominent features, rhizotomy may also be useful, as in cases of spinal cord injury with a radicular distribution of allodynia at the level of the cord lesion. If a limb is to be denervated, even with a single level rhizotomy, the accompanying loss of position sense must be considered, and this is best assessed at the time of the essential diagnostic root blockade. Multiple consecutive rhizotomies are more risky.

The technique consists of identifying the correct root(s) to be denervated by clinical means and diagnostic local blocks. Then, with the patient either under general anesthesia without paralysis or under intravenous sedation, a suitable electrode such as that used for thermocoagulation of the trigeminal nerve (see Fig. 32-1) is introduced into the dorsal portion of the appropriate intervertebral foramen, aided by image intensification suitably angled so as to reveal the foramen "face-on" (see Chapter 11, Fig. 11-2). The electrode is stimulated first at 2 and then 100 Hz and positioned so as to avoid motor contractions. If done under local anesthesia, paresthesias should be induced with currents below 0.5 v in the appropriate site. A graded RF lesion is then made, as already described, until the desired sensory deficit is induced.

At C2 the needle is introduced 1 cm below the mastoid in the midpoint of the foramen in a rostral-caudal direction and in its dorsal one-third. If CSF flow is obtained, the needle is withdrawn 1 mm. Stimulation at 2 Hz should produce motor contractions in trapezius at less than 1 v, and sensory stimulation should produce a response at less than 0.5 v.

Needles aimed at thoracic roots should be aligned from below upward into the foramen, heading from the tip of the lower transverse process to the base of the one above. In the lumbar area the needle is introduced into the dorsal one-third of the foramen from a point 4 cm from the midline, with the patient positioned painful side up in the lateral recumbent position. At L5 the needle is introduced, with the patient prone, from laterally and inferiorly into the space between the transverse process of L5 and the ala of the sacrum, aimed at the neck of the L5 transverse process of L5. Progress is often impeded here by lumbarization or osteophytes. Sacral roots are reached through appropriate dorsal sacral foramina, bringing the electrode tip to the ventral foramina. Here one must be alert to the risks of causing bladder and sexual dysfunction (see Chapter 9, Fig. 9-2 and Chapter 11, Fig. 11-4).

Uematsu and his colleagues[330–332] reported seven excellent and two good results out of 17 patients operated upon for various pain syndromes. Pagura[224] reported 76% pain relief in 50 patients, 13 suffering from cancer and 37 from disk disease, with a 4% incidence of temporary postoperative paresis.

Dubuisson[57] lists the data quoted in Table 32-3. Of the patients reported by van Kleef et al.,[334] 13 suffered from degenerative disk disease in the C4–C6 region; of these, 75% enjoyed pain relief after 3 months and 50% after 6 months. After test blocks, they inserted an electrode with a 2-mm bare tip into the dorsal portion of the foramen between its middle and caudal thirds to avoid the motor root and vertebral artery. In a correct position, paresthesias occurred with 50 Hz stimulation between 0.2 and 1.2 v. At 2 Hz, no motor effects should be elicited between 1.5 v and the sensory threshold. Omnipaque, 0.5 ml, was then injected to identify and avoid any intradural penetration, and a 60-second 67°C lesion made. Patients were monitored with electromyelograms (EMGs) and somatosensory evoked potentials, only one showing abnormalities of the latter. Appropriately, dermatomal burning from iatrogenic deafferentation occurred in 12 patients (60%) but did not persist past 3 weeks; decreased sensation was seen in 7 (35%) but disappeared after 6 weeks; no motor or reflex deficits were seen.

Gybels and Sweet[82] collected the following published data: of 192 patients with noncancerous pain, 69% were enjoying useful pain relief; of six with pain caused by cancer, all were relieved; follow-ups were short.

The complications of rhizotomy, other than failure and pain recurrence, include iatrogenic loss of proprioception, iatrogenic neuropathic pain, weakness, and the risk of cord infarction (see Chapter 7, Figs. 7-10 and 7-11).

CRANIAL NERVE PROCEDURES

Table 32-4 summarizes percutaneous destructive procedures available for pain in the distribution of the cranial nerves, of which tic douloureux is the most prevalent.

TABLE 32-3. *Results of percutaneous RF dorsal rhizotomy*

Authors	Levels treated	Initial relief	Late relief	Mortality	No. of cases
Uematsu *et al.* (1974)[332]	Spinal roots	39%	?	0	13
Lazorthes *et al.* (1976)[135]	Spinal roots	65%	?	0	20
Nash (1986)[206]	Spinal ganglia	58%	50%	0	26
van Kleef *et al.* (1993)[334]	Spinal ganglia	75%	39%	0	20

RF, radiofrequency.

From Dubuisson, D.: Root surgery. *In* Wall, P.D., and Melzack, R. (eds.): Textbook of Pain, 3rd Ed. pp. 1055. Edinburgh, Churchill Livingstone, 1994.

TABLE 32-4. *Percutaneous surgery of the cranial nerves*

Tic douloureux	
Trigeminal nerve	
Alcohol injection:	
Supraorbital nerve	
Infraorbital nerve	
Meckel's cave	
Glycerol injection:	
Percutaneous RF coagulation: Meckel's cave	
Microcompression: Meckel's cave	
IX–X Cranial nerve	
Percutaneous RF coagulation	
Nociceptive cancer pain	
Percutaneous RF coagulation V, lower cranial nerves	
Migrainous cephalgia	
Percutaneous RF coagulation V nerve	
Neuropathic pain	
?Allodynia and hyperpathia, percutaneous RF coagulation V nerve	

RF, radiofrequency.

Tic Douloureux

Tic douloureux is a unique pain syndrome nearly always affecting cranial nerve V, rarely nerves IX and X or VII. The diagnosis is based solely on the patient's description of the pain. In trigeminal territory, this pain affects the sexes approximately equally (45% males), the right side possibly more frequently, while the incidence increases with age. It can affect any or all portions of the territory supplied by the nerve V, but the lower face is preferentially affected, tic being most common in V2 and V3 together, next most common in V3 then V2 and rarest in V1. In 3% the disease becomes bilateral. The typical diagnostic features of the pain include abrupt onset of severe intermittent lancinating pain consistently affecting a particular portion of the trigeminal territory, interrupted by periods of remission, with the pain gradually becoming more severe and frequent with time and often slowly spreading to adjacent trigeminal territory. Triggering always arises from ipsilateral stimulation, most commonly in the nose and mouth region, not necessarily in the field of pain; occasionally, triggering occurs from outside trigeminal territory, including the C2, C3 dermatomes. The pain can be triggered by touching the face, talking, swallowing, brushing the teeth, washing the face, or drafts of wind.[115,157–159,329] Usually no abnormality is detectable on neurologic examination or by imaging. In a small number of patients, typical tic accompanies multiple sclerosis. Occasionally, an underlying lesion appears to be responsible, particularly a schwannoma, rarely an AVM, and exceptionally hydrocephalus.[325] Although many processes, both central and peripheral, have been advocated as the underlying cause of tic, especially compression of the nerve's dorsal root entry zone by an arterial or, less often, venous loop,[111] the etiology remains uncertain.

Treatment of Tic Douloureux

When treatment with carbamazepine fails, surgical therapy is often required, most of the currently practiced surgical modalities being accomplished percutaneously except for microvascular decompression of the root in the posterior fossa. Tic is unique in that denervation of the field to which the pain is referred always stops the pain, though recurrence is common because of regeneration; thus, several of the surgical techniques advocated for its treatment involve trigeminal denervation by various means at various levels.

A variety of compression and/or decompression procedures also can result in relief of the pain without accompanying sensory loss, including (i) the Sheldon[262,263] and Taarnhöj[290] procedures, which are now probably of historical interest, in which the roots of the nerve are either lightly traumatized (compressed) or dissected free of arachnoid adhesions (decompressed) in the middle fossa, (ii) the Mullan microcompression[201] technique, and (iii) microvascular decompression.[2,111] The mechanism of action of these procedures relevant to the underlying pathophysiology of tic is highly debated. It is important to reiterate that these procedures, so successful for tic, are inappropriate in most other types of craniofacial pain.

Furthermore, despite the fact that tic douloureux is a unique type of chronic intractable pain for which by far the most successful medical and surgical treatment available for any chronic pain syndrome exists, two of the most popular surgical modalities—percutaneous radiofrequency coagulation of the gasserian ganglion and/or its roots and microvascular decompression in the posterior fossa—yield about 20% (after 10 years) and 50% (after 15 years) long-term relief, respectively.[158] Though tic is one of the most common pain syndromes for which surgery is performed, outcome data are seldom published since the procedures used have been known for a long time.

Percutaneous Denervation of the Supraorbital or Infraorbital Nerves

The simplest percutaneous techniques for treating tic are percutaneous denervation of supraorbital or infraorbital nerves by the injection of absolute alcohol. Though simple and perhaps indicated in the very elderly or very ill with well-defined tic in the appropriate territory, any benefit is reversed within a few months to a year by nerve regeneration; the risk of blindness and oculomotor palsy has been mentioned. Rarely do such peripheral denervations, more effectively performed by open operation, result in neuropathic pain despite the fact that traumatic damage to the infraorbital nerve in facial fracturing is a common cause of deafferentation pain (see Chapter 15, Fig. 15-3).

Radiofrequency Coagulation of the Trigeminal Nerve

The treatment of choice for trigeminal tic douloureux after failure of medical treatment with carbamazepine is, in my

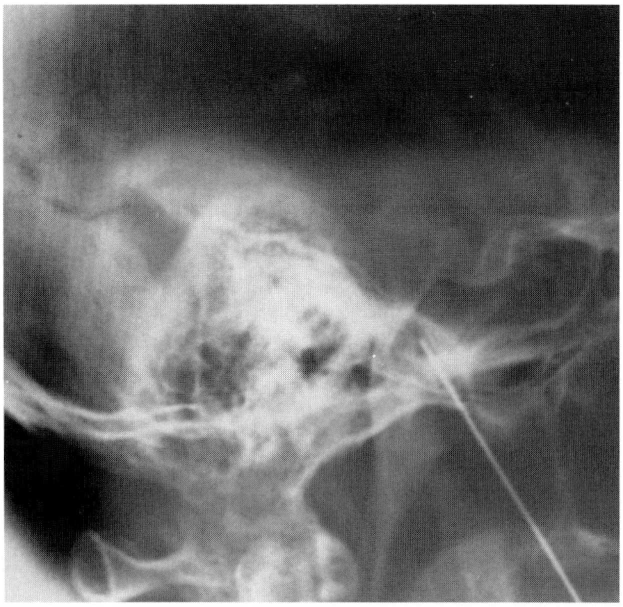

FIG. 32-5. Lateral x-ray showing electrode for conventional thermocoagulation of the trigeminal nerve inserted where stimulation and lesion-making produced effects in V3.

opinion, percutaneous radiofrequency coagulation, by which pain relief can be achieved at a risk a fraction of that faced with decompression of the trigeminal root entry zone in the posterior fossa.

Conventional Procedure

The conventional technique will be discussed first. Based on the original work of Kirshner[119] and Härtel,[85] the technique required certain refinements, including radiofrequency lesion-making as described by Sweet and Wepsic,[287] before precision became great enough and risks low enough for general acceptance.

Technique. The patient is positioned supine, head precisely in "anatomic" position (see Fig. 15-5A, Chapter 15), with lateral image intensification, under brief periods of intravenous sedation with analgesia. A suitable varnish-insulated electrode with a 3-mm noninsulated tip fashioned from a No. 16 lumbar puncture needle (see Fig. 32-1) is used. This needle is introduced into the symptomatic side of the face one fingerbreadth lateral to the lateral angle of the mouth and advanced toward the intersection of the sagittal plane through the pupil of the eye and the coronal plane through the middle of the zygoma (see Fig. 15-5A), avoiding the buccal cavity by having one finger inside the patient's mouth. The needle is advanced and followed radiographically, "walking" off the pterygoid plates or base of the skull into the foramen ovale, where a sudden contraction of jaw muscles or an exacerbation of pain heralds its arrival. Although, theoretically, the needle can now be advanced until it impinges on the vault of the skull, the tip should not rise above the line connecting the crest of the petrous ridge and the posterior clinoid as its progress is followed on the image intensifier. For third-division (V3) tic, the tip should lie relatively low on this trajectory, as shown in Figure 32-5; for first division tic (V1), relatively high, as shown in Figure 32-6. If CSF flow occurs, a more permanent and often more complete denervation is likely, since the electrode lies among preganglionic rootlets. In V3 tic this situation need not be sought, for the procedure is easily repeated in the event of recurrence when a postganglionic lesion is made. It may not be radiographically apparent when the electrode lies in alternate adjacent foramina except for the jugular, as shown in Figure 32-7—hence the importance of physiologic localization. If

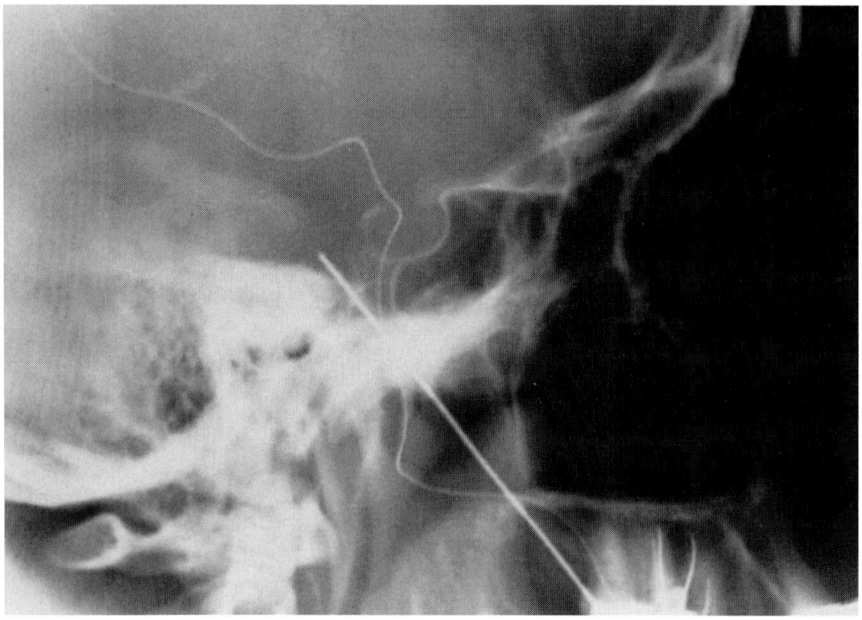

FIG. 32-6. Lateral x-ray, as in Figure 32-5, where stimulation produced paresthesias in the forehead.

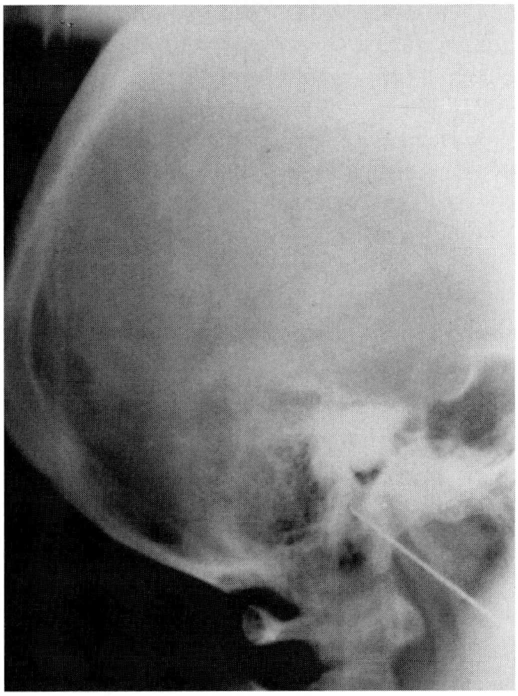

FIG. 32-7. Lateral x-ray, as in Figure 32-5, for thermocoagulation of glossopharyngeal nerve in jugular foramen.

arterial blood is encountered in foramen lacerum, the needle need only be withdrawn and reinserted. In proper position, stimulation at 1 to 5 Hz may elicit ipsilateral masticatory muscle contractions at thresholds under 2 to 3 v. There is no need to reposition the electrode to try to avoid these, for any weakness induced is likely to be transient, and unilateral permanent weakness is seldom apparent; however, bilateral RF coagulation should be approached with caution. The patient is now awakened, and stimulation at 50 to 100 Hz carried out. This should induce paresthesias in the area where the pain occurs, preferably at less than 0.5 v, certainly at no more than 1 v. Under repeated intravenous sedation, a radiofrequency lesion is now made, progressively increasing current flow and needle tip temperature to 150 to 250 mA (average, 175–200) and 70° to 90°C, respectively, over 30 to 90 seconds. Too hurried a current and temperature rise, producing early fall-off of current, will prevent significant lesion-making owing to the insulation from boiling at the needle tip. A visible flush will often appear in the denervated part of the face. Our current practice is to push lesion-making only to the point of inducing analgesia without loss of appreciation of touch in the painful area of the face. Unexpected, massive sensory loss, even spreading beyond the confines of the patient's pain, may still occur despite all attempts to avoid it.

Selective Procedure. A modification of the above-described technique is referred to as the selective technique,[218,322] in which the electrode described above is replaced by a finer 0.4-mm electrolytically sharpened stainless steel wire with a 2-mm bare tip, similar to a cordotomy electrode (described below), whose tip is angulated at about a 45° angle to the shaft of the introductory No. 18 lumbar puncture (LP) needle (see Fig. 32-4). This has two advantages over the conventional technique: (i) since the electrode and its tip are smaller, a smaller and more selective lesion can be made, and is better tailored to selectively induce analgesia in the area of pain; (ii) the electrode tip can be withdrawn into the introductory needle and rotated, like the hands of a clock, and readvanced to sample a large area of adjacent nerve fibers with a single LP needle position until the ideal lesion site is found. Lesion parameters are similar to those used for cordotomy, often 80 to 90 mA for 60 seconds. Using this technique, Tew and his colleagues[321,322] found their results to be better than with the conventional technique. Complications consisted of a 9% incidence of masseter weakness, 11% unpleasant paresthesias, no diplopia, and 2% keratitis. Our experience has been that recurrence is more likely when the selective method is used.

Results. Tew and colleagues[321] reported 93% excellent-to-good results in 400 patients with tic after using the conventional technique. Fourteen percent complained of unpleasant sensory effects; in 1% these were so severe as to lead to excoriation of the face, nostril, or scalp. Only 2% developed keratitis, although 30% had corneal analgesia. Two percent exhibited transient diplopia and 22% paresis in the distribution of the motor root, which was usually transient. The latter was occasionally associated with complaints referred to the ear because of paralysis of the tensor veli palatini or tensor tympani. Over 1 to 8 years, tic recurred in 14%, and 9% underwent a second operation. In a subsequent review,[322] Tew and associates reported 76% excellent, 17% good, 6% fair, and 1% poor results with 700 procedures, also performed in the conventional way, over a 10-year period; of the 24% with recurrence, 9% underwent reoperation. Complications in this larger series using the conventional method consisted of a 24% incidence of masseter weakness, 27% unpleasant paresthesias, 2% diplopia, and 4% keratitis.

Latchaw and co-workers[129] reported 52% good results with the conventional method without recurrence in 96 patients with tic, particularly if the patient had not been previously exposed to open surgery and particularly if dense sensory loss was achieved. All patients without persistent sensory loss suffered recurrence. Twenty-six percent had depressed and 13% absent corneal reflexes, 2% keratitis, 5% masseter paresis, 42% unintended sensory loss, 26% unpleasant sensory effects, and 1% anesthesia dolorosa. The severity of the latter was related to the degree of sensory loss. Latchaw's useful literature review suggests a 7% to 22% incidence of corneal anesthesia, 0 to 5% keratitis, 1% to 19% dysesthesia, and 15% to 50% unintended sensory loss. Recurrences were reported in these series in 6% to 46% over 2 to 2 1/2 years, 9% to 53% over 4 to 5 years, 18% to 22% over 7 to 8 years, and 80% in longer follow-ups.

Turnbull[329] reported his experience in 41 patients in a graphic and particularly interesting way. Anesthesia in at least part of the face occurred in the only patient with V1 tic, four of nine with V1–V2 tic, six of 14 with V2 tic, three of nine with V2–V3 tic, and two of 11 with V3 tic. Pain was relieved in all, but recurred in five patients over 0 to 4 years. Motor weakness occurred in nine, keratitis in two, and corneal areflexia in eight, six of whom did not have V1 tic to start with. Five developed dysesthesia and one anesthesia dolorosa. Anesthesia occurred in facial areas not afflicted with tic in 0 of one patients with V1 tic, one of nine with V1–V2 tic, five of 14 with V2 tic, one of nine with V2–V3 tic, and 0 of 11 with V3 tic. Analgesia occurred in unafflicted areas, in one of one, two of nine, nine of 14, two of nine, and two of 11 patients with V1, V1–V2, V2, V2–V3, and V3 tic, respectively.

Whatever the technique, the chief disadvantages of radiofrequency thermocoagulation of nerve V are that it deliberately produces sensory loss with an unavoidable incidence of neuropathic pain and, if the patient is followed long enough, recurrence of tic (80% in 10 years).[156,157] "Anesthesia dolorosa" is more likely to occur the older the patient, the greater the degree of sensory loss induced and the higher in the face it occurs. Sweet[284] noted that, after RF coagulation of nerve V, early relief was reported in 96% to 100% of cases, reoperation being needed after 1 to 13 years in 7% to 31%. In larger series, the most significant complication was deafferentation pain occurring in 0.2% to 7.9%. Corneal anesthesia affected 1% to 35%, keratitis 0.4% to 20%, motor weakness 13% to 40%, and oculomotor palsy 0.2% to 6.5% in large series. Complications were somewhat different in smaller series. Epilepsy from temporal lobe damage, dry eye (3%), nasal wetness (23%), and increased (17%) or decreased (3%) salivation also occur (see Tables 32-5 and 32-6).

Sweet[284] advises abandoning the procedure till another day, should the carotid artery be punctured, though I have uneventfully completed the procedure after needle replacement at the same sitting in a number of cases; serious sequelae occur, however, if an RF lesion is made in the foramen lacerum. Sweet mentions that the foramina of Vesalius and Arnold as well as anomalous ones may also be entered, making careful attention to physiologic monitoring essential lest complications occur. Finally, damage to the trochlear nerve may occur, even with a correctly placed lesion, due to heat spread, but it usually recovers after 3 months; damage to the temporal lobe can similarly take place. X-ray monitoring should prevent entry into supraorbital fissure or jugular foramen.

Bilateral RF lesions in bilateral tic should be undertaken with caution for fear of the devastating complication of bilateral trigeminal motor root paralysis. Since the motor root also supplies the tensor tympani and tensor veli palatini, RF tic damage to the motor root can produce aberrations of function of the middle ear musculature or eustachian tube resulting in various, fortunately usually temporary, auditory perversions or ear pain.

Although percutaneous thermocoagulation of the trigeminal nerve is still a procedure with low morbidity and mortality, I am aware of (i) two incidences of fatal hemorrhage unrelated to the lesion, one in a personal case, possibly caused by acute hypertension induced by needle introduction and preventable by appropriate premedication, (ii) one case of bacterial meningitis, (iii) one of temporal lobe abscess, and (iv) reported cases of stroke following carotid artery puncture and of carotid cavernous fistula; Sweet[284] reviews these problems in some detail (see Table 32-7).

Alcohol injection

Though probably of historical interest today, the injection of absolute alcohol into the CSF of Meckel's cave was popular well past the middle of the twentieth century but has probably been replaced by other procedures.

Percutaneous Injection of Glycerol

Håkansson[83] has introduced the treatment of tic by the injection, through a 22-gauge needle, of 0.2 to 0.4 ml of glycerol into the CSF of Meckel's cave under local anesthesia, using a technique similar to that employed for radiofrequency coagulation. CSF is drained and metrizamide slowly injected in 0.2- to 0.4-ml increments until the cistern is filled and dye starts to empty into the posterior fossa. Cisternal metrizamide is emptied by head positioning to uncover the parts of the root intended to be affected by glycerol (see Fig. 15-5B). The calculated volume of the cistern is used to estimate the volume of glycerol needed. If the entire cistern is exposed to glycerol, all three divisions will be affected; leaving metrizamide in place to cover rootlets uninvolved with tic will protect them from the injection. In 15% of Håkansson's cases, the first attempt failed, pain recurred in 18% over a period of 2 to 48 months, and 60% noted slight facial numbness for the first postoperative week. None suffered from dysesthesia, and alteration of facial sensation was barely detectable in "the majority." Eighty-six percent of 75 patients were totally free of their pain, half immediately and half within 4 to 6 days. One patient died of pulmonary embolism.

Sweet and Poletti[285] note that Håkansson's recurrence rate was 31% over 1 to 6 years in 100 patients. They themselves treated 31 patients, 27 suffering from tic, three from atypical facial pain, and one from post-traumatic pain. Pain was relieved in 24 of the 27 with tic. The only failures were in patients who did not develop analgesia during or after the injection, and 16 of their patients had persistent sensory loss, including nine who developed dysesthesia and five reduced corneal reflexes.

Lunsford and Bennett[168] reported 67% complete and 23% partial control of tic in 112 patients followed from 4 to 28 months. Seventy-three percent had no sensory loss, 3% developed aseptic meningitis, and 3.6% had severe postoperative dysesthesia. None of their patients developed motor weakness, oculomotor disturbance, or keratitis.

Sweet[284,285] and Gybels and Sweet[82] have exhaustively studied the published results with glycerol injection (see

TABLE 32-5. *Trigeminal thermal rhizotomy: 31 services with less than 600 procedures*

Author[a]	No. of pts.	No. of RF ops	Early complete relief[b]	Follow-up period Range	Follow-up period Average	% Recurrence not requiring reoperation	% Recurrence requiring reoperation	Anesthesia, analgesia hypalgesia dolorosa	Dysesthesias controlled with drugs	Keratitis	Corneal anesthesia	Masticator paralysis	Oculomotor paresis temp.
Apfelbaum	48	51	88%	0–36 mo	19 mo	10%	12%	12%			14%	2%	
Brandt	229	~325		1–13 yr		23%	28%	3.5%			8%	3%	1%
Browne	106	121	100%	0–4 yr			14%				5% in 50% of pts with V1 pain		1 pt 1%
Burchiel	78	92	77%		56 mo	41%	23%	4%		3%			
Campos	72	79	93%	6 mo–3 yr		6%	12%	3–3.5%	10%	2.5%	20%	25%	1 pt
Eiras	36	?40	98%	3–23 mo			6%	0%			6%	0%	0%
Ferguson	55	58		1–50 mo	30 mo	31%	11%	2%	0%	0%	7%	30%	0%
Fraioli	481				4.2 yr		9%		11%				
Galbraith	102	120	92%	1–7 yr	3 yr		20%	0%					0%
Graziussi	205	219	93%	6 mo–5 yr	3 yr		20% {65% 1st yr, 23% 2nd yr} 6% 3rd & 4th yr	6%	62%	4%	4%	15%	0.4%
Guidetti	167	173	99.4%	2 yr				0.6%		0%	4%	3.4%	0.6%
Hitchcock	47	70	98%	Up to 40 mo		13%	28%	4%		2%	2%	8%	0%
Kanpolat	256	290	94% of 240 pts (final)				12% of 256	1.8%			5%		
Lahuerta	30	35	97%	15–26 mo				10%	7%	3%	19%		2 pts = 6%
Latchaw	96	135	100%	2–8 yr	5 yr	8%	48% at 5 yr	2%	32%	3%	19%	5%	
Mittal	216	267	91%	3 mo–8 yr	3.8 yr		21%	9%	6%	4%			3 pts = 1%
Onofrio	135	140	97%	Up to several yr		6%	6% (16 pts slight sensory loss —recurrence 2 wk–14 mo)	1.5%		1.5%	8%	15%	0.8%
Penzholz	232		85%	1–9 yr		7%	24%	1.3%	5%				
Perez Calvo	50	57	100%	0.5–5 yr	11 mo		6% in <1 yr	2%					2%
Pertuiset	100	113	100%	Longest 3 yr	11 mo		13%		5%	0%	3%	2%	1%
Philippon	50	60		2–6 yr	3 yr		>40% after 3 yr	0	4%	2%	17%	25% Gone in 6 mo	1 pt
Salar	46	?50	100%	More than 1 yr			7%			0%	0%	0%	0%
Schürmann	282	351 413	100%	1963–1975			22% or 193 pts >3-yr follow-up	1 pt	10%	0%		12%	0%
Schvarcz	400	411		1–6 yr in 75%	4 yr		9%	0%			3%		0%
Sengupta	39		92%	2–20 mo		6%	3%			5%	15%		
Silverberg	38		95%	2–36 mo			14%	0%		0%	0%	0%	0%
Spincemaille	53		85%	6–42 mo	2 yr		5%	0	8%	0%			
Steude	194		100%	10–50 mo			11%	0.5%		0%		0%	0%
Thiry	225	(1950–1960)	100%	Up to 23 yr			17%			3%	9%		3%
	140	(1960–1970)	98%	Up to 13 yr			27%			1%	4%		3%
Turnbull	41		100%	6 mo–3 yr		5%	7%	2.5%	10%	5%	22%	22%	0%
Turner	51	64	92%				26%	2%		2%	6%		0%

[a] For complete References, see source of Table (Sweet[284]).
[b] Includes those relieved after early operation.
RF, radiofrequency.

From Sweet, W.H.: Treatment of trigeminal neuralgia by percutaneous rhizotomy. *In* Youmans, J.R. (ed.): Neurological Surgery. A Comprehensive Reference Guide to the Diagnosis and Management of Neurosurgical Problems, 3rd ed. Philadelphia, Saunders, 1990, p. 3888.

TABLE 32-6. *Trigeminal thermal rhizotomy: 11 services with 600 or more procedures*

Author[a]	No. of pts.	No. of RF ops	Early complete relief	Follow-up period range-average	No. of recurrences not requiring reoperation	No. of recurrences requiring reoperation	Anesthesia, analgesia hypalgesia dolorosa	Dysesthesias controlled with drugs	Keratitis	Corneal anesthesia	Masticator paralysis	Oculomotor paresis temp.	Oculomotor paresis temp.
Broggi	1000		100%	1–10 yr		13%	7.9% "often unbearable"		Tarsorr. 0.4%	Reduced or absent 21%	10%		0.3%
Frank	939		100%	6 mo–5 yr		21%	0.6%	11.6%		1%	1%		
Maxwell	unstated	>600					2%		1%				
Nugent	643	~800		4.7 yrs		23%	1%	5%	0.5%	2% last 600 ops 1 loss of eye		10%	0.25%
Rhoton	unstated	~1500											
Rovit	550	600				19%	0.2%	0.7%		4%			0.2%
Siegfried	1000		100%	135 pts followed 5½–8 yr	4%	21% at 5½–8 yr	3%	24% at 5½–8 yr	0.8%	2.8%	15%	25%	4%
Sindou	609		100%	1–13 yr		7%		25% "painful"	20%	35%	Lasting 2% Temp. 25%		6.5%
Sweet	702	1119	99%	1–33 yr avg 5.6 yr	6%	31%	2.1%	6%	3% Tarsorr. 1.5%	9%	25%	40%	0.4%
Tew	1100		98%	1–18 yr avg 8 yr	9%	8%	1%	9%	3%			13% (curved electrode)	1.5%
Thurel	890	1150	96%			23%	0.6%	7%	2%	6%		25%	0.7%

[a] For complete References, see source of Table (Sweet[284]).

[b] Includes relief after early reoperation

RF, radiofrequency

From Sweet, W.H.: Treatment of trigeminal neuralgia by percutaneous rhizotomy. *In* Youmans, J.R. (ed.): Neurological Surgery. A Comprehensive Reference Guide to the Diagnosis and Management of Neurosurgical Problems. 3rd ed. pp. 3888. Philadelphia, Saunders, 1990.

TABLE 32-7. *Complications of percutaneous radiofrequency trigeminal rhizotomy*[a]

	Number of cases
Central retinal artery occlusion	1
Optic nerve lesion	
Blindness, ipsilateral, permanent	2
Amblyopia, ipsilateral, transient	1
Blindness, complete, permanent	4
Myocardial infarction	
Death (91-year-old patient)	1
Recovery	1
Intracerebral abscess	
Death	3
Mental impairment, permanent	1
Recovery	3
Meningitis	
Death	1
Recovery	21
Hemorrhages	
Related to needle puncture	
Subdural, infratemporal	
Recovered	1
Intracerebral	
Death	2
Recovered	1
Disabled, permanent	1
Not related to needle puncture	
Intracerebral	
Death	8
Disabled, permanent	4
Hemiplegia, transient	3
Hemiparesis	
Transient	1
Permanent	1
Subarachnoid hemorrhage	
Death	3
Recovered	2
Neuroparalytic keratitis	18
Carotid cavernous fistulas	5
Meningeal reaction	
Negative cultures	8
Oculomotor palsy	
Temporary	16
Permanent	2
Seizure, intraoperative	2
Psychosis, postoperative	
Transient	1

[a] Reported from 92 services with over 7000 patients. Not all services gave the number of patients, and as a result not all are included in the figure of 7000 patients; however, the complications they reported are included in this Table.

From Sweet, W.H.: Treatment of trigeminal neuralgia by percutaneous rhizotomy. *In* Youmans, J.R. (ed.): Neurological Surgery. A Comprehensive Reference Guide to the Diagnosis and Management of Neurosurgical Problems. 3rd Ed. pp. 3888. Philadelphia, Saunders, 1990.

Table 32-8). They note that initial failure ranges from 4% to 18%, that early relief is often delayed up to a week, and that the first attempt yields 69% to 96% relief, with 9% to 30% of patients requiring reoperation. They note that corneal anesthesia, though rare, does occur.

It appears that the technique exposes patients to the same risks, including neuropathic pain, as RF coagulation, that it requires more attention to detail to perform (radical head positioning after the needle has been inserted), and that its somatotopic selectivity is not established. Its great advantage is that it can be used to treat V1 tic without the need to produce significant sensory loss in V1 territory, with its ensuing risk of keratitis and the greater chance of neuropathic pain than that seen after denervation of the lower face.

Percutaneous Compression of Trigeminal Nerve

Harking back to the technique of open compression or decompression of Meckel's cave advocated by Taarnhoj[290] and Sheldon and their associates[263] for the treatment of tic, Mullan and Lichtor[201] have introduced a method for percutaneous compression of the nerve. Under general anesthesia, with the patient intubated, and using biplanar imaging, a No. 4 (0.75–1.0 ml capacity) Fogarty balloon catheter inserted to the tip of a liver biopsy needle is passed through the foramen ovale by the method described above, after filling its air space with Conray. The catheter is now advanced 1 cm and slowly inflated with Conray diluted to a manageable viscosity until the balloon fills Meckel's cave and begins to assume a pear shape by slowly expanding into the posterior fossa. The balloon is held inflated 3 to 10 minutes with 0.5 to 1 ml Conray, then collapsed and withdrawn. Difficulties may be encountered in patients with a scarred cave, including rupture of the balloon (not a dangerous occurrence). In 50 patients with tic, 49 obtained immediate relief, six experienced recurrence in 6 to 31 months, three suffered from dysesthesia, four from analgesia, and one from trochlear nerve palsy. All patients experienced subjective numbness and ipsilateral motor paralysis; some experienced sensory loss persisting 4 to 6 months.

According to Gybels and Sweet[2,8] Bricolo and Dalle Ore[24] performed the procedure in 51 patients, all of whom experienced pain relief; a few suffered sensory loss, and pain recurred in 22% in a year. Fraioli et al.[69] reported 90% early relief in 125 patients, a 10.6% recurrence over a mean 2.5-year follow-up; 57% had minimal sensory loss. Lobato et al.[156] reported three recurrences in 100 patients in 7 to 11 months; 29% still had sensory loss after 1 year, while 18% had minor and 3% significant dysesthesia. Meglio et al.[181] noted frequent recurrence but no dysesthesia in 25 patients. Belber and Rak[12] recorded 100% initial pain relief in 33 patients, 24% experiencing recurrence over 7 years; 1 patient had mild dysesthesia.

Radiofrequency Coagulation of Trigeminal Nerve for Pain Other Than Tic

The conventional percutaneous thermocoagulation technique can also be used to treat trigeminal pain caused by cancer and also migrainous pain that consistently afflicts one part of the trigeminal territory, although it should be avoided

TABLE 32-8. *Trigeminal glycerol rhizotomy: 16 services*

Author[a]	No. of patients	Initial failure	Days to relief	Relief 1st op	Relief 2nd op	Average follow-up	Recurrence: reoperation not needed	Recurrence: reoperation needed	Corneal anesthesia	Sensory status
Arias	100	5%	2–4 days in 6%			6–36 mo			0	Never more than 30% loss in any division
Beck	58	17%		69%	72%	2–40 mo Avg 18 mo	16%	9%	1%	17%-? intraganglion inj. in 1 1 lasting total analgesia
Burchiel	48	12%					Mean time to recurrence 5 mo in 43% of 46 ops		7%	Sensory loss >1 mo in 72%
Dieckmann	51					78% relief at 1 yr				40% anesthesia dolorosa 2%
Håkansson	100	4%	4–6 days in 50%	96%		1–6 yr	16%	15%	0	Never more than mild No dysesthesias
Igarashi	27		Up to 1 wk						Decreased with more than 0.4 ml	Hypalgesia at 8 wk 30% 3 high-grade dysesthesias
Lunsford	73	14%	Avg 5 days up to 21 days	86%	90%	Up to 3 yrs Avg 15 mo	10% of 73 19% of 62 pts	13% of 73 15% of 62 pts		6% dysesthesias 0 anesthesia dolorosa
Lunsford	225						Pain-free at follow-up 65%			
Rappaport	43		Relief at once 54%: 46% relief in avg 3 days—max 14 days	81%	97%		Recurrence rate 25% at 1 yr		0	Hypalgesia 38%; of 7 recurrences 6 did not have sensory deficit
Saini	412		Relief in 2–42 hr							3.4% anesthesia dolorosa 13% dysesthesias
Shetter	64	14%		86%		2–45 mo Avg 18 mo	61% pain-free at avg 18 mo 11%	28%	3%	Analgesia 1 of 64; dysesthesia bothers about 5%
Slettebo	60	10%		90%		Avg 24 mo		30% at avg 2 yr		Higher proportion sensory deficits than in earlier articles
Sweet	88	18%	Up to 1 wk in 24%	82%		Avg 2.9 yr 1–8½ yr		22%	14% 50% of 14 V1 trigger zones	27 hyp; 49 analg; 4 anesth (2 anesth dol; 1 hyp dol; 0 hyp dol since 1983; 0 analg dol since 1980; 0 anesth dol since 1983)
Takusagawa	122	10%		79%		1–3 yr	58% pain-free; 17% improved; 25% in pain			Anesth dol 2 pts 1.5%; hypesthesia 80%; dysesthesias 35%
Thurel	50			75%		Avg 15 mo		15%	2%	1 anesthesia complete V1, V2 at 5 mo but no major dysesthesias
Waltz	184	18%		70%	81%	1–52 mo	12%	17%		Hypesthesia 67%; "sensory deficit mild with one exception"
Young	157	6%					Pain-free 79%		5%	67% significant sensory loss 0% anesthesia dolorosa 2% dysesthesias

[a] For complete References, see source of Table (Sweet[284]).

From Sweet, W.H.: Treatment of trigeminal neuralgia by percutaneous rhizotomy. *In* Youmans, J.R. (ed.): Neurological Surgery. A Comprehensive Reference Guide to the Diagnosis and Management of Neurosurgical Problems. 3rd Ed. pp. 3888. Philadelphia, Saunders, 1990.

in atypical facial pain, deafferentation pain, and postherpetic neuralgia unless intended for the control of allodynia or hyperpathia alone.

In cancer, pain is rarely confined to the trigeminal territory, so that trigeminal denervation alone is nearly always unsuccessful and cancerous destruction of the base of the skull may prevent needle positioning. In those few selected suitable candidates, denervation for the relief of cancer pain should be as complete as possible. Siegfried and Broggi[266] relieved pain in 10 of their 20 patients who had pain caused by cancer. Maxwell[176] relieved all eight of his patients with migrainous neuralgia, although pain eventually recurred in three. Watson and colleagues[345] reported pain relief in eight of 13 patients with cluster headache treated by percutaneous thermocoagulation. One developed anesthesia dolorosa, and five suffered from recurrence, one of whom did not respond to repeated coagulation. Pain relief required sensory loss in the area of pain.

Gybels and Sweet[82] note that denervation in migrainous face pain results in a greater incidence of dysesthetic pain than in tic, that a greater degree of sensory loss is necessary than in tic to achieve pain relief, and that, in six of their own patients, pain relief did not accompany sensory loss in the painful area. They quote the results of Onofrio and Campbell[222] with 11 early failures and one recurrence after 6 months in 22 patients.

Few data have been recorded for glycerol injection in migrainous pain.

Glossopharyngeal Neuralgia

Glossopharyngeal neuralgia, first recognized by Sicard and Robineau in 1920, requires special attention, not because it is common (its incidence is 1:40 to 1:250 that of trigeminal tic), but because it is so rare that it is unfamiliar to many and in danger of being confused with other craniofacial pain syndromes. Inappropriate treatment may be *disastrous*. The peak age incidence is 40 to 60 years, incidence is equal for the two sexes, and it is more common on the left side; 10% to 30% of cases co-exist with trigeminal tic, and in up to 25% of cases, it occurs bilaterally. The same etiologies have been suggested as for trigeminal tic except that it has not apparently been recognized in multiple sclerosis. It tends to be less severe than trigeminal tic, 67% of patients suffering a single episode (29% in trigeminal tic) and 42% requiring no treatment, (9% in trigeminal tic).[33,114,115,118,250,273]

Like trigeminal tic, the condition can be diagnosed only on the basis of the history of the pain in the absence of neurologic or imaging abnormalities, a difficult exercise since the symptomatology is complex. Apart from rare purely syncopal attacks, most patients complain of pain, though syncopal attacks, first described in 1942 by Riley, may accompany the pain.[115,237] The pain may be of two main types, typical (tic-like lancinating) and atypical. Atypical pain can be dull, aching, burning, or a sense of pressure or swelling. Even typical pain may be preceded by itching, tickling, tingling, a feeling of sticking, choking or scratching of a foreign body, and, as in trigeminal tic, may be followed by an afterpain.

Both types of pain begin either (i) in the ear, mandibular angle, eustachian tube, or front of the ear or (ii) in the pharynx, tonsil, or posterior tongue and may project from either to the other site. Rarely, pain spreads over the mastoid and adjacent occipital area. Triggering is sometimes seen, induced by swallowing, especially of cold fluids, yawning, chewing, coughing, sneezing, clearing the throat, blowing the nose, talking, or turning the head, or by touching the gingivae, external canal of the ear, tongue, periaural skin, tonsillar pillars, or pharynx; sometimes triggering occurs from outside glossopharyngeal-vagal territory. It may be accompanied by tinnitus, by soreness in the cheek or mandible, and, like trigeminal tic, occasionally by sensory loss. Still more atypical are accompanying voluntary gestures, involuntary coughing, dyspnea, hoarseness, sweating, dryness of the mouth, salivation, choking, hiccups, flushing, mydriasis, and tearing. In 10% of patients, bradycardia, hypotension, asystole, syncope, or fits accompany the pain, sometimes resulting in sudden death.

When surgical therapy becomes necessary, the chief options are: open section of cranial nerve IX and the upper one-quarter to one-third of the roots of cranial nerve X, microvascular decompression of these nerves, or percutaneous RF thermocoagulation. In this condition, open surgery may be preferable to avoid the indiscriminate damage to other lower cranial nerves that may follow the percutaneous technique, causing hoarseness and cardiovascular instability.[25,26,104,136,223,250,253,273,322]

The percutaneous technique consists of introducing a needle into the external, pars nervosa portion of the jugular canal in which the vein lies laterally. This site lies in line with, but posterior to, the foramen ovale in line with the pupil of the eye and a point 3 cm anterior to the tragus, behind the temporomandibular joint and anterior to the occipital condyle, medial to the carotid artery. The needle is passed 20° posterior and 5° to 10° medial to the course used to enter the foramen ovale, the x-ray film (see Fig. 32-7) showing a more posterior position. Electrocardiogram and blood pressure should be monitored to avoid problems associated with alterations in vagus nerve function; correct positioning is indicated when 0.1 to 0.3 v stimulation produces paresthesias, some say pain, in the external auditory meatus or the ipsilateral side of the pharynx. Trapezius contractions and alterations in blood pressure and cardiograph should be avoided. After a test lesion to avoid untoward effects, a 60- to 90-second RF lesion is made starting at 60°C, with 5°C increments, watching for alterations in pulse or blood pressure; if these occur, repositioning of the electrode is necessary. The lesion is enlarged until the tonsillar pharynx is analgesic and the gag reflex is lessened. Since vocal cord paralysis may occur, the percutaneous technique is better suited to cases of cancer than to those of tic.

Isamat and associates[104] used this procedure in four patients with glossopharyngeal tic without complications, although pain recurred in two. The procedure was successfully repeated in one. Tew and co-workers[322] and Lazorthes and Verdie[136] relieved pain in three patients, but dysarthria and dysphasia were postoperative problems. Broggi[25] treated six patients with tic, three having good results and one fair results. Salar and colleagues[253] treated three patients with tic by a lateral approach, all of whom were relieved, although 75% showed transient vagal dysfunction. Tew and associates[322] treated nine patients with cancer in glossopharyngeal distribution, eight of whom were relieved. Broggi[25] used the procedure in five patients with cancer, with two excellent results and two recurrences successfully managed by reoperation. Salar and co-workers[253] treated five patients with cancer in their series. Pagura and colleagues[225] relieved 11 of 15 patients with cancer pain at the expense of glossopharyngeal dysfunction in all. Dubuisson[57] summarized reported experience, as shown in Table 32-9. Sindou et al.[273] reviewed 15 cases from the literature and three of his own treated by thermocoagulation, finding complications greater than in cases treated by open means. In 18 patients operated upon, one procedure was not completed because of coronary ischemia and one that was completed led to cardiac arrest; 14 (78%) enjoyed excellent and two (11%) partial pain relief. Complications affected 10 (56%); in addition to the above-mentioned cardiac complications, seven patients suffered sensory loss, six suppression of gag reflex, five transient dysphagia, one persistent dysphagia, and one deafness. Ori et al.[223] reported thermocoagulation in nine patients, in one of whom two repetitions were required; 6 of 11 procedures caused cardiac dysrhythmia or over a 50% fall in blood pressure or heart rate, causing syncope in two cases and seizures in one.

A lateral cervical approach is also available, as described by Salar et al.[253] The needle is introduced anterior to the mastoid process below the external auditory meatus perpendicular to skin and is advanced until the styloid process is reached at a depth of 1.5 to 2 cm. The needle is pulled back and pushed across the styloid posteriorly for 2 cm, when the tip will lie tangential to and below the lateral part of jugular foramen (see Chapter 15, Fig.15-7). After x-ray confirmation of the needle's location pointing toward the medial pars nervosa, stimulation induces slightly painful paresthesias in the retropharyngeal-tonsillar area as well as in the external meatus. Suprathreshold stimulation may cause laryngeal muscle contraction. Vagal hyperactivity may also be seen with a fall in blood pressure and heart rate, in which case the needle must be repositioned. Then a thermal lesion is made as before.

SYMPATHECTOMY

The use of sympathectomy has a long and varied history, being employed in the past to treat a vast array of problems from epilepsy through pain to vascular disease. Currently, the indications appear to include hyperhydrosis, vascular insufficiency, and pain. Under the latter indication it is used in patients with visceral pain including that from cancer of the pancreas, pain associated with vascular insufficiency in the limbs, reflex sympathetic dystrophy, and sympathetically maintained pain. In general, sympathectomy is less useful in controlling intractable "nonmalignant" pain than that of cancer, though the sympathetic dystophic changes that sometimes accompany deafferentation pain may be relieved[307,311] without affecting the underlying pain. This occurs despite the fact that local sympathetic blockade proximal or distal to the causative lesion may temporarily relieve the deafferentation pain,[161,162] especially if allodynia is present, just as proximal and distal local somatic blockade usually do[117,209,211] (see Chapter 27).

Apparently there are two types of neuropathic pain for which sympathectomy may be effective. The first is complex regional pain syndrome type II, so-called "major causalgia,"[209,311] usually resulting from incomplete lesions of the sciatic nerve or its divisions, the median nerve, or the medial portion of the brachial plexus. Such lesions, usually the result of low-velocity gunshot wounds, are rare in peacetime, so that contemporary experience is limited. The second is sympathetically maintained pain,[15] a type of neuropathic pain associated with allodynia in which the pain can be

TABLE 32-9. *Results of percutaneous RF coagulation of IX nerve*

Authors	Levels treated	Initial relief	Late relief	Mortality	N
Lazorthes and Verdie (1979)[136]	Ninth/tenth cranial (cancer)	?	73%	0	11
	(glossopharyngeal neuralgia)	?	100%	0	1
Isamat *et al.* (1980)[104]	Ninth/tenth cranial (glossopharyngeal neuralgia)	100%	75%	0	4
Tew (1982)[322]	Ninth/tenth cranial (cancer)	56%	?	0	9
	(glossopharyngeal neuralgia)	100%	?	0	2
Giorgi and Broggi (1984)[76]	Ninth/tenth cranial (cancer)	100%	100%	0	5
	(glossopharyngeal neuralgia)	100%	60%	0	5

RF, radiofrequency.

From Dubuisson, D.: Root surgery. *In* Wall, P.D., and Melzack, R. (eds.): Textbook of Pain. 3rd Ed. pp. 1055. Edinburgh, Churchill Livingstone, 1994.

shown to be dependent on sympathetic function, but in which overt nerve injury is minimal or absent.

Various open and percutaneous techniques are available for sympathectomy[313] (see Chapters 13 and 27).

Gybels and Sweet[82] review the development of percutaneous lumbar sympathectomy with phenol,[18] usually for relief of symptoms of peripheral vascular disease, which are reviewed in Chapter 13. They quote results of Reid et al.[239]—77% initial and 60% longer-term relief of ischemic rest pain in 189 men. Dondelinger and Kurdziel[53] suppressed pain in 60%, but vascular improvement occurred in only 33%. Cross and Cotton[43] recorded a 67% reduction in rest pain persisting for 6 months. Gybels and Sweet note the confusion as to whether the procedure achieved its results in patients with peripheral vascular disease by virtue of vasodilation or of pain fiber interruption. Cousins et al.[42a] reported that 80% of 386 patients with rest pain had complete or partial pain relief, with a mean duration of 6 months, regardless of changes in blood flow.

Wilkinson[348] has described a percutaneous radiofrequency technique for upper thoracic sympathectomy. With the patient prone under local anesthesia, a needle is introduced 6 to 7 cm from the midline and directed toward three sites. The most caudal site is lesioned first to best retain the pupillary response as a guide to lesion-making. An 18-gauge needle with a 10-mm bare tip is inserted within a 16-gauge needle between the third and fourth ribs medial to the scapular margin and aimed at a point 2 to 5 mm lateral and rostral to the midpoint of the T3 vertebra. The electrode tip is positioned at the ventral edge of T3 in the lateral x-ray image under the head of the third rib. The next lesion is made by passing the electrode between the second and third ribs to reach just lateral to the T2–T3 interspace. The third lesion is made through the same rib space, but the tip is directed to the midportion to rostral portion of T2 body beneath the head of the second rib. When each needle is properly positioned, stimulation is carried out and positioning effected so as to avoid a somatic motor or sensory response below 0.5 v. This avoids damage to the somatic roots. A test lesion at 60°C for 60 seconds is now made to guard against Horner's syndrome, while plethysmography and hand temperature monitoring indicate whether sympathetic interruption is occurring. When all criteria have been satisfied, a 90°C 180-second lesion is made and enlarged by withdrawing the tip 8 to 10 mm. Twenty procedures on 27 sides produced 24 instances of sympathetic denervation. Two patients suffered from pneumothorax, three from brachial neuralgia, and one from unwanted Horner's syndrome.

Gybels and Sweet[82] collected 65 cases treated by upper thoracic percutaneous RF sympathectomy; postoperatively, eight suffered initial and one delayed failure (14%), one developed pneumonia, and four developed new pain syndromes.

In the case of visceral somatic pain, pain fibers use the sympathetic system as a scaffold to reach the somatic afferent pathways, so that sympathetic denervation of a painful viscus, such as the pancreas, usually performed percutaneously also produces nociceptive interruption. The pain caused by cancer of abdominal viscera may also be alleviated by open or percutaneous injection of alcohol into the celiac plexus as in the experience of Moore,[197] who reported 94% excellent-to-good results in 168 patients undergoing 186 blocks. Complications included hypotension, iatrogenic pain, and inadvertent somatic nerve damage with the theoretic possibility of subarachnoid and intravisceral alcohol injection. Gybels and Sweet[82] concluded that phenol or 50% alcohol injections into the celiac plexus carried an unusually high (15%) mortality. They quote the initial relief rate of 88% persisting for a mean 4.3 months in 41 cancer patients treated by Flanigan and Kraft.[64] Gardner and Solomon[73] reported 70% pain relief till the patients' deaths, at the expense of a 5% mortality in 37 cancer patients. They commented upon difficulties from the poor radiologic landmarks, the diffuse spread of agent, and the complex widespread anatomy of the target. However, others have reported a high success rate with an acceptable complication rate (see Chapter 14).

INTRATHECAL ALCOHOL, PHENOL INJECTION TECHNIQUE

This technique to treat pain is discussed in Chapter 31.

PERCUTANEOUS DESTRUCTIVE PROCEDURES ON THE SPINAL CORD

Percutaneous procedures aimed at the spinal cord for the control of intractable pain are listed in Table 32-10; of these, percutaneous cordotomy is most often employed. Since the spinal cord can readily be approached percutaneously only at the occipital C1 and the C1–C2 interspaces, the available techniques are limited.[302]

Open versus Percutaneous Cordotomy

Although there are still advocates of open cordotomy, a careful review of the situation reveals few indications for the open procedure. Pathologic and anatomic abnormalities virtually never interfere with the percutaneous approach, so that the lesser impact and increased precision of the latter should give it priority, except when a surgeon capable of performing the procedure is not readily available to a sick patient who cannot travel. If a patient's inability to cooperate pre-

TABLE 32-10. *Percutaneous procedures for pain relief in the spinal cord*

Percutaneous cordotomy
Lateral high cervical approach
Dorsal high cervical approach
Low anterior approach
Percutaneous cervical myelotomy
Percutaneous trigeminal nucleotomy/tractotomy

TABLE 32-11. *Differential effect of surgical procedures on different elements of central pain of spinal cord origin*

	% of Patients significantly relieved	
Pain element	Destructive surgery[a]	Chronic stimulation[b]
Steady, causalgic dysesthetic, aching	26	36
Intermittent shooting	89	0
Allodynia and hyperpathia	84	16

[a] Cordotomy, cordectomy, dorsal root entry zone (DREZ).
[b] Dorsal column, deep brain stimulation producing paraesthesias in pain area.

cludes local anesthesia, percutaneous cordotomy can be performed under general anesthesia without muscle paralysis.[110,304,305,309] Percutaneous cordotomy is the operative procedure of choice in cancer pain whenever it is not contraindicated.[230,234,296,297,347]

Percutaneous Cordotomy

Percutaneous cordotomy, modeled after the open operation of Spiller and Martin,[276] was first employed by Mullan et al.[200] by the lateral approach between C1 and C2, using a radiostrontium source to make the lesion. In a short time, the procedure was perfected by the addition of myelography[221] to guide electrode position, electrical impedance monitoring[74] to guide cord penetration, RF lesion-making[246,247,288] to replace the radioactive source, physiologic corroboration,[92,294,295,314,318] and computed tomography (CT) guidance.[113] Meanwhile, Hitchcock[87,88] and others[44] developed a dorsal approach in the occiput–C1 space requiring the use of a stereotactic frame, while Lin et al.[143] introduced a low anterior cervical approach to avoid potential damage to the pathways responsible for respiratory control. Of these, the lateral high cervical method has been most popular.

Indications. Percutaneous cordotomy by the lateral high cervical approach is indicated in cases of nociceptive pain below the C5 dermatome, above which level lasting analgesia cannot be achieved. The usual cause of the pain is cancerous involvement of lumbosacral plexus, for which it is the procedure of choice, though it may rarely be indicated for nociceptive pain caused by noncancerous disease. The lancinating element of central pain of cord origin, so common with thoracolumbar injuries, and allodynia or hyperpathia associated with neuropathic pain in the lower extremities are also indications[306,316] (see Table 32-11).

In general, severe pain in a single lower extremity is the best indication; bilateral lower limb pain requiring bilateral cordotomy exposes the patient to the risk of bladder dysfunction and respiratory complications. Bilateral lower truncal-pelvic-perineal pain is a poor indication,[188] partly because it responds poorly—possibly because elements of neuropathic pain are present caused by previous surgery and/or radiation—and partly because it requires bilateral operation. Intraspinal morphine infusion may be superior here.

Respiratory contraindications require special comment.[13,14,66,91,199,212,248,320] Voluntary respiration, in response to the command "take a deep breath," is controlled by the corticospinal tract, rarely damaged during percutaneous cordotomy. Unconscious respiration on the other hand, as in sleep or during reading, is mediated by the strictly ipsilaterally distributed reticulospinal tracts. Since these lie adjacent to the cervical dermatomes of the spinothalamic tract, they are easily damaged by a cordotomy lesion that achieves high levels of cervical analgesia. This is of no concern if both lungs and their innervation are functioning normally. However, if, for example, an apical carcinoma has destroyed the

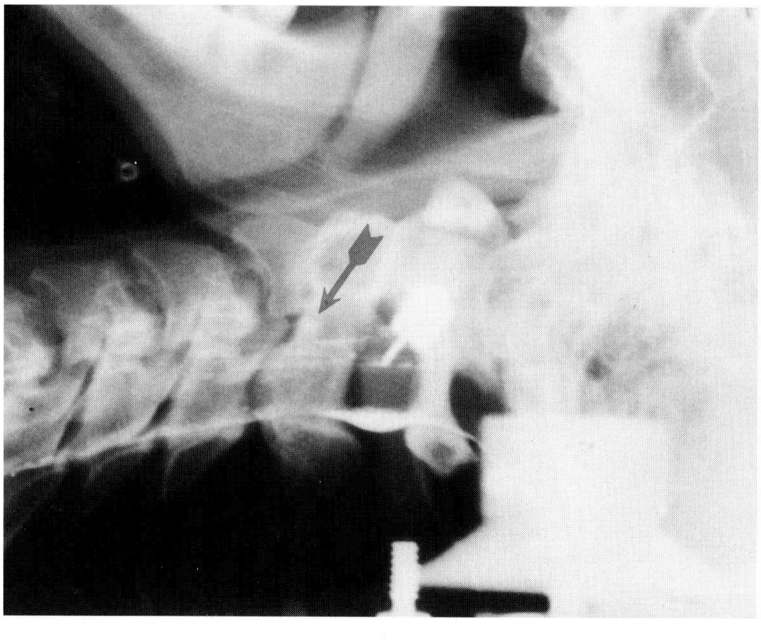

FIG. 32-8. Lateral x-ray of neck during percutaneous cordotomy. A drop of contrast medium *(arrow)* lies on the anterior cord margin. The ventral root line and dorsal dura are well outlined. The electrode tip is impaling the cord at the level of the dentate ligament, where a lesion produced analgesia up to T6 without complications.

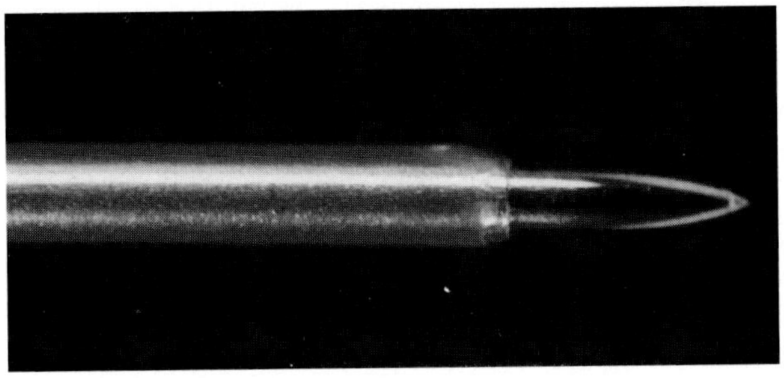

FIG. 32-9. Tip of cordotomy electrode. ×15.

phrenic nerve on one side and a cordotomy is being contemplated on the other to produce analgesia into the upper cervical dermatomes, the remaining reticulospinal tract will be interrupted and unconscious respiration abolished with fatal results. In such situations, cordotomy is either contraindicated or fraught with much risk. The same issues apply if a previous cordotomy has interrupted the tract and a new cordotomy is now being considered on the second side. Lema and Hitchcock[140] found that respiratory function (measured as the forced expiratory volume in 1 second) was interfered with to a greater degree by high dorsal percutaneous cordotomy than by percutaneous myelotomy or trigeminal tractotomy.

Other contraindications such as anomalies or disease in the C1–C2 area virtually never interfere, and in children or confused patients who cannot cooperate, general anesthesia may be used.

The choice of percutaneous technique depends upon the surgeon's experience and preferences. The dorsal[44,87,88] approaches requiring a stereotactic frame can achieve a slightly higher level of analgesia than the lateral high cervical approaches but appear to have been little exploited. The low anterior approach[143] has two disadvantages: it achieves a low level of analgesia and requires first traversing the cervical disk and part of the cord with the electrode before the spinothalamic tract is reached. Thus, small changes of electrode position require first withdrawal of the electrode through the disk and then reinsertion.

Technique: Lateral High Cervical Cordotomy. The lateral high cervical procedure is usually carried out under local anesthesia with intravenous sedation, but as mentioned, it can be performed under general anesthesia without paralysis when only the guidance of the sensory effects elicited by 100 Hz stimulation as described below[298] is lost. With the patient positioned supine, an LP needle is introduced into the middle of the C1–C2 space under lateral image intensification (see Fig. 32-8). When the subarachnoid space is entered, a small volume of a mixture of CSF, air, and contrast medium is forcefully injected in the hope of visualizing the dentate ligament. Oil-based contrast medium, which is superior to the evanescent water-soluble types, is now difficult to obtain. The cordotomy electrode (see Fig. 32-4) is now introduced into the LP needle, replacing the latter's stylette. This is a monopolar sharpened wire with a 2-mm bare tip insulated with shrunk-fit Teflon, which locks into the LP needle so that 2 mm of Teflon, in addition to the bare tip, projects beyond the tip of the LP needle (Fig. 32-9). It is grounded against an indifferent electrode in the ipsilateral upper arm. These dimensions ensure the optimum 2-mm penetration of the cord for lesioning the spinothalamic tract and provide standard impedance measurements. The electrode/needle assembly is directed toward the image of the dentate ligament and advanced so as to penetrate the cord at that site, penetration being signaled by an impedance rise from the 400 w characteristic of CSF to the 800–1200 w of cord (Fig. 32-10). Stimulation is now

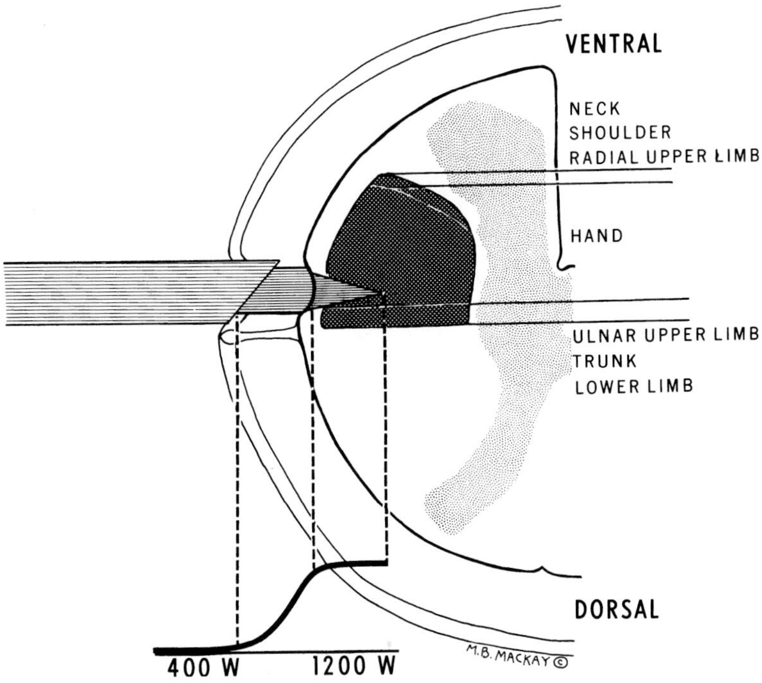

FIG. 32-10. Diagram illustrating technique of percutaneous cordotomy by the lateral high cervical approach, including impedance changes on cord impalation and anatomic organization of the region.

TABLE 32-12. *Published success after unilateral percutaneous cordotomy (% patients)*

Pain relief (% of patients)		
Complete	Significant	References
63		O'Connell (1969)[220]
75	96	Lorenz (1976)[166]
77	89	Grote and Roosen (1976)[a79]
75	83	von Schröttner (1978)[a340]
79	—	Meglio and Cioni (1981)[178]
—	68	Kühner (1981)[123]
75	—	Lipton (1981)[153]
—	79.1 50% after 3 mos.	Ventafridda, DeConno and Fochi (1982) (literature review)[335]
71	82.3	Tasker (1982)[298]
—	75	Siegfried Kühner and Sturm (1984)[269]
	80	Lipton (1984)[154]
—	71	Ischia *et al.* (1984)[109]
64	87	Lahuerta Lipton and Wells (1985)[126]
76	92.5	Ischia *et al.* (1985)[106]
—	89	Farcot *et al.* (1988)[62]
74.5	87.8	Tasker (1988)[304]
90—immediately 84—@ 3 months 61—@ 1 year 43—1-5 years 37—5-10 years		Rosomoff *et al.* (1990)[249]
64	82	Amano *et al.* (1991)[1]
	59–96	Tasker (1993) (literature review)[308]
72	84	Tasker (1995)[309]
	81.1	Ischia *et al.* (1984)[108]

[a] Mostly cancer pain and unilateral cordotomy.

carried out. If the electrode is correctly positioned, 2 Hz stimulation should produce muscle contractions in the ipsilateral neck, and sometimes the upper limb, while 100 Hz stimulation should produce no tetanization but rather contralateral warm or cold sensations. If these are felt in the lower limb, the electrode tip lies in the distal dermatomes of the spinothalamic tract; if in the hand, it lies in the proximal dermatomes. When all parameters are satisfactory, a test (20–30 mA for 60 seconds) and then a graded permanent (up to 60–70 mA for 60 seconds) RF lesion is made until the desired level and degree of analgesia are achieved. Otherwise, the electrode must be repositioned and the various steps repeated.

If cordotomy is to be performed on the second side, an interval of at least a week should intervene. Extreme caution must be observed to avoid respiratory complications; persisting unconscious respiration on the first side should be confirmed radiologically preoperatively, and the patient should be observed in an intensive care unit postoperatively, with monitoring of blood gases to detect a rising arterial CO_2 level forewarning of respiratory arrest. A significant risk of bladder dysfunction must be anticipated after bilateral cordotomy.

Results. The results of percutaneous cordotomy are perhaps best displayed in tabular form. Table 32-12 summarizes published results of unilateral procedures; Table 32-13 summarizes those of bilateral cordotomy; and Table 32-14 summarizes complications.

In a personal series of 244 cases,[298] the procedure was completed in 99% of patients, achieving spinothalamic interruption in 92.4%. In unilateral cases, effective pain relief was obtained in 94.4% at the time of discharge from hospital and in 82.3% in longer-term follow-up. Incidence of pain relief after bilateral cordotomy obeys the P-squared rule and is therefore lower than for unilateral cordotomy (82.3% × 82.3% = 67.7%). Recurrence of the nociceptive pain for which the procedure was performed virtually never occurs in an area of persisting analgesia. Nevertheless, persistent or recurrent pain after cordotomy can result from a variety of causes: (i) technical failure of the procedure, (ii) spread of cancer beyond the site involved at the time of the cordotomy (6% of our 244 cases developed pain above their cordotomy

TABLE 32-13. *Published success after bilateral percutaneous cordotomy (% patients)*

Relief		
Complete	Significant	Reference
58	77	Rosomoff (1969)[245]
—	71.4	Tasker (1982)[298]
47	59.5	Ischia *et al.* (1984)[107]
76	95	Amano *et al.* (1991)[1]
	47	Tasker (1993) (literature review)[308]

TABLE 32-14. *Reported complications of percutaneous cordotomy (% of patients)*

Complication	Unilateral																	Bilateral						
References	220	79	152	180	123	335	269	109	154	126	106	62	226	249	308	309	283	245	123	121	107	1	308	309
Death (most respiratory)		1.5			4.5			1.4	6.2	5	4.2		0.6		0–6	0.3	3.3	2	9.9	27.2		0	→27	1.6
Severe respiratory failure		2	6.2	9		.5–20							0.6	1	2.6–27		0.8	2		29.2		0	→36	
Mild respiratory problems					5.7						3.9			3		1.2			27.0	4.5		0		1.6
Transient respiratory problems		3.2		7.9		1–15							2.4	2		0.3			18.1					3.2
Significant paresis or ataxia	5.5	2	2.5	10.5	6	2–100	8	10.1	8–20	4	3.9	16		6	1–2	1.0	1.5	5		13.6	2.8	0		1.6
Mild or transient paresis or ataxia	11 1	2.9	20		48.5		100		100	69	31	4.7	4.3	25	→100	17.9		39		67.8	36.1		→67	29.5
Significant worsening micturition	13	3.2		5.3	4	2–35		7.2		3	8.7			2	→19	3.5	1.1	2	9.9	18.1	58	6.7		21.3
Mild, transient worsening micturition	18				8					19		10.5	6.1	10	0–8.7	7.0		15	36.3				→100	9.8
Transient bowel incontinence																2.1								9.8
Transient hypotension				2.6	8.7											1.8		4	54.5		36.1		40	8.1
Contralateral limb weakness										6						0								0
Postcordotomy dysesthesia		14.1 0.7 severe			3	1–50		8.7		6	6.8	16		1	→20	8.3	0.7							
Horner's syndrome					75			94	100	100	most	42	most		→100	23.0 ½ persist				59	100	common		23¼ persist
Neck pain					50					26		58				2.4								1.6
Other significant																0.3								1.6
Other transient, minor																0.6								1.6

level), (iii) presence or development of neuropathic pain from plexus destruction,[303] and (iv) development of, or intensification of, ipsilateral or "mirror" pain (41% of our 244 cases). The latter is particularly interesting. Once thought to be the result of unmasking of lesser pain on the other side of the body, it now seems more likely to be the result of opening up of previously inactive ipsilateral spinothalamic cord synapses after successful cordotomy, allowing painful stimuli applied to the now analgesic site to be appreciated in the mirror position on the other side of the body.[22,105,203–205,210] In those patients in whom cordotomy is performed for other than malignant disease,[306] levels of analgesia tended to fade with time and pain recurred. In six of our 24 paraplegics undergoing cordotomy, this happened after 1, 1 1/12, 4, 5, 13, and 21 years, pain relief being restored in two patients after 5 and 21 years, respectively, by repetition of the cordotomy.

It is unfortunate that percutaneous cordotomy has been so nearly supplanted in many centers by the subcutaneous infusion of morphine using an external pump or by intrathecal/epidural administration of opioid and non-opioid drugs (see Chapter 29). Because of tolerance, the latter therapy may result in enormous daily dosages of morphine, with their inevitable secondary effects, and continual attendance may be required at a medical facility. In selected patients, particularly with lower limb pain, cordotomy, a once-only procedure, may achieve sufficient ongoing pain relief so that the patient may require only small doses of oral analgesics postoperatively until the terminal stages of the illness.

Other Cord Procedures

Hitchcock[89] has evolved a high cervical dorsal percutaneous technique in the occipital–C1 space for central myelotomy, a substitute for longitudinal myelotomy done by open laminectomy. This latter curious procedure, introduced by Armour,[3] was originally intended to interrupt decussating spinothalamic fibers in the anterior commissure and thus to raise the analgesic level achieved by a cordotomy at the same level. The open operation also achieved the same effect as cordotomy if performed over many levels; when performed in the cervical area, it avoided the risk of respiratory complications. Hitchcock's percutaneous operation, however, performed in the upper cervical spine, can relieve pain at any level in the cord, and any analgesia induced bears no somatotopographic relationship to the level of the pain relieved. Thus it is thought to interrupt an extralemniscal pain pathway whose nature is unclear and which is distinct from the spinothalamic tract.[41,257] The procedure is an option in patients with pain caused by cancer, whereas its role in those with deafferentation pain needs further observation. It is a useful alternative to intrathecal or epidural opiate instillation in patients with midline or bilateral trunk pain in the lower body.

High cervical commissurotomy is performed percutaneously under local anesthesia through the occipital-C1 interspace with the patient sitting, using a suitable frame. A cisternal Conray myelogram outlines the dorsal and ventral aspects of the medulla and cord. A sharpened 0.5-mm electrode is introduced under impedance control with stimulation for physiologic localization. It is passed toward a point 5 mm anterior to the dorsal cord margin in the midsagittal plane. As the electrode enters the cord, stimulation of dorsal columns produces paresthesias in both feet. More deeply near the central canal, stimulation effects are referred to more dorsal aspects of the lower limbs. At the central canal region paresthesias occur in the soles, spreading to the dorsal aspects of the legs as the current is increased. Sometimes paresthesias affect the whole face, crossed limbs, or bilateral upper limbs, or else burning in the trunk occurs. Lesions are made as in cordotomy, just anterior to or at the sites of distal lower limb responses. Lesions produce subjective analgesia without clinically demonstrable sensory loss unrelated in location to areas of pain relief.

Results. Hitchcock[89] reported 10 excellent and two good results in 14 patients with cancer pain and excellent results in three with deafferentation pain, associated with unpredictable bilateral alterations in the appreciation of pinprick. Eiras and co-workers[60] reported good initial results in patients with cancer pain, with recurrence in some patients. Side effects consisted of dysmetria and ataxia for up to 2 weeks in all patients. Schvarcz[257] reported 78% satisfactory pain relief in patients with midline and bilateral pelvic cancer pain. These patients experienced varying degrees of alteration of appreciation of pinprick. Postoperative gait ataxia was reported as "common." Papo[227] found the pain relief from the procedure to be short-lived. Gybels and Sweet[82] compiled outcome data in 260 cases of percutaneous cervical RF myelotomy in patients with noncancerous pain syndromes; 66% derived useful relief. In 141 patients with pain caused by cancer, 63% were relieved.

Percutaneous Tractotomy of the Caudal Nucleus and Descending Tract of Trigeminal Nerve

Percutaneous tractotomy of the trigeminal nerve has been performed at both the lower medullary[45,46,67,68,255,256,323] and the upper cervical[87–90,93] levels. Unlike the previously discussed destructive techniques aimed at interrupting nociception in the management of nociceptive pain, this procedure at the cord level has been directed toward the management of deafferentation pain in the face, though the mechanism of this relief is unknown. Possibly it is similar to that in the so-called dorsal root entry zone introduced by Hyndman[100] and elaborated by Sindou and co-workers[272] in the treatment of cancer pain, by Nashold and Ostdahl[207] for deafferentation pain at the cord level, and by Nashold et al.[208] for deafferentation pain affecting the trigeminal nerve. Crue and colleagues[45,46,323] first performed trigeminal medullary tractotomy primarily for the treatment of nociceptive pain; Fox[67,68] introduced radiographic localization.

Technique

Medullary. The patient is positioned prone under local anesthesia. A No. 18 lumbar puncture needle is introduced between occiput and C1 into the midline of the cisterna magna, and 1 ml of Pantopaque emulsified with 1 ml of CSF is injected under lateral image intensification, outlining the floor of the fourth ventricle, the dorsum of the brain stem, and the obex, the latter appearing as a step in the shadow of the contrast medium. Four centimeters lateral to the midline, a second 18-gauge thin-wall lumbar puncture needle is passed over C1 lamina and aimed toward cisterna magna, terminating 12 mm from the midline as measured uncorrected on the posteroanterior film and 8 mm caudal to obex at the level of the dorsum of the brain stem on the lateral film (also uncorrected). These x-rays are achieved with a 30-inch tube to target and a 40-inch tube to film distance so as to afford reproducible measurements. A second electrode, such as the stylet of a 22-gauge 4 1/2-inch lumbar puncture needle insulated with vinyl tubing, except for a 3-mm bare tip, is passed through the laterally placed guide needle into the brain stem under impedance control at a site 0 to 10 mm from the midline of the odontoid on the uncorrected posteroanterior film, and at, or just caudal to, the obex and 4 mm anterior to the level of the floor of the fourth ventricle on the lateral film. In proper position, 50 Hz stimulation should cause ipsilateral facial sensation, whereupon a graded radiofrequency lesion up to 50 mA for 10 to 60 seconds is made with serial sensory testing.

Cervical. Hitchcock and Schvarcz[93] performed the procedure, with the patient in the sitting position, under local anesthesia using a stereotactic frame. A needle is passed through the occipital C1 interspace in the midsagittal plane, and 50% Conray is injected to outline the anterior/posterior aspects of the cord and the cisterna magna. The caudal dermatomes of the spinal tract of the fifth nerve at this location are said to lie 3 to 4 mm anterior to the posterior aspect of the cord and 6 mm lateral. Rostral dermatomes lie more laterally and anteriorly, and intermedius, ninth, and tenth dermatomes more posteriorly and medially. A 0.5-mm sharpened varnish-insulated electrode with a 2-mm bare tip enclosed in a nylon tube is advanced under radiologic and impedance control using monopolar stimulation until stimulation induces sensation in the face, said to be paresthetic[255] or painful.[93] Stimulation of the dorsal columns or their nuclei may induce ipsilateral sensory effects; stimulation of the spinopthalamic tract, contralateral sensory effects; the trigeminal effects are ipsilateral. At the level of C1, all of the trigeminal fibers, including those for the circumoral dermatomes, are present, the latter not being represented more distally. As soon as satisfactory positioning is achieved, a graded radiofrequency lesion is made.

Results. Fox[67] operated on eight patients with cancer, two with postherpetic neuralgia, one with tic, and one with questionable iatrogenic deafferentation facial pain. Analgesia of the fifth, seventh, ninth, and tenth nerves occurred in seven, V2–V3 analgesia in the rest. Complications included transient ipsilateral ataxia (common), three instances of contralateral body analgesia, and "nearly all patients suffered from postoperative hyperpyrexia of 101° to 102°F."

Schvarcz[255,256] reported 53 procedures in 52 patients with 87.5% relief of postherpetic neuralgia, 56% of anesthesia dolorosa, and 74% of "dysesthetic pain." He reported 83.8% relief of pain in 31 cancer patients. Complications consisted of contralateral hypalgesia and ipsilateral ataxia. Full evaluation of this interesting technique awaits wider experience.

TECHNIQUES THAT MODULATE PAIN

Modulating procedures can be separated into those that appear to modulate nociceptive pain and those that affect deafferentation pain. The former include techniques for the epidural or intrathecal instillation of opiates, PVG stimulation, and percutaneous hypophyseal alcohol injection. The latter include various techniques of chronic stimulation, of which only those at the spinal epidural and trigeminal level can be considered as percutaneous. Opiate infusions are discussed in Chapter 29; PVG stimulation is not within the subject of this book.

Hypophyseal Alcohol Injection

It is difficult to classify hypophyseal alcohol injection as to whether it is a destructive or a modulatory procedure. Hypophysectomy was originally directed toward treating hormone-dependent cancers of breast and prostate using open transfrontal and various percutaneous or stereotactic and transphenoidal means. Morrica[198] popularized the use of percutaneous injection of alcohol into the pituitary by a trans-sphenoidal approach for the treatment of pain caused by hormone-dependent and non-hormone-dependent cancer alike. The method by which this treatment affects cancer pain, although unknown, presumably is a modulatory one affecting the processing of noxious afferent input. It is not related to pituitary destruction, involvement of hypothalamus, or manipulation of levels in blood or CSF of any recognizable substance, including enkephalins and endorphins, and the effect is not reversed by naloxone.[35,291,292]

Technique. The procedure is performed under neuroleptanalgesia. After preparing the nasal cavity with cocaine paste, a 16-gauge 12-cm needle is introduced into the right nostril under biplanar x-ray control and through the sphenoid sinus, which is sterilized, until it impinges on sella. A 19-gauge needle of greater length is now introduced through the first needle and hammered through the sellar floor. Aspiration is applied to be sure that blood or CSF return is not obtained. A total of 1.0 to 2.4 ml (average 2.0 ml) pure ethanol is introduced by means of one to two such punctures, with the radiologically localized needle tip lying in the midline almost against the posterior sellar wall. The needles are removed after 5 minutes and the nose packed. Pupillary responses and eye movements are monitored during the injections (see Chapter 31, Figs. 31-10 to 31-13).

Results. Miles[192–194] achieved 41% to 43% excellent and 30% partial pain relief in 122 patients, although relief persisted for 3 months or more in only 21%. Eight of his patients died, and five suffered from visual or oculomotor disturbances, two from hypopthalamic destruction, and 10% to 20% from CSF leakage and 1% from meningitis. There was a 60% incidence of diabetes insipidus, complications usually being transient. Madrid's patients[169] experienced 67% immediate relief of pain at the expense of 3% CSF rhinorrhea, 0.3% meningitis, and 3% visual-oculomotor disturbances. Takeda and his colleagues[291,292] observed 80% immediate pain relief in 102 patients overall; there was 95% success in the 43% with hormone-dependent cancer and 69% in the rest. Cancer in the hormone-dependent group sometimes regressed. Complications included an almost universal transient euphoria and polyphagia, 10% visual and 4% oculomotor disturbances, and a 50% incidence of diabetes insipidus. A review of other publications on the subject suggests that pain recurrence after 3 to 4 months, a 2% mortality, rhinorrhea, 2% visual complications, transient headache, diabetes insipidus, hyperthermia, and polyphagia are regular features of the operation. Levin and co-workers,[141] using a stereotactic technique, reported relief of thalamic pain in three patients following this procedure. A subsequent review by Miles[194] of 250 personal cases showed that pain relief persisted in 21% past 3 months at the expense of a 2.4% mortality, an 0.8% incidence of visual field defect, and a 0.4% incidence of persistent CSF rhinorrhea. His literature review is summarized in Table 32-15.

Gybels and Sweet[82] record 62% significant relief in 709 cases reported in the literature.

Percutaneous Chronic Stimulation for the Treatment of Deafferentation Pain

Chronic stimulation can be applied to peripheral nerves, the spinal cord, and the brain, only the former two of which will be discussed here. In order to relieve pain, the stimulation must induce paresthesias in the area of the patient's pain.

Peripheral and Trigeminal Nerve Stimulation

Although the first trials of chronic stimulation were applied to peripheral nerves,[286,344] this usually requires an open procedure beyond the scope of this chapter. The only peripheral nerve that can be stimulated percutaneously and with which there is published experience is the trigeminal. Sheldon[262] originally conceived the idea, but Meyerson and Håkansson[190] first performed trigeminal stimulation to treat deafferentation pain by inserting a plate electrode on Meckel's cave at craniotomy; Steude developed a percutaneous technique.[274,278] The indication is steady neuropathic pain in trigeminal distribution. Because only an unpredictable 50% of apparently appropriate candidates show even a short-term response, in common with all paresthesia-producing stimulation techniques, it is advisable to first carry out a trial of test stimulation.

Technique. Under local anesthesia with IV sedation, as for percutaneous RF coagulation of nerve V, a suitably sized Tuohy needle is passed through the foramen ovale, its progress monitored by lateral image intensification. When CSF return occurs, the stylet is replaced by a single monopolar test electrode. The cathether (Fig. 32-11)[235] (available from Racz Lec Tro Cath, Medical Evaluation Devices & Instruments Corp., Gloversville, NY) is suitable for this purpose provided the threaded lock is tightened to prevent CSF leakage. The electrode is advanced to at least the level of the line joining the apex of the petrous ridge and the top of the posterior clinoid. The Tuohy needle is removed, leaving the electrode in place, and the latter is tunneled with the Tuohy needle to a site on the side of the neck remote from the original insertion. Stimulation at 30 to 100 Hz is then carried out using an indifferent electrode on the ipsilateral upper arm. The electrode is carefully withdrawn until paresthesias are reported in the patient's area of pain and then anchored to the skin with tape; the two wounds are sutured. During several days' trial, the patient decides whether the stimulation produces 50% or more pain relief and then the test electrode is removed. In the event of a successful trial, the patient is readmitted after the wounds have healed for insertion of a permanent device under general anesthesia. For this we find the Medtronic DBS or sacral root electrode satisfactory, placed at the same x-ray-documented site as the original Racz catheter (Fig. 32-12). It can be activated by either an RF coupled implant (Fig. 32-13) or a battery-powered totally programmable stimulator (Fig. 32-14) placed in an infraclavicular subcutaneous pocket to which the electrode is connected with a cable. It is important to anchor the electrode to the fascia of the maxilla to avoid

TABLE 32-15. *Comparative efficiency of alcohol injection into the pituitary gland in relieving pain*

	Patients	Injections	Excellent	Some	None
Morrica, 1977[198]	822	1900	809	12	1
Katz and Levin, 1977[a]	13	15	6	7	0
Lipton, 1978[152]	106	155	38	28	26
Madrid, 1979[169]	329		220	89	20

[a] Katz J. and Levin A. B.: Treatment of diffuse metastatic cancer pain by instillation of alcohol into the sella tursica. Anesthesiology, *46*: 115, 1977.

From Miles, J.: Pituitary destruction. *In* Wall, P.D., and Melzack, R. (eds.): Textbook of Pain. 3rd Ed. pp. 1159. Edinburgh, Churchill Livingstone, 1994.

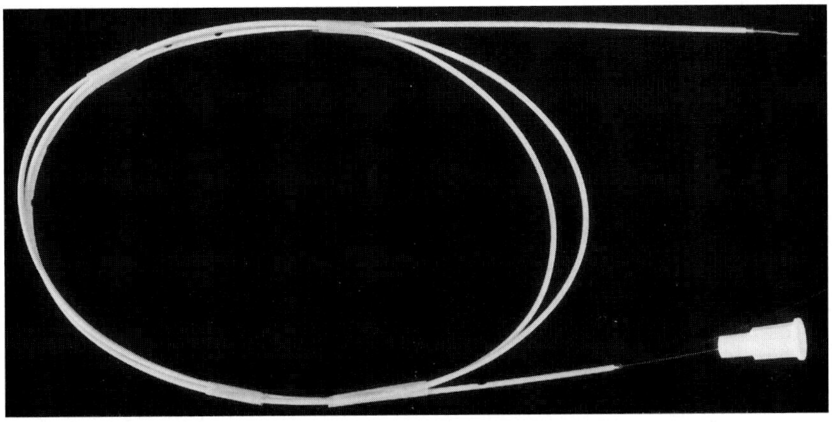

FIG. 32-11. Catheter and monopolar stimulating electrode available from Medical Evaluation Devices & Instruments Corp. (Racz Lec Tro Cath.)

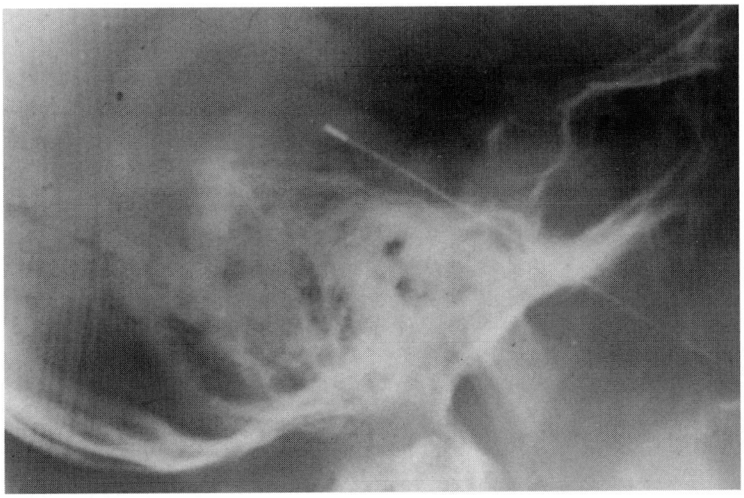

FIG. 32-12. Lateral x-ray showing Medtronic straight "PISCES"-type electrode introduced into Meckel's cave via foramen ovale and beginning to enter the posterior fossa.

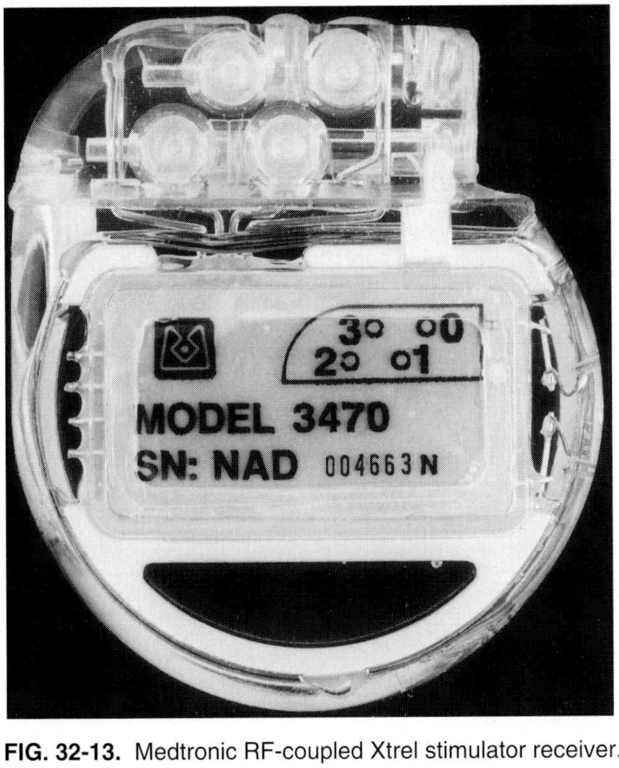

FIG. 32-13. Medtronic RF-coupled Xtrel stimulator receiver.

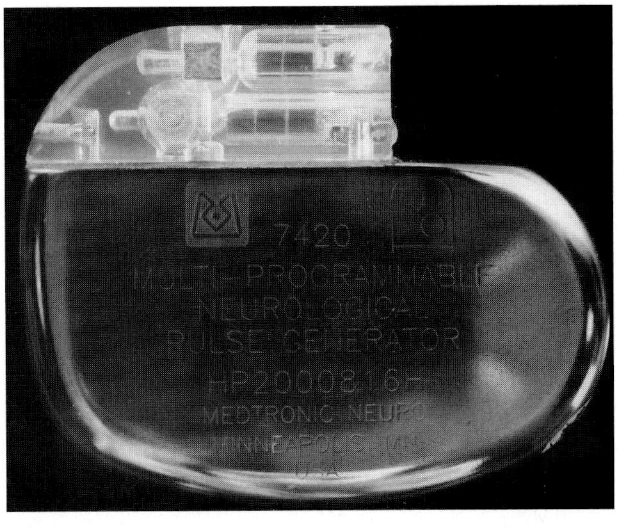

FIG. 32-14. Medtronic battery powered totally programmable Itrel stimulator.

TABLE 32-16. *Percutaneous trigeminal stimulation for neuropathic pain*

Diagnosis	No. of patients	Successful trial % of patients	Longer term >50% pain relief % all cases treated
Trigeminal nerve damage	20 19 iatrogenic	50 1—no paresthesias	40
Postherpetic neuralgia	3	33	0
Central lesions of trigeminal tract	6	83	83
Unknown	1	0	0

electrode movement when the jaw opens and closes. In order to minimize the high rates of superficial infection seen after permanent internalization, we believe it important to insert the permanent system at a single sitting under general anesthesia several weeks after the stimulation trial, with scrupulous attention to sterility and antibiotic coverage.

Results. To date little has been published concerning this technique. Meyerson and Håkansson[190] found that 56% of their 25 patients "passed" the stimulation test, of whom six were implanted by open means, all with satisfactory pain relief. They preferred 50 to 100 Hz stimulation, producing paresthesias in the painful area. Steude[278] reported three of his 10 patients with atypical facial pain relieved. We have employed Steude's percutaneous technique in 30 patients (Tables 32-16 and 32-17). Curiously, central pain syndromes appear to respond well. Unfortunately, this simple procedure is marred by a high risk of infection, all (fortunately) superficial, whose incidence has been substantially lessened by the two-stage procedure described. However, such infections usually require removal and later replacement of the equipment.

Dorsal Column Stimulation (DCS)

Dorsal column stimulation for the relief of intractable pain was introduced by Shealy[258–261] as a natural extension of peripheral nerve stimulation, initially by open surgery. Gradually, it was realized that it was effective mainly for the steady element of neuropathic pain,[307,316] so that, after a percutaneous technique was introduced,[55,61,96] it has become a very popular method for treating that problem; there is little evidence of its usefulness in nociceptive pain caused by cancer.

Mechanism of Action. Despite the length of time the technique has been used, its mechanisms of action remains unclear. The subject is discussed by Barolat,[7] implicating both centrifugal and centripetal neural and neurochemical mechanisms from stimulation that could arise in dorsal roots, dorsal root entry zone,[101] or dorsal columns.[27,34,56,58,65,70,72,84,86,128,144,145,146,149,150,151,175,189,219,238,240,251,264,271,279,280–282] To me it seems likely that DCS in some way inhibits unknown central mechanisms responsible for the steady component of neuropathic pain.[164,187,195,324,333] The notion that it functions by suppressing conduction in pain fibers seems unjustified since it may suppress pain associated with complete interruption of peripheral input.

One of the problems with DCS, or any other technique for chronic stimulation, is the inability to identify in advance the approximately 50% of patients who will respond. Many workers screen prospective patients psychologically,[23,47,125] but there is no consensus as to the efficacy of such studies. Although we have had the impression that pain relief with transcutaneous electrical nerve stimulation (TENS) suggested a good prognosis, LeDoux and Langford[139] found no significant relationship between the effects of the two modalities. A number of observers have shown that DCS and cutaneous nerve stimulation suppress, particularly, the late events in the somatosensory evoked potential,[16,78,254,319] and we have very preliminary data that suggest that such suppression occurs particularly in patients who enjoy pain relief. This suppression may reflect the mechanisms by which DCS suppresses pain, a subject on which a variety of other related observations are of interest. Gildenberg and Murthy[75] found that DCS suppressed the late events of the evoked potentials in the intralaminar nucleus of thalamus in man but not in ventrobasal complex. Tsubokawa and Moriyasu[324] found that stimulating the lemniscal pathway in the ventrocaudal nucleus suppressed nociceptor activity in the medial thalamus. Modesti and Waszak[195] (in man) and Nishimoto et al.[214] and Nyquist and Greenhoot[219] (in cats) found that DCS suppressed neuronal firing in intralaminar nuclei. Augustinsson et al.[4,5] found that DCS suppressed late events of the somatosensory evoked potential in the ventrocaudal nucleus in man, while Dong and Wagman[54] showed that DCS suppressed neural firing in the cat's posterior thalamic group nuclei. Mertens et al.[186] found DCS was more effective in patients with normal somatosensory evoked potentials, while Coffey et al.[38] described a technique for monitoring evoked potentials elicited by an RF coupled DCS. Iacono et al.[101,102] and Yingling and Hosobuchi[352] use cortical and spinal evoked potentials from nerve stimulation to help position the electrode for dorsal root entry zone stimulation.

TABLE 32-17. *Complications of percutaneous stimulation of trigeminal nerve*

Complication	% of 30 cases
Superficial infection	23
Electrode migration and other technical problems	23
Minor damage to V nerve	10 7% with increase in pain
Transient diplopia	7

Hosobuchi et al.[99] examined the usefulness of studies of evoked potentials in explaining failures of DCS.

Clinical Features. After experimentation with DCS on the dorsal and ventral surfaces of the cord for the treatment of various types of pain,[95,127,138,301] it appeared that the technique was most useful if applied over the dorsal surface so as to produce paresthesias in the distribution of the patient's pain. However, efficacy is difficult to determine for a variety of reasons: (i) any pain relief achieved is partial, (ii) only about half the patients selected for treatment report relief even at the outset, (iii) a further group escape from control despite continuing technically successful stimulation over the first few months of treatment, possibly reflecting a placebo effect,[342] and (iv) efficacy varies with the type of neuropathic pain treated.

In the case of neuropathic pain, it has been our experience that chronic stimulation is most effective for treating the steady, often causalgic, dysesthetic element and that it is not effective for the neuralgic element.[112,316] Jones[112] found a less than 20% reduction in shooting pain, 60% to 90% in steady aching and burning.

Its role in the treatment of allodynia and hyperpathia is unclear and presents a rather intriguing opportunity for clinical investigation. Meyerson et al.[191] have demonstrated that DCS reduces allodynia in a rat model. Overall, the success of DCS is much less in the treatment of evoked pain in central pain of cord origin than it is for steady pain,[316] and the same applies to paresthesia-producing brain stimulation in central pain,[306,312] where it may be perceived as painful,[299,300] especially in the presence of allodynia or hyperpathia. We are uncertain of the incidence of relief by DCS of allodynia and hyperpathia in peripheral neuropathic pain; there are patients in whom it is effective, steady and evoked pain being abolished together, but other patients with allodynia and hyperpathia perceive DCS as painful when applied to the same dermatomes as those in which evoked pain occurs, just as natural stimulation is. The explanation of these phenomena would doubtless clarify the mechanisms of control of neuropathic pain by chronic stimulation.

Another area of controversy is the role of DCS in other than neuropathic pain. Although it is generally thought to be ineffective for nociceptive pain, there is new evidence that it may be effective for the relief of low back pain, perhaps through a different technique than that used in neuropathic pain (mentioned below under Failed Back).

DCS is most effective for the pain associated with peripheral vascular disease (PVD) in the lower limbs; this is the best indication for DCS. While there is conflicting evidence concerning its usefulness for the healing of ischemic ulcers, the effect on pain is dramatic, although it remains uncertain whether this effect is a direct one on the pain or the result of improved vascular perfusion (see under Peripheral Vascular Disease). Similar questions apply to the use of DCS to treat angina pectoris (see under Angina).

One issue is the safety of chronic stimulation for pain in patients with heart pacemakers. Romano et al.[244] reported 10 patients with heart pacemakers who underwent DCS. Interference was minimized if a bipolar or multiprogrammable heart pacemaker was used, but regardless of equipment used, problems did not occur as long as output voltage of the DCS was limited so that the product of its voltage × pulse duration was below 1.9 to 2.

Cost Effectiveness. It may be argued that the high cost of DCS equipment coupled with the reported modest incidence of success is not cost-effective. Bel and Bauer[11] reported that 700,000 patients are treated annually in Germany for the pain of degenerative lumbar disk disease, with a related loss of 13×10^6 work days. In Switzerland this condition has been estimated to cost 600×10^6 Swiss francs (SWF) and in the U.S. 12×10^9 U.S. dollars (USD) annually. Bel and Bauer followed the courses of 14 patients treated by DCS, 12 of whom were still working. Drug costs fell from an average of 3553 German marks (DM) to 400DM per patient postoperatively. The cost of the DCS equipment averaged 11761 DM and of the necessary hospitalization 10700DM per patient. These costs were more than compensated for by increased earning capacity postoperatively. However, relatively few of my patients returned to work as a result of treatment with DCS, so that cost-effectiveness in them would have to depend on drug intake reductions (3153DM/patient/year in the German series) and any reduced costs of medical attention.

Kupers et al. have carried out a cost-efficacy study of DCS in Belgium. From 1983 to 1992, about 700 devices were implanted in a population of less than 10 million people, 61.4% for failed back surgery. Less than 5% of these patients returned to work after 1 year; 52% of a different group of patients regarded the results of DCS to be good or very good after 3.5 years, men particularly. Psychiatric screening seemed to be useful in increasing success rate, and results seemed better when DCS was done in university teaching hospitals.

Choice of Techniques

Various techniques have been employed for DCS. The earliest was the intradural implantation of a plate-type electrode by laminectomy, but this was associated with serious complications, particularly cord compression and CSF leakage, leading to the modern practice of inserting one or more plate-type electrodes of varying configurations epidurally at laminotomy, a technique beyond the scope of this chapter.

Though many surgeons prefer the use of such plate-type electrodes, the introduction of percutaneously introduced electrodes was a major advance; after all, when a technique is only partially successful in half the patients treated, the surgical impact should be minimal. Various types of percutaneous electrodes are available from a variety of sources (Fig. 32-15), ranging from monopolar, such as the Medtronic "sigma," to multipolar with varying numbers of terminals, used singly or in combinations. These can be activated by RF coupled stimulators such as the Medtronic "Xtrel" (see Fig. 32-13) or by totally programmable battery-powered devices

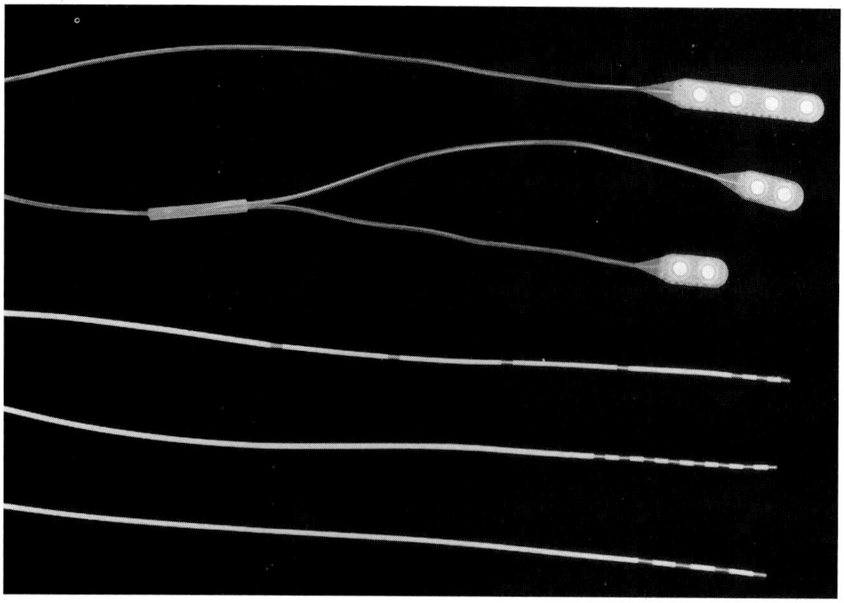

FIG. 32-15. Electrodes available from Neuromed (Fort Lauderdale, FL) for DCS. From above downward: two models of plate electrode, three of percutaneously introduced electrodes, the lowest being the Multistim model.

such as the Medtronic "Itrel" (see Fig. 32-14) and Neuromed "Time" (Fig. 32-16); the latter can also be driven by RF coupling. Perhaps the most popular electrodes are the 4-pole Medtronic "Quad" (Fig. 32-17) and Neuromed "Multistim" (Fig. 32-15). Whereas all our early experience was with percutaneously inserted monopolar electrodes, there is no question that multipolar electrodes are to be preferred:[215,216] (i) They are sturdier and less likely to migrate after implantation than are monopolar electrodes; (ii) if they do migrate, changing pole selection may recapture adequate stimulation; (iii) choice of different selections of poles allows coverage of larger portions of the body; and (iv) although it is difficult to assess the relative usefulness of monopolar versus bipolar or more complex patterns of stimulation, there are claims that the latter may be more effective in certain situations. Law[130] and North et al.[216] have developed a patient interactive computer program to manage the multiple variables. These developments have helped to achieve the important aim of matching the area of stimulation with the painful areas in the patients pain diagram.

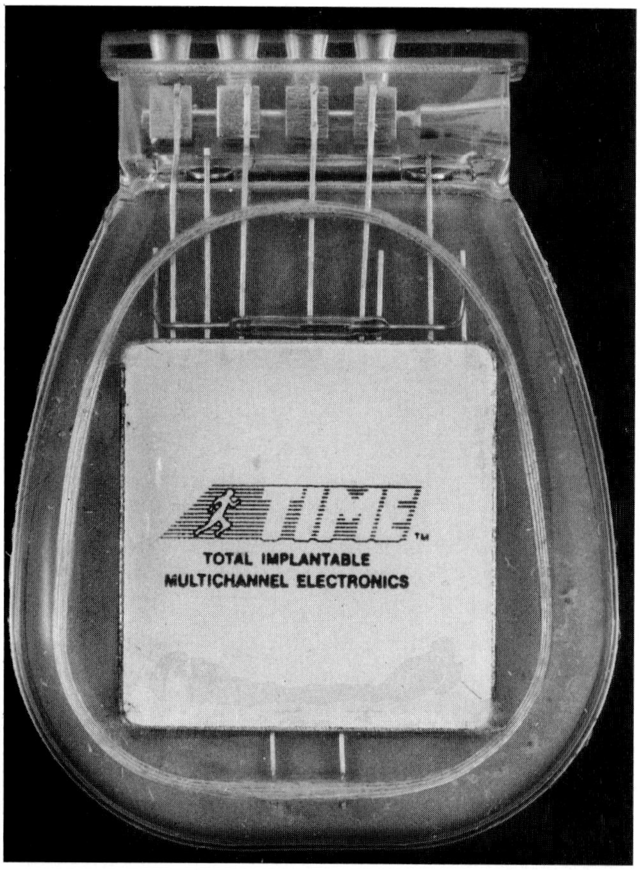

FIG. 32-16. Neuromed Time stimulator.

Trial Stimulation

The excellent available equipment is expensive, and only half the patients selected for DCS respond. It seems clear that reason dictates a pre-implantation trial of test stimulation using expendable equipment.[98] For this purpose, various devices are available; we have found the inexpensive percutaneous monopolar electrode-catheter (the same as used in trial of trigeminal stimulation), available from Racz (see Fig. 32-11), to be most satisfactory. Delayed implantation of the

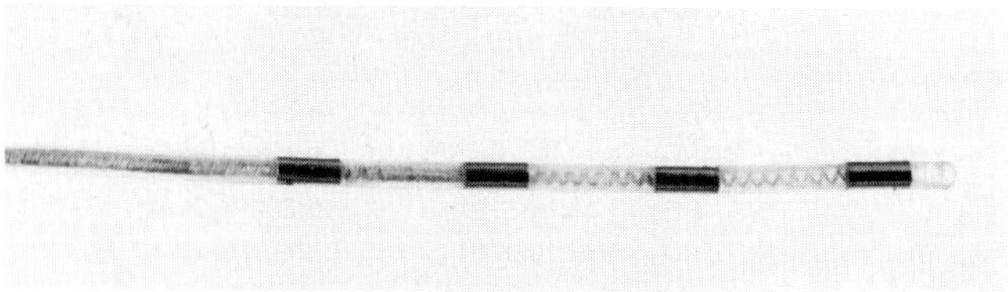

FIG. 32-17. Medtronic Quad electrode for DCS.

entire permanent system at one sitting, as in trigeminal stimulation, reduces the incidence of infection. Temporary quadropole electrodes are also available (e.g., from Medtronic or Neuromed) and provide a more accurate assessment of the potential efficacy of definitive implantation.

Evaluation of the results of the trial procedure must include: careful charting of the areas where satisfactory stimulation is obtained and comparison with the pre- and post-test pain diagram; charting of visual analogue (or other) pain scores; recording of analgesic consumption; and appropriate pre- and post-test measures of physical function, with emphasis on those functions limited by pain.

The success, or otherwise, of trial stimulation should be judged as objectively as possible on the basis of improved function resulting from pain relief, preferably not only on the patient's report of pain relief. Assessment of all of the foregoing measures usually takes at least 2 to 3 days; thus, temporary electrodes need to be carefully secured so that they function reliably during the entire trial period.

In some pain centers, the DCS trial continues during a 3-week cognitive-behavioral program, to permit rigorous evaluation of changes in physical and psychological indices of function. This certainly permits a thorough evaluation and may decrease the chance of implanting in inappropriate patients. However, this advantage has to be weighed against the costs of the program and the increased risk of infection, although the latter is decreased by tunneling the temporary electrode prior to exteriorizing it.

Location of Electrode

Since the procedure depends on the induction of paresthesias in the area of the patient's pain, it must be planned so that the active poles of the electrode end up at appropriate sites over the spinal cord. For lower limb stimulation, placement within one vertebra of bony level T10 is usually adequate. Barolat[7] and Barolat et al.[10] suggest that lateral placements are more likely to induce paresthesias in anterior aspects of the lower limbs, and midline placements in posterior aspects. For upper limb stimulation, electrode placement over bony levels C4–C7, whether midline or lateral, are adequate; Barolat[7] suggests lateral placements for pain in C2 distribution. For trunk stimulation, somatotopically appropriate intermediate levels are used; Barolat[7] suggests midline placements for midline pain, lateral for chest and abdominal wall pain. If it is agreed that DCS is useful for low back pain, the best locations are said to be bony T5–T6.

Tolerance

Another issue is the possibility that patients might develop tolerance to DCS as they do to opiates. However, a review of our own patients and those reported in the literature does not support this concern, nor would it be expected to do so, since the mechanism of action of DCS, effective as it is primarily for steady neuropathic pain, is not likely to involve opiate systems that are known to develop tolerance.

Technique

The operation is performed with the patient prone and the spine flexed to facilitate electrode insertion under local anesthesia with intravenous sedation and anteroposterior image intensification (Fig 32-18.1 to 32-18.2). The back is prepared and draped at the expected level of introduction, which is about 15 cm below the intended target (Fig 32-18.3); the greater the length of electrode inserted in the epidural space the more stable its positioning. If the patient is right-handed, the electrode should be brought out to the surface for testing to the left of midline, and vice versa. A 15 gauge Tuohy needle is introduced at as low an angle as possible (Fig 32-18.4 and 32-18.5) to facilitate cephalad electrode introduction into the selected interspace and cautiously advanced under image intensification. Entry into the epidural space is monitored by loss of resistance technique (see Chapter 8) or by retraction of a drop of normal saline into the hub of the needle, followed by cautious introduction of a suitable spring guide wire (Fig. 32-18.6). Intrathecal penetration is carefully avoided; if it occurs, a new level must be selected. Epidural adhesions may impede introduction in the lumbar area while previous nearby spinal surgery does so at any level. Once the epidural space has been entered, a suitable track for the electrode is developed with the guide (close to mid-dorsal for limb stimulation) (Fig 32-18.7). The electrode is now introduced and test stimulated, if monopolar against an indifferent skin electrode, and the position adjusted until paresthesias are produced in the desired site (Figs 32-18.8 and 32-18.9). The electrode is then tunneled a short distance to the right or left, depending upon handedness, and brought out to the skin for trial stimulation. The patient is instructed to stimulate for 2 hours, then rest for one, over the next several days, and to decide: (i) Is the stimulation acceptable? (ii) Are there untoward effects such as muscle contraction? (iii) Does DCS reduce the pain by 50% or more? As noted above, objective measures of function and analgesic consumption are also made. At this stage the test electrode is withdrawn and discarded. If a permanent electrode was used for trial stimulation, the patient is returned to the operating room and the transcutaneous connector removed. The electrode is tunneled around the body to the site of implantation of the stimulator, using local anesthetic and intravenous sedation. For lower body pain, the latter is placed in a subcutaneous pocket in the lower quadrant of the abdomen; for upper limb and neck pain, below the clavicle. Some devices require an intermediate connector between electrode and stimulator; in others, electrodes connect directly to the stimulator. If a trial electrode was used, the patient is discharged and subsequently readmitted for insertion of a permanent system as in trigeminal stimulation. Prophylactic antibiotics are advisable during permanent implants.

For permanent implantation, the technical steps can be

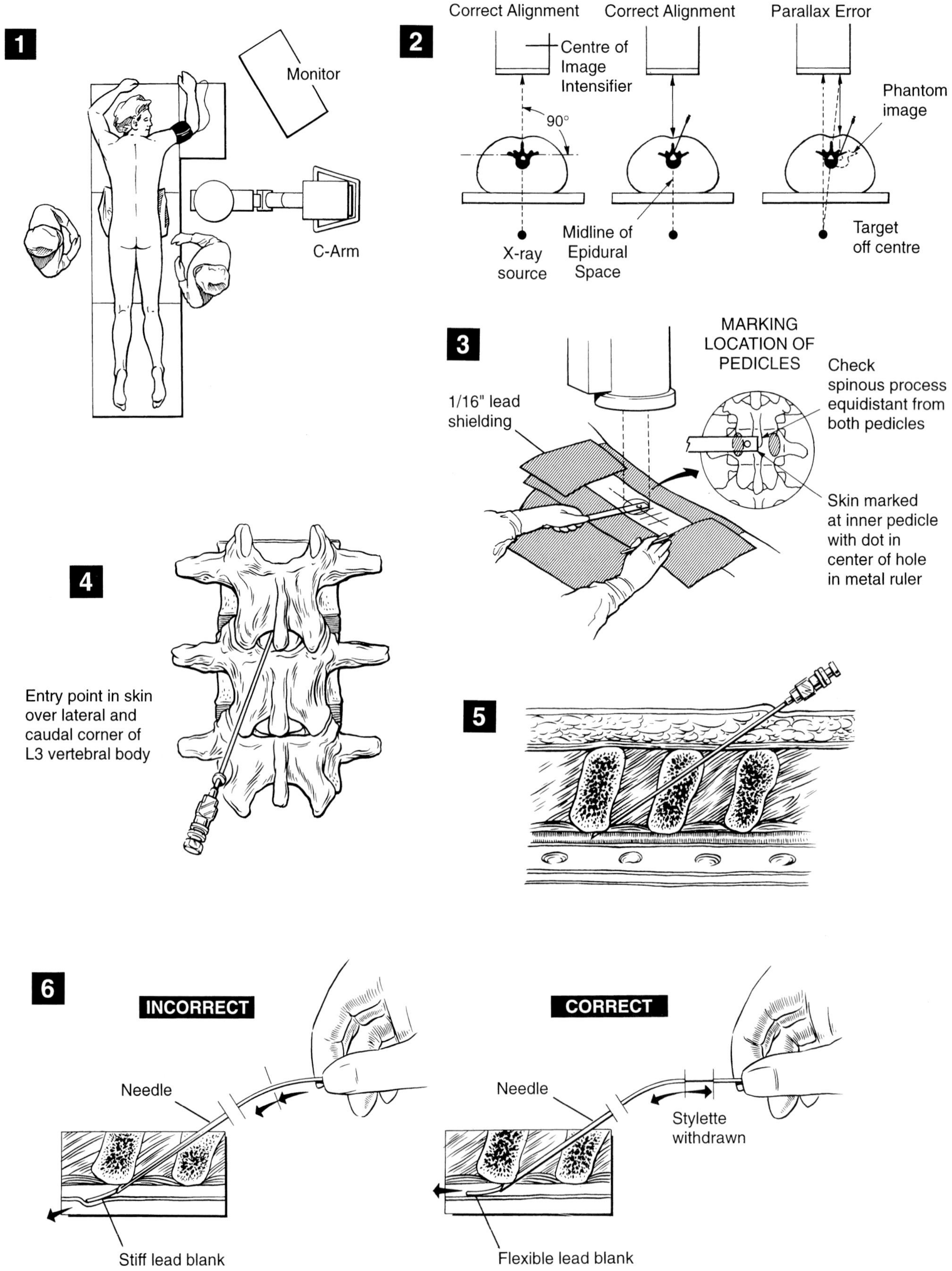

FIG. 32-18. Steps in implantation of DCS. (See text.)

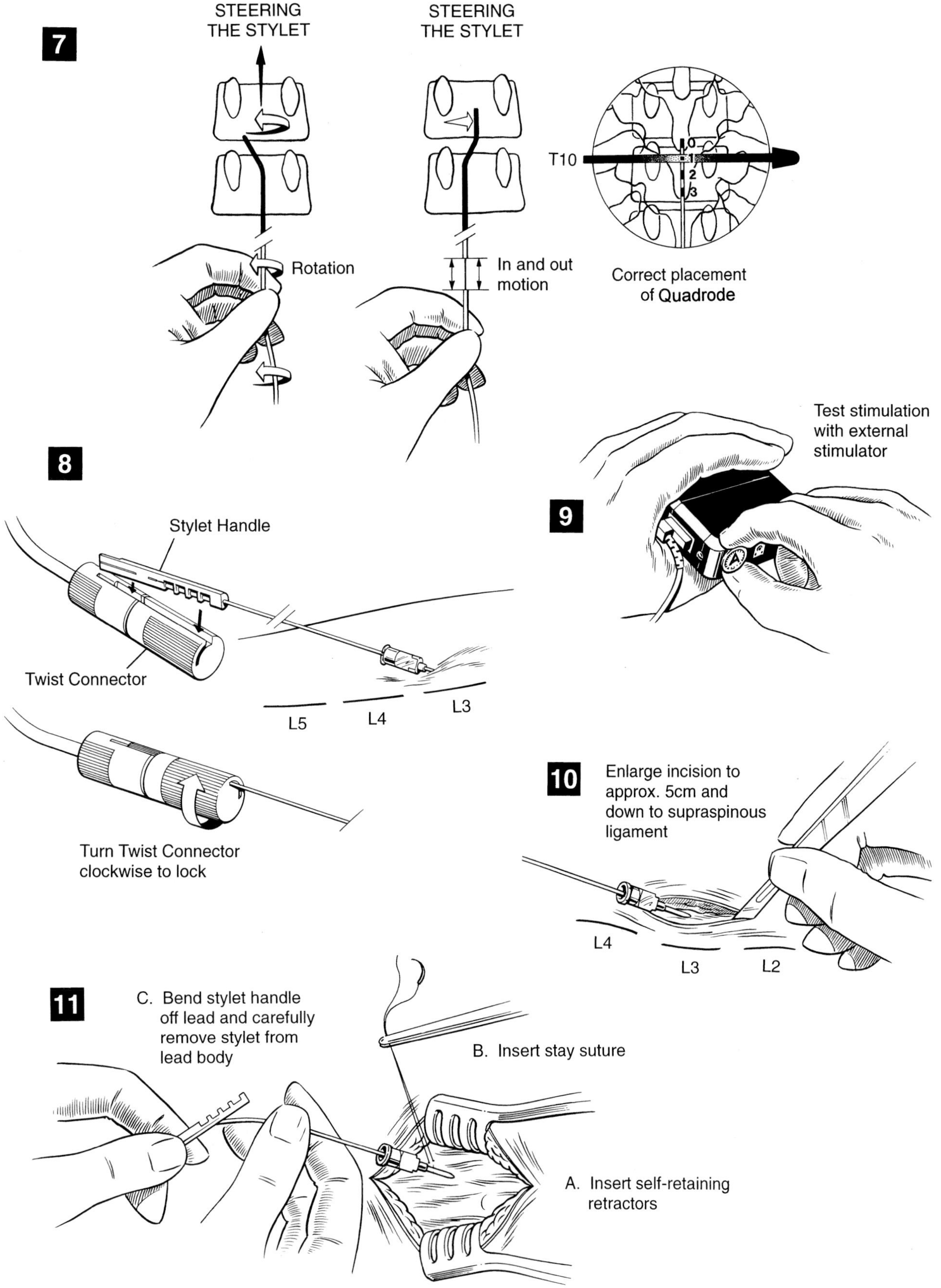

FIG. 32-18. *Continued.*

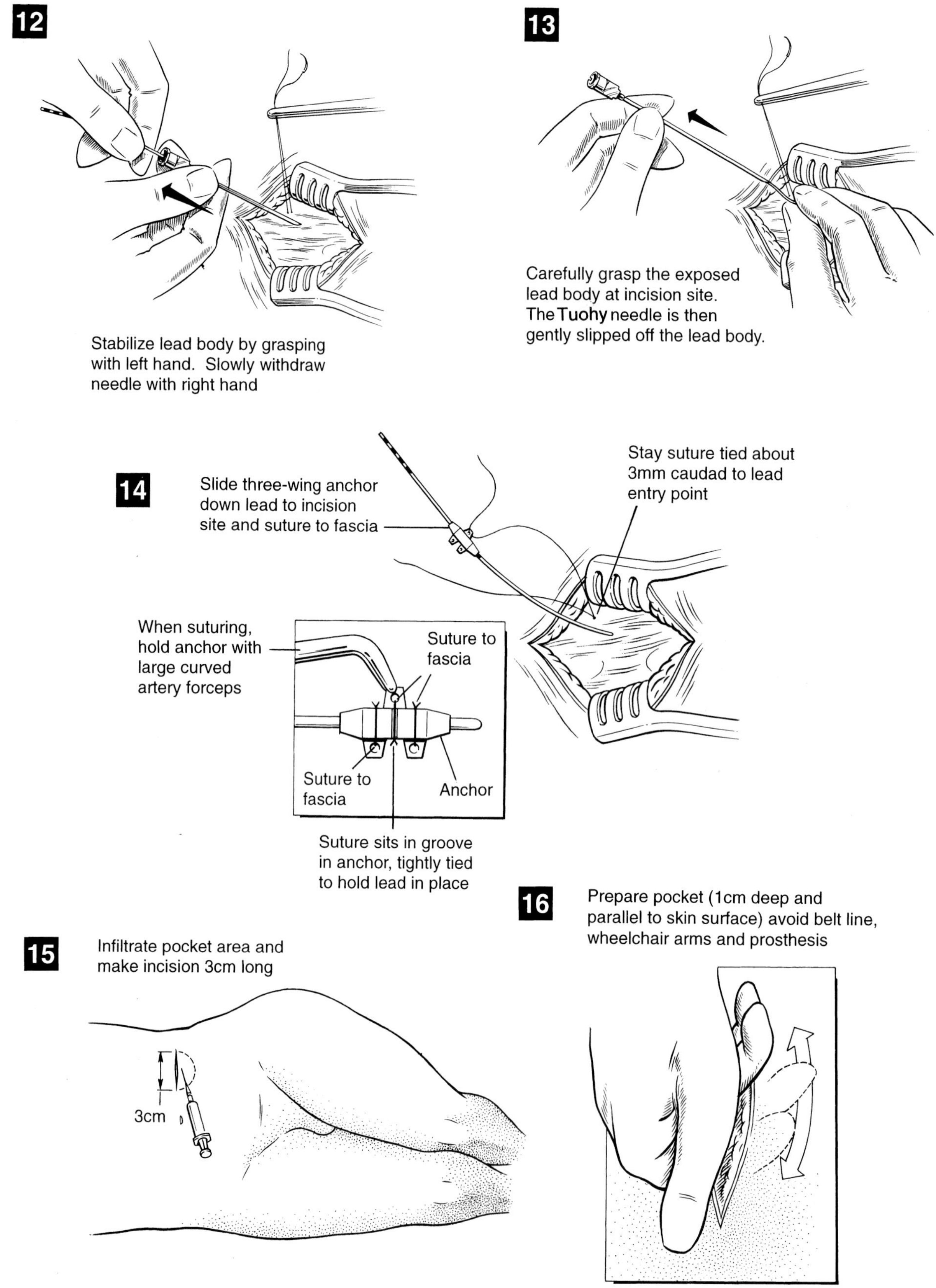
12
Stabilize lead body by grasping with left hand. Slowly withdraw needle with right hand
13
Carefully grasp the exposed lead body at incision site. The Tuohy needle is then gently slipped off the lead body.
14
Slide three-wing anchor down lead to incision site and suture to fascia
Stay suture tied about 3mm caudad to lead entry point
When suturing, hold anchor with large curved artery forceps
Suture to fascia
Suture to fascia
Anchor
Suture sits in groove in anchor, tightly tied to hold lead in place
15
Infiltrate pocket area and make incision 3cm long
3cm
16
Prepare pocket (1cm deep and parallel to skin surface) avoid belt line, wheelchair arms and prosthesis

FIG. 32-18. *Continued.*

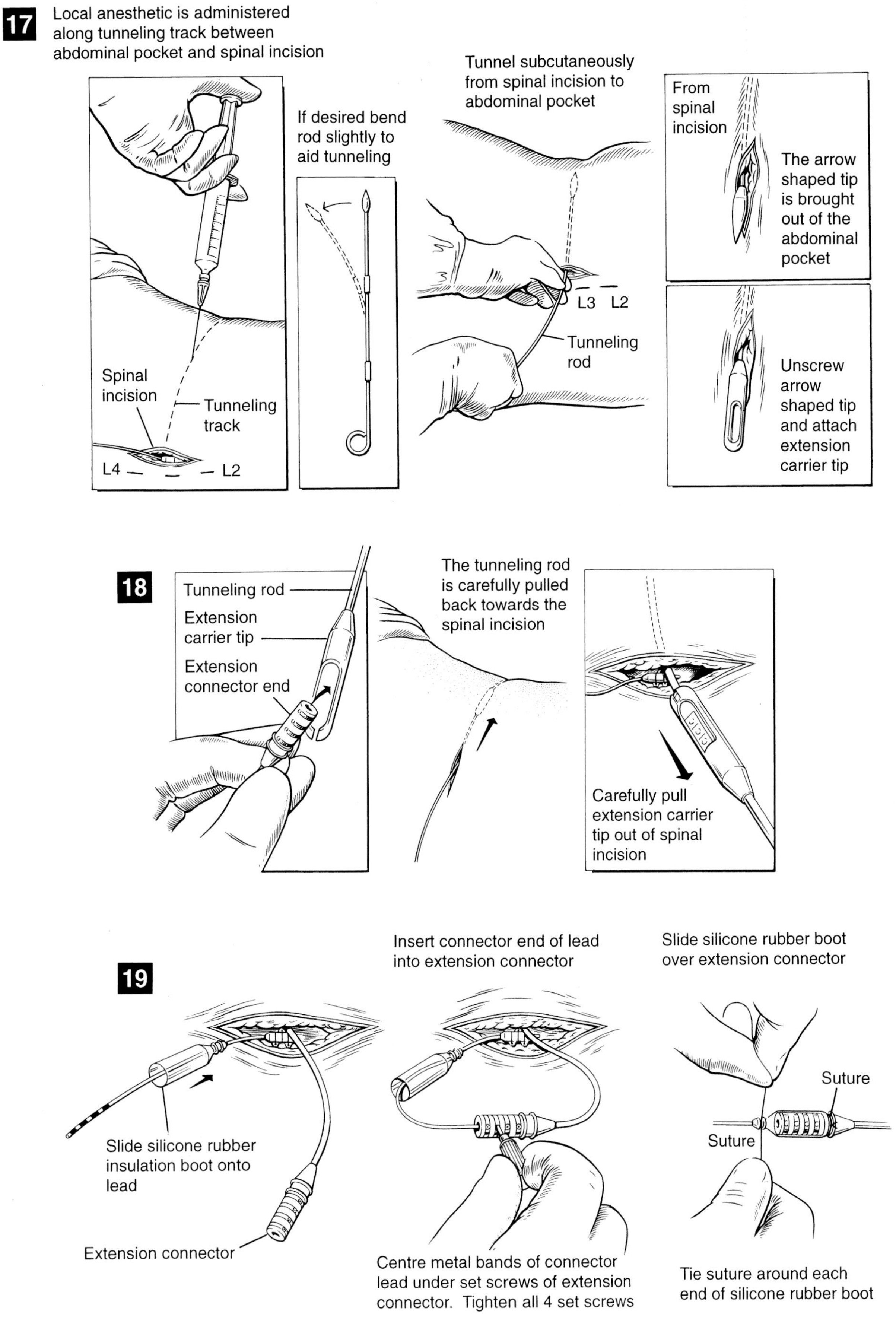
17
Local anesthetic is administered along tunneling track between abdominal pocket and spinal incision
Spinal incision
Tunneling track
L4
L2
If desired bend rod slightly to aid tunneling
Tunnel subcutaneously from spinal incision to abdominal pocket
L3 L2
Tunneling rod
From spinal incision
The arrow shaped tip is brought out of the abdominal pocket
Unscrew arrow shaped tip and attach extension carrier tip
18
Tunneling rod
Extension carrier tip
Extension connector end
The tunneling rod is carefully pulled back towards the spinal incision
Carefully pull extension carrier tip out of spinal incision
19
Insert connector end of lead into extension connector
Slide silicone rubber boot over extension connector
Slide silicone rubber insulation boot onto lead
Extension connector
Centre metal bands of connector lead under set screws of extension connector. Tighten all 4 set screws
Suture
Suture
Tie suture around each end of silicone rubber boot

FIG. 32-18. *Continued.*

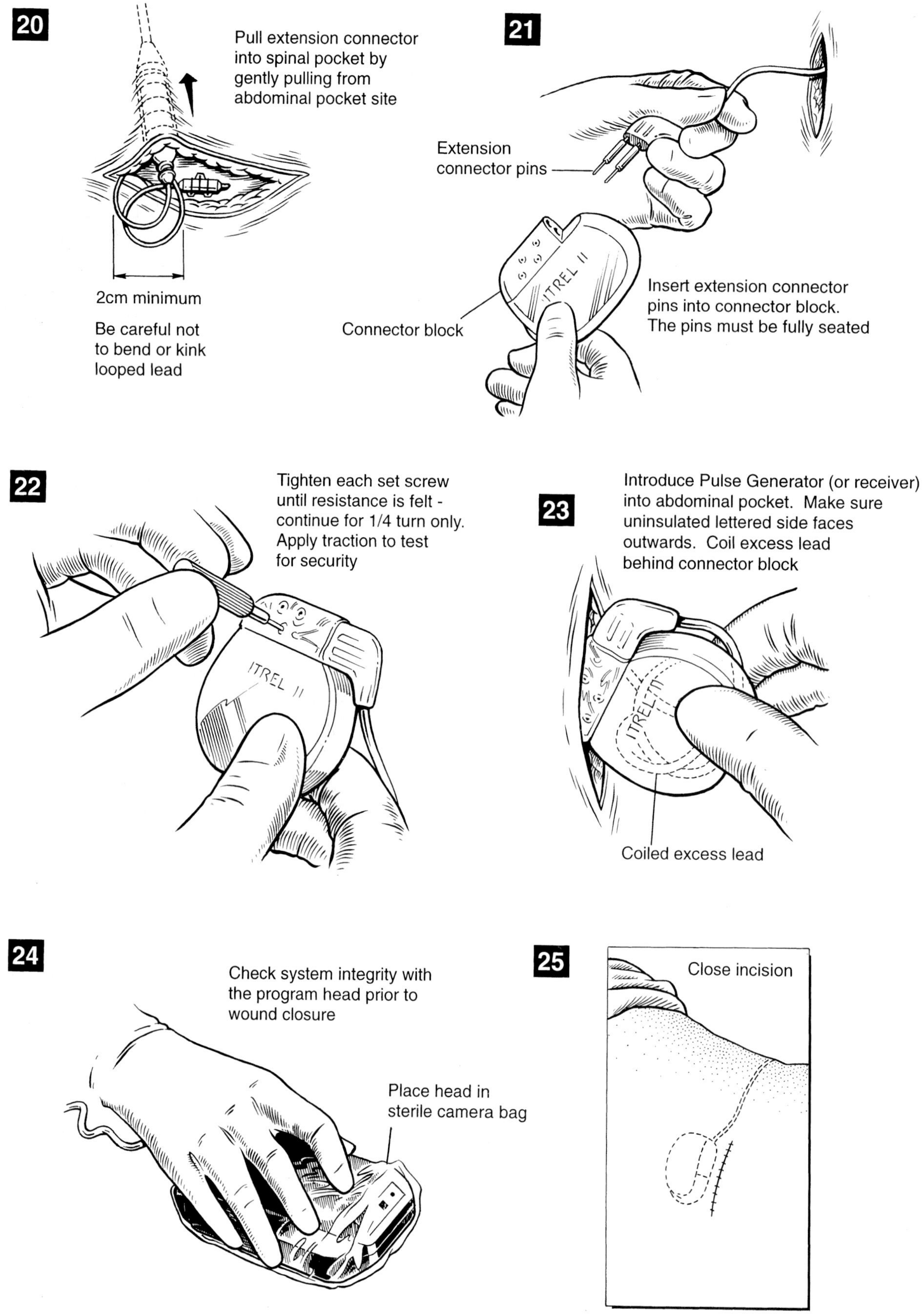
20
Pull extension connector into spinal pocket by gently pulling from abdominal pocket site
2cm minimum
Be careful not to bend or kink looped lead
21
Extension connector pins
Connector block
Insert extension connector pins into connector block. The pins must be fully seated
ITREL II
22
Tighten each set screw until resistance is felt - continue for 1/4 turn only. Apply traction to test for security
ITREL II
23
Introduce Pulse Generator (or receiver) into abdominal pocket. Make sure uninsulated lettered side faces outwards. Coil excess lead behind connector block
Coiled excess lead
24
Check system integrity with the program head prior to wound closure
Place head in sterile camera bag
25
Close incision

FIG. 32-18. *Continued.*

picked up at Figure 32-18.10. Up to this point, the procedure for trial and that for permanent DCS are identical. For permanent implant, the initial insertion of the Tuohy needle must be via a small vertical "stab" incision; this facilitates the step shown in Figure 32-18.10, where the incision is enlarged and extended down to the deep fascia so that the supraspinous ligament can be palpated. Prior infiltration with epinephrine or octapressin containing local anesthetic is essential. It is convenient to have working space both cephalad and caudad to the needle; however, the majority of the space is needed caudad to the entry point of the Tuohy needle through the deep fascia; because of the oblique angle of the needle, this will be achieved if the incision is enlarged equally at skin level cephalad and caudad.

As shown in Figure 32-18.11, a self-retaining retractor (e.g. Mollison's) greatly facilitates the placement of stay sutures. Although a single suture is shown in Figure 32-18.11, it is helpful to insert up to three sutures. The placement of the sutures can be checked by holding the "anchoring device" with a large curved artery forceps (see Fig 32-18.14), in its intended position. At least one of the stay sutures must take a "bite" through the supraspinous ligament. Thus, the Tuohy needle should be inserted using a "paraspinous" rather than a "lateral" technique (see Fig. 8-30, Chapter 8).

The stylet handle, used for test stimulation (Fig. 32-18.8), and stylet must be removed prior to removal of the Tuohy needle (Fig. 32-18.12). Great care must be exercised, when removing the Tuohy needle, to maintain the position of the DCS electrode. It may be helpful to advance the DCS electrode a short distance in the epidural space and then to stabilize the lead and withdraw the epidural needle toward the fixed left hand (Fig. 32-18.12). Once the Tuohy needle is clear of the deep fascia, the DCS lead should be grasped, while the Tuohy needle is gently removed over the metal bands of the DCS lead (Fig. 32-18.13); subsequently the DCS lead may need to be withdrawn into optimal position (see below).

As shown in Fig 32-18.14, the anchoring device is now slid over the DCS lead, and the previously placed sutures are threaded through the eyelets of the wings of the device. It is then optional as to whether a loose tie is made prior to threading the anchor to deep fascia, or the anchor is threaded first and the suture tied while it is *in situ*. It greatly facilitates securing the anchor if it is held in place with a large curved artery forceps while the sutures are tied; otherwise the DCS lead may be unintentionally withdrawn. However, prior to tying the central tie in the anchor groove, to "lock" the DCS lead in the anchor, the position of the DCS lead must be checked. This is particularly so if the lead was advanced prior to removal of the Tuohy needle, in which case it is withdrawn to precisely the level where test stimulation identified satisfactory placement.

Checking the DCS electrode position can be done by "storing" the test position image or by obtaining a hard copy by printer, Polaroid camera, or other device. This also serves

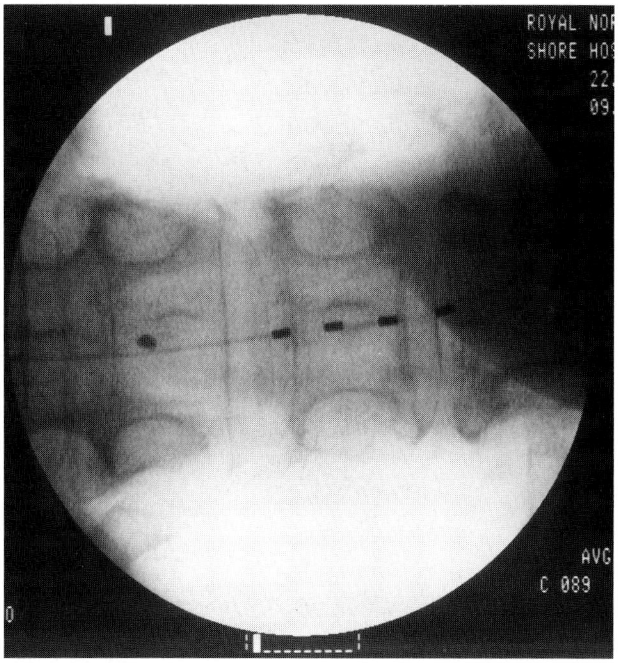

FIG. 32-19. X-ray showing "Quad" DCS lead correctly placed. Note the electrode placed midway between the pedicles (oval-shaped structures equidistant laterally from spinous process). The four electrodes straddle the vertebral body (T10).

as a useful record for subsequent management (Fig. 32-19).

A pocket area is now prepared, either for the totally implanted pulse generator (e.g. Itrel-11) or for the receiver for an external antenna and stimulation transmitter (Figs. 32-18.15 and 32-18.16).

The abdominal site shown in Fig 32-18.15 is frequently used; however, another alternative is below the line of the iliac crest, just above the hip-pocket position. As is the case with the spinal incision, prior infiltration with epinephrine or octapressin containing local anesthetic is essential to provide analgesia and to reduce vascularity of the area.

Tunneling is now performed between the spine incision and the pocket area. The track from spinal site is enlarged laterally for about 5 cm while the tunneling rod is still in place. This can be achieved with blunt dissecting scissors. Subsequent threading of the DCS connector is greatly helped by this step (see following). The extension cord, which will connect DCS lead with pulse generator (e.g. Itrel II) or alternative, is pulled through from the pocket area to the spinal site (Figs. 32-18.17 to 32-18.18).

It is now important to slide the silicone rubber insulation boot onto the DCS lead, prior to inserting the DCS lead into the extension connector (Fig. 32-18.19). It is vital that the metal bands of the DCS lead are positioned under the screws of the extension connector. This is checked by looking through the clear plastic of the extension connector and confirming that the metal bands cannot be seen, and are thus positioned under the set screws. All four screws are tightened with the "torque" screw driver which prevents overtightening. The silicone boot is now slid into position and sutured in place (Fig. 32-18.19). The extension connector can now be pulled laterally into the previously enlarged portion of the lateral tunnel (Fig. 32-18.20). This step is very difficult if the tunnel track has not been opened up as described above, since the bulky extension connector will "catch" posteriorly and will tend not to pull through. Vigorous pulling from the pocket area should not be done since it may damage the DCS system. It is preferable to leave only a gentle curve of DCS lead in the spinal incision area, rather than the several loops often recommended.

The extension connector is now inserted into the connector block of the pulse generator or alternative device and the screws tightened (Figs. 32-18.21 to 32-18.22). The print on the device should face outward. The excess lead is coiled under the device before placing it in the pocket (Fig. 32-18.23).

Finally the function of the stimulator is checked prior to suturing the pocket and spine areas (Fig. 32-18.25).

Results

All reported series of DCS thus far appear to be retrospective, though in some a third party evaluated the results. Most patients treated have suffered from pain derived from lumbar degenerative disk disease. In most series with an unspecified mix of pain syndromes, 40% to 50% of patients reported relief during trial stimulation, and the subsequently implanted devices usually delivered 60% to 84% continuing significant pain relief for an overall success rate of 50% to 65%. There is gradual attrition of relief over time despite continuing adequate technical performance of the device.[315] Complications consisted of electrode migration in up to 61% (average 25%), requiring repositioning or reintroduction, infection in 1% to 7%, incisional pain in up to 58%, electrode breakage in 4% to 23%, receiver failure in 0.5%, transmitter failure in 5%, and antenna failure in 100% within several years; skin irritation or breakdown at the antenna site occurred in 1% to 5% of patients. Tulgar and colleagues[326–328] have carried out an interesting study of the parameters used by DCS patients.

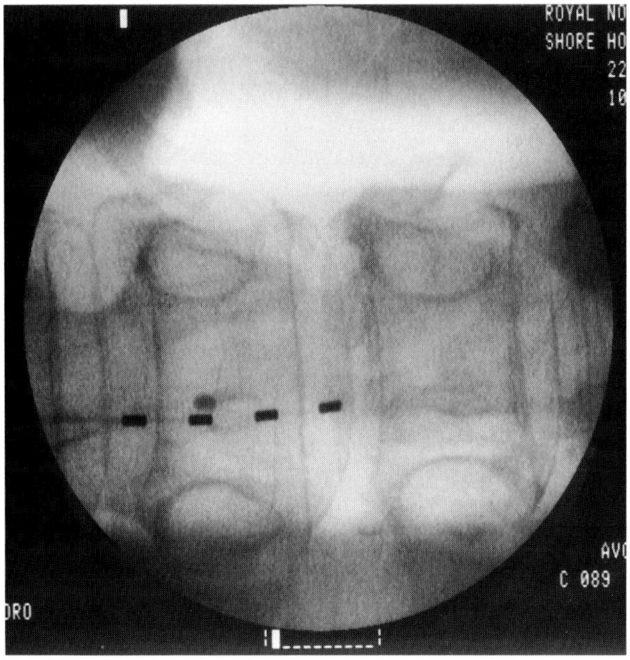

FIG. 32-20. X-ray showing "Quad" DCS lead. In this x-ray there is a parallax error; the midline spinous process is not equidistant from the lateral pedicles. Thus it is not possible to be certain of the position of the electrodes in the midline or laterally.

Table 32-18 lists published data for incidence of permanent implantation of DCS equipment after a trial of stimulation by diagnosis from a review by Tasker and Parrent.[315] Table 32-19 summarizes the longer-term follow-up after implantation of a permanent device, and Table 32-20 lists the complications (see also prospective study[354]).

It is clear that success varies markedly with the diagnosis; central pain of brain and cord origin and phantom limb pain yield the poorest results, and peripheral vascular disease and peripheral nerve injury the best. My own data,[315] collected between 1972 and 1990, are comparable to those of other series. Other conditions that may respond poorly are postherpetic neuralgia[159] and post-thoracotomy syndrome. Problems with phantom and cord central pain in part derive from the technical difficulty of producing paresthesias in the area of pain, since the associated massive deafferentation results in dieback of the dorsal columns to their nuclei. Krainick et al.[122] found that only 23% of 61 amputees enjoyed a good level of long-term pain relief.

When complications (Table 32-20) are reviewed, our incidence of electrode migration, failure, and fracture is higher than in other series since all our procedures were done with a Medtronic monopolar Sigma or straight electrode, with which these problems are more frequent. Moreover, all patients underwent trial stimulation and, if successful, internalization with the same test electrode, yielding a 7% superficial infection rate, which lies at the high end of the spectrum for reported series. Since adoption of the two-stage procedure described above, all these problems have become much less frequent; 22 or 41% of our failures after internalization occurred in the first 3 months despite the fact that paresthesias continued to be felt in the patient's area of pain, suggesting that the initial pain relief in these patients might have been a placebo effect.[165] Other authors[233] have also noted the highest recurrence rate in the first year.

The choice of parameters for DCS does not seem important. Most of our patients used their device through most of the waking day since their pain soon recurred once stimulation stopped; exceptional cases could derive long-lasting relief after an hour or two of DCS. Most patients selected 30 to 50 Hz stimulation and pulse-widths in the range of 0.2 to 0.6 msec. Increasing pulse-width was the most effective strategy for increasing the area of the body in which paresthesias were felt. North et al.[217] found that patients stimulated 0.5 to

TABLE 32-18. *Stimulator implantation after stimulation trial*[a]

	PHN	PVD	FBS	PN	RSD	Amp	Phant	Stump	BPA	Plexus	SCI	Cord	Brain
Barolat *et al.* (1987)[8]					13/16								
Barolat *et al.* (1989)[9]					15/18								
Broggi *et al.* (1987)[28]		31/140			4/6								
Broseta *et al.* (1982)[31]				3/3				5/5	1/1	2/2			
Broseta *et al.* (1986)[29]		37/41											
Cioni *et al.* (1995)[37]												9/25	
Cole *et al.* (1991)[39]	2/4										0/4		
De La Porte and Siegfried (1983)[49]			38/94										
De La Porte and van de Kelft (1993)[50]			64/78										
Demirel *et al.* (1984)[51]			7/11			5/6				6/9	4/8	3/3	
Fiume (1983)[63]		12/21											
Garcia-March *et al.* (1987)[71]									6/6				
Groth (1985)[80]		101/115											
Hood and Siegfried (1984)[94]									5/13	8/8			
Kumar *et al.* (1991)[124]	0/1	4/5	57/66	4/5	2/3	0/2					1/2	10/11	
Meglio and Cioni (1982)[179]	1/3												
Meglio *et al.* (1989)[184]		32/40	13/19										
Meglio *et al.* (1989)[182]	10/15			3/9									
North *et al.* (1993)[217]			133/153										
Richardson *et al.* (1979)[242]			8/9	3/3		2/3							1/1
Richardson *et al.* (1980)[241]											5/7	1/3	
Robaina *et al.* (1989)[243]		3/3			8/8								
Sanchez-Ledesma *et al.* (1989)[252]	4/6			11/13	8/11		3/6	4/5	6/8				
Siegfried and Cetinlap (1981)[267]					11/25					6/15	1/10		
Siegfried and Lazorthes (1982)[268]			89/191										
Spiegelmann and Friedman (1991)[275]	1/3	2/2	12/18	5/6					2/2			4/6	
Tallis *et al.* (1983)[293]		5/10											
Tasker and Parrent (in press)[315]	2/4	4/5	34/43	13/19			2/9	3/7	2/3	7/12		11/31	6/12
Urban and Nashold (1978)[333]	1/2	2/3	3/10	1/1					0/1	0/1	2/2		
Vogel *et al.* (1986)[339]	0/2		16/29				1/3	4/4				0/3	
Waisbrod and Gerbershagen (1985)[341]			16/16										
Wester (1987)[346]	1/2		10/11		1/1		5/5				3/3	4/7	
Winkelmuller (1981)[350]		2/10	56/64			9/12					2/10	1/3	0/1
Totals	22/42	132/170	493/743	43/59	62/88	16/23	11/23	16/21	22/34	29/47	18/46	34/64	6/14
	52%	**77%**	**66%**	**77%**	**70%**	**70%**	**48%**	**76%**	**65%**	**62%**	**39%**	**53%**	**43%**

[a] Number of patients implanted compared to number receiving stimulation trial.

PHN, postherpetic neuralgia; PVD, peripheral vascular disease; FBS, failed back syndrome; PN, peripheral nerve injury; RSD, reflex sympathetic dystrophy; Amp, post-amputation pain (not specified); Phant, phantom limb pain; Stump, post-amputation stump pain; BPA, brachial plexus avulsion; Plexus, plexus injury; SCI, spinal cord injury (traumatic); Cord, pain from other cord lesions; Brain, pain after brain lesions.

TABLE 32-19. *Follow-up after stimulator implantation*[a]

	PHN	PVD	FBS	PN	RSD	Amp	Phant	Stump	BPA	Plexus	SCI	Cord	Brain
Barolat *et al.* (1987)[8]					7/13								
Barolat *et al.* (1989)[9]					11/15								
Broggi *et al.* (1987)[28]		31/31			2/4								
Broseta *et al.* (1982)[31]				3/3				1/5	1/1	2/2			
Broseta *et al.* (1986)[29]		29/37											
Cioni *et al.* (1995)[37]												4/25	
De La Porte and Siegfried (1983)[49]			13/38										
De La Porte and van de Kelft (1993)[50]		94/101	35/64										
Demirel *et al.* (1984)[51]	0/2		3/7			1/5				1/6	0/4	0/3	
Devulder *et al.* (1991)[52]		3/4	24/43	6/11		3/5			1/2		0/3	1/1	
Fiume (1983)[63]		12/12											
Garcia-March *et al.* (1987)[71]									3/6				
Groth (1985)[80]													
Hood and Siegfried (1984)[94]									0/5	2/8			
Krainick *et al.* (1980)[122]						14/61							
Kumar *et al.* (1991)[124]		4/4	37/57	3/4	1/2						0/1	8/10	
Lazorthes and Verdi (1985)[137]			29/57	4/10			0/3	2/3			0/4	3/6	
Long (1981)[163]			18/24	1/1			1/1						
Meglio and Cioni (1982)[179]	1/1											1/1	
Meglio *et al.* (1989)[184]		32/32	2/9								3/5		
Meglio *et al.* (1989)[182]	9/10			3/3									
North *et al.* (1991)[215]			26/50								2/5		
Probst (1990)[233]			62/92										
Ray *et al.* (1982)[236]			27/50										
Richardson *et al.* (1979)[242]			8/8	3/3		2/2							1/1
Richardson *et al.* (1980)[241]											1/5	1/1	
Robaina *et al.* (1989)[243]		3/3			7/8								
Sanchez-Ledesma *et al.* (1989)[252]	3/4			11/11	8/8		1/3	3/4	3/6				
Siegfried and Cetinlap (1981)[267]					4/9					3/4	0/1		
Siegfried (1991)[265]	7/21	12/19	71/123	116/127		13/19					13/17	21/56	
Spiegelmann and Friedman (1991)[275]	0/1	2/2							1/2			3/4	
Tallis *et al.* (1983)[293]		5/5											
Tasker and Parrent (in press)[315]	1/2	4/4	21/34	8/10			0/1	2/2	1/2	3/7		0/10	1/6
Urban and Nashold (1978)[333]	0/1	0/2	2/3	1/1							1/2		
Vogel *et al.* (1986)[339]			4/11				1/1	3/3					
Waisbrod and Gerbershagen (1985)[341]			12/16										
Wester (1987)[346]	1/1		6/8		1/1		2/5				1/3	0/4	
Totals	22/43	134/151	257/450	153/173	40/60	30/87	5/14	11/17	9/22	11/26	11/47	37/85	2/7
	51%	89%	57%	88%	68%	34%	36%	65%	41%	42%	23%	44%	29%
% of all patients tested	**27%**	**69%**	**38%**	**68%**	**48%**	**24%**	**17%**	**49%**	**27%**	**26%**	**9%**	**23%**	**12%**
Tasker and Parrent % all patients tested	25%	80%	49%	42%	—	—	0%	29%	33%	—	—	0	8%

[a] Number of patients with successful outcome compared to total number implanted.

PHN, postherpetic neuralgia; PVD, peripheral vascular disease; FBS, failed back syndrome; PN, peripheral nerve injury; RSD, reflex sympathetic dystrophy; Amp, post-amputation pain (not specified); Phant, phantom limb pain; Stump, post-amputation stump pain; BPA, brachial plexus avulsion; Plexus, plexus injury; SCI, spinal cord injury (traumatic); Cord, pain from other cord lesions; Brain, pain after brain lesions.

TABLE 32-20. *Complications and technical problems with spinal cord stimulation*

	Patients	Lead extrusion	Lead migration	Infection	Hardware pain	Electrode fracture/failure	Receiver failure
Barolat *et al.* (1989)[9]	18		6%	0%	22%	17%	
Broseta *et al.* (1986)[29]	41		24%				
De La Porte and Siegfried (1983)[49]	38	24%	55%	26%	11%	5%	5%
De La Porte and van de Kelft (1993)[50]	35		13%	7.8%		9.3%	
Demirel *et al.* (1984)[51]	33		33%	0%		9%	
Koeze *et al.* (1987)[120]	26		77%	38%		38%	
Kumar *et al.* (1991)[124]	94		27%	9%		12%	2%
Law and Kirkpatrick (1992)[134]	241		5%	2%	8%		
Lazorthes and Verdi (1985)[137]	93	22%	25%	8%		3%	1%
Meglio and Cioni (1982)[179]	26		4%	0%			
Meglio *et al.* (1989)[184]	109		3%	3%			
North *et al.* (1991)[215]	62		2%	11%		13%	
Probst (1990)[233]	42		22%	3%		8%	
Racz *et al.* (1989)[235]	26		69%	8%		23%	12%
Richardson *et al.* (1979)[242]	36		14%	3%			
Sanchez-Ledesma *et al.* (1989)[252]	36	3%	3%	0%			
Simpson (1991)[270]	60		27%	5%		7%	12%
Spiegelmann and Friedman, (1991)[275]	43		3%	7%		13%	
Tasker and Parrent (in press)[315]	101		48%	7%	9%	19%	
Wester (1987)[346]	35		37%	6%	3%		

24 (mean 11.5±8.1) hours daily. Pain relief followed onset of stimulation with a latency of 0 to 60 (mean 8.3±15.7) minutes and outlasted stimulation 0 to 60 (mean 2.0±6.6) hours. Frequency used ranged from 8 to 200 (mean 62.7±54.2) Hz, only one patient stimulating below 25 Hz.

"Failed Back" Pain

The pain associated with chronic degenerative lumbar disk disease consists of a variable mixture of psychogenic, nociceptive, spondylogenic, radicular, and deafferentation pain syndromes associated with root damage, whether produced by disease or previous surgery (see also Chapter 28). Treatment strategies in these patients may include several different modalities tailored to the patients' needs after careful identification of the clinical problem (see also Chapters 27 and 33). First, treatable conditions such as root compression, skeletal instability, and spinal stenosis must be recognized and dealt with. Then a decision must be made on the need for psychotherapy, supportive therapy, TENS, "facet rhizotomy" (rarely, if ever, rhizotomy), and chronic spinal epidural stimulation. DCS has been used mainly to treat the associated leg pain since most authors have found it relatively ineffective for back pain. Probst,[233] for example, reported 67% "very good and good" results in 92 patients for their "radicular" pain, but only 25% for back pain, though occasional very good relief occurred. However, some authors also find DCS useful for treating low back pain,[7,50,51,350] but point out that special efforts are needed to produce persistent paresthesias in the back.[7] Law[130–134] recommends the use of two octopolar electrodes placed parallel to one another near the midline (Fig. 32-21).

Angina

The role of DCS in treating angina pectoris is intriguing but has had relatively little exposure. According to Gonzales-Darder et al.[77], Mannheimer first used TENS and then DCS to treat angina starting in 1982,[170–174] and Murphy and Giles[202] first reported long-term relief in six out of 10 cases, though three died cardiac deaths. These authors treated 12 patients with angina at rest or caused by minimal effort with a DCS electrode inserted at C2 to the left of midline. Stimulation caused paresthesias in the left neck, shoulder, upper thorax, upper extremity, and hand. A trial of over 3 to 5 days using a Medtronic Quad percutaneous electrode was followed by internalization. In all patients, the frequency of angina attacks fell; one patient died suddenly, one developed pulmonary edema when the stimulator battery failed, and one died of renal failure; one electrode became displaced. Staal et al.[277] examined DCS in refractory angina in an open randomized study involving 22 patients with percutaneous monopolar epidural electrodes, finding subjective and objective evidence for benefit that included reduction of both pain and cardiac ischemia. One patient suffered five electrode displacements. Others[17] have presented evidence that high cervical DCS improves carotid and cerebral blood flow in the laboratory and in man,[32,48,97,183] but it is still not certain whether the effect of DCS in angina is on pain, perfusion, or both.[59,171]

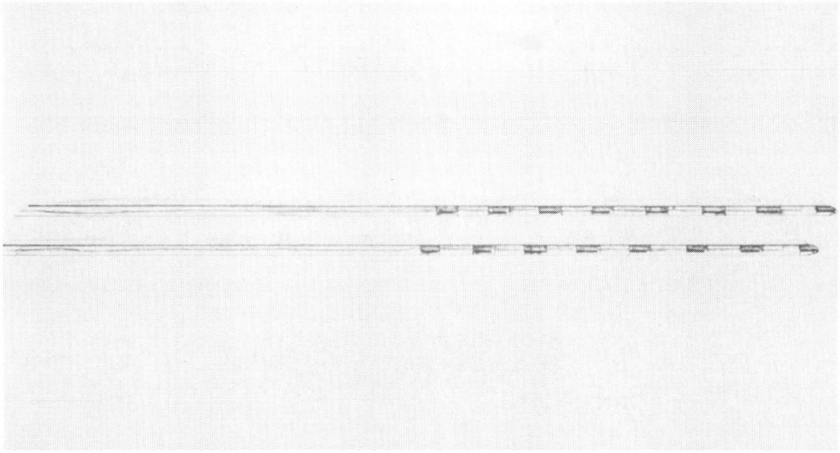

FIG. 32-21. Neuromed dual octrode DCS equipment for treating low back pain.

Peripheral Vascular Disease

The use of DCS to treat the pain of PVD has similarly been attributed both to direct effects on pain and to vasodilation,[4,5,30,147,148,180,293] but the benefit of DCS in this condition is undisputed; PVD is the best indication for DCS,[42,80,180] though most authors do not find a true limb-saving effect. Naver et al.[213] present an interesting case study of a woman whose contralateral arm became cyanotic and cold after a high sympathectomy with removal of stellate and thoracic ganglion down to T4. After 2 years, DCS at C5–C6 had an immediate vasodilating effect on the arm with a 10-fold, Doppler-measured, increase in blood flow. They present evidence that the effect is sympathetically mediated. Polisca et al.[231] treated 11 patients with PVD for 15 months, noting pain reduction but not improvement in gangrenous changes, despite 40% increase in exercise tolerance. Groth[80] found not only reduction in pain, but also increased claudication distance and evidence for increased blood flow (increase in toe pressure, foot skin temperature, blood flow in the skin of the foot, and blood flow in muscle at rest).

Sacral Plexus Stimulation

A new application of chronic stimulation is the percutaneous stimulation of the sacral plexus. Electrodes are introduced through first the dorsal and then the ventral sacral foramina into the plexus.[6] The technique is useful for the relief of unspecified chronic rectal and lower limb pain, though accompanying motor contractions make the technique impractical in leg pain.

CONCLUSION

The treatment of intractable pain first requires that the pain problem be dissected into its various components such as psychogenic, deafferentation, and nociceptive problems. Treatment techniques must then be selected starting with the simplest, using percutaneous techniques whenever possible. Progression to more complex techniques is pursued as far as the disability caused by the pain, and not the underlying disease, and the risks warrant, keeping in mind the likelihood of success. Both interruptive and modulatory procedures are available for both nociceptive and deafferentation pain syndromes. Of those discussed here, the treatment of choice for nociceptive pain is percutaneous cordotomy, and for deafferentation pain, chronic spinal epidural or trigeminal stimulation. For tic douloureux, selective percutaneous radiofrequency thermocoagulation of the roots in Meckel's cave is one of the most satisfactory approaches.

REFERENCES

1. Amano, M., Kawasura, H., Tanikawa, T., *et al.*: Bilateral versus unilateral percutaneous high cervical cordotomy as a surgical method of pain relief. Acta Neurochi., 52(suppl.):143, 1991.
2. Apfelbaum, R.I.: Surgical management of disorders of the lower cranial nerves. *In* Schmidek, H.H., and Sweet, W.H., (eds.): Operative Neurosurgical Techniques. Indications, Methods and Results. 2nd Ed. pp. 1097 Orlando, Grune & Stratton, 1988.
3. Armour, D.: Surgery of the spinal cord and its membranes. Lancet, *ii:*691, 1927.
4. Augustinsson, L.-E., Carlsson, C.-A., and Leissner, P.: Effect of dorsal column stimulation on pain-induced intracerebral impulse patterns. Appl. Neurophysiol., *42:*212, 1979.
5. Augustinsson, L.E., Holm, J., Carlsson, C.A., and Jivegård, L.: Epidural electrical stimulation in severe limb ischaemia. Evidences of pain relief, increased blood flow and a possible limb-saving effect. Ann. Surg., *202:*104, 1985.
6. Barolat, G.: Percutaneous retroperitoneal stimulation of the sacral plexus. Stereotact. Funct. Neurosurg. *56:*250, 1991.
7. Barolat, G.: Spinal cord stimulation for persistant pain management. *In* Gildenberg, P.L., and Tasker, R.R. (eds.): Stereotactic and Functional Neurosurgery. pp. 1519–1537. New York, McGraw Hill, 1998.
8. Barolat, G., Schwartzmann, R., and Woo, R.: Epidural spinal cord stimulation in the management of reflex sympathetic dystrophy. Appl. Neurophysiol., *50:*442, 1987.
9. Barolat, G., Schwartzmann, R., and Woo, R.: Epidural spinal cord stimulation in the management of reflex sympathetic dystrophy. Stereotact. Funct. Neurosurg., *53:*29, 1989.
10. Barolat, G., Zeme, S., and Ketcik, B.: Multifactorial analysis of epidural spinal cord stimulation. Stereotact. Funct. Neurosurg., *56:*77, 1991.

11. Bel, S., and Bauer, B.L. Dorsal column stimulation (DCS): Cost to benefit analysis. Acta Neurochir. Suppl. *52:*121, 1991.
12. Belber, C.J., and Rak, R.A.: Balloon compression rhizolysis in the surgical management of trigeminal neuralgia. Neurosurgery, *20:*908, 1987.
13. Belmusto, L., Brown, E., and Owens, G.: Clinical observations on respiratory and vasomotor disturbances as related to cervical cordotomies. J. Neurosurg., *20:*225, 1963.
14. Belmusto, L., Woldring, S., and Owens, G.: Localization and patterns of potentials of the respiratory pathways in the cervical spinal cord in the dog. J. Neurosurg., *22:*277, 1965.
15. Bennett, G.J.: The role of the sympathetic nervous system in painful peripheral neuropathy. Pain, *45:*221, 1991.
16. Blair, R.D.G., Lee, R.G., and Vanderlinden, G.: Dorsal column stimulation. Its effect on the somatosensory evoked response. Arch. Neurol., *32:*826, 1975.
17. Blomberg, S., Emanuelsson, H., and Ricksten, S.E.: Thoracic epidural anesthesia and central hemodynamics in patients with unstable angina pectoris. Anesth. Analg. *69:*558, 1989.
18. Boas, R.A., Hatangdi, V.S., and Richards, E.G.: Lumbar sympathectomy - a percutaneous chemical technique. *In* Bonica, J.J., and Albe-Fessard, D.G. (eds.): Advances in Pain Research and Therapy. Vol 1. pp. 685. New York, Raven, 1976.
19. Blume, H.G.: Radiofrequency denervation in occipital pain: A new approach in 114 cases. *In* Bonica, J.J., and Albe-Fessard, D.G., (eds.): Advances in Pain Research and Therapy. Vol 1. pp. 691. New York, Raven, 1976.
20. Blume, H., and Fromm, S.: Radiofrequency denervation in occipital pain: A new approach. Sixth International Congress of Neurologic Surgeons. International Congress Series, *148:*221, 1977.
21. Boureau, F., Doubrère, J.F., and Luu, M.: Study of verbal description in neuropathic pain. Pain, *5:*(Suppl.)S465, 1990.
22. Bowsher, D.: Contralateral mirror-image pain following anterolateral cordotomy. Pain, *33:*63, 1988.
23. Brandwin, M.A., and Kewman, D.G.: MMPI indicators of treatment response to spinal epidural stimulation in patients with chronic pain and patients with movement disorders. Psychol. Rep. *51:*1059, 1982.
24. Bricolo, A., and Dalle Ore, G.: Percutaneous microcompression of the gasserian ganglion for trigeminal neuralgia; preliminary results. Acta Neurochir. *69:*102, 1983.
25. Broggi, G.C.: Surgical treatment of glossopharyngeal neuralgia and pain from cancer of the nasopharynx. J. Neurosurg. *61:*952, 1984.
26. Broggi, G.C., and Siegfried, J.: Percutaneous differential radiofrequency rhizotomy of glossopharyngeal nerve in facial pain due to cancer. *In* Bonica, J.J., and Ventafridda, V. (eds.): Advances in Pain Research and Therapy. Vol 2. pp. 469. New York, Raven, 1979.
27. Broggi, G., Franzini, A., *et al.*: Neurochemical and structural modifications related to pain control induced by spinal cord stimulation. *In* Lazorthes, Y., and Upton, A. (eds.): Neurostimulation: An Overview. pp. 87. New York, Futura Publishing, 1985.
28. Broggi, G., Servello, D., Franzini, A., *et al.*: Spinal cord stimulation for treatment of peripheral vascular disease. Appl. Neurophysiol., *50:*439, 1987.
29. Broseta, J., Barbera, J., De Vera, J.A., *et al.*: Spinal cord stimulation in peripheral arterial disease. A cooperative study. J. Neurosurg., *64:*71, 1986.
30. Broseta, J., Garcia-March, G., Sanchez, M.J., and Gonzáles, J.: Influence of spinal cord stimulation on peripheral blood flow. Appl. Neurophysiol., *48:*367, 1985.
31. Broseta, J., Roldan, P., González-Darder, J., *et al.*: Chronic epidural spinal cord stimulation in the treatment of causalgic pain. Appl. Neurophysiol., *45:*190, 1982.
32. Broseta, J., Sánchez-Ledesma, M.J., Silva, I., *et al.*: High cervical spinal cord electrical stimulation in brain infarction: Experimental basis and preliminary clinical experience. Acta Neurochir., *117:*95, 1992.
33. Bruyn, C.W.: Glossopharyngeal neuralgia. Cephalalgia, *3:*143, 1983.
34. Campbell, J.N.: Examination of possible mechanisms by which stimulation of the spinal cord in man relieves pain. Appl. Neurophysiol. *44:*181, 1981.
35. Capper, S.J., Conlon, J.M., Lahuerta, J., *et al.*: Peptide concentrations in the CSF following injection of alcohol into the pituitary gland. Pain, *2*(Suppl):S316, 1984.
36. Cassinari, V., and Pagni, C.A.: Central Pain: A Neurosurgical Survey. Cambridge, Harvard, 1969.
37. Cioni, B., Meglio, M., Pentimalli, L., and Visocchi, M.: Spinal cord stimulation in the treatment of paraplegic pain. J. Neurosurg., *82:*35, 1995.
38. Coffey, R.J., Krieger, D.N., and Sclabasse, R.J.: Evoked potential recording using radiofrequency-coupled stimulation of internalized dorsal column stimulation electrodes in pain patients. Stereotact. Funct. Neurosurg., *59:*20, 1992.
39. Cole, J.D., Illis, L.S., and Sedgwick, E.M.: Intractable central pain in spinal cord injury is not relieved by spinal cord stimulation. Paraplegia, *29:*167, 1991.
40. Condouris, G.A.: Local anesthetics as modulators of neural information. *In* Bonica, J.J., and Albe-Fessard, D.G. (eds.): Advances in Pain Research and Therapy. Vol 1. pp. 663. New York, Raven, 1976.
41. Cook, A.W., Nathan, P.W., and Smith, M.C.: Sensory consequences of commissural myelotomy. A challenge to traditional anatomical concepts. Brain, *107:*547, 1984.
42. Cook, A.W., Oygar, A., Baggenstos, P., *et al.*: Vascular disease of extremities. New York State J. Med., *76:*366, 1976.
42a.Cousins, M.J., Reeve, T.S., Glynn, C.J., *et al.*: Neurolytic lumbar sympathetic blockade: duration of denervation and relief of rest pain. Anaesth. Intens. Care, *7:*121, 1979.
43. Cross, F.W., and Cotton, L.T.: Chemical lumbar sympathectomy for ischemic rest pain. A randomized prospective controlled clinical trial. Am. J. Surg., *150:*341, 1985.
44. Crue, B.L., Todd, E.M., and Carregal, E.J.A.: Posterior approach for high cervical percutaneous radiofrequency cordotomy. Confin. Neurol., *30:*41, 1968.
45. Crue, B.L., Todd, E.M., and Carregal, E.J.: Percutaneous radiofrequency stereotactic trigeminal tractotomy. *In* Crue, B.L. (ed.): Pain and Suffering. pp. 69 Springfield, Ill., Charles C. Thomas, 1970.
46. Crue, B.L., Jr., Todd, E.M., Carregal, E.J.A., and Kilham, O.: Percutaneous trigeminal tractotomy. Case report utilizing stereotactic radiofrequency lesion. Bull. Los Angeles Neurol. Soc., *32:*86, 1967.
47. Daniel, M., Long, C., Hutcherson, M., and Hunter, S.: Psychological factors and outcome of electrode implantation for chronic pain. Neurosurgery, *17:*773, 1985.
48. De Landsheere, C., Rigo, P., and Kulbertus, H.E.: Epidural spinal cord stimulation: any effect on regional myocardial perfusion? Int. Congr. Epidural Spinal Cord Stimulation, Groningen, 1989.
49. De La Porte, C., and Siegfried, J.: Lumbar spinal fibrosis (spinal arachnoiditis)—its diagnosis and treatment by spinal cord stimulation. Spine, *8:*593, 1983.
50. De La Porte, C., and Van de Kelft, E.: Spinal cord stimulation in failed back surgery syndrome. Pain, *52:*55, 1993.
51. Demirel, T., Braun, W., and Reimers, C.D.: Results of spinal cord stimulation in patients suffering with chronic pain after a two-year observation period. Neurochirurgia, *27:*47, 1984.
52. Devulder, J., Vermeulen, H., De Colvenaer, L., *et al.*: Spinal cord stimulation in chronic pain: Evaluation of results, complications, and technical considerations in sixty-nine patients. Clin. J. Pain, *7:*21, 1991.
53. Dondelinger, R., and Kurdziel, J.C.: Percutaneous phenol neurolysis of the lumbar sympathetic chain with computed tomography control. Ann. Radiol., *27:*376, 1984.
54. Dong, W.K., and Wagman, I.H.: Modulation of nociceptive responses in the thalamic posterior group of nuclei. *In* Bonica, J.J., and Albe-Fessard, D. (eds.): Advances in Pain Research and Therapy. pp. 455. New York, Raven, 1976.
55. Dooley, D.M.: A technique for the epidural percutaneous stimulation of the spinal cord in man. Presented Annual Meeting AANS, Miami Beach, 1975.
56. Dubuisson, D.: Effect of dorsal-column stimulation on gelatinosa and marginal neurons of cat spinal cord. J. Neurosurg., *70:*257, 1989.
57. Dubuisson, D.: Root surgery. *In* Wall, P.D., and Melzack, R. (eds.): Textbook of Pain. 3rd Ed. pp. 1055 Edinburgh, Churchill Livingstone, 1994.
58. Duggan, A.W., and Foong, F.W.: Bicuculline and spinal inhibition produced by dorsal column stimulation in the cat. Pain, *22:*249, 1985.
59. Eliasson, T., Jern, S., Leijon, M., *et al.*: Clinical effects of epidural electrical stimulation (ESES) in angina pectoris. Effect on arrhythmia, myocardial perfusion and clinical long-term effects. Pain, S235, 1990.
60. Eiras, J., Garcia, J., Gomez, J., *et al.*: First results with extralemniscal myelotomy. Acta Neurochir., *30*(Suppl.):377, 1980.
61. Erickson, D.L.: Percutaneous trial of stimulation for patient selection for implantable stimulating electrodes. J. Neurosurg., *43:*440, 1975.

62. Farcot, J.-M., Mercky, F., Tritschler, J.-L., and Schaeffer, F.: Cordotomies cervicales percutanées dans les douleurs cancéreuses thoraciques primitives ou secondaires (a propos de 19 cas). Agressologie, *29:*87, 1988.
63. Fiume, D.: Spinal cord stimulation in peripheral vascular disease. Appl. Neurophysiol., *46:*290, 1983.
64. Flanigan, D.P., and Kraft, R.O.: Continuing experience with palliative chemical splanchnicectomy. Arch. Surg., *113:*509, 1978.
65. Foreman, R.D., Beall, J.A., Applebaum, A.E., *et al.*: Effects of dorsal column stimulation on primate spinothalamic tract neurons. J. Neurophysiol., *39:*534, 1976.
66. Fox, J.L.: Localization of the respiratory pathway in the upper cervical spinal cord following percutaneous cordotomy. Neurology, *19:*1115, 1969.
67. Fox, J.L.: Delineation of the obex by contrast radiography during percutaneous trigeminal tractotomy. Technical note. J. Neurosurg., *36:*107, 1972.
68. Fox, J.L.: Percutaneous trigeminal tractotomy. Variations in delineation of the obex using emulsified pantopaque. Confin. Neurol., *36:*97, 1974.
69. Fraioli, B., Esposito, V., and Santoro, A.: Treatment of trigeminal neuralgia by percutaneous techniques: therapeutic protocol. Pain, *4*(Suppl.):S126, 1987.
70. Franck, J., Brodin, E., and Fried, G.: Differential release of endogenous 5-hydroxytryptamine, substance P, and neurokinin A from rat ventral spinal cord in response to electrical stimulation. J. Neurochem., *61:*704, 1993.
71. Garcia-March, G., Sanchez-Ledesma, M.J., Diaz, P., *et al.*: DREZ lesions versus spinal cord stimulation in the management of pain from brachial plexus avulsion. Acta Neurochir., *39*(Suppl.):155, 1987.
72. Garcia-Larrea, L., Sindou, M., and Mauguiere, F.: Nociceptive flexion reflexes during analgesic neurostimulation in man. Pain, *39:*145, 1990.
73. Gardner, A.M.N., and Solomou, G. Relief of the pain of unresectable carcinoma of pancreas by chemical splanchnicectomy during laparotomy. Ann. Roy. Coll. Surg. Engl., *66:*409, 1984.
74. Gildenberg, P.L., Zanes, C., Flitter, M.A., *et al.*: Impedance monitoring device for detection of penetration of the spinal cord in anterior percutaneous cervical cordotomy. Technical note. J. Neurosurg., *30:*87, 1969.
75. Gildenberg, P.L., and Murthy, K.S.K.: Influence of dorsal column stimulation upon human thalamic somatosensory-evoked potentials. Appl. Neurophysiol., *43:*8, 1980.
76. Giorgi, C., and Broggi, G.: Surgical treatment of glossopharyngeal neuralgia and pain from cancer of the nasopharynx. A 20-year experience. J. Neurosurg., *61:*952, 1984.
77. González-Darder, J.M., Canela, P., and Gonzáles-Martinez, V. High cervical spinal cord stimulation for unstable angina pectoris. Stereotact. Funct. Neurosurg., *56:*20, 1991.
78. Grieshop, I., Goldstein, F.P., and Larson, S.J.: Spinal electroanaesthesia. Its relationship to somatosensory cerebral evoked potentials. *In* Electrotherapeutic Sleep and Electroanaesthesia. Amsterdam, Excerpta Medica, 1990.
79. Grote, W., and Roosen, C.W.: Die percutane chordotomie. Langenbecks Arch. Chir., *342:*101, 1976.
80. Groth, K.E.: Spinal cord stimulation for the treatment of peripheral vascular disease. *In* Fields, H.L., *et al.* (eds.): Advances in Pain Research and Therapy. Vol 9. pp. 861. New York, Raven, 1985.
81. Gybels, J.M.: Analyses of clinical outcome of a surgical procedure. Pain, *44:*103, 1991.
82. Gybels, J.M., and Sweet, W.H.: Neurosurgical treatment of persistent pain; physiological and pathological mechanisms of human pain. *In* Gildenberg, P.L. (ed.): Pain and Headache. Basel, Karger, 1989.
83. Håkansson, S.: Trigeminal neuralgia treated by the injection of glycerol into the trigeminal cistern. Neurosurgery, *9:*683, 1981.
84. Handwerker, H.O., Iggo, A., and Zimmermann, M.: Segmental and supraspinal actions on dorsal horn neurons responding to noxious and non-noxious stimuli. Pain, *1:*147, 1975.
85. Härtel, F.: Die Leitungsanästhesie und Injections—behandlung des Ganglion Gasseri und der Trigeminusstäme. Arch. Klin. Chir., *100:*193, 1912.
86. Hillman, P., and Wall, P.D.: Inhibitory and excitatory factors influencing the receptive fields of lamina 5 spinal cord cells. Exp. Brain Res., *9:*284, 1969.
87. Hitchcock, E.R.: An apparatus for stereotactic spinal surgery. Lancet, *i:*705, 1960.
88. Hitchcock, E.R.: Stereotactic spinal surgery. A preliminary report. J. Neurosurg., *31:*386, 1969.
89. Hitchcock, E.R.: Stereotactic cervical myelotomy. J. Neurol. Neurosurg. Psychiatry, *33:*224, 1970.
90. Hitchcock, E.R.: Stereotactic trigeminal tractotomy. Ann. Clin. Res. *2:*131, 1970.
91. Hitchcock, E.R., and Leece, B.: Somatotopic representation of the respiratory pathways in the cervical cord of man. J. Neurosurg., *27:*320, 1967.
92. Hitchcock, E.R., and Tsukamoto, Y.: Distal and proximal sensory responses during stereotactic spinal tractotomy in man. Ann. Clin. Res., *5:*68, 1973.
93. Hitchcock, E.R., and Schvarcz, J.R.: Stereotaxic trigeminal tractotomy for post-herpetic facial pain. J. Neurosurg., *37:*412, 1972.
94. Hood, T.W., and Siegfried, J.: Epidural vs thalamic stimulation for the management of brachial plexus lesion pain. Acta Neurochir., *33:*(suppl)451, 1984.
95. Hoppenstein, R.: Electrical stimulation of the ventral and dorsal columns of the spinal cord for the relief of chronic intractable pain. Preliminary report. Surg. Neurol., *4:*180, 1975.
96. Hoppenstein, R.: Percutaneous implantation of chronic spinal cord electrode for control of intractable pain. Preliminary report. Surg. Neurol., *4:*195, 1975.
97. Hosobuchi, Y.: Electrical stimulation of the cervical spinal cord increases cerebral blood flow in humans. Appl. Neurophysiol., *48:*372, 1985.
98. Hosobuchi, Y., Adams, J.E., and Weinstein, P.R.: Preliminary percutaneous dorsal column stimulation prior to permanent implantation. Technical note. J. Neurosurg., *37:*242, 1972.
99. Hosobuchi, Y., Rutkin, B., Neilson, D., and Adams, J.E.: Evoked potential study of dorsal column stimulator—a potential explanation for DCS failures. *In* Hosobuchi, Y., and Corbin, T. (eds.): Indications for Spinal Cord Stimulation. pp. 97. Amsterdam, Excerpta Medica, 1981.
100. Hyndman, O.R.: Lissauer's tract section. A contribution to chordotomy for the relief of pain. (Preliminary report.) J. Int. Coll. Surg. *5:*394, 1942.
101. Iacono, R.P., Boswell, M.V., and Guthkelch, A.N.: Placement of spinal cord stimulators using spinal anaesthesia and monitored by cortical evoked potentials obtained from spinal cord stimulation. Pain, *5:*S234, 1990.
102. Iacono, R.P., Guthkelch, A.N., and Boswell, M.V.: Dorsal root entry zone stimulation for deafferentation pain. Stereotact. Funct. Neurosurg., *59:*56, 1992.
103. Inbal, R., Devor, M., Tuchendler, O., and Lieblich, I.: Autotomy following nerve injury: Genetic factors in the development of chronic pain. Pain, *9:*327, 1980.
104. Isamat, F., Ferrán, E., and Acebes, J.J.: Selective percutaneous thermocoagulation rhizotomy in essential glossopharyngeal neuralgia. J. Neurosurg., *55:*575, 1981.
105. Ischia, S., and Ischia, A.: A mechanism of new pain following cordotomy (letter). Pain, *32:*383, 1988.
106. Ischia, S., Ischia, A. Luzzani, A., *et al.*: Results up to death in the treatment of persistent cervicothoracic (Pancoast) and thoracic malignant pain by unilateral percutaneous cervical cordotomy. Pain, *21:*339, 1985.
107. Ischia, S., Luzzani, A., Ischia, A., and Maffezzoli, G.: Bilateral percutaneous cervical cordotomy immediate and long-term results in 36 patients with neoplastic disease. J. Neurol. Neurosurg. Psychiatry, *47:*141, 1984.
108. Ischia, S., Luzzani, A., Ischia, A., *et al.*: Subarachnoid neurolytic block (L5-S1) and unilateral percutaneous cervical cordotomy in the treatment of pain secondary to pelvic malignant disease. Pain, *20:*139, 1984.
109. Ischia, S., Luzzani, A., Ischia, A., and Pacini, L.: Role of unilateral percutaneous cervical cordotomy in the treatment of neoplastic vertebral pain. Pain, *19:*123, 1984.
110. Izumi, J., Hirose, Y., and Yazaki, T.: Percutaneous trigeminal rhizotomy and percutaneous cordotomy under general anesthesia. Stereotact. Funct. Neurosurg., *59:*62, 1992.
111. Jannetta, P.J.: Arterial compression of the trigeminal nerve at the pons in patients with trigeminal neuralgia. J. Neurosurg., *26:*159, 1967.
112. Jones, M.W.: Effects of dorsal column stimulation on three aspects of pain: burning, shooting and steady aching. Acta Neurochir., *117:*95, 1992.

113. Kanpolat, Y., Deda, H., Akyar, S., and Bilgic, S.: CT-guided percutaneous cordotomy. Acta Neurochir. *46:*(suppl.)67, 1989.
114. Katusic, S., Williams, D.B., Beard, C.M., *et al.*: Incidence and clinical features of glossopharyngeal neuralgia. Rochester, Minnesota, 1945–1984. Neuroepidemiology, *10:*266, 1991.
115. Katusic, S., Williams, D.B., Beard, C.M., *et al.*: Epidemiology and clinical features of idiopathic trigeminal neuralgia and glossopharyngeal neuralgia: Similarities and differences. Rochester, Minnesota 1945–1984. Neuroepidemiology, *10:*276, 1991.
116. Katz, J.: Current role of neurolytic agents. *In* Bonica, J.J. (ed.): Advances in Neurology. Vol 4. pp. 471. New York, Raven, 1974.
117. Kibler, R.F., and Nathan, P.W.: Relief of pain and paraesthesia by nerve block distal to a lesion. J. Neurol. Neurosurg. Psychiatry, *23:*91, 1960.
118. King, J.: Glossopharyngeal neuralgia. Clin. Exp. Neurol., *24:*113, 1987.
119. Kirschner, M.: Elektrokoagulation des Ganglion Gasseri. Zentralbl. Chir., *47:*2841, 1932.
120. Koeze, T.H., de Williams, A.C., and Reiman, S.: Spinal cord stimulation and the relief of chronic pain. J. Neurol. Neurosurg. Psychiatry, *50:*1424, 1987.
121. Koulousakas, A., and Nittner, K.: Bilateral C1-C2 cordotomies. Can complications be avoided? Appl. Neurophysiol., *45:*500, 1982.
122. Krainick, J.U., Thoden, U., and Riechert, T.: Pain reduction in amputees by long-term spinal cord stimulation. J. Neurosurg., *52:*346, 1980.
123. Kühner, A.: La cordotome percutanée. Sa place actuelle dans la chirurgie de la douleur. Anesth. Analg., *38:*357, 1981.
124. Kumar, K., Nath, R., and Wyant, G.M.: Treatment of chronic pain by epidural spinal cord stimulation: a 10 year experience. J. Neurosurg., *75:*402, 1991.
125. Kupers, R.C., Van den Oever, R., Van Houdenhove, B., *et al.*: Spinal cord stimulation in Belgium: A nation-wide survey on the incidence, indications and therapeutic efficacy by the health insurer. Pain, *56:*211, 1994.
126. Lahuerta, T., Lipton, S., and Wells, J.C.D.: Percutaneous cervical cordotomy: Results and complications in a recent series of 100 patients. Ann. Roy. Coll. Surg. Engl. *67:*41, 1985.
127. Larson, S.J., Sances, A., Cusick, J.F., *et al.*: A comparison between anterior and posterior spinal implant systems. Surg. Neurol., *4:*180, 1975.
128. Larson, S.J., Sances, A. Jr., Riegel, D.H., *et al.*: Neurophysiological effects of dorsal column stimulation in man and monkey. J. Neurosurg., *41:*217, 1974.
129. Latchaw, J.P., Jr., Hardy, R.W., Jr., Forsythe, S.B., and Cook, A.F.: Trigeminal neuralgia treated by radiofrequency coagulation. Neurosurgery, *59:*479, 1983.
130. Law, J.: Spinal stimulation: Statistical superiority of monophasic stimulation of narrowly separated longitudinal bipoles having rostral cathodes. Appl. Neurophysiol., *46:*129, 1983.
131. Law, J.D.: A new method for targeting a spinal stimulator: Quantitatively paired comparisons. Appl. Neurophysiol., *50:*436, 1987.
132. Law, J.D.: Spinal stimulation in the "failed back surgery syndrome": Comparison of technical criteria for palliating pain in the leg vs. in the low back. Acta Neurochir., *117:*95, 1992.
133. Law, J.D.: Targeting a spinal stimulator to treat the "failed back surgery syndrome." Appl. Neurophysiol., *50:*437, 1987.
134. Law, J.D., and Kirkpatrick, A.F. Update: spinal cord stimulation. A.J.P.M., *2:*34, 1992.
135. Lazorthes, Y., Verdie, J.C., and Lagarrigue, J.: Thermocoagulation percutanée des nerfs rachidiens à visée analgésique. Neurochirurgie, *22:*445, 1976.
136. Lazorthes, Y., and Verdie, J.C.: Radiofrequency coagulation of the petrous ganglion in glossopharyngeal neuralgia. Neurosurgery, *4:*512, 1979.
137. Lazorthes, Y., and Verdie, J.C.: Technical evolution and long-term results of chronic spinal cord stimulation. *In* Lazorthes, Y., and Upton, A. (eds.): Neurostimulation: An overview. pp. 67. New York, Futura Publishing, 1985.
138. Lazorthes, Y., Verdie, J.-C., and Arbus, L.: Stimulation analgésique medullaire antérieure et postérieure par technique d'implantation percutanée. Acta Neurochir., *40:*253, 1978.
139. Le Doux, M.S., and Langford, KH.: Spinal cord stimulation for the failed back syndrome. Spine, *18:*191, 1993.
140. Lema, J.A., and Hitchcock, E.: Respiratory changes after stereotactic high cervical cord lesions for pain. Appl. Neurophysiol., *49:*62, 1986.
141. Levin, A.B., Ramirez, L.F., and Katz, J.: The use of stereotaxic chemical hypophysectomy in the treatment of thalamic pain syndrome. J. Neurosurg. *59:*1002, 1983.
142. Levitt, M., and Levitt, J.H.: The deafferentation syndrome in monkeys: Dysesthesias of spinal origin. Pain, *10:*129, 1981.
143. Lin, P.M., Gildenberg, P.L., and Polakoff, P.P.: An anterior approach to percutaneous lower cervical cordotomy. J. Neurosurg., *25:*553, 1966.
144. Lindblom, U., and Meyerson, B.A.: Influence on touch, vibration and cutaneous pain of dorsal column stimulation in man. Pain, *1:*257, 1975.
145. Lindblom, U., Tapper, N., and Wiesenfeld, Z.: The effect of dorsal column stimulation on the nociceptive response of dorsal horn cells and its relevance for pain suppression. Pain, *4:*133, 1977.
146. Linderoth, B.: Dorsal column stimulation and pain: Experimental studies of putative neurochemical and neurophysiological mechanisms. Thesis Karolinska Inst, Stockholm, 1992.
147. Linderoth, B., Fedorcsak, I., and Meyerson, B.A.: Is vasodilation following dorsal column stimulation mediated by antidromic activation of small diameter afferents? Acta Neurochir. *46:*(suppl.)99, 1989.
148. Linderoth, B., Fedorcsak, I., and Meyerson, B.A.: Peripheral vasodilation after spinal cord stimulation: animal studies of putative effector mechanisms. Neurosurgery, *28:*187, 1991.
149. Linderoth, B., Gazelius, B., Franck, J., and Brodin, E.: Dorsal column stimulation induces release of serotonin and substance P in the cat dorsal horn. Neurosurgery, *31:*289, 1992.
150. Linderoth, B., Stiller, C.-O., Gunasekera, L., *et al.*: Release of neurotransmitters in the CNS by spinal cord stimulation: survey of present state of knowledge and recent experimental studies. Stereotact. Funct. Neurosurg., *61:*157, 1993.
151. Linderoth, B., Stiller, C., Gunasekera, L., *et al.*: Gamma-aminobutyric acid is released in the dorsal horn by electrical spinal cord stimulation: An in vivo microdyalisis study in the rat. Neurosurgery, *34:*484, 1994.
152. Lipton, S.: Percutaneous cervical cordotomy and the injection of the pituitary with alcohol. Anaesthesia, *33:*953, 1978.
153. Lipton, S.: Percutaneous cervical cordotomy. Acta Anaesthesiol. Belg., *32:*81, 1981.
154. Lipton, S.: Percutaneous cordotomy. *In* Wall, P.D., and Melzack, R. (eds.): Textbook of Pain. pp. 632. Edinburgh, Churchill Livingstone, 1984.
155. Livingston, W.K.: Pain Mechanisms: A Physiologic Interpretation of Causalgia and Its Related Causes. 2nd Ed. New York, Plenum, 1976.
156. Lobato, R.D., Rivas, J.J., Sarabia, R., and Madrid, J.L.: Percutaneous compression of the Gasserian ganglion for trigeminal neuralgia. Pain, *4:*(Suppl.)S129, 1987.
157. Loeser, J.D.: Tic douloureux and atypical face pain. *In* Wall, P.D., and Melzack, R. (eds.): Textbook of Pain, 2nd Ed. pp. 535. Edinburgh, Churchill Livingstone, 1989.
158. Loeser, J.D.: Tic douloureux and atypical face pain. *In* Wall, P.D., and Melzack, R. (eds.): Textbook of Pain. pp. 699. 3rd Ed. Edinburgh, Churchill Livingstone, 1994.
159. Loeser, J.D.: Herpes zoster and postherpetic neuralgia. Pain, *25:*149, 1986.
160. Loeser, J.D., Ward, A.A., and White, L.E.: Chronic deafferentation of human spinal cord neurons. J. Neurosurg., *29:*48, 1968.
161. Loh, L., and Nathan, P.W.: Painful peripheral states and sympathetic blocks. J. Neurol. Neurosurg. Psychiatry, *41:*664, 1978.
162. Loh, L., Nathan, P.W., and Schott, G.D.: Pain due to lesions of central nervous system removed by sympathetic block. Br. Med. J., *282:*1026, 1981.
163. Long, D.: Patient selection and results of spinal cord stimulation for chronic pain. *In* Hosobuchi, Y., and Corbin, T. (eds.): Indications for Spinal Cord Stimulation. pp. 1. Amsterdam, Excerpta Medica, 1981.
164. Long, D.M., and Hagfors, N.: Electrical stimulation in the nervous system: The current status of electrical stimulation of the nervous system for relief of pain. Pain, *1:*109, 1975.
165. Long, D.M., Uematsu, S., and Kouba, R.B.: Placebo responses to medical device therapy for pain. Stereotact. Funct. Neurosurg., *53:*149, 1989.
166. Lorenz, R.: Methods of percutaneous spinothalamic tract section. *In* Krayenbühl, H. (ed.): Advances and Technical Standards in Neurosurgery. Vol 3. pp. 123. Vienna, Springer Verlag, 1976.
167. Lozano, A.M.: Microsurgical C2 ganglionectomy for chronic intractable occipital pain. Presented at the 62nd Annual Meeting, AANS, San Diego, April 9–14, 1994.

168. Lunsford, L.D., and Bennett, M.H.: Percutaneous retrogasserian glyerol rhizotomy for tic douloureux. Part 1. Technique and results in 112 patients. Neurosurgery, *14:*424, 1984.
169. Madrid, J.L.: Chemical hypophysectomy. *In* Bonica, J.J., and Ventafridda, V. (eds.): Advances in Pain Research and Therapy. Vol 2. pp. 381. New York, Raven, 1979.
170. Mannheimer, C., Augustinsson, L., Carlsson, C., *et al.*: Epidural spinal electrical stimulation in severe angina pectoris. Eur. Heart J., *59:*56, 1988.
171. Mannheimer, C., Augustinsson, L.-E., Eliasson, T., *et al.*: Myocardial release of endogeneous opioids in human heart and the effect of epidural electrical stimulation (ESES) in pacing-induced angina pectoris. Pain, *5*(Suppl.):S82, 1990.
172. Mannheimer, C., Carlsson, C.A., Emanuelsson, H., *et al.*: The effects of transcutaneous electrical nerve stimulation in patients with severe angina pectoris. Circulation, *71:*308, 1985.
173. Mannheimer, C., Carlsson, C.A., Eriksson, K., *et al.*: Transcutaneous electrical nerve stimulation in severe angina pectoris. Eur. Heart J., *3:*297, 1982.
174. Mannheimer, C., Carlsson, C.-A., Vedin, A., and Wilhelmsson, C.: Transcutaneous electrical nerve stimulation in severe angina pectoris: a controlled long-term study. *In* Fields, H.L., Dubner, R., and Cervero, F. (eds.): Advances in Pain Research and Therapy. Vol 9. pp. 853 New York, Raven, 1985.
175. Marchand, S., Bushnell, M.C., Molina-Negro, P., *et al.*: The effects of dorsal column stimulation on measures of clinical and experimental pain in man. Pain, *45:*249, 1991.
176. Maxwell, R.F.: Surgical control of chronic migrainous neuralgia by trigeminal ganglio-rhizolysis. J. Neurosurg., *57:*459, 1982.
177. Mayer, D.J., and Price, P.D. Central nervous system mechanisms of analgesia. Pain, *2:*379, 1976.
178. Meglio, M., and Cioni, B.: The role of percutaneous cordotomy in the treatment of chronic cancer pain. Acta Neurochir., *59:*111, 1981.
179. Meglio, M., and Cioni, B.: Personal experience with spinal cord stimulation in chronic pain management. Appl. Neurophysiol., *45:*195, 1982.
180. Meglio, M., Cioni, B., Dal Lago, A., *et al.*: Pain control and improvement of peripheral blood flow following epidural spinal cord stimulation. J. Neurosurg., *54:*821, 1981.
181. Meglio, M., Cioni, B., D'Annunzio, V., and Rossi, G.F.: A comparison of the results of treatment of trigeminal neuralgia using gasserian ganglion percutaneous microcompression and selective thermocoagulation. J. Neurosurg. Sci., *29:*166, 1985.
182. Meglio, M., Cioni, B., Prezioso, A., and Talamonti, G.: Spinal cord stimulation in the treatment of postherpetic pain. Acta Neurochir. *46*(suppl):65, 1989.
183. Meglio, M., Cioni, B., Rossi, G.F., *et al.*: Spinal cord stimulation affects the central mechanisms of heart rate. Appl. Neurophysiol., *49:*139, 1986.
184. Meglio, M., Cioni, B., and Rossi, G.F.: Spinal cord stimulation in management of chronic pain—a 9 year experience. J. Neurosurg., *70:*519, 1989.
185. Melzack, R., and Wall, P.D.: Pain mechanisms. A new theory. Science, *150:*971, 1965.
186. Mertens, P., Sindou, M., Gharios, B., *et al.*: Spinal cord stimulation (SCS) for pain treatment. Prognostic value of somesthetic evoked potential (SEP). Acta Neurochir., *117:*90, 1992.
187. Meyerson, B.A.: Electrostimulation procedures: Effects, presumed rationale, and possible mechanisms. *In* Bonica, J.J., Lindblom, U., and Iggo, A. (eds.): Advances in Pain Research and Therapy. Vol 5. pp. 495 New York, Raven, 1983.
188. Meyerson, B.A., Arnér, S., and Linderoth, B.: Pros and cons of different approaches to the management of pelvic cancer pain. Acta Neurochir., *33*(Suppl.):407, 1984.
189. Meyerson, B.A., Brodin, E., and Linderoth, B.: Possible neurohumeral mechanisms in CNS stimulation for pain suppression. Appl. Neurophysiol., *48:*175, 1985.
190. Meyerson, B.A., and Håkansson, S.: Alleviation of atypical trigeminal pain by stimulation of the gasserian ganglion via an implanted electrode. Acta Neurochir., *30*(Suppl.):303, 1980.
191. Meyerson, B.A., Herregodts, P., and Linderoth, B.: Enhanced flexor reflex in the mononeuropathic rat is attenuated by spinal cord stimulation. Acta Neurochir., *117:*88, 1992.
192. Miles, J.: Chemical hypophysectomy. *In* Bonica, J.J., and Ventafridda, V. (eds.): Advances in Pain Research and Therapy. Vol 2. pp. 373. New York, Raven, 1979.
193. Miles, J.: Pituitary destruction. *In* Wall, P.D., and Melzack, R. (eds.): Textbook of Pain. pp. 656. Edinburgh, Churchill Livingstone, 1984.
194. Miles, J.: Pituitary destruction. *In* Wall, P.D., and Melzack, R. (eds.): Textbook of Pain. 3rd Ed: pp. 1159. Edinburgh, Churchill Livingstone, 1994.
195. Modesti, L.M., and Waszak, M.: Firing pattern of cells in human thalamus during dorsal column stimulation. Appl. Neurophysiol., *38:*251, 1975.
196. Moore, D.C.: Role of nerve block with neurolytic solutions for pelvic visceral cancer pain. *In* Bonica, J.J., and Ventafridda, V. (eds.): Advances in Pain Research and Therapy. Vol 2. pp. 593. New York, Raven, 1979.
197. Moore, D.C.: Celiac (splanchnic) plexus block with alcohol for cancer pain of the upper intra-abdominal viscera. *In* Bonica, J.J., and Ventafridda, V. (eds.): Advances in Pain Research and Therapy. Vol 2. pp. 357. New York, Raven, 1979.
198. Morrica, G.: Chemical hypophysectomy for cancer pain. *In* Bonica, J.J. (ed.): Advances in Neurology. Vol 4. pp. 707. New York, Raven, 1974.
199. Mullan, S., and Hosobuchi, Y.: Respiratory hazards of high cervical percutaneous cordotomy. J. Neurosurg., *28:*291, 1968.
200. Mullan, S., Harper, P.V., Hekmatpanah, J., *et al.*: Percutaneous interruption of spinal pain tracts by means of a strontium-90 needle. J. Neurosurg., *20:*931, 1963.
201. Mullan, S., and Lichtor, I.: Percutaneous microcompression of the trigeminal ganglion for trigeminal neuralgia. J. Neurosurg., *59:*1007, 1983.
202. Murphy, D.F., and Giles, K.E.: Dorsal column stimulation for pain relief from intractable angina pectoris. Pain, *28:*365, 1987.
203. Nagara, T., Amakawa, K., Arai, T., and Ochi, G.: Ipsilateral referral of pain following cordotomy. Pain, *55:*275, 1993.
204. Nagara, T., Amakawa, K., Kumura, S., and Arai, T.: Reference of pain following percutaneous cervical cordotomy. Pain, *53:*205, 1993.
205. Nagara, T., Kimura, S., and Arai, T.: A mechanism of new pain following cordotomy; Reference of sensation. Pain, *30:*89, 1987.
206. Nash, T.P.: Percutaneous radiofrequency lesioning of dorsal root ganglia for intractable pain. Pain, *24:*67, 1986.
207. Nashold, B.S., and Ostdahl, R.H.: Dorsal root entry zone lesions for pain relief. J. Neurosurg., *51:*59, 1979.
208. Nashold, B.S., Lopez, H., and Chodakiewitz, J.: Trigeminal DREZ for facial pain. *In* Samii, M. (ed.): Surgery in and Around the Brain Stem and the Third Ventricle. pp. 54. Berlin, Springer-Verlag, 1986.
209. Nathan, P.W.: On the pathogenesis of causalgia in peripheral nerve lesions. Brain, *70:*145, 1947.
210. Nathan, P.W.: Reference of sensation at the spinal level. J. Neurol. Neurosurg. Psychiatry, *19:*88, 1956.
211. Nathan, P.W.: Improvement in cutaneous sensitivity associated with relief of pain. J. Neurol. Neurosurg. Psychiatry, *23:*202, 1960.
212. Nathan, P.W.: The descending respiratory pathway in man. J. Neurol. Neurosurg. Psychiatry, *26:*487, 1963.
213. Naver, H., Augustinsson, L.E., and Elam, M. The vasodilating effect of spinal cord stimulation is mediated by sympathetic nerves. Clin. Auton. Res., *2:*41, 1992.
214. Nishimoto, H., Tsubokawa, T., Yamamoto, T., *et al.*: Inhibitory effect of dorsal column stimulation upon thalamic noxious neurons. Appl. Neurophysiol., *43:*336, 1980.
215. North, R.B., Ewend, M.G., Lawton, M.T., and Piantadosi, S.: Spinal cord stimulation for chronic intractable pain: Superiority of "multi-channel" devices. Pain, *44:*119, 1991.
216. North, R.B., Fowler, K., Nigrin, D.J., and Szymanski, R.: Patient-interactive computer-controlled neurological stimulation system: Clinical efficacy in spinal cord stimulator adjustment. J. Neurosurg., *76:*967, 1992.
217. North, R.B., Kidd, D.H., Zahurak, M., *et al.*: Spinal cord stimulation for chronic intractable pain: Experience over two decades. Neurosurgery, *32:*384, 1993.
218. Nugent, G.R., and Berry, B.: Trigeminal neuralgia treated by differential radiofrequency coagulation of the gasserian ganglion. J. Neurosurg., *40:*517, 1974.
219. Nyquist, J.K., and Greenhoot, J.H.: Responses evoked from the thalamic centrum medianum by painful input: Suppression by dorsal funicular conditioning. Exp. Neurol., *39:*215, 1973.
220. O'Connell, J.E.A.: Anterolateral chordotomy for intractable pain in carcinoma of the rectum. Proc. Roy. Soc. Med., *62:*31, 1969.

221. Onofrio, B.M.: Cervical spinal cord and dentate delineation in percutaneous radiofrequency cordotomy at the level of the first to second cervical vertebrae. Surg. Gynecol. Obstet., *133:*30, 1971.
222. Onofrio, B.M., and Campbell, J.K.: Surgical treatment of chronic cluster headache. Mayo Clin. Proc., *61:*537, 1986.
223. Ori, C., Salar, G., and Giron, G.P.: Cardiovascular and cerebral complications during glossopharyngeal nerve thermocoagulation. Anesthesia, *40:*433, 1985.
224. Pagura, J.R.: Percutaneous radiofrequency spinal rhizotomy. Appl. Neurophysiol., *46:*138, 1983.
225. Pagura, J.R., Schnapp, M., and Passarelli, P.: Percutaneous radiofrequency glossopharyngeal rhizolysis for cancer pain. Appl. Neurophysiol., *46:*154, 1983.
226. Palma, A., Hozer, J., Cuadra, O., and Palma, J.: Lateral percutaneous spinothalamic tractotomy. Acta Neurochir., *93:*100, 1988.
227. Papo, I.: Spinal posterior rhizotomy and commissural myelotomy in the treatment of pain. *In* Bonica, J.J., and Ventafridda, V. (eds.): Advances in Pain Research and Therapy. Vol 2. pp. 439. New York, Raven, 1979.
228. Papo, I., and Visca, A.: Phenol subarachnoid rhizotomy for the treatment of cancer pain: a personal account on 290 cases. *In* Bonica, J.J., and Ventafridda, V. (eds.): Advances in Pain Research and Therapy. Vol 2. pp. 339. New York, Raven, 1979.
229. Parrent, A., Lozano, A., Tasker, R.R., and Dostrovsky, J.: Periventricular gray stimulation suppresses allodynia and hyperpathia in man. Stereotact. Funct. Neurosurg., *59:*82, 1992.
230. Poletti, C.E.: Open cordotomy medullary tractotomy. *In* Schmidek, H.H., and Sweet, W.H. (eds.): Operative Neurosurgical Techniques: Indications, Methods and Results. 2nd Ed. pp. 1155. Orlando, Grune & Stratton, 1988.
231. Polisca, R., Domenichini, M., Signoretti, P., and Marchi, P.: SCS (spinal cord stimulation) nelle gravi ischeme degli arti inferiori. Minerva Anestesiol., *58:*419, 1992.
232. Portenoy, R.K.: Issues in the management of neuropathic pain. *In* Basbaum, A.L., and Besson, J.-M. (eds.): Towards a New Pharmacotherapy of Pain. pp. 393. New York, Wiley & Sons, 1991.
233. Probst, C.: Spinal cord stimulation in 112 patients with epi/intradural fibrosis following operation for lumbar disc herniation. Acta Neurochir. (Wien), *107:*147, 1990.
234. Probst, C.L.: Microsurgical cordotomy in 20 patients with epi/intradural fibrosis following operation for lumbar disc herniation. Acta Neurochir., *107:*30, 1990.
235. Racz, G.B., McCarron, R.F., and Talboys, P.: Percutaneous dorsal column stimulation for chronic pain control. Spine, *14:*1, 1989.
236. Ray, C.D., Burton, C.V., and Lifson, A.: Neurostimulation as used in a large clinical practice. Appl. Neurophysiol., *45:*160, 1982.
237. Reddy, K., Hobson, D.E., Gomori, A., and Sutherland, G.R.: Painless glossopharyngeal "neuralgia" with syncope: A case report and literature review. Neurosurgery, *21:*916, 1987.
238. Rees, H., and Roberts, M.H.: Antinociceptive effects of dorsal column stimulation in the rat: Involvement of the anterior pretectal nucleus. J. Physiol., *417:*375, 1989.
239. Reid, W., Watt, J.K., and Gray, T.G.: Phenol injection of the sympathetic chain. Br. J. Surg., *57:*45, 1970.
240. Richardson, D.E., and Dempsey, C.W.: Monoamine turnover in CSF of patients during dorsal column stimulation for pain control. Pain, *2*(suppl):224, 1984.
241. Richardson, R.R., Meyer, P.R., and Cerullo, L.J.: Neurostimulation in the modulation of intractable paraplegic and traumatic neuroma pains. Pain, *8:*75, 1980.
242. Richardson, R.R., Siqueira, E.B., and Cerullo, L.J.: Spinal epidural neurostimulation for treatment of acute and chronic intractable pain: Initial and long-term results. Neurosurgery, *5:*344, 1979.
243. Robaina, E.J., Dominguez, M., Diaz, M., *et al.*: Spinal cord stimulation for relief of chronic pain in vasospastic disorders of the upper limbs. Neurosurgery, *24:*63, 1989.
244. Romano, M., Zucco, F., Baldini, M.R., and Allara, B.: Technical and clinical problems in patients with simultaneous implantation of a cardiac pacemaker and spinal cord stimulator. Pace, *16:*1639, 1993.
245. Rosomoff, H.L.: Bilateral percutaneous radiofrequency cordotomy. J. Neurosurg., *31:*41, 1969.
246. Rosomoff, H.L.: Percutaneous radiofrequency cervical cordotomy for intractable pain. Sixth International Congress of Neurologic Surgeons. International Congress Series. Amsterdam, Excerpta Medica, *148:*110, 1977.
247. Rosomoff, H.L., Carroll, E., Brown, J., and Sheptak, P.: Percutaneous radiofrequency cervical cordotomy: Technique. J. Neurosurg., *23:*639, 1965.
248. Rosomoff, H.L., Krieger, A.J., and Kuperman, A.S.: Effects of percutaneous cervical cordotomy on pulmonary function. J. Neurosurg., *31:*620, 1969.
249. Rosomoff, H.L., Papo, I., Loeser, J.D., and Bonica, J.J.: Neurosurgical operations on the spinal cord. *In* Bonica, J.J. (ed.): The Management of Pain. 2nd Ed. pp. 2067. Philadelphia, Lea & Febiger, 1990.
250. Rushton, J.G., Stevens, C., and Miller, R.H.: Glossopharyngeal (vasoglossopharyngeal) neuralgia. A study of 217 cases. Arch. Neurol., *38:*201, 1981.
251. Saade, N.E., and Jabbur, S.J.: Dorsal column influence, through the brain stem, on spinal nociceptive input. *In* Rowe, M. and Willis, W.D. (eds.): Development, Organization, Processing in Somatosensory Pathways. pp. 367–373. Allan R Liss Inc, 1985.
252. Sanchez-Ledesma, M.J., Garcia-March, G., Diaz-Cascajo, P., *et al.*: Spinal cord stimulation in deafferentation pain. Stereotact. Funct. Neurosurg., *53:*40, 1989.
253. Salar, G., Ori, C., Baratto, V., *et al.*: Selective percutaneous thermolesions of the ninth cranial nerve by lateral cervical approach: Report of eight cases. Surg. Neurol., *20:*276, 1983.
254. Satran, R., and Goldstein, M.N.: Pain perception: Modification of threshold of intolerance and cortical potentials by cutaneous stimulation. Science, *180:*1201, 1973.
255. Schvarcz, J.R.: Spinal cord stereotactic techniques re trigeminal nucleotomy and extralemniscal myelotomy. Appl. Neurophysiol., *41:*99, 1978.
256. Schvarcz, J.R.: Stereotatic spinal trigeminal nucleotomy for dysesthetic facial pain. *In* Bonica, J.J., Liebeskind, J.C., and Albe-Fessard, D.G. (eds.): Advances in Pain Research and Therapy. Vol 3. pp. 331. New York, Raven, 1979.
257. Schvarcz, J.R.: Stereotactic high cervical extralemniscal myelotomy for pelvic cancer pain. Acta Neurochir., *33*(Suppl):341, 1984.
258. Shealy, C.N.: Pain suppression through posterior column stimulation. *In* Fields, W.S. (ed.): Neural Organization and its Relevance to Prosthetics. pp. 251. New York, Intercontinental Medical Book Corp, 1973.
259. Shealy, C.N., Mortimer, J.T., and Hagfors, N.R.: Dorsal analgesia. J. Neurosurg., *32:*560, 1970.
260. Shealy, C.N., Mortimer, J.T., and Reswick, J.B.: Electrical inhibition of pain by stimulation of the dorsal columns—preliminary clinical report. Anesth. Analg., *46:*489, 1967.
261. Shealy, C.N., Tashitz, N., Mortimer, J.T., and Becker, D.P.: Electrical inhibition of pain: Experimental evaluation. Anesth. Analg., *46:*299, 1967.
262. Sheldon, C.H.: Depolarization in the treatment of trigeminal neuralgia: Evaluation of compression and electrical methods; clinical concept of neurophysiological mechanisms. *In* Knighton, R.S., and Dumke, P.R. (eds.): Pain. pp. 373. Boston, Little Brown, 1966.
263. Sheldon, C.H., Pudenz, R.H., Freshwater, D.B., *et al.*: Compression rather than decompression for trigeminal neuralgia. J. Neurosurg. *12:*123, 1955.
264. Shetter, A.G., and Atkinson, J.R. Dorsal column stimulation: Its effect on medial bulboreticular unit activity evoked by noxious stimuli. Exp. Neurol., *54:*185, 1977.
265. Siegfried, J.: Therapeutic neurostimulation—indications reconsidered. Acta Neurochir., *52*(Suppl.):112, 1991.
266. Siegfried, J., and Broggi, G.: Percutaneous thermocoagulation of the gasserian ganglion in the treatment of pain in advanced cancer. *In* Bonica, J.J., and Ventafridda, V. (eds.): Advances in Pain Research and Therapy. Vol 2. pp. 463. New York, Raven, 1979.
267. Siegfried, J., and Cetinlap, E.: Neurosurgical treatment of phantom limb pain: A survey of methods. *In* Siegfried, J., and Zimmermann, M. (eds.): Phantom and Stump Pain. pp. 148. New York, Springer-Verlag, 1981.
268. Siegfried, J., and Lazorthes, Y.: Long-term follow-up of dorsal column stimulation for chronic pain syndrome after multiple lumbar operations. Appl. Neurophysiol., *45:*201, 1982.
269. Siegfried, J., Kühner, A., and Sturm, V.: Neurosurgical treatment of cancer pain. Recent results. Cancer Res. *89:*148, 1984.
270. Simpson, B.A.: Spinal cord stimulation in 60 cases of intractable pain. J. Neurol. Neurosurg. Psychiatry, *54:*196, 1991.
271. Simpson, R.K., Jr., Robertson, C.S., Goodman, J.C., and Halter, J.A.:

Recovery of amino acid neurotransmitters from the spinal cord during posterior epidural stimulation: A preliminary study. J. Am. Paraplegia Soc., *14:*3, 1991.
272. Sindou, M., Fischer, G., Goutelle, A., and Mansuy, L.: La radicellotomie postérieure sélective. Premiers résultats dans la chirurgie de la douleur. Neurochirurgie, *20:*391, 1974.
273. Sindou, M., Henry, J.F., and Blanchard, P.: Névralgie essentielle du glossopharyngien étude d'une série de 14 cas et revue de la littérature. Neurochirurgie, *37:*18, 1989.
274. Spaziante, R., Ferone, A., and Cappabianca, P.: Simplified method to implant chronic stimulating electrode in the gasserian ganglion. Appl. Neurophysiol., *49:*1, 1986.
275. Spiegelmann, R., and Friedman, W.A.: Spinal cord stimulation: A contemporary series. Neurosurgery, *28:*65, 1991.
276. Spiller, W.G., and Martin, E.: The treatment of persistent pain of organic origin in the lower part of the body by division of the anterolateral column of the spinal cord. J.A.M.A., *58:*1489, 1912.
277. Staal, M., de Jongste, M., and Zijlstra, G.: Spinal cord stimulation for intractable angina pectoris. Acta Neurochir., *117:*95, 1992.
278. Steude, V.: Radiofrequency electrical stimulation of the gasserian ganglion in patients with atypical trigeminal pain. Acta Neurochir., *33*(Suppl.):481, 1984.
279. Stiller, C.O., O'Connors, W., and Linderoth, B.: PAG-microdialysis in the awake, freely moving rat during spinal cord stimulation: Release of GABA. Acta Neurochir., *117:*87, 1992.
280. Struijk, J.J., Holsheimer, J., van Veen, B.K., and Boom, H.B.K.: Epidural spinal cord stimulation: Calculation of field potentials with special reference to dorsal column nerve fibers. IEEE Trans. Biomed. Eng., *38:*104, 1991.
281. Struijk, J.J., Holsheimer, J., van der Heide, G.G., and Boom, H.B.: Recruitment of dorsal column fibers in spinal cord stimulation: Influence of collateral branching. IEEE Trans. Biomed. Eng., *39:*903, 1992.
282. Struijk, J.J., Holsheimer, J., and Boom, H.B.: Excitation of dorsal root fibers in spinal cord stimulation: a theoretical study. IEEE Trans. Biomed. Eng., *40:*632, 1993.
283. Stuart, G., and Cramond, T.: Role of percutaneous cervical cordotomy for pain of malignant origin. Med. J. Australia, *158:*667, 1993.
284. Sweet, W.H.: Treatment of trigeminal neuralgia by percutaneous rhizotomy. *In* Youmans, J.R. (ed.): Neurological Surgery. A Comprehensive Reference Guide to the Diagnosis and Management of Neurosurgical Problems. 3rd ed. pp. 3888. Philadelphia, Saunders, 1990.
285. Sweet, W.H., and Poletti, C.E.: Retrogasserian glycerol injection as treatment for trigeminal neuralgia. *In* Schmidek, H.H., and Sweet, W.H. (eds.): Operative Neurosurgical Techniques. Indications, Methods and Results. pp. 1107. New York, Grune & Stratton, 1982.
286. Sweet, W.H., and Wepsic, J.G. Treatment of chronic pain by stimulation of fibres of primary afferent neuron. Trans. Am. Neurol. Assoc., *93:*103, 1968.
287. Sweet, W.H., and Wepsic, S.G.: Controlled thermocoagulation of trigeminal ganglion and results for differential destruction of pain fibres. J. Neurosurg., *29:*143, 1974.
288. Sweet, W.H., Mark, V.H., and Hamlin, H.: Radiofrequency lesions in the central nervous system of man and cat, including case reports of eight bulbar pain tract interruptions. J. Neurosurg. *17:*213, 1960.
289. Swerdlow, M.: Subarachnoid and extradural neurolytic blocks. *In* Bonica, J.J., and Ventafridda, V. (eds.): Advances in Pain Research and Therapy. Vol 2. pp. 325. New York, Raven, 1979.
290. Taarnhöj, P.: Decompression of the trigeminal root and the posterior part of the ganglion as treatment in trigeminal neuralgia. Preliminary communication. J. Neurosurg., *9:*288, 1952.
291. Takeda, F., Fujii, T., Uki, J., *et al.*: Cancer pain relief and tumor regression by means of pituitary neuroadenolysis and surgical hypophysectomy. Neurol. Med. Chir. Tokyo, *23:*41, 1983.
292. Takeda, F., Uki, J., Fujii, T., *et al.*: Pituitary neuroadenolysis to relieve cancer pain: Observations of spread of ethanol installed into the sella turcica and subsequent changes of the hypothalamopituitary axis at autopsy. Neurol. Med. Chir. Tokyo, *23:*50, 1983.
293. Tallis, R.C., Illis, L.S., Sedgwick, E.M., *et al.*: Spinal cord stimulation in peripheral vascular disease. J. Neurol. Neurosurg. Psychiatry, *46:*478, 1983.
294. Taren, J.A.: Physiologic corroboration in stereotactic high cervical cordotomy. Confin. Neurol., *33:*285, 1971.
295. Taren, J.A., Davis, R., and Crosby, E.C.: Target physiologic corroboration in stereotactic cervical cordotomy. J. Neurosurg., *30:*569, 1969.
296. Tasker, R.R.: The merits of percutaneous cordotomy over the open operation. *In* Morley, T.P. (ed.) Current Controversies in Neurosurgery. pp. 496. Philadelphia, Saunders, 1976.
297. Tasker, R.R.: Open Cordotomy. *In* Krayenbühl, H., Maspes, P.E., and Sweet, W.H. (eds.): Progress in Neurological Surgery. Pain, Its Neurosurgical Management. Pt 11. Vol 8. pp. 1. Basel, Karger, 1977.
298. Tasker, R.R.: Percutaneous cordotomy—the lateral high cervical technique. *In* Schmidek, H.H., and Sweet, W.H. (eds.): Operative Neurosurgery Techniques. Indications, Methods and Results. pp. 1137. New York, Grune & Stratton, 1982.
299. Tasker, R.R.: Identification of pain processing systems by electrical stimulation of the brain. Hum. Neurobiol., *1:*261, 1982.
300. Tasker, R.R.: Deafferentation. *In* Wall, P.D., and Melzack, R. (eds.): Textbook of Pain. pp. 119. Edinburgh, Churchill Livingstone, 1984.
301. Tasker, R.R.: Safety and efficacy of chronic neural stimulation. Contract with Canada Dept. Health and Welfare, 1984.
302. Tasker, R.R.: Surgical approaches to the primary afferent and the spinal cord. *In* Fields, H.L., Dubner, R., and Cervero, F. (eds.): Advances in Pain Research and Therapy. Vol 9. pp. 799. New York, Raven, 1986.
303. Tasker, R.R.: The problem of deafferentation pain in the management of the patient with cancer. J. Palliat. Care, *2:*8, 1987.
304. Tasker, R.R.: Percutaneous cordotomy: The lateral high cervical techniques. *In* Schmidek, H.H., Sweet, W.H. (eds.): Neurosurgical Techniques. Indications, Methods and Results. 2nd ed. pp 1191. Orlando, Grune & Stratton, 1988.
305. Tasker, R.R.: Percutaneous cordotomy. *In* Youmans, J.R. (ed.): Neurological Surgery. A Comprehensive Reference Guide to the Diagnosis and Management of Neurosurgical Problems. 3rd ed. pp. 4045. Philadelphia, Saunders, 1990.
306. Tasker, R.R.: Pain resulting from central nervous system pathology (central pain). *In* Bonica, J.J. (ed.): The Management of Pain. 2nd Ed. pp. 264. Philadelphia, Lea & Febiger, 1990.
307. Tasker, R.R.: Deafferentiation pain syndromes: Introduction. *In* Nashold, B.S., Jr., and Ovelmen-Levitt, J. (eds.): Advances in Pain Research and Therapy. Vol 19. Deafferentation Pain Syndromes, Pathophysiology and Treatment. pp. 241. New York, Raven, 1991.
308. Tasker, R.R.: Ablative central nervous system lesions for control of cancer pain. *In* Arbit, E. (ed.): Management of Cancer-Related Pain. pp. 231. Mt. Kisco, N.Y., Futura, 1993.
309. Tasker, R.R.: Percutaneous cordotomy. *In* Schmidek, H.H., and Sweet, W.H. (eds.): Operative Neurosurgical Techniques. Indications, Methods and Results. 3rd ed. pp. 1595. Philadelphia, Saunders, 1995.
310. Tasker, R.R.: The recurrence of pain after neurosurgical procedures. Qual. Life Res., *3*(Suppl. 1):543, 1994.
311. Tasker, R.R., and Dostrovsky, J.O.: Deafferentation and central pain. *In* Wall, P.D., and Melzack, R. (eds.): Textbook of Pain. 2nd Ed. pp. 154. Edinburgh, Churchill Livingstone, 1989.
312. Tasker, R.R., and Vilela Filho, O.: Deep brain stimulation for the control of intractable pain. *In* Youmans, J.R. (ed.): Neurological Surgery. 4th Ed. pp. 3512–3527. Philadelphia, Saunders, 1995.
313. Tasker, R.R., and Lougheed, W.M.: Neurosurgical techniques of sympathetic interruption. *In* Stanton-Hicks, M. (ed.): Pain and the Sympathetic Nervous System. pp. 165. Boston, Kluwer, 1990.
314. Tasker, R.R., and Organ, L.W.: Percutaneous cordotomy. Physiological identification of target site. Confin. Neurol. *35:*110, 1973.
315. Tasker, R.R., and Parrent, A.G.: Surgery for movement disorders and pain. *In* Swash, M., and Wilden, J. (eds.): Outcomes of Neurosurgical Disorders. Cambridge, Cambridge, in press.
316. Tasker, R.R., de Carvalho, G.T.C., and Dolan, E.J.: Intractable pain of spinal cord origin: Clinical features and implications for surgery. J. Neurosurg. *77:*373, 1992.
317. Tasker, R.R., Organ, L.W., and Hawrylyshyn, P.: Deafferentation and causalgia. *In* Bonica, J.J., (ed.): Pain. pp. 305. New York, Raven, 1980.
318. Tasker, R.R., Organ, L.W., and Smith, K.C.: Physiological guidelines for the localization of lesions by percutaneous cordotomy. Acta Neurochir., *21*(Suppl.):111, 1974.
319. Tasker, R.R., Tsuda, T., and Hawrylyshyn, P.: Clinical neurophysiological investigation of deafferentation pain. *In* Bonica, J.J., Lindblom, U., and Iggo, A. (eds.): Advances in Pain Research and Therapy. Vol 5. pp. 713. New York, Raven, 1985.
320. Tenicela, R., Rosomoff, H.L., Feist, J., and Safar, P.: Pulmonary function following percutaneous cervical cordotomy. Anesthesiology, *29:*7, 1968.
321. Tew, J.M., Jr., Keller, J.T., and Williams, D.S.: Functional surgery of

the trigeminal nerve: Treatment of trigeminal neuralgia. *In* Rasmussen, T., and Marino, R. (eds.): Functional Neurosurgery. pp. 129. New York, Raven, 1979.

322. Tew, J.M., Jr., and Tobler, W.D.: Percutaneous rhizotomy in the treatment of intractable facial pain (trigeminal, glossopharyngeal, and vagal nerves). *In* Schmidek, H.H., and Sweet, W.H. (eds.): Operative Neurosurgical Techniques. Indications, Methods and Results. pp. 1083. New York, Grune and Stratton, 1982.
323. Todd, E.M.J., Crue, B.L., and Carregal, E.J.A.: Posterior percutaneous tractotomy and cordotomy. Confin. Neurol., *31:*106, 1969.
324. Tsubokawa, T., and Moriyasu, N. Follow-up results of centre median thalamotomy for relief of intractable pain. Confin. Neurol., *37:*280, 1975.
325. Tucker, W.S., Fleming, R., Taylor, F.A., and Schutz, H. Trigeminal neuralgia in aqueduct stenosis. Can. J. Neurol. Sci., *5:*331, 1978.
326. Tulgar, M., Barolat, G., and Ketak, B.: Analysis of parameters for epidural spinal cord stimulation. 1. Perception and tolerance thresholds resulting from 1,100 combinations. Stereotact. Funct. Neurosurg., *61:*129, 1993.
327. Tulgar, M., Barolat, G., and Ketak, B.: Analysis of parameters for epidural spinal cord stimulation. 2. Usage ranges resulting from 3000 combinations. Stereotact. Funct. Neurosurg., *61:*140, 1993.
328. Tulgar, M., He, J., Barolat, G., *et al.*: Analysis of parameters for epidural spinal cord stimulation. Topographical distribution of paresthesiae—A preliminary analysis of 266 combinations with contacts implanted in the midcervical and midthoracic vertebral levels. Stereotact. Funct. Neurosurg., *61:*146, 1993.
329. Turnbull, I.M.: Percutaneous rhizotomy for trigeminal neuralgia. Surg. Neurol., *2:*385, 1974.
330. Uematsu, S., Udbarhelyi, G.B., Benson, D.W., and Siebens, A.A.: Percutaneous radiofrequency rhizotomy. Surg. Neurol., *2:*319, 1974.
331. Uematsu, S.: Percutaneous electrothermocoagulation of spinal nerve trunk, ganglion, and rootlets. *In* Schmidek, H.H., and Sweet, W.H. (eds.): Operative Neurosurgical Techniques. Indications, Methods, and Results. pp. 1177. New York, Grune and Stratton, 1982.
332. Uematsu, S., Udbarhelyi, G.B., Benson, D.W., and Siebens, A.A.: Percutaneous radiofrequency rhizotomy. Surg. Neurol., *2:*319, 1974.
333. Urban, B.J., and Nashold, B.S.: Percutaneous epidural stimulation of the spinal cord for the relief of pain. J. Neurosurg., *48:*323, 1978.
334. Van Kleef, M., Spaans, F., Dingemans, W., *et al.*: Effects and side effects of a percutaneous thermal lesion of the dorsal root ganglion in patients with cervical pain syndrome. Pain, *52:*49, 1993.
335. Ventafridda, V., De Conno, F., and Fochi, C.: Cervical percutaneous cordotomy. *In* Bonica, J.J., Ventafridda, V., and Pagni, A. (eds.): Advances in Pain Research and Therapy. Vol 4. Management of superior sulcus syndrome (Pancoast Syndrome) pp. 185. New York, Raven, 1982.
336. Ventafridda, V., Fochi, C., Sganzerla, E.P., and Tamburami, M.: Neurolytic blocks in perineal pain. *In* Bonica, J.J., Ventafridda, V. (eds.): Advances in Pain Research and Therapy. Vol 2. pp. 597. New York, Raven, 1979.
337. Ventafridda, V., and Martino, G. Clinical evaluation of subarachnoid neurolytic blocks in intractable cancer pain. *In* Bonica, J.J., and Albe-Fessard, D. (eds.): Advances in Pain Research and Therapy. Vol 1. pp. 699. New York, Raven, 1976.
338. Ventafridda, V., and Spreafico, R.: Subarachnoid saline perfusion. *In* Bonica, J.J. (ed.): Advances in Neurology. pp. 477. New York, Raven, 1974.
339. Vogel, H.P., Heppner, B., Humbs, N., *et al.*: Long-term effects of spinal cord stimulation in chronic pain syndromes. J. Neurol., *233:*16, 1986.
340. Von Schröttner, O.: Die perkutane zervikale anterolaterale Chordotomie. Wien. Klin. Wochenschr. *90:*372, 1978.
341. Waisbrod, H., and Gerbershagen, H.U.: Spinal cord stimulation in patients with a battered root syndrome. Arch. Orthop. Trauma Surg., *104:*62, 1985.
342. Wall, P.D.: The placebo effect: An unpopular topic. Pain, *51:*1, 1992.
343. Wall, P.D.: Introduction. *In* Wall, P.D., and Melzack, R. (eds.): Textbook of Pain. pp. 1. Edinburgh, Churchill Livingstone, 1984.
344. Wall, P.D., and Sweet, W.H.: Temporary abolition of pain in man. Science, *155:*108, 1967.
345. Watson, C.P., Morley, T.P., Richardson, J.C., *et al.*: The surgical treatment of chronic cluster headache. Headache, *23:*289, 1983.
346. Wester, K.: Dorsal column stimulation in pain treatment. Acta Neurol. Scand., *75:*151, 1987.
347. White, J.C., and Sweet, W.H.: Pain and the Neurosurgeon. A forty-year experience. pp. 435. Springfield, Charles C. Thomas, 1969.
348. Wilkinson, A.: Percutaneous radiofrequency upper thoracic sympathectomy: A new technique. Neurosurgery, *15:*811, 1984.
349. Willis, W.D.: The pain system. The Neural Basis of Nociceptive Transmission. *In* Gildenberg, P.L. (ed): The Mammalian Nervous System Pain and Headache. Vol 8. Basel, Karger, 1985.
350. Winkelmuller, W.: Experience with the control of low back pain by the dorsal column stimulation system and by the peridural electrode system. *In* Hosobuchi, Y., and Corbin, T. (eds.): Indications for Spinal Cord Stimulation. pp. 34. Amsterdam, Excerpta Medica, 1981.
351. Woolf, C.J.: Excitability changes in central neurons following peripheral damage; role of central sensitization in the pathogenesis of pain. *In* Willis, W. (ed.): Hyperalgesia and Allodynia. pp. 221. New York, Raven, 1992.
352. Yingling, C.D., and Hosobuchi, Y.: Use of antidronic evoked potentials in placement of dorsal cord disc electrodes. Appl. Neurophysiol., *49:*36, 1986.
353. Zimmermann, M.: Peripheral and central nervous mechanisms of nociception, pain, and pain therapy: Facts and hypotheses. *In* Bonica, J.J., Liebeskind, J.C., and Albe-Fessard, D. (eds.): Advances in Pain Research and Therapy. Vol 3. pp. 3. New York, Raven, 1979.

*354. Ohnmeiss, D.D., Rashbaum, R.F., and Bogdanaffy, G.M.: Prospective outcome evaluation of spinal cord stimulation in patients with intactable leg pain. Spine, *21:*1344, 1996.

*Editors Note: Reference 354 has been added as the only *prospective* evaluation of spinal cord stimulation.

Neural Blockade in Clinical Anesthesia and Management of Pain, Third Edition,
edited by M.J. Cousins and P.O. Bridenbaugh.
Lippincott–Raven Publishers, Philadelphia © 1998.

CHAPTER 33

Evolution of the Speciality of Pain Medicine and The Multidisciplinary Approach to Pain

J. David Haddox and John J. Bonica*

For three-quarters of a century, neural blockade was used widely for the relief of acute and chronic pain syndromes. Its widespread use was related to the pre-eminent concepts of pain during the same period. An equally important fact was that, besides systemic analgesics, neural blockade represented the only nonsurgical treatment modality for pain control. Before, during, and after World War II, this trend was further engendered by the development of nerve block clinics in many parts of Australia, the United States, Britain, and Continental Europe.

In recent years, a marked increase in pain research has resulted in a great deal of new information on the physiologic, biochemical, and psychological substrates of acute pain, and the findings from research in the behavioral and basic sciences have added new dimensions to our view of chronic pain. These advances have markedly enhanced our knowledge of sensory coding and sensory modulation and have effected a significant change in our conceptualization of clinical pain and pain therapy, particularly with regard to chronic pain syndromes. As one example, these advances have encouraged many physicians and other health professionals to become involved in managing patients with chronic pain within the context of multidisciplinary/interdisciplinary pain clinics/centers. They have also markedly changed the role of neural blockade in managing these patients. Indeed, some authorities state that neural blockade currently has little or no role in managing patients with chronic pain. On the other end of the spectrum there are those who, because of their extensive experience with these techniques, firmly believe that neural blockade can be used to advantage, particularly within the setting of the multidisciplinary/interdisciplinary pain center.

Why should so much time, effort, and text be dedicated to the treatment of pain? This volume includes numerous chapters designed to instruct the reader in methods of pain control for a variety of conditions. This particular chapter focuses primarily on chronic pain. While pain clinicians are convinced that chronic pain presents a serious health problem, many health care providers and the lay public do not have any sense of the magnitude of the problem.

In 1985, Louis Harris and Associates conducted a survey of pain in the United States that was commissioned by the Bristol-Myers Company. A report analyzing this survey was published in 1986 by Richard A. Sternbach.[56] The survey used a demographically representative sample of 1254 people 18 years of age or older who were interviewed by telephone via a structured item set. The sampling error was calculated to be on the order of 3%. The results of this survey indicated that headaches, backaches, muscle pains, joint pains, stomach pains, pain associated with menses, and dental pains accounted for 94% of all pain experienced by those interviewed. Seventy-three percent of the sample had experienced at least one headache in the preceding 12 months. Other figures are listed in Table 33-1. Note that 34% of the sample had experienced at least one type of pain for more than 101 days in the preceding 12 months. This cut-off was used to define chronic pain for study purposes.

When projected to the 1985 U.S. population of 174 million, pain accounted for 4,063,000,000 lost work days. Using nominal assumptions for the full-time employees in the sample, this translated to 55 billion dollars in lost productivity to the U.S. economy in that year alone.

*Dr. John J. Bonica wrote this chapter in previous editions. He had agreed to co-author this revision but, to the great sorrow of the international pain community, he died before he was able to make any new contribution to this work. Accordingly, parts of his previous chapter are reproduced herein, with occasional modification, as his observations and comments remain in many instances relevant and representative of current thought and practice in the field of Pain Medicine.

J. D. Haddox: Center for Pain Medicine, Emory University Medical Center, Atlanta, Georgia 30322.

J. J. Bonica: Department of Anesthesiology, University of Washington, Seattle, Washington 98195.

TABLE 33-1. *Pain experienced by Americans in the past 12 months*

	%	101 days or more (%)
Headaches	73	5
Backaches	56	9
Muscle pains	53	5
Joint pains	51	10
Stomach pains	46	3
Premenstrual or menstrual pains	40	<0.5
Dental pains	27	1
Other types of pain	6	1

Adapted from Sternbach, R.A.: Survey of pain in the United States: The Nuprin pain report. Clin. J. Pain, *2*:49, 1986.

Dr. Bonica was asked to comment at a round-table discussion on another study conducted by Louis Harris and Associates.[29] This study, entitled Pain and Absenteeism in the Work Place, was commissioned by Ortho McNeil Pharmaceutical and was conducted between December 5, 1995 and February 18, 1996. The methodology was similar to, although improved over, the previous study. It was based on computer-assisted telephone interviews of a demographically representative cross-section sample of 1007 full-time employees and 300 employee benefit managers from companies employing 150 people or more. The United States currently has approximately 120 million full-time employees. Two-thirds of the full-time work force say they suffer from conditions that cause pain. Headaches and pain related to menses each accounted for 33% of the reports, with low back pain accounting for 30%. The remaining pains were muscle pain, neck pain, sprains, strains, fractures, arthritis, carpal tunnel syndrome, and other upper extremity disorders. When asked if they suffer pain on a chronic basis, 19% of the sample agreed. This extrapolates to 15 million workers in the U.S. with some type of chronic pain.

In an effort to understand the cost of this pain, this study focused only on "casual absenteeism." That is, the study did not address long-term disability or Worker's Compensation losses, but focused solely on full-time employees who missed work periodically as a result of pain. They found that pain accounted for one-fourth of all sick days in the preceding 12 months or the equivalent of 50 million lost work days in 1995. Since 69% of the full-time employees reported that they received 100% compensation for sick days, this translates into 3.3 billion dollars in wages paid out while employees were at home sick. The average number of sick days for pain was 3, and 14% of the full-time work force missed some work because of pain during the preceding year. It is important to note that this study did not attempt to calculate the cost of hiring replacement workers, the lost productivity due to having inefficient or inexperienced workers temporarily replacing a worker who was out sick, the medical costs associated with sick days or any other costs associated with

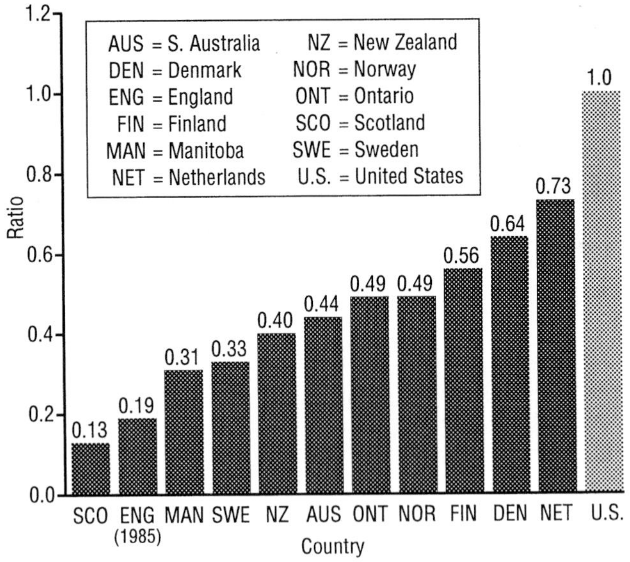

FIG. 33-1. Ratios of back surgery rates in selected countries to back surgery rate in the United States (1988–1989). (From Cherkin, D.C., Deyo, R.A., Loeser, J.D. *et al.* An international comparison of back surgery rates. Spine, *19*:1201, 1994.)

this phenomenon. Therefore, one can readily see that pain is a major medical and economic problem in the United States. While studies of this magnitude do not exist in other nations, it would be reasonable to assume that this is a phenomenon that applies to all developed nations.

In a study of 3020 volunteer workers of a large aircraft manufacturer, Bigos and others found during 4 years of study that 279 subjects reported acute back problems.[5] When analyzing factors that predicted reporting of back injuries, only job task dissatisfaction and distress, as determined by MMPI, were statistically significant. This raised the notion

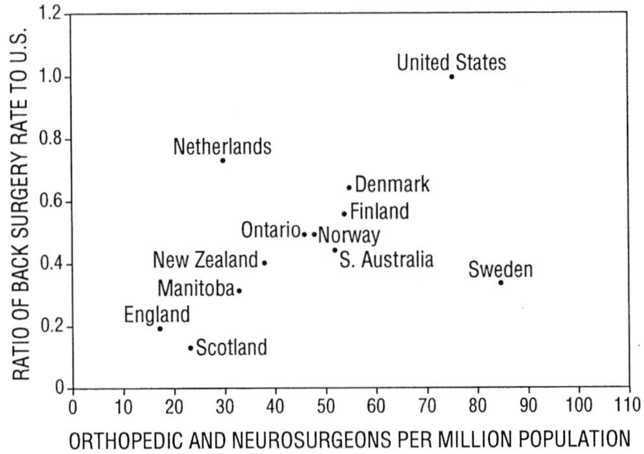

FIG. 33-2. Relationship between relative supply of orthopedic surgeons and neurosurgeons in a country and that country's back surgery rate. (From Cherkin, D.C., Deyo, R.A., Loeser, J.D., *et al.* An international comparison of back surgery rates. Spine, *19*:1201, 1994.)

TABLE 33-2. *Annual low back nonsurgical hospitalization rates per 100,000 adults by diagnosis—1979–1990[a]*

Principal diagnosis	Years				Rate ratio
	1979–1981	1982–1984	1985–1987	1988–1990	1988–1990/ 1979–1981
Herniated disk	70.0	84.6	86.1	52.6	0.75
Degenerative changes	57.7	60.1	46.0	24.5	0.42
Spinal stenosis	2.3	4.8	9.6	8.1	3.52
Possible instability	15.2	13.9	9.2	4.8	0.32
Closed fractures	12.6	10.0	13.2	15.1	1.20
Nonspecific conditions	218.5	195.1	131.7	66.1	0.30
All diagnoses	376.2	368.5	295.7	171.0	0.45

[a] All rates are age- and sex-adjusted to the 1990 U.S. population.

From Taylor, V.M., Deyo, R.A., Cherkin, D.C., and Kreuter, W.: Low back pain hospitalization: Recent United States trends and regional variations. Spine, *19*:1207, 1994.

that clinically important nonphysical factors may have significant impact on the reporting of back injuries or affect the response of individuals to medical treatment for back pain. This study indicated not only the magnitude of the problem, but set the stage for re-conceptualization of back pain, which will be discussed later in this chapter.

In 1994, Cherkin et al. reported on a comparison of back surgery rates throughout the world.[12] They studied 11 developed countries and found that the rate of back surgery in the U.S. was at least 40% higher than in any other country and was more than five times the rate of England and Scotland (Fig. 33-1). Further, the back surgery rate showed a nearly linear relationship with the per capita supply of back surgeons (Fig. 33-2). Countries with higher back surgery rates also had high rates of other elective procedures such as tonsillectomy, cholecystectomy, inguinal hernia repair, prostatectomy, hysterectomy, and lens operations. Despite this high surgical rate, however, the U.S., as the Harris polls indicate, still suffers significant costs from low back pain. If Worker's Compensation and long-term disability costs were factored into the data obtained by the surveys, these figures would be startlingly higher. In a companion article, Taylor et al. investigated trends in hospitalization for low back pain in the U.S.[57] They analyzed data from the National Hospital Discharge Survey from 1979 through 1990. They noted that nonsurgical hospitalizations for low back pain decreased dramatically, while low back operation rates increased markedly (Tables 33-2 and 33-3). Surgery and hospitalization rates were highest in the south and lowest in the west. Owing to their study design, they felt the rates they reported were probably under-representing the actual rates. Taken together, the data from these studies argue that pain and, in particular, chronic pain account for a tremendous societal cost to developed nations. The interested reader can draw no other conclusion than that traditionally accepted medical means of treating chronic pain appear to be inadequate.

This chapter will discuss the evolution of pain concepts that led to the inevitable birth and development of a separate medical endeavor—the speciality of Pain Medicine (algology). The chapter will then continue with the discussion of credentials for the pain physician, accreditation of pain treatment facilities, and a review of some of the organizations with which a modern pain practitioner should become familiar. It will then discuss the concept of multidisciplinary pain treatment, both from an organizational standpoint and from clinical applicability.

TABLE 33-3. *Annual low back surgery rates per 100,000 adults, by diagnosis—1979–1990[a]*

Principal diagnosis	Years				Rate ratio
	1979–1981	1982–1984	1985–1987	1988–1990	1988–1990/ 1979–1981
Herniated disk	77.4	96.5	109.4	107.3	1.39
Degenerative changes	10.7	13.7	13.4	10.6	0.99
Spinal stenosis	4.0	8.9	14.0	17.7	4.43
Possible instability	4.6	5.1	6.1	4.3	0.93
All diagnoses[b]	102.6	131.7	150.9	146.8	1.43

[a] All rates are age- and sex-adjusted to the 1990 U.S. population.
[b] Includes nonspecific diagnoses.

From Taylor, V.M., Deyo, R.A., Cherkin, D.C., and Kreuter, W.: Low back pain hospitalization: Recent United States trends and regional variations. Spine, *19*:1207, 1994.

EVOLUTION OF PAIN CONCEPTS

The evolution of pain concepts has been reviewed in detail in previous versions of this chapter. In brief, the understanding of pain proceeded along linear thought processes until very recently, with all attention focused on the sensory aspects of the experience and little credence given to the emotional, behavioral, or cognitive concomitants (Table 33-4).

With such a "telegraphic" notion of pain as merely a special type of sensation that was transmitted along the known neural pathways, it was inevitable that techniques and drugs utilized for the temporary interruption of these pathways in the surgical setting would be tried on patients suffering from more chronic forms of pain. Clinical experience has shown that many patients with persistent pain derive little benefit from neural blockade, and this realization initially caused consternation on the part of pain practitioners. As more modern concepts of pain evolved, however, the reasons for these failures became apparent.

To further this discussion, it is useful to review the definition of *pain* set forth by the International Association for the Study of Pain (IASP): "an unpleasant sensory and emotional experience associated with actual or potential tissue damage, or described in terms of such damage."[38] There are four key elements to that definition. First, pain is unpleasant. It is feared and avoided. Second, it clearly has a sensory dimension, as has been known for centuries. However, it *always* has an emotional element, which is why the definition reads "sensory *and* emotional" where *and* is used in a Boolean sense. Finally, it is an experience and, as such, cannot be adequately quantified. One can ask patients what they are experiencing and, from the answer, make inferences about their pain, but pain cannot be objectively measured any more than can hunger or love.

TABLE 33-4. *Evolution of pain concepts: Early history*

320 B.C. Aristotle	Increased body heat in "flesh" conveyed by blood to heart *(sensorium commune)* Opposed unsuccessfully by Galen, Vesalius, da Vinci, Descartes—all favored brain as center where pain was felt
1810–1820 Bell and Magendie	Dorsal roots sensory Ventral roots motor
1840 Muller	"Doctrine of specific nerve energies." Pain (and other senses) each had a specific *form of energy* carried from sensory organ to brain
1858 Schiff	"Specificity theory"—specific pain pathway to brain ("Private Line" Telephone Cable System)
1894 Von Frey	Specific pain receptors connected to pathways
1840 Henle and Weber	"Intensive theory" (originated by Erasmus Darwin in 1790)
1894 Goldscheider	Stimulus *intensity* and central summation are critical determinants of pain.

Many have attempted to define "chronic pain syndrome." None of the attempts thus far has gained universal acceptance. This is undoubtedly due to the fact that patients who complain of unremitting pain are not a homogeneous group. There are common features that most would agree upon, however. The "typical" patient with chronic pain has pain complaints that are out of proportion to the degree of physical findings and abnormalities noted on conventional diagnostic testing. Their complaints outlast the expected period of healing. They usually have a great deal of disability, that is, perceived limitations of task-specific activity, with little or moderate impairment or objective decrement in functional ability. Often, mood disorders of the depressive or anxiety type ensue. This cluster of findings is found in an individual in whom pain has a substantial negative impact upon quality of life.

Within the population of patients complaining of chronic pain, there are some who have a significant nociceptive substrate for their pain experience. These may well benefit from interventions designed to interrupt or modulate neural traffic. The clinical reality is, however, that it is often difficult to discern which patients will respond to neural blockade prospectively, especially when it is customary for the pain specialist to become involved late in the process, after the chronic pain syndrome has become manifest.

As Loeser and Cousins articulately opine, "The concepts one utilises are determinants of the physician's diagnostic and therapeutic approaches to the patient."[31] Therefore, much thought has gone into the exploration of the way clinicians conceptualize pain, since this will guide their clinical endeavors. Loeser and Cousins, with the influence of Fordyce, have used a four-part diagram to illustrate one way of conceptualizing pain patients (Fig. 33-3). The components of this array of encompassed eccentric circles are nociception, pain, suffering, and pain behavior. They argue that the first three elements are totally subjective and can only be inferred by another individual. Pain behavior, on the other hand, can be observed and quantified by others. They further describe that nociception is a physiologic process that has a well-defined neural basis. Pain is a perception, generally believed to be in response to the noxious stimulus. However, nociception does not necessarily lead to pain, nor does all pain rely upon a nociceptive substrate. Suffering occurs when the individual perceives pain. This is a negative affective response, however, which does not always require the presence of pain or occur predictably in the presence of pain, as suffering can have many other causes.

Pain behavior can describe a number of seemingly different entities, from moaning, splinting, limping, complaining of pain, visiting doctors for pain, avoiding work, and seeking succor from others to seeking compensation. Fordyce had the vision to understand that pain behaviors, like any other

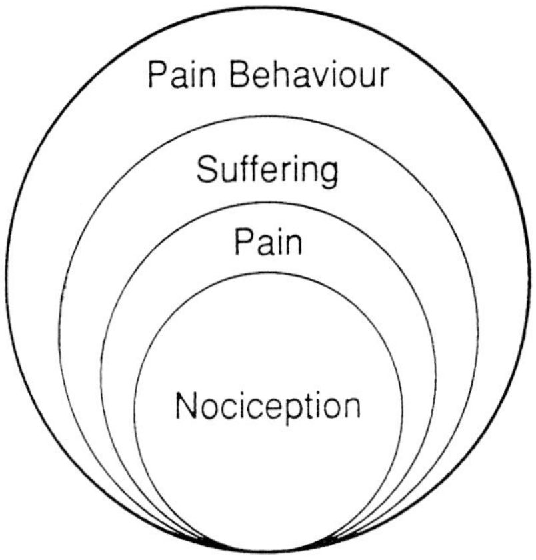

FIG. 33-3. A conceptual approach to the components of pain. (From Loeser, J.D., and Cousins, M.J.: Contemporary pain management. Med. J. Aust., *153*:208, 1990.)

behavior, can be manipulated in an operant paradigm. Pain behaviors, however, may occur in the absence of pain-induced suffering and may not necessarily occur in the presence of pain-induced suffering. Therefore, instead of the commonly seen version of the figure, in which each larger circle entirely subsumes all smaller circles, one could alternatively redraw the figure to show intersecting circles, indicating a less rigid cause and effect relationship between components (Fig. 33-4).

Another way of conceptualizing pain, especially as an educational tool, involves a graphic representation of the IASP definition.[25] This "conceptual model of pain" involves mentally placing an individual upon a Cartesian coordinate system that factors interactions of the affective, behavioral, and cognitive factors of the pain experience with the somatesthetic or sensory substrate for the pain experience. By "plotting" an individual situation upon this diagram, which has no specified units on the axes by design, one can convey to others the justification for a given combination of treatment approaches to facilitate moving the individual closer to the origin point (Fig. 33-5). Points further from the origin represent greater complaints of pain. Two points the same distance from the origin, but in different areas of the model, show how similar complaints of pain arise from different aspects of the pain experience, with one person's pain predominantly due to somatic factors, while another's is predominantly influenced by affective, behavioral, or cognitive factors.

The most recent re-conceptualization of pain involves nonspecific low back pain (NSLBP), a major cause of disability compensation in the United States and other countries. The IASP has released a report of the Task Force on Pain in the Work Place, chaired by Fordyce, which reconceptualizes NSLBP not as a medical problem, but as a problem of activity intolerance.[19] This was published to emphasize work site-based interventions as a method for minimizing/limiting disability; to structure medical management of NSLBP on a time-contingent basis, rather than a pain-contingent basis; to limit permanent disability status to situations in which objective impairment exists, while defining the period of temporary disability as not requiring impairment; to avoid excess disability; to establish vocational redirection programs for those individuals in whom NSLBP does not resolve, and to spark reanalysis of disability policies.

The evolution of the construct of pain is ongoing. Numerous factors contribute to this process: (i) better basic science understanding of nociceptive processes, (ii) further inquiries by behavioral scientists into the concomitants of nociception, (iii) frustration on the part of clinicians with treatment failures employing current strategies, and (iv) societal pressure, both political and popular, to better manage pain and its social and economic sequelae.

THE SPECIALITY OF PAIN MEDICINE

In the previous version of this chapter, one can read in detail the history of the development of medical thought regarding pain treatment. An excellent review of this was written by Madigan and Raj.[232] In essence, the concepts of therapy parallel the pain constructs that were prevalent at the time. Therefore, early interventions, based on the specificity theory, were surgical in nature (Table 33-5). As clinical experience accumulated, Bonica and others began conceiving of a closely knit group of different physician and non-physician specialities working in concert to evaluate patients and construct coincident, parallel treatment plans to effect change in somatic, psychological, and social aspects of pain problems. At about this same time, new medical specialities

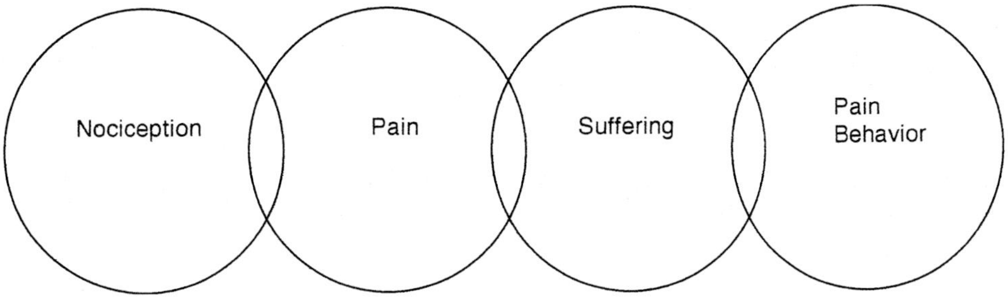

FIG. 33-4. An alternative representation of relationships between aspects of the pain experience.

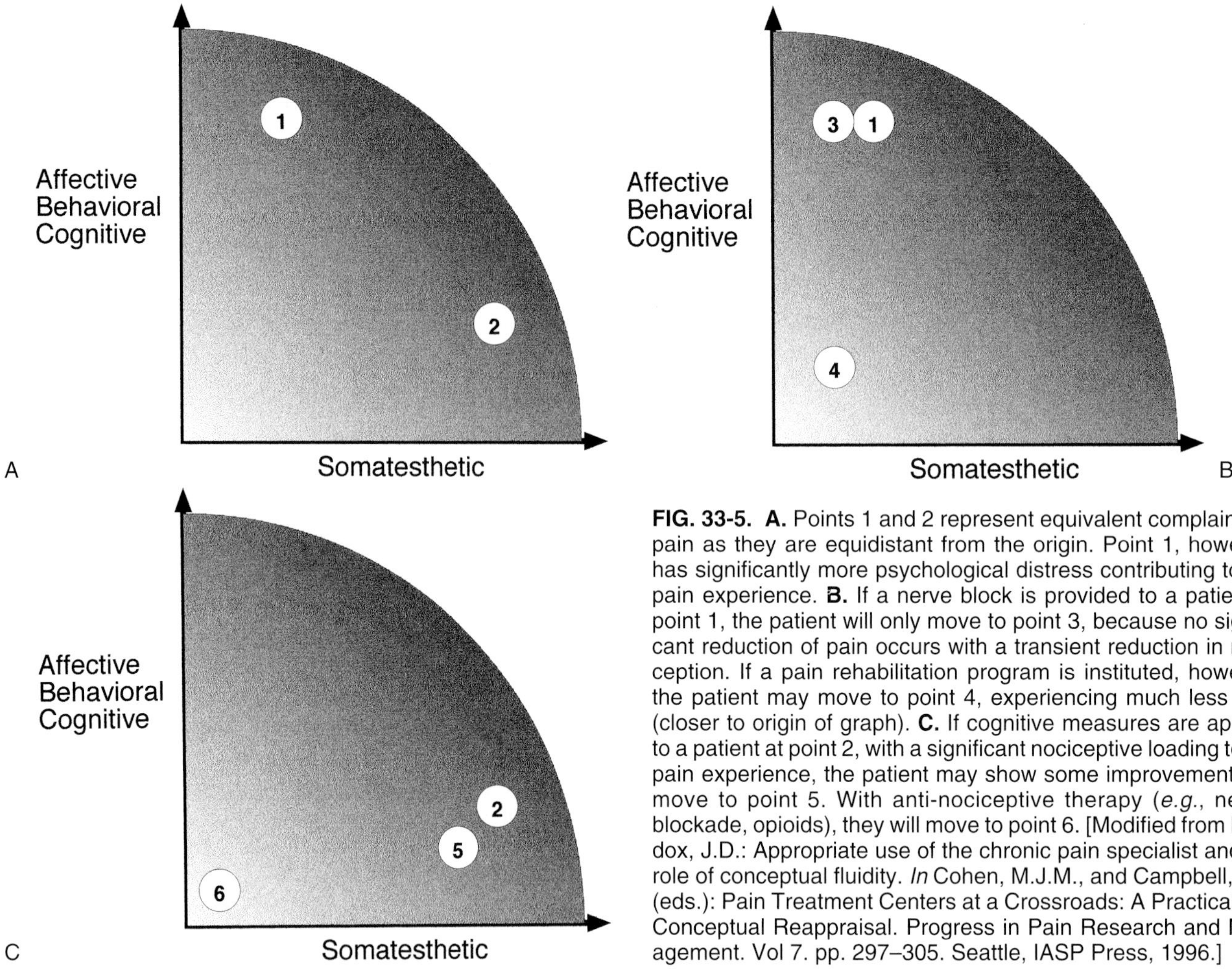

FIG. 33-5. A. Points 1 and 2 represent equivalent complaints of pain as they are equidistant from the origin. Point 1, however, has significantly more psychological distress contributing to the pain experience. **B.** If a nerve block is provided to a patient at point 1, the patient will only move to point 3, because no significant reduction of pain occurs with a transient reduction in nociception. If a pain rehabilitation program is instituted, however, the patient may move to point 4, experiencing much less pain (closer to origin of graph). **C.** If cognitive measures are applied to a patient at point 2, with a significant nociceptive loading to the pain experience, the patient may show some improvement and move to point 5. With anti-nociceptive therapy (*e.g.*, neural blockade, opioids), they will move to point 6. [Modified from Haddox, J.D.: Appropriate use of the chronic pain specialist and the role of conceptual fluidity. *In* Cohen, M.J.M., and Campbell, J.N. (eds.): Pain Treatment Centers at a Crossroads: A Practical and Conceptual Reappraisal. Progress in Pain Research and Management. Vol 7. pp. 297–305. Seattle, IASP Press, 1996.]

TABLE 33-5. *Evolution of pain concepts: recent history*

1860s–?1950s		Preeminence of specificity theory
1930s–40s	Leriche, Livingstone, Ruth, Rovenstine	WW II, nerve block clinics, writings of value of nerve blocks
1946	Bonica Alexander	Concept of Multidisciplinary Pain Management Group
1953	Bonica	*Management of Pain*—published. Neural blockade described in context of multidisciplinary approach to pain management
1960	Bonica	Multidisciplinary Pain Clinic (Washington)
1960	Crue	Multidisciplinary Pain Clinic (California)
1966	Melzack and Wall	Gate control theory of pain published, questioning "telegraphic" pain models
1974	Bonica et al.	IASP founded
1975	IASP	*Pain* published, first journal devoted to the topic
1981	CARF	Standards for Pain Rehabilitation Programs developed
1983	Crue et al.	American Academy of Pain Medicine founded
1991	Parris et al.	American Board of Pain Medicine founded
1993	AMA	Recognition of Pain Medicine as a designated specialty

IASP, International Association for the Study of Pain; CARF, Commission for the Accreditation of Rehabilitation Facilities; AMA, American Medical Association.

were evolving from primary specialities, based on new technology or new approaches to disease management.

In 1974, the IASP was founded by Bonica and others to serve as an international forum for study of these phenomena. This quickly gave rise to national chapters, such as the American Pain Society. The parent organization and the national chapters became active with numerous publications in journal, newsletter, and book form, and began holding respected scientific meetings.

In 1983, the American Academy of Pain Medicine (AAPM) was formed, under the initial name American Academy of Algology. This group was initially meant to be a forum for medical directors of pain programs, but quickly evolved into the physician organization representing those practicing the emerging speciality of pain medicine. In 1991, with support from the American Academy of Pain Medicine, the American Board of Pain Medicine (ABPM) was founded as the American College of Pain Medicine, the name being changed in 1994 to better reflect the credentialing aspects of the ABPM. In 1993, the American Medical Association (AMA) officially recognized Pain Medicine as a designated speciality for physician practice. The American Academy of Pain Medicine maintains a seat in the AMA House of Delegates and is thus influential in numerous aspects of organized medicine policy development.

In 1995, both the AAPM and the ABPM adopted the following definition:

> The Speciality of Pain Medicine is concerned with the prevention, evaluation, diagnosis, treatment and rehabilitation of painful disorders. Such disorders may have pain and associated symptoms arising from a discrete cause, such as postoperative pain or pain associated with a malignancy, or may be syndromes in which pain constitutes the primary problem, such as neuropathic pains or headaches. The diagnosis of painful syndromes relies on interpretation of historical data; review of previous laboratory, imaging and electrodiagnostic studies; behavioral, social, occupational, and avocational assessment; interview and examination by the pain specialist; and may require specialized diagnostic procedures, including central and peripheral neural blockade or monitored drug infusions. The special needs of the pediatric and geriatric populations are considered when formulating a comprehensive treatment plan for these patients.
>
> The pain physician serves as a consultant to other physicians but is often the principal treating physician and may provide care at various levels, such as direct treatment, prescribing medication, prescribing rehabilitative services, performing pain relieving procedures, counselling of patients and families, direction of a multidisciplinary team, coordination of care with other health care providers and consultative services to public and private agencies pursuant to optimal health care delivery to the patient suffering from a painful disorder. The pain physician may work in a variety of settings and is competent to treat the entire range of pain problems encountered in the delivery of quality health care.

Thus, this field is developing, much like the specialty of emergency medicine did, in that currently one must enter the specialty of pain medicine via another primary specialty, such as anesthesiology, just as one would have entered the practice of emergency medicine from medicine, pediatrics, or surgery a few decades ago. Now, however, major medical centers offer specific training in emergency medicine that, while building upon the foundation provided by the contributions of other specialities, has a unique body of knowledge and defined characteristics of practice.

Since the speciality of pain medicine is also evolving beyond the scope of other contributing specialities, the American Academy of Pain Medicine and American Board of Pain Medicine formed a joint Task Force on Graduate Medical Education in 1995, which was chaired by Dr. Kim J. Burchiel. The results of this task force have been compiled into a document that outlines the requisite training for physicians wishing to practice Pain Medicine. It discusses the current status, that is, training in a primary residency followed by fellowship training, such as occurs in the United States in anesthesiology, via fellowship programs that are recognized by the Accreditation Council on Graduate Medical Education (ACGME). However, it further outlines an educational plan by which an individual could enter the field of Pain Medicine as his primary residency choice in the future. It recognizes that a transition period will be needed. The proposed training outline includes significant training in primary care and should produce, at the end of a 4-year postgraduate curriculum, a competent practitioner of the speciality of pain medicine. The report recognizes that this endeavor will require considerable time and resources, but both organizations feel that this is a viable vision for the future.

Along similar lines, though not quite as involved, the University of Sydney, Australia is now offering a Masters of Science degree in Pain Medicine to various types of health care practitioners, not limited to those at the doctoral level. Individuals who complete this program will have gained special knowledge through didactic and practical curriculum in the various aspects of pain medicine.

Credentialing and Accreditation

As the field of pain medicine has evolved, it has been recognized that there is a public interest in determining that practitioners and programs meet certain standards. "Credentialing" refers to the awarding of a certificate to an individual to attest that he has a particular status. In medicine, this has come to mean certification by a board, which is an entity chartered for the improvement of quality medical education and medical care. Boards function to evaluate candidates in a medical field and to certify as diplomates those who are qualified to practice a particular speciality by virtue of education, experience, and performance on comprehensive examinations. In the United States, 24 Boards are members of a federation known as the American Board of Medical Specialities (ABMS). The ABMS is generally recognized as being the standard of credentialing by the American Medical Association, hospitals, the courts, and the public. There are, however, over 100 boards not affiliated with the ABMS, some of which are recognized as being comparable in quality to ABMS Boards.

In the United States, there are currently two boards that have procedures designed solely for examining and credentialing physicians in pain medicine: The American Board of Anesthesiology (ABA) and the ABPM. While similar in some respects, their programs do have some significant differences which bear comment.

The ABA was formed as an affiliate of the American Board of Surgery, Inc. in 1937 by a Committee composed of members of the American Society of Anesthetists, Inc. (now the American Society of Anesthesiologists, Inc.), the American Society of Regional Anesthesia, Inc., and the Section on Surgery of the American Medical Association. In 1941, the Advisory Board for Medical Specialities approved the establishment of the ABA as a separate primary board within the ABMS. In 1991, the ABMS allowed the ABA to issue a Certificate of Added Qualifications (CAQ) in pain management. A CAQ is a mechanism whereby a primary board may recognize qualifications that are seen to be *addition* to the primary board certificate. This presumes that the knowledge demonstrated by holders of this credential is an extension of the fund of knowledge and skills required by the primary certificate. This is in contrast to a Certificate of Special Qualifications (CSQ), such as that awarded by the ABA and several other boards in critical care medicine. A CSQ is also an extension of skills and knowledge but is felt not to be the purview of a single ABMS member board.

To receive the CAQ in pain management from the ABA, an applicant must first be a diplomate of the ABA and must hold an unconditional, unrestricted and unexpired license to practice medicine or osteopathy in one state or jurisdiction of the U.S. or Canada. The candidate must also fulfill the ABA's Continuum of Education in Pain Management and pass a 4-hour examination. If these criteria are fulfilled, the applicant will be awarded a certificate that is valid for 10 years.

The Australian and New Zealand College of Anaesthetists (ANZCA) has also commenced a Certificate in Pain Management, beginning in 1996. This is available to those who have passed the ANZA final examination, and who have completed a further year of training in an ANZCA-approved Multidisciplinary Pain Centre. Additional requirements include: a log-book of clinical experience (with mandatory targets in acute, chronic, and cancer pain), "a mini-thesis," and reports of Pain Centre Staff, based upon in-training assessment.

The American Board of Pain Medicine conceptualizes pain medicine as an emerging specialty, not a subspecialty of a pre-existing specialty. The ABPM, while not yet a member of ABMS, is functioning in a fashion analogous to ABMS member boards. Unlike the ABA, however, the ABPM does not limit examination eligibility to diplomates of any one board, but allows applicants to sit for examination if they are diplomates of any ABMS member board that has identifiable training in pain medicine as part of its educational requirements. Candidates must also possess a valid, unrestricted, and current license to practice medicine or osteopathy in one of the states of the United States of America, its territories or possessions, a branch of the United States Uniformed Services, or one of the provinces or territories of Canada. They also must have satisfactorily completed an ACGME approved residency program and be certified by the ABA, the American Board of Neurological Surgery, the American Board of Psychiatry and Neurology, or the American Board of Physical Medicine and Rehabilitation *or* be certified by another member of the ABMS and be able to document identifiable training in pain medicine within an ACGME-accredited training program. Candidates must also have been practicing pain medicine for at least 2 years after the completion of formal residency training and must have completed a minimum of 50 hours of Category I CME relevant to pain medicine and approved by the Accreditation Council on Continuing Medical Education (ACCME) or the Canadian equivalent.

The 8-hour ABPM examination is broad in scope and is designed to test knowledge important to the competent practice of pain medicine as determined by a field-based survey followed by expert deliberation. In February of 1996, the Medical Board of California determined that ABPM credentials are equivalent to those offered by members of the ABMS. As California licenses approximately 20% of the physicians in the U.S., this represents a significant recognition of the legitimacy of the ABPM. As of June 1996, over 600 physicians had successfully completed the ABPM examination process.

As credentialing is important for physician practitioners, so is accreditation important for the public and payers in identifying programs that have met established criteria. In 1966, two organizations that had been providing similar services merged to become the Commission for the Accreditation of Rehabilitation Facilities (CARF). The current mission statement reads "the mission of CARF is to serve as the pre-eminent standards-setting and accrediting body, promoting the delivery of quality of services to people with disabilities and others in need of rehabilitation."[10] CARF is a not-for-profit organization that is financed by survey fees, grants, sales of publications, and contributions from the sponsoring and associate members. CARF is composed of full-time staff and volunteer surveyors who conduct site visits to: (i) determine whether an organization applying for accreditation meets current standards and (ii) serve in a consultant role to assist the applicant organization in achieving compliance with standards. All policy decisions, standards for accreditation, and decisions regarding the individual organization's accreditation status are determined by the Board of Trustees. This Board is composed of representatives from "sponsoring" members who are interested entities who apply for membership on the Board. The American Academy of Pain Medicine, the American Pain Society, the American Hospital Association, and others comprise this group (Table 33-6). Each sponsoring member may designate one trustee. This group is then complemented by an equal number of Board-appointed at-large trustees.

TABLE 33-6. *Sponsoring members of CARF*

American Academy of Neurology
American Academy of Orthopaedic Surgeons
American Academy of Orthotists and Prosthetists
American Academy of Pain Medicine
American Academy of Physical Medicine and Rehabilitation
American Hospital Association
American Network of Community Options and Resources
American Occupational Therapy Association, Inc.
American Pain Society
American Physical Therapy Association
American Psychological Association
American Rehabilitation Association
American Speech-Language-Hearing Association
American Spinal Injury Association
American Therapeutic Recreation Association
Association of Rehabilitation Nurses
Brain Injury Association, Inc.
Federation of American Health Systems
Goodwill Industries International, Inc.
International Association of Jewish Vocational Services
International Association of Psychosocial Rehabilitation Services
Paralyzed Veterans of America
United Cerebral Palsy Associations

CARF concerns itself with the entire field of rehabilitation, not just pain (Table 33-7). In 1977, Bonica recommended to the IASP that it encourage national chapters to develop criteria, guidelines, and the mechanisms for evaluating pain clinics/centers on a voluntary basis. In 1981, with prompting from several prominent members of the American Pain Society, CARF began the formulation of standards for accreditation of programs that provided rehabilitation for chronic pain patients. These standards have undergone continual revision, with pain-related standards being most recently revised at the National Advisory Committee conference sponsored by CARF in 1994. The structure of these conferences consists of several-day meetings between numerous invited experts in the relevant field of interest, and these are facilitated by CARF staff. The goal of these meetings is to create and revise standards that reflect the current thinking in the field of pain rehabilitation. Conference attendees review, in detail, (i) the critiques from facilities that have been surveyed since the last new set of standards, (ii) new developments in treatment approaches, and (iii) ways in which the field is responding to external influences such as health care reform; they then synthesize these into a revised set of standards for accreditation.

The 1994 conference was a seminal one in that, for the first time in its history, CARF departed from promulgating standards for chronic adult pain rehabilitation only. The 1995 standards manual contains accreditation programs for *comprehensive pain management programs*. Relevant to this chapter, these standards state that "a comprehensive pain management program provides coordinated, goal-oriented, interdisciplinary team services to improve functioning and decrease the dependence on health care systems by persons with pain. The program is applicable to those persons who have limitations that interfere with their physical, social, and/or vocational functioning."[10] Core program areas identified in the manual are acute, chronic, and cancer- related programs for organizations operating in a comprehensive pain management model, with either pediatric or adult populations.

To become accredited, an organization must meet standards in a hierarchial fashion. If, for example, an organization's pain program meets all of the specific program standards but does not meet the standards applicable to all medical rehabilitation programs, it will not be accredited. Thus the standards are, in a sense, nested. A program must meet all general accreditation criteria first, then standards relating to the promotion of organizational quality, then those applicable to program quality, then the standards on management and outcome measurement, then the overall program standards, and then finally, must be in substantial compliance with the specific program standards to achieve accreditation. While this may seem like a daunting task, CARF develops the standards from input from the field and, prior to formal publication of revised standards, sends them out for review to surveyors, consumers, consumer groups, professional organizations, third-party purchasers, and others. CARF estimates that approximately 10,000 people have had the opportunity to review and comment upon proposed standards before they are put in effect. It is beyond the scope of this chapter to venture into a detailed listing of every relevant standard, but it is absolutely essential to understand that CARF standards apply only to programs that emphasize rehabilitation, not other treatment models. Lack of this understanding has caused many practitioners in the U.S. to feel that they were being unfairly discriminated against, after being deemed ineligible for accreditation under CARF standards. Standards manuals are available from CARF and should be consulted by anyone who wishes to seek accreditation or who wishes to utilize a blueprint for establishment or refinement of a pain treatment facility. As of August 1996, there are currently 11,510 rehabilitation programs with some form of CARF accreditation, with 199 accredited pain reha-

TABLE 33-7. *CARF programs*

Comprehensive Inpatient Medical Rehabilitation
Spinal Cord Rehabilitation
Comprehensive Pain Management
Brain Injury
Outpatient Medical Rehabilitation
Home- and Community-Based Rehabilitation
Occupational Rehabilitation
Employment Services
Community Support Services
Early Childhood Services
Alcohol and Other Drug Programs
Mental Health Programs

CARF, Commission for the Accreditation of Rehabilitation Facilities.

bilitation programs in the United States. Of these, 45 are inpatient chronic pain rehabilitation programs, 146 are outpatient chronic pain programs, six are comprehensive multidisciplinary acute pain rehabilitation programs, and two programs treat cancer pain in this model.

Training in Pain Medicine

Pain fellowships are currently offered in many anesthesiology training programs in the United States. These are examined periodically by the Residency Review Committee (RRC) composed of members of the ABA, the ASA, and the AMA's Council on Medical Education. The ACGME, composed of five members (ABMS, the American Hospital Association, AMA, the Association of American Medical Colleges, and the Council on Medical Speciality Societies), promulgates standards termed "essentials" for graduate medical training in pain management. The RRC for anesthesiology adapted those essentials, modifying them to be specifically applicable to anesthesiology training programs. These are called "Special Requirements for Residency Education in Pain Management." Although somewhat confusing, the ABA and other ABMS boards eschew the terms fellow and fellowship, so that the special requirements all contain the term *residency* where educational vernacular would employ *fellowship*. These requirements specify a training period of 12 months and dictate the curriculum, in detail, with regard to didactic and clinical exposure.

Other fellowship opportunities exist in different disciplines. Departments of neurology, psychiatry, and oncology are currently offering graduate medical training in pain. If sufficient numbers of programs exist within one specialty, usually about 40 programs, the ACGME will allow the RRC for that specialty to adapt the essentials for training in pain management into special requirements for residency education in that particular specialty.

PAIN ORGANIZATIONS

International Association for the Study of Pain

Founded in 1974 by Dr. John J. Bonica, the IASP was the first world-wide organization of individuals interested in the study and treatment of pain. It is set up to foster interaction among its members and is dedicated to cross-discipline interchange. Its members, numbering nearly 5800 in 85 countries, are physicians, psychologists, basic scientists, nurses, and a variety of other therapists, all of whom are students of the field of pain. It publishes the journal *Pain* and the *IASP Newsletter*, and has begun a book publication arm, the IASP press. It holds World Congresses on Pain every 3 years, with the most recent one being in Vancouver, British Columbia, in August 1996. These interdisciplinary congresses enjoy an attendance by several thousand individuals. The IASP also encourages the formation of national chapters to carry out its mission.

American Pain Society

The APS is the U.S. Chapter of the IASP. Its mission is to serve people in pain by advancing research, education, treatment, and professional practice through a joint and interactive effort among basic scientists and health professionals. Its membership is of a similar composition to that of the IASP and numbers over 3000. Anesthesiologists comprise the largest percentage of membership (27%), followed by psychologists (15%) and nurses (13%) with the remaining 45% made up of other disciplines. It has recently become active in the public policy arena, with several committees and task forces that are targeting public and professional education about pain, analyzing health reform legislative initiatives, providing input to regulators regarding the use of opioids and pain treatment, and drafting model legislative language for inclusion in upcoming federal and state laws. Its publications include the *APS Bulletin* and *Pain Forum*, a journal devoted to airing scientific opinions on controversies in the field. Other national IASP chapters function along similar lines.

American Academy of Pain Medicine

The AAPM consists solely of physicians who have an interest in the practice of pain medicine. Its mission is to "provide for quality care to patients suffering with pain, through the education and training of all physicians, through research and through the advancement of the specialty of pain medicine." Its membership is now close to 1000, with considerable growth in the past few years. The majority of its members are also anesthesiologists. It is concerned with scientific, economic, social, and political aspects of pain medicine. It has been influential, as a designated specialty society within the AMA, in revisions of the Current Procedural Terminology (CPT), which is the accepted reimbursement coding scheme for physician services in the United States. It publishes a newsletter, *Pain Medicine Network,* and the *Clinical Journal of Pain*, a peer-reviewed and indexed journal.

The American Society of Regional Anesthesia

This organization is comprised almost entirely of anesthesiologists who have an interest in the use of regional anesthetic techniques in surgery, obstetrics, and pain control. It currently numbers about 7000 members. It produces a newsletter and the peer-reviewed, indexed journal, *Regional Anesthesia.*

American Society of Pain Management Nurses

Founded in 1992, this group of nurses who have an interest in all aspects of pain management is the most rapidly growing pain organization in the United States. It is composed of nurse anesthetists, ward and office nurses, nurses who are part of a multidisciplinary team treating chronic and acute pain, and nurses who are research oriented. The 1995 membership is approximately 1100. The ASPMN publishes a newsletter called *Pathways*.

MULTIDISCIPLINARY FACILITIES—ORGANIZATIONAL CONSIDERATIONS

Dr. John J. Bonica is credited with developing the concept of a multidisciplinary approach to pain problems. In late 1946, he put the concept of a multidisciplinary facility for the diagnosis and therapy of complex chronic pain problems into practice in Tacoma General Hospital in the state of Washington. This group consisted of an anesthesiologist, neurosurgeon, orthopaedist, psychiatrist, and radiation therapist, all of whom had a special interest and some expertise in pain. Despite problems inherent in individual private practice, for 13 years the group was successful in its objectives and goals, a fact that further strengthened his conviction of the value of the multidisciplinary approach. At approximately the same time, Dr. F. Duncan Alexander had independently developed the same concept, initiating a multidisciplinary pain diagnostic and therapeutic program at the Veteran's Administration Hospital in McKinney, Texas in 1947. Shortly thereafter, Dr. William K. Livingston established the third multidisciplinary pain facility in the U.S. at the University of Oregon in Portland. He worked in collaboration with the Anesthesiology Department to diagnose and manage complex pain problems. Notably, his was the first multidisciplinary pain research program supported by the National Institutes of Health of the U.S. Bonica strongly emphasized the rational use of neural blockade in the multidisciplinary setting, as described in Chapter 31 of the second edition of this text.

In 1960, Dr. Bonica assumed the chair of the Department of Anesthesiology at the University of Washington and began to develop a multidisciplinary pain facility there. This facility evolved into a group of some 20 individuals from 14 different medical specialties and clinical disciplines who participated in the program. Also in 1960, Dr. Benjamin Crue, a neurosurgeon, initiated a multidisciplinary pain program at the City of Hope Medical Center in Duarte, California.

The salient feature of these initial centers, many of which still function actively, is their ability to bring a number of specialists who are contributing unique knowledge and skills to the resolution of various aspects of a presenting problem. These individuals work in close daily contact with each other to ensure maximum communication and facilitation of the overall treatment plan. This approach, initially unique in medicine, has been modeled in several other aspects of medical practice, including certain disciplines within pediatric medicine, psychiatry, and rehabilitation medicine. The multidisciplinary approach, by its very nature, embodies the understanding that chronic debilitating pain, in most instances, is not simply reducible to a single irritated nerve that will respond to neural blockade, stimulation, or resection. Rather, this approach utilizes the more broad-based conceptualizations discussed earlier in this chapter and employs a variety of individual talents to achieve resolution of a patient's problem in an effort to maximize patient function.

Owing to a number of factors, including growth of knowledge and increased interest in treating pain, the world experienced a great proliferation of pain programs during the 1980s. These programs varied considerably in their expertise, focus, treatment philosophy, and personnel composition. The IASP, recognizing the confusion that was arising from the lack of a standard nomenclature, convened a task force for Guidelines for Desirable Characteristics for Pain Treatment Facilities. The task force released the results of its deliberations in 1990.[30] They chose the term *Pain Treatment Facility* (PTF) to apply, in a generic sense, to all forms of pain treatment delivery systems, regardless of personnel or patient types. They stated that the term *pain unit* was synonymous with PTF. They then listed a group of terms and definitions, as well as an amplified listing of desirable characteristics for each form of service delivery. Implicit in the definitions is the concept that an *isolated solo practitioner* cannot be considered to constitute a clinic or a center.

A *modality-oriented clinic* is the simplest of this classification scheme. This facility employs a single type of therapy and does not provide comprehensive assessment or management. By definition, regardless of the number of practitioners, it does not qualify as multidisciplinary. It does not provide services in an integrated, comprehensive fashion. Common examples include nerve block clinics, biofeedback clinics, work-hardening clinics, etc. The salient feature is provision of a single treatment approach. Such facilities are at risk of falling victim to the "carpenter's syndrome," wherein, when all you have is a hammer, all the world begins to look like a nail. Some patients will undeniably benefit from a single intervention, yet many patients suffering with pain, especially in a chronic form, will not benefit from a single intervention and, indeed, may be worsened by blind adherence to a traditional medical/surgical model of pain intervention, instead of the more comprehensive biopsychosocial model.

A *pain clinic* is the next most complex type of health care delivery system focusing on those suffering with chronic pain. It may be specialized with regard to body regions (e.g., headache) or diagnoses (e.g., herpetic pain syndromes). Pain clinics may be comprised of a few or many practitioners. A single practitioner in a large medical complex where other consultative and therapeutic services can easily be arranged could qualify, provided there is regular access to an interaction with at least three medical specialities, including a practitioner of behavioral sciences.

Next in complexity is the *multidisciplinary pain clinic*. This is a delivery facility that is composed of different physicians and other health care providers who specialize in the diagnosis and management of patients with chronic pain. This may include inpatient and outpatient capabilities. The team must function in an integrated manner, performing a multidisciplinary assessment of patients, developing and providing a comprehensive treatment plan, and communicating regularly about each patient's progress. An array of specialists is required to address the specific needs of the population being served by the clinic and may include various medical disciplines, nursing, psychology, physical therapy, occupational therapy, vocational rehabilitation, and others.

The most complex facility is a *multidisciplinary pain center*. This encompasses all of the characteristics and functions of the *multidisciplinary pain clinic*, but also includes an active teaching and research program. This facility will serve patients suffering from both acute and chronic pain syndromes. It will exist most commonly as a component of a teaching hospital or medical school. A detailed analysis of the organization of a multidisciplinary pain center is beyond the scope of this chapter. The reader is referred to several excellent reviews of the subject.[1,6–8,21] It is imperative, however, if one wishes to endeavor to treat patients in this manner, that a clear analysis of the target patient population be made. One may wish, for instance, to develop a multidisciplinary program that is limited to a general condition, such as pelvic pain or temporomandibular disorders.[15,20,39,40] One may wish a broader population, such as patients suffering from cancer-related pain syndromes.[3,4] Or one may wish to focus on work-related or industrial injuries only. Finally, one could create a multidisciplinary center in which all painful entities can be managed by that approach. Clearly, the physical equipment and space requirements, as well as personnel structure, will logically follow from the analysis of the target population. Likewise, "product lines" or specific services should be analyzed, based on needs of target populations. A facility may offer, for example, forensic activities, wherein multidisciplinary evaluation is used for legal or administrative purposes, whereas some centers may serve only as a patient advocate, arranging for impairment ratings and other forensic services that may present conflicts of interest to be provided elsewhere.

The team must have a leader. This individual should be someone who is competent, is recognized in the field, and is able to administer a program involving contributions from multiple departments. In the United States, there are currently no academic pain programs that are discrete "department equivalents." All programs are joint ventures between numerous existing departments or are "owned" by a single department. Unfortunately, with physician and other reimbursement being tied to the department level, this creates inevitable conflicts in the administration of a truly multidisciplinary center. Individual participants are financially beholden to their department of origin rather than the center *per se*. As academic medicine re-evaluates its service delivery models, in the face of tremendous pressures from "health care reform" legislation and managed care delivery systems, this "product line" or "center" model might be seen as feasible. Private practice entities, recognizing the potential for fluid operation when all participants are under one fiscal entity, have typically been functioning much more efficiently than their academic counterparts. After identification of target populations, their service needs, and the administrative, financial, and logistic requirements, the team should set about the task of developing a mission statement. This should include an overall statement of "vision," or an articulation of the direction in which the team would like to see the program evolve. The mission statement then should proceed naturally from that and be a clearly articulated statement of purpose. This is increasingly valuable for organizational clarity, as well as to effectively communicate the function of a particular unit to the consumer, payers, and referral base.

Quality assurance or continuous quality improvement is best initiated at the inception of a PTF. This will ensure that outcome data will be available in a relatively short time. These outcome data, while quite useful internally for addressing quality issues and highlighting processes that can be improved, are becoming increasingly important for external purposes. CARF, for instance, requires a quality improvement program to be ongoing, as well as program evaluation procedures which evaluate outcome. As the future of health care changes, outcome-based treatment is likely to take priority over any other treatment, no matter how empirically or scientifically sound. Therefore, it is crucial that outcome data be collected in a contemporaneous manner.

MULTIDISCIPLINARY PAIN TREATMENT—CLINICAL CONSIDERATIONS

Numerous attempts have been made to conceptualize chronic pain patients in an effort to guide therapy. Rene Cailliet stated in 1979 that an acute phase of pain must logically precede a chronic phase.[9] He felt that chronic pain patients become chronic because their participation in recovery is not requested or encouraged. He argued that the physician should become an educator rather than remain only a therapist. He argued for a thorough clinical examination to conceptualize clinical aspects of the patient's presentation followed by effective communication to the patient and enlisting the patient in his own therapy. He laid out a plan for chronic pain treatment which included cessation of drug intake and dependence, the utilization of modalities such as nerve blocks to interrupt nociceptive pathways, encouragement of activity and exercises with recording of time spent being active as a measure of improvement, group therapy, extinguishing pain behavior, and resumption of vocational activities. He concluded with "it can be truly stated that if acute pain were approached more astutely, there would be less chronic pain."

Numerous other authors have looked at the problem of unremitting pain. Issy Pilowsky has promulgated the notion that pain can be considered abnormal illness behavior[47,48] and has devised an instrument to assess this construct.[49,50] He suggests that the concept of a sick role, which carries certain obligations and privileges, can be adopted by a patient and should be addressed in the clinical conceptualization of a particular presentation. He further develops Mechanic's concept of illness behavior and describes several examples. Illness behavior can be generally defined as an individual's reaction or response to disease. It is well known that individuals with the same viral upper respiratory infection (VRI) will respond or react differently to the condition. For example, some individuals will attend work, despite the VRI, whereas others will stay home. He states that chronic pain frequently constitutes a leading symptom in abnormal illness behavior syndromes, and that these syndromes may, at times, take the form of recognizable psychiatric entities in which there are conscious motivations and conscious control of illness behavior (malingering and Munchausen syndrome) or predominantly unconscious motivation for abnormal illness behavior, such as hypochondriasis or conversion reactions.

Characterizing the Chronic Pain Experience

The Illness Behavior Questionnaire (IBQ) quantifies certain aspects of the way individuals respond to and experience their health status.[49,50] It includes a number of scales which range from concepts of hypochondriasis to disease conviction to psychological versus somatic perception of illness. This provides one way of conceptualizing patients with chronic pain that may give rise to therapeutic strategies. A detailed analysis of the factor structure, validity, reliability, and interpretation of the IBQ is beyond the scope of this chapter. Whatever psychometric critiques are raised of the instrument itself, the construct of abnormal illness behavior is often useful in attempting to understand patients with complaints of chronic pain.

Chronic pain patients are noted to have a number of factors that influence their behavior. Mendelson studied measures of conscious symptom exaggeration in 157 patients with chronic pain who were involved in personal injury litigation and compared this to 106 patients not seeking compensation.[37] All patients were attending a multidisciplinary pain clinic. Of the litigating patients, 84 were related to motor vehicle accidents and 73 were involved in Worker's Compensation claims. He used several validated psychometric tests including assessments of anxiety, personality style, hostility, depression, and the IBQ. A conscious exaggeration scale was developed from the IBQ which was also employed in the study. He found that the conscious exaggeration scale could not distinguish chronic pain patients involved in litigation related to their pain or those receiving compensation payments from those who did not receive pain-contingent financial gain. He did, however, demonstrate a high correlation between the conscious exaggeration scale and personality factors such as propensity toward anxiety, state anxiety, depression, and hostility. He suggested that this cluster of factors, which would clearly be evident at some level in a clinician-patient interaction, may adversely influence a physician's view of the patient's veracity. The data in this study would suggest that, on the basis of clinical interaction or psychometric instruments employed in this study, concluding that a patient is exaggerating symptoms for material gain is invalid.

Guest and Drummond further investigated the effect of compensation on emotional state and disability in chronic back pain patients.[24] They compared 19 patients in active compensation programs to 18 who had settled their low back pain claim. They noted that compensation recipients showed more signs of emotional distress, reported pain as being more disruptive, and had greater difficulty coping with pain than those who had settled. They noted, however, that even after settlement, clear evidence of emotional distress remained. This would call into question the commonly held notion that once a compensation claim is settled, the patient will necessarily be comfortable and relatively unaffected by his pain.

Greenough and Fraser compared eight different psychometric instruments in an unselected population of low back pain patients and found the IBQ, Waddell's signs and symptoms, and the pain drawing to be the least useful in discriminating psychological disturbances in patients with low back pain.[22] They found pain, employment status, and compensation status to influence the performance of various instruments. The Modified Perception Questionnaire and the Zung depression scale formed a combination that was relatively immune to the effect of pain, social group, compensation, and migrant status, although unemployment did affect these two devices disproportionately. They suggested that this combination could be useful in evaluating the psychological disturbances of patients with low back pain.

Villard et al., in 1986, conducted an interesting study looking at psychosomatic variables after first-time lumbar disk surgery, in 27 low back pain patients who had not had previous contact with psychiatry.[60] This study design was implemented to control for previous studies which were based largely on psychological factors in low back pain patients that had been referred for psychiatric evaluation. They employed a structured interview, a questionnaire assessing physical and mental state, and a psychometric evaluation using a variety of the McGill Pain Questionnaire (MPQ), the pain drawing test, and the 16 PF, all of which were completed during a 4-hour period approximately 4 years after diskectomy. On the personality structures, there were no major abnormal findings with the exception that both the good- and bad-outcome groups tended to be somewhat suspicious and distrustful. The poor-outcome group reported more inattention, irritability, and restlessness than are found in normal populations. Whether this is a predictive factor or a resultant factor from their poor outcome is not clear. They did find some variation in the pain drawing analysis, in that good-outcome groups tended to have pain patterns conforming to known neuroanatomic patterns, whereas the poor-outcome group did not. Not surprisingly, the poor-outcome group endorsed more items on the modified MPQ. They concluded by stating that poor outcome might be predicted by: (i) difficulty in perceiving feelings and expressing affect coupled with a tendency to deny psychological conflicts, (ii) financial compensation on a pain-contingent basis, and (iii) a high rating on pain assessment tests.

In a more recent analysis of psychological factors in chronic low back pain patients, Klapow and associates demonstrated that all chronic low back pain patients are not psychologically similar, but rather could be clustered according to psychosocial factors such as coping strategies, stress, and satisfaction with social supports.[28] Thus, the literature begins to reflect the notion that "chronic pain" is not a single thing, but is a diverse spectrum of presentations which, intuitively, should be treated with different strategies, depending upon the details of a particular patient's presentation.

Fear also plays an important role in the chronic pain experience. Waddell and colleagues developed a tool to assess fear in patients.[62] The Fear-Avoidance Beliefs Questionnaire (FABQ) focuses on patients' beliefs about how activity will effect their pain. The authors were motivated by the studies alluded to previously, which failed to account for disability on the basis of medical factors alone. The FABQ is based on fear theory and fear-avoidance cognitions and also includes the concept of disease conviction put forth in the IBQ. They were able to demonstrate test-retest stability and patient understanding of the individual items. Results clustered into two factors that are largely independent of any biomedical measures of pain. Fear-avoidance beliefs, as measured by the FABQ, explained a highly significant portion of the variance in disability and work loss even when accounting for severity of pain. Their study of 184 patients also concluded that there was little direct relationship between pain and disability, in that severity of pain accounted for only 14% of the variance in disability with regard to activities of daily living. The various biomedical measures combined to explain only 5% of the variance in work loss. They were able to demonstrate that both work loss and disability in activities of daily living were strongly related to fear-avoidance beliefs about work. Fear-avoidance beliefs about other physical activities strongly related to fear-avoidance beliefs about work and explained additional variance. They postulate a model (Fig. 33-6) of causal pathways operated between low back pain and disability. They argue that the relationship between fear-avoidance beliefs and disability has implications for the management of low back pain, emphasizing that inappropriate fear-avoidance beliefs need to be recognized and dealt with early in an effort to prevent chronicity.

Vlaeyen and colleagues studied 103 chronic low back pain patients, exploring the relationship of kinesophobia with demographic, pain-related, and affective variables.[61] They found that fear of reinjury or fear of movement correlated with those individuals whose coping style is characterized as catastrophizing, those who were depressed, and those who experienced social phobia, agoraphobia or other fears of injury, illness, and death. When analyzing these and other variables, catastrophizing coping styles and depression most accurately predicted fear of movement or fear of reinjury.

In another study reported in the same paper, 33 chronic low back pain patients were asked to lift and hold a 5.5-kg bag. The time was measured to a maximum of 300 seconds. Heart rate and skin conductance level were measured at baseline, several seconds after hearing verbal instructions (anticipation phase), at the beginning of the task, at the end of the task, and 30 to 50 seconds following the task. The kinesophobia scale, a visual analogue fear scale, and the State Trait Anxiety Inventory (STAI) were also administered. The results indicated that patients with high scores on the kinesophobia scale performed less well on this simple motor task. No significant correlation or trends were found between the psychophysical variables and the kinesophobia scale or performance on the motor task. Significant correlations were noted between the fear VAS and the kinesophobia scale and between the kinesophobia scale and STAI state. Patients who reported fear of movement or reinjury were more anxious after being exposed to the stimulus than during the preparatory phase of the experiment. This study points out in a systematic fashion how fear can influence behavioral aspects of the chronic pain experience.

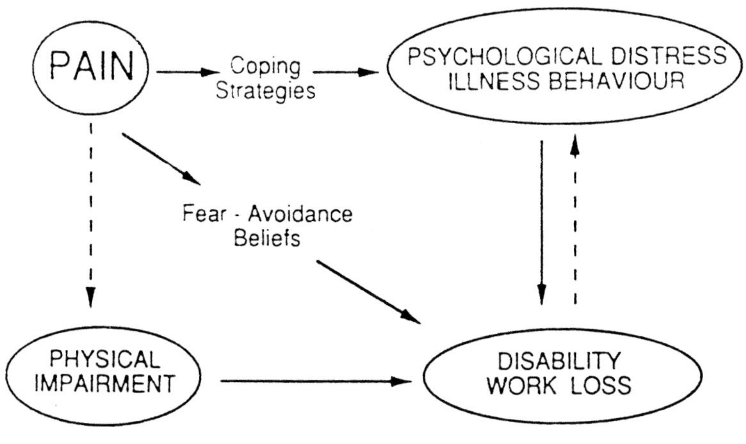

FIG. 33-6. The major cognitive, affective, and behavioral pathways postulated between low back pain and disability. [From Waddell, G., Newton, M., Henderson, I., *et al.*: A fear-avoidance beliefs questionnaire (FABQ) and the role of fear-avoidance beliefs in chronic low back pain and disability. Pain, *52*:157, 1993.]

Issues Accompanying Chronic Pain

In addition to trying to understand the dimensions of the chronic pain experience, one must also be cognizant of the common concomitants that occur in the setting of chronic pain. Maruta and colleagues, in 1979, reported 144 patients with chronic nonmalignant pain, noting that 24% were drug dependent and 41% were drug abusers, by their criteria.[33] They found that non-abusers had significantly better outcome and suggested that early detection and treatment of drug abuse could minimize some of the difficulties involved in treating these otherwise recalcitrant pain presentations. There is currently a reassessment of the tenets regarding the use of analgesics in chronic pain. Many physicians are beginning to accumulate experience that indicates that opioids can be used safely over long periods of time and still be efficacious in some chronic pain patients. This area of controversy is evolving and is beyond the scope of this chapter, but may influence multidisciplinary pain treatment in the future.

As alluded to previously, depression is a frequent accompaniment of pain. Haythornthwaite and colleagues published a study comparing depressed and nondepressed chronic pain patients.[26] They found that depressed individuals suffering from chronic pain were likely to report greater pain intensity, exhibit more pain behaviors, and report greater interference in life activities due to pain than their nondepressed counterparts. They suggested that clinicians must incorporate an understanding of depression into the conceptualization and treatment of chronic pain.

Jamison and colleagues have commented on significant weight gain in chronic pain patients.[27] Not surprisingly, there was a significant relationship between weight gain of more than 15 pounds since onset of pain and decreased physical activity. Increased weight was also associated with increased emotional distress and accident liability. These authors suggested, and many have followed their advice, that weight management be part of a multidisciplinary rehabilitation pain program.

Finally, when conceptualizing chronic pain patients, one must be aware that this condition is not limited to the identified patient, but affects the entire family. Studies have indicated that the spouse of a chronic pain patient suffers from increased rates of psychological and affective problems and have demonstrated significant marital distress in couples in which one spouse suffers from chronic pain. Chun, Turner, and Romano have studied the negative effects of chronic pain patients on their children.[13] They found that children of parents with chronic pain had significantly greater school behavioral problems and less social skills in the school environment than children of healthy controls. Thus, there is the need to consider family therapy services as part of a multidisciplinary pain program.

Cognitive Behavioral Aspects of Treatment

In 1995, the U.S. National Institutes of Health sponsored a Technology Assessment Conference on the Integration of Behavioral and Relaxation Approaches into the Treatment of Chronic Pain and Insomnia.[44] These two conditions were chosen because they afflict millions of Americans and do have some interrelationship. Additionally, similar strategies may be useful in treating both conditions. The conference reviewed data on the relative merits of specific interventions and identified biological and psychological factors that might predict outcome. The members of the panel also examined mechanisms by which behavioral and relaxation approaches could lead to more satisfactory clinical outcome in these conditions. The final statement, published in 1996, concluded that there was strong evidence for the effectiveness of relaxation techniques in reducing chronic pain. Hypnosis also had strong evidence supporting it, whereas cognitive behavioral therapies and biofeedback had moderate evidence supporting their use in the treatment of pain. A consistent positive effect with "multimodal" treatment was demonstrable. The panel warned that for any particular patient, one approach might be more appropriate than another.

In 1978 Newman, Painter, and Seres reported on the concept of a therapeutic milieu for patients suffering from chronic pain.[43] They felt that the atmosphere in a pain center could be structured to encourage reduction of pain behaviors by employing a multidisciplinary approach. They provided an analysis of various pain and psychologic models and how the milieu could be constructed to address pain and pain behavior while encompassing a variety of pain conceptualizations.

Moore and colleagues, in 1984, studied 51 patients completing an inpatient multidisciplinary pain program.[42] They noted group effects at 6-month follow-up with patients who had gone through the program in a single group tending to fair better or worse in concert with other members of their treatment group. They commented on the importance of understanding social factors in maintaining chronic pain behavior and suggested that therapeutic programs should attempt to exploit social factors to therapeutic advantage. Those involved in multidisciplinary programs frequently employ group activities for physical therapy, education, and psychological groups and recognize a powerful group effect. This effect appears to be enhanced when individual patients enter the program in a staggered fashion, so that the group is constructed of patients in various stages of therapy. Patients who are more advanced in their therapy tend to exert a positive peer effect on newer patients, thus facilitating progress of these individuals while instilling some sense of self-worth and value in the more senior patients. In a study of cognitive behavioral treatment groups on an outpatient basis, Skinner and colleagues reported significant decrement in physical disability and analgesic consumption coupled with improvements in mood and coping skills over a 7-week period, utilizing one afternoon session per week in which the patients were involved in a multidisciplinary team setting.[55]

Williams and Keefe have demonstrated that patients' use of cognitive coping strategies can be dependent upon their belief systems.[63] Therefore, one must structure psychological therapies individually to achieve optimum benefit. In a review of the efficacy of cognitive therapies for chronic low back pain patients, Turner and Jensen compared outpatient group cognitive therapy, relaxation training, and a combination of both to a waiting list control in a total of 102 low back pain patients.[59] At 12-month follow-up, pain intensity had decreased significantly for patients in all three treatment conditions, but not in the waiting list group. Depressive symptoms and disability improved in all conditions, including the waiting list, with no statistically significant differences among the treatments. The study suggested that cognitive therapy, especially involving identification and modification of negatively distorted thoughts, might be equivalent to relaxation, but did not necessarily provide greater results when coupled with relaxation. The authors felt that more studies should be aimed at attempting to elucidate mechanism of action of behavioral therapies.

A component of many multidisciplinary programs is education. This may diminish fear, provide some cognitive benefits by counteracting distorted or unrealistic notions of disease, and provide a cost-effective way to facilitate pain rehabilitation. In a review of educational strategies for low back pain patients, Cohen et al. found that there was insufficient evidence to recommend group education for people with low back pain.[14] This study is quoted because it is counterintuitive to the "typical" multidisciplinary models that are prevailing today.[51]

Roy stated that, since chronic pain is a complex phenomenon, negative outcome could be due to neglect of social factors.[54] He emphasized, again, the need for individualization of treatment utilizing an eclectic approach. He opined that interventions should be determined on the basis of specific problem identification in the medical, social, and psychologic realms.

Physical Aspects of Treatment

The physical aspects of chronic pain patients have been explored as part of the rehabilitation program. Edwards et al. reported in 1992 on the results of 54 patients taking part in a predominantly physical reconditioning program for low back pain.[17] The program involved mobilizing physical therapy, physical reconditioning, work hardening, and isokinetic testing. This program also included an educational component. They found that 56% of patients successfully completing the 4-week program remained at work at one-year follow-up. Anxiety scores, despite any specific psychological therapies, tended to decrease throughout the program. No variables predicted successful outcome.

Davis and colleagues were able to document objective enhancement in fitness indices at the conclusion of a multidisciplinary program.[16] Their subjects, 46 patients, were studied using computer-assisted ergometric devices. The variables included maximum oxygen uptake, work rate, respiratory exchange ratio, maximum heart rate, and minute ventilation. This study found significant increases in various objective measures of physical performance as a result of a pain rehabilitation program. Using U.S. Department of Labor categories, the group, as a whole, moved from performance consistent with the "sedentary" level to the "light" level. This equates to an objective improvement in employability because moving between these two work levels exposes the patient to a significantly greater number of potential jobs.

MULTIDISCIPLINARY PAIN MANAGEMENT—EFFICACY

The multidisciplinary approach to pain management is considered to be labor intensive. Various practitioners of differing, but complimentary, health fields need to be involved in a particular patient's care in order to effect a reasonable outcome. This premise, however, is often challenged by those individuals and entities who prefer a more simplistic approach for economic reasons. A major goal of practitioners of pain medicine is to convince payers that most complex long-term presentations of chronic pain are not amenable to a "quick fix" with a nerve block or two, a few pills, or a few more surgeries. There are, at present, significant numbers of patients for whom a "cure," in the traditional sense, is not possible. Therefore, one must have realistic expectations when undertaking to treat such patients. If one uses return to work as the only success criterion, the multidisciplinary approach to pain management, especially in later stages, may not appear to be efficacious. However, the realistic practitioner must also set realistic goals, given the entry status of a particular patient. Return to work may not be a viable goal in many instances. Rather, improved quality of life, stabilization of pain, reduction of pain behaviors, enhanced coping skills, and appropriate health care utilization may be more realistic, desirable, and attainable goals.

In the past decade, numerous authors have attempted to quantify efficacy of the multidisciplinary pain management approach. This is important for obvious clinical reasons and, in the climate of health care "reform," is becoming more important for economic reasons as health care systems are demanding more evidence of efficacy before authorizing payment for a particular treatment. In 1985, Guck and Colleagues compared the long-term efficacy of a multidisciplinary approach to pain by studying 20 treated patients with 20 patients who were not eligible to participate in the program because of lack of insurance coverage.[23] It should be noted that the control patients met the program's entry criteria and expressed a desire to undergo treatment. They used a follow-up period of at least one year and, in some cases, up to 5 years. Entry criteria were (i) chronic pain that was not associated with an active disease process, (ii) other interventions, either medical or psychiatric, were not considered to be appropriate, (iii) pain of at least 6 months' duration, (iv) patient's desire to participate, and (v) willingness of a family member or significant other to be involved in the patient's treatment. The program was 4-week inpatient style with weekends out of the program. The program involved gradual reduction and eventual elimination of all opioid, nonopioid and psychotropic medications used for pain. It also involved progressive increase of daily exercise and physical activity in a group setting. Finally, an attempt to resolve psychosocial issues related to the clinical presentation was made. Treatment was delivered in group sessions, by educational lectures, through individual counseling and psychotherapy, through conferences with family members, through training in biofeedback and relaxation, and via vocational counseling. Follow-up data regarding hospitalizations and surgeries, medication use, further interactions with health care systems, employment status, litigation and compensation, mood, and perception of pain were obtained on all patients. Success was defined by employment status, lack of compensation for pain problems, absence of pain-related hospitalization or surgery, and absense of prescription opioid or psychotropic medications.[53]

Of the 20 subjects that were treated, 12 (60%) met all success criteria, compared to none of the control group meeting all criteria. The treated group reported less pain on good and bad days, had significantly more "up time," demonstrated significantly less depression, and had fewer pain-related hospitalizations than the control group. The difficulty with no-treatment control groups had been a significant problem in studies predating this one. The authors of this study did their best to compare two groups that, except for insurance approval, were equal. Pitfalls of choosing control groups, as well as other factors in outcome studies, were discussed in detail by Turk and Rudy in an article in 1990.[58] The *caveats* they listed were, for the most part, considered by Guck et al. as lending credence to their conclusions that inpatient multidisciplinary pain treatment was efficacious and had long-term benefit.

A group of 702 consecutive patients admitted to a large multidisciplinary treatment program for chronic low back pain were accessed at admission, discharge, and initial follow-up (one month) with a variety of psychological and functional performance measures.[35] The authors used simple measures of endurance, truncal and lower extremity strength, flexibility, muscle tension, and sitting tolerance. They also assayed pain behavior, assertiveness, comprehension regarding the program and its goals, and comprehension of the relationship between pain and anxiety. Additionally, they administered the Wechsler Adult Intelligence Scale (WAIS) and the MMPI to all subjects at admission and at one-month follow-up.

In an effort to describe this population demographically, they found that their group was dominated by middle-aged, middle-class Caucasians experiencing severely disabling low back pain for more than 4 years. Slightly over half of their subjects were males, and virtually all had sought medical treatment prior to selecting the multidisciplinary pain program, with one-third having undergone at least one surgical intervention for back pain. A third of these patients had undergone psychological treatment. One-third had concurrent chronic medical conditions and 2/3 had been engaged in litigation related to their back pain. Only 6% were considered to be employable at the time of admission. At discharge from the program, 2/3 of the patients showed improvement in the physical and psychological measures. Not surprisingly, completers significantly outpaced those who dropped out, suggesting that modification of behavior and attitude, one of the program's goals, was occurring. Using principle components analysis, the behavior change scores clustered in two factors, one involving cognitive aspects of behavior and the other involving physical abilities. Interestingly, the first factor accounted for nearly 48% of the variance between success and failure, while the second factor accounted for 12% of the variance. Program completers also reported a 41% reduction in VAS scores. At one-month follow-up, seven of the parameters showed further improvement beyond discharge while two—muscle tension while sitting and sitting tolerance—demonstrated no further improvement. Self ratings of pain at one month were relatively stable to slightly improved.

Analysis of WAIS scores demonstrated average intelligence, comparable to full-scale values seen in nonchronic populations. MMPI results reflected a profile that is now considered typical in the chronic pain population, distinguished by high elevations on the Hs, De, and Hy scales, with the De elevation being slightly less than the other two, the inappropriately named "conversion V." Other scales (Pd, Pt, Sc, and M) were also significantly elevated. Interestingly, the male subgroup of this population had significantly higher scores than did the females. Also, the Hy scale was significantly elevated for those engaged in litigation, while the Hs scale was significantly elevated for those who had concurrent other chronic medical problems. At initial follow-up, dramatic improvements were demonstrated, so that 64% showed an increased number of scales in the nonimpaired range, compared to their scores on admission. Specifically, the first three scales were often significantly reduced.

The authors analyzed these data in an effort to predict successful outcome by initial behavioral, psychological, and psychometric assessment. No single variable or combination of measures obtained in admissions predicted accurately whether a given patient would complete the program. Patients who left the program early, however, did not show any significant gains in behavioral or functional status.

The same authors performed long-term follow-up on 210 program completers over a period of 6 months to 5 years.[36] Using telephone interviews, attempts were made to contact program completers at 6 months and at 1, 2, 3, 4, and 5 years following discharge. Thirty items were presented in a structured interview format requiring 12 minutes. Six items were selected for analysis, based on the authors' assertion that these factors represented specific outcome goals of this program or had a significant relationship to outcome assessed at short-term follow-up. They report on: (i) return to work, (ii) litigation status, (iii) self report of pain, (iv) pain interference with activity, (v) analgesic use, and (vi) pain-related hospitalizations. Univariate analysis of variance (ANOVA) demonstrated increased return to work and decreased interference of activities from pain. Two hundred and ten patients were contacted at the 6-month follow-up, 161 were contacted at 12 months, 100 at 24 months, and so on, with 24 being contacted at 60 months. At the 2-year follow-up contact, 9% of patients reported favorable outcome on all six variables, compared to 5% reporting unfavorable outcome on all six variables. At 5 years, 17% reported completely favorable outcome and 8% reported completely unfavorable outcome. At 6-month follow-up, 33% of respondents had successfully returned to gainful employment. This number continued to improve over the follow-up period in a linear fashion. Percent of patients in litigation remained relatively constant throughout the study, showing some slight decrease at the 60-month follow-up. Pain ratings tended to decrease over time as did pain interference with activity and medication use. Hospitalizations for pain increased slightly from the 6-month to 5-year follow-up. While this information provides useful data in an aggregate fashion, the authors were again unable to predict individual variability with much success. Nonetheless, long-term efficacy, as demonstrated by stability of indicators of program success over time, was demonstrated.

In what is surely one of the most interesting papers published in this area, Cassisi, Sypert, and colleagues published a review of patients with severe chronic low back pain who were treated at a single facility over a 5-year period.[11] What made this paper unique was that the authors had no connection with the program being evaluated, nor did the multidisciplinary team itself have any knowledge of this evaluation. This study, therefore, constitutes perhaps the best blinded study ever conducted in this area. Two hundred and thirty-six patients referred by one physician to the pain rehabilitation program constituted the initial sample. Of these, 61%, or 143 patients, were able to be contacted and given a structured telephone interview followed by receipt of the McGill Pain Questionnaire and the Oswestry Low Back Pain Disability Questionnaire in the mail. The average time from referral to interview was 22 months. The patients comprised five groups: (i) 39 patients who completed the 4-week inpatient program, (ii) 30 patients who were denied entry into the program because of failure of the insurance company to authorize treatment, (iii) 36 patients who had insurance approval but declined participation, (iv) 14 who participated in other programs, and (v) 14 patients who dropped out of the program being studied. Eighty-five patients originally referred to the program were not able to be contacted for inclusion in this study. Demographic variables of all groups at entry were similar and resembled, in general, demographics published of chronic low back pain patients. Myofascial pain syndrome was the predominant pre-referral medical diagnosis, comprising about 80% of each group. The mean pain rating varied between groups from 7.2 to 8.3 on a scale of 10. About half of each group had prior surgery, with the mean number of surgeries being 1.1 to 1.7 across the groups. Prereferral employment status, interestingly, was significantly *lower* in group 1 than in groups 2 and 3. Approximately an equal number of patients in each group were litigants.

Data from the follow-up interview was interesting in that the average self-reported pain intensity for the preceding month was 5.9 in group 1 and was not significantly different among the other groups. There was, however, a significant difference in the percent decrease in pain intensity from prereferral levels in group 1 (27%) compared to the other groups. Group 4, those who participated in other programs, reported no decrease in pain intensity. Group 1 patients had fewer subsequent physician visits, hospitalizations, and surgeries than the other groups. Sixty-nine percent of group 1 patients were employed at follow-up. This was significantly greater than in groups 2, 3 and 5. Global level of functioning was also higher in group 1 patients than in groups 2 or 3.

Fifty-four percent of group 1 and 50% of groups 2 and 3, considered the nonparticipant group for the analysis, returned the questionnaires. Group 1 had a significantly lower score on all three scales of the MPQ, but had no significant difference in total score or number of words chosen. On the Oswestry instrument, group 1 patients reported significantly fewer problems lifting heavy weights than the other groups, but otherwise did not score differently than the nonparticipant group. This study clearly indicated the efficacy of a multidisciplinary approach to the management of chronic low back pain and associated disability. Done in a truly blinded fashion, it demonstrates that on significant quality of life measures, patients suffering from chronic low back pain may benefit from a multidisciplinary approach.

In 1990, Maruta, Swanson, and McHardy extended their original analysis of long-term efficacy of their multidisciplinary pain center.[34] They studied 408 patients who were admitted to their program between 1979 and 1982. Eighty-two were initially rejected because of lack of motivation, and 44 patients rejected the program, even though the evaluators felt that they were rehabilitation candidates. Of those remaining, 249 completed the program and 33 were early drop-outs. The demographics of the 249 program completers were not dissimilar from other published data, with a mean duration of pain of 6.7 years, an average of two previous pain-related surgical procedures, and participation in a multitude of single-modality pain treatment approaches. Forty-three percent were receiving Worker's Compensation, and the group averaged 2 years away from full-time work. Few patients were involved in litigation.

The authors defined drug abuse or dependency as more than the "recommended" dose for a month or more. This definition, of course, does contain a significant bias against the use of pain-related medications in the context of a multidisciplinary approach to pain. This notion, as mentioned earlier, appears to be evolving somewhat over time. Forty-two percent of patients met the authors' criteria for abuse or dependency.

MMPI profiles were similar to those in other published reports. The intelligence quotient, as determined by the Shipley Institute of Living Scale, was within normal range for the population at large. On admission to the program, the Hamilton rating scale for depression (Ham-D) averaged 15.0, suggesting subclinical depression.

The program involved an average of 23 days of hospitalization, during which the self-reported pain level did not change significantly. The Ham-D scale, however, averaged 6.3 on discharge. Success was determined by change on three parameters: (i) attitude, (ii) reduction in medication use, and (iii) improved physical functioning. A five-point scale of change is completed by an independent rater for each of the three parameters, with the program coordinator rating attitudinal change, the staff physician rating reduction of medication, and physical function being rated by the physical therapist. Success required a rating of moderate or marked improvement in all categories. Failure was determined by lack of modest improvement in any category, and partial success was determined by values between those two extremes. Seventy percent (174 patients) were considered successful, while 7% were considered failures. Twenty-three percent were considered partial successes.

Follow-up was made at 3 years on all but 10 of the original program completers. Eighty-seven percent responded to either mailed questionnaires or follow-up telephone calls by an independent reviewer. The same success criteria were used to determine maintenance of treatment effect. Thirty-nine percent (81 patients) maintained improvement in all categories and were classified as final successes, with 36% being partial successes and 23% considered to have failed treatment due to lack of long-term maintenance of treatment effect. No significant differences were discernible in the demographics between those who had long-term success and those who did not. The outcome of 39% long-term maintenance of treatment effect is, given the entry population, both statistically and clinically significant. The authors could not determine any predictive variables, consistent with other studies of this nature.

In 1992, Flor, Fydrich, and Turk published a meta-analysis of the literature dealing with multidisciplinary pain management approaches.[18] They analyzed 65 studies that reported on multidisciplinary approaches for chronic back pain. Studies included had empirical data, described treatment in a multidisciplinary program, and were published from 1960 to 1990. Three hundred studies were reviewed to determine whether they met inclusion criteria for this meta-analysis. Data from 3089 patients were included in this report, with an average of 61 subjects reported per study. Mean demographic variables indicated an even split between male and female, pain duration of 85 months, with 34% of subjects working and 51% of subjects on compensation. The mean number of surgeries was 1.76, while 85% of the subjects used pain-related medications. Twenty-one percent of the subjects were involved in litigation. Thus, the demographic variables were consistent with what most clinicians see in their practices.

The majority of treatments were a combination of psychological interventions, medical treatments, and physical/occupational therapies, with an average duration of 7 weeks (1–31 weeks). Fifty percent were performed in inpatient settings and 28% were performed in outpatient settings, while the remainder were either mixed or did not provide information on the treatment location. Treatments were divided into short-term follow-up (less than 6 months) or long-term follow-up. Overall, the results of this analysis indicate that, even at long-term follow-up, patients who were treated in a multidisciplinary pain management program function better than 75% of samples that are untreated or are treated by conventional unimodal approaches. Treatment effect sizes compared to controls were not significantly different, whether the control group was composed of patients for whom insurers declined payment, was a waiting list control group, or other purely medical treatment control group. More importantly, in today's environment, the treatment effects were not limited simply to subjective variables but included objective data. Patients treated in this manner returned to work at a 68% rate, compared to a 36% rate in the untreated/conventionally treated groups. Taken another way, 43% more patients were working after treatment than were working before treatment. The authors note that, while this figure may not seem impressive at first glance, when the duration of pain and the extent of disability with their associated costs are considered, this represents a tremendous savings to society.

As health care delivery changes, more procedures are being done on an outpatient basis to reduce costs. Much of the early work in multidisciplinary pain treatment was done in an inpatient model, and this influenced program design even until today. As financial pressures increase, the need to demonstrate value, that is, acceptable outcome at acceptable cost, has forced many programs to restructure to an outpatient basis.

Two groups have questioned whether treatment outcome is the same with inpatient program delivery as with outpatient modes. Intuitively, following the operant conditioning paradigm, inpatient programs might be expected to have better outcome since the reinforcements from the environment could presumably be better controlled. The first randomized control trial testing this thesis was published in 1990 by Peters and Large.[45] They studied 85 patients of 132 who consented to random assignment to inpatient management (IN), outpatient management (OUT), or a no-treatment control condition (CON). Allowing for dropouts for various reasons, the first groups were comprised of 29, 23, and 16 members, respectively.

The inpatient program was cognitive-behaviorally focused with a graded exercise component and was conducted on a general medical ward, 5 days a week for 4 weeks. The outpatient program consisted of nine 2-hour sessions conducted weekly by a team with a similar, but not exact, composition as the inpatient team. The controls were assessed four times in one year and had the ability to receive standard medical treatment if needed, but were not allowed to participate in formal pain management. The demographics of the groups were similar to other published studies, except that there was a slight female preponderance (61.2%).

Measures included a number of accepted tools, such as the pain drawing, General Health Questionnaire (GHQ), BDI, MPQ, and Sickness Impact Profile (SIP), as well as measures of physical performance and surface EMG muscle tension data. Patients were assessed at entry and at near conclusion of the inpatient and outpatient programs, with controls being assessed at entry and at the eleventh week. Inpatient BDI scores were higher than those of the other groups, and psychological distress over health issues (GHQ) was higher in the IN than in the OUT group, with the CON group mean in between. Otherwise, other variables did not differ between groups.

At the conclusion of follow-up: (i) SIP scores were lower in both treatment conditions than in controls, (ii) health concerns decreased in both IN and OUT to similar levels, (iii) IN and OUT both showed decreased pain behaviors, and there were time-dependent changes in many of the psychometrics. Measures of function improved in both IN and OUT groups. Significant treatment effects were not found on measures of depression, although the BDI scores did improve with time in all groups. Likewise, treatment did not appear to affect the regions or amount of the body involved with pain.

Since the initial scores on some measures were higher in the IN groups, some of the improvement may be attributed to regression to the mean. Nonetheless, the authors did demonstrate treatment-related effects in psychological distress associated with pain and illness behavior in *both* in- and outpatient multidisciplinary management of chronic pain.

In a second article studying the same subjects, the authors reported results of follow-up at 9 to 18 months of 22 IN, 18 OUT, and 12 CON members.[46] Using similar measures, they concluded that 68% of the IN group, 61% of the OUT group, and 21% of the CON group were successes at follow-up. Both treatment groups had increased numbers of subjects working at follow-up, and three more control group patients were not working. They concluded that pain management programs, whether in- or outpatient, were beneficial to society in terms of cost, and to patients in terms of quality of life.

Pither, Williams, and colleagues have recently published work of a similar nature, but attempted to design their study so that the only variable was inpatient versus outpatient treatment.[52] They randomly allocated 121 chronic pain patients to either treatment groups or waiting list control. The program content, which consisted of cognitive-behavioral approaches coupled with gradually increasing physical activity, was kept identical, and both treatment groups ran in parallel. The inpatient arm (IN) consisted of 4 weeks of 4.5 hours of treatment/day, 5 days a week (90 hours total treatment exposure). The outpatient arm (OUT) consisted of 3.5 hours per week over 8 weeks (28 hours total). The setting, written program materials, recording forms, and staff were identical. Assessments occurred at pre-treatment, at one month, and at one year. Instruments included the BDI, the Multidimensional Pain Inventory (MPI), and the Pain Self-Efficacy Questionnaire (PSEQ), SIP, STAI and others. Physical measures were also included. Demographic variables were not significantly different than expected.

Accounting for treatment dropouts and the like, 41 patients constituted the IN, 42 comprised the OUT, and 31 patients made up the waiting list control group. At one-month follow-up, 93% of IN and 81% of OUT subjects were available for analysis. At one year, 78% of each group was available for study. Controls did not change significantly over time. At one month, IN made more gains than OUT, but both improved more than controls, in regard to pain impact, physical performance, depression, and catastrophizing. At one year, these treatment effects were largely maintained, with the exception of pain intensity. Again, IN showed more improvement than OUT. No variables predicted successful outcome.

The differences in treatment outcome between IN and OUT may be due to a number of factors, including peer relationships formed during a longer treatment time, more exposure to therapies, or tighter environmental control. Thus, the overwhelming evidence leads to two conclusions regarding chronic pain management in a multidisciplinary setting: (i) it is effective, with demonstrable maintenance of treatment effect, whether performed in an inpatient or an outpatient setting, and (ii) it is not always effective for every patient. Clearly, research is needed to identify ways of more productive matching particular patient needs to specific programmatic elements to enhance outcome in a cost-effective manner.

Neural blockade techniques may contribute to management of individual patients in the multidisciplinary setting. However, as is the case with other ingredients of multidisciplinary pain management, rigorous evaluation of the specific contribution of neural blockade techniques is largely lacking. It is the observation of a number of experienced pain clinicians that interventional techniques such as spinal cord dorsal column stimulation (SCS) and intrathecal drug administration systems may achieve pain relief in appropriately selected patients (see Chapters 27, 28, 29, and 32). However, it is also observed that a substantial percentage of patients do not improve in terms of objective indices of physical and mental functioning, and the important end point of return to work. In such situations patients need the added help of a cognitive behavioral program. Molloy et al. report that when this is done, objective indices of function do improve.[2,41]

SUMMARY

This chapter has reviewed the parallel evolution of: (i) the conceptualization of pain, (ii) the multidisciplinary approach to treatment of pain, and (iii) the speciality of pain medicine. These events, while discussed separately, are inextricably interrelated. Were it not for changes in how pain is conceptualized, the multidisciplinary approach and the speciality of pain medicine would never have arisen. The increasing sophistication of understanding pain on a psychological and neurophysiologic basis, coupled with better understanding of treatment efficacy for a variety of pain conditions discussed in this text, has given rise to a discrete body of knowledge that is encompassed in the specialty of pain medicine. Explicit in the definition of pain medicine is the concept of the multidisciplinary approach to many chronic pain presentations. This approach recognizes the essential contribution of non-physician practitioners in the evaluation, analysis, and treatment of those suffering from complex chronic pain problems.

The current economic, political, and social climate in the United States and other countries has brought an unprecedented pressure to demonstrate treatment efficacy in health care. Fortunately, the data reviewed in this chapter argue convincingly that the multidisciplinary approach to pain treatment can be effective. The challenge for the next decade is to demonstrate that it is not only efficacious but cost-effective. Only cost-effective methods of approaching health problems are likely to be reimbursed in the future. Cost-effectiveness, however, comprises a number of factors; indirect costs, as well as human suffering, must be figured into any analysis. As the specialty of pain medicine and other disciplines practicing in a multidisciplinary pain management setting mature, our attention should be directed to interventions that improve quality of life in a manner that is financially acceptable to society.

REFERENCES

1. Aronoff, G.M., and McAlary, P.W.: Organization and personnel functions in the pain clinic. *In* Ghia, J.N. (ed.): The Multidisciplinary Pain Center: Organization and Personnel Functions for Pain Management. pp. 21–43. Boston, Kluwer, 1988.
2. Asghari, A., Nicholas, M.K., Molloy, A.R., and Cousins, M.J.: Outcomes following intrathecal opioid therapy. Abstracts of the 11th World Congress of Anesthesiology, Sydney, 1996.
3. Banning, A., Sjøgren, P., and Henriksen, H.: Pain causes in 200 patients referred to a multidisciplinary cancer pain clinic. Pain, *45:*45, 1991.
4. Banning, A., Sjøgren, P., and Henriksen, H.: Clinical section. Treatment outcome in a multidisciplinary cancer pain clinic. Pain, *47:*129, 1991.
5. Bigos, S.J., Battie, M.C., Spengler, D.M., *et al.*: A longitudinal, prospective study of industrial back injury reporting. Clin. Orthop., *279:*21, 1992.
6. Brena, S.F.: Pain control facilities: Patterns of operation and problems of organization in the United States. *In* Brena, S.F., and Chapman, S.L. (eds.): Chronic Pain: Management Principles. Clinics in Anesthesiology. pp. 183–195. Philadelphia, W.B. Saunders, 1985.
7. Brena, S.F.: Pain clinics around the world. An overview. *In* Brena, S.F., and Chapman, S.L. (eds.): Chronic Pain: Management Principles. Clinics in Anesthesiology. pp. 75–80. Philadelphia, W.B. Saunders, 1985.
8. Bullingham, R.E.S., McQuay, H.J., and Budd, K.: Pain Control Centers: Problems of Organization and Operation in the UK. *In* Brena, S.F., and Chapman, S.L. (eds.): Chronic Pain: Management Principles. Clinics in Anesthesiology. pp. 211–221. Philadelphia, W.B. Saunders, 1985.
9. Cailliet, R.: Chronic pain: Is it necessary? Arch. Phys. Med. Rehabil., *60:*4, 1979.
10. CARF: Standards Manual and Interpretive Guidelines for Medical Rehabilitation. Tucson, CARF, 1996.
11. Cassisi, J.E., Sypert, G.W., Salamon, A., and Kapel, L.: Independent evaluation of a multidisciplinary rehabilitation program for chronic low back pain. Neurosurgery, *25:*877, 1989.
12. Cherkin, D.C., Deyo, R.A., Loeser, J.D., *et al.*: An international comparison of back surgery rates. Spine, *19:*1201, 1994.
13. Chun, D.Y., Turner, J.A., and Romano, J.M.: Children of chronic pain patients: Risk factors of maladjustment. Pain, *52:*311, 1993.
14. Cohen, J.E., Goel, V., Frank, J.W., *et al.*: Group education interventions for people with low back pain: An overview of the literature. Spine, *19:*1214, 1994.
15. Cooper, B.C., and Cooper, D.L.: Multidisciplinary approach to the differential diagnosis of facial, head and neck pain. J. Prosthet. Dent., *66:*72, 1991.
16. Davis, V.P., Fillingim, R.B., Doleys, D.M., and Davis, M.P.: Assessment of aerobic power in chronic pain patients before and after a multidisciplinary treatment program. Arch. Phys. Med. Rehabil., *73:*726, 1992.
17. Edwards, B.C., Zusman, M., Hardcastle, P., *et al.*: A physical approach to the rehabilitation of patients disabled by chronic low back pain. Med. J. Aust., *156:*167, 1992.
18. Flor, H., Fydrich, T., and Turk, D.C.: Efficacy of multidisciplinary pain treatment centers: A meta-analytic review. Pain, *49:*221, 1992.
19. Fordyce, W.E.: Back pain in the work place: Management of Disability in Nonspecific Conditions. Seattle, IASP Press, 1995.
20. Gambone, J.C., and Reiter, R.C.: Nonsurgical management of chronic pelvic pain: A multidisciplinary approach. Clin. Obstet. Gynecol. *33:*205, 1990.
21. Ghia, J.N.: Development and organization of pain centers. *In* Raj, P.P. (ed.): Practical Management of Pain. 2nd Ed. pp. 16–39. St. Louis, Mosby–Year Book, Inc., 1992.
22. Greenough, C.G., and Fraser, R.D.: Comparison of eight psychometric instruments in unselected patients with back pain. Spine, *16:*1068, 1991.
23. Guck, T.P., Skultety, F.M., Meilman, P.W., and Dowd, E.T.: Multidisciplinary pain center follow-up study: Evaluation with a no-treatment control group. Pain, *21:*295, 1985.
24. Guest, G.H., and Drummond, P.D.: Effect of compensation on emotional state and disability in chronic back pain. Pain, *48:*125, 1992.
25. Haddox, J.D.: Appropriate use of the chronic pain specialist and the role of conceptual fluidity. *In* Cohen, M.J.M., and Campbell, J.N. (eds.): Pain Treatment Centers at a Crossroads: A Practical and Conceptual Reappraisal. Progress in Pain Research and Management, Vol 7. pp. 297–305. Seattle, IASP Press, 1996.
26. Haythornthwaite, J.A., Sieber, W.J., and Kerns, R.D.: Depression and the chronic pain experience. Pain, *46:*177, 1991.
27. Jamison, R.N., Stetson, B., Sbrocco, T., and Parris, W.C.V.: Effects of significant weight gain on chronic pain patients. Clin. J. Pain, *6:*47, 1990.
28. Klapow, J.C., Slater, M.A., Patterson, T.L., *et al.*: Psychosocial factors discriminate multidimensional clinical groups of chronic low back pain patients. Pain, *62:*349, 1995.
29. Leitman, R., Cooner, E., and Schiffman, S.: Pain and Absenteeism in the Workplace: A Study of Full-Time Employees and Employee Benefit Managers. New York, Louis Harris and Associates, Inc., 1996.
30. Loeser, J.D.: Desirable Characteristics for Pain Treatment Facilities and Standards for Physician Fellowship in Pain Management. Seattle, IASP, 1990.
31. Loeser, J.D., and Cousins, M.J.: Contemporary pain management. Med. J. Aust., *153:*208, 1990.
32. Madigan, S.R., and Raj, P.P.: History and current status of pain management. *In* Raj, P.P. (ed.): Practical Management of Pain, 2nd ed. pp. 3–15. St. Louis, Mosby–Year Book, Inc., 1992.
33. Maruta, T., Swanson, D.W., and Finlayson, R.E.: Drug abuse and dependency in patients with chronic pain. Mayo Clin. Proc., *54:*241, 1979.
34. Maruta, T., Swanson, D.W., and McHardy, M.J.: Three-year follow-up of patients with chronic pain who were treated in a multidisciplinary pain management center. Pain, *41:*47, 1990.
35. McArthur, D.L., Cohen, M.J., Gottlieb, H.J., *et al.*: Treating chronic low back pain. I. Admissions to initial follow-up. Pain, *29:*1, 1987.
36. McArthur, D.L., Cohen, M.J., Gottlieb, H.J., *et al.*: Treating chronic low back pain. II. Long-term follow-up. Pain, *29:*23, 1987.
37. Mendelson, G.: Measurement of conscious symptom exaggeration by questionnaire: A clinical study. J. Psychosom. Res., *31:*703, 1987.

38. Merskey, H., and Bogduk, N.: Classification of Chronic Pain: Descriptions of Chronic Pain Syndromes and Definitions of Pain Terms. 2nd Ed. Seattle, IASP Press, 1994.
39. Milburn, A., Reiter, R.C., and Rhomberg, A.T.: Multidisciplinary approach to chronic pelvic pain. Obstet. Gynecol. Clin. North Am., *20:*643, 1993.
40. Mohler, S.N., and Tarrant, J.D.: Multidisciplinary treatment of chronic craniomandibular disorder: A preliminary investigation. J. Craniomandib. Pract. *9:*29, 1990.
41. Molloy, A. Muir, A., Sharp, T., *et al.*: Comparison of responders and non-responders to intrathecal testing with morphine. Abstracts of the 8th World Congress on Pain. pp. 39. IASP Press, 1996.
42. Moore, M.E., Stephen, N.B., and Nypaver, A.: Chronic pain: Inpatient treatment with small group effects. Arch. Phys. Med. Rehabil., *65:*356, 1984.
43. Newman, R.I., Painter, J.R., and Seres, J.L.: A Therapeutic Milieu for Chronic Pain Patients. J. Hum. Stress, *4:*8, 1978.
44. NIH Technology Assessment Panel. Integration of behavioral and relaxation approaches into the treatment of chronic pain and insomnia. J.A.M.A., *276:*313, 1996.
45. Peters, J.L., and Large, R.G.: A randomised control trial evaluating in- and outpatient pain management programmes. Pain, *41:*283, 1990.
46. Peters, J.L., Large, R.G., and Elkind, G.: Follow-up results from a randomised control trial evaluating in- and outpatient management programmes. Pain, *50:*41, 1992.
47. Pilowsky, I.: Pain as abnormal illness behaviour. J. Hum. Stress, *4:*22, 1978.
48. Pilowsky, I.: Abnormal illness behaviour (dysnosognosia). Psychother. Psychosom., *42:*76, 1986.
49. Pilowsky, I., Bassett, D., Barrett, R., *et al.*: The illness behavior assessment schedule: Reliability and validity. Int. J. Psychiatry Med., *13:*11, 1983.
50. Pilowsky, I., Spence, N., Cobb, J., and Katsikitis, M.: The illness behavior questionnaire as an aid to clinical assessment. Gen. Hosp. Psychiatry, *6:*123, 1984.
51. Pither, C.E., and Nicholas, M.K.: Psychological approaches in chronic pain management. Br. Med. Bull., *47*(3):743, 1991.
52. Pither, C.E., Williams, A.C. de C., Richardson, P., *et al.*: Inpatient vs outpatient pain management: Results of a randomised controlled trial. Pain, *66:*13, 1996.
53. Roberts, A.H., and Reinhardt, L.: The behavioral management of chronic pain: Long-term follow-up with comparison groups. Pain, *8:*151, 1980.
54. Roy, R.: Pain clinics: Reassessment of objectives and outcomes. Arch. Phys. Med. Rehabil., *65:*448, 1984.
55. Skinner, J.B., Erskine, A., Pearce, S., *et al.*: The evaluation of a cognitive behavioural treatment programme in outpatients with chronic pain. J. Psychosom. Res., *34:*13, 1990.
56. Sternbach, R.A.: Survey of pain in the United States: The nuprin pain report. Clin. J. Pain, *2:*49, 1986.
57. Taylor, V.M., Deyo, R.A., Cherkin, D.C., and Kreuter, W.: Low back pain hospitalization: Recent United States trends and regional variations. Spine, *19:*1207, 1994.
58. Turk, D.C., and Rudy, T.E.: Neglected factors in chronic pain treatment outcome studies—referral patterns, failure to enter treatment, and attrition. Pain, *43:*7, 1990.
59. Turner, J.A., and Jensen, M.P.: Efficacy of cognitive therapy for chronic low back pain. Pain, *52:*169, 1993.
60. Villard, H.P., Imbeault, J., and Duguay, M.: Low back pain: A Psychosomatic clinical study. Psychother. Psychosom., *45:*78, 1986.
61. Vlaeyen, J.W.S., Kole-Snijders, A.M.J., Boeren, R.G.B., and van Eek, H.V.: Fear of movement/(re)injury in chronic low back pain and its relation to behavioral performance. Pain, *62:*363, 1995.
62. Waddell, G., Newton, M., Henderson, I., *et al.*: A fear-avoidance beliefs questionnaire (FABQ) and the role of fear-avoidance beliefs in chronic low back pain and disability. Pain, *52:*157, 1993.
63. Williams, D.A., and Keefe, F.J.: Pain beliefs and the use of cognitive behavioral coping strategies. Pain, *46:*185, 1991.

Neural Blockade in Clinical Anesthesia and Management of Pain, Third Edition,
edited by M.J. Cousins and P.O. Bridenbaugh.
Lippincott–Raven Publishers, Philadelphia © 1998.

CHAPTER 34

New Horizons

An Essay

Patrick D. Wall

The readers of this book have digested a rich banquet of many chapters, and they may question, as I do, the function of a final chapter. In the beginning, the editors provided an introduction which not only summarized the contents of the subject today, but pointed to the future. Perhaps this last chapter should be simply a blank page with a large full stop, since the editors and authors have completed their best efforts. But I am challenged to look to the future and cannot resist.

Last chapters of this type can be pretty embarrassing when future readers check on the validity of the predictions. One would expect such a chapter to start with a precise definition of the present and then to launch into a science fictional extrapolation of what the future will hold. Our present situation is dominated by reductionism. By reductionism, I mean the strategy that takes each problem and reduces it to its fundamentals, preferably its single indivisible component. In the life sciences today, that strategy involves a search to define the problem and its solution in molecular terms. This hugely successful approach can forge a route through the old obscurities of complex whole bodies and interacting systems to target individual molecules.[4–6,9,11] The future of this "high tech" technique is assured and involves even higher "tech," the meat for great science fiction. I will not explore this avenue but will propose that it will be necessary to explore in parallel the *biologic* nature of the mechanism with which we are dealing.[10] By biologic I do not mean something that is obscure and mystical. I mean that biologic systems have evolved to incorporate integration and reaction which is as precise and as crucial as any one molecule. By disease or by genetic error or by drug application, a system may be perturbed by the appearance of a single novel type of molecule. All biologic systems, in contrast to inorganic systems, always react to a single perturbation in an active energy-consuming manner (Table 34-1). I propose to explore the consequences of this fact first in relation to local anesthetics and then in relation to the local application of drugs.

One could parody the profession of most of the readers of this book by saying that it has two characteristics. One is that they are addicted to injecting into others drugs with names ending in "-caine." The other is that they have developed extraordinary skills in inserting needles and catheters into hidden parts of the body. To move from the joke to the serious, this chapter should ask about the future of the local anesthetics and the future of the localized application of drugs. I hope I will be able to show that both of these futures are remarkable and powerful.

THE FUTURE OF LOCAL ANESTHETICS

An examination candidate asked to define the action of local anesthetics would give a satisfactory answer to almost all examiners if he or she replied that local anesthetics act by blocking nerve impulse propagation, which they do by stabilizing sodium channels in the nerve membrane (see Chapter 2). That answer is more than adequate since it includes the reductionist aim of defining the crucial target, i.e., the sodium channel. Furthermore, the three-dimensional structure and the molecular content of the sodium channel is precisely understood. One might reasonably conclude that, with this degree of precision, we were approaching full understanding and that future developments would involve the discovery of only a few minor details. I hope to persuade the reader that this is far from the truth and that local anesthetics are in fact a powerful probe into a number of crucial unsolved questions. Let us start with the nerve membrane itself.

P. D. Wall: Department of Physiology, United Medical and Dental Schools, St. Thomas Campus, London SE1 7EH United Kingdom.

TABLE 34-1. *Biologic consequences of local application of drugs*

Biologic systems possess *integration and reaction*
Locally applied drug molecule, etc. → Perturbation
↓
Biologic system *reacts*

The Nerve Membrane As Target

One might reasonably conclude that after a century of development of a large family of molecules related to cocaine, there is little reason to explore further. It is obvious that a variety of highly efficient local anesthetics exist and that they are safe, convenient, and effective. However, as we shall see, there are numerous other effects of these compounds which are potentially useful or unwanted. This means that it will be of interest to produce compounds that only stabilize the nerve membrane and do not have direct effects on other structures. It would seem unlikely that further exploration of the cocaine family would achieve this end. However, it is tempting to speculate that the present knowledge of the structure of the target sodium channel would permit the construction of a tailor-made antagonist molecule that would be precisely targeted on the channel. The most obvious candidate would be an antibody. Antibodies are huge molecules, and they can be effective antagonists in *in vitro* situations. In practice, *in vivo*, it is unlikely that antibodies could be applied with sufficient precision to allow the agent to penetrate to the desired location. However, molecular biologists are becoming skilled at identifying that part of the large molecule which is active in achieving the specificity of control. Examples of these much smaller molecules are already being identified and used to neutralize the effect of the antigen. This opens the possibility of an entirely new family of sodium channel blockers, which have been shaped to affect nerve membrane alone. The hope that such molecules would be more specific than the present local anesthetics is encouraged by the fact that the detailed chemistry of nerve membrane sodium channels differs from that of the ubiquitous sodium channels that are present in all types of cell.

However, we already have naturally occurring compounds that imitate sodium channel blocking local anesthetics in some respects. These include (i) tetrodotoxin (TTX), which occurs in puffer fish and newts, (ii) saxitoxin, which is found in a dinoflagellate and infects clams, and (iii) muculotoxin, which comes from the salivary glands of an Australian octopus. TTX is 100,000 times more potent than cocaine in blocking nerve impulses. That in itself is not interesting except for those who like the Guinness Book of Records. What is interesting is that it blocks impulses at such a low concentration that there are not enough TTX molecules to go around, one for each sodium channel. That, in turn, shows that there are single receptors present in nerve membrane, each of which can influence the stability of many nearby sodium channels. TTX is a small but complex molecule and is difficult to synthesize. It points to the possibility of a local anesthetic from an entirely new family, which is free of some of the other effects of local anesthetics we are about to discuss.

Other Effects of Local Anesthetics

Our ideal examination candidate would, of course, inform the examiners that there are systemic toxic effects of local anesthetics when the blood level reaches concentrations far beyond the levels needed for successful regional anesthesia. These toxic effects of gross overdosage would seem to be of no basic interest. For reasonable therapeutic doses, the candidate and his examiners would consider all effects other than sensory anesthesia to be the consequence of the inevitable blocking of motor fibers and autonomic fibers and possibly a direct effect on conducting membranes within the heart. They would be wrong.

To illustrate this, I will quote from a remarkable paper. In 1990, Arner, Lindblom, Meyerson, and Molander wrote a paper entitled "Prolonged relief of neuralgia after regional anesthetic blocks. A call for further experimental and systematic clinical studies."[1] This paper appears to have sunk without trace in spite of being written by the most distinguished group from the Karolinska in Stockholm. Their call for further studies seems to have fallen on deaf ears in spite of potential future consequences of their findings for practical therapeutics and the other evidence that therapeutic doses of local anesthetics were having long-term and long-range effects. They examined 38 consecutive patients with neuralgia after peripheral nerve injury and blocked the damaged nerve with 5 to 10 ml 0.5% bupivacaine without adrenaline. All patients experienced an initial total relief of ongoing pain, relief lasting at least 4 to 12 hours. By 12 hours, there is every reason to believe that the peripheral nerve block had disappeared. However, 26 of the 38 experienced pain relief beyond 12 hours. This lasted from 12 to 48 hours in 18 patients and for 2 to 6 days in another five. Even more puzzling, in eight patients there was a second period of analgesia lasting 4 hours to 6 days within 12 hours of the recurrence of the pain. No wonder the paper has been ignored. Who wants to consider such bizarre results when accepted dogma insists that the action of local anesthetics is adequately explained by their temporary block of transmitted nerve impulses? I want to consider these results because I believe they contain a clue for other useful effects of local anesthetics, which could be exploited. In order to do that, let us first ask if local anesthesia has direct or indirect effects on structures other than the nerve membrane that is blocked, and then we will return to the Arner et al. phenomenon.

Distant Effects of Blocking Sensory Nerve Impulses

Immediate Effects. We have all experienced an example of this effect. The common dental local anesthetic produces anesthesia of one quadrant of the mouth. On leaving the dentist while the block remains, one is aware not just of a numb lip, but of an apparently swollen lip, which attracts the attention and provokes palpation. That is a phantom lip. A phantom limb is dramatically provoked by a brachial plexus block. The effect has been repeatedly studied on single cells in the sensory pathways of animals. It has been observed in the dorsal horn, dorsal column nuclei, ventral posterior lateral nucleus of the thalamus, and the primary sensory cortex. In the simplest example, a cell is located and its cutaneous receptive field is identified. Then the receptive field in the skin is infiltrated with local anesthetic, and obviously the cell no longer responds to any stimuli to that area. However, many cells immediately begin to respond to a neighboring area of skin to which the cell was previously unresponsive. This common phenomenon has important practical implications. It means that there is a steady tonic input from the periphery which is in part inhibitory. When that input is blocked, central cells expand their receptive fields and immediately begin to respond to novel inputs and increase their excitability (see Chapter 27). This is an example of the homeostatic control of sensory cells. When a normal input fails, there is a compensatory increase of excitability, perhaps by a decrease of inhibition. This phenomenon is the beginning of the troublesome consequences of deafferentation. This raises the question of the origin of the tonic afferent input from the peripheral nerve that is blocked by local anesthetic. With the special exception of the muscle spindle afferents, most myelinated sensory afferents are silent in the absence of stimulation. This suggests that the unmyelinated fibers might be the source of the tonic input since it is true that a number of unmyelinated C fibers have a low level of ongoing activity (Table 34-2). The possibility that the C fibers are the source of the input is reinforced by the effect of a cuff occlusion of a limb (see Chapter 27). After 20 to 30 minutes, there is a complete block of myelinated fibers, but some C fibers are still conducting past the block. In this situation there is no phantom, even though the distal limb appears almost completely anesthetized. This emphasizes that the phantom only appears with a complete block and presumably explains why phantoms are rare with spinal anesthesia, which is unlikely to produce complete blockade of all afferents.[3] I introduce this phenomenon and the other "side" effects to be listed below not because they are scientific trivial curiosities, but because they could be used to advantage. Furthermore, as we understand the multiple effects of these hugely powerful local anesthetics, it may be possible to select molecules that exaggerate or diminish these secondary effects. One thinks of this family mainly as blockers, and yet here is a secondary consequence in which the activity of some nerve cells increases, a factor that could be therapeutically useful or deleterious (see Chapter 27).

Pre-emptive Effects. This topic has been examined in depth in Chapter 5 by Kehlet and in Chapter 26 by Sinatra. Briefly, the arrival in the spinal cord of a volley of impulses, particularly in unmyelinated fibers, triggers an immediate response in dorsal horn cells, which is followed by prolonged increases of excitability. The afferent fibers release excitatory amino acids and peptides. These not only excite cells but trigger a cascade of changes in the cell membrane and in the cytoplasm and nucleus. These prolonged changes include the entry of calcium ions, the unmasking of N-methyl-D-aspartate (NMDA) receptors, and the appearance of nitric oxide and of novel proteins.[2] These changes last for many hours in animals and are associated with a marked increase of excitability.[3,5] They prompted me to propose that these changes could be prevented in the practical situation of surgery if peripheral or central blocks were introduced before surgery began. Specifically, I proposed that a fraction of postoperative pain was the consequence of the lighting up of the spinal cord by the afferent barrage produced by the surgery during the operation (see Chapter 23.1). The powerful long-term effect of pre-emptive analgesia is clear in animals. The effect in man remains under investigation and is discussed in Chapter 26.

Chronic Effects. For reasons that I will discuss below, we need to consider the consequences of long-term impulse blockade lasting for days, weeks, and months. In the fetus and neonate, there is clear evidence in the visual somatosensory and auditory systems that nerve impulse transmission in the input is a critical component in establishing the final adult form of the system. In the early stages of development of the fetus, the general plan of the nervous system appears to be laid down by developmental mechanisms that are independent of nerve impulses. However, in the neonate—best studied in the visual system of cat, monkey, and other animals—there is a critical period during which the fine tuning of final connections is critically de-

TABLE 34-2 *Local anesthetics: Possible effects*

A. Nerve block effects
   1. Blockade of transmission of peripheral nerve impulses
   2. "Phantom" phenomena in area of blocked nerve(s)
      - Expansion of receptive field of central neurons
      - Increased central neuronal excitability: ?by decreased inhibition, normally activated by "tonic" input, ?from C Fibers
   3. "Pre-emptive effects" of nerve block
      - ?↓ Peripheral and central sensitization

B. Effects of local anesthetics at site of application or via systemic absorption
   1. Anti-inflammatory
   2. ↓ Ectopic impulses in damaged nerve
   3. ↓ Ectopic impulses in dorsal root ganglion
   4. ↓ Slow and rapid axonal transport systems
   5. ?↓ Norepinephrine re-uptake in spinal cord (?→ analgetic effects at spinal level)
   6. Cardiac: Membrane stabilization in muscle and nerve
   7. CNS: High concentrations → convulsions
      Low concentrations → ↓ hyperalgesia

pendent on the presence of patterned impulses in the input. For example, in the normal striate visual cortex, cells receive a convergent input from both eyes, which is accurately timed so that the two inputs originate from precisely homologous functional areas of the two retinas. This exact binocular overlap is achieved by linking together on single cells those inputs that fire together. Any maneuver that disturbs the synchrony of firing of the two inputs such as a squint in one eye, or rearing in the dark, results in grossly abnormal binocular responses. In the adult, there is one obvious example of impulse-dependent integrity of structure in the form of disuse atrophy of muscle. Perhaps surprisingly, it is not at all certain whether a similar phenomenon exists in sensory systems. The main reason for this uncertainty is that it is rarely clear whether maneuvers that affect nerve impulses do not also affect the transport system within nerve fibers. We will return to this crucial subject. Simple manipulations such as tenotomy, which produces a short muscle and therefore a silent proprioceptive input, result in a radical change of the entire reflex circuit supplying the affected muscle. Even in this situation, there may be changes in the chemicals transported from and to the muscle as well as the obvious changes of impulse pattern. We do not know nearly enough about the long-term consequences of changes of nerve impulse pattern in the adult. Obviously, there are some structures, such as the hippocampus, that are treated as special cases because obvious learning and memory changes take place as a result of changes in input pattern. We need to know the extent to which these changes occur in the adult in other structures because they could be manipulated for therapeutic reasons.

Local Anesthetic Effects on Phenomena Other Than Conducted Nerve Impulses

Inflammation. Local anesthetics have an anti-inflammatory action other than the obvious effect on pain. The mechanism has not been studied, amazingly, but there are three obvious possibilities, all of which might be acting simultaneously. First, sensory unmyelinated fibers play a role in the inflammatory process. These fibers contain a variety of peptides, such as substance P, which leak from the nerve fibers into the surrounding tissue when the nerves are excited.[5] These substances produce vasodilatation and swelling and sensitization of nerve endings by separate processes. Local anesthetics would reduce the amount of secreted peptide by blocking the nerve impulses that trigger some of the peptide release. Second, it is becoming apparent that sympathetic fibers play a role in inflammation by mechanisms other than the obvious release of noradrenaline and effects on blood vessels. Local anesthetics would reduce this effect by blocking efferent nerve impulses in the sympathetic axons. A third aspect of inflammation is the invasion of cells from the blood stream and from nearby tissue. This invasion of cells involves an active infiltration by cell movement. Although it has not been investigated, I guess that local anesthetics might influence the mobility of the white cells. One reason for that guess is by analogy with the dramatic effect of colchicine on gout, which is attributed to the paralysis of monocytes, which are thereby prohibited from invasion. As we shall see, there are some shared properties between colchicine-like drugs and local anesthetics. After a century of relative inactivity, the study of inflammation is now the center of fascinating advances, which are surely likely to produce revolutionary therapies.

Damaged Nerve. When nerve membrane is damaged, it takes on new properties, which are not observed in the normal tissue.[3,7] The membrane becomes mechanically sensitive, responds to the alpha action of adrenaline, and becomes spontaneously active. In transected and ligated nerves, these changes in myelinated fibers take days to develop fully and last for weeks. In unmyelinated fibers, the changes develop more slowly but remain indefinitely. The ectopic impulses, which are associated with an increase of sodium channels, occur spontaneously in irregular trains or high-frequency bursts. This generator of ectopic impulses is silenced by systemic lidocaine at levels far below those that block transmission in normal axons. Here we see local anesthetics taking on a new property, which is not apparent in intact tissue (see Table 34-2).

I will insert here a crucial discussion of the meaning of the word "block," which relates to the entire chapter. As the concentration of a local anesthetic *in vitro* around a peripheral nerve is raised, the first effect that is observed is a prolongation of the refractory period. That is to say, it takes longer for the membrane to become re-excitable after it has generated one action potential. An inevitable consequence of this low-level effect is that the axon is no longer capable of transmitting a high-frequency burst of impulses even though it can still transmit at a low frequency. Block is therefore not an all-or-none phenomenon, but a gradual loss of the ability to carry repetitive impulses until, in the extreme, it is unable to transmit even a single impulse, i.e., it is totally blocked (see Chapter 2). This can have practical consequences if some sensations such as pain or itch can only be provoked by high-frequency bursts, while other sensations such as touch may be provoked by single impulses. This could in turn mean that the famous ability of local anesthetics to abolish pain while touch can still be detected is not because local anesthetics pick out a special kind of fiber, but because they selectively limit the frequency of impulse transmission over a wide range of dosages before achieving a complete block at a high dose. Similar considerations would make spontaneously occurring ectopic impulses more sensitive than the normally evoked action potentials.

Dorsal Root Ganglion Cells. These cells are normally stable and silent when isolated from the periphery. However, if the peripheral axon has been damaged, the cells, like the damaged membrane, become a source of ectopic impulses.[3] Therefore, with damaged nerve, the spinal cord receives an abnormal input originating from two sources in the same axon, one from the area of damage and the other from the dorsal root ganglion cell. Similarly, these cells become mechanosensitive and react to adrenaline by alpha action. This source of ectopic impulses is even more sensitive to circulating lidocaine than is the peripheral area of damage and many times more sensitive than transmission in normal nerve membrane. It remains to be seen whether these cells are crucially important in peripheral neuropathies, but their extreme sensitivity to local anesthetics offers one way to determine their role.

Transport In Nerve Fibers. We come now to a generally ignored factor that may dominate one aspect of the future of local anesthesia. In addition to nerve membrane excitable properties, all nerve cells contain another quite different communication system within their cytoplasm. This is the chemical transport system, which moves large molecules from one part of the cell to another. There are slow and fast transport systems, which need energy to move molecules often on the surface of neurotubules. The cell body and its nucleus is the site of synthesis of many molecules, particularly proteins, which are required for the integrity and function of all parts of the cell. The transport system moves these molecules from the cell body down the axon to supply the nerve membrane and terminals. When an axon is cut or ligated, there is a massive accumulation of transported protein and peptide molecules on the proximal side of the ligation. The axon distal to the ligation is now starved of its normal steady supply of replacement molecules synthesized in the cell body. That is the cause of Wallerian degeneration (see Chapter 30).

At the same time, the same transport systems are operating in the reverse direction. They normally carry material from the distal axon to the cell body, including substances that have been picked up by the terminals. This is the basis of the modern transport methods of following nerve connections. If a foreign marker molecule such as horseradish peroxidase (HRP) is injected into peripheral tissue or a cut nerve, it is transported to the cell body. If the marker molecule is injected into the cell body, it is transported to the distal parts of the axon. More interesting to the animal or human, the distal peripheral nerves are normally picking up compounds present in tissue and moving them back to the cell body, where they act as signals to change the nature of the cell's metabolism. These signaling compounds are the neurotrophins, the most famous being nerve growth factor (NGF). Eight of these neurotrophins have been identified and there are more to come. They are active in low concentrations, they signal to the cell the nature of the tissue in which the axon terminates, and they change the cell's metabolism appropriately. They clearly have a crucial function in the embryo, but their role in the adult is becoming more apparent. For example, when a peripheral axon is cut, there are gross changes in its cell body. For the dorsal root ganglion cell, many of these changes are caused because the cell is cut off from its normal supply of NGF. An artificial supply of NGF to the cut end of the nerve prevents many of the changes. In the presence of pathology in peripheral tissue, the supply of neurotrophins changes, and it may be that novel pathologic molecules are also inserted. This traffic is a particular speciality of unmyelinated C fibers, and I believe they will turn out to be the chemical pathologists of the body, literally tasting the nature of the tissue in which they terminate and thereby signaling the appropriate changes of central response. This may well be the reason for the apparent duplication of the peripheral nerves into the A and C families, since I propose that the C fibers are in charge of slow reactions, including those triggered by chemical transport of neurotrophins.

Local anesthetics block transport as well as impulses (see Chapter 2). This makes the subject highly relevant to this book and to the future. *In vitro*, a low concentration of local anesthetic blocks impulses without affecting transport, perhaps because of easier access of externally applied local anesthetics to membrane. However, a small increase of concentration blocks slow transport, and a further small increment blocks fast transport. This means that, in practical circumstances of *in vivo* nerve infiltration, both impulses and transport are fully blocked.

The most famous transport blockers are colchicine and its slightly less toxic relatives, the vinca alkaloids such as vinblastine and vincristine. These are antimitotic agents and also transport blockers because the same protein that pulls apart the chromosomes in mitosis is also a crucial protein for transport along axons. This in turn explains why the limiting factor in the dosage of these anticancer drugs is peripheral nerve degeneration, since by blocking transport they starve the peripheral axons to death. It is possible to give a single low dose of vinblastine, which blocks some transport for 4 days without degeneration, but if the dose is raised or prolonged, degeneration results. Turning back to local anesthesia of the cocaine family, it will now be seen why there is a time-dose limit on local anesthesia. It is inevitable that degeneration will result if doses are raised or if lower doses are prolonged over days. This establishes an important limit on the future of this family in one respect and opens new possibilities in others. A much more practical aspect is that TTX, as we have said, blocks membranes by a different mechanism, but it does *not* block transport. Therefore, if one were to desire prolonged block lasting over weeks, one should turn away from the otherwise excellent cocaine family to another family such as TTX and its relatives (see Table 34-2).

Blood Vessels. A trivial and unimportant effect of local anesthetics contains a hint of something much more interesting. Low levels of the drugs produce vasoconstriction, whereas high levels produce vasodilatation (see Chapter 3). The high-level effect is expected since there is a paralysis of smooth muscle contraction and a block of sympathetic fibers. However, the low-level effect is unexpected. A likely and interesting explanation is that at low levels the drugs inhibit the re-uptake of catecholamine by the nerve fibers. When a sympathetic fiber emits noradrenaline, part of the termination of the effect is produced by the re-uptake of the amine. Therefore, when a local anesthetic is present, the duration of the extracellular presence of noradrenaline is increased, and therefore the amount of constriction is increased. If this effect occurs in the central nervous system (CNS) and there are signs that cocaine is particularly effective, it could explain part of the mood effect. Much more interesting for us is the fact that adrenaline is released in the spinal cord and has an analgesic effect, and therefore these agents might have a central analgesic effect by increasing the availability of adrenaline by re-uptake inhibition (see Table 34-2).

The Heart. Local anesthetics have both useful therapeutic actions on the heart and toxic effects. There is every reason to accept a common action by the membrane stabilizing action of local anesthetics, both on nerve membrane and on heart muscle and conducting bands. Although this is not a serious practical problem with the common uses of local anesthetics, it can be in other situations. For example, tocainide, which we will discuss in the next section because of its promising effects on the CNS, is not usable because of its dangerous blood and cardiac toxicity. Therefore, it would be of interest to separate cardiac from neural effects. It is possible that the subtle differences of the ion channels found in these structures might allow tailoring of drugs to affect one more than the other.[5]

The Central Nervous System. The actions of local anesthetics on the central nervous system are normally discussed in terms of blocking nerve fibers in roots with local application, or in terms of light-headedness, confusion, and convulsions with high toxic systemic doses. However, animal studies of hyperexcitable cord cells and reflex circuits following bombardment from peripheral unmyelinated afferents show a striking reduction of hyperexcitability with low systemic levels of lidocaine. A number of clinical reports also record an improvement of the hyperalgesic responses in postherpetic neuralgia and other conditions with low levels of intravenous lidocaine[8] (see Table 34-2). With the same rationale, Arner et al., in the paper quoted earlier in this chapter,[1] gave a dose of 250 mg tocainide intravenously and a placebo injection to seven of their peripheral nerve injury neuralgia patients. Four of the seven had a striking reduction of their pain with tocainide and none with placebo. Subsequent trials were stopped because of the reported cardiac and hematologic dangers discussed above. I take all of this to offer promising indications for the future. A safe relative of tocainide, mexiletine, which is orally active, has not yet received clear support as an effective substitute. I would hope that the central action of these drugs can be isolated from their peripheral and toxic reactions (see Chapter 27).

Summary of Possible Future Developments of Local Anesthesia

Regional anesthesia has a hundred-year history of steady development to its present status as a highly effective safe therapy. It seems to me that it has been so successful in its main aim to achieve the temporary block of nerve impulses that I can suggest no major future advance that is needed. I am sure the wonderful ingenuity of its practitioners will continue to hone this fine tool.

I do suggest, however, that in their dedicated concentration on the stated aim, a number of attractive babies have been thrown out with the bath water. A startling example is the paper of Arner et al., which reported that two-thirds of their patients experienced pain relief beyond the period of nerve block.[1] That report makes no sense to those who "know" as fundamental dogma that pain is generated by nerve impulses in peripheral nerves and that the analgesic action of local anesthetics is to briefly block those impulses. Since the report makes no sense to the dogmatists, they can forget it or ignore it or declare it to be a placebo response. Placebo responses are always those that the patient expects. Perhaps the patients expected a longer relief than the doctors. However, neither doctors nor patients expected the pain to return and then go away a second time. That is *not* a placebo reaction. As an aside, one can point out that if the one-mechanism enthusiasts insisted on a placebo trial, it would be extremely difficult to design. A saline injection would be a useless placebo since anyone would detect a difference between bupivacaine and saline. A bupavicaine block of a neighboring uninjured nerve would be interesting, but since nerves interact, it is possible that it would produce a "true" effect. However, the Stockholm group did just such a test in normal subjects and showed that local block of one nerve did not affect sensation in the territory of a neighboring nerve.

Returning to the Arner et al. phenomenon, the authors (and I) do not understand it, but they and I have a number of suggestions which I believe should be explored and which might open a novel future for local anesthesia. I have listed a series of consequences of local anesthetics other than nerve blocks. Some are immediate and long-term and long-range secondary effects of nerve block. Some are other effects of the powerfully active drugs which, although counted as unwanted side effects, could be useful if isolated and exploited.

Starting with explanations in the periphery, it is possible that the damaged nerve has foci that are abnormally sensitive to block. Moving centrally, it is possible that pathologically hyperexcitable mechanisms need to be continually fed by nerve impulses to keep the fire burning (see Chapter 27). If they are given a holiday, the fire dies down and takes time to burst out again. This raises the question of time and the possibility of prolonged holidays, which are at present not possible because of the chronic toxicity of the blockers. Since the blocks are affecting transport as well as nerve impulses, it is possible that the long-term effects, especially the "two-phase analgesia" effects, are produced by chemical changes within the nerve. This suggests the need to explore manipulation of both prolonged *impulse block* and, separately, *transport block.* Finally, there is the appealing evidence for *direct central effects* other than block, which calls for urgent exploration of safe ways to manipulate this mechanism (see Table 34-2).[4]

THE FUTURE OF LOCALIZED THERAPY

The other great success of regional anesthesia has been to implant needles or catheters in almost any structure in the body (see Chapters 26 through 32). This brought the therapy to the target, and one may speculate on the future of this obviously worthy aim. It has been used with three intentions, each with a different future. One use was to destroy tissue either by cold or by heat electrolysis or by chemicals. Judging by present trends, destructive methods will sink to a low level of use. The reason is that irreversible lesions fail to face the reactive integrated nature of the nervous system, which can recreate pathologically functional systems by reassigning novel roles to the remaining nerve cells (see Chapters 23.1, 24, 27, 31, and 32). The second use has been electrical stimulation. I played some role in initiating this method, and I believe it has a limited future, particularly when more than one target is stimulated and when electrodes are moved from the surface into the depths (see Chapter 32). I will not explore that method further in order to concentrate on the future of the third most common use, which was to deliver drugs. Obviously the future depends on how compounds can be more precisely targeted with defined spatial and temporal parameters.

Mechanical Delivery System. Present methods in man are limited to open-ended tubes (see Chapter 29). This represents a point source of the drug, which then reaches the target by diffusion and flow, which is a sloppy route. Furthermore, the tubes are normally placed on the surface of the target structure. Yet metal electrodes are commonly inserted chronically into the depths in the middle of the target (see Chapter 32). It would seem reasonable to develop this method for drug delivery tubes. This has been done for brief test periods of localized local anesthesia prior to stereotactic lesions in neurosurgical operations. It will surely be developed for more chronic indwelling purposes.

Methods have been developed in animals for the inserting of lengths of dialysis tubes through central nervous tissue. These fine continuous tubes can be used both to deliver drugs and to sample the tissue fluid. A striking advantage of the system is that it gets away from the point source of an open tube and substitutes a line source, which can be made as long as is appropriate. Furthermore, there is no net volume injected into the tissue. The tubes can be inserted as a continuous line from one side of the structure to the other or as loops or as a single tube with an internal division, permitting fluid to pass to the closed tip and back along the other half of the tube (Table 34-3).

Target-Seeking Molecules. This phrase is, of course, a physical impossibility, but as the specificity of the drug-receptor interaction increases, the end result makes it look as though it is happening. When the reactive combination of drug and receptor is made highly specific and when the time of sticking of drug to receptor is prolonged, the presence of receptors can sweep a solution clear of the drug. This moves the system to one where the normal equilibrium pharmacodynamics no longer apply. Botulinum toxin therapy is an example. A combination of pharmacologic design and a therapeutic demand that has defined the biologic nature of the target will surely change the nature of available drugs.

Transport Systems. As I have described in the section of this chapter on local anesthetics, each nerve cell contains an internal active chemical transport mechanism. Molecules, including proteins, which are present in the cell body are transported from the cell body to all parts of the cell, including the dendrites, and to the axon and the axon terminals. In the opposite direction, molecules in the axon terminals are transported retrogradely to the cell body. The rate of transport is slow, in the millimeters-per-hour range, but eventually the molecules get to their destination. This process is critical to the survival of the cell. It has been extensively used for experimental purposes to mark the anatomy of cells. Why not use it for therapeutic purposes (Table 34-3). Each axon could be considered as a catheter, which is exactly what occurs in certain pathologies. In herpes zoster, an explosive duplication of the varicella virus in a dorsal root ganglion is followed by the transport of the virus to the distal terminals of the axons, where it emerges in the skin to produce the characteristic rash. The rash marks the dermatome supplied by the ganglion from which the virus originates. In the opposite direction, the route by which the poliomyelitis virus penetrates the central nervous system is by motor axons, which transport them back to the motor neurons where they duplicate and may kill the cell. This effect has been used experimentally with single types of molecules. For example, ricin, which is a powerful neurotoxin, has been placed on single peripheral nerves followed by transport to the cells of origin of the axons, where those cells are destroyed. This destructive technique takes advantage of the steady reliable transport system to force the unwitting cells to commit a form of suicide. Surely it can be used for more creative purposes.

The question of how to make foreign molecules penetrate cells has been extensively investigated. The crude method is simply to flood the region of the cell bodies with the desired molecule. Some molecules penetrate or are transported

TABLE 34-3. *Future of localized drug treatment of pain*

?Selective A-delta and C-fiber blockade (e.g., butamben)
"Slow release" formulations (e.g. microspheres)
Traditional local anesthetics
?Biotoxins and other agents
Epidural/intrathecal "dialysis" type tubes: "line-source" delivery
Target-seeking molecules
Transport systems
Via axonal transport
Via endocytotic cell membrane transport
Via "vectors" to "active" CNS cells
Analgesic-molecule producing cells
Tissue cultured cells in closed dialysis "packets"

across the membrane to penetrate the cytoplasm and reach the transport distribution system. Direct injection into single cells is of great experimental interest but clearly of no practical therapeutic value. When axons are cut, there is a brief period in which cytoplasm is exposed to interstitial fluid. This method has been used experimentally in the peripheral and central nervous system to flood cell bodies with marker molecules. A much more interesting practical way of penetrating the inside of a nerve cell takes advantage of another inherent property of nerves. At axon terminals, substances are secreted by the process of exocytosis. Vesicles fuse with the cell membrane, pass through, and dump their contents in the extracellular space. The remnants of these vesicles are taken up again by the nerve membrane as part of the re-uptake process. In this movement across the otherwise intact membrane, they insert into the cytoplasm whatever garbage may be lying about in the extracellular fluid. These molecules are then transported and distributed throughout the cell.

Even more interesting from a potentially useful therapeutic viewpoint, this endocytotic transport across cell membranes is greatly accelerated by cell activity. In this way, it is possible to mark experimentally those systems that are most active. One can immediately see the therapeutic possibilities of delivering therapeutic compounds to cells that are particularly active. Active peripheral nerve terminals pick up more material from the extracellular space than quiescent terminals. What about central synapses? We are taught quite correctly that synapses are unidirectional so that presynaptic action potentials produce postsynaptic changes, but that postsynaptic changes do not leak back onto the synaptic end bulbs. This is approximately true and is the basis of the classic neurophysiology of cell connectivity. However, this one-way synaptic activity is achieved by the asymmetric distribution of the presynaptic source of neurotransmitters and the postsynaptic location of the receptors for the neurotransmitters. On both sides of the synapse, the endocytotic penetration of the cell membrane is in progress. A practical consequence of this has produced a novel experimental technique. First, motor neurons were heavily loaded with the foreign marker molecule HRP, which was introduced into the cells by soaking the cut ends of their axons in HRP. Then the animal and its spinal cord was allowed to operate for some time in its normal unanesthetised fashion. Finally, the spinal cord was searched for cells containing HRP. Of course, the motor neurons whose axons had been treated were heavily labeled, but the active interneurons, which had been driving the motor neurons into activity, were also labeled. This is a method of tracing active pathways by labeling them while the cells not involved in that pathway were not affected. Is that not exactly an ideal of restorative therapy?

Let me return to the question of viral spread within the central nervous system. This is of therapeutic interest for two reasons. Genetic engineering is faced with exactly the same problem as the one we are discussing here, i.e., how to insert large fragile molecules into a cell. Great skill and ingenuity have been mobilized to insert deoxyribonucleic acid (DNA) into cells. As this technique develops, it would seem reasonable to utilize the present skills of regional anesthetists. The vector that has been most commonly used is a virus, particularly herpes virus. Strains of herpes virus have been selected which spread in the nervous system but which produce no overt chronic pathology in monkeys. The second interest of these viruses is that they appear to spread along active pathways in strong preference over inactive or neighboring pathways. They have been used to trace chains of active neurons whose activity is sequentially driven. In this way, the virus spreads across synapses and invades those cells that are driven by the donor-infected axons. One could imagine the insertion of therapeutic molecules which would be actively spread through an interlinked chain of neurons (see Table 34-3)[6,10]

Cells that produce useful molecules. There is intense investigation in progress on the insertion of cells that would produce a steady supply of a therapeutic compound. There has been massive publicity for the early clinical attempts to transplant local concentrations of fetal cells to provide a steady source of L-DOPA in Parkinsonian patients and to transport pancreatic islet cells producing insulin in diabetics. I will illustrate the state of the art with reference to increasing the concentration of adrenaline in the spinal cord. It has been known for a long time that adrenaline exerts a powerful inhibitory effect on nociceptive systems in the spinal cord. In animal experiments, it was shown that transported fragments of adrenal medulla could survive on the surface of cord and produced an analgesia in neuropathic models limited to the segments involved. In man, a slurry of adrenaline-producing cells was injected intrathecally in cancer patients, combined with immune suppression to prevent rejection of the transported cells. Now a newer technique has been extensively developed in animals and is under clinical trial in man. Cells that have been grown in tissue culture are inserted into closed packets of dialysis membrane (see Chapter 29). These "ravioli" permit the diffusion in and out of small molecules while preventing the transfer of large molecules such as proteins. This permits the maintenance of a supply of molecules such as adrenaline without triggering immune rejection (see Table 34-3).

Invasive Restoration. I will illustrate what is meant by this phrase by summarizing the present exciting situation with respect to repair of spinal cord injury. Over the past 10 years it has become apparent that the classic certainty that the axons of central nerve cells were incapable of regeneration is no longer true. If cut central axons are permitted contact with Schwann cells of peripheral origin, they regenerate. This discovery has released an intense new area of research divided into solving a series of problems. Immediately after injury, at the site of the damage, inflammatory invasion takes place which needs analysis and control. The cells whose axons have been cut begin to deteriorate because they are starved of the neurotrophic molecules normally supplied by their target regions and they need an alternative supply. Outgrowing fibers from the cut axon encounter inhibitory molecules on the surface of surround cells, and these "stop" molecules can be neutralized. The advancing sprouts need their supply of nutrient and attractant molecules. Finally, the surface on which the regenerating axons grow must be compatible. One problem that does not exist is the preservation of the target markers, which allowed the correct connections to be made in the embryo, and which remain in the adult. All of this means that successful regeneration could be achieved if the five precisely identified factors could be provided. Four of these five needs could be satisfied by a local supply of soluble molecules. That is the specialty of the readers of this book. The fifth requirement of a compatible solid state surface is obviously the most difficult to achieve in practice. Could existing cells be persuaded to change their surface molecules? Alternatively, could cells with a surface friendly to growing axons be introduced or even trained to invade? Each of these factors is now under intense investigation with the remarkable power of modern molecular biology.[10] That leaves the problem of how to locate the identified molecules in the right place where they may exercise their properties.

Summary of the Future of Localized Therapy

Regional anesthetists are the experts in delivering active molecules to small areas. The future of many general therapies depends on an extension of the ability to localize. Finer needles and more delicate catheters will generate a limited improvement. I have suggested that if the regional anesthetist recruits the biology of the tissue as an ally, the tissue itself may help in the localization of therapy. Instead of dominating tissue by an overwhelming flood of drug, the technique could move to the setting up of a reservoir, while the final task of delivery to precise targets is carried out by virtue of the inherent property of the cells themselves.

REFERENCES

1. Arner, S., Lindblom, U., Meyerson, B.A., and Molander, C.: Prolonged relief of neuralgia after regional anesthetic blocks. A call for further experimental and systemic clinical studies. Pain, *43:*287, 1990.
2. Basbaum, A. Memories of pain. Sci. Med., *3:*22, 1996.
3. Devor, M.: Pain mechanisms and pain syndromes. *In* Campbell, J.N. (ed.): Pain 1996: An Updated Review. pp. 89–96. Seattle, IASP Press, 1996.
4. Dickensen, A.H.: Pharmacology of pain transmission and control. *In* Campbell, J.N. (ed.): Pain 1996: An Updated Review. pp. 113–122. Seattle, IASP Press, 1996.
5. Dray, A.: Pharmacology of analgesics for peripheral targets. *In* Campbell, J.N. (ed.): Pain 1996: An Updated Review. pp. 370–374. Seattle, IASP Press, 1996.
6. Iadarola, M.J.: Functional analysis of cloned genes and regulation of gene expression: Examples of pain-related studies. *In* Campbell, J.N. (ed.): Pain, 1996: An Updated Review. pp. 533–548. Seattle, IASP Press, 1996.
7. Wall, P.D.: The mechanisms by which tissue damage and pain are related. *In* Campbell, J.N. (ed.): Pain 1996: An Updated Review. pp. 123–128. Seattle, IASP Press, 1996.
8. Wall, P.D., and Melzack, R. (eds.): Textbook of Pain. 3rd Ed. Edinburgh, Churchill Livingstone, 1994.
9. Willis, W.D.: Signal transduction mechanisms. *In* Campbell, J.N. (ed.): Pain, 1996: An Updated Review. pp. 527–532. Seattle, IASP Press, 1996.
10. Woolf C.J.: Molecular neurobiology. *In* Campbell, J.N. (ed.): Pain 1996: An Updated Review. pp. 549–558. Seattle, IASP Press, 1996.
11. Yaksh, T.L.: Intrathecal and epidural opiates: A review. *In* Campbell, J.N. (ed.): Pain 1996: An Updated Review. pp. 381–396. Seattle, IASP Press, 1996.

Subject Index

Note: Pages numbers followed by f indicate figures; those followed by t indicate tables.

G

O

U

V

W